1981
CURRENT THERAPY
1981

CONSULTING EDITORS:

W. B. SAUNDERS COMPANY/Philadelphia / London / Toronto / Sydney

1981
1981
1981
1981
1981
1981

CURRENT THERAPY

LATEST APPROVED METHODS OF TREATMENT FOR THE PRACTICING PHYSICIAN

EDITED BY HOWARD F. CONN, M.D.

1981
1981
1981

W. B. Saunders Company: West Washington Square
Philadelphia, PA   19105

1 St. Anne's Road
Eastbourne, East Sussex BN 21 3UN, England

1 Goldthorne Avenue
Toronto, Ontario M8Z 5T9, Canada

9 Waltham Street
Artarmon, N.S.W. 2064, Australia

Library of Congress Cataloging in Publication Data

Current therapy; latest approved methods of treatment for
the practicing physician. 1949–

v. 28 cm. annual.

Editors: 1949–   H. F. Conn and others.

1. Therapeutics.   2. Therapeutics, Surgical.   3. Medicine—
   Practice.   I. Conn, Howard Franklin, 1908–   ed.

RM101.C87   616.058   49–8328 rev*

Current Therapy   ISBN   0-7216-2709-9

Last digit is the print number: 9   8   7   6   5   4   3   2   1

Consulting Editors

NOTICE

Extraordinary efforts have been made by the authors, the editors, and the publisher of this book to insure that dosage recommendations are precise and in agreement with standards officially accepted at the time of publication.

It does happen, however, that dosage schedules are changed from time to time in the light of accumulating clinical experience and continuing laboratory studies. This is most likely to occur in the case of recently introduced products.

It is urged, therefore, that you check the manufacturer's recommendations for dosage, *especially if the drug to be administered or prescribed is one that you use only infrequently or have not used for some time.*

THE PUBLISHER

Preface

This is the thirty-third in a series of annual editions designed to bring to the practicing physician current and authoritative information on the treatment of those diseases he or she is most likely to encounter in practice. The format and editorial policies of previous editions have been continued in response to the wishes of the contributors and of the physicians who use this book. The articles have been written to give concise, accurate, and sufficiently detailed information unhampered by material not directly related to the therapy proposed.

A correct diagnosis is assumed to have been made before the book is consulted, although in some instances a brief definition or discussion may be given if in the opinion of the author it is necessary.

The term "method of" preceding the author's name in most articles does not imply that the author necessarily was the originator or discoverer of the method described. The use of the term denotes that if the author were faced with the problem of treating a patient having the particular disease in question, his or her current management would be that given in the discussion.

It is assumed that the physicians using this volume have intimate knowledge of the detailed information available in the manufacturer's official publications for each drug before prescribing the drug for their patients. The therapeutic use of most drugs mentioned is under continuous clinical evaluation, and, from time to time, new uses, changes in dosage, and the appearance of unexpected contraindications and adverse reactions are reported. Official announcements and product circulars should be followed to keep abreast of these changes. Sometimes a larger dose than that usually recommended is advised for patients under exceptional circumstances or in cases of serious or life-threatening illness. In these instances, the use of a dose or drug becomes a matter of the physician's own clinical judgment and depends on knowledge obtained by consulting official drug information sources.

Over 90 per cent of the articles in this edition are new, and all of the articles carried over from the previous editions have been reviewed and revised as needed by the authors.

The editor wishes to thank the contributors and consultants for their invaluable assistance; the greatest share of credit for the success of this book must be given to them. The editor also wishes to express his appreciation to the staff of the W. B. Saunders Company for their wise guidance and help and to Mr. C. F. Robinson and Mrs. Franklin Cole for their valuable assistance in the preparation of this book.

HOWARD F. CONN, M.D., F.A.C.P.
Uniontown, Pennsylvania

Contributors

MICHAEL B. AINSLIE, M.D.

Pediatrician and Pediatric Endocrinologist, St. Louis Park Medical Center; Clinical Instructor, University of Minnesota Department of Pediatrics; Staff Pediatrician, Methodist Hospital, St. Louis Park, Minnesota
Diabetes Mellitus in Childhood and Adolescence

ROBERT H. ALFORD, M.D.

Professor of Medicine, Vanderbilt University School of Medicine; Chief, Infectious Diseases Section, Veterans Administration Medical Center, Nashville, Tennessee
Histoplasmosis

EDWARD A. ALLEN, M.B., F.R.C.P.(C.), F.C.C.P.

Director, Division of Tuberculosis Control, Province of British Columbia, Canada
Tuberculosis and other Mycobacterial Diseases

H. V. ALLINGTON, M.D.

Senior Staff, Samuel Merritt Hospital, Peralta Hospital, Providence Hospital, Alameda County Hospitals, Oakland, California
Warts

F. P. ANTIA, M.D., M.S., F.R.C.P. (Lond.)

Chief Physician and Gastroenterologist, Tata Memorial Hospital, Bombay; Emeritus Professor of Medicine and Gastroenterology, T.N. Medical College and B.Y.L. Nair Hospital; Consultant Physician, Radiation Medicine Center, B.D. Petit Parsee General Hospital, Jerbai Wadia Hospital for Children, Bombay India
Amebiasis

JAY M. ARENA, M.D. B.S.M.

Professor of Pediatrics, Duke University School of Medicine; Director, Poison Control Center, Duke University Medical Center, Durham, North Carolina
Acute Miscellaneous Poisoning

HENRY H. BALFOUR, JR., M.D.

Professor, Department of Laboratory Medicine and Pathology, and Professor of Pediatrics, University of Minnesota Medical School; Attending Pediatrician, University of Minnesota Medical Health Sciences Center, Minneapolis, Minnesota
Rubella

ROBERT W. BALOH, M.D.

Associate Professor, University of California, Los Angeles, School of Medicine, Department of Neurology and Surgery/Head and Neck (Otolaryngology), Los Angeles, California
Episodic Vertigo

CAMERON C. BANGS, M.D.

Clinical Instructor of Medicine, University of Oregon Health Science Center, Portland; Willamette Falls Community Hospital, Oregon City, Oregon
Disturbances Due to Cold

LARRY J. BARAFF, M.D.

Assistant Professor of Pediatrics, University of California, Los Angeles; Chief, Pediatric Emergency Medicine, University of California, Los Angeles School of Medicine, Los Angeles, California
Pertussis (Whooping Cough)

DONALD A. G. BARFORD, M.D., M.R.C.O.G.

Assistant Professor, Case Western Reserve University School of Medicine; Attending Physician, Cleveland Metropolitan Hospital, Cleveland, Ohio
Pregnancy-Induced Hypertension

JOHN G. BARTLETT, M.D.

Professor of Medicine, Johns Hopkins School of Medicine; Chief, Infectious Diseases Division, The Johns Hopkins Hospital, Baltimore, Maryland
Primary Lung Abscess

FRANK J. BAUMEISTER, JR., M.D.

Clinical Associate Professor of Medicine, University of Oregon Health Sciences Center; Gastroenterologist, Good Samaritan Hospital, Portland, Oregon
Peptic Ulcer

OLIVER H. BEAHRS, M.D., F.A.C.S.

Department of General Surgery, Mayo Clinic, Rochester, Minnesota
Thyroid Malignancy

WILLIAM B. BEAN, M.D.

Sir William Osler Professor of Medicine, University of Iowa Department of Internal Medicine, College of Medicine; Consulting Physician, University of Iowa Hospitals and Veterans Hospital, Iowa City, Iowa
Scurvy and Vitamin C Deficiency

RICHARD P. BENDEL, M.D.

Associate Professor, Department of Obstetrics and Gynecology, University of Minnesota Medical School; Assistant Chief, Department of Obstetrics and Gynecology, Hennepin County Medical Center, Minneapolis, Minnesota
Antepartum Care

ROBERT M. BENNETT, M.D., M.R.C.P. (Lond.)

Associate Professor of Medicine and Head, Section of Rheumatology, University of Oregon Health Sciences Center, Portland, Oregon
Ankylosing Spondylitis

GARY S. BERGER, M.D., F.A.C.O.G., F.A.C.P.M.

Clinical Assistant Professor of Obstetrics and Gynecology, Adjunct Professor of Maternal and Child Health, University of North Carolina Schools of Medicine and Public Health, Chapel Hill; Attending Physician, Durham County General Hospital, Wake County Medical Center, and Raleigh Community Hospital, Raleigh, North Carolina
Contraception

GERSON CHARLES BERNHARD, M.D., M.S., B.S.

Clinical Professor of Medicine, Medical College of Wisconsin; Chief of Rheumatology Division, Columbia Hospital; Attending Staff, Milwaukee County Hospital, Milwaukee, Wisconsin
Osteoarthritis

CHRISTOPHER R. BLAGG, M.D., F.A.C.P.

Professor, Department of Medicine, University of Washington Medical School; Director, Northwest Kidney Center, Seattle, Washington
Acute Renal Failure

MARY BLAINE, B.Sc., R.D.

Clinical Dietitian, Grand Forks Clinic Ltd., Grand Forks, North Dakota; Formerly Consulting Dietitian, Massachusetts General Hospital, Boston, Massachusetts
Diabetes Mellitus in Adults

TOMAS S. BOCANEGRA, M.D.

Senior Fellow in Rheumatology, University of South Florida College of Medicine, Tampa, Florida
Juvenile Rheumatoid Arthritis

HUBERTO BOGAERT, M.D.

Professor of Dermatology, Medical School, Universidad Autonoma de Santo Domingo; Medical Director of Dominican Dermatological Institute, Santo Domingo
Granuloma Inguinale; Lymphogranuloma Venereum

GIANNI BONADONNA, M.D.

Director, Division of Medical Oncology, Istituto Nazionale Tuitori, Milan, Italy
Non-Hodgkin's Lymphomas

ALFRED M. BONGIOVANNI, B.S., M.D., F.A.C.P.

Professor of Pediatrics and Pediatrics in Obstetrics, University of Pennsylvania School of Medicine; Director, Perinatal Endocrinology, Pennsylvania Hospital; Senior Physician, Children's Hospital, Philadelphia, Pennsylvania
Adrenocortical Insufficiency

THOMAS A. BORDEN, M.D.

Professor and Chairman, Division of Urology, Associate Professor of Pediatrics and Director, Urology Residency Program, University of New Mexico School of Medicine; Chief, Director of Urology, Veterans Administration Hospital, Albuquerque, New Mexico
Genitourinary Tumors

JOHN M. BOYCE, M.D.

Assistant Professor of Medicine, Internal Division of Infectious Diseases, University of Mississippi Medical Center; Attending Physician and Hospital Epidemiologist, University Hospital, Jackson, Mississippi
Plague

WILLIAM H. BOYCE, M.D.

Professor and Chairman, Section of Urology, Bowman Gray School of Medicine and Wake Forest University; Attending Staff, North Carolina Baptist Hospital, Winston-Salem, North Carolina
Renal Calculi

WILLIAM E. BRENNER, M.D.

Professor, Department of Obstetrics and Gynecology, University of North Carolina School of Medicine, Chapel Hill, North Carolina
Abortion

HAROLD BROWN, M.D.

Professor and Deputy Chairman, Department of Internal Medicine, Baylor College of Medicine, Houston, Texas
Malignant Carcinoid Syndrome

ANTHONY BRYCESON, M.D., F.R.C.P.E., D.T.M.&H.

Senior Lecturer, London School of Hygiene and Tropical Medicine; Consultant Physician, Hospital for Tropical Diseases, London
Relapsing Fever

JOHN G. BURFORD, M.D.

Assistant Professor of Medicine, Louisiana State University School of Medicine in Shreveport; Medical Director of Respiratory Care, Veterans Administration Medical Center, Shreveport, Louisiana
Blastomycosis

IRVING M. BUSH, M.D.

Professor of Urology, the Chicago Medical School/University of Health Sciences, Chicago; Senior Consultant, Center for the Study of Genitourinary Diseases, Burlington; Attending Physician, Cook County Hospital, Chicago; St. Joseph Hospital and Sherman Hospital, Elgin; Sycamore Municipal Hospital, Sycamore, Illinois
Genitourinary Tract Trauma

WILLIAM W. BUSSE, M.D.

Associate Professor of Medicine, University of Wisconsin Medical School; Attending Staff, University of Wisconsin Hospital and Clinics, Madison, Wisconsin
Allergic Reactions to Insect Stings

JOHN E. BYFIELD, M.D., Ph.D.

Professor of Radiology and Medicine, School of Medicine, University of California, San Diego; Consulting Physician, La Jolla Veterans Administration Hospital, Balboa Naval Hospital, San Diego Tumor Institute
Hodgkin's Disease – Radiation Therapy

LOUIS A. CANCELLARO, Ph.D., M.D.

Professor of Psychiatry, Professor of Anatomy, East Tennessee State University Quillen-Dishner College of Medicine; Associate Chairman, Department of Psychiatry and Chief of Psychiatry, Veterans Administration Medical Center, Mountain Home; Consulting Medical Staff, Indian Path Hospital, Kingsport; Courtesy Medical Staff, Johnson City Medical Center, Johnson City, Tennessee
Psychoneurosis

LOUIS R. CAPLAN, M.D.

Associate Professor of Neurology, University of Chicago Pritzker School of Medicine, Chairman, Department of Neurology, Michael Reese Hospital, Chicago, Illinois
Acute Ischemic Cerebrovascular Disease

LARRY C. CAREY, M.D.

Robert M. Zollinger, Professor and Chairman, Department of Surgery, Ohio State University College of Medicine; Attending Surgeon, Ohio State University Hospital, Children's Hospital, and Grant Hospital, Columbus, Ohio
Cholelithiasis and Cholecystitis

HARRY W. CARLOSS, M.D.

Assistant Professor of Clinical Medicine, University of Louisville School of Medicine; Attending Hematologist, Lourdes Hospital, Paducah, Kentucky
Immune Hemolytic Anemia

IVOR CARO, M.D.

Clinical Assistant Professor of Medicine (Dermatology), University of Washington School of Medicine; Attending Dermatologist, University of Washington Hospitals, The Mason Clinic, and Virginia Mason Hospital, Seattle, Washington
Dermatomyositis/Polymyositis

WILLIAM J. CASHORE, M.D.

Assistant Professor of Pediatrics, Brown University Program in Medicine; Attending Neonatologist, Women and Infants Hospital of Rhode Island; Attending Pediatrician, Rhode Island Hospital, Providence, Rhode Island
Normal Infant Feeding

AGUSTIN CASTELLANOS, M.D.

Professor of Medicine, University of Miami School of Medicine; Director of Electrophysiology, Jackson Memorial Hospital, Miami, Florida
Premature Beats

HYMAN CHAI, M.D., F.R.C.P.(E), D.Ch.

Associate Clinical Professor of Pediatrics, University of Colorado School of Medicine; Director of Clinical Services, West Campus National Jewish Hospital/National Asthma Center; Director, Pediatric Allergy Clinic, University Hospital, Denver, Colorado
Asthma in Children

CHARLES H. CHESNUT, III, M.D.

Associate Professor of Medicine and Radiology, University of Washington School of Medicine; Director, Harborview Medical Center Nuclear Medicine Laboratories; Attending Physician, University Hospital, Seattle, Washington
Osteoporosis

ROBERT CHILCOTE, M.D.

Assistant Professor, University of Chicago School of Medicine (Hematology-Oncology, Department of Pediatrics), Chicago, Illinois
Vitamin K Deficiency

LUIS A. CISNEROS, M.D.

Fellow in Infectious Diseases, University of Maryland School of Medicine, University of Maryland Hospital, Baltimore, Maryland
Typhoid Fever

JAY D. COFFMAN, M.D.

Professor of Medicine, Boston University School of Medicine; Visiting Physician, Section Head, Peripheral Vascular Department, University Hospital, Boston University Medical Center, Boston, Massachusetts
Thrombophlebitis in Obstetrics and Gynecology

BRUCE M. COHEN, M.D., Ph.D

Assistant Professor, Harvard Medical School, Boston; Assistant Psychiatrist, McLean Hospital, Belmont, Massachusetts
Schizophrenia

PATRICK J. CONDRY, M.D.

Private Practice, Weirton, West Virginia
Herpes Simplex

REX B. CONN, M.D.

Professor of Pathology and Laboratory Medicine, Emory University School of Medicine, Atlanta; Director, Clinical Pathology Laboratories, Emory University Hospital, Atlanta, Georgia
Laboratory Reference Values of Clinical Importance

JOHN E. CONNOLLY, M.D.

Professor of Surgery, University of California at Irvine; Chief, Cardiovascular and Thoracic Surgery, University of California at Irvine Medical Center, Orange, California
Varicose Veins

MARCEL E. CONRAD, M.D.

Professor of Medicine, Director of Hematology and Oncology, School of Medicine, University of Alabama in Birmingham; Attending Physician, University of Alabama Hospitals, Birmingham, Alabama
Malaria

GIBBONS G. CORNWELL, III, M.D.

Professor of Medicine, Chief, Section of Hematology and Oncology, Dartmouth Medical School, Hanover; Staff Physician, Mary Hitchcock Memorial Hospital, Hanover, New Hampshire; Consultant, Veterans Administration Hospital, White River Junction, Vermont
Multiple Myeloma

E. DAVID CRAWFORD, M.D.

Assistant Professor, Department of Surgery, Division of Urology, University of New Mexico School of Medicine; Chief of Urology, Cancer Research Treatment Center; Director GU Oncology, University of New Mexico School of Medicine; Attending Urologist, Veterans Administration Hospital, Albuquerque, New Mexico
Genitourinary Tumors

DUDLEY SETH DANOFF, M.D., F.A.C.S.

Clinical Faculty, Department of Surgery-Urology, University of California, Los Angeles, School of Medicine; Attending Urologist, Cedars-Sinai Medical Center and University of California, Los Angeles Medical Center Hospital and Clinic, Los Angeles, California
Genitourinary Tuberculosis

FAITH B. DAVIS, M.D.

Clinical Associate Professor of Medicine, State University of New York at Buffalo; Staff Endocrinologist, Erie County Medical Center, Buffalo, New York
Hypothyroidism

PAUL J. DAVIS, M.D.

Professor of Medicine, State University of New York at Buffalo; Vice-Chairman, Department of Medicine, Erie County Medical Center; Chief, Medical Services, Head Endocrinology Division, Buffalo Veterans Administration Medical Center, Buffalo, New York
Hypothyroidism

ROBERT L. DEATON, M.D.

Assistant Professor of Obstetrics and Gynecology, Indiana University Medical Center, Indianapolis; Obstetrician and Gynecologist, Methodist Hospital, Indianapolis, Indiana
Preoperative and Postoperative Care for Elective Gynecologic Surgery

FLOYD W. DENNY, JR., M.D.

Professor and Chairman, Department of Pediatrics, University of North Carolina School of Medicine, Chapel Hill; Chief, Department of Pediatrics, North Carolina Memorial Hospital, Chapel Hill, North Carolina
Viral Pneumonia; Mycoplasma Pneumonia

JOHN H. DIRCKX, M.D.

Medical Director, C. H. Gosiger Health Center, University of Dayton, Dayton, Ohio
Infectious Mononucleosis

W. EDWIN DODSON, M.D.

Associate Professor of Pediatrics and Neurology, Washington University School of Medicine; Attending Staff, St. Louis Children's Hospital and Barnes Hospital, St. Louis, Missouri
Epilepsy in Childhood

MARGARET C. DOUGLASS, M.D.

Clinical Assistant Professor of Dermatology, University of Michigan Medical School; Staff Physician, Department of Dermatology, Henry Ford Hospital, Detroit, Michigan
Diseases of the Nails

THOMAS M. DREW, M.D.

Clinical Assistant Professor, Brown University Medical School; Cardiologist, Rhode Island Hospital, Providence, Rhode Island
Angina Pectoris

EDMUND L. DUBOIS, M.D.

Clinical Professor of Medicine, University of Southern California School of Medicine, Los Angeles, California
Lupus Erythematosus

DAVID L. DUNNER, M.D.

Professor, Department of Psychiatry and Behavioral Sciences, University of Washington, Seattle; Chief of Psychiatry, Harborview Medical Center, Seattle, Washington
Affective Disorders

ISADORE DYER, M.D.

Professor Emeritus, Obstetrics and Gynecology, Tulane University Medical School; Attending Physician, Touro Infirmary, Charity Hospital, New Orleans, Louisiana; Consultant, U.S. Air Force Medical Center, Keesler Air Force Base, Biloxi, Mississippi
Hemorrhage in Late Pregnancy

ANTHONY J. EDIS, M.D., F.A.C.S.

Department of General Surgery, Mayo Clinic, Rochester, Minnesota
Thyroid Malignancy

YNGVE EDLUND, M.D., Ph.D.

Professor of Surgery, University of Göteborg; Chairman Surgical Department III, Sahlgrenska sjukhuset, Göteborg, Sweden
Acute Pancreatitis

MERRILL W. EDMONDS, M.D., F.R.C.P.(C.)

Assistant Professor of Internal Medicine, University of Western Ontario; Director of Medical Education, Director of Metabolic Education Centre, Victoria Hospital Corporation, London, Ontario, Canada
Thyroiditis

E. CHRISTOPHER ELLISON, M.D.

Clinical Instructor in Surgery, Ohio State University College of Medicine; Resident in Surgery, Ohio State University Hospitals, Columbus, Ohio
Cholelithiasis and Cholecystitis

KENNETH ENG, M.D.

Associate Professor of Surgery, New York University School of Medicine; Attending Physician, University Hospital, Bellevue Hospital, and Manhattan Veterans Administration Hospital, New York, New York
Diverticula of the Alimentary Tract

NORMAN H. ERTEL, M.D.

Professor of Medicine, College of Medicine and Dentistry of New Jersey Medical School, Newark; Chief, Medical Service, Veterans Administration Medical Center, East Orange, New Jersey
Pheochromocytoma

LUIS R. ESPINOZA, M.D.

Associate Professor of Medicine, University of South Florida College of Medicine; Attending Rheumatologist, Tampa General Hospital and James A. Haley Veterans Administration Medical Center, Tampa, Florida
Juvenile Rheumatoid Arthritis

STEPHEN A. ESTES, M.D.

Assistant Professor of Dermatology, University of Cincinnati; Attending Dermatologist (Full-Time Staff), University of Cincinnati Medical Center Children's Hospital, and Holmes Hospital, Cincinnati, Ohio
Scabies

DONNELL D. ETZWILER, M.D.

Clinical Associate Professor, Department of Pediatrics, University of Minnesota Medical School; Pediatrician, St. Louis Park Medical Center and Methodist Hospital, Minneapolis, Minnesota
Diabetes Mellitus in Childhood and Adolescence

HOWARD E. FAUVER, Jr., M.D.

Assistant Clinical Professor of Surgery (Urology), University of Colorado; Chief, Urology Service, Fitzsimons Army Medical Center, Aurora, Colorado
Pyelonephritis

ROBERT FEKETY, M.D.

Professor of Internal Medicine, University of Michigan Medical School; Chief, Infectious Diseases Service, University Hospital, Ann Arbor, Michigan
Diphtheria

ROBERT G. FELDMAN, M.D.

Professor of Neurology and Pharmacology, Chairman, Department of Neurology, Boston University School of Medicine; Chief of Neurology Services, University Hospital and Boston Veterans Administration Medical Center, Boston, Massachusetts
Epilepsy in Adolescents and Adults

BRIAN G. FIRTH, M.D., D.Phil.

Assistant Professor of Internal Medicine, University of Texas Southwestern Medical School; Associate Director, Cardiac Catheterization Laboratory, Parkland Memorial Hospital, Dallas, Texas
Acute Myocardial Infarction

JOHN F. FISHER, M.D.

Assistant Professor of Internal Medicine, Medical College of Georgia, Augusta, Georgia
Rocky Mountain Spotted Fever

LESLIE R. FLEISCHER, M.D.

Former Senior Cardiology Fellow, Division of Cardiology, University of Vermont College of Medicine, Burlington, Vermont; Attending Cardiologist, St. Joseph's Hospital, Lancaster, Pennsylvania
Tachycardia

FREDERICK J. FLEURY, M.D.

Clinical Assistant Professor of Obstetrics and Gynecology, Southern Illinois University School of Medicine; Attending Staff, Memorial Medical Center and St. John's Hospital, Springfield, Illinois
Vulvovaginitis

BOY FRAME, M.D.

Clinical Professor of Medicine, University of Michigan Medical School, Ann Arbor; Chief, Bone and Mineral Metabolism Division, Henry Ford Hospital, Detroit, Michigan
Rickets and Osteomalacia

ERNEST W. FRANKLIN, III, M.D.

St. Joseph Hospital, Atlanta, Georgia
Carcinoma of the Vulva

ROBERT J. FREEARK, M.D.

Professor and Chairman, Department of Surgery, Stritch School of Medicine of Loyola University; Surgeon-in-Chief, Foster G. McGaw Hospital of Loyola University, Chicago, Illinois
Intestinal Obstruction

NORBERT FREINKEL, M.D.

Kettering Professor of Medicine; Director, Center for Endocrinology, Metabolism, and Nutrition; Chief, Section of En-

docrinology, Metabolism, and Nutrition, Northwestern University Medical School; Attending Physician and Director, Endocrine/Metabolic Clinic, Northwestern Memorial Hospital; Consultant, Veterans Administration Lakeside Hospital, Chicago, Illinois
Reactive Hypoglycemias

ELI A. FRIEDMAN, M.D.

Professor, Department of Medicine, State University of New York Downstate Medical Center College of Medicine, Brooklyn; Chief, Division of Renal Diseases, Kings County Hospital, State University Hospital, Brooklyn, New York
Chronic Renal Failure

WESLEY FURSTE, M.D., F.A.C.S.

Clinical Professor of Surgery, Ohio State University, Columbus, Ohio
Tetanus

J. WILLIAM FUTRELL, M.D.

Professor and Chief of Plastic Surgery, University of Pittsburgh School of Medicine, Pittsburgh, Pennsylvania
Disorders of the Mouth (Malignant)

JOHN T. GALAMBOS, M.D.

Professor of Medicine (Digestive Diseases), Emory University School of Medicine, Atlanta, Georgia
Bleeding Esophageal Varices

WESLEY KING GALEN, M.D.

Assistant Professor, Section of Dermatology, Department of Medicine, Tulane University School of Medicine; Attending Staff, Tulane Medical Center Hospital, Children's Hospital, Hotel Dieu, New Orleans, Louisiana
Pruritus Ani and Vulvae

PIERCE GARDNER, M.D.

Professor of Medicine and Pediatrics, Director of Infectious Diseases Training Program, University of Chicago, Chicago, Illinois
Coccidioidomycosis

MARILYN H. GASTON, M.D.

Assistant Clinical Professor, Howard University; Deputy Branch Chief, Sickle Cell Disease Branch, National Institutes of Health, Bethesda, Maryland
Sickle Cell Disease

WILLIAM A. GAY, Jr., M.D.

Professor of Surgery, Cornell University Medical College; Chief, Division of Cardiothoracic Surgery, The New York Hospital, New York, New York
Acquired Diseases of the Aorta

SAUL M. GENUTH, M.D.

Professor of Medicine, Case Western Reserve University School of Medicine; Director, Saltzman Institute for Clinical Investigation, Mount Sinai Hospital, Cleveland, Ohio
Obesity

RONALD B. GEORGE, M.D.

Professor of Medicine, Louisiana State School of Medicine in Shreveport; Chief, Medical Service, Veterans Administration Medical Center, Shreveport, Louisiana
Blastomycosis

JOSEPH E. GERACI, M.D.

Professor of Medicine, Mayo Graduate School of Medicine; Attending Staff, Mayo Clinic and Affiliated Hospitals, Rochester, Minnesota
Infective Endocarditis

ALBERT B. GERBIE, M.D.

Professor of Obstetrics and Gynecology, Northwestern University Medical School, Chicago; Attending Obstetrician and Gynecologist, Prentice Women's Hospital and Maternity Center of Northwestern Memorial Hospital, and Children's Memorial Hospital, Chicago, Illinois
Myoma of the Uterus

BERNARD F. GERMAIN, M.D.

Associate Professor of Medicine, Assistant Professor of Pediatrics, University of South Florida College of Medicine; Attending Rheumatologist, Tampa General Hospital and James A. Haley Veterans Administration Medical Center, Tampa, Florida
Juvenile Rheumatoid Arthritis

JAMES JEROME GIBSON, M.D., M.P.H.

Assistant Professor of Preventive Medicine and Clinical Assistant Professor of Medicine, University of South Carolina School of Medicine; Consultant, Richland Memorial Hospital and Veterans Administration Hospital, Columbia, South Carolina
Intestinal Parasites

HARRIET S. GILBERT, M.D.

Associate Professor of Internal Medicine, Mount Sinai School of Medicine of City University of New York; Associate Attending in Medicine, the Mount Sinai Hospital, New York; Consultant, Bronx Veterans Administration Hospital, Bronx, New York
Polycythemia Vera, Erythrocytosis, and Relative Polycythemia

MICHAEL E. GLASSCOCK, III, M.D., F.A.C.S.

Associate Professor of Surgery, Vanderbilt University School of Medicine; Otologist, Baptist Hospital, Nashville, Tennessee
Meniere's Disease

FRANZ GOLDSTEIN, M.D.

Professor of Medicine, Jefferson Medical College of Thomas Jefferson University; Chief, Division of Gastroenterology, Lankenau Hospital, Philadelphia, Pennsylvania
Gaseousness

ROBERT C. GOLDSZER, M.D.

Research Fellow in Medicine (Renal Division), Peter Bent

Brigham Hospital, and Boston Hospital for Women, Harvard Medical School, Boston, Massachusetts
Glomerular Disorders

HARVEY M. GOLOMB, M.D.

Associate Professor, Division of the Biologic Sciences of the Pritzker School of Medicine; Associate Professor, Section of Hematology/Oncology, Department of Medicine, the University of Chicago, Chicago, Illinois
Hodgkin's Disease — Chemotherapy

JAMES T. GOOD, Jr., M.D.

Assistant Professor of Medicine, University of Colorado Medical Center; Codirector of Respiratory Therapy, Denver General Hospital, Denver, Colorado
Pleural Effusions and Empyema Thoracis

JOSEPH H. GRAZIANO, Ph.D.

Associate Professor of Pediatric Pharmacology, Columbia University College of Physicians, New York, New York
Thalassemia

MARTIN H. GREENBERG, M.D., F.A.A.P., F.A.C.O.G.

Professor, Department of Pediatrics, Medical College of Georgia, Augusta; Director of Pediatrics, Memorial Medical Center, Savannah, Georgia
Care of the Low Birth Weight Infant

PETER GREENBERG, M.D., Ph.D., F.R.A.C.P.

Senior Associate in Medicine, University of Melbourne Department of Medicine, Royal Melbourne Hospital; Physician, Royal Melbourne Hospital, Victoria, Australia
Hyper- and Hypoparathyroidism

JAMES F. GREGORY, M.D.

Assistant Clinical Professor of Dermatology in Medicine, St. Louis University School of Medicine; Attending Staff, St. Elizabeth's Hospital and Memorial Hospital, Belleville Illinois
Acne Rosacea

ROBERT L. GRISSOM, M.D.

Professor of Internal Medicine, University of Nebraska College of Medicine; Attending Physician, University of Nebraska Hospital, Omaha, Nebraska
Brucellosis

PAUL R. GROSS, M.D.

Clinical Assistant Professor of Dermatology, University of Pennsylvania School of Medicine; Chief Dermatology Sections, Pennsylvania Hospital and Methodist Hospital, Philadelphia, Pennsylvania
Lichen Planus

HELEN E. GRUBER, Ph.D.

Research Instructor, Medicine, University of Washington School of Medicine, Seattle; Research Instructor, Mineral Metabolism Laboratories, Veterans Administration Hospital, Tacoma, Washington
Osteoporosis

KENNETH M. GRUNDFAST, M.D.

Assistant Professor, George Washington University School of Medicine; Chairman, Department of Otorhinolaryngology, Children's Hospital National Medical Center, Washington, District of Columbia
Acute Otitis Media

STEFAN GRZYBOWSKI, M.D.

Professor of Medicine, University of British Columbia; Senior Active Staff, Head, Respiratory Division, Vancouver General Hospital, Vancouver, British Columbia, Canada
Tuberculosis and Other Mycobacterial Diseases

RICHARD L. GUERRANT, M.D.

Associate Professor of Medicine, University of Virginia School of Medicine; Head, Division of Geographic Medicine, University of Virginia Hospital, Charlottesville, Virginia
Food Poisoning

PATRICK GUINAN, M.D., M.P.H.

Associate Professor of Surgery (Urology), Abraham Lincoln School of Medicine, The University of Illinois; Chairman, Division of Urology, Cook County Hospital, Chicago, Illinois
Genitourinary Tract Trauma

JOHN C. HALL, M.D.

Professor (Associate, Teaching), University of Missouri at Kansas City; Associate Teaching at Children's Mercy Hospital; Full Time Staff (Dermatology), St. Luke's Hospital; Courtesy Staff, St. Mary's Hospital, Kansas City, Missouri
Pseudofolliculitis Barbae

WILLIAM J. HALL, M.D.

Associate Professor of Medicine and Pediatrics, Co-head Pulmonary Disease Unit, University of Rochester School of Medicine, Rochester, New York
Acute Respiratory Failure

BRUCE W. HALSTEAD, M.D.

Director, International Biotoxicological Center, World Life Research Institute, Colton, California
Portuguese Man-of-War (Jellyfish) Stings

ROBERT E. HARRIS, M.D., Ph.D.

Clinical Assistant Professor of Obstetrics and Gynecology, Adjunct Associate Professor of Microbiology, University of Texas Health Science Center at San Antonio; Obstetrics/Gynecology Staff, Methodist Hospital, San Antonio, Texas
Urinary Tract Infections During Pregnancy

DANIEL E. HATHAWAY, M.D.

Assistant Professor of Medicine, University of Minnesota Department of Medicine; Chief, Rheumatology Section, St.

Paul-Ramsey Medical Center, Minneapolis, Minnesota
Rheumatoid Arthritis

EDGAR A. HAUNZ, M.D., M.Sc. (MED.), D.Sc. (HON.), F.A.C.P.

Emeritus Professor of Medicine, University of North Dakota School of Medicine; Senior Consultant, Diabetes Division, Grand Forks Clinic; Consulting Diabetologist, the United Hospital, Grand Forks, North Dakota
Diabetes Mellitus in Adults

LEON M. HEBERTSON, M.D.

Director of Public Health, County of Kern, Bakersfield, California
Measles (Rubeola)

PAUL B. HELLER, M.D., LT. COL M.C.

Assistant Professor of Obstetrics and Gynecology, Uniformed Services University of the Health Sciences; Chief, Gynecologic Oncology Service, Walter Reed Army Medical Center, Washington, District of Columbia
Cancer of the Uterus

DANIEL HIER, M.D.

Assistant Professor of Neurology, University of Chicago Pritzker School of Medicine; Neurologist, Michael Reese Hospital, Chicago, Illinois
Acute Ischemic Cerebrovascular Disease

L. DAVID HILLIS, M.D.

Assistant Professor of Internal Medicine, University of Texas Southwestern Medical School; Director Cardiac Catheterization Laboratory, Parkland Memorial Hospital, Dallas, Texas
Acute Myocardial Infarction

NORBERT HIRSCHHORN, M.D.

Staff Associate, John Snow Public Health Group, Inc., Boston, Massachusetts
Cholera

JOHN E. HODGKIN, M.D.

Associate Professor of Medicine, Loma Linda University School of Medicine; Chief, Pulmonary Section, Jerry L. Pettis Memorial Veterans Hospital, Loma Linda, California
Chronic Bronchitis, Bronchiectasis, and Emphysema

A. V. HOFFBRAND, D.M., F.R.C.P., F.R.C.PATH.

Professor of Haematology, Royal Free School of Medicine; Honorary Consultant, Royal Free Hospital, Bond Street, London, England
Pernicious Anemia and Other Megaloblastic Anemias

LARRY H. HOLLIER, M.D.

Assistant Professor of Surgery (Peripheral Vascular Surgery), Mayo Medical School and Mayo Graduate School, University of Minnesota; Staff Member and Consultant, St.

Mary's Hospital, Rochester Methodist Hospital, and Rochester State Hospital, Rochester, Minnesota
Degenerative Arterial Disease

RICHARD R. HOOPER, M.D., M.P.H.

Epidemiologist, Naval Regional Medical Center, Oakland, California
Gonococcal Infection

WILLIAM HOROWITZ, M.D., F.A.C.P., F.A.C.C.

Assistant Clinical Professor of Medicine, Albert Einstein College of Medicine of Yeshiva University, New York City; Attending Physician, Bronx Veterans Administration Medical Center; Adjunct Physician, Montefiore Hospital and Medical Center; Associate Visiting Physician, St. Agnes Hospital, White Plains, New York
Cardiac Arrest

ROBIN P. HUMPHREYS, M.D., F.R.C.S. (C.)

Assistant Professor, Department of Surgery (Neurosurgery), Faculty of Medicine, University of Toronto; Staff Neurosurgeon, Hospital for Sick Children; Consulting Neurosurgeon, Ontario Crippled Children's Centre, and North York General Hospital, Toronto, Canada
Brain Abscess

ROBERT JACKSON, M.D., F.R.C.P. (C.)

Associate Professor of Medicine (Dermatology), University of Ottawa; Dermatologist, Ottawa Civic Hospital, Ottawa, Ontario, Canada
Decubitus Ulcer

W. DAVID JACOBY, JR., M.D.

Associate in Internal Medicine (Dermatology), University of Arizona College of Medicine; Attending Dermatologist, University of Arizona Hospital, Tucson Medical Center, and St. Joseph's Hospital; Consultant, Davis-Monthan Air Force Base Hospital, Tucson, Arizona
Inflammatory Eruptions of the Hands and Feet

MELVIN E. JENKINS, M.D., F.A.A.P.

Professor and Chairman, Department of Pediatrics and Child Health, Howard University College of Medicine; Chairman, Chief Pediatrician, and Pediatric Endocrinologist, Department of Pediatrics and Child Health, Howard University Hospital, Washington, District of Columbia
Childhood Enuresis

LAWRENCE F. JOHNSON, M.D.

Professor of Medicine, Uniform Services University of Health Sciences; Chief, Gastroenterology Service, Walter Reed Army Medical Center, Washington, District of Columbia
Dysphagia and Esophageal Obstruction

LENNART A. JUHLIN, M.D.

Professor of Dermatology, University of Uppsala; Head, Department of Dermatology and Venereology, University Hospital, Uppsala, Sweden
Urticaria and Angioedema

GUNTER KAHN, M.D.

Director Pediatric Dermatology Seminars, Parkway Hospital Medical Plaza, North Miami Beach, Florida
Sunburn and Photosensitivity

WILLIAM S. KAMMERER, M.D.

Associate Professor of Medicine, Pennsylvania State University College of Medicine; Attending Physician, M. S. Hershey Medical Center, Hershey, Pennsylvania
Echinococcosis (Hydatid Disease)

SOLOMON A. KAPLAN, M.D.

Professor of Pediatrics, University of California at Los Angeles School of Medicine; Head, Division of Pediatric Endocrinology and Metabolism, University of California at Los Angeles Center for Health Sciences, Los Angeles, California
Fluid Therapy in Children

A. B. A. KARAT, M.D., F.R.C.P. (London), F.R.C.P. (Edin.)

Consultant Physician, The Royal Infirmary, Sunderland, United Kingdom
Leprosy

RICHARD J. KATZ, M.D.

Assistant Professor of Medicine, George Washington University School of Medicine; Director, Cardiographics Laboratory and Attending Cardiologist, George Washington Medical University Center, Washington, District of Columbia
Congestive Heart Failure

CHUICHI KAWAI, M.D., D. MED. SC.

Professor of Medicine, Faculty of Medicine, Kyoto University; Director, Third Division, Department of Internal Medicine, Kyoto University Hospital, Kyoto, Japan
Beriberi

DONALD KAYE, M.D.

Professor and Chairman, Department of Medicine, Medical College of Pennsylvania; Chief of Medicine, Hospital of Medical College of Pennsylvania; Consultant, Philadelphia Veterans Administration Hospital, Philadelphia, Pennsylvania
Salmonellosis (Other than Typhoid Fever)

HAROLD L. KAYE, M.D.

Clinical Assistant Professor, University of Texas Health Science Center at Dallas; Attending Physician, Presbyterian Hospital, Dallas, and Richardson Medical Center, Richardson, Texas
Menopause

LOUIS G. KEITH, M.D.

Professor of Obstetrics and Gynecology, Northwestern University Medical School; Attending Physician, Prentice Women's Hospital and Maternity Center, Chicago, Illinois
Contraception

JOHN R. KELSEY, JR., M.D.

Clinical Professor of Medicine, Baylor College of Medicine, Houston, Texas
Constipation

JAMES W. KENDIG, M.D.

Fellow in Neonatal-Perinatal Medicine, The Milton S. Hershey Medical Center of the Pennsylvania State University, Hershey, Pennsylvania.
Hemolytic Disease of the Newborn

CHARLES D. KIMBALL, M.D.

Former Clinical Associate Professor of Obstetrics and Gynecology, University of Washington; Attending Staff, Virginia Mason Hospital, Northwest Hospital, and Swedish Hospital; Affiliated Member, Virginia Mason Research Center, Seattle, Washington
Postpartum Care

DAVID B. KING, M.D., B.Sc.

Assistant Professor of Medicine, Dalhousie University; Attending Neurologist, Victoria General Hospital; Consulting Neurologist, Dartmouth General Hospital, Halifax Infirmary, Camp Hill Hospital, Nova Scotia Rehabilitation Hospital, Halifax, Nova Scotia, Canada
Rehabilitation of the Paraplegic Patient

LORRAINE C. KING, M.D., F.A.C.O.G.

Assistant Clinical Professor, Obstetrics and Gynecology, Jefferson Medical College of Thomas Jefferson University, Philadelphia; Attending Physician, Thomas Jefferson University Hospital, Philadelphia, Pennsylvania
Dysfunctional Uterine Bleeding

LOWELL R. KING, M.D.

Professor of Urology and Surgery, Northwestern University Medical School; Attending Urologist, Children's Memorial Hospital and Northwestern Memorial Hospital, Chicago, Illinois
Bacterial Infections of the Urinary Tract (Female Children)

LESTER A. KLEIN, M.D.

Associate Professor, Harvard Medical School; Chief, Division of Urology, Beth Israel Hospital, Boston, Massachusetts
Prostatitis

ROBERT S. KLEIN, M.D.

Assistant Professor of Medicine, Albert Einstein College of Medicine; Assistant Attending Physician, Division of Infectious Diseases, Montefiore Hospital and Medical Center and North Central Bronx Hospital, Bronx, New York
Bacterial Pneumonia

G. ERIC KNOX, M.D.

Associate Clinical Professor of Obstetrics and Public Health, University of Minnesota; Perinatologist, Abbott-Northwestern Hospital, Minneapolis, Minnesota
Pelvic Infections

FRANK C. KORANDA, M.D.

Assistant Professor of Dermatology, University of Iowa
School of Medicine; Director, Cutaneous Surgery Section,
Chief, Contact Dermatitis Clinic, University of Iowa Hospitals, Iowa City, Iowa
Occupational Dermatoses

NICHOLAS T. KOUCHOUKOS, M.D.

Professor of Surgery, University of Alabama in Birmingham;
Attending Surgeon, University Hospitals, Birmingham Veterans Administration Hospitals, Birmingham, Alabama
Atelectasis

MICHAEL J. KOWERTZ, M.D.

Kaiser-Permanente Medical Center, Santa Clara, California
Contact Dermatitis

EDWARD A. KRULL, M.D.

Clinical Professor of Dermatology, University of Michigan
Medical School; Chairman, Department of Dermatology,
Henry Ford Hospital, Detroit, Michigan
Diseases of the Nails

BAYLOR KURTIS, M.D.

Assistant Professor of Dermatology, Baylor University College of Medicine; Assistant Chief, Dermatology Service,
Houston Veterans Administration Hospital, Houston, Texas
Bacterial Diseases of the Skin

PEARON G. LANG, JR., M.D.

Assistant Professor of Dermatology, Medical University of
South Carolina; Attending Physician, Hospital of the Medical
University of South Carolina, Charleston, South Carolina
Polyarteritis Nodosa

JAMES W. LANGLEY, M.D.

Medical Director, South Texas Regional Blood Bank; Clinical
Assistant Professor of Pathology, University of Texas Health
Science Center at San Antonio; Attending Immunohematologist, Bexar County Teaching Hospital and Audie Murphy
Veterans Hospital, San Antonio, Texas
Therapeutic Use of Blood Components

THOMAS J. LAWLEY, M.D.

Senior Investigator, Dermatology Branch, National Cancer
Institute, National Institutes of Health, Bethesda, Maryland
*Herpes Gestationis; Pruritic Urticarial Papules and Plaques of
Pregnancy*

J. MICHAEL LAZARUS, M.D.

Associate Professor of Medicine, Harvard Medical School;
Associate-in-Medicine, Peter Bent Brigham Hospital and
Boston Hospital for Women, Boston, Massachusetts
Glomerular Disorders

MYRON M. LEVINE, M.D., D.T.P.H.

Associate Professor, Infectious Diseases, Associate Professor,
Preventive Medicine, University of Maryland School of

Medicine; Attending Physician, University of Maryland
Hospital, Baltimore, Maryland
Typhoid Fever

ARTHUR M. LEVY, M.D.

Professor of Medicine and Pediatrics, Director of Division
of Cardiology, University of Vermont College of Medicine;
Attending Cardiologist and Director, Division of Cardiology, Medical Center Hospital of Vermont, Burlington, Vermont
Tachycardia

ERIC CHUN-YET LIAN, M.D.

Associate Professor of Clinical Medicine, University of
Miami School of Medicine; Director of the Miami Comprehensive Hemophilia Center at Jackson Memorial Hospital;
Attending Hematologist, University of Miami Hospitals and
Veterans Administration Hospital, Miami, Florida.
*Disseminated Intravascular Coagulation (DIC); Thrombotic
Thrombocytopenic Purpura*

PHIL LIEBERMAN, M.D.

Professor of Internal Medicine, Chief, Division of Allergy-
Immunology, University of Tennessee Center for the
Health Sciences, College of Medicine; Active Staff, Baptist
Memorial Hospital, William F. Bowld Hospital, Memphis,
Tennessee
Anaphylaxis and Serum Sickness

CHARLES S. LINCOLN, JR., M.D.

Associate Clinical Professor of Dermatology, University of
California Medical School, San Francisco, California
Cancer of the Skin

JOHN A. LINFOOT, M.D.

Clinical Professor of Medicine, University of California,
Davis; Director of Endocrine-Metabolic Service, Director of
the Pituitary Center, Alta Bates Hospital, Berkeley; Consultant, Veterans Administration Hospital, Martinez, California
Acromegaly

JOSEPH F. LIPINSKI, M.D.

Assistant Professor, Harvard Medical School; Assistant Psychiatrist, McLean Hospital, Belmont, Massachusetts
Schizophrenia

S. ARTHUR LOCALIO, M.D.

Professor of Surgery, New York University School of Medicine; Attending Physician, University Hospital, Bellevue
Hospital, and Manhattan Veterans Administration Hospital,
New York, New York
Diverticula of the Alimentary Tract

JOHN D. LOESER, M.D.

Associate Professor, Department of Neurological Surgery,
University of Washington School of Medicine; Attending
Physician, University Hospital, Harborview Medical Center,
Veterans Administration Hospital, Children's Orthopedic
Hospital, Seattle, Washington
Trigeminal Neuralgia

DONALD P. LOOKINGBILL, M.D.

Assistant Professor of Medicine, Pennsylvania State University College of Medicine, Hershey; Chief of Dermatology, Hershey Medical Center, Hershey, Pennsylvania
Seborrheic Dermatitis

JOYCE H. LOWINSON, M.D.

Associate Clinical Professor of Psychiatry, Albert Einstein College of Medicine of Yeshiva University, New York; Director, Substance Abuse Service, Albert Einstein College of Medicine; Attending Psychiatrist, Bronx Municipal Hospital Center, Bronx, New York
Narcotic Poisoning

EDMUND D. LOWNEY, M.D.

Professor of Dermatology, Ohio State University College of Medicine; Attending Staff, Ohio State University Hospitals, Columbus, Ohio
Dermatitis Herpetiformis

JEANNE M. LUSHER, M.D.

Professor of Pediatrics, Wayne State University School of Medicine; Director, Department of Hematology-Oncology; Director, Regional Hemophilia Treatment Center, Children's Hospital of Michigan, Detroit, Michigan
Hemophilia and Related Disorders

SEAN R. LYNCH, M.D.

Associate Professor of Medicine, University of Kansas; Attending Physician, University of Kansas Medical Center, Kansas City, Kansas, and Veterans Administration Hospital, Kansas City, Missouri
Anemia Due to Iron Deficiency

JOSHUA LYNFIELD, M.B., B.Ch. Cantab.

Professor of Clinical Pediatrics, New York University School of Medicine; Attending Physician, University Hospital, New York University; Visiting Physician, Bellevue Hospital, New York, New York
Rheumatic Fever

MORELLY L. MAAYAN, M.D., Ph.D., F.A.C.P.

Associate Professor of Nuclear Medicine, State University of New York, Downstate Medical Center; Chief, Nuclear Medicine Service, Veterans Administration Medical Center, Brooklyn, New York
Simple Goiter

JAMES D. MABERRY, M.D.

Clinical Instructor of Dermatology, John Peter Smith Hospital; Attending Dermatologist, Harris Hospital, All Saints Hospital, Saint Joseph Hospital, Fort Worth, Texas
Hidradenitis Suppurativa

GORDON MacDONALD, M.D.

Lecturer Emeritus, University of Southern California School of Medicine; Attending Staff, Department of Medicine, Riverside Community Hospital, Riverside, California
Herpes Zoster

M. JEFFREY MAISELS, M.B., B.Ch.

Professor of Pediatrics and Obstetrics and Gynecology, the Milton S. Hershey Medical Center of the Pennsylvania State University, Hershey, Pennsylvania
Hemolytic Disease of the Newborn

JOHN C. MAIZE, M.D.

Associate Professor of Dermatology and Pathology, Medical University of South Carolina; Attending Dermatologist, Medical University of South Carolina Hospital, Charleston, South Carolina
Pemphigus and Pemphigoid

DOUGLAS J. MARCHANT, M.D.

Professor of Obstetrics and Gynecology, Tufts University School of Medicine; Director, the Cancer Center, New England Medical Center Hospital, Boston, Massachusetts
Diseases of the Breast

FRAY F. MARSHALL, M.D.

Associate Professor of Urology, the Johns Hopkins University School of Medicine; Attending Staff, the Johns Hopkins Hospital, Baltimore, Maryland
Epididymitis

KENNETH P. MATHEWS, M.D.

Professor of Internal Medicine, University of Michigan Medical School; Head, Division of Allergy, Department of Internal Medicine, University of Michigan; Consultant in Allergy at Wayne County General Hospital and Ann Arbor Veterans Administration Hospital, Ann Arbor, Michigan
Adverse Reactions to Drugs: Hypersensitivity

SHARON G. McDONALD, M.D.

Associate Professor of Dermatology, Abraham Lincoln School of Medicine, University of Illinois, Chicago, Illinois
Pityriasis Rosea

RICHARD B. McELVEIN, M.D.

Associate Professor of Surgery, University of Alabama in Birmingham Veterans Hospitals, Birmingham, Alabama
Atelectasis

KEVIN M. McINTYRE, M.D.

Assistant Professor of Medicine, Harvard Medical School; Assistant Chief of Cardiology, Veterans Administration Medical Center, West Roxbury, Massachusetts
Pulmonary Embolism

DONALD S. McLAREN, M.D., Ph.D., M.R.C.R.E.

Reader in Clinical Nutrition, Edinburgh, Scotland; Consultant, Department of Medicine, Royal Infirmary
Hypo- and Hypervitaminosis

DAVID G. McLONE, M.D., Ph.D.

Associate Professor, Northwestern University Medical School; Chairman, Division of Neurosurgery, Children's Memorial Hospital, Chicago, Illinois
Head Injuries in Children

ROBERT McMILLAN, M.D.

Scripps Clinic and Research Foundation, La Jolla, California
Immune Hemolytic Anemia

THOMAS A. MEDSGER, Jr., M.D.

Associate Professor of Medicine, University of Pittsburgh
School of Medicine; Active Staff, Presbyterian-University
Hospital; Consultant Staff, St. Margaret Memorial Hospital,
Pittsburgh, Pennsylvania
Scleroderma (Systemic Sclerosis)

ROBERT G. MENY, M.D.

Assistant Professor, College of Medicine and Dentistry of
New Jersey Rutgers Medical School; Director, Neonatal In-
tensive Care, St. Peters Medical Center, New Brunswick,
New Jersey
Resuscitation of the Newborn

RONALD P. MESSNER, M.D.

Professor of Medicine, University of Minnesota Department
of Medicine; Chief, Section of Rheumatology/Clinical Immunology, University of Minnesota Hospitals, Minneapolis,
Minnesota
Rheumatoid Arthritis

BOYD E. METZGER, M.D.

Professor of Medicine, Member, Center for Endocrinology,
Metabolism, and Nutrition, Northwestern University Medi-
cal School; Attending Physician, Northwestern Memorial
Hospital; Consultant Attending Physician, Veterans Admin-
istration Lakeside Hospital, Chicago, Illinois
Reactive Hypoglycemias

HENRY M. MIDDLETON, III, M.D.

Associate Professor of Medicine, Medical College of Georgia; Assistant Chief, Gastroenterology Service, Veterans Administration Medical Center (Downtown Division), Augusta,
Georgia
Chronic Pancreatitis

DONALD J. MIECH, M.D.

Assistant Clinical Professor of Dermatology, University of
Minnesota and University of Wisconsin; Attending Derma-
tologist, St Joseph's Hospital, Marshfield, Wisconsin
Pruritus

AARON MILLER, M.D.

Assistant Clinical Professor of Neurology, Albert Einstein
College of Medicine of Yeshiva University, Bronx, New
York
Multiple Sclerosis

DENIS R. MILLER, M.D.

Enid A. Haupt Professor and Chairman, Department of Pe-
diatrics, Memorial-Sloan Kettering Cancer Center; Professor
of Pediatrics, Cornell University Medical College; Attending
Pediatrician, Memorial Hospital and New York Hospital-
Cornell Medical Center, New York, New York
Childhood Acute Leukemia

DAVID MINKOFF, M.D.

Associate Physician, Pediatric Infectious Diseases, University
of California at San Diego; Attending Physician, Pediatric
Infectious Disease, University of California at San Diego
Hospital and Children's Hospital, San Diego, California
Mumps

ROBERT S. MODLINGER, M.D.

Associate Professor of Medicine, College of Medicine and
Dentistry-New Jersey Medical School, Newark; Chief, Hy-
pertension Section, Veterans Administration Medical
Center, East Orange, New Jersey
Pheochromocytoma

JAY P. MOHR, M.D.

Professor and Chairman, Department of Neurology, Col-
lege of Medicine, University of South Alabama; Attending
Staff, University Medical Center, Mobile, Alabama
Parenchymatous Hemorrhage of the Brain

JOSEPH MOLDAVER, M.D.

Clinical Professor of Neurology, Columbia University, College of Physicians and Surgeons, New York, New York
Acute Peripheral Facial Paralysis (Bell's Palsy)

WILLIAM C. MOLONEY, M.D.

Professor Emeritus, Harvard Medical School; Attending
Physician, Peter Bent Brigham Hospital and Boston Hospi-
tal for Women, Boston, Massachusetts
The Chronic Leukemias

WILLIAM W. MONAFO, M.D. F.A.C.S.

Professor of Surgery, Washington University School of
Medicine; General Surgeon and Director of Hartford Burn
Center at Barnes Hospital, St. Louis, Missouri
Burns

CECIL MORGAN, Jr., M.D., F.A.C.S.

Clinical Assistant Professor of Surgery (Urology), University
of Alabama School of Medicine, Birmingham; Attending
Staff, St. Vincent's Hospital, University Hospital, Children's
Hospital, Baptist Medical Centers, Brookwood Hospital,
Birmingham, Alabama
Urethral Stricture

WILLIAM K. C. MORGAN, M.D.

Professor of Medicine, University of Western Ontario;
Director, Chest Disease Service, University Hospital, Lon-
don, Ontario, Canada
Coal Workers' Pneumoconiosis and Silicosis

MAURICE A. MUFSON, M.D.

Professor and Chairman, Department of Medicine, Marshall
University School of Medicine; Acting Associate Chief of
Staff for Research, Veterans Administration Medical
Center; Attending Physician, Cabell Huntington and St.
Mary's Hospitals, Huntington West Virginia
Toxoplasmosis

THOMAS F. MURPHY, M.D.

Fellow, Pediatric Infectious Diseases, University of North Carolina School of Medicine, Chapel Hill, North Carolina
Viral Pneumonia; Mycoplasma Pneumonia

YVES NAJEAN, M.D., Sc.D.

Professor of Hematology, Faculty of Medicine-University Paris-VII; Head of the Department of Nuclear Medicine, Hospital Saint Louis, Paris, France
Aplastic Anemia

JAY S. NEMIRO, M.D.

Fellow, Reproductive Endocrinology, Georgetown University School of Medicine, Washington, District of Columbia
Dysmenorrhea

RICHARD B. ODOM, M.D., Col., M.C.

Associate Clinical Professor, University of California, San Francisco; Chief, Dermatology Service, Letterman Army Medical Center, San Francisco, California
Chancroid

PAUL L. OGBURN, Jr., M.D.

Assistant Professor, University of Minnesota Medical School; Attending Staff, Department of Obstetrics and Gynecology, University of Minnesota Hospitals, Minneapolis, Minnesota
Abortion

WILLIAM OH, M.D.

Professor of Pediatrics and Obstetrics, Brown University Program in Medicine; Pediatrician in Chief, Women and Infants Hospital of Rhode Island; Attending Pediatrician, Rhode Island Hospital, Providence, Rhode Island
Normal Infant Feeding

PHYLLIS A. OILL, M.D.

Assistant Professor of Internal Medicine, University of California, Los Angeles; Attending Internist, Veterans Administration Wadsworth Medical Center, Los Angeles, California
Streptococcal Pharyngitis

DONALD R. OLSON, M.D.

Clinical Professor of Neurosurgery, University of Nevada School of Medical Science; Attending Neurosurgeon, Sunrise Hospital, Southern Nevada Memorial Hospital, and Valley Hospital, Las Vegas, St. Mary's Hospital, Reno, Nevada, and Moffitt Hospital, University of California, San Francisco, California
Brain Tumors

NORMAN ORENTREICH, M.D.

Clinical Associate Professor of Dermatology, New York University School of Medicine; Attending Staff, University Hospital of New York University School of Medicine, New York, New York
Alopecia

THOMAS D. PALELLA, M.D.

Rheumatology Fellow, University of Michigan Medical School; Resident in Internal Medicine, University of Michigan Hospital, Ann Arbor, Michigan
Hyperuricemia and Gout

HILLEL PANITCH, M.D.

Assistant Professor of Neurology, University of California, San Francisco, School of Medicine; Staff Physician, Veterans Administration Medical Center, San Francisco, California
Viral Meningoencephalitis

ROBERT C. PARK, M.D.

Professor of Obstetrics and Gynecology, Uniformed Services University of the Health Sciences; Chief, Department of Obstetrics/Gynecology, Walter Reed Army Medical Center, Washington, District of Columbia
Cancer of the Uterus

C. LOWELL PARSONS, M.D.

Assistant Professor of Surgery/Urology, School of Medicine, University of California, San Diego; Assistant Professor of Surgery/Urology, University of California Medical Center, San Diego; Chief, Urology Section, San Diego Veterans Administration Hospital, San Diego, California
Bacterial Infections of the Urinary Tract (Male)

ROBERT O. PASNAU, M.D.

Professor of Psychiatry, University of California, Los Angeles, School of Medicine; Chief, Adult Psychiatry Division, University of California, Los Angeles, Neuropsychiatric Institute, Los Angeles, California
Delirium

WILLIAM C. PATTON, M.D.

Associate Professor of Obstetrics and Gynecology; Chief, Section of Reproductive Endocrinology, Loma Linda University School of Medicine, Loma Linda, California
Amenorrhea

GEORGE W. PAULSON, M.D.

Clinical Professor of Neurology, Ohio State University; Senior Attending Staff, Riverside Methodist Hospital, Columbus, Ohio
Tetanus

ZBIGNIEW S. PAWLOWSKI, M.D., D.T.M.&H.

Professor of Medical Parasitology, Academy of Medicine, Poznan, Poland; World Health Organization, Parasitic Diseases Programme, Geneva, Switzerland
Trichinellosis

CARL J. PEPINE, M.D.

Professor of Medicine, University of Florida Department of Medicine; Chief of Cardiology, Veterans Administration Medical Center, Gainesville; Director of Adult Cardiac Catheterization Laboratories, University of Florida and Veterans Administration Medical Center, Gainesville, Florida
Pericarditis

THOMAS L. PERRY M.D.

Clinical Assistant Professor of Dermatology, University of Oregon School of Medicine, Portland, Oregon; Attending Staff, Yakima Valley Memorial Hospital, Yakima, Washington
Miliaria (Prickly Heat)

DAVID A. PEURA, M.D.

Assistant Professor of Medicine, Uniform Services University of Health Sciences; Assistant Chief, Gastroenterology Service, Walter Reed Army Medical Center, Washington, District of Columbia
Dysphagia and Esophageal Obstruction

SERGIO PIOMELLI, M.D.

Professor of Pediatrics, Columbia University College of Physicians and Surgeons; Director, Pediatric Hematology/Oncology; Attending Physician, Babies Hospital, New York, New York
Thalassemia

ROBERT T. PLUMB, M.D.

Clinical Professor of Surgery/Urology, University of California, San Diego; Senior Staff, Mercy Hospital, Sharp Hospital, Children's Hospital, San Diego, Coronado Hospital, Coronado, California
Balanitis and Balanoposthitis

PETER E. POCHI, M.D.

Professor of Dermatology, Boston University School of Medicine; Visiting Dermatologist, University Hospital; Visiting Physician, Dermatology, Boston City Hospital, Boston, Massachusetts
Acne Vulgaris

JOHN L. POOL, M.D.

Associate Clinical Professor of Surgery Emeritus, Yale University Medical School; Consultant Surgeon, Memorial Sloan Kettering Cancer Center, New York, New York; Honorary Surgeon, Norwalk Hospital, Norwalk, Connecticut
Primary Lung Cancer

PAUL J. POPPERS, M.D.

Professor and Chairman, Department of Anesthesiology, State University of New York Health Sciences Center, Stony Brook; Anesthesiologist-in-Chief, University Hospital, Stony Brook; Consultant in Anesthesiology, Veterans Administration Medical Center, Northport, New York
Anesthetic Care of the Obstetric Patient

JOHN M. PORTER, M.D.

Professor of Surgery, Head, Division of Vascular Surgery, University of Oregon Health Sciences Center, Portland, Oregon
Massive Deep Vein Thrombosis of the Lower Extremities

BERTRAM E. PORTIN, M.D.

Associate Clinical Professor of Surgery, Chairman, Division of Colon and Rectal Surgery, State University of New York at Buffalo School of Medicine; Chief, Division of Colon and Rectal Surgery, Buffalo General Hospital, Deaconess Hospital, Erie County Medical Center, and Sisters of Charity Hospital, Buffalo, New York
Hemorrhoids, Anal Fissure, Anorectal Abscess, Anorectal Fistula

HARVEY D. PREISLER, M.D.

Chief Deputy, Medical Oncology, Boswell Park Memorial Institute, Buffalo, New York
Acute Leukemia in Adults

W. PRYSE-PHILLIPS, M.D., M.R.C.P., F.R.C.P. (C.)

Professor of Medicine (Neurology), Memorial University of Newfoundland; Attending Staff, Health Sciences Centre, St. John's, Newfoundland, Canada
Headache

SUDHAKER D. RAO, M.B., B.S., F.A.C.P.

Visiting Instructor, Endocrine Teaching Faculty, Wayne State University School of Medicine, Detroit; Staff Physician, Bone and Mineral Metabolism, Research Associate, Bone and Mineral Research Laboratory, Henry Ford Hospital, Detroit, Michigan
Rickets and Osteomalacia

P. SYAMASUNDAR RAO, M.B., B.S., D.C.H., F.A.C.C.

Professor of Pediatrics, Associate Director of Section of Pediatric Cardiology, Assistant Professor of Physiology, Medical College of Georgia, Augusta; Pediatrician and Pediatric Cardiologist, Eugene Talmadge Memorial Hospital and University Hospital; Consultant Pediatric Cardiologist, Dwight D. Eisenhower Army Medical Center, Fort Gordon, and Savannah Memorial Center, Savannah, Georgia
Congenital Heart Disease

MORTON I. RAPOPORT, M.D.

Professor of Medicine, University of Maryland School of Medicine, Baltimore, Maryland
Tularemia

JONATHAN I. RAVDIN, M.D.

Fellow, Division of Infectious Diseases, University of Virginia School of Medicine, Charlottesville, Virginia
Food Poisoning

CHARLES E. REED, M.D.

Professor of Medicine, Mayo Medical School; Consultant in Internal Medicine and Allergic Diseases, Mayo Clinic, Rochester, Minnesota
Hypersensitivity Pneumonitis

ROBERT H. RESNICK, M.D.

Associate Clinical Professor of Medicine, Harvard Medical School; Lecturer in Medicine, Tufts University Medical School; Associate Visiting Physician, Beth Israel Hospital; Senior Physician, Lemuel Shattuck Hospital, Boston, Massachusetts
Cirrhosis

RONALD A. RESTIFO, M.D., F.A.C.P.

Arthritis and Connective Tissue Disease Medical Clinic, San Jose, California
Bursitis and Calcific Tendinitis

RICHARD J. REYNOLDS, M.D.

Assistant Professor of Medicine, Louisiana State University School of Medicine in Shreveport; Medical Director of Pulmonary Diagnostic Laboratories, Veterans Administration Medical Center, Shreveport, Louisiana
Blastomycosis

PETER A. RICE, M.D.

Assistant Professor of Medicine, Boston University School of Medicine, The Maxwell Finland Laboratory for Infectious Diseases, Boston City Hospital; Assisting Physician, Boston City Hospital; Associate Staff (Infectious Diseases) University Hospital; Consultant in Medical Oncology and Microbiology, Sidney Farber Cancer Institute, Boston, Massachusetts
Bacterial Meningitis

DOUGLAS D. RICHMAN, M.D.

Assistant Professor of Pathology and Medicine, University of California, San Diego, Medical School; Attending Staff, San Diego Veterans Administration Medical Center, San Diego, California
Viral Respiratory Infections

BASIL M. RIFKIND, M.D., F.R.C.P.

Chief, Lipid Metabolism Branch, National Heart, Lung, and Blood Institute, Bethesda, Maryland
Hyperlipoproteinemia

HUGH P. ROBINSON, M.D.

Associate Chief, Urology, Maine Medical Center, and Mercy Hospital, Portland, Maine
Benign Prostatic Hyperplasia

JAMES A. ROLLER, M.D.

Private Practice, Hannibal, Missouri
Spider Bites and Scorpion Stings

RANDOLPH W. ROLLER, M.D.

Clinical Assistant Professor of Obstetrics and Gynecology, Southern Illinois University School of Medicine, Springfield; Attending Staff, Memorial Medical Center and St. John's Hospital, Springfield, Illinois
Vulvovaginitis

E. WILLIAM ROSENBERG, M.D.

Professor of Dermatology, University of Tennessee College of Medicine, Memphis, Tennessee
The Erythemas

DAVID S. ROSENTHAL, M.D.

Associate Professor of Medicine, Harvard Medical School; Clinical Director of Hematology, Peter Bent Brigham Hospital and Boston Hospital for Women, Boston, Massachusetts
The Chronic Leukemias

RICHARD R. ROSENTHAL, M.D.

Assistant Professor of Medicine, Johns Hopkins School of Medicine; Chief, Allergy Section, The Fairfax Hospital, Fairfax, Virginia; Active Staff, Johns Hopkins Hospital, Baltimore Maryland
Asthma in Adults

ALLAN M. ROSS, M.D.

Professor of Medicine and Chief, Division of Cardiology, George Washington University School of Medicine; Attending Staff, George Washington University Medical Center, Washington, District of Columbia
Congestive Heart Failure

AVRON H. ROSS, M.D.

Professor of Pediatrics, State University of New York at Stony Brook School of Medicine; Dean, Clinical Campus Attending Pediatrician, Nassau County Medical Center, East Meadow, New York
Chickenpox (Varicella)

GERALD ROTHSTEIN, M.D.

Associate Professor of Medicine, University of Utah College of Medicine, Salt Lake City, Utah
Neutropenia

JOHN J. ROZANSKI, M.D.

Assistant Professor of Medicine, University of Miami School of Medicine; Director of Electrophysiology, Miami Veterans Administration Hospital, Miami, Florida
Premature Beats

FREDERICK L. RUBEN, M.D.

Associate Professor of Medicine, University of Pittsburgh School of Medicine; Associate Head of Infectious Diseases, Montefiore Hospital, Pittsburgh, Pennsylvania
Epidemic Influenza

ROBERT H. RUBIN, M.D.

Associate Professor of Medicine, Harvard Medical School; Associate Physician, Infectious Disease and Transplantation Units, Massachusetts General Hospital, Boston, Massachusetts
Leishmaniasis

ANDREW H. RUDOLPH, M.D.

Associate Professor, Baylor College of Medicine; Chief, Dermatology Service, Veterans Administration Medical Center, Houston, Texas
Superficial Fungus Infections of the Skin

JOHN F. RYAN, M.D.

Associate Professor of Anaesthesia, Harvard Medical School; Director, Pediatric Anesthesia, Massachusetts General Hospital, Boston, Massachusetts
Disturbances Due to Heat

ALFRED J. SAAH, M.D.

Division of Infectious Diseases, University of Maryland School of Medicine, Baltimore, Maryland
Typhus Fever

HOWARD L. SALYER, M.D.

Clinical Instructor, Vanderbilt University School of Medicine; Attending Dermatologist, St. Thomas Hospital, Baptist Hospital, and Park View Hospital, Nashville, Tennessee
Pediculosis

DON M. SAMPLES, M.D.

Clinical Associate Professor of Medicine, Tulane University; Associate Chairman, Department of Medicine, and Head,

Section of Hematology-Medical Oncology, Ochsner Clinic; Attending Staff, Ochsner Foundation Hospital, New Orleans, Louisiana
Hemochromatosis and Hemosiderosis

ARTHUR A. SASAHARA, M.D.

Professor of Medicine, Harvard Medical School; Chairman, Department of Medicine, Veterans Administration Medical Center, West Roxbury, Massachusetts
Pulmonary Embolism

TERRY K. SATTERWHITE, M.D.

Associate Professor of Medicine, University of Texas Medical School at Houston; Attending Staff, Hermann Hospital, Houston, Texas
Rat Bite Fever

ANTHONY J. SCHAEFFER, M.D.

Assistant Professor of Urology, Northwestern University Medical School; Associate Attending, Northwestern Memorial Hospital, Chicago, Illinois
Bacterial Infections of the Urinary Tract (Female Adults)

IRWIN J. SCHATZ, M.D.

Professor of Medicine and Chairman, Department of Medicine, University of Hawaii John A. Burns School of Medicine; Program Director, University of Hawaii Integrated Medical Residency Program, Honolulu, Hawaii
Stasis Dermatitis and Ulcers

LABE SCHEINBERG, M.D.

Professor of Neurology and Rehabilitation Medicine, Albert Einstein College of Medicine of Yeshiva University, Bronx, New York
Multiple Sclerosis

TORE SCHERSTEN, M.D., Ph.D.

Professor of Surgery, University of Göteborg; Chairman, Surgical Department I, Sahlgrenska sjukhuset, Göteborg, Sweden
Acute Pancreatitis

ADRIAN M. SCHNALL, M.D.

Assistant Clinical Professor of Medicine, Case Western Reserve University School of Medicine; Attending Physician and Consultant in Endocrinology, University Hospitals of Cleveland and Cleveland Veterans Administration Hospital, Cleveland, Ohio
Cushing's Syndrome

J. SPALDING SCHRODER, M.D.

Professor of Medicine (Digestive Diseases), Emory University School of Medicine; Attending Physician, Emory University Hospital and Grady Memorial Hospitals, Atlanta, Georgia
Acute and Chronic Hepatitis

MICHAEL J. SCOTT, M.D.

Seattle Dermatology Center, Seattle, Washington
Neurodermatitis

STEPHEN L. SEAGREN, M.D.

Assistant Professor of Radiology and Medicine, School of Medicine, University of California, San Diego; Consulting Physician, La Jolla Veterans Hospital, Balboa Naval Regional Medical Center, San Diego, California
Hodgkin's Disease — Radiation Therapy

JOHN B. SELHORST, M.D.

Associate Professor, Department of Neurology, Medical College of Virginia, Richmond, Virginia
Optic Neuritis or Neuropathy

G. V. R. K. SHARMA, M.D.

Assistant Professor of Medicine, Harvard Medical School; Director, MICU-CCU, Veterans Administration Medical Center, West Roxbury, Massachusetts
Pulmonary Embolism

THOMAS W. SHEEHY, M.D., M.S. (MED.)

Professor, University of Alabama School of Medicine; Chief of Medicine, Birmingham Veterans Administration Medical Center; Attending Physician, University of Alabama Hospitals, Birmingham, Alabama
The Malabsorption Syndrome

E. DORINDA SHELLEY, M.D.

Professor and Chair, Department of Dermatology, Peoria School of Medicine, University of Illinois; Physician/Consultant, Methodist Hospital, Peoria, Pekin Hospital, Pekin, Lincoln Development Center, Lincoln, and Veterans Administration Outpatient Clinic, Peoria, Illinois
Pityriasis Rosea

PAUL SHERLOCK, M.D.

Professor of Clinical Medicine, Cornell University Medical College, Chairman, Department of Medicine, Memorial Sloan-Kettering Cancer Center, New York, New York
Tumors of the Colon and Rectum

BARRY M. SHERMAN, M.D.

Professor of Internal Medicine, University of Iowa College of Medicine; Director, Clinical Research Center, Iowa City, Iowa
Hypopituitarism; Hyperprolactinemia

ROY G. SHORTER, M.D.

Professor of Medicine and Pathology, Mayo Medical School, Rochester; Consultant Physician, Mayo Clinic, Rochester, Minnesota
Crohn's Disease

DAVID N. SILVERS, M.D.

Associate Clinical Professor of Dermatology and Pathology, Director, Section of Dermatopathology, the College of Physicians and Surgeons of Columbia University, New York, New York
Pigmentary Disturbances

RICHARD L. SIMMONS, M.D.

Professor of Surgery, University of Minnesota; University of Minnesota Hospitals, Veterans Administration Hospital, Minneapolis, Minnesota
Gas Gangrene and Similar Anaerobic Soft Tissue Infections

MICHAEL N. SKAREDOFF, M.D.

Assistant Professor of Anesthesiology, State University of New York Health Sciences Center, Stony Brook; Attending Anesthesiologist and Head, Division of Obstetric Anesthesia, University Hospital, Stony Brook, New York
Anesthetic Care of the Obstetric Patient

ALBERT H. SLEPYAN, M.D.

Professor Emeritus, Abraham Lincoln School of Medicine of University of Illinois; Senior Attending Physician, Highland Park Hospital, Highland Park, Lake Forest Hospital, Lake Forest, Illinois
Poison Ivy Dermatitis

SHERRILL J. SLICHTER, M.D.

Associate Professor of Medicine, University of Washington School of Medicine, Seattle; Medical Director, Puget Sound Blood Center, Seattle, Washington
Bleeding Disorders Secondary to Platelet Abnormalities

RICHARD SNEPAR, M.D.

Instructor in Medicine, Medical College of Pennsylvania, Philadelphia, Pennsylvania
Salmonellosis (Other than Typhoid Fever)

ROBERT J. SOKOL, M.D.

Associate Professor, Case Western Reserve University School of Medicine; Associate Obstetrician/Gynecologist, Cleveland Metropolitan General Hospital, Cleveland, Ohio
Pregnancy-Induced Hypertension

JOSEPH S. SOLOMKIN, M.D.

Instructor, University of Minnesota Health Sciences Center, University of Minnesota Hospitals, Minneapolis, Minnesota
Gas Gangrene and Similar Anaerobic Soft Tissue Infections

FREDERICK T. SPORCK, M.D.

Assistant Professor, Department of Otolaryngology, School of Medicine of West Virginia University; Attending Staff, West Virginia University Medical Center, Morgantown, West Virginia
Sinusitis

PHILIP M. SPRINKLE, M.D.

Professor and Chairman, Department of Otolaryngology, School of Medicine of West Virginia University; Attending Staff, West Virginia Medical Center, Morgantown, West Virginia
Sinusitis

JOHN J. STANGEL, M.D., F.A.C.O.G.

Clinical Associate Professor and Director of the Section of Reproductive Endocrinology and Infertility, Department of Obstetrics and Gynecology, New York Medical College, Valhalla; Attending and Director of Reproductive Endocrinology and Infertility, Westchester County Medical Center, Valhalla, and Metropolitan Hospital Center, New York, New York
Ectopic Pregnancy

DAVID STATE, M.D.

Professor of Surgery, University of California at Los Angeles School of Medicine; Chairman, Department of Surgery and Acting Chief, Division of General Surgery, Harbor University of California at Los Angeles Medical Center, Torrance, California
Tumors of the Stomach

SAMUEL J. STEGMAN, M.D.

Assistant Clinical Professor of Dermatology, University of California Medical School, San Francisco; Active Staff, Ralph K. Davies Hospital, Herbert C. Moffitt Hospital, and Peninsula Medical Center, California
Keloids

NEAL H. STEIGBIGEL, M.D.

Professor of Medicine, Albert Einstein College of Medicine of Yeshiva University; Attending Physician, Head, Division of Infectious Diseases, Montefiore Hospital and Medical Center, Bronx, New York
Bacterial Pneumonia

HERMAN STEINBERG, M.D.

Clinical Professor of Medicine, Cornell University College of Medicine; Attending Physician, New York Hospital, New York, New York
Ulcerative Colitis

RICHARD H. STERNS, M.D.

Assistant Professor of Medicine, University of Rochester College of Medicine; Attending Nephrologist, Rochester General Hospital and Strong Memorial Hospital, Rochester, New York
Diabetes Insipidus

ROBERT J. STILLMAN, M.D.

Assistant Professor, Obstetrics and Gynecology, George Washington University School of Medicine and Health Sciences; Co-Director, Division of Reproductive Endocrinology and Fertility and Consultant in Adolescent Gynecology, Children's Hospital National Medical Center, Washington, District of Columbia
Dysmenorrhea

WILLIAM B. STRONG, M.D.

Charbonnier Professor of Pediatrics, Chief of Section of Pediatric Cardiology, Medical College of Georgia, Augusta, Georgia
Congenital Heart Disease

DONALD L. SWEET, M.D.

Assistant Professor, Section of Hematology/Oncology, Department of Medicine, The University of Chicago, Chicago, Illinois
Hodgkin's Disease — Chemotherapy

FRANCIS J. TEDESCO, M.D.

Associate Professor, Chief of Gastroenterology, Medical College of Georgia, Augusta, Georgia
Acute Infectious Diarrhea

PATRICK O. TENNICAN, M.D.

Assistant Professor, University of Washington Medical School, Seattle; Director, Internal Medicine, Sacred Heart Medical Center and Deaconess Hospital, Spokane, Washington
Psittacosis (Ornithosis)

HEIN J. TER POORTEN, M.D.

Clinical Assistant Professor, Division of Dermatology, University of Texas Southwestern Medical School; Attending Staff, Medical, Parkland Memorial Hospital, Dallas, and Richardson Medical Center, Richardson, Texas
Precancerous Lesions of the Skin and Mucous Membranes

JOSEPH EDWARD TETHER, M.D.,
F.A.C.P.

Associate Professor of Neurology, Indiana University School of Medicine; Attending Staff, Internal Medicine and Neurology, Indiana University Medical Center; Staff, Internal Medicine, Winona Hospital and Methodist Hospital, Indianapolis, Indiana
Myasthenia Gravis

GEORGE T. TINDALL, M.D.

Professor of Surgery, Chairman, Division of Neurosurgery, Emory University School of Medicine; Attending Neurosurgeon, Emory University Hospital, Atlanta, Georgia
Acute Head Injuries in Adults

SUZIE C. TINDALL, M.D.

Resident, Emory University Affiliated Hospitals, Emory University School of Medicine, Atlanta, Georgia
Acute Head Injuries in Adults

MARGARET TIPPLE, M.D.

Assistant Professor of Pediatrics, University of Chicago School of Medicine, Chicago, Illinois
Coccidioidomycosis

PETER V. TISHLER, M.D.

Assistant Professor of Medicine, Harvard Medical School; Associate Chief of Staff/Education, Veterans Administration Medical Center, Brockton, Massachusetts; Associate in Medicine, Peter Bent Brigham Hospital and Boston Hospital for Women, Boston, Massachusetts
The Porphyrias

EDMUND C. TRAMONT, M.D.

Associate Professor of Medicine, Uniformed Services University of the Health Sciences Medical School; Chief, Division of Infectious Diseases, Walter Reed Army Medical Center, Washington, District of Columbia
Syphilis

CHARLES C. TSAI, M.D., F.A.C.O.G.

Associate Professor of Obstetrics/Gynecology, Medical University of South Carolina; Staff, Medical University Hospital and Charleston County Hospital; Consultant, Veterans Administration Hospital, Charleston, South Carolina
Endometriosis

ARVID A. UNDERMAN, M.D.

Assistant Professor of Medicine, University of Southern California School of Medicine; Attending Physician, Communicable Disease Division, Los Angeles County-University of Southern California Medical Center, Los Angeles, California
Q Fever

CONDON R. VANDER ARK, M.D.

Associate Professor of Internal Medicine, Head Cardiovascular Section, University of Wisconsin Medical School; Staff Cardiologist, University of Wisconsin Hospitals and Clinics, Madison, Wisconsin
Atrial Fibrillation

FRANK B. VASEY, M.D.

Assistant Professor of Medicine, University of South Florida College of Medicine; Attending Rheumatologist, Tampa General Hospital and James A. Haley Veterans Administration Medical Center, Tampa, Florida
Juvenile Rheumatoid Arthritis

VICTOR VERTES, M.D.

Professor of Medicine, Case Western Reserve University School of Medicine; Director, Department of Medicine, the Mount Sinai Hospital, Cleveland, Ohio
Obesity

FRANCISCO VILARDELL, M.D., D.Sc.
(MED.), D.Sc. (HON.)

Professor of Medicine, Universidad Autonoma, Barcelona; Director, Gastroenterology Service, Hospital Santa Cruz y San Pablo, Barcelona, Spain
Gastritis

RICHARD W. VILTER, M.D., M.A.C.P.

Professor of Medicine, University of Cincinnati College of Medicine; Attending Physician, University of Cincinnati Medical Center Hospitals; Consultant on Staffs of Christ, Jewish, Deaconess, Good Samaritan, and Veterans Administration Hospitals, Cincinnati, Ohio
Pellagra

ROBERT VOLPÉ, M.D., F.R.C.P. (C.),
F.A.C.P.

Professor, Department of Medicine, University of Toronto; Physician-in-Chief, The Wellesley Hospital, Toronto, Ontario, Canada
Hyperthyroidism

ERIC C. VONDERHEID, M.D.

Associate Professor of Dermatology, Temple University

School of Medicine; Attending Staff, Skin and Cancer Hospital, Philadelphia, Pennsylvania
Mycosis Fungoides and the Sézary Syndrome

MORRIS WAISMAN, M.D.

Clinical Professor of Medicine (Dermatology) and Clinical Professor of Pharmacology, University of South Florida College of Medicine; Adjunct Professor of Dermatology, University of Miami School of Medicine; Attending Dermatologist, Tampa General Hospital and St. Joseph's Hospital, Tampa; Consultant in Dermatology, Veterans Administration Hospital, Bay Pines, Florida
Atopic Dermatitis

WILLIAM WATSON, M.D.

Associate Professor of Clinical Dermatology, Stanford University School of Medicine; Attending Dermatologist, Stanford University Hospital, Stanford, California
Psoriasis

STEPHEN B. WEBSTER, M.D.

Associate Professor of Dermatology, University of Minnesota Medical School, Minneapolis; Staff, La Crosse Lutheran Hospital, Gunderson Clinic, Ltd., La Crosse, Wisconsin
Sarcoidosis

ALLAN J. WEINSTEIN, M.D.

Clinical Assistant Professor of Medicine, Department of Medicine, Case Western Reserve University School of Medicine; Attending Staff, Cleveland Clinic Foundation, Department of Infectious Disease, Cleveland, Ohio
Bacteremia

HARRY S. WEISBERG, M.D.

Clinical Professor of Pathology, University of Wisconsin Medical School, Madison, and Medical College of Wisconsin, Milwaukee, Wisconsin; Visiting Professor, of Medicine, Chicago Medical School, Chicago; Illinois Director, Division of Biochemistry (Department of Pathology), Mount Sinai Medical Center, Milwaukee, Wisconsin
Parenteral Fluid and Electrolyte Therapy in Adults

WILLIAM A. WELTON, M.D.

Professor and Chairman, Dermatology Department, West Virginia University Medical Center, Morgantown, West Virginia
Herpes Simplex

NANETTE K. WENGER, M.D.

Professor of Medicine (Cardiology), Emory University School of Medicine; Director, Cardiac Clinics, Grady Memorial Hospital, Atlanta, Georgia
Rehabilitation of the Patient After Myocardial Infarction

CHARLES L. WHITFIELD, M.D.

Associate Professor of Medicine, Associate Professor of Family Medicine, Assistant Professor of Psychiatry, NIAAA/NIDA Career teacher in Substance Abuse, Director, Alcoholism and Drug Abuse Education, University of Maryland School of Medicine and Professional Schools at Baltimore, Maryland
Alcoholism

W. C. WIEDERHOLT, M.D.

Professor and Chairman, University of California, San Diego, School of Medicine, La Jolla; Chief of Neurology, University of California, San Diego, Medical Center, San Diego, California
Peripheral Neuropathy

KENNETH R. WILCOX, JR., M.D., DR. P.H.

Chief, Bureau of Disease Control and Laboratory Services, Michigan Department of Public Health, Lansing, Michigan
Rabies

H. OLIVER WILLIAMSON, M.D.

Professor of Obstetrics and Gynecology, Medical University of South Carolina; Staff, Medical University Hospital and Charleston County Hospital; College Affiliate, Roper Hospital; Consultant, Veterans Administration Hospital, Charleston, South Carolina
Endometriosis

PARK W. WILLIS, IV, M.D.

Instructor in Internal Medicine, University of North Carolina; Attending Cardiologist, North Carolina Memorial Hospital, Chapel Hill, North Carolina
Heart Block

PARK W. WILLIS, III, M.D.

Professor of Medicine, Michigan State University College of Human Medicine; Attending Cardiologist, Ingham Medical Center, Lansing, Michigan State University Clinical Center, East Lansing, Michigan
Heart Block

WALTER R. WILSON, M.D.

Assistant Professor of Internal Medicine and Microbiology, Mayo Graduate School of Medicine; Attending Staff, Mayo Clinic and Affiliated Hospitals, Rochester, Minnesota
Infective Endocarditis

SIDNEY J. WINAWER, M.D.

Professor of Clinical Medicine, Cornell University Medical College; Chief, Gastroenterology Service, Department of Medicine, Memorial Sloan-Kettering Cancer Center, New York, New York
Tumors of the Colon and Rectum

JOHN S. WOLFSON, M.D. PH.D.

Clinical and Research Fellow, Harvard Medical School; Fellow, Infectious Disease Unit, Department of Internal Medicine, Massachusetts General Hospital, Boston, Massachusetts
Leishmaniasis

JAMES W. WOODS, M.D.

Professor of Medicine, University of North Carolina School of Medicine, Senior Attending Staff, North Carolina Memorial Hospital, Chapel Hill, North Carolina
Hypertension

MELVIN D. YAHR, M.D.

Professor and Chairman, Department of Neurology, Mount Sinai School of Medicine of the City University of New York; Neurologist in Chief, Mount Sinai Hospital, New York, New York
Parkinson's Disease

MEYER YANOWITZ, M.D.

Clinical Professor of Dermatology, University of Miami School of Medicine; Attending Dermatologist, Jackson Memorial Hospital, Miami; Consultant in Dermatology, Cedars of Lebanon Hospital, Miami, Florida
Creeping Eruption

C. THOMAS YARINGTON, Jr., M.D., F.A.C.S.

Clinical Professor of Otolaryngology, University of Washington, Seattle; Chief, Otolaryngology and Facial Plastic Surgery, the Mason Clinic and the Virginia Mason Hospital, Seattle, Washington
Disorders of the Mouth (Benign)

RALPH ZALUSKY, M.D.

Professor of Internal Medicine, Mount Sinai School of Medicine of City University of New York; Chief, Division of Hematology/Oncology, Beth Israel Medical Center, New York, New York
Hemolytic Anemia — Nonimmume

SALVADOR ZAMORA, M.D.

Assistant Professor of Surgery (Urology), Abraham Lincoln School of Medicine of the University of Illinois; Attending Physician in Urology, Cook County Hospital, Chicago, Illinois
Genitourinary Tract Trauma

LAWRENCE ZASLOW, M.D., F.A.C.P.

Associate Clinical Professor of Medicine, Tulane University School of Medicine; Visiting Physician, Charity Hospital of Louisiana, New Orleans; Attending Physician, Allergy, Veterans Administration Hospital, New Orleans; Medical Staff, Department of Medicine, Touro Infirmary, New Orleans, East Jefferson General Hospital, Metairie, and West Jefferson Hospital, Marrero, Louisiana
Nasal Allergy Due to Inhalant Factors

MURRAY C. ZIMMERMAN, M.D.

Clinical Professor of Medicine (Dermatology), University of Southern California School of Medicine, Los Angeles, California
Nevi (Moles)

THOMAS F. ZUCK, M.D., Col. M.C.

Clinical Professor, Uniformed Services University of Health Sciences, Bethesda, Maryland; Chief, Department of Pathology, Walter Reed Army Medical Center, Washington, District of Columbia
Adverse Reactions to Blood Transfusions

Contents

SECTION 1. THE INFECTIOUS DISEASES

Amebiasis 1
F. P. Antia

Bacteremia 3
Allan J. Weinstein

Brucellosis 10
Robert L. Grissom

Chickenpox (Varicella) 11
Avron H. Ross

Cholera 14
Norbert Hirschhorn

Diphtheria 19
Robert Fekety

Echinococcosis (Hydatid Disease) 21
William S. Kammerer

**Gas Gangrene and Similar Anaerobic
Soft Tissue Infections** 22
Joseph S. Solomkin and
Richard L. Simmons

Food Poisoning 23
Jonathan I. Ravdin and
Richard L. Guerrant

Epidemic Influenza 32
Frederick L. Ruben

Leprosy (Hansen's Disease) 34
A. B. A. Karat

Leishmaniasis 39
John S. Wolfson and
Robert H. Rubin

Malaria 40
Marcel E. Conrad

Measles (Rubeola) 42
Leon M. Hebertson

Bacterial Meningitis 44
Peter A. Rice

Infectious Mononucleosis 52
John H. Dirckx

Mumps 54
David Minkoff

Plague 55
John M. Boyce

Psittacosis (Ornithosis) 56
Patrick O. Tennican

Q Fever 57
Arvid Underman

Rabies 58
Kenneth R. Wilcox, Jr.

Rat Bite Fever 62
Terry K. Satterwhite

Relapsing Fever 63
Anthony Bryceson

Rheumatic Fever 66
Joshua Lynfield

Rocky Mountain Spotted Fever 69
John F. Fisher

Rubella 71
Henry M. Balfour, Jr.

**Salmonellosis (Other than Typhoid
Fever)** 73
Richard Snepar and
Donald Kaye

Tetanus 75
Wesley Furste and
George W. Paulson

Toxoplasmosis 82
Maurice A. Mufson

Trichinellosis 84
Zbigniew S. Pawlowski

Tularemia 85
Morton I. Rapaport

Typhoid Fever 86
Myron M. Levine and
Luis Cisneros

Typhus Fever 88
Alfred J. Saah

Pertussis (Whooping Cough) 89
Larry J. Baraff

SECTION 2.   THE RESPIRATORY SYSTEM

Acute Respiratory Failure 93
William J. Hall

Atelectasis 99
Nicholas T. Kouchoukos and
Richard B. McElvein

**Chronic Bronchitis, Bronchiectasis,
and Emphysema** 102
John E. Hodgkin

Primary Lung Cancer 109
John L. Pool

Coccidioidomycosis 115
Pierce Gardner and
Margaret Tipple

Histoplasmosis 117
Robert H. Alford

Blastomycosis 119
John G. Burford,
Richard J. Reynolds, and
Ronald B. George

**Pleural Effusions and Empyema
Thoracis** 120
James T. Good

Primary Lung Abscess 121
John G. Bartlett

Acute Otitis Media 123
Kenneth M. Grundfast

Bacterial Pneumonia 128
Robert S. Klein and
Neal H. Steigbigel

Viral Pneumonia 132
Thomas F. Murphy and
Floyd W. Denny

Mycoplasma Pneumonia 133
Thomas F. Murphy and
Floyd W. Denny

Pulmonary Embolism 134
G. V. R. K. Sharma,
Kevin M. McIntyre, and
Arthur A. Sasahara

Sarcoidosis 137
Stephen B. Webster

**Coal Workers' Pneumoconiosis and
Silicosis** 138
W. K. C. Morgan

Hypersensitivity Pneumonitis 141
Charles E. Reed

Sinusitis 142
Philip M. Sprinkle and
Frederick T. Sporck

Streptococcal Pharyngitis 144
Phyllis A. Oill

**Tuberculosis and Other Mycobacterial
Diseases** 145
Stefan Grzybowski and
Edward A. Allen

Viral Respiratory Infections 153
Douglas D. Richman

SECTION 3.   THE CARDIOVASCULAR SYSTEM

Acquired Diseases of the Aorta 157
William A. Gay

Angina Pectoris 160
Thomas M. Drew

Cardiac Arrest 164
William Horowitz

Atrial Fibrillation 167
Condon R. Vander Ark

Premature Beats 171
John J. Rozanski and
Agustin Castellanos

Heart Block 173
Park W. Willis IV and
Park W. Willis III

Tachycardia 178
Leslie R. Fleischer and
Arthur M. Levy

Congenital Heart Disease 185
P. Syamasundar Rao and
William B. Strong

Congestive Heart Failure 209
Richard J. Katz and
Allan M. Ross

CONTENTS

Infective Endocarditis 213
   Walter R. Wilson and
   Joseph E. Geraci

Hypertension 219
   James W. Wood

Acute Myocardial Infarction 223
   L. David Hillis and
   Brian G. Firth

Rehabilitation of the Patient After
Myocardial Infarction......................... 233
   Nanette K. Wenger

Pericarditis 237
   Carl J. Pepine

Degenerative Arterial Disease................. 241
   Larry H. Hollier

Massive Deep Vein Thrombosis of
the Lower Extremities 246
   John M. Porter

Varicose Veins 249
   John E. Connolly

SECTION 4.   THE BLOOD AND SPLEEN

Aplastic Anemia 251
   Yves Najean

Anemia Due to Iron Deficiency............... 256
   Sean R. Lynch

Immune Hemolytic Anemia 259
   Harry W. Carloss and
   Robert McMillan

Hemolytic Anemia—Nonimmune............ 261
   Ralph Zalusky

Pernicious Anemia and Other
Megaloblastic Anemias 263
   A. V. Hoffbrand

Thalassemia 265
   Joseph H. Graziano and
   Sergio Piomelli

Sickle Cell Disease 269
   Marilyn H. Gaston

Neutropenia 272
   Gerald Rothstein

Hemolytic Disease of the Newborn 274
   James W. Kendig and
   M. Jeffrey Maisels

Hemophilia and Related Conditions........ 278
   Jeanne M. Lusher

Bleeding Disorders Secondary to
Platelet Abnormalities 287
   Sherrill J. Slichter

Disseminated Intravascular
Coagulation (DIC)............................... 293
   Eric Chun-Yet Lian

Thrombotic Thrombocytopenic
Purpura... 294
   Eric Chun-Yet Lian

Hemochromatosis and Hemosiderosis 295
   Don M. Samples

Hodgkin's Disease: Chemotherapy 296
   Harvey M. Golomb and
   Donald L. Sweet

Hodgkin's Disease: Radiation
Therapy... 302
   Stephen L. Seagren and
   John E. Byfield

Acute Leukemia in Adults..................... 306
   Harvey D. Preisler

Childhood Acute Leukemia.................... 309
   Denis R. Miller

The Chronic Leukemias.......................... 318
  David S. Rosenthal and
  William C. Moloney

Non-Hodgkin's Lymphomas.................. 320
  Gianni Bonadonna

Mycosis Fungoides and the Sézary
Syndrome 329
  Eric C. Vonderheid

Multiple Myeloma................................ 333
  Gibbons G. Cornwell III

Polycythemia Vera, Erythrocytosis,
and Relative Polycythemia..................... 336
  Harriet S. Gilbert

The Porphyrias................................... 342
  Peter V. Tishler

Therapeutic Use of Blood
Components 347
  James W. Langley

Adverse Reactions to Blood
Transfusions 352
  Thomas F. Zuck

SECTION 5.   THE DIGESTIVE SYSTEM

Bleeding Esophageal Varices.................. 361
  John T. Galambos

Cholelithiasis and Cholecystitis 364
  Larry C. Carey and
  E. Christopher Ellison

Cirrhosis... 366
  Robert H. Resnick

Constipation....................................... 372
  John R. Kelsey

Dysphagia and Esophageal Obstruction ... 374
  Lawrence F. Johnson and
  David A. Peura

Diverticula of the Alimentary Tract 378
  Kenneth Eng and
  S. Arthur Localio

Crohn's Disease 382
  Roy G. Shorter

Hemorrhoids, Anal Fissure, Anorectal
Abscess, Anorectal Fistula..................... 387
  Bertram A. Portin

Gastritis... 390
  Francisco Vilardell

Gaseousness 392
  Franz Goldstein

Acute and Chronic Hepatitis.................. 396
  J. Spalding Schroder

The Malabsorption Syndrome................. 398
  Thomas W. Sheehy

Intestinal Obstruction........................... 405
  Robert J. Freeark

Acute Pancreatitis................................ 406
  Yngve Edlund and
  Tore Schersten

Chronic Pancreatitis............................. 409
  Henry M. Middleton III

Peptic Ulcer....................................... 411
  Frank J. Baumeister, Jr.

Tumors of the Stomach.......................... 415
  David State

Tumors of the Colon and Rectum 416
  Sidney J. Winawer and
  Paul Sherlock

Acute Infectious Diarrhea 421
  Francis J. Tedesco

Intestinal Parasites 423
  James J. Gibson

**Ulcerative Colitis (Chronic Ulcerative
Colitis, Proctocolitis)** 428
  Herman Steinberg

SECTION 6.   METABOLIC DISORDERS

**Beriberi (Thiamine [Vitamin B₁]
Deficiency)** 435
  Chuichi Kawai

Hypo- and Hypervitaminosis A 436
  Donald S. McLaren

Diabetes Mellitus in Adults 437
  E. A. Haunz and
  Mary Blaine

**Diabetes Mellitus in Childhood
and Adolescence** 452
  Michael B. Ainslie and
  Donnell D. Etzwiler

Hyperuricemia and Gout 459
  Thomas D. Palella

Hyperlipoproteinemia 463
  Basil M. Rifkind

Reactive Hypoglycemias 470
  Boyd E. Metzger and
  Norbert Freinkel

Obesity 472
  Saul Genuth and
  Victor Vertes

Pellagra 475
  Richard W. Vilter

Rickets and Osteomalacia 476
  Sudhaker D. Rao and
  Boy Frame

Scurvy and Vitamin C Deficiency 482
  William B. Bean

Vitamin K Deficiency 483
  Robert Chilcote

Osteoporosis 485
  Robert H. Chesnut III and
  Helen E. Gruber

**Parenteral Fluid and Electrolyte
Therapy in Adults** 488
  Harry F. Weisberg

Fluid Therapy in Children 501
  Solomon A. Kaplan

SECTION 7.   THE ENDOCRINE SYSTEM

Acromegaly 509
  John A. Linfoot

Adrenocortical Insufficiency 514
  Alfred M. Bongiovanni

Cushing's Syndrome 515
  Adrian M. Schnall

Diabetes Insipidus 519
  Richard H. Sterns

Simple Goiter 522
  Morelly L. Maayan

Hyper- and Hypoparathyroidism 525
  Peter Greenberg

Hypopituitarism 528
  Barry M. Sherman

Hyperprolactinemia 531
  Barry M. Sherman

Hyperthyroidism 533
  Robert Volpé

Hypothyroidism 540
  Paul J. Davis and
  Faith B. Davis

Thyroid Malignancy...................... 543
  Anthony J. Edis and
  Oliver H. Beahrs

Pheochromocytoma....................... 546
  Norman H. Ertel and
  Robert S. Modlinger

Thyroiditis............................. 550
  Merrill W. Edmonds

Malignant Carcinoid Syndrome 551
  Harold Brown

SECTION 8. THE UROGENITAL TRACT

Bacterial Infections of the Urinary
Tract (Male) 555
  C. Lowell Parsons

Bacterial Infections of the Urinary
Tract (Female Adults)..................... 557
  Anthony J. Schaeffer

Bacterial Infections of the Urinary
Tract (Female Children)................... 560
  Lowell R. King

Childhood Enuresis...................... 561
  Melvin E. Jenkins

Epididymitis 563
  Fray F. Marshall

Balanitis and Balanoposthitis 563
  Robert T. Plumb

Glomerular Disorders.................... 564
  Robert C. Goldszer and
  J. Michael Lazarus

Pyelonephritis......................... 568
  Howard E. Fauver, Jr.

Genitourinary Tract Trauma 570
  Irving M. Bush,
  Patrick Guinan, and
  Salvador Zamora

Benign Prostatic Hyperplasia 576
  Hugh P. Robinson

Prostatitis 581
  Lester A. Klein

Acute Renal Failure 582
  Christopher R. Blagg

Chronic Renal Failure 588
  Eli A. Friedman

Genitourinary Tuberculosis.................. 594
  Dudley Seth Danoff

Genitourinary Tumors.................... 597
  E. David Crawford and
  Thomas A. Borden

Urethral Stricture 610
  Cecil Morgan, Jr.

Renal Calculi 612
  William H. Boyce

SECTION 9.   THE VENEREAL DISEASES

Chancroid 617
    Richard B. Odom

Gonococcal Infection 618
    Richard R. Hooper

Granuloma Inguinale 620
    Huberto Bogaert

Lymphogranuloma Venereum 621
    Huberto Bogaert

Syphilis 621
    Edmund C. Tramont

SECTION 10.   DISEASES OF ALLERGY

Anaphylaxis and Serum Sickness 625
    Phil Lieberman

Asthma in Adults 629
    Richard R. Rosenthal

Asthma in Children 634
    Hyman Chai

**Nasal Allergies Due to Inhalant
Factors** 643
    Lawrence Zaslow

**Adverse Reactions to Drugs:
Hypersensitivity** 647
    Kenneth P. Mathews

Allergic Reactions to Insect Stings 651
    William W. Busse

SECTION 11.   DISEASES OF THE SKIN

Acne Vulgaris 655
    Peter E. Pochi

Pseudofolliculitis Barbae 658
    John C. Hall

Alopecia 659
    Norman Orentreich

Cancer of the Skin 662
    Charles S. Lincoln, Jr.

Creeping Eruption 665
    Meyer Yanowitz

Decubitus Ulcer 666
    Robert Jackson

Contact Dermatitis 666
    Michael J. Kowertz

**Dermatitis Herpetiformis (Duhring's
Disease)** 667
    Edmund D. Lowney

Atopic Dermatitis 668
    Morris Waisman

Neurodermatitis 670
    Michael J. Scott

Poison Ivy Dermatitis 672
    Albert H. Slepyan

Seborrheic Dermatitis 673
    Donald P. Lookingbill

Stasis Dermatitis and Ulcers 674
    Irwin J. Schatz

Dermatomyositis/Polymyositis 676
    Ivor Caro

The Erythemas 677
   E. William Rosenberg

Superficial Fungus Infections of
the Skin 678
   Andrew H. Rudolph

Herpes Simplex 682
   Patrick Condry and
   William Welton

Hidradenitis Suppurativa 684
   James D. Maberry

Keloids 685
   Samuel J. Stegman

Lichen Planus 687
   Paul R. Gross

Sunburn and Photosensitivity 687
   Guinter Kahn

Lupus Erythematosus 690
   Edmund L. Dubois

Disorders of the Mouth (Benign) 695
   C. Thomas Yarington, Jr.

Disorders of the Mouth (Malignant) 709
   J. William Futrell

Diseases of the Nails 712
   Margaret C. Douglass and
   Edward A. Krull

Nevi (Moles) 719
   Murray C. Zimmerman

Occupational Dermatoses 721
   Frank C. Koranda

Pediculosis 723
   Howard L. Salyer

Pigmentary Disturbances 724
   David N. Silvers

Pemphigus and Pemphigoid 726
   John C. Maize

Pityriasis Rosea 728
   E. Dorinda Shelley and
   Sharon G. McDonald

Polyarteritis Nodosa 729
   Pearon G. Lang

Precancerous Lesions of the Skin and
Mucous Membranes 731
   Hein J. Ter Poorten

Miliaria (Prickly Heat) 733
   Thomas L. Perry

Pruritus 734
   Donald J. Miech

Pruritus Ani and Vulvae 736
   Wesley King Galen

Psoriasis 738
   William Watson

Inflammatory Eruptions of the Hands
and Feet 743
   W. David Jacoby, Jr.

Bacterial Diseases of the Skin 745
   Baylor Kurtis

Acne Rosacea 747
   James F. Gregory

Scabies 748
   Stephen A. Estes

Scleroderma (Systemic Sclerosis) 749
   Thomas A. Medsger

Urticaria and Angioedema 752
Lennart Juhlin

Warts 755
H. V. Allington

Herpes Zoster 757
Gordon MacDonald

Herpes Gestationis 757
Thomas J. Lawley

Pruritic Urticarial Papules and
Plaques of Pregnancy 758
Thomas J. Lawley

SECTION 12. THE NERVOUS SYSTEM

Brain Abscess 759
Robin P. Humphreys

Parenchymatous Hemorrhage of the
Brain 762
J. P. Mohr

Acute Ischemic Cerebrovascular
Disease 763
Louis R. Caplan and
Daniel B. Hier

Rehabilitation of the Hemiplegic
Patient 766
David B. King

Epilepsy in Adolescents and Adults 772
Robert G. Feldman

Epilepsy in Childhood 781
W. Edwin Dodson

Headache 788
W. Pryse-Phillips

Episodic Vertigo 793
Robert W. Baloh

Meniere's Disease 796
Michael E. Glasscock, III

Viral Meningoencephalitis 797
Hillel Panitch

Multiple Sclerosis 799
Labe Scheinberg and
Aaron Miller

Myasthenia Gravis 803
J. E. Tether

Trigeminal Neuralgia 808
John D. Loeser

Optic Neuritis or Neuropathy 809
John B. Selhorst

Acute Peripheral Facial Paralysis
(Bell's Palsy) 812
Joseph Moldaver

Parkinson's Disease 814
Melvin D. Yahr

Peripheral Neuropathy 818
W. C. Wiederholt

Acute Head Injuries in Adults 822
George T. Tindall and
Suzie C. Tindall

Head Injuries in Children 829
David G. McLone

Brain Tumors 834
Donald R. Olson

SECTION 13.   THE LOCOMOTOR SYSTEM

Rheumatoid Arthritis 839
   Daniel E. Hathaway and
   Ronald P. Messner

Juvenile Rheumatoid Arthritis............... 843
   Bernard F. Germain,
   Tomas S. Bocanegra,
   Frank B. Vasey, and
   Luis R. Espinoza

Ankylosing Spondylitis......................... 846
   Robert M. Bennett

Bursitis and Calcific Tendinitis 848
   Ronald A. Restifo

Osteoarthritis 849
   Gerson C. Bernhard

SECTION 14.   OBSTETRICS AND GYNECOLOGY

Antepartum Care 853
   Richard P. Bendel

Abortion 861
   Paul Ogburn and
   William E. Brenner

Resuscitation of the Newborn................. 865
   Robert G. Meny

Ectopic Pregnancy 868
   John J. Stangel

Hemorrhage in Late Pregnancy 871
   Isadore Dyer

Pregnancy-Induced Hypertension........... 873
   Donald A. G. Barford and
   Robert J. Sokol

**Anesthetic Care of the Obstetric
Patient**.. 877
   Paul J. Poppers and
   Michael N. Skaredoff

Postpartum Care 886
   Charles D. Kimball

Care of the Low Birth Weight Infant....... 887
   Martin H. Greenberg

Normal Infant Feeding 893
   William J. Cashore and
   William Oh

Diseases of the Breast........................... 896
   Douglas J. Marchant

Endometriosis 902
   Charles C. Tsai and
   H. O. Williamson

Dysfunctional Uterine Bleeding.............. 904
   Lorraine C. King

Amenorrhea 906
   William C. Patton

Dysmenorrhea....................................... 912
   Jay S. Nemiro and
   Robert J. Stillman

Menopause.. 913
   Harold L. Kaye

Vulvovaginitis 914
   Frederick J. Fleury and
   Randolph Wm. Roller

**Urinary Tract Infections During
Pregnancy**... 918
   Robert E. Harris

Pelvic Infections..................... 921
  G. Eric Knox

Myoma of the Uterus........................... 923
  Albert B. Gerbie

Cancer of the Uterus......................... 925
  Paul B. Heller and
  Robert C. Park

Carcinoma of the Vulva...................... 930
  Ernest W. Franklin, III

Preoperative and Postoperative Care
for Elective Gynecologic Surgery............ 934
  Robert L. Deaton

Thrombophlebitis in Obstetrics and
Gynecology.................................. 937
  Jay D. Coffman

Contraception...................................... 940
  Gary S. Berger and
  Louis G. Keith

SECTION 15. PSYCHIATRY

Alcoholism............................... 943
  Charles L. Whitfield

Narcotic Poisoning............................ 949
  Joyce H. Lowinson

Psychoneurosis..................................... 951
  Louis A. Cancellaro

Delirium................................... 955
  Robert O. Pasnau

Affective Disorders 956
  David L. Dunner

Schizophrenia...................................... 965
  Bruce M. Cohen and
  Joseph F. Lipinski

SECTION 16.   PHYSICAL AND CHEMICAL INJURIES

Burns.. 973
  William J. Monafo

Disturbances Due to Cold 981
  Cameron C. Bangs

Disturbances Due to Heat 988
  John F. Ryan

Spider Bites and Scorpion Stings 990
  James A. Roller

Portuguese Man-of-War (Jellyfish)
Stings.. 991
  Bruce W. Halstead

Acute Miscellaneous Poisoning............... 992
  Jay M. Arena

SECTION 17. APPENDICES AND INDEX

Tables of Metric and Apothecaries'
Systems 1014

Tables of Height and Weight for Men
and Women... 1015

Glossary of American Drug Names
and International Synonyms.................... 1016

Laboratory Reference Values of
Clinical Importance 1018
   Rex B. Conn

Reference Values in Hematology 1020

Reference Values for Blood, Plasma,
and Serum 1022

Reference Values for Urine.................... 1026

Reference Values for Therapeutic
Drug Monitoring.................................. 1028

Reference Values in Toxicology 1030

Reference Values for Cerebrospinal
Fluid 1030

Reference Values for Gastric Analysis..... 1031

Gastrointestinal Absorption Tests 1032

Reference Values for Feces 1032

Reference Values for Semen Analysis...... 1033

Pancreatic (Islet) Function Tests............. 1033

Reference Values for Immunologic
Procedures... 1034

Index 1037

SECTION 1

The Infectious Diseases

AMEBIASIS

method of
F. P. ANTIA, M.D.
Bombay, India

Amebiasis is the state of harboring *Entamoeba histolytica*. It has a worldwide distribution. Many Europeans and North Americans fear going to a tropical country or are obliged to leave a tropical country because of "amebophobia." This is a fear created by friends or physicians because of persistence of abdominal complaints not related to amebiasis. The diagnosis of amebiasis and its eradication are relatively simple.

The stool examination may be negative during or soon after a course of antiamebic therapy. More commonly, untrained technicians mistakenly report as amebae other organisms seen on stool examination. False positive reports perpetuate amebophobia.

"Chronic Amebiasis"

Many physicians also mistakenly label almost any chronic abdominal symptom which cannot be relieved as "chronic amebiasis" despite a negative stool examination. If amebae persist in the stool despite adequate therapy, the source of infection from food or water should be searched for and eradicated.

Emetine Hydrochloride

Emetine hydrochloride is the most effective drug for acute amebic dysentery, ameboma, and hepatic amebiasis. In the aged an electrocardiogram may be taken prior to and during emetine therapy whenever indicated. The patient should be allowed to visit the bathroom and the dining table. *Contraindications* include myocardial infarction, congestive heart failure, and cardiac arrhythmias.

Dosage. Emetine causes tissue necrosis; hence intramuscular injections are very painful.

Deep subcutaneous injections given in different sites in the upper and outer quadrant of the gluteal region are painless. Prior to such injection the pulse rate, rhythm, and blood pressure should be recorded. The daily dosage is 60 mg for those over 60 kg, 45 mg for those between 45 and 60 kg, and 30 mg for those between 30 and 45 kg of body weight. A total of up to 10 injections are given.

Toxicity and Tolerance. Great care must be taken in diabetics to avoid injection abscess. The myocardial effects may be tachycardia, premature beats, and hypotension. Electrocardiographic changes are flattening or inversion of the ST segment and the T waves, which may not necessitate abandoning therapy. The electrocardiogram reverts to normal after a few weeks. Skeletal muscle weakness may occur. Strenuous exercise is forbidden for 4 to 6 weeks.

Response. After three or four injections, in *acute dysentery* the blood, mucus, and frequency of stools decrease, and in *liver abscess* the pain, tenderness, and the liver size decrease.

Dehydroemetine. Dehydroemetine is a synthetic emetine more rapidly excreted than emetine hydrochloride (investigational in the United States). Daily dosage is 60 mg, but a higher dosage of 90 to 120 mg is sometimes advocated. The indications, contraindications, and toxicity are the same as for emetine hydrochloride. It is not as potent as emetine hydrochloride.

Metronidazole

Metronidazole is relatively nontoxic, well tolerated, and effective for amebic dysentery, cyst passers, and hepatic amebiasis. To avoid nausea, metronidazole is administered after food ingestion. The patient may notice a metallic or bitter taste. The usual adult dose is 400 mg three times a day (1200 mg daily) for 10 days. Some use a higher dosage: 750 mg three times daily for 5 to

1

10 days. Because it is suspected to be teratogenic, the drug is avoided in pregnant women.

Broad-Spectrum Antibiotic

For their growth *Entamoeba histolytica* organisms require other intestinal bacteria. Tetracyclines help alleviate acute dysenteric symptoms by suppressing intestinal bacterial growth. For amebic abscess tetracycline is used only during secondary bacterial infection (rather uncommon). The usual dosage is 250 mg four times daily or 500 mg three times daily for 7 to 10 days.

Chloroquine

Chloroquine is rapidly absorbed and hence not effective in intestinal amebiasis. Its concentration in the liver makes it effective in hepatic amebiasis.

Toxicity. Nausea and vomiting are minimized by administering chloroquine after meals. Temporary difficulty of visual accommodation, muscular twitchings, convulsions, and psychic stimulation sometimes occur. Corneal opacities and retinal changes are possibilities with prolonged administration (as for rheumatoid arthritis).

Dosage. Each tablet contains 150 mg chloroquine base. In hepatic amebiasis the initial dose is 2 tablets twice a day (600 mg daily) for 2 days, and then 1 tablet twice a day (300 mg) for 20 days. If a patient is nauseated, intramuscular injections of chloroquine (Aralen, Nivaquine) are used.

Prophylactic Use. In intestinal amebiasis, 1 tablet (150 mg) of chloroquine twice a day for 10 days is used as prophylaxis against hepatic amebiasis. (This specific use of chloroquine is not listed in the manufacturer's official directive.)

Diloxanide Furoate (Furamide)

Diloxanide furoate,* a synthetic amebicide, is used for intestinal amebiasis. It has no action on hepatic amebiasis. The dose is 500 mg (1 tablet) three times daily for 10 days. It is relatively nontoxic.

Halogenated Hydroxyquinoline Compounds

Diiodohydroxyquinoline (Yodoxin) is a halogenated compound that is poorly absorbed and hence useful for less severe forms of colonic amebiasis. A dosage of 650 mg three times daily for 10 days is well tolerated.

Subacute myelo-opticoneuropathy (SMON) has been described in Japanese patients after large doses and prolonged administration of iodochlorhydroxyquinoline (Entero-Vioform) or diiodohydroxyquin derivatives. Clinically, there is paresthesia, peripheral neuropathy of the lower limbs, myelopathy, optic neuritis, and optic atrophy. Whether the drug or another virus is responsible is debated, but SMON is rare outside Japan.

MANAGEMENT OF INTESTINAL AMEBIASIS

Acute and Subacute Amebic Dysentery

Rest at home. Bland diet, including egg, meat, chicken, bread, biscuits, and liberal fluid intake.

Initial Treatment. *Any one* of the following three schedules: (1) emetine hydrochloride or dehydroemetine,* daily deep subcutaneous injections 60 mg, for 10 days; *or* (2) metronidazole, 400 mg three times daily for 10 days, *or* (3) tetracycline, 250 mg four times daily for 10 days, *and* diloxanide furoate (Furamide),* 1 tablet three times daily for 10 days.

Subsequent Treatment. (1) Diloxanide furoate,* 500 mg three times daily for 10 days (if not given during the aforementioned initial treatment), *or* metronidazole, 400 mg three times daily for 10 days (if not given during the aforementioned initial treatment). (2) Chloroquine, 150 mg twice a day for 10 days.

Milder Forms of Colonic Amebiasis and Cyst Passers

For those passing two or three unformed stools and for cyst passers, the following three courses should be given consecutively. *First 10 days:* Metronidazole, 400 mg three times daily. *Subsequent 10 days:* Diloxanide furoate (Furamide),* 1 tablet three times daily. *Final 10 days:* Chloroquine, 1 tablet twice daily.

Cyst Passers (Asymptomatic Amebiasis; Carriers)

Cyst passers are more common in Western countries, where a relatively bland diet is consumed. In the tropics, with pungent spiced food, symptomatic amebiasis is more common. Asymptomatic cyst passers are treated to prevent hepatic amebiasis and also spread of infection to others. The treatment schedule is the same as for milder forms of colonic amebiasis.

Entamoeba coli, Iodamoeba buetschlii, and *Endolimax nana* are other amebae that produce flatulence and diarrhea with pungent and spiced

---

*Investigational in the United States. Further information may be obtained from the Center for Disease Control, Atlanta, Georgia 30333 (404–329–3670).

*Investigational in the United States. Further information may be obtained from the Center for Disease Control, Atlanta, Georgia 30333 (404–329–3670).

food. The symptoms are relieved with diloxanide furoate (Furamide) and halogenated hydroxy-quinoline compound.

Ameboma

Amebomas commonly occur in the rectosigmoid or the cecum. *Initial 10 days:* inject emetine or dehydroemetine,* 60 mg daily, *and* tetracycline, 250 mg four times daily. *Subsequent 10 days:* diloxanide furoate,* 500 mg three times daily, *and* chloroquine, 150 mg twice a day.

For *rectosigmoid ameboma* repeated sigmoidoscopy and biopsies are necessary until the ameboma heals or the mass is proved to be either malignant or due to other disease. Detection of amebae in the stool does not exclude malignancy.

Prevention of Recurrence

Food when served should be boiling hot. Cold salads, puddings, and unboiled water should be avoided.

HEPATIC AMEBIASIS

Hepatic amebiasis is common in alcoholics. The following three drugs are used for hepatic amebiasis: (1) Emetine hydrochloride or dehydroemetine,* 60 mg deep subcutaneous daily for 10 days. (2) Metronidazole, 400 mg three times a day for 10 days. (3) Chloroquine, 2 tablets twice a day (600 mg chloroquine base) for 2 days and then 1 tablet twice daily (300 mg) for 20 days.

For *more severe* hepatic amebiasis the initial therapy should be both emetine and metronidazole for the first 10 days. This is followed by a course of chloroquine. For *milder* hepatic amebiasis the initial therapy is metronidazole and a subsequent course of chloroquine. Tetracycline is not administered unless secondary bacterial infection is suspected by toxicity and high fever.

Aspiration of Liver Abscess

A few patients with hepatic amebiasis require aspiration of a liver abscess. *Indications:* (1) To establish the diagnosis of liver abscess. (2) Threat of rupture of the abscess when pointing through intercostal spaces, epigastrium, or diaphragm as seen on x-ray. (3) Deteriorating condition despite therapy. (4) Inadequate response to therapy.

Surgical Drainage

Surgical drainage is rarely required. It is considered after the failure of drug therapy or abscess aspiration.

---

*Investigational in the United States.

OTHER FORMS

Cutaneous and pulmonary amebiasis should be treated with a course of emetine and metronidazole. In *amebic brain abscess* the response to drug therapy is poor, as emetine does not penetrate the brain barrier. Metronidazole intravenously (investigational in the United States) can be tried.

BACTEREMIA

method of
ALLAN J. WEINSTEIN, M.D.
Cleveland, Ohio

General Principles

Although bacteremia is frequently a condition with a grave prognosis, a systematic approach to this infection will assist in early recognition and prompt treatment. It is possible to identify those patients who are at greatest risk for the development of bacteremia, the clinical situations in which it is most likely to occur, the organisms that most frequently produce it, the course that it may take, and the appropriate therapy.

It is uncommon for an otherwise healthy person to develop bacteremia. Many patients with this condition have pre-existing abnormalities of local or systemic host defenses. These include individuals at the extremes of age; hospitalized patients; those who suffer from immunodeficiency or a malignant disease; those receiving immunosuppressive, cytotoxic, or antibiotic therapy; patients being treated with a special device or procedure; narcotic addicts; and those who have recently undergone surgery.

Gram-negative bacteremia has been described as a "disease of medical progress." While it is now possible to prolong the survival of many patients with diseases such as the leukemias, lymphomas, and other malignancies that formerly were rapidly fatal, and to surgically repair formerly uncorrectable cardiac valvular and joint abnormalities, the therapy that is employed for these conditions often predisposes the patient to gram-negative infection. Although the infection initially may be localized, it may quickly disseminate.

In hospitalized patients, one of the most important factors associated with the development of both gram-positive and gram-negative bacteremia is the administration of broad-spectrum antibiotics. Use of these agents may alter the normal microflora of the patient, leading to colonization and subsequent infection with antibiotic-resistant gram-positive and gram-negative organisms. Other factors commonly associated with the development of bacteremia include the presence of kidney stones; intestinal or other organ obstruction; the use of devices or instruments, such as a urinary catheter, cystoscope, or intravenous catheter for drug infusion or hyperalimentation; and surgical procedures.

The clinical manifestations of bacteremia may be nonspecific. The presence of both fever and hypotension is common, but renal failure, tachypnea, hypotension alone, hyperthermia alone, or hypothermia may be the only signs that are present, and similar abnormalities may be observed in other noninfectious conditions. Because the clinical findings may be nonspecific, the diagnosis of bacteremia often depends on the high index of suspicion of the physician. The signs and symptoms of gram-negative bacteremia may be indistinguishable from those that are observed in gram-positive bacteremia caused by staphylococci or streptococci.

The patient with suspected bacteremia must undergo a careful physical examination, because identification of the origin of the bacteremia may provide important information concerning the microorganism(s) most likely to be responsible for the infection. If the origin is the urinary tract, the organism most probably involved is *Escherichia coli*, provided that the patient has not previously received antimicrobial therapy and does not have a urinary catheter in place. In such situations, other aerobic gram-negative bacteria assume prominence. If the primary focus of infection is an intra-abdominal abscess, anaerobic gram-positive and gram-negative bacteria or aerobic gram-negative organisms are likely to be present. Anaerobic bacteria also are commonly isolated from infections originating in the female genitourinary tract. Bacteremia emanating from the central nervous system is most commonly produced by *Streptococcus pneumoniae*, *Neisseria meningitidis*, and *Hemophilus influenzae*. When infection of the skin and soft tissues has been complicated by bacteremia, *Staphylococcus aureus* and group A beta-hemolytic streptococci may be responsible. With knowledge of the primary focus of infection and the microorganisms most commonly responsible for infections in that site, rational antimicrobial therapy may be instituted.

Hypotension in gram-negative bacteremia is due initially to hypovolemia. Fluid (preferably blood, plasma, or an albumin or dextran preparation) should be administered first. A central venous or Swan-Ganz catheter must be utilized to measure the effect of fluid administration. With aggressive volume replacement, many patients with bacteremia-related hypotension will respond dramatically, and further therapy to elevate blood pressure will not be required. If it becomes necessary to employ other therapeutic agents to treat hypotension, vasopressors such as levarterenol bitartrate and metaraminol bitartrate should be avoided, since they restrict renal blood flow and may compound the renal failure that frequently develops in patients with bacteremia. Compounds such as dopamine and dobutamine, which are myocardial stimulants and maintain renal blood flow, should be administered. Digitalis preparations must be employed when clinically indicated. The role of corticosteroids remains controversial, but some physicians administer large doses of methylprednisolone to all patients with presumed bacteremia.

After examination of the patient, blood cultures must be obtained and antibiotic therapy instituted.

Selection of Antibiotics (Table 1)

The choice of antimicrobial therapy for the patient with presumed or documented bacteremia must be derived from an understanding of the principles upon which antibiotic selection is based.

1. The agent administered must be known or proved by susceptibility testing to be among the most effective agents available for eradication of the isolated organism.

2. If several agents are equally effective, the one with the lowest potential for producing untoward effects must be chosen. A compound that has previously produced a severe reaction in the patient must not be readministered to that patient, even if it has been shown in vitro to be highly effective against the organism.

3. The use of a combination of antibiotics cannot substitute for precise clinical and laboratory diagnosis. Although some combinations may produce a broad-spectrum effect, the effect of other combinations may be inferior to that produced by a single antibiotic.

4. If there is a choice between equally effective and safe agents, the physician should choose the compound that is least expensive.

5. A bactericidal antibiotic is preferable to a bacteriostatic compound in the treatment of bacteremia.

6. Antibiotics in oral form should not be administered to patients with bacteremia.

7. Since susceptibility patterns of microorganisms vary from city to city and from institution to institution, it is imperative that the physician be aware of patterns of antimicrobial

susceptibility in his hospital. This knowledge will influence the selection of antibiotics for patients with bacteremia.

8. Knowledge of the pharmacokinetic properties of antibiotics is important in the selection of agent(s) for the treatment of bacteremia. If the focus from which the bacteremia has originated can be identified, an antibiotic which diffuses well into that site should be selected. Thus, compounds with biliary penetration should be administered in bacteremia which has originated in the biliary tract, and antibiotics, such as penicillins and chloramphenicol, should be utilized when infection has originated in the central nervous system. Conversely, cephalosporin antibiotics, clindamycin, and the aminoglycosides, which penetrate the blood-brain barrier poorly, are contraindicated in such infections.

TABLE 1. **Recommended Doses and Potential Toxicity of Antimicrobial Agents Used in Treatment of Bacteremia***

ANTIMICROBIAL AGENT	USUAL TOTAL DAILY DOSE	USUAL INTERVAL BETWEEN DOSES	MAJOR SIDE EFFECTS
Amikacin	15 mg/kg/day	q8–12h	Ototoxicity (primarily hearing loss), nephrotoxicity, neuromuscular blockade (rare)
Ampicillin	100–200 mg/kg/day	q6h	Hypersensitivity, rash, diarrhea
Carbenicillin	500 mg/kg (*P. aeruginosa*) 200 mg/kg (non–*P. aeruginosa* infections)	q4h	Hypersensitivity, sodium overload, hypokalemia, alkalosis, leukopenia, CNS toxicity in uremia, bleeding disorder, interstitial nephritis (rare), hepatitis (rare)
Cefamandole	100–200 mg/kg/day	q4–6h	Resembles cephalothin
Cefazolin	50–80 mg/kg/day (2–6 grams/day)	q6h	Hypersensitivity, CNS toxicity in uremia, thrombophlebitis, possible nephrotoxicity with aminoglycosides
Cefoxitin	100–200 mg/kg/day	q4–6h	Resembles cephalothin
Cephalothin	100–200 mg/kg/day	q4–6h	Hypersensitivity, thrombophlebitis, nephrotoxicity with aminoglycosides, leukopenia, hemolytic anemia (rare)
Cephapirin	100–200 mg/kg/day	q4–6h	Hypersensitivity, thrombophlebitis, possible nephrotoxicity with aminoglycosides
Chloramphenicol	40–100 mg/kg/day	q6h	Hematopoietic toxicity (dose-related; aplasia rare), gray baby syndrome
Clindamycin	30–40 mg/kg/day	q6h	Diarrhea, pseudomembranous colitis
Colistimethate†	2.5–5.0 mg/kg/day	q8h	Nephrotoxicity, circumoral and acral paresthesias
Erythromycin	30–60 mg/kg/day (2–4 grams/day)	q6h	Diarrhea, nausea and vomiting, transient deafness (rare), thrombophlebitis
Gentamicin	3–5 mg/kg/day	q8h	Nephrotoxicity, ototoxicity (primarily vestibular), neuromuscular blockade (rare)
Kanamycin	15 mg/kg/day	q8–12h	Ototoxicity (primarily hearing loss), nephrotoxicity, neuromuscular blockade (rare)
Methicillin	100–200 mg/kg/day	q4–6h	Hypersensitivity, interstitial nephritis
Nafcillin	100–200 mg/kg/day	q4–6h	Hypersensitivity, leukopenia, interstitial nephritis (rare)
Oxacillin	100–200 mg/kg/day	q4–6h	Hypersensitivity, hepatotoxicity, leukopenia, interstitial nephritis (rare)
Penicillin G	150,000–300,000 units/kg/day	q4h	Hypersensitivity, CNS toxicity in uremia, leukopenia
Polymyxin B†	1.5–2.5 mg/kg/day	q8h	Nephrotoxicity, neuromuscular blockade
Streptomycin	15–30 mg/kg/day (1–2 grams/day)	q12h	Vestibular toxicity, fever, eosinophilia
Sulfonamides	100 mg/kg/day	q6h	Rash, nephrotoxicity, anemia, neutropenia, Stevens-Johnson syndrome
Tetracycline	15–30 mg/kg/day (1–2 grams/day)	q6h	Diarrhea, nausea and vomiting, nephrotoxicity, hepatotoxicity
Ticarcillin	300 mg/kg/day (*P. aeruginosa*)	q4h	Hypersensitivity, anemia, leukopenia, thrombocytopenia, CNS toxicity in uremia
Tobramycin	3–5 mg/kg/day	q8h	Nephrotoxicity, ototoxicity (vestibular and cochlear)
Trimethoprim-sulfamethoxazole‡	—	q12h	Pancytopenia (trimethoprim) rash, nephrotoxicity, anemia, neutropenia Stevens-Johnson syndrome (sulfamethoxazole)
Vancomycin	30 mg/kg/day (2 grams/day)	q6–12h	Thrombophlebitis, ototoxicity (hearing loss), nausea, hypersensitivity, and tinnitus

*Certain doses in this table may be higher than listed in the manufacturer's official directive.
†Rarely indicated in bacteremia.
‡Intravenous preparation investigational. This use of this combination is not listed in the manufacturer's official directive.

9. Knowledge of those host factors which influence antibiotic efficacy is important in the selection of an agent for the treatment of the patient with bacteremia. Since renal excretion of penicillins may be delayed in very young infants, such antibiotics must be administered in lower dose to these individuals. Chloramphenicol must be administered with great caution in newborns, since "standard doses" may be associated with the production of the "gray baby" syndrome and kernicterus. In diabetes mellitus, there is diminished absorption of penicillin from intramuscular sites, and this antibiotic must be administered intravenously if bacteremia has developed in a diabetic patient. Chloramphenicol and tetracyclines, which are metabolized and/or excreted by the liver, must be administered with caution to patients with pre-existing hepatic dysfunction, and penicillins, aminoglycosides, cephalosporins, and vancomycin must be administered in modified dose to individuals with disordered renal function.

Bacteremia in Which the Infecting Organism Is Unknown

Antibiotics. When the patient is critically ill, it is most reasonable to administer more than one antibiotic. Approximately 85 per cent of all cases of gram-negative bacteremia are caused by *Escherichia coli*, Klebsiella, Pseudomonas species, and Proteus species, and initial antimicrobial therapy must include agents with a broad spectrum of antibacterial activity directed against these microorganisms. If the patient has had a previously documented infection, or the focus of bacteremia is readily evident, more specific antibiotic therapy may be administered.

Because it is frequently difficult to distinguish gram-positive from gram-negative bacteremia, the initial therapy of patients with presumed bacteremia usually includes combinations of agents effective against staphylococci and streptococci, as well as against aerobic gram-negative bacilli. In most centers a penicillinase-resistant penicillin, such as nafcillin or oxacillin, or a cephalosporin antibiotic is combined with an aminoglycoside antibiotic, such as gentamicin, tobramycin, or amikacin. When culture results become available, it is frequently found that the infecting organism can be inhibited with a less toxic antibiotic, and the physician should not hesitate to change therapy to a safer drug.

The initial antibiotic therapy of bacteremia must also be based on knowledge of the organisms most likely to be responsible for infection in a particular community or hospital. Thus, in some hospitals it is recognized that certain strains of bacteria, such as ampicillin-resistant *Escherichia*

coli and gentamicin-resistant *Pseudomonas aeruginosa*, may be resistant to certain antibiotics, and the initial therapy of the bacteremic patient must take this into account. If bacteremia develops in a patient residing in an area of a hospital, such as an intensive care unit, where nosocomial infection with a particular microorganism has been documented, the presumptive antimicrobial therapy of the patient must include agents directed against such a species.

Prognosis. It is possible to define important prognostic factors in patients with bacteremia. These relate to the underlying disease of the patient, the degree of debility associated with the bacteremia, the duration of illness, and the original focus of infection. Among all patients with bacteremia, the prognosis is most favorable in women whose infection emanates from the pelvic organs. Prognosis also is favorable in individuals whose bacteremia originates in the respiratory tract or from an intravenous catheter. The prognosis is least favorable in patients in whom the source of bacteremia is the abdominal cavity.

Patients with underlying diseases, such as malignancy, that are ultimately fatal, have a significantly poorer prognosis than individuals with bacteremia superimposed upon conditions that are not lethal. Patients whose hypotension is profound have a much poorer prognosis than those with minimal decreases in blood pressure. The duration of illness is another important prognostic indicator. The individual who has had bacteremia for 7 days or longer is at greater risk of death than one who has had the infection for a shorter period of time. Patients with urinary tract or intra-abdominal infection occasionally may have intermittent bacteremia lasting for many days or weeks prior to establishment of a diagnosis; the prognosis is poor in such patients.

Although prognosis depends to a large extent on the patient's underlying state of health, early diagnosis and appropriate therapy of bacteremia, including fluid replacement, blood pressure management, and antibiotic administration, may serve to increase the prospects for success.

Treatment of Specific Types of Bacteremia
(Table 2)

Group A Streptococcal Infections. Bacteremia caused by group A streptococcus occasionally emanates from pharyngeal infection, but in the modern era is most commonly associated with infections of the skin and soft tissues. Penicillin G is the agent of choice for such infections. In the penicillin-allergic patient, who has not reacted in an immediate (anaphylactic) fashion to penicillin, a cephalosporin may be utilized. If the individual is unable to tolerate either a penicillin or cephalo-

TABLE 2. Antimicrobial Agents for Treatment of Bacteremia Caused by Susceptible Pathogens*

ORGANISM	DRUGS OF CHOICE	ALTERNATIVES (IN ORDER OF PREFERENCE)
Gram-positive cocci		
Staphylococcus aureus	Penicillin G	Cephalosporin, vancomycin
Staphylococcus aureus (penicillin-resistant)	Nafcillin or oxacillin	Cephalosporin, vancomycin
Staphylococcus aureus (methicillin-resistant)	Vancomycin	Gentamicin plus cephalosporin
Staphylococcus epidermidis	Penicillin G	Cephalosporin, vancomycin
Staphylococcus epidermidis (penicillin-resistant)	Nafcillin, oxacillin, or cephalosporin	Vancomycin
Staphylococcus epidermidis (methicillin-resistant)	Vancomycin	Cefamandole
Streptococcus pyogenes (Group A)	Penicillin G	Cephalosporin, erythromycin, clindamycin
Streptococcus, Groups B, C, G	Penicillin G	Cephalosporin, erythromycin, clindamycin, vancomycin
Streptococcus, Group D	Ampicillin or penicillin G plus gentamicin or tobramycin	Vancomycin plus gentamicin or tobramycin
Streptococcus bovis, Group D	Penicillin G plus or minus streptomycin	Cephalosporin, vancomycin
Viridans streptococcus	Penicillin G	Cephalosporin, vancomycin, clindamycin
Peptostreptococcus species (anaerobic streptococci)	Penicillin G	Cephalosporin, vancomycin, erythromycin, clindamycin, chloramphenicol
Streptococcus pneumoniae (pneumococcus)	Penicillin G	Erythromycin, cephalosporin, clindamycin
Gram-negative cocci		
Neisseria gonorrhoeae (gonococcus)	Penicillin G	Ampicillin, tetracycline, erythromycin, cefoxitin
Neisseria meningitidis (meningococcus)	Penicillin G	Ampicillin, chloramphenicol, sulfonamide†
Gram-positive bacilli		
Clostridium perfringens	Penicillin G	Chloramphenicol, cephalosporin, tetracycline
Listeria monocytogenes	Ampicillin plus or minus gentamicin	Penicillin, erythromycin, tetracycline
Gram-negative bacilli		
Escherichia coli	Ampicillin,‡ cephalosporin, gentamicin§	Carbenicillin or ticarcillin, chloramphenicol
Klebsiella pneumoniae	Cephalosporin‡ plus or minus gentamicin§	Chloramphenicol, tetracycline
Enterobacter species	Cefamandole†	Carbenicillin or ticarcillin, chloramphenicol, gentamicin, tobramycin, amikacin
Proteus mirabilis	Ampicillin	Cephalosporin, chloramphenicol
Proteus species (indole-positive) (*P. morganii, P. vulgaris, P. rettgeri*)	Cefoxitin† or cefamandole†	Chloramphenicol, carbenicillin or ticarcillin, tobramycin, gentamicin, amikacin
Pseudomonas aeruginosa	Tobramycin plus carbenicillin or ticarcillin	Amikacin, gentamicin
Providencia stuartii	Kanamycin or amikacin	Carbenicillin or ticarcillin, cefoxitin†
Salmonella typhi	Chloramphenicol	Ampicillin, trimethoprim-sulfamethoxazole
Salmonella species other than *typhi*	Ampicillin	Chloramphenicol, trimethoprim-sulfamethoxazole
Brucella species	Tetracycline plus streptomycin	Chloramphenicol plus streptomycin, trimethoprim-sulfamethoxazole
Bacteroides fragilis	Chloramphenicol	Clindamycin, cefoxitin, metronidazole (investigational), carbenicillin,† doxycycline
Bacteroides species other than *B. fragilis* (head and neck source)	Penicillin G	Clindamycin, chloramphenicol, cefoxitin, tetracycline
Serratia marcescens or *Serratia liquefaciens*	Gentamicin	Chloramphenicol, carbenicillin or ticarcillin, cefoxitin,† tobramycin
Shigella species	Ampicillin	Chloramphenicol, trimethoprim-sulfamethoxazole
Hemophilus influenzae	Chloramphenicol	Cefamandole, ampicillin,† trimethoprim-sulfamethoxazole, tetracycline
Citrobacter species	Gentamicin	Chloramphenicol

*Bactericidal drugs alone or in combination recommended for endocarditis.
†Susceptibility testing results required.
‡Hospital-acquired strains may be resistant.
§Tobramycin may be substituted for gentamicin. For enteric gram-negative rod bacteremia, amikacin may be used if organisms are resistant to tobramycin and gentamicin but susceptible to amikacin.

sporin antibiotic, vancomycin may be given. Erythromycin and clindamycin are alternatives.

Group B Streptococcal Infections. Group B streptococcus *(Streptococcus agalactiae)* has been increasingly recognized to be responsible for bacteremia both in neonates and in women of child-bearing age. This organism may be associated with neonatal sepsis and meningitis and infections of the female genital tract. Penicillin G is the agent of choice for treatment of group B streptococcal infections. If this antibiotic cannot be administered, cephalosporin antibiotics, vancomycin, erythromycin, or clindamycin may be utilized.

Staphylococcus Aureus Infections. *Staphylococcus aureus* may produce bacteremia as the result of infections of the skin, upper respiratory tract (including paranasal sinuses, mastoids, and peritonsillar or retropharyngeal areas), lungs, or, rarely, the genitourinary tract. *Staphylococcus aureus* is responsible for the majority of cases of osteomyelitis and septic arthritis, and has become important in the pathogenesis of infective endocarditis in individuals who abuse intravenous narcotics.

There are many antibiotics available for the treatment of staphylococcal infections. A bactericidal, penicillin-like drug, such as penicillin G, is preferable, but the initial choice must be an agent that is penicillinase-resistant, since most strains of *Staphylococcus aureus* which produce infection in the hospital, and almost as many in the community, are resistant to penicillin G. If antibiotic susceptibility tests demonstrate that the organism is sensitive to penicillin G, this agent is preferable, since it is the most convenient and inexpensive to administer. If the patient is able to tolerate cephalosporins, these provide effective and safe alternatives to penicillins. If penicillins and cephalosporins cannot be administered, vancomycin, clindamycin, or erythromycin may be utilized.

Staphylococcus Epidermidis Infections. *Staphylococcus epidermidis* usually is a nonpathogen. However, this organism may be associated with the production of both localized and disseminated infections in individuals in whom prosthetic devices have been implanted. Individuals at risk for the development of *Staphylococcus epidermidis* bacteremia include those who have undergone cardiac valve replacement, the insertion of prosthetic orthopedic devices, and the placement of ventriculoatrial or ventriculoperitoneal shunts for hydrocephalus. Susceptibility patterns of *Staphylococcus epidermidis* vary, depending on the institution in which the organism has been isolated. Many strains of this organism remain susceptible to penicillin G. Those that are not susceptible to penicillin G may be effectively eradicated

by cephalosporin antibiotics or by penicillinase-resistant penicillins, such as nafcillin or oxacillin. In the patient who is unable to tolerate penicillins or cephalosporins, vancomycin may be administered.

Enterococcal Infections. Enterococcal bacteremia may emanate from the genitourinary tract, the gastrointestinal tract, or the endocardium. The enterococcus is important in the pathogenesis of urinary tract infections, and may produce bacteremia from sites in the upper and lower urinary tract. Enterococcal bacteremia has been associated with abnormalities of the lower gastrointestinal tract, including diverticulitis, inflammatory bowel disease, and malignancy. The enterococcus has recently been recognized to have been responsible for an increasing percentage of cases of infective endocarditis.

Penicillin (or ampicillin), in conventionally administered dose ranges, provides only bacteriostatic activity against enterococci. It has long been recognized that the combination of penicillin (or ampicillin) and an aminoglycoside antibiotic is necessary to provide synergism, resulting in bactericidal activity against the enterococcus. Although the combination of penicillin (or ampicillin) and streptomycin formerly was utilized for the therapy of enterococcal bacteremia, the increasingly frequent isolation of enterococci resistant to streptomycin has led to the use of other aminoglycoside antibiotics in combination with penicillin (or ampicillin). At present, a combination of penicillin (or ampicillin) and gentamicin or tobramycin provides the greatest possibility of bactericidal activity against enterococci. In the penicillin-allergic patient, a combination of vancomycin and an aminoglycoside (gentamicin or tobramycin) must be administered.

Gram-Positive Anaerobic Infections. Bacteremia caused by anaerobic streptococci (peptococci, peptostreptococci) usually originates from the upper respiratory or the gastrointestinal tract. Anaerobic streptococci are susceptible to penicillin G. In those who are unable to tolerate penicillin G, cephalosporins, vancomycin, erythromycin, clindamycin, or chloramphenicol may be substituted.

Pneumococcal Infections. Pneumococcal bacteremia most commonly emanates from infections of the respiratory tract. These may be manifest by otitis media, sinusitis, mastoiditis, or pneumonia. Penicillin G provides the greatest efficacy against pneumococci. In the penicillin-allergic patient, a cephalosporin antibiotic, vancomycin, erythromycin, or clindamycin may be utilized.

Gonococcal Infections. Disseminated gonococcal infections (arthritis-dermatitis syndrome) have been recognized with increasing frequency in recent years. This syndrome usually develops in women, particularly at the time of the menstrual period or during pregnancy, and is associated with the production of monarticular or polyarticular arthritis, fever, and purpuric or pustular skin lesions. Penicillin G and ampicillin are effective in the treatment of disseminated gonococcal infection. In the penicillin-intolerant patient, erythromycin, tetracycline, or a cephalosporin antibiotic may be administered.

Meningococcal Infections. Meningococcal bacteremia develops in individuals with meningococcal meningitis and in the syndrome of chronic meningococcemia. Penicillin G or ampicillin may be administered to patients with meningococcal bacteremia. Substitutes for penicillin include ampicillin and chloramphenicol.

Clostridial Infections. Clostridial bacteremia is observed in individuals who have undergone serious trauma, either accidental or surgical. Clostridial bacteremia usually emanates from the gastrointestinal or female genital tracts, but may be associated with wounds, particularly those resulting from trauma, such as that sustained in industrial or automobile accidents. Penicillin G is the agent of choice for the treatment of clostridial infections. Cephalosporin antibiotics, chloramphenicol, and tetracycline provide effective alternatives.

Listeria Monocytogenes Infections. *Listeria monocytogenes* most commonly produces infection in compromised hosts, particularly those with malignant disease such as the lymphomas and Hodgkin's disease. Bacteremia caused by *Listeria monocytogenes* is frequently associated with the presence of bacterial meningitis. Ampicillin provides greatest activity against *Listeria monocytogenes*. It has been suggested that ampicillin and gentamicin may produce synergism against *Listeria monocytogenes,* and that such a combination should be utilized for the treatment of bacteremia (and meningitis) in immunocompromised patients. Penicillin G and erythromycin are alternatives for the treatment of *Listeria monocytogenes* infections in individuals who are unable to tolerate ampicillin.

Gram-Negative Anaerobic Infections. Bacteremia produced by Bacteroides species, particularly *Bacteroides fragilis*, emanates from infections of the female genital tract, the lower gastrointestinal tract, and, occasionally, the lower respiratory tract. A number of antibiotics may be effective in the treatment of Bacteroides bacteremia. These include clindamycin, chloramphenicol, carbenicillin, cefoxitin, and the tetracyclines, particularly doxycycline. Patterns of antimicrobial susceptibility of *Bacteroides fragilis*

differ in various institutions, and the selection of one of the compounds must depend on knowledge of the susceptibility patterns in a particular hospital. In many hospitals, the greatest percentage of *Bacteroides fragilis* species are susceptible to chloramphenicol and clindamycin, and these should be selected first. Cefoxitin has the lowest potential for untoward effects. Chloramphenicol is associated with the possible production of abnormalities of the blood-forming elements. Clindamycin rarely may produce pseudomembranous enterocolitis, and carbenicillin administration is occasionally associated with sodium overload and functional platelet abnormalities. Doxycycline is particularly useful in the individual with abnormal renal function, since this compound is excreted by a hepatic mechanism.

Gram-Negative Infections

Escherichia Coli Infections. Formerly, the majority of *Escherichia coli* isolates were susceptible to ampicillin. Recently, there has been the emergence of ampicillin-resistant *Escherichia coli* in many institutions. In some hospitals, 20 to 40 per cent of *Escherichia coli* strains may be resistant to ampicillin. Many of these strains are susceptible to cephalosporins. Similarly, carbenicillin and chloramphenicol possess activity against most *Escherichia coli* strains. Aminoglycoside antibiotics (gentamicin, tobramycin, and amikacin) are extremely useful in the treatment of *Escherichia coli* infections, but are associated with the potential for producing untoward effects involving the kidney and eighth cranial nerve. The selection of an antibiotic for the treatment of *Escherichia coli* bacteremia must depend on knowledge of the susceptibility patterns in a particular institution. If it is recognized that significant ampicillin resistance is present, cephalosporins, chloramphenicol, or aminoglycosides should be selected.

Klebsiella Infections. *Klebsiella pneumoniae* may produce infections of the urinary and lower respiratory tracts which serve as foci for the development of bacteremia. The majority of *Klebsiella pneumoniae* isolates are susceptible to cephalosporin antibiotics. It has been suggested that cephalosporins and aminoglycoside antibiotics, such as tobramycin, gentamicin, and amikacin, are synergistically active against *Klebsiella pneumoniae,* and concomitant cephalosporin-aminoglycoside therapy has been recommended in *Klebsiella pneumoniae* bacteremia.

Proteus Mirabilis Infections. The majority of isolates of *Proteus mirabilis* are susceptible to ampicillin and to the cephalosporin antibiotics, and these should be administered for the treatment of *Proteus mirabilis* bacteremia. If ampicillin or cephalosporin resistance is present, chloramphenicol or an aminoglycoside antibiotic may be utilized.

Indole-Positive Proteus Infections. The advent of the newer cephalosporin antibiotics ("second generation" cephalosporins — cefamandole and cefoxitin) has provided safe and effective therapy for the majority of indole-positive Proteus infections. Cefamandole is active against most strains of *Proteus inconstans*, *Proteus morganii*, and *Proteus rettgeri*. Cefoxitin is active against the majority of *Proteus inconstans*, *Proteus morganii*, *Proteus rettgeri*, and *Proteus vulgaris* isolates. Since the cephalosporins provide a measure of safety greater than that of chloramphenicol and the aminoglycosides, which also are active against indole-positive Proteus species, cefamandole and cefoxitin should be considered to be the agents of first choice for the treatment of infections produced by these organisms.

Pseudomonas Aeruginosa Infections. The aminoglycoside antibiotics, and carbenicillin and ticarcillin, are active against *Pseudomonas aeruginosa*. Comparative assessments of the aminoglycosides suggest that tobramycin is the most active and least toxic of these compounds. Extensive in vitro and in vivo investigations have indicated that combinations of antibiotics are most useful in the treatment of *Pseudomonas aeruginosa* bacteremia. Such combinations should include an aminoglycoside (tobramycin) and either ticarcillin or carbenicillin. Gentamicin or amikacin may be utilized, but these agents are somewhat less active against *Pseudomonas aeruginosa* than is tobramycin.

Hemophilus Influenzae Infections. *Hemophilus influenzae* may be associated with localized infections of the upper respiratory tract (including sinusitis and otitis media) and pneumonia, and may also produce bacteremia and meningitis. There has been increasing awareness of the importance of ampicillin-resistant *Hemophilus influenzae* in the production of serious infections. Accordingly, ampicillin cannot be recommended as the agent of first choice for the treatment of *Hemophilus influenzae* infections, particularly when it has been recognized that ampicillin-resistant *Hemophilus influenzae* are present in a community. Chloramphenicol provides the greatest activity against *Hemophilus influenzae* strains, whether sensitive or resistant to ampicillin. This antibiotic is effective not only in the localized infections produced by *Hemophilus influenzae*, but also when bacteremia develops. Cefamandole, a "second generation" cephalosporin, is active against both ampicillin-sensitive and ampicillin-resistant *Hemophilus influenzae*, and may be utilized in the treatment of *Hemophilus influenzae* bacteremia. Cefamandole, as other cephalo-sporins, is ineffective in the treatment of infections of the central nervous system, and should not be utilized when bacteremia produced by this organism emanates from meningeal infection.

Salmonella Infections. Typhoid fever is uncommon in urban populations, but is occasionally recognized in individuals in the underdeveloped countries and in travelers. Chloramphenicol provides greater activity than ampicillin against *Salmonella typhi*, and is the agent of choice for the treatment of typhoid fever. In Salmonella infections produced by species other than *Salmonella typhi*, ampicillin remains highly active and should be selected before chloramphenicol.

Shigella Infections. Shigella bacteremia occasionally develops in individuals with intestinal shigellosis. Both ampicillin and chloramphenicol are highly active against Shigella species, and can be effectively utilized in the treatment of Shigella bacteremia. Since ampicillin is less commonly associated with significant untoward effects, it should be selected first. If ampicillin-resistant shigellae, which frequently are resistant to chloramphenicol, have been identified in a community, trimethoprim-sulfamethoxazole should be administered.

Serratia Infections. *Serratia marcescens* and *Serratia liquefaciens* have recently been recognized to be important in the pathogenesis of nosocomial infections. These bacteria have been associated with the production of urinary and respiratory tract infections and bacteremia in hospitalized individuals. The aminoglycosides possess greatest activity against Serratia species, and gentamicin is the most active of the aminoglycosides. Chloramphenicol, carbenicillin, ticarcillin, and cefoxitin, although less active than gentamicin, may also be utilized in the treatment of infections produced by Serratia species.

BRUCELLOSIS

method of
ROBERT L. GRISSOM, M.D.
Omaha, Nebraska

Acute Brucellosis

Acute brucellosis is most often a self-limited disease in which the outstanding symptoms of fatigue and weakness are best relieved by bed rest. Most persons who acquire the disease are not aware they have it. It should be suspected in younger persons, especially men, following exposure to animal tissues (cattle, hogs, goats, even dogs and cats, and some wild animals) and in whom fever and arthralgias develop without diagnostic findings in the clinical or routine laboratory examination. The disease is reportable to the Health Department. However, its prevalence is only a small fraction of its occurrence in the 1930's and 1940's in our country, although we continue to have one to four cases every year. It is desirable to know the type, mainly for prognosis, although all respond to the same management. Most cases are identified by serologic testing with only a minority of 10 to 20 per cent by culture. The majority affected are packing house workers, but over the years eradication in animals and improved sanitation have reduced the incidence of new cases. In the United States, midwestern states have most of the cases; it is more common abroad.

The infection is effectively managed in the majority of patients by use of one of the tetracyclines. The WHO/FAO Expert Committee has recommended 2 to 3 grams daily for 3 weeks, given in 0.5 gram doses every 4 to 6 hours. The course may be repeated if relapse occurs. Along with appropriate rest and nursing care, this suffices in the usual case. However, in most patients streptomycin, in 0.5 gram doses every 12 hours intramuscularly, is also recommended for 2 to 3 weeks. In one series of 308 patients the relapse rate was less than 3 per cent. When brucellosis has been recognized and treated, the mortality rate should be zero. Several authors have emphasized the importance of psychotherapy, with reiteration to the patient and his family as to the eventual full recovery from illness. Complications such as abscess and involvement of bone and other organs should be managed by an appropriate course of antibiotics before any operative approach is considered.

There appears to be no obvious benefit from the use of corticosteroids except in the rare patient who exhibits marked toxicity. Occasionally a severe reaction occurs after the early administration of antibiotics, and this reaction may be ameliorated by the use of the steroid. Aspirin has helped considerably in the control of fever and of rheumatic symptoms.

Although vaccine is used in animals, it is generally agreed that it has no value in humans. Indeed its use may be hazardous because of the development of hypersensitivity reactions. Accidental injection of the animal vaccine into humans (e.g., in a veterinarian) should be treated with tetracycline. The skin test may complicate the problem of diagnosis and should not be used.

Part of the resistance to therapy arising from

Brucella infection is related to the organism's intracellular position, which gives it partial protection from the action of antibiotics. When the organisms emerge from the host's cells, they may then cause a relapse and the patient may need another course of treatment. Fever results from endogenous pyrogen release from the leukocytes harboring the organisms.

Chronic Brucellosis

Therapy of a patient with chronic brucellosis can pose a difficult problem. It is essential to establish the diagnosis firmly before treatment. In former years, chronic brucellosis was a popular diagnosis which appears to have been made more often than warranted. Therapy by antibiotics of chronic brucellosis is much less successful than that of acute brucellosis. Nevertheless, a similar though somewhat longer course of antibiotic treatment should be given.

Prevention

The only satisfactory long-term solution to prevention is improved sanitation and the eradication of the disease among animals. Brucellosis from milk products is uncommon in the United States because of almost universal pasteurization. Goat's milk cheese is the major remaining food hazard, although the organism does not survive well over 2 to 3 months or with refrigeration. Travelers take warning! Most patients who acquire the disease get it from contact with slaughtered animals that are infected; but in properly managed meat processing plants, human infection is very uncommon. Handling of cultures in the laboratory may be dangerous, and all specimens for culture must be plainly marked: "Possible brucella." Vaccination of animals has much to recommend it, but eradication of the disease by removal of infected animals from herds is the only completely satisfactory solution. Man-to-man transmission is most unusual.

CHICKENPOX
(Varicella)

method of
AVRON H. ROSS, M.D.
East Meadow, New York

Introduction

Chickenpox is the primary clinical form of varicella-zoster (VZV) infection. It may occur at any age, least often in fetal life and after age 50. Spread is chiefly airborne, seeded in winter and spring by children in kindergarten through third grade. Highest attack rate is at home — 87 per cent of exposed susceptible children. One attack confers lifelong immunity, and regularly precedes the secondary form, shingles or herpes zoster (HZ), probably always endogenous. HZ is seen chiefly in healthy children and adults, and rarely recurs except in lymphoma patients. Apparent recurrences in well patients usually are due to herpes simplex virus (HSV). Ordinarily mild, chickenpox may run a complicated or fatal course, especially in risk groups defined below.

Modalities of Prevention and Treatment

Symptomatic. ISOLATION. Rarely effective at home; prevention undesirable in childhood, as adult varicella is frequently more severe and may include pneumonia.

BED REST. Unnecessary if patient feels well.

PREVENTION OF SECONDARY INFECTION. Clip nails short. Quick detergent bath at onset; no rubbing. Wash fingertips three times daily with hexachlorophene.

FEVER, HEADACHE, MALAISE. Acetaminophen may give some relief. As aspirin does not seem to prevent temperature spikes, and as most children with Reye's syndrome have conscientiously taken it before onset, a moratorium on aspirin in varicella is in order to see if this will largely eliminate the varicella-associated syndrome.

PRURITUS AND RESTLESSNESS. Warm the calamine-antihistamine lotion for local use. Cyproheptadine HCl (Periactin) is a good antihistamine with a mild sedative property for pruritus: from 1 mg (2.5 ml syrup) for a 1-year-old infant to 4 mg (1 tablet) for a child 7 years of age or older, two to three times daily.

MUCOUS MEMBRANE POX. Oropharyngeal pox cause transient dysphagia. Conjunctival pox are benign. Laryngeal pox may cause edema, rarely necessitating airway assistance.

RESIDUAL SKIN LESIONS. Permanent facial pitting is the natural outcome of large vesicles, not of scratching or picking. Small keloids likewise will persist. Pigmentation and depigmentation are temporary.

LYMPH NODES. Small cervical and occipital nodes, often visible for weeks, arouse parental anxiety.

SCHOOL. Return in 1 week if no new pox for 2 days. Scabs, as well as thick-walled residual vesicles on palms and soles, are not infectious.

Immunization. Passive or active immunization may be considered in nonimmune subjects, preferably after testing for unremembered or subclinical prior immunity. Complement-fixation (CF) test is limited because antibody rapidly disappears. Research laboratories do FAMA or VZMA test, highly accurate in detecting immunity acquired at any past time.

ZOSTER IMMUNE GLOBULIN (ZIG). ZIG, not yet licensed, has been extensively tested in our program. It is remarkably effective in attenuation or prevention (these overlap with same dosage) if given within 9 days after initial exposure, in dosage given on page 13. It holds for the second round in the family. VZIG is an alternative form developed at the Sidney Farber Cancer Institute. (For information call 617–732–3121.)

IMMUNE SERUM GLOBULIN (ISG). For moderate to marked modification: 0.2 to 1.2 ml per kg. Use 20 gauge needle, fixed firmly to avoid leakage. Doses of 0.8 ml per kg or above, if divided into two sites, cause little immediate pain, but muscle spasm occurs hours later. Preferably given within 3 days of exposure.

ZOSTER IMMUNE PLASMA (ZIP). If no ZIG is obtainable. Seven ml per kg, with VZV CF titer $\geq$ 1:32, by intravenous drip, within 6 days after exposure. May prevent or attenuate. Crossmatch. Prior tests for HB_sAg, VDRL, Coombs, sterility. One frozen unit (250 ml) of each major blood type should be kept on hand. Small risk of serum hepatitis.

VARICELLA VACCINE. Varicella vaccine, developed by the Japanese, has been experimentally used for leukemic children with favorable results, and merits careful study in high risk patients.

Antiviral Chemotherapy. *Vidarabine (adenine arabinoside, Vira-A, Ara-A)* has been under therapeutic trial for active VZV complications. In our experience it appears dramatically effective in 36 to 48 hours, in a regimen of 10 mg per kg per day in a 12-hour infusion once daily for about 5 days. Solubility limit is 1 mg per 2 ml of intravenous fluid, which may be warmed to dissolve residual crystals. Side effects, all reversible, rare in children, include anorexia, nausea, vomiting, generalized tremors, acute weight loss, asthenia, megaloblastosis in erythroid series in bone marrow, and local thrombophlebitis.

Interferon and *acyclovir (acycloguanosine)* are major agents with potential to be explored.

Exposure and Susceptibility

Exposure means simultaneous presence in a confined indoor space of a susceptible human and one with varicella or zoster not over 24 hours before onset or later than the drying of vesicles.

Site of Exposure: In evaluating effectiveness of preventive measures, the attack rates in differing situations for exposed susceptible children should be considered. The rate for household members is about 87 per cent, for social contacts about 13 per cent, and for pediatric inpatients other than those sharing the room of the index case about 4 per cent.

Susceptibility is probable if there is neither a history of disease nor intimate prior exposure to varicella or zoster. A typical facial pit is consistent with probable immunity. When time permits, serologic tests are the most accurate.

Risk Groups — Attenuation or Prevention

Normal Individuals. Healthy exposed susceptible infants and children do not require preventive measures. Exceptional social needs — such as final examinations or marriage — may engender justifiable requests.

Age-Related Risk. ADOLESCENTS AND ADULTS. Chief risk is varicella pneumonia, which may develop in healthy individuals — figures vary widely for percentages — and be mild, serious, or fatal. Only 44 per cent of adolescents and 23 per cent of adults well screened for a negative history have developed varicella after home contact. For modification, presumed susceptibles may be given 0.2 ml per kg of ISG. While this tends to reduce toxicity, the effect in preventing complications is unknown. If available, 0.02 ml per kg of ZIG gives striking attenuation and apparently prevents severe pneumonia.

PREGNANCY. Risk of varicella pneumonia is as for other adults. Congenital varicella syndrome is a very rare complication; risk to the fetus is exceedingly low. There is no evidence that prophylactic measures might alter this.

Debilitated Patients. Severe eczema, furunculosis, keloid tendency, seizure disorder, diabetes, systemic lupus, or debilitation from other illness or handicap may make modification desirable. Use 0.6 ml per kg of ISG, or 0.02 ml per kg of ZIG when available, within 9 days of exposure.

High Risk. CONGENITAL EXPOSURE. If the mother has developed varicella 4 days or less prior to delivery, the infant is in a group with a high fatality rate. At birth give 0.10 ml per kg of ZIG. Maternal varicella with onset 5 days or more before delivery generates effective transplacental antibodies, and no prophylaxis is thought to be required. If the mother is a susceptible exposed within 21 days before birth but without clinical disease, ZIG should be similarly given to the newborn. Exposure of the neonate after birth is probably not dangerous; for now, give 0.6 ml per kg of ISG.

IMMUNOSUPPRESSED PATIENTS. Progressive varicella ($\geq$ 5 days of fever with accelerating eruption) tends to develop regularly in this special group. Although some may come through unscathed, others may go on to major complications or fatality. Parents of such children are often unaware of the danger of chickenpox or herpes zoster exposure and should always be so forewarned! Chemotherapy for cancer or leukemia is responsible for much of the compromised resistance. Patients include those with (1) leukemia or other malignancy — even if in remission; (2) congenital or acquired immunologic deficiency; (3) other diseases treated with antimetabolites, other chemotherapeutic agents, corticosteroids, and/or ionizing radiation; and (4) severe hematologic disorders. They should receive 0.10 mg per kg of ZIG within 9 days of exposure. Steroids should be adjusted, when the disease condition permits, to physiologic maintenance (20 ± 10 mg of cortisol per square meter per day), or reinstituted at that level in patients from whom they have been withdrawn if the patients have had 2 weeks or more of steroid therapy within the preceding 6 months. Other therapy should be suspended during the course of the varicella.

Complications

Viral. Five principal serious viral manifestations are described. Various other systems and organs have also been rarely involved.

PROGRESSIVE VARICELLA. In high risk immunosuppressed and in age-related risk patients who have not had ZIG prophylaxis, this is the usual form of viremia seen prior to contracting localized viral complications. It has not occurred, in our extensive experience, in ZIG-modified varicella, although reported by others. By the fifth day or even sooner, hundreds to thousands of fine early maculopapules and vesicles are blooming at an accelerated rate and fever remains high. Vidarabine, 10 mg per kg per day, should be started at once. (This use of vidarabine is not listed in the manufacturer's official directive.) There is a turn-around time of 36 to 48 hours.

PNEUMONIA. This ranges from disease so mild as to be detected only on x-ray in adults or high risk patients to symptomatic pneumonia (tachypnea, cyanosis, hemoptysis) which has a high fatality rate, warrants immediate vidarabine therapy, and requires oxygen and life support systems.

ENCEPHALOMYELITIS. This is an entity separate from the encephalopathy of Reye's syndrome. The cerebral type, which is rare, may cause meningeal signs, focal signs, and increase in cerebrospinal fluid (CSF) cells and protein. Virus may be present and vidarabine* should be used, 15 mg per kg per day for 10 days as in herpes simplex virus encephalitis (HSVE). The cerebel-

---

*See manufacturer's official directive before using.

lar form is more common, usually benign, and self-limited.

REYE'S SYNDROME — HEPATIC INVOLVEMENT WITH ENCEPHALOPATHY. Repeated vomiting is not a normal feature of varicella, and Reye's syndrome should be suspected at once! If the vomiting is due to intercurrent unrelated virus infection, only gastrointestinal symptoms occur and the liver is nontender with normal size and chemistries. If there is any liver abnormality plus disorientation or lethargy, treatment for Reye's syndrome (discussed elsewhere) should be instituted on an emergency basis! As it is unknown whether virus is present in the affected tissues, and since vidarabine has central nervous system (CNS) side effects, its empirical use here is debatable.

PURPURA FULMINANS. This dangerous manifestation, with hemorrhagic pox and purpura, is due to disseminated intravascular coagulation (DIC), requiring laboratory confirmation. Vidarabine,* 10 mg per kg per day, should be given, along with supportive measures such as infusion of low molecular weight dextran, 10 ml per kg of 10 per cent solution. The value of heparinization is controversial. Idiopathic thrombocytopenic purpura is a less serious complication and may be treated with prednisone.

Bacterial. *Cellulitis,* often staphylococcal or streptococcal, starts in areas accessible to scratching — face, neck, anterior trunk — during eruption, on the second to fourth day. Infected pox, tender in contrast to uninfected, call for immediate culture and sensitivities and prompt systemic antibiotic therapy. If topical therapy alone is used, cellulitis may result in sepsis and metastatic localization.

Impetigo occurs toward the end of eruption, with rapid peripheral enlargement of vesicles to as much as 3 to 5 cm in diameter. Use systemic antibiotics.

Nosocomial Exposure

This may occur in ambulatory facilities, newborn nurseries, or inpatient services. Clinic exposure, like social exposure, has a low "take" rate. Our experience with many nursery exposures by house staff, nursing staff, and laboratory technicians at work unaware of their own varicella has shown that they do not usually infect the newborns under such circumstances. On hospital wards, as noted above, there is in most instances a very low incidence of secondary transmission except for occupants of the same room. However, this is dependent upon air flow pressure gradients between rooms spreading airborne infected droplets. All exposed susceptibles should be discharged as rapidly as possible and none admitted while the index case is infectious except if urgent. Isolation of the index case means keeping the door closed, the room air vented away from patient areas, and susceptible personnel out. Gowns, masks, and gloves probably give no protection to the wearer, and are warranted only to keep secondary infection from the patient. Even with the low inpatient attack rate, high risk patients deserve 0.1 ml per kg of ZIG and debilitated patients 0.02 ml per kg, because of the serious consequences if they should contract varicella.

CHOLERA

method of
NORBERT HIRSCHHORN, M.D.
Boston, Massachusetts

Definition

Cholera is an acute diarrheal disease caused by *Vibrio cholerae* which multiply profusely in the small intestine and release an enterotoxin. The organism remains in the lumen. The enterotoxin binds to cell membranes and by stimulation of adenyl cyclase, and hence cyclic AMP, induces salt and water secretion. The diarrhea may be mild, simulating nonspecific enteritis, or severe with stool outputs of 500 to 1000 ml per hour. In the latter instance the stool is nonfecal and opalescent with flecks of mucus (hence the classic term, "rice-water stool"). Without treatment one third to one half of patients with serious disease may die of hypovolemic shock or its consequences.

The manifestations of severe cholera are due almost entirely to the loss of stool containing water, sodium (100 to 140 mEq per liter), bicarbonate (30 to 50 mEq per liter), and potassium (15 to 30 mEq per liter), with an osmolarity close to that of plasma. Salt and water loss produce signs of volume depletion and shock; bicarbonate loss produces metabolic acidosis; and potassium loss of 10 to 20 per cent or more of body stores may cause cardiac arrhythmias, muscular weakness, and ileus, especially in children.

Any diarrheal disease which stimulates small intestinal secretion can produce volume depletion and thus simulate cholera; the treatment for volume loss is much the same. Any episode of severe diarrhea or an outbreak should be reported immediately to public health authorities.

Vibrio cholerae and related organisms have been found on all continents. In the United States, a recent outbreak in Louisiana, related to the ingestion of raw seafood, displays the potential for an epidemic anywhere.

*See manufacturer's official directive before using.

Objectives of Treatment

1. Rehydration. Rapidly replace water, salt, bicarbonate, and potassium losses with a polyelectrolyte solution.

2. Maintenance. Replace ongoing stool losses and provide water for evaporative loss and urinary water requirement.

3. Shorten the duration of diarrhea with antimicrobials.

Objectives 1 and 2 are critical; objective 3 is useful. On the average the disease lasts 3 to 5 days without antimicrobials and 1 to 2 days with antimicrobials. Patients in shock, unable to drink, or with ileus must receive polyelectrolytic fluids intravenously. Patients not in shock, strong enough to drink, and with bowel sounds may be given a glucose-electrolyte solution by mouth, or by nasogastric tube (see Oral Maintenance, below).

Electrolyte Solutions

Worldwide experience, considerably documented, indicates that a single intravenous solution and a single oral glucose-electrolyte solution may be successfully used for all age groups with cholera and with noncholera volume-depleting diarrhea as well. The composition of the intravenous polyelectrolyte solution has latitude but should contain, per liter, sodium (110 to 140 mEq), potassium (10 to 15 mEq), and base (30 to 50 mEq), with chloride as the other anion. Several commercial products are available with electrolyte composition in these ranges. Ringer's lactate solution is most widely available but requires addition of 10 mEq per liter of potassium chloride, especially when used in children. A good ad hoc intravenous solution may be composed as follows:

500 ml 0.9% sodium chloride (isotonic saline)
+500 ml 5% dextrose in water
+50 ml 1 molar sodium lactate (or sodium bicarbonate) (1 ml = 1 mEq)
+8 ml 2 molar potassium chloride (1 ml = 2 mEq)

1058 ml yields (mM/L)

Na$^+$	120
K$^+$	15
Base	47
Cl$^-$	88
Glucose	131

A single *oral* solution for all age groups as recommended by the World Health Organization may be prepared by weight as follows:

grams per liter solution

Sodium chloride	3.5
Sodium bicarbonate	2.5
Potassium chloride	1.5
Glucose	20.0

which yields (mM/L)

Na$^+$	90
K$^+$	20
HCO$_3^-$	30
Cl$^-$	80
Glucose	111

A good approximation of the latter may be had with the use of United States Standard (cooking) spoons with *level* measurements of the *crushed, dry* chemicals as follows:

teaspoons per 900 ml solution

Sodium chloride	0.5
Sodium bicarbonate	0.5
Potassium chloride	0.25
Glucose	4.0

which yields approximately in mM/L (±5%)

Na$^+$	89
K$^+$	20
HCO$_3^-$	31
Cl$^-$	78
Glucose	102

Amount, Route, and Speed of Fluid Administration

Rehydration. Acute fluid loss, expressed as per cent of body weight is associated with clear physical signs (Table 1).

The majority of the moderate and nearly all of the mild group may be rehydrated by the oral route (see below). The severe group requires intravenous fluid replacement. Example: A 60 kg person with acute diarrhea, shock, and/or signs of severe dehydration has lost approximately 6 kg (or 6 liters) of isotonic body fluid. Intravenous replacement with 6 liters of an isotonic polyelectrolyte fluid is required. A 10 kg child in shock would require 1 liter of rehydration fluid. The first half of the replacement should be given over 1 hour, and the balance within 4 hours. Simple

TABLE 1.

	MILD	MODERATE	SEVERE
Loss of body weight	0–3% (Ave. 1%)	3–8% (Ave. 5%)	8–12% (Ave. 10%)
	Thirst	Thirst	Shock, coma, or stupor
		Postural cardiovascular changes	Weak or absent radial pulse
		Some impairment of skin turgor	Dry mucous membranes
			Poor skin turgor
			Severe muscle cramps

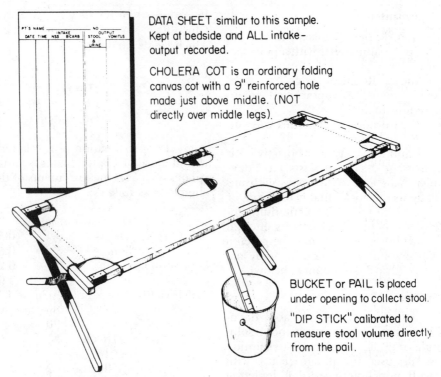

DATA SHEET similar to this sample. Kept at bedside and ALL intake-output recorded.

CHOLERA COT is an ordinary folding canvas cot with a 9" reinforced hole made just above middle. (NOT directly over middle legs).

BUCKET or PAIL is placed under opening to collect stool.

"DIP STICK" calibrated to measure stool volume directly from the pail.

Figure 1.   Cholera bed. (From Phillips, R. A.: Fed. Proc. *23*:705, 1964.)

bedside guides to adequacy of hydration are state of well-being, resolution of signs, return to maintenance of stable body weight and cardiovascular status, and urine output (the latter is frequently delayed for several hours).

Glucose stimulates salt and water absorption by the intestine. Those strong enough to drink, and without ileus, can take an oral glucose-electrolyte solution for rehydration, on the order of 75 ml per kg body weight within 4 hours. Most adults and children, if continuously encouraged to drink, will replace existing and ongoing losses on an ad libitum basis. The hypotonic solution (with respect to electrolytes) supplies adequate water for evaporative and urinary requirements. During sleep the solution may be given by nasogastric tube. Vomiting (less than twice per hour) is usually not an impediment to oral therapy, especially once volume and electrolyte deficits are near total repair.

Maintenance.   Ongoing losses should be replaced by measuring stool output and replacing losses on a volume-for-volume basis, using 1 to 6 hour intake and output balances. A "cholera bed" permits easy collection and provides better hygiene besides (Fig. 1). Any simple bed is easily modified for this purpose. A 9 inch hole is cut in the mattress beneath the patient's buttocks. The bed is covered with a rubber sheet, with a central sleeve (9 inch diameter) passing through the hole in the mattress into a plastic bucket beneath the bed. The bucket can be calibrated in 500 ml

quantities to permit easy measurement of stool volume. Patients should be given bedpans or urinals and instructed to pass urine separately from stool. Children's beds can be similarly modified, although separation of urine and stool for small children is often impossible. A bedside record should be maintained, showing the amounts of intravenous or oral solutions given and the volume of stool output.

INTRAVENOUS MAINTENANCE.   The same solution used for rehydration should be used to replace stool losses on a one-volume for one-volume basis. During the first 24 hours patients should be evaluated at least every 4 hours to be certain that the rate of fluid administration is adjusted to equal the changing rate of stool loss. Water must be given freely by mouth as soon as vomiting ceases, which is usually within 2 to 3 hours. Small children who cannot ask for it must be offered water at 2 to 3 hour intervals.

ORAL MAINTENANCE.   The aim of oral maintenance is to provide an amount equaling about 1.5 times the stool volume. This satisfactorily replaces stool losses and provides water for evaporative and urinary losses as well.

After rehydration, adults with serious diarrhea should drink, or be given by nasogastric tube, about 800 ml per hour during the first 4 to 6 hours (about 10 to 15 ml per kg per hour). Those with mild diarrhea may be given less (e.g., 5 ml per kg per hour), whereas those with profuse diarrhea require more (e.g., 25 ml per kg per hour). During this period the rate of stool output in most patients will become apparent. In each subsequent 4 to 6 hour period oral replacement should be about 1.5 times the output of the preceding period.

After rehydration, children with serious diarrhea should receive about 10 ml per kg per hour during the first 4 to 6 hours. This may be increased to 15 ml per kg per hour for severe diarrhea, or be reduced to 5 ml per kg per hour for mild diarrhea. During subsequent 4 to 6 hour periods, the volume given is based upon the output of the preceding period, as described above. Some individuals may drink 50 ml per kg per hour or more for 6 to 8 hours, but about half of those purging stool at a rate of over 15 ml per kg per hour are unable to drink enough oral fluid to keep up with losses.

Bedside signs of adequacy of hydration evaluated every 4 hours, especially when coupled to, ad libitum use of oral glucose-electrolyte solution, are often just as satisfactory a way of following fluid requirements.

A very few patients, usually malnourished children, seriously malabsorb glucose. Glucose intolerance in the course of oral therapy may be detected by voluminous, watery stool whose output matches or exceeds intake; failure to maintain hydration; a high concentration of glucose in the stool; and rapid reduction (in hours) of stool output on cessation of oral intake. Treatment with intravenous fluids (including glucose), a carbohydrate-free formula, and broad-spectrum antibiotics is necessary. The condition may clear in a few days but has a high associated mortality. A normal diet for age may be resumed as soon as vomiting ceases and the patient is hungry, which often happens on the first day of treatment. There is no reason to withhold food until diarrhea stops. Children may not tolerate cow's milk during acute diarrhea.

Antimicrobials

Tetracycline, furazolidone, or chloramphenicol eliminates *V. cholerae* from stool within 24 to 48 hours and terminates diarrhea within 48 to 72 hours. Total stool output in patients with severe disease is reduced by over 50 per cent.

Antimicrobials may be started when the patient can take them by mouth, ordinarily after rehydration is completed.

Parenteral antibiotics offer no advantage over the oral route. The doses are shown in Table 2.

In one study, doxycycline, in a single dose of 300 mg, was nearly as effective as the 48 hour tetracycline regimen.

Attempts to reduce transmission of cholera by antimicrobial prophylaxis to family contacts have produced variable results. The appearance of vibrios resistant to antimicrobials in recent outbreaks makes prophylaxis an unlikely method of control.

The Course of Cholera During Optimal Therapy

With rapid rehydration marked shivering can occur, sometimes sufficient to dislodge the needle. This reaction is most often due to rapid infusion of fluids considerably colder than body temperature and can be eliminated by using warmed fluids. True pyrogenic reactions are accompanied by shaking chills and high fever. When these occur the infusion bottle should be changed immediately. Soon after completion of rehydration, muscular cramps abate, bowel sounds return, vomiting ceases, the patient develops a sense of well-being, and he often falls asleep.

The signs of volume depletion should have disappeared. Children who are stuporous or comatose at the start of treatment may remain lethargic for 12 to 18 hours.

Stool output may be suppressed for 2 to 4 hours after an episode of severe hypovolemia but can recur in remarkable volume thereafter. Urine output is often suppressed for up to 12 hours after initiation of rehydration. Moderate elevations in temperature are seen only occasionally in adults but occur commonly in children under 2 years of age. Temperature returns rapidly to normal with adequate rehydration.

Complications of Cholera

Virtually all complications of cholera are prevented by adequate replacement of water and electrolytes and by provision of calories. If replacement is inadequate, the following may occur:

1. Persistence or recurrence of signs of hypovolemia, dehydration, or shock. In a patient with cholera the cause is always inadequate fluid replacement.

2. Persistence of nausea or vomiting. Most

TABLE 2.

DRUG	ADULTS	CHILDREN
Tetracycline	500 mg every 6 hours for 48 hours	25–50 mg/kg per day in divided doses for 2 days
Furazolidone	100 mg every 6 hours for 72 hours	5 mg/kg per day in divided doses for 3 days
Chloramphenicol (do *not* use the palmitate suspension)	500 mg every 6 hours for 72 hours	50–75 mg/kg per day in divided doses for 3 days

often the cause is uncorrected acidosis or hypovolemia.

3. Renal failure. Inadequate fluid therapy with prolonged or repeated episodes of hypotension precedes renal failure. The initial episode of hypovolemia, if promptly and fully corrected, rarely causes renal failure.

4. Hypokalemia. Potassium loss uncommonly causes symptoms in adults, but in children abdominal distention, paralytic ileus, cardiac arrhythmias, and weakness are often seen.

5. Overhydration. Puffy eyes are first seen when an excess of intravenous fluid is given, amounting to 3 per cent of body weight more than needed. Volume replacement in excess of need greater than this is manifest by distended neck veins, a slow, full pulse, and, eventually, frank cardiac failure. Acute pulmonary edema is induced far more readily, however, during intravenous rehydration if acidosis is uncorrected.

6. Hypoglycemia. A small percentage of children who do not receive glucose or food have hypoglycemic seizures. It may be prevented by inclusion of 1 per cent glucose in the intravenous infusion used for children.

7. Abortion. Stillbirths often occur in women in the third trimester of pregnancy. There should be no maternal mortality, however.

Atherosclerosis

Most clinical studies of cholera have been done in children and young adults, or with older patients from populations in which severe atherosclerosis is far less common than in western nations. Myocardial infarction and stroke are rare complications of hypovolemic shock in such patients. There is, however, scant information on how patients with advanced atherosclerosis would respond to the rapid volume depletion of cholera. It is likely that a considerable number would sustain strokes, myocardial infarctions, and other vascular complications. Rapid and complete rehydration would appear to provide the best means of protecting against such vascular complications. Close attention to clinical signs, electrocardiographic changes, and blood electrolytes and acid-base values would be especially important in this setting.

Useless Remedies

A number of treatment measures occasionally employed are useless or even dangerous. They frequently detract from the major objectives of treatment: prompt restoration and maintenance of normal hydration and electrolyte balance. Included are the following:

1. Cardiotonics such as nikethamide (Coramine) and epinephrine, and agents that elevate blood pressure such as levarterenol (noradrenalin), or adrenal steroids. Hypotension results from hypovolemia and requires water and electrolyte replacement only.

2. Oxygen. Cyanosis often accompanies hypovolemic shock and is therefore treated by water and electrolyte replacement.

3. Plasma volume expanders such as dextran, plasma, or blood. Isotonic water and electrolyte replacement is the ideal "plasma volume expander" for cholera.

4. Kaolin, pectin, bismuth, paregoric, or charcoal. These do not stop the diarrhea. Charcoal actually interferes with the effectiveness of tetracycline.

Newer Remedies

Based on an understanding of the subcellular mechanisms by which cholera toxin causes diarrhea, several chemical agents have been proposed that could potentially shut off intestinal secretion, thereby reducing total fluid loss and duration of illness. Aspirin, propranolol, loperamide, nicotinic acid, and chlorpromazine have all been suggested on the basis of in vitro experiments. Chlorpromazine, in a single, small clinical trial in cholera patients, significantly reduced stool output compared to a control group. The doses used were 1 to 4 mg per kg of body weight, intramuscularly or orally. More data from larger clinical trials are needed before any recommendations for these (or other) remedies may be made. None can replace fluid therapy, which is lifesaving.

Summary of the Treatment of Cholera

1. The patient is admitted, the diagnosis of dehydrating diarrhea is made with reasonable certainty, and the patient is weighed.

2. For adults, place a 16 to 18 gauge needle into a large, peripheral vein. For children, use a scalp-vein needle. (a) Use femoral or external jugular when no peripheral vein is found. (b) Use several sites at once if necessary to deliver large volume rapidly.

3. Severe dehydration — give approximately 10 per cent body weight in intravenous fluids over a 4 hour period, one half in the first hour. Moderate dehydration — give approximately 5 per cent body weight in intravenous fluids over a 4 hour period (or see 4 below).

4. Oral therapy may be started when shock is remedied and the patient is alert, and is given ad libitum.

5. Follow clinical signs, urine output, and stool volume to determine adequacy of hydration and fluid needs. A cholera cot is helpful for

hygienic collection of excreta and ready measurement of losses. Replace continuing stool losses on a one-volume for one-volume basis with intravenous polyelectrolyte solution, or 1.5 times the volume if using the oral glucose-electrolyte solution.

6. Water by mouth and food as desired after vomiting ceases.

7. Supplemental potassium to be given by mouth, if not in intravenous solution.

8. Antibiotics (tetracycline, furazolidone, or chloramphenicol) given for 2 to 3 days.

DIPHTHERIA

method of
ROBERT FEKETY, M.D.
Ann Arbor, Michigan

Diphtheria is an infrequent but still serious disease in the United States, where about 250 cases are reported each year, and about 10 per cent are fatal. It is remarkable that the case fatality rate for diphtheria has not declined despite the use of antitoxin and antibiotics. Antitoxin is the most important therapeutic modality, but it is most beneficial *early* in the disease. Once the disease is fully developed and the toxin is bound to tissues, antitoxin is of little benefit. The disease is most common in the southern part of the United States, in nonwhites, in children between the ages of 1 and 9, and in unimmunized persons. Selective media are needed for isolation of the organism. The disease may be seen in fully immunized persons, in whom it is usually mild and rarely fatal. Cutaneous diphtheria classically presents as "punched-out" ulcers, but recently impetiginous and eczematous forms of the disease have been recognized in the northwestern part of the United States in Indians and skid-row alcoholics.

General Management

1. The patient with diphtheria should be hospitalized.

2. Absolute bed rest is important for about 14 to 21 days because of the frequency of myocardial involvement.

3. If thrombocytopenia (which is associated with a poor prognosis) or signs of cardiac involvement are present, the cardiac rate and rhythm should be monitored.

4. Strict isolation precautions should be instituted.

5. Unless there is trouble with swallowing or breathing, parenteral feeding is not necessary.

Specific Management

Antitoxin. Antitoxin is most important in the treatment of diphtheria. It should be given to all patients in whom diphtheria is seriously considered, including those who have been fully immunized. Since antibiotics may stop toxin production and prevent spread of the organism, an appropriate antibiotic (see later) should be given.

PREVENTION OF REACTIONS TO THE ANTITOXIN. Tests for hypersensitivity to horse serum are mandatory before diphtheria antitoxin is injected.

1. A syringe containing 1 ml of 1:1000 epinephrine must be available for immediate treatment of reactions.

2. Skin tests are performed with an intradermal injection of 0.1 ml of antitoxin diluted 1:100 with isotonic saline solution. A positive wheal and flare reaction will reach its maximum in 15 to 20 minutes. A control injection of 0.1 ml of isotonic saline solution should be given. Undiluted toxin will produce a reaction in almost everyone.

3. The conjunctival test may be used in doubtful cases. One drop of a 1:10 saline dilution of antitoxin is instilled into the conjunctival sac, and one drop of isotonic saline solution is instilled into the other eye as a control. Suffusion, itching, tearing, and edema appearing within 30 minutes in the test eye constitute a positive reaction.

ANTITOXIN DOSAGE. If tests for hypersensitivity are negative, antitoxin should be administered without delay. The dose is empiric. Intramuscular injection of 10,000 to 20,000 units will control early or mild cases, both in adults and children. Patients with severe or late cases should be given 40,000 to 100,000 units (Table 1). If the patient is not hypersensitive to horse serum, up to 10,000 or 20,000 units may be given intramuscularly; if there is no reaction within 30 minutes, the rest may be given by slow intravenous infusion in 200 to 300 ml of isotonic saline solution or 5 per cent glucose. Epinephrine should be available.

ANTITOXIN IN THE HYPERSENSITIVE PATIENT. If the patient is allergic to horse serum,

TABLE 1. **Suggested Diphtheria Antitoxin Dosages**

LOCATION	CHILD	ADULT
Anterior nasal	5000 units	10,000 units
Mild pharyngeal	10,000 units	20,000 units
Laryngeal	10,000 units	20,000 units
Moderate pharyngeal	40,000 units	80,000 units
Two sites, severe, or late cases	40,000 units	100,000 units

antitoxin may be administered following desensitization; or, if it can be obtained, diphtheria immune globulin of human origin may be used instead.

DESENSITIZATION TO HORSE SERUM. 1. Antitoxin should be given with extreme caution and never intravenously to these patients.

2. Antihistaminic drugs should be administered parenterally before beginning desensitization.

3. Epinephrine 1:1000 must be ready in a syringe for immediate administration should reactions occur. An intravenous infusion should be in place for the rapid and certain administration of emergency medication. Equipment for providing an airway should be immediately available in case laryngospasm occurs.

4. The following steps may be taken at 20-minute intervals to desensitize the patient to horse serum: (a) 0.1 ml of a 1:20 dilution of antitoxin subcutaneously; (b) 0.1 ml of undiluted antitoxin subcutaneously; (c) 0.3 ml of undiluted antitoxin intramuscularly; (d) 0.5 ml of undiluted antitoxin intramuscularly; (e) if no reactions have occurred, the rest of the antitoxin dose may then be given intramuscularly (Table 1); (f) if a reaction occurs at any of the aforementioned steps, go back to the previous dose and start over; consider the use of diphtheria immune globulin instead of horse antitoxin if reactions are alarming.

DIPHTHERIA IMMUNE GLOBULIN. Commercially available immune and hyperimmune globulin preparations have low diphtheria antitoxin titers and are not useful. There is an investigational preparation that may be useful in special circumstances. It consists of a high-titer gamma globulin preparation made from blood of persons with high titers of antitoxin. It was intended for use in prophylaxis but should be considered for treatment of markedly allergic individuals. It may be given safely to persons who are allergic to horse serum. It is obtainable from the Communicable Disease Division, State Department of Public Health, Lansing, Michigan. The dose for treatment has not been established. This preparation should never be given intravenously.

Antibiotic Treatment. Antibiotics are believed to have little effect on the clinical course of diphtheria of the respiratory tract, but they may terminate the production of toxin by the organisms and benefit some patients. They may be useful in treatment of associated infections, will hasten clearance of the carrier state, and prevent spread of the organism to others. Cutaneous diphtheria responds to antibiotics, not antitoxin.

Penicillin is the drug of choice. Intramuscular procaine penicillin, 600,000 units twice daily

for 7 to 14 days, is usually adequate. Oral penicillin V can be substituted after the third day with uncomplicated infections. Penicillin G may be incorporated into intravenous solutions in a dose of 4 to 6 million units per 24 hours. If the patient is allergic to penicillin, erythromycin may be used (25 to 50 mg per kg per day for 10 to 14 days). The organism is usually sensitive to ampicillin, clindamycin, tetracycline, and rifampin. It is frequently resistant to cephalexin, colistin, lincomycin, and oxacillin. The latter antibiotics should not be relied upon in treating diphtheria. Erythromycin resistance has been seen in some recent outbreaks. Cultures and sensitivity tests may be helpful in special cases.

The Diphtheritic Membrane. The membrane will usually slough away cleanly and spontaneously during convalescence. It is generally best to leave it alone.

Management of Complications

Laryngotracheal Obstruction. Tracheostomy or endotracheal intubation under direct vision should be provided early. Adrenal corticosteroids have been advocated for patients with marked toxicity, laryngeal obstruction, shock, or myocarditis, but their efficacy is unproved.

Myocarditis. The majority of patients with diphtheria show myocarditic changes on the electrocardiogram, but only 10 per cent develop clinical evidence of myocarditis. Myocarditis is the most important cause of death.

The most important feature of the management of diphtheritic myocarditis is monitoring the heart and specific treatment of arrhythmias, which are more frequent than cardiac failure. Digitalis is not indicated unless congestive heart failure is apparent or unless needed for treatment of arrhythmias. Prednisone may be useful.

Neurologic Complications. Palatal paralysis may require a nasogastric tube, intravenous feedings, or tracheostomy. Mechanical respiratory assistance may be necessary.

Bleeding. The importance of thrombocytopenia in fatal diphtheria has recently been recognized. Platelet transfusions and possibly adrenal steroids may be useful in these patients. Other clotting factors have been normal.

Prophylaxis of Contacts

1. Case contacts who have been previously immunized should be given a booster.

2. For those not previously immunized, the intramuscular administration of 2000 units of diphtheria antitoxin is recommended after appropriate skin and eye tests. Diphtheria immune globulin (human) may be useful in hypersensitive patients (see earlier).

3. Cultures should be obtained from contacts, and, if positive, penicillin or erythromycin may be given as for the acute disease.

Management of the Carrier State

The use of antibiotics in the same schedules as for the disease is the most effective method of managing carriers. Benzathine penicillin is preferred when compliance is doubtful. Repeat cultures should be obtained no sooner than 48 hours after treatment. Three negative cultures are required before the person is no longer considered a carrier.

Prevention

Everyone should be immunized. The best time is during infancy, with combined diphtheria toxoid, tetanus toxoid, and pertussis vaccine (DPT). Three doses must be given at intervals. A booster should be given at approximately 18 months of age, just prior to starting school, and every 5 to 10 years thereafter. For adults, combined diphtheria-tetanus toxoid (dT) may be used for primary immunization or recall immunizations every 10 years.

ECHINOCOCCOSIS
(Hydatid Disease)

method of
WILLIAM S. KAMMERER, M.D.
Hershey, Pennsylvania

Human hydatid disease is caused by the cystic larval stage of four different species of Echinococcus: *E. granulosus*, of global distribution; *E. multilocularis*, confined to the Northern Hemisphere; and *E. vogeli* and *E. oligarthus*, found in Central and South America. Eggs passed in the feces of dogs and other carnivores are ingested and penetrate the bowel wall to develop into cysts in the liver and lungs primarily but, on occasion, in a number of other organs, most notably brain, eye, heart, and bone. Patients may come to the attention of physicians with symptoms related to the cyst mass (especially with brain or eye cysts), or with allergic and toxic reactions to degenerating or ruptured cysts, but most commonly are referred, often without symptoms, following serologic or radiographic screening programs associated with control campaigns and epidemiologic surveys.

Therapy

While the natural history of small or asymptomatic cysts has not been clearly defined, the risks of anaphylactic reactions, of dissemination following rupture, and of relentless growth making later therapy more difficult or impossible argue strongly for therapy.

Whenever possible, surgery remains the treatment of choice. When cysts cannot be removed intact, the surgical field should be isolated with packs saturated with a 20 per cent solution of sodium chloride, and the cysts cautiously aspirated and flushed for 5 minutes with one of several effective protoscolicidal solutions. The most practical and effective are 0.5 per cent silver nitrate, saturated solution of sodium chloride, or 1 per cent cetrimide (cetyltrimethyl ammonium bromide). Peritoneal and pleural lavage with 0.5 per cent cetrimide is also effective in diminishing the risk of dissemination following cyst rupture at surgery, although a chemical peritonitis has been reported with this procedure. One to 2 days prior to surgery, mebendazole should be started at a dosage of 30 mg per kg per day orally. If no spillage has occurred, mebendazole can be stopped; otherwise, mebendazole should be continued for 3 weeks at the same dose. (This use of mebendazole is not listed in the manufacturer's official directive. See final paragraph of this article before using.)

Frequently, because of the extent or location of cysts, the patient's general condition, or the lack of surgical facilities or expertise, surgery may be impractical or impossible. Under such conditions, mebendazole may offer the patient the only possible therapy. While mebendazole therapy in animal models has been promising, results with humans have been less predictable, and a number of adverse reactions have been reported. Pulmonary cysts of *E. granulosus* seem to respond best, hepatic cysts less dramatically, and cysts in other locations, particularly brain, bone, and eye, poorly or not at all. Cysts of *E. multilocularis* are probably not destroyed by mebendazole but may cease to grow further while therapy is continued. No information is available for *E. vogeli* or *E. oligarthus* infections. While the optimal dose of mebendazole has not been determined, prolonged high-dose therapy appears necessary. For *E. granulosus*, 40 to 50 mg per kg per day for 3 months is probably the minimal effective dose, with many patients requiring repeated courses or continuous therapy for up to 18 months. The drug is best given in two to three divided doses with meals, as this tends to reduce gastrointestinal side effects and to enhance absorption. Higher doses do not seem to increase effectiveness. For *E. multilocularis*, continuous therapy at 30 mg per kg per day for 1 to 3 years, or perhaps indefinitely, is required.

Adverse reactions generally occur within the

first month of therapy and may include febrile and anaphylactic reactions, glomerulonephritis, and leukopenia, requiring particularly close patient observation during this time.

In addition to clinical and radiologic follow-up, serologic tests may be helpful in determining treatment efficacy. Those correlating best with treatment results are the disappearance of the arc-5 band by immunoelectrophoresis, and a decrease in titer of hydatid specific IgE.

While mebendazole remains readily available commercially, it has not been approved by the Food and Drug Administration for the treatment of human hydatid disease, and the manufacturer, Janssen Pharmaceutica, has withdrawn IND support for its use for this condition. Therefore, physicians must rely upon their professional judgment, on an individual basis, to determine whether its use is appropriate.

GAS GANGRENE AND SIMILAR ANAEROBIC SOFT TISSUE INFECTIONS

method of
JOSEPH S. SOLOMKIN, M.D.,
and RICHARD L. SIMMONS, M.D.
Minneapolis, Minnesota

Soft tissue infections in which anaerobic organisms play the predominant role are uncommonly encountered but may have a fulminating course requiring immediate and extensive operation to salvage the patient. The dilemma posed by the presence of gas in a soft tissue infection is whether radical excisional operation is required or whether simple incision and drainage will suffice. A classification scheme based on this differentiation is provided in Table 1, along with nonanaerobic soft tissue infections which can closely mimic the anaerobic infections and which require similar therapy. The toxicity and rapidity of spread of the anaerobic infections is related to dense growth in the presence of devitalized or devascularized (diabetic) tissue and to production of exotoxins by Clostridium species (particularly lecithinase by *C. welchii*). The role of synergistic aerobic organisms is unclear, but these often play an important role in the pathogenesis of infection.

Diagnosis

Accurate diagnosis is crucial in determining the timing and extent of operation, and adjuvant antibiotic therapy. Important factors are (1) type of trauma producing devitalized tissue, (2) location of the primary lesion, (3) toxicity of the patient, (4) presence of crepitance and skin changes, and (5) Gram smear results of exudate. It must be stressed that antibiotic therapy cannot control these infections and is used only as an adjuvant to prompt operation.

In the presence of crepitance and serious toxicity, urgent surgical operation (1 to 2 hours) is mandatory. Patients with clostridial myonecrosis, cellulitis, or synergistic gangrene are often hypotensive and may require aggressive fluid and electrolyte therapy.

Operative Therapy

Incisions must be planned so that adequate debridement can be performed while salvaging as much usable skin cover as possible. The long-term functional consequences of a poorly placed incision are not justified by the gravity of the patient's condition. If the skin overlying crepi-

TABLE 1.

SYNDROME	OFFENDING ORGANISM	CLINICAL SETTING	FINDINGS
Necrotizing cellulitis	Hemolytic streptococci	Minor extremity wounds	Red, rapidly advancing borders, with bleb formation
Necrotizing fasciitis	Mixed gram-negative rods and gram-positive cocci	Operative or traumatic wounding	Ulcer with wide subcutaneous dissection; hypesthesia with extreme toxicity
Clostridial cellulitis	Clostridium species	Minor trauma	Creptitant or noncrepitant with bleb formation; extreme toxicity
Nonclostridial anaerobic gangrene	Mixed gram-negative rods and anaerobes	Diabetics with peripheral vascular disease	Distal ulceration, gas in the subcutaneous tissue planes, moderate toxicity
Synergistic gangrene	Micro-aerophilic streptococci plus aerobic staphylococci or gram-negative rods	Delayed appearance post-wounding	Central necrosis with satellite ulcers; incision and drainage required
Clostridial myonecrosis	Clostridium species	Operative or traumatic wounding	Rapidly spreading crepitance; extreme toxicity; incision and drainage required

tance appears intact, long transverse parallel skin incisions may be made, particularly over the abdominal wall. In the extremities, longitudinal incisions are made as for escharotomies, and continued until obviously normal skin and fascia have been encountered.

In the presence of Clostridium species, as determined by Gram smear, myonecrosis must be sought by fasciotomy, and all questionably viable tissue must be resected. Failure to achieve complete debridement will greatly increase the chance of recurrent infection. Pale, noncontractile, or nonbleeding muscle must be resected, and a margin of normal tissue must be removed to ensure adequate excision. Over the abdomen full thickness excision of the peritoneum and muscle may be necessary, with Marlex repair of the fascial defect. In the extremity, the surgeon must be prepared to proceed to amputation if the toxicity of the patient and extent of infection are severe.

Once thoroughly debrided, these wounds are drained with suction drains if flaps are left. In this case, continuous wound irrigations with antibiotic solutions may be of value. If no flaps are left, the wound is treated as a burn with topical silver sulfadiazine application.

In both clostridial and nonclostridial infections, wounds should be left open. If large skin flaps are left following fasciotomy for fasciitis or myonecrosis, return to the operating room for careful inspection of the wound, redebridement, and dressing changes, which should be done during the first and second postoperative days. Nonclostridial anaerobic gangrene, probably the most common soft tissue anaerobic infection, is seen in diabetic legs and must be distinguished from clostridial infections because radical operation is not required. The crepitance distant from the initial wound does not have the same significance as in clostridial infections.

Adjuvant Therapy

Because most anaerobic infections are nonclostridial, antibiotic therapy must initially be guided by Gram smear results. If clostridia are identified, high dose penicillin (4 million units every 4 hours intravenously) is begun. If clostridia are not identified, an assumption of a mixed infection is made and therapy with tobramycin (80 mg intravenously every 8 hours) and clindamycin (600 mg intravenously every 6 hours) is begun. Tobramycin is used because Pseudomonas species may be present. Speciation and antibiotic sensitivity testing are important because of increasing clindamycin resistance in both Clostridium and Bacteroides species. Recurrent infection does not represent antibiotic fail-

ure, and therapy for recurrence is operative. Since hemolytic staphylococci may be present, nafcillin, 1 gram every 4 hours intravenously, should be added if Gram smear shows gram-positive cocci. The role of hyperbaric oxygen is unclear; the value of such therapy may reside more in the experienced personnel associated with such a unit. Hyperbaric therapy requires patient transfer, and definitive surgical therapy must be done prior to transfer. Gas gangrene antitoxin is of unproved value, and we have not used it.

FOOD POISONING

method of
JONATHAN I. RAVDIN, M.D.,
and RICHARD L. GUERRANT, M.D.
Charlottesville, Virginia

Food poisoning is a disease state, most often with gastrointestinal or neurologic manifestations, resulting from the ingestion of food or water containing pathogenic organisms or substances toxic to man.

The most commonly recognized causes of food poisoning are bacterial agents, followed by chemical, parasitic, and viral agents. These diseases are underdiagnosed because the majority are self-limiting illnesses of short duration. However, proper management can be accomplished only after specific diagnosis is made, which is crucial in the life-threatening syndromes. Over 300 outbreaks of foodborne disease per year have been reported to the Center for Disease Control during a 5 year period (1972 to 1977).

Understanding pathogenic mechanisms of these diseases aids in prevention, management, and assessment of public health significance. Foodborne disease caused by bacteria can be due to ingestion of a preformed toxin (i.e., S. aureus, B. cereus, C. botulinum), toxin production by bacteria infecting the intestinal tract (i.e., C. perfringens, enterotoxigenic E. coli, V. cholerae), direct tissue invasion (i.e., Shigella sp., invasive E. coli), or a combination of toxin production and tissue invasion (i.e., V. parahaemolyticus, Y. enterocolitica, and possibly Salmonella or Shigella sp.). Chemical intoxication can be due to contamination of food (i.e., heavy metals, mercury), the food itself being toxic to man (i.e., mushrooms, puffer fish), or an accumulation of toxic material in a normally safe food (i.e., paralytic shellfish poisoning, Ciguatera poisoning). Protozoan and viral agents often spread by food or water that has been contaminated with feces or with an intermediate stage in the parasite's life cycle. Characterizations of toxins, as heat-stable or heat-labile, gives information as to whether proper cooking of food can prevent illness. Clues to etiology are suggested by the implicated food, with beverages, fish, mushrooms, and Chinese food causing most chemical food poisoning, while implicated meat, salads, and desserts suggest infectious agents (bacterial or parasitic). Clues to pathogenesis are often provided by the incubation periods and symptom complexes. Rapid onset of upper or lower gastrointestinal or neurologic symptoms suggests possible chemical or preformed toxin causes, while most infections or toxico-infections require longer incubation periods for multiplication of the organisms or production of toxins in the bowel. Agents not covered in detail in this article that can be transmitted in food but that do not give an acute "food poisoning"–like illness include brucellosis, Group A streptococcal disease, toxoplasmosis, tapeworm, paragonimiasis, Q fever, tularemia, anthrax, and tuberculosis.

The key to management is diagnosis of the specific cause of a food poisoning syndrome (see Tables 1 to 4).

1. Characterize the illness by gastrointestinal manifestations (upper or lower tract, absence or presence of leukocytes in a fresh fecal specimen), neurologic manifestations (paresthesias and/or paralysis), and a careful epidemiologic history (travel, identification of common meal or source, attack rate among persons sharing meal, incubation period) to provide clues to a specific diagnosis (see Tables 1 to 4).

2. Obtain specimens of suspected foods, serum, vomitus, and feces if possible for specific cultures or toxin assays. To implicate a specific food as a cause of food poisoning in a common source outbreak, one should first define the illness and then record the attack rate for each food consumed (number of people who became ill per total number who ate each food), as shown in example given in Table 5, which implicates meat. Attack rates should be high among those who ate the implicated food and low among those who did not. If two foods are suspected, they can be separated by the "cross table analysis," comparing attack rates when each implicated food is eaten alone or in combination with the other.

Notify the local Department of Health, which can aid in processing of specimens and conducting an epidemiologic investigation.

3. Institute supportive care consisting of maintenance of fluid balance, correcting metabolic alkalosis (vomiting) or acidosis (diarrhea), following respiratory status in neurologic syndromes (monitor vital capacity every 4 hours, cranial nerve function) and following renal and hepatic function. When managing diarrheal illnesses, one must first correct and maintain full isotonic hydration, which is usually possible with oral glucose- or sucrose-containing electrolyte solutions, as recommended by the World Health Organization: NaCl 3.5, NaHCO$_3$ 2.5, KCl 1.5, and glucose 20 or sucrose 40 grams per liter of clean or boiled water to give Na 90, Cl 80, K 20, HCO$_3$ 30, glucose 110 mMol per liter. Checking electrolytes of vomitus and stool can guide replacement therapy, which can be intravenous or oral, depending on whether oral fluids can be tolerated.

4. Clear toxins from gut. Emetics (ipecac syrup 15 to 20 ml orally) or gastric lavage should be used only if the patient is alert with intact bulbar function. Enemas and cathartics (magnesium sulfate, 15 grams orally) are used as well.

5. Avoid antiperistaltic agents; they are potentially deleterious in invasive bacterial syndromes. Atropine is useful only for muscarine and organic phosphate poisoning. Bismuth subsalicylate (Pepto-Bismol), 30 ml orally every 30 minutes over 2 to 4 hours, may aid in the control of diarrhea.

6. Specific antimicrobial or antiparasitic therapy is indicated only in invasive syndromes (i.e., shigellosis, *S. typhi*, *C. fetus*), in parasitic infections (*Giardia lamblia*, *Entamoeba histolytica*, *Strongyloides stercoralis*, anisakiasis), or when it is known to shorten duration of illness of toxin disease (i.e., *V. cholerae*). See Tables 1 to 4 for specific drugs and dosages.

7. Use specific antitoxin or toxin antagonist, especially in neurologic syndromes (see Tables 1 to 4).

8. Limit spread and morbidity of agent; this may include patient isolation (i.e., shigellosis), prophylaxis of exposed persons (i.e., hepatitis A), proper handling of food (refrigeration, adequate cooking, cleaning of fish, avoidance of contaminated mollusks, identification of contaminated food handlers), and proper sanitation and notification of authorities (health department, Center for Disease Control). The most common, avoidable errors made in food preparation relate to time-temperature abuse. The amount of time that foods are left at medium temperatures (i.e., between cooking and refrigeration) should be

TABLE 1. Food Poisoning Syndromes: Primarily Gastrointestinal Symptoms

AGENT	FOODS	INCUBATION PERIOD	CLINICAL PRESENTATION AND DURATION OF ILLNESS	DIAGNOSIS	THERAPY	PREVENTION
A. Upper Gastrointestinal Symptoms Predominate						
Bacterial						
Staph. aureus enterotoxin (heat-stable)	Meats, cream, desserts (high protein)	1–6 hours	Nausea, vomiting, watery diarrhea; fever uncommon; duration 12–24 hours	(a) Coagulase (+) Staph. aureus in vomitus, feces, food ($>10^5$ organisms per gram) (b) Toxin in food (RIA, gel precipitation)	Supportive	Avoid temperatures of 8–45 C for food, food handler contamination
Bacillus cereus toxin (heat-stable)	Fried rice	1–6 hours	Vomiting, abdominal cramps, occasional diarrhea; duration <12 hours	Food with $>10^5$ organisms per gram	Supportive	Avoid reheated rice
Heavy metals						
Zinc, copper, tin, cadmium	Acid beverages (pH 5) in metallic containers, tubing, nitrate-containing foods	5 minutes–2 hours	Nausea, vomiting, cramps, headache, diarrhea (zinc, tin); duration 2–24 hrs	Clinical syndrome, metal in food or beverage	Supportive	Prolonged storage of acid beverages in metal containers or tubing should be avoided
Protozoan						
Anisakiasis (eosinophilic gastritis)	Raw fish	Days–months	Abdominal pain, intestinal obstruction, heme (+) stool, eosinophilia	Gastroscopy	(a) Remove larvae via gastroscopy (b) Surgery	(a) "Gut" fish and refrigerate prior to use (b) Thorough cooking
B. Lower Gastrointestinal Symptoms Predominate, No Fecal Leukocytes						
Bacterial						
Clostridium perfringens enterotoxin (heat-labile) release in gut	Meats, gravies, poultry, fish	8–16 hours	Watery diarrhea, cramps, nausea (30–50%); duration 24 hours	(a) Food and stool for C. perfringens ($>10^5$/gm) (+) (b) Enterotoxin in stool (CIEP) (c) Rise in serum antibody to enterotoxin	Supportive	Eat or store food rapidly after preparation; 15–50 C permits growth
Bacillus cereus enterotoxin (heat-labile) release in gut	Raw meats, vegetables, dried foods	8–16 hours	Watery diarrhea, nausea, cramps; fever rare; duration 48 hours	(a) Stool (+) for B. cereus (b) Enterotoxin activity in stool, food (rabbit ileal loop)	Supportive	Avoid prolonged warming of food

TABLE 1. **Food Poisoning Syndromes: Primarily Gastrointestinal Symptoms** (*Continued*)

AGENT	FOODS	INCUBATION PERIOD	CLINICAL PRESENTATION AND DURATION OF ILLNESS	DIAGNOSIS	THERAPY	PREVENTION
Enterotoxigenic *Escherichia coli* (heat-labile and heat-stable enterotoxins; LT and ST)	Water-borne; salads, raw vegetables	1–4 days	Travel history, watery diarrhea, fever in children, nausea, vomiting, muscle ache; duration 1–5 days	Enterotoxin assay LT:tissue culture (CHO or Y1 adrenal) or immunoassay ST:suckling mouse	Supportive (oral glucose electrolyte solutions)	Avoid incriminated foods, water
Vibrio cholerae enterotoxin secreted in small intestine	Water-borne; contaminated foods, Gulf region shellfish	24–72 hours	Travel history, achlorhydria, explosive and painless watery diarrhea, hypovolemia, acidosis	(a) Rapidly motile comma-shaped bacteria on dark field of stool (b) TCBS culture of stool	(a) Oral electrolyte solutions; 3.5 gm NaCl, 2.5 gm NaHCO$_3$, 1.5 gm KCL, 20 gm glucose in 1 liter H$_2$O (b) IV replacement (c) Tetracycline 10 mg/kg PO q6H × 2 days if sensitive	Avoid infected water; vaccine for travel to endangered area (60–80% efficacy × 3–6 months)
Protozoan *Entamoeba histolytica*	Water-borne; fecal contamination of foods	2–7 days	Gradual onset diarrhea (dysentery-like); abdominal pain, fever 30%; can be chronic	(a) Stool exam, trichrome stain for trophozoite (b) Indirect hemagglutination (CDC) (+) 80–90% (c) Proctoscopy, scraping of ulcers	Metronidazole, 750 mg PO tid × 10 days (if shorter duration of therapy, follow with diloxanide furoate* 500 mg PO tid × 10 days) (CDC)	Adequate sanitation
Giardia lamblia	Water-borne (Rocky Mountains) (Leningrad)		Travel history, persistent diarrhea, malabsorption, abdominal bloating, nausea	(a) Stool exam × 3 (b) Enterotest (examine duodenal contents)	Quinacrine, 100 mg PO tid × 10 days	Sanitation; avoid surface water
C. **Lower Gastrointestinal Symptoms Predominate, Fecal Leukocytes Present**						
Bacterial						
Salmonella (enterotoxin effect and invasion)	Poultry, beef, ice cream	6–48 hours	Diarrhea (watery or dysentery-like), fever, cramps, hypovolemia; duration 2–7 days	(a) Stool culture (b) Positive blood cultures rare	(a) Supportive (b) Avoid antibiotics (don't alter course, prolong carrier state) unless systemic fever, chronic bacteremia, abscess)	(a) Adequate cooking and refrigeration (b) Identify carriers (c) Isolate active cases

Organism	Source	Incubation period	Symptoms	Diagnosis	Treatment	Prevention
Salmonella typhi (typhoid fever) (also *S. paratyphi*, *S. schottmülleri*, *S. hirschfeldii*—paratyphoid fever)	Fecal contamination; water, milk	10–14 days	Travel history, fever, malaise, headache, chills, constipation or diarrhea, cough, sore throat, rose spots, hepatosplenomegaly; duration 3–4 weeks	(a) (+) Blood culture (1st week) (+) stool culture not definitive (b) Serology (Widal 50% rise) (c) Leukocytosis, ↑SGOT, ↑LDH, monocytes in stool	(a) Chloramphenicol, 50 mg/kg/day PO, divided 4 doses × 4 days; if resistant, ampicillin, 100 mg/kg/day PO or IV qid × 14 days, or trimethoprim-sulfamethoxazole, 2–4 (80/400 mg) tablets PO q 12 h × 14 days (b) Avoid antipyretics (c) Supportive (d) Monitor Hct, stools for blood	(a) As above (b) Immunization increases infective dose of bacteria
Shigella enterotoxin and invasion	Potato, egg salads; fecal contamination, water-borne	36–72 hours	Fever, abdominal cramping, watery diarrhea followed by bloody mucoid stools, nausea, vomiting; duration, average 7 days	(a) Abundant fecal leukocytes (b) Stool culture on selective media	(a) Supportive (b) Ampicillin, 50 mg/kg/day in 4 divided doses PO × 5–6 days; if resistant, trimethoprim + sulfamethoxazole, 2 (80/400 mg) tablets PO q 12h × 5 days	(a) Adequate sanitation (b) Hand washing (c) Isolate active cases
Vibrio parahemolyticus enterotoxin (heat-labile) + invasion	Bivalve mollusks, crabs, raw saltwater fish (Japan); untreated seawater	12–24 hours	Explosive watery diarrhea, cramps, nausea, headache, fever 20% or dysentery, abdominal pain; duration up to 10 days	Culture stool, food (TCBS media) (Kanagawa, hemolysin (+) stain in stool)	(a) Supportive (b) If dysentery or prolonged illness, ampicillin, 100 mg/kg/day PO or IV qid × 5–7 days, or tetracycline, 500 mg PO qid × 5–7 days	(a) Proper cooking of seafood (b) Rapid refrigeration
Yersinia enterocolitica	Milk, ice cream, meat, mussels; water-borne	16–48 hours	Fever, diarrhea, abdominal pain, mesenteric adenitis, arthritis, erythema nodosum; duration 1–3 weeks	(a) Stool culture (b) Blood culture (c) Serology	Supportive unless septicemia; then gentamicin, 5 mg/kg/day IV, or chloramphenicol, 50 mg/kg/day PO or IV	None specific
Invasive *Escherichia coli*	Cheese, meats	24–72 hours	Dysentery, fever, malaise, myalgia, abdominal cramps	Sereny test	Supportive	None specific
Non-0-1 *V. cholerae* ("noncholera vibrio")	Seafood, water-borne	24 hours	Travel, diarrhea, abdominal cramps, nausea, vomiting, fever (58%), biliary disease	Stool culture on TCBS agar	(a) Supportive (b) Antibiotic— ampicillin, 100 mg/kg/day PO or IV qid 7–14 days, if sensitive organism	Proper cooking of seafood
Campylobacter fetus spp. jejuni	Water-borne; poultry, raw milk, farm animal, canine exposure; ?garden vegetables	72 hours	Bloody diarrhea, cramps, fever, vomiting; duration 1–4 days; relapse common	(a) Special stool culture in selective media, reduced pO₂ at 42 C (b) Blood culture	(a) Supportive (b) Erythromycin, 500 mg PO qid × 7 days (longer therapy if bacteremic syndrome develops)	Avoid raw milk, farm animal contamination

*Investigational drug. Available from Center for Disease Control, Atlanta, Georgia.

Table 2. Food Poisoning Syndromes: Gastrointestinal Plus Neurologic Symptoms

AGENT	FOODS	INCUBATION PERIOD	CLINICAL PRESENTATION AND DURATION OF ILLNESS	DIAGNOSIS	THERAPY	PREVENTION
A. Without Paresthesias						
Bacterial						
Clostridium botulinum neurotoxin (A, B, E, heat-labile) ingestion	Low acid home-canned vegetables, fruits; <10% of cases from commercial foods—vichyssoise, peppers, beef stew, mullet	18–36 hours	Nausea, vomiting, diarrhea (25%), followed by constipation and descending symmetrical motor weakness (cranial nerves initially); duration weeks–months	(a) Presence of toxin and *C. botulinum* in food and stool (mouse test with antisera) (b) Electromyography, facilitation of action potential with repetitive stimuli	(a) Respiratory support, tracheostomy if needed (b) Emetics/cathartics to remove unabsorbed toxin (c) Botulinal antitoxin if severe case (20% side effects, R/O horse serum allergy) (d) ? Guanidine hydrochloride, 35 mg/kg/day PO, improves eye/limb weakness only (e) Report CDC: 404-329-3753 or 404-329-3644 (nights, weekends)	(a) pH <4.5 home-canned foods (b) Boil prior to ingestion (c) Store food < 10 C (d) Nitrites are inhibitory
Clostridium botulinum, infants: neurotoxin released in gut	Honey, ?soil, dust		Age 2–26 weeks, constipation, poor feeding, descending motor paralysis (weak cry, "floppy baby"), 20% respiratory arrest; duration weeks–months	Clinical picture plus above	(a) Supportive (b) Antitoxin not required for recovery (c) Guanidine no longer recommended	Unknown
Chemical						
Organic phosphates (insecticides), cholinesterase inhibitors	Sugar, flour, bread, cereals, pastries	15 minutes–2 hours	Parasympathetic hyperactivity, cramps, nausea, vomiting, diarrhea, blurred vision, urinary/fecal incontinence, respiratory failure; 30% fatality	Clinical presentation plus low red cell and plasma cholinesterase levels	(a) Gastric lavage (b) Atropine, 0.4 mg IV q6h as needed (c) Pralidoxime, 1 gram IV, can be repeated × 1	Avoid insecticide use close to harvest
Solanine (potato poisoning)	Potato "eyes," sprouts, skin	7–19 hours	Abdominal pain, vomiting, diarrhea, fever, confusion, hallucinations, visual alterations; duration 1–2 days	(a) Clinical presentation (b) Solanine dose >25 mg in food	Supportive	(a) Toxin water soluble, removed by boiling (b) If eating >1 lb potatoes, peel and boil

B. With Pareshesias

	Source	Onset	Symptoms	Diagnosis	Treatment	Prevention
Fish toxins						
Scromboid (histamine, saurine)	Tuna, mackerel bonito, skipjack	5 minutes–1 hour	Histamine reaction, cramps, nausea, vomiting, diarrhea, flushing, oral burning, paresthesias, urticaria, bronchospasm, pruritus; duration hours	Histamine in fish >100 mg/100 grams	(a) Antihistamines (b) Emetic and cathartic (c) Treat bronchospasm, epinephrine or aminophylline	(a) Avoid storage of fish at 20–30 C (68–86 F) (b) Avoid fish with bitter, peppery taste
Puffer fish tetrodotoxin (heat-stable)	Puffer fish	10–45 minutes	Paresthesias of lip, tongue, and extremities; nausea, vomiting, cramps, loss of proprioception, flaccid paralysis, respiratory failure; 40–50% mortality	Tetrodotoxin bioassay (food)	(a) Supportive (b) Emetic and enemas	Avoid puffer fish served in Japan
Ciguatera fish ciguatoxin (heat-stable)	400 species: barracuda, red snapper, larger fish; 90% Hawaii or Florida	1–6 hours	Abdominal cramps, nausea, vomiting, watery diarrhea, paresthesias of lips and tongue, metallic taste, dry mouth, visual disturbance, transient blindness, sensation of loose and painful teeth, reversal of hot-cold sensation, hypotension, respiratory paralysis; duration days; residual years	(a) Bioassay for toxin (b) RIA toxin assay in food	(a) Supportive (b) Enemas (c) Analgesics (d) Atropine, 0.4 mg IV q6h, for CNS and GI manifestations	(a) Avoid fish liver, intestine, ovary ingestion (b) Clean fish immediately
Neurotoxic shellfish *Gymnodinium breve* (dinoflagellate), heat-stable toxins (red tide)	Oysters, clams, mussels (Gulf coast)	5 minutes–4 hours	Paresthesias of mouth and lips, reversal of hot-cold sensation, no paralysis, nausea, vomiting, diarrhea; can get respiratory syndrome; duration hours-days	Toxin in food	Supportive	Avoid possible contaminated bivalves
Paralytic shellfish *Gonyaulax catenella* (Pacific coast), *Gonyaulax tamarensis* (Atlantic coast), saxitoxin and other neurotoxins (heat-stable) red tide (summer, fall)	Oysters, clams, mussels, scallops	5 minutes–4 hours, dose-dependent	Paresthesias of mouth and lips, paralysis, respiratory insufficiency (first 12 hours), nausea, vomiting, diarrhea; duration hours-days	(a) Mouse bioassay of toxin in food (b) Dinoflagellates in seawater	(a) Cathartic, gastric lavage (b) Supportive	(a) Mollusks can be toxic without red tide (b) Avoid possible contaminated bivalves
Chemical						
Monosodium-L-glutamate	Wonton soup (absorption increased when stomach empty)	1 hour	Paresthesias; burning of neck, chest, arms; chest pain, headache, flushing, lacrimation, nausea, cramps, thirst; duration hours	MSG in food (>4 grams total dose)	None needed	Susceptible individuals should avoid MSG, especially on empty stomach

TABLE 3. **Food Poisoning Syndromes: Gastrointestinal Plus Other Systemic Diseases**

AGENT	FOODS	INCUBATION PERIOD	CLINICAL PRESENTATION AND DURATION OF ILLNESS	DIAGNOSIS	THERAPY	PREVENTION
Mushroom poisoning						
Muscarine	Inocybe, clitocybe species	<2 hours	Parasympathetic hyperactivity, salivation, diarrhea, diaphoresis, bradycardia, bronchospasm; duration 24 hours	Mushroom identification	(a) Atropine, 0.4 mg IV q6h, as needed (b) Supportive	Use commercial mushrooms only
Disulfiram-like	Coprinus atramentus plus/minus alcoholic beverages up to 48 hours after mushroom ingestion	<2 hours	Nausea, vomiting, flushing, palpitations, tachycardia; duration 24 hours	As above	Supportive	As above
General gastrointestinal irritants	Many species	<2 hours	Nausea, vomiting, cramps, diarrhea	As above	Supportive	As above
Amatoxins, phallotoxins	Amanita phalloides, Amanita verosa, Amanita verna, Galerina autumnalis, Galerina marginata, Galerina venenata	6–24 hours	Abdominal cramps, watery diarrhea for 24 hours, then hepatic and/or renal failure—hypoglycemia, metabolic acidosis, cardiomyopathy; 30% mortality; duration days	(a) As above (b) Renal/hepatic abnormalities	Supportive, including dialysis and metabolic correction; consider thioctic acid (experimental)	As above
Gyromitrin	Helvella species	6–24 hours	Cramps, diarrhea, followed by hepatic failure	Identify mushroom	Supportive	As above
Parasite						
Trichinosis	Pork, bear	1 week	Often asymptomatic; intestinal phase—malaise, anorexia, cramps, vomiting; muscle invasion—bilateral orbital edema, myalgias, fever, urticaria for 1–3 weeks, then convalescence, fatigue, listlessness; duration 3–10 weeks	(a) Deltoid or gastrocnemius muscle biopsy (b) Serology (c) Eosinophilia increased LDH, CPK	95% spontaneous recovery (a) Thiabendazole, 25 mg/kg bid × 5 days in early stages (b) Prednisone up to 60 mg PO qd for <2 weeks to treat severe symptoms	(a) Freeze food (b) Cook pork to internal temperature > 70 C (c) Use cuts of pork <6″ thick
Viral						
Hepatitis A	Mollusks, salads, cole slaw, sandwiches; waterborne	14–49 days	Fever, malaise, headache, anorexia, nausea, vomiting, then hepatomegaly, jaundice; duration 3–24 weeks	(a) Elevated SGOT, bilirubin (b) Hepatitis A particle in stool by IEM (c) Anti-hepatitis A (fourfold rise) in serum	Supportive	(a) Human immune globulin (0.02 ml/kg IM) if known contaminated ingestion within 6 weeks and asymptomatic or travel to endemic area (b) Isolation of cases (c) Handwashing (d) Eliminate primate spread

Table 4. Food Poisoning Syndromes: Neurologic Symptoms Alone

AGENT	FOODS	INCUBATION PERIOD	CLINICAL PRESENTATION AND DURATION OF ILLNESS	DIAGNOSIS	THERAPY	PREVENTION
Mushroom						
Ibotenic acid, muscimol	*Amanita muscaria, Amanita pantherina*	1–2 hours	Confusion, restlessness, visual disturbance; duration 24 hours	Mushroom identification	(a) Supportive (b) Physostigmine, 1 mg IV, for anticholinergic symptoms	Use commercial mushrooms only
Psilocybin, psibcin	Psilocybe species	<2 hours	Psychotic reaction, hallucinations; duration 12 hours	Mushroom identification	Supportive	As above
Chemical						
Alkyl mercury	Pork, grain, fish, shellfish	<2 hours or chronic exposure	Ataxia, agitation, visual impairment, hyperreflexia, coma; duration months	Increased mercury in food, serum, hair	(a) Supportive (b) Dimercaprol (BAL), 0.5 mg/kg IM q4h × 2 days; q12h × 1 day; qd × 5–10 days	Avoid alkyl mercury–treated grain or animal feed

TABLE 5. **Example of Food-Specific Attack Rates***

	ATE	DID NOT EAT
Meat	9/10	0/4
Potatoes	6/9	3/5
Salad	7/12	2/2

*Number ill per total number eating or not eating each food.

kept at a minimum to avoid multiplication of bacteria that may then cause disease by making a toxin (i.e., *Staph. aureus, B. cereus, C. botulinum*), by degrading tissue (i.e., scromboid fish poisoning), or by multiplying to a large infectious inoculum (Salmonella, *C. perfringens, Vibrio parahaemolyticus*, et al.).

EPIDEMIC INFLUENZA

method of
FREDERICK L. RUBEN, M.D.
Pittsburgh, Pennsylvania

Background Information

Epidemic influenza occurs from infection with type A or B influenza virus. Major antigenic changes or shifts in the type A virus' surface antigens, the hemagglutinin (H) and the neuraminidase (N), have been accompanied by pandemics of influenza. Examples of major antigenic shifts of influenza A in recent years include the 1957 H_2N_2 virus, in 1968 the H_3N_2 virus, and in 1977 the H_1N_1 virus. In years between these major alterations, minor changes in the H and N antigens, known as antigenic drift, have resulted in somewhat less extensive epidemics. The major antigenic shifts and minor drifts in the virus' surface antigens are important, because in each instance a portion of the population becomes susceptible to infection. Antibodies to the earlier virus strains provide lesser protection from the newly emerging strains. Exceptions to this have been noted in persons living at the turn of the century, who, prior to exposure to the H_3N_2 virus in 1968, had antibodies against this strain. Presumably in their childhood these people were infected with a strain of influenza A closely related or identical to the 1968 H_3N_2 virus. Influenza B viruses have shown much less of a tendency to shift or drift, although recently the B type virus has drifted, resulting in a significant epidemic in 1980.

Treatment of an Uncomplicated Case

The treatment of typical symptoms of influenza is directed at reducing or alleviation of the discomfort of the patient.

1. Reduction of activity and, frequently, bed rest are necessary for the duration of the fever. Hydration with water, carbonated beverages, or fruit juices is required and helps keep the respiratory secretions thin. Alcohol should be avoided, since it can reduce clearance of secretions. Smoking is harmful, since it interferes with normal ciliary function.

2. A cool mist vaporizer or air humidifier may help reduce the irritation to the respiratory tract mucosa.

3. Fever, sore throat, myalgias, and headache can be treated with aspirin, or, when aspirin is contraindicated, acetaminophen. For adults the aspirin dose is 0.6 gram every 4 hours, and for children 5 to 12 years old the dose is 0.15 to 0.3 gram every 4 hours. For adults the dose for acetaminophen is 625 mg every 4 hours, and for children 5 to 12 years up to 325 mg every 4 to 6 hours.

4. Cough is best reduced with hydration and humidification. To this may be added codeine phosphate. For adults tablets of 10 mg every 6 hours, and for children 5 to 12 years a dose of 5 to 10 mg of elixir every 6 hours, are appropriate. Less effective but still useful are any number of non-narcotic proprietary preparations.

5. Amantadine (Symmetrel) can be used in the management of symptoms caused by influenza A (not B, however) virus strains. It should be started within 24 to 48 hours of the onset of illness and continued for up to 3 days after the disappearance of symptoms. It is available in 100 mg capsules and in syrup form with 50 mg per 5 ml teaspoonful. For persons 13 years and older the dose is 200 mg a day given by mouth, either as two divided doses or as a single dose. Children 9 to 12 are given 200 mg a day as two divided doses. Children 1 to 9 years may be given 2 to 4 mg per pound (0.45 kg) in divided doses, not to exceed 150 mg per day. Use of amantadine in pregnancy requires weighing the possible risks to the fetus against the benefits to the mother, since at higher dosages than are given to man it was teratogenic in rats. Amantadine is secreted in breast milk and should be avoided in nursing mothers. Dosage reductions are required in patients with impaired renal function, since the drug may accumulate in the patient. Side effects are a significant problem with amantadine, and are mainly related to the central nervous system. The worst symptoms are depression, dizziness, psychosis, and urinary retention. Other symptoms have been described as well (see Physician's Desk Reference, 34th edi-

tion). These side effects may force discontinuation of the drug; however, the effects are reversible after the drug is stopped.

Complicated Cases

Bacterial pneumonia is a serious complication of influenza. It tends to occur more frequently in elderly or debilitated people. There is no evidence that prophylactic antibiotics can prevent this complication. Chest x-ray, sputum Gram stain and culture, and blood cultures are helpful in selecting an appropriate antibiotic if bacterial pneumonia is present.

Pneumonia may also be a pure viral pneumonia. Primary viral pneumonia is frequently quite severe and may necessitate the use of ventilatory assistance. In respiratory failure, correction of hypoxemia and suctioning of excess secretions may be lifesaving.

Encephalitis and myelitis are complications that require supportive care, because no specific measures are currently available.

Myocarditis occurs rarely and is best managed by supportive measures and careful monitoring and therapy for any heart failure or arrhythmias that occur.

Reye's syndrome is a serious disease closely associated with epidemic influenza B, although it is also known less frequently to accompany influenza A. It occurs primarily in children, but cases have been seen in adults. It follows a seemingly uncomplicated case of influenza when, in the recovery period, the patient begins to vomit uncontrollably. This is followed by lethargy and then coma. It is most important to recognize this syndrome early, since appropriate management can be lifesaving. The diagnosis can be made by obtaining the aforementioned history for any stage of the progression of symptoms, and performing laboratory tests showing abnormality of liver function (e.g., serum glutamic oxaloacetic transaminase [SGOT]), blood glucose, and, if available, blood ammonia. The suspected child or adult should be immediately referred to a medical center where one of several highly sophisticated forms of treatment may be begun (see Trauner, D. A.: Annals of Neurology 7:2–4, 1980).

Prevention

Avoiding exposure to influenza during epidemic periods is probably impossible, and isolation of cases in hospitals is of no practical value in preventing the spread of influenza.

Vaccines offer the best current means of preventing disease and have been up to 80 per cent effective in this role. Persons at greatest risk for developing fatal complications of influenza are people 65 years of age or older and people with rheumatic heart disease or any one of many other chronic debilitating conditions such as arteriosclerotic and hypertensive heart disease, chronic bronchopulmonary disease, and diabetes mellitus. Immunization is recommended for these people, and to be effective it should be given annually. It is controversial as to whether pregnant women are at greater risk from complications of influenza, and therefore their vaccination must be left to individual discretion. Vaccines can also be recommended for use in persons such as physicians, hospital workers, and closed military personnel, and for groups in which morbidity poses great consequence.

All licensed influenza vaccines are of the killed or inactivated type. Antigens for use in the vaccines are derived from virus which was grown in embryonated chicken eggs. The final vaccine, which is highly purified, may be one of two types: a whole virus preparation, or a so-called split or disrupted virus vaccine. Vaccines are now standardized as to the micrograms of hemagglutinin (one of two virus surface antigens) in one dose.

The formulation (meaning virus strains to be included in the vaccine), potency (meaning micrograms of each hemagglutinin type), and schedule for influenza vaccines are revised annually by the United States Public Health Service Advisory Committee on Immunization Practices. Their decisions reflect the best estimates of the virus strains which are expected to circulate during the coming influenza season. Since formulation, potency, and schedule may vary each year, one must refer to the vaccine package insert for this information.

Vaccine should be given each fall, using an up-to-date formulation and schedule. Vaccine is contraindicated in persons who have previously had severe reactions to influenza vaccines and in persons with known allergy to eggs. It may be given in conjunction with pneumococcal vaccine (see p. 132). Up to 20 per cent of vaccine recipients may note 1 to 2 days of local soreness, erythema, or induration at the site of injection, but this may be reduced by using an intramuscular injection. These reactions probably reflect true reactions to the virus antigens and not to the negligible vaccine impurities. Up to 5 per cent of vaccine recipients may develop brief systemic symptoms such as headache, malaise, or fever which usually subside over a day or two, and may respond to aspirin treatment.

During the 1976 swine flu immunizations, there was a definite association between receiving the swine flu vaccine and the occurrence of Guillain-Barré syndrome. Since that time surveillance has been reassuring by demonstrating no further association between the more recent vaccines and the syndrome. When Guillain-Barré syndrome was associated in 1976, it occurred at a rate of 1 in 100,000 vaccinees and mainly in younger healthy individuals for whom vaccine is not routinely recommended. Thus there seems to be little or no risk for the syndrome to occur after current vaccines are given to high risk groups.

An adjunct to vaccines, or an alternative in allergic persons, is amantadine (Symmetrel). The dosage, side effects, and contraindications have been described under Treatment, above. It must be emphasized that this drug is effective only against influenza A strains. To be effective prophylactically it must be given before or as soon as possible after potential exposure to influenza, and continued until after the virus is no longer prevalent in the community. Used in this way amantadine itself is possibly 70 per cent effective in preventing influenza A. It has an additive effect in conjunction with influenza vaccine. It may be given along with vaccine without impairing the antibody response to the vaccine, thereby providing protection during the 2 to 3 weeks required for the acquisition of vaccine-induced antibodies.

LEPROSY
(Hansen's Disease)

method of
A. B. A. KARAT, M.D.
Sunderland, England

Leprosy occurs throughout the world, though the majority of patients are found in tropical and subtropical countries of the third world. Leprosy was known in prehistoric and Biblical times and has been demonstrated in Egyptian mummies. It was endemic in the western countries between the sixteenth and nineteenth centuries, and then for some as yet unexplained reason, practically disappeared from the western world during the second half of the nineteenth and first two decades of the twentieth century, long before specific antileprosy therapy was discovered. The World Health Organization estimates the current global prevalence of leprosy at about five million, which is probably a significant underestimation of the magnitude of the problem.

The successful management of leprosy depends crucially on the recognition of a concept of leprosy in which there is a spectrum of immunologic and prognostic significance. There are two polar types of leprosy, tuberculoid (TT) and lepromatous (LL). The majority of cases lie in between these polar types almost in a continuous spectrum, between borderline-tuberculoid (BT) and borderline-lepromatous (BL) types. Host-parasite relationship with particular reference to immunologic competence or noncompetence determines the type of leprosy. The tuberculoid end of the spectrum represents the "high immunity" group with competent cell-mediated immunity, and the lepromatous end of the spectrum represents "low immunity" group with little or no cell-mediated immunity to *Mycobacterium leprae*.

Without an accurate diagnosis of leprosy itself and the precise location of a patient in the "leprosy spectrum," no rational therapy can be initiated.

Management of Leprosy

Effective treatment of leprosy patients must consist of:
1. Treatment of the bacterial infection.
2. Correction of deformities and re-education for resettlement, which should include training in caring for anesthetic limbs.
3. Prevention of progression of existing deformities and of the appearance of new deformity and disability once the patient has been started on specific antileprosy therapy.

In no other disease is the care of the "whole patient" so imperative for a successful outcome. One must avoid the paradoxical result of complete bacterial clearance and arrest of the disease but with the development of deformities and disabilities that render the patient incapable of looking after himself and make him a burden on his family and the society. "What the limbs cannot feel, the eye must feel" is a lesson to be learned and taught in the rehabilitation of the leprosy patient. A team approach is therefore essential in the care of patients with anesthetic limbs and deformity. Orthopedic and plastic surgery plays a major part in the management of deformities in leprosy, with support from physical therapy to enable the patient to relearn the activities of daily living.

Chemotherapy of Leprosy

There are widely divergent views about the dose, duration of treatment, and choice of drug for various types of leprosy and their complications. The views expressed here are largely based on my personal experience.

Dapsone (diaminodiphenylsulfone, DDS) is the drug of choice for all types of leprosy in all the age groups except in patients who either are sensitive to sulfone or have sulfone-resistant *M. leprae*. It is the cheapest and most effective drug available to date, is easy to administer in a single daily oral dose, has relatively few side effects when administered in the correct dosage, and has no demonstrable teratogenic effect. It is therefore safe in pregnancy and childhood. The average adult dose is 100 mg daily (6 to 10 mg per kg body weight) given as a single dose. Children below 5 years may be given 10 mg daily; between 5 and 12 years, 25 mg daily; and over 12 years, the adult dose according to body weight (these doses may be higher than those listed in the manufacturer's official directive).

Indeterminate and Polar Tuberculoid Leprosy Patients. These patients are treated with full dosage of dapsone for 3 years after *all* evidence of clinical activity of the disease in the skin lesion or the affected nerve has become quiescent (static) or for a total of 5 years, whichever is longer. It is important to ensure that the patients take the drug regularly — every day — for the duration of the treatment. Those patients with indeterminate leprosy who are lepromin negative, especially if they are below 12 years of age, may also be given BCG vaccination since there is some evidence that BCG may "boost" their cell-mediated immunity.

Borderline-Tuberculoid Leprosy (BT or BT/TT). Dapsone in full dosage is continued for a minimum of 5 years (where practicable for 10 years) after the cutaneous and nerve lesions have become quiescent and inactive.

Borderline, Borderline/Lepromatous, and Lepromatous Leprosy (BB and BL, BL/LL, LI, LL). The decision as to when to stop treatment in patients at the borderline-to-lepromatous end of the spectrum is rather more complex and debatable. On the available evidence, there appears to be a relatively high risk of relapse/recrudescence of leprosy in this group when specific chemotherapy is withdrawn even after 10 years of bacterial clearance from the skin and inactivity of the disease. The current thinking would favor lifelong treatment with full doses of dapsone.

When dapsone is administered in the dose mentioned above, serious complications are rare. In patients with glucose-6-phosphate dehydrogenase deficiency, dapsone may cause hemolytic anemia even in relatively small doses. Methemoglobinemia, exfoliative dermatitis, toxic psychosis, and insomnia are other rare side effects of dapsone therapy.

Sulfone-Resistant Leprosy

Sulfones were first introduced as specific therapy for leprosy in the early 1940s, and after nearly 40 years we are beginning to see the specter of emergence of sulfone-resistant leprosy (primary and secondary resistance). A large measure of responsibility for this catastrophic development must be laid on experimental workers who, through the 1960s and even the early 1970s, encouraged clinicians to develop a therapeutic policy of "low-dose" dapsone therapy (1 mg to 10 mg daily). This was based on the laboratory finding of the infinitely small dose of dapsone (0.0001 per cent W/W dietary dapsone) needed to produce an inhibitory effect on the multiplication of *M. leprae* in the footpads of mice. Despite a few lonely dissenting voices, low-dosage dapsone therapy became accepted as the rational approach to control and cure of leprosy throughout the world. Another cause of resistance was intermittent therapy. There was an association between ingestion of dapsone, killing of *M. leprae,* and the development of "reactions" (exacerbated states) in leprosy, and in the past there has been very little effective therapy for such reactions. Until recently the majority of clinicians recommended interruption of dapsone therapy during these periods of moderate to severe reactions. Once the reaction subsided, "low-dosage" dapsone therapy was recommenced in the erroneous belief that these reactions were dose-related phenomena. These two unfortunate therapeutic policies — low-dosage regimen and interrupted therapy — have been responsible for the emergence of secondary resistance. In the recent past a small number of primary resistant cases have been identified.

Apart from the clinical observation of gradual deterioration of the patient, appearance of fresh skin lesions and a rising bacterial index or morphologic index, the only means of detecting and confirming strains of *M. leprae* resistant or partially resistant to dapsone is by the use of mouse footpad system. It is fortunate that a significant number of strains so tested have only shown partial resistance and were susceptible to the full dose (equivalent of 100 mg daily in man) of dapsone. It would therefore appear logical to increase the dose of dapsone to 100 mg daily if sulfone resistance is suspected in a given patient who either has been on low doses for a prolonged period or has had frequent interruption of therapy for whatever reason. As a further precaution, polytherapy may be considered in such patients — Dapsone, 100 mg daily, with thiacetazone (thiosemicarbazone),* 150 mg daily, and isoniazid (INH),† 200 mg daily. On the other hand, if development of brownish-black pigmentation and ichthyosis of the skin is no bar to therapy, clofazimine (Lamprene),* 100 mg daily, is the alternative therapy of choice. It can safely

---

*Not available in the United States or is investigational.

†This use of this agent is not listed in the manufacturer's official directive.

be combined with dapsone, 100 mg daily, with thiacetazone, 150 mg daily, or with INH, 200 mg daily. In patients who show complete resistance to dapsone, either clofazimine alone or rifampicin (rifampin),* 600 mg daily, with either thiacetazone, 150 mg daily, isoniazid (INH), 200 mg daily, or clofazimine, 100 mg daily, can be used. The main limiting factor as far as rifampicin is concerned is the cost of the drug (about $500 to $600 per annum per patient). Hepatotoxicity, gastrointestinal intolerance, thrombocytopenia, and "flu-like" syndrome are relatively uncommon side effects of rifampicin. The latter two side effects are more frequently associated with intermittent therapy than when the drug is administered continuously.

Treatment of Reactions in Leprosy

The most frequent complication of leprosy is reaction or exacerbation. These reactions occur in 10 to 20 per cent of untreated patients and in 25 to 50 per cent of patients on chemotherapy. These reactions are essentially a manifestation of hypersensitivity to the mycobacterial antigens of dead *M. leprae*. There are two main types of reactions, and each of them presents a different management problem.

Erythema Nodosum Leprosum (ENL) Reaction:
Lepromatous Lepra Reaction

This type of reaction occurs only in bacilliferous patients toward the lepromatous end of the leprosy spectrum — BB/BL, BL, BL/LL, LL, LI, and rarely borderline (BB) leprosy. Although well recognized before the introduction of sulfones and other specific antileprosy drugs, there has been dramatic rise in the incidence and severity of ENL reactions in patients given specific antileprosy therapy. Nearly 50 per cent of treated lepromatous leprosy patients develop ENL during the first year of treatment. In severe ENL reactions, circulating immune complexes can be demonstrated. In a significant proportion of cases, the ENL reactions tend to be recurrent or chronic, and they are often associated with ENL acute peripheral neuritis, ENL lymphadenitis, ENL iridocyclitis, ENL orchitis, ENL arthropathy, and ENL nephropathy. The management of these patients, especially those with the severe recurrent/chronic ENL, can be very demanding. Specific therapy with dapsone should be continued uninterruptedly and appropriate antireaction therapy should be instituted. *Clofazimine* (Lamprene), 300 mg daily, is probably the treatment of choice if pigmentation can be tolerated.

---

*This use of this agent is not listed in the manufacturer's official directive.

This dose may be continued for 12 to 24 weeks, and then the dose can be reduced to 100 mg daily. At the end of 24 weeks, dapsone, 100 mg daily, may be continued alone with comparatively small risk of further reactions. *Thalidomide,* 300 to 400 mg daily in divided doses, effectively controls most ENL manifestations in 48 hours (investigational in the United States). The specific antileprosy drug (e.g., dapsone, 100 mg daily) should, of course, be continued. Thalidomide is contraindicated in females of childbearing age because of its teratogenic effect. There is a tendency for "rebound phenomenon" to occur if thalidomide is withdrawn too rapidly, and often it is necessary to keep patients on a small maintenance dose (e.g., 100 mg daily) for several months.

Steroids

Steroids are very effective in controlling the symptoms of ENL, especially in relieving the pain of acute ENL neuritis and reducing the risk of development and progression of neurologic deficit. Thirty to 60 mg per day of prednisolone will control the symptoms of ENL within 2 to 3 days. It should only be used concurrently with full doses of dapsone (e.g., 100 mg daily). The dose of steroids may then be gradually reduced over a 4 to 12 week period by giving the steroid on alternate days. This reduces the chance of suppression of the adrenopituitary feedback mechanism. Steroids are particularly valuable in three situations: (1) acute neuritis, (2) acute ocular complications during ENL where sight is threatened, and (3) ENL in puerperium. Steroids can be combined with clofazimine to take advantage of the rapid action of steroids, and they can be withdrawn in 2 to 4 weeks, while continuing with clofazimine.

Ocular complications of ENL include acute anterior uveitis (iridocyclitis), acute keratitis, and acute scleritis. They respond to the systemic antireaction therapy. Local application of mydriatics, e.g., 2 per cent homatropine eye drops twice daily, and betamethasone eye ointment (if available) during the acute phase is recommended. Protection from strong light (e.g., dark glasses, eyeshades) will add to the comfort of these patients. Prolonged use of topical steroids may predispose to the development of "steroid cataracts." In patients with recurrent or chronic (continuing) ENL, a careful search for a precipitating cause can be rewarding in that its elimination will stop the vicious circle. The most common precipitating causes are tuberculosis of the lungs and lymph glands, recurrent chest or urinary infections, and emotional upheaval or crises (e.g., rejection by the family, loss of job, social ostracism). It is also worth noting that if a patient suffering from ENL should become pregnant, she may have acute recurrence of severe ENL 7 to 14 days after delivery.

Reversal (Upgrading) Reactions

These occur over the whole of the leprosy spectrum except at the two polar ends (TT and LL). They occur by and large in the treated nonlepromatous patients, and represent delayed type hypersensitivity reaction to antigens of dying or dead M. leprae. They are characterized by the appearance of grossly edematous, swollen, erythematous, tender leprous lesions, and these develop over a period of days or weeks and are often associated with onset of acute neuritis and accompanied by systemic upset. They settle slowly over weeks or months. During the reversal reactions, the patients tend to shift toward the tuberculoid end of the spectrum — hence the term "upgrading" reaction. The development and progression of acute neurologic deficit is the main hazard, and it is imperative to treat these patients with adequate doses of steroids, e.g., 45 to 90 mg prednisolone daily, while ensuring that they continue on full doses of dapsone. Thalidomide is relatively ineffective in this condition. Clofazimine, 300 to 600 mg daily, is a useful therapeutic regimen, although in the first 2 to 4 weeks of clofazimine treatment, 30 to 60 mg of prednisolone a day must be added when reversal reaction is associated with acute peripheral neuritis. In fact, this is the only absolute indication for using steroids in leprosy.

Reversal reactions usually result in accelerated bacterial clearance by the efficient cell-mediated immune mechanism.

Lepromatous Mother and Pregnancy, Delivery, and Puerperium

Pregnancy itself does not appear to influence the course of the bacillary types of leprosy (borderline group and lepromatous group), so long as the patient is on specific antileprosy treatment. There is a tendency for an increased incidence of folate-deficiency megaloblastic anemia in pregnant women with leprosy, and the administration of dapsone exacerbates the situation. Hence it would be advisable for pregnant women with leprosy on dapsone therapy to have supplements of folic acid, 5 mg daily, along with oral iron. As mentioned earlier, there is a definite risk of reaction occurring 7 to 14 days after delivery, especially in borderline and lepromatous types of leprosy. This risk is reduced if patients have been on full doses of dapsone throughout pregnancy and the puerperium. Prompt recognition of reactions and institution of antireaction therapy can save the patient from catastrophic neurologic deficit and development of a chronic reactional state.

To date there is no conclusive evidence of transplacental transmission of leprosy in utero. Breast-feeding would be an advantage in this situation since therapeutic levels of dapsone are secreted in human breast milk and thus provide effective chemoprophylaxis to the infant. There is some evidence that neonatal BCG vaccination produces an immunoprophylactic effect. There is no indication for separating infants from leprous mothers on treatment, and these mothers should be encouraged to breast-feed their babies.

Prophylaxis

Immunoprophylaxis. The prophylactic value of BCG in reducing the incidence of new cases of leprosy is somewhat controversial. In view of the divergent results and inconsistent protection against leprosy, BCG immunoprophylaxis cannot be recommended for universal application. However, since tuberculosis and leprosy run parallel in tropical and subtropical countries, there may be some advantage in using BCG prophylaxis for children who are in contact with an index leprosy patient in the expectation that it may, in addition to protecting against tuberculosis, at least offer partial protection against M. leprae by augmenting cell-mediated immunity sufficient to prevent the development of the "malignant" form of the disease, namely, lepromatous leprosy. There is already some very promising work being done toward the development of a vaccine against leprosy from M. leprae harvested from armadillos infected with human leprosy bacillus. We can reasonably look forward to the production of an effective vaccine against leprosy during the next decade.

Chemoprophylaxis. The real value of chemoprophylaxis against the development of lepromatous leprosy remains unproved. The duration of such treatment and the dosage of dapsone required are, as yet, unresolved. Therefore, a firm recommendation regarding chemoprophylaxis cannot be made at this stage.

Other Antileprosy Drugs

Thiambutosine, thiacetazone, and long-acting sulfonamides have their advocates. However, on balance they do not appear to confer any particular advantage over dapsone and hence are not recommended for monotherapy of leprosy. There is reasonably good evidence to suggest that secondary resistance to these drugs begins to develop between 18 and 36 months from initiation of monotherapy with them. They may be useful in polytherapy, which is considered later in this discussion.

Clofazimine (Lamprene, B 663)

There are three special indications for the use of clofazimine in leprosy: (1) sulfone-resistant leprosy (primary or secondary), (2) recurrent/chronic reactions in leprosy, (3) dapsone intolerance. Clofazimine is the drug of choice for management of sulfone-resistant leprosy in a dose of 100 mg daily. If reactions should occur while the patient is on clofazimine, they are quickly controlled by increasing the dose to 200 to 300 mg, without the need for any other antireaction therapy, since clofazimine is an effective anti-inflammatory agent under these circumstances. The major disadvantage of clofazimine is the development of brownish-black pigmentation of the skin, often associated with ichthyosis. The pigmentation and ichthyosis are reversible on withdrawal of the drug, although it may take several months to 2 years to clear. Rarely, a variety of "granulomatous ileitis" may occur, especially in patients on the larger doses for more than 12 weeks. This condition is also reversible on withdrawal of the drug. Sweat, breast milk, urine, and semen also appear pigmented.

Rifampicin (Rimactan, Rifampin)

This well-known antituberculous drug is rapidly bactericidal for *M. leprae*, but has no effect on the rate of elimination of *M. leprae* from the human body. Therefore, its rapid bactericidal effect has not conferred any major therapeutic advantage over dapsone in clinical practice. In certain situations, from the epidemiologic point of view, there may be a case for short-term treatment (say for 4 weeks) of hitherto untreated or sulfone-resistant leprosy concurrently with another effective antileprosy drug to reduce the risk of transmission of leprosy in the community. The recommended dose is 450 to 600 mg daily in a single dose, depending on the weight of the patient. Rifampicin is also effective in rapidly relieving symptoms of leprous rhinitis and laryngitis. For this purpose, treatment for 2 to 4 weeks seems adequate.

The major disadvantage of rifampicin is its prohibitive cost, particularly in developing countries, where unfortunately most cases of leprosy occur. In addition, following monotherapy with rifampicin, the development of secondary resistance has been noted over a 3 to 4 year period. Therefore, if rifampicin is used in leprosy, it should be used *only* in combination with another effective antileprosy drug. Side effects include hepatotoxicity and a flu-like syndrome. When rifampicin is administered intermittently, the risks of thrombocytopenia and renal failure resulting from immune complex deposition need to be borne in mind.

Streptomycin*

Another active antituberculous drug, streptomycin, has been used in leprosy. Dosage has varied from 1.0 gram intramuscularly daily to 1.0 gram intramuscularly three times a week. Resistance develops in 6 to 36 months if used as monotherapy. A short course (1 gram daily for 2 to 4 weeks) has been used with considerable benefit in patients with upper respiratory involvement and in patients with acute leprous ulcerations of the skin. Streptomycin should always be used in combination with dapsone or another active antileprosy drug.

Ethionamide*

This drug is active against *M. leprae* in doses of 250 to 750 mg daily. If used as monotherapy, resistant strains begin to emerge in 3 to 4 years. Hence, ethionamide should be used only in polytherapy of leprosy. Gastrointestinal intolerance and hepatotoxicity are well-recognized side effects.

Combination Therapy (Polytherapy)

Following emergence of sulfone-resistant leprosy, clinicians have been debating the role of combination therapy in leprosy similar to the situation with treatment of tuberculosis. It must be emphasized that, as yet, there is no convincing evidence of the development of sulfone resistance in patients on continuous uninterrupted treatment with dapsone, 100 mg daily. This may be an opportune moment to conduct carefully planned trials of combination therapy versus full dosage of dapsone therapy. On theoretic and economic grounds, dapsone, 100 mg, with thiacetazone, 150 mg, daily with or without isoniazid (INH), 200 mg daily, may be worthwhile. Clofazimine, 100 mg daily, with dapsone, 100 mg daily, or rifampicin, 450 to 600 mg daily, with dapsone, 50 to 100 mg daily, is another combination worthy of trial.

In the present state of knowledge, the role of such combination therapy must remain experimental and speculative.

---

*This use of this agent is not listed in the manufacturer's official directive.

LEISHMANIASIS

method of
JOHN S. WOLFSON, M.D.,
and ROBERT H. RUBIN, M.D.
Boston, Massachusetts

Leishmaniasis is a disease caused by flagellated tissue protozoa of the genus Leishmania. It is transmitted from animals, and sometimes man, to man by the bite of the sandfly, Phlebotomus. Only three autochthonous cases have been reported in the United States, all from Texas. However, the disease is an important worldwide problem, afflicting many millions of persons. Leishmaniasis may take visceral, mucocutaneous, or cutaneous forms. Treatment varies with the form, extent, and geographic source of the disease. Because of the importance of geographic exposure, a careful epidemiologic history is essential in evaluating the patient with possible leishmaniasis.

Visceral Leishmaniasis (Kala-azar)

This form of the disease is caused by *Leishmania donovani*, with endemic areas well defined in India, China, the Middle East, Africa, and Latin America. Kala-azar resembles lymphoma in presentation, with chronic recurrent fevers, splenomegaly, weight loss, pancytopenia, and hyperglobulinemia. Treatment includes supportive care, treatment of other complicating illnesses, and specific chemotherapy. For chemotherapy, the mainstay is the pentavalent antimony compounds. In the United States, the only available agent, and then only through the Parasitic Diseases Drug Service of the Center for Disease Control (telephone 404–329–3670 during working hours, 404–329–4644 for emergency drug use, day or night), is sodium antimony gluconate (Pentostam). This drug is given intramuscularly or slowly intravenously in a dose of 10 mg per kg, with the daily dose not to exceed 0.6 gram (6 ml), each day for 6 days for Indian kala-azar, and each day for 30 days in other forms. Adverse reactions to sodium antimony gluconate are uncommon and usually mild, consisting of cough, gastrointestinal upset, arthralgias, myalgias, headache, rash, pruritus, fever, transient electrocardiogram changes, hypotension, and syncope. Cardiac, renal, or hepatic disease constitutes a relative contraindication to antimony therapy. The pentavalent antimonial antimony-N-methyl glucamine (Glucantime), used in Latin America and in French-speaking countries, is felt to be clinically indistinguishable from sodium antimony gluconate in terms of efficacy and toxicity.

When antimonials fail in the treatment of kala-azar, the aromatic diamidines, pentamidine isethionate and hydroxystilbamidine isethionate, can be used. The dose of pentamidine is 2 to 4 mg per kg per day intramuscularly up to 15 doses. Solutions of this drug should be protected from light to avoid the production of hepatotoxic compounds. Although effective, pentamidine is frequently quite toxic. Adverse effects include hypotension, tachycardia, nausea, vomiting, and facial flushing as immediate effects; azotemia, hypoglycemia, liver damage, rash, and rarely hyperglycemia or a Herxheimer reaction as later onset problems; and pain, abscess, and necrosis at the injection site as local toxicities. Pentamidine, like sodium antimony gluconate, is available in the United States only from the Center for Disease Control. Hydroxystilbamidine is available in the United States only from Merrell-National by special order. Because of problems of resistance to antimonials, kala-azar from the Sudan is sometimes initially treated with an aromatic diamidine.

An alternative to the diamidines for kala-azar is amphotericin B. The treatment course is similar to that for deep mycoses, with a dose of 0.25 to 0.5 mg per kg by intravenous infusion over 4 hours, each day or every other day, for a total dose of 1.5 to 2.0 grams.

With therapy, response is for the most part prompt, with a great reduction in the untreated mortality of 95 per cent in adults and 80 per cent in children. Relapses occur in 5 to 15 per cent of cases and should be treated in the same way as the initial illness. A fortunately rare sequela, post-kala-azar dermal leishmaniasis, is difficult to treat, often not responding to antimonials, diamidines, or amphotericin B.

Mucocutaneous Leishmaniasis

American mucocutaneous leishmaniasis, caused by *Leishmania brasiliensis*, includes two diseases, uta and espundia. Uta, which occurs in cooler elevated climates of South and Central America, is characterized by a single or multiple lesions on the nose and lips, with mucosal spread uncommon. In tropical Latin America, a different variety of *L. brasiliensis* causes espundia, a disease in which skin lesions enlarge, often become secondarily infected, and spread to mucosal surfaces of the mouth and nose, which can be destroyed. Treatment consists of antibiotics for superinfection and a 6- to 10-day course of a pentavalent antimonial in doses used for kala-azar; sometimes treatment must be repeated. Treatment failures require amphotericin B. Early lesions respond well, but in espundia heal quite slowly.

Cutaneous Leishmaniasis

American cutaneous leishmaniasis (Chiclero ulcer), caused by *Leishmania mexicana,* is characterized by a single nonulcerating cutaneous lesion on the face, ear, or hand. Spontaneous healing usually occurs within 6 months. Nonhealing or ear lesions, because of the destructive nature, should be treated with a 6- to 10-day course of pentavalent antimony, in doses used for kala-azar. Alternative drugs are amphotericin B and cycloguanil pamoate in oil (Camolar). Cycloguanil pamoate, a repository, is given as a single intramuscular injection, 350 mg base for adults, 280 mg for children aged 1 to 5 years, and 140 mg for infants. If necessary, the dose can be repeated after 1 month. Prior to injection, the vial should be warmed and well shaken to ensure complete dispersion of drug in the oil. Adverse reactions to cycloguanil pamoate are minimal and include occasional local tenderness at the injection site, and rare allergic reactions or blood dyscrasias. The drug is not available in the United States.

Old World leishmaniasis (Oriental sore) is caused by *Leishmania tropica. L. tropica major* causes a rural disease, with ulcers on the extremities and regional lymphadenopathy, which spontaneously heal in 3 to 6 months. *L. tropica minor* leads to the urban (dry) type of disease, with a purplish, pruritic facial nodule that enlarges and breaks down in about 4 months. Healing often takes a year. Treatment includes antibiotics and hot soaks for bacterial superinfection. It is possible that infrared heat therapy is of value. If lesions are single or few and not cosmetically significant, local or topical therapy is preferred. However, when necessary, systemic treatment can be given with sodium antimony gluconate in the same way as for American cutaneous leishmaniasis. Some doses of the drug may be injected locally in 0.6 gram amounts three or four times on alternate days. For patients who live in endemic regions, antimony therapy should not be initiated until ulceration occurs, since this allows for the development of protective immunity against future infections.

Prophylactic measures for the individual against leishmania include the use of insect repellent on exposed skin, fine mesh screens in dwellings, and fine mesh nets around beds. Drug prophylaxis does not exist. Vaccines also are not available. With respect to new drugs, currently allopurinol and allopurinol derivatives, which interfere selectively with RNA metabolism in leishmaniads, are being evaluated for possible future use as anti-leishmanial therapeutic agents.

MALARIA

method of
MARCEL E. CONRAD, M.D.
Birmingham, Alabama

Malaria is an infection with a parasite of the genus Plasmodium. Although it is usually a mosquito-transmitted disease of tropical and semitropical areas, it also occurs in many temperate zones of the world and can be transmitted by blood transfusion, by sharing of contaminated hypodermic syringes and needles, and by the transplacental route. The diagnosis should be considered in every febrile patient and in all persons with coma, shock, or acute renal failure who have recently traveled in a tropical area, have received a blood transfusion, or are suspected of being addicts. The diagnosis should be established by microscopic examination of thick and thin smears of blood before treatment is begun.

Most human cases of malaria are caused by *P. vivax* and *P. falciparum. P. malariae* and *P. ovale* are less commonly encountered infections. Mixed infections with more than one parasite are not unusual. Rarely, certain simian malarial strains infect man, and cases of babesiosis may be difficult to differentiate from malaria without expert laboratory aid.

From a therapeutic viewpoint, it has become important to identify *P. falciparum* infections not only because they cause a more dangerous disease but also because many Asian and South American strains have become resistant to the synthetic antimalarial drugs used for both chemoprophylaxis and therapy. Clinical manifestations which make the diagnosis of *P. falciparum* probable in patients with malaria include renal or neurologic manifestations, sustained low grade fever between paroxysms, moderate or severe anemia (hematocrit, <30 per cent), and thrombocytopenia (<100,000 cells per cu mm). Simple morphologic characteristics of *P. falciparum* are the occurrence of only ring forms in peripheral blood with an absence of schizonts and mature trophozoites, multiple infection of erythrocytes with ring forms, double chromatin dots in ring forms, invasion of both large basophilic young erythrocytes and smaller, older red blood cells with parasites, the finding of characteristic banana- or sausage-shaped gametocytes in circulating erythrocytes, and the frequent finding of accolé or appliqué forms on the margin of red blood cells.

Prophylaxis

An individual entering an area where malaria remains endemic should avoid contact with mosquitoes and systematically take drug prophylaxis. Either 500 mg of chloroquine diphosphate (300 mg base) or 520 mg (400 mg base) of amodiaquine dihydrochloride should be taken weekly by adults, with proportionately smaller dosages for children. Prophylaxis should be initiated 2 weeks prior to entering a malarious area and continued for 6 weeks after departure. In addition, upon leaving an area where malaria is endemic, primaquine phosphate (15 mg base) should be taken daily for 14 days to eradicate the exoerythrocytic stages of plasmodia infections. Primaquine should not be administered to individuals with glucose-6-phosphate dehydrogenase (G-6-PD) deficiency because it will cause hemolytic anemia.

Weekly prophylaxis with either chloroquine or amodiaquine may be ineffective in areas where chloroquine-resistant falciparum malaria is endemic. Although there is no antimalarial prophylaxis that may be recommended in their place in the United States, combinations that have been effectively utilized elsewhere include either pyrimethamine, 25 mg, plus sulfadoxine, 500 mg, once weekly, or chloroguanide hydrochloride, 100 mg, plus dapsone, 25 mg, once daily.

Since malaria-carrying mosquitoes bite in the evening and night, the traveler should be advised to seek screened areas during these portions of the day with appropriate use of insecticides and repellents such as N,N-diethyltoluamide.

Chemotherapy

The preferable treatment for acute malaria in nonimmune subjects (except for *P. falciparum* infections in geographic areas where drug-resistant forms of this disease are prevalent) is either chloroquine or amodiaquine. Doses are expressed in terms of the free base and are provided for a 70 kg adult. Children and adults weighing less than 40 kg should be given a proportionately smaller dose. One of the following regimens is recommended: (1) chloroquine, 600 mg initially, 300 mg 6 hours later, and 300 mg on each of the next 2 days; *or* (2) amodiaquine, 600 mg initially and 400 mg on each of the next 2 days.

Whenever possible, these drugs should be given after meals to diminish their irritating effect on the gastrointestinal tract. These regimens should abolish the fever of malaria and parasitemia within 3 days. Persistence of either fever or parasitemia or an increase in parasitemia with therapy makes infection with a drug-resistant strain of *P. falciparum* likely. Occasionally, parenteral therapy with chloroquine is necessary because of severe vomiting. Then 200 mg of chloroquine hydrochloride (Aralen) should be dissolved in 5 ml of sterile water and given intramuscularly. This dose of chloroquine base should not be repeated more frequently than

every 8 hours, and the patient should be placed on oral therapy as soon as possible.

Chloroquine and amodiaquine do not cure the exoerythrocytic forms of the malaria parasite. Therefore it is necessary to treat all patients with *P. vivax*, *P. ovale*, and *P. malariae* with primaquine in a daily dose of 15 mg of base for 14 days in order to provide a radical cure. This is not useful for the treatment of *P. falciparum* infections, because this form of malaria does not have a secondary exoerythrocytic stage of disease.

Drug-resistant strains of *P. falciparum* have been found with increasing frequency in Southeast Asia and South and Central America. They have been imported into the United States by both servicemen and travelers. Drug-resistant malaria is likely in any patient with *P. falciparum* malaria who has traveled in a known endemic area within the last 2 years or acquired the infection while taking prophylactic drugs and when parasitemia is not reduced by treatment with chloroquine or amodiaquine. Combination drug therapy is the method of choice for the treatment of drug-resistant falciparum malaria. The most successfully proved regimens consist of triple treatment with quinine, a dihydrofolate reductase inhibitor (pyrimethamine or trimethoprim), and either a sulfonamide (sulfadiazine, sulforthomidine,* sulfisoxazole, or sulfalene*) or a sulfone (dapsone*). A method of combination oral therapy that has proved successful includes quinine sulfate, 650 mg every 8 hours for 10 days; pyrimethamine, 25 mg twice daily for 3 days; and a sulfonamide (sulfisoxazole or sulfadiazine) 0.5 gram every 6 hours for 5 days.

Parenteral treatment of drug-resistant falciparum infections may be required if the patient is comatose or has intense parasitemia (>100,000 parasites per cu mm of blood). Quinine dehydrochloride is available for parenteral administration. Single doses should not exceed 650 mg of base and should be diluted in either saline or glucose solution for slow intravenous administration by drip infusion. A patient with renal failure should not receive more than one third of this dose. No more than three doses should be given within 24 hours, and oral therapy should be initiated as soon as possible.

Toxicity of Antimalarial Drugs

Quinine. Cinchonism occurs with overdosage and is most frequent when renal function is compromised. Symptoms of cinchonism may be difficult to differentiate from those caused by falciparum malaria and necessitate the perfor-

---

*Investigational for this use in the United States.

mance of quinine blood levels. Patients receiving repeated courses of therapy or prolonged therapy with quinine have developed either acute hemolytic anemia with hemoglobinuria or thrombocytopenia. Quinine therapy must be stopped when these complications are believed to be caused by treatment.

Chloroquine and Amodiaquine. These are safe drugs in the dosage recommended. Overdosage can cause convulsions and death.

Primaquine, Sulfones, and Sulfonamides. These drugs can cause a self limited hemolytic anemia in patients with glucose-6-phosphate dehydrogenase (G-6-PD) deficiency and methemoglobinemia and in patients with heterozygous deficiency of NADH methemoglobin reductase in their erythrocytes. The hemolytic process is usually mild and does not persist with continued therapy in the Type A G-6-PD deficiency commonly found in black persons. It is more severe with other forms of G-6-PD deficiency and requires a modification of therapy. Sulfones and sulfonamides rarely cause agranulocytosis.

Pyrimethamine. As with other antifolic drugs, bone marrow suppression with megaloblastic changes can occur with repeated therapy.

General Therapy and Complications

As a guide to chemotherapy and the early recognition of complications, body temperature should be measured every 4 hours, a parasite count performed twice daily, body weight and a hematocrit obtained daily, and a careful record of intake and output of fluid maintained during the acute stage of disease. Serious complications are unusual in all forms of malaria except that caused by *P. falciparum*.

Overhydration must be avoided because renal failure and pulmonary edema are serious complications of falciparum malaria; a weight loss of half a pound (0.23 kg) daily should be expected during the acute illness. A sudden fall in urinary output should be treated with early use of mannitol therapy, careful fluid management, and a reduction in dosage of antimalarial drugs. Sudden gains in weight signal fluid retention that can lead to pulmonary edema. Fluid restriction, diuretic therapy, and even peritoneal dialysis or hemodialysis or phlebotomy may be required.

Scrutiny of the patient's behavior and mental status should be ascertained every 4 hours. In cerebral malaria, phenytoin, 400 mg daily, has been used to control convulsions and dexamethasone sodium phosphate, 3 mg every 8 hours, has been recommended to reduce cerebral edema. The level of parasitemia is not too helpful in following the effectiveness of chemotherapy in

patients with cerebral malaria because the parasitized erythrocytes are sequestered in peripheral blood vessels. Evidence of disseminated intravascular coagulation should be sought in these patients. Whether or not anticoagulation with heparin will prove useful is unknown because an insufficient number of humans have been studied.

A sudden decrease in the hematocrit or the occurrence of hemoglobinuria is indicative of an acute hemolytic reaction and may herald the onset of renal complications. If transfusion is required, packed red cells should be used. Corticosteroid therapy should be employed, coagulation studies performed for disseminated intravascular coagulopathy, and quinine therapy reconsidered if the drug is believed to be important in the cause of the anemia. The moderate anemia that occurs after an attack of falciparum malaria often responds to folic acid therapy.

MEASLES
(Rubeola)

method of
LEON M. HEBERTSON, M.D.
Bakersfield, California

Measles is an acute viral disease characterized by coryza, conjunctivitis, high fever, "Koplik's spots," and a maculopapular rash which usually appears the fourth or fifth day after the onset of symptoms. The disease is highly contagious and is transmissible from the earliest onset of symptoms until the fourth or fifth day after the appearance of the rash. Prior to the advent of effective measles vaccine, widespread measles epidemics occurred in preschool and young school age children. Most older children and adolescents were immune by virtue of naturally acquired infection. Since measles vaccine was introduced in 1963, outbreaks in the United States have become more limited, and currently over 60 per cent of cases occur in inadequately immunized older children, adolescents, and young adults. Greater attention to the immunization status of these persons is now required. Center for Disease Control (CDC) officials estimate that there are now fewer than 200 measles transmission chains extant in the entire country at any one time, and because sufficient containment resources are available, a nationwide effort has been launched to eliminate the disease or at least make it exceedingly rare in the United States. Containment is dependent on immediate telephonic reporting of all proved or suspect cases, aggressive management of contacts to cases, and continuing efforts to vaccinate all susceptible persons who can safely be immunized.

Prevention

Active Immunization. Active immunization is accomplished with a single dose of live attenuated measles vaccine given subcutaneously in the volume specified by the manufacturer. Measles vaccine should normally be given at 15 months of age when optimal antibody response has been shown to occur. Infants as young as 6 months old may be vaccinated when there is risk of exposure to measles, but they should be revaccinated at 15 months of age. There is no increased risk of revaccinating a previously immunized child. Older children, adolescents, and adults should also be vaccinated unless there is reliable evidence of immunity from natural infection or prior immunization with *live* measles vaccine given *after* the age of 1. Persons vaccinated before 12 months of age and persons uncertain of their age of vaccination should be reimmunized.

Between 1963 and 1967, large numbers of persons received *inactivated* measles virus vaccine which failed to produce lasting immunity to measles. Such persons are susceptible to measles and may develop severe atypical disease. Individuals vaccinated prior to 1968 should also be revaccinated unless it is known that they received live measles virus vaccine after 1 year of age.

To ensure there is no loss of potency, measles vaccine must be maintained at a temperature between 2 and 8 C (35.6 and 46.4 F). It must also be protected from light and discarded if not used within 8 hours after reconstitution. When properly handled, measles vaccine will produce durable immunity in 95 per cent of children 15 months of age and older. It is available as a monovalent vaccine (measles only) or in combined form with other vaccines: measles-rubella (MR), and measles-mumps-rubella (MMR). Either the monovalent or a combination vaccine may be used in situations in which measles vaccination is indicated, and it is customary to use a combined form (MR or MMR) when immunization against mumps and/or rubella is also needed.

Side effects of measles vaccine include local tenderness and slight fever or rash occurring 7 to 10 days after vaccination in about 15 per cent of children. Encephalitis or encephalopathy occurs about once per million doses of vaccine administered. Local edema, induration, lymphadenopa-thy, and fever are sometimes seen following vaccination of persons previously vaccinated with inactivated measles vaccine. The possibility of such reactions should be explained before vaccine is administered.

Contraindications. Contraindications to the use of live attenuated measles virus vaccine are discussed in each manufacturer's package insert, which should always be reviewed. These include pregnancy, conditions of altered immunity, and allergy to certain trace antibiotics as noted in the labeling information.

Allergy to penicillin, eggs, chicken, or feathers is not a contraindication. Vaccination should be postponed in persons with acute febrile illness but need not be deferred because of minor upper respiratory infections.

Live attenuated measles vaccine has not been reported to exacerbate active tuberculosis, and routine tuberculin testing is not a necessary prerequisite to measles vaccination. Measles vaccine may cause temporary anergy to tuberculin reagent; if there are reasons to suspect tuberculosis, skin testing should be done before or at the time of measles vaccination and read in 72 hours. Further investigation and/or treatment of tuberculosis can be accomplished if indicated.

Treatment

Management of Exposed Susceptibles. The danger of a measles outbreak exists whenever a case of measles occurs. Prompt telephonic reporting to local health agencies and immediate steps to identify exposed susceptible individuals should be initiated. All contacts without documented history of measles or evidence of appropriate vaccination should receive live measles vaccine *or* immune serum globulin (ISG), 0.25 ml per kg of body weight (maximum dose 15 ml). Considerable discretion should be exercised in deciding which of these measures to use.

Live measles vaccine given within 3 days of first exposure may prevent measles. Even when the interval since first exposure exceeds 3 days, live measles vaccine is usually preferable in healthy school age children since the vaccine will protect the individual from other cases in the community if the current exposure does not result in disease.

ISG will prevent or modify measles when given within 6 days of first contact, but it cannot be relied on to prevent disease from future exposure. ISG should be used when protection from measles is required for persons for whom live measles vaccine is contraindicated. It may also be indicated for susceptible household contacts, particularly infants, for whom the risk of complications is greatest. Persons given ISG should guard against re-exposure to other measles cases in the community and should receive live attenuated measles vaccine in approximately 3 months when passive measles antibodies have disappeared. ISG should not be used to control outbreaks of measles in the community. Vaccination and/or exclusion of susceptible school contacts is more effective.

Treatment of Active Disease. The disease is best managed at home unless the child is desperately ill. The symptoms of cough, fever, and anorexia predominate and become increasingly severe through the prodromal and eruptive stages of the disease. Rapid improvement generally occurs on the sixth or seventh day of illness when the rash has completely covered the body. Antipyretics, antitussives, bed rest, and liquids high in carbohydrate are generally prescribed. Humidification and tepid water baths will help relieve cough and fever during the height of the illness. Reduced light and simple eye care are helpful in relieving conjunctival irritation. Antibiotic ophthalmic preparations are rarely needed.

The chief complications of measles are otitis media, pneumonia, and encephalitis. Myocarditis also occurs. Otitis media is usually bacterial in origin and should be treated with antibiotics. Pneumonia occurs in about 10 per cent of cases and may be either an interstitial type caused by the measles virus itself or a superimposed bacterial bronchopneumonia. Streptococcus, pneumococcus, and *Hemophilus influenzae* are the common invading organisms. Antibiotics are indicated if secondary bacterial infection is suspected. Measles encephalitis and parainfectious encephalitides are observed in 0.1 to 0.2 per cent of cases. Such complications are potentially fatal and may lead to permanent brain damage. However, residual neurologic sequelae cannot be correlated with the severity of disease. Patients with severe encephalitis may completely recover and should receive intensive supportive care.

Atypical Measles. Atypical measles is an unusual and severe form of measles seen in persons who were vaccinated with inactivated measles virus vaccine. The disease is characterized by high fever and a centripetal rash consisting of papules, blisters, wheals, and pinpoint hemorrhages into the skin. Peripheral edema and pulmonary infiltrates are common. The diagnosis is suspected from the history and clinical findings and confirmed by a fourfold rise between acute and convalescent antibody titers or a single high reciprocal convalescent titer. Treatment is symptomatic and supportive.

BACTERIAL MENINGITIS
method of
PETER A. RICE, M.D.
Boston, Massachusetts

Bacterial meningitis is a life-threatening infection that must be recognized early in order to avert a catastrophic result. Prior to the advent of effective antimicrobial therapy, bacterial meningitis was almost uniformly fatal; however, with prompt recognition and correct antimicrobial therapy and supportive care, both the case fatality rate and neurologic sequelae can be greatly reduced. In order to make a rapid diagnosis, the clinician must suspect bacterial meningitis in patients with fever and altered mental status; meningeal signs are usually, though not invariably, present. A lumbar puncture must be performed rapidly in patients suspected of having bacterial meningitis, since confirmation of the diagnosis and guidance on initial antimicrobial therapy can only come from the evaluation of cerebrospinal fluid. Patients who have a questionable clinical diagnosis of bacterial meningitis and who have signs of increased cerebrospinal fluid pressure accompanied by focal neurologic signs may need alternative neurologic evaluation in the form of brain scan, computed tomography (CT), or angiography performed immediately to exclude other neurologic disorders when lumbar puncture may be contraindicated. However, if these ancillary studies do not rapidly provide an alternative diagnosis, the lumbar puncture must be performed even in the face of increased cerebrospinal fluid pressure.

Antibiotic Therapy

Antibiotic therapy should be started as soon as the presumptive diagnosis of bacterial meningitis is made. Usually, this is before bacteriologic results are available. The initial drug regimen chosen depends on Gram's stain of the cerebrospinal fluid (CSF) sediment and the patient's associated clinical problem. Subsequent bacteriologic findings and the patient's clinical response may dictate later changes in the treatment regimen. Table 1 lists antibiotic regimens useful in treating bacterial meningitis when the results of Gram's stain (initial) and culture (usually later) are known. Table 2 lists the recommended intravenous dosage regimens for antibiotics used in bacterial meningitis in patients of all ages who have normal renal function. The package insert should be consulted for dosage modifications when renal function is impaired.

When one of the penicillins would ordinarily

TABLE 1. **Meningitis Pathogens, Antibiotic Therapy, and Duration of Treatment**

GRAM STAIN	PATHOGEN	PREFERRED ANTIBIOTIC	ANTIBIOTIC FOR PENICILLIN-ALLERGIC PATIENT	DURATION OF THERAPY
Gram-positive diplococci only (confirm as pneumococci by quellung reaction if available)	Streptococcus pneumoniae	Penicillin	Chloramphenicol	10–14 days
Gram-negative diplococci only (confirm as meningococci by quellung reaction if available)	Neisseria meningitidis	Penicillin	Chloramphenicol	7–10 days
Gram-negative coccobacilli only (confirm as Hemophilus influenzae with quellung reaction if available)	Hemophilus influenzae	Chloramphenicol*	Chloramphenicol	10–14 days
Gram-positive cocci in clumps only	Staphylococcus aureus	Oxacillin, bacitracin† (IT‡ if necessary)	Vancomycin	≥4 weeks
Gram-positive cocci in pairs (confirm as *not* being pneumococci by quellung reaction if available)	Group B streptococcus	Penicillin	—	10–14 days
Gram-positive bacilli	Listeria			
	Normal host	Penicillin or ampicillin	See text	14 days
	Immunosuppressed or relapse	Penicillin or ampicillin plus gentamicin IV (and IT* if necessary)		4 weeks
Gram-negative bacilli	Enteric bacilli			
	Unknown susceptibility	Gentamicin IV *and* IT‡	—	10–14 days after cultures are negative and fever gone
	Known to be susceptible to chloramphenicol	Chloramphenicol	—	10–14 days after cultures are negative and fever gone
	Resistant to gentamicin or likely to be so§	Amikacin IV *and* IT‡	—	10–14 days after cultures are negative and fever gone
	Pseudomonas	Carbenicillin with gentamicin IV *and* IT‡	—	10–14 days after cultures are negative and fever gone
Gram-positive cocci in clumps only	Staphylococcus epidermidis	Penicillin or oxacillin or vancomycin (depending on susceptibility)	Vancomycin	14 days after removal of shunt
Gram-positive cocci in pairs	Enterococcus	Penicillin with gentamicin IV (*and* IT‡ if necessary)	Vancomycin with gentamicin	10–14 days

*If beta-lactamase test proves negative, switch to ampicillin.
†Adjunctive therapy (optional).
‡IT, intrathecal (lumbar or ventricular). The intrathecal use of bacitracin, gentamicin, or amikacin is not listed in the manufacturer's official directive. Intrathecal (lumbar or ventricular) plus parenteral administration of aminoglycosides in the initial management of neonatal gram-negative meningitis has not proved superior to parenteral therapy alone.
§Based upon susceptibilities of bacterial flora in the hospital.

TABLE 2.   **Intravenous Dosage Regimens Used in Bacterial Meningitis***

ANTIBIOTIC	DAILY ADULT DOSAGE	DAILY PEDIATRIC DOSAGE	DAILY NEONATAL (8–30 DAYS) DOSAGE	DAILY NEONATAL (<7 DAYS) DOSAGE
Penicillin G	24 million units (8–12 doses)	300,000 units/kg (6–8 doses)	150,000 units/kg (3 doses)	100,000 units/kg (2 doses)
Ampicillin	12 grams (8–12 doses)	400 mg/kg (6–8 doses)	200 mg/kg (3 doses)	100 mg/kg (2 doses)
Chloramphenicol	4 grams (4 doses)	100 mg/kg (4 doses)	Rarely used; 50 mg/kg (3 doses)	Rarely used; 25 mg/kg (1 dose)
Oxacillin	12 grams (6 doses)	200 mg/kg (4 doses)	150 mg/kg (3 doses)	100 mg/kg (2 doses)
Gentamicin				
Intravenous	5 mg/kg (3 doses)	7.5 mg/kg (3 doses)	7.5 mg/kg (3 doses)	5 mg/kg (2 doses)
Intrathecal†	6 mg every 24 hours	4 mg every 24 hours	4 mg every 24 hours	4 mg every 24 hours
Amikacin				
Intravenous	15 mg/kg (2 doses)	15 mg/kg (2 doses)	15.0 mg/kg (2 doses)	15.0 mg/kg (2 doses)
Intrathecal†	15 mg every 24 hours	10 mg every 24 hours	10 mg every 24 hours	10 mg every 24 hours
Vancomycin	2 grams (4 doses)	40 mg/kg (4 doses)	Infants <2000 grams body weight: 100 mg/kg initial dose 400 mg/kg (4 doses) 225 mg/kg (3 doses) Infants >2000 grams body weight: 100 mg/kg initial dose 400 mg/kg (4 doses) 300 mg/kg (4 doses)	
Carbenicillin	30–40 grams (6 doses)	500 mg/kg (6 doses)		
Bacitracin (intrathecal†)	10,000 units/24 hours	10,000 units/24 hours		

*Some doses listed in this table are higher than those usually recommended. See manufacturer's official directives.

†Data on appropriate doses are very limited; CSF obtained prior to each dose should be assayed for antibiotic and bactericidal levels. Administer in 1 to 3 ml saline over 5 to 10 minutes after withdrawing equal volume of spinal fluid; periodically withdraw CSF during administration to confirm location of needle. The intrathecal use of gentamicin, amikacin, or bacitracin is not listed in the manufacturer's official directives.

be the drug of choice in a patient with a history of immediate or accelerated hypersensitivity reaction to penicillin G or one of its semisynthetic derivatives, the risk of a severe reaction must be balanced against the need for penicillin. Ordinarily, chloramphenicol is an effective alternative to penicillin G or ampicillin in the treatment of bacterial meningitis.

When the initial examination of CSF fails to provide an etiologic diagnosis, then therapy must be instituted empirically; the choice of drugs should be influenced by the history, knowledge of epidemiologic factors, age of the patient, and presence of underlying disease. The antibiotic therapy should be as specific as possible. If the initial examination of CSF is negative but the culture is positive, results may still be delayed 24 to 36 hours. For this period, the clinician is in a quandary for which there is no easy answer, but Table 3 offers guidelines for the management of these patients.

Hemophilus Meningitis

Currently, a major problem of clinicians is the patient with *Hemophilus influenzae* type b meningitis, which may be caused by a strain resistant to ampicillin. Rapid tests for beta-lactamase production are available, and they should be performed. If the initial Gram stain is positive for gram-negative coccobacilli (confirmed as Hemophilus by quellung reaction if possible) the results of the beta-lactamase test will be available within a matter of hours and the patient should be treated with chloramphenicol until the results of the test are known. Thereafter, therapy can be changed to ampicillin if the test is negative.

Pneumococcal Meningitis

Penicillin G in high dosage for 10 to 14 days is the preferred treatment; history of immediate skin rash, bronchospasm, or anaphylaxis after penicillin should prompt the use of chloramphenicol. A prompt, thorough search for an otitic, sinusal, or pulmonary focus should be undertaken to allow surgical drainage if necessary. Recurrent pneumococcal meningitis strongly suggests a cerebrospinal fluid leak or associated immunologic disorder.

Meningococcal Meningitis

Penicillin G for 7 to 10 days is optimal therapy, with alternative of chloramphenicol for patients with a history of serious hypersensitivity to penicillin. If shock or the appearance of petechiae, purpura, or hemorrhage occurs as a result of disseminated intravascular coagulation, corticosteroids or heparin, or both, have been recommended, although the use of these agents

TABLE 3. **Guide to Initial Therapy of Presumed Bacterial Meningitis Without an Identified Etiologic Agent**

CLINICAL SETTING	REGIMEN*
Otherwise healthy infant aged 0–1 month	Ampicillin and gentamicin
Otherwise healthy child aged 1 month–10 years	Chloramphenicol and ampicillin
Otherwise healthy adult	Penicillin G†
After neurosurgery or lumbar puncture:	
If patient is stable	Oxacillin‡ and gentamicin (IV and IT [lumbar])
If patient is comatose	Oxacillin‡ and gentamicin (IV and IT [ventricular])
After recent head or spinal trauma	
0–3 days post trauma	Penicillin G†
≥4 days post trauma	
If patient is stable	Oxacillin‡ and gentamicin (IV and IT [lumbar])
If patient is comatose	Oxacillin‡ and gentamicin (IV and IT [ventricular])
History of chronic CSF rhinorrhea, recurrent meningitis, or both	Penicillin G†
Immunosuppressed host	
If patient is stable	Gentamicin (IV and IT [lumbar]) and chloramphenicol
If patient is comatose	Gentamicin (IV and IT [ventricular]) and chloramphenicol
Known or believed antecedent staphylococcal infection	
If patient is stable	Oxacillin‡ and bacitracin (IT—lumbar)
If patient is comatose	Oxacillin‡ and bacitracin (IT—ventricular)
Known or believed antecedent gram-negative bacillary infection	
If patient is stable	Penicillin† and gentamicin (IV and IT [lumbar])
If patient is comatose	Penicillin† and gentamicin (IV and IT [ventricular])

*See Table 2 for recommended dosage schedule.

†If the patient has a history of severe or immediate allergic reaction to penicillins, substitute chloramphenicol.

‡If the patient has a history of severe or immediate allergic reaction to penicillins, treat initially with vancomycin and consider skin testing and possible desensitization to oxacillin as described in the text.

in this setting is disputed. Appropriate fluid replacement (including fresh frozen plasma for clotting factors if indicated) and control of the infection with antibiotics constitute the mainstay of therapy.

Staphylococcal Meningitis

Oxacillin should be used for at least a month. Chloramphenicol is the alternative when the organism is sensitive to this drug, but most strains of *Staphylococcus aureus* are currently resistant to chloramphenicol.

A particularly difficult dilemma exists when a patient likely to be allergic to penicillin develops meningitis caused by potentially or definitely chloramphenicol-resistant staphylococci. Skin testing with benzylpenicilloyl polylysine (Pre-Pen) may be helpful in assessing the risk of penicillin administration. A cautious method for administering penicillin in graduated doses to permit desensitization has been outlined (Green et al.: Ann. Intern. Med., 67:235, 1967). The applicability of benzylpenicilloyl polylysine testing and the optimal approach to desensitization before administering a penicillinase-resistant semisynthetic penicillin (oxacillin) for staphylococcal meningitis, however, have not been established; hence, for patients with potentially life-threatening penicillin allergy, infected with a suspected or definitely chloramphenicol-resistant Staphylococcus, vancomycin is indicated, but nephrotoxicity, fever, and rash occur frequently. The use of intrathecal bacitracin as adjunctive therapy may be particularly well suited to this situation, since vancomycin does not diffuse well across the blood-brain barrier. Patients should have an identifiable reason for the occurrence of staphylococcal meningitis, usually trauma, which may require surgical therapy; if the reason is endocarditis, potentially repairable brain abscesses or arterial aneurysms should be sought and, of course, antibiotic treatment should be continued 4 to 6 weeks.

Meningitis Due to Enteric Gram-Negative Bacteria

Because up to 25 per cent of enteric gram-negative organisms are resistant to chloramphenicol, initial therapy pending identification and susceptibility determination will usually consist of parenteral gentamicin in addition to intrathecal gentamicin (the use of gentamicin intrathecally is not listed in the manufacturer's official directive), administered initially by the lumbar route in adult patients whose conditions are stable. To date intrathecal (lumbar and ventricular) therapy added to intravenous aminoglycoside therapy has not proved superior to parenteral therapy alone in the management of neonatal enteric gram-negative meningitis, and initial therapy for this disease need not include intrathecal therapy in these young patients. However, if the patient (adult or neonate) worsens and there is no improvement of the CSF with repeat lumbar punctures at 24 hours (sugar is not higher than that obtained on admission, and cultures of fluid remain positive), or if in the adult there is reason to suspect impairment of spinal fluid circulation from the lumbar area, gentamicin should be given by cisternal tap or into the ventricles via an Ommaya reservoir (this use of gentamicin is not listed in the manufacturer's official directive). Prior cultures may suggest modification of this initial regimen, e.g., if a prior urinary tract isolate is resistant to gentamicin, amikacin should be substituted; or if Pseudomonas is suspected, parenteral carbenicillin should be added. Susceptibilities of the spinal fluid isolate will determine subsequent therapy; chloramphenicol should be used if susceptibility is demonstrated. Therapy should continue at least 10 to 14 days after the cultures have become negative. Delayed recovery and relapse are frequent. Surgical repair of dural defects or leaks can be considered after cultures are negative. (The high frequency of resistance to kanamycin among these bacteria in most hospitals dictates against using it in initial therapy.)

Some patients with enteric gram-negative meningitis being treated initially with chloramphenicol (organism sensitive) will clinically and bacteriologically *relapse,* with the same strain having become resistant to chloramphenicol. It is particularly important, therefore, to monitor these patients closely and to perform lumbar punctures at appropriate intervals in order to recognize this situation as quickly as possible. In these cases, therapy should be switched to gentamicin (intravenous and intrathecal). Chloramphenicol is rarely indicated in neonates and then only when the responsible organism has been demonstrated to be resistant to aminoglycosides. Recommended dosages are listed in Table 2; however, frequent monitoring of blood levels is essential in these young patients; despite apparently safe levels clinically, the risk of "gray syndrome" is still present.

Group B Streptococcal Meningitis. This infection of neonatal infants should be treated with high doses of penicillin for 10 to 14 days.

Listeria Meningitis. *Listeria monocytogenes* is often confused with diphtheroids or corynebacteria and streptococci; the distinction is important because some patients will relapse after treatment for 14 days with recommended doses of penicillin or ampicillin, perhaps because these drugs are only bacteriostatic against Listeria.

If the patient has impaired host defenses or has relapsed after initial penicillin therapy, eradication of the infection may require penicillin or ampicillin for 4 weeks with the addition of gentamicin intravenously and intrathecally for part of that period. (The use of gentamicin intrathecally is not listed in the manufacturer's official directive.) In a truly penicillin-allergic patient, tetracycline (15 mg per kg daily, in four doses intravenously) probably should be used, although spinal fluid levels may be erratic; chloramphenicol may also be effective.

Staphylococcus Epidermidis Meningitis. This infection occurs in patients with indwelling spinal fluid shunts or reservoirs, which must be removed or replaced to achieve successful treatment. Because of frequent resistance to penicillin and semisynthetic penicillins, initial therapy pending susceptibility results must consist of intravenous vancomycin or intravenous and intrathecal gentamicin. (The use of gentamicin intrathecally is not listed in the manufacturer's official directive.) Subsequent treatment, preferably with penicillin or a semisynthetic penicillin, should continue 14 days after shunt removal.

Enterococcal Meningitis. This infection, which usually occurs in patients with endocarditis or an evident genitourinary focus, requires parenteral penicillin and gentamicin (the use of gentamicin intrathecally is not listed in the manufacturer's official directive) for 10 to 14 days. Penicillin hypersensitivity requires its substitution by vancomycin; some cures have been achieved using parenteral vancomycin without gentamicin.

General Therapeutic Measures

Patient Care. Most patients should be admitted to the intensive care unit initially, with at least 2-hourly monitoring by nurses of vital signs and neurologic functions (alertness and focal weakness in face, arms, or legs). Nothing should be given by mouth until the patient is clearly alert and stable. Maintenance fluid and electrolytes should be administered and any plastic intravenous catheter changed every 2 days. Fluid intake and output should be monitored, as excess fluid intake may contribute to cerebral edema. An indwelling bladder catheter should not be used to assist output determination unless the patient is hypotensive. The possibility of seizures and potential need for respiratory support should be made clear to those caring for the patient. No sedatives, tranquilizers, or sleep medication should be administered. Antipyretics should not be given—since monitoring the temperature response to treatment is very helpful—unless the fever may result in seizures (in children), hyperthermic brain damage (greater than 104 F [40 C]), or cardiac compromise. Under these circumstances, regular doses of antipyretics will provide better control than irregular doses (PRN) and may allow observation of the residual fever.

The physician should examine the patient at least twice daily for changes in mental status, the appearance of rash or focal neurologic signs, evidence of associated disease (such as endocarditis or sinusitis), and the occurrence of complications such as hospital-acquired infections. Daily measurement of head circumference in young infants will detect the development of hydrocephalus.

Three times weekly the following laboratory studies should be performed: hematocrit, white cell count, platelet count and examination of the peripheral smear, urinalysis, serum electrolytes, and urea nitrogen or creatinine. Prothrombin time (PT), partial thromboplastin time (PTT), liver function tests, and chest radiograph should also be monitored one to three times weekly, depending upon the clinical situation. Conditions to keep in mind when reviewing these results are electrolyte imbalance from inappropriate antidiuretic hormone (ADH) (hyponatremia) or from inappropriate fluid and electrolyte administration, aminoglycoside nephrotoxicity, chloramphenicol marrow suppression, and nosocomial pneumonia or urinary infection.

Monitoring Therapy. After 24 to 36 hours of therapy, a repeat lumbar puncture with cerebrospinal fluid (CSF) examination is necessary. This procedure is second in importance only to the initial diagnostic lumbar puncture. *The Gram stain of the CSF sediment should be negative for microorganisms, and there should be no growth on the cultures.* Occasionally, the Gram stain may contain demonstrable microorganisms, but by this time testing for sensitivity and, in the case of *H. influenzae* type b, beta-lactamase production, should be completed. If the microorganism is susceptible, and the beta-lactamase assay for *H. influenzae* type b is negative, therapy may be continued. If the culture as well as the Gram stain remains positive, the possibility of parameningeal foci or subdural effusions should be excluded. If these studies prove negative, perform yet another lumbar puncture following an additional 24 hours of therapy. If there still is persistence of a positive Gram stain or culture, alternative therapy should be considered.

The CSF cell count and protein of the 24 hour lumbar puncture may be the same or greater than the initial admission values. This is predictable and should not be a cause for alarm. On the other hand, if therapy is effective, the CSF glucose level should be higher than on admission. A normal value, however, will not be achieved until the third or fourth day of effective therapy and, 1 to 2 days thereafter, cell counts and protein level will begin to fall. Repeat the lumbar puncture on the seventh day of therapy in order to follow these changes.

In neonatal and gram-negative meningitis in adults, the foregoing rapid responses do not apply. Rather, a delayed response is to be expected for all variables. Nevertheless, if the causative organism is a gram-negative enteric bacterium, and the CSF Gram stain and cultures remain positive, daily intrathecal administration of the most appropriate aminoglycoside should be considered. Persistence of gram-negative bacteria often is associated with a concomitant ventriculitis. Ventricular instillation of the drug is believed to be superior to the lumbar route in that the latter rarely will give adequate enough ventricular levels to treat an associated ventriculitis. The ultimate usefulness of this form of therapy has not yet been proved, although it is based on sound pharmacokinetic information. Adults appear to benefit most from intrathecal therapy, whereas neonates have only minimally improved survival at the cost of profound residua.

Discontinuing Therapy

With the exception of neonatal meningitis and, in older patients, meningitis caused by the "unusual organisms," treatment is continued until the patient has been afebrile for a minimum of 5 days. At this time, a repeat lumbar puncture is performed and, if the cell count is less than 30 to 50 cells, the CSF glucose level is normal, and the protein is less than 60 mg per dl (100 ml), therapy may be discontinued and the patient observed for 24 to 48 hours before discharge. If these criteria are not met, one should again evaluate for parameningeal foci. Occasionally a patient's cell count and protein level will remain elevated even with additional therapy. In these patients, if a good clinical response has been made, treatment may be discontinued and the patient observed.

Complications

Shock. Fluid therapy is initiated to reverse the systemic effects of hypotension and shock. Sufficient colloid or crystalloid is given to restore perfusion pressure and urine output. Thereafter, minimal maintenance fluids are administered (1000 ml per square meter of surface area per 24 hours) for the first 24 to 36 hours. This may decrease cerebral edema and the possibility of herniation. With continued improvement, normal maintenance fluids are given (1500 ml per square meter per 24 hours). Since antibiotics are salts and massive doses are administered, one should include the amount of Na^+ and K^+ contained in them when calculating electrolyte maintenance (ampicillin, 3.4 mEq Na^+ per gram; benzyl penicillin, 1.7 mEq Na^+ or 0.20 mEq K^+ per million units). Serum electrolyte levels and renal function should be monitored regularly.

The vast majority of patients will require only fluid therapy to maintain cardiac output and circulatory volume. However, in some patients, especially the elderly, a pressor or cardiotonic agent may be necessary. In these patients, monitoring with a central venous pressure catheter should be done in order to eliminate any hypovolemic component of hypotension. If, however, the patient is in congestive heart failure or has an element of gram-negative shock, pulmonary artery wedge pressures are more accurate, and a Swan-Ganz type of catheter may be required.

If a vasopressor is needed, use dopamine in doses beginning at 2 micrograms per kg per minute and increase incrementally. Use of levarterenol should be avoided. Levarterenol, as well as dopamine, may worsen ischemic damage of the extremities and digits in patients with meningococcemia.

Seizures. Seizures accompanying meningitis usually occur in infants; these may be "febrile" seizures and do not necessarily imply the existence of a focal intracranial process. Seizures should be treated aggressively medically: initial interruption with slow intravenous doses of diazepam (5 to 10 mg in adults and older children, 0.04 mg to 0.2 mg per kg in younger children, over 2 to 3 minutes), then suppression with phenytoin and phenobarbital parenterally. Respiratory and cardiac depression may occur, so resuscitation and ventilatory support equipment should be at hand. Until seizures are controlled, the patient should be positioned on his side or abdomen with head down to prevent aspiration. If seizures are difficult to control, persist after improvement in the meningitis, or occur in adults, specific treatable causes should be sought, such as hyponatremia from inappropriate secretion of antidiuretic hormone, brain abscesses, subdural empyema or hematomas, and other focal lesions.

Focal Neurologic Signs. Focal neurologic signs, particularly transient ones, may accompany or follow seizures occurring with meningitis and may have no specific anatomic basis. However, prominent or persistent local signs indicate the presence of a significant pathologic process other than or in addition to meningitis: (1) increased intracranial pressure may affect function of the third or sixth cranial nerves (for treatment, see above); (2) meningitis may only be one part of a process with a focal lesion, such as a brain abscess "leaking" into the CSF; endocarditis with arterial aneurysm, abscess, or embolism, subdural empyema; or malignant otitis externa; (3) venous thrombosis may complicate meningitis, causing focal signs or seizures; (4) some nonbacterial processes may mimic meningitis with focal signs, such as herpes simplex encephalitis, producing temporal lobe signs and CSF pleocytosis with red cells.

Coma. The patient should be positioned in the lateral decubitus position with his face turned downward to minimize the risk of aspiration of vomitus. The patient should be turned to the opposite side every 1 to 2 hours around the clock to prevent decubitus ulcers. An oral airway should be placed and the patient's mouth and pharynx suctioned frequently. Careful attention should be given to the adequacy of the airway and ventilation. Oxygen supplementation may be given as needed. If mechanical ventilation is required, soft cuffed tubes are desirable in that they may obviate the need for subsequent tracheostomy. Children rarely require intubation even though their respirations appear labored. In adults, a volume respirator allows more adequate control of ventilation and prevents excessive hypocapnia and its effect on the acid-base status.

The eyes should be taped shut under gauze pads to prevent corneal injury. An indwelling bladder catheter connected to closed drainage with or without bladder lavage should be inserted if urinary retention occurs. In males the tubing should run cephalad and be taped to the abdomen, not the thigh, to prevent pressure necrosis of the urethra.

The patient should be given nothing by mouth. Parenteral fluids, electrolytes, and water-soluble vitamins should be administered as needed, monitoring intake and output and blood chemistries. Giving protein hydrolysates and glucose intravenously can partially supply requirements for essential amino acids and calories. If coma is prolonged, supplement the parenteral fluids with tube feedings via nasogastric tube or gastrostomy. Nasogastric tube insertion in a comatose patient should not be permitted until an inflated, cuffed endotracheal tube is first in place.

Arterial blood gas determinations and chest x-rays should be performed daily at first to monitor for microatelectasis or gross atelectasis causing shunting and requiring intubation and assisted ventilation.

Cerebral Edema. Preventive measures include avoiding hypoxia and hyponatremia and treating coexisting hypertension.

In the event of threatened transtentorial or

tonsillar herniation or progressive rostrocaudal deterioration in neurologic status, emergency countermeasures may be tried. None is known to help in purulent meningitis:

1. Twenty per cent mannitol, 7.5 to 10 ml per kg intravenously through a filter over 30 to 60 minutes, may be tried, but it may induce hyponatremia or vascular overload, especially in the setting of renal or cardiac dysfunction.

2. Dexamethasone, 10 mg intravenously immediately and 4 mg intravenously every 6 hours, is of questionable benefit. Its use involves all the risks attending adrenocorticosteroid therapy.

3. On largely theoretic grounds, intubation and controlled ventilation on a respirator (with paralysis as necessary with succinlycholine or pancuronium bromide) to lower arterial P_{CO_2} to 25 to 35 mm Hg and maintain a high-normal arterial P_{O_2} has been suggested. This might counteract the intracerebral lactic acidosis of bacterial meningitis. This measure is potentially hazardous; its efficacy is not established.

Hyponatremia. Inappropriate antidiuretic hormone (ADH) secretion may produce hyponatremia, particularly in children. It is rarely severe and usually responds to withholding hypotonic fluids, such as drinking water and 5 per cent glucose infusions.

Severe hyponatremia (serum sodium <110 mEq per liter) with convulsions or other significant neurologic symptoms may be treated by administering a 3 per cent NaCl solution intravenously with or without concomitant furosemide and supplemental KCl. The initial dose of hypertonic saline can be calculated as follows: ml of 3 per cent NaCl = $0.58 \times (125 -$ patient's serum Na in mEq per liter) $\times$ patient's weight in kg.

Adjust further treatment by monitoring the patient's neurologic status, serum Na and K, urine output, and urinary Na and K. Restoration of serum Na concentration to 125 mEq per liter usually suffices. Overly complete or rapid correction of hyponatremia may cause vascular overload or neurologic deterioration.

Paralysis. This may be due to cortical venous thrombosis. Re-evaluate the patient for possible brain abscess or parameningeal focus in sinuses, ears, mastoids, skull, or subdural or epidural space.

Physical therapy should be employed for active and passive exercises and splinting to avoid contractures. Nursing care should be ensured to prevent decubitus ulcers.

Subdural Effusions. Subdural effusions usually are sterile but may be infected in a few patients (i.e., subdural empyema). The incidence of subdural effusions is related directly to the vigor with which they are sought, ranging from as low as 5 per cent of cases to as high as 50 per cent. Clinically significant effusions are few. If the appearance of significant subdural effusion is demonstrated by transillumination or scanning techniques, daily subdural taps should be performed. Fluid should not be aspirated but should be allowed to drip spontaneously to a maximum of 15 ml per side per day. Reaccumulation of subdural fluid beyond 2 weeks may require neurosurgical intervention, but this is rare.

Renal Failure. This may occur during the course of meningitis for a number of reasons. High doses of penicillin in the face of renal failure can cause myoclonic muscle twitching and generalized seizures; hence, with severe oliguria or serum creatinine greater than 3.0 ml per dl, the doses of penicillin and the penicillinase-resistant penicillins should be halved; the dose of carbenicillin should be reduced to 4 to 6 grams per day to prevent platelet dysfunction and bleeding. Reduction in the parenteral maintenance doses of all aminoglycosides and vancomycin must accompany any diminution in renal function, guided by the package insert recommendations. Chloramphenicol dosage need not be altered in renal failure.

Continued Fever. If unchanged after 24 to 48 hours of therapy, continued fever suggests that (1) the meningitis is not bacterial — viral, fungal and tuberculous causes should be reconsidered; (2) the bacteria are not susceptible to the antibiotic regimen chosen (very unlikely for pneumococcal or meningococcal meningitis treated with penicillin or chloramphenicol; more likely for enteric bacillary meningitis); (3) the antibiotics are not being administered properly (i.e., orally or irregularly); (4) there is localized, undrained infection, particularly in paranasal sinuses, middle ear, intracranial abscess, paramenigeal osteomyelitis of the cranium or vertebrae, or subdural abscess; the choice of CT brain scan, bone scan, sinus films, cerebral arteriogram, or direct exploration as a means of diagnosis will depend upon how quickly each can be accomplished: very prompt drainage can be lifesaving; (5) in enteric bacillary meningitis being treated by parenteral and lumbar intrathecal aminoglycosides, ventriculitis may not be reached by either route of drug administration; in this case, intraventricular aminoglycoside must be given via an indwelling Ommaya reservoir; or (6) drug-induced fever may be present, which should be the last cause to be considered, as the only definitive diagnosis is accomplished by changing antibiotics, and there are often only one or two adequate choices.

Fever Relapse. Relapse of fever after an initial response to treatment may be due to any of the aforementioned reasons or to the occurrence of nosocomial infection, most commonly urinary tract (if a catheter has been present), pulmonary (if intubation or aspiration has occurred), or thrombophlebitis (from indwelling plastic catheters).

Otitis and Mastoiditis. Otitis or mastoiditis commonly precedes meningitis. If associated with persistent fever, relapse, or brain abscess, surgical intervention is required; this ranges from simple myringotomy to mastoidectomy or operative drainage of a sinus. The last two procedures should be delayed until convalescence, unless progressive localizing signs, neurologic deterioration, or local suppuration necessitates emergency surgery.

Other Complications. Septic arthritis may occur as a complication of the bacteremic phase in any of the three major kinds of bacterial meningitis. In addition, a nonsuppurative pauciarticular arthritis occasionally occurs during convalescence from meningococcal disease and is thought to be immunologically mediated. Endocarditis and pneumonia are associated with pneumococcal disease. Pericarditis and myocarditis may result from meningococcal infection, and supervening congestive heart failure should alert the clinician to these complications. Cerebrovascular occlusion can be the result of venous sinus thrombosis or arteriolar vasculitis in bacterial meningitis of all types.

Chemoprophylaxis

Secondary cases of pneumonococcal meningitis have not been reported. The incidence of secondary cases that occur in young siblings of patients with meningitis caused by *H. influenzae* type b has been recently shown to approximate that of meningococcal disease. Although antimicrobial prophylaxis for household contacts has not been deemed necessary in the past, the high rate of secondary cases in household contacts and recent reports of epidemics of meningitis caused by *H. influenzae* type b in closed populations will in the future result in alteration of this position. However, the antimicrobial agent, dosage, and duration of prophylaxis for such individuals less than 5 years of age have not yet been defined.

The frequency and severity of coprimary and secondary cases among close contacts of patients with meningococcal disease are well known, with the highest established secondary attack rate at 5.9 per cent. The secondary case rate is inversely proportional to age (11.8 per cent risk for the group 1 to 4 years of age). This knowledge, coupled with the known effectiveness of sulfonamides in the reduction of nasopharyngeal carrier rates and the prevention of meningococcal disease caused by susceptible strains among military recruits, justifies prophylaxis. Nearly every antibiotic has been tried for chemoprophylaxis. Resistance to sulfonamides has negated their routine use, although in specific instances (infections with group Y meningococci) they still may be effective. The use of minocycline has been abandoned by most physicians because of its vestibular side effects, although, in combination with rifampin, it has been shown to reduce nasopharyngeal carrier rates by 100 per cent. Currently, rifampin (5 mg per kg in children 1 year of age, 10 mg per kg in older children, or 600 mg in adults) given every 12 hours for four doses is an acceptable agent for eradication of meningococci from the nasopharynx. Rifampin-resistant strains of meningococci occur, and undoubtedly will be isolated with increasing frequency if use of the drug increases. The efficacy of groups A and C meningococcal vaccines warrants their use for immunizing close household contacts who are at risk for exposure to either of these two serogroups. These vaccines are particularly useful for long-lasting protection, since antimicrobial prophylaxis is short-lived and does not necessarily protect against exposure to meningococci.

Current prophylactic agents will not reliably abort incipient meningococcemia; hence, close observation of household contacts is of utmost importance. With the first sign of fever, sore throat, otitis, rash, or meningitis, patients should be hospitalized and effective therapy instituted pending cultures. Casual contacts need not receive prophylaxis. Likewise, medical personnel do not normally require prophylaxis unless they have given mouth-to-mouth resuscitation or have had prolonged close contact with a patient prior to institution of therapy.

INFECTIOUS MONONUCLEOSIS

method of
JOHN H. DIRCKX, M.D.
Dayton, Ohio

Introduction

Infectious mononucleosis (IM) is an acute, communicable, lymphoproliferative disease caused by the Epstein-Barr herpesvirus and characterized by fever, lymph node enlargement, and the presence in the blood of mononuclear cells ("atypical lymphocytes") and heterophil antibodies. Specific antibodies are also formed, conferring lifelong immunity to future attacks. Onset may be abrupt or insidious. Fever occurs in virtually all cases, as well as generalized, painless enlargement of lymph nodes, of which those in the posterior cervical chains may be especially prominent. Infection in children is typically but not always mild, and heterophil antibodies may not appear. The dominant features of IM after puberty are usually lethargy and a painful, exudative tonsillopharyngitis, although either or both of these may be absent. Secondary bacterial infection often increases throat symptoms and induces painful anterior cervical lymphadenitis. Palatal petechiae, swelling of the eyelids, palpable splenomegaly, and transient subclinical disturbance of liver function are seen in 25 to 75 per cent of patients. Less common are pericarditis and myocarditis (usually benign), morbilliform or urticarial rash, jaundice, hemolysis, thrombocytopenia, neurologic involvement, and rupture of the spleen. Any of these may, on occasion, be the presenting feature. Transmission of IM is usually salivary, through kissing or sharing of food or eating utensils; rarely by transfusion of blood or fresh plasma. The incubation period is 4 to 8 weeks. Complete, spontaneous recovery in 10 to 25 days is the rule. The disease is uncommon after age 30.

General Measures

Acetylsalicylic acid or acetaminophen, with or without codeine, should be prescribed in conventional dosage for pain and fever. Hot saline gargles or irrigations relieve pharyngeal pain better than anesthetic lozenges or sprays. When dysphagia is severe, intravenous supplementation of oral fluid intake may be indicated.

The febrile or lethargic patient will usually stay in bed of his own accord. When he feels well enough to be up and around, enforced bed rest is not beneficial, and may lead to deconditioning and apparent prolongation of illness. Although a student will usually miss some classes, uncomplicated IM almost never justifies withdrawal from school or college for a whole term.

The patient should not engage in *strenuous* physical activity until he feels perfectly fit (usually 2 to 3 weeks after onset of illness). He should avoid contact sports, and other pursuits in which the spleen may be injured, for a full 4 weeks. I show him where his spleen is and instruct him to seek medical attention at once if he feels definite pain there, especially after injury to the trunk. After recovery from IM, activities such as running, weight lifting, and competitive athletics should be resumed *gradually*.

Diet may be left up to the patient, but the use of alcohol is to be discouraged. Vitamin supplements and central nervous system stimulants have no place in the treatment of IM. Effective management may include patiently and tactfully dispelling myths and misconceptions about the severity and expected duration of illness, the need for bed confinement, and the likelihood of recurrence.

Antibiotics

Specific antiviral therapy is not available. Secondary infection with beta-hemolytic streptococci is, however, a common complication of IM. Hence, the viral etiology of the primary disease should not dissuade the physician from using antibiotic therapy just as he would in any other severe pharyngitis with edema, exudate, and fever. When clinical and laboratory findings indicate infection with beta-hemolytic streptococci, the patient should receive a 10-day course of oral penicillin V or erythromycin, 250 mg every 6 hours (unless a parenteral route is indicated). On no account should ampicillin be given, since it will cause a rash in about 95 per cent of IM patients.

Adrenocortical Steroid

Steroid promptly reduces fever and relieves pharyngeal pain and swelling. Although the risks are small with short-term therapy, I use steroid in uncomplicated IM only when other measures cannot adequately control pain and fever. A proved regimen is as follows: first day, prednisone 80 mg or the equivalent, orally, in divided doses; second day, 60 mg; third day, 40 mg; fourth day, 20 mg; fifth day, 10 mg. When there is threat of airway obstruction, parenteral steroid is urgently indicated.

Treatment of Complications

Autoimmune phenomena (hemolysis, thrombocytopenia) and neurologic involvement (meningoencephalitis, seizures, polyneuritis of the Guillain-Barré type) occur infrequently but may be life threatening. Steroid therapy is indicated in these complications, in addition to obvious supportive measures.

Transient disturbance of liver function, indicated by abnormal laboratory studies and occasionally by jaundice, is a feature of *uncomplicated* IM. Persistence of jaundice for more than a week, or a total bilirubin of 8 mg per dl or more, suggests an unusually severe liver involvement, an indication for adrenocortical steroid. As in hepatitis A and B, enforced rest and dietary restrictions are of dubious value unless physical signs and blood ammonia level raise the threat of hepatic coma. This is a very rare development. In discussing liver involvement with the patient or his family, it is best to avoid the term "hepatitis," which often arouses undue anxiety.

Splenic rupture probably does not occur without at least mild trauma (though it has been reported after vigorous diagnostic palpation). A dull sense of fulness in the left upper quadrant of the abdomen is not unusual in IM, but pain there, particularly if it radiates to the shoulder or is accentuated by inspiration, suggests hemorrhage from a ruptured spleen. The patient must be closely observed. Any evidence of internal bleeding (rising pulse at rest, falling hematocrit, positive tilt test, or positive peritoneal tap) demands immediate laparotomy.

Prevention of Spread

Transmission of IM is usually by direct, intimate oral contact. Some patients continue to shed live virus for 18 to 24 months after recovery. For these reasons, isolation and other measures intended to prevent the spread of IM are probably futile. By all indications, an IM patient very seldom transmits the disease to a roommate or classmate. Neither active nor passive immunization is available.

Prognosis

Fatalities, which are very rare (<0.05 per cent), have usually been due to respiratory paralysis, splenic rupture, or secondary infection. Hepatic involvement does not culminate in cirrhosis. Complete recovery of health and strength in less than 1 month is to be expected. When illness is protracted beyond that period, another diagnosis, perhaps psychiatric, must be sought. Laboratory tests are of *no* value in estimating severity or duration of uncomplicated disease, or in monitoring convalescence. Relapse or recurrence of IM is so exceedingly rare as not to merit consideration in the patient with an unimpaired immune system.

MUMPS

method of
DAVID MINKOFF, M.D.
La Jolla, California

Mumps (paramyxovirus parotitis) is a contagious disease usually characterized by a mild febrile course accompanied by painful parotid enlargement. However, a spectrum of manifestations ranging from inapparent infection (in 30 per cent) to clinical involvement of multiple organ systems with a tropism for glandular and neuronal tissue may occur during the course of, or shortly following, the viral infection. After exposure to aerosol droplet or direct contact from the respiratory tract, an incubation period of 12 to 21 days ensues during which there is viral replication in the upper respiratory tract with spread to regional lymph nodes, followed by viremia and infection of liver, kidney, pancreas, ovaries or testicles, spleen, lung, and central nervous system. Late in the incubation period, virus may be found in blood, urine, cerebrospinal fluid (CSF), and saliva. Clinically apparent disease is a result of organ infection, inflammation, and hypersensitivity reaction to viral structural components. Infectivity has been demonstrated as much as 7 days before symptoms of parotid swelling and until 7 to 10 days after, but the actual communicable period is probably shorter.

After infection, lasting immunity develops whether or not clinical symptomatic infection was present and is reliably demonstrated by the presence of specific viral neutralizing antibody. Other tests, including the complement fixation (CF), hemagglutination inhibition (HI), and mumps skin test, have variable correlation with host immunity to mumps.

Clinical Illness

After an incubation period of 12 to 21 days, 60 to 70 per cent of patients have clinically evident infection, with the parotid most frequently involved. Bilateral involvement occurs in 75 per cent of cases. Parotitis usually presents with painful "ear ache" and swelling located anterior to the ear lobe and over the parotid gland. Pain is accentuated by chewing movement and sour foods. Over 48 hours there is rapid increase in size and displacement of the ear lobe outward and upward. Swelling of the hemilateral pharynx is common and Stenson's and Wharton's ductal orifices may show reddening and edema.

Meningoencephalitis

Mumps meningoencephalitis in children is the second most common manifestation, after parotitis, and occurs symptomatically in 10 per cent of cases. But, in greater than one half of the patients who have clinical parotitis without overt central nervous system (CNS) symptoms, a spinal tap will reveal lymphocytic pleocytosis. Atypically, polymorphonuclear leukocyte predominance and hypoglycorrhachia have been described. In 10 per cent of symptomatic cases, clinical meningitis may precede parotitis by 1 to 5 days. Clinical illness is manifested by fever, headache, and nuchal rigidity. The usual course is that of benign aseptic meningitis without sequelae.

Orchitis

Orchitis occurs in 14 to 35 per cent of postpubertal males, and in 25 per cent of these the disease is bilateral. Along with fever and lower abdominal pain, there is painful and tender testicular swelling that may reach four times normal testicular size. Epididymal inflammation accompanies orchitis in 85 per cent of cases. No true sterility or impotence has been documented as a sequela. Oophoritis in the postpubertal female may mimic acute appendicitis and should be considered in the differential diagnosis of acute abdominal pain and surgical abdomen.

Treatment

Mumps, orchitis, and oophoritis are self-limited, and treatment is aimed at analgesia. Ice packs may offer local relief. Occasionally, incision of the tunica albuginea may relieve the pain in cases in which the testicle is massively swollen. In severe cases, short-term high dose steroid may be beneficial to reduce inflammation. In the adult, a dose of dexamethasone, 2.5 mg every 6 hours for eight consecutive doses, may represent an adequate therapeutic trial. If effective, it may be continued for 5 to 7 days and tapered. Steroids do not prevent contralateral involvement. Orchitis before puberty is very rare, is usually mild, and requires only analgesia.

Pancreatitis, nephritis, arthritis, thyroiditis, myocarditis, and nerve deafness have all been reported with mumps, but are quite rare.

Vaccine

Since its introduction in 1967, more than 40 million doses of live mumps vaccine have been given in the United States. The vaccine produces a subclinical noncommunicable infection in greater than 90 per cent of persons immunized. Susceptibles develop measurable antibody which, although of lower titer than that following natural infection, correlates with protective immunity which is long lasting. Vaccine-associated side effects are rare and of little clinical significance. Live vaccine is recommended for all children after 12 months of age. It should not be given to younger infants, because persisting maternal antibody may interfere with seroconversion. Equal efficacy of seroconversion is achieved when mumps vaccine is given alone or in combination with measles and/or rubella vaccine. When combined with measles antigen, it should not be given until the child is 15 months or older to achieve a maximal rate of measles conversion. Vaccine use is contraindicated in pregnancy and in immunodeficient or immunosuppressive conditions.

PLAGUE

method of
JOHN M. BOYCE, M.D.
Jackson, Mississippi

Plague is an endemic disease of rodents caused by *Yersinia pestis*, a bipolar staining gram-negative bacillus. The disease occurs worldwide, but in the continental United States only animal populations in 15 western states have been affected. In the period 1970 through 1979, 105 human plague cases occurred in New Mexico, Arizona, California, Colorado, Oregon, Utah, Nevada, and Wyoming. *Y. pestis* is usually transmitted to man via the bite of an infected rodent flea. However, in recent years about 15 to 20 per cent of human cases in the United States occurred following direct contact with plague-infected mammals.

Bubonic plague, which accounts for about 90 per cent of cases, is characterized by fever and painful lymphadenopathy with or without overlying erythema and edema. The lymph nodes most commonly involved are inguinal or femoral, axillary, and cervical. Septicemic plague accounts for about 5 to 10 per cent of cases and causes a gram-negative septicemia without detectable lymphadenopathy. Primary pneumonic plague is a very rare form of the disease caused by direct inhalation of *Y. pestis*. Pneumonic plague may occur in persons exposed to (1) patients with bubonic or septicemic plague complicated by secondary pneumonia, (2) patients with primary pneumonic plague, or (3) *Y. pestis* cultures or animals with experimentally induced plague.

The most common complications of bubonic or septicemic plague are disseminated intravascular coagulation, meningitis, and pneumonia. The mortality rate in untreated plague is 50 to 60 per cent. In the last decade 15 per cent of cases acquired in the United States have been fatal.

Antibiotics

Antibiotic therapy should be instituted as soon as possible after appropriate diagnostic procedures (Gram stain and culture of bubo aspirate and blood cultures) have been performed. Streptomycin is the drug of choice. Adults should receive 30 mg per kg per day in divided doses given intramuscularly for 10 days. Children should be treated with 20 to 30 mg per kg per day intramuscularly in two divided doses.

Streptomycin-induced vestibular or renal toxicity is uncommon following the short courses of therapy used in treating plague. The newer aminoglycosides such as gentamicin, tobramycin, amikacin, and netilmicin are more nephrotoxic than streptomycin and have not been proved to be efficacious in treating plague. Renal function should be monitored during therapy, especially in patients with preceding vestibular, auditory, or renal dysfunction. Concomitant administration of potent diuretics (e.g., furosemide) or other nephrotoxic drugs should be avoided if possible. In mild renal failure the dose of streptomycin should be reduced to 1.5 grams per day. In severe renal failure a 1 gram loading dose should be followed by 0.5 gram intramuscularly every 3 days.

Tetracycline hydrochloride is also of proved efficacy in the treatment of plague, and may be used in patients who are allergic to streptomycin or in situations in which field conditions make the administration of intramuscular medications impractical. Adults should receive 30 to 50 mg per kg per day (maximum, 4 grams per day) orally in four divided doses for 10 days. Tetracycline therapy is contraindicated in children less than 8 years old, pregnant women, and patients with renal failure.

Chloramphenicol is preferred in patients with profound hypotension, which makes absorption of intramuscular medications unreliable, and in patients with diarrhea, which decreases the absorption of oral tetracycline. Chloramphenicol is the drug of choice for patients with plague meningitis (about 5 per cent of cases) since the drug penetrates well into the cerebrospinal fluid. Patients should be given a loading dose of 25 mg per kg intravenously, followed by 50 to 75 mg per kg per day intravenously in four divided doses. When the patient has been afebrile for several days, chloramphenicol may be given orally at a reduced dosage (30 mg per kg per day) until a total course of 10 days has been completed. The hematocrit, white blood cell count, and platelet count should be monitored during chloramphenicol therapy since reversible marrow suppression may occur. The irreversible type of bone marrow suppression associated with chloramphenicol is rare (approximately two to three cases per 100,000 patients), and should not dissuade physicians from using chloramphenicol to treat potentially fatal infections such as plague.

There is little information regarding treatment of plague in pregnant women. Administration of either streptomycin or chloramphenicol would appear to be reasonable (see manufacturers' official directives).

Sulfonamides, trimethoprim-sulfamethoxazole, and kanamycin have also been used to treat plague, but none of these drugs appear to be as safe and effective as streptomycin, tetracycline, or chloramphenicol.

Supportive Care

Volume depletion caused by fever, vomiting or diarrhea, and endotoxemia caused by Y. pestis may result in profound hypotension. Hemodynamic monitoring and administration of 0.9 or 0.45 per cent saline solutions are important adjuncts to antimicrobial therapy. If vasopressor drugs are required, dopamine is probably the drug of choice. Many patients with plague have laboratory evidence of disseminated intravascular coagulation, but clinically significant bleeding is uncommon. Heparin therapy is not indicated. There is no evidence that corticosteroids are beneficial in treating plague.

Buboes do not require incision and drainage unless they become fluctuant. Even with optimal therapy buboes take several weeks to resolve.

Prevention

All hospitalized patients with plague should be placed in strict isolation. In the absence of plague pneumonia, strict isolation may be discontinued after 48 to 72 hours of specific antimicrobial therapy. Wound precautions should be continued if a draining bubo or plague carbuncle is present. Laboratory personnel who handle specimens from patients with suspected plague should be informed so that appropriate precautions will be observed.

All strongly suspected cases of plague should be reported promptly to state health department officials, who can help identify persons in the community who may be at risk and might require observation or chemoprophylaxis. Diagnostic, therapeutic, and epidemiologic advice is also available from the Plague Branch, Center for Disease Control, Fort Collins, Colorado (303–482–0213).

A formalin-killed plague vaccine is available in the United States, but it is indicated only for persons with high risk occupations in plague-endemic areas and laboratory workers exposed to Y. pestis or animals with plague.

PSITTACOSIS
(Ornithosis)

method of
PATRICK O. TENNICAN, M.D.
Spokane, Washington

Introduction

The causative agent of psittacosis is *Chlamydia psittaci,* an obligatory intracellular pathogen which is structurally related to gram-negative bacteria. The chlamydial infection is established by the elementary body, which attaches to susceptible cells, is phagocytized, reproduces intracellularly, and then lyses the host phagocytic cells. In humans the incubation period from exposure to clinical symptoms is 7 to 14 days.

Treatment

Supportive Therapy. 1. Fever, which may persist for 1 to 3 weeks, usually can be controlled by either acetaminophen, 325 to 650 mg every 4 to 6 hours, or aspirin, 300 to 600 mg every 4 to 6 hours in the average adult.

2. If the patient has headache, myalgias, pleurodynia, or excessive cough, judicious use

of codeine, 15 to 45 mg every 4 to 6 hours, should be adequate.

3. If the patient presents with volume depletion and hypotension, intravenous fluids (initially isotonic or one half isotonic saline solution) may be required to replete the plasma volume.

Specific Antimicrobial Therapy. 1. Although many patients with a mild influenza-like illness may be treated at home, more seriously ill patients with hyperpyrexia, respiratory, cardiovascular, or central nervous system impairment, or underlying systemic diseases should be treated with bed rest in the hospital.

2. The drug of choice for adults with psittacosis is tetracycline, 500 mg orally four times a day for 10 to 14 days or, in seriously ill patients, 250 mg intravenously every 6 hours. Although fever and systemic symptoms often subside 2 to 3 days after treatment, tetracycline therapy should be continued for 7 days after defervescence to prevent relapse and retreatment.

3. In adults with renal failure, doxycycline, 100 mg twice a day for 14 days, has been used successfully.

4. Since children and pregnant women should not receive tetracycline drugs, chloramphenicol can be given orally or intravenously at 30 to 50 mg per kg of body weight per day divided in four equal portions once every 6 hours for 14 days and at least 7 days after defervescence.

Complications

1. Hyperpyrexia may require cooling blanket treatment in addition to antipyretic therapy.

2. Interstitial or lobar pneumonia caused by psittacosis may require oxygen therapy by nasal cannula or mask; rarely, severe hypoxemia demands intubation and respirator management.

3. Encephalitic symptoms are more common in severe psittacosis. Sustained delirium and stupor portend a poor prognosis, and good supportive therapy is necessary.

4. Endocarditis, myocarditis and pericarditis have all been reported in severe systemic infection. These specific etiologies should be differentiated from the fulminant syndrome associated with generalized toxemia and acute renal failure. In this setting placement of a Swan-Ganz catheter and monitoring of the pulmonary artery and arteriolar wedge pressures will facilitate optimal fluid replacement.

5. In acute renal failure caused by toxemia, acute tubular necrosis, or glomerulonephritis, volume overload, hyperkalemia, and metabolic acidosis should be prevented by careful monitoring and supportive therapy.

Prevention

The majority of human cases of psittacosis occur in the adult, predominantly male, population through occupational or avocational exposure to infected avian species. Identification and isolation of obviously infected birds would reduce transmission, but apparently healthy birds may shed chlamydiae in their cloacal contents and remain a source of human infection.

Spread from imported exotic birds could be controlled by the 30-day quarantine and chlortetracycline impregnated feed treatment required by current United States Public Health Service regulations. Although a well supervised treatment regimen with chlortetracycline in a closed facility has been shown to eradicate the chlamydial infection in psittacine birds, exposure to other infected birds and therapeutic inconsistencies have resulted in the distribution of many infected psittacines. The problem with eradicating psittacosis in turkeys is even greater because of their exposure to infected feral (wild) birds.

In the hospital setting, acutely ill patients should be placed in strict respiratory isolation until the cough has subsided and then on secretion precautions. Although person-to-person transmission of psittacosis is uncommon, hospital outbreaks in nursing personnel and other close contracts have resulted in serious illness. Doxycycline, 100 mg once a day for 10 days (not approved by the Food and Drug Administration for this indication), appears to be an effective prophylaxis for adult nonpregnant close contacts. For epidemiological investigation and control of spread, all cases of psittacosis should be reported promptly to local and state public health authorities.

Q FEVER

method of
ARVID UNDERMAN, M.D.
Los Angeles, California

Introduction

Q fever is a systemic disease caused by the zoonotic rickettsial pathogen *Coxiella burnetii*. For most individuals this illness is acute and self-limited. Rarely, it becomes chronic with endocarditis occurring 3 to 20 years after the initial infection, usually in those with antecedent valvular heart disease.

Treatment

Supportive Measures. Acute Q fever is uncommonly diagnosed outside areas of endemicity or without a strong contact history to livestock. It is commonly misdiagnosed as a "flu syndrome." Symptomatic therapy includes the following measures:

1. *Antipyretics, analgesics, and antitussives:* The complaints of severe headache, fever, and cough can be best managed by aspirin or acetaminophen in combination with codeine. Antipyretics are generally avoided except in severe pyrexia (105 F [40.5 C] or greater).

2. *Hydration and nutrition:* Diet and activity should be ad libitum. Copious fluid intake (3 to 4 liters per day) is desirable. If nausea or vomiting precludes oral intake, then parenteral maintenance fluids must be given. Urinary output and serum electrolytes should be monitored.

3. *Nursing requirements:* Isolation procedures are not required since human-to-human transmission is rare and poorly documented. Nevertheless, a private room is warranted, and the patient's secretions and fomites should be regarded as potentially infectious.

4. *Pulmonary therapy:* In severe pneumonia, supplemental oxygen should be administered to maintain oxygenation. Chest clapping, intermittent positive pressure breathing (IPPB), and postural drainage may be helpful.

Specific Therapy. Available agents are rickettsiostatic, not rickettsicidal. Tetracycline is the cornerstone of therapy. Chloramphenicol is effective but potentially toxic. Rifampin possesses powerful in vitro activity against *Coxiella burnetii*. Lincomycin and trimethoprim-sulfamethoxazole have been used in chronic Q fever but experience is limited. No other available antibiotics are effective for the treatment of Q fever.

ACUTE Q FEVER. Tetracycline administered within the first 3 days of illness has significant effect. The response is less favorable in those who are begun on therapy later. Patients with valvular heart disease are at higher risk for developing chronic Q fever and should probably always receive treatment. Oral therapy is 2 grams per day in four divided doses. If intravenous therapy is indicated, doxycycline is preferable. The dose is 100 mg given twice 12 hours apart, then 50 mg every 12 hours thereafter. Oral administration is reinstituted as soon as feasible. In renal insufficiency, doxycycline should be used: 50 mg orally every 12 hours. In pregnancy, tetracycline is contraindicated and chloramphenicol is substituted: 500 mg orally

every 6 hours, making sure to monitor for hematologic toxicity. In general, therapy is continued until the patient has been afebrile 5 to 7 days (usually a 10- to 14-day course).

CHRONIC Q FEVER. The therapy of Q fever endocarditis is difficult. Tetracycline, 2 grams daily, or doxycycline, 200 mg daily, should be given in conjunction with rifampin, 600 mg daily. (This use of rifampin is not listed in the manufacturer's official directive.) Treatment must be continued for at least 12 to 18 consecutive months. Serologic monitoring of Phase I and Phase II antibodies to *Coxiella burnetii* is mandatory during and subsequent to therapy. Treatment should be reinstituted if signs of reactivation occur. Surgical valvulectomy and replacement is indicated only if hemodynamic decompensation supervenes or if major emboli occur or seem imminent.

Prevention

The prevention of Q fever is impractical. Potentially manufacturable human and livestock vaccines are not considered cost effective. Because *Coxiella burnetii* is so widespread in nature, it is impossible to avoid, except for obvious high risk situations such as contact with the parturitional products of infected animals. Seroepidemiologic studies suggest that ingestion of raw milk may cause asymptomatic infection.

RABIES

method of
KENNETH R. WILCOX, JR., M.D.
Lansing, Michigan

One of the most vexing decisions faced by the clinician is whether or not to recommend antirabies treatment for an animal bite. On the one hand, there is the fear of almost inevitable death if rabies should occur. On the other hand is the cost, discomfort, and sometimes danger of antirabies treatment. The emotional aura surrounding this situation makes it essential that the physician make a clear decision as to the course recommended for the patient and be in a position to reassure the patient.

It is important to realize that rabies infection is a consequence of inoculation of the virus into the flesh and migration of the virus to nerves.

The infection is not generalized or extended beyond the nervous system, although the virus may migrate to other organs, such as the eye or salivary gland. Therefore, the primary principle of treatment is to prevent the invasion of the nervous system by the virus by either removing the virus or neutralizing it before it enters nerve tissue. Since the virus appears to be absorbed over time, there is a race between the time taken for the virus to find and fix in the nerve endings and the time taken to either remove the virus or neutralize it. Obviously if antibody is circulating through the body prior to the bite, the patient has a head start. However, under ordinary circumstances one is faced with attempting to stimulate the antibody system fast enough to win the race. It is important, therefore, to begin the treatment as promptly as possible after exposure.

Pre-Exposure Immunization

Before going on to the treatment of bite exposures, a few words are necessary concerning pre-exposure immunization. It is wise to give active immunization to those who run a high risk of being bitten by an animal that is likely to be or suspected of being rabid. The availablity of less reactive vaccine has made this common practice in the past few years. If tissue culture rabies vaccine, such as Human Diploid Cell Rabies Vaccine (HDCV), is available, an immunization course of three injections on days 0, 7, and either 21 or 28 provides consistently high antibody titers to vaccine recipients. An alternative if tisssue culture vaccine is not available is rabies vaccine (duck embryo). This vaccine also is given in three doses, the first two of which are given 1 month apart, and the third dose 6 to 7 months after the second dose. If desired, the immunization can be given as three injections of duck embryo vaccine at weekly intervals, with the fourth dose 3 months later. In any case, individuals having pre-exposure rabies immunization should have their rabies serum titer checked to be sure that an adequate titer has been reached. Generally, a titer of 1:16 or at least 0.5 international unit is considered adequate. This test is available through state health departments. If an adequate antibody titer is not reached, two booster doses of duck embryo vaccine on days 0 and 7 can be given, with serum again collected for testing 2 to 3 weeks later. If the antibody response is still inadequate, tissue culture vaccine should be used. Notify your local or state health department or contact the Communicable Disease Center in Atlanta, Georgia, for information concerning this vaccine if it is not available on the market. Serum titers should be checked every 2 years and a booster dose given if the titer is inadequate.

Potential Rabies Exposure

After a potential exposure to rabies the physician is faced with two types of decisions: first, was the person exposed to rabies or was he likely to be exposed to rabies; and second, if so, what treatment is necessary? The question of whether the person was exposed to rabies must be handled in two parts: first, was there an opportunity for virus to penetrate the skin and thus be in contact with nerve endings if rabies was present; and, second, was the animal demonstrated to or likely to have rabies? The following are the steps that must be considered in the decision of whether or not to recommend treatment to prevent rabies.

First, it must be determined whether or not there was actually penetration of the skin by the tooth of the animal or whether or not virus-contaminated saliva (or other potentially infectious material, such as brain tissue) from a rabid animal contaminated scratches, abrasions, open wounds, or mucous membranes. Casual contact, such as petting an animal that turned out to be rabid or being in the same room with it, does not constitute an exposure and is not an indication for rabies treatment. There have been two instances of airborne rabies in laboratories handling concentrated rabies virus and two probable instances from visiting caves infested with bats; but aside from these circumstances of intense exposure, respiratory transmission of rabies has not been described. If there was actual opportunity for the virus to penetrate the skin and come in contact with nerve endings, one must proceed to determine whether or not the animal in question was likely to be rabid.

Second, the likelihood of the animal having rabies must be determined. The first step in considering the biting animal as a possible source of rabies is to obtain identification by accurate history of exactly what animal is involved. If the animal can be positively identified, every effort should be made to capture and contain it. If the animal is captured, there is clearly an opportunity to determine whether or not it was rabid. One must be careful, of course, that the animals are identified properly, particularly in the case of children who have been bitten but who may not be completely accurate reporters.

If the animal is a domesticated dog or cat that is behaving normally, particularly when it has been not vaccinated, it is justifiable to observe the animal for the next 10 days to be certain that it remains normal. If it becomes sick, it should be examined promptly for rabies. In most parts of the country, particularly those with dog immunization laws, the spread of virus by domesticated dogs and cats is very uncommon.

If the animal is other than a dog or cat or is a dog or cat that is acting abnormally or is a stray, the animal should be examined promptly for rabies. The animal should be killed humanely in a manner that preserves the contents of the skull, and the head submitted to the state or local public health laboratory performing such examinations. Information on the details of specimen submission will be available from local veterinarians or state or local health departments. If the examination is negative, this means that the person was not exposed to rabies. The decision whether or not to submit the animal head for examination should depend upon the local circumstances of rabies. Sometimes a clear knowledge of the biting animal may help guide the decision if other information is lacking. If the biting species is almost never rabid or is not rabid in the area of the country in question, one may be justified in not considering rabies as a potential problem. For example, rabies has not been found in rodents such as squirrels, hamsters, gerbils, mice, or rats in most parts of the country. There has also never been a case of human rabies transmitted by such animals. In these instances the persons bitten may be reassured that they were not exposed to rabies on the basis of the history of the species and geographic location. On the other extreme, persons exposed to abnormally behaving wild vectors of rabies such as bats, skunks, and foxes may best be started on treatment while the animal is being sent for examination, if there is any significant delay in getting results. Thus, if the animal turns out to be rabid, treatment has been instituted early, and if it is not, the treatment can be stopped with very little risk of reaction having accrued to the patient.

If the animal cannot be located and captured, one must make a decision depending upon the circumstances of the biting animal. As indicated above, if it is a rodent in most areas, unless there are special circumstances, treatment would not be indicated. If the animal acted relatively normally, rabies is not present in the area in question, and the species is seldom or never rabid, circumstances may dictate a decision not to treat the individual. However, if the animal has been sick and in an area where the species has been known to be rabid, it is almost mandatory to initiate treatment. The fact of whether or not the animal was provoked into the bite may assist in determining whether or not the animal was acting normally but is not the sole deciding factor. In most cases it will be necessary to consult with the local or state health departments to determine what the incidence of rabies has been in the various species in the area. If the rabies status of the animal is unknown and there is a recent history of rabies in the area, it generally is desirable to complete the treatment, particularly in view of the improved nature of the treatment tools.

Postexposure Treatment

The treatment of rabies-suspected wounds consists of three parts: (1) treatment of the wound, (2) passive antibody treatment, and (3) active immunization. Persons having successful preexposure immunization should receive only wound treatment and a reduced immunization series (see below). The event necessary for rabies to occur is for virus to have access to nerves; if virus can be inactivated or removed from the wound promptly, this should be the first course of action. Washing the wound thoroughly with soap and water is the mandatory immediate step, particularly in severe bites. In some experimental circumstances this treatment alone offers substantial protection.

Since the objective of therapy is to neutralize virus before it gets to nerve cells, the use of passive antibody shortly after the bite has been shown to be of benefit. The product of choice for passive rabies treatment is rabies immune globulin, human (RIG). This product comes in either 2 ml or 10 ml vials containing 150 IU per ml. It is important that immune globulin be administered only once at the beginning of antirabies prophylaxis; further administration will inhibit antibody formation and may put the patient in greater risk of eventually contracting rabies. It should be given as soon as possible in a recommended dose of 20 units per kg or approximately 9 units per pound of body weight. If possible, up to half the dose of RIG should be thoroughly infiltrated in the area around the wound to neutralize the virus before it attacks and enters the nerve cells, and the rest should be given intramuscularly. If rabies immune globulin is not available, equine antirabies serum (ARS) may be used. It comes in vials containing approximately 1000 units per vial, and the recommended dose is 40 units per kg or approximately 18 units per pound or 1000 units per 55 pounds of body weight. The ARS is given in the same manner as RIG, but the general precautions associated with giving a horse serum product must be observed.

The third part of the treatment is to administer inactivated rabies vaccine to promote the formation of host antibody through active immunization as quickly as possible. The vaccines of choice for this purpose are those derived from tissue culture, such as the Hamster Diploid Cell Rabies Vaccine (HDCV). Such vaccines are in the process of being licensed and may be available by the time of the publication of this volume. Five 1 ml doses of tissue culture vaccine should be given intramuscularly in various appropriate sites. The first dose should be given as soon as possible after exposure at the same time the passive antibody therapy is given, and the subsequent doses on days 3, 7, 14, and 28, after the first dose. The World Health Organization currently recommends a sixth dose 90 days after the first dose. A serum specimen for rabies antibody testing should be collected on day 28 when the last dose is given or 2 to 3 weeks after the last dose. Although tissue culture vaccines have given uniformly successful results to date, it is important to measure the rabies antibodies to be sure that the individual patient did in fact respond to the vaccine. This can be arranged through the state health department.

If tissue culture rabies vaccine is not available, duck embryo vaccine (DEV) may be used. DEV is used in a 23 dose course that should be administered as 21 daily 1 ml doses, or, in the case of severe exposures, 14 1 ml doses (two per day) in the first 7 days followed by seven 1 ml daily doses. The doses should be given subcutaneously at separate sites on the abdomen and back or lateral aspect of the thighs. The site should be rotated to assure that injections are not given at the site of previous injections. Following the 21 doses, one booster should be given 10 days after the 21 doses and a second 10 days later. It is particularly important to measure the antibodies by collecting sera at the time of the second booster. If no antibody is detected, it is imperative that tissue culture vaccine be obtained and that three doses on days 0, 7, and 14 be given. In prior studies, from 10 to 20 per cent of individuals did not respond adequately to a normal course of DEV. It should be noted that one rabies vaccine can be used to complete postexposure prophylaxis begun with another vaccine. For example, if treatment must be begun with DEV and the tissue culture vaccine becomes available, the immunization may be completed with the latter. If three or less doses of DEV have been given, a normal course of tissue culture vaccine should follow; if four to seven doses of DEV have been given, four doses of tissue culture vaccine, omitting the day 3 dose, should be given; after eight or more doses of DEV, three doses of tissue culture vaccine (days 0, 7, and 14) may be given. Naturally serum should be collected for antibody testing 2 weeks after the last dose has been given.

Persons who have attained an adequate titer after pre-exposure immunization may be presumed to have antibodies and should not be given antibody preparations (e.g., RIG). The wound should be cleansed, and an abbreviated course of vaccine should be given. If tissue culture vaccine is available, two doses should be given: the first immediately and the second 3 days later. If DEV is used, five daily doses plus a booster dose 20 days after the fifth dose should be used. Serum rabies antibodies should be checked 2 to 3 weeks after the last dose with either schedule.

Live Rabies Vaccine Exposures

Occasionally veterinarians or other persons caring for animals will inadvertently prick themselves with a needle containing live rabies virus vaccine manufactured for animal use. Most such vaccines are considered innocuous for man, but some of them are not. If faced with this problem of an accidentally inoculated person, the best recourse is to obtain the exact name of the vaccine and, if it is made from live, attenuated virus, to call the state health department or the Center for Disease Control for the latest information on the vaccine in question.

Adverse Reactions and Responses

Rabies immune globulin (RIG) treatment has the same risk of reaction as any immune serum globulin (ISG) preparation. Local aching and pain are not uncommon, and low-grade fever may occur. In rare instances angioedema, nephrotic syndrome, and anaphylaxis have been reported following ISG use. It is important that the RIG not be given intravenously. Such administration is thought to be associated with most significant reactions to ISG.

Equine antirabies serum (ARS) produces serum sickness in at least 40 per cent of adult recipients and a lesser reaction rate in children. Other serious allergic reactions, such as generalized urticaria and anaphylaxis, may occur. If ARS must be used, patients should be tested for sensitivity to the product with the realization that anaphylaxis or other allergic manifestations may occur in sensitive individuals to the test dose alone.

By comparison with prior vaccines, tissue culture rabies vaccines are relatively free of significant reactions. Even so, with the human diploid cell vaccine (HDCV) one can expect about 25 per cent of persons receiving five doses to have local reactions, such as pain, erythema, and swelling or itching at the injection sites. As many as 20 per cent may have mild systemic symptoms, such as headache, nausea, abdominal pain, muscle aches, and dizziness. No serious reactions have been reported, but additional experience is needed to assess more accurately whether such reactions may occur as rare events.

Local reactions to DEV are very common.

Most patients experience pain, erythema, and induration at injection sites, and these tend to increase with subsequent injections. Systemic symptoms occur in about one third of patients, usually after five to eight doses. Anaphylactic reactions may occur in 1 per cent or less of patients, sometimes after the first dose. Rarely patients may develop abdominal pain, hematuria, or generalized urticaria. Neuroparalytic reactions occur rarely (approximately 1 per 25,000 patients) and may include encephalopathy, cranial or peripheral neuropathy, or transverse myelitis.

Management of Adverse Reactions

Persons administering rabies treatment must be prepared for serious allergic reactions even though they are rare. Epinephrine should always be readily available, and it is preferable to have oxygen available. The patient should wait for 20 minutes after each injection before leaving. Arrangements for transportation to an emergency facility must be clearly established should a serious reaction occur. If a person with suspected hypersensitivity to a treatment component must be treated, antihistamines may be given with the treatment to minimize reactions. Steroids, however, should be avoided, because they depress the antibody formation and may prevent the development of a measurable serum titer, particularly if DEV is used.

Once rabies vaccine has been started, the series should not be interrupted because of local or mild systemic reactions. Antihistamines and anti-inflammatory and antipyretic agents, such as aspirin, may be used to decrease the discomfort. Serious systemic reactions, including anaphylaxis and neuroparalytic reactions, pose a serious problem, particularly those arising early in the treatment course. It is vital to obtain a serum rabies antibody titer as quickly as possible. The chances of the patient developing rabies, the risk associated with further treatment, and the availability of alternative vaccine must be carefully weighed in making the decision as to how to proceed. If steroids are felt to be indicated because of the nature of the reaction, the problem is further complicated by the depressing effect on the rabies response. Advice on the management of such situations may be sought from the state health department or the Center for Disease Control, Atlanta, Georgia (404–329–3727 or 404–329–3644) if consultation of an experienced infectious disease expert is not readily available.

Treatment of Rabies

Once the symptoms of rabies have started, the outlook for the patient is bleak. Two persons have survived rabies, but one of those had had preexposure immunization some time prior to exposure. Such patients should be sent immediately to a medical center capable of maintaining respiration and intensive relaxant therapy. Although there is frequent concern for the safety of medical care personnel treating rabid patients, rabies has not been a practical problem, and there is a question as to whether person-to-person transmission has ever really occurred. Only those persons with definite and appropriate, exposures, such as bites or contaminated skin wounds, should be considered for rabies prophylaxis.

RAT BITE FEVER

method of
TERRY K. SATTERWHITE, M.D.
Houston, Texas

Streptobacillus moniliformis and *Spirillum minus* are the causative agents of rat bite fever. Man usually acquires the disease from a rat bite, but other animals such as cats, squirrels, and weasels may also transmit the disease. Epidemic disease has occurred from contaminated raw milk. Up to 50 per cent of rats may carry the streptobacillus in their oropharynxes, and the risk of infection following a rat bite is estimated to be 10 per cent.

These organisms produce a similar febrile illness characterized by chills, myalgias, headache, and rash. The streptobacillary form of the illness has an incubation period of less than 10 days, and a morbilliform rash that may become petechial is found in 75 per cent of patients. Arthritis is present in about half the patients.

The spirillary disease has an incubation period of more than a week, a macular rash is present in about three fourths of patients, and arthritis is unusual. Unlike *S. moniliformis,* in which the bite usually heals promptly, the infection caused by *S. minus* usually has induration with ulceration or eschar formation at the bite site.

Rat bite fever may be confused with other diseases, including viral exanthems, Rocky Mountain spotted fever, pyogenic arthritis, and acute rheumatic fever.

Therapy

Bacterial cultures should be obtained prior to antibiotic administration. The streptobacillus must be grown in media enriched with blood, serum, or ascitic fluid. Since spirilla cannot be grown in culture, a Wright or Wayson stain of blood should be done in addition to a darkfield examination to find the organisms. Other studies should be done to exclude viral, other bacterial, and rickettsial infections.

General Measures. The patient will usually require hospitalization to facilitate diagnostic tests and symptomatic therapy. Should the patient be dehydrated, intravenous therapy may be necessary, especially if vomiting is part of the clinical picture.

Antibiotics. The drug of choice for both *S. moniliformis* and *S. minus* is penicillin. The usual dose is 600,000 units of procaine penicillin intramuscularly every 12 hours for 7 days. After improvement occurs, the patient may have the penicillin changed to phenoxymethyl penicillin, 500 mg orally every 6 hours. The penicillin-allergic patient may be treated with tetracycline, 500 mg orally every 6 hours for 7 days, or streptomycin, 7.5 mg per kg intramuscularly every 12 hours for 7 days. Children should not receive tetracycline. Chloramphenicol, 50 mg per kg per day in three or four divided doses, has been used and should be considered in those patients in whom the differential diagnosis includes Rocky Mountain spotted fever and meningococcemia. Sulfonamide drugs are not used in the therapy of these infections.

Complications. Endocarditis may rarely occur with either of these organisms. High doses of penicillin G in the order of 15 to 20 million units a day should be given intravenously for 4 weeks. Sensitivity testing of the streptobacillus must be performed to guide antibiotic selection. As in other causes of endocarditis, minimal bacteriostatic and bactericidal concentrations of the antibiotic being used in therapy may be helpful. Streptobacillary abscesses and septic joints may need drainage. Should the fever be prolonged with the usual doses of penicillin and no complication found, persistent infection caused by streptobacillary L-forms should be considered and tetracycline or streptomycin substituted for penicillin.

Prevention

Prevention of rat bites by rodent control and wearing protective gloves is clearly indicated. Isolation of patients is not necessary.

Prophylaxis

Wounds of rat bites should be carefully cleansed with soap and water. Since some estimate that up to 10 per cent of those bitten may acquire the disease, oral penicillin or tetracycline administration seems reasonable.

RELAPSING FEVER
method of
ANTHONY BRYCESON, M.D.
London, England

Principles

The three principles of treatment are as follows: (1) kill the spirochete; (2) manage the complications of the disease and the reaction which follows treatment; and (3) prevent relapses.

These principles apply both to louse-borne and to tick-borne disease, but there are differences between the two diseases which may modify their practice in individual patients. Louse-borne disease is more severe: its mortality varies from 4 per cent to over 40 per cent, being greatest in epidemics. It tends to kill in the first attack. Target organs and systems, especially liver, spleen, brain, myocardium, blood vessels, and coagulation, are more severely damaged, and the crisis which characterizes the response to treatment or naturally terminates each attack is worse. Tick-borne disease shows a greater tendency to relapse, and the relapses are harder to prevent. It kills mainly during relapses because of the cumulative effects of the attacks. Neurological complications, especially during relapses, are more common. Some species of tick-borne Borrelia are resistant to penicillin.

General Management

Bed Rest. The onset and progression of relapsing fever are more rapid than in almost any other infectious disease. Few patients are able to walk; many are confused. Even in patients with apparently mild early disease the complications of myocarditis and shock that so commonly follow treatment make bed rest essential for all patients for at least 72 hours after their first dose of antibiotics. The patient should not leave hospital until the effects of the more serious complications have passed off. Because of the hepatitis the patients usually have a gradual convalescence.

Fluid and Diet. Thirst is compelling and anorexia usually total. In early disease the patient can drink all that is required. If there is vomiting, or the patient presents already dehydrated, intravenous rehydration is indicated, using 0.18 per cent saline in 4.3 per cent dextrose. Rehydration may be complicated by the presence of myocardial failure, and it is essential to monitor the jugular venous pressure and listen for signs of pulmonary edema. As the disease is short lived, diet is unimportant and intravenous feeding is not needed. There is no consistent pattern of disturbed electrolytes, and their estimation is not routinely indicated.

Nursing Care. The usual care for debilitated, febrile, or unconscious patients may be needed. In particular at the crisis, when there may be rigors (chills), extreme restlessness, delirium, convulsions, vomiting, incontinence of urine, diarrhea, and hyperpyrexia, skilled nursing is a help.

Relief of Pain. Rapid enlargement of liver and spleen may be painful, but seldom requires treatment. Splenic infarction and headache are painful and call for paracetamol (acetaminophen). 1 gram every 4 hours, which also helps control the fever. In view of the bleeding tendency a nonsalicylate analgesic is preferred. Severe pain in the left hypochondrium, followed by generalized abdominal pain, tenderness, and rigidity, indicates splenic rupture. This is managed with opiates, e.g., morphine, 15 mg every 6 hours, and blood transfusion, but if the blood pressure falls and pulse rate rises, splenectomy may be necessary.

Specific Treatment

Louse-Borne Disease. The organism is sensitive to penicillin, tetracycline, and chloramphenicol, which have replaced the arsenicals. The more rapidly the spirochetes are killed, the worse is the reaction that ensues. Oral medications are often vomited. A slow-acting injectable antibiotic is therefore indicated. The best treatment has not yet been established, but it is probably procaine penicillin, 300,000 units by intramuscular injection. This clears the blood of spirochetes in a mean time of 8 to 9 hours, as compared with 1 to 2 hours with intravenous tetracycline or 4 to 5 hours with oral tetracycline. Penicillin aluminum monostearate* may be even more safe. It clears the blood in a mean time of 17 hours after a single intramuscular injection of 600,000 units. Only one patient in ten is said to experience a clinical reaction.

As the drug-induced crisis is worse than the natural one, there is a case for delaying specific treatment in patients with severe disease who are approaching the end of their first attack. This requires judgment and courage which few physicians possess.

The relapse rate after penicillin, even if given for 3 days, is about 5 per cent. There are probably no relapses after oral tetracycline, 500 mg given once, and it is therefore recommended that oral tetracycline be given the day after peni-

---

*Not available in the United States.

cillin is given or as soon after that as the patient can tolerate it.

Tick-Borne Disease. Some strains of spirochetes are reported insensitive to penicillin, which is also ineffective in eradicating organisms dormant during remission in the central nervous system. Tetracycline is the drug of choice. The optimal dosage is not known and presumably varies with the strain of organism. The recommended dose is 250 mg orally every 6 hours until the patient is afebrile and then 500 mg every 6 hours for 7 days. Alternatively after the initial response, 2 grams can be given weekly for 4 weeks, after which time the patient is unlikely to relapse.

In patients who are vomiting, 250 mg of tetracycline can be given intravenously over a period of 5 minutes, but a severe reaction can be expected within 2 hours.

Complications of the Disease

Hemorrhage. Petechial hemorrhages that occur early in the disease result from capillary damage by spirochetes, are not serious, and do not call for treatment despite the associated thrombocytopenia.

Later severe liver damage is accompanied by prothrombin deficiency and a tendency to extensive purpura and severe epistaxis. For this reason vitamin K_1, 20 mg, is usually given by intramuscular injection. The prothrombin and partial thromboplastin times, which can be used as an index of the bleeding tendency, usually return to normal within 3 days of antibiotic treatment, and there is no evidence that this is accelerated by the administration of vitamin K_1. Severe hemorrhage is treated with blood transfusion.

Hepatic Failure. All patients with relapsing fever. have some degree of hepatitis. No special treatment is called for in most cases because the liver recovers rapidly and completely. Some patients present with signs of liver failure, namely, deep jaundice, coma, and grossly elevated serum glutamic oxaloacetic transaminase levels. The management of acute hepatic failure is detailed on pages 396 to 398.

Myocardial Failure. There is evidence of myocardial damage in about one-third of patients with relapsing fever. Signs which should be looked for as possible pointers to impending failure are hypotension, gallop rhythm, multiple ventricular ectopic beats, electrocardiographic evidence of acute right heart strain, and a prolonged QTc or PR interval. Frank cardiac failure with raised jugular venous pressure or pulmonary edema may be present when the patient is first seen, but more commonly complicates the reaction to treatment. If cardiac failure is present, the patient is supported in a sitting-up position and given digoxin, 1 mg intravenously followed by 0.5 mg orally twice daily, until failure is controlled. Diuretics should not be used, because there is usually an associated depletion of extracellular fluid volume. The patient is kept in bed until the electrocardiogram has returned to normal. Long-term treatment is not needed, because the myocardium recovers rapidly.

Disseminated Intravascular Coagulation. In a few patients thrombocytopenia, low plasma fibrinogen levels, and raised fibrin degradation products have suggested the presence of intravascular coagulation. The changes become more marked immediately after the reaction to treatment. These investigations would be indicated in a patient in coma and shock unresponsive to the measures outlined below. If suggestive, the use of heparin could be considered; 100 units per kg is given by intravenous injection, followed by 15 units per kg per hour. These doses should be halved if the platelet count is under 50,000 per cu mm. If bleeding develops or worsens, heparin is neutralized by protamine sulfate, 1.5 mg per 100 units of heparin given in the past 4 hours. There is very little experience with the use of heparin in relapsing fever.

Intercurrent Infection. In epidemics of louse-borne relapsing fever, patients have often been found to be suffering also from Salmonella infections or from typhus. Diarrhea is seldom a feature of relapsing fever and suggests a complicating intestinal infection which must be identified because it may not respond to tetracycline. Relapsing fever can unmask latent infections such as malaria or kala-azar, which should be looked for if the temperature does not return to normal within 48 hours of treatment or relapses in the face of adequate treatment.

Natural Termination by Crisis. This is managed in the same way as the reaction after treatment.

Complications of Treatment:

Jarisch-Herxheimer Reaction

Four phases are recognizable during the reaction to treatment, and must be carefully looked for. The prodromal phase is uneventful until just before the rigors, when there are sharp increases in blood pressure, heart rate, and cardiac output, and the complications listed under Nursing Care may develop. These are transient and do not usually call for medical treatment. Rigors characterize the chill phase, oxygen consumption and cardiac output increase rapidly, peripheral vasoconstriction is intense, and the temperature rises rapidly by 1 to 2 C. The danger of hyperpyrexia continues into the flush phase

which follows, when rectal temperatures may reach 41 to 43 C (106 to 110 F). There is profound peripheral and splanchnic vasodilatation, and the brachial artery mean pressure falls below 60 mm Hg and remains low for about 8 hours. Pulmonary artery pressure is increased and cardiac output remains high at about 10 liters per minute. There is a metabolic acidosis. After about 8 hours, the recovery phase begins and physiologic changes return toward normal. There is therefore a sequence of potentially lethal complications which may require treatment. It is not possible to reduce the severity of the reaction by the use of corticosteroids, even in large doses.

Hyperpyrexia. As soon as specific treatment is given, it is necessary to take the patient's temperature every 15 minutes (after tetracycline) or 30 minutes (after penicillin). If the oral temperature rises through 40 C (104 F) (40.5 C rectal, 39.5 C axillary), the patient should be sponged with tepid water and fanned vigorously until the temperature falls to 38.5 C (101.5 F). Chlorpromazine is not indicated because of its hypotensive action.

"Shock." The blood pressure and pulse rate should be taken every 30 minutes from the start of specific treatment until the recovery phase has been entered. The continuing demand to dissipate heat in the flush phase often produces a state of low blood pressure with warm extremities in a patient who is misleadingly calm. The classic state of shock with cold extremities in a restless patient is seldom seen. If the systolic pressure falls below 60 mm Hg, the foot of the bed should be raised and fluid intake by mouth strenuously encouraged. If this is inadequate to maintain the systolic pressure, fluids (e.g., 0.18 per cent saline in 4.3 per cent dextrose) are given intravenously at such a rate that the pressure is maintained. If the extremities are warm, but not if they are cold, a vasoconstrictor such as metaraminol bitartrate, 10 mg by intramuscular injection, should be tried, but its use could interfere with heat loss. If intravenous fluids are given, it is imperative to monitor the central or jugular venous pressure, preferably via a catheter passed into the right atrium of the heart. If this is not possible, the patient should be propped up at a 45 degree angle and the jugular venous pressure observed. At the same time signs of pulmonary edema (restlessness, cough, frothy sputum, and crepitations on auscultation of the lungs) should be sought; if found, treatment is given as detailed under Myocardial Failure.

Myocardial Failure. If this develops, it is managed in the manner already described.

Lactic Acidosis. This develops in the flush

phase as the result of tissue hypoxia. It is unnecessary to routinely measure blood gases, arterial
pyruvate, and lactate levels. The hypoxia and
acidosis can be prevented by allowing the patient
to breathe "100 per cent" oxygen during the
reaction. The possible benefit of this is uncertain,
but it may speed convalescence.

Cerebral Edema. This should be suspected
in any patient who becomes unconscious in the
chill phase and fails to recover consciousness
rapidly in the flush phase. The usual measures
are instituted.

Public Health Measures

Management of an Epidemic. Individual
cases are treated in the usual way. Mass control is
instituted, with the use of insecticides applied to
clothing for louse-borne disease or to huts for
tick-borne disease, and with one injection of
long-acting penicillin, such as penicillin aluminium monostearate, 1 megaunit, to the whole
population at risk.

Personal Prophylaxis. Clothes of lousy patients are disinfested by puffing with insecticide
dust, such as 5 per cent carbaryl, 0.5 per cent
malathion, or 2 per cent gamma benzene hexachloride. Most strains of lice are resistant to
DDT. In areas of endemic tick-borne disease,
clothing, especially stockings and socks, may be
impregnated with 5 per cent dimethyl phthalate
in 2 per cent oil emulsion, and insect repellents
applied to the skin. Where the disease is sporadic,
focal sites such as caves, burrows, or old campsites
should be avoided. In the Rocky Mountains summer cabins should be rodent proof and the wood-
en walls and floors treated with creosote. In the
spring bedding should be treated with insecticide.
The blood of patients may remain infective for
up to 4 days outside the body and should not be
allowed to spill on the skin even if the epithelium
is intact. Surgical gloves should be worn while
taking blood at venipuncture. If there is any risk
of a medical attendant having accidentally been
inoculated with the spirochete, he should take
tetracycline, 500 mg orally once.

RHEUMATIC FEVER

method of
JOSHUA LYNFIELD, M.D.
New York, New York

Acute rheumatic fever is a self-limited disease that has tended to be milder and shorter
than it used to be 20 years ago. To ensure optimal

therapy, therapeutic plans should be tailored to
the manifestations of the disease encountered in
the individual patient. This applies particularly to
the duration of bed rest.

Most patients with acute rheumatic fever are
hospitalized. However, home care immediately or
after a short period of hospitalization in patients
with uncomplicated acute rheumatic polyarthritis
or carditis may be very satisfactory. During the
first week of the illness, the diagnosis should be
established, the severity of the disease assessed,
treatment initiated, and the response to therapy
evaluated. Carditis usually becomes evident
within a week or, rarely, somewhat longer after
the appearance of polyarthritis. Careful records
of the pulse should be kept, especially the sleeping pulse. Tachycardia out of proportion to the
fever or after the fever has subsided, particularly
during sleep in the afebrile patient, should lead
to evaluation of the heart for a significant murmur.

Rebounds are more likely to appear in patients with severe carditis than in patients with
polyarthritis or mild carditis.

The aims of therapy include the eradication
of the causal streptococcal infection, treatment
and suppression of the acute inflammatory manifestations and cardiac complications if present,
the prevention of recurrences, and the return of
the patient to normal activities.

Aspirin is the mainstay of therapy for the
anti-inflammatory treatment of polyarthritis and
mild carditis. Steroids and aspirin are used together in the treatment of the patient with more
severe carditis. In the case of a monarticular
arthritis or when the diagnosis is in doubt, it is
wise to withhold aspirin and to use propoxyphene (Darvon) so that the development of
polyarthritis is not masked and the diagnosis does
not remain permanently in doubt. Neither aspirin nor steroids appear to reduce cardiac damage
or to shorten the duration of the illness. However, they do control fever, arthritis, and tachycardia, reduce the sedimentation rate, and result in
the disappearance of the C-reactive protein;
steroids act more rapidly than aspirin.

Eradication of Infection

It is mandatory to eradicate the streptococcal
infection even while the results of laboratory tests
are pending if the clinical picture is characteristic.
In older children and adults, 1.2 million units of
long-acting benzathine penicillin (Bicillin) should
be given intramuscularly; 600,000 units of benzathine penicillin (Bicillin) should be adequate
for children under 5 years of age. Oral penicillin
should be used if there is some good reason for
not using the intramuscular preparation. An initial dose of 800,000 units (500 mg of penicillin V

potassium) should be followed by 400,000 units four times per day for 10 days. The oral suspension, 400,000 units per 5 ml, is suitable for children and the tablets containing 400,000 units per tablet for adults. For patients allergic to penicillin, erythromycin, 250 mg four times per day, may be given for 2 weeks. Sulfonamides should not be used for eradication of the streptococcal infection because they are bacteriostatic rather than bactericidal. Continuous prophylaxis to prevent recurrences should be started immediately after the streptococcal infection has been eradicated.

Anti-Inflammatory Treatment

Polyarthritis. Aspirin is the drug of choice for rapid relief of the symptoms of arthritis and fever, which usually respond in 24 to 72 hours. A dose of 100 mg per kg of body weight is given in six divided doses per day for the first 3 days. The dose may then be reduced to 64 mg per kg of body weight for 24 hours given in four divided doses for 1 to 2 weeks. The dose is then further reduced to 32 mg per kg of body weight for 24 hours and given in divided doses for about a week, after which it is discontinued if all signs of activity remain absent. Occasionally larger doses of aspirin may be needed, especially in adults, to control the joint pains. Aspirin up to 160 mg per kg of body weight per day may be given, but the dosage should be reduced as outlined above as soon as symptoms are under control. There is no need for routine blood salicylate levels. However, they should be obtained with inadequate relief of symptoms or if toxic side effects occur such as vomiting, tinnitus, hyperpnea, or bleeding. Appropriate adjustments in the dosage should then be made. Salicylate levels of 20 to 25 mg per 100 ml are considered to be in the therapeutic range. Aspirin is best taken after meals or with milk to decrease gastric irritation.

The patient should be carefully evaluated following completion of therapy with aspirin to ensure that all evidence of activity is absent and that no significant murmur has appeared. Should mild fever or polyarthralgia recur, they will usually subside without further therapy. If arthritis recurs, therapy should be resumed and continued for 1 week after all signs of activity have disappeared. Therapy does not have to be continued until the sedimentation rate is normal.

Treatment of Patients with Mild Carditis (Without Cardiac Enlargement). Treatment is similar to the treatment of patients with polyarthritis, but the duration of therapy is generally longer. Treatment is started with 100 mg per kg of body weight of aspirin in divided doses for 1 week. If temperature drops and tachycardia subsides, the dose is reduced to 60 mg per kg per day in divided doses for about 3 weeks. Further reduction to 30 mg of aspirin per kg for 24 hours in divided doses is then continued for 1 week. The dosage is then further reduced to 0.6 gram per day for a few days, and therapy is then stopped. The patient is observed off therapy. Should the temperature and heart rate increase for more than a few days, treatment has to be reinstituted and aspirin therapy will have to be tapered more gradually.

Treatment of Patients with Carditis and Cardiac Enlargement or Congestive Heart Failure. Patients should be treated with prednisone, starting with a dose of 2 mg per kg per day in divided doses for children under 12. In the adolescent or adult, prednisone in doses of 40 or 60 mg per day is used. If this is not enough to suppress the signs of inflammatory activity, the dose must be increased according to severity. From 80 to 160 mg per day or even more may be necessary. The initial effective dose is maintained for 1 week. The dose is reduced to three quarters for 1 week, and if improvement is maintained, half the initial dose is used for 1 week. At this point, when the dose of prednisone is halved, "overlap therapy" with aspirin is introduced to minimize the incidence of rebound. Aspirin is given in a dose of 60 mg per kg per 24 hours in divided doses. At the end of 1 week, the daily dose of prednisone is reduced by 5 mg every 3 or 4 days until it is discontinued. When steroids have been discontinued, the dose of aspirin is tapered off over 2 or 3 weeks and then discontinued. If signs of activity reappear during tapering, it is advisable to go back to the previous dosage at which signs of activity were controlled and to delay further reduction for a week or two. Patients must be observed for 2 or 3 weeks after termination of therapy for reappearance of signs of activity. Laboratory or clinical rebounds are best left untreated unless severe, because treatment may result in further rebounds.

In some patients, the erythrocyte sedimentation rate may remain elevated for months after completion of treatment. This is a benign phenomenon. Steroids should be avoided in patients who have not had chickenpox if carditis occurs in the chickenpox season.

Treatment of Congestive Heart Failure

Prompt therapy is most important. Tachypnea may be the earliest manifestation of heart failure, preceding signs of systemic circulatory congestion. Diuretic therapy with furosemide (Lasix) is effective. One mg per kg of body weight is given intravenously. For adolescents and adults, 40 to 80 mg may be used. Further administration is dictated by the clinical course of the disease. Oxygen is indicated in the presence of dyspnea and cyanosis. Digitalization should be performed if tachycardia and signs of circulatory congestion persist after diuretic therapy has been tried. Care should be taken to avoid digitalis intoxication. Evaluation of the sleeping pulse is important in assessing activity. Diet should be salt restricted.

Rarely, the patient may remain in chronic congestive heart failure due to the mechanical burden or severe mitral insufficiency. Such patients may be improved by surgical therapy. Mitral valve annuloplasty is the operation of choice and has resulted in dramatic improvement in congestive heart failure.

Treatment of Complete Heart Block

Complete heart block complicated by Stokes-Adams attacks occurs very rarely and should be treated with temporary transvenous pacing.

Regulation of Physical Activity

Polyarthritis. Bed rest is necessary until joint symptoms disappear and the fever subsides. Then ambulation is begun and activities are increased. If the patient remains asymptomatic, he may be discharged from the hospital at the end of the first week to continue medications at home and return for re-evaluation at weekly intervals. School may be resumed 1 week after completion of therapy if the patient remains asymptomatic. Competitive sports and strenuous physical activities should be deferred for a further month.

Mild Carditis. The patient should be at bed rest during the acute phase, but bathroom privileges are allowed. Once the temperature has subsided and the pulse returns to normal, progressive ambulation is begun. In fact, treatment may be completed at home, and if findings of rheumatic activity remain in abeyance, the patient may return to school 2 weeks after completion of therapy. School sports may be resumed 2 to 3 months after completion of therapy.

Carditis with Cardiac Enlargement. A similar program may be followed for the patient with cardiac enlargement. However, it is advisable to wait for 1 month after conclusion of therapy before returning to school. It may be wise at first to try a half day at school prior to returning to a full-time school program. Gymnastics and strenuous activities should be avoided until 2 to 3 months after heart size has returned to normal.

The patient in congestive heart failure should remain on bed rest until signs of congestive heart failure disappear. Ambulation and return to activities should be more gradual than described above. If cardiac enlargement persists after return to school, he should be encouraged to lead as normal a life as possible but to avoid exertion entailing undue dyspnea.

A program of home instruction should be arranged with the school authorities in order to provide continuity of education and minimize the emotional trauma of the illness.

Chorea. Bed rest is necessary during the acute stage in the patient with severe chorea. However, ambulation and return to normal life are advisable as soon as possible.

Management of Chorea

Chorea is a self-limiting disease which usually subsides over a period of 2 to 3 months without residua. It is important to stress this to patient and parents in order to allay their fears. Streptococcal infection must be eradicated and continuous prophylaxis instituted. Rest, reassurance, and patience are required in the care of patients with chorea. Treatment with phenobarbital in anticonvulsant doses of about 1.5 to 3 mg per kg per day may be effective. For the excessively disturbed patient, chlorpromazine (Thorazine) may be tried, starting with doses of 25 mg three times daily and gradually increasing this to 50 mg three times daily. Therapy is continued until symptoms subside.

Erythema Marginatum

Erythema marginatum occurring with other manifestations of rheumatic fever requires no additional treatment. Antistreptococcal treatment is required if it occurs as an isolated finding.

Follow-up and Prevention of Recurrences

Recurrences of rheumatic fever can be prevented in the overwhelming majority of patients by strict adherence to an appropriate antibiotic prophylaxis program. Continuous prophylaxis must be started immediately after eradication of the streptococcal infection. The most effective protection is obtained by intramuscular injection of 1.2 million units of long-acting benzathine penicillin every 4 weeks. For children under 6 years of age, 600,000 units is adequate. For those who can be relied upon to take the drug by mouth, penicillin V potassium, 400,000 units, is also effective. However, oral prophylaxis is less reliable than repository penicillin prophylaxis. It may be used in patients with minimal or no heart disease. However, intramuscular injections of long-acting penicillin every 4 weeks are better for patients with well established heart disease and for those who have had a recurrence while on oral penicillin.

Oral sulfadiazine in a dose of 1 gram per day, and 0.5 gram per day for patients under 30 kg of body weight, may be slightly superior to oral penicillin. The patient should be carefully monitored for signs of sulfonamide toxicity or allergy, especially during the first month of therapy. Severe side effects are unusual.

For the exceptional patient who is sensitive to both penicillin and sulfonamides, oral erythromycin, 250 mg twice daily, is used. Prophylaxis for those patients with cardiac involvement should be continued indefinitely. Prophylaxis for patients who have had polyarthritis but no carditis may be discontinued at age 20, provided that there have been no recurrences of rheumatic fever in the preceding 5 years. The risk of discontinuing prophylaxis should be explained to the patient. During periods of increased risk, prophylaxis may be reinstated. In the patient who has had carditis, but in whom there is no residual heart disease and who has had no recurrences, prophylaxis should be continued indefinitely. If this is not possible, prophylaxis should be reinstated during periods of increased risk and throat cultures obtained when pharyngitis occurs so that a beta-hemolytic streptococcal infection can be appropriately treated.

Patients with chronic rheumatic heart disease must also be protected by antibiotics when exposed to risk factors which may result in bacterial endocarditis. These include dental extractions, oral surgical procedures, tonsillectomy, adenoidectomy, bronchoscopy, incision and drainage of abscess, dilatation and curettage, instrumentation of the genitourinary tract, and childbirth.

ROCKY MOUNTAIN SPOTTED FEVER

method of
JOHN F. FISHER, M.D.
Augusta, Georgia

Introduction

Rocky Mountain spotted fever (RMSF) is a potentially life-threatening febrile illness caused by a rickettsial organism, *Rickettsia rickettsii*. Although numerous tick species may harbor the organism, the disease is generally transmitted by the bite of one of three hard-shelled (ixodid) ticks capable of being efficient vectors for man: *Dermacentor variabilis* (American dog tick), *D. andersoni* (wood tick), and *Amblyomma americanum* (Lone Star tick). Approximately 5 per cent of ticks are infected. The disease occurs over a wide geographic area from Washington State to Massachusetts, but the largest number of cases are reported from the central and south Atlantic states, especially North Carolina and Virginia.

Specific Therapy

Antimicrobial Agents. Tetracycline (Achromycin) and chloramphenicol (Chloromycetin) are considered to be equally effective in arresting the multiplication of rickettsiae but must be given early in the disease for rapid defervescence, clearing of rickettsemia, and prevention of complications.

Selection of one of these agents over another has been often a matter of individual physician preference and to some extent is likely to remain so.

TETRACYCLINE. Tetracyclines can result in hepatotoxicity, particularly in patients with compromised renal function, since the drug is eliminated largely by renal excretion. Newborn infants with immature renal clearance mechanisms and pregnant women with renal disease are vulnerable to this side effect, and use of tetracycline in these patients should be avoided altogether.

A newer agent, doxycycline (Vibramycin), a derivative of chlortetracycline, has a prolonged half-life and can be given at 12-hourly intervals. Although more experience is needed, this agent would be expected to be of similar efficacy to tetracycline in RMSF. In addition, improved patient compliance might be anticipated because of the dosing interval. The lack of dependence on a renal route of excretion makes doxycycline the agent of choice if a tetracycline must be given to a patient with kidney disease.

Physicians may be reluctant to use tetracycline because of the demonstration that tetracyclines can stain deciduous or permanent teeth if a fetus is exposed in the last 2 trimesters of pregnancy or if the drugs are given to children under 12 years of age. Although this effect is most clearly related to protracted therapy with large doses, it has been reported after minimal exposure. Moreover, the disfigurement may be pronounced and result in severe emotional difficulties in affected patients. Recent techniques in cosmetic dentistry are encouraging, however. Unfortunately, safer alternative drugs for the treatment of RMSF are not available.

CHLORAMPHENICOL. The physician must weigh the potential development of untoward reactions to tetracycline with that of chloramphenicol. Chloramphenicol has a dual effect on the hematopoietic system. The first of these, a reversible dose-related bone marrow suppression, is by far the more common of the two reactions. In one report this complication developed in 2 of 20 patients who received 2 grams per day and 18 of 21 patients given 6 grams per day of the drug. In contrast, an irreversible idiosyncratic aplastic anemia with high mortality has occurred in between 1 in 25,000 and 1 in 40,000 patients receiving chloramphenicol.

CLINICAL APPLICATION. Because of the foregoing considerations, it has become the author's preference to prescribe oral tetracycline in a dose of 30 to 50 mg per kg daily in four divided doses for most patients in the early stages of RMSF if vomiting is not present and the drug is being tolerated. For the critically ill patient or in those unlikely or unable to tolerate oral therapy, intravenous chloramphenicol in a dosage of 50 to 100 mg per kg per day is preferred. Alternatively, intravenous tetracycline in a dosage of 250 mg at 6-hourly intervals in adults and 10 to 20 mg per kg per day in four divided doses in children should be sufficient. Although precise data on the duration of therapy are unavailable, treatment should probably be continued for several days after signs of toxicity such as fever, chills, anorexia, and sense of ill being have disappeared.

Supportive Care. Significant morbidity and mortality from RMSF are more likely to occur with fulminating infections or if antibiotics have been delayed. Supportive therapy is generally aimed at treating complications that are present or anticipated. These include hypotension and inadequate tissue perfusion; myocarditis and resulting congestive heart failure; renal insufficiency; the syndrome of inappropriate antidiuretic hormone secretion; thrombocytopenia, disseminated intravascular coagulation (DIC), and hemorrhage; major neurologic deficit; and nosocomial infection. Assiduous attention should therefore be given to the type and volume of intravenous fluids administered because of the danger of pulmonary edema and decreased renal perfusion. A balloon-tipped, flow-directed catheter for measuring pulmonary arterial and wedge pressures (Swan-Ganz catheter) will guide volume expansion in the critically ill hypotensive patient. Although the administration of platelets and transfusions of clotting factors are appropriate in profoundly thrombocytopenic or actively bleeding patients, the use of heparin to counteract DIC remains controversial and is not recommended.

When used as an adjunct to appropriate antibiotics, severely toxic patients with evidence of vascular collapse may benefit from large doses of corticosteroids such as 30 mg per kg of methylprednisolone (Solu-Medrol) intravenously given 6 hours apart for two to four doses. Controlled observations, however, using these agents in RMSF are lacking.

Critically ill patients with RMSF are subject to suppurative complications such as bacterial pneumonia, parotitis, otitis media, infection of infarcted skin, and infections related to indwelling vascular and bladder catheters. Repeated physical examination, urinalyses, and inspection of vascular access sites may obviate the need for additional antibiotics. If early evidence of nosocomial infection is found, major infectious complications may be avoided by the initiation of prompt treatment based on appropriate stains and cultures. Sulfonamides, however, should not be given, because treatment with these agents may aggravate RMSF.

Prevention. The most effective prophylaxis for RMSF is the avoidance of ticks. When this is impossible for occupational or other reasons, the wearing of protective clothing such as boots and a one-piece outer garment in wilderness areas is prudent. Regular inspection of the entire integument for ticks, with special attention to the scalp and intertriginous areas, is extremely important. When a tick is discovered, it is best removed by continuous gentle traction with forceps until the intact vector is removed. Forceful tugging, squeezing, or burning of the tick may actually increase the risk of disease. According to some authors, the application of petrolatum and certain organic solvents (e.g., turpentine, nail polish) to the body of the arachnid facilitates detachment of the mouthparts.

The acquisition of RMSF by canines suggests that these animals are important reservoirs of infection for man in addition to their role as carriers of the vectors. The use of tick repellents and careful inspection of dogs for ticks and cautious removal of the vectors are simple but highly effective maneuvers in preventing RMSF.

A vaccine of killed rickettsiae is available but yields a short-lived immunologic response. Thus, the efficacy of the vaccine is limited and only persons who are at risk in research laboratories or who frequent highly endemic areas should be considered for vaccination.

Prophylactic antibiotics after tick exposure are not effective.

RUBELLA

method of
HENRY H. BALFOUR, JR.
Minneapolis, Minnesota

Rubella (German measles or 3-day measles) is a mild exanthematous disease of little consequence except when acquired during pregnancy. If a pregnant woman contracts rubella, particularly during the first trimester, major congenital malformations may result. Therefore, patients with rubella must be identified and managed appropriately in order to prevent spread of infection to susceptible, pregnant women.

Management of Acquired Rubella

For uncomplicated cases of acquired rubella, specific therapy is neither available nor needed. Patients should avoid contact with pregnant women for 2 weeks. Headache, sore throat, or arthralgia may be treated symptomatically with aspirin in the usual doses. Rubella arthritis is often confused with rheumatoid arthritis and has been treated with steroids. There is no proof that steroids are useful in rubella arthritis. Management of rubella encephalitis is similar to that of other postinfectious encephalitides, involving careful attention to maintenance of blood pressure, respiration, and fluid and electrolyte balance. Although thrombocytopenic purpura usually remits spontaneously, it may be severe enough to require platelet transfusions and steroids.

Prevention of Rubella Exposures During Pregnancy

1. Women of childbearing years should have a rubella antibody test. A positive result, that is, a standard hemagglutination-inhibiting (HI) antibody titer of 8 or greater, indicates immunity. Approximately 75 per cent of postpubertal women in the United States are immune and do not require surveillance for rubella exposures during pregnancy. Those who lack immunity should be vaccinated after assurances have been obtained that they are not pregnant and will practice contraception for at least 3 months after vaccination. (See also Rubella Control, below.) If we know that a patient either has natural immunity or has been vaccinated appropriately, rubella exposures during pregnancy will not be a problem.

2. Patients suspected of having rubella should be advised to avoid contact with pregnant women for 2 weeks. This is because rubella virus can be recovered from the pharynx as long as 14 days after development of rash.

3. If patients with suspected or known rubella are admitted to the hospital, they should be placed in strict isolation. Rubella virus is spread easily by the respiratory route and is particularly dangerous in obstetrical areas where many pregnant women might be exposed.

Management of Pregnant Patients Exposed to Rubella

1. If the exposed patient is known to be immune by previous antibody tests or has been vaccinated properly, she can be reassured. Congenital rubella is extraordinarily rare in offspring of women with natural or vaccine-induced immunity.

2. If rubella immune status is not known or if the patient is known to be seronegative, order a rubella hemagglutination-inhibiting (HI) titer as soon as possible after exposure. If serum is collected within a week of the exposure and the HI titer is 8 or greater, I would consider the patient immune because of past infection and would reassure her that the present exposure was inconsequential. If she was exposed more than a week before testing and has a titer of 8 or more, a second sample must be collected 2 to 4 weeks later in order to determine if the titer is rising. A fourfold or greater boost in titer, if the specimens are tested simultaneously, would indicate recent infection. An unchanging titer is consistent with an infection prior to pregnancy. If a pregnant woman has a titer less than 8, regardless of when the exposure occurred she should be retested 2 to 4 weeks later. If the titer remains negative, I would consider that the exposure did not result in transmission of rubella. Should a fourfold or greater rise in antibody titer be found, the patient has laboratory evidence of acute rubella. The probabilities of fetal malformation are approximately 50 per cent if rubella infection occurs during the first month of pregnancy, 20 per cent during the second, 10 per cent during the third, and 5 per cent during the fourth. Even after the fourth month of pregnancy there is a possibility of deafness or psychomotor retardation resulting from maternal rubella. If acute rubella is documented during pregnancy, the probabilities of congenital defects should be explained and consideration given to therapeutic abortion.

3. At the time antibody tests are performed on the mother, it is useful to do virologic studies on the index case as well to determine if rubella is present in your community. Except during recognized rubella epidemics, most rashes clinically diagnosed as rubella are due to adenoviruses, enteroviruses, or erythema infectiosum. Never-

theless, the consequence of congenital rubella is so grave that these exanthems should be considered rubella until proved otherwise.

4. The efficacy of immune serum globulin after exposure to rubella remains controversial. The recommended dose is 20 ml intramuscularly and is most likely to be effective when given as soon as possible after the exposure. I recommend it only for women who categorically would refuse therapeutic abortion. If immune serum globulin is given, it is important to order rubella antibody titers as outlined above to detect subclinical rubella. Documentation of acute rubella despite injection of immune globulin might prompt the parents to reconsider therapeutic abortion.

Management of Congenital Rubella

Congenital rubella should be suspected in infants who are small for gestational age, since rubella virus causes cells to divide less frequently than normal, giving rise to small babies with small organs. Principal targets are the eye, ear, heart, and central nervous system, but virtually every organ and tissue may be involved. Long bones, especially the distal femur and proximal tibia, may have damage to the metaphyses, resulting in a "chewed celery stalk" appearance on x-ray. The clinical impression of congenital rubella must be confirmed by one of the following laboratory criteria:

1. Fourfold or greater rise in maternal rubella antibody titer during pregnancy. For the rise to be valid, paired serum specimens must be tested simultaneously.

2. Presence of rubella-specific IgM antibody in infant's serum at birth.

3. Isolation of rubella virus from infant (virus can be recovered from throat, urine, cerebrospinal fluid, and stool).

4. Rubella antibody titer that remains elevated in infant's serum for at least 6 months after birth.

Once the diagnosis has been established, management requires a team approach, involving (1) careful ophthalmologic examination with attention to recognition of congenital glaucoma and cataracts; (2) cardiac evaluation with corrective surgery for symptomatic defects; (3) appropriate hearing examination, with follow-up studies necessary for 2 to 4 years since hearing loss can be ongoing; and (4) neurologic follow-up for at least 4 years to pinpoint deficits and help the parents to deal with these at the preschool and elementary school levels. Infected infants continue to shed virus for months or even years after birth and therefore represent a risk to susceptible pregnant women. Thus, hospitalized infants suspected of congenital rubella should be placed in strict isolation until they are shown not to be excreting virus.

If a mother has delivered a child with congenital rubella, she can be assured that subsequent infants born to her will not have congenital rubella. Immunity conferred by rubella is long lasting, and no woman has given birth to babies successively infected with rubella virus.

Rubella Control

Control of rubella is attainable by the appropriate use of live, attenuated rubella vaccines. The only vaccine now distributed in the United States is the RA27/3 strain. RA27/3 rubella vaccine appears excellent since it elicits an immune response that closely resembles natural rubella. The rubella vaccine program in the United States has aimed at achievement of herd immunity to protect susceptible pregnant women. This is implemented by immunizing children during routine "well baby" visits. Although vaccination of young children is a reasonable approach to rubella control, children should not be vaccinated before the age of 15 months. Optimal active rubella immunity may not develop if children are immunized when younger than 15 months because of interference by passively transferred maternal antibody.

In addition to vaccinating toddlers when 15 months or older, I recommend obtaining a rubella HI titer on all preadolescent girls and women of childbearing age whether or not they have been vaccinated. Those found to lack antibody should be offered rubella vaccine after informed consent has been obtained stating that the vaccinee is not pregnant and will use contraception for at least 3 months. Since rubella vaccine strains have been shown to cross the placenta, vaccination of a pregnant woman or one who becomes pregnant within 3 months is a risk to the fetus, and therapeutic abortion should be considered in such instances. No term infant is known to have been damaged by rubella vaccine, but the potential exists.

If rubella antibody tests are not readily available, I would recommend revaccinating all preadolescent girls and women because rubella antibody titers 4 years after primary immunization have been found to be low or absent in 10 to 30 per cent of vaccinees. These vaccinees appear to have some degree of protection despite low antibody titers, but I would rather be safe than sorry and would reimmunize them.

Women who are pregnant and lack rubella immunity should be offered rubella vaccination after delivery. The immediate postpartum period is an excellent time for vaccination because the probability of conception is relatively low at that time.

SALMONELLOSIS (OTHER THAN TYPHOID FEVER)

method of
RICHARD SNEPAR, M.D.,
and DONALD KAYE, M.D.
Philadelphia, Pennsylvania

The genus Salmonella consists of three species: *S. typhi* (one serotype), *S. choleraesuis* (one serotype), and *S. enteritidis* (over 1700 serotypes). This article will cover infection with the latter two species. The Kauffmann-White schema divides the salmonellae into groups according to their somatic (O) antigens, the majority of which fall into groups A through E. Each group consists of various serotypes on the basis of both somatic and flagellar (H) antigens.

The nontyphoidal salmonellae are widespread among animals and infect man via the oral route. Poultry, eggs, meat, dairy products, and pets are important sources of infection. Person-to-person spread, although less common, does occur, primarily in nurseries and institutions.

While infections from *Salmonella typhi* are declining in incidence in the United States, the incidence of nontyphoidal salmonellosis has been constant or slightly increasing. Infections follow a seasonal pattern, peaking from July to November. More than 50 per cent of the cases are in children under 5 years of age, and the attack rates are highest in the first year of life.

The development of disease after contact with salmonella depends on the virulence of the organism (e.g., *S. anatum* usually causes asymptomatic disease, while *S. choleraesuis* generally causes bacteremia), the number of organisms ingested, and the status of the host (e.g., sickle cell disease, lymphoma, prior gastric surgery).

Infection with salmonella results in four clinical syndromes: acute gastroenteritis, bacteremia (with or without focal infection), enteric fever, and the carrier state (including asymptomatic infection, the convalescent carrier, and the chronic carrier). Before discussing these syndromes and their specific management, some general points regarding antibiotic therapy for salmonella infection should be stressed: (1) There is incomplete correlation between in vitro and in vivo effectiveness of antibiotics. A number of antibiotics inhibit growth in vitro but are ineffective in vivo. (2) The antibiotics useful in salmonellosis are chloramphenicol, ampicillin (and its congener amoxicillin), and trimethoprim-sulfamethoxazole. (3) While chloramphenicol resistance has been rare, ampicillin resistance (mediated by R factors) has been common (especially in isolates of *S. typhimurium*).

Acute Gastroenteritis

This is the most common clinical expression of salmonellosis in humans. It occurs 8 to 48 hours after the ingestion of contaminated food. Initially there is nausea and vomiting, followed by abdominal cramps and diarrhea. Diarrhea is generally watery, ranging from a few to over 20 bowel movements per day. In rare cases it can be cholera- or dysentery-like. Temperature elevation occurs in most patients and may be very high. Diarrhea and fever usually subside in 2 to 7 days. Bacteremia is uncommon. Gastroenteritis occurs with increased frequency in patients with achlorhydria or previous gastrectomy because of delivery of a larger viable inoculum into the small intestine.

Management. In mild cases, no specific therapy is indicated. In cases in which symptoms are more pronounced, the following measures are observed: (1) The patient should be at bed rest with weight, blood pressure, and intake and output carefully monitored. (2) Attention must be directed toward adequate replacement of fluid and electrolyte losses. If the patient can take fluids by mouth, broths, juices, and carbonated beverages are usually sufficient. If vomiting and diarrhea are severe, intravenous replacement with 5 per cent glucose in water and isotonic saline supplemented with potassium chloride may be necessary. Careful monitoring of serum electrolytes, blood urea nitrogen (BUN) and creatinine, and the parameters mentioned above should be maintained. (3) Nausea and vomiting in adults can be controlled with prochlorperazine (Compazine), 5 to 10 mg orally or intramuscularly every 6 hours or 25 mg rectally every 12 hours. Trimethobenzamide hydrochloride (Tigan), 200 mg orally, intramuscularly, or rectally four times daily, is an alternative. (4) Antidiarrheal and antiperistaltic drugs such as tincture of opium or diphenoxylate hydrochloride with atropine (Lomotil) may delay clearing of organisms from the stool and should be avoided if possible. However, for relief of severe cramping use of the aforementioned agents is reasonable. (5) Antibiotic therapy is not recommended in uncomplicated gastroenteritis. Antibiotics have been shown to prolong excretion of salmonella in the stool and to be ineffective in reducing the severity or duration of symptoms. Antibiotics should be considered in neonates and elderly patients because of the higher rate of bacteremia. Treatment might also be considered in patients with high fever who have underlying leukemia or lymphoma, sickle cell anemia, or other hemolytic disorders, or who are taking steroids or have other serious illnesses. Antibiotic therapy would be similar to that discussed below.

Bacteremia and Focal Infection

The syndrome of salmonella bacteremia is one of intermittent prolonged fever and chills, associated with sustained bacteremia. Metastatic foci are common, most often in bone. Gastrointestinal manifestations are usually absent. *Salmonella typhimurium* accounts for the majority of cases of bacteremia; however, *S. choleraesuis* is the serotype most likely to result in bacteremia or focal infection. The bacteremia syndrome is associated with such underlying diseases as neoplasia, lymphoma, leukemia, and sickle cell disease or administration of corticosteroids. Metastatic localized infection may result in osteomyelitis (sickle cell disease), arthritis, pneumonia, empyema, pyelonephritis, meningitis (infants), endocarditis, and endarteritis, as well as abscesses at any site.

Management. (1) The nature of the bacteremia should be investigated with multiple blood cultures at intervals. Continuous bacteremia may suggest an intravascular focus. (2) Evidence of metastatic spread should be sought with x-rays, radionuclide scans, and ultrasound. If continuous bacteremia is present, echocardiography and, if negative, angiography (especially of the abdominal aorta) should be considered to localize an intravascular site of infection. (3) Abscesses should be surgically drained, and intravascular foci may have to be surgically resected. (4) Therapy should be initiated with chloramphenicol intravenously at a daily dose of 50 mg per kg per day in adults and children in divided doses every 6 hours. Children under 1 month of age should receive no more than 25 mg per kg per day to avoid the gray syndrome. Chloramphenicol should not be used intramuscularly because of poor absorption. Hematologic parameters should be monitored closely in all patients receiving chloramphenicol for evidence of development of bone marrow toxicity. If the organism is found to be susceptible, ampicillin at a dose of 150 to 200 mg per kg per day in adults (200 to 400 mg per kg per day in children) in divided doses every 4 hours intravenously should be substituted. Duration of therapy for uncomplicated bacteremia is 14 days, but localized sites such as osteomyelitis and endocarditis require 4 to 6 weeks of therapy or longer.

Trimethoprim-sulfamethoxazole (80 mg of trimethoprim and 400 mg of sulfamethoxazole per tablet), 4 to 8 tablets, two to three times per day orally, has been shown to be effective in bacteremic salmonella infections. It is not recommended as primary therapy but may be considered if the aforementioned antibiotics cannot be used or organisms resistant to chloramphenicol and ampicillin are isolated. (This use of trimethoprim-sulfamethoxazole is not listed in the manufacturer's official directive.)

Enteric Fever

Enteric fever is the typhoid fever syndrome caused by *S. typhi* or by salmonella other than *S. typhi.* It is characterized by prolonged fever, sustained salmonella bacteremia, splenomegaly, rose spots, and leukopenia. Species other than *S. typhi* most commonly responsible for this syndrome are *S. paratyphi A, S. paratyphi B (S. schottmülleri),* and *S. paratyphi C (S hirschfeldii).* However, any salmonella can cause the enteric fever syndrome. Although nontyphoidal enteric fever may be clinically indistinguishable from typhoid fever, it is usually milder with fewer complications, and is of shorter duration.

Management. (1)Supportive measures as described for gastroenteritis should be employed. (2) Chloramphenicol is the antibiotic of choice and initially should be given intravenously and continued for at least 14 days. Ampicillin is also effective if the organism is found to be sensitive. Antibiotic dosages are those described above for bacteremia. Trimethoprim-sulfamethoxazole should be used for the same indications as listed above. Defervescence usually requires 3 to 5 days, and relapse may occur when antibiotics are stopped. Relapse is related to persistence of salmonella in tissue and not antibiotic resistance. Treatment of a relapse is the same as for initial therapy. (3) Although controversial, a 3-day course of corticosteroid therapy may be useful in the occasional patient with profound systemic toxicity.

Carrier State

All patients with salmonella gastroenteritis and enteric fever excrete salmonella in the feces for variable periods of time. Following gastroenteritis, approximately 90 per cent of patients have recoverable organisms at 2 weeks, 40 per cent at 4 weeks, and 5 per cent at 20 weeks. Children less than 1 year of age tend to excrete salmonella for more prolonged periods of time. A "chronic carrier" is an individual who excretes organisms in the stool for more than 1 year after the initial infection. Following infection with *Salmonella typhi,* 3 per cent of patients become chronic fecal carriers. With nontyphoidal salmonella the chronic carrier state is less than 1 per cent.

Management. (1) Generally no specific therapy is recommended other than instructing the patient in good personal hygiene. The patient is considered cured when three successive monthly cultures are negative. The patient should not work as a food handler and should be restricted from working in hospital nurseries and obstetrical services. (2) If restrictions from nursing or food handling cause undue hardship to the patient, eradication of the carrier state can be attempted with ampicillin, 1.5 grams, plus 0.5 gram of probenecid four times daily orally for 6 weeks. However, there is no proof of efficacy, and cure is unlikely in patients with cholelithiasis.

TETANUS

method of
WESLEY FURSTE, M.D.,
and GEORGE W. PAULSON, M.D.
Columbus, Ohio

PROPHYLAXIS

Adequate tetanus prophylaxis is based on (1) proper use of tetanus toxoid, (2) immediate surgical care of all wounds of violence, (3) proper employment of antitoxin (heterologous equine antitoxin) and more recently tetanus immune globulin (human), and (4) proper use of emergency medical identification devices. *These principles of prophylaxis — as outlined in the following guide — can prevent tetanus.*

General Principles

1. Triple responsibility: Physicians, public health officials, and patients are responsible for the prevention of tetanus.

2. Professional liability problems: To protect the medicolegal rights of the patient, of nonphysician personnel involved in the care of the patient, and of all physicians associated with the care of the patient, record the history and complete care of the patient, including all skin or other sensitivity tests performed and all injections on permanent and available records.

3. Basic immunization and nonwound booster immunization: Basic immunization for tetanus with adsorbed tetanus toxoid requires three injections, with the first two administered 4 to 6 weeks apart and the third given 6 to 12 months after the second injection. A booster of adsorbed tetanus toxoid is indicated 10 years after the third injection or 10 years after an intervening booster.

All individuals, including pregnant women, should have basic immunization and booster injections when indicated. Neonatal tetanus is preventable by active immunization of the mother before or during the first 6 months of pregnancy. This immunization can be achieved by two intramuscular injections of adsorbed toxoid given 6 weeks apart. In the event that a neonate is borne

by a nonimmunized mother without adequate obstetrical care, the infant should receive 250 units or more of tetanus immune globulin (human) (TIG H). Active and passive immunization for the mother should also be initiated.

4. Individualization of wounded patients: The attending physician must determine for each patient what is required for adequate prophylaxis against tetanus.

5. Surgical wound care: Regardless of the status of the active immunization of the patient, for all wounds render immediate optimal surgical care, including removal of all devitalized tissue and foreign bodies.

6. Toxoid and antitoxin at the time of injury: Whether or not to provide active immunization with tetanus toxoid and passive immunization with TIG(H) must be decided individually for each patient. The characteristics of the wound, conditions under which it was incurred, its treatment, its age, and the previous active immunization status of the patient must be considered. *The patient's stating that he has had a significant reaction to tetanus toxoid may be a contraindication to the injection of toxoid, and requires investigation.*

7. Emergency medical identification devices: To every wounded patient, give a written record of the immunization provided, instructing him to carry the record at all times, and, if indicated, to complete active immunization. For precise tetanus prophylaxis, an accurate and immediately available history regarding previous active immunization against tetanus is required or rapid laboratory titration to determine the patient's serum tetanus antitoxin level is necessary.

8. Antibiotics: The effectiveness of antibiotics for prophylaxis of tetanus remains unproved.

Specific Measures for Patients with Wounds

1. Wounded persons who have received no previous injections or whose immunization history is unknown are considered for the following: (a) For non-tetanus-prone wounds (clean and/or minor), give 0.5 ml of toxoid* (initial immunizing dose) and instructions for completion of the basic

---

*With different preparations of adsorbed toxoid, the volume of a single booster dose should be modified as stated on the package label.

The Public Health Service Advisory Committee on Immunization Practices in 1977 recommended DTP (diphtheria and tetanus toxoids combined with pertussis vaccine) for basic immunization in infants and children from 2 months through the sixth year of age, and Td (combined tetanus and diphtheria toxoids: adult type) for basic immunization of those over 6 years of age. For the latter group, Td toxoid was recommended for routine or wound boosters; but if there is any reason to suspect hypersensitivity to the diphtheria component, tetanus toxoid (T) should be substituted for Td.

series. (b) For tetanus-prone wounds (severe, neglected, or more than 24 hours old), give 0.5 ml of toxoid* (initial immunizing dose), instructions for completion of the basic series, and 250 or more units of TIG(H).†

2. Wounded persons who have been given an indeterminate number of tetanus toxoid injections are considered for the following: (a) For non-tetanus-prone wounds, give a booster dose of toxoid* unless the patient has received his last dose during the previous 5 years. (b) For tetanus-prone wounds, give a booster dose of toxoid* unless the patient has received his last dose within the previous year. (c) For tetanus-prone wounds, give a booster dose of toxoid* and 250 or more units of TIG(H)† when the patient has received his last dose of toxoid more than 10 years previously.

3. Wounded persons who have received at least *four unequivocally documented doses of tetanus toxoid* with the last given more than 10 years previously are considered for the following: (a) For non-tetanus-prone wounds, give 0.5 ml of toxoid.* (b) For tetanus-prone wounds, give 0.5 ml of toxoid* and possibly 250 or more units of TIG(H)†

4. Wounded persons who have received at least *four unequivocally documented doses of tetanus toxoid* with the last given within 10 years are considered for the following: (a) For non-tetanus-prone wounds, no booster dose is indicated. (b) For tetanus-prone wounds, give 0.5 ml of toxoid* unless the patient has received a booster dose within the previous 5 years.

TREATMENT

At the time of the Civil War and immediately thereafter, little was known about the prevention and treatment of tetanus. By our standards, wound care at its best was poor, consisting primarily of analgesics, attempts at hemostasis, nonspecific ointments, and amputation. During the Civil War, in 280,040 admissions for wounds and

injuries, there were 505 cases of tetanus, with 451 deaths (89.3 per cent). In the 1863 *Manual of Military Surgery for the Army of the Confederate States* appeared this statement: "To enumerate the means used for the relief of tetanus would require a volume; to record those entitled to confidence does not require a line."

In contrast to such a statement of 1863, it may be stated now that the treatment of tetanus is complex but successful. It requires devoted and exhausting attention by all echelons of physicians and hospital personnel. It is truly a team effort that can best be carried out in a tetanus center in which many cases of tetanus have been treated successfully or in the intensive care unit of a large general hospital where all the modern medical and surgical advances can be directed toward overcoming a terrible disease associated with horrible pain for the unfortunate patient.

The confident evaluation of various forms of therapy is particularly difficult for tetanus. The following parable indicates how the relationship between a cause and an effect may be incorrectly interpreted:

FIDO AND THE SUNRISE

One morning Fido awoke earlier than usually. For unknown reasons, he barked. The sun rose. Then Fido discovered that each morning after he barked, the sun appeared. He had discovered, he thought, a cause and effect.

One morning Fido overslept; and when he awakened, the sun was in the sky.

Fido, to his chagrin, learned that his barking did not cause the sun to appear in the sky.

If methods of therapy are to be evaluated correctly, there should be developed a uniform system of grading of tetanus. If such a system is not developed, cases of mild tetanus with a naturally low mortality rate may be wrongly compared with cases of severe tetanus which would be expected to have a high mortality rate.

The therapeutic recommendations that follow are those that have been generally accepted by those particularly interested in the management of tetanus. They have been discussed in detail at the five International Conferences on Tetanus in India in 1963, Switzerland in 1966, Brazil in 1970, Sénégal in 1975, and Sweden in 1978. Their initiation is based on the establishment of a diagnosis of tetanus. Obviously, they constitute only a guide that is to be altered according to the experience and personal judgment of the attending physician.

Some of the methods of treatment can have adverse as well as beneficial effects. Hence, when any treatment is initiated, a quotation of Hippocrates should be remembered: "Primum non nocere." His advice, liberally translated, is: "As to

---

*With different preparations of adsorbed toxoid, the volume of a single booster dose should be modified as stated on the package label.

The Public Health Service Advisory Committee on Immunization Practices in 1977 recommended DTP (diphtheria and tetanus toxoids combined with pertussis vaccine) for basic immunization in infants and children from 2 months through the sixth year of age, and Td (combined tetanus and diphtheria toxoids: adult type) for basic immunization of those over 6 years of age. For the latter group, Td toxoid was recommended for routine or wound boosters; but if there is any reason to suspect hypersensitivity to the diphtheria component, tetanus toxoid (T) should be substituted for Td.

†Use different syringes, needles, and sites of injection for toxoid and TIG(H).

diseases, make a habit of two things — to help, or at least to do no harm."

The following recommendations for management are given in order of chronologic priority.

Complete History and Physical Examination

Obtain a complete medical and surgical history of the patient, and perform a complete physical examination. In particular, inquire about the date of injury, the circumstances of injury, the depth of the injury below the skin, and allergies. Such information forms a baseline for the recognition of such complications as atelectasis, pneumonia, traumatic glossitis, fractures of the vertebrae, decubital ulcers, and fecal impaction.

Antitoxin

Intramuscular Injection. As soon as the diagnosis of tetanus is made, give deeply intramuscularly 500 to 10,000 units of tetanus immune globulin (human).

In a report to the Fourth International Conference on Tetanus, Blake et al. summarized a study of the influence of tetanus antitoxin on the outcome of human tetanus. For this study, they analyzed 545 cases, using data collected by the United States Public Health Service Center for Disease Control, in cooperation with state epidemiologists, from 1965 to 1971. Patients treated with antitoxin had a significantly lower case-fatality ratio than untreated patients, and the effect of serotherapy was not modified significantly by confounding effects such as age, race, sex, immunization history, and incubation period. Antitoxin of equine origin and TIG(H) were equally effective. Their data on the effect of different doses of TIG(H) suggest that 500 units may be as effective as the dose of 3000 to 10,000 units that was being recommended in 1975.

Since TIG(H) causes no hypersensitivity phenomena when injected intramuscularly and since it appears to be at least equal in efficacy to equine antitoxin, TIG(H) should be given instead of the heterologous tetanus antitoxin (equine).

TIG(H) is to be given intramuscularly in the proximal portion of the extremity in which is the wound responsible for tetanus, or in the gluteal muscles when the wound is not in an extremity or when the causative wound cannot be found.

In the United States, where there are now adequate supplies of TIG(H), there are no indications for the administration of heterologous tetanus antitoxin (equine), which has been responsible for serum sickness, myocardial infarction, peripheral neuritis, and anaphylactic shock with death. Moreover, in the human being, the life span of the heterologous antitoxin cannot be predicted with certainty.

In countries in which TIG(H) is not available, heterologous tetanus antitoxin (equine) is still being used. A dosage of 10,000 units is considered to be adequate. No significant lowering of the mortality rate has been found for doses ranging from 5000 units to 60,000 units of equine antitoxin in adults. Fifteen hundred units of heterologous tetanus antitoxin (equine) appears to be as effective as a larger dose in neonates.

Intrathecal Injection of a Mixture of Antitoxin and Prednisolone. Consider the intrathecal injection of a mixture of antitoxin and prednisolone. For a number of years, intrathecal serotherapy of tetanus has not been performed. There has been a fear that such therapy can contribute to a fatal outcome by causing excitement, serum meningitis, and possibly cerebral or medullary edema. At the 1970, 1975, and 1978 International Conferences on Tetanus, Ildirim of Turkey, Diop Mar of Sénégal, and others presented stimulating and provocative papers which strongly indicate intrathecal injections. At the present time, serious considerations should be given to simultaneous single injections of TIG(H) and prednisolone intrathecally and of TIG(H) intramuscularly. For neonatal tetanus, 250 units of TIG(H) and 12.5 mg of prednisolone are administered intrathecally and 250 units of TIG(H) is given intramuscularly. For adults, the dose of TIG(H) for the intrathecal route is increased to 1000 units and for the intramuscular route to 1000 units. Complications of intrathecal administration are believed to be due to the preservatives rather than to the antitoxin itself.

Laboratory Tests

Order the following tests:

1. Complete blood cell count with differential white blood cell count.

2. Urinalysis.

3. Serologic test for syphilis.

4. Prothrombin time and partial thromboplastin time.

5. Blood chemistry tests: urea nitrogen, creatinine, electrolytes, serum protein electrophoresis, bilirubin, calcium, glucose.

6. Arterial blood gases.

7. Chest roentgenogram.

8. Electrocardiogram.

9. Electroencephalogram.

10. Wound and — if the patient is febrile — blood cultures.

11. If necessary for diagnosis, cerebrospinal fluid for culture, smear, cells, and chemistry tests.

12. Diazepam levels of serum.

Nursing Care

Provide 24-hour constant nursing care. A resident or intern immediately available for complications, particularly respiratory problems such as respiratory arrest, will greatly increase the patient's chance for recovery from tetanus.

Analgesics

Administer analgesics, which will relieve the pain associated with the tonic contractions of tetanus but which will not cause respiratory depression.

Codeine, meperidine (Demerol), and meperidine with promethazine (Phenergan) are suitable drugs.

Sedatives and Muscle Relaxants

Use sedatives and muscle relaxants correctly. *A most important consideration is that the physician know how to use safely the sedatives and muscle relaxants that he orders for the patient with tetanus and that he use those with which he obtains the best results.*

The mildest cases of tetanus can be sedated adequately with phenobarbital, pentobarbital, secobarbital, or paraldehyde.

In the more severe cases, thiopental sodium (Pentothal) may be administered intravenously in a very dilute solution (0.5 to 1.0 gram per 1000 ml) at a rate of 20 to 25 drops per minute in an effort to lower the patient's threshold of irritability to external stimuli and to reduce the number and severity of seizures and respiratory arrests. Care is taken to avoid overdosage. The optimal level of continuous sedation is obtained when the patient remains sleepy but still can be aroused by moderate external stimuli sufficiently to obey commands. Objectively, the best indication of this level is when the rectus muscles of the abdomen lose their hypertonic state and have only a normal degree of resistance to palpation. When a severe convulsive seizure occurs, with respiratory arrest, 2 to 8 ml of a 2.5 per cent solution of thiopental sodium is injected intravenously immediately and as necessary. This usually produces muscle relaxation within 30 to 45 seconds, and permits spontaneous re-establishment of the respiratory cycle.

Some centers have been enthusiastic about the use of muscle-relaxant drugs to control convulsive seizures. Such drugs are difficult to manage and have not prevented death from respiratory arrest. Drugs more commonly suggested for such use are diazepam (Valium), d-tubocurarine, succinylcholine (Anectine), and pancuronium (Pavulon). The margin of safety with these drugs is narrow; they seem best designed for patients excessively difficult to manage — and then only under careful observation of an experienced anesthesiologist.

Surgical Wound Care

Carry out optimal surgical care of wounds in accordance with the following concepts:

1. The wounds are taken care of at the earliest possible moment.

2. Aseptic technique, with the use of gloves, gowns, masks, sterile instruments, and the application of proper solutions to prepare the skin before the necessary operative procedures at the injured site, is observed.

3. During skin preparation, the wound should be covered with gauze to prevent further contamination.

4. Proper lighting, so that the surgeon can exactly identify and protect vital structures such as nerves and vessels, is provided.

5. Adequate instruments and adequate help, so that there is the best possible and gentle retraction of structures in wounds, are available.

6. Hemostasis, with delicate instruments and with fine suture material so that there is a minimum of necrotic tissue left in wounds, is effected.

7. Tissues are handled gently at all times so that necrotic tissue is not produced.

8. Complete debridement, with scalpel excision of necrotic tissue and with removal of foreign bodies so that no pabulum is left on which any unremoved bacteria can propagate, is carried out.

9. The wound is irrigated copiously with large amounts of physiologic salt solution to wash out minute avascular fragments of tissue and to eliminate foreign bodies.

10. If there is any doubt concerning a wound providing anaerobic conditions so that the tetanus bacillus can grow and produce its lethal toxin in it, the wound is left widely open and drainage is instituted when necessary.

Antibiotics

Consider the administration of antibiotics for the treatment of the infectious complications of tetanus.

In vitro, penicillin is effective against the tetanus bacillus. It is not surprising, however, that antibiotic therapy is clinically disappointing insofar as it is directed against the tetanus disease itself. Tetanus is not a bacteremia, for the bacillus remains at the place of its entry. By the time antibiotic therapy is begun, the wound often has been excised; and the toxins are already spread in the circulation. When the site of infection is not known and the antibiotic effect would be particularly desired, there is little probability that the bacteria are reached by parenteral administration of an antibiotic owing to avascular conditions in a concealed, closed puncture wound. Despite the in vitro effects of penicillin, a noticeable, specific therapeutic reaction cannot be expected.

On the other hand, the antibiotics do play their part in the therapy plan. They are irreplaceable in the care of infectious complications of tetanus, especially in combating pneumonia or secondary, invasive, wound infections. A combination of clindamycin phosphate injection, 600 mg every 6 hours, and gentamicin sulfate injection, 80 mg every 8 hours, may be given intravenously. An antibiotic with a broad-spectrum effect, such as a cephalosporin, may be administered intravenously. Penicillin and colistin have been injected down the tracheostomy tube with considerable success in neonatal tetanus.

The possible complications that may develop with antibiotic therapy must be given particular attention in the case of tetanus patients. Especially in the more severe cases, in which nourishment is accomplished through less than ideal methods, there will be a tendency toward gastrointestinal disturbances.

Tracheostomy

Perform tracheostomy when indicated if personnel and facilities are available to care adequately for the tracheostomy.

If the incubation period has been only a few days so that the patient may have very severe tetanus, a tracheostomy probably will be necessary, and can be performed with general anesthesia when extensive wound debridement is necessary, with local anesthesia, or with a combination of local and general anesthesia.

Tetanus patients in whom a tracheostomy is necessary also will need, in most cases, continuous artificial respiration. Such respiration is facilitated by attaching with a gas-tight adapter a tracheostomy tube with double inflatable cuffs to a volume-controlled respiration unit.

Nursing care of the seriously ill tracheostomy patient is not easy. Inspired air must be moist. If the patient can breathe spontaneously, moisturizing apparatus is set up in the patient's hospital room; if, however, the patient is being given artificial respiration, the respirator used must be one that continuously moistens the gas mixture. Dehydration of the respiratory tract can lead to severe hemorrhagic tracheobronchitis, which can be fatal. Even with absolutely correct conditioning of the inspired air, secretions can collect in the airway. A suction machine always must be at the patient's bedside. Patients with paralyzed respiratory muscles must be suctioned every hour. Also of extreme importance is the cleanliness of the tracheostomy tube; dehydrated secretions, pseudomembranes, and crusts can form on the inner margin of the cannula, and may lead to narrowing of the respiratory airway. The tracheostomy tube should be changed whenever it cannot be made to function correctly by cleaning and manipulation.

An improperly cared-for tracheostomy may be worse than none.

Tracheostomy may be poorly tolerated in the newborn infant, and decannulation may be quite difficult. In infants, particularly those with neonatal tetanus, before performing a tracheostomy, consider endotracheal intubation by insertion of an endotracheal tube through the nose, or, less preferably, through the mouth.

Iatrogenic Problems

Be constantly on the alert to avoid iatrogenic problems. For example, if rectal probes are left in place for constant recording of temperature, they must be checked carefully to prevent trauma to the rectal mucosa and anorectal veins during convulsions.

Private, Dark, Quiet Room

Place the patient in a private, dark, quiet room. Efforts should be made to reduce as much as possible all external stimuli. Visitors should be limited to the absolute minimum. It should be pointed out that, with adequate sedation and muscle relaxation, some patients no longer require the dark, quiet room.

Proper Environment for Infants

Place infants with neonatal tetanus in an incubator in which the oxygen partial pressure, environmental temperature, and a nebulized atmosphere of distilled water can be monitored and maintained.

Roentgenograms

Order indicated roentgenograms. These may be for (1) fractures associated with the initial injury, (2) determination of pulmonary problems such as atelectasis and pneumonia, (3) fractures or avulsions of muscle insertions produced by the tonic muscle contractions of tetanus, and (4) evaluation of resulting osteoarthropathies. Compression fractures of the vertebrae may be the result of the intense paroxysms that characterize the disease, and their diagnosis may be easily missed without roentgenograms.

Padded Tongue Depressor

By insertion of a padded tongue depressor, protect the tongue from being bitten during tonic contractions.

Oral Hygiene

Clean the lips, teeth, tongue, and oral cavity daily to lessen the possibility of growth of pathologic bacteria and viruses. Remove all loose debris from the oral and nasal cavities.

Nutrition

Give correct amounts of nourishment by oral, nasogastric tube, gastrostomy tube, or intravenous routes. The relaxed patient is totally dependent on artificial nourishment. Initially, tube feedings through a soft nasogastric or nasojejunal tube are indicated. If difficulties are encountered with the tube feedings, it may be necessary to resort to intravenous supplements. Central venous pressure systems using the subclavian vein provide an excellent route for feeding, including hyperalimentation. Transfusions of blood, plasma, and human albumin can be supplemented with electrolyte solutions of glucose, alcohol, fructose, and protein hydrolysates. The infusions can be further supplemented with high doses of vitamins C and B complex. Serum protein and electrolytes should be checked repeatedly. Nothing is given by mouth until improvement begins. In choosing a diet, the fact that the patient on occasion may feel pain when he eats and endeavors to open his mouth should be taken into consideration.

Alimentary Tract Elimination

Provide for adequate gastrointestinal elimination. Spontaneous defecation usually is absent. Defecation can be controlled by saline laxatives given orally or into the nasogastric tube and by enemas as required.

Urine Elimination

When necessary, provide for elimination of bladder urine by the insertion of a Foley catheter. Remove the catheter at the earliest possible time to reduce the possibility of urinary tract infections.

Intake and Output Records

Record intake and total output, and alter intake as indicated.

Protection of the Eyes

Protect the eyes. Particular attention must be given to incomplete closure of the eyelids. Without prophylactic measures, exsiccation, keratitis, and corneal ulcer can develop. An ophthalmic ointment may be applied, and the eyes covered with a moist gauze sponge.

Prevention of Decubital Ulcers

Keep the patient's skin dry, and cushion pressure points to avoid decubital ulcers.

Blood Dyscrasias and Bleeding Problems

If there is a possibility of blood problems, order complete blood cell counts, promptly investigate the clotting mechanisms, and render treatment.

Prevention of Pulmonary Emboli

Carry out indicated procedures, including ordering of heparin.

Prevention of Cardiac Exhaustion and Circulatory Disruption Which Can Result from Sympathetic Overstimulation

Advances during the past decade have indicated the importance of proper use of alpha and beta blockers for sympathetic overactivity as may be manifested by tachyarrhythmias and hemodynamic instability.

Consideration of Temporary Endocardial Pacemaker in Cases with Severe Bradycardic Episodes

A temporary endocardial pacemaker may be indicated for patients with severe, medically refractory bradycardia of unknown cause.

Prevention of Muscle Contractures

As the patient improves, prevent muscle contractures with resulting deformities, such as foot drop. Use foam-rubber padding, pillows, sandbags, and splints as indicated. When necessary for muscle imbalance, physiotherapy should be instituted as soon as possible.

Electroencephalograms

Order electroencephalograms when it is technically possible to obtain them and when their procurement will not interfere with the patient's recovery. Such records may be of considerable importance in the long-range evaluation and care of the patient, particularly as regards the possibility of brain damage.

Steroid Therapy

Consider steroid therapy if there is a possibility of adrenal gland exhaustion. Although not used routinely, steroid therapy has been employed in a few patients with severe tetanus in

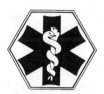

EMERGENCY MEDICAL IDENTIFICATION

Department of Health Education
Communications Division
American Medical Association
535 North Dearborn Street
Chicago, Illinois 60610

Why You Should Carry Emergency Medical Identification

An emergency medical identification card is your protection in an emergency. If you are not able to tell your medical story after an accident or sudden illness, the information entered on this card can save your life.

You may have health problems which can affect your recovery from an emergency. You may have a problem which is no emergency but often is treated as one, such as epilepsy. Even if you do not have a health problem, the information on this card can be of valuable assistance to the first aid attendant.

Why You Should Wear an Emergency Medical Signal Device

In an emergency, you may be separated from your pocket card. Possibly you are one who has a medical problem so critical that it must be immediately known to those who help you. If so, a signal device of durable material should be worn around your neck or wrist so that it can be present at all times, even while swimming.

The device should be fastened to the person wearing it with a strong nonelastic cord or chain so designed that it does not become an accident hazard in itself.

On this device there should be:

• The symbol of emergency medical identification
• The name of your major health problem
• For children and the aging, the name and address of a responsible relative and a telephone number, including area code.

Carry Your Card and Wear Your Signal Device at All Times!

to put E.M.I. to work for you...

fill in both sides of this card. **For example,** under

Immunizations

The date is important. If you note immunization over three years old, ask your doctor about a booster immunization. For tetanus toxoid, note the date of your first immunization as well as your last.

Present Medical Problems

Epilepsy	Tracheotomy (neck
Diabetes	breather)
Glaucoma	Pneumothorax
Hemophilia	Pneumoperitoneum
Chorea	Colostomy

Dangerous Allergies

Drug allergies	Feathers (pillows)
Horse serum (as in	Common foods
tetanus antitoxin)	Penicillin sensitivity

Medicines Taken Regularly

Anticoagulants	When noting drugs, ask
Cortisone or ACTH	your doctor for the name
Heart drugs such as	to use that will be easy to
digitalis or nitrites	identify in an emergency.
Thyroid preparation	

Other information

Scuba diver	Speak no English (note the
Recurring uncon-	language you speak)
sciousness	Wearing contact lenses
Hard of hearing	

Price: Single copy, 20c; 50-99, 18c each;
100-499, 16c each; 500-999, 14c each;
1000 or more, 12c each.

971-100M-OP2   *Prices are subject to change*

Emergency Medical Identification

My name Is _____

_____

_____

Please call _____

My Doctor is _____

_____

_____

Fig. 1

Medical Information

Last Immunization Date

diphtheria _____ mumps _____ tetanus toxoid _____

German measles _____ polio Sabin _____

measles _____ small pox _____ typhoid _____

Present Medical Problems _____

_____

Medicine Taken Regularly _____

_____

Dangerous Allergies _____

_____

Other Information _____

_____

Fig. 2

Figure 1.   Front of the A.M.A. emergency medical identification card.
Figure 2.   Back of the A.M.A. emergency medical identification card.

which the prolonged course of the disease was thought to exhaust the adrenal glands.

Tetanus Toxoid

At the end of the hospital treatment of tetanus, give 0.5 ml of adsorbed tetanus toxoid intramuscularly for active immunization, 1 month later another dose, and 6 months from this latter dose one more dose to complete the basic active immunization. Then, routine tetanus toxoid boosters are given every 10 years. Such immunization is necessary because *an attack of tetanus does not produce antibodies to prevent another attack.*

Emergency Medical Identification Devices (EMID)

At the time of discharge from the hospital, give the cured patient a completed EMID, such as the American Medical Association card (Figs. 1 and 2), and instruct him to complete his active immunization with tetanus toxoid to prevent recurrent tetanus.

Hyperbaric Oxygen

Hyperbaric oxygen is not recommended in view of no or minimal good effects and in view of the complications of such treatment. Tetanus is a toxemic state, and is not due to bacteria that are spreading throughout the body and which might be acted on by oxygen in the circulating blood.

Control of Body Temperature

Carry out necessary procedures to lower excessively high body temperatures. Tetanus per se does not cause fever, but the complications of tetanus cause fever. Hence, tetanus and its complications should be treated, not the fever itself.

Recording of Data

In view of professional liability problems, record completely and accurately the progress and treatment and especially significant reasons for giving or not giving drugs.

FINAL THOUGHT

At best, the results of therapy of tetanus are not as good as desired.

In World War II, United States military personnel were given complete tetanus toxoid prophylaxis. There were only four cases of tetanus among 2,734,819 United States officers and men who had received complete tetanus toxoid prophylaxis and who were admitted to United States Army hospitals for wounds. Such data proved unequivocally the efficacy of tetanus toxoid. The need for therapy of tetanus — as valuable as such therapy can be — indicates a failure to prevent an eminently preventable disease. *If all persons had the benefit of basic tetanus toxoid immunization and of the indicated booster toxoid injections, tetanus would no longer occur, and would indeed be a disease of only historical significance.*

TOXOPLASMOSIS

method of
MAURICE A. MUFSON, M.D.
Huntington, West Virginia

Toxoplasmosis, a worldwide parasitic infection of man caused by the coccidian sporozoan, *Toxoplasma gondii*, exhibits protean manifestations. It is transmitted by ingestion of cysts in contaminated, uncooked meat or, in some instances, by ingestion of mature oocysts transmitted by infected domestic cat feces. Naturally acquired infection can present a wide clinical spectrum, including subclinical infection, acute localized or generalized lymphadenitis, isolated ocular disease, or ocular disease associated with disseminated disease of the brain, heart, lungs, and other organs. Subclinical infection may occur in as many as 50 to 60 per cent of the general population. Immunodeficient individuals are uniquely susceptible to developing disseminated disease from infection with *T. gondii*, either by naturally acquired infection or reactivation of a latent infection. The normal adult rarely develops serious disease.

The pregnant woman must be protected from acquiring infection with *T. gondii* during all of pregnancy because the organism can be transmitted vertically, resulting in congenital infection which occurs at a high rate, approximately 1 case per 2000 to 5000 births. Congenital toxoplasmosis represents a major outcome of maternal infection during pregnancy, although the naturally acquired infection in the pregnant female will be minimal or subclinical. The fetus infected in utero usually develops disease of most of the solid organs, including the eyes, brain, heart, lungs, liver, spleen, and skin; the disseminated nature of congenital toxoplasmosis probably reflects the inability of the fetus to react immunologically to the infection. Five to 15 per cent of these infected infants fail to come to term or they die soon after birth. One fourth to one half of women in the childbearing age groups have chronic latent toxoplasmosis infection; however, these chronically infected women do not transmit the encysted organism to the fetus.

Treatment

Treatment of toxoplasmosis varies with the type and extent of clinical involvement. Subclinical infection or minimally symptomatic naturally acquired infection in the normal host usually does not require specific drug therapy. These infections may be detected incidentally by routine antibody determinations. Clinical symptoms may be waning by the time the infection can be confirmed by laboratory procedures, obviating the need to use specific drug therapy. Ocular and disseminated disease and congenital disease require drug treatment, as does infection in the pregnant woman. The cyst form of the parasite, which is present in chronic latent toxoplasmosis, is refractory to any treatment regimen.

The recommended therapy of choice for clinical disease is the combination of sulfadiazine and pyrimethamine (Daraprim). This combination of chemotherapeutic agents is particularly effective because both drugs act synergistically to block sequential steps in the synthesis of tetrahydrofolate. Other drug regimens have been used in the treatment of toxoplasmosis, and some are less toxic than sulfadiazine and pyrimethamine, but controlled studies of the use of other drugs are lacking. These drugs include trimethoprim-sulfamethoxazole and clindamycin. Spiramycin. which has been used in Europe, is not available in the United States.

Ocular Disease Alone or in Combination with Disseminated Disease in the Immunodeficient or Normal Host. These infections must be treated vigorously with the combination of sulfadiazine and pyrimethamine. In the adult, the dosage of sulfadiazine is 100 to 125 mg per kg per day (to a maximum of 8 grams per day) orally in four divided doses, and the dose of pyrimethamine is 100 to 200 mg loading dose orally (this dose may be higher than that listed in the manufacturer's official directive) on the first day of treatment and then 25 to 50 mg per day. The duration of therapy should be from 4 to 6 weeks. Since pyrimethamine antagonizes folate, folinic acid (leucovorin) should be given also in doses of 2 to 6 mg intramuscularly three times weekly. It is especially recommended when the platelet count drops below 100,000 cells per cu mm. Complete blood counts and platelet counts should be performed twice weekly and the dosage of pyrimethamine adjusted accordingly if counts fall. For patients with ocular disease, prednisone, 80 to 160 mg per day, should be given concomitantly with the sulfadiazine and pyrimethamine. Although the use of steroids in the treatment of systemic toxoplasmosis remains somewhat controversial, they may diminish the hypersensitivity reaction which is thought to contribute to the pathogenesis of ocular disease.

Congenital Infection. Although some infants manifest disease at birth, in others the disease will not become evident until months or even years later. Congenitally infected children must be treated with pyrimethamine and sulfadiazine. Usually these two drugs are given daily for several 3 week treatment periods separated by 30 to 45 day periods of spiramycin therapy (not available in the United States). Treatment should be administered for at least 1 year. The dose of pyrimethamine is 2 mg per kg on the first day and then 1 mg per kg per day afterward, and for sulfadiazine the daily dose is 100 mg per kg.

Naturally Acquired Infection in a Pregnant Woman. Treatment of toxoplasmosis in the pregnant woman must not include pyrimethamine because it is teratogenic. Therapy can include trimethoprim-sulfamethoxazole (this use of this combination is not listed in the manufacturer's official directive). The dosage is 160 mg orally twice a day of trimethoprim and 800 mg orally twice a day of sulfamethoxazole for 3 months. Alternatively, clindamycin, 600 mg orally per day for 1 month, can be used. Clindamycin has been reported to be effective in the treatment of toxoplasmosis; however, no controlled studies have been conducted. Since clindamycin does not cross the blood brain barrier, it should not be used in patients with central nervous system infection. When an acute toxoplasmosis infection is identified in a pregnant woman, she should be advised early in the course of the pregnancy of the likelihood of congenital infection of the fetus, and the option for a therapeutic abortion should be offered to her because one third of these children who come to term will be infected.

Prevention of Toxoplasmosis in Pregnant Women. Toxoplasmosis infection in pregnant women must be prevented. The following measures should be followed carefully throughout the pregnancy to prevent toxoplasmosis infection: (1) avoid eating uncooked or partially cooked meat; (2) wash hands thoroughly after handling uncooked meats; (3) all meats for consumption should be cooked first; (4) avoid domestic cats, including contact with pet cats, stray cats, cat litter boxes, or sand which cats use as a litter box; (5) if cats are kept as household pets, do not allow the cats to go outdoors because they can become infected with *T. gondii*; (6) have someone else in the household attend to the cat and clean litter boxes daily; (7) sterilize cat litter boxes before disposing; and (8) cover children's sandboxes when not in use (also prevents visceral and cutaneous larva migrans).

TRICHINELLOSIS

method of
ZBIGNIEW S. PAWLOWSKI, M.D.
Geneva, Switzerland

The efficacy of treatment of human trichinellosis depends on the intensity of infection, the strain of infecting *Trichinella spiralis*, the duration of infection (early infection, acute disease, late phase of disease), and the character and intensity of the host response.

Intestinal Infection

The production of newborn *T. spiralis* larvae which migrate to the muscle tissue of the human host is stopped by ridding the small intestine of *T. spiralis* adults. Therefore, treatment against intestinal Trichinella is obligatory in any case of infection, irrespective of whether or not it is symptomatic, severe or light, early or late (up to 6 weeks after ingestion of infected meat). Nowadays, widely used drugs are pyrantel (10 mg per kg of body weight per day for 4 days) and mebendazole (200 mg per day for 4 days). (This use of pyrantel is not listed in the manufacturer's official directive.) Mebendazole is not given to pregnant women.

T. spiralis larvae have been sporadically identified in animals a short time after infected meat has been eaten raw. When the time lapse after ingestion is only a few hours, induced vomiting or stomach wash-out, alcoholic drinks, or purgatives may reduce the infective dose. In the few days after ingestion of infected meat, thiabendazole, given orally in a daily dose of 50 mg per kg for 5 days, has been reported to prevent symptomatic trichinellosis. In intense infections it is suggested that treatment with thiabendazole be repeated after a week. Piperazine, tetramisole, pyrantel, and mebendazole would probably have a similar effect, but this has not been proved satisfactorily in human infections.

Acute Severe Trichinellosis

In acute trichinellosis symptoms common to some other infections are found, such as fever, myalgia, and general weakness, in addition to characteristic allergic signs, i.e., periorbital edema, conjunctival hemorrhages, and high eosinophilia. Corticosteroids are the drugs of choice in acute trichinellosis because of their anti-inflammatory, anti-allergic, and anti-shock action. The usual dose is 40 to 60 mg of prednisolone per day, taken until the fever and allergic signs disappear. Severe cases may require higher doses of corticosteroids given in conjunction with tetracycline as well as supportive drugs. Bed rest is always necessary, and any cardiac, circulatory, neurologic, or pulmonary complications may need additional, intensive, specific treatment.

Thiabendazole has been used in severe trichinellosis but with very controversial effects: dramatic clinical improvement was observed by some authors and no beneficial action by others. By destroying muscle larvae and liberating antigenic substances, thiabendazole can provoke a systemic hypersensitivity response and may be a potential hazard to patients already suffering from an allergy. However, a combination of thiabendazole or mebendazole and corticosteroids was reported to be highly effective in severe trichinellosis caused by sylvatic or polar strains of *T. spiralis*, which may respond poorly to corticosteroids alone.

Moderate or Mild Trichinellosis

Corticosteroids prolong the intestinal infection and increase the number of larvae parasitizing the muscle tissue by depressing the natural inflammatory and immune response of the host to *T. spiralis*. The use of corticosteroids is therefore justified only in patients with fever, allergic symptoms, high leukocytosis, and eosinophilia. The dosage of corticosteroids depends on the intensity of the signs and symptoms and does not usually exceed 40 mg of prednisolone per day. In mild infections corticosteroid therapy is not necessary, as antipyretic and analgesic treatment alone give a satisfactory result.

Late Phase of Trichinellosis

From the third week of the disease, metabolic and circulatory disorders dominate the clinical picture of severe trichinellosis. Profound hypoalbuminemia may require replacement human serum therapy. Some cardiac symptoms caused by hypokalemia are controlled by restoration of the correct electrolyte balance.

Trichinellosis is a self-limiting disease in both intestinal and muscular phases, and complete recovery usually occurs within a few months. In sporadic cases, some symptoms have been known to persist for several years. It is generally agreed that there is no justification for the use of larvicidal drugs if the acute phase of infection occurred some months before the time of diagnosis.

TULAREMIA

method of
MORTON I. RAPOPORT, M.D.
Baltimore, Maryland

Tularemia, caused by the gram-negative coccobacillus *Francisella tularensis*, is an acute bacterial infection with remarkable similarity to plague. The disease is encountered worldwide and is epizootic and enzootic in numerous species of animals, particularly rabbits (cottontail and jackrabbits). In addition, a variety of insects, including ticks and deer flies, have been established as vectors in the transmission of the disease. The National Center for Disease Control (NCDC) has reported less than 200 cases per year for the last 5 years. Human infection usually occurs by virtue of direct contact with infected animals or tissues. Hunting and trapping activities are the customary factors associated with infection, and cutaneous inoculation as well as aerosol infection are the common modes of transmission. Sporadic outbreaks of waterborne disease, either by ingestion of contaminated water or by direct invasion through the skin, have been reported. The major forms of the disease include the ulceroglandular, oculoglandular, enteric or typhoidal, and pulmonary. Most human infections are of the ulceroglandular type, although pulmonary infections are frequently encountered.

Diagnosis

The diagnosis may be suspected clinically, but signs and symptoms are dependent on the form of the disease. Laboratory confirmation involves isolation of the organism from culture material obtained from ulcers, secretions, and biopsy specimens using selected media. Serologic diagnosis may be extremely useful even in the early diagnostic process. Indeed, significant increases in agglutinating antibodies may be detected within the first 10 to 14 days of clinical illness. As with most serologic studies, the diagnosis is established using paired or sequential sera. In diagnosis of tularemia, the importance of sequential or paired sera is underscored by virtue of the fact that antibodies persist for many years.

Management

General Measures. Most patients require hospitalization, particularly those with constitutional symptoms. Patients with ocular involvement require ophthalmologic consultation, when available. Suppuration of lymph nodes is uncommon, and aspiration and drainage are rarely required. Constitutional symptoms and headache are usually treated with non-narcotic analgesics. There is no evidence that corticosteroids are useful in patients with any form of tularemia.

Antibiotic Therapy. Streptomycin remains the treatment of choice for this disease. The drug is given intramuscularly in two daily divided doses, totaling 15 to 30 mg per kg for 10 days. Children are generally treated with the lower dose. There is minimal risk for the vestibular, auditory, or renal complications of streptomycin therapy when treatment is limited to 10 days. Doses should be reduced in patients with renal failure.

Other aminoglycoside antibiotics, including gentamicin and kanamycin, have been used with increased frequency. However, there is no evidence that any of these antibiotics are superior to streptomycin.

Tetracycline and Chloramphenicol. Both these drugs are bacteriostatic, and both are associated with relapses at a higher rate than that observed in those patients receiving streptomycin. Surprisingly, relapse occurs more frequently in those patients in whom therapy is initiated early. The mechanism for relapse in these patients is most likely due to incomplete eradication of the organisms in association with a blunted antibody response, usually to reduced antigenic stimulus.

Tetracycline may be given in a dose of 2 to 4 grams per day for 14 days, or chloramphenical may be given in a dose of 3 to 4 grams per day for 14 days. Both these drugs have been recommended for patients in whom streptomycin is found inappropriate. Common complications of tetracycline treatment include gastrointestinal tract signs and symptoms such as nausea and vomiting and diarrhea, cutaneous eruptions, photosensitivity, hepatotoxicity, and nephrotoxicity.

Chloramphenicol may be associated with impaired hemoglobin synthesis and very rarely with agranulocytosis.

Prevention and Prophylaxis

Patients with suspected tularemia should be reported to local health departments. Since human-to-human infection has not been reported, there is no need for respiratory isolation, although handling of cultural and infected material should be done with care in recognition of its potential infectivity. Laboratory personnel experiencing accidental exposure should receive prophylaxis with streptomycin for 10 days in the same dose recommended for treatment. It should be obvious that meat from rabbits should be well cooked before eating, and care should be taken when handling wild game or dead animals. Tick searches in tick-infested areas are appropriate, since this may be an occasional source of infection.

TYPHOID FEVER

method of
MYRON M. LEVINE, M.D.,
and LUIS CISNEROS, M.D.
Baltimore, Maryland

Typhoid fever is an enteric fever that occurs 8 to 14 days following ingestion of *Salmonella typhi*. The disease is characterized by generalized infection of the reticuloendothelial system, including the lymphoid tissue of the small intestine. Man is the reservoir of infection, which is usually transmitted by contaminated food and water. At the turn of the century in the United States typhoid fever was a common cause of morbidity and mortality in both urban and rural settings. In ensuing decades, consequent to improved sanitation, food hygiene, and water quality, transmission of *S. typhi* greatly decreased, typhoid fever incidence plummeted, and the prevalence of carriers diminished. Typhoid fever is now only rarely acquired indigenously within the United States, but several hundred cases per year still occur in travelers to less-developed areas of the world where the disease is still highly endemic.

The diagnosis should be bacteriologically confirmed by isolation of *S. typhi* from blood, stool, or bone marrow cultures and the strain examined for its antibiotic sensitivity pattern.

Historically the therapy of typhoid fever can be divided into three eras: (1) Prior to 1948, when specific effective antibiotic therapy was unavailable and case fatality was approximately 10 per cent. (2) The period from 1948 to 1972, during which oral chloramphenicol was shown to be a highly efficacious, practical, and economical therapy, particularly in less-developed areas of the world. (3) From 1973 to the present, wherein, as a result of increasing prevalence of chloramphenicol-resistant strains of *S. typhi* and the advent of trimethoprim/sulfamethoxazole and amoxicillin, alternative drugs appeared to challenge the pre-eminent role of chloramphenicol as the mainstay of therapy of typhoid fever.

Therapy

It is helpful to divide the management of acute typhoid fever into three categories: (1) specific antibiotic therapy, (2) general supportive measures, and (3) treatment of the more common life-endangering complications.

Antimicrobial Agents. Chloramphenicol has been the mainstay of specific therapy of typhoid fever since its first demonstration of efficacy in 1948. While many other antibiotics of the 1950s had impressive in vitro activity against *S. typhi* (such as tetracycline, streptomycin, kanamycin, and colistimethate sodium [Coly-Mycin]), only chloramphenicol was effective in patients. Chloramphenicol remains the drug of choice in less-developed countries because of its practical-ity, relative inexpensiveness, and effectiveness when administered orally. Chloramphenicol has reduced typhoid fever from a 3 to 4 week illness with 10 per cent case fatality to an illness of 1 week or less with a case fatality below 1 per cent. However, a number of observations make chloramphenicol a less than ideal drug: (1) relapse occurs in approximately 8 to 15 per cent of patients; (2) it causes irreversible aplastic anemia in approximately 1 in 40,000 recipients; (3) occasional patients treated with this drug develop "toxic crises" (Herxheimer-like reactions); (4) in recent years the duration of therapy required until an afebrile state occurs has increased; (5) the drug is not impressive in preventing development of chronic carriers; and (6) epidemics caused by chloramphenicol-resistant strains have occurred (as in Mexico in 1972 and Vietnam in 1973).

The regimen we prefer involves giving 750 mg of chloramphenicol every 6 hours to adults (50 mg per kg to children) until the fever subsides (usually 3 to 7 days), followed by 500 mg 6-hourly in adults (50 mg per kg in children); the drug is continued for a total of 14 days. If the patient is unable to take oral medication, the drug should be given intravenously until the switch to oral medication can be made. Chloramphenicol should not be given intramuscularly because only poor blood levels are achieved. Occasional patients develop a "toxic crisis" following the first doses of drug; it is postulated that this may result from a sudden release of endotoxin secondary to death of the bacteria.

If the *S. typhi* isolate is known to be resistant to chloramphenicol or if epidemiologic data make such infection likely, there exist two highly effective alternatives, trimethoprim/sulfamethoxazole and amoxicillin, both of which are administered orally.

Amoxicillin, a congener of ampicillin, shows superior intestinal absorption. Adults are given 1.0 gram (and children 100 mg per kg) 6-hourly for 14 days. During the 1972 Mexican epidemic caused by chloramphenicol-resistant *S. typhi*, strains began to appear bearing plasmid-mediated resistance to amoxicillin as well. Infections with such strains can be successfully treated with oral trimethoprim/sulfamethoxazole. The dose is 2 tablets of 80 mg trimethoprim/400 mg sulfamethoxazole twice daily for 14 days. Children should receive 8 mg per kg trimethoprim and 40 mg per kg sulfamethoxazole daily in two divided doses (this use of trimethoprim/sulfamethoxazole is not listed in the manufacturer's official directive). A large experience with trimethoprim/sulfamethoxazole therapy of typhoid fever caused by chloramphenicol-sensitive strains has shown that it is comparable in efficacy to chloramphenicol in approximately 90 per cent of cases. In 8 to 10 per cent of infected persons, however, the therapeutic response is retarded, requiring 10 or more days for the temperature to become normal.

Irrespective of the aforementioned antibiotics selected, the clinical response in typhoid fever is not dramatic. Usually 2 full days of therapy are required before the fever begins to abate, and a normal temperature is usually not reached for 5 to 7 days.

General Supportive Measures. Because of the high fever, maintenance requirements for water and electrolytes are greatly increased so the patient should be encouraged to drink fluids liberally. If the patient is too ill to maintain hydration via oral fluids, intravenous fluids must be given; daily maintenance requirements should be increased by 10 per cent for each degree of fever above 99 F (37.2 C).

Salicylates should not be given to patients with typhoid fever, since they can induce wide swings in temperature, hypotension, and even shock. The temperature should be lowered by sponging with tepid water.

Laxatives and enemas should, in general, not be employed because of the danger of precipitating intestinal hemorrhage. If constipation requires relief, oral lactulose should be used. This nonabsorbable disaccharide is a gentle physiologic softener of stool, and the short-chain fatty acids produced as a result of its metabolism by normal enteric flora are probably inhibitory for salmonellae.

Complications. In the preantibiotic era typhoid fever was a disease marked by a wide array of complications involving virtually every organ system, including intestinal perforation, intestinal hemorrhage, myocarditis, empyema of the gallbladder, encephalopathy, bronchitis, pneumonia, parotitis, osteomyelitis, hepatitis, meningitis, septic arthritis, and orchitis. Since the advent of specific antimicrobial therapy, most of these complications are now rare. Nevertheless, a few complications are still encountered with some frequency and are discussed below.

A few patients with acute typhoid fever present with severe toxemia. A 2 or 3 day course of prednisone (60 mg per day) is indicated in this instance. The fever lyses and toxemia is reduced. The use of steroids should be reserved for this rare situation only and otherwise plays no role in therapy of typhoid fever.

Despite adequate therapy with appropriate antibiotics, 5 to 15 per cent of patients manifest relapse. The clinical syndrome is comparable, but all signs and symptoms are milder in nature. The treatment is the same as for the initial episode.

Two dreaded complications of typhoid fever are still encountered: intestinal hemorrhage and perforation. When a definitive diagnosis of typhoid fever is made, a unit of blood should be typed and cross-matched as a precaution. Hemorrhage occurs late in the course, often in the second or third week, when the patient is often feeling better. The management of hemorrhage is conservative, utilizing repeated transfusion, unless there is evidence of intestinal perforation. In the preantibiotic era intestinal perforation was almost universally fatal. Current consensus favors combined medical and surgical intervention. Most surgeons experienced in typhoid fever prefer simple closure of the ulcer. This must be accompanied by additional antibiotics, such as cefoxitin and gentamicin, to combat peritoneal contamination by normal enteric flora including anaerobes.

Carrier State

A few persons with acute typhoid fever become chronic biliary carriers. The propensity to become a carrier increases with age at the time of initial *S. typhi* infection and is greater in females. Most all chronic carriers have cholecystitis with stones; carriers lacking gallbladders manifest chronic pathology and infection in the intrahepatic biliary system.

If indicated because of economic or social factors, and if the patient is sturdy enough to withstand surgery, cholecystectomy accompanied by 4 weeks of combined intravenous ampicillin and oral amoxicillin therapy can cure the carrier state in approximately 85 per cent of instances. When this is not feasible, 3 weeks of high dose intravenous ampicillin therapy has also shown promising results. Most recently a high success rate has been reported by long-term (at least 4 weeks) amoxicillin therapy (3 to 6 grams per day), accompanied by probenecid.

Prevention

In multiple controlled field trials in endemic areas, acetone-killed *S. typhi* parenteral vaccine has been shown to confer 75 to 90 per cent protective efficacy against typhoid fever. The protection afforded to persons from nonendemic areas appears to be somewhat less. Furthermore, the vaccine causes fever or adverse local reactions (heat, swelling, erythema) in 25 per cent of recipients. Nevertheless, for persons traveling to highly endemic areas, immunization with two 0.5 ml doses 1 month apart is recommended. It should be recognized that the diagnostic value of the Widal test in immunized persons is nil.

TYPHUS FEVER

method of
ALFRED J. SAAH, M.D.
Baltimore, Maryland

The typhus fever group of diseases caused by rickettsia consist of epidemic typhus (louse-borne) and its recrudescent form, Brill-Zinsser disease, caused by *Rickettsia prowazekii*, murine typhus (flea-borne, endemic) caused by *R. typhi*, and scrub typhus caused by *R. tsutsugamushi*. Tick typhus, a term used to describe illness caused by the spotted fever group of organisms, is considered elsewhere. Murine typhus occurs in areas of the United States where exposure to rats and their ectoparasites is heavy, e.g., seaports, granaries, or food storage facilities. Serologic evidence of indigenous acquisition of epidemic typhus in the eastern United States has been reported. Infection may be related to flying squirrels, but as yet infection has not been confirmed by Koch's postulates. Brill-Zinsser disease occurs primarily in immigrants who became infected in eastern Europe during World War II. Scrub typhus does not occur in the United States.

A rash is frequently found on the trunk in murine and epidemic typhus and spreads distally; the converse is true in Rocky Mountain spotted fever. Murine typhus and Brill-Zinsser disease are milder than epidemic typhus, which may result in death.

Therapy

Chloramphenicol or tetracycline is effective against these rickettsiae and results in dramatic improvement within 48 hours. These agents should not be used in combination to treat typhus. Delay in therapy is the most frequent cause of a poor outcome in serious rickettsial infections; therapy should begin when the diagnosis is considered likely. Naturally occurring drug resistant strains are not known.

Oral therapy is preferred but may be impossible because of delirium or vomiting. Intravenous therapy is then recommended for drug administration and for hydration. Symptoms of myalgia and/or headache are difficult to treat but are fortunately short lived with effective therapy. If the patient requires hospitalization, isolation is not necessary. Delousing should be done if lice are found.

Specific Therapy. Specific therapy consists of either chloramphenicol or tetracycline (including its congeners). Other routinely used antibiotics are not effective.

Oral therapy is preferred when possible. In children less than 8 years old, chloramphenicol should be used because of tetracycline-associated staining of teeth. The following regimen is recommended for oral therapy in adults and children:

Tetracycline: 25 mg per kg of body weight per day divided into four equal doses each day.

Chloramphenicol: 50 mg per kg of body weight per day divided into four equal doses each day.

When intravenous treatment is indicated, chloramphenicol sodium succinate may be preferable because of the thrombophlebitis that frequently complicates intravenous tetracycline therapy.

Chloramphenicol sodium succinate: 50 mg per kg of body weight per day divided into four equal doses (one dose infused every 6 hours).

Tetracycline: 15 mg per kg of body weight per day divided into four equal doses (one dose infused every 6 hours).

In severely ill patients an initial loading dose (tetracycline, 25 mg per kg of body weight; chloramphenicol, 50 mg per kg of body weight) of the selected antibiotic should be given, and subsequent doses given according to the schedule above. The initial loading dose is the same for oral or intravenous administration.

Antibiotic therapy should continue for 2 to 3 days following defervescence. An occasional patient will recrudesce if specific therapy is initiated early in illness (prior to the fourth day of fever) because the antibiotics are rickettsiostatic; repeating the course of therapy suffices. In scrub typhus, relapses are more common and may be eliminated by continuing antimicrobial therapy for 7 to 14 days or, if antibiotics are stopped after 2 days without fever, the adult patient should receive chloramphenicol, 3 grams by mouth as one dose, 6 days after ending the primary course of therapy.

If the patient with typhus has renal failure, the use of full dose chloramphenicol is preferred because experience with doxycycline is limited. Under adverse field conditions, one dose of doxycycline, 100 mg by mouth or by intramuscular injection, seems to be effective in treating epidemic typhus.

Therapy of Complications. If antimicrobial therapy is started before the patient is moribund, fatalities are infrequent. Hypotension is frequently due to dehydration, which should be corrected intravenously. Azotemia also responds to rehydration. Adjunctive therapy such as oxygen should be used when indicated.

Disseminated intravascular coagulopathy may occur in epidemic typhus; the use of heparin in this situation is controversial. Corticosteroids used briefly in high doses may be beneficial in the unstable, toxic-appearing patient.

Prevention

In general, prevention is accomplished by minimizing or eliminating exposure to the insect vectors — the human body louse (epidemic typhus), the rat flea (murine typhus), and the mite (scrub typhus). A vaccine is available only for epidemic typhus; it does not protect against murine or scrub typhus. Vaccine is not recommended for travelers unless close contact with the indigenous population is planned and typhus is endemic in the area. Medical personnel caring for patients ill with epidemic typhus in areas where the disease occurs and laboratory personnel working with *R. prowazekii* should also receive vaccine.

When epidemic typhus occurs and lousiness is identified, delousing the patient's family and close contact neighbors is indicated. Health authorities will conduct the delousing after susceptibility of the lice is shown. The agents used include chlorophenothane (DDT), lindane, and malathion mixed with talc. The epidemiology of epidemic typhus suspected of being acquired in the United States is not sufficiently defined to identify preventive measures. No preventive measure is known for Brill-Zinsser disease other than prevention of the primary infection.

Murine typhus is best prevented by controlling rats and their ectoparasites. If the density of ectoparasites is high, control of this population should be accomplished before rats are killed. Rat ectoparasites should be tested for susceptibility to the agents being used for environmental application.

Prevention of scrub typhus involves avoiding the natural habitat of the mite in endemic areas, or applying miticidal agents, such as dibutyl phthalate, dimethyl phthalate, and benzyl benzoate, to clothes and insect repellent to skin. Chemoprophylaxis with chloramphenicol is effective but should be restricted to special circumstances in which the risk of infection is high, the period of exposure limited to a few weeks, and the need to prevent the disease critical. Chloramphenicol is given by mouth as one 3 gram dose weekly, and continued for 1 month after the last exposure.

Cases of typhus fever should be reported to local and/or state health departments. The health department can also help in the serodiagnosis of suspected cases.

PERTUSSIS
(Whooping Cough)

method of
LARRY J. BARAFF, M.D.
Los Angeles, California

Approximately 2000 cases of pertussis are reported annually in the United States. Forty to 50 per cent of recognized cases occur in infants less than 1 year of age. The overall mortality rate is 5 per 1000 with most deaths in infants. Pertussis is significantly under-reported, as most cases are not diagnosed.

Since the use of pertussis vaccine became widespread in 1950, there has been a steady decline in the incidence of this illness. However, the efficacy of pertussis vaccine is not comparable to that of other childhood immunizations, e.g., polio, tetanus, measles. Immunity associated with this vaccine declines rapidly after early childhood and seldom lasts longer than 10 years; 10 to 20 per cent of immunized children remain susceptible. Adults rarely have protective antibody titers in their sera; therefore, transplacental transfer of protective antibodies to the newborn is uncommon. This explains the high proportion of cases in infants, and the need to immunize this population as early as possible. Waning vaccine-induced immunity is responsible for infections which occur in older children and adults. Hospital personnel attending to children with whooping cough are susceptible, and several nosocomial outbreaks have occurred, including spread to infants in the newborn nursery.

Modified Pertussis. Adults and older children who have been immunized and therefore are partially immune may not manifest the characteristic paroxysms of coughing. Household contacts of infants with the characteristic paroxysms of pertussis frequently have a history of a severe cough of 2 or more weeks' duration. They seldom have characteristic lymphocytosis or chest radiograph findings. However, such patients may be symptomatic carriers of organisms and a threat to infants who are not immune and should receive antimicrobial therapy.

Bordetella pertussis is the responsible etiologic agent for the majority of cases of clinical pertussis. Other Bordetella species (parapertussis and bronchiseptica) in addition to some viral agents, notably adenovirus, may be responsible for a similar clinical syndrome. Because of the difficulty in culturing *B. pertussis,* it is suggested that all patients who present with the characteristic symptoms of cough for greater than 1 week, associated with whoop, vomiting, or cyanosis, should be considered to have pertussis.

Treatment

The therapy of pertussis has four components: supportive care, antimicrobial· therapy, therapy of complications, and prevention of communicability.

Supportive Care. Infants less than 6 months of age, older children with convulsions or significant post-tussive cyanosis, or patients with inability to maintain hydration because of coughing episodes should be admitted to a hospital for close observation and supportive care.

The importance of close observation by experienced nursing personnel cannot be overemphasized. Hospitalized infants less than 6 months of age, or patients experiencing post-tussive cyanosis, should be in a setting in which they can be carefully observed. The patient should be isolated until at least 5 days following initiation of appropriate antimicrobial therapy to eliminate nosocomial spread of the disease. During a coughing paroxysm, an infant should be placed on his stomach in a head down position and be given supplemental oxygen. The oropharynx should be suctioned, using a bulb syringe; hypopharyngeal suction with a catheter should be avoided, as this may induce excessive vagal tone and reflex bradycardia. Infants who experience frequent paroxysms of coughing associated with cyanosis should have continuous cardiac monitoring for bradyarrhythmias. If exhaustion results from a paroxysm, bag-valve-mask ventilation may be temporarily required. Placing an infant in a croup tent is not advised as it is of no demonstrable benefit and interferes with careful observation. Continuous oxygen therapy is indicated only when pulmonary complications result in persistent hypoxemia.

Infants with whooping cough tend to vomit their feedings with coughing episodes; therefore, they should be fed in small quantities after each paroxysm. If the child vomits after a coughing paroxysm, he should be refed. The majority of children may be maintained with oral feedings. Intravenous hydration or alimentation is necessary only in very young infants with severe paroxysms and vomiting. The duration of hospitalization of infants with pertussis is usually 1 to 3 weeks, and it is impractical to maintain an intravenous line during this period.

Antitussives or sedatives should not be prescribed. They are seldom effective in reducing either the frequency or severity of coughing paroxysms. Furthermore, coughing clears the airway of the thick, tenacious secretions associated with this illness and should not be suppressed. Pertussis immune globulin has been shown to be of no therapeutic value in the management of patients with pertussis.

Corticosteroids have been reported to significantly alter the severity and duration of pertussis, even when given after the paroxysmal stage. Hydrocortisone sodium succinate (Solu-Cortef) should be given in an initial dose of 20 mg per kg per day for 2 days and then tapered to complete a total course of 1 week's therapy.

Prolonged convulsions should be treated immediately with intravenous diazepam, 1 mg per year of age at the rate of 1 mg per minute until the convulsions stop. If convulsions recur, intramuscular phenobarbital, 5 mg per kg initially, and then 5 mg per kg per day, should be given for the duration of the illness.

Infants should be hospitalized until parents and nursing staff feel that they can be cared for at home. This usually means that post-tussive cyanosis and significant post-tussive vomiting which may lead to aspiration are no longer a problem. Adults with classic pertussis should be discouraged from operating dangerous machinery or driving an automobile. Adults have been known to be severely incapacitated and to even lose consciousness during paroxysms of coughing.

Antimicrobial Therapy. No antibiotic has been demonstrated to significantly affect the severity or duration of symptoms once paroxysmal coughing has begun. However, such therapy does decrease the duration of respiratory shedding of the organism, and therefore will reduce communicability. The antibiotic of choice in treating patients with pertussis is erythromycin, given orally, 40 mg per kg per day in four divided doses for 10 days. This will usually eradicate *B. pertussis* from respiratory secretions within 5 days, thereby rendering patients noninfectious. Tetracycline is a suitable alternative antibiotic for adults, but should not be used for infants or young children. Ampicillin, though effective in the laboratory, does not eradicate the organisms in vivo.

Patients should be isolated from susceptible contacts for a minimum of 5 days after antibiotic therapy has been begun. If laboratory facilities are available to identify *B. pertussis*, then tests should be performed to confirm eradication of the organism 5 days after initiation of therapy.

Respiratory Complications. *B. pertussis* infects the respiratory epithelium of the tracheobronchial tree. Pneumonia is usually due to superinfection and is suggested by the appearance of interparoxysmal respiratory distress, i.e., tachypnea or retractions and fever. At this time, a polymorphonuclear leukocytosis should be present and the chest radiograph should demonstrate a lobar or bronchopneumonia. Antibiotic therapy should be aimed at the most likely superinfecting organisms, including pneumococci, staphylococci, *Hemophilus influenzae*, and gram-negative aerobic organisms. A Gram stain of tracheal secretions may be helpful in determining which antibiotic to use. In general, oxicillin, ampicillin, or an aminoglycoside is indicated, depending on the results of the Gram stain. In the past, bronchiectasis was reported as a sequela of pertussis; this is seldom seen in the era of antimicrobial therapy.

Infants and small children with pertussis are also susceptible to otitis media. Patients with fever should be examined using pneumatic otoscopy to determine if an acute inflammation exists in the middle ear. Such infections are usually secondary to pneumococci or *H. influenzae* and should respond to therapy with erythromycin, sulfisoxazole (Gantrisin), or trimethoprim-sulfamethoxazole (Bactrim).

Neurologic Complications. Neurologic complications are secondary to hypoxia, small intracerebral hemorrhages, or cerebral edema. Catastrophic central nervous system hemorrhage is virtually nonexistent. Convulsions and encephalopathy are also very rare and are usually due to hypoxia. The administration of oxygen during coughing paroxysms in association with the maintenance of an adequate airway should lessen the risk of these complications.

Other Complications. Subconjunctival hemorrhage, epistaxis, ulceration of the lingual frenulum, and petechiae of the face and neck are secondary to the increase in intrathoracic and intra-abdominal pressures associated with coughing paroxysms. No therapy is required.

Therapy of Contacts

All patient contacts should be treated with a 5 day course of erythromycin, 40 mg per kg per day in four divided doses, not to exceed 250 mg four times a day. Postexposure vaccination with DTP vaccine is not indicated, especially in patients more than 6 years of age. Pertussis immune globulin has not been demonstrated to be of any value in the prevention of pertussis in contacts. Unimmunized infants and small children are at extreme risk. Antibiotic treatment during the incubating or preparoxysmal stage of the illness may abort the development of paroxysmal coughing episodes.

In the hospital setting, patients with pertussis should be strictly isolated, using techniques to prevent microdroplet (aerosol) transmission. All patients exposed to an unrecognized case of pertussis should be treated as noted above with erythromycin for 5 days. All hospital personnel with symptoms suggestive of pertussis should be barred from further patient contact until adequately treated. It should be recognized that the paroxysmal phase of the illness will last from 2 to 4 weeks, long after treated patients have become culture negative and are no longer communicable.

SECTION 2

The Respiratory System

ACUTE RESPIRATORY FAILURE

method of
WILLIAM J. HALL, M.D.
Rochester, New York

The major function of the respiratory system is to maintain levels of arterial oxygenation adequate for the energy needs of body tissues and to facilitate elimination of carbon dioxide, the principal by-product of cellular metabolism. Proper functioning of this system requires extraordinary integration of central nervous system control mechanisms, respiratory muscles, and the gas exchanging surface of the lung parenchyma. "Failure" of the respiratory system, therefore, may involve any portion of this complex integrative system.

All forms of respiratory failure are always characterized by hypoxemia, but only sometimes by carbon dioxide retention. Arterial blood gas determination, therefore, is the single most important tool in developing a therapeutic approach to respiratory failure. Respiratory failure may be diagnosed when, in a patient breathing room air, arterial blood gas determination demonstrates an arterial partial pressure of oxygen (Pao_2) of less than 50 mm Hg or a partial pressure of carbon dioxide ($Paco_2$) of greater than 50 mm Hg. A few basic physiologic principles, which can be understood painlessly without resorting to complex formulas, form the basis of our approach.

Carbon Dioxide Retention. Carbon dioxide produced by cellular metabolism equilibrates with inspired gas in the alveoli and is eliminated by ventilation. Carbon dioxide retention takes place under only two circumstances. First, if total ventilation is depressed because of an abnormality of central nervous system regulation (drug overdose, trauma, or stroke) or muscular weakness (myasthenia gravis, myopathies, fatigue), alveolar and, therefore, arterial carbon dioxide tension ($Paco_2$) will rise. Second, certain common pulmonary disorders, chief among them ob-

structive lung disease, result in an increase in "dead-space" ventilation, that is, ventilation distributed to non-gas-exchanging portions of damaged lung. If total ventilation cannot be proportionately increased to compensate for this wasted ventilation, carbon dioxide retention ensues (alveolar hypoventilation). Note that although carbon dioxide retention is the common denominator here, in the first instance minute ventilation (the amount of air exchanged per minute as measured at the mouth) is decreased, and in the second instance it is actually increased above normal. This difference will have obvious therapeutic importance.

Carbon dioxide retention will have significant but variable clinical sequelae. Rapid rise of $Paco_2$ to extremely high levels of 80 to 90 mm Hg has a direct narcotizing effect on central nervous system function, including ventilatory regulation and level of consciousness. Depending on the acuteness of $Paco_2$ elevation, pH will fall. If the rise is rapid and immediate, acute respiratory acidosis will be a major problem, while if the rise is over a period of weeks, relatively little change in pH will be noted because of efficient renal compensatory mechanisms. A less obvious sequela of hypoventilation, but one that is often of most important immediate therapeutic concern, is the effect of hypoventilation on the arterial oxygen tension (Pao_2). As alveolar carbon dioxide tension ($P_{A}co_2$) rises in this setting, there is a corresponding drop in the alveolar oxygen tension ($P_{A}o_2$) and, therefore, a drop in the Pao_2. This relationship may be quantitated by use of a modified form of the alveolar air equation:

$$P_{A}o_2 = 150 - Paco_2 \times 1.2$$

This equation states that at sea level, and with a patient breathing room air, the alveolar oxygen tension is a function of the inspired oxygen tension (150 mm Hg) less the arterial (or alveolar) carbon dioxide tension modified by a small correction factor. For example, a patient admitted following an acute drug overdose might have a $Paco_2$ of 80 mm Hg and a Pao_2 of 50 mm Hg. His estimated $P_{A}o_2$ would be 54 mm Hg, a value very similar to the observed Pao_2 of 50 mm Hg. A conventional way of expressing this relationship is to simply calculate the difference, or "gradient" between the computed $P_{A}O_2$ value (54 mm Hg) and the measured Pao_2 (50 mm Hg). In this instance, the alveolar-arterial gradient would be 4 mm Hg, which is a normal value (the usual alveolar-arterial gradient is less than 10 mm Hg). A normal alveolar-arterial gradient rules out intrinsic lung disease, and suggests in this case that the hypoxemia is related to an abnormality of the control mechanism, rather than of the lung parenchyma. Therefore, the appropriate therapeutic approach to this form of hypoxia is not primarily supplemental oxygen administration but rather ventilatory support. Failure to recognize this difference can lead to incorrect and potentially fatal therapeutic decisions. Most blood gas laboratories are now routinely calculating and reporting the alveolar-arterial oxygen gradient on arterial blood gas determinations. Physicians ordering this test must have a working knowledge of its utility.

Other Mechanisms of Hypoxia. All other clinically important forms of hypoxemia are associated with an abnormal alveolar-arterial oxygen gradient and imply intrinsic lung damage. Two important types must be distinguished: hypoxemia resulting from mismatching of ventilation to perfusion (more specifically characterized by areas of lung with diminished ventilation and relatively well-preserved perfusion); and shunting of blood through the pulmonary capillary tree without contacting a ventilated, gas-exchanging surface.

Ventilation-Perfusion Abnormalities. In a numerical sense, ventilation-perfusion mismatching is by far the most common physiologic mechanism for hypoxemia encountered in adult patients. Such common entities as pneumonia, congestive heart failure, exacerbations of bronchitis, and asthma all have ventilation-perfusion mismatching as a primary or contributing cause of hypoxemia. Two important therapeutic corollaries bear mentioning. First, in marked contrast to hypoxemia associated with shunting, hypoxemia resulting largely from ventilation-perfusion imbalance is usually substantially correctable by means of supplemental oxygen therapy and rarely in and of itself will be an indication for intubation. Second, ventilation-perfusion mismatching usually implies reversible airway disease amenable to therapy (such as bronchospasm, secretions, or interstitial edema).

Shunting. In contrast, when hypoxia is due primarily to shunt mechanisms, substantial alterations in alveolar capillary permeability are present, the degree of hypoxia is much more severe, and supplemental oxygen therapy will be a less effective treatment modality. Another less well emphasized consideration with shunt mechanisms is the effect of alterations in cardiac output on the Pao_2 in the setting of significant intrapulmonary shunting. In most clinical settings, a diminution in cardiac output will not influence the measured arterial Pao_2. As cardiac output falls, greater peripheral extraction of oxygen from hemoglobin ensues, resulting in a lowered partial pressure of oxygen in mixed venous blood re-turning to the right ventricle. Under normal circumstances despite the lower mixed venous oxygen level, the blood is well oxygenated in the lung, and the Pao_2 remains unchanged. However, when a large portion of that mixed venous blood with lower partial pressure of oxygen is being shunted through the lungs, it will mix with the arterialized blood and result in a lowered oxygen content and Pao_2.

TREATMENT

From a clinical standpoint we recognize three therapeutically distinct forms of acute respiratory failure: (1) respiratory failure in patients with previously normal lungs, (2) respiratory failure complicating established chronic obstructive pulmonary disease or asthma, and (3) respiratory failure attributable to abnormalities in ventilatory control or neuromuscular function.

Respiratory Failure in Patients with Previously Normal Lungs

For some years it has been recognized that acute pulmonary injury characterized by extreme degrees of hypoxemia can develop in the course of a wide variety of seemingly unrelated diseases. These have all collectively become identified as the "adult respiratory distress syndrome" (ARDS). This term is justified not in the sense that it defines a common cause, but that it groups widely disparate clinical entities in which a common pathophysiologic mechanism of lung injury exists. The mechanism of injury in turn determines our therapeutic approach. ARDS of any cause is characterized physiologically by increased permeability of the alveolar capillary membrane with resultant interstitial and, at times, alveolar edema. Second, there is marked instability of terminal airways and acinar units so that airway closure may occur prematurely in exhalation. These two phenomena create a classic shunt mechanism through the lung with sequelae as previously outlined. The disorder rarely presents in a subtle fashion — patients are acutely dyspneic, often have a pulmonary edema pattern on chest roentgenogram, and have marked hypoxemia resistant to supplemental oxygen administration. In addition to pulmonary edema caused by left ventricular failure, a number of specific causes of noncardiogenic pulmonary edema have been documented. These include shock, especially when associated with gram-negative sepsis, pulmonary aspiration, pancreatitis, viral pneumonia, uremia, and trauma.

Therapeutic Approach to ARDS. ADEQUATE OXYGENATION. The most immediate threat to the patient with ARDS is irreversible end-organ damage secondary to tissue hypoxia. In particular, the subendocardial portion of the myocardium, brain, and kidneys are susceptible to serious damage. Therefore, the first therapeutic goal is to ensure adequate levels of oxygenation, keeping in mind that the determinants of tissue oxygenation include oxygen loading in the lung, oxygen carrying capacity of the blood, and maintenance of adequate blood flow to critical capillary beds. The initial step in this process is to improve oxygen exchange at the alveolar-capillary membrane. Our therapeutic goal in this setting is to maintain a Pao_2 of 60 mm Hg at the least risk to the patients. At this Pao_2, approximately 90 per cent of available hemoglobin is saturated with oxygen. Raising the Pao_2 to higher levels results in a less than 5 to 6 per cent increase in oxygen content, a marginal gain since one is generally forced to use far more complicated therapy to achieve this additional increment in Pao_2. If adequate oxygenation can be achieved with supplemental oxygen alone, there is no reason to proceed to mechanical ventilation. However, because of the unpredictable fulminant potential of ARDS, serial determinations of arterial blood gases are mandatory.

MECHANICAL VENTILATION. If an adequate Pao_2 cannot be maintained or other indications for intubation develop (such as fatigue or alteration in consciousness), an artificial airway should be established and mechanical ventilation instituted. These patients are usually quite agitated and have very little oxygen reserve — factors which complicate intubation. Therefore, intubation should be carried out in as controlled a fashion as possible. The presence of the best trained personnel available, meticulous attention to oxygenation during the procedure, and judicious use of sedation and neuromuscular blocking agents are all important. A large bore (usually 7 to 8 mm internal diameter) tube equipped with a soft, low compliance cuff should be utilized. We prefer a nasotracheal over an orotracheal insertion since the nasotracheal placement is much more stable and causes fewer problems with oral secretions and patient comfort.

We feel strongly that only volume-cycled ventilators should be used in the setting of ARDS. Pressure-cycled machines generally deliver unpredictable tidal volumes in the setting of ARDS because of the fluctuating changes in lung compliance which characterize this disorder. Relatively large tidal volumes are usually chosen, in the range of 10 ml per kg of body weight. An initial respiratory rate of 10 to 14 is usually sufficient.

Assuming successful establishment of an airway, several important therapeutic decisions now must be made. With the cuffed tube and ventilator it is possible to deliver virtually any concentration of oxygen desired. However, the sustained use of greater than 50 per cent oxygen leads to oxygen toxicity with damage to the alveolar-capillary membrane similar to that already existing in ARDS. We utilize a rule of thumb, the "50-rule," to resolve this dilemma: any patient requiring greater than 50 per cent oxygen to maintain a Pao_2 of 50 mm Hg for longer than 50 hours is at high risk of oxygen toxicity and should be treated with the use of positive end-expiratory pressure (PEEP).

Positive end-expiratory pressure refers to a treatment modality first developed by neonatologists for treating babies with the respiratory distress syndrome. It has been observed that if airway pressures are not permitted to return to baseline atmospheric pressure during the expiratory phase of breathing, a higher resting lung volume is obtained, there is greater stability of airways against terminal closure, and there is a better distribution of ventilation. Most important, this relatively simple modification of ventilatory pattern results in improvement in Pao_2 without resorting to higher concentrations of oxygen. This elegantly simple technique has been one of the most important therapeutic advances in respiratory therapy. We generally start with 5 cm H_2O end-expiratory pressure and increase in increments up to 15 to 20 cm H_2O, always guided by our initial goal of achieving a Pao_2 greater than 50 mm Hg utilizing less than 50 per cent oxygen. Some experts utilize higher levels of end-expiratory pressure, but this should probably be done only at specialized centers. Significant side effects are always possible, particularly at higher levels of PEEP. Elevated intrathoracic pressures are transmitted to the mediastinum and may adversely affect venous return to the heart, thereby leading to decreased cardiac output. High distending pressures coupled with a damaged lung enhance the potential for spontaneous pneumothorax. These pneumothoraces are often under tension, and can be fatal within minutes. A complete thoracostomy set should be at the bedside of any patient being managed with PEEP.

Patients being treated in this manner are often agitated, and the addition of PEEP generally enhances this anxiety. In the past sedation and neuromuscular blockers have been used with success. More recently we have preferred to use a further modification of the ventilator to permit the patient to set his own ventilatory pattern — a system generally known as intermittent mandatory ventilation (IMV). In this system, the patient, the ventilator, and a reservoir bag make up a closed system in which continuous positive airway pressure may be maintained. Patients are allowed to generate spontaneous breaths, and at designated intervals a machine-cycled breath can also be synchronized with the patient's own breathing pattern. This system will often negate the need for potentially dangerous sedative agents.

ASSESSMENT AND CORRECTION OF HEMODYNAMIC ABNORMALITIES. As previously mentioned, establishing an adequate Pao_2 is but one phase of avoiding tissue hypoxia. A variety of factors involved in ARDS make the clinical evaluation of cardiac function and oxygen delivery very difficult. ARDS is frequently associated with hypotension and some degree of renal and possibly cardiac failure. Usually wide fluctuations in fluid balance have taken place, and the use of high distending pressures may adversely affect cardiac function. The best available monitoring plan to guide subsequent therapy is to place a pulmonary artery (Swan-Ganz) catheter and monitor pulmonary capillary wedge pressure, pulmonary artery pressures, and cardiac output. These data allow rational decisions about use of diuretics and fluid administration, and monitor potential harmful effects of ventilatory therapy on cardiac function.

FLUID ADMINISTRATION. Our first priority in administration of fluids is to normalize hemoglobin, thereby maximizing oxygen carrying capacity. Subsequently fluid decisions must be guided by hemodynamic data. Two factors are of special importance. First, ARDS is characterized by an abnormally permeable alveolar-capillary membrane. Therefore, a different relationship may exist between hydrostatic and oncotic pressures, generally favoring capillary leak. Second, it is profoundly difficult in most hospital settings not to have somewhat overhydrated patients with ARDS because of needs for constant medications and the elimination of insensible water loss via the respiratory tract once a patient is being treated with a ventilator equipped with a modern humidification system. Both these factors generally suggest that patients will be relatively overhydrated and in most settings will benefit from diuresis and fluid restriction. The pulmonary artery catheter will often confirm these observations. Careful intake-output charts and daily weights are mandatory.

NUTRITION. Patients with ARDS are generally not previously malnourished and may sustain several days of relative starvation without adverse effect. However, in patients with pre-existing nutritional disorders or those who are in a hypermetabolic state, enteral or peripheral alimentation should be instituted. Modern preparations generally allow this to be done without undue difficulty. One note of caution is that the me-

tabolism of carbohydrate loads in such patients may result in marked increases in CO_2 production which are at times of clinical significance.

CARDIAC MEDICATIONS. There is no convincing evidence that digitalis in the absence of left ventricular failure has a role in the treatment of ARDS. Arrhythmias, particularly atrial tachyarrhythmias, are quite common but are generally related to combined metabolic effects and often quite resistant to antiarrhythmic therapy. Our approach is to not treat with antiarrhythmics unless hemodynamically significant events occur.

SUPERINFECTION. Superinfection is a potentially serious problem. Serial Gram stains and bacterial cultures should be done. We tape initial Gram stain slides in the chart for later comparison.

STEROIDS. The role of steroids is controversial. We tend to use high dose therapy, 40 mg of methylprednisolone sodium succinate (Solu-Medrol) equivalent four times a day, in those patients in whom we judge that a significant inflammatory reaction has occurred.

Withdrawal of Ventilatory Support. Even under the best circumstances the treatment of ARDS may lead to significant complications. It is often not a question of if but rather when a potentially life-threatening complication will ensue. Therefore, constant reassessment of a patient's need for various levels of ventilatory support is mandatory. When a patient stabilizes, it is best to make changes one at a time. We prefer the following schema:

1. If it has been necessary to use greater than 50 per cent oxygen, this should be reduced to approximately 40 per cent inspired oxygen, but no lower.

2. Reduce PEEP in small increments monitoring arterial blood gases carefully.

3. When the patient no longer requires PEEP, ask if any other indications for an artificial airway exist (coma, secretions, need for an imminent surgical procedure). If this is the case, little is to be gained by withdrawal of ventilatory support.

4. Utilize the IMV mode on the ventilator, gradually allowing the patient to control the rate and depth of ventilation. The one danger associated with the use of IMV is its potential to unnecessarily prolong the withdrawal phase. At this stage with a T-piece set up, we measure spontaneous minute ventilation. Usually, minute ventilation will be higher than predicted values owing to increased physiologic dead space. If this value is consistently greater than 10 liters per minute, the patient may not be able to maintain adequate gas exchange without ventilatory sup-

port and may require a tracheostomy if the endotracheal tube has been in place more than 7 to 10 days. If minute ventilation is low, usually also associated with a tendency toward carbon dioxide retention, our attention is drawn to potential extra-pulmonary complications (inadvertent use of sedative drugs, malnutrition, severe metabolic alkalosis, central nervous system disease, hypothyroidism).

5. Patients are generally ready for extubation if adequate levels of oxygenation (Pa_{O_2} >60 mm Hg) can be maintained with less than 50 per cent supplemental oxygen administration, and a normal Pa_{CO_2} is maintained with a minute ventilation less than 10 liters per minute.

Acute Respiratory Failure Complicating Pre-existing Obstructive Lung Disease or Asthma

Based on the pathophysiologic mechanism of respiratory failure in patients with obstructive lung disease, a very different therapeutic approach is followed. In contrast to ARDS, hypoxemia in this setting is generally caused by mismatching of ventilation to perfusion. As previously outlined, this mechanism implies airway disease, often of a reversible nature; most importantly in the acute setting, hypoxemia caused by ventilation-perfusion mismatching is responsive to administration of supplemental oxygen. Put another way, the emphasis in ARDS is to proceed to aggressive ventilator therapy as one of the first orders of business, whereas in the setting of exacerbations of COPD one tries very much to avoid intubation altogether.

The pathophysiology of these exacerbations follows a predictable course. Airway obstruction develops as a result of retained secretions and bronchospasm. The work of breathing is increased, ventilation-perfusion mismatching is exaggerated, and Pa_{O_2} falls. In marked contrast to systemic capillary beds, hypoxemia produces vasoconstriction in the pulmonary capillary bed. The resultant pulmonary hypertension increases the work load of the right ventricle, which has only marginal reserve and quickly fails. This is the setting of cor pulmonale. Initially, although CO_2 production is increased, the patient can compensate by increasing minute ventilation. At some point, variable between individual patients, carbon dioxide retention occurs, resulting in respiratory acidosis.

Therapeutic Approach to Respiratory Failure Complicating Pre-existing Lung Disease. ESTABLISHMENT OF CHRONOLOGY AND PHYSIOLOGIC SEVERITY OF PRESENT ILLNESS. The most pressing problem for the patient, as in all other forms of respiratory failure, is the deleterious effects of hypoxia on various end-organs. Peripheral signs such as cyanosis are useless, and arterial blood gas determinations should be done at the outset. Some assessment of the acuteness versus chronicity of the abnormalities should be assessed. Another "50 rule" is useful. The majority of patients with chronic obstructive lung disease in a stable state, not seeking emergency medical treatment, will not have a Pa_{CO_2} much greater than 55 mm Hg or a Pa_{O_2} less than 50 mm Hg. Further elevations of Pa_{CO_2} will result in more hypoxemia and the entire series of events leading to cor pulmonale will ensue, requiring fairly immediate medical attention. Therefore, one may assume superimposed acute (therefore, potentially reversible) disease in a patient presenting, for example, with a Pa_{CO_2} of 60 and a Pa_{O_2} of 40.

TREATMENT OF HYPOXEMIA. First we establish our therapeutic goal: to achieve a Pa_{O_2} greater than 50 mm Hg at least risk to the patient. In the past there has been hesitation in some circles regarding prompt oxygen therapy. Patients with chronic elevations of Pa_{CO_2} tend to have a blunted ventilatory response to further elevations of Pa_{CO_2}. Their primary stimulus to respiration is hypoxemia. If hypoxemia is suddenly reversed with oxygen therapy, respiratory drive may cease, and the patient will retain carbon dioxide to the point of becoming narcotized. While this phenomenon can occur, it is largely a problem of injudicious use of oxygen, and it should in no way militate against the use of supplemental oxygen to raise the Pa_{O_2} up from virtually life-threatening levels. The judicious use of low flow oxygen has considerably reduced the potential of oxygen-induced carbon dioxide narcosis. Because hypoxemia caused by ventilation-perfusion imbalance is so sensitive to oxygen therapy, most patients will respond satisfactorily to increments in the range of 24 to 40 per cent. Face masks utilizing the Venturi principle are readily available and can precisely deliver 24, 28, 35, and 40 per cent oxygen. We generally start at the 24 per cent level and adjust upward, depending on arterial blood gas determinations. In patients who find these masks uncomfortable, a nasal cannula with oxygen flowing at 1 to 2 liters per minute will in most circumstances result in approximately 30 per cent oxygen. Gradual increments in Pa_{CO_2} can be tolerated as long as adequate supervision of the patient by a trained nursing staff is available.

ASSESSMENT AND TREATMENT OF CAUSE OF CLINICAL EXACERBATION. *Unusual causes of exacerbation*: Consider the possibility of drug intoxication, especially alcohol. A careful perusal of the initial chest x-ray should be done to rule out a small spontaneous pneumothorax, which is often very easy to overlook.

Bronchospasm: Some degree of bronchial hyperreactivity characterizes most exacerbations of COPD and is the chief reversible factor in those with a predominantly asthmatic pattern. Theophylline remains the mainstay of treatment. Important modifications of dose schedules have been developed in the past year. In the past continuous intravenous administration of aminophylline at a rate of 0.9 mg per kg per hour was the standard recommendation. Recent literature has suggested that this is often a dangerous, potentially fatal dose level in the types of patients we are describing. There is extraordinary variability in theophylline kinetics. The serum half-life ranges from 3 to 13 hours in adults, and is unpredictably prolonged in the setting of fever, congestive heart failure, infection, and hepatic dysfunction — all commonly associated with exacerbations of obstructive lung disease. Therefore, determination of serum theophylline levels is important in guiding therapy. One should aim for levels between 10 and 20 micrograms per ml. Therapy should be individualized. However, a loading dose of 6 mg per kg of aminophylline (equivalent to 80 per cent anhydrous theophylline) is the usual intravenous starting dose in a patient not previously being treated with aminophylline. This dose is based on the expectation that each 0.5 mg per kg of theophylline will result in a 1 microgram per ml increase in serum theophylline concentration. Maintenance therapy thereafter should be at 0.6 mg per kg per hour for the first 12 hours, and 0.3 mg per kg per hour thereafter by continuous intravenous infusion. In patients with congestive heart failure or liver disease, this maintenance dose may have to be halved.

Some form of beta-adrenergic drug is also useful. In the hospital setting we prefer the use of aerosolized isoproterenol, 0.5 ml of 1:200 aqueous solution in 5 ml of saline solution, or isoetharine, 0.5 ml in 5 ml of saline solution, administered via an oxygen-powered nebulizer. Administration of aerosolized bronchodilators via IPPB affords no therapeutic advantage and may be a source of superinfection. We initially avoid orally administered beta-adrenergic agents such as terbutaline because of uncertainties of oral absorption in ill patients and the tendency toward significant muscle tremors in patients not previously treated with these agents. In most instances, refractory bronchospasm should be treated with corticosteroids in the range of 60 mg of prednisone equivalent daily.

Infection: Bacterial infection is a common cause of exacerbation of obstructive pulmonary disease. Sputum Gram stains should be evaluated and sputum cultured. Antibiotics effective against *Hemophilus influenzae* are generally used, such as ampicillin or amoxicillin. Other respiratory-borne organisms such as *Legionella pneumophila* may become more important as the clinical features of these illnesses are better defined. Most infected patients will benefit from physiotherapy such as postural drainage and induced coughing to assist in mobilization of secretions. We avoid use of mucolytic agents because of their potential tendency to exacerbate bronchospasm.

Diuretics: Most patients with acute exacerbations of obstructive disease will have significant fluid retention secondary to cor pulmonale. Diuretic therapy, particularly the use of intravenous furosemide, will often be beneficial. We usually start with small doses, approximately 20 mg intravenously, since restoration of adequate arterial oxygen levels often improves cardiac output and renal blood flow so that a spontaneous diuresis ensues. Overzealous use of parenteral furosemide may cause a transient decrease in blood volume and hypotension.

Digitalis: Digitalis glycosides do not have a major role to play in the therapy of right-sided congestive heart failure. Atrial arrhythmias are almost invariably related to hypoxemia and sometimes are a manifestation of aminophylline toxicity. Antiarrhythmics should be reserved for hemodynamically significant events.

MECHANICAL VENTILATION IN ACUTE RESPIRATORY FAILURE COMPLICATING CHRONIC OBSTRUCTIVE PULMONARY DISEASE. Although the majority of patients will not require intubation and mechanical ventilation, some will, and some specialized problems not encountered in treating patients with previously normal lungs may develop. The most common indication in our experience is the patient's inability to adequately clear secretions over a sustained period of time. Other patients will develop carbon dioxide retention resulting in narcosis or acute respiratory acidosis. These patients are usually somewhat somnolent, and intubation is readily accomplished. If some sedation is required, we prefer very small doses of morphine (1 to 4 mg) given intravenously. Institution of mechanical ventilation in these patients can be extremely hazardous, even fatal, if certain physiologic principles are overlooked. Some degree of carbon dioxide retention has almost invariably been present long enough for renal compensatory mechanisms to have partially compensated for respiratory acidosis, primarily by retention of bicarbonate. If a patient is over-ventilated, the precipitous drop in $Paco_2$ in the setting of increased buffer stores in the blood may result in a profound respiratory alkalosis. Transient redistribution of systemic blood flow then ensues, in particular resulting in decreases in cerebral and subendocardial blood flow. Fatal seizures and arrhythmias are common in this setting. Our initial ventilatory settings are generally in the range of 10 ml per kg tidal volume at a rate of 10 to 12 breaths per minute. Blood gases are checked, and all further changes are made based on serial arterial blood gas measurements. We aim for Pao_2 value in the 55 to 60 mm Hg range and $Paco_2$ approximating the patient's preillness steady state, usually being a $Paco_2$ in the 50 to 55 range.

In assessing the patient for withdrawal of ventilatory support we follow many of the steps previously outlined. Assessment of need for artificial airway is made irrespective of the need for mechanical ventilation. Minute ventilation is measured, again recognizing that most patients will not be able to maintain a minute ventilation greater than 10 liters per minute for indefinite periods of time. IMV offers a quantitative approach to this stage of management. This withdrawal process is often more protracted than is the case with previously normal lungs. Whatever process or technique is used, we find it useful to re-establish a day-night cycle for patients. Generally, patients are allowed complete rest at night with no unnecessary ventilator adjustments.

Some patients will be particularly difficult to withdraw from ventilatory support. Usually they will remain hypercarbic despite careful attention to appropriate Pao_2 levels and meticulous attention to relieving airway obstruction. These patients will often be found to have a metabolic alkalosis superimposed on a respiratory acidosis. As a rule of thumb, an arterial pH value of greater than 7.45 with any degree of elevation of $Paco_2$ suggests this type of mixed acid-base disturbance. More precise documentation is available in the form of convenient nomograms expressing "confidence bands" for respiratory versus metabolic alterations in acid-base balance. In this setting ventilatory response to elevated $Paco_2$ is blunted by an alkalotic blood and cerebrospinal fluid. The key feature of this alkalosis is that it is often not self-correcting, primarily because of a lack of a readily available anion, namely chloride, to exchange for bicarbonate in the renal tubules. Aggressive replacement of chloride with potassium chloride, often in the range of 100 mEq daily for 5 to 7 days, is required. Chloride can also be administered in the form of ammonium chloride tablets.

Respiratory Failure Attributable to Abnormalities in Ventilatory Control or Neuromuscular Function

A large diverse group of patients will require ventilatory support not because of any intrinsic abnormality of lung function, but rather because of neuromuscular disease. Examples of varying clinical entities include drug overdoses, neurologic catastrophes such as intracerebral bleeds and trauma, myasthenia gravis, and ascending paralysis. Previous guidelines are largely applicable, keeping in mind that alveolar hypoventilation will be the primary physiologic mechanism involved. Several important pointers peculiar to the management of respiratory failure in patients with muscular disease bear emphasis. Respiratory failure in this setting is very unpredictable, often sudden and catastrophic. If a decision to intubate such patients is deferred, we closely monitor vital capacity at the bedside. A falling vital capacity is usually an indication to intubate. When these patients are being mechanically ventilated, much smaller tidal volumes are used, thus approximating their own stable tidal volumes. Utilization of higher volumes makes withdrawal from assisted ventilation very difficult. Finally, these patients may aspirate, and an abnormal alveolar-arterial oxygen gradient may be an early sign, prior to frank hypoxemia or chest roentgenogram changes.

ATELECTASIS

method of
NICHOLAS T. KOUCHOUKOS, M.D.,
and RICHARD B. McELVEIN, M.D.
Birmingham, Alabama

Atelectasis may be defined as a loss of pulmonary volume resulting from progressive alveolar collapse. It commonly has a segmental or lobar distribution. Occasionally it is a more diffuse process (microatelectasis). Common causes of atelectasis include inflammation, hypoventilation, congestion, emboli, decreased surfactant, and reflex phenomena. If atelectasis persists, fluid accumulation, hemorrhage, areas of hyperinflation, and infection may develop. The resulting hypoxemia and hypercarbia may result in respiratory insufficiency. The diagnosis of atelectasis should be considered when fever, tachypnea, tachycardia, and hypoxemia are present. Characteristic chest roentgenographic findings are not always present. Therapy is directed toward measures to re-expand and maintain aeration of the involved segments.

Compressive Atelectasis

Collapse of pulmonary alveoli can occur from external pressure, and the bronchial tree generally remains patent. A variety of conditions may cause compressive atelectasis: congenital diaphragmatic hernia, eventration of the diaphragm, severe gastrointestinal dilatation, cardiac enlargement or pericardial effusion, large tumors of the chest wall, aneurysms, pneumothorax, hemothorax, pleural effusion, emphysema, congenital or acquired cystic disease of the lung, and intrathoracic tumors. Each of these conditions has its specific therapy.

1. Diaphragmatic or gastrointestinal causes are treated by surgical correction or intestinal decompression.

2. Chest wall, intrathoracic, and intrapulmonary tumors and thoracic aneurysms are treated surgically when possible.

3. Air and fluid are removed from the pleural space by needle or tube thoracostomy and occasionally by thoracotomy.

4. Increased bronchial secretions may result from compressive atelectasis and should be managed appropriately (see below).

Obstructive Atelectasis

This is the most common form of atelectasis and usually results from some degree of obstruction in the bronchial tree, with subsequent absorption of air from alveoli distal to the obstruction. Major causes of obstruction include endobronchial tumors, aspirated foreign bodies, inflammatory stenosis, bleeding and clot formation in a bronchus, and inspissated mucus after chest trauma or major thoracic or abdominal surgical procedures when coughing is ineffective.

The most common cause of obstructive atelectasis is alteration in the ventilatory pattern postoperatively, with persistent shallow respirations and absence of the deep inspiratory and expiratory excursions necessary to maintain alveolar inflation and ventilation.

Treatment. Obstructing tumors and other endobronchial lesions require surgical intervention. Irradiation of unresectable tumors may relieve the associated atelectasis. Foreign bodies, blood clots, or mucous plugs can be removed by bronchoscopy.

Postoperative atelectasis can be anticipated in many patients (e.g., those who are obese, elderly, or heavy smokers, or who have known bronchopulmonary disease) who undergo thoracic or upper abdominal procedures.

PREOPERATIVE TREATMENT. Atelectasis and other postoperative pulmonary complications can be minimized by measures instituted preoperatively.

1. Cessation of smoking for 7 to 10 days before operation to reduce bronchitis and secretions.

2. Coughing and deep breathing exercises with emphasis on forced inspiration (incentive spirometry, sighing) and forced expiration.

3. Expectorants such as potassium iodide or glyceryl guaiacolate (Robitussin) to liquefy thick secretions and promote expectoration. Postural drainage is also helpful.

4. Adequate hydration of the patient and humidification of inspired air.

5. Specific antibiotic therapy if pulmonary infection is present.

6. Bronchodilators and mucolytic agents may be given to patients with significant chronic obstructive lung disease by inhaler or intermittent positive pressure breathing (IPPB).

INTRAOPERATIVE TREATMENT. Operative procedures should be planned to keep anesthesia time to a minimum and should be performed expeditiously. An adequate airway must be maintained with frequent aspiration of secretions. Deep inspiratory volumes should be delivered intermittently to prevent microatelectasis.

POSTOPERATIVE TREATMENT. 1. Postoperatively, patients should be turned hourly, alternating between supine and right and left 90 degree lateral positions. This promotes uneven ventilation and minimizes alveolar collapse.

2. Coughing and deep breathing exercises every 3 to 4 hours or more frequently as necessary. Manual percussion of the chest wall promotes coughing and loosens secretions. Postural drainage is of value when secretions are excessive. Intermittent inhalation of ultrasonically nebulized water or isotonic saline solution also promotes coughing and liquefies secretions.

3. Small doses of narcotics (morphine, meperidine, codeine) at frequent intervals to control pain and permit effective coughing and ventilation. Large doses may depress respiration and should not be used. Intercostal nerve block with 1

to 2 ml of 1 per cent lidocaine (Xylocaine) every 4 to 6 hours can be performed for relief of pain after thoracotomy or chest trauma.

4. Oxygen by nasal catheter or face mask should be administered if arterial hypoxemia is present. The inspired oxygen concentration should be adjusted to obtain an arterial Po_2 of 100 to 150 mm Hg. In patients with chronic obstructive pulmonary disease, a lower arterial Po_2 is desirable (70 to 80 mm Hg) to avoid respiratory depression. Inspired gases should be humidified with distilled water, saline, or prophylene glycol to prevent drying of secretions.

5. Routine intermittent positive-pressure breathing (IPPB) treatments do *not* decrease the incidence of postoperative atelectasis and pneumonitis.

6. Endotracheal suctioning with a nasotracheal catheter should be used only if other methods to promote coughing and expectoration of secretions are unsuccessful. Suction on the catheter should be brief and intermittent to avoid reduction of arterial Po_2.

7. If coughing is ineffective, needle puncture of the cricoid membrane with passage of a polyethylene catheter into the trachea permits instillation of saline and will stimulate coughing.

8. A mucolytic agent such as N-acetylcysteine (Mucomyst) may occasionally be helpful in patients with thick secretions. It can be administered by IPPB or by direct instillation into the tracheobronchial tree. This agent may produce profuse secretions and should be used cautiously in patients who have a depressed coughing reflex.

9. Bronchodilators — isoproterenol (Isuprel), racemic epinephrine (Vaponefrin), or phenylephrine (Bronkosol) — can be administered by nebulizer or IPPB when bronchospasm is present. Aminophylline may be administered intravenously (250 mg over 10 to 15 minutes). These agents should be used cautiously in patients with cardiac disease.

10. If the secretions are purulent, culture and sensitivity studies should be obtained and appropriate antibiotics administered for 7 to 10 days.

11. Bronchoscopy with rigid or fiberoptic instruments is occasionally indicated when the atelectasis is refractory to the measures listed above.

12. Abdominal distention is relieved by insertion of a nasogastric tube and early removal of restrictive bandages.

13. Endotracheal intubation or tracheostomy with ventilatory support may be necessary for patients with persisting respiratory insufficiency.

Congestive Atelectasis (Adult Respiratory Distress Syndrome)

The adult respiratory distress syndrome is seen after major trauma or surgery associated with multiple transfusions or administration of large volumes of intravenous fluid, with hypotension, and with sepsis or septic shock. It can also be seen after cardiac surgical procedures, renal transplantation, and severe burns. Clinically, there may be tachypnea, tachycardia, dyspnea, and cyanosis. Roentgenographic features are variable, and initially there may be no evidence of pulmonary infiltration. As the disorder becomes more severe, hypoxemia becomes progressive, with evidence of severe ventilation-perfusion abnormalities. In severe cases, hypoxemia becomes unresponsive to a high inspired oxygen concentration, and death may result. The major histologic features are a marked increase in lung water, interstitial and intra-alveolar hemorrhage, and vascular congestion. Varying degrees of alveolar edema and alveolar collapse are present. The term congestive atelectasis has been used to describe these pathologic findings.

Treatment. Mechanical ventilatory support with positive end-expiratory pressure is essential for therapy of most patients with the acute respiratory distress syndrome. This should be continued until the respiratory failure is corrected and ventilation and oxygenation return to normal.

1. Positive end-expiratory pressure is essential to maintain the functional residual capacity of the lungs above the critical closing volume and, thereby, to minimize atelectasis and alteration in ventilation-perfusion ratios.

2. The arterial Po_2 should be maintained above 60 to 70 mm Hg, and the inspired oxygen concentration should be adjusted to achieve this value. High concentrations of oxygen should be avoided to minimize the possibility of oxygen toxicity.

3. Fluid volume overload, a contributing factor to this entity, should be avoided. When excessive fluid is present, diuresis with furosemide (Lasix) or ethracrynic acid (Edecrin) intravenously can result in an increase in arterial Po_2 and a decrease in the aveolar-arterial oxygen gradient.

4. Specific antibiotics to treat known pulmonary or other infections are necessary.

5. Tracheostomy may be indicated if prolonged ventilatory support is required.

6. Prolonged extracorporeal support with a pump-oxygenator has been successfully applied in some cases, but it is considered experimental at present.

CHRONIC BRONCHITIS, BRONCHIECTASIS, AND EMPHYSEMA

method of
JOHN E. HODGKIN, M.D.
Loma Linda, California

The term chronic obstructive pulmonary disease (COPD) refers to those diseases characterized by increased resistance to flow in the airways of the lungs, generally resulting in dyspnea, wheezing, and cough productive of sputum. This term includes such entities as chronic bronchitis, emphysema, asthma, and bronchiectasis.

Chronic bronchitis has been defined as a disease characterized by daily productive cough for at least 3 months each year for 2 successive years when there are no other diseases present to account for these symptoms. *Emphysema* is characterized morphologically by an increase in alveolar size associated with destruction of the walls of the air spaces distal to the terminal bronchioles. Terms commonly applied to the chronic bronchitic and to the emphysema patient are blue bloater and pink puffer, respectively; however, the majority of patients have a combination of these entities rather than solely one or the other pathologic process.

Bronchiectasis is characterized by dilation of the segmental or subsegmental bronchi. This dilation may be reversible, as occurs following pneumonia; however, with repeated infections permanent destruction of the integrity of the wall of the bronchi occurs with resultant permanent cylindrical or saccular dilation. Common manifestations of bronchiectasis include cough productive of copious amounts of mucopurulent sputum (particularly in the morning), hemoptysis, and recurrent lower respiratory infections.

This article will deal with the management of patients with obstructive airway disease. Since patients usually have a combination of these disorders, the management described is generally applicable regardless of the precise etiology and pathogenesis of the airway obstruction.

FUNDAMENTALS OF MANAGEMENT

General Measures

Patient and Family Education. A patient's compliance should be enhanced by carefully explaining to the patient and key persons responsible for the patient's care information regarding the disease process and treatment recommended. The patient should be told what type of pulmonary disorder is present and how that disease affects function. Each component of the patient's comprehensive care program — for example, reasons for the medications prescribed, their side effects and proper administration — should be discussed.

Determination of Goals. Realistic goals for the patient should be determined after a thorough evaluation of the patient's problems. The patient should be told what areas of impaired function are likely with his or her degree of disability. Helping the patient and others understand what goals are reasonable is essential so that discouragement does not develop as a result of unrealistic expectations.

Avoidance of Smoking. Not only is smoking a major factor in the etiology of chronic obstructive pulmonary disease, it also aggravates symptoms and signs of the respiratory disorder. Each patient should be strongly encouraged to stop smoking as an integral part of the treatment plan. Cessation of smoking usually results in decreased airway inflammation, less sputum, reduced cough, improvement in appetite, and sometimes improvement in pulmonary function.

Encouraging the patient to make a definite commitment to quit is important in achieving smoking cessation. A variety of programs aimed at smoking cessation are available. The usual success rate for continued nonsmoking at the end of 1 year for most programs averages around 20 to 30 per cent. Probably the most effective technique is for the patient's physician to provide strong encouragement and support for avoidance of smoking. Although for most smokers it is best to break the habit abruptly, a gradual reduction in consumption may work for others.

Constant nagging is counterproductive and often leads to patient frustration and hostility. The physician should never refuse to take care of a patient because the patient is unable to quit smoking, since most persons can be helped significantly even if they are not able to quit totally.

Cooperation and support by family members is essential. It is particularly difficult for the patient to quit smoking if another member of the family smokes.

If the patient is unable to stop smoking completely, at least the risk can be reduced by (1) choosing a cigarette with less tar and nicotine, (2) taking fewer draws on each cigarette, (3) decreasing the depth of inhalation, (4) throwing away the cigarette before smoking it all the way down, and (5) reducing the number of cigarettes smoked per day.

Avoidance of Other Inhaled Irritants. A careful history is important to discover other forms of inhaled pollutants which may cause airway irritation. Exposure to dust, fumes, mists, and gases not only irritates the airway but can add to the health hazards of cigarette smoking.

When air pollution levels are particularly high, the patient should avoid outdoor physical activity and stay indoors with the doors and windows closed. In areas where air pollution or inhaled particulates are prevalent, the use of filtering systems should be considered. High efficiency particulate air (hepa) filters and electrostatic filters help remove particulate matter from the air. Offending fumes, odors, or gas pollutants, e.g., oxides of nitrogen and ozone, can be removed by activated charcoal filters. If possible, it is, of course, advisable for a patient with obstructive airway disease to move out of a highly polluted area.

Avoidance of Infection. Since respiratory infections may not only exacerbate a patient's status but produce irreversible damage, patients with chronic obstructive pulmonary disease (COPD) should avoid exposure to those with respiratory tract infections. When influenza or other respiratory infections are prevalent, it is best to avoid large gatherings. Since influenza is particularly prone to produce respiratory deterioration in COPD patients, it is advisable for the patient to get an annual influenza immunization (unless the patient is allergic to eggs or has had a previous allergic reaction to the vaccine). Since pneumococcal pneumonia can also result in significant respiratory distress, the COPD patient should receive the vaccine against *Streptococcus pneumoniae* (pneumococcus). A pneumococcal vaccine should probably not be administered more frequently than every 3 years to avoid significant reactions to the vaccine.

Proper Environment. Patients residing in very hot or very cold environments are more likely to be symptomatic. An air conditioner is helpful for patients exposed to hot weather, while a cold weather mask or scarf may help patients who must go outside during excessively cold weather. Exceptionally dry or humid climates also lead to increased symptoms. A humidifier should be used during the winter in cold climates (since heating the air also results in drying of the air) and also in hot, dry areas. The optimal humidity for mucociliary function is approximately 30 to 50 per cent.

Since high altitude results in a lower inspired oxygen tension, patients with significant hypoxemia may benefit by moving to a lower altitude. If the patient intends to fly in a commercial airliner, the physician should remember that such travel exposes persons to an altitude equivalent to 5000 to 8000 feet, so supplemental oxygen might be required.

Adequate Hydration. Adequate fluid intake is probably the best method for liquefying sputum. Those patients who are dehydrated or who are having difficulty clearing sputum should be encouraged to increase their daily fluid intake. A trial of 8 to 10 glasses (2 to 2½ quarts) of fluid per day seems reasonable. The physician, of course, must always be alert to the possibility of fluid overload. Excessively hot or cold fluids should be avoided, since they can lead to exacerbations of airway obstruction.

Proper Nutrition. Patients with COPD commonly complain of anorexia as a result of air swallowing associated with dyspnea and ingestion of medications that impair the appetite. A reducing diet for obese patients can help decrease the work of breathing. In those patients with progressive weight loss associated with their COPD, a high protein diet with multiple small feedings (between-meal feedings and a bedtime snack) will help improve caloric intake. In any patient in whom nutritional intake seems to be impaired, supplemental vitamins should be considered. In the patient who develops significant dyspnea while eating, supplemental oxygen may help to relieve the dyspnea, thus allowing for improved food intake. A dietitian can recommend a proper nutritional pattern after carefully evaluating the patient's dietary habits.

Immunotherapy. The use of immunotherapy (also called desensitization) has been promoted for years. Immunotherapy involves treating allergic respiratory disease by injections of extracts of those antigens thought to be responsible for the illness. Nonspecific immunizations against molds, dust, and bacterial antigens have never been demonstrated to be effective and are not recommended. Immunotherapy is not helpful for the usual patient with chronic bronchitis, emphysema, bronchiectasis, or adult onset asthma, and should only be considered when there is definite evidence that the allergens to be used in the injections indeed contribute to the disease.

Medications

Bronchodilators. A trial of bronchodilators should be intitiated in any patient with obstructive airway disease. Their administration should not be reserved for acute attacks but should be used on a chronic basis, since significant airway obstruction often persists even though the patient is virtually asymptomatic. A wide variety of bronchodilator drugs are available, with these medications divided into several categories:

BETA-AGONIST SYMPATHOMIMETIC PREPARATIONS. Sympathomimetic preparations activate adenyl cyclase, leading to increased production of cyclic AMP. The increased level of cyclic AMP results in relaxation of smooth muscle in the wall of the airway, as well as inhibition of the release of mediators of bronchospasm such as histamine and SRS-A. Beta-agonist drugs have also been shown to enhance tracheal mucus velocity, which should help with clearance of airway secretions.

Sympathomimetic preparations which stimulate beta$_2$ sympathetic receptor sites are preferable, since they result in bronchodilation while avoiding beta$_1$ cardiovascular side effects. Certain of the new beta$_2$-type stimulators, e.g., metaproterenol and terbutaline, are resistant to the enzyme catechol-O-methyl transferase (COMT), thus resulting in a longer duration of action than the older beta-agonist agents.

Those sympathomimetic medications with more beta$_2$ effect than ephedrine (which has been in bronchodilator preparations for many years) are as follows:

1. Isoetharine mesylate. Available as: (a) Cartridge inhaler. Usual dose: 1 to 2 whiffs every 3 to 4 hours. (b) Solution for aerosolization. Usual dose: 0.25 to 0.5 ml per 3.0 ml H$_2$O every 3 to 4 hours.

2. Metaproterenol sulfate. Available as: (a) Cartridge inhaler. Usual dose: 1 to 2 whiffs every 3 to 4 hours. (b) Tablets (10 mg, 20 mg). Usual dose: 10 to 20 mg three to four times daily. (c) Liquid (10 mg per teaspoonful). Usual dose: 10 to 20 mg three to four times daily.

3. Terbutaline sulfate. Available as: (a) Tablets (2.5 mg, 5.0 mg). Usual dose: 2.5 to 5 mg three times daily. (b) Injectable (1 mg per ml; 2 ml amp). Usual dose: 0.25 ml subcutaneously every 4 to 6 hours (not to exceed 0.5 ml per 4 hours).

4. Certain purer beta$_2$ stimulators, such as salbutamol and fenoterol, are being used elsewhere in the world. It is hoped that they will soon be available in the United States, since they produce sustained bronchodilation while minimizing undesirable cardiovascular side effects.

Since beta$_2$ receptor sites are also present in skeletal muscle, some beta$_2$ stimulators, e.g., terbutaline sulfate, result in tremor. This problem can usually be minimized by reducing the dose of the medication and continuing therapy for several weeks.

XANTHINE COMPOUNDS. Xanthine or aminophylline-like preparations inhibit the enzyme phosphodiesterase, thus blocking the breakdown of cyclic AMP. Theophylline preparations, then, have a synergistic effect when used with sympathomimetic agents, since they enhance cyclic AMP levels by a different mechanism. The major toxic side effects of xanthine drugs include nausea, vomiting, anorexia, irritability, personali-

ty changes, and seizures. Optimal bronchodilation, while avoiding undesirable side effects, is achieved when the serum or plasma theophylline level is in the range of 10 to 20 micrograms per ml. A blood theophylline level should be checked in any patient whose bronchospasm does not seem to be relieved satisfactorily or whenever side effects suggestive of theophylline toxicity are present.

Certain factors affect the amount of theophylline required to achieve optimal blood levels. The dose required is reduced by such things as old age, congestive heart failure, liver disease, and antimicrobials such as erythromycin and oleandomycin, while increased doses are needed in young people, smokers, and those taking barbiturates.

Numerous salts of aminophylline are available, which may help to avoid gastric irritation resulting from aminophylline. The development of pure anhydrous theophylline preparations represents a significant advance in bronchodilator therapy. Not only do these preparations result in a more constant blood level of theophylline, thus minimizing peaks and valleys in the theophylline effect, but they have a longer duration of action so that the preparation need only be taken two or three times daily. See Tables 1 and 2 for recommended dosages for intravenous and oral aminophylline/theophylline therapy.

PARASYMPATHOLYTIC AGENTS. Parasympatholytic agents such as atropine and its derivatives have been used in other countries as bronchodilators. When atropine derivatives that avoid some of the undesirable side effects of atropine do become available, they may offer another avenue for bronchodilator therapy.

The use of medications containing a combination of ingredients is no longer desirable. Ephedrine is the sympathomimetic agent commonly included in combination preparations and, in addition to its being a weak bronchodilator, it results in such undesirable side effects as insomnia, cardiovascular stimulation, tremor, and urinary retention in elderly males with prostatic hypertrophy. In addition, combination preparations do not allow one to increase or decrease the amount of aminophylline being administered in order to achieve an optimal blood theophylline level. Furthermore, the combination preparations usually include a barbiturate or tranquilizer to calm down the adverse stimulation of the ephedrine.

Bronchodilators are particularly beneficial in patients with bronchospasm who have spirometrically demonstrated bronchodilator improvement; however, every patient with chronic obstructive pulmonary disease deserves a trial of

TABLE 1. **Dosage Guidelines for Theophylline Products: Intravenous Aminophylline Dosage for Patients Not Currently Receiving Theophylline Preparations***

	LOADING DOSE†	MAINTENANCE DOSE† FOR NEXT 12 HOURS	MAINTENANCE DOSE† BEYOND 12 HOURS
Children 6 months to 9 years	6 mg/kg	1.2 mg/kg/hr	1.0 mg/kg/hr
Children age 9–16 and young adult smokers	6 mg/kg	1.0 mg/kg/hr	0.8 mg/kg/hr
Otherwise healthy nonsmoking adults	6 mg/kg	0.7 mg/kg/hr	0.5 mg/kg/hr
Older patients and patients with cor pulmonale	6 mg/kg	0.6 mg/kg/hr	0.3 mg/kg/hr
Patients with congestive heart failure or liver disease	6 mg/kg	0.5 mg/kg/hr	0.1–0.2 mg/kg/hr

*From FDA Drug Bulletin, *10*:1, 4–6, February 1980.
†Based on estimated lean (ideal) body weight.

bronchodilators whether or not the spirogram shows acute improvement after bronchodilator inhalation. If there is no subjective or objective evidence of benefit from bronchodilator medication after several months of use, it would then be justifiable to reserve their use for acute exacerbations.

Inhalation of sympathomimetic agents has the advantage of a quicker response to the drug, while avoiding some of the systemic side effects of oral ingestion of the same agent. A logical approach to initial bronchodilator therapy would be to combine an inhaled sympathomimetic-type agent with a long-acting anhydrous theophylline oral preparation. If this combination of agents does not seem to be providing satisfactory relief from the effects of the airway obstruction, it would then be legitimate to add an oral beta$_2$-type sympathomimetic agent.

Expectorants. Water is the safest and least expensive agent available to help liquefy secretions. Guaifenesin (glyceryl guaiacolate), 100 to 200 mg four times daily, and saturated solution of potassium iodide (SSKI), 10 to 20 drops in juice four times daily, have been used for a long time with little scientific evidence to support their use. Both drugs can produce gastric irritation, and SSKI has other significant side effects such as skin rash, swelling of salivary glands, and precipitation of hypothyroidism. If in spite of adequate hydration and good bronchodilator therapy the patient is still having difficulty expectorating sputum, a trial of guaifenesin for several weeks would be warranted. However, it should not be continued indefinitely unless there is evidence for therapeutic efficacy.

Although preparations that suppress cough, e.g., codeine-containing compounds, may impair clearance of secretions and so should be prescribed cautiously, they are sometimes helpful for those with a persistent hacking cough that results in increasing airway inflammation and trouble sleeping. Antihistamines may dry airway secretions, making sputum expectoration more difficult; however, in some patients with allergic rhinitis they can be beneficial in minimizing nasal congestion and postnasal drainage.

Antimicrobials. Although sputum in patients with acute respiratory infections commonly grows out "usual flora," *Hemophilus influenzae*, or *Streptococcus pneumoniae*, antimicrobial therapy is often beneficial. At the first sign of a respiratory infection involving the airway, e.g., increase in sputum production and purulence, change in sputum color to yellow or green, or increased cough, antimicrobial agents should be initiated. Agents useful in treating these acute respiratory infections include the following:

1. Tetracycline, 500 mg four times daily for 2 days, then 250 mg four times daily for 5 to 8 days.

2. Ampicillin, 500 mg four times daily for 2 days, then 250 mg four times daily for 5 to 8 days.

3. Amoxicillin, 500 mg three times daily for 2 days, then 250 mg three times daily for 5 to 8 days.

TABLE 2. **Dosage Guidelines for Theophylline Products: Oral Anhydrous Theophylline Dosage for Patients Not Currently Receiving Theophylline Preparations***

1. Starting dose:† Begin with a dose of 16 mg/kg/day or 400 mg/day, whichever is less.
2. Maintenance dose:† Increase dose, if tolerated, in approximately 25 per cent increments at 3 day intervals, to age-related levels needed for therapeutic effects. Dosage should not be exceeded without measurement of serum theophylline levels.

Age < 9 years	24 mg/kg/day
Age 9–11 years	20 mg/kg/day
Age 12–16 years	18 mg/kg/day
Age > 16 years	13 mg/kg/day or 900 mg/day, whichever is less

*From Physicians' Desk Reference. Oradell, N.J., Medical Economics Company, 1980.
†Based on estimated lean (ideal) body weight, and generally divided into every 12 hour doses.

4. Doxycycline hyclate (Vibramycin), 100 mg every 12 hours on the first day, then 100 mg daily for 6 to 9 days.

5. Trimethoprim and sulfamethoxazole (Bactrim, Septra), 1 double-strength tablet every 12 hours for 7 to 10 days.

Antimicrobials should be taken an hour before or 2 hours after meals or milk or antacid ingestion to avoid interference with absorption of these agents. Taking the medication with small amounts of food, e.g., crackers, helps to avoid the abdominal discomfort which sometimes occurs.

If the patient does not seem to be responding to empiric antimicrobial therapy or appears acutely ill with high fever, hemoptysis, or chest pain, a sputum Gram stain and culture should be obtained. In this situation one should also consider analyzing the sputum for eosinophils, e.g., with a wet-mount preparation or Wright stain, since yellow-green sputum may signify allergy rather than infection.

Corticosteroids. Corticosteroids are especially helpful in those persons with intermittent attacks of bronchospasm, particularly when associated with blood or sputum eosinophilia. For an acute exacerbation related to allergy, it would be appropriate to start out with 60 mg of prednisone daily for several days, e.g., until significant improvement has occurred, with the dose being tapered by decrements of 5 mg per day until none is given; however, in some patients with obstructive airway disease, particularly those with asthma, it is necessary to maintain low maintenance doses of prednisone, e.g., 5 to 10 mg per day for weeks to months to provide satisfactory relief from symptoms. Using alternate day prednisone, e.g., giving two to three times the daily dose every other morning, has been shown to significantly reduce systemic side effects. A major advance in corticosteroid therapy for patients with asthma occurred with release of beclomethasone dipropionate for inhalation. This provides the benefit of steroids but significantly reduces systemic side effects. Beclomethasone will be discussed further under Aerosol Therapy.

Long-term corticosteroid therapy for patients with stable chronic bronchitis or emphysema without bronchospasm is of no demonstrable value and increases the risk for opportunistic infection in addition to other serious systemic side effects. A short-term trial of prednisone may be warranted in COPD patients with exacerbations who are not responding to such measures as adequate hydration, bronchodilators, and antimicrobials.

Cromolyn Sodium. Cromolyn sodium may reduce the need for corticosteroids in younger patients with asthma. Inhalation of this agent apparently stabilizes mast cells, thus preventing the release of mediators of bronchospasm. The recommended dosage is inhalation of powder from a 20 mg capsule four times daily with at least a 1 month trial. This agent is not helpful in patients with stable pulmonary emphysema and chronic bronchitis and is generally not beneficial for patients with adult-onset asthma. Inhalation of a bronchodilator 5 to 10 minutes prior to cromolyn sodium inhalation can lessen the potential for coughing induced by inhalation of the cromolyn and may result in improved deposition.

Digitalis. Digitalis is definitely helpful for those patients with left ventricular failure; however, there is little evidence to support its use for pure cor pulmonale. This drug should be given cautiously to patients with COPD, since hypoxemia enhances the risk of digitalis toxicity. Digoxin is an ideal form of digitalis to use, since its effects are not as long-lasting as other preparations, e.g., digitoxin, in case digitalis toxicity develops. A usual maintenance dose for digoxin in the COPD patient would be 0.125 to 0.25 mg per day. Blood digoxin levels can be monitored, with the therapeutic range considered to be 1 to 2 nanograms per ml; however, digitalis toxicity can occur in spite of normal or even reduced digoxin blood levels, so these only provide a guide to digoxin administration.

Diuretics. Diuretics are helpful in patients with left ventricular or right ventricular decompensation. Certain medications such as thiazides and furosemide (Lasix) may precipitate hypokalemia, hypochloremia, and metabolic alkalosis. Both hypokalemia and metabolic alkalosis increase the risk of digitalis toxicity and cardiac arrhythmias. Metabolic alkalosis may also result in compensatory hypoventilation. The combination of triamterene (Dyrenium) with a thiazide helps conserve potassium, thus lessening the risk of hypokalemia and metabolic alkalosis.

Certain foods with increased amounts of potassium, e.g., raisins, prunes, avocados, bananas, oranges, apricots, squash, and potatoes, if eaten regularly, will diminish the problem of potassium depletion. Numerous potassium chloride supplements are available; however, most of these have an undesirable taste and can result in nausea and gastric distress. In any patient receiving diuretic therapy, serum electrolytes should be measured to make certain that potassium depletion does not occur.

Psychopharmacologic Agents. The use of psychopharmacologic agents may be necessary when a patient's emotional disturbance does not respond to usual counseling, reassurance, and emotional support. Many of these agents can result in diminished ventilation from respiratory center depression. Certain antidepressants, i.e., amitriptyline (Elavil, Amitril) and protriptyline (Vivactil), may dry secretions because of anticholinergic and antihistaminic effects. These two antidepressants may also cause cardiac arrhythmias. Desipramine (Pertofrane, Norpramin) and doxepin HCl (Sinequan) have much less anticholinergic effect and are thus safer in elderly COPD patients.

Anxiolytic agents, e.g., chlordiazepoxide HCl (Librium), hydroxyzine HCl (Atarax, Vistaril), and diazepam (Valium), may be helpful in the patient who is anxious, nervous, and emotionally upset.

As a general rule, the older the patient, the lower the dose of psychopharmacologic agent that is advisable. In many elderly COPD patients, the dose of psychoactive medication will be one third or less of that normally prescribed. The dosage range, therapeutic indications, and significant side effects should be reviewed in the appropriate literature by any physician ordering these preparations.

Respiratory Therapy Techniques

Respiratory therapy techniques which are commonly used for patients with pulmonary disease include aerosol therapy, intermittent positive pressure breathing (IPPB) treatments, and oxygen therapy. Each of these will be discussed individually.

Aerosol Therapy. BRONCHODILATORS. Inhalation of bronchodilators is particularly effective in patients with bronchospasm. A variety of devices are available for aerosolization of bronchodilators, including metered-dosage cartridge inhalers, hand-bulb nebulizers, compressor pumps, and IPPB machines.

Cartridge inhalers containing a variety of different sympathomimetic agents are available. Although inhalation of strong $beta_1$ stimulators, e.g., epinephrine and isoproterenol, can work very quickly to reverse bronchospasm, inhalation of $beta_2$-type agents such as metaproterenol may result in a more sustained bronchodilating effect while avoiding adverse cardiovascular side effects of the $beta_1$ agents. Cartridge inhalers are very convenient to use; however, they should be prescribed only for patients judged to be responsible for correct use, since overuse can result in a high concentration of the drug being inhaled with resultant cardiovascular side effects.

Hand-bulb nebulizers are inexpensive and allow for varying the dosage of bronchodilator to be administered; however, muscle fatigue or lack of hand coordination can be a limiting factor in elderly patients. A compressor pump nebulizer allows for alteration in the dose of bronchodilator

being administered; i.e., the concentration and amount of drug to be administered can be varied. This device is much less expensive than an IPPB machine and works satisfactorily to aerosolize bronchodilator in patients able to take deep breaths spontaneously.

BLAND MIST SOLUTIONS. Aerosolization of bland mist is commonly used, particularly in the hospital in an attempt to liquefy thick secretions. Solutions containing 3 to 5 per cent saline, 3 to 6 per cent sodium bicarbonate, or 3 to 10 per cent propylene glycol have been commonly used in an attempt to deposit liquid in the airways, thus assisting in sputum liquefaction. A variety of devices ranging from heated nebulizers to ultrasonic equipment have been used.

There is very little evidence that inhalation of bland mist does indeed liquefy airway secretions, aiding in their mobilization. A trial of bland mist inhalation is warranted in those patients having trouble expectorating thick, tenacious sputum. Unless such a trial is shown to have definite therapeutic benefit, bland mist aerosol generators should not be sent home with patients. These nebulizers are particularly prone to contamination with bacteria and, if used, the equipment must be regularly cleaned.

MUCOLYTIC AGENTS. Inhalation of acetylcysteine (Mucomyst) has been used in an attempt to liquefy thick sputum. Once again, there is little scientific evidence to support the use of this modality. A trial of acetylcysteine inhalation may be warranted in patients not responding to good hydration, bronchodilator therapy, antimicrobials, and physical therapy techniques. If used, the acetylcysteine should always be inhaled along with a bronchodilator, since aerosolization of this medication alone can provoke bronchospasm.

CORTICOSTEROIDS. Inhalation of beclomethasone dipropionate is a major advance in the treatment of patients with reactive airway disease. This agent provides the topical benefit of corticosteroid therapy while virtually eliminating systemic side effects. Monilia infection of the mouth and throat has been observed in a small number of patients inhaling corticosteroid aerosols. Gargling with water immediately after inhalation of the steroid may help decrease the tendency for Monilia infection and topical irritation from the steroid. Nystatin oral suspension along with cessation of the steroid inhalation rapidly clears up any oral Monilia infection. Hoarseness has also been occasionally reported and is reversed on cessation of steroid inhalation. The usual dose for beclomethasone inhalation is one or two inhalations from the cartridge inhaler three to four times per day (initially starting with two inhalations four times daily). With the implementation of beclomethasone inhalation, many patients who were previously prednisone dependent have been able to eliminate the oral corticosteroid completely or at least get by satisfactorily on alternate day or low dose daily prednisone therapy, thus eliminating significant systemic side effects.

ANTIMICROBIALS. Aerosolization of antimicrobials should be used only rarely. This method of administration does not take the place of oral or parenteral use, and there is no evidence that combining it with systemic therapy is of value in treating respiratory infections. Occasionally, a patient with significant obstructive airway disease, e.g., bronchiectasis or cystic fibrosis, may develop recurrent Pseudomonas pneumonias with the sputum remaining infected with the organism in spite of parenteral therapy. In this type of patient, aerosolization of gentamicin may eliminate the Pseudomonas colonized in the airway, helping reduce the frequency of Pseudomonas respiratory infections. (This use of gentamicin is not listed in the manufacturer's official directive.) This form of therapy can result in the development of resistant organisms and should only rarely be considered.

Intermittent Positive Pressure Breathing (IPPB). IPPB has been promoted for the prevention or treatment of atelectasis as well as for aerosolization of medications. There is no evidence that IPPB is helpful with prevention or treatment of atelectasis in patients who are able to take deep inhalations spontaneously. In those with difficulty taking deep breaths, e.g., patients with prominent obesity, neuromuscular disturbances, and restrictive disorders, a trial of IPPB would be indicated when other measures have not been successful in preventing or reversing atelectasis.

There is no scientific evidence that IPPB more effectively delivers bronchodilator medication than simpler aerosol devices in the usual patient with COPD. IPPB for medication administration should be considered only in patients who are unwilling to take or incapable of taking deep breaths spontaneously. In those patients with severe airway obstruction caused by a large amount of thick, tenacious secretions or severe bronchospasm, IPPB may help them inhale the bronchodilator more effectively than they can with spontaneous effort alone. When IPPB is ordered, tidal volumes in the range of 12 to 15 ml per kg of body weight should be achieved with the IPPB device. The tidal volume being delivered should be measured to ensure that the IPPB device is indeed delivering tidal volumes in this range. IPPB should be considered only for bronchodilator aerosolization in those patients in whom less expensive devices have been shown to be unsuccessful.

Oxygen Therapy. Oxygen should be considered for patients with an arterial oxygen tension (Pao_2) less than 55 mm Hg, particularly when associated with polycythemia, pulmonary hypertension, or cor pulmonale. A reduction in Pao_2 is the primary reason for the development of pulmonary hypertension and cor pulmonale in patients with COPD. Patients with obstructive airway disease associated with prominent hypoxemia (Pao_2 less than 55 mm Hg) have shown improvement in psychologic testing, motor coordination, and sleep pattern with the addition of continuous low concentration oxygen to their program. Oxygen has also been demonstrated to be helpful in those patients unable to exercise because of hypoxemia-induced arrhythmias or lactic acid accumulation. Continuous long-term low-flow oxygen has been shown to prolong the life span of hypoxemic patients with associated polycythemia and carbon dioxide retention.

One should remember that a patient's Pao_2 is often considerably lower when asleep than when awake. Such complaints as sleeplessness, irritability, and headache may be indicative of severe hypoxemia at night. Sleep-induced apnea episodes caused by upper airway obstruction, central neurologic causes, or a combination of these may also lead to severe hypoxemia at night. If the Pao_2 is less than 50 mm Hg, the patient should be considered for continuous low-flow oxygen therapy.

The risk of oxygen flows greater than 2 liters per minute or an inspired oxygen concentration (FIo_2) greater than 28 per cent in patients with chronic CO_2 retention should be explained to the patient and the family, since these patients may be dependent upon a hypoxic drive to breathe. In the presence of chronic CO_2 retention, one should strive to establish a Pao_2 in the range of 55 to 60 mm Hg so as to eliminate severe hypoxemia and yet maintain a hypoxic drive. Higher Pao_2s may lead to increased hypoventilation, worsening respiratory acidosis, and respiratory deterioration.

The most convenient device for administration of oxygen is the nasal cannula (nasal prongs). More precise levels of oxygen can be administered by using Venturi-type masks; however, these are less acceptable to the patient, since they cover both the nose and mouth. Portable oxygen using liquid oxygen or an E-cylinder on wheels can allow the patient with severe hypoxemia to get out of the house for activities. Devices that extract nitrogen from the air, thus resulting in increased amounts of oxygen in the air, are available. In patients using oxygen continuously, particularly when high flows of oxygen are involved, these devices may be more economical than using cylinders of oxygen.

It is presently thought that oxygen is needed for at least 12 to 15 hours per day in order to prevent or reverse pulmonary hypertension and cor pulmonale. Further studies are in progress to help answer this question more definitively.

Physical Therapy Techniques

Relaxation Techniques. A variety of techniques have been proposed to help the patient relax. Such things as consciously attempting to relax muscles while in a comfortable position in a quiet room or listening to soothing music with the eyes closed may help the patient relax, thus reducing stress.

Breathing Retraining. Inhalation through the nose while relaxing the abdominal muscles, followed by a slow expiration through pursed lips aided by abdominal muscle contraction, can improve ventilation, reduce respiratory rate, and decrease the alveolar to arterial oxygen difference. This slowing of the respiratory rate can help the patient with COPD during episodes of dyspnea and during exercise.

Chest Percussion and Postural Bronchial Drainage. In those patients with excessive amounts of thick, tenacious sputum, i.e., greater than 30 ml per day, chest percussion techniques in combination with postural positioning may assist in expectoration of the sputum. A variety of techniques for accomplishing chest percussion are available, including clapping with cupped hands and vibration with the hands or a mechanical device. A variety of positions have been described to assist in draining specific lung areas. Preceding the postural drainage with inhalation of bronchodilator and bland mist may aid in clearance of the secretions.

Conditioning Exercises. Exercise training has been repeatedly demonstrated to improve physical endurance of patients with obstructive airway disease. Patients with COPD should definitely be encouraged to exercise to prevent their muscles from becoming progressively weaker, resulting in increased disability. An exercise program should be prescribed, with the patients instructed to exercise for 20 to 30 minutes several days each week at an intensity that approximates 60 to 80 per cent of their maximal oxygen consumption (about 70 to 85 per cent of their achievable maximal heart rate).

IN-HOSPITAL MANAGEMENT OF COPD

When the patient with COPD is sick enough to require hospital admission, all the measures discussed in the preceding paragraphs should be applied intensively. Parenteral therapy should be considered, rather than oral administration, in the acutely ill patient, to ensure adequate blood levels of the medications. Vigorous chest physiotherapy in conjunction with nasotracheal suctioning can improve gas exchange in those patients with airways plugged with thick secretions.

In an occasional COPD patient with acute respiratory failure, intubation and assisted ventilation become necessary. Vigorous application of the therapeutic modalities already discussed is generally sufficient to reverse the respiratory deterioration; however, the following would suggest that intubation is indicated: (1) arrhythmias or cardiovascular collapse; (2) decreasing level of consciousness; (3) worsening muscle fatigue in spite of vigorous therapy; (4) increasing acidosis (decreasing pH) in spite of vigorous therapy; (5) inability to oxygenate the patient adequately on low-flow oxygen; (6) inability to remove secretions from obstructed airways in spite of nasotracheal suctioning, chest physiotherapy, and/or flexible fiberoptic bronchoscopy.

The services of allied health personnel, important in the outpatient setting, are crucial for successful management of the hospitalized patient with respiratory decompensation.

PRIMARY LUNG CANCER

method of
JOHN L. POOL, M.D.
Wilton, Connecticut

The worldwide epidemic of lung cancer is a phenomenon of this century and increasing year by year. The ratio of male to female approaches one to one, and within 5 years primary lung cancer will be the leading cause of cancer deaths in both sexes. Cigarette smoking is the major etiologic factor in over 80 per cent of patients and greatly increases the co-carcinogen effect of such industrial pollutants as asbestos fibers and coke furnace emissions. As the overall 5 year survival is less than 10 per cent, prevention by correcting the smoking habits of all patients seen by physicians is just as important as treating the established disease. People listen to what physicians say to them directly and individually, and of course the doctor and his office staff should practice what he advocates.

Surveys of high risk populations by chest x-ray and sputum cytology of men over 45 years who smoke two packages of cigarettes a day have yielded 7 cancers per 1000 examinations initially, and 3 per 1000 yearly thereafter. Five year surgical salvage for asymptomatic cancer approaches 80 per cent, but is only 8 to 10 per cent after hemoptysis or other respiratory complaint. Positive sputum cytology in a patient with a negative chest x-ray leaves the expectant surgeon in a quandary because he does not know where the cancer is, and, of course, the malignant cell could come from the nasopharynx, the larynx, the trachea, or anywhere in the lower respiratory tract. Careful bronchoscopic exploration of all major branches of both lungs must be carried out. Washings, brushings, and biopsies in an orderly way are mandatory, and no thoracotomy can be undertaken until the surgeon exactly identifies the site of the malignant cells.

When a coin lesion is found in the parenchyma of the lung, its identification becomes a detective job. First, the previous films must be compared to see if this lesion is new or has been previously present. Change in size can indicate rate of growth. The primary lung cancer of low malignancy may change very little in a 5 year span, but this is unusual. On the other hand, such a benign lesion as a hamartoma also enlarges. The radiographic characteristics of the coin lesion are important. Rigler pointed out that a crescent toward the hilum of the lung is suggestive of primary as opposed to metastatic lung cancer and the S curve of an atelectatic lobe or segment identifies hilar adenopathy concomitant with atelectasis. The coin lesion contour may be absolutely smooth in granulomas and cysts and mucous plugs. In cancer, it is usually slightly crenelated. The presence of calcium within the coin lesion as determined tomographically can identify granuloma only when there is a true central nidus or onion skin periphery. Cancer occurs in scars which may have calcifications eccentric to the shadow. Computerized tomography (CT) helps identify the location and multiplicity of coin lesions within the lung substance but cannot determine histology.

When lung cancer is suspected in a patient, diagnosis must be established. This can be done about 80 per cent of the time by sputum cytology. It can also be accomplished by bronchoscopic biopsy or bronchial washing or brushing and by aspiration biopsy through the intact chest wall under fluoroscopy, by biopsy of a metastatic deposit such as an enlarged cervical node, or by open thoracotomy. Treatment has a sound basis only when a histologic diagnosis has been achieved. Primary and secondary cancer can usually be differentiated. Histologic characteristics influence prognosis. The well-differentiated

epidermoid carcinoma offers the best prognosis; terminal bronchiolar carcinoma and adenocarcinoma, which are more prone to hematogenous spread, offer a poorer prognosis; oat cell carcinoma is practically incurable by any method currently available.

The International Union Against Cancer and the American Joint Commission on Cancer Staging and End Result Reporting have developed a staging system to improve accuracy of diagnosis and comparability of diagnostic and therapeutic measures (Tables 1 and 2). The tumor size and location, the presence of intrathoracic nodal metastases, and the presence of other metastases are charted as T, N, and M, and combinations provide three stages of increasing tumor burden. In the lung clinical staging is defined to include history, physical, review of all types of chest x-rays, bronchoscopy, neck node biopsy, mediastinoscopy, bone scan, brain scan, blood chemistries (especially of liver function),

TABLE 1. **The Definitions of T, N, and M Categories for Carcinoma of the Lung**

T: Primary Tumors

T0 No evidence of primary tumor.

TX Tumor proved by the presence of malignant cells in bronchopulmonary secretions but not visualized roentgenographically or bronchoscopically.

TIS Carcinoma in situ.

T1 A tumor that is 3.0 cm or less in greatest diameter, surrounded by lung or visceral pleura and without evidence of invasion proximal to a lobar bronchus at bronchoscopy.

T2 A tumor more than 3.0 cm in greatest diameter, or a tumor of any size which invades the visceral pleura or, with its associated atelectasis or obstructive pneumonitis, extends to the hilar region. At bronchoscopy the proximal extent of demonstrable tumor must be within a lobar bronchus or at least 2.0 cm distal to the carina. Any associated atelectasis or obstructive pneumonitis must involve less than an entire lung, and there must be no pleural effusion.

T3 A tumor of any size with direct extension into an adjacent structure such as the chest wall, the diaphragm, or the mediastinum and its contents; or bronchoscopically demonstrated to involve a main bronchus less than 2.0 cm distal to the carina; any tumor associated with atelectasis or obstructive pneumonitis of an entire lung or pleural effusion.

N: Regional Lymph Nodes

N0 No demonstrable metastasis to regional lymph nodes.

N1 Metastasis to lymph nodes in the peribronchial and/or the ipsilateral hilar region (including direct extension).

N2 Metastasis to lymph nodes in the mediastinum.

M: Distant Metastasis

M0 No distant metastasis.

M1 Distant metastasis such as in scalene, cervical, or contralateral hilar lymph nodes, contralateral lung, brain, bones, liver.

TABLE 2. **The Stages in Carcinoma of the Lung**

Occult carcinoma	
TX N0 M0	An occult carcinoma with bronchopulmonary secretions containing malignant cells but without other evidence of the primary tumor or evidence of metastasis to the regional lymph nodes or distant metastasis.
Stage I	
TIS N0 M0	Carcinoma in situ.
T1 N0 M0	A tumor that can be classified T1 without
T1 N1 M0	any metastasis or with metastasis to the
T2 N0 M0	lymph nodes in the ipsilateral hilar region only, or a tumor that can be classified T2 without any metastasis to nodes or distant metastasis. *Note:* TX, N1, M0 and T0 N1 M0 are also theoretically possible, but such a clinical diagnosis would be difficult if not impossible to make. If such a diagnosis is made, it should be included in Stage I.
Stage II	
T2 N1 M0	A tumor classified as T2 with metastasis to the lymph nodes in the ipsilateral hilar region only.
Stage III	
T3 with any N or M	Any tumor more extensive than T2, or
N2 with T or M	any tumor with metastasis to the lymph nodes in the mediastinum, or with distant
M1 with any T or N	metastasis.

and bone marrow biopsy. Not necessarily all these areas must be examined in order to stage a particular patient with lung cancer, but they may be employed in a clinical staging. Surgical staging includes all of the above plus an exploratory thoracotomy, and pathologic staging includes all of the above plus examination of the removed primary site or an autopsy investigation.

Surgery is without question the treatment of choice for cancer confined to one lung or part of that lung. Prior to contemplated surgery, careful history, repeated physical examinations, and some laboratory tests will determine the possibility of extrathoracic spread. X-ray studies of the chest in various projections, particularly as compared with prior films if any exist, help determine the extent of the gross pathologic condition. CT scan is invaluable in demonstrating invasion of mediastinum or chest wall and the presence of small effusions. I do not believe that bone x-rays are worthwhile unless the patient has a specific bone-related complaint. Scanning techniques may detect metastatic deposits in brain and vertebrae, the most common sites of extrathoracic spread, although fairly large deposits can remain

undetected until the passage of time and serial scans clarify the issue. Abnormal blood chemistry findings pinpoint the need for further evaluation of a given organ or area. Exploratory laparotomy in search of metastatic lung cancer need be done only if there is evidence of some abnormality in the history or laboratory findings. When in doubt, more sophisticated studies combining tomography, arteriography, and ultrasonography will prove reliable. The same is true for diagnostic x-rays of other organ systems.

The extent of endobronchial disease can be determined at bronchoscopy, and routine biopsy of the mucosa of the main carina may reveal unsuspected submucosal lymphatic cancer in 4 per cent, precluding "cure" by resection.

Scalene nodes, when palpable, will almost always show metastatic cancer, but when impalpable, metastasis is found in only 5 per cent of nodes microscopically examined. Mediastinoscopy or anterior mediastinotomy can detect invasion of mediastinal tissue and contralateral node metastasis, which would also preclude cure by resection. Contrast visualization of the vena cava as well as the pulmonary artery and veins in frontal and lateral projections is vital in determining the hilar and mediastinal extent of the cancer. Pulmonary veins can be evaluated only by cinefluorography. All these special diagnostic studies are reserved for problem cases of marginal resectability. Pulmonary function must be evaluated so that the surgeon will know the maximal amount of lung tissue he can resect without leaving his patient incapacitated.

Treatment prior to surgery includes (1) cessation of smoking and (2) proper instruction in breathing and coughing. Postural drainage may be required. Bronchial spasm may be relieved by oral bronchodilators and expectorants such as oxtriphylline and guaifenesin (Brondecon), 1 tablet four times daily. Cleansing of the lower respiratory tract can be aided by aerosol inhalations with a current of compressed air or oxygen via ultrasonic nebulizer or intermittent positive pressure apparatus. In the presence of bronchial spasm, bronchodilators and sympathomimetic amines will often open the bronchus to allow passage of mucolytic agents. Isoetharine (Bronkosol), 0.5 ml in 1.5 ml saline solution aerosol for 3 minutes, serves well. Acetylcysteine in 5 to 20 per cent solution in saline or freshly prepared pancreatic dornase delivered in this manner will help liquefy thick secretions. Each treatment should not last more than 10 minutes; it can be repeated four or five times a day. Appropriate antibiotic therapy after determination of bacteria in sputum culture and their sensitivity is important. Before cultural characteristics are known, oxytetracycline (Terramycin), 100 mg in 1 ml of isotonic saline added to the aerosol, can speed clearing of infection from major bronchial tubes. With pulmonary resection contemplated, even in the absence of positive sputum culture, antibiotic treatment over the period of surgery is advisable. At present, cephalothin is most likely to protect against the most probable contaminants. A suggested course is to give 500 mg intravenously 6 hours prior to surgery, at the time of surgery, and every 6 hours thereafter for 48 hours, and then stop.

Preoperative treatment with radiation has not proved valuable statistically when cancericidial doses of 4000 R or more have been employed, and surgical complications have more than doubled. Studies by Bromley and Szur and by Roswit and Shields demonstrate that radiation can destroy the lung cancer and that the resected specimen shows no residual neoplasm, but that 3 years later there is no increased salvage over patients treated by surgery alone. There is some evidence that 2000 or 2400 R of high voltage radiation to the tumor site and adjacent pulmonary hilum followed by resection provides a setting in which fewer distant metastases appear. In the special superior sulcus position of lung cancer, preoperative radiation appears to enhance the long-term survival of the resected patients.

The overall 5 year survival after resectional surgery across the country is about 25 to 30 per cent. Some factors that enhance the chance for long survival in the individual patient are as follows: (1) chance-found, asymptomatic cancer; (2) a slow rate of growth as seen on serial x-rays, especially a doubling time of more than 12 months; (3) small size, that is, less than 3 cm in diameter; (4) a low-grade squamous or epidermoid cancer even though in a major bronchus; (5) a polypoid cancer; (6) location of the cancer in the substance of the lung rather than near the hilum or periphery; and (7) cancer in an upper rather than lower lobe. Factors which are adverse include (1) size, especially over 7 cm in diameter; (2) undifferentiated cancer; (3) oat cell cancer; (4) short duration of symptoms, especially pain; (5) rapid change in chest x-ray; and (6) invasion of the chest wall, though still resectable. Factors which do not appear to influence the outcome of surgery include the side involved, the sex, and the patient's age.

The extent of surgery performed in relation to that particular patient's cancer influences the long-term results. Evidence is beginning to accumulate that a careful block removal of the mediastinal lymph nodes draining the involved lung or lobe adds to the chance of survival. The patients benefited are those in whom pulmonary nodes contain metastasis but the mediastinal nodes are free. In 295 resections, some comparisons seem valid. When the cancer could be removed by lobectomy and no mediastinal node dissection was carried out, the salvage was 30.2 per cent at 5 years when the intrapulmonary nodes contained no metastasis and 7.7 per cent when such nodes were positive. Those patients who had a concomitant mediastinal node dissection showed comparable figures of 60.0 per cent and 38.8 per cent. At pneumonectomy when no mediastinal dissection was carried out, the figures were 54 per cent with nodes negative and 10 per cent with nodes positive. Finally, when a careful pulmonary and mediastinal cleanout was accomplished in one specimen, the salvage was 50.0 per cent when no nodes contained cancer, but fell to 28.8 per cent when nodes did contain cancer. There is even a 12 per cent 5 year survival for patients subjected to radical pneumonectomy or lobectomy in whom some mediastinal nodes contain metastatic disease. Extension of metastatic cancer to contralateral mediastinal nodes, as is sometimes discovered at mediastinoscopy, means that cure cannot be achieved. Resection should be carried out when the chest wall is invaded in an area that is technically removable, including the entirety of involved ribs, as spread occurs along the marrow. About a 10 per cent 5 year salvage will ensue. Similarly, invasion of the pericardium in a resectable area will yield some salvage. Sleeve resection of a main bronchus or even a short tracheal segment allows removal of some hilar cancers with preservation of better pulmonary reserve and a one in four chance of long-term life. In essence, lobectomy with appropriate mediastinal node dissection remains the standard procedure with additions for special circumstances.

Palliative Treatment for the Primary Site

Not every patient with proved lung cancer is a candidate for pulmonary resection. Unfortunately, less than 40 per cent of all patients can be offered surgery. Of those offered surgery three quarters or more actually have resection. The contraindications to exploratory thoracotomy are (1) evidence of extrathoracic metastasis, (2) superior vena caval blockage or angiographic evidence of direct invasion of the superior vena cava, (3) pleural fluid containing cancer cells, (4) paralysis of either vocal cord, (5) paralysis of the diaphragm when the phrenic nerve involvement is not on a resectable portion of the pericardium, (6) invasion of the paranodal tissues of the mediastinum, (7) direct invasion of the esophagus, (8) invasion of the vertebral body except in the special instance of superior sulcus tumor, (9) proved coronary occlusion within 3 months, and (10) insufficient pulmonary reserve to support the patient after the necessary resection. When the lung cancer is invading the superior vena cava, the esophagus, and the direct tissues of the superior mediastinum, heroic resection will not yield worthwhile palliation. On the other hand, palliative resection is worthwhile in a few situations in which the total cancer cannot be resected, as in the presence of a lung abscess distal to a stenotic bronchus where the mediastinum is frozen, or in the presence of severe hemoptysis, even though this may be from oat cell cancer not otherwise considered worthwhile to remove.

Palliation of symptoms of a nonresectable primary lung cancer is achieved principally with radiation therapy. I believe that practically all lung cancers that are not resected should receive a course of supervoltage radiation carefully limited to the primary site and the lymph node drainage area within the mediastinum. When first diagnosed, even though the patient is asymptomatic, a dose of not more than 4500 R in 4 weeks should be administered. The disagreeable complications of radiation esophagitis, tracheitis, and dermatitis that ensue from too rapid or too intense treatment can be avoided. Radiation pneumonitis and pulmonary fibrosis may be prevented by treatment planning that excludes normal lung tissue. The rate of growth at the primary site can be checked. Blocked bronchi will often open, and at least some of the pain of chest wall and mediastinal invasion can be alleviated. Another method of palliation at the primary site is the implantation of a radioactive isotope such as 125-iodine when resection cannot be done. Ten per cent of such patients will survive 5 years, and in practically all those treated in whom the primary site is less than 7 cm in diameter, worthwhile tumor shrinkage is achieved and the median survival rises to 14 months as compared to 9 for those receiving radiation externally and 5 for exploratory thoracotomy alone.

Malignant Pleural Effusion

The identification of cancer cells in an effusion complicating lung cancer means a fatal outcome, because the cancer cells will have already spread into the lymphatics leading to the prevertebral space along the intercostal route. Thoracentesis with complete removal of the fluid, which may require more than one tap if the volume is more than 1500 ml, and the immediate instillation of a sclerosing agent can produce pleural seal and stop this aspect of the cancer activity. The lung must be able to expand to fill the space as the fluid is withdrawn. In my experience nitrogen mustard, 10 to 20 mg freshly prepared in 30 ml

of water, is most efficacious. This drug is destroyed if shaken vigorously and should be used within 5 minutes of preparation. Right after injection, turning the patient in different positions will spread the medication. If all the fluid cannot be readily aspirated, perhaps because of fibrin balls or a concomitant air leak, closed thoracotomy and high suction (30 to 60 cm of water) until no more fluid is drained and the lung is fully expanded will almost always be effective. The nitrogen mustard is then instilled through the tubing, and pleural adhesion can be expected to occur. The tube is left clamped for 2 hours, and then high suction is applied once again until no fluid is withdrawn and the tube can be removed. Tetracycline (1.0 to 1.5 grams in 100 ml of water) may also be used, but other agents have not done as well in my hands. In a patient whose lung is captive by a surface layer of cancer cells or fibrin and whose general health is strong, decortication and partial parietal pleurectomy to eliminate the pleural effusion can be most satisfactory.

Superior Vena Caval Blockage

The presence of severe edema of face and orbits, distention of neck veins, and head and neck cyanosis, accompanied by respiratory embarrassment and severe blockage of the superior vena cava or innominate veins, is life-threatening. Limitation of salt intake to 2 grams a day and the use of diuretics (hydrochlorothiazide, 50 mg twice a day) and steroids (prednisone, 40 to 60 mg a day) give temporary relief, but irradiation to the involved mediastinum is the most important treatment. I do not believe that the addition of chemotherapeutic agents speeds tumor shrinkage. Thrombus forms readily in the occluded superior vena cava and may propagate through the innominate veins as far as the axillary and block the developing collateral, seriously aggravating the symptoms of venous obstruction. Preventive measures include adequate water intake and meticulous care of the upper extremities, with special attention to the nails and axillae to prevent infection. Venipuncture should not be practiced in either arm. In my opinion anticoagulant therapy should be employed prophylactically from the moment superior vena caval obstruction is diagnosed. Rapid heparinization by the intravenous route can be accomplished by using a dose between 5000 and 10,000 units every 4 to 6 hours and aiming for a clotting time of 30 minutes at 3 hours after the heparin injection, and after a few days by concomitantly introducing an oral agent such as bishydroxycoumarin (Dicumarol) in a dose of 275 mg (100 mg, 100 mg, 75 mg) the first day, and then a maintenance dose of 25 to 75 mg a day to maintain a prothrombin time of 25 seconds. A surgical bypass graft of saphenous vein to axillary vein has been reported successful.

Hormone-Producing Lung Cancers

Certain lung cancers alter the patient's metabolic climate. Their recognition is important, both because a hormone abnormality may herald unsuspected lung cancer and because treatment of lung cancer may relieve the symptoms and dangers of the hormone overproduction. Adrenal cortical hyperplasia caused by tumor production of ACTH and leading to the cushingoid syndrome can be abated by removal or destruction of the primary cancer or by bilateral adrenalectomy. The symptoms of an antidiuretic hormone, often with neurologic complaints and demonstrated by hyponatremia, is controlled by water restriction. Unrecognized hypercalcemia resulting from parahormone production by the tumor or parathyroid hyperplasia is the hormone abnormality most likely to be exaggerated when the cancer is treated by radiation or chemotherapy. Psychic symptoms, anorexia, and changes in urinary habits are suggestive, and the calcium level should be brought down to 12 mg per 100 ml before starting radiation, especially to bone metastases. Hyperuricemia must also be looked for during radiation therapy; it is best handled with allopurinol, 200 mg two or three times a day.

Neurologic manifestations, myopathies, and Guillain-Barré syndrome are at times not due to metastasis and in such instances removal of the primary neoplasm dramatically corrects the neuromuscular deficits.

Extrathoracic Metastases

The physician following a patient with known primary lung cancer, whether resected or not, must be constantly alert to the subtle development of extrathoracic organ metastasis, especially to brain and bones. Examination at monthly intervals for the first year and at longer intervals thereafter is important in this regard. Serial scans are helpful in spotting metastasis, and when suspected can be confirmed by arteriography and needle biopsy.

Metastasis or new primary cancer occurs in the second lung in nearly one fifth of patients surviving 5 to 10 years after a successful resection and can occasionally be removed. Otherwise, treatment must be symptomatic.

Brain metastases are so universally multiple that resectional techniques have not proved useful, and radiation should include the entire brain. There is a 70 per cent chance that worthwhile palliation will follow. Relief of bone pain by accurately placed radiation is dramatic and need not wait scan or x-ray verification of bone destruction. Similar treatment for liver metastasis has been fraught with more complications than value except in instances of severe pain caused by rapid growth of the hepatic deposits.

Treatment of Oat Cell Carcinoma

The usual presentation of this histologic type is with a small primary site, huge mediastinal node metastases, and early extension to brain, bone marrow, and throughout the body. After definite establishment of the histologic type, radiation therapy to known disease has been the practice with rapid shrinkage, but prompt recurrence of incompletely destroyed cancer. Combination chemotherapy recently offers median survival of over a year and some patients alive and disease free at 3 years. One such program includes cyclophosphamide, doxorubicin, vincristine, CCNU, VP-16, procarbazine, cisplatin, and methotrexate. Radiation therapy is reserved for prophylactic total brain irradiation and treatment after chemotherapy failure.

Chemotherapy and Immunotherapy in Non–Oat Cell Carcinoma

Prophylactic chemotherapy after successful surgery for cure has not yielded increased numbers of survivors, but McKneally has found intrapleural bacille Calmette-Guérin (BCG) leads to fewer and later recurrences. Single agent chemotherapy is less effective than multiple agent regimens in relieving symptoms for inoperable lung cancer patients. The latter may produce significant objective response in half the patients treated with a definite improved performance status at the penalty of drug reactions. There are no complete responders. On the other hand, steroids (prednisone, 45 to 125 mg a day) relieve laryngeal and lower respiratory tract and brain edema dramatically, even though long-range use has demonstrated a slightly shortened life span. Analgesics must be rotated and varied. Mood elevators such as amitriptyline (Elavil), 25 mg three to four times a day, can be helpful. The most important aspect of long-term comfort for the patient with fatal lung cancer is the continued concern of his physician and the maintenance of care by one physician so that the patient does not feel shunted among internist, surgeon, and radiation therapist.

COCCIDIOIDOMYCOSIS

method of
PIERCE GARDNER, M.D.,
and MARGARET TIPPLE, M.D.
Chicago, Illinois

Judgments regarding therapy revolve around an understanding of the pathophysiology and natural history of coccidioidomycosis. It is estimated that each year 35,000 people living in the semiarid regions of the southwestern and western United States become infected by the fungus *Coccidioides immitis.* With rare exceptions the infection occurs by inhalation of dust containing *C. immitis* arthrospores, which evoke an inflammatory response in the terminal bronchioles and alveoli. This response is generally so mild that in the majority of infections no clinical disease is recognized. When symptomatic respiratory infection occurs, the illness most commonly resembles mild influenza, although a spectrum of illnesses, including severe bronchopneumonia, may be seen. In approximately 2 per cent of patients with pulmonary infections residual solid or cavitary lesions persist on subsequent roentgenologic examination.

Dissemination of endospores from the lung to extrapulmonary sites via the bloodstream is a serious but rare event, occurring in approximately 0.05 to 0.2 per cent of primary infections. The mortality of untreated disseminated coccidioidomycosis approaches 50 per cent, with skin, bone, central nervous system, and abdominal viscera being the most frequently involved organs.

Race, sex, and age appear to be important variables in the host response to infection by *C. immitis.* The risk of severe pneumonia and disseminated disease appears to be greatly increased among blacks and Filipinos, among males (and pregnant females), and among the very young, the elderly, and the immunocompromised. The incidence of allergic manifestations (erythema nodosum, arthralgia, fever) appears to be greatest among Caucasian women.

General Measures

1. Bed rest during symptomatic illness.
2. Patients with pulmonary coccidioidomycosis need not be isolated, because endospores in the sputum are not infectious for man. However, in patients with disseminated coccidioidomycosis with draining wounds or osteomyelitis, there is a small risk of fomite transmission owing to the formation of arthrospores in dressings or cast material; therefore, medical personnel should wear masks during cast or dressing changes.
3. Symptomatic relief of cough and pain.
4. Symptomatic relief of allergic manifestations (erythema nodosum, arthralgia, fever). Although a short course of corticosteroids (40 mg of prednisone per day tapered over 7 days) may provide dramatic relief of symptoms in patients with severe symptoms, relief usually can be obtained with safer drugs such as aspirin.
5. Although coccidioidomycosis is generally not considered to be one of the "opportunistic" fungi, in patients with severe pulmonary or disseminated coccidioidomycosis a search should be made for underlying disease such as diabetes mellitus, malignancy, or problems with immune response (especially cell-mediated delayed immunity).
6. In patients receiving immunosuppressive therapy for any reason, attempts should be made to reduce such therapy to the lowest level consistent with adequate treatment of the underlying problem.

Specific Therapy

Indications for Therapy. Although the great majority of patients with coccidioidomycosis recover spontaneously, specific antifungal therapy should be administered to patients who have severe forms of infection or who are at high risk of developing serious infections. These patients include virtually all patients with disseminated coccidioidomycosis as well as patients with severe progressive primary pulmonary disease. High risk patients, such as blacks, Filipinos, pregnant women, infants, and the elderly and debilitated, should be considered for therapy early in the course of illness. Prior to initiation of specific antifungal therapy a bone scan and cerebrospinal fluid examination to evaluate the most common sites of disseminated infection should be considered.

Amphotericin B. Amphotericin B remains the primary drug in the treatment of *C. immitis* infections, although both its toxicity and its less than uniform success rate have encouraged continued search for better drugs.

METHOD OF ADMINISTRATION. Amphotericin B is an antibiotic with both fungistatic and fungicidal activity against fungi with sterol-containing cell membranes. It is poorly absorbed from the gastrointestinal tract, so intravenous administration is required for the therapy of systemic fungal disease. In addition to its inherent toxicity, the drug (a lyophilized powder which is relatively insoluble) is difficult to administer. In order to minimize problems of administration, the following procedure is recommended:

1. Dissolve the contents of the vial (50 mg) in 10 ml sterile distilled water. This requires great patience and vigorous shaking.

2. Add the contents of the vial to 500 ml 5 per cent dextrose in water (final concentration 0.1 mg per ml). Do not use saline solutions or distilled water with preservatives, because these may cause precipitation of the antibiotic. If precipitation is visible, discard the bottle and begin again. Addition of sterile phosphate buffer to correct the initial acid pH of some commercial 5 per cent dextrose in water (D5/W) preparations may help avoid problems of precipitation. The solution should be protected from direct sunlight, although wrapping with foil is generally unnecessary.

3. In order to minimize the risk of thrombophlebitis, administer the drug through a pediatric scalp vein needle; inject 10 mg hydrocortisone succinate directly into the intravenous tubing prior to infusion; and flush the tubing with D5/W following the infusion.

4. In order to minimize the acute adverse effects of amphotericin B (fever, chills, nausea, vomiting, headache, flushing, anxiety), premedicate the patient with aspirin, 0.6 gram orally, and an antiemetic (promethazine, 25 mg orally or intramuscularly) approximately one half hour prior to beginning the infusion.

5. The recommended time for infusion is 4 to 6 hours (although some reports suggest no greater incidence of adverse reactions with shorter infusion periods, 45 to 60 minutes). If in-line membrane filters are used for the intravenous infusion of amphotericin B, they should not be less than 1.0 micron in order to assure passage of the drug.

DOSAGE. Following a test dose of 1 mg, 0.25 mg per kg is administered on the first day, followed by daily increments of 0.25 mg per kg until the full daily dose of 0.5 to 0.7 mg per kg is reached.

CHRONIC TOXICITY. Since decreased renal function occurs in approximately 80 per cent of patients receiving intravenous amphotericin B, renal function tests (creatinine clearance, blood urea nitrogen) and urine sediment should be monitored closely. Hypokalemia resulting from increased urinary potassium loss generally can be corrected by oral potassium supplements, and alkali therapy is indicated in patients who develop renal tubular acidosis. Normochromic normocytic anemia is common but rarely requires transfusions. Although acute toxic hepatitis is uncommon, when it occurs amphotericin B must be discontinued.

DURATION OF THERAPY AND FOLLOW-UP. The usual total dose of amphotericin B is 2 to 3 grams, although larger doses (up to 7 grams) may be required in difficult cases. The most useful parameters to follow are the clinical course and the immunologic status. Successful therapy is usually accompanied by the appearance of a positive skin test to coccidioidin (1:100) and a decrease in complement fixing antibody titer to less than 1:32. Early or late dissemination or relapse may occur and is generally preceded by a rising complement fixing antibody titer. Therefore, this test should be performed regularly in patients who have had severe coccidioidomycosis; if a rise in titer is noted, retreatment with amphotericin B should be considered.

LOCAL THERAPY. Local irrigation of wounds and sinuses with 10 mg of amphotericin B in 5 per cent dextrose in water has been a useful adjunct to systemic therapy, allowing a greater concentration of drug in the infected sites without increasing the systemic toxicity. (This specific use of amphotericin B is not listed in the manufacturer's official directive.)

Combined intravenous and intrathecal (investigational for this use) amphotericin B offers the best hope of recovery from coccidioidal meningitis. The drug is irritating to the meninges, and in order to minimize arachnoiditis the drug (0.5 mg in 5 ml cerebrospinal fluid) should be injected into the cisterna magna or into the lateral ventricle via a reservoir. Duration of therapy is decided by the clinical course and immunologic status, but intrathecal therapy (at lengthening intervals) is often necessary for 3 or more years.

Miconazole. Miconazole is an imidazole drug with activity against *C. immitis*. Favorable experience in humans with severe coccidioidomycosis has been reported, but a high relapse rate has limited its usefulness. In patients with severe renal toxicity, excessive side effects, or failure to respond to amphotericin B, miconazole is the alternative drug of choice. When used to treat coccidioidal meningitis, the poor cerebrospinal fluid penetration of miconazole requires that the drug be administered intrathecally as well as intravenously. No serious renal or hepatic toxicity has been reported, although phlebitis, pruritus, nausea, and fever and chills are common. Hyponatremia, anemia, thrombocytosis, rouleaux formation, interactions with coumarin drugs, and hyperlipidemia have been reported.

ADMINISTRATION AND DOSAGE. The dose of miconazole for coccidioidomycosis is 1800 to 3600 mg per day (in children, 20 to 40 mg per kg per day) administered intravenously in divided every 8 hour doses, each infusion given over a 30 to 60 minute period (a dose of 15 mg per kg per infusion should not be exceeded). The duration of therapy has not been established, but 3 to 12 weeks or longer has been suggested, depending on the type of infection and the clinical response.

Surgical Therapy. Surgical resection is indicated for residual pulmonary lesions that are cavitary and cause significant hemoptysis, rupture into the pleural cavity, or produce severe local symptoms. Likewise, nodular lesions suggesting malignant disease should be removed for diagnostic purposes. Surgical drainage or resection of local skin or bone infections is often a valuable adjunct to systemic and local use of amphotericin B.

Future Possibilities. Ketoconazole is a recently developed imidazole drug which appears to be about five times more active than miconazole in vitro against *C. immitis* and has shown promise in some patients with coccidioidomycosis. Toxicity studies indicate that liver function test abnormalities may result, and the drug has not yet been approved by the Food and Drug Administration. Transfer factor from sensitized to human T cells has reportedly been successful in treating certain patients with disseminated coccidioidomycosis. These potential advances in the treatment of disseminated coccidioidomycosis are undergoing further evaluation but must be considered experimental at present.

HISTOPLASMOSIS

method of
ROBERT H. ALFORD, M.D.
Nashville, Tennessee

Clinical Manifestations

Initial Infection. In highly endemic areas, initial Histoplasma infections usually occur during childhood, but are more likely later in life in less endemic regions. Initial infections, although usually asymptomatic, may cause a flu-like illness. Areas of patchy granulomatous pneumonitis may develop with associated regional hilar or paratracheal adenopathy. Self-limited dissemination is the rule, judging by the prevalence of healed Histoplasma granulomas in autopsied spleens from the endemic area. Heavy inocula can produce multiple areas of pneumonitis which may eventually calcify, resulting in inconsequential "buckshot" calcification on chest radiographs. After a 10 to

18 day incubation period, very large inocula can cause acute pulmonary illness with fever, nonproductive cough, dyspnea, and infrequently pulmonary insufficiency to the point of cyanosis. Even highly symptomatic cases are usually self-limited, so that antifungal chemotherapy is not required. However, extremely heavy inocula, immunologic immaturity (infants), and immunologic incompetence (e.g., lymphomas), may promote rapidly progressive primary infection with dissemination and a fatal outcome without therapy.

Reinfection. Reinfection with Histoplasma causes disease modified by the degree of persisting fungal immunity. Illness resembling initial infection may result. After a shorter incubation period (7 to 10 days), heavy inocula may still cause pneumonitis, which is usually self-limited over days to weeks, having an acute onset of cough, fever, malaise, dyspnea, and rarely impaired oxygen diffusion. Large inocula in the fully immune person may produce diffuse hypersensitivity-like pneumonitis with less hilar adenopathy than initial infections, occasionally with smaller discrete granulomatous foci which may give a miliary appearance on x-ray.

Progressive Histoplasmosis. Progressive histoplasmosis is usually chronic in nature with the unusual exceptions mentioned above. Chronic pulmonary histoplasmosis, the most frequently encountered symptomatic form of the disease, develops uncommonly almost exclusively in middle-aged white males with underlying chronic obstructive pulmonary disease. Episodes of destructive segmental or lobar (usually upper) granulomatous pneumonitis which have a tendency to cavity formation, contraction, fibrosis, and compensatory emphysema tend to recur often in adjacent lung segments. Rarely, chronic progressive disseminated histoplasmosis evolves in adults of either sex and all races, with fever; weakness; weight loss; hepatosplenomegaly; leukopenia; mucous membrane ulceration involving oropharynx, tongue, and larynx; and, in up to 50 per cent, eventual adrenal insufficiency.

Treatment

The only antifungal agent currently approved and recommended for therapy of histoplasmosis is amphotericin B (Fungizone, intravenous).

Patient Selection and Dosage. Total amphotericin B dosage varies according to difficulty in eradicating the different types of Histoplasma infections and with the likelihood of relapse. Forms of histoplasmosis requiring therapy and their dosages are as follows: (1) Serious acute initial or reinfection pulmonary disease, especially when symptomatic beyond 2 weeks or associated with progressive diffusion abnormalities, requires 250 to 500 mg of amphotericin B over 2 to 3 weeks. (2) Patients with exacerbation of chronic pulmonary histoplasmosis should receive 2.0 grams of amphotericin B over a period of 2 months. (3) Patients with acute or chronic disseminated infection require 2.0 to 3.0 grams of amphotericin B over 2 to 3 months. (4) Persons with Histoplasma endocarditis not undergoing valvular resection should be treated with 4.0 grams of amphotericin B.

Amphotericin B, a toxic colloidal polyene, is solubilized with sodium desoxycholate for intravenous injection. Its common toxicities are local phlebitis; systemic reactions, including chills, fever, aching, nausea, and vomiting; reversible renal toxicity; hypokalemia; and anemia. Infrequently, anaphylaxis, marrow suppression, and cardiovascular and hepatic toxicity develop.

The drug is provided in vials containing 50 mg of dry powder initially diluted in 10 ml of preservative-free water for injection or 5 per cent dextrose in water. Subsequent dilutions are made only in 5 per cent dextrose in water because sodium chloride and various other salts will cause precipitation of the colloidal suspension. The final volume for infusion is usually 500 or 1000 ml but can be limited to 50 ml per 5 mg if fluids must be restricted. Infusions should be administered over 1 to 6 hours according to patient tolerance — usually 2 hours is satisfactory. Diluted amphotericin B needs not be shielded from light. It should be infused through small bore (20 or 22 gauge) butterfly-type metal needles which are removed after each infusion. Daily infusions in differing sites, beginning with the most peripheral arm veins, will preserve venous access. Occasionally it is necessary to administer the drug through indwelling central venous lines (preferably subclavian) which are changed only once or twice during the course of therapy.

A 1 mg test dose is mandatory, as anaphylactoid shock can occur with the initial dose. If that dose is well tolerated, the next (usually 5 mg) may be administered immediately. Usually increments of 5 to 10 mg daily are given as tolerated until a daily dose of 40 to 50 mg is reached. Nausea, vomiting, chills, fever, and aching frequently occur initially but diminish as patients appear to become tolerant despite a steady dose or even during gradually increasing dosage. In my opinion, there is no advantage in exceeding 50 mg daily. Usually this dose is administered daily for 2 to 4 weeks, and then an every other day or 3 to 5 times weekly regimen is initiated. Intermittent regimens are often better tolerated late in therapy, and are also rational because amphotericin B remains in the body for relatively long periods.

Systemic toxicity usually can be lessened by premedication with 600 mg of aspirin with 25 to 50 mg of diphenhydramine (Benadryl) or pro-

methazine (Phenergan) or 10 mg of prochlorperazine (Compazine) orally. In an attempt to minimize phlebitis, heparin, 10 mg, and hydrocortisone succinate (Solu-Cortef), 20 to 50 mg, added to infusions have sometimes been of benefit. If systemic intolerance is excessive, the daily dosage should be temporarily decreased or suspended, restarting at a lower dose.

Azotemia, which is largely reversible, regularly occurs upon amphotericin B administration. The level of azotemia should be monitored by biweekly blood urea nitrogen (BUN) or serum creatinines. A BUN of greater than 40 or creatinine nearing 3.0 indicates a need to consider temporary reduction or cessation of drug administration allowing improvement of the azotemia and continuation of therapy. The dose does not necessarily have to be modified in persons with *pre-existing* renal disease, because amphotericin B is cleared chiefly by extrarenal means. Serum potassium concentration also should be determined twice weekly, and hypokalemia treated with oral potassium chloride supplementation. Anemia is frequent, usually stabilizing at a hematocrit of 25 to 35 per cent. Transfusion with packed red blood cells should be reserved for patients with anemia-aggravated congestive heart failure or angina pectoris.

Other Therapeutic Modalities. Convalescence is prolonged in some patients with histoplasmosis and requires extensive rest for control of symptoms. Some authorities have advocated moderate dosage prednisone (60 mg) in addition to amphotericin B for severe acute disease with respiratory insufficiency, since its pathogenesis is in part that of a hypersensitivity pneumonitis. Too rapid tapering of prednisone in this situation may lead to precipitous exacerbation of respiratory insufficiency. Corticosteroids are contraindicated in other forms of histoplasmosis.

Resective pulmonary surgery is rarely needed. It is required only for patients with adequate pulmonary reserve and residual cavities who are unable to tolerate amphotericin B. In Histoplasma endocarditis in which vascular incompetence or major embolic events supervene, affected valves must be replaced. In such patients, at least 1.5 grams of the total amphotericin B dose should be given post-surgery.

Ketoconazole, an orally well absorbed imidazole, is currently under investigation. It has produced gratifying results in disseminated histoplasmosis. When released, this agent may be useful alone in selected cases or as adjunctive oral therapy after initial control of the illness with amphotericin B.

BLASTOMYCOSIS

method of
JOHN G. BURFORD, M.D.,
RICHARD J. REYNOLDS, M.D.,
and RONALD B. GEORGE, M.D.
Shreveport, Louisiana

Although blastomycosis is more common and was originally recognized in North America, it is by no means restricted to this continent. Several reports have shown that the disease is also probably quite common in Africa and that the disease is also found in South America. Thus the name "blastomycosis" is preferred to the former term, "North American blastomycosis." Most cases in North America are from the South Central United States and the Mississippi, Ohio, and St. Lawrence River valleys, including several Canadian provinces. The causative agent is the dimorphic fungus, *Blastomyces dermatitidis*. After inhalation of infective spores, the fungus grows as a yeast, causing an inflammatory process which is initially polymorphonuclear leukocytic and later a noncaseating granulomatous process.

While there have been several reports of acute pulmonary blastomycosis having a self-limited course and requiring no specific therapy, endogenous reactivation may occur as late as several years later. Because of the serious prognosis associated with disease dissemination, we continue to treat all patients in whom the diagnosis is established. The role of surgery in the management of blastomycosis is minimal and is primarily restricted to the drainage of abscesses. Rarely a patient with empyema and bronchopleural fistula may require surgical correction in combination with chemotherapy.

Treatment

Amphotericin B. Amphotericin B (Fungizone) continues to be the most effective commercially available agent for the treatment of blastomycosis. The drug is toxic, and the combination of immediate and dose-related side effects often creates major problems in the administration of the drug (Table 1). The more common immediate reactions to the infusion of amphotericin B are nausea, vomiting, chills, fever, and headache. Giving the infusion of amphotericin B over approximately 1 to 2 hours and premedication of patients with aspirin and diphenhydramine (Benadryl) results in fewer and less severe reactions. Fortunately, the reactions usually decrease in frequency and intensity as therapy continues. Phlebitis may occur, and attempts should be

TABLE 1. Guidelines for Amphotericin B Therapy

Laboratory	Obtain CBC, serum potassium, BUN, and creatinine prior to therapy, twice weekly during the first 4 weeks of treatment, then weekly until the drug is discontinued.
Premedication	Give 600 mg aspirin and 50 mg diphenhydramine (Benadryl) orally 60 minutes before infusion is started.
Administration of infusion	Give each infusion intravenously over 1 to 2 hours. Add 2500 units of heparin to each infusion. If immediate reactions are not controlled by premedication, add 25 to 50 mg of hydrocortisone to infusion.
Amphotericin B dosage	Give 10 mg as initial dose. Add 10 mg daily until 50 mg dose is reached. After 50 mg dose is reached, switch to alternate day or three times per week schedule. Total dose should be 2 grams.
Monitoring	If BUN rises above 40 or creatinine above 3, reduce or temporarily discontinue amphotericin B. If hypokalemia develops, treat with oral KCl. After treatment has stabilized, patient may be treated as an outpatient.

made to lessen the incidence of this complication by using carefully placed scalp vein needles, alternating infusion sites, and adding 2500 units of heparin to each infusion.

The most important limitations of amphotericin B are the dosage-related renal toxicity and anemia associated with its protracted use. A decrease in the 24 hour endogenous creatinine clearance, with an increase in the blood urea nitrogen and creatinine, can be expected in most patients. The hematocrit frequently falls to a level of 22 to 35 per cent secondary to decreased erythrocyte production; however, transfusion is rarely required. Significant urinary losses of potassium occur in most patients and may result in severe hypokalemia and rhabdomyolysis. Oral potassium chloride supplementation is needed in virtually all patients taking amphotericin B. Less common side effects include renal tubular acidosis, cylindruria, thrombocytopenia, hepatic dysfunction, and allergic reactions.

Amphotericin B is administered in a solution of 5 per cent dextrose in water in a concentration of 0.1 mg per ml (10 ml for each mg). Saline should not be used as the diluting vehicle as it causes precipitation of the drug. The infusion mixture is stable at room temperature and need not be protected from light. The drug should be administered the same day it is added to the glucose solution.

We usually initiate amphotericin therapy with a dose of 10 mg. The dose is increased by 10 mg daily until a level of 50 mg is reached. At this time we switch to either every other day or three times weekly administration of the 50 mg dose. We occasionally accelerate this regimen in severely ill patients by giving an initial dose of 0.25 mg per kg of body weight, 0.5 mg per kg on the second day, and then using the schedule as noted above.

During treatment, an increase of blood urea nitrogen (BUN) or serum creatinine is expected and, by itself, does not necessitate discontinuation of therapy. Once the alternate day or three times weekly schedule is established, the BUN and creatinine will often stabilize and present no further problems with the administration of the drug. However, some patients will show a continued deterioration of renal function. If the BUN rises above 40 mg per dl (100 ml) and/or the creatinine above 3 mg per dl, we decrease the dose by 10 mg until the renal function has stabilized. If the BUN rises above 50 mg per dl, we temporarily discontinue the drug until the renal function improves and again stabilizes. In almost all cases, the impaired renal function will return to pretreatment levels within 6 months after discontinuation of therapy.

We currently recommend a total dose of 2 grams of amphotericin B for the treatment of blastomycosis provided that the clinical response is acceptable. Relapse occurs in 10 to 15 per cent of patients within 5 years after completion of treatment; in these instances, retreatment with amphotericin is effective.

2-Hydroxystilbamidine Isethionate. 2-Hydroxystilbamidine isethionate is a less toxic agent than amphotericin; unfortunately, it is also less effective. We generally restrict the use of this drug to those patients having limited pulmonary involvement without evidence of cavitation or dissemination, who have demonstrated significant toxicity with the use of amphotericin. Treatment failures and relapses are relatively frequent after 2-hydroxystilbamidine therapy. The toxicity of the drug is primary hepatic and most often limited to mild to moderate rises in serum glutamic oxaloacetic transaminase levels. On occasion jaundice occurs, and deaths secondary to liver failure have been reported. The drug is given daily in doses of 225 mg diluted in 250 ml of 5 per cent dextrose in water or saline infused over a 1 hour period. We recommend a 12 gram total dose in most cases. However, as most reported experience has been with a 16 gram dose, and it has been shown that 8 grams can effect cures in some instances, the extent of disease involvement and the nature of the therapeutic response should be considered in determining whether an adequate total dose has been given.

PLEURAL EFFUSIONS AND EMPYEMA THORACIS

method of
JAMES T. GOOD, JR., M.D.
Denver, Colorado

Etiology

Pleural effusions result from disorders which cause either increased fluid formation (capillary leak) or decreased fluid absorption (visceral pleural capillary and lymphatic blockage). Traditionally effusions are classified as either transudates (pleural fluid protein less than 3 grams per 100 ml, lactic dehydrogenase [LDH] less than 200 units per ml, and specific gravity more than 1.016) or exudates (high protein, LDH, and specific gravity). Transudates are usually the result of abnormalities in salt and water accumulation and are commonly found in congestive heart failure, cirrhosis, and nephrotic syndrome. The cause of the transudate can usually be established on clinical grounds alone. However, multiple causes of exudative effusions frequently require several pleural fluid analyses, including Gram stains, cultures, cytology, glucose, pH, lipid profiles, and cell counts with differentials to establish a specific cause. Recently it has been reported that a low pH (less than 7.30) and low glucose (less than 60 mg per deciliter [100 ml]) limit the differential of the exudate to six possibilities: (1) malignancy, (2) empyema, (3) collagen vascular disease, (4) esophageal rupture, (5) tuberculosis, and (6) massive hemothorax, the last-named diagnosis usually being clinically obvious. Additionally, in the setting of parapneumonic effusion a low pH (less than 7.30) has been used to distinguish the empyema (which requires tube drainage) from the uncomplicated parapneumonic effusion (which will resolve with antibiotics alone). Appropriate management of a pleural effusion obviously requires establishing a correct diagnosis. Therapy may range from treatment of the underlying disorder to open drainage for empyema or sclerosis of the pleural space for a malignant effusion.

Treatment of Empyema

Empyema (infection of the pleural space) usually results from an underlying pneumonia but may result from bacterial contamination of the pleural space by either direct or hematogenous inoculation. The goals of therapy are to control the infection, reduce patient discomfort, and prevent a fibrothorax.

Thoracentesis (a Diagnostic Procedure). 1. The clinical diagnosis of pleural effusion should be confirmed by a chest roentgenogram; if this is equivocal, a lateral decubitus film should be obtained. Ultrasound for localization of a loculated effusion may be of value.

2. A small syringe with a 22 gauge needle is used. The skin is anesthetized with 1 per cent lidocaine (Xylocaine) and the needle advanced with infiltration of tissue. Once pleural fluid is localized, the needle is withdrawn.

3. A 19 gauge needle is attached to a 20 ml syringe rinsed with 0.1 ml of heparin (1000 units per ml), and 15 ml of pleural fluid is collected anaerobically.

4. The fluid obtained is observed and sent to the laboratory for protein, LDH, pH, glucose, cell count, Gram stain, aerobic and anaerobic cultures, and acid-fast bacteria (AFB) smear and culture.

5. The findings of (a) gross pus, (b) positive Gram stain or culture, or (c) low pH (less than 7.30) and low glucose (less than 60 mg per deciliter) in the clinical setting of a parapneumonic effusion identifies an empyema which will require drainage.

6. When the diagnosis of empyema is clinically suspected but not proved and the pleural fluid pH is greater than 7.30 and glucose greater than 60 mg per deciliter, a repeat thoracentesis should be performed within 6 to 8 hours. If the effusion develops a low pH or low glucose, the patient should be treated as having an empyema.

Antibiotic Selection. Initially parenteral antibiotics should be used to treat empyema in addition to drainage of the pleural space. The most common causes of bacterial empyema include (1) anaerobic bacteria (mouth flora), (2) *Staphylococcus aureus,* and (3) *Streptococcus pneumoniae.* Gram-negative organisms, including *Escherichia coli,* Klebsiella, and Pseudomonas, may account for 20 per cent of empyemas. When there is no clue as to the specific bacterial organism, the patient should be treated with both an aminoglycoside, gentamicin (Garamycin), 3 to 5 mg per kg per 24 hours intravenously, and a cephalosporin, cephradine (Velosef), 1 gram every 6 hours intravenously. If it clinically appears likely to be an empyema caused by *S. pneumoniae,* treat with 1.2 million units of procaine penicillin intramuscularly twice daily. Treatment for anaerobic empyema requires 1.5 to 2 million units of aqueous penicillin intravenously every 4 hours. Parenteral therapy should be continued 48 to 72 hours after the patient is afebrile. The appropriate oral antibiotic should be administered for 10 to 14 days after discontinuing parenteral treatment (e.g., penicillin VK, 500 to 750 mg orally four times daily for anaerobic empyema). As a general rule pleural fluid culture and sensitivity data should direct one's choice of antibiotics.

Tube Thoracostomy (Therapeutic Procedure). Adequate drainage of an infected pleural space is imperative for control of infection. Once a diagnosis of empyema is established, all patients should have one or more chest tubes placed into the pleural space for adequate drainage.

1. Infiltrate skin and intercostal tissue with 1 per cent lidocaine (Xylocaine) and administer systemic analgesia such as morphine, 4 to 8 mg intramuscularly.

2. Locate fluid with an aspiration needle; make a ¾ to 1 inch skin incision and use blunt dissection to reach the pleural space.

3. Introduce a No. 36 French catheter into the pleural space with Kelly forceps and suture tube to chest wall after making certain of adequate drainage.

4. Connect to an underwater seal and apply negative suction of 20 cm H_2O pressure.

5. When the patient is afebrile, the fluid is no longer purulent, and drainage is less than 100 ml per 24 hours, the tube may be removed.

Rib Resection. When loculations prevent adequate chest tube drainage (often manifested by persistent fever), open drainage with rib resection should be performed by an experienced thoracic surgeon. Adequate exploration with digital manipulation and breakdown of the fibrinous adhesions should be performed to insure complete drainage.

Decortication. Decortication should be reserved for longstanding empyema which could not be adequately drained, or situations in which empyema has resulted in a trapped lung, causing a significant restrictive ventilatory impairment. Fortunately, early chest tube drainage with good antibiotic coverage has made this procedure unnecessary treatment in most patients with empyema.

PRIMARY LUNG ABSCESS

method of
JOHN G. BARTLETT, M.D.
Boston, Massachusetts

Lung abscess refers to lung suppuration with parenchymal necrosis caused by bacteria other than mycobacteria. Lung abscesses may be "primary" or "secondary," depending on predisposing conditions. Primary lung abscesses are usually found in patients who are prone to aspiration, or they may occur in previously healthy persons. Secondary abscesses represent complications of a local lesion, such as a pulmonary malignancy or a systemic disease which compromises immunologic defenses. The usual method to detect this type of lesion is with a chest x-ray showing a cavity with an air-fluid level within a pulmonary infiltrate. Other diagnoses to be considered with this type of x-ray change are a cavitating neoplasm, cavitating pulmonary infarction, Wegener's granulomatosis, an infected pulmonary cyst or bullae, a loculated empyema with an air-fluid level, or infection caused by mycobacteria, Nocardia, or fungi.

Bacteriologic Diagnosis

The most common bacterial pathogens in primary lung abscess are anaerobic bacteria which represent the normal flora of the gingival crevice. A usual mechanism is aspiration of these microbes during a period of compromised consciousness (e.g., alcoholism, general anesthesia, seizure disorder, drug overdose) or as a result of dysphagia (esophageal disorder or neurologic deficit). Most patients with infections caused by anaerobic bacteria have associated oral sepsis such as pyorrhea or gingivitis. Approximately 60 per cent of patients with primary lung abscess caused by oral anaerobic bacteria have putrid-smelling sputum which is regarded as diagnostic of anaerobic infection. The most common aerobic bacteria that cause suppurative pulmonary infections are *Staphylococcus aureus* and *Klebsiella pneumoniae*. Less common are *Streptococcus pyogenes, Streptococcus pneumoniae, Hemophilus influenzae, Pseudomonas aeruginosa* and enteric gram-negative bacilli other than *K. pneumoniae*. Primary lung abscess involving aerobic gram-negative bacilli are most common in patients with hospital-acquired infections and in the immunologically compromised host.

Antimicrobial Selection

Antimicrobials are the mainstay of treatment for primary lung abscess, and suggested regimens for initial treatment are summarized in Table 1. As noted above, the most common organisms are penicillin-sensitive anaerobes derived from the normal flora of the upper airways. Aqueous penicillin G is considered the drug of choice for initial treatment. This recommendation should be modified if penicillin-resistant pathogens are recovered in a reliable specimen source such as transtracheal aspiration, pleural fluid, or blood culture. Penicillin should be given intravenously until fever resolves and there is definite clinical improvement. At this time, the drug should be continued with intramuscular or oral administration for an extended period of time based on findings with follow-up chest x-rays. It is our practice to continue oral penicillin G, penicillin V, or ampicillin (500 mg orally every 6 hours) until the x-rays show complete clearing of the pulmonary infiltrate or a small stable scar. The purpose of the prolonged course of treatment is to prevent relapses. Carbenicillin and ampicillin are considered equivalent to penicillin G in activity against anaerobic bacteria; however, semisynthetic penicillins which

TABLE 1. **Antimicrobial Treatment of Primary Lung Abscess**

PATHOGEN	ANTIMICROBIAL REGIMEN	ALTERNATIVES
Anaerobic bacteria	Aqueous penicillin G, 1–2 million units IV q6h	Clindamycin, 600 mg IV q8h Cephalothin,* 1–2 grams IV q6h
Staphylococcus aureus	Oxacillin or nafcillin 1.5–2 grams q6h	Cephalothin,* 2 grams IV q6h Clindamycin, 600 mg IV q8h
Gram-negative bacilli†	Gentamicin, 1.5 mg/kg q8h, *plus* Cephalothin,* 2 grams IV q6h, *or* Carbenicillin, 5 grams IV q6h	

*Other parenteral cephalosporins are considered equally efficacious.

†The preferred agent or combination of agents is determined by in vitro sensitivity tests.

are resistant to penicillinase are less active and should not be substituted for the regimen specified. Alternative regimens for patients with anaerobic lung abscess who have a contraindication to penicillin are cephalosporins or clindamycin. Drugs within the cephalosporin class are considered equally active against anaerobes, except for cefoxitin, which would be preferred for infections involving *B. fragilis*. It should be noted that the published experience with any cephalosporin in the treatment of primary lung abscess is limited. These drugs are included because they may be preferred for situations in which the identification of the causative agent is unclear, and likely possibilities include *S. aureus* or Klebsiella as well as anaerobes. A penicillin or clindamycin would be preferred for pulmonary infections that are definitely due to anaerobic bacteria.

Most patients treated with penicillin for a primary lung abscess will show clinical improvement within 3 to 7 days, and the fever resolves over 1 to 2 weeks. Improvement as shown by chest x-rays lags behind the clinical response, but a progression of the cavity size of the infiltrate after 1 to 2 weeks of treatment is distinctly unusual. If patients with anaerobic infections show an inadequate response to penicillin, therapy should be changed to clindamycin. An alternative is to use a regimen that is active against potentially pathogenic aerobes as well as anaerobes on the assumption that there is a mixed aerobic-anaerobic infection requiring therapy directed at both components of the infection.

The drugs of choice for pulmonary infections involving *Staphylococcus aureus* are nafcillin or oxacillin. Alternatives for patients with a contraindication to penicillins or for mixed infections involving other microbes are a cephalosporin or clindamycin. The drug regimen of choice for lung abscesses involving aerobic gram-negative bacilli is best determined by in vitro susceptibility tests of isolates in expectorated sputum or, preferably, a transtracheal aspirate. A combination of an aminoglycoside (gentamicin, tobramycin, or amikacin) with either a cephalosporin or carbenicillin may be used for seriously ill patients until this information is available.

Other Therapeutic Measures

Drainage is facilitated by appropriate positioning based on the pulmonary segment involved and by chest physical therapy.

Bronchoscopy may be performed to detect an underlying lesion such as a bronchogenic neoplasm or foreign body, and to facilitate drainage. In the past, an accepted dictum was to perform a bronchoscopy of virtually all patients with a primary lung abscess. It has become common practice in more recent years to reserve this procedure either for patients who have an atypical presentation or for those who show a suboptimal response to appropriate therapy.

Most patients with primary lung abscess respond well to treatment, and the overall prognosis with antibiotic treatment is excellent. Factors associated with a relatively poor prognosis are abscess in association with an obstructed bronchus, extremely large abscess size, abscesses which have been present for an extended period before treatment, and abscesses caused by gram-negative bacilli. Additional considerations in patients who fail to respond are inadequate antimicrobial coverage necessitating a change in the treatment, empyema formation necessitating a surgical drainage procedure, or inadequate host defense mechanisms.

The major indications for surgical drainage or resection of a lung abscess in former years was delayed resolution based on the persistence of the cavity on chest x-ray at 4 to 6 weeks after initiating antimicrobial treatment. Recent studies indicate that most of these patients will eventually have abscess closure if antimicrobials are continued for an extended period. The failure to demonstrate progressive improvement remains an indication for surgery, provided that alternative therapeutic options noted above have been considered, but this is unusual. Additional indications for surgery are severe or life-threatening hemoptysis and resectable bronchogenic neoplasms. The usual procedure for lung abscess refractory to medical management is lobectomy. Patients with an inadequate pulmonary reserve

may undergo wedge resection or an external drainage procedure. An alternative to thoracotomy is percutaneous drainage using a tube inserted under fluoroscopic control.

ACUTE OTITIS MEDIA

method of
KENNETH M. GRUNDFAST, M.D.
Washington, D.C.

General Considerations

Acute otitis media (AOM) is the rapid development of a middle ear effusion. It usually is caused by a pyogenic infection of the mucoperiosteal lining of the middle ear. Sharp pain and a conductive hearing loss in the affected ear are characteristic symptoms, and a bulging eardrum that is erythematous or yellowish is often observed. Sometimes there is an associated fever. Supposedly, the natural history of untreated AOM leads eventually to spontaneous recovery from the infection either with or without rupture of the eardrum.

In recent years, antimicrobial therapy has become the mainstay of initial treatment for AOM. Although advertisements prepared by pharmaceutical manufacturers tend to give the impression that the key to successful therapy lies in the critical choice of a single *most effective* antimicrobial agent, in a more realistic sense the rational approach to the treatment of AOM encompasses a continuum of management decisions. Thus, therapy for AOM should be considered as more than a simplistic matter. Goals of therapy are *rapid* resolution of the infection, *minimal* discomfort during the infection, and *avoidance* of late sequelae by early identification of complications. Since the pathogenesis and microbiology of AOM differ at varying stages in life, recommendations for therapy are described according to the relative age of the patient.

Neonates

Diagnosis — Tympanocentesis. The small size of the ear canal, the angulation of the eardrum, inability to readily assess hearing thresholds, and inability to elicit a specific history regarding onset of otologic symptoms make diagnosis of AOM in an infant during the first 6 weeks of life extremely difficult. Further, when a neonate develops AOM, more often than not the eardrum may be neither red nor bulging. Therefore, when a neonate presents with signs and symptoms indicative of sepsis and it is found that one or both eardrums move poorly with pneumo-massage, then AOM must be considered as a possible source of infection, and *tympanocentesis** *is warranted* both for the purpose of making a definitive diagnosis and for the purpose of obtaining a specimen for culture.

Antimicrobial Therapy. Once it has been determined that a neonate (less than 6 weeks of age) has AOM, antimicrobial therapy should be initiated. Although it had been reported several years ago that AOM in neonates is likely to be caused by gram-negative enteric organisms or staphylococci, more recent studies indicate that the generally healthy, nonhospitalized neonate is *not* likely to have AOM caused by these pathogens. Therefore, in the selection of therapy for AOM, a differentiation should be made between therapy for neonates hospitalized in a neonatal intensive care unit and therapy for those neonates seen in an outpatient setting.

The nonhospitalized, generally healthy neonate with AOM should be treated initially with amoxicillin, 30 to 50 mg per kg per day in three divided doses for 10 days, and neither hospitalization nor aminoglycoside therapy is warranted provided that the infant is able to feed adequately and shows no signs of severe sepsis or increasing lethargy, and provided that close communication with the parent is maintained.

Infants hospitalized in a neonatal intensive care unit, especially preterm and low birth weight infants, are more likely to have AOM caused by staphylococci or gram-negative enteric bacteria than are those infants who are healthy enough to be brought home from the maternity hospital at the time the mother was discharged. Thus, as soon as an infant hospitalized in a neonatal intensive care unit is diagnosed as having AOM, antisepsis of the ear canal followed by tympanocentesis to obtain a specimen for culture and Gram stain is warranted, and parenteral aminoglycoside therapy should be initiated while culture and sensitivity results are pending. For neonates less than 1 week of age recommended initial therapy is gentamicin, 5 mg per kg per day, along with ampicillin, 100 mg per kg per day, both given intravenously every 12 hours. For neonates older than 1 week of age, the gentamicin dose is 7.5 mg

per kg per day and that for the ampicillin is 100 to 150 mg per kg per day, both given intravenously every 8 hours. When it is known or suspected that the causative organism is staphylococcus, then recommended treatment is methicillin, 100 mg per kg per day given every 12 hours for neonates less than 2 weeks of age, and 200 mg per kg per day given every 6 hours for neonates older than 2 weeks of age (see also manufacturer's official directive).

Follow-up. The neonate undergoing treatment for AOM, either in the hospital or at home, requires frequent general health assessment. The appearance of the eardrum per se is not always a good parameter of the efficacy of therapy. When a neonate develops AOM, it may take several weeks before the middle ear space becomes aerated and the eardrum is seen to move briskly with gentle pneumomassage. Further, sterile middle ear effusion may persist after resolution of an acute infection. Therefore, the persistence or subsidence of constitutional symptoms, rather than appearance of the eardrum, should be utilized in monitoring the efficacy of therapy for AOM in the neonate. When initial antimicrobial therapy has been effective, symptoms such as poor feeding, irritability, or listlessness should subside within 48 to 72 hours.

If the nonhospitalized neonate has failed to respond appropriately within 48 hours after beginning use of orally administered antimicrobial therapy, then the infant should be hospitalized for observation and further treatment. Usually, definitive results of culture and sensitivity testing on the specimen obtained at the time of tympanocentesis (prior to initiating therapy) will be available within 48 hours so that modifications in type of antimicrobial therapy can be based on culture results.

In addition, if it appears that a nonhospitalized neonate is becoming more severely ill while receiving orally administered antimicrobial therapy for AOM, then a complete physical examination should be repeated and an attempt should be made to uncover a source of infection other than the middle ear. Of course, lumbar puncture may be necessary to rule out a source of infection in the cerebrospinal fluid. That is, realizing the difficulty that can be encountered in assessing the appearance of a neonate's eardrum and realizing that the presence of fluid in the middle ear does not necessarily indicate that there is active infection in the middle ear mean that the neonate being treated for AOM who manifests signs of worsening sepsis warrants *thorough* evaluation even though one or both eardrums appear abnormal.

---

*There is a subtle difference in the meaning of the terms tympanocentesis and myringotomy. *Tympanocentesis* is a puncture of the eardrum with suction aspiration of liquid from the middle ear through a hollow needle, while *myringotomy* involves the making of an incision in the eardrum with a surgical blade; usually the incision is of sufficient size to allow fluid contained in the middle ear to exude at the incision site.

Infants and Young Children

Diagnosis — Tympanocentesis. The two periods during which children are particularly prone to developing AOM are below the age of 2 years, and around 5 or 6 years of age. When AOM develops in children over 1 year of age, history and physical findings usually make the diagnosis evident. Pneumatic otoscopy provides the best method of observing changes in the appearance and mobility of the eardrum that will lead to proper diagnosis. Also, use of the electroacoustic impedance bridge (tympanometer) enables the physician to make objective and recordable assessments of physical properties of the eardrum in children over 4 months of age. Thus, the combination of pneumatic otoscopy and tympanometry affords the optimal method for diagnosis of AOM in children. In fact, while tympanocentesis may be a determining factor in diagnosing AOM in neonates, in older children tympanocentesis is usually *not* required for purely diagnostic purposes. Further, sufficient studies have already been reported delineating the microbiology of AOM (see below), so that treatment can be initiated, in most cases, without tympanocentesis for the purpose of determining the specific causative organism.

Antimicrobial Therapy. The organisms most frequently causing AOM in children are *Streptococcus pneumoniae* (pneumococcus) and *Hemophilus influenzae*. Recently, there have been reports of an increasing percentage of beta-lactamase producing (ampicillin resistant) strains of *H. influenzae* recovered from culture of middle ear fluid present during AOM. However, since resistant organisms are identified in a relatively small number of cases of AOM, ampicillin or amoxicillin remains the single most useful agent in the *initial* therapy for AOM. Ampicillin, 50 to 100 mg per kg per day, administered orally in four divided doses for 10 days, is recommended. Amoxicillin, 25 to 30 mg per kg per day, administered orally for 10 days, has the advantage of being effective when given in *three* divided doses, and it has less of a tendency to cause diarrhea than ampicillin. If the child is allergic to penicillin, then a combination of erythromycin, 40 to 50 mg per kg per day, along with sulfisoxazole, 100 mg per kg per day, administered orally in four divided doses for 10 days, is recommended. The combination of erythromycin and sulfonamide can be given as two separate medications, or in the form of a newly marketed fixed combination, erythromycin and sulfisoxazole (Pediazole). The combination of trimethoprim and sulfamethoxazole (Bactrim, Septra) can be given to children allergic to penicillin, although its efficacy in the treatment of AOM caused by Group A beta-hemolytic streptococci is uncertain. When utilizing Bactrim or Septra, the dose is calculated according to the required amount of the sulfamethoxazole component — 40 mg per kg per day given orally in two divided doses for 10 days is recommended. Cefaclor is a newly introduced cephalosporin that may become useful in the treatment of AOM. It is administered orally in three divided doses totaling at least 40 mg per kg per day, with a maximum of 1 gram, for 10 days. Though it is more costly to the patient than therapy with ampicillin, amoxicillin, or erythromycin and sulfonamides, cefaclor has the advantage of being effective against ampicillin resistant strains of *H. influenzae* (in vitro) as well as against Group A beta-hemolytic streptococci, and since cefaclor is not a sulfa derivative the chance of a child's developing an untoward reaction to sulfa medication is avoided.

Adjunctive Therapy. There is no evidence to indicate that the administration of a systemic decongestant and/or an antihistamine specifically hastens the resolution of AOM. Such medications may ameliorate symptoms of rhinorrhea, coryza, and rhinitis that are manifest if an upper respiratory infection is occurring concomitantly with AOM. Pseudoephedrine hydrochloride, 30 mg given orally three to four times daily for children 6 months to 6 years of age, and 60 mg given orally three to four times daily for 3 to 4 days for older children, can be utilized for symptomatic relief of nasal congestion.

For relief of severe otalgia associated with AOM, topical or systemic analgesics can be administered or a myringotomy can be done. An otic solution containing the analgesics benzocaine and antipyrine in dehydrated glycerine (Auralgan) can provide relief of ear pain when 4 drops warmed to body temperature are instilled in the ear canal every 3 to 4 hours or as needed. This otic solution, available without prescription, does not blanch or mask the eardrum and therefore does not render otoscopic findings inaccurate. Since some children may be frightened by the instillation of an otic solution in the painful ear, a systemically administered analgesic is sometimes preferable. An elixir containing acetaminophen and codeine phosphate (Tylenol with codeine) can be administered in pediatric doses based on weight.

When there has been spontaneous rupture of the eardrum and mucopurulent discharge fills the external ear canal, then the administration of an antibiotic–anti-inflammatory otic suspension may be indicated. A suspension containing polymyxin B, neomycin, and hydrocortisone (Cortisporin otic suspension), can be given, 4 drops in the affected ear three to four times daily for 3 days or until the ear discharge has noticeably diminished. Two cautions are noteworthy when recommending use of this otic medication for topical use. First, the pharmaceutical manufacturer produces *two* otic preparations, both with the same name — one is a *solution* and the other a *suspension*. The solution (clear liquid) tends to be extremely irritating to middle ear mucosa, and therefore use of the suspension (milky white liquid) is preferred when an eardrum perforation is present. Second, some patients are sensitive to neomycin. When redness, dry scaling, itching, and swelling of the ear canal occur after the administration of a neomycin-containing otic suspension, the medication should be promptly discontinued.

Monitoring Therapy. Antimicrobial therapy alone is not always sufficient therapy for AOM. When there has been neither symptomatic relief nor defervescence within 48 hours after initiating antimicrobial therapy, the child should be re-examined. Poor compliance in administering medications, resistant organisms, or sequestered infection can be causes for AOM recalcitrant to therapy. If there is persistent fiery red erythema with bulging of the eardrum and associated significant ear pain, then myringotomy is indicated. In such instances, the myringotomy is both diagnostic and therapeutic; a sample of the middle ear fluid is collected with sterile technique for culture, and, as a consequence of the release of accumulated purulent fluid from within the middle ear, the pressure exerted on the eardrum is lessened, thereby diminishing pain in the ear. When symptoms of AOM and fever persist more than 48 hours after initiating therapy with ampicillin or amoxicillin, it must be considered that beta-lactamase producing strains of *H. influenzae* could be causing the AOM. In such instances, myringotomy may be indicated, and it is advisable to switch to therapy with erythromycin and triple sulfonamides, trimethoprim/sulfamethoxazole, or cefaclor while awaiting the results of culture and sensitivity on the specimen obtained from the middle ear during myringotomy.

Ordinarily, it is acceptable to schedule a child with AOM for re-examination in the office 10 days to 2 weeks after the onset of symptoms. However, it is important to realize that the child undergoing treatment for AOM requires prompt re-examination and re-evaluation *whenever* new symptoms develop. In fact, the key factor in avoiding serious sequelae of AOM is the matter of making the parents aware of the danger signals that mean a potential complication could be in the process of developing. Recrudescence of fever, lethargy, and severe headache could mean that there has been intracranial spread of infection. Redness, tenderness, and bulging behind the affected ear may mean that mastoiditis is developing. Dysequilibrium and vertigo are indicative of labyrinthitis. Ipsilateral facial weakness means that inflammation is involving the facial nerve. The parent should be instructed to contact the physician immediately if any of the previously mentioned signs or symptoms are noticed. If there is evidence of the development of such complications as mastoiditis, facial paralysis, meningitis, cerebritis, lateral sinus thrombosis, or cerebral abscess, then the patient should be hospitalized and an otolaryngologist should be consulted to provide assistance with further management.

When it seems that initial therapy for AOM has been successful, as judged by alleviation of symptoms, lack of fever, and lack of the development of new symptoms, the child is re-examined 10 days to 2 weeks after the onset of AOM in order to assess the condition of the affected ear.

Two Week Follow-up. When fever and otalgia subside promptly after initiating antimicrobial therapy, a follow-up examination 2 weeks after the onset of AOM is warranted so that the affected eardrum can be inspected. If the eardrum appears normal and pneumatic otoscopy and tympanometry findings are within normal limits, then there is no need for further therapy. If there is partial aeration of the middle ear as evidenced by an observable air-fluid level or bubbles seen within a middle ear effusion, or if there is persistent middle ear effusion filling the middle ear, then it may be helpful to forcibly aerate the middle ear, utilizing the technique originally described by Adam Politzer, i.e., politzerization.

Politzerization involves the application of positive pressure to one nostril with a rubber bulb while the other nostril is occluded by finger pressure and the soft palate is elevated by asking the child to sip water. Contraction of the tensor veli palatini muscle during the swallow aids in opening the eustachian tube lumen, and the elevation of the soft palate separates the nasopharynx from the oropharynx so that the applied bolus of air does not escape into the oral cavity. A 3 ounce size Davol infant nasal aspirator can be utilized instead of the old-fashioned rubber bulb introduced by Politzer. Alternatively, an apparatus specifically designed for aeration of the middle ear in children can be utilized. The device, called a Mathes Middle Ear Inflator, consists of a plastic nozzle that fits into the nostril and a hollow tube that can be attached to the common type of rubber balloon. The apparatus is inexpensive and comes with complete instructions.

Prior to attempting forcible aeration of the middle ear, it is important to make sure that the nose and nasopharynx are free of purulent secretions. Otherwise, there is significant risk of forcing bacteria-containing mucus into the middle ear instead of air. It is advisable to utilize a topical vasoconstrictor such as phenylephrine (Neo-Synephrine) ¼ per cent, three drops, or three sprays, in each nostril about 5 minutes prior to beginning a middle ear aeration procedure.

Four Week Follow-up. When middle ear effusion persists for 4 weeks following the onset of AOM, despite attempts to forcibly aerate the middle ear, the question often arises as to whether a second course of antimicrobial therapy may be helpful in promoting resolution of the effusion. Although it is rational to assume that persistence of viable pathogens within the middle ear is the underlying cause of persistent middle ear effusion following AOM, there is no clear evidence to prove the assumption. Therefore, it is *as justifiable* to continue attempts at forcible inflation, or merely observe with repeated examinations, as it is to treat with a second course of antimicrobial therapy. When a decision is made to utilize another course of antimicrobial therapy, the antibiotic prescribed should be different from the one utilized initially. If ampicillin or amoxicillin was utilized initially, then erythromycin with a sulfonamide (Pediazole) is recommended for the second course of antimicrobial therapy. If erythromycin and a sulfonamide had been given initially, then a second course with trimethoprim-sulfamethoxazole or cefaclor is recommended.

Chronic Middle Ear Effusion. In some children, middle ear effusion persists despite all types of medical therapy. When middle ear effusion persists longer than 12 weeks despite appropriate therapy, surgical evacuation of the effusion and possibly insertion of a tympanostomy (ventilating) tube should be considered. When the persistent effusion is unilateral and there is no history of frequently recurring episodes of AOM, tympanocentesis with aspiration of the middle ear fluid, utilizing iontophoresis for local anesthesia, should be considered. When there is bilateral longstanding middle ear effusion, history of frequently recurring episodes of AOM, or both, bilateral myringotomy, aspiration of the middle ear fluid, and insertion of tympanostomy tubes under general anesthesia may be indicated.

Prophylaxis. Since some children experience frequent repeated episodes of AOM, prophylactic therapy is sometimes warranted. In an attempt to diminish the frequency of episodes of AOM, sulfisoxazole can be administered once or twice daily at a total dose equal to approximately half the usual therapeutic dose for 2 to 3 months. Although such therapy reportedly is effective in the prevention of frequently recurring AOM, the physician prescribing prophylactic antimicrobial therapy should be aware that prolonged administration of antimicrobials for prevention of AOM is not a Food and Drug Administration–approved indication for the use of these agents.

Adolescents and Adults

Diagnosis. When adolescents or adults complain of pain in the ear, AOM should be suspected. Usually an erythematous bulging drum is observed, and pneumatic otoscopy reveals the presence of middle ear effusion. Tympanocentesis is not necessary for the purpose of making a diagnosis.

Antimicrobial Therapy. Since *S. pneumoniae* was the organism most frequently reported as causing AOM in adults, traditional therapy for AOM has been phenoxymethyl penicillin, 250 to 500 mg given orally four times daily for 10 days. However, in recent years, there have been reports of an increasing proportion of AOM caused by *H. influenzae* in adolescents and even young adults. Therefore, although a course of therapy with phenoxymethyl penicillin will probably be effective in most cases, amoxicillin, 250 mg given orally three times daily for 10 days, is recommended, especially for treatment of AOM in adolescents.

Follow-up. Since eustachian tube dysfunction and concomitant problems with middle ear ventilation predominantly occur during childhood, adolescents and adults do not have the propensity that children do for developing repeated bouts of AOM or persistent middle ear effusion. When an adult develops AOM, it is usually an isolated illness that does not recur. Thus, it is usually sufficient to re-examine the affected ear 2 to 3 weeks following the onset of AOM. In most cases, a single course of antimicrobial therapy will result in resolution of the infection and the middle ear will become aerated within 2 to 3 weeks. If effusion persists and the patient finds the accompanying conductive hearing loss annoying, then forcible aeration of the middle ear can be attempted as an office procedure or the patient can be taught autoinflation techniques such as the Toynbee maneuver (swallowing while the nostrils are pinched shut) or the Valsalva maneuver (blowing the nose against closed nostrils with the mouth closed). If the effusion persists despite attempts to aerate the middle ear, then the effusion can be evacuated from the middle ear by tympanocentesis, utilizing local infiltration of lidocaine (Xylocaine) for analgesia.

Thus, the treatment of AOM and even persistent middle ear effusion in adults is relatively straightforward. However, it must be remembered that the presence of a unilateral middle ear effusion in an adult may be the result of eustachian tube dysfunction caused by a tumor in the nasopharynx. Therefore, when an adult has a unilateral persistent middle ear effusion, nasopharyngeal tumor should be suspected and the nasopharynx *must* be adequately examined.

BACTERIAL PNEUMONIA

method of
ROBERT S. KLEIN, M.D.
and NEAL H. STEIGBIGEL, M.D.
Bronx, New York

In the rational management of pneumonia one should consider that the majority of the infections that develop outside the hospital are nonbacterial, caused by viral agents or *Mycoplasma pneumoniae*. In hospitalized patients, pneumonias are more often bacterial, and most of them developing before hospital admission are due to *Streptococcus pneumoniae* (pneumococcus). The other important bacterial pulmonary pathogens are *Staphylococcus aureus, Klebsiella pneumoniae,* and *Hemophilus influenzae,* and these generally cause pneumonia in association with typical clinical settings. Staphylococcal pneumonia may be associated with influenza or with staphylococcal septicemia or endocarditis, or it may develop in a debilitated hospitalized patient. Klebsiella pneumonia developing in the community is typically encountered in alcoholics or diabetics; it is also a common nosocomial pneumonia. Pneumonia caused by *Hemophilus influenzae* is common in infants and young children, but may be seen in adults, especially those with chronic bronchopulmonary disease. Aspiration pneumonia commonly is a mixed infection, often involving species of anaerobic mouth flora. Pneumonia caused by infection with enteric gram-negative bacilli (*Escherichia coli,* Proteus species, Enterobacter-Serratia group) or *Pseudomonas aeruginosa* is most often acquired in hospitals, and is especially associated with prior antimicrobial therapy, aspiration, tracheostomy, contaminated ventilatory equipment, or an immunosuppressed patient. Pneumonia caused by the agent of legionnaires' disease (*Legionella pneumophila*) occurs in epidemiologic clusters or in a sporadic form in adults, particularly those with chronic pulmonary or other debilitating illness. The "Pittsburgh pneumonia agent" is a newly described pathogen which causes pneumonia in immunosuppressed patients, especially after renal transplantation and high dose corticosteroid therapy. The clinical picture is often similar to that of pneumonia caused by *Legionella pneumophila.*

Bacterial pneumonia is often more satisfactorily treated in the hospital because diagnostic facilities are readily available, and the occasional severe complications can be quickly noted and treated. The principles of treatment of bacterial pneumonia include the use of antimicrobial agents aimed at the most likely pathogens (therefore a working diagnosis of the most likely etiologic agent or agents is important); antibiotics given to assure adequate antibacterial activity in pulmonary tissue (parenteral therapy using agents known to achieve such activity is always preferred); maintenance of a clear airway and adequate pulmonary gas exchange; drainage of any closed space infection; maintenance of adequate hydration; treatment of infectious complications (such as septic shock, extreme fever, consumption coagulopathy, lactic acidosis, extrapulmonary infection); and relief of pleuritic chest pain.

Antimicrobial Therapy

Whenever possible the antibiotic used should be aimed specifically at the known pathogen; the use of antimicrobial therapy with broad antibacterial activity or in excessive dosage may increase the chances for bacterial superinfection. The use of more than one antibiotic is only occasionally indicated, as in the treatment of a mixed infection of the lungs, when antibiotic synergy is desired in a very ill patient or when definition of a single causative bacterial species is not possible in a seriously ill patient. Table 1 indicates the drugs useful in the treatment of the major causes of bacterial pneumonia. Full parenteral doses are generally preferred. The duration of antibiotic therapy cannot be stated categorically for every patient. In uncomplicated pneumococcal pneumonia, therapy continued until the patient has been afebrile for 2 to 5 days is adequate. When empyema or endocarditis occurs, treatment should be continued for 3 to 4 weeks. Staphylococcal or Klebsiella pneumonia is generally treated for 4 to 6 weeks, depending on the extent and presence of complications. Such patients may remain febrile for more than 1 week; this need not indicate inappropriate treatment or presence of complications. Signs of consolidation and radiologic abnormalities may persist for several weeks after any bacterial pneumonia has been successfully treated. Prolonged persistence of these pulmonary signs beyond this period may require a search for bronchial obstruction. The adequacy of therapy can be judged by the clinical response of the patient, including defervescence, loss of toxicity, return of appetite and sense of well-being, return of white blood cell count to normal, and decrease in purulence of the sputum.

The choice of antibiotic therapy for acute bacterial pneumonia should not be delayed until bacterial culture reports are available, but should be made on the basis of the clinical background of the patient and the findings in Gram stain of the sputum. Occasionally sputum is not produced by the patient; sputum induction by use of a nebulizer, or transtracheal aspiration, may prove invaluable in making a diagnosis in such cases. When the Gram stain does not sufficiently differentiate among the possible gram-positive cocci as to which is the likely pulmonary pathogen, selection of one of the penicillinase-resistant penicillins (nafcillin or oxacillin) will be effective against the pneumococcus, staphylococcus, and streptococcus. Gram-negative rod pneumonia involving hospital-associated organisms is most consistently responsive to gentamicin or tobramycin; ticarcillin or carbenicillin should be added when *Pseudomonas aeruginosa* is a likely pathogen. In a severely ill patient with acute bacterial pneumonia, the pathogen may occasionally not be defined despite the use of proper diagnostic maneuvers; when this occurs, particularly in a debilitated, alcoholic, or diabetic patient, treatment for both gram-positive coccal and gram-negative rod pneumonia should be initiated with a penicillinase-resistant penicillin or a cephalosporin combined with gentamicin or tobramycin, pending further laboratory confirmation of the cause. Anaerobic pneumonia or lung abscess caused by aspiration of mouth organisms, as typically seen in the alcoholic, is well treated with parenteral crystalline penicillin G. Some studies demonstrate excellent response to as little as 2.4 million units per day, but in the seriously ill patient we suggest beginning with 2 to 3 million units every 4 to 6 hours. After initial response, dosage may be reduced. Treatment should continue for several weeks after initial clinical improvement; antibiotics given by mouth are satisfactory in the later phase of treatment. Clindamycin is an alternative to penicillin G in this setting.

Supportive Therapy

Bed rest in the hospital is preferred for the acutely ill patient. A soft diet is tolerated best. Hydration by mouth must often be supplemented with intravenous fluids because of the increased insensible water loss as a result of fever and tachypnea.

Adequate clearance of pulmonary secretions is essential and is probably best promoted by adequate hydration and use of a steam vaporizer or water nebulizer (precautions must be taken to maintain the sterility of the latter) and certainly by encouraging coughing. Excessive sedation with its suppression of coughing and respiration should be avoided. Expectorants are of questionable benefit, and mucolytic agents with their occasional severe hypersensitivity reactions are rarely helpful. When appreciable bronchospasm is present, the use of 500 mg of aminophylline given intravenously over several hours or isoproterenol by nebulizer is helpful. When large volumes of secretions are pooled in an area (as in an abscessed or bronchiectatic lobe), postural drainage for 5 to 10 minutes three to four times daily is most helpful, especially when supervised by a skilled pulmonary physiotherapist. When the aforementioned measures fail to clear secretions, nasal tracheal suction using sterile technique or bronchoscopy may be needed. The latter procedure is also useful to rule out foreign bodies, carcinoma, or other obstruction impairing drainage. When even these measures are unable to promote a clear airway and adequate gas exchange, endotracheal intubation or tracheostomy should be performed without delay and before the clinical condition has markedly deteriorated.

An excessive, debilitating cough should be partially suppressed with codeine, 45 to 60 mg as needed. Codeine may also relieve pleuritic pain; however, when it is very severe, an intercostal nerve block may be needed. There is usually no need to treat moderate degrees of fever, and the routine use of aspirin should be avoided. However, when temperature elevations are poorly tolerated, as in patients with myocardial ischemia or mitral stenosis, or with elevations of 105 F (40.5 C) or greater, 0.6 gram of aspirin every 4 to 6 hours should be given. Sudden drops of temperature may be accompanied by chills and hypotension. Gastric dilatation or ileus that may occur with pneumonia should be treated with nasogastric suctioning and insertion of a rectal tube.

When there is hypoxia, as indicated by central cyanosis, arterial blood gas determinations, or deterioration of mental status, oxygen therapy is indicated. The flow of gas should be through a moisturizer; high flows (6 liters per minute) through nasal cannulas are satisfactory for patients who do not have a background of chronic lung disease. However, in patients with a history of respiratory insufficiency, the essential supplemental oxygen must be given cautiously in con-

Text continued on page 132

TABLE 1. **Antimicrobial Therapy of Bacterial Pneumonia**

PATHOGEN	DRUG (ALTERNATIVES IN ORDER OF PREFERENCE)	DOSE[1] (ADULTS)	ROUTE
Streptococcus pneumoniae (pneumococcus)			
Severe pneumonia	Penicillin G, crystalline[2]	600,000 units q6h	IV or IM
Mild pneumonia[3] or after good initial response	Penicillin V	250–500 mg q6h	PO
Alternatives[4]	Erythromycin[2]	250–500 mg q6h	PO
	Cephalothin	500 mg q6h	IV
	Cefazolin	500 mg q8h[5]	IM or IV
	Vancomycin	500 mg q6h[5]	IV
Staphylococcus aureus[6]			
Penicillinase-producing	Nafcillin or oxacillin	1–3 grams q4h	IV or IM[7]
Nonpenicillinase-producing	Penicillin G, crystalline[8]	1 million units q4h	IV or IM[7]
Alternatives	Cephalothin	1–2 grams q4h	IV or IM[7]
	Vancomycin	500 mg q6h[5]	IV
	Clindamycin	600–900 mg q8h	IV or IM
Klebsiella pneumoniae[6]	Gentamicin or tobramycin[9]	1–1.5 mg/kg q8h[5, 10]	IM or slowly IV
Alternatives	Kanamycin or amikacin[9]	7.5 mg/kg q12h[5, 10]	IM or slowly IV
	Cephalothin	1–2 grams q4h	IV
	Cefazolin	500 mg–1 gram q6–8h[5]	IM or IV
	Chloramphenicol	500 mg–1 gram q6h	IV or PO
Hemophilus influenzae[6]	Ampicillin[11]	1 gm q4–6h	IM, IV, or PO
Alternatives	Chloramphenicol	500 mg q6h	IV or PO
	Tetracycline	0.5 gram q6h[5]	PO
		250 mg q6h[5]	IV
	Trimethoprim-sulfamethoxazole	160 mg TM/800 mg SMX q12h	PO
Escherichia coli[6]	Gentamicin or tobramycin	Same as for Klebsiella	
Alternatives	Kanamycin or amikacin	Same as for Klebsiella	
Strains acquired outside the hospital often sensitive to:	Ampicillin	1 gram q4h	IV or IM[7]
	Cephalothin	1 gram q4h	IV
	Cefazolin	1 gram q8h[5]	IM or IV
Proteus species[6, 12]	Gentamicin or tobramycin[13]	Same as for Klebsiella	
alternatives	Kanamycin or amikacin[13]	Same as for Klebsiella	
	Cefoxitin	1–2 grams q4–6h	IV or IM
Enterobacter species[6]	Tobramycin or gentamicin[13]	Same as for Klebsiella	
Alternatives	Amikacin[13]	Same as for Klebsiella	
	Cefamandole	1–2 grams q4–6h	IV or IM
	Chloramphenicol	Same as for Klebsiella	
Legionella pneumophila (legionnaires' disease)	Erythromycin[14, 15]	500 mg–1 gram q6h	IV or PO
Pittsburgh pneumonia agent	Erythromycin[14–16]	500 mg–1 gram q6h	IV or PO
Alternative	Trimethoprim-sulfamethoxazole[14, 16]	160 mg trimethoprim/800 mg sulfamethoxazole q12h	PO
Serratia marcesens[6]	Gentamicin[13]	Same as for Klebsiella	
	Amikacin[13]	Same as for Klebsiella	
	Cefoxitin	Same as for Proteus	
Acinetobacter species (Mima, Herrellea)	Gentamicin or tobramycin	Same as for Klebsiella	
Alternatives	Kanamycin or amikacin	Same as for Klebsiella	
Pseudomonas aeruginosa[6, 17]	Gentamicin or tobramycin	1–1.5 mg/kg q8h[5, 10]	IM or slowly IV
	and carbenicillin	2–3 grams q2h	IV
	or ticarcillin	2 grams q3–4h	IV
Alternative	Amikacin (plus carbenicillin or ticarcillin).	7.5 mg/kg q12h[5, 10]	IM or slowly IV
Group A Streptococcus[18]	Same as for *S. pneumoniae*		
Bacteroides species			
Mouth strains	Penicillin G, crystalline	2–3 million units q4h[19]	IV
Alternatives	Clindamycin	600 mg q8h	IV or IM
	Tetracycline	250–500 mg q6h[5, 20]	IV or PO
	Erythromycin	500 mg–1 gram q6h	IV
Gastrointestinal strains	Clindamycin[21]	Same as for mouth strains	
Alternatives	Chloramphenicol	Same as for mouth strains	
	Cefoxitin	Same as for Proteus	

[1]Dosage for adults with normal renal function; significant modifications are required in the presence of complications, including meningitis, endocarditis, empyema, and abscess. Dosage for children is reduced proportionately according to body weight; further modifications must often be made in dosage for neonates because of immature renal and hepatic function. See package insert for all drugs.

[2]Resistant strains have been isolated rarely from patients who had prior treatment with one of these drugs.

[3]It may be preferable to begin treatment with crystalline penicillin G intravenously for a few doses until definite improvement is noted.

[4]Antibiotics of the penicillin group (i.e., ampicillin, oxacillin, cloxacillin, dicloxacillin, nafcillin) that are primarily used for treatment of infections caused by organisms other than the pneumococcus are also effective in treating pneumococcal pneumonia.

[5]Major alterations of dosages or dosage intervals must be made in the presence of renal insufficiency.

[6]Antibiotic-resistant strains, especially associated with hospital-acquired infections, occur. In vitro sensitivity testing should always be performed so that initial drug choice may then be readjusted if necessary.

[7]Intravenous route usually required for such dosage.

[8]Used only if the isolated strain has been found sensitive to penicillin G by reliable laboratory testing.

[9]Synergy of aminoglycosides and cephalosporins against some strains of *Klebsiella pneumoniae* has been demonstrated in vitro. Cephalosporins in full parenteral doses should be added to gentamicin or tobramicin in therapy of patients who are seriously ill.

[10]Whenever possible, aminoglycoside serum levels should be monitored and therapy adjusted to maintain therapeutic levels.

[11]Penicillin-resistant strains are increasingly being found. In the severely ill patient, chloramphenicol should be considered the drug of first choice until ampicillin sensitivity is documented by reliable in vitro sensitivity tests.

[12]*Proteus mirabilis* strains, especially those acquired outside the hospital, are often sensitive to ampicillin and cephalosporin antibiotics.

[13]In severely ill patients, carbenicillin or ticarcillin may be added to the aminoglycoside antibiotic in dosages recommended for *Pseudomonas aeruginosa*.

[14]Not approved for this indication by the Food and Drug Administration.

[15]In patients who do not respond to erythromycin alone, rifampin, 600 mg daily in a single oral dose, should be added.

[16]Optimal therapy for this newly described pathogen is not yet established. Recommendation should be considered preliminary and may need revision.

[17]Gentamicin or tobramycin together with ticarcillin or carbenicillin is often synergistic in vitro against *Pseudomonas aeruginosa* and should generally be used together in full doses in severe cases of pneumonia. The penicillins should not be mixed in the same bottle as the aminoglycosides nor run simultaneously through one intravenous line.

[18]Treatment should continue for at least 10 days. Initial therapy with penicillin G should employ 5 to 10 million units per 24 hours in seriously ill patients.

[19]High-dose penicillin is generally recommended initially for aspiration pneumonia in a seriously ill patient. Lower dosage may be used if the pneumonia is mild (see text). After initial improvement, dosage may be lowered to that of pneumococcal pneumonia.

[20]The higher dose of tetracycline should not be given intravenously if an alternative regimen is available.

[21]Strains of *Bacteroides fragilis* commonly show in vitro resistance to penicillin. However, good clinical response of aspiration pneumonia to penicillin is usually seen even with such isolates.

trolled concentrations (as by Ventimask, providing 24 to 28 per cent inspired oxygen, or by nasal prongs at a flow rate of 1 to 2 liters per minute) to avoid suppression of the hypoxic drive, with resulting dangerous hypoventilation. If necessary, oxygen may be given by mechanically assisted respiration.

The treatment of septic shock has not yet been adequately defined. Measures that may be useful are the correction of any hypovolemia with albumin solution, the intravenous administration of sodium bicarbonate in lactic acidosis, intravenous dopamine, and possibly digitalis to improve organ perfusion. Preliminary evidence suggests that a large dose of glucocorticoids, equivalent to methylprednisolone, 30 mg per kg intravenously, may improve survival.

Extrapulmonary manifestations of pneumonia are not uncommon. Sterile pleural effusions often accompany pneumococcal pneumonia and are associated with more prolonged fever; a thoracentesis should be undertaken to differentiate such an effusion from empyema. Closed space infections such as empyema, purulent pericarditis, and septic arthritis require early and aggressive drainage procedures, which should be repeated often enough to prevent reaccumulation of pus. When possible, infected pleural fluid should be drained by repeated needle aspiration; however, viscous fluid usually requires the use of indwelling chest tube drainage or occasionally an open surgical procedure, especially when the fluid is loculated. Antibiotics need not be instilled into the drained space at the completion of the thoracentesis because penetration of a systemically administered drug is usually adequate. A pulmonary abscess will usually drain spontaneously through the bronchial tree, especially when aided by postural drainage. Meningitis and endocarditis require treatment with higher doses of antibiotics over more prolonged periods than does pneumonia.

Clinical improvement of the pneumonia patient may be slow in certain situations. This is true for alcoholics, elderly patients, and those with underlying lung disease or extensive pneumonia. Staphylococcal or Klebsiella pneumonia resolves more slowly than pneumococcal pneumonia. Bronchial obstruction (by mucus, tumor, foreign body, or enlarged, inflamed lymph nodes) and atelectasis delay resolution of the pneumonia. Empyema, pulmonary abscess, or metastatic infection will also be characterized by a slower response to therapy. Superinfection of the lung with new pathogens may complicate recovery; this implies clinical evidence of renewed or continued infection, such as recurrence of fever,

purulent sputum, leukocytosis, or other signs, and not just the identification of new organisms in the sputum. The latter finding of mere colonization of the sputum in a recovering patient is very common and is not an indication for the addition of new antibiotics. Antibiotic hypersensitivity reactions may also complicate the course of therapy and require substitution of alternative drugs. When none of the above account for a poor response of the patient after the first 48 hours, the initial etiologic diagnosis of the pneumonia and choice of therapy should be reconsidered.

Immunization

A vaccine containing capsular polysaccharides of the 14 most common types of *Streptococcus pneumoniae* has been shown to be effective in preventing pneumococcal pneumonia and other severe pneumococcal disease in subjects older than 2 years of age. We recommend this vaccine for use in all high-risk patients over 2 years old, including those with chronic cardiorespiratory problems, sickle cell anemia, anatomic or functional asplenia, nephrotic syndrome, alcoholism, diabetes mellitus, or immunosuppression caused either by disease or by chemotherapeutic agents. Side effects are minor and consist of local soreness and erythema. Because fever occasionally occurs with vaccination, the immunization should be delayed in the febrile patient. Although the exact duration of immunity is not known, protection probably lasts several years.

VIRAL PNEUMONIA

method of
THOMAS F. MURPHY, M.D.,
and FLOYD W. DENNY, M.D.
Chapel Hill, North Carolina

In the general population, the incidence of pneumonia varies with age. The peak attack rate (40 cases per 1000 children per year) occurs in children less than 5 years old; after decreasing in school age children to 5 cases per 1000 children per year, the rate stabilizes in adults until about 60 years of age, after which the rate again increases. Table 1 demonstrates the relative importance of several nonbacterial agents as causes of pneumonia in patients within different age groups. In children less than 5 years of age, respiratory syncytial virus (RSV) is the predominant agent. RSV is responsible for yearly midwinter

TABLE 1. **Relative Importance of Respiratory Tract Pathogens as Causes of Pneumonia in Patients of Different Ages**

	AGE IN YEARS			
	≦ 5	6–20	21–60	> 60
Respiratory syncytial virus	+++*	+	−	+
Parainfluenza virus type 1	++	−	−	−
Parainfluenza virus type 3	++	+	−	+
Adenoviruses	+	+	+	−
Influenza A virus	+++	+	++	+++
Mycoplasma pneumoniae	+	+++	++	−

```
*    −:A rare cause of pneumonia.
     +: An occasional cause of pneumonia.
    ++: A relatively common cause of pneumonia.
   +++: A regular cause of pneumonia.
```

to early spring epidemics of wheezing and pneumonia; such epidemics usually last 6 to 8 weeks. In contrast, influenza A viruses, while also causing epidemics of pneumonia in young children, do not have the same propensity to cause wheezing as does RSV. Parainfluenza virus type 3 (P3) tends to be endemic in nature, while parainfluenza virus type 1 (P1) is usually associated with fall outbreaks of croup. With increasing age, the relative importance of these agents changes. In general, RSV, P1, and P3 are less important during the adult years. Influenza A, however, becomes increasingly more significant during adult life; it has a major effect on morbidity and mortality rates in the elderly and in individuals with underlying cardiovascular and/or metabolic diseases. RSV and P3 also have been shown to cause sporadic epidemics of pneumonia in closed populations of elderly people. Finally, the importance of adenoviruses should be appreciated. Adenovirus types 1, 2, and 5 can cause moderate to severe illness in infants and young children; types 4, 7, and 21 are commonly associated with epidemics of pneumonia in military recruits.

Treatment

There is no specific therapy available for patients with viral infection of the lower respiratory tract, with the possible exception of influenza. In a patient suspected of having viral pneumonia, the following supportive measures may be indicated:

1. *Bed rest.* During the acute illness, bed rest is usually necessary; duration should be dictated by the patient's needs.

2. *Fluids.* Maintenance of an adequate intake of fluids is essential. Parenteral administration may be necessary in infants and the elderly.

3. *Antitussives.* Antitussives should be em-

ployed to control the dry, hacking cough which may occur.

4. *Hospitalization.* Although rarely necessary, hospitalization may be required in the patient who is hypoxemic, who develops evidence of inadequate fluid intake, or in whom secondary bacterial infection is suspected (usually associated with influenzal pneumonia).

5. *Oxygen.* The need for oxygen supplementation should be determined by arterial blood gas analysis. The method of administering oxygen should depend upon patient age and available facilities, while serial arterial blood samples should be used to monitor arterial oxygen saturation.

The use of amantadine hydrochloride has been recommended as a prophylactic agent for influenza A infection in certain high risk groups. Its use, however, should be restricted to situations in which both epidemiologic and virologic evidence of influenza A infection within the community are available. Therapy may also be of some value if initiated within 48 hours after onset of symptoms; in particular it should be considered in the patient felt to have influenza A pneumonia.

Complications

Bacterial superinfections in patients with viral pneumonia are unusual; prophylactic antibiotics are not indicated. Appropriate antibiotics should be selected after adequate microbiological evaluation in the patient who is felt to have a bacterial superinfection.

Vaccines

At present, influenza vaccine is available for general use. Specific recommendations are published yearly by the Center for Disease Control. Vaccines for RSV, P1, and P3 are not commercially available.

MYCOPLASMA PNEUMONIA

method of
THOMAS F. MURPHY, M.D.,
and FLOYD W. DENNY, M.D.
Chapel Hill, North Carolina

Mycoplasma pneumoniae (M. pn.) is a common cause of upper and lower respiratory tract disease in humans. While asymptomatic infection or upper respiratory tract symptoms predominate in children less than 5 years of age, tracheobronchitis and pneumonia are the characteristic forms of illness in older children and adults. The majority of pneumonias caused by *M. pn.* occur between the ages of 5 and 30 years, while peak attack rates are noted in 5- to 15-year-old children. Pneumonia caused by *M. pn.* is rare beyond 55 years of age. During an epidemic period of *M. pn.* activity, up to 60 per cent of all pneumonias in the 5- to 20-year-old group can be shown to be caused by *M. pn.* At least 15 per cent of all cases of pneumonia in adults can be related to *M. pn.* infections even during periods when disease activity is endemic in nature.

Treatment

Specific. Although the clinical course of untreated *M. pn.* infection may be prolonged, recovery is the rule. *M. pn.* has been shown to be sensitive in vitro to tetracycline and erythromycin. Clinical studies have demonstrated that both clinical manifestations of illness and radiographic evidence of disease disappear more quickly in patients treated with these antimicrobial agents. These drugs will not, however, alter the carriage of the organism in the respiratory tract. Erythromycin would be the drug of choice in children, while either drug would be acceptable in adults. Therapeutic doses should be continued until the patient is afebrile for at least 2 to 3 days; the usual course would be 10 to 14 days in duration. Since this organism lacks a cell wall, penicillin therapy has no effect on clinical illness caused by *M. pn.*

Nonspecific. For recommendations on nonspecific treatment of patients with *M. pn.* pneumonia, refer to page 133.

Complications

Complications associated with *M. pn.* pneumonia are uncommon. Bacterial superinfection of the lung is rare. Bullous myringitis, meningoencephalitis, myocarditis, and Stevens-Johnson syndrome/erythema multiforme have also been reported to occur in conjunction with *M. pn.* infection of the respiratory tract.

Vaccine

Vaccine trials involving both inactivated and live attenuated vaccines have yielded variable degrees of protection in recipients. Administration of an alum-adsorbed mycoplasma preparation to military recruits resulted in a reduction in the occurrence of tracheobronchitis and pneumonia caused by *M. pn.*; vaccine recipients experienced no untoward adverse effects. Other trials have yielded less promising results. At present a vaccine for *M. pn.* is not available commercially.

PULMONARY EMBOLISM

method of
G. V. R. K. SHARMA, M.D.,
KEVIN M. McINTYRE, M.D.,
and ARTHUR A. SASAHARA, M.D.
Boston, Massachusetts

A comprehensive approach to the therapy of pulmonary embolism must include early recognition, indications for medical and surgical therapy, the treatment of acute cor pulmonale when present, and the recognition and treatment of recurrent pulmonary embolism. Since prevention of pulmonary thromboembolism is certainly preferable to treatment of an acute event, recognition and control when possible of factors predisposing to venous thrombosis constitute the approach of choice to thromboembolism and accordingly deserve special consideration.

Early Recognition of Pulmonary Thromboembolism

The first and most consistently helpful step in the early recognition of pulmonary thromboembolism is the awareness of patient predisposition to deep vein thrombosis. Among the more important predisposing factors are immobilization for trauma (especially hip fracture), the postpartum and postoperative periods, congestive heart failure, chronic venous insufficiency of the legs, obesity, and oral contraceptive agents. Since deep vein thrombosis may be present with no clinical evidence in half the cases, physical signs cannot be relied upon to exclude this diagnosis.

It is important to appreciate that the clinical manifestations of pulmonary thromboembolism may be nonspecific or suggestive. When hemoptysis, pleuritic chest pain, or a pleural friction rub occurs acutely as the result of pulmonary embolism, the diagnosis of embolism can usually be established quickly by the usual studies and treatment instituted promptly. Frequently, however, clinical manifestations are nonspecific: dyspnea, tachycardia, tachypnea, and fever — signs and symptoms consistent with a number of cardiopulmonary processes. When embolism manifests itself in such nonspecific terms in patients with underlying heart or lung disease, embolism as a cause of these symptoms can be easily overlooked. Accordingly, the unexplained development of such symptoms in patients under treatment for symptomatic heart or lung disease should raise the question of superimposed pulmonary embolization. The acute development of nonspecific cardiopulmonary symptoms in a patient with clinically recognizable thrombophlebitis should be considered to be due to thromboembolism until that diagnosis is excluded.

Diagnosis of pulmonary embolism is usually established in the young patient with no prior cardiopulmonary disease by the finding of arterial hypoxemia, signs of pulmonary infarction on chest x-ray, and an abnormal perfusion lung scan. In the patient with prior cardiopulmonary disease, however, all these abnormalities are nonspecific. Lung scanning, with an objective assessment of the leg veins for deep vein thrombosis or selective pulmonary angiogram, should be done to confirm the diagnosis.

Therapy of Acute Pulmonary Embolism

Anticoagulant Therapy: Submassive and Massive Thromboembolism. The primary treatment of acute pulmonary embolism is clearly medical, and the cornerstone of medical treatment is intravenous heparin. The patient should be at bed rest. Heparin can be given every 4 or every 6 hours in dosage sufficient to maintain clotting times at 2 to 2.5 times the control level, an hour before the next dose. When a 4-hourly schedule is employed, 5000 to 6000 units of heparin is usually required. On a 6-hourly regimen, 7500 to 10,000 units is generally needed. It is recommended that clotting tests (activated partial thromboplastin time or the Lee-White clotting time) be performed as often as necessary to achieve the desired dosage range and thereafter on a daily basis. There is evidence that continuous heparin administration by infusion pump may minimize bleeding complications while maintaining the clotting times smoothly within the therapeutic range, once the rate of administration necessary for the desired level of anticoagulation has been achieved.

The duration of heparin therapy should be regulated according to clinical improvement. It appears, however, that 7 to 10 days may be required before thrombi in deep veins fix firmly to the vessel wall. It is recommended that bed rest be maintained over this period to minimize the risk of re-embolization from those sources. Gradual ambulation may be started at or after the seventh day. Coumarin derivatives may be started several days before ambulation. Heparin therapy can usually be reduced with institution of oral anticoagulants, because the interaction of the latter agents with heparin usually results in a prolonged clotting or partial thromboplastin time. The prothrombin time is usually less affected by combined use. Alternatively, coumarin derivatives may be instituted when heparin is

begun, providing a longer period for adjustment or oral anticoagulant dosage.

Effective oral anticoagulant therapy (warfarin) requires achievement and maintenance of a dosage level which will prolong the Quick one-stage prothrombin time to about two times the control level. Warfarin should be given in dosages of 15 mg per day for 3 days initially and regulated thereafter by the prothrombin time. A "loading dose" need not be given, because it may excessively depress factor VII and result in bleeding. In addition to a decrease in factor VII, depression of factors II, IX, and X must be achieved to retard coagulation. Depression of these factors requires 3 to 4 days of therapy and may not be hastened by employing a "loading dose" of warfarin. Before therapy is begun, the patient's medications should be examined for those that interact with warfarin.

Anticoagulation should usually be maintained for at least 3 months and preferably for 6 months, even if the predisposing factor has been eliminated. If the predisposition is chronic, indefinite oral anticoagulation is recommended. When contraindications to anticoagulant therapy are present, including evidence of active bleeding, significant liver disease, independent abnormalities of the clotting system, recent surgery, or unreliability of the patient, consideration must be given to an inferior vena caval interruption.

Thrombolytic Therapy. A major new development in the treatment of extensive pulmonary embolism is the use of the thrombolytic agents urokinase and streptokinase. Both drugs have been shown to lyse fresh (<7 days old) thromboemboli to restore the circulation to normal. Lung perfusion and reversal of the hemodynamic disturbances are also hastened by thrombolysis. They are also effective in resolution of proximal deep vein thrombosis and restoration of venous valve function to normal. However, prior to the consideration of thrombolytic therapy, it must be recognized that there are risks associated with this form of therapy, particularly bleeding. It is therefore important, before urokinase or streptokinase is used, (1) that the diagnosis be firmly established; (2) that the severity of the clinical problem exceed the risk of bleeding, which can be minimized by careful patient selection; (3) that proper care be taken in handling the patient and in avoidance of any but absolutely essential invasive procedures; and (4) that there be clear understanding of the details of therapy, including monitoring, management of bleeding complications, and the control of subsequent anticoagulation.

In the absence of major contraindications, urokinase is administered intravenously in a loading dose of 2000 units per pound (4400 units per kg) in 10 minutes, followed by a maintenance dose of 2000 units per pound (4400 units per kg) per hour for 12 hours. Streptokinase is administered in a loading dose of 250,000 units over a 30 minute period, followed by a maintenance dose of 100,000 units per hour intravenously for at least 24 hours. Heparin should be stopped prior to initiating thrombolytic therapy and restarted within 24 hours after therapy has been completed and the clotting times have returned to normal. During the infusion of urokinase or streptokinase, lytic status should be monitored by measurement of thrombin time (TT) or by whole blood euglobulin lysis time (WBELT). If the latter is not available, the PT or PTT may be used. Subsequent anticoagulation with intravenous heparin and warfarin (after completion of lytic therapy) is continued according to the conventional method (outlined above).

Treatment of Acute Cor Pulmonale

Although the great majority of patients with massive or submassive embolism can be satisfactorily treated with the medical regimen detailed earlier, there may be a few patients with massive embolism and shock who require intensive medical therapy consisting of oxygen, intravenous isoproterenol (useful for both its inotropic and its vasodilator effects), vasopressors, and heparin. It is recommended that isoproterenol be given by drip (2 to 4 mg per 500 ml of 5 per cent dextrose in water) to increase cardiac output and, ideally, restore systemic arterial pressure. If hypotension persists after isoproterenol administration, dopamine (5 micrograms per kg per minute) may be used. Occasionally, when central venous pressure is low, administration of intravenous fluids may be helpful in improving the hemodynamic status. It is important to treat such coexisting causes of hemodynamic impairment as may be present, e.g., left heart failure, with such agents as digitalis, glycosides, and intravenous diuretics as indicated clinically.

A number of patients with hypotension or shock secondary to massive embolism will quickly stabilize and be candidates for thrombolytic therapy. A few, however, may have persistent hypotension and may require mechanical removal of emboli to survive. Pulmonary embolectomy with cardiopulmonary bypass is indicated in this situation once pulmonary arterial obstruction has been shown by angiography to be massive and to be sufficiently proximal to be surgically accessible. Pulmonary embolectomy carries a high mortality risk and is therefore infrequently employed.

Adjunctive Therapy

Adjunctive therapy plays an important role in acute pulmonary embolism. Since most patients with clinically detectable pulmonary embolism will have some degree of hypoxemia, oxygen therapy is an important adjunct. Since hypoventilation is rarely a cause of hypoxemia in pulmonary embolism, oxygen may be administered comfortably by nasal catheter without fear of suppressing ventilation.

In patients who complain of severe pleuritic pain or who exhibit apprehension, intravenous morphine sulfate administered slowly 1 mg at a time (up to 5 to 10 mg) may be very helpful. Apprehension is lessened, and ventilation is frequently improved. Codeine sulfate (30 to 60 mg) may be given for lesser pain.

Recognition of Recurrence of Thromboembolism

The recognition of "true" recurrence during the acute phase of pulmonary embolism is a difficult problem which cannot be resolved without the aid of lung scanning and/or pulmonary angiography. Only by angiography can the distinction between recurrent pulmonary embolism and fragmentation with distal migration of the original clot be made. The importance of this distinction lies in the therapy. Should true recurrence happen during a period when adequate anticoagulation with intravenous heparin has been maintained, the patient may be considered a "heparin failure" and caval interruption indicated. The fragmentation and migration process, on the other hand, requires only continuation of heparin.

If recurrence takes place during well controlled oral anticoagulation in the recovery period or during long-term anticoagulation, management depends on the cardiopulmonary status of the patient, the magnitude of recurrence, the status of the deep veins, and the nature of the predisposing event. If the underlying cardiopulmonary status is satisfactory, the embolic episode submassive (i.e., less than 40 per cent of total pulmonary vasculature affected), the deep veins minimally abnormal, and the predisposing event temporary (e.g., leg trauma), retreatment with intravenous heparin may be carried out, following the same time course as in the initial event. However, if the underlying cardiopulmonary status is unstable, the recurrence massive, the deep veins grossly abnormal, or the predisposing condition chronic (e.g., varicose veins), caval interruption is recommended.

Interruption of Inferior Vena Cava

Currently, the procedure is indicated in the following conditions: (1) presence of contraindications to anticoagulation, (2) recurrence during adequate anticoagulation, (3) septic pelvic thrombophlebitis with embolism, (4) recurrent pulmonary emboli, and (5) as an adjunct to pulmonary embolectomy.

The majority of patients requiring inferior vena caval interruption are those in whom contraindications to anticoagulation exist. These include severe systemic hypertension with Grade III or IV retinopathy; presence of an actively bleeding lesion in the gastrointestinal or genitourinary tract (symptomatic lesions without active bleeding are considered relative contraindications); craniotomy or a cerebrovascular accident within the prior 2 months; evidence of a lesion known or suspected to be associated with intracranial hemorrhage, including malignancy; presence of an uncontrolled hypocoagulable state, including coagulation factor deficiencies, platelet abnormalities, or other spontaneous hemorrhagic or purpuric phenomena; and severe renal or hepatic insufficiency. Relative contraindication must be considered on an individual patient basis, weighing the risk and impact of bleeding against the morbidity of venous interruption.

Although interrupting the inferior vena cava will prevent further embolization in the acute period, recurrences are possible. In addition, the mortality and morbidity of such procedures under general anesthesia have limited their use. The introduction of the inferior vena cava "umbrella filter" by Mobin-Uddin, as well as other filters which can be placed under fluoroscopy with local anesthesia, has minimized the hazards of inferior vena caval interruption. The procedure is associated with a negligible recurrence rate and complications.

SARCOIDOSIS

method of
STEPHEN B. WEBSTER, M.D.
La Crosse, Wisconsin

Sarcoidosis is an acute granulomatous disease of unknown cause. Intrathoracic involvement is most common with involvement of hilar lymph nodes and lung parenchyma. Other areas commonly involved are the skin, eyes, and peripheral lymph nodes, followed by salivary glands, bones, muscles, heart and the nervous system. Complete evaluation of each patient is important, and generally the diagnosis is made by demonstrating involvement of more than one organ system, usually by biopsy and histopathologic examination. Therapy depends on the degree of involvement and progression of the disease. It should be remembered that a significant number of patients with sarcoidosis will run a benign course, and therapy will not be required.

Clinical Features

Involvement of the lungs and hilar and mediastinal nodes are the most common manifestation of sarcoidosis. Definite parenchymal changes with or without hilar adenopathy are seen in 50 to 90 per cent of the patients. The extent and chronicity of the pulmonary involvement can be classified on roentgenologic evaluation as listed below:

Stage I — Hilar adenopathy with no parenchymal change.

Stage II — Hilar adenopathy with diffuse parenchymal changes.

Stage III — Diffuse parenchymal changes without hilar adenopathy.

Indications for Therapy

A high percentage of patients with sarcoidosis have an asymptomatic and self-limited form and require no specific therapy. It is estimated that only 30 per cent of patients with sarcoidosis will require treatment. The general indications for therapy in sarcoidosis are progression of the granulomatous process to serious involvement of a vital organ or the possibility of late fibrosis and impairment of function. Specific indications for therapy of sarcoidosis are as follows: (1) ocular lesions; (2) persistent or progressive pulmonary involvement; (3) central nervous system involvement; (4) hypercalcemia or hypercalciuria with renal damage; (5) myocardial involvement; (6) hypersplenism; (7) grossly disfiguring skin lesions; (8) evidence of progressive involvement of salivary glands, lymph nodes, upper respiratory mucosa, muscles, or joints; and (9) persistent toxic symptoms indicating systemic involvement.

It should be remembered that although therapy is indicated in these instances and may be highly effective, the course of sarcoidosis is highly unpredictable and relapses are frequent.

Therapy

Adrenal Corticosteroids. In general, the adrenal corticosteroids are the primary agents used in the treatment of sarcoidosis. Corticosteroids will prevent the progression of the disease but do not necessarily affect the ultimate outcome of the process, and recurrences are frequent when the dosage is reduced. In patients requiring treat-

138   COAL WORKERS' PNEUMOCONIOSIS AND SILICOSIS

ment, earlier initiation of therapy may produce better results.

Intrathoracic disease is the most common reason for the institution of systemic therapy. A commonly quoted system for the initiation of corticosteroids is based on the staging of the intrathoracic disease by x-ray as listed previously. Stage I disease does not require therapy but requires only careful follow-up. Stages II and III should be observed for 6 months; if there is no improvement, corticosteroids should be initiated, utilizing 40 mg of prednisone equivalent every other day. Re-evaluation is undertaken at 3 months; if there is improvement, the dosage is decreased by 10 mg and a repeat re-evaluation done 3 months later. If there is no improvement, the same dosage is continued for another 3 months. The 3 month re-evaluation periods are continued with reduction of the dosage to 0 in 15 months if progress has been satisfactory. It should be emphasized that a long period of therapy will be required, and careful observation is necessary to watch for possible recurrences as the dosage is reduced. Maintenance therapy may be necessary in some patients. The usual precautions with the use of corticosteroids should be followed.

The use of corticosteroids for other indications will follow a similar course. In some cases, daily dosage of the equivalents of 30 to 40 mg of prednisone may be required, but the use of the alternate-day therapy will cut down the incidence of side effects and is effective in most patients. Dosages should be tapered slowly and maintenance therapy is often necessary. Rarely will it be possible to use a course of therapy shorter than 8 months; the average course is 12 to 24 months.

Topical Corticosteroids. In anterior involvement of the eye with iridocyclitis, topical corticosteroids are effective and may be combined with local subconjunctival injections. If there is a lack of improvement or posterior uveal involvement develops, high dosage systemic steroids are indicated.

In cutaneous involvement, the use of high potency topical steroid creams such as triamcinolone acetonide 0.1 per cent can be used under plastic wrap occlusion. If occlusive wrapping is not practical in the area of the body involved, a very high potency cream such as triamcinolone acetonide 0.5 per cent can be rubbed into the lesions three times a day.

Intralesional Corticosteroids. These are generally used in cutaneous lesions. Triamcinolone acetonide, 10 mg per ml, may be diluted with 1 per cent lidocaine (Xylocaine) to 5 mg per ml for the larger plaques and to 2 mg per ml for smaller

papules. It should be remembered that although regression of the lesion occurs with this therapy, there may be some atrophy, and in pigmented skin depigmentation may develop. If this is a problem, such as with lesions on the face, topical steroid creams as listed above should be tried.

Other Therapeutic Modalities. In some patiens chloroquine has been utilized, as has immunosuppressive therapy with methotrexate. Both these drugs are considered investigational for use at this time. They have a limited use in patients in whom corticosteroids cannot be utilized; however, these are very rare and unique cases.

COAL WORKERS' PNEUMOCONIOSIS AND SILICOSIS

method of
W. K. C. MORGAN, M.D.
London, Ontario, Canada

COAL WORKERS' PNEUMOCONIOSIS

Definition

The International Labour Organization (ILO) has defined coal workers' pneumonconiosis (CWP) as the deposition of coal dust in the lungs and the tissue's reaction to its presence. This definition has received widespread acceptance by the medical and scientific communities, but not by politicians. The term black lung, although popular with those running for office, has little to commend it in that it has come to mean the presence of any respiratory symptoms or disease which occur in a coal miner, irrespective of the cause.

Etiology

CWP is a distinct entity and should not be regarded as a form or variant of silicosis. It exists in two forms: simple and complicated. Simple CWP is a reaction to coal dust alone and is diagnosed on the bases of a suitable history of exposure, namely at least 10 years underground, plus the presence of certain fairly distinctive radiographic features, in particular an abnormal number of small rounded opacities in the chest radiograph. The simple form of the disease is divided into categories 1, 2, and 3, according to the profusion of small opacities in the chest film. Unlike simple silicosis, simple CWP does not progress in the absence of further dust exposure; however, it must be remembered that complicated

CWP may develop once the lung has been primed by a sufficiently high dust burden.

Complicated pneumoconiosis or progressive massive fibrosis (PMF) is a reaction to dust plus some other factor or factors as yet not identified. PMF or complicated CWP may progress in the absence of further exposure, and indeed may develop after exposure to coal dust has ceased. Not all subjects with PMF progress, and in this sense the term PMF is a misnomer. It is subdivided into stages A, B, and C, according to the size of the opacities. Those who are interested in the further details of the ILO/UC Classification should consult Medical Radiography and Photography, 48:67, 1972.

Clinical Features

Simple CWP is not associated with either symptoms or signs. Coincident industrial bronchitis is common, and often leads to the presence of cough and sputum. PMF in its early stages, viz., A and early B, is likewise without symptoms, but the later stages, advanced B and C, are almost invariably associated with progressive shortness of breath, cough, and sputum. For the most part the cough and sputum are a consequence of coincident industrial bronchitis. As the large opacities increase in size, they encroach on and obliterate the pulmonary vascular bed and airways. This leads first to the development of pulmonary hypertension on exercise, and later as the disease advances, to pulmonary hypertension at rest, and finally to overt clinical cor pulmonale.

Category 1 simple CWP is unassociated with any detectable respiratory impairment; however, categories 2 and 3 may lead to minor abnormalities of the distribution of inspired gas. The abnormalities are manifested by a slight increase in the alveolar to arterial gradient for oxygen (A-aO$_2$), a slight reduction in the diffusing capacity of subjects with the p type of small opacity, and exceptionally a minimal reduction of the arterial oxygen tension. Simple CWP is not associated with a decreased life expectancy. In contrast, stages B and C PMF are associated with several abnormalities of pulmonary function. Lung volumes are decreased and the decrement is related to the size of the opacity. Airways obstruction is frequent in stages B and C, and in addition the diffusing capacity is reduced in proportion to the degree of encroachment the large opacities make on the vascular bed. Ventilation-perfusion inequalities may lead to a reduction in the arterial oxygen tension of the blood and occasionally to desaturation. The large masses lead to increased stiffness of the lungs and an increased recoil pressure at total lung capacity. The distribution of inspired gas is abnormal. PMF is associated with a decreased life expectancy.

Prevention

Prevention is the only effective method of dealing with the problem of CWP. If categories 2 and 3 simple CWP can be prevented, then the likelihood of PMF developing is remote. Studies from Great Britain and Germany have shown that effective dust control lessens the risk of CWP, and moreover, if the dust level can be kept below 3.5 mg per cubic meter, then less than 3.5 per cent of new entrants in coal mining will develop category 2 or above with 35 years of underground exposure. In this regard the present United States standard is 2 mg per cubic meter, and provided the dust levels remain in effect, the incidence of PMF should fall to near zero. This is a consequence of the fact that PMF develops only on a background of categories 2 and 3, that is to say when the lungs have been primed by a high dust burden. The use of masks has a strictly limited role in the prevention of the disease and should not be used as a substitute for adequate control.

Treatment

No treatment for simple CWP is known. Smoking should be discouraged since there is little doubt that should PMF develop, the additional insult of cigarette smoke places the miner in double jeopardy. In this regard the hazards of cigarette smoking alone should be enough to deter any wise person from the habit. Cough and sputum, when caused by industrial bronchitis, usually clear up or improve when dust exposure ceases. Airways obstruction when present is mainly due to cigarette smoking and emphysema and exceptionally due to industrial bronchitis. If the obstruction is severe and associated with shortness of breath, oral bronchodilators are occasionally helpful. In this regard oxtriphylline, 200 mg three times daily, or another beta stimulant such as metaproterenol, 20 mg three times daily, or salbutamol, should the Food and Drug Administration ever release it, 4 mg three times daily, may be used in lieu of ephedrine or related drugs. A metaproterenol or salbutamol inhaler is also helpful. The standard treatment is as for bronchitis and emphysema, and the reader should consult pages 102 to 109.

The early stages of PMF, since they are asymptomatic, do not require treatment, but as the disease progresses symptomatic relief should be attempted in those patients who have severe shortness of breath and other related symptoms. The treatment of complicated CWP is identical to the management of conglomerate silicosis and the reader is referred to the article below on silicosis. When significant pulmonary impairment is present, especially if obstruction is prominent each autumn, it is advisable to give the patient polyvalent influenza vaccine. Finally, it may well also be worthwhile giving him polyvalent pneumococcal vaccine in order to prevent the development of pneumonia.

SILICOSIS

Definition

Silicosis is best defined as the deposition of silica (SiO_2) in the lungs and tissue's reaction to it. The inhalation of silicates, viz., talc, kaolin, asbestos, may also lead to pneumoconiosis, but the pathophysiological effects of silicates differ markedly from those of silicosis. The latter, as in CWP, can be recognized in life by a history of exposure and certain fairly distinctive radiographic features.

Etiology

Silicosis is due to the deposition and retention of silica particles of between 0.5 and 5 microns in size. Although occasionally seen in coal miners, the disease must be differentiated from coal workers' pneumoconiosis. The latter condition is caused by the inhalation of coal mine dust and leads to radiographic appearances that are usually indistinguishable from those of silicosis; however, the presence of egg shell calcification in the hilar nodes is strong presumptive evidence of the latter. The silica content of the lungs of most coal miners is not significantly increased; however, there are two exceptions to this rule in that motor men and roofbolters may still develop classic silicosis. The former put sand on the rails in order to obtain traction for the wheels of their cars, and the latter drill through adjacent rock strata which often have a high silica content. Silicosis is seen in a variety of other occupations, including iron and metal miners, foundry workers, potters, sand blasters, tunnelers, and bentonite miners.

In general the disease has a slow onset, but exceptionally it may appear in as little as 6 months. The acute fulminant variety of silicosis may be fatal in as little as 2 years and may be associated with pulmonary alveolar proteinosis.

Silica is not itself fibrogenic. The deposited silica particle is ingested by an alveolar macrophage, and as such has a toxic effect on the cell leading to its death. It is the toxic breakdown products liberated by the disruption and death of the macrophage that induce fibrogenesis.

Prevention

Prevention is the only effective way of dealing with the problem of silicosis. This is best done by cutting down the generation of dust, by providing adequate ventilation, and by wearing masks or respirators when the ambient air is contaminated by silica. Mouth breathers are probably more susceptible to the condition because they are deprived of the nasal filter. Thus workers with nasal polyps or other causes of nasal obstruction should not be allowed to work in dusty atmospheres. Serial chest radiographs should be carried out to monitor dust exposure, and to detect those workers who are showing most rapid radiographic progression.

Aerosolized aluminium, which used to be given to prevent pneumoconiosis, is ineffective, and indeed may itself induce pulmonary fibrosis and a toxic encephalopathy.

Respiratory Impairment in Silicosis

The inhalation of silica may lead to both restrictive and obstructive impairment. All of the obstruction seen in simple silicosis is due to a nonspecific dust-induced occupational bronchitis which is due to larger particles settling in the dead space. Restrictive impairment is often accompanied by evidence of obliteration of the pulmonary vascular bed, and is significant only in complicated silicosis. Simple silicosis leads either to no detectable pulmonary impairment or to a minimal increase in the stiffness of the lungs. The excellent preservation of function is a consequence of the silicotic nodules being separated from each other by large areas of normal lung. Complicated silicosis has similar effects on pulmonary function to complicated CWP (see above).

Treatment

No really effective treatment is known. The subject with acute fulminating silicosis should be put on steroids and isonicotinic acid hydrazine (INH). There is no clear-cut evidence that these measures prolong life, but they may provide symptomatic relief. Prednisone, 60 mg daily for 3 days, is recommended. The drug should be gradually tapered over the next 7 to 10 days so that the subject is maintained on 15 to 20 mg per day. INH should be given in a dose of 300 mg per day. When the histologic appearances of the condition show concomitant pulmonary alveolar proteinosis, it may be worthwhile considering pulmonary lavage. Lung transplantation has been used in silicosis with survival for several months.

There is no known treatment for the chronic forms of either simple or complicated silicosis. Symptomatic relief of concomitant bronchitis may be effected by means of oral bronchodilators such as oxtriphylline, 200 mg three times daily, or terbutaline, 2.5 mg three times daily. In some patients the dose of terbutaline can be increased to 5 mg three times daily. Indeed, the treatment of bronchitis occurring with silicosis is no different from that of naturally occurring chronic bronchitis, and the reader is referred to the article on that subject (pp. 102 to 109). Cigarette smoking should be discouraged.

When conglomerate silicosis leads to cor pulmonale and hypoxia, oxygen therapy may be helpful. If the arterial Po_2 is less than 50 mm, supplementary oxygen is often helpful, especially at night. Three to 4 liters of oxygen per minute through nasal prongs may lead to a significant increase in the patient's well-being and exercise tolerance. Portable oxygen apparatus is also available and may be worthwhile. Before a patient is given oxygen at home, it is advisable to see that he does not have carbon dioxide retention, although this is unusual in complicated silicosis or PMF. If he does, he may well be worsened by uncontrolled oxygen therapy. If a subject with complicated silicosis or PMF develops right heart failure with edema and a congested liver, digitalis and diuretics should be given, but are seldom effective for long.

Tuberculosis is seen as a complication of silicosis and occurs three to five times more commonly in silicotics than in the general population. Every subject who has conglomerate silicosis should have his sputum examined for *Mycobacterium tuberculosis*. Repeat sputum cultures are indicated if the conglomerate opacity is increasing in size. When silicosis and tuberculosis occur together the patient should be treated as if he has tuberculosis only. The response of silicotuberculosis to antituberculosis therapy is often slow, and therefore a three drug regimen is recommended (INH, ethambutol, and rifampin) for the first 6 months. Two drugs should be continued for at least 2 years and there are those who feel INH should be continued indefinitely. The presence of a positive tuberculin test of 10 mm or more in a silicotic patient is an indication for prophylactic INH which should be continued for life. Silica permanently impairs lung macrophage function, and since the latter is partly responsible for the lung's defenses against tuberculosis, the predisposition remains.

HYPERSENSITIVITY PNEUMONITIS

method of
CHARLES E. REED, M.D.
Rochester, Minnesota

Inasmuch as the most important principle of treatment is to stop exposure, the first step is to establish the diagnosis.

Hypersensitivity pneumonitis (extrinsic allergic alveolitis) is a diffuse, granulomatous, fibrosing, interstitial, inflammatory disease of the lung predominantly involving the respiratory bronchioles and alveoli owing to allergy to finely-divided organic dusts.

No single clinical feature or laboratory test is diagnostic for the disease. Diagnosis is made from the combination of a history of exposure to one of the agents in Table 1 and appropriate symptoms, physical findings, x-ray abnormalities, pulmonary function tests, and immunologic tests, especially precipitins to the offending antigen. The onset may be acute or insidious. When exposure is relatively heavy but intermittent, symptoms begin abruptly 4 to 6 hours later. Chills, fever of 101 to 104 F (38.3 to 40 C), malaise, and dyspnea predominate. A dry cough may occur. The fever subsides in 8 to 24 hours, but cough, dyspnea, and easy fatigue may persist for several weeks. With repeated exposure, weight loss of 10 to 20 pounds is usual. Involvement of the airways is exceptional, though occasional patients do develop both asthma and hypersensitivity pneumonitis.

When the exposure is relatively less intense but more continuous, chills and fever may not occur. Exertional dyspnea, cough with scanty mucopurulent sputum, easy fatigue, and weight loss are the usual symptoms.

Loud late inspiratory crackling rales may be heard only at the peak of an acute illness or may persist for weeks or months. Wheezing or prolonged expiration occurs in occasional patients allergic to birds and a few other antigens but does not occur with exposure to thermophilic actinomycetes. Ankle edema and enlargement of the liver indicate complicating right-sided heart failure.

Other aspects of the physical examination serve mainly to exclude other diagnoses. Clubbing of the fingers occurs in less than 1 per cent of patients. Peripheral lymphadenopathy does not occur, and hilar adenopathy is most unusual.

TABLE 1. **Common Antigens Causing Hypersensitivity Pneumonitis**

AGENT	TYPICAL EXPOSURE
Thermophilic actinomycetes	
Micromonospora faeni *Thermoactinomyces vulgaris* *Thermoactinomyces saccharai*	Moldy hay, fodder, or bedding in dairy farming; mushroom compost; bagasse
Others, chiefly *T. candidus*	Air conditioners Home humidifiers
Molds	
Cryptostroma corticale	Maple bark, paper, or sawmills
Alternaria	Paper mills and sawmills
Graphium, Aureobasidium	Redwood sawdust
Aspergillus clavatus and *A. fumigatus*	Malt processing
Penicillium casei	Cheese washing
Animal dusts	
Bird droppings	Breeding pigeons or parakeets, pet birds
Fur dust	Sewing furs
Pituitary powder	Treatment of diabetes insipidus
Mist type humidifier (microorganism unidentified)	Cold water spray type home or industrial air humidifiers

Complicating arthritis or skin rashes are not observed.

During the acute febrile episodes there is a polymorphonuclear leukocytosis of 15,000 to 25,000 and a lymphopenia of less than 1000. Eosinophilia is exceptional. Serum electrophoresis shows elevation of gamma globulins in the range of 2 to 3 grams per 100 ml. Rheumatoid factor test is often positive.

The chest x-ray typically shows diffuse micronodular infiltrates 1 to 5 mm in diameter. Occasionally these areas become confluent and present patchy areas of infiltrate several centimeters in diameter. Often the x-ray appears quite normal.

Pulmonary function tests show decreased lung volumes and decreased diffusing capacity. Typically, there is no airway obstruction.

Arterial blood gases show decreased Pao_2 with either slight respiratory alkalosis or normal pH and $Paco_2$. In mild cases or during convalescence, the hypoxemia may occur only during exercise.

Skin tests with bird sera and some of the mold antigens may evoke a dual positive skin test. A positive response consists of an immediate wheal-and-erythema reaction followed 3 to 8 hours later by an area of dermal and subcutaneous swelling several centimeters in diameter. Other antigens such as thermophilic actinomycetes are not suitable for skin tests, for they evoke an inflammatory response in everyone.

Precipitin tests, usually performed by double diffusion in agar gel, are exceedingly useful. Caution is required in their interpretation. Artifacts must be distinguished from true positive reactions. The precipitin test may become negative several weeks or months after exposure ceases. Some persons develop precipitins from exposure to the antigens but have no signs or symptoms of lung disease. Thus, a positive precipitin test may indicate only exposure to the antigen, not necessarily lung disease.

In doubtful cases lung biopsy may be required to establish the anatomic diagnosis. The characteristic histology serves to distinguish hypersensitivity pneumonitis from other interstitial lung diseases. Bronchial lavage fluid contains lymphocytes and macrophages similar to the finding in sarcoidosis and quite different from the neutrophils that predominate in other diffuse interstitial lung diseases.

Inhalation testing in the pulmonary function laboratory with aerosolized antigen may reproduce an acute attack with fever, rales, and a drop in diffusing capacity 4 to 6 hours after the exposure. Such testing is advised only for research purposes, for exposure may cause severe illness. At times the diagnosis can be established by observing the consequence of a deliberate repetition of natural exposure.

In most industrial outbreaks, it has been possible to change the plant process to eliminate or greatly reduce exposure. Obviously the particular changes required vary with the particular process. Occasionally when only one or two workers are affected, it is more practical to transfer them to a different job. The remaining workers should be followed to identify insidiously developing hypersensitivity pneumonitis before extensive and disabling pulmonary fibrosis occurs.

As a result of improvements in the industrial process, bagassosis and maple bark stripper's diseases have disappeared. After they dispose of their birds, patients with bird fancier's disease usually recover within a few weeks to months. Exposure to thermophilic actinomycetes on the farm is more difficult to control, and long-term studies of patients with farmer's lung show a high frequency of progressive pulmonary fibrosis. In theory, respirators should provide protection, but in practice few patients will wear them regularly.

Treatment of a mild acute episode requires only rest. Antibiotics are not helpful. In severe episodes, prednisone, 20 mg four times a day for 2 to 3 weeks, is indicated to hasten recovery and perhaps to reduce fibrosis. Supportive care with oxygen, fluids, and cough suppressants is useful as symptoms warrant.

SINUSITIS

method of
PHILIP M. SPRINKLE, M.D.,
and FREDERICK T. SPORCK, M.D.
Morgantown, West Virginia

Sinusitis in our era of mass media advertising has become a very popular complaint among the general public. It is many things to many people and so needs to be defined. At present headaches and most nasal problems, including normal postnasal discharge, allergic rhinitis, vasomotor rhinitis, and nasopharyngitis, all are attributed to sinusitis.

Sinusitis by definition is an inflammatory change in the mucosal lining of one or more of the paranasal sinuses. There are four pairs of paranasal sinuses in the human: the maxillary, frontal, ethmoid, and sphenoid. The ethmoid and maxillary are the most commonly involved with sinusitis, followed by the frontal and sphenoid in that order. Involvement may be unilateral or bilateral or both, and may involve one group or all. Involvement of the sphenoid alone is very rare and, in older age groups, should call to mind a malignancy. We will deal mainly with maxillary sinusitis and touch briefly on frontal sinusitis.

Etiology

Most cases of sinusitis probably follow a viral insult to the upper respiratory tract such as the common cold. If the disease remains viral, no treatment other than symptomatic management is necessary. Frequently, however, there is a secondary bacterial involvement. Because the sinus is a closed cavity, it is difficult to isolate a pure culture. Cultures taken from the nose may be contaminated by local flora. In most series in which pure cultures were obtained by antral aspiration, the predominant organisms have been *Diplococcus pneumoniae, Hemophilus influenzae, Staphylococcus aureus,* and *Strepotococcus pyogenes.*

Contributing factors may be changes in pressure from forcible nose blowing, swimming and diving in contaminated water, facial trauma, and dental disease. Nasal allergy with or without nasal polyps can certainly be implicated. As we learn more about immunology, it appears that some cases of chronic sinusitis may be a type III immune-complex disease.

Treatment

The aim of treatment of sinusitis is to establish drainage of the involved sinus and eradication of the infecting organism by appropriate antibiotic therapy.

Acute Maxillary Sinusitis. 1. Topical decongestants are useful during the acute phase of sinusitis (2 per cent ephedrine, 0.25 per cent phenylephrine (Neo-Synephrine), and oxymetazoline). These must be used judiciously, however, because of their ability to produce a rebound phenomenon and rhinitis medicamentosa. They probably should not be used more than 5 to 7 days in succession.

2. Systemic decongestants or antihistamines alone or in combination play an important part in the management of acute sinusitis. There continues to be controversy regarding the use of these two types of drugs in combination. Some studies have suggested that alpha-adrenergic drugs may have the effect of increasing histamine release. Other studies indicate that adrenergic agents may act synergistically with antihistamines.

Decongestants should of course be used with caution in patients with glaucoma, hypertension, and diabetes and in those taking monoamine oxidase inhibitors and tricyclic antidepressants. If decongestants alone are used, ephedrine and the pseudoephedrines are probably the most effective.

Antihistamines are divided into five classes, and some patients may respond better to one class than another. Generally speaking, the propylamine class is the most commonly used (chlorpheniramine, brompheniramine, pyrrobutamine, and triprolidine).

In our practice we generally use a combination drug in those patients in whom there is no contraindication to the decongestant component.

We like to use these for 3 to 4 weeks after the symptoms have resolved so that the ostia will remain patent and obstruction does not recur.

3. As the predominant organisms in most series are *H. influenzae* and *D. pneumoniae,* we prefer to use a broad-spectrum antibiotic such as ampicillin. The dosage varies from 250 to 500 mg, depending on the patient and the severity of the disease. In penicillin-sensitive patients, erythromycin is a good choice. For chronic infections tetracycline is usually our choice. We normally use a 10 to 14 day course of antibiotics in most instances and longer if symptoms do not resolve in that period of time.

4. In many cases aspirin or acetaminophen will provide sufficient analgesia. If not, we generally use a combination of one of these with codeine or propoxyphene.

5. The place of antral puncture and irrigation is currently somewhat controversial, with many recommending that it not be done until the patient has had several days of antibiotic therapy to reduce the danger of producing an osteomyelitis. In our practice we find that a certain number of patients who are particularly symptomatic experience a good deal of relief with acute antral puncture and irrigation. There is little question that in patients in whom there has been little resolution of symptoms or findings after a week to 10 days of appropriate medical therapy, antral puncture and irrigation is in order.

6. The application of moist heat over the involved sinus is also recommended for symptomatic relief and to help resolve the inflammation. Humidification of the environment is also thought to be helpful, and adequate fluid intake is a necessity.

Acute Frontal Sinusitis. Involvement of the frontal sinus with an air fluid level and pain and tenderness over the involved frontal sinus is a serious problem, as this indicates that the nasofrontal duct is occluded. If allowed to go unchecked, the infection may spread through the posterior table via the veins of Breschet to the epidural space with the danger of intracranial complications.

Immediate treatment consists of large doses of antibiotics, preferably intravenously, infracturing of the middle turbinate, and spot suctioning in an attempt to open the ostium. The other steps outlined for acute maxillary sinusitis also hold true here. If symptoms fail to resolve within 24 to 48 hours, trephination through the floor of the frontal sinus is done with insertion of a drainage and irrigation catheter. This is irrigated two to three times a day with an antibiotic solution until spontaneous drainage begins via the nasofrontal duct.

Acute Ethmoiditis. In uncomplicated ethmoiditis the management is similar to that for acute maxillary sinusitis. When ethmoiditis becomes complicated with extension into the orbit, periorbital abscess, and ensuing ocular complications, it becomes an acute surgical emergency, and an external ethmoidectomy must be done.

Chronic Sinusitis. Chronic sinusitis is a more difficult problem. Many of these patients will have a strong allergic component to their disease and should be skin tested and desensitized. They should also be evaluated for food allergies with rotational diets. Those with nasal polyps usually require polypectomy, although we have found that the use of dexamethasone sodium phosphate (Decadron Turbinaire) two to three times daily results in marked improvement and sometimes resolution of polyps in many of our patients.

In those patients in whom long-term medical management with antihistamines, decongestants, antibiotics, and allergic management fails to produce a response, surgical management becomes a necessity. The aims of such management are to restore a functioning nasal airway, restore more normal drainage for the sinus, eradicate diseased tissue, and prevent complications of sinus disease.

The surgery usually done for chronic maxillary disease is a nasoantral window either alone or in combination with a Caldwell-Luc procedure.

For chronic frontal sinusitis an osteoplastic frontal flap is done through either a spectacle or coronal incision. The mucosal lining is removed, the nasofrontal duct is plugged with fascia, and the cavity is filled with a free abdominal fat graft.

In chronic ethmoiditis the ethmoidectomy may be done either through an external approach or intranasally, with the external approach probably being more popular today.

STREPTOCOCCAL PHARYNGITIS

method of
PHYLLIS A. OILL, M.D.
Los Angeles, California

The management of group A streptococcal pharyngitis includes the general measures of bed rest, soft or liquid diet if pharyngeal discomfort is severe, and the institution of appropriate antimicrobial therapy.

There are several goals in the use of antimicrobial agents:

1. Eradication of the streptococcus and prompt control of pharyngeal and upper respiratory infection.
2. Reduction of the incidence of suppurative complications such as otitis media, mastoiditis, and sinusitis.
3. Prevention of nonsuppurative complications, particularly rheumatic fever.
4. Elimination of the carrier state and prevention of the spread of the organism to contacts.

These goals are best accomplished with antimicrobial agents which eradicate the organism. A relationship has been shown between duration of therapy and eradication of the organism.

Management

The most difficult problem in managing patients with sore throats is determining which of these are due to group A streptococci. It is impossible to accurately differentiate viral from streptococcal pharyngitis on clinical grounds. Recent exposure to streptococcal infection, tonsillar or pharyngeal exudate, tender or enlarged anterior cervical nodes, scarlatiniform rash, and high fever (>101F [38.3 C]) suggests streptococcal infection. However, no combination of clinical findings is a perfect predictor. Similarly, most laboratory data, including Gram stain analysis of pharyngeal smears, are of limited value. Because of these limitations and a number of cost-effectiveness studies, several protocols and algorithms have been proposed. Unfortunately, most of these have difficulties which preclude general acceptability.

In the selection of patients for throat culture, priority should be given to the following groups:

1. Those with a high risk of rheumatic fever (patients between the ages of 5 and 25 years).
2. Patients with a history of rheumatic fever.
3. Patients over 25 years of age with clinical findings suggestive of streptococcal pharyngitis (see above).
4. Diabetics. These patients combat bacterial infections poorly and, thus, are at particular risk from streptococcal pharyngitis.

Streptococcal *infection* is defined as a positive culture plus an antibody response to streptococcal antigens; the *carrier state* is a positive culture without an antibody response. Thus, the etiologic diagnosis of streptococcal pharyngitis rests on a rising titer of immunologic response (such as a four-fold rise in antistreptolysin O antibody) and

TABLE 1. **Antibiotic Therapy for Streptococcal Pharyngitis**

ANTIBIOTIC	DOSE	REGIMEN
Penicillins		
Benzathine penicillin G	Adults and children >60 lbs (27 kg)—1.2 million units	1 dose, intramuscularly
	Children <60 lbs (27 kg)—600,000 units	
Buffered penicillin G	Adults and children—250,000 units tid or qid	10 days, orally
Alpha-phenoxymethylpenicillin	Adults and children >60 lbs (27 kg)—250 mg tid or qid	10 days, orally
(penicillin V)	Children <60 lbs (27 kg)—125 mg tid or qid	
Erythromycin*	Adults—250 mg qid	10 days, orally
	Children—40 mg/kg/day in 3 or 4 equal doses	

*Erythromycin should be used only in patients with known or suspected penicillin allergy. The amount given to children should not exceed the adult dose.

culture of the organism. The former is not timely and cannot be used when the patient is first seen. Therefore, throat culture is relied upon for diagnosis. Unfortunately, a positive culture alone cannot distinguish between "infection" and the "carrier state." This dilemma is best resolved by treating all patients with a positive culture for group A streptococci even though many of these patients will be uninfected carriers.

Treatment

The data in Table 1 are modifications of the recommendations of the American Heart Association.

1. *Benzathine penicillin G* is the antibiotic of choice. Mixtures containing shorter-acting penicillins in addition to benzathine penicillin have not been shown to be superior to benzathine penicillin alone. If such a mixture is used, it must contain benzathine penicillin in the doses recommended.

2. In patients *allergic to penicillin,* erythromycin should be used. Limited clinical evaluations have suggested that oral cephalosporins, clindamycin, and lincomycin are effective in 10 day treatment courses. Tetracyclines and sulfonamides should not be used because of poor effectiveness.

3. The *risk of spread of infection* to contacts is limited to 2 to 3 days after starting antibiotics. At this time, the patient may return to school or work, if afebrile.

4. *Follow-up* strategy includes repeating cultures 7 to 10 days after completion of a course of orally administered antibiotics or 4 to 5 weeks after an injection of benzathine penicillin G. Follow-up cultures are particularly important in high-risk patients, especially in all patients with a history of rheumatic fever and in patients who have received oral therapy only. If these cultures are positive, a second course of benzathine penicillin G should be given (or a second course of erythromycin if patients are allergic to penicillin).

5. Household members or other intimate *contacts* of patients with streptococcal pharyngitis who become symptomatic, or asymptomatic persons who are at high risk (history of rheumatic fever or indigent people living in crowded conditions), should have throat cultures. If the cultures are positive, these patients should be treated.

TUBERCULOSIS AND OTHER MYCOBACTERIAL DISEASES

method of
STEFAN GRZYBOWSKI, M.D.,
and EDWARD A. ALLEN, M.B.
Vancouver, British Columbia, Canada

Introduction

Tuberculosis has been declining slowly but steadily over many decades; consequently most of the public health programs directed toward early detection of this disease have been abandoned, and most cases of tuberculosis are now diagnosed by general practitioners or by internists. Unfortunately, this highly curable disease is sometimes forgotten in differential diagnosis, and serious cases are not infrequently diagnosed late, sometimes only at postmortem examination. In certain forms of the disease, such as tuberculous meningitis, serious permanent sequelae are the result of late diagnosis. It remains important, therefore, to think of tuberculosis in the differential diagnosis of many complex clinical problems.

Diseases caused by nontuberculous (atypical) mycobacteria are being recognized more frequently in recent years, and indeed their incidence may be increasing; however, as these mycobacteria are only slightly pathogenic, the frequency of these diseases is never likely to match that of true tuberculosis, although their relative importance is increasing. Leprosy, another mycobacterial disease, will not be discussed here (see pp. 34 to 38).

General Principles

The physician undertaking the treatment of a case of active tuberculosis must establish an excellent rapport with the patient. The patient must understand at the onset that treatment will extend for many months and that perseverance and attention to detail are necessary; he must realize that his chances for a complete recovery are excellent if he takes the prescribed medications faithfully. Both doctor and patient must be aware that this disease is infectious, and therefore the aim of treatment is not only to restore the patient to health but also to protect the community. Because of this public health aspect, it is the physician's responsibility to arrange follow-up visits and the patient's duty to attend regularly. It is desirable, with the patient's permission, to discuss the disease and details of treatment with the patient's spouse, whose collaboration may make the difference between success and failure of therapy.

Hospital or Ambulatory Treatment

The decision to hospitalize the patient with active tuberculosis is often difficult and must take into account factors individual to that patient. Traditional concepts of the preantibiotic era often weigh in favor of hospitalization. The questions which should be asked are: What are the indications for hospitalization of this patient? What benefits will he derive? At what price? Unnecessary hospital admission or prolonged hospital stay not only constitutes an unjustified burden on the resources of the community; it may also be harmful to the patient.

It has been said, with more than a grain of truth, that all patients with active tuberculosis require antimicrobial therapy, those who are infectious need to be isolated, and those who feel ill should have bed rest. Hospitals, particularly sanatoria, usually provide an excellent way of isolating an infectious patient and, above all, impressing upon him the potential seriousness of his condition. On the other hand, these objectives can often be achieved without admission, but this requires the time and attention of the attending physician.

In most cases the choice between hospital or outpatient therapy is based on three factors: (1) infectiousness of the patient and the danger he presents to those around him, (2) the degree of cooperation expected, and (3) severity of illness. Closely connected with the first two are a variety of socioeconomic factors.

Infectivity

Tuberculosis is not a highly infectious disease. For practical purposes, only patients with pulmonary tuberculosis with positive sputum on microscopy should be considered infectious; even they do not transmit infection readily, as evidenced by the fact that two thirds of small children living with parents with smear positive tuberculosis remain uninfected. During the initial assessment patients with pulmonary tuberculosis should have microscopic examination and culture of at least three specimens of sputum. If there are acid-fast bacilli seen on direct smear, such patients must be considered to be potential sources of infection; they must be quickly isolated from the tuberculin negative members of the community. Usually this means prompt admission to hospital, although in some instances, satisfactory isolation can be achieved at home. If it is decided to hospitalize the patient, but for one reason or another that is not possible immediately, antimicrobial treatment should be started, as it will render the patient less infectious within a few weeks. Furthermore, any reasonable individual who is told that he has tuberculosis will immediately become concerned about the possibility of transmitting infection to others and will adopt appropriate precautions if he is suitably instructed.

If several sputum smears are negative for acid-fast bacilli, the patient is unlikely to be a source of infection even if subsequent cultures reported 6 to 8 weeks later prove to be positive. Such patients may present a slight danger, and it is usually advisable to have them stop work during this initial 6 weeks' period of bacteriologic assessment, particularly if they are in intimate contact with the public, such as school teachers, practicing physicians, dentists, barbers, and hairdressers; such patients must not be allowed to resume work until there is definite proof that their sputum is consistently negative for tubercle bacilli.

When the patient denies expectoration of sputum, bacteriologic examination must be done on bronchial secretions induced by heated aerosols (20 per cent prophylene glycol in 15 per cent saline solution); gastric lavage and laryngeal swab are somewhat less effective alternatives. Specimens obtained at fiberoptic bronchoscopy often lead to diagnosis; it must be remembered, however, that local anesthetic agents are sometimes lethal to tubercle bacilli. Request for sensitivity studies to the main antimicrobial drugs should accompany the specimens sent for initial cultures.

Examination of the Contacts

Examination of the family and other close contacts of patients with tuberculosis must be of direct concern to the physician undertaking treatment. While certain phases of such examinations are often delegated to special agencies, such as public health departments, it is necessary in the thorough assessment of the patient to attempt to answer two questions: first, where was the infection acquired, and second, who else has been infected? The answer to the first of these questions, while obtainable only in the minority, may affect the choice of drugs if the probable source of infection is known to harbor organisms resistant to certain drugs. The tuberculin status of contacts of the patient, particularly when they are known (or can be reasonably presumed) to have been previously negative reactors, provides a direct measurement of the patient's infectivity. It should be remembered that the incubation period of tuberculous infection is 6 to 8 weeks and tuberculin negative close contacts of the patient should be re-examined in about 2 months. In contact examination it is worthwhile to remember that only smear positive cases of pulmonary tuberculosis are really infectious and that the patient is likely to infect first those closely associated with him — his household contacts. If these are shown to have escaped infection, examination of more casual contacts such as workmates and friends is usually unnecessary, for it only results in unwarranted anxiety.

Education

Tuberculosis is a serious disease, and it is essential for every sufferer to know the fundamental facts about it, about treatment, and about the dangers of spread of infection to others. The patient must realize the importance of continuity of treatment and should have a fair knowledge of the drugs which he is taking. With an intelligent patient who is not highly emotional, it is often wise to ask him to report immediately their occurrence. The patient should fully appreciate the fact that he may be infectious to others and should be instructed as to disposal of sputum, covering his face while coughing, avoidance of kissing, and so forth. On the other hand, some patients as well as their families and friends suffer unnecessarily as a result of an exaggerated fear of infection, particularly in the later stages of treatment; it is for instance unnecessarily cruel to forbid a grandmother to visit her grandchildren when she is taking her treatment well and when her sputum has been consistently negative.

Antimicrobial Treatment of Tuberculosis

The last few years have seen a revolution in the chemotherapy of tuberculosis. Our understanding of the action of individual drugs, the introduction of short courses of chemotherapy, realization of the importance of rifampin in treatment, and an appreciation that an old drug, pyrazinamide, is both more effective and less toxic than was thought previously are all the product of research done in the 1970's. While many investigators of many nations share the credit for this progress, undoubtedly the most important role has been played by the British Medical Research Council Tuberculosis Unit, which conducted many studies in developing countries.

Antituberculous Drugs

Table 1 lists the antimicrobial agents used in treatment of tuberculosis.

The drugs are divided into "most effective" and "other (supportive) drugs" categories. The drugs in the first group are bactericidal and are capable of killing even those organisms with a very low rate of metabolism ("persisters"), while

TABLE 1. **Antimicrobial Drugs**

MOST EFFECTIVE DRUGS		OTHER (SUPPORTIVE) DRUGS	
Drug	Usual Daily Dose	Drug	Usual Daily Dose
Isoniazid (INH)	300 mg by mouth	Ethambutol (EMB)	1–1.5 grams by mouth
Rifampin (RF)	600 mg by mouth	Para-aminosalicylic acid (PAS)	12 grams by mouth
		Capreomycin	1 gram/day intramuscularly
Pyrazinamide (PZA)	1.5–2 grams	Cycloserine	0.5–1 gram/day by mouth
		Ethionamide	0.75–1 gram/day
Streptomycin (SM)	1 gram intramuscularly	Thiacetazone (not available in the United States)	150 mg by mouth

those among the other (supportive) drugs are mainly bacteriostatic, although they have some bactericidal activity.

Side-Effects of Antituberculous Drugs

The main side effects are shown in Table 2. Although the list of various untoward reactions shown in Table 2 is quite formidable and could readily be supplemented by a large number of uncommon reactions, it must be emphasized that most patients with tuberculosis take their treatment with no difficulty whatsoever. It is customary to divide the side effects of the drugs into three groups: those resulting from local effects (e.g., gastrointestinal irritation caused by PAS or ethionamide), those resulting from hypersensitivity (e.g., rash and fever caused by streptomycin), and those resulting from toxicity (e.g., eighth nerve damage caused by streptomycin). While such a division is helpful in clinical management (for example, hypersensitivity reactions can be suppressed by corticosteroids, while the toxic reactions are dose related and the offending drug must be discontinued or at least the dose appreciably diminished), the fact remains that the mechanisms underlying some of the aforementioned side effects have still to be elicited with certainty. It should be noted that only one of the drugs listed in Table 2 must be given in divided doses, cycloserine (250 mg twice to four times a day). It is preferable to give all other drugs in one daily dose usually taken first thing in the morning, as this combats forgetfulness and is likely of some therapeutic benefit. It is sometimes necessary to divide the dose of drugs such as PAS or ethionamide into two or three smaller doses when gastric irritation is a problem. These drugs are seldom used now.

Isoniazid

Isoniazid (INH) is one of the most effective antituberculous agents used today. It is also the cheapest. The usual adult dose is 300 mg a day. The daily dose for children is 5 to 10 mg per kg of body weight. It is practically the only drug used for chemoprophylaxis. Hepatitis is a serious but fortunately rare side effect, although slight elevation of liver enzymes, particularly SGOT, is common and usually not significant. The incidence of hepatitis is age related; it is virtually unknown in children, particularly younger children, but it may reach a figure of 2 or 3 per cent in older age groups.

At the 300 mg dosage level isoniazid does not cause neuropathy in persons with normal nutrition. Neuropathy is due to a deficiency of pyridoxine (vitamin B_6) and is induced by urinary loss of this substance when isoniazid is taken. In most cases it is unnecessary to give pyridoxine supplements with isoniazid. In patients with poor nutritional status (e.g., chronic alcoholics) a small supplement of pyridoxine (10 mg daily) may be prescribed; when symptoms suggestive of neuropathy arise, larger doses of pyridoxine (100 to 250 mg a day) should be given. Isoniazid alone practically never gives rise to hypersensitivity reactions. Psychotic reactions may rarely be caused by usual doses of isoniazid in patients with previous psychiatric disturbances. Massive overdosage, taken accidentally or with suicidal intent, causes seizures, coma, and death. This is particularly common among young North American Indians; giving a small supply of the drug at a time would, at least in part, prevent these tragedies as well as assure better compliance with treatment.

The genetically determined characteristic of rapid or slow INH inactivation has little practical importance to treatment of tuberculosis or the occurrence of side effets. The only known exception is intermittent chemotherapy regimens in which drugs are given once a week; studies in India have shown that the therapeutic results in rapid inactivators are poorer than in slower inac-

TABLE 2. **Side Effects of Antituberculous Drugs**

DRUG	MAIN SIDE EFFECTS	USUAL MONITORING	REMARKS
Isoniazid	Hepatitis, neuropathy due to B_6 deficiency, rash	Liver function tests, SGOT, bilirubin	Rare; B_6 supplement necessary only if nutrition is poor
Rifampin	Hepatitis, neutropenia, flu syndrome	Liver function tests	Flu syndrome only in intermittent therapy
Pyrazinamide	Hepatitis, elevation of uric acid, arthralgia	Liver function tests	
Streptomycin	Rash, eighth nerve damage (vestibular)		Eighth nerve toxicity; common with renal impairment
Capreomycin	Rash, eighth nerve damage (vestibular)		Eighth nerve toxicity; common with renal impairment
Ethambutol	Optic neuritis	Snellen's chart	
Cycloserine	Convulsion, psychosis		Given in divided doses
Ethionamide	Gastric irritant, hepatitis		
Thiacetazone	Gastrointestinal symptoms, hepatitis, renal failure, agranulocytosis		Not used in the United States or Canada

tivators; however, this regimen is not used in North America, and these differences are not apparent in twice weekly intermittent regimens.

Rifampin

Rifampin is a powerful antituberculous agent with a potency at least equal to that of isoniazid. Introduction of rifampin to treatment of tuberculosis has enabled us to shorten considerably the total duration of chemotherapy. Side effects are uncommon. Hepatitis probably occurs in less than 1 per cent of patients; the underlying mechanisms are unknown, and it is possible that in most instances rifampin simply facilitates the development of INH-induced hepatitis. Treatment should be stopped if hepatitis develops, but when liver function comes back to normal it may be resumed with careful monitoring of the liver function. Skin rashes caused by rifampin occur but are usually quite mild; occasional patients complain of stomach irritation, and in these cases it is justifiable to give rifampin with meals. Purpura has been described but is extremely uncommon; it necessitates discontinuation of rifampin permanently. When rifampin is taken intermittently, either by design as in intermittent courses of treatment or because of irregular taking of medication by the patient on daily treatment, a number of immunologic reactions may occur. The most common is the so-called "flu" syndrome, which can be dealt with by resuming the daily treatment. Very rarely more severe reactions such as shock, acute attacks of breathlessness, hemolytic anemia, or renal failure occur; in intermittent treatment they require cessation of rifampin treatment. These reactions are never seen when the ordinary 600 mg dose of rifampin is used three times a week and are very uncommon with that dose in twice weekly regimens. They become somewhat more common with larger doses of rifampin or with once weekly treatment schedule.

Rifampin interferes with the action of contraceptive pills. While teratogenetic effects have been described in experimental animals, an extensive human experience suggests that rifampin does not cause fetal abnormalities. Rifampin renders body secretions (saliva, urine) pink; this is harmless but may cause worry if the patient is not told about it.

Pyrazinamide

Pyrazinamide (PZA) has been known for close to 30 years, but has in the past been used as a "second line" drug in the treatment of patients with resistant tubercle bacilli. It is a bactericidal drug acting on intracellular organisms, and recently it has been shown to be a powerful drug in a number of short chemotherapy trials. It is particularly effective when given along with streptomycin.

Pyrazinamide is particularly valuable in the early phases of treatment. Apart from usually mild gastrointestinal effects, pyrazinamide occasionally causes hepatotoxicity. Elevation of uric acid, sometimes to quite high levels, is common, but overt gout rarely occurs. Arthralgia occurs and is unrelated to the uric acid elevation.

Streptomycin

Streptomycin is another very effective antituberculous drug. It is given in a dose of 1 gram a day by intramuscular injection; in people over the age of 50 the dose should be smaller (0.5 to 0.75 gram a day). At times, pain at the site of injection creates a problem. An occasional patient complains of a reaction consisting of the sensation of numbness around the mouth associated with a general feeling of "fuzziness" or inability to concentrate; this reaction is usually quite innocuous, occurring an hour or two after injection and lasting several hours; changing the preparation of streptomycin is sometimes helpful. Eighth (vestibular) nerve toxicity is much more serious; vestibular toxicity is related to the dose; some streptomycin is eliminated by the kidneys, and a patient with impaired renal function is particularly liable to develop this toxicity. Assessment of renal function is therefore necessary when one embarks on a prolonged course of streptomycin. The earliest manifestation of vestibular toxicity is a complaint of dizziness and vertigo; this occurs before any objective signs of impairment of vestibular function can be elicited. Dizziness is therefore an indication that treatment with streptomycin should be discontinued or interrupted. Hypersensitivity reactions, usually manifested by fever, skin rash, or both, occur in about 5 per cent of patients, usually during the first few months of treatment, often some 3 to 4 weeks after starting on a course of streptomycin.

Ethambutol

Ethambutol (EMB) is a relatively weak antituberculous agent, and its chief role in treatment is that of "resistance prevention" when given with more powerful bactericidal drugs. The only important toxicity is optic neuritis, but this very seldom occurs when the currently recommended dose of 15 mg per kg per day is used. There is very little justification for using a larger dose; until relatively recently a dose of 25 mg per kg per day was used in the early stages of treatment.

Para-aminosalicylic Acid

Para-aminosalicylic acid (PAS) is another mainly bacteriostatic agent probably somewhat stronger than ethambutol. It is infrequently used now except in children. Gastrointestinal symptoms are common. Hypersensitivity reactions (skin rashes and fever) are also relatively common. Hepatitis, a syndrome resembling infectious mononucleosis, and transient pulmonary infiltrations have all been described.

Treatment Regimens

The degree of cooperation likely to be expected from the patient should be a primary consideration in choosing the treatment regimen.

Regimen for "Cooperative" Patients. All these patients are placed on isoniazid, 300 mg a day, rifampin 600 mg a day, and ethambutol, approximately 15 mg per kg of body weight per day, for the initial 2 months or so of chemotherapy. Approximately at that time the results of sensitivity studies become available, and if, as is usually the case, the bacilli are found to be sensitive to all the antimicrobial agents, then ethambutol should be discontinued, as it will have fulfilled its role of preventing the organisms from becoming resistant to rifampin in those few patients who are found to harbor INH-resistant bacilli. Treatment is often continued with daily isoniazid and rifampin. The total duration of treatment should be 9 months, except in that very small group of patients with very advanced disease whose sputum converts slowly. In these cases, treatment should be given for 5 months after sputum conversion.

Treatment of Potentially "Uncooperative" Patients. During the initial phase of treatment these patients should receive isoniazid, 300 mg a day, rifampin, 600 mg a day, pyrazinamide, 1.5 to 2 grams a day, and streptomycin, 0.75 to 1 gram a day. Some of these patients, particularly alcoholics, may require a small supplement of pyridoxine (vitamin B_6). This regimen can generally be discontinued when the results of the sensitivity tests of their tubercle bacilli become available, to be replaced by a completely supervised regimen consisting of isoniazid, 15 mg per kg of body weight, rifampin, 600 mg, and pyridoxine (vitamin B_6), given three times per week. The total duration of treatment is the same as in the first regimen: 9 months, or 5 months after sputum conversion in the "slow converters." The initial treatment with four bactericidal drugs is the most powerful treatment available, and it is likely that further study will reveal that total duration of therapy can be shortened. The reason for giving intermittent treatment three times rather than twice a week is two-fold: first. to eliminate the "immunologic" side effects of rifampin; and second, and more important, to give effective chemotherapy in spite of the frequent lapses which occur in this group of patients.

The treatment regimens recommended above are intended for advanced, smear positive cases of pulmonary tuberculosis. Minimal, smear negative pulmonary tuberculosis, pleural effusion, and other forms of disease in which the total bacterial population is rather small should be given shorter courses of chemotherapy. At present it is safe to reduce it to 6 months, and possibly further studies will reveal that it may be curtailed even further.

These regimens are recommended for patients in the developed countries such as the United States or Canada, where the aim is to achieve almost 100 per cent success with no relapses and where the cost of treatment is a relatively minor consideration. In developing countries, where the cost of drugs is often of more importance, it is justifiable to reduce the total duration of treatment of advanced cases to 6 months and accept a relapse rate of under 10 per cent. Patients who relapse can be retreated with the same regimen in these circumstances.

It is not justifiable to extend the treatment of far advanced cases beyond 9 months except in the rare cases of slow converters, as the risk of side effects, although small, is greater than the probably nonexistent benefits derived by the patients. The continuation phase of the treatment for cooperative patients (daily isoniazid and rifampin) should be carefully monitored; it is wise to see such patients twice a month throughout the course of treatment, and if there is any doubt about compliance, they should be transferred to the intermittent, supervised regimen. Patients on such intermittent supervised regimens with high doses of isoniazid should be given a vitamin B_6 supplement. Occasionally streptomycin, 0.75 to 1 gram, may be added to three times a week INH and rifampin; while it is uncertain that this addition substantially strengthens the regimen, the psychologic effect of receiving needles occasionally assures better compliance. It should be appreciated that the three times a week regimen with a high dose of isoniazid is as potent as the daily INH and rifampin regimen, and it is quite permissible to transfer patients from one to the other as circumstances demand. To assure compliance with intermittent supervised chemotherapy it is necessary to make such treatment as convenient as possible for the patient: e.g., evening clinics, home visits, and the like.

In a relatively small minority of patients the regimens outlined above cannot be applied because of serious side effects or are inappropriate because of initial drug resistance. In INH resistant cases the treatment should be continued with two drugs, e.g., rifampin and ethambutol (and sometimes another drug if the bacterial population is large), for 18 to 24 months. When such other drugs are used on an intermittent basis, the dose should be adjusted upward two to three times in the case of isoniazid, ethambutol, and pyrazinamide, but should remain the same as the daily dose in the case of streptomycin and rifampin.

Sputum Conversion

Conversion of sputum from positive to negative depends on a number of factors. Generally patients with extensive lesions and a large bacterial population show slower conversion than those with less extensive disease. The character of the lesion is also of some importance; those with a lot of fibrosis (e.g., silicotuberculosis) tend to convert more slowly. However, the vast majority of smear positive cases of pulmonary tuberculosis become negative on microscopic examination in 2 to 8 weeks. Before the introduction of rifampin, culture conversion from positive to negative occurred fairly regularly some 4 weeks following smear conversion, but now with the regimens containing rifampin, culture conversion not infrequently occurs at the time of smear conversion or even earlier. This has been variously interpreted as signifying that the bacilli seen on smear are not viable or that sputum in such cases contains a high enough concentration of rifampin to inhibit their growth (inadvertent sensitivity test).

It is often claimed that even 2 weeks of intensive chemotherapy renders the patient non-infectious. While the number of bacilli in the sputum undoubtedly falls precipitously during the initial stages of chemotherapy and while the patient, knowing that he has tuberculosis, commonly takes extra precautions, it is, until conclusively proved otherwise, probably wiser to consider any patient who excretes enough bacilli in his sputum for them to be visible under the microscope to be still potentially infectious.

Resistance

Primary drug resistance of tubercle bacilli is uncommon when infection has been acquired in the United States or Canada. Probably well below 5 per cent of cases arising from such infections show primary resistance to isoniazid or to streptomycin, while resistance to rifampin and ethambutol is even less common. This proportion of patients, harboring resistant bacilli, is appreciably higher with infections acquired in developing countries, but even there the vast majority of patients harbor sensitive bacilli. This is particularly true of older patients who acquired their infection many years ago before the current

resistance patterns developed. It is because of this risk of primary resistance, small as it is, that the initial treatment of tuberculosis should be with three or more drugs.

Secondary resistance — that occurring in patients who have previously received chemotherapy for tuberculosis — is much more common. It should always be assumed when prescribing chemotherapy that the patient is resistant to all the drugs which he received previously. While it is justified to include in the treatment regimen some or all of those drugs, *two* new drugs must always be added; the regimen may then be modified appropriately when results of sensitivity studies become available. In actual practice, this seldom modifies the regimens recommended above, as at present we see practically no relapses among patients who received rifampin and very few among those who received ethambutol or pyrazinamide during previous chemotherapy. It should be added that the regimens outlined above are not producing resistance as the patient who completes a 9 months' course practically never relapses, while those who abandon treatment earlier are fully sensitive and can be placed back on the same regimen.

Supervision and Follow-up

Follow-up examination of outpatients on treatment must be quite frequent. Those who are started on chemotherapy without initial hospitalization should be seen at least once a week during the first 8 weeks. During the continuation phase of treatment follow-up visits should be arranged at 2 week intervals irrespective of whether or not the patient was hospitalized for his initial care. While the initial therapy is of great importance, there often seems to be a discrepancy between the effort devoted to the initial period of treatment in the hospital and the relative neglect of the continuation phase of treatment.

If the patient is on an unsupervised regimen, he should be questioned carefully at each of the follow-up examinations about the way in which he takes his drugs, and the total dosage should be compared with the number of pills remaining from the previous prescription. Urine tests for INH derivatives should be done from time to time. Brief inquiry for the possible side effects of the drugs should be included. Chest x-rays and bacteriologic investigation are indicated at monthly intervals during the first few months of treatment; then if the patient responds satisfactorily to treatment, x-ray should be taken at intervals of 2 or 3 months but sputum should be examined monthly. It is unnecessary to stop treatment during the period of collection of bacteriologic specimens.

When 9 months' treatment has been completed and medication was taken regularly, the chances of relapse are very small, and therefore no further regular follow-up is necessary. However, patients should understand that they must report if and when systemic or respiratory symptoms develop. In patients in whom there is doubt, a 2 year follow-up period with x-rays and bacteriology done every 6 months should be undertaken.

Corticosteroid Therapy

Corticosteroids are known to reactivate latent tuberculous foci. They can, however, be of considerable benefit in certain clinical situations when combined with an effective antimicrobial regimen. Indications for corticosteroid therapy are few, chief among them being a severe tuberculous illness; in such cases a combination of antimicrobial therapy and corticosteroids can be lifesaving. In certain cases of tuberculous meningitis with exudate blocking or threatening to block cerebrospinal circulation, corticosteroids are effective and should be used. Similarly corticosteroids are helpful in management of obstructive lesions of the ureters in genitourinary tuberculosis. The dose of steroids in all those situations probably does not need to be very large; we usually use between 20 and 40 mg of prednisone daily initially, and taper it over a period of weeks.

The Place of Surgery in Pulmonary Tuberculosis

While surgery contributed a great deal to the treatment of this disease in the past, currently available antimicrobial treatment is so powerful that it has all but eliminated surgery from a role in treatment. A persistent cavity which fails to close in spite of sputum conversion should be left alone, as such "open negative cases" seldom relapse. Occasional indications for surgery result from the sequelae of tuberculosis such as severely damaged lung with gross bronchiectasis; however, the indications for resection arise from the severity of symptoms, e.g., repeated profuse hemoptysis, gross suppurative lung disease, recurrent pneumonia, and not from the radiologic appearance per se. Surgery could have a place in unilateral disease in patients with complete bacterial resistance to all the antimicrobial agents, but with the exception of certain atypical mycobacterial infections one rarely meets such cases at present.

Extrapulmonary Tuberculosis

The principles of antimicrobial treatment of tuberculous meningitis, genitourinary tuberculosis, skeletal tuberculosis, tuberculous cervical adenitis, and so forth are in essence the same as those discussed above in connection with pulmonary tuberculosis. The treatment of these patients should be a joint responsibility of a physician versed in the treatment of tuberculosis and a specialist in the diseases of the system which is involved. Unless close cooperation of this kind is forthcoming, these patients may receive inadequate antimicrobial treatment.

Childhood Tuberculosis

Tuberculosis in children is now uncommon in the United States and Canada, particularly among the Caucasian population. The principles of treatment are the same as those discussed for adults. Children take all antimicrobial agents with relative impunity; side effects are less common than in adults. The doses of the drugs are adjusted to weight. Isoniazid is given at a dose of between 5 and 10 mg per kg of body weight and rifampin at 10 to 20 mg per kg. The bacterial population in most forms of tuberculosis in children is small, and the outlook for all but hematogenous forms of tuberculosis was good even in the preantimicrobial era. Thus, although there have been no extensive chemotherapy trials, it would appear that in cases of primary tuberculosis, segmental and lobar lesions ("epituberculosis"), and primary pleural effusions, 6 months' chemotherapy utilizing the regimens outlined above should be quite sufficient. Forms of disease resulting from hematogenous dissemination, particularly miliary tuberculosis and meningitis, should be treated somewhat longer, for 9 months.

It should be remembered that segmental and lobar lesions complicating primary tuberculosis are fairly common, particularly in younger children, and they resolve very slowly. These lesions are relatively benign and do not require resection unless there are severe symptoms caused by bronchiectasis or bronchostenosis and secondary bacterial infection.

Chemoprophylaxis

Chemoprophylaxis (preventive treatment) substantially diminishes the risk of developing tuberculosis in infected individuals. Hepatotoxicity of isoniazid, low as it is, has made widespread public health programs of INH prophylaxis less acceptable. Furthermore, the realization that tuberculin reaction is somewhat less reliable than was previously believed has curtailed a number of the rather broad indications for chemoprophylaxis. It is realized now that not all positive reactors have been infected with tubercle bacilli; nor are all the conversions due to recent infection with these organisms. Chemoprophylaxis should therefore be used only in well documented situations in which there is a high risk of tuberculosis.

From the point of view of practicing physicians there are two main indications for chemoprophylaxis. The first is the contacts of sputum positive (smear positive) cases of tuberculosis. Such individuals, if recently infected as indicated by skin test, have a very high risk of disease, and this can be appreciably diminished by a course of isoniazid. The second indication relates to patients with inactive tuberculosis or scarring of the lungs, presumably caused by old tuberculosis, who are placed on corticosteroids or immunosuppressive agents for the treatment of other disorders. A number of other indications for chemoprophylaxis which fall into the domain of public health programs are being currently reassessed and need not be discussed here.

A course of chemoprophylaxis consists of isoniazid taken at the usual dose of 300 mg a day daily for 1 year. It is somewhat anomalous that treatment of active disease recommended now lasts 9 months, while the course of prophylaxis actually takes longer. It seems likely that shorter courses of prophylaxis, particularly in infected contacts, will prove to be effective, but this has yet to be documented.

Individuals receiving chemoprophylaxis should be aware of the very slight danger of isoniazid toxicity; they should be seen at monthly intervals.

Bacille Calmette-Guérin (BCG) Vaccination

Various trials of this vaccine produced widely different results, with effectiveness varying from 0 to 80 per cent. From the standpoint of the practicing physician there are practically no indications for BCG vaccination. The only exceptions are tuberculin negative contacts of sputum positive patients with tuberculosis who harbor bacilli with multiple resistance; such cases are, however, very few. In our judgment, BCG should also be given to tuberculin negative individuals leaving for countries with a considerable tuberculosis problem; this should apply to those likely to come into very close contact with the local population such as Peace Corps volunteers.

Atypical Mycobacterioses

Atypical mycobacterioses are uncommon. These organisms are much less pathogenic than tubercle bacilli, and this is the main reason why these diseases are uncommon in the face of the fairly high prevalence of atypical infection in the population. While all the groups affected by tubercle bacilli may be affected by atypical mycobacteria, only two entities which are seen with any frequency need to be considered here. These are pulmonary mycobacteriosis and cervical adenitis.

Pulmonary (Atypical) Mycobacteriosis. This is usually caused by either of two types of organisms: *Mycobacterium kansasii* or the intracellulare-avium group. *M. kansasii* is usually sensitive to a number of antituberculosis drugs, and appropriate chemotherapy can be prescribed and achieve a cure. Initial treatment should be similar to that given for pulmonary tuberculosis; when sensitivity study results are available, other agents may have to be added. Mycobacteria from the intracellulare-avium group are usually completely resistant to most antimicrobial agents, with the usual exception of cycloserine and ethionamide. Because of this resistance pattern, we often have no specific treatment to offer these patients; it was recently shown that chemotherapy with five or six of the antituberculosis drugs (see Table 1) is effective in some of these cases. These claims, while likely true, are not based on controlled studies and do not take into account the intrinsic tendency of mycobacterioses (including tuberculosis) to heal.

Cervical Adenitis Due to Atypical Mycobacteria. This form of disease is often seen in small children, presenting with enlargement of a lymph node in the neck, which on biopsy is shown to contain caseating granuloma with acid-fast bacilli. In the Vancouver area, atypical mycobacteria are usually responsible for cervical adenitis in Caucasian children under the age of 10, tubercle bacilli being a very uncommon cause of this condition in this group of children. While differential skin tests (using tuberculin antigens derived from atypical mycobacteria) are helpful, definite proof comes from culture of the biopsy. The condition is benign, the organism is usually resistant, and usually chemotherapy is both ineffective and unnecessary.

VIRAL RESPIRATORY INFECTIONS

method of
DOUGLAS D. RICHMAN, M.D.
San Diego, California

Viral respiratory infection represents the most common illness experienced by patients in any age group. Such infections represent the most frequent single cause of visits to physicians and of absenteeism from work or school. Viral respiratory infections may range in severity from the mild "common cold," characterized by afebrile rhinorrhea and perhaps pharyngitis, to fatal pneumonitis. The specific identification of the etiologic agent of a viral respiratory infection is difficult in practice. There are over 200 serologically distinct respiratory viruses that are members of such structurally different families as the myxoviruses, paramyxoviruses, coronaviruses, picornaviruses, herpesviruses, and adenoviruses. No single clinical syndrome can be attributed to a single agent or even a single group of closely related agents. Diagnostic virology is not widely available, and even if available, virus isolation takes at least a few days and a diagnostic seroconversion takes at least a week or two to document. Rapid viral diagnosis is a rapidly developing field with promise for application to viral respiratory infections in the future.

The pressure to make a specific diagnosis is not yet great, because only influenza A infections are amenable to specific chemoprophylaxis and therapy with amantadine. Readily available information about influenza epidemiology can increase the index of suspicion of the probability of an influenza infection. The approach to the patient with viral respiratory infection requires appreciation of the fact that most of these infections are both uncomplicated and self-limited. Consequently, with the exception of influenza A infections, the role of the physician caring for a patient with a viral respiratory infection is to provide reassurance, to avoid potentially toxic and unnecessary therapy, to recommend measures that relieve symptoms, and to remain alert for serious and treatable complications.

General Symptomatic Therapy

The age-old recommendation of rest, fluids, and aspirin remains the mainstay of management. Fluid intake should be encouraged to compensate for diminished appetite and for increased loss owing to fever. The avoidance of irritants, such as tobacco smoke, is obviously recommended. Since over-the-counter cold preparations contain many of the drugs for symptomatic relief that are listed below, it is important to establish the fact with the patient in order to avoid duplication of medication. Since these medications are for symptomatic relief and do not hasten the resolution of the infectious process, they should be used for as short a period as possible and should be discontinued when any untoward side effect is suspected.

Antipyretics-Analgesics. ACETYLSALICYLIC ACID. The dose is 650 mg (2 tablets of 325 mg) orally every 4 hours. For children give 40 to 60 mg of chewable baby aspirin (60 to 80 mg per tablet) for every year of age under 10, every 4 to 6 hours.

ACETAMINOPHEN. For patients who cannot tolerate aspirin or who are taking anticoagulant

medications, give 650 mg (2 tablets of 325 mg) every 4 hours. Eighty mg chewable tablets and an elixir are available for children; give 16 to 32 mg every 4 to 6 hours for infants under 1; 60 to 120 mg every 4 to 6 hours for children 1 to 3 years old; 120 to 240 mg for children 3 to 6 years old; and 240 to 325 mg for children 6 to 12 years old.

Decongestants. LOCAL NASAL DECONGESTANTS. Local drops or spray provides substantial local effects with negligible systemic absorption. The readily appreciable nasal decongestion produced may result in excessive or prolonged use by patients. Such misuse can result in a rebound vasodilatation of constricted mucosal vessels, and this may perpetuate the nasal congestion. The only cure for this "rebound congestion" is withdrawal of the drug. Longer acting local decongestants are less likely to produce this complication, and are also more convenient to use. Consequently, I recommend xylometazoline (Otrivin) or oxymetazoline (Afrin) over the shorter acting agents. The use of a dropper or spray nozzle by more than one individual should be avoided. The nasal decongestants should be administered only when needed and should be avoided after 3 or 4 days. The adult dosages are provided except where specifically indicated.

Xylometazoline HCl (Otrivin) 0.1 per cent, 2 drops or sprays two to three times daily. For children use a 0.05 per cent solution, 2 drops per dose for 6 to 12 years old, and 1 drop per dose for 2 to 6 years old.

Oxymetazoline HCl (Afrin) 0.05 per cent, 2 drops or sprays two to three times daily. For children 6 to 12 years old, a 0.025 per cent solution is available.

Naphazoline HCl (Privine) 0.05 per cent, 1 to 2 drops or sprays every 4 to 6 hours. For children 6 to 12 years old use a 0.025 per cent solution, 1 to 2 drops or sprays every 6 hours.

Phenylephrine HCl (Neo-Synephrine) 0.5 per cent, 2 drops or sprays every 4 hours. The 0.25 per cent solution should be used for children 6 to 12 years old and the 0.125 per cent solution for children 2 to 6 years old.

Ephedrine HCl or sulfate 0.5 per cent, 2 drops or sprays every 4 hours.

ORAL DECONGESTANTS. Oral decongestants are less effective than topical decongestants for the relief of nasal congestion. Whether one or the other is superior in relieving obstruction of the eustachian tubes, if in fact either is effective, has not been demonstrated. Oral decongestants may induce sympathomimetic side effects such as nervousness, sleeplessness, and tachycardia. Although they are available over the counter, oral decongestants should not be used by patients with hypertension, cardiac disease, diabetes mellitus, or hyperthyroidism without medical supervision. In addition, patients taking monoamine oxidase inhibitors should avoid taking oral decongestants. The adult dose should be halved for children between the ages of 6 and 12 and quartered for children between the ages of 2 and 6.

Phenylephrine HCl, 10 mg every 4 hours.

Phenylpropanolamine HCl, 25 mg every 4 hours or 50 mg every 8 hours.

Pseudoephedrine HCl (Sudafed), 60 mg every 4 hours. For children less than 4 months, give 15 mg every 8 hours; for children ages 4 months to 6 years, give 30 mg every 6 to 8 hours.

Antihistamines. There is evidence indicating that antihistamines may have an antitussive effect through central action and may reduce rhinorrhea in common colds. There is marked patient variability in the susceptibility to the sedative and other central nervous system side effects of antihistamines; dosing and patient cautioning should be made accordingly. Antihistamines are contraindicated in patients with glaucoma or urinary retention. Although many antihistamines are available, only three of the more frequently utilized in respiratory infection are listed:

Chlorpheniramine maleate (Chlor-Trimeton), 4 mg every 6 hours for adults; 2 mg every 6 hours for children 6 to 12 years old; 1 mg every 6 hours for children 2 to 6 years old; and 1 mg every 8 hours for infants under 2 years.

Diphenhydramine HCl (Benadryl), 25 mg every 4 hours for adults; 12.5 mg every 4 hours for children 6 to 12 years old, and 6.25 mg every 4 hours for children 2 to 6 years old.

Brompheniramine maleate (Dimetane), 4 mg every 4 to 6 hours for adults; 2 mg every 6 hours for children 6 to 12 years old; 1 mg every 6 hours for children 2 to 6 years old; and 1 mg every 8 hours for infants under 2 years.

Many combinations of antihistamines and decongestants are available: Actifed, Drixoral, Dimetapp, and others. These have the advantage of convenience, but the potential disadvantages of providing an unnecessary drug and of not titrating the patient to the ideal ratio of each drug.

Antitussives. The cough reflex is important in clearing the bronchial tree of excessive secretions and other materials. The cough of viral infections, however, may often reflect only mucosal irritation. The nonproductive cough in viral respiratory infection is often a frustrating

and debilitating symptom rather than a beneficial reflex. Accordingly, suppression of such a cough will provide much relief.

The centrally acting antitussives include opiate narcotics, of which codeine is the most widely used, and non-narcotics such as dextromethorphan and antihistamines (see above). The narcotic antitussives are the most effective but should be administered with caution because of their potential for abuse, for central respiratory depression (a special concern for patients with lung disease associated with a tendency to retain CO_2), and for impairment of motor skills (a special concern for operators of machinery and motor vehicles).

All antitussives should be limited to use for less than 1 week because persistent cough may indicate serious disease and thus merits medical evaluation. The doses listed are for adults and older children. These dosages should be halved for children between 6 and 12 years of age and quartered for children between 2 and 6 years of age.

Codeine phosphate, 15 to 30 mg orally every 4 to 6 hours not to exceed 120 mg in 24 hours.

Dextromethorphan, 15 to 30 mg orally every 4 to 6 hours not to exceed 120 mg in 24 hours.

Expectorants. Expectorants are generally used in an attempt to reduce the viscosity of secretions and to aid in their formation. The most valuable approach in achieving this goal is clearly to prevent or relieve dehydration. Hydration is thus of great importance, and I am unconvinced that any additional measures presently available offer benefits in the mobilization of respiratory secretions. The most commonly prescribed expectorant, guaifenesin (glyceryl guaiacolate), has little demonstrated toxicity, except for inhibition of platelet function in experimental situations; however, efficacy has never been demonstrated in any clinical situations or in animal models. Its use thus appears to be more a medical ritual than a therapeutic intervention.

Recognition and Treatment of Complications

The serious complications of viral respiratory infections can be divided into the life-threatening lower respiratory tract processes directly produced by virus infection and the complications caused by secondary bacterial infection. In adults viral pneumonitis is seen, especially with influenza. The most frequent victims of serious, pure virus infections are infants less than 6 months old. They are subject to laryngotracheobronchitis (croup), bronchiolitis, and pneumonitis. Signs of respiratory impairment from any of these syndromes merits hospitalization to maintain hydration, to observe the respiratory status closely, to monitor blood gases, to administer oxygen as needed, and to provide endotracheal intubation and respiratory support if necessary. The role of bronchodilators and steroids in these illnesses has not been established.

The most common bacterial complications of viral infections are acute otitis media, acute purulent sinusitis, and bacterial pneumonia. These complications may accompany the viral infection, often overshadowing the viral syndrome itself, or they may follow the viral syndrome. The specific therapeutic approach to each of these problems is considered in separate articles.

Specific Antiviral Chemotherapy

The only specific antiviral agent currently available for respiratory infections is amantadine HCl (Symmetrel). Amantadine has been shown to be efficacious only for infection with type A influenza virus. Originally approved for chemoprophylaxis of influenza A virus infection, it has been recently approved for therapeutic use as well. Regarding prophylaxis, it should be borne in mind that effective killed influenza vaccines are available for both type A and B influenza virus infection and that vaccination is protective for at least a year or two. Prophylaxis with amantadine is effective only for as long as it is administered. When an influenza A epidemic develops, amantadine is indicated for patients at high risk for complications (underlying cardiopulmonary disease, old age) or for medical personnel. For these indications killed influenza vaccine should be administered as well, if vaccine containing the appropriate antigens is available.

Amantadine has been shown to reduce the height and duration of fever and several other symptoms of the influenza syndrome. The reduced dynamic compliance caused by influenza virus infection as measured by pulmonary function testing has also been shown to resolve more rapidly in patients treated with amantadine. Although amantadine has not been systematically studied in patients with pneumonitis, the early use of the drug is probably indicated in any patient with documented or highly suspected influenza A infection that is neither mild nor clearly resolving. The dosage of amantadine for either prophylaxis or therapy is 100 mg orally twice daily in adults and children over 40 kg. For children below 40 kg the dose is 5 mg per kg orally in two divided doses but not to exceed 150 mg per day. A small percentage of patients will experience mild central nervous system symptoms, including insomnia, anxiety, confusion, and dizziness. These symptoms are reversed upon discontinuation or reduction of the dosage of the drug. Since amantadine is excreted via the kidney, modification of the dosage is indicated for patients with renal impairment.

The Cardiovascular System

ACQUIRED DISEASES OF THE AORTA

method of
WILLIAM A. GAY, Jr., M.D.
New York, New York

Arteriosclerosis of the Aorta

As the body's major arterial conduit the aorta is a prime target for the most common disease which affects the arterial tree, arteriosclerosis. Whereas obstruction to flow is the chief manifestation of significant arteriosclerotic involvement in most arteries, expansion up to, and including, rupture also may commonly result from arteriosclerosis of the aorta.

Preventive Measures and Medical Treatment

Since little is known regarding the precise cause of arteriosclerotic disease, no absolute preventive regimen exists. Nonetheless, certain risk factors are able to be controlled by the patient and his doctor. Among these are obesity, tobacco use, hypertension, diabetes, certain hyperlipidemias, and some endocrine disorders. Some individuals will develop significant arteriosclerosis of the aorta in spite of their diligence and the expert attentiveness of their physician, as there are unknown and uncontrollable factors also involved.

Patients with arteriosclerotic aortic disease, proved or suspected, should certainly avoid tobacco, control their weight, and abstain from foods high in cholesterol and animal fats. The use of pharmacologic agents aimed at lipid control has been of help in small numbers of patients with highly specific metabolic or endocrine disorders up to this date. Severely regimented dietary programs have, likewise, been of limited success, perhaps not because of ineffectiveness but lack of patient compliance. Although salicylates and other agents to reduce platelet adhesiveness have been widely used, their potential benefits are largely theoretical.

In brief, because so little is known regarding the precise cause and pathogenesis of aortic atherosclerosis, prevention or reversal of the actual disease process is not possible in most instances. Instead we are called upon to treat the results of the disease, obstruction, expansion, or rupture. The treatment of these conditions is most often operative.

Operative Management

The operative treatment of acquired aortic disease is directed toward the alleviation of obstructive symptoms or the prevention, or treatment, of rupture.

Obstruction

The abdominal aorta at its bifurcation is the most common site of chronic progressive atherosclerotic occlusion. This site is also the area where embolic occlusion of the aorta most frequently occurs. The latter condition is best managed by embolectomy. This is a quick and simple procedure which may be done under local anesthesia. Bilateral femoral arteriotomies are done and Fogarty balloon embolectomy catheters are passed retrograde into the abdominal aorta and the clot extracted. The extracted material should always be sent for pathologic confirmation, since an occasional atrial myxoma may present in this fashion.

Most often atherosclerotic obstruction of the aorta will have a more insidious onset, and symptoms will usually be of a chronic nature. Atherosclerotic occlusion of the distal aorta requires

157

surgical treatment when symptoms become significant. Two forms of surgical therapy are available, bypass grafting and endarterectomy. The choice of operations depends largely upon the extent of arteriosclerotic involvement of both the aorta and the iliofemoral system. In either event the transperitoneal approach via a midline xiphoid to pubis incision is usually preferred. In instances in which entry into the peritoneal cavity is undesirable, a unilateral retroperitoneal approach can be made, using a flank incision.

If the occlusive defect in the aorta is well localized over a distance of 8 cm or less, endarterectomy is the preferred treatment. When the aorta is exposed, 5000 units of heparin is given intravenously and the aorta is cross-clamped just below the renal arteries. A longitudinal incision is made through the adventitia of the aorta and a plane developed subintimally. The atheromatous core is removed and the distal intima tacked to the aortic wall with several fine horizontal mattress sutures. The distal arterial tree is then flushed with heparinized saline and the aortic adventitia closed with a continuous simple suture, taking care not to narrow the aortic lumen any more than necessary. Extreme care should be exercised during the procedure not to allow thrombotic, atherosclerotic debris from entering the distal arterial tree. If there is any question of this, Fogarty embolectomy catheters may be passed into both distal arterial systems.

Most patients with aortic obstructive disease requiring operation will need bypass grafting rather than endarterectomy, because the disease, in most, is not well localized to a short segment. In some of these, however, a localized endarterectomy may be necessary in order to prepare a site on the aorta suitable for graft placement. A bifurcation graft of appropriate size is nearly always indicated, since iliac disease, when present, is usually bilateral. Our preference is to use the end-to-side approach to the aortic anastomosis as well as those to the common femoral arteries. This allows preservation of what little flow there is and may result in better perfusion of pelvic organs following bypass grafting.

Aneurysms of the Aorta

The inelasticity of the aortic wall caused by arteriosclerosis may result in aneurysm formation. The most common location for aortic aneurysms is the abdominal aorta between the level of the renal arteries and the bifurcation. When an abdominal aneurysm is 7 cm or larger in its transverse diameter, surgical resection and grafting is warranted unless there are other serious coexisting conditions. Among these are serious coronary heart disease, cerebral vascular disease,

extensive peripheral vascular disease, or severe pulmonary disease. Any of these conditions would significantly increase the risk of resection, and consideration should be given to close, frequent follow-up examinations in these patients. Surgical intervention may then be undertaken when the size of the aneurysm exceeds 10 cm, if there is evidence of rapid expansion or the development of symptoms felt to be due to the aneurysm.

Elective resection of an abdominal aneurysm should be preceded by effective mechanical bowel preparation. Preoperative adminstration of broad-spectrum antibiotic with antistaphylococcal activity should assure an effective blood level at the time of operation. At the time of operation the bladder is catheterized with an indwelling catheter, and monitoring of systemic arterial and pulmonary arterial pressures is accomplished with appropriate catheters. Electrocardiographic monitoring is also done. The lower chest, entire abdomen, and both legs down to the knees are prepped and included in the operative field. A xiphoid to pubis midline incision is made and the aorta approached transperitoneally. Five thousand units of heparin is given intravenously just prior to aortic clamping, except in cases of ruptured aneurysm where no heparin is given. A vascular clamp is placed across the aorta several centimeters proximal to the origin of the aneurysm — usually just below the level of the left renal vein. The positioning of the distal clamps depends upon the extent of the aneurysm, but most often these vascular clamps are placed upon the common iliac arteries. Caution is necessary to avoid injury to the vena cava, the iliac veins, and the ureters. The aneurysm is entered and all thrombotic material is evacuated. Culture of this material is advisable, since, occasionally, graft infections may arise from infected clot present preoperatively. Lumbar arteries are oversewn with nonabsorbable material. A woven Dacron graft of appropriate size and configuration is selected and sutured into place with nonabsorbable sutures, placing the proximal suture line first. It is our practice to place a vascular clamp on the graft itself and release the proximal aortic clamp at this time in order that the proximal anastomosis might be inspected in its entirety prior to proceeding with the distal suture lines. The aorta is not transected either proximally or distally, and the entire suture line, except for the anterior-most sutures, lies within the lumen of the aorta, thereby tucking the graft into the remnants of the aneurysm sac. When a straight graft is used, the distal anastomosis is done in a manner similar to that described above. In cases in which a bifurcation graft is necessary, an end-to-end reconstruction is preferred, dividing the proximal iliac (femoral) artery and oversewing its end whenever possible. That portion of the graft lying within the bed of the opened aneurysm is covered by sewing together the walls of the aneurysm sac. The cross-clamps are released slowly, and extreme care is taken to avoid dislodgment of thrombotic debris into the distal arterial tree. It is our practice to flush the distal vessels with heparinized saline solution prior to unclamping. Slow, gradual release of the clamps along with the assurance of adequate blood volume replacement will lessen the risk of hypotension at this time. In the event of severe, persistent hypotension occurring at the time of clamp release, the clamp may be reapplied and measures taken to ensure an adequate pressure on the subsequent release.

When operation is undertaken for ruptured abdominal aneurysm, the procedure must be done without delay; therefore bowel preparation may not be accomplished. Most often these patients present with hypotension and severe abdominal pain to an emeregency room and are found to have a ruptured aneurysm. The natural tendency is to institute blood transfusion in an attempt to restore the blood pressure to normal. While blood should certainly be typed and cross-matched in adequate quantities, transfusion should be avoided if possible until the patient is in the operating room. Our policy is to rapidly transport the patient to the operating room, where general anesthesia is induced. Sometimes relaxation of the abdominal musculature coincident with the administration of a muscle relaxant results in an abrupt fall in an already low, but previously stable, blood pressure. This generally means aortic rupture has occurred, and the abdomen must be opened with haste in order to secure control of the aorta. When aortic rupture has occurred, the entire abdomen may be filled with blood, or, more commonly, the retroperitoneal area is the site of a large hematoma. In either case the usual intra-abdominal anatomy may be obscured. Rapid proximal control of the aorta may be gained by placement of a clamp across the aorta superior to the lesser curvature of the stomach through the lesser peritoneal sac. In some instances a large Foley catheter (No. 24 or larger) with a 30 ml balloon may be inserted directly into the aortic defect, passed a short distance proximally, and the balloon inflated. Distal control may usually be accomplished in a more methodical manner and followed by accurate placement of the proximal clamp so as not to compromise flow to the renal arteries. Once the aorta has been controlled, rapid transfusion should be undertaken to replace the estimated

shed volume. Additionally, it is our practice to administer an osmotic diuretic (usually 12.5 grams of mannitol) at this time to stimulate continued urine flow. The remainder of the procedure is similar to that described above for elective aneurysm resection.

While aneurysms of the abdominal aorta are most common, arteriosclerotic disease in other areas may result in aneurysm formation.

Aneurysms of the Ascending Aorta

Although most aneurysms in this location result from arteriosclerosis, cystic disease of the aortic media and congenital sinus of Valsalva aneurysms also are causative factors. Cardiopulmonary bypass is required. Our practice is to lower body temperature to 28 C and induce further cardiac hypothermia by bathing the heart in iced saline (4 C solution). The ascending aorta is clamped just proximal to the arch vessels and the aneurysm opened. Five hundred ml of hyperkalemic cardioplegic solution at 4 C is infused into the coronary ostia by means of a Spencer coronary perfusion catheter. In some instances, replacement of the aortic valve is necessary and may be carried out with a suitable prosthesis by itself or incorporated into a composite graft if valve replacement and aortic root replacement are both necessary. In these instances the coronary ostia are removed from the aorta with a button of aortic tissue for reimplantation. The graft of tightly woven Dacron is then sutured into place, cardiac end first, with continuous, simple nonabsorbable sutures. After the distal anastomosis has been completed, the aneurysm sac is closed over the graft, the clamps removed, and cardiopulmonary bypass discontinued.

Aneurysms of the Transverse Arch

The great majority of these aneurysms are of arteriosclerotic origin. Surgical resection is a formidable undertaking, but, because of the usual grave consequences of nonsurgical management, represents the treatment of choice. Cardiopulmonary bypass is required with special provisions made for maintenance of cerebral perfusion during the temporary interruption of carotid flow required for their reimplantation. Our approach is to place a large caliber tightly woven Dacron graft from the ascending aorta to the descending aorta, using partially occlusive clamps, at least on the ascending aortic side. Once this graft has been placed, the aorta may be excluded between the two extremes of the aneurysm and an elliptical segment of the transverse arch excised, which includes the origins of the arch vessels. This ellipse is then implanted into the graft in a defect created for this purpose.

Aneurysms of the Descending Aorta

Although traumatic aneurysms occur most commonly at the site of the ligamentum arteriosum, most aneurysms of the descending aorta are arteriosclerotic. Expansion and threatened, or actual, rupture indicate surgical resection. Our practice is to utilize a heparin-coated shunt placed either from the proximal descending aorta or the left ventricular apex to the femoral artery during the period of aortic cross-clamping necessary for resection and graft insertion. Use of this shunt obviates the need for total body heparinization as required for cardiopulmonary bypass when that technique is used. A left posterolateral thoracotomy is used to approach this portion of the aorta, generally resecting the fourth or fifth rib. Care should be exercised in selecting a tightly woven graft to minimize blood loss. Reapproximation of the edges of the aneurysm sac over the graft also helps to minimize intraoperative bleeding. Although the reapproximation of the aortic ends in some instances of traumatic aortic transection without use of a graft may be tempting if the tissues appear normal, our policy has been to use a short segment of graft in all these cases.

Thoracoabdominal Aneurysms

Virtually all thoracoabdominal aneurysms are of the arteriosclerotic type. Rapid expansion or the presence of symptoms referable to the aneurysm makes surgical resection mandatory. A left thoracoabdominal incision is the one most likely to afford the best exposure. The aorta is exposed above the diaphragm by retracting the lung anteriorly. Below the diaphragm all the abdominal viscera may be reflected anteriorly and to the right. Hypertension is avoided during aortic clamping by the intravenous administration of nitroprusside (a solution of 50 mg nitroprusside in 1000 ml of 5 per cent dextrose in water). The aneurysm is opened after securing proximal and distal control and clamps have been applied. An autotransfusion apparatus may be useful in these patients, since back bleeding from visceral arteries may be brisk. The visceral branches are removed from the native aorta individually with a button of aortic tissue and are reimplanted into the graft at appropriate locations. Since prolonged deprivation of renal blood flow is likely, administration of 12.5 to 25 grams of mannitol prior to aortic clamping seems prudent. A tightly woven Dacron graft of appropriate size should be used.

Dissecting Aneurysms

Dissection of the aorta usually results from an intimal tear in the aorta occurring in a patient with disease of the media and, most commonly, hypertension. Most tears occur just above the aortic value and result in dissection of the aorta from this level down to the bifurcation of the abdominal aorta or below (Type I). Occasionally the dissection is confined to the ascending aorta (Type II). Aortic valve incompetence not uncommonly accompanies these two types. Type III dissections originate from a tear in the proximal descending thoracic aorta at or near the level of the ligamentum. While aortic tears may occur at any location, most are in the above-described locations. Operative treatment will most likely be required for all patients with aortic dissections, but is necessary early in those with involvement of the ascending aorta (Types I and II). Initial stabilization of the patient with intravenous nitroprusside infusion (50 mg in 1000 ml 5 per cent dextrose in water) to a systolic blood pressure in the 90 to 100 mm Hg range and the use of small intravenous doses (0.5 to 2.0 mg) of propranolol is followed by aortography to confirm the diagnosis. In Types I and II operation should be undertaken without delay and consists of insertion of a tightly woven Dacron graft into the proximal ascending aorta, closing the minimally disturbed aneurysm sac over the graft. Aortic valve replacement and/or coronary reimplantation is rarely necessary in our experience. Type III dissections may be treated with antihypertensive therapy as described above during the acute period and the patient placed on strict antihypertensive treatment and followed with frequent (every 3 months) chest x-rays and examinations. At the first sign of progressive aortic enlargement or the development of symptoms referable to the aneurysm, operation should be advised. Operation is carried out in a manner similar to that for arteriosclerotic aneurysms of the descending thoracic aorta. Patients with dissections of the aorta require close lifelong medical management with strict attention to blood pressure control.

ANGINA PECTORIS

method of
THOMAS M. DREW, M.D.
Providence, Rhode Island

Introduction

Angina pectoris is generally diagnosed by the characteristic history. However, before embarking on a course of treatment one should consider the following in the differential diagnosis: (1) chest pain from noncardiac sources (e.g., cervical disc disease, esophageal spasm); (2) expression of myocardial ischemia caused by other cardiac conditions, such as dilated cardiomyopathy, aortic stenosis, aortic insufficiency, hypertrophic subaortic stenosis, and pulmonary hypertension.

Classic angina pectoris in coronary heart disease is precipitated by an increase in oxygen demand in the setting of a restricted fixed supply resulting from coronary atherosclerosis. Thus the historic findings of exertional or emotional induced symptoms are explained by concomitant increase in heart rate, blood pressure, or sympathetic tone, which increases myocardial oxygen demand. Symptom relief with rest represents reversal of that process. Variant angina, however, is due to proximal spasm of the coronary arteries with a concomitant decrease in blood flow and secondary myocardial ischemia. This may occur in the setting of normal coronary arteries or proximal fixed atherosclerotic lesions. Historically, variant angina is suspected when symptoms occur in the absence of these precipitating causes, very often at rest or during the early morning hours.

Once the diagnosis has been established, careful screening for any exacerbating conditions should be undertaken:

1. Complicating cardiac conditions, such as aortic stenosis–aortic insufficiency or idiopathic hypertrophic subaortic stenosis, which increase myocardial oxygen demand and may coexist with symptomatic coronary artery disease.

2. Noncardiac disorders which may increase myocardial oxygen demand or decrease supply: thyrotoxicosis, hypertension, anemia, hyperviscosity.

3. Concomitant use of drugs which increase myocardial oxygen demand, in particular sympathomimetic agents used for nasal congestion or drugs such as amphetamines.

Coronary angiography may be necessary to confirm or exclude the diagnosis of angina pectoris.

Management of Risk Factors

Of risk factors classically associated with coronary heart disease, hypertension, diabetes, hypercholesterolemia, and tobacco abuse can be altered. The importance of discontinuation of smoking and lowering blood pressure to a physiologic range is well established. Careful control of diabetes and dietary lowering of an abnormal cholesterol, while not yet proved, are appropriate in the management of coronary heart disease. Maintenance of reasonable body weight will help normalize carbohydrate metabolism, lower a mildly elevated blood pressure, and help lower cholesterol.

Pharmacologic Intervention

Nitroglycerin. Trinitroglycerin is the cornerstone of anginal management. The mechanism of action of the trinitroglycerin is complex: (1) It causes peripheral arteriolar dilatation, which results in lowering blood pressure and a decrease in myocardial oxygen demand. (2) Peripheral venous dilatation results in decreased venous return with a decrease in left ventricular end diastolic volume and therefore decreased myocardial oxygen demand. (3) Coronary blood flow is redistributed from normal to ischemic zones, improving the ratio of oxygen supply to oxygen needed. It is a combination of these effects which results in the relief of pain.

Trinitroglycerin is available in strengths of from 0.15 to 0.6 mg for sublingual absorption. In the administration of the trinitroglycerin several points should be kept in mind:

1. The patient should be advised to administer the drug to him/herself quickly at the outset of an attack, rather than waiting for worsening of symptoms. In fact, prophylactic use of nitroglycerin when angina is predictable is very effective in reducing the frequency of angina and increasing the ability of most patients to undertake a more active life style.

2. The drug is not habit forming, and patients will not develop "tolerance" to the drug, even when long-acting nitrates are being used.

3. The side effects of the drug should be carefully described to the patient: burning under the tongue and headache and/or pounding sensation in the head. These not only are expected but also help define the pharmacologic effect for a given dose of nitroglycerin.

4. Patients must be cautious of outdated nitroglycerin. In as little as 3 to 4 months after opening the bottle, the drug may become ineffective, particularly if not stored in a dark container.

5. Poor response to the drug at any given time (especially when side effects document the pharmacologic effectiveness of the preparation) may represent worsening ischemia or frank infarction and demands the physician's attention.

Long-Acting Nitrates. Oral nitrates have documented hemodynamic effects for several hours and provide subjective relief of angina pectoris for up to 3 to 4 hours. In stable patients a regimen such as isosorbide dinitrate, 20 to 40 mg every 6 hours or every 4 hours, is easily followed and effective in decreasing the number of anginal attacks. The initial dose should be lower (5 mg every 6 hours), as some patients experience side effects even at a low dose. Sublingual nitrates such as isosorbide dinitrate, while clearly effective in controlling symptoms, have a shorter duration of action, requiring a more frequent dosage schedule which is less easily followed. Nitroglycerin ointment (2 per cent) can be applied to the skin and covered by a protective covering. It will provide a sustained antianginal effect and can be used as little as three times daily with excellent results. The dosage will vary greatly (0.5 inch to 3 inch strips [1.25 to 7 cm]). The dosage schedule may be increased up to six times daily to obtain good symptomatic relief.

Sublingual nitrates and nitroglycerin ointment are most effective in acute situations when a patient has unstable or rest angina. In this setting, a therapeutic effect is sought as rapidly as possible and the dosage can be increased on a rapid schedule (every hour) by following the hemodynamic response.

All long-acting nitrates have potential side effects of significant hypotension and severe headaches. The hypotension is generally postural, resolving with the patient in the supine position. Gastrointestinal intolerance with oral nitrates may be confused with worsening angina and provides a diagnostic dilemma. It should be considered if the patient's symptoms occur shortly after oral nitrate administration.

Beta-Adrenergic Blocking Agents. There are two types of beta-adrenergic blocking receptors: Beta 1 receptors are located in the myocardium and mediate increased contractility and heart rate. Beta 2 receptors are located in the smooth muscle of the bronchial tree, gut, and arterial wall. The usefulness of beta blockers in the treatment of angina relates to blocking beta 1 receptors.

Propranolol (Inderal) is a nonselective beta blocker and is the most popular beta-blocking drug in use presently. It is an extremely effective antianginal agent when adequate beta blockade is obtained. It may in fact be effective not only in symptomatic improvement but also in preventing subsequent morbidity or mortality following myocardial infarction. The dosage of propranolol should be low initially, 20 mg four times daily. The dose can be increased at weekly intervals (or more frequently) while monitoring pulse to determine the effective level. Complete beta blockade can be considered present not only when the heart rate is lowered to 60 at rest but when effective blunting of exercise-induced increase in heart rate (usually no more than 10 beats per minute increase with mild exercise) is also present. The effective dose of beta blockade can vary tremendously. A usual dose is 160 to 320 mg daily (40 to 80 mg four times daily), but much higher doses, even 800 mg daily, may be necessary for effective beta blockade. (This dose may be higher than that listed in the manufacturer's official directive.)

Several aspects relating to treatment with beta blockers should be considered:

1. Despite potential symptomatic relief with low doses, more myocardial protection is offered if the dosage schedule is increased as tolerated to reach a full therapeutic level.

2. Monitoring of the heart rate response to exercise can be accomplished by exercise testing, by simulating patient activities at the time of an office visit, or possibly by self-monitoring of the pulse by the patient.

3. Congestive heart failure is unusual in the absence of significant predisposing left ventricular dysfunction. If no prior myocardial infarction has occurred (or no other cause for myocardial dysfunction is present), the dose of propranolol (Inderal) adequate to obtain chronotropic block is usually well tolerated. If doubt exists concerning left ventricular function appropriate assessment with chest x-ray, echocardiogram and/or heart pool scan should be undertaken prior to initiation of therapy.

4. Abrupt propranolol withdrawal has been associated with an increased incidence of acute cardiac events: myocardial infarction and/or sudden death. While the explanation for this phenomenon is not completely clear, it is appropriate to taper propranolol therapy over 2 weeks whenever possible and advise patients to limit activity during that period.

5. It is clear that beta blockers may have some long-term protective effect in coronary heart disease, especially in patients who have had a myocardial infarction. Until the final data have been assessed, it is appropriate to continue beta-blocking agents in patients with angina pectoris even in clinical remission, as long as the drug is well tolerated.

Side effects: (1) Left ventricular failure in previously compromised patients. (2) Exacerbation of bronchospasm. Propranolol is contraindicated in patients with a history of adult asthma and should be used with extreme caution in patients with significant chronic obstructive pulmonary disease. (3) Propranolol may mask the sympathetic manifestations of hypoglycemia. Therefore, in diabetes careful attention to insulin dose should be paid. (4) Gastrointestinal symptoms, depression, nightmares, and fatigue may occur even with small doses. The fatigue is apparently unrelated to full beta blockade and may limit the usefulness of the drug. (5) Occasional severe bradycardia may occur. Careful monitoring with initial administration of the drug is appropriate.

Metoprolol is a relatively selective beta 1 blocker which has been approved by the Food and Drug Administration for use in hypertension. It may prove useful as an antianginal agent in selected patients intolerant of propranolol. Other selective beta-blocking agents can be expected in the near future.

Digitalis. There are two major uses of digitalis in angina pectoris: (1) Treatment of arrhythmias such as supraventricular tachycardia which can precipitate angina by increasing heart rate, thereby increasing myocardial oxygen demand. (2) Treatment of congestive heart failure.

By decreasing left ventricular size and left ventricular wall tension, vigorous treatment of congestive heart failure will reduce myocardial oxygen consumption. Nocturnal angina may be a manifestation of incipient congestive heart failure in coronary heart disease, and digitalis may prove to be effective therapy.

Calcium-Blocking Agents. Calcium-blocking agents have been established as effective therapy for angina caused by coronary spasm. Drugs such as nifedipine have been studied extensively and are available in this country only on an investigational basis. They have also been shown to be effective in classic stable angina, increasing exercise tolerance when compared to treatment with placebo. The additional clinical value of calcium-blocking agents in the treatment of patients with chronic angina already treated pharmacologically is not yet established.

Antiplatelet Drugs. Heparin and sodium warfarin (Coumadin) have not been shown to be effective in the treatment of angina pectoris. Antiplatelet drugs, however, have been effective in the treatment of coronary heart disease. Sulfinpyrazone appears effective in decreasing subsequent infarction or death in patients with prior myocardial infarction. Although antiplatelet drugs have not been shown to be effective in the symptomatic treatment of angina, they may be appropriate adjunctive therapy in chronic long-term management.

Exercise Conditioning

Exercise programs for patients with angina pectoris provide conditioning which allows patients to exercise more vigorously before developing symptoms. In addition, it may be helpful in reducing stress, lowering the blood pressure, and aiding weight reduction. Exercise and cardiovascular conditioning may also help develop collateral blood supply to ischemic myocardium.

Exercise programs must be developed carefully with the level of activity defined by ambulatory monitoring or prior exercise testing. Aerobic exercise (e.g., swimming, jogging, walking) is preferred to isometric exercise.

Catheterization and Surgical Considerations

Coronary artery bypass grafting has become one of the most common operations presently performed. With improved techniques of myocardial preservation and perioperative care, mortality and perioperative morbidity have been significantly reduced, making the operation an appropriate and safe alternative to continued medical therapy. The efficacy of coronary artery bypass grafting and the relief of angina is well established, with up to 90 per cent of patients reporting improvement in symptoms and up to 70 per cent being completely pain-free following operation. Improvement in postoperative mortality compared to medical therapy is well established for left main coronary artery stenosis and may apply to other anatomic subsets as well. Consideration for surgical intervention should be given in chronic stable angina if the patient's symptoms are poorly controlled on adequate medical therapy and/or if the patient's life style is severely limited by symptoms.

A strongly positive exercise test (3 mm depression or significant ST depression with symptoms at very low level exercise) may be a marker for left main coronary artery stenosis. Consideration for cardiac catheterization should be given in those patients in whom surgery is otherwise being considered, and in those with strongly positive exercise tests.

Unstable Angina

1. Patients should be treated with bed rest and sedation, most often in the hospital setting. Appropriate studies should be performed to rule out myocardial infarction.

2. Vigorous medical management should be undertaken. Beta blockade (if not contraindicated) should be accomplished with propranolol in increasing doses on every 4 hour regimen. The dose should be increased by 20 mg with each dose until the heart rate is maintained below 60 beats per minute.

3. Nitrate therapy should be instituted. Sublingual isosorbide can be started at 2.5 mg and increased every 2 hours by 2.5 mg until adequate blood pressure response has been obtained. In previously normotensive patients one should aim for a systolic pressure of 100 to 110 mm Hg. The end point must be adjusted in previously hypertensive patients or those with cerebrovascular disease. An alternative approach is the use of nitroglycerin paste, starting with 1 inch (2.5 cm) and a new dosage applied every 4 hours, increasing by ½ inch with each dose (remove prior dose of paste with each subsequent administration).

4. If the patient cannot be stabilized with the aforementioned measures and continues to have angina at rest, consideration should be given to insertion of the intra-aortic balloon pump. While this is an effective measure of decreasing afterload and thereby decreasing myocardial oxygen consumption, it should be approached with caution because of significant associated side effects.

5. Consideration should be given to cathe-

terization, preferably after stabilization of the patient, which decreases the risk of catheterization. Risk of catheterization will vary, depending on the experience of the laboratory and skill of the catheterizer. Timing of catheterization should be individualized according to the patient's clinical response to medical therapy.

6. Consider coronary artery bypass grafting if amenable surgical lesions are defined. If the patient can be stabilized medically, there appears to be no urgency in proceeding with immediate bypass grafting.

Variant Angina

Angina occurring without exertion, especially in the setting of ST segment elevation, raises the possibility of coronary artery spasm, either in the setting of a normal vessel or superimposed on significant proximal disease. Patients with variant angina should be hospitalized to exclude myocardial infarction. They should be monitored for arrhythmias and heart block. Treatment should consist of nitrates as defined above. Propranolol may in fact exacerbate coronary artery spasm. Patients with recurrent coronary spasm should undergo diagnostic cardiac catheterization, possibly accompanied by provocative testing (e.g., ergonovine administration or cold pressor test). Coronary artery bypass grafting may be effective for those patients with spasm superimposed on proximal fixed lesions. Coronary artery bypass grafting is not effective for spasm with normal coronaries. Treatment should consist of nitrates. Calcium-blocking agents can be used if nitrates are ineffective.

CARDIAC ARREST

method of
WILLIAM HOROWITZ, M.D.
Bronx, New York

Cardiac arrest is the sudden and/or unexpected cessation of an effective cardiac ouptut. When the circulation is arrested, consciousness is lost in 6 or 7 seconds. In 20 to 30 seconds there is complete absence of cortical activity on the electroencephalogram (EEG). After 3 to 4 minutes irreversible changes develop in the more sensitive areas of the brain.

Diagnosis

(1) Sudden loss of consciousness *with* (2) absence of heart sounds and all peripheral pulsations *and* (3) absence of respiration and/or increasing cyanosis.

Mechanisms

(1) Asystole — cardiac standstill; (2) ventricular fibrillation; (3) electromechanical dissociation — unobtainable blood pressure and pulse while QRS and T persist (exsanguination; pericardial tamponade).

Causes

(1) Acute myocardial infarction; (2) cardiac arrhythmias: (a) heart block, (b) ventricular fibrillation; (3) anaphylaxis or lesser allergic reactions; (4) fear, apprehension, nightmares; (5) intubation, extubation, tracheal suction; (6) manipulations during surgery, especially on the heart, gallbladder, peritoneum, or eye; (7) cardiac catheterization, angiography, pyelography; (8) vagovagal reflex; (9) electrocution, drowning.

MANAGEMENT

Management of cardiac arrest is a matter of urgency. Do it fast. Do what you are trained to do. Worry later.

Cardiopulmonary Resuscitation (CPR)

Face up (supine position on a firm surface).

Cardiac thump — one sharp blow with the closed fist to the lower half of the sternum.

Start basic life support immediately if there are no signs of life — spontaneous breathing and/or carotid artery pulsation.

A — Airway. Lift neck with one hand beneath neck. Press head backward with other hand pressing forehead (*omit if there is question of a neck injury*). If head tilt does not clear airway, use *jaw thrust* by pushing lower jaw forward with fingers. If airway remains obstructed, swing one or two fingers through the mouth from one side to the other. If patient is choking, apply Heimlich maneuver (forceful bearhug to upper abdomen).

B — Breathing — Artificial Respiration. *Mouth to mouth* — Close off nose with fingers; rescuer takes a quick deep breath; apply mouth firmly to victim, making a tight seal; blow out hard; remove your mouth, allowing victim to exhale; repeat maneuver every 5 seconds.

Mouth to nose — Jaw thrust seals lips; after deep breath, close lips around nose of victim; blow out hard; remove mouth, allowing victim to exhale; repeat at 5 second intervals.

Mouth to stoma — Blow directly into stoma, sealing mouth and lips.

C — Circulation — External Cardiac Compression (ECC). Technique of ECC — heel of one hand positioned on lower half of sternum 1 inch above xiphoid; other hand placed on top of first hand; keeping arms straight with shoulder over sternum, vertical downward pressure is exerted; depress lower sternum 1½ to 2 inches; release immediately after compression, keeping heel of hand on sternum. *Compression* and *relaxation* should be *regular, smooth, and rhythmic.*

One rescuer — Two quick lung inflations, followed by 15 chest compressions; lung inflations must be done rapidly within 6 seconds. This does not allow time for full exhalation, so that 60 compressions per minute are achieved.

Two rescuers — Get on opposite sides of victim; one at side of victim performs chest compression, 60 per minute; one at head of victim tilts head back and performs artificial ventilation after every five chest compressions; on tiring, rescuers switch positions without interrupting rhythm. *Pupillary reactions* (dilated, unresponsive to light — ominous signs) and *carotid pulsation* should be checked without interruption of rhythmic cardiac compression and artificial ventilation by other observers or on changes of rescuers.

Basic life support is continued without interruption until advanced life support is established.

Advanced Life Support

Adjunctive Equipment and Techniques. *Airway and Ventilation:* Oxygen; airway — oropharyngeal, nasopharyngeal; bag, mask, valve units; endotracheal intubation — *only by trained personnel;* pressure-cycled automatic resuscitators (IPPB, time-cycled); suction equipment; nasogastric tube for gastric decompression.

Circulation: Central venous line; electrocardiographic monitoring; arterial blood gas monitoring.

Ventricular Fibrillation. Thump.

Ventricular Defibrillation. Application of DC countershock, 400 watt-seconds, applied with precautions by experienced personnel. If unsuccessful by ECG, repeat one more shock.

If ventricular fibrillation persists on ECG, give intravenous or intracardiac epinephrine 0.5 or 1 ml (1:1000) or 5 or 10 ml (1:10,000). Injection should be given with 22 needle (3 inches) in fifth left interspace just to left of sternum at a slant.

Repeat countershock.

If ECG shows continued ventricular fibrillation, repeat epinephrine injection, making sure blood is withdrawn into the syringe. May repeat in 3 minutes.

Lidocaine bolus, 75 mg, may be repeated every 5 minutes. Do not exceed 200 mg per hour.

If ventricular fibrillation continues on ECG, give propranolol (Inderal), 1 mg intravenously. Repeat countershock.

For digitalis toxicity use phenytoin (Dilantin)* instead of lidocaine. Phenytoin, 100 mg

intravenously in 5 minutes, followed by countershock. Repeat dose in 5 minutes, followed by countershock.

After sinus rhythm is restored, continue lidocaine intravenously at 4 mg per minute.

Ventricular Tachycardia. Thump. Lidocaine bolus, 100 mg (2 per cent) intravenously. Procainamide bolus, 100 mg intravenously. Propranolol (Inderal), 2 mg intravenously with lidocaine bolus.

Asystole. Thump. Epinephrine intracardiac, 1 ml (1:1000) or 10 ml (1:10,000). Calcium chloride, 10 ml (10 per cent solution). Isoproterenol (Isuprel), 2 mg in 500 ml 5 per cent dextrose in water.

Electromechanical Dissociation. Pericardiocentesis for pericardial tamponade. Calcium chloride, 10 ml (10 per cent solution) intravenously or intracardiac. Atropine, 1 mg intravenously for bradycardia. If central venous pressure (CVP) is less than 5 cm, infuse 500 ml fluid rapidly (in less than 10 minutes). Plasma or isotonic saline for blood loss. Five per cent dextrose in water for pulmonary edema. Isotonic saline or 5 per cent dextrose in saline for hyponatremia caused by vomiting or diuretics. Corticosteroids (Methylprednisolone), 2 grams intravenously.

Drugs for Maintenance of Life Support. Sodium bicarbonate for metabolic acidosis, 1 mEq per kg bolus *or* continuous infusion. Prefilled syringe, 50 ml (8.4 per cent) = 50 mEq). Ampule, same. Infusion bottle, 500 ml (5 per cent) = 297.5 mEq.

Epinephrine intravenously or intracardiac, 0.5 or 1 ml (1:1000) or 5 or 10 ml (1:10,000).

Atropine sulfate, 0.5 to 0.8 ml (1 ampule = 0.4 mg).

Lidocaine, 75 mg bolus; 1.5 mg per kg slow intravenous bolus (50 to 100 mg), then 1 to 4 mg per minute. Two grams per 500 ml = 4 mg per ml.

Procainamide (Pronestyl), 100 mg intravenously slowly every 5 minutes up to 1000 mg, then 1 to 4 mg per minute or 250 to 500 mg orally every 4 hours. Two grams per 500 ml = 4 mg per ml.

Phenytoin (Dilantin),* 100 mg intravenously slowly every 5 minutes up to 750 mg, then 300 mg per day intravenously or orally.

Bretylium (Bretylol), 5 mg per kg intravenously, with increments up to maximum of 30 mg per kg. Then 5 to 10 mg per kg every 6 to 8 hours, or 1 to 2 mg per minute. (Comes in 500 mg ampules.) Two grams per 500 ml = 4 mg per ml.

Propranolol (Inderal), 0.5 mg intravenously

---

*This use of phenytoin is not listed in the manufacturer's official directive.

*This use of phenytoin is not listed in the manufacturer's official directive.

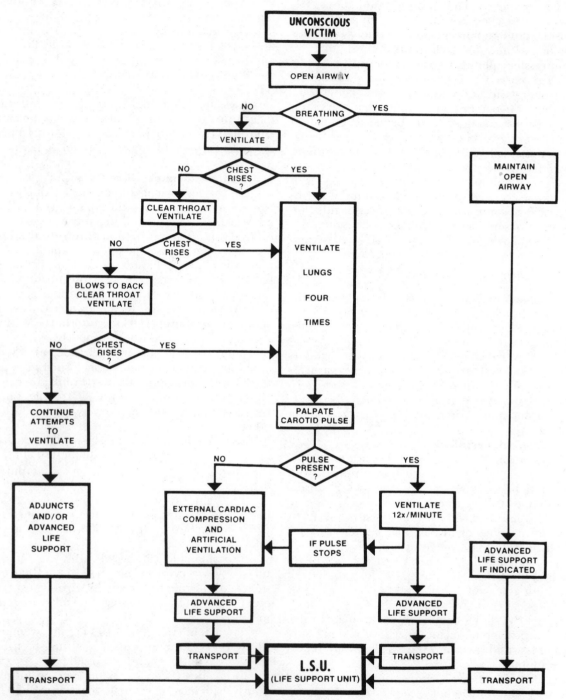

Figure 1. Life support decision tree (unwitnessed arrest). (Reprinted from the Supplement to Journal of the American Medical Association, February 18, 1974. Copyright 1974, the American Medical Association. Reprinted with permission from the American Heart Association.)

slowly every 5 minutes up to maximum of 10 mg.

Dopamine (Intropin), 1 to 50 micrograms per kg per minute. Four hundred mg per 500 ml = 800 micrograms per ml.

Dobutamine (Dobutrex), 1 to 10 micrograms per kg per minute. Two hundred and fifty mg per 500 ml = 500 micrograms per ml.

Norepinephrine (Levophed, levarterenol), 2 to 8 micrograms per minute. Four mg per 500 ml = 8 micrograms per ml.

Calcium chloride, 5 ml (10 per cent solution).

Isoproterenol (Isuprel), 2 to 8 micrograms per minute or 0.2 mg intravenous bolus. Four mg per 500 ml = 8 micrograms per ml.

Metaraminol (Aramine), 0.01 to 1.0 mg per minute intravenously. One hundred mg per 500 ml = 0.2 mg per ml.

Furosemide (Lasix), 40 to 80 mg intravenously.

Corticosteroids: methylprednisolone, 5 mg per kg, or dexamethasone, 1 mg per kg.

Internal Cardiac Compression. In the operating room with open chest. Penetrating wound of the heart and/or other thoracic injuries.

Postcardiac Arrest for Control of Cerebral Edema. Hypothermia; hyperventilation.

Complications of CPR

Rib fractures; sternal fractures; pneumothorax; hemothorax; fat embolism, air embolism; lung contusions and lacerations; lacerations of liver; costochondral separations; aspiration pneumonitis.

Late Complications of CPR

Anoxic encephalopathy; sepsis; renal failure.

Termination of CPR

This is always a difficult decision.

1. A flat ECG persisting after 20 minutes of continuous CPR.

2. If ECG is not available: fixed dilated pupils; absence of any arterial pulsations and blood pressure; absence of spontaneous respirations; and deep unconsciousness.

3. If the patient is hypothermic (less than 90 F or 32.2 C) or has taken drugs, continue CPR for several hours.

Annually in the United States more than 350,000 sudden cardiac deaths occur outside the hospital. A program to extend the teaching of CPR into the school, workplace, and community should save a significant number of lives.

ATRIAL FIBRILLATION

method of
CONDON R. VANDER ARK, M.D.
Madison, Wisconsin

Atrial fibrillation is most often associated with ischemic heart disease, hypertension, rheumatic mitral valve disease, thyrotoxicosis, chronic obstructive lung disease, and pericarditis. It is also a common arrhythmia following cardiac and pulmonary surgery. Although less common, its association with hypertrophic cardiomyopathy and Wolff-Parkinson-White type pre-excitation may produce unique life-threatening emergencies. The therapeutic decisions required in the proper management of atrial fibrillation are largely determined by the underlying heart disease and the hemodynamic consequences of this common atrial arrhythmia. The hemodynamic effects of atrial fibrillation result from the rapid ventricular rate which decreases diastolic filling time and from the loss of atrial contraction which would normally contribute to ventricular filling in late diastole. The ideal goal of therapy is to reestablish normal hemodynamics. This is accomplished by controlling the ventricular rate, followed by restoring sinus rhythm with atrial contraction. It is then important to take measures to prevent recurrence of atrial fibrillation.

Rapid Ventricular Rates

The initial step in successful management of atrial fibrillation is a careful assessment of the patient's hemodynamic status. The rapid ventricular rate may produce angina pectoris in patients with ischemic heart disease who do not tolerate the increased myocardial oxygen demand and decreased coronary perfusion pressure. Patients with mitral valve stenosis require prolonged diastolic filling time which is severely compromised by the rapid rate and may thus result in acute left heart failure. Patients with noncompliant hypertrophy of the left ventricle as seen with systemic hypertension or hypertrophic cardiomyopathy (asymmetric septal hypertrophy) may develop acute left heart failure and/or anginal pain as a result of the rapid rate and loss of the atrial contribution to ventricular filling. Patients with the Wolff-Parkinson-White type pre-excitation have extremely fast ventricular rates (frequently >300 beats per minute) and wide bizarre QRS complexes with varying configurations because of fusion of impulses transmitted over both the AV node and an accessory pathway. These patients may develop ventricular fibrillation because of the dual input to the ventricle and decreased myocardial perfusion. Digitalis facilitates accessory pathway conduction and is therefore absolutely contraindicated.

The majority of patients may be treated medically with the aim of controlling the ventricular rate. A small minority, however, will require emergency DC cardioversion. Almost all patients with atrial fibrillation and a rapid ventricular rate will be symptomatic. If these symptoms are tolerated reasonably well, the initial management should be to slow AV conduction and decrease the ventricular rate. Digitalis is the drug of choice and digoxin is the preferred glycoside. If the atrial fibrillation is of recent onset, the administration of 1.0 mg of digoxin intravenously over 2 to 3 minutes may convert the rhythm to normal. If this fails to convert the arrhythmia, it will usually decrease the ventricular rate. This 1.0 mg dosage of digoxin should not be used if there is any question of prior digitalis administration or possible hypokalemia, as may occur in patients receiving potassium-depleting diuretics. If the atrial fibrillation has been present for several days or if any of the aforementioned concerns are present, a more modest initial intravenous dose of 0.5 mg should be used. In either situation, one may follow the initial dose with the administration of 0.25 mg every 2 to 3 hours until a total dose of 1.5 mg has been given or the ventricular rate has slowed to <100 beats per minute. Serum potassium should be determined; if this is >4 mEq per liter, a total digoxin dose of 2.0 mg over a 24 hour period is reasonable.

Patients who have increased levels of catecholamines may not slow adequately with digitalis. One should then consider the addition of a beta receptor blocking agent before risking potentially toxic doses of digitalis. These patients are particularly prone to digitals-induced tachyrhythmias. They usually respond well to beta receptor blockade. This group includes patients with hyperthyroidism, those with febrile illnesses, postoperative patients, and patients with other forms of stress in which one might expect sinus tachycardia if atrial fibrillation were not present. In such instances, propranolol may be given intravenously with an initial dose of 1.0 mg and repeated doses of 1.0 mg given at 5 to 10 minute intervals until the rate is controlled, hemodynamic changes occur, or a total dose of 10.0 mg is reached. If more time is available, the propranolol may be given orally with an initial dose of 20 mg followed by 20 to 40 mg every 2 hours to achieve a ventricular rate of <100 beats per minute. It is preferable not to exceed a total dosage of 320 mg in a 24 hour period.

Propranolol should not be used in patients with congestive heart failure resulting from myocardial insufficiency or in patients with obstructive lung disease with bronchospasm. Patients with obstructive lung disease but no congestive heart failure may tolerate the use of metoprolol (Lopressor), 50 mg orally every 6 to 8 hours. (This use of metoprolol is not listed in the manufacturer's official directive.) Propranolol may be used very effectively in the face of left heart failure when the pulmonary congestion is due to the combination of atrial fibrillation with either mitral valve stenosis or obstructive hypertrophic cardiomyopathy. One should be very certain of the underlying hemodynamic mechanisms before propranolol is used. In the patient with obstructive hypertrophic cardiomyopathy, propranolol may be more effective than digoxin and may be considered to be the drug of choice.

Emergency QRS synchronized DC cardioversion should be used for those patients with Wolff-Parkinson-White type pre-excitation and those patients in whom atrial fibrillation has produced hypotension with impairment of cerebral function, signs or symptoms of acute left heart failure, and/or prolonged anginal type chest pain. Digitalis should not be given if emergency DC cardioversion is required, as its administration only increases the risk of postconversion arrhythmias. If an anesthesiologist is not immediately available to administer a short-acting barbiturate, a modest dose (10 to 20 mg) of diazepam (Valium) may be given intravenously in these hemodynamically critical situations. If normal sinus rhythm is not maintained after the initial DC cardioversion, the intravenous infusion of procainamide at a rate of 50 mg per minute to achieve a total dose of 250 mg may be used before repeating the DC cardioversion. This process may be repeated a second time if necessary. A procainamide dosage exceeding 500 mg is usually not used except with the Wolff-Parkinson-White pre-excitation syndrome. A total dose of 1.0 gram may be used for patients with Wolff-Parkinson-White type pre-excitation. The higher doses of procainamide may slow the ventricular rate by prolonging the refractory period of the accessory pathway as well as facilitating maintenance of normal sinus rhythm. Propranolol, 1.0 mg intravenously every 5 to 10 minutes to achieve a total dose of 5 mg, may be added if procainamide alone has failed to control the arrhythmia.

Slow Ventricular Rates

Some patients will present with untreated atrial fibrillation and ventricular rates of <100 beats per minute. These patients are most likely to be over 60 years of age, and one must suspect underlying SA and AV node disease. No immediate therapy is required. These patients should have a 24 hour Holter recording made with particular attention to changes in ventricular rates with activity and detection of slow regular ventricular rates that may indicate complete AV block. Conversion of atrial fibrillation to normal rhythm may reveal the "sick sinus syndrome" with an unstable atrial mechanism as evidenced by sinus pauses and/or nodal escape rhythms. Digitalis should be administered with caution in those patients who have excessive ventricular rate responses to activity or if there is evidence of a low cardiac output syndrome or congestive heart failure. These patients may develop excessively slow ventricular rates when receiving digitalis. Demand ventricular pacing may be necessary if slow ventricular rates are seen initially or are produced as a result of the drug treatment of the tachyrhythmia.

Systemic Thromboembolism

The onset of atrial fibrillation is associated with a significant increase in systemic embolic events in patients with rheumatic mitral stenosis. This risk is independent of the severity of the valve lesion, functional class, and patient age. The highest risk is in the first few days and weeks after the onset of atrial fibrillation. Restoration of normal sinus rhythm greatly reduces the risk of systemic emboli.

A clear association of increased frequency of thromboembolic events associated with atrial fibrillation in other forms of heart disease has not been conclusively shown.

Nevertheless, there are significant thromboembolic events in patients with cardiomyopathies, left atrial enlargement, and congestive heart failure of any cause. The onset of atrial fibrillation may increase embolic events in these patients, particularly in the first few days or weeks following conversion. It has also been observed that paroxysmal atrial fibrillation may have a higher incidence of systemic emboli than sustained fibrillation. It has been reported that 27 per cent of elderly patients who present with systemic emboli have paroxysmal atrial arrhythmias — often atrial fibrillation.

Anticoagulation is recommended for chronic atrial fibrillation in patients who have rheumatic mitral stenosis, left atrial enlargement, congestive heart failure, or cardiomyopathy. This same group should be anticoagulated for 2 to 3 weeks before attempts to convert atrial fibrillation to normal sinus rhythm. Patients with paroxysmal atrial fibrillation should be anticoagulated unless, as rarely occurs, all paroxysms are suppressed.

Conversion to Normal Sinus Rhythm

Restoration of normal sinus rhythm is the ideal therapeutic goal in all patients but cannot be achieved in a significant number. Reduction of the risks of systemic thromboembolism is probably the major reason to attempt restoration and maintenance of normal rhythm. There are also hemodynamic benefits for some patients. Stroke volume is most likely to be increased in those patients with noncompliant and hypertrophied left ventricles in which an active "atrial kick" may take advantage of the Frank-Starling mechanism. In the dilated heart where passive filling fully utilizes the Frank-Starling mechanism, little hemodynamic improvement can be expected.

The decision as to whether or not to convert atrial fibrillation to normal must therefore take into consideration the benefits to be gained, the risk of embolic episodes with conversion, the likelihood of maintaining normal rhythm, and the risk of the drug maintenance program. There is a greater risk in switching back and forth between atrial fibrillation and normal rhythm than in the case of properly maintained chronic atrial fibrillation.

Some consideration of when to convert atrial fibrillation in the time course of an individual's disease is important. Atrial fibrillation precipitated by a correctable acute illness or stress such as acute pericarditis, myocarditis, pneumonitis, hyperthyroidism, or major surgery can be converted and maintained with relative ease provided that conversion is postponed until after the acute illness or stress has been resolved. The ventricular rate in these situations should be controlled as previously outlined until a stable clinical state has been achieved. Patients with advanced valvular disease may be considered for cardioversion 2 to 3 months after surgical therapy when hemodynamic stability has been achieved. Atrial fibrillation which has been present for more than 2 years is unlikely to be maintained in normal rhythm unless some real change has been made in the patient's underlying disease state.

Atrial fibrillation may be converted to normal rhythm with quinidine sulfate or with elective QRS synchronized DC shock. The risk of systemic emboli is similar with either method of conversion. There may be some increased risk of serious ventricular arrhythmias with quinidine conversion. This risk cannot be totally eliminated with either method, as both require drug therapy to maintain normal rhythm. DC cardioversion is quicker and more convenient that the pharmacologic method which requires the physician to evaluate the patient and obtain an electrocardiogram before each dose of quinidine.

Patients should be properly prepared for elective DC cardioversion and the procedure carried out as follows:

1. Those patients with a high risk of post-conversion embolic episodes should be anticoagulated as previously outlined.

2. Digitalis should be withheld for a time equal to 1½ to 2 half-lives of the glycoside (usually 2 to 3 days with digoxin).

3. The patient should receive nothing orally for 12 hours before conversion.

4. Informed consent should be obtained.

5. Quinidine sulfate, 300 mg, or disopyramide (Norpace), 200 mg, should be given 2 hours before cardioversion.

6. The patient should be in an intensive care unit with an intravenous line, a cuff in place for monitoring blood pressure, and oxygen delivered by nasal prongs or mask.

7. The electrocardiogram (ECG) must be continuously monitored and properly synchronized to the defibrillating unit. A record of the arrhythmia should be recorded.

8. Anesthesia may be accomplished with a short-acting barbiturate such as methohexital sodium (Brevital) administered by an anesthesiologist. Intravenous diazepam in a dose of 10 to 40 mg to produce satisfactory sedation and amnesia is an acceptable alternative.

9. DC shock should be applied using a posterior paddle placed between the tip of the left scapula and the spine and an anterior paddle just to the right of the lower third of the sternum. The QRS synchronized shock should be 100 watt-seconds initially, with rapid progression to 200 watt-seconds or 400 watt-seconds if required.

10. Following cardioversion an ECG should be recorded. Food and drugs can be resumed as soon as the patient is alert.

11. In some instances patients can be discharged after 6 to 8 hours of postconversion observation, but 24 hours is preferred.

There is a substantial body of data on quinidine protocols used to induce conversion of atrial fibrillation but virtually no data on using other Class I antiarrhythmic drugs for this purpose. Quinidine conversion has certain risks which can be reduced but not eliminated by careful attention to details. Patients must be adequately digitalized to control the ventricular rate, which may increase under the "vagolytic" effect of quinidine. Prior anticoagulation of the high risk group of patients noted earlier should be carried out. The serum potassium should be measured and should be normal (preferably >4.0 mEq/per liter). The patient should have continuous ECG monitoring in an intensive or intermediate care unit. The ECG-monitored lead should not be changed so that the QRS and QTU interval can be measured before the first and all subsequent doses of quinidine. Several quinidine dosage schedules have been proposed. I prefer a 1 day program of 400 mg of quinidine sulfate every 2 hours to a maximum of seven doses. This protocol is stopped when the patient converts to normal rhythm or has severe gastrointestinal side effects, the QRS interval increases by 30 per cent or more compared with control, or new ventricular arrhythmias develop. True dose-related toxicity is uncommon with this protocol. "Quinidine syncope," characterized by a prolonged QTU interval with paroxysms of ventricular tachycardia or ventricular fibrillation, is reported in up to 4.4 per cent of quinidine-attempted cardioversions. This is a major complication which is not dose related and precludes ever using quinidine in the patient again. Management of "quinidine syncope" requires that quinidine be stopped and the ventricular arrhythmia controlled with 300 mg of bretylium tosylate intravenously and/or temporary ventricular pacing. This complication clears within 24 hours of discontinuing quinidine. One may expect conversion with this protocol in about 75 per cent of patients. If conversion does not occur, no further trials of quinidine are used. The patient is then scheduled for elective DC cardioversion.

Prevention of Atrial Fibrillation

The prevention of recurrent atrial fibrillation requires the use of a Class I antiarrhythmic drug. Quinidine has been the standard for many years, but early reports suggest that disopyramide may be equally effective. Procainamide is the least effective agent. Maintenance quinidine therapy has been reported to result in unexpected sudden death in 0.5 per cent of cardioverted patients. This is probably due to quinidine-induced delayed repolarization arrhythmias (quinidine syncope). Similar arrhythmias have been reported with disopyramide, but the true incidence, though apparently quite low, is unknown. The usual side effects of these drugs may preclude effective therapy in some patients.

Those patients who are converted to normal rhythm after resolution of an acute illness or stress may be maintained on quinidine or disopyramide for 4 to 6 weeks and then have the drug discontinued. Recurrence of atrial fibrillation in such cases is rare. In patients with more chronic disease the maintenance program may have to be maintained indefinitely. Several studies indicate that atrial fibrillation recurs within 1 year in up to 75 per cent of this group.

Quinidine sulfate may be used in a dose of

200 to 400 mg every 6 to 8 hours. Long-acting quinidine preparations may also be used in a dose of 300 to 400 mg every 8 hours. Disopyramide may be given in a dose of 150 to 300 mg every 6 to 8 hours. Procainamide in a dose of 500 mg every 4 to 6 hours is less effective, requires more frequent administration, and eventually will induce a positive antinuclear antibody test or overt "lupus-like syndrome." If one of these programs is ineffective alone, beta-blocking agents may be added. Propranolol added to disopyramide has a significant incidence of myocardial depression and in general should be avoided. A combination of quinidine and propranolol has been effective when each has failed alone. This combination is particularly effective in the difficult patient with the Wolff-Parkinson-White pre-excitation syndrome. The usual dose of propranolol in combination with quinidine is 20 to 40 mg every 6 to 8 hours.

PREMATURE BEATS

method of
JOHN J. ROZANSKI, M.D.,
and AGUSTIN CASTELLANOS, M.D.
Miami, Florida

Introduction

The cornerstone of therapy of premature beats rests on whether they are supraventricular or ventricular. Premature beats may be considered supraventricular if they originate in the atria or junctional tissue, or ventricular if they originate below the bifurcation of the His bundle. This distinction is more than academic, since in general premature beats of ventricular origin are much more serious than atrial premature beats.

Supraventricular Beats (APBs)

Normal Persons Without Heart Disease. Although nearly all healthy individuals have (at one moment or another of their lives) APBs, they are not always bothersome enough to warrant intensive antiarrhythmic therapy. A careful history will usually reveal predisposing factors such as heightened anxiety with or without overuse of coffee, cigarettes, alcohol, cocaine, and sympathicomimetic agents (used for weight reduction or for the control of nasal or bronchial diseases). Under these circumstances temporary elimination or judicious regulation of the precipitating factors coupled with supportive therapy (reassurance) will usually suffice. When pharmacologic treatment appears clinically indicated, it seems best to use minor tranquilizers cautiously (diazepam, 2 to 5 mg two or three times daily for 7 to 10 days) rather than specific antiarrhythmic drugs, since the APBs are benign and easily controlled. If the person has an additional tendency to sinus tachycardia, then propranolol, 10 mg three times daily for 10 to 14 days, may be required. Quinidine sulfate, procainamide, and disopyramide phosphate all have inevitable side effects. Their use is reserved for patients with organic heart disease or severe symptoms. As a principle, the less medication used in normal persons, the better.

Organic Heart Disease. In patients with organic heart disease and APBs the clinician should first consider the underlying problems. In this manner drugs which are not specifically antiarrhythmic agents may have the effect of reducing APBs. For example, antihypertensive drugs by lowering afterload and therefore myocardial work may reduce APBs. Antianginal drugs may reduce APBs in ischemic heart disease. Likewise in congestive heart failure (CHF) treatment with diuretics, vasodilating agents, or oral digoxin (0.125 to 0.5 mg daily) might reduce the number of APBs. Finally, the smallest therapeutic doses of quinidine sulfate (200 mg four times daily) or quinidine gluconate (324 mg twice daily) or disopyramide phosphate (100 mg four times daily) should be used for APBs. One must be mindful of the significant myocardial depressant effects of disopyramide.

Chronic Lung Disease. In patients with chronic lung disease, resistant APBs and multifocal atrial rhythms may occur with very rapid atrioventricular (AV) conduction caused by heightened sympathetic tone. All antiarrhythmic agents are likely to prove ineffective if the underlying causes are not corrected. Treatment of hypoxia, maximization of pulmonary function and cardiac hemodynamics, minimization of xanthine or sympathomimetic agents (which provoke these arrhythmias and speed AV conduction), and correction of hypercarbia, hypokalemia, and acidosis are cornerstones of therapy.

Pre-excitation Syndromes. In Wolff-Parkinson-White (WPW) and Lown-Ganong-Levine (LGL) syndromes (short PR interval and paroxysmal supraventricular tachycardia) medical treatment is best individualized, based on the results of a careful electrophysiologic study. For example, empirical treatment with digoxin may be dangerous in certain patients with WPW syndrome prone to develop atrial fibrillation with rapid ventricular rates (with AV conduction occurring almost exclusively through the Kent bundle), since severe ventricular arrhythmias can be induced. When APBs trigger atrial fibrillation or reciprocating AV tachycardias, quinidine sulfate, 200 mg orally four times daily, with or without propranolol, 40 to 100 mg orally every 6 hours, can be used.

Acute Myocardial Infarction. APBs complicating acute myocardial infarction (MI) are frequently due to acute pump failure and may herald atrial fibrillation. Other causes of APBs in this setting are pericarditis, atrial or right ventricular infarction, and pulmonary embolism. Treatment is addressed first to optimization of cardiac hemodynamic function and oxygenation. Quinidine sulfate or quinidine gluconate can be used as previously outlined. Other agents such as disopyramide (100 mg orally three times daily) can be tried provided that there is minimal or no heart failure. The role of digoxin is still very controversial. It can be used in severe heart failure or when APBs lead to atrial fibrillation with a rapid ventricular response. Digoxin in doses ranging between 0.125 and 0.25 mg daily is used for the treatment of APBs only, but not for atrial fibrillation. (For the treatment of atrial fibrillation, see the article immediately preceding this one.)

Premature Ventricular Beats (VPBs)

Characteristically VPBs are premature and have a wide (bizarre) QRS complex with ST-T vector which is opposite the QRS axis. Usually the sinus node is not reset; therefore a full compensatory pause is present. VPBs may be due to reentry or automaticity. At present this distinction has little clinical relevance, since antiarrhythmic agents affect both mechanisms. The prevalence of VPBs increases with age. In general, the seriousness of VPBs in any given patient is directly proportional to the severity of the underlying heart disease. Such host factors are frequently more important than the specific types of ventricular arrhythmias present.

VPBs are classed solely for purposes of description as follows: occasional VPBs — less than 30 per hour; frequent — more than 30 per hour or 1 per minute; complex — occurring in multiple forms, bigeminy, early VPBs (R-on-T phenomenon), couplets (2 VPBs in a row), and salvos of VPBs.

Specific Syndromes

Individuals Without Detectable Heart Disease. The best approaches for asymptomatic patients without clinical, radiologic, or echocardiographic evidence of heart disease (or in persons having mitral valve prolapse without mitral insufficiency) are reassurance and supportive therapy. In patients (with or without mitral valve prolapse) who have palpitations, anxiety, and chest wall pain of undetermined origin, mild sedatives (diazepam or analgesics — aspirin) or small doses of propranolol (as outlined for APBs) can be added. However, in any patient with VPBs a thorough cardiovascular evaluation is warranted, including 24 hour Holter monitoring and echocardiography. The role of exercise stress testing is still controversial in this regard because of nonreproducibility of the results. In all cases one must weigh the risks of antiarrhythmic therapy against the expected benefits.

Drug-Induced VPBs. It is important to note that antiarrhythmic agents themselves can be the cause of severe ventricular arrhythmias. At present it seems as if the most frequent offender in this regard is quinidine, not digoxin. This can occur even with therapeutic doses and normal or subtherapeutic serum levels. Frequently, the initial stage of drug-induced multiform VPBs is missed (especially if there were pre-existing VPBs from other foci). Quinidine syncope may be recognized by the occurrence of a "polymorphic" ventricular tachycardia (now called "torsades de pointes") in the setting of QT interval prolongation. Awareness that this can occur is the most important consideration. Lidocaine (see below) is the treatment of choice for quinidine-induced VPBs.

Digoxin in some patients with severe congestive heart failure and cardiomegaly may have antiarrhythmic effects, possibly by decreasing ventricular size. Hypokalemia must be watched for in all patients on digoxin, since VPBs or other ventricular arrhythmias may be precipitated.

Recently, quinidine has been shown to raise serum digoxin levels by a factor of 2. Currently, all patients receiving both agents should have serum digoxin levels carefully monitored.

Mild hypokalemia should be treated with oral potassium chloride supplementation (20 mEq orally four times daily). Severe hypokalemia should be treated with intravenous potassium chloride (40 mEq in 500 ml of 5 per cent glucose) given slowly over a 4 hour period. The latter (slow infusion method) will prevent the rare possibility of paradoxical potassium-induced AV block. All patients with digitalis toxicity should be monitored in the coronary care unit. Digoxin-induced VPBs can be treated with lidocaine (see below).

Patients with Vasospastic or Prinzmetal's Angina. VPBs are very common and frequently herald ventricular tachycardia or fibrillation. Treatment is best directed toward prevention of coronary vasospasm by nitrates or new experimental slow channel calcium-blocking agents such as verapamil or nifedipine.

VPBs in Patients with Stable Chronic Coronary

Heart Disease. Even in these cases care should be taken to exclude VPBs produced by administered stimulants as well as certain other arrhythmogenic drugs such as quinidine, digoxin, phenothiazines, and tricyclic antidepressants. Although all current antiarrhythmic agents are not without potentially serious side effects, we believe that in this clinical setting malignant VPBs should be treated. Commonly used agents and their side effects are as follows: procainamide, 250 to 1000 mg orally four times daily or every 4 hours (lupus-like syndrome, positive ANA); disopyramide, 100 to 300 mg orally four times daily (glaucoma, congestive heart failure, urinary retention); propranolol, 10 to 80 mg orally four times daily (asthma, congestive heart failure); quinidine sulfate or gluconate, 200 to 400 mg orally four times daily (gastrointestinal distress).

End points of therapy are frequently difficult to ascertain, since there is wide spontaneous variability in frequency and complexity of arrhythmias from one 24 hour period to the next. Holter monitoring for assessment of therapy is therefore fraught with hazard. In general, in symptomatic patients not at risk of sudden death, relief of symptoms is a reasonable end point. Complete abolition of VPBs, while desirable, is frequently impossible. The practical goal is reduction both in total frequency and in complexity.

Acute Myocardial Infarction. Although any VPB may be significant in patients with acute myocardial infarction, in most coronary care units around the country treatment with lidocaine is still instituted only when the patient develops so-called warning arrhythmias, namely (1) more than five VPBs per minute; (2) VPBs falling on the antecedent T wave; (3) two or more VPBs in a row; and (4) multifocal (or multiform) VPBs.

Because the distribution half-life of lidocaine is 8 minutes and the elimination half-life 120 minutes, loading doses (2 boluses of 75 mg each, given at 8 to 10 minute intervals) should be given first before starting a drip infusion at a rate of 3 mg per minute. These dosages should be halved in patients with severe heart failure, cardiogenic shock, or liver disease and in patients over 70 years of age. Contraindications are AV block and severe sinus bradycardia (rates under 50 per minute). Some authors consider that ventricular fibrillation in acute myocardial infarction is unpredictable and is related more to the time of appearance of VPBs after the onset of the myocardial infarction than to the presence of malignant features. This has led to the still unanswered controversy over whether lidocaine should be used prophylactically in all patients with acute myocardial infarction. At present there is an increasing

trend toward doing this. Several points are noteworthy: (1) lidocaine should be started as soon as the diagnosis of MI is made (in the emergency room, preferably); (2) trained personnel should be available to decide if lidocaine is contraindicated or if the dose has to be reduced; and (3) continuous monitoring of the ECG and observation of the patient are required. In institutions where these conditions cannot be met, it is preferable to continue conventional (not prophylactic) treatment. In any case the risk of ventricular fibrillation falls off rapidly after several hours post-MI. Hence we feel that prophylaxis is of dubious benefit after this very early high risk period.

Chronic Phase of Myocardial Infarction. Although there is still much controversy, patients discharged from the hospital after an MI should probably be treated if the predischarge Holter shows frequent VPBs (>30 per hour), couplets or salvos of VPBs, or other complex forms. Since VPBs are almost universal post-MI, we do not treat a patient with only occasional VPBs at the time of discharge. Treatment (as outlined for patients with chronic stable coronary disease) when instituted is frequently maintained for 12 months and the patient re-evaluated at that time, since many transient ischemia-related arrhythmias will resolve by then.

Sudden Death Survivors. This group is at high risk of subsequent sudden death. Patients resuscitated from out-of-the-hospital ventricular fibrillation and whose condition does not evolve into a myocardial infarction have a particularly high risk of recurrent ventricular fibrillation. We generally recommend vigorous treatment of all sudden death survivors in an attempt to suppress VPBs. If complete suppression fails, as it quite frequently does, we at least attempt to maintain high constant blood levels of the antiarrhythmic agents being employed. Liberal use of 24 hour Holter recording is recommended. Major poor prognostic factors are functional Class IV, cardiomegaly, and new left bundle branch block.

HEART BLOCK

method of
PARK W. WILLIS, IV, M.D.,
Chapel Hill, North Carolina
and PARK W. WILLIS, III, M.D.
East Lansing, Michigan

Heart block is a nonspecific term applied to delay in conduction at different sites within the heart. Three types of heart block are most important: abnormal conduction between the sinus node and right atrium (SA block), between the atria and the ventricles (AV block), and within the ventricles (intraventricular block). Unless modified, the term heart block in this article refers to AV block.

General Considerations

Proper management of the patient with heart block depends upon accurate diagnosis and usually requires objective evidence that a patient's symptoms are associated with the abnormality identified. The presence of heart block may be suspected clinically, but the type of conduction disturbance is determined from the electrocardiogram (EKG). As far as this is possible, the cause of impaired impulse transmission should be identified. Knowledge of the natural history of a specific type of heart block is important in making decisions about long-term therapy, but acute management is more often determined by the effective ventricular rate and the hemodynamic consequences of the conduction disturbance.

Pharmacologic Therapy

Stopping Previous Drug Treatment. Digitalis glycosides, beta-receptor blocking agents, quinidine preparations, procainamide, disopyramide phosphate, or verapamil may depress cardiac conduction and impulse formation and should be discontinued in a patient who develops significant heart block. Antihypertensive drugs such as guanethidine, reserpine, and methyldopa may aggravate heart block by depleting myocardial catecholamine stores and interfering with sympathetic activation of the heart.

Atropine. This vagolytic drug may be useful when there is a disturbance of sinus node function or of conduction through the atrioventricular (AV) junction. Increased vagal tone can have a profound effect at these sites, and under such circumstances atropine will increase the atrial rate and enhance AV conduction. Vagal influence is minimal in the distal ventricular conduction system, and atropine is of no use for block below the AV node. Atropine should be given in an initial dose of 0.5 mg intravenously. The onset of action is rapid and an effect should be evident within 2 minutes. If conduction has not improved by this time, repeated doses of 0.5 mg should be given every 2 or 3 minutes. The total dose should not exceed 2.0 mg in 10 to 15 minutes. Additional doses are unlikely to produce a satisfactory response, may produce untoward effects, and may delay more effective therapy. The duration of action of atropine is from 1 to 4 hours, and in many acute situations, even with

acute infarction, a single dose may suffice because the block is often transient.

Long-term atropine therapy, 0.5 to 1.0 mg intravenously every 3 to 4 hours, can be effective treatment for AV heart block or severe sinus bradycardia, but since there is a high prevalence of side effects, including gastric and urinary retention, mental confusion, and acute glaucoma, atropine should be reserved for acute treatment.

Isoproterenol. This drug is a synthetic catecholamine and is a beta-receptor agonist (stimulator). It increases atrial rate, enhances AV conduction, and increases the rate of escaped junctional or ventricular rhythm in complete heart block (CHB). Intravenous administration is preferred in acute situations. Preparations for sublingual administration are available, but are not useful for the treatment of heart block. For intravenous use, 1 mg of isoproterenol is diluted in 500 ml of 5 per cent dextrose in water to yield a concentration of 2.0 micrograms per ml. The drug should be administered continuously, using a microdrip infusion set or, preferably, an infusion pump. The initial infusion rate should be 0.5 ml (1.0 microgram) per minute. The onset of action is rapid, and the effect of the drug can be assessed in 2 or 3 minutes. If the infusion rate is inadequate, it should be increased 0.5 ml (1.0 microgram) per minute every 2 to 3 minutes until the desired effect is achieved. Most patients will respond to doses of 1 to 5 micrograms per minute, but as much as 10 micrograms per minute may be necessary.

Isoproterenol infusions require frequent adjustment to achieve the desired heart rate (60 to 80 beats per minute) while avoiding the undesirable side effects of the drug such as sinus tachycardia or ventricular arrhythmia. If these occur, the infusion should be stopped and then started at a slower rate when the arrhythmia has disappeared. Isoproterenol is contraindicated for most patients with acute myocardial infarction.

Pacemakers. Electronic pacemakers provide the most reliable control of cardiac rate and rhythm, but with a certain amount of associated risk. Temporary and permanent transvenous pacemakers should be placed by those experienced with the techniques.

In an acute situation it is essential that medical therapy be initiated while preparations are being made for temporary pacemaker placement. During this short interval drug therapy will usually provide an adequate heart rate and satisfactory systemic perfusion.

A temporary pacing catheter may be inserted percutaneously via a subclavian, internal jugular, or femoral venipuncture. Alternatively, an antecubital vein cutdown may be used. In general, the subclavian approach provides the most stable catheter position, and right-sided veins are preferable because they provide a more direct route to the right ventricle. With direct fluoroscopic visualization, the tip of the pacing catheter should be advanced so that the tip is at the apex of the right ventricle. When the position is satisfactory and the catheter seems stable, the catheter should be connected to a demand pacemaker unit, which can be activated to pace or "capture" the ventricle. It may be necessary to reposition the catheter a number of times before the ventricle responds regularly to each electrical stimulus; repositioning should always be carried out with the help of fluoroscopic visualization. When a satisfactory position has been achieved, the pacing threshold must be measured. If the threshold is acceptable (less than 1.0 mA), the catheter should be sutured to the skin and a sterile dressing applied. The generator should be set at the desired pacing rate (usually 70 to 80 beats per minute) and at the stimulus strength required (usually three times threshold and less than 5 mA). It is important to measure the pacing threshold and inspect the pacemaker position by fluoroscopy after the catheter has been secured and the dressing applied, because these tasks may result in displacement of the catheter tip within the right ventricle, which, if not corrected, may result in later loss of capture of the ventricle by the pacemaker.

In an emergency situation, it is possible to insert a temporary pacemaker without the aid of fluoroscopy. The catheter may be advanced transvenously with electrocardiographic monitoring by connecting a precordial electrode to the pacing catheter. This technique requires experience, skill, and luck. A more direct approach for emergency pacing is the transthoracic technique. This can be accomplished by a direct puncture of the right ventricle through the third or fourth intercostal space at the left sternal edge. A long intracardiac or spinal needle with a large bore can be advanced in a direction perpendicular to the chest wall, until aspiration yields free-flowing unoxygenated blood, indicating that the needle is in the cavity of the right ventricle. A pacing catheter can then be passed through the needle into the right ventricle. The needle should then be removed and the catheter attached to a pacing unit. This technique may be associated with serious complications and should be used only in emergency situations when fluoroscopy is not available and other methods to establish an adequate cardiac rhythm have failed.

Permanent pacing can be established by means of endocardial or epicardial electrodes.

The most common technique is the transvenous approach, which requires local anesthesia to insert the pacemaker catheter through the cephalic, subclavian, external jugular, or internal jugular vein. The battery-powered impulse generating unit is usually implanted subcutaneously, superficial to the pectoral muscles. The endocardial pacing catheter can perforate the ventricle; stable electrode position may be difficult or impossible to maintain; and, rarely, the catheter tip may serve as a nidus for important thrombus formation or infection. The placement of epicardial electrodes requires general anesthesia and a limited thoracotomy and is associated with a higher complication rate than the endocardial technique. The principal advantage of this approach is electrode stability, and this method may be particularly useful for patients with right ventricular dilatation and tricuspid regurgitation, as well as those who wish to have unlimited mobility of their arms and shoulders.

Atrial, coronary sinus, and AV sequential pacing techniques are available, but at present are much less often used than ventricular demand pacemakers.

Most ventricular pacemakers in use today are of the demand (synchronous) rather than fixed rate (asynchronous) type. Demand units are preferred because, under normal circumstances, they will not discharge during the vulnerable period of the cardiac cycle. The most consistently used demand unit is the ventricular inhibited type, which does not fire as long as normal QRS complexes occur at a rate rapid enough to suppress the pacemaker.

Late complications of permanent pacemakers are battery failure, lead breakage, electrode dislodgment, and infection at the site of the lead or in the pacemaker pocket. Ventricular arrhythmias can occur during the first 24 to 48 hours after implantation but rarely require treatment. Patients should be monitored for the first 24 to 48 hours so that, if necessary, lidocaine can be administered intravenously.

Electrocardiograms and periodic electronic analysis must be obtained at regular intervals on patients who have permanent pacemakers, since subtle rate or artifact duration changes are the earliest signs of battery depletion. Currently available techniques allow telephone transmission of the patient's EKG to a central location. Impending battery failure may be suspected when there is a gradual fall in the rate of the pacemaker discharge. Most modern pacemakers have lithium power sources which should last for at least 8 years; but even so, failure can occur without warning.

Treatment for Specific Forms of Heart Block

Heart Block Complicating Acute Myocardial Infarction. Acute myocardial infarction (AMI) is one of the most frequent causes of impaired conduction. The AV block is reversible in most cases, and the proper initial therapy is usually pharmacologic. Nevertheless, temporary pacing is often necessary during AMI.

In the early stages of AMI, the drug of choice for pain is intravenous morphine sulfate in doses of 2 to 4 mg every 5 to 10 minutes until pain is relieved. Morphine has vagotonic effects; if there is sinus bradycardia or AV block associated with the pain, atropine should be given simultaneously in order to prevent more profound slowing of the ventricular rate. It is not uncommon, especially in patients with inferior MI (commonly associated with high degrees of vagal tone), for AV block to disappear with relief of pain.

The proper management of patients with AMI who show persistent AV block depends upon the effective ventricular rate and the hemodynamic consequences of the block, the type of conduction disturbance, and the site of the infarction. The goal of therapy is to maintain an adequate heart rate and prevent sudden bradycardia and other serious cardiac arrhythmias. Initial therapy should include intravenous atropine.

Patients who develop complete heart block (CHB) with a wide QRS complex and a ventricular escape rhythm with a slow rate require a temporary transvenous pacemaker regardless of the site of infarction. Occasionally, patients with inferior AMI progress from first degree AV block to Mobitz I second degree AV block and finally to CHB with a normal QRS complex, which is identical to that present prior to the onset of the conduction disturbance. If the ventricular rate is greater than 50 beats per minute and there are no symptoms or signs of hypoperfusion or congestive heart failure, these patients need not be paced. However, if symptoms of pulmonary venous congestion or hypotension develop, a temporary transvenous pacemaker should be placed promptly. In patients with anterior myocardial infarction, CHB is usually associated with a slow ventricular rate (30 to 40 beats per minute), abnormally wide QRS complexes, and evidence of inadequate cardiac output. Temporary pacing is indicated for these individuals, but they have a high mortality rate even with pacing.

With AMI the occurrence of Mobitz II second degree AV block with a wide QRS complex or left anterior or posterior fascicular block (LAFB or LPFB) may precede the sudden development of CHB. This is especially likely with anterior myocardial infarction, and these patients should be treated prophylactically with a temporary pacemaker, since 50 per cent of patients with anterior AMI and de novo bifascicular block progress unexpectedly to complete AV block. Patients with 2:1 AV block, normal QRS complex, adequate ventricular rate, and satisfactory systemic perfusion present difficult therapeutic decisions. Those with inferior MI usually have reversible block at the level of the AV node, and no treatment is necessary unless hemodynamic complications occur. It is uncommon for patients with anterior wall MI to develop this type of conduction disturbance, and it is difficult to define appropriate management. However, it is our practice to use a temporary pacemaker for these patients, since they are likely to have distal conduction system disease and are prone to the sudden development of CHB with possible catastrophic consequences.

Mobitz I second degree AV block (Wenckebach phenomenon) or first degree AV block occurring after AMI usually requires no treatment. These conduction defects are most common with inferior MI and are usually temporary and well tolerated by most patients.

Patients with AMI and acute or pre-existing bundle branch or fascicular block require special attention, since they may be prone to the sudden development of CHB. The onset of right bundle branch block (RBBB) in a patient with inferior AMI is not an indication for a temporary pacemaker. However, patients with anterior MI and acute RBBB should be paced. Those with AMI and old or indeterminate age RBBB do not require temporary pacing unless there is a more advanced conduction disturbance associated with the bundle branch block. For example, patients with transmural AMI who have RBBB and LAFB or LPFB are at increased risk of sudden CHB and should receive a temporary pacemaker. Temporary pacing is also indicated for patients with AMI and left bundle branch block (LBBB) that is acute or of indeterminate age. A pacemaker is not necessary for the patient with pre-existing LBBB who does not show other evidence of seriously impaired AV conduction, such as second or third degree heart block.

Decisions regarding permanent pacemaker placement in patients who develop transient CHB during the course of AMI are often difficult. Permanent pacing is not necessary for patients with inferior MI who have shown the common progression from first degree to Mobitz I second degree to CHB during the acute phase of illness with subsequent restoration of AV conduction during recovery. However, there is a higher than expected incidence of later sudden death in patients with anterior MI who had transient CHB during the acute illness. Permanent pacemakers are indicated for these individuals.

Furthermore, recent evidence has suggested that permanent pacing is indicated for patients with AMI and bundle branch block who develop transient high grade AV block, defined as Mobitz II second degree AV block or CHB (sudden or preceded by Mobitz II second degree block).

Hyperkalemia. Immediate medical therapy is necessary for advanced heart block resulting from hyperkalemia.

Intravenous calcium gluconate quickly reverses the cardiac toxicity of hyperkalemia in most cases. However, it should not be given to individuals receiving digitalis except in life-threatening situations.

The usual dose is 5 to 10 ml of a 10 per cent solution given over a 2 minute period. This may be repeated in 5 minutes if the EKG shows no change for the better. If there is no response after two doses of calcium gluconate, it is unlikely that more will be effective.

Sodium bicarbonate ($NaHCO_3$) causes potassium to move rapidly from extracellular to intracellular spaces. For the treatment of heart block resulting from hyperkalemia, $NaHCO_3$ may be given intravenously in a dose of 45 mEq over a 5 minute period. The dose may be repeated 10 to 15 minutes later if EKG abnormalities persist. Large quantities of $NaHCO_3$ can cause intravascular volume overload.

Although effective acutely, calcium gluconate and $NaHCO_3$ each have a short duration of action. A glucose infusion can be used to achieve a more sustained reduction in the serum potassium level; 200 to 300 ml of a 20 per cent glucose solution given over 30 to 60 minutes will usually produce an increase in plasma insulin and an intracellular shift of potassium. Chronically debilitated or malnourished patients may show a blunted insulin response to the glucose load, and in these individuals 1 unit of regular insulin should be given intravenously with each 4 grams of glucose.

Cation exchange resins lower serum potassium more slowly than the treatments described above, but they reduce the total body potassium stores. Sodium polystyrene sulfonate (Kayexalate) may be given orally in a dose of 20 to 50 grams dissolved in 100 to 200 ml of 20 per cent sorbitol solution every 3 to 4 hours until the serum potassium has returned to normal. The drug may also be given rectally as a retention enema. The dose is 50 grams of sodium polystyrene sulfonate (Kayexalate) and 50 grams of sorbitol in 200 ml of water. The enema should be retained for 30 to 60 minutes, and repeated doses may be given hourly if necessary to lower the serum potassium level.

Dialysis may be necessary to control hyperkalemia in some patients.

Drug Toxicity. Heart block may be caused by digitalis glycosides, beta-blockers, procainamide, quinidine preparations, disopyramide phosphate, or verapamil. Drug toxicity is reversible when the medication is discontinued, and in an asymptomatic patient without ventricular arrhythmia no further therapy is necessary. If the heart block is associated with hemodynamic failure or a complex ventricular arrhythmia, medical therapy with atropine and isoproterenol or a temporary transvenous pacemaker may be necessary. It is important to remember that although supplemental potassium may be a useful treatment in hypokalemic patients with ventricular arrhythmias resulting from digitalis intoxication, AV block caused by digitalis is potentiated by high serum potassium levels.

Sinoatrial Block and Sinus Node Dysfunction. Sinoatrial (SA) block is relatively uncommon. First degree SA block, prolonged conduction of the impulse from the sinus node to atrial muscle, cannot be recognized in the surface EKG. Second degree SA block is present when one or more sinus node impulses fail to cause atrial depolarization. This is manifested in the EKG by the absence of an expected sinus P wave; the usual associated QRST complex is also absent, but a junctional or ventricular escape beat may occur before the next sinus beat. Complete SA block is manifested by absence of P waves and is usually associated with a slow junctional or idioventricular escape rhythm. Although SA block may be caused by high vagal tone, it is usually due to cardiac disease (such as myocardial ischemia or myocarditis) or to drug toxicity. If the patient is taking a drug that might be responsible, it should be discontinued. Atropine and isoproterenol may be effective in restoring SA conduction acutely, but patients with chronic symptomatic SA block usually require a permanent pacemaker.

Another form of heart block, characterized by sinus node dysfunction, has been named the "sick sinus" or "tachycardia-bradycardia" syndrome. This may be manifested as sinus arrest, SA block, marked sinus bradycardia, prolonged sinus pauses, or paroxysmal ectopic atrial tachycardia or fibrillation followed by prolonged pauses. Proper management of this syndrome requires a search for correctable causes of sinus node dysfunction such as drug intoxication, thyrotoxicosis, or hyperkalemia. After these have been excluded, it is important to establish that important symptoms are associated with the disorder. Sinus node dysfunction frequently occurs in older individuals who have vague symptoms such as dizziness and fatigue. A long-term EKG recording with careful notation of symptoms by the patient is essential to establish that a relationship exists between symptoms and impaired function of the sinus node. Electrophysiologic study using abrupt cessation of rapid atrial pacing with measurement of the time required for the SA node to recover may confirm the presence of sinus node dysfunction in questionable cases. This measurement, the sinus node recovery time, is abnormal in about two thirds of patients with the "sick sinus" syndrome, and then is of help in making the decision about permanent pacing. Unfortunately, a normal sinus node recovery time does not exclude sinus node dysfunction, and in this situation therapeutic decisions must be based on clinical assessment and the long-term (24 to 72 hours) EKG. Patients who have sinus node dysfunction require no treatment unless symptoms develop. Patients with important symptoms require permanent pacemakers. In addition, therapy with digitalis or propranolol is frequently necessary to control arrhythmias.

Chronic (AV) Block. Chronic AV block may be congenital or acquired. Prolongation of the PR interval to 0.21 second or more (first degree AV block) and Mobitz I second degree AV block may occur in normal subjects and can be caused by increased vagal tone. Diseases most commonly responsible for first and second degree AV block include chronic ischemic heart disease and myocarditis. Chronic first degree AV block requires no treatment. Chronic second degree AV block is not usually symptomatic and does not require treatment unless marked bradycardia produces hemodynamic compromise. In the absence of remedial cause such as drug intoxication or electrolyte disturbance, a permanent pacemaker may be necessary. Chronic complete AV block (CHB), especially of congenital origin, may be associated with an adequate ventricular rate, a narrow QRS deflection, and an absence of symptoms. If a long-term (Holter) EKG shows no periods of marked bradycardia, there may be no need for therapy. However, if there is associated angina, effort intolerance, congestive heart failure, near syncope, or syncope, permanent pacing is necessary. Symptoms such as dizziness, fatigue, and impaired mental function are often difficult to sort out in elderly patients with coincidental chronic CHB. In such instances, it is important to establish a cause and effect relationship between the patient's symptoms and the slow heart rate. A trial of temporary pacing with serial observations of hemodynamic response and symptoms may be

useful in making the decision regarding permanent pacing for these patients.

Chronic Intraventricular Block. In recent years, there has been a great deal of interest in chronic bifascicular block (RBBB and LAFB, RBBB and LPFB, alternating LBBB and RBBB, LBBB and AV block). There is no indication for treatment of the asymptomatic patient with these conduction disturbances; temporary pacemakers are not necessary during operative procedures. Patients who report symptoms suggesting profound bradycardia, asystole, or serious cardiac arrhythmia should be thoroughly evaluated. Permanent pacemakers should be reserved for those in whom serious symptoms remain unexplained despite a thorough medical evaluation.

TACHYCARDIA

method of
LESLIE R. FLEISCHER, M.D.,
and ARTHUR M. LEVY, M.D.
Burlington, Vermont

The field of tachycardias generated great interest in the last decade because new electrophysiologic techniques produced an explosion of information concerning the mechanism of these rhythm disturbances. The decade from 1980 to 1989 will almost certainly continue this trend, as it appears that many new drugs and pacemaker techniques will become available for treating these disturbances, still as a result of this information. Thus, an annual review of this particular topic will be especially useful, as will an understanding of at least the rudiments of physiology and pharmacology of these fascinating arrhythmias. While shotgun therapy was a frequently successful method of treating tachyrhythmias in the past, new information has shown that this approach is frequently ineffective and occasionally hazardous, either in itself or as more correct therapy is withheld.

The ideal situation today is to identify the type of tachycardia exactly and respond accordingly. This article will be written in broad terms of regular and irregular narrow QRS and broad QRS tachycardias. Nonetheless, making an exact diagnosis will often be helpful. The reason shotgun therapy has been effective in supraventricular tachycardias is that with rare exceptions the pathway in some way involves the atrioventricular (AV) node, the heart's marvelous built-in safety mechanism for rate control. Therefore, digitalis glycosides and propranolol, both of which primarily affect the AV node, can be counted on to slow or stop most of these tachycardias. One can totally avoid the selective process with regard to antiarrhythmic agents by using cardioversion as the primary antiarrhythmic agent and worrying later about the type of arrhythmia and its prevention. Problems with both approaches will be discussed under each type of arrhythmia.

A few general principles should be mentioned before outlining the therapy for individual tachycardias. In terms of drug use a single drug may be insufficient to control the tachycardia and a second or even third drug must be added. However, as this is done, there must be more and more awareness of potential side effects. A totally unexpected recent finding after years of using quinidine and digitalis together is that *the addition of quinidine to an already digitalized patient will significantly increase the serum level and may produce manifest digitalis toxicity.* (Adverse effects previously described in this setting were frequently ascribed to quinidine rather than digitalis toxicity.) So-called Class I antiarrhythmic agents (e.g., disopyramide, procainamide, quinidine) can prolong the QT interval and actually worsen ventricular arrhythmias rather than produce the desired alleviation.

In treating a patient with tachycardia, one must develop from the beginning a conscious consideration of the time frame in which one must act. Significant hemodynamic impairment calls for immediate therapeutic results and usually militates for the use of DC cardioversion. However, just as important, one must be careful not to exclude future therapeutic avenues as one chooses initial treatment — i.e., before fully digitalizing a patient with a tachycardia one should set a decision-making point after giving half or three-quarters of the digitalis dose, since DC cardioversion following full digitalization may produce digitalis-toxic rhythms.

Treatment Schedules for Adults with Tachycardia

The following treatment schedules will be referred to in the text, some of them multiple times. To avoid redundancy we shall refer to these schedules each time a specific therapeutic modality is mentioned.

Carotid Sinus Massage. While monitoring an electrocardiogram, massage the right carotid with steady pressure and circular motion for 10 to 15 seconds. If unsuccessful, repeat with the left carotid. Use carotid massage with caution in elderly patients because of possible carotid flow compromise.

Cardioversion. Principles of cardioversion include the following:

1. Cardioversion should be attempted using the least energy necessary.

2. In emergency situations, unless ventricular fibrillation is present, the synchronous mode should be utilized; but if there is failure of output, one should switch to asynchronous mode.

3. Patients with permanent pacemakers can be cardioverted, but the paddles should not be placed over the generator and the generator should be checked after cardioversion.

4. One should be cautious about cardioverting fully digitalized patients and especially cardioverting patients on both digitalis and quinidine, since this combination produces higher than average serum digoxin levels

CARDIOVERSION SCHEDULE A. Give initial shock of 25 to 50 watt-seconds, then double succeeding shocks (100–200–400 watt-seconds).

CARDIOVERSION SCHEDULE B. Initial attempt at 100 watt-seconds, followed by 200 and 400 watt-seconds if unsuccessful. If the patient is on digitalis, start at 10 to 25 watt-seconds and if premature ventricular contractions (PVC's) are produced by this initial stimulus, significant digitalis toxicity could be manifest postcardioversion.

Propranolol Schedule. Initial total intravenous dose should be set at 0.1 mg per kg. Initially, give 0.5 mg intravenously and then give in 1.0 mg increments every 1 to 5 minutes to reach total. If slowing has occurred but tachycardia perists and the patient shows no side effects, give three more 1.0 mg increments or a new total of 0.15 mg per kg.

Digoxin Schedule. Give 0.5 mg of intravenous digoxin as first dose. Follow with another 0.25 mg in 2 hours. After another 2 hours, make a decision with regard to attempting cardioversion as opposed to continuing digoxin therapy. If the decision is against use of cardioversion, give more digoxin in 0.25 mg increments to a total of 1.0 to 1.25 mg. If the dose exceeds 0.75 mg, no cardioversion should be attempted until at least 2 hours after the last dose, and then a test dose of 10 to 25 watt-seconds should be used to see if any signs of digitalis toxicity are brought out, namely ventricular premature contractions.

Quinidine Sulfate Schedule. Give 200 mg orally every 4 hours times six doses for a maximum of 1.2 grams.

Procainamide Schedule. Give 100 mg intravenously every 2 minutes up to a total of 800 to 1000 mg.

Lidocaine Schedule. Give 75 to 100 mg in an intravenous bolus, followed by 50 to 100 mg 15

minutes later to reach a total bolus dose of approximately 200 mg. Start a lidocaine drip at 2 mg per minute following the first bolus.

Bretylium Tosylate Schedule. Give 5 mg per kg intravenously slowly over 10 minutes, followed by a drip at 1 to 2 mg per minute.

Edrophonium (Tensilon) Schedule. Give a 2 mg test dose, then 8 mg more intravenously over 10 minutes. (This use of edrophonium is not listed in the manufacturer's official directive.)

Regular Narrow QRS (Supraventricular) Tachycardia

Sinus Tachycardia. This tachyrhythmia is usually not a clinical problem. It is almost always a physiologic response to some other derangement or to catecholamine stimulation for whatever reason. Re-entrant or circus movement tachycardias involving the SA node do exist but are uncommon. It is, however, important to be able to recognize sinus tachycardia, since occasionally therapy aimed at breaking the tachycardia, including cardioversion, is attempted by mistake. Specific therapy for sinus tachycardia is rarely necessary, although propranolol is occasionally used to slow this rhythm in patients with angina pectoris or thyrotoxicosis. This form of tachycardia is recognized by observing P waves similar to the sinus P waves on or after the T wave. A 12 lead electrocardiogram (ECG) to look at P and QRS morphology may add to the information on a long lead II. Carotid sinus stimulation may slow this tachycardia, which speeds up when stimulation has stopped. The rate should be under 200 beats per minute and usually is in the 100 to 160 range.

Paroxysmal Supraventricular Tachycardia. The terminology associated with regular supraventricular tachycardia has become confusing, especially with the common use of the term paroxysmal atrial tachycardia (PAT) in the past. The term paroxysmal supraventricular tachycardia seems to cover the situation best. The great majority of these regular tachycardias (excluding for now atrial flutter) are circus movement or synonymously re-entrant tachycardias. Once initiated, the tachycardia persists by stimulating the ventricles each time this circus movement enters the ventricular conduction system. The circular path may be within the AV node (micro re-entry) or may include the AV nodal His system and a bypass tract such as a Kent bundle (macro re-entry). The P waves (usually inverted) may or may not be visualized as the atria are depolarized in a retrograde fashion.

Since conduction velocities and recovery periods of each portion of this loop are crucial in allowing the circus movement to continue, any method of changing one or both of these parameters in any portion of the loop could break the tachycardia.

CAROTID SINUS STIMULATION. This should be step number one. If done properly, it may break as many as 80 per cent of these most common supraventricular tachycardias. One should repeat carotid massage after each unsuccessful stage of drug therapy, as it may break the tachycardia with the new physiologic milieu produced by the drugs. Since these are re-entry tachycardias, the vagal effects of carotid massage on the AV node will not produce 2:1 or higher block, as this is not possible with circus movements. If indeed 2:1 or higher block is produced, a different physiologic mechanism must be operative.

DRUG THERAPY. Propranolol is our drug of choice in patients without contraindication for its use (see Propranolol Schedule, p. 179). If, during the course of intravenous propranolol therapy, there is no measurable lengthening of RR intervals, one should suspect re-entry is not present. Our second choice (in adults) is edrophonium (Tensilon) (see above). The treatment of paroxysmal supraventricular tachycardia in the pediatric age group is discussed at end of this article. One should try carotid sinus stimulation immediately after the use of edrophonium if the tachycardia persists. One should not use edrophonium in patients with acute myocardial infarction and should use it with caution in patients who are already on digitalis or who have coronary artery disease. If both propranolol and edrophonium have been unsuccessful, one can add either *digoxin* (see Digoxin Schedule, p. 179) or a vasopressor. The intravenous use of pressor agents should be monitored with a goal of raising the blood pressure to a maximum of 30 to 50 mm Hg above normal.

It is possible that *verapamil*, a calcium antagonist, will be released for the intravenous therapy of supraventricular tachycardia during the 1980–81 period. This drug has been shown to be almost uniformly successful with paroxysmal supraventricular tachycardia in European trials. It may well replace the other agents listed above as the primary drug, although there will be some contraindications such as the use of previous beta blocker therapy and suspected digitalis toxicity.

DC CARDIOVERSION. One can interrupt the drug schedule outlined above at any time by turning to cardioversion. However, cardioversion should not be attempted after full doses of digoxin have been given, at least without the realization that it may rarely produce resistant ventricular fibrillation under these circumstances. One should decide to use cardioversion (see Cardioversion Schedule B, p. 179) before completing a full digitalization regimen.

RAPID ATRIAL PACING. An additional mode of therapy for re-entrant supraventricular tachycardia (as well as for atrial flutter) is to attempt to break into the re-entry cycle by utilizing a *temporary pacer wire* in the right atrium. Having confirmed that the tip of the bipolar catheter is definitely against the right atrial wall and not in the right ventricle, one can give brief bursts of rapid stimuli (300 to 1000 per minute). It is important to give brief bursts, since one can stop and restart the tachycardia with longer bursts without realizing it. It may be necessary to place the tip of the catheter in various positions in the right atrium to be successful. This method of overdrive stimulation for breaking the tachyrhythmia is really a simple and very frequently successful one, and the patient does not have to be sedated as for cardioversion.

Atrial Flutter. Atrial flutter is listed under the regular narrow QRS tachycardias since it is usually very regular. However, variable AV block may make it appear to be irregular. The most common situation is 2:1 flutter with a ventricular rate of almost exactly 150 per minute. A 12 lead ECG may be of significant help in finding the characteristic saw-toothed flutter waves. One wave usually distorts the T wave, but the other or a portion of the other may be seen just after the QRS. Higher grades of block than 2:1 are easily diagnosed, and 1:1 flutter at a rate of 300 is extremely rare.

CAROTID SINUS STIMULATION. Carotid sinus stimulation will help to make the diagnosis if it is not clear by producing increased AV block and unmasking the rapid flutter waves.

CARDIOVERSION (see Cardioversion Schedule A, p. 179). This is the *method of choice* for breaking atrial flutter in the uncomplicated situation, i.e., the patient not on multiple antiarrhythmic agents. This is because of its high success rate with very small amounts of electrical energy. Again, one should be cautioned about problems of digitalis and digitalis plus quinidine as noted in the discussion of cardioversion under Paroxysmal Supraventricular Tachycardia.

RAPID ATRIAL PACING. Again this is mentioned ahead of drug therapy because of its effectiveness and also because of the relative ineffectiveness of the available drugs for treating atrial flutter. The pacing can be done in two ways: (1) as mentioned above under Paroxysmal Supraventricular Tachycardia, with short bursts of rapid (300 to 1000 stimuli per minute) stimulation; or (2) by slowly increasing the pacing rate, starting below the atrial rate at about 150 per minute and progressing up to a rate faster than

the flutter rate (300 to 350 per minute), to capture the atria. With successful capture, one should see a sudden change in the axis of the P wave, following which the pacing rate can be slowed and stopped.

DRUG THERAPY. *Digoxin* and *propranolol* are not good drugs in this situation. Both will increase the degree of AV block so that if the patient is not tolerating a rate of approximately 150 the ventricular response can be slowed. Conversion can be effected with these drugs, particularly with digoxin, but not in a high percentage (see Digoxin Schedule and Propranolol Schedule, p. 179). Quinidine can be used to break atrial flutter (see Quinidine Sulfate Schedule, p. 179). It is commonly cautioned to use digoxin prior to quinidine, as quinidine alone may increase the ventricular rate. Propranolol can be substituted for digoxin prior to using quinidine to help prevent this sudden increase of ventricular rate. In resistant cases of atrial flutter, one should not overlook possible contributing factors such as pericarditis or theophylline overdosage.

Ectopic Atrial Tachycardia (PAT). This form of regular narrow QRS supraventricular tachycardia is associated with visible upright P waves, demonstrating that conduction is not retrograde from low atrium to high atrium as in the previously described paroxysmal supraventricular tachycardia. The rate of the P waves usually varies from 150 to approximately 240. There frequently is 2:1 or variable AV block. The older term paroxysmal atrial tachycardia (PAT) can probably be used in this situation, since these rhythms are probably ectopic (are not re-entry) and do originate in the atria. Certainly digitalis toxicity should be ruled out when making this diagnosis by looking at serum levels of digoxin and potassium. In the face of proved or suspected digitalis toxicity, *cessation of the drug* is the obvious first step and may be all that is necessary to treat this arrhythmia. If the patient is in difficulty from the rhythm, intravenous *procainamide* can be used (see Procainamide Schedule, p. 179). Propranolol could be used to increase AV block and slow the rate if necessary. In the absence of digitalis toxicity, ectopic atrial tachycardias can be treated with either oral *quinidine* or intravenous *procainamide,* depending on the urgency of the situation (see Quinidine Sulfate Schedule and Procainamide Schedule, p. 179).

Irregular Narrow QRS Tachycardias

While atrial tachycardia with variable block or atrial flutter with variable block may appear irregular, the atrial activity is very regular, and these can be separated from atrial fibrillation and multifocal atrial tachycardias, which are the two truly irregular narrow beat tachycardias discussed here.

Paroxysmal Atrial Fibrillation. Atrial fibrillation may in fact not be a tachycardia in terms of ventricular response, as many people have normal or even slow ventricular rates, although obviously it is always a tachycardia in terms of the atrial rates. Given a particularly slow response in the absence of any antiarrhythmic therapy, one should consider tachy-brady syndrome.

CAROTID SINUS STIMULATION. This is not useful to break this tachyrhythmia, but if one does carotid sinus stimulation and finds high grade AV block with very slow ventricular response, one might be more cautious in giving AV nodal blocking agents such as digoxin or propranolol.

CARDIOVERSION. This can be used as a primary treatment (see Cardioversion Schedule B, p. 179). However, if there is any question about the patient having chronic atrial fibrillation, the patient should be anticoagulated first. In addition, if there is monitor evidence that the patient is going in and out of this arrhythmia spontaneously, there is no reason to consider cardioversion. In this setting, the problem is *keeping* the patient in sinus rhythm and *not putting* the patient into sinus rhythm. (This is true of all the rhythms mentioned thus far.) Atrial fibrillation, in the setting of an acute myocardial infarction, is especially harmful, and cardioversion is definitely the treatment of choice in this situation.

RAPID ATRIAL PACING. Not useful (rare exceptions).

DRUG THERAPY. As in paroxysmal atrial flutter, *digoxin* (see Digoxin Schedule, p. 179), followed by *quinidine* (see Quinidine Schedule, p. 179), is the drug therapy of choice. Digoxin therapy itself may result in conversion to normal sinus rhythm. Digoxin can be used in higher doses than outlined, since one can follow the rate response rather than an absolute dosage schedule. However, once again adding quinidine therapy to high dose digoxin may produce digoxin toxicity, which may be manifest after conversion to normal sinus rhythm is effected.

Multifocal Atrial Tachycardia. This is defined as a supraventricular tachycardia with more than two different P wave contours and variable P-P intervals. It is most often found in patients with severe pulmonary insufficiency. This problem is seen with increasing frequency as more patients with end stage lung disease are being supported by mechanical ventilation. It is essential to treat the pulmonary insufficiency and to attempt to decrease serum theophylline levels. Digitalis is poorly tolerated by these patients and is usually ineffective in either converting the

arrhythmia or decreasing the ventricular response. In view of the additional confusion with digitalis toxicity that exists with this arrhythmia, digitalis, if used at all, should be given in very low doses. Cardioversion is contraindicated, and carotid sinus and other drug therapies are not indicated.

Other supraventricular tachycardias are seen with pulmonary insufficiency, including sinus tachycardia, ectopic atrial tachycardia, and atrial flutter. Only the last of these should be treated with cardioversion, but a particularly useful method of therapy may be overdrive atrial pacing (see Atrial Flutter, p. 181). In a desperate situation intravenous edrophonium (Tensilon) has been used at a dose of 5 to 10 mg, followed by an intravenous drip of 0.25 to 2.0 mg per minute to slow ventricular response. (This use of edrophonium is not listed in the manufacturer's official directive.) We have had limited experience with this method.

Regular Broad QRS Tachycardia

Any of the aforementioned regular tachycardias can have a wide QRS, either because of pre-existing conduction abnormalities (i.e., bundle branch block) or because of aberration (an intermittent form of conduction abnormality). There is no foolproof way to separate this group of supraventricular tachycardias (SVT) from ventricular tachycardia (VT). However, there are some useful clues as well as many described clues which are relatively useless. Useful clues used to separate ventricular tachycardia from supraventricular tachycardia with aberration include the following:

1. AV *association* (1:1 or 2:1 P:QRS ratios) can be present with SVT or VT, but AV *dissociation* (no obvious relationship between P and QRS) is most likely VT.

2. The presence of capture beats (normal QRS) or fusion beats without coexisting sudden rate change strongly suggests VT.

3. Known pre-existing bundle branch block with the same QRS configuration as the tachycardia strongly suggests SVT.

4. Utilizing a 12 lead ECG if time allows, marked right or left axis deviation and a similar QRS configuration from V1-V6 strongly suggest VT.

Essentially useless clues are those related to rate, degree of regularity, type of bundle branch block, and similarity between the initial deflection of the broad QRS and the patient's normal QRS.

The supraventricular tachycardias with wide QRS should be treated exactly as those with narrow QRS, as mentioned previously.

Ventricular Tachycardia. The initial response to ventricular tachycardia should be *DC cardioversion* using 200 watt-seconds. Higher energy settings may be used in patients larger than 100 kg. The synchronous mode should be used if time allows. *Lidocaine,* 75 to 100 mg intravenous push, can be given before countershock if (1) the patient is tolerating the tachycardia adequately, or (2) an intravenous line can be started simultaneously with preparations for DC countershock. With serious hemodynamic compromise, countershock should be used immediately. Following conversion, the *lidocaine* treatment schedule, as outlined on page 179, should be followed to prevent recurrence. In the event of lidocaine failure in preventing recurrence, intravenous *procainamide* as outlined on page 179 is most often utilized as the second line drug. However, *bretylium tosylate* appears to be a very potent agent in this situation, and consideration of its use as outlined on page 180 should be given early on. As one acquires more experience with this drug, one may begin to use it before procainamide as second choice to lidocaine. A fourth drug to be occasionally considered is phenytoin, 100 mg intravenously over 2 minutes to a total of 1000 mg, followed by an intravenous infusion. (This use of phenytoin is not listed in the manufacturer's official directive.) One mg doses of propranolol intravenously and atrial pacing at a rate of 100 to 120 may also help prevent relapse. Obvious electrolyte imbalance, hypoventilation, or pH abnormalities should be corrected.

While not a broad QRS *regular* tachycardia, an unusual form of ventricular tachycardia called *torsade des pointes* should be mentioned. It is particularly a problem in polypharmacy situations with worsening of the arrhythmias. The hallmarks of this form of ventricular tachycardia are (1) prolonged QT of the sinus beat, (2) tachycardia frequently initiated by a late diastolic PVC, and (3) complete reversal of the QRS and T deflections during the tachycardia, leading to what appears to be a modulated sign curve or "twisting around a point."

Initiators of this rhythm include Type I antiarrhythmic agents (usually quinidine, disopyramide, procainamide), hypomagnesemia, hypokalemia, the long QT syndrome itself, and phenothiazine therapy. Recognition of this uncommon form of tachycardia should lead to the correction of underlying abnormalities if possible, including *withholding of all previously used antiarrhythmic agents* and the slow infusion of *isoproterenol,* 2 micrograms per minute, to attempt to shorten the QT interval. There is limited experience suggesting that bretylium tosylate may be helpful, and in a desperate situation this drug could be tried.

Irregular Broad QRS Tachycardias

Atrial Fibrillation with Broad QRS. While ventricular tachycardia can on occasion be very irregular, the primary tachycardia here is atrial fibrillation with wide QRS. This wide QRS can be due to aberrancy; if so, one can sometimes notice that as the R-R interval varies, there is resultant variation in the degree of aberration (minor QRS changes).

ATRIAL FIBRILLATION WITH WIDE QRS AND SLOW VENTRICULAR RESPONSE (UP TO 150 PER MINUTE). This arrhythmia can be treated exactly like paroxysmal atrial fibrillation with a narrow QRS (see p. 182). However, the wide QRS may be due to conduction over a Kent bypass tract which circumvents the AV node and allows the atrial stimuli to enter ventricular muscle directly. In this instance digoxin will be ineffective and may actually increase the rate.

ATRIAL FIBRILLATION WITH WIDE QRS AND RAPID VENTRICULAR RESPONSE. This tachycardia is of most importance in this discussion. If the response is very rapid with any R-R intervals being near 0.20 second, one should diagnose atrial fibrillation in the setting of Wolff-Parkinson-White (WPW) syndrome, i.e., the fibrillatory waves are being rapidly conducted down a Kent bypass tract to the ventricle without the normal AV nodal filtering system. This tachycardia is potentially dangerous, as ventricular fibrillation may ensue from bombardment of the ventricle by the rapid impulses. The usual therapy used with atrial fibrillation to slow ventricular response (propranolol or digitalis) either is useless or, in the case of digitalis, may even be dangerous. While digitalis is not absolutely contraindicated in all patients with WPW, *it is absolutely contraindicated* in patients with rapid atrial fibrillation and WPW. Thus patients with rapid atrial fibrillation and wide QRS should be treated as though they have WPW, with the following rules utilized:

1. Carotid sinus stimulation is of no help.

2. Digitalis is contraindicated (may speed the rate and lead to ventricular fibrillation).

3. Propranolol is of no help (since it acts primarily on the AV node and the AV node is being bypassed).

4. Lidocaine may convert the atrial fibrillation and should be used as with ventricular tachycardia (see Lidocaine Schedule, p. 179). However, there is one recent report of lidocaine increasing the ventricular response in this setting, and this should be carefully watched for. If the rate appears to become even faster with lidocaine therapy, one should immediately institute DC cardioversion.

5. Disopyramide, quinidine, and procaina-

mide may break the tachycardia, but only procainamide can be given intravenously in this relatively urgent situation.

6. Cardioversion should be instituted right away or immediately after an attempt with lidocaine.

Miscellaneous Problems Concerning Tachycardias

Tachycardias in Patients with Known WPW Syndrome. As just discussed above, a patient with *rapid* irregular broad-beat tachycardia should be considered to have atrial fibrillation associated with a Kent bypass tract (WPW syndrome). It must be recognized that this can deteriorate to ventricular fibrillation and that digoxin (and perhaps lidocaine) can make this more likely by increasing the ventricular response. However, *the patient with known WPW,* presenting with atrial fibrillation with wide QRS and modest ventricular rates, allows one to utilize some simple physiologic and pharmacologic principles, namely that propranolol and digoxin are relatively ineffective because the AV node is not being utilized; that quinidine, procainamide, and disopyramide can produce slowing by effects on the Kent tract, which is made up of atrial muscle; that the latter three drugs can convert the atrial fibrillation to sinus rhythm; and that cardioversion is effective. Slow ventricular response does not seem to be any more dangerous than ordinary atrial fibrillation that does utilize the AV node.

The most common arrhythmia with WPW, however, is paroxysmal supraventricular tachycardia (see p. 180). The only difference when there is a Kent bundle in the circus movement pathway is that again quinidine, procainamide, and disopyramide can be effective in breaking the tachycardia because of their effects on atrial muscle, whereas they are relatively ineffective when the re-entry is totally within the AV node.

Pediatric Tachycardias. A brief discussion of this topic is important in light of the newer electrophysiologic information. The great majority of pediatric tachycardias are paroxysmal supraventricular tachycardias, i.e., narrow beat rapid regular tachycardia. As in adults, these may be AV nodal re-entry or may utilize a Kent bundle as well as the AV nodal–His system in the tachycardia circuit (WPW). The latter is quite common in infancy and may later disappear or at least become inoperative.

The following principles and concepts are important:

1. Fairly rapid attempts to convert are important, as infants usually are in congestive heart failure when the arrhythmia is finally diagnosed.

2. Digoxin and propranolol are the best available drugs. They should be given intravenously, first one and then the other. The order is not that important, but we prefer digoxin and then propranolol if time permits.

3. Digoxin dose (intravenous) in newborns and infants (under 1 year) is 0.02 mg per pound (0.04 mg per kg) as total dose, given in three increments ($\frac{1}{2}$, $\frac{1}{4}$, $\frac{1}{4}$). After 1 year of age, one must be careful in calculating the total dose, e.g., in a 60 pound child 60×0.02 mg $= 1.2$ mg, more than the adult dose suggested in the previous discussions.

4. Digoxin should not be given orally in this situation (patient may vomit) or intramuscularly (cannot be sure of absorption).

5. Propranolol can be given in the same total dose as for adults (0.1 mg per kg), but in small increments, i.e., a 5 kg baby has a calculated total dose of 0.5 mg. This is given in five doses of 0.1 mg — all intravenously. As in adults, if some slowing is seen but the rhythm persists and no side effects are noted, this total can be modified to reach a 0.15 mg per kg total dose.

6. Cardioversion is rarely necessary, but as with adults one should decide upon the necessity before full digitalization.

7. Regular broad beat tachycardias in infants are probably not supraventricular with aberrancy, as aberrancy appears to be very rare in this age group. One should consider ventricular tachycardia, which fortunately is also uncommon in this age group.

Tachy-brady Syndrome. Whenever tachycardias are seen in adults, especially elderly adults, one should consider possible tachy-brady syndrome. Holter monitoring will often confirm this with multiple types of tachycardia seen over the prolonged monitoring period (atrial tachycardia, atrial fibrillation, atrial flutter) as well as various forms of bradycardia such as sinus arrest, sinus pauses, sinus exit block, and intermittent AV block. Obviously, this is a very diffuse disease, but it is mentioned since the treatment of tachycardias can be more worrisome in the face of an unstable underlying pacemaker and AV node. Digoxin, while theoretically contraindicated, appears to be safe and often useful. The Type 1 drugs (quinidine, procainamide, disopyramide) can be used with caution, as they may worsen the bradycardic aspects. In the presence of either a temporary or permanent pacemaker, they can be tried safely. Finally, cardioverting a tachycardia in this setting could result in sudden bradycardia. One should consider this possibility before choosing this mode of therapy as well as monitoring carefully to make certain the patient is not going in and out of the tachycardia on his own, for in this instance cardioversion has no place.

CONGENITAL HEART DISEASE*

method of
P. SYAMASUNDAR RAO, M.B.,
and WILLIAM B. STRONG, M.D.
Augusta, Georgia

TABLE 1.

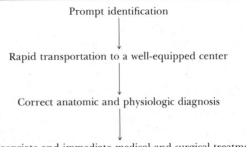

Prompt identification

↓

Rapid transportation to a well-equipped center

↓

Correct anatomic and physiologic diagnosis

↓

Appropriate and immediate medical and surgical treatment

The incidence of congenital heart disease is about 8 per 1000 live births. Each year approximately 25,000 infants with cardiac defects are born in the United States. Twenty per cent of these infants will present with symptoms in the first week of life. Significant advances in the diagnostic and therapeutic aspects of congenital heart defects have occurred in the past three decades; many of these are equally applicable to neonates. Therefore, in this article management of infants and children as well as that of the neonates will be discussed.

MANAGEMENT OF THE NEONATE WITH SUSPECTED SERIOUS HEART DISEASE

Neonates with distress caused by a cardiac malformation may die if not treated appropriately and rapidly. They must all be considered acute emergency problems. If we are to increase the survival rate in this age group, it is necessary that these infants be promptly recognized and treated. Table 1 indicates the steps essential to the management of these neonates. Prompt identification and initial management of these infants is the responsibility of the primary physician caring for the newborn. Rapid and safe transportation of the infants with suspected serious heart disease to a *regional pediatric cardiology center* equipped with facilities for diagnosis and treatment is the next logical step. Accurate anatomic diagnosis and appropriate medical and/or surgical treatment are in the realm of the pediatric cardiologist and cardiovascular surgeon.

Prompt Identification

Efforts on the part of the general practitioner or the pediatrician to make an exact anatomic diagnosis of neonatal heart disease are, for the most part, inaccurate and unnecessary and represent an avoidable source of frustration and delay. Even the experienced pediatric cardiologist often cannot make an accurate anatomic diagnosis

prior to specialized cardiac studies such as echocardiography, cardiac catheterization, and selective cineangiography. Therefore, attempts by the primary physician to make an anatomic diagnosis in a neonate will often cause unnecessary delay in referral and loss of precious time while the infant's status deteriorates. The realistic (and achievable) goal of the neonatal primary care is the prompt recognition of a *functional abnormality* of the cardiovascular system. The major signs indicative of serious problem are cyanosis, signs of congestive heart failure, respiratory distress (tachypnea or hyperpnea), and lethargy or lack of spontaneous movement.

Cyanosis of the central type (bluish discoloration not only of the extremities but also of the buccal and labial mucous membranes) is one of the most important and helpful findings in the detection of the neonate with congenital heart disease. Cyanosis beyond 20 minutes of age in a resting or sleeping newborn requires an explanation; usually, this will not improve with further "careful observation." Arterial blood gas analysis will confirm the clinical suspicion; hypoxemia is considered to be present when arterial Po_2 is less than 60 mm Hg before 24 hours of age or less than 75 mm Hg after 24 hours of age.

Congestive heart failure may manifest with signs of pulmonary or systemic venous congestion or altered myocardial function. Pulmonary venous congestion may present only with tachypnea. Rales and wheezing are uncommon in the neonate, but irritability and difficulty in feeding and sleeping are common. Hepatomegaly is the hallmark of systemic venous congestion in the newborn. In normal infants, the liver is normally palpable 1 to 3 cm below the right costal margin in the midclavicular line and should not be interpreted as hepatomegaly. Other signs of systemic venous congestion such as neck vein distention and edema are only occasionally observed in the infant, and the latter when present may be atypical in distribution (periorbital or sacral). Finally,

---

*The manufacturers' official directives may not list doses for children for some agents mentioned in this article.

185

the signs of impaired myocardial function — tachycardia, cardiomegaly, gallop rhythm, and decreased arterial pulses — when identified should focus attention to a cardiac cause.

Tachypnea (increased respiratory rate with normal or decreased tidal volume), hyperpnea (increased rate and depth of respiration), and retractions may suggest a cardiac, respiratory, or metabolic problem. Although lethargy and lack of spontaneous movement can be caused by metabolic acidosis secondary to hypoxia of cardiac origin, they are frequently seen with serious intracranial pathology, hypoglycemia, sepsis, or shock.

Rapid Transportation to a Well-Equipped Center

Selection of Infants for Transfer. As soon as the distressed infant has been recognized and congenital heart disease is suspected, immediate transfer to a regional pediatric cardiology center is mandatory. In general, the indications for emergency cardiac catheterization relate primarily to the potential need for early surgery or balloon atrial septostomy to sustain life. Virtually all neonates with cyanosis, with or without heart failure, appearing soon after birth should have prompt investigation. Infants with minimal or no cyanosis but with signs of left or right heart failure are also candidates for catheterization on an urgent basis. Of course, the babies with respiratory distress are obviously candidates for further study.

Infants with the murmur of a small ventricular septal defect, patent ductus arteriosus or peripheral pulmonic stenosis (more common in premature infants), decreased femoral pulses, an abnormal electrocardiogram, or an abnormal x-ray finding, but without signs of impaired cardiac function, are not necessarily candidates for immediate transfer. These infants should be referred to a pediatric cardiologist when between 2 and 6 weeks of age. If at all possible, the parents of these infants should be spared the anxiety, expense, and inconvenience of transfer of their babies soon after birth. In addition to these guidelines, early and frequent use of phone consultation with a pediatric cardiologist at the referral center should help clarify problem cases and result in the appropriate timing of cardiac evaluation. However, if any doubt exists as to the infant's cardiovascular function, the infant should be transferred immediately.

Transportation. If there are no adequate facilities for immediate and safe transportation of the sick neonate from the community hospital to the medical center, early identification of the distressed newborn is futile. Because of a trend in many areas toward the development of regional newborn special care centers for high-risk infants, the use of specialized infant transport services has become increasingly common. The transportation can generally be arranged through the pediatric cardiology center. The pediatric cardiology centers are on "round-the-clock" call 365 days per year. Therefore, do not wait to call until morning or, if on a weekend, until Monday. The type of transportation used, helicopter or ambulance, is dependent upon the distance and the type of transportation available in a given area. The type of vehicle is not important, but what it provides in the way of facilities for monitoring vital signs and for resuscitation is important. A sick infant should *never* have to be transferred by private automobile in the arms of a distressed parent or relative. The infant should be accompanied by a nurse, paramedic, or physician.

Before and During Transfer. Upon identification of an infant with cardiac distress, the primary physician should have telephone consultation with his or her pediatric cardiologist and make arrangements for referral. A summary as well as copies of all the infant's and mother's records should be sent with the baby. Most of the infants are likely to require blood transfusion, and therefore 5 ml of clotted maternal blood must accompany the infant. A thorough explanation to the parents of the need for the transfer of the baby and the procedures that the infant is likely to undergo at the medical center is the responsibility of the referring physician. The primary physician should also have the parents see and touch the baby and have the appropriate religious rites performed before the transfer to the medical center.

Before and during the transfer, monitoring the infant's temperature and maintenance of a neutral thermal environment are extremely important. Metabolic acidosis (pH less than 7.25), if any, should be corrected with sodium bicarbonate (usually 1 mEq per kg diluted half and half with 5 per cent dextrose solution) immediately. Respiratory acidosis should be cared for by appropriate suctioning, intubation, and assisted ventilation. In hypoxic infants, ambient oxygen (less than 40 per cent) should be administered. Hypoglycemia is a significant problem; therefore, the infant's serum glucose should be monitored and the infant should receive 10 per cent dextrose in water intravenously. If there is hypoglycemia (less than 30 mg per 100 ml), 15 per cent dextrose solution should be administered. Any other medications that may be needed (e.g., digitalis and diuretics) should be administered after consultation with the pediatric cardiologist under whose care the infant is to be transferred.

During transport — apart from facilities to monitor heart rate, infant's and incubator's temperature, and inspired oxygen concentration — facilities for suction, cardiorespiratory resuscitation, including intubation, and intravenous medication should be available. Only when meticulous care is given to the neonate prior to and during the transfer, can the infant be in an optimal condition to successfully undergo the diagnostic and therapeutic procedures. Only then will there be improvement in the survival of these babies. The potential for cure of 80 per cent of distressed neonates is now available.

Correct Anatomic and Physiologic Diagnosis

Discussion of the diagnosis of specific cardiac defects is beyond the scope of this article.

Appropriate and Immediate Treatment

Discussion of the treatment of all the specific cardiac defects seen in neonates is beyond the scope of this article. Some defects will be discussed subsequently. Here, only the management of some derangements will be discussed.

Cyanosis. The treatment of cyanosis largely depends upon its cause. Cyanosis is caused by disorders of the respiratory, cardiac, or central nervous system as well as by a large number of miscellaneous conditions. With the use of usual clinical and laboratory data, the diagnosis of the cause of cyanosis can be established. However, there will remain a significant number of infants in whom it is difficult to differentiate severe pulmonary disease from a congenital cyanotic heart defect. The following may be used to differentiate these. Respiratory cause is suggested if there were complications of pregnancy and/or delivery, maternal fever prior to birth, prematurity, inappropriate size for gestational age, asphyxia neonatorum, meconium staining, low Apgar score, and onset of cyanosis within a few hours after birth. Chest x-ray will be of help in excluding surgical and parenchymal causes of respiratory disorders (e.g., pneumothorax, diaphragmatic hernia). The arterial blood gas analysis is of some help in separating cardiac from pulmonary disorders; the $Paco_2$ may be elevated with respiratory problems, which is not uniformly so in the cyanosis of cardiac origin. The response of arterial Po_2 to 100 per cent oxygen and continuous positive airway pressure (CPAP) may be of help.

HYPEROXIC TEST. 1. Obtain a blood sample from the right radial artery (or temporal artery) while the infant is in room air (or at whatever ambient level of oxygen the infant was in at the time of first examination) for determination of Pao_2.

2. Administer 100 per cent oxygen for 10 to 15 minutes.

3. Determine simultaneous Po_2 from the right radial (or temporal) artery and umbilical artery. Infants with cardiac cyanosis show no significant increase in Po_2 (< 10 mm Hg) with 100 per cent oxygen. Infants with pulmonary causes usually increase Po_2 significantly. A Pao_2 higher than 150 mm Hg is highly suggestive of respiratory disease. A higher Po_2 in the radial artery than umbilical artery is suggestive of a right-to-left ductal shunting commonly seen with persistent fetal circulation.

CPAP TEST. Although a lack of Po_2 response to 100 per cent oxygen most likely suggests a cardiac origin of cyanosis, some infants with severe meconium aspiration and/or hyaline membrane disease may not show a significant increase in Po_2. In these infants the CPAP test may be indicated:

1. After No. 3 above, apply 8 to 10 cm H_2O continuous positive airway pressure with 100 per cent oxygen for 10 to 15 minutes via a face mask or transnasally. If the infant seems to deteriorate or respiratory distress increases, discontinue the CPAP test.

2. Obtain a radial or temporal artery sample for blood gas analysis. A significant increase (>10 mm Hg) of Po_2 is indicative of pulmonary disease. A decrease or a lack of increase of Po_2 is highly suggestive of cardiac disease. When the Po_2 in room air and in 100 per cent oxygen is less than 50 mm Hg, a Po_2 in 100 per cent oxygen with CPAP greater than 50 mm Hg suggests pulmonary disease and less than 50 mm Hg suggests cyanotic heart disease.

TREATMENT OF CYANOSIS. 1. No more than 40 per cent humidified oxygen is necessary in infants with cyanotic heart disease.

2. Correct metabolic acidosis (pH less than 7.25), hypoglycemia, hypocalcemia, and anemia, if present.

3. In infants with severe right ventricular outflow tract obstruction, the pulmonary flow is ductal dependent. The ductus arteriosus may be kept patent by an infusion of prostaglandin E_1 or E_2 (PGE_1, PGE_2). Various cardiac defects with ductal dependent pulmonary blood flow in which prostaglandins are useful are listed in Table 2. The current recommendations are for infusion of PGE_1, 0.05 to 0.1 microgram per kg per minute into the aorta at the level of ductus. Although the drug appears to be effective even with intravenous infusion, the preferred method is intra-aortic. Although PGE_1 has been used in infants from 1 day to 99 days, it is more likely to be effective the earlier in life it is begun. It appears that a small ductus may be made to dilate

TABLE 2. **Lesions with Ductal Dependent Pulmonary Blood Flow**

Pulmonary atresia with intact ventricular septum
Pulmonary atresia with ventricular septal defect
Severe tetralogy of Fallot
Complex cyanotic heart disease with pulmonary atresia or
   severe stenosis
Tricuspid atresia
Critical pulmonary stenosis
Ebstein's anomaly of tricuspid valve
Hypoplastic right ventricle

but an already closed ductus cannot be reopened. PGE_1 is currently available for investigational use only. Side effects include apnea (in 10 per cent), elevation of temperature (10 per cent), muscular twitching, and severe flushing. The side effects have not posed substantial management problems.

The major use of the drug lies in its benefit to keep the infants in reasonable condition so that a well planned catheterization and angiography, as well as palliative or corrective surgery, can be performed with relative safety because of higher Po_2 and corrected metabolic acidosis. Also, the infusion of PGE_1 can be maintained during and immediately after the shunt operation so that the blood flow across the ductus could be beneficial while the surgical shunt is being established.

4. If the cause of cyanosis is transposition of the great arteries, perform balloon atrial septostomy.

5. Treat heart failure, if present.

6. If there is marked hypercarbia ($Paco_2$ >60 mm Hg) or respiratory depression, intubation and mechanical ventilation are indicated.

7. If the cause of cyanosis is persistent fetal circulation, see that text heading, below.

8. Other types of treatment are dependent upon the specific cause of the cyanosis and may require palliative or corrective surgery.

Congestive Heart Failure. The treatment of congestive heart failure is discussed beginning on page 190. Of particular importance is the use of PGE_1 in the neonate with heart failure in conditions in which the systemic perfusion to the lower part of the body is ductal dependent, as in severe coarctation of the aorta or interruption of the aortic arch. The dosage and method of administration of PGE_1 are the same as described above (0.05 to 0.1 microgram per kg per minute).

Polycythemia. Significant degrees of polycythemia may cause cyanosis, heart failure, or respiratory distress. Polycythemia is considered to be present if the central hematocrit is greater than 65 per cent. Specific treatment of polycythemia is exchange transfusion with plasma (for details see p. 204).

Methemoglobinemia. When severe cyanosis in the absence of distress is seen, methemoglobinemia should be suspected. These infants appear ruddy and have a peculiar lavender color. The blood from heel stick is chocolate colored and does not become pink when exposed to room air. The Po_2s may be normal, but the O_2 saturation by direct oximetry will be markedly reduced. Methemoglobinemia may be either hereditary in origin or acquired from exposure to agents such as nitrites in contaminated well water or from aniline derivatives.

1. Exclude other causes of cyanosis.

2. Confirm diagnosis by spectrophotometric analysis of blood for methemoglobin; it has a characteristic absorption peak at 634 μ.

3. Give methylene blue, 1 to 2 mg per kg intravenously, which should promptly eliminate cyanosis. Follow this by either 3 to 5 mg per kg of methylene blue orally or 200 to 500 mg of ascorbic acid orally.

Persistent Fetal Circulation. In some neonates, markedly increased pulmonary vascular resistance causes severe right-to-left shunting across the patent foramen ovale and/or patent ductus arteriosus with resultant severe hypoxemia. This may be secondary to pulmonary disease or to a variety of other causes. In many infants, a specific cause cannot be determined.

1. The diagnosis must first be established. This can be done with the usual history, physical examination, and laboratory studies. Simultaneous right radial (temporal) artery and umbilical artery Po_2 in 100 per cent oxygen will reveal lower umbilical artery Po_2. However, such a difference may not be seen if a major right-to-left atrial shunt exists. Echocardiography is helpful in identifying all cardiac chambers and valves, thus assuring that there is no structural heart disease. It is also helpful in estimating pulmonary artery pressure; increased right-sided pre-ejection period to ejection time ratio (PEP/ET) suggests elevated pulmonary pressures. Pulmonary valve time interval ratio is also useful to monitor the effectiveness of the treatment. If doubt remains regarding the diagnosis, cardiac catheterization is indicated.

2. Ambient humidified oxygen to maintain $Pao_2 \geq 50$ mm Hg.

3. Prompt correction of hypothermia, hypoglycemia, acidosis, polycythemia, and hypocalcemia.

4. Treatment with digoxin and diuretics if heart failure is present.

5. Intubation and mechanical ventilation may sometimes be beneficial. Hyperventilation to decrease the arterial Pco_2 to 25 to 30 mm Hg has been helpful in some infants. Occasionally the use of positive end expiratory pressure (PEEP), 6 to

10 cm H_2O, may improve oxygenation. One should be cautious, however, because it may occasionally cause clinical deterioration.

6. Tolazoline (Priscoline) is a potent vasodilator; 1 to 2 mg per kg may be infused over 10 minutes with a beneficial effect to many infants. (This specific use of tolazoline is not listed in the manufacturer's official directive). The drug also produces systemic vasodilatation and causes systemic hypotension. Therefore, it should be given intravenously from an arm or neck vein to encourage delivery of the drug into the pulmonary circulation, taking advantage of the fetal circulatory pathways. Administration of the drug in the pulmonary artery is most effective; however, even from this site of administration right-to-left shunting across the ductus arteriosus or via intrapulmonary shunts may make it futile. If effective by either route, it should be continued as an infusion at a rate of 1 to 2 mg per kg per hour. If no improvement occurs or hypotension develops, tolazoline should be discontinued. Some workers have added systemic vasoconstrictors to the regimen to counter the hypotension but with little benefit.

7. Recent reports suggest that dopamine, 2 to 5 micrograms per kg per minute, is effective in the treatment of persistent fetal circulation. Further experience with this modality of treatment is necessary before it can be recommended for routine use.

8. Theoretically PGE_1 and PGE_2 should be effective by acting as pulmonary vasodilators, but limited experience thus far has not shown any consistent benefit. Currently, studies with the use of prostaglandin I_2 are being performed to evaluate its effect on dilating pulmonary arterioles.

Patent Ductus Arteriosus in the Premature Infant. Premature infants with hyaline membrane disease may have an open ductus arteriosus with a large left-to-right shunt, which can cause further deterioration of respiratory function and delay the expected timely recovery from hyaline membrane disease.

1. In premature infants with hyaline membrane disease with a patent ductus arteriosus, instead of the expected recovery, there will be a greater requirement of inspired oxygen concentration and a greater need for ventilatory support. A cardiac murmur may appear; hyperdynamic precordium and bounding pulses may also be observed. Chest x-ray may reveal cardiomegaly. Echocardiograms may show enlarged left atrium and left ventricle, increased left atrium to aortic root (LA/Ao) ratio, and normal or increased left ventricular shortening fraction. These findings are indicative of a significant ductus. At this time a trial of fluid restriction (<

70 ml per kg per day), diuretics (furosemide, 1 mg per kg per dose intravenously), and perhaps digoxin is indicated.

2. If no improvement occurs in 24 to 48 hours or worsening of the signs listed in No. 1 takes place, and on a repeat echocardiogram further enlargement of left atrium and ventricle occurs and left ventricular shortening fraction diminishes, further measures to close the ductus should be undertaken.

PHARMACOLOGIC CLOSURE. Since it has been shown that prostaglandins are necessary to keep the ductus open, administration of prostaglandin synthesis inhibitors may result in constriction of the ductus arteriosus. This concept has been applied by several groups of workers, and it is now clearly shown that indomethacin, a potent inhibitor of prostaglandin synthesis, can cause constriction and closure of the ductus and result in abatement in the symptoms caused by the ductus.

Indomethacin may be administered either via a gastric tube or by retention enema in a dose of 0.1 to 0.2 mg per kg. (This use of indomethacin is not listed in the manufacturer's official directive.) If no clinical improvement occurs, it may be repeated at a dose of 0.2 mg per kg in 6 to 8 hours and repeated in 6 to 12 hours if no improvement occurred after the second dose. Beneficial effect of indomethacin appears to be age related. It is most effective when the infant's actual age (gestational plus chronologic) is less than 36 weeks. Indomethacin seems to be less effective when the infant is more than 10 days post partum.

Potential complications of indomethacin therapy include impairment of renal function (oliguria, increase in blood urea nitrogen [BUN] and creatinine, and reduction in urinary sodium concentration) and altered platelet function. Therefore, one should be sure of normality of renal and coagulation functions in these infants prior to giving indomethacin.

SURGICAL CLOSURE. Surgical ligation of the patent ductus arteriosus may be performed in infants who are unresponsive to pharmacologic closure and in those in whom indomethacin is contraindicated.

Cardiomyopathy in the Infants of Diabetic Mothers. Infants of diabetic mothers (IDM) have been known to have a high incidence of postnatal complications. These include macrosomia, hypoglycemia, hypocalcemia, hyperbilirubinemia, polycythemia and the hyperviscosity syndrome, transient tachypnea of the newborn, hyaline membrane disease, persistent fetal circulation, cardiomyopathy, renal vein thrombosis, and an increased incidence of congenital anomalies. The incidence of cardiac involvement may be as high as 50 per cent. Two basic forms of cardiomyopathy have been recognized in IDM, a congestive cardiomyopathy and an obstructive cardiomyopathy.

CONGESTIVE CARDIOMYOPATHY. This may be related to (or secondary to) the hematologic, metabolic, or respiratory problems listed above, or it may occur independent of them.

1. When present, treat hypoglycemia, hypocalcemia, polycythemia, or other problems listed above.

2. Digitalis, diuretics, and other measures as listed under Congestive Heart Failure (see below).

OBSTRUCTIVE CARDIOMYOPATHY. This group of infants has been described to have findings similar to those of patients classified as having hypertrophic obstructive cardiomyopathy (HOCM). Their echocardiogram reveals a thickened interventricular septum, increased septal to left ventricular free wall ratio (> 1.3), and systolic anterior motion of the anterior leaflet of the mitral valve. Cardiac catheterization data reveal a systolic pressure gradient across the subaortic region. Left ventricular angiography reveals a thickened interventricular septum bulging into the left ventricular outflow tract; a finding similar to that is characteristically observed in HOCM.

1. The administration of digitalis and diuretics, the standard treatment of most cases of congestive heart failure, is contraindicated in HOCM. Digitalis may accentuate the left ventricular outflow obstruction and can cause clinical deterioration.

2. Treat metabolic, hematologic, and respiratory problems, if present.

3. Administer propranolol, 1 to 4 mg per kg per day orally in three to four divided doses. (This use of propranolol is not listed in the manufacturer's official directive.) Start with 1 mg per kg per day and increase until clinical responsive.

4. The HOCM of IDM improves with time; echocardiographic findings may revert to normal within 6 months. Propranolol may be discontinued once the echographic abnormalities revert to normal.

CONGESTIVE HEART FAILURE

About 20 per cent of children born with congenital heart disease will develop congestive heart failure (CHF). Ninety per cent of those who develop CHF are likely to do so within the first year of life. The management of CHF is aimed at providing exogenous support for the failing myocardium and reducing the work load placed upon the failing heart.

Digitalis

Digitalis is a positive inotropic agent which enhances myocardial contractility. The mechanism of action of digitalis is not clearly understood; it is presumed to act by inhibiting sodium-potassium ATPase. Of the two major preparations of digitalis, namely digitoxin and digoxin, digoxin is almost exclusively used in pediatric patients. Commonly used digoxin forms are listed in Table 3. It has been a practice to administer a loading (digitalizing) dose followed by maintenance doses. These doses are calculated on the basis of age and weight and are listed in Table 4. From this table, oral total digitalizing dose (TDD) for initial digitalization can be calculated. One half of the TDD should be administered immediately. We believe that infants with CHF should receive the first dose intravenously; in infants with moderate to severe CHF, the absorption of oral or intramuscular digoxin may be markedly delayed because of edema and diminished cardiac output. When given intravenously three fourths of the calculated oral dose should be given. The second and third doses (one quarter of the TDD each) may be administered at 6 to 8 hour intervals (Table 5). However, when treating severe CHF, one or both intervals may be reduced to 1 or 2 hours. Prior to the third dose, the cardiac rhythm and rate should be evaluated, preferably by an electrocardiographic (ECG) rhythm strip. Twelve hours following the TDD, maintenance digoxin should be started. The maintenance dose is one quarter of the TDD per day. This is usually administered orally in two equally divided doses (one eighth of the TDD, two times a day). It should be noted that the maintenance dose is arbitrary and can be increased gradually until full therapeutic effect is attained or toxicity symptoms appear.

Most if not all infants with CHF are treated in the manner described above. But a few infants and children who have minimal signs of CHF may not need hospitalization and rapid digitalization. These babies can be started on maintenance

TABLE 3. **Digoxin Preparations**

Oral	Digoxin (Lanoxin) elixir	0.05 mg/ml
	Digoxin (Lanoxin) tablets	0.125 mg (yellow)
		0.25 mg (white)
		0.5 mg (green)
Injectable	Digoxin (Lanoxin)	0.1 mg/ml (pediatric)
		0.25 mg/ml (adult)

TABLE 4.   **Total Digitalizing Dose (TDD), Digoxin (Oral)***

Preterm infants	0.03 mg/kg body weight
Newborn infants, 0–6 weeks	0.04 mg/kg
6 weeks–2 years	0.06–0.08 mg/kg
2–5 years	0.04–0.06 mg/kg
5 years and older	0.03–0.04 mg/kg†

*This dose is for oral digitalization only. If digitalis is administered parenterally, give three fourths of the oral dose.

†If the total calculated dose exceeds the average adult dose (1.0 mg), give only the average adult dose.

doses of digoxin (one eighth of the TDD, twice a day). By this method, the infant is completely digitalized within 5 to 7 days.

Contraindications. Digitalis is contraindicated in children with paroxysmal hypoxemic spell syndrome seen in patients with tetralogy of Fallot or similar lesions, idiopathic hypertrophic subaortic stenosis, and ventricular tachycardia. Overzealous administration of digoxin in patients with cor pulmonale or myocarditis may result in toxicity, and therefore one should be cautious with these patients.

Digoxin Toxicity. There is a narrow margin between therapeutic and toxic effects of digoxin; the therapeutic dose represents 65 per cent of the toxic dose. Furthermore, there is considerable individual variation in the tolerance to digoxin. The most common manifestations of digoxin toxicity are premature ventricular contractions and varying degrees of atrioventricular block, including prolongation of the PR interval. Any arrhythmia beginning after the institution of digoxin therapy must be attributed to it until proved otherwise. Other rhythm disturbances associated with digoxin toxicity are marked sinus arrhythmia with wandering atrial pacemaker, severe sinus bradycardia (excessive vagal tone), supraventricular or ventricular tachycardia, and atrial flutter or fibrillation. Anorexia, nausea, and vomiting may accompany digoxin toxicity. Central nervous system signs of toxicity such as

TABLE 5.   **Schedule of Initial Digitalization**

First dose	1/2 TDD stat, intravenous (3/4 of oral dose)
Second dose	1/4 TDD 6–8 h,* intravenous or oral
Third dose†	1/4 TDD 6–8 h,* usually given orally

*The time interval between first and second as well as second and third doses could be reduced to 2 hours or even 1 hour if severe heart failure or pulmonary edema is present.

†Prior to the third dose, the patient's cardiac rhythm and rate should be evaluated, preferably by an ECG rhythm strip.

TDD = Total digitalizing dose (see Table 4).

headache, fatigue, malaise, drowsiness, mental confusion, and blurred vision are not common in pediatric patients. Depression of the ST segment and inversion of the T wave, the so-called digitalis effect on the ECG, do not necessarily imply digoxin toxicity, nor do they indicate adequacy of digitalization.

Digoxin Levels. Serum digoxin levels by radioimmunoassay are now readily available. The theoretic basis for clinical use of serum digoxin levels rests on the constant relationship between tissue and serum levels and the fairly uniform serum concentration over several hours of postabsorptive phase. It is now known that the ratio of digoxin concentration between the heart and serum is rather constant at about 30:1. But there is a wide range (Table 6) of digoxin levels in patients receiving digoxin, and routine digoxin levels cannot separate toxic from nontoxic patients. Therefore, we would not recommend obtaining routine digoxin levels on all patients on digoxin therapy. There are two major indications for obtaining digoxin levels: (1) if clinical signs of toxicity are present; then, even if the digoxin level is in the borderline range, one might consider the patient to be digoxin intoxicated and reduce the dosage; and (2) if there is a strong suspicion that the infant (or child) has not been receiving the prescribed digoxin. Digitalis levels should also be obtained in patients with accidental digitalis poisoning and in patients with renal disease. Finally, it should be remembered that the digoxin level should be obtained about 6 hours after the last dose was given so as to avoid determining the serum level prior to its equilibration with the tissues.

Treatment of Digoxin Toxicity. 1. Discontinue further digoxin whenever digitalis toxicity is suspected.

2. If an excessive amount was administered by mouth, it is desirable to induce vomiting or to attempt gastric lavage.

3. Serum potassium levels should be determined. If serum potassium level is normal or decreased, potassium may be administered intravenously 40 to 80 mEq per 1000 ml of 5 per cent dextrose in water. Rate of administration of potassium should not exceed 0.5 mEq per kg per hour. The total daily dose of potassium should not be above 2 to 3 mEq per kg. The favorable effect of potassium is nonspecific, and it has relatively little influence on the toxic and inotropic actions of digitalis when this is administered after binding of the glycoside to the myocardium. This is the usual situation encountered in clinical practice. Potassium pretreatment with increased serum levels reduces the uptake of digitalis by the heart, thus diminishing electrical

TABLE 6. **Toxic and Nontoxic Levels of Serum Digoxin (ng/ml)**

	INFANTS AND CHILDREN LESS THAN 2 YEARS	CHILDREN ABOVE 2 YEARS
Nontoxic levels	< 2.0	< 1.0
Borderline levels	2.0–5.0	1.0–2.0
Toxic levels	> 5.0	> 2.0

toxicity of subsequently administered digitalis. It should be remembered that when digitalis toxicity inhibits the potassium uptake by skeletal muscle, a significant rise in serum potassium may result from the administration of small amounts of this cation.

Potassium depresses atrioventricular conduction, and therefore it is contraindicated in patients with atrioventricular block secondary to digitalis intoxication.

4. Minor arrhythmias will resolve with simple discontinuation of the digoxin. Severe arrhythmias need further treatment.

Phenytoin (Dilantin) has been shown to be capable of reversing digitalis-induced tachyrhythmias. This drug depresses the enhanced ventricular automaticity without any significant depression of conduction. It may be given intravenously in a dose of 3 to 5 mg per kg over a 5 minute period. If necessary, it may be repeated in 10 to 15 minutes. (This use of phenytoin is not listed in the manufacturer's official directive.) Phenytoin is contraindicated in bradyrhythmias or atrioventricular block. It should be mentioned that it is a short-acting agent, and thus it is not suitable in treating the sustained and recurrent tachyrhythmia.

Propranolol is useful in the treatment of both supraventricular and ventricular arrhythmias secondary to digitalis toxicity, and it has been most successful in terminating premature ventricular extrasystoles. Propranolol, 0.1 to 0.15 mg per kg, may be given intravenously over a period of 10 minutes with great caution and constant ECG monitoring, since this potent adrenergic blocking agent could suppress all pacemaker activity and depress cardiac contractility, resulting in either cardiac standstill or sudden cardiocirculatory collapse with hypotension. (See manufacturer's official directive.) This drug should not be used in the presence of significant congestive heart failure. If effective, propranolol may later be continued orally, 1 to 4 mg per kg per day in three to four divided doses.

Other drugs such as lidocaine, quinidine, and procainamide may be useful when the afore-

mentioned treatment is not effective. Dosages of these drugs are listed in Table 7.

Electrical conversion for the treatment of digitalis-induced arrhythmias may be hazardous, since serious ventricular arrhythmias have occurred after countershock even with nontoxic doses of digitalis. Cardioversion should be used only when all other measures have failed to control sustained arrhythmias induced by digitalis. Pretreatment with phenytoin prior to cardioversion may reduce postconversion ventricular arrhythmias. In newborns and infants low energy levels of countershock should be used, 1 to 2 watt-seconds per kg.

5. Impending heart block or symptomatic complete heart block should be immediately treated.

Atropine, 0.01 to 0.03 mg per kg intravenously, may be given with a maximum of 0.4 mg per dose in treating conduction disturbances induced by digitalis. It would appear that atropine may be effective in atrioventricular block produced by the excessive vagal action of the digitalis if the ventricular pacemaker is junctional or in the high His bundle. However, the therapeutic success is unpredictable.

Isoproterenol, 0.1 to 0.5 microgram per kg per minute in 5 per cent dextrose in water, may be given in complete heart block (while preparing for pacemaker insertion) and the dose adjusted to the response. However, the drug may have certain disadvantages in digitalis-induced conduction disturbances because of increased incidence

TABLE 7. **Drugs Commonly Used in the Management of Arrhythmias**

DRUG	DOSE AND ROUTE OF ADMINISTRATION
Phenytoin* (Dilantin)	3–5 mg/kg/dose IV given over a 5 minute period
Lidocaine (Xylocaine)	1 mg/kg IV as a bolus May be repeated in 20–60 minutes or start continuous IV infusion, 20–50 micrograms/kg/min
Quinidine	6 mg/kg PO or IM qid (loading dose, 3–6 mg/kg q2–3h, five doses, and 12 mg/kg q2–3h, five additional doses)
Procainamide (Pronestyl)	6 mg/kg IM qid 15 mg/kg PO qid
Propranolol (Inderal)	0.05 to 0.1 mg/kg IV; dilute in 50 ml of D5W, infuse slowly while monitoring ECG 1 mg/kg/day PO in 3 to 4 divided doses; then increase as needed (2–4 mg/kg/day)

*This use of this agent is not listed in the manufacturer's official directive.

of ventricular ectopic rhythms associated with its use in the presence of toxic levels of digitalis.

Transvenous pacemaker insertion may be necessary in patients with a high degree of atrioventricular block; this may be particularly useful in patients who have accidentally ingested large doses of digoxin.

Diuretics

Diuretics are a useful pharmacologic adjunct in the management of infants with CHF. Digitalis and rest may be all that is necessary in order to treat mild or even moderate CHF. Severe forms of CHF require diuretic therapy. Sodium and water retention, increased blood volume, increased preload, and augmented cardiac output occur in sequence in patients with CHF and are significant compensatory mechanisms. Therefore, we feel that diuretics should not be used as the first drugs in the treatment of CHF unless pulmonary edema is evident. Barring this exception, digitalis should precede the administration of diuretics. The adequacy of diuresis is often estimated better by daily weights than by urine outputs, since the latter values are notoriously inaccurate owing to inadequate collection methods in infants and children.

Furosemide (Lasix), 1 mg per kg intravenously, is our first choice. Ethacrynic acid (Edecrin) has similar actions and may be used in a similar fashion; see manufacturer's official directive before using. Furosemide may be given one or more times a day, depending upon the patient's response. Once the infant is stable, furosemide may be given orally, 2 to 5 mg per kg per day as a single dose. We usually give furosemide three times a week (Monday, Wednesday, and Friday). This intermittent therapy usually does not produce the electrolyte imbalance which is often observed with continuous diuretic therapy; therefore there is no need for potassium supplement.

We personally have had little success with thiazide diuretics. If additional diuretics are needed, especially in chronic CHF, spironolactone (Aldactone), 3 to 5 mg per kg per day in three divided doses, may be given.

Other Therapeutic Measures

Position. Propping the patient to elevate the head and shoulders to 45 degrees may be beneficial. This position probably encourages peripheral pooling in the inferior portion of the body rather than in the lungs.

Rest and Sedation. Exercise and activity require an increase in cardiac output. Therefore, this extra burden should be avoided on the compromised heart. In the older children, bed rest is recommended during the acute phase. Thereafter, the patient should be slowly allowed to resume normal activity as the cardiac function improves with treatment. In the infant, parenteral feeding enables the infant to refrain from sucking and utilizing excessive energy. Intravenous fluids should be adjusted to replace insensible and other losses (approximately 50 to 60 ml per kg per day) and should contain 10 per cent dextrose because of possible hypoglycemia. Potassium maintenance should be given, but sodium chloride should not be added because of the elevated total body sodium.

If the patient is restless and agitated, sedation with morphine sulfate, 0.1 mg per kg, should be given subcutaneously. Apart from sedation, morphine has some other beneficial effects, the nature and mechanism of which are not clearly defined. However, one should observe the patient for signs of respiratory depression.

Oxygen. Increasing the ambient oxygen concentration overcomes the pulmonary component of hypoxia and enables systemic arterial Po_2 to rise. Forty per cent humidified oxygen should be given initially to all infants and children with acute CHF. The oxygen should be discontinued after improvement with CHF.

Diet. In a sick infant feeding should be withheld to avoid aspiration. As the infant improves, start feeding with 10 per cent dextrose in water. Formula and solid foods can then be added to provide adequate calories. For infants and children who continue to be in chronic CHF, salt restriction may be necessary. In young babies, low-salt-containing formulas such as SMA, Similac PM 60-40, or Lonalac may be used. In children, avoiding salt-containing snacks (e.g., chips, pretzels) and restricting added salt to food may be necessary.

Other Measures. Other measures such as rotating tourniquets and venisection are rarely necessary now because of the availability of potent diuretic drugs.

Treatment of Underlying Conditions

Treatment of the associated and/or underlying abnormalities will be of help in the management of CHF. Maintenance of a neutral thermal environment in the neonate is important. Packed red blood cells for anemia, glucose for hypoglycemia, calcium for hypocalcemia, substitution therapy for other metabolic disorders, antihypertensive medications for hypertension, countershock or antiarrhythmic drugs for arrhythmias, steroids for severe carditis, respiratory toilet for cystic fibrosis, and tonsillectomy with adenoidectomy for chronic upper airway obstruction syndrome may be necessary.

If all the aforementioned treatment is not successful in controlling CHF, specific palliative or corrective surgery for the underlying cardiac defect should be undertaken.

Other Drugs Used in Refractory Failure

In patients with severe CHF not responding to conventional treatment, additional drugs may be used. These can be subdivided into other inotropic agents and afterload reducing agents.

Other Inotropic Agents. ISOPROTERENOL. Infuse 0.1 to 0.5 microgram per kg per minute intravenously. Mix 0.2 to 0.4 mg of isoproterenol in 250 ml of 5 per cent dextrose in water and adjust the rate to the desired effect. The drug markedly increases the heart rate and may also produce arrhythmias.

The severely distressed infant who is a candidate for catheterization and/or surgery and who is deteriorating rapidly can sometimes be transiently assisted by an infusion of isoproterenol in 30 ml of 20 per cent dextrose and 20 ml of sodium bicarbonate. Isoproterenol should be added to deliver 0.2 microgram per kg per minute by an infusion pump.

EPINEPHRINE. Infuse 0.25 to 1.0 microgram per kg per minute in 5 per cent dextrose in water intravenously. Adjust the rate according to response.

DOPAMINE. This new drug is preferable to isoproterenol and epinephrine because it does not have the chronotropic effect when used at low doses. Additionally, it selectively dilates the renal vessels (see manufacturer's official directive). When only oliguria is present, infuse 2 to 5 micrograms per kg per minute in 5 per cent dextrose in water intravenously. When both oliguria and hypotension are present, a dosage of 5 to 10 or even 20 micrograms per kg per minute may be given. Since dopamine is inactivated by sodium bicarbonate, do not add it to an infusion containing dopamine.

Afterload Reducing Agents. Conventional treatment regimens of congestive heart failure have relied on manipulation of the preload (diuretics, salt restriction) and contractile state (digoxin and other inotropic agents) of the heart. Over the past several years significant advances in the understanding of afterload manipulation have occurred and will be briefly discussed here. What is afterload? It is the load against which the heart has to contract during systole. It is proportional to the systolic pressure in the aorta and the size or diameter of the ventricle and inversely related to the thickness of the ventricular wall. Systemic vascular resistance is a better indicator of the afterload than the systolic pressure. This can be calculated if mean blood pressure (BP) and cardiac index (CI) are known:

$$\text{Resistance} = \text{mean BP/CI}$$

In heart failure, both acute and chronic, despite a decrease in cardiac output, near normal blood pressure is maintained; this is done by elevating the systemic vascular resistance. The cardiac size is also larger in heart failure. As can be seen, this is a perfect set-up for increased afterload on the left ventricle. It is suggested that if the afterload is reduced with vasodilator agents, the myocardial function will improve:

1. Sodium nitroprusside, 1 to 8 micrograms per kg per minute in 5 per cent dextrose in water, intravenously by a constant infusion pump. Since this drug is inactivated by light, the infusion syringe and tubing should be covered with aluminum foil.

2. Nitroglycerine, 0.1 to 0.4 microgram per kg per minute in 5 per cent dextrose in water, intravenously by a constant infusion pump.

Because of the vasodilatation produced by these drugs, circulatory blood volume redistributes into the periphery. Left ventricular filling pressure should be maintained by careful transfusion of blood or other colloid. Continuous measurement of blood pressure and of pulmonary arterial wedge or end-diastolic pressure and intermittent determinations of cardiac index to calculate the systemic vascular resistance are essential for accurately adjusting the dosage of the vasodilator agents. The use of these vasodilator agents in infants and children is still experimental and is reserved for patients with heart failure refractory to conventional treatment.

PULMONARY EDEMA

If signs of pulmonary edema are present, immediate treatment should be instituted:

1. Prop the patient at approximately 45 degrees.

2. Morphine sulfate, 0.1 mg per kg intravenously.

3. Furosemide (Lasix), 1 mg per kg intravenously.

4. Rapid digitalization by the intravenous route over a 2 to 4 hour period.

5. Humidified oxygen in high concentration may be administered via a face mask or a hood. Continuous positive airway pressure (CPAP), 6 to 8 cm H_2O with oxygen, may be instituted in severe cases. Very severely ill infants with pulmonary edema and elevated $Paco_2$ (> 60 mm Hg) require endotracheal intubation and mechanical

ventilation. Positive end-expiratory pressure (6 to 8 cm H₂O) on the ventilator may be beneficial.

6. In severe pulmonary edema, rotating tourniquets may be beneficial, especially when the other methods are not effective. Blood pressure cuffs may be placed around three of the four extremities and cuffs inflated with a pressure midway between systolic and diastolic blood pressure. Rotate the tourniquets every 15 to 20 minutes.

7. If significant improvement is not observed with the aforementioned measures, treatment listed under Other Drugs Used in Refractory Failure, above, should be instituted, particularly dopamine or nitroprusside.

PAROXYSMAL HYPOXEMIC SPELLS
(HYPERCYANOTIC SPELLS)

The spell syndrome has variously been described by several names, including anoxic spells, hypoxic spells, paroxysmal hyperpnea, blue spells, tetralogy spells, paroxysmal hypoxic attacks, and hypercyanotic episodes. These spells are most common in patients with tetralogy of Fallot, although they can occur in patients with tricuspid atresia or any lesion with severe pulmonary outflow tract obstruction and a systemic-to-pulmonary communication. The spells are most commonly seen between 1 and 12 months of age, with a peak frequency in 2- to 3-month-old children. The spells can occur at any time of the day but are most common in the morning after awakening from sleep; defecation, crying, and feeding are common precipitating factors. The hypoxemic spells are characterized by increased rate and depth of respiration and increased cyanosis progressing to limpness and syncope but usually with subsequent recovery. Occasionally, the spells terminate with convulsions, cerebrovascular accident, or, rarely, death. During the spell, the previously heard murmur either disappears or markedly diminishes in intensity. The exact cause of the spell syndrome is not known, but numerous hypotheses have been advanced. The two most possible mechanisms are right ventricular outflow tract spasm precipitated by acute increase in catecholamines and any stimulus producing hyperpnea. The treatment of the spells should be as follows:

Milder Spells

1. The infant should be placed in the knee-chest position. The reason for its effectiveness appears to be related to its effect in increasing the systemic vascular resistance and thus decreasing the right-to-left shunt and improving the pulmonary blood flow.

2. Humidifed oxygen via a face mask should be administered. Since the major defect in the spell syndrome is pulmonary oligemia rather than alveolar oxygenation, the oxygen administration has limited usefulness. If the infant is unduly disturbed by the face mask, discontinue oxygen therapy.

3. Morphine sulfate, 0.1 mg per kg subcutaneously, may be effective in aborting the spell. The mechanism of action is not clearly delineated, but its effect on the central nervous system respiratory drive (thus reducing hyperpnea) and sedation of the infant may be important in its favorable effect.

4. Once the physical examination is completed (and the limited but important laboratory studies are obtained), leave the infant undisturbed and let the infant rest; this in itself may improve the infant's condition.

5. Correct metabolic acidosis (with sodium bicarbonate or THAM), anemia (by blood transfusion), and dehydration, if present.

More Severe Spells

6. If the spell continues, vasopressors to increase the systemic vascular resistance and thus increase the pulmonary blood flow may be tried. In our experience, methoxamine (Vasoxyl), an alpha agonist, has been most helpful. Administer 20 to 40 mg in 250 ml of 5 per cent dextrose in water intravenously and adjust the rate of infusion to increase the systolic blood pressure by 15 to 20 per cent.

7. Beta blockade with propranolol, 0.1 mg per kg body weight, diluted in 50 ml of 5 per cent dextrose in water, may be administered intravenously while monitoring the heart rate (by ECG if possible). Should there be any marked bradycardia, the propranolol should be stopped. Once it is found to be effective, the infant may be switched to 1 to 4 mg per kg per day orally in three to four divided doses.

8. Infrequently, general anesthesia may be necessary to break the spell.

9. If the infant improves with the management outlined above, total surgical correction of the cardiac defects, if anatomically feasible, or a systemic-to-pulmonary shunt to improve the pulmonary blood flow on an elective basis within the next several days may be performed. An alternative to surgery is oral propranolol (dose as above), which may help postpone surgery by several months to years. If the infant does not improve with any of the aforementioned measures, an emergency systemic-to-pulmonary artery shunt

(we prefer Blalock-Taussig anastomosis) should be performed. Occasionally, total correction, if the anatomy is adequate, may be performed on an emergency basis. The important principle is that the infant requires more pulmonary blood flow.

ARRHYTHMIAS

Sinus Arrhythmia

Both phasic and nonphasic types of sinus arrhythmia are normal phenomena and do not require therapy.

Wandering Atrial Pacemaker

This term is applied when there is a change in the P wave configuration and/or a variation in the PR interval. This is usually seen in subjects with extreme degrees of sinus arrhythmia and is not considered pathologic. No treatment is necessary.

Sinus Tachycardia

Treat the cause of sinus tachycardia, namely fever, anemia, or thyrotoxicosis. Digitalis should not be used to treat sinus tachycardia.

Sinus Bradycardia

Sinus bradycardia can be seen with breath-holding, depression of the tongue, overdistention of the stomach (particularly in the premature infant), jaundice, increased intracranial pressure, and myxedema, as well as in well trained athletes. Again, treat the primary cause, if need be. Occasionally, sinus bradycardia is seen with digitalis intoxication.

If the heart rate is less than 50 beats per minute and hypotension is present, the sinus bradycardia may be treated with atropine, 0.01 to 0.02 mg per kg subcutaneously. If the patient does not improve or deteriorates, a transvenous pacemaker should be inserted. However, an intravenous infusion of isoproterenol (Isuprel), 0.5 to 1.0 microgram per kg per minute (Table 8), should first be attempted.

Premature Contractions

Premature beats may be of atrial, junctional, or ventricular origin. Infants and younger children are more likely to have premature atrial contractions, and older children to have premature ventricular contractions (PVCs). Because many normal children will have premature contractions and have no significant problems, no therapy is necessary. The characteristics of these benign premature beats are (1) unifocal beats, (2)

fixed coupling with the preceding R wave, (3) no association with structural heart disease, and (4) disappearance with exercise. If there are any associated symptoms (questionable episodes of tachycardia), or if they occur very frequently (more than 10 to 15 per minute) or present as bigeminy, these children should have exercise electrocardiography and a 24 hour Holter monitoring to see if there is any evidence for 3 or more consecutive PVCs (short bursts of ventricular tachycardia). If these are not present, no therapy is warranted. Follow-up electrocardiograms at 1 to 2 year intervals may be obtained for the child with frequent ectopic beats. If these tests detect bursts of three or more consecutive PVCs, propranolol (1 to 4 mg per kg per day in three to four divided doses) or quinidine (see Table 7) may be tried to suppress the arrhythmia.

If the PVCs are multifocal in origin, increase with exercise, or occur in runs of three or more, treatment may be indicated. Propranolol (see above), quinidine, or procainamide (Table 7) may be used.

If the PVCs are associated with (1) digitalis intoxication, (2) congenital or acquired heart disease (especially in the postoperative patient), (3) myocarditis, (4) electrolyte imbalance, or (5) prolonged Q-T interval, therapy is indicated.

1. If the PVCs are related to digitalis toxicity, treat digitalis toxicity (see above).

2. In the immediate postoperative period, lidocaine, 1 mg per kg per dose, may be given intravenously, followed by a continuous infusion of 25 to 50 micrograms per kg per minute. In the late postoperative period, because of the recent reports of sudden death, careful Holter monitoring and exercise electrocardiography are indicated. If runs of three or more consecutive PVCs are detected, treatment with propranolol (see above) or other antiarrhythmic drugs (Table 7) is indicated.

3. If the PVCs are associated with cardiomegaly and/or congestive heart failure, treatment of congestive failure with digitalis preparations (see above) may improve PVCs.

4. If the PVCs are associated with myocarditis, careful observation and perhaps lidocaine (see above) on an acute basis may be necessary.

5. If the PVCs are associated with electrolyte imbalance, treat the electrolyte imbalance. Temporary suppression of the ectopic beats may be undertaken with lidocaine (see above).

6. If the PVCs are associated with prolonged Q-T syndrome, mitral prolapse, or congenital or acquired heart disease without signs of heart failure, propranolol, 1 to 4 mg per kg per day orally in three to four divided doses, may be administered.

TABLE 8.   An Alphabetical List of Drugs Commonly Used in the Management of Pediatric Patients with Heart Disease*

DRUG	DOSE AND ROUTE OF ADMINISTRATION
Allopurinol (Zyloprim)	Mild hyperuricemia, 200–300 mg/day PO
	Severe hyperuricemia, 300–600 mg/day PO in two divided doses
Aminophylline	3–5 mg/kg/dose IV (may be given over ½ h during expected peak action of another diuretic agent)
Atropine sulfate	0.01–0.03 mg/kg/dose IV or subcutaneous; may be repeated in 4–6h
Calcium gluconate	2–4 ml of 10% solution IV very slowly
Chloral hydrate	20–40 mg/kg (maximum 1 gram) PO or rectal, may be repeated in 6–8h
Chlorothiazide (Diuril)	20–40 mg/kg/day PO in 2 divided doses
Chlorpromazine	0.6 mg/kg (maximum 15 mg) IM as part of a sedative cocktail with meperidine (Demerol) and promethazine (Phenergan)
Diazepam (Valium)	0.1 to 0.2 mg/kg IV
Digoxin (Lanoxin)	See Tables 3, 4, and 5
Dopamine (Intropin)	1–10 micrograms/kg/min IV
Epinephrine	0.25–1.0 microgram/kg/min IV
	or
	1–2 mg in 250 ml D5W; administer IV and adjust the rate to the desired effect
Furosemide (Lasix)	1–2 mg/kg/day IV
	2–5 mg/kg/day PO
Indomethacin (Indocin)	0.1 to 0.2 mg/kg PO
Isoproterenol (Isuprel)	1–2 micrograms/kg/min IV
	or
	0.2–0.4 mg in 250 ml D5W; administer IV and adjust the rate to the desired effect
Lidocaine (Xylocaine)	See Table 7
Meperidine (Demerol)	1–2 mg/kg (maximum 50 mg) IM; can be given alone or as part of a sedative cocktail with chlorpromazine (Thorazine) and promethazine (Phenergan)
Methoxamine (Vasoxyl)	40 mg in 250 ml D5W; infuse IV and adjust the rate to increase the systolic blood pressure by 15–20%; closely monitor the blood pressure
Morphine sulfate	0.1–0.2 mg/kg IV or subcutaneously
Neostigmine (Prostigmin)	0.05 mg subcutaneoulsy for a young infant
Nitroglycerin	0.1–0.4 microgram/kg/min IV by constant IV infusion pump
Phenylephrine (Neo-Synephrine)	0.005–0.01 mg/kg/dose IV
	or
	10 mg in 250 ml D5W; administer IV and adjust the rate to increase the systolic blood pressure by 15–20%; monitor the blood pressure
Phenytoin (Dilantin)	See Table 7
Potassium chloride	1–1.5 mEq/kg/day PO in 2–3 divided doses
Procainamide (Pronestyl)	See Table 7
Promethazine (Phenergan)	0.6 mg/kg IM, given as part of a sedative cocktail along with the chlorpromazine (Thorazine) and meperidine (Demerol)
Propranolol (Inderal)	See Table 7
Prostaglandin E_1	0.05 to 0.1 microgram/kg/min IV
Quinidine sulfate	See Table 7
Sodium bicarbonate	1–2 mEq/kg, diluted half and half with 10% D5W, IV
Sodium nitroprusside (Nipride)	1–8 micrograms/kg/min IV
Spironolactone (Aldactone)	3–5 mg/kg/day PO in three divided doses
Tolazoline (Priscoline)	1–2 mg/kg IV infusion over a period of 10 minutes, followed by 1–2 mg/kg/h as a continuous IV infusion
Tromethamine (THAM)	Weight in kg × base deficit = dose in ml of 0.3 molar solution
Warfarin sodium (Coumadin)	Initial, 10–30 mg/day PO
	Maintenance, 1–5 mg/day PO; adjust dose to maintain prothrombin time 2–2½ times the control value

*The authors have taken sufficient care to ensure that the drug dosages listed are accurate and are in line with accepted recommendations at the time of publication. However, the reader is urged to verify this information from the package insert of each drug.

Paroxysmal Supraventricular Tachycardia (PST)

Infants. PST is a medical emergency in an infant; the infant may develop congestive heart failure within hours of onset of PST and may die within 48 to 72 hours. Most frequently, the PST infants have no associated cardiac defects.

MODERATE TO SEVERE HEART FAILURE, SHOCK, OR EXTREME ILLNESS. In these infants, DC cardioversion should be performed. Start with low energy level, 1 to 2 watt-seconds per kg of body weight and increase stepwise until a response is effected (maximum is probably in the range of 5 to 10 watt-seconds per kg). The DC shock should be synchronized with the QRS complex. Unless the infant is moribund and unconscious, the infant should be completely sedated with diazepam (Valium), 0.2 mg per kg intravenously. General supportive measures such as oxygen administration and correction of metabolic acidosis and abnormalities in glucose and electrolyte concentration should be undertaken. Once cardioversion occurs, the infant should receive digitalis to prevent recurrences.

Insertion of a transvenous pacemaker and overdrive atrial stimulation to suppress the arrhythmia may be necessary, especially when the paroxysms are frequent.

NO HEART FAILURE OR MILD HEART FAILURE. 1. Vagal stimulating maneuvers, though sometimes effective in older children and adults, are usually not effective in converting PST to normal rhythm in infants and young children. Submerging the baby's face in ice water to simulate the "diving reflex" has been reported to be occasionally effective.

2. Sedation. Once the physical examination and limited but important laboratory studies are obtained, leave the infant undisturbed. If the infant is markedly restless, chloral hydrate, 25 mg per kg, may be given orally (or rectally) as a single dose. Rarely is it necessary to administer drugs such as morphine or meperidine (Demerol).

3. Digitalis is the drug of choice for PST in infants. For the dosage (Table 4) and the method of administration (Table 5), see above. We usually administer the first two doses intravenously. After the first dose, carotid sinus massage (only one side at a time) may be tried. Ninety-five per cent of the infants with PST will respond to digitalis alone.

4. If there is no response to digitalization, vasopressors to increase the systemic vascular resistance, and thus indirect vagal action, may be tried. In our experience, methoxamine (Vasoxyl), an alpha agonist, has been most helpful. Administer 20 to 40 mg in 250 ml of 5 per cent dextrose in water intravenously and adjust the rate of infusion to increase the systolic blood pressure by 15 to 20 per cent. Alternatively, 1 per cent phenylephrine hydrochloride (Neo-Synephrine) solution may be administered intravenously. The rate of infusion should be adjusted in a manner similar to that described for methoxamine.

5. Other antiarrhythmic drugs such as propranolol, quinidine, procainamide, or lidocaine (Table 7) may be tried next. We have used propranolol almost exclusively over the last several years with good success. It may be given in a dose of 0.1 mg per kg diluted in 50 ml of 5 per cent dextrose in water and administered slowly by intravenous route while monitoring the ECG. If there is marked slowing of the heart rate, propranolol should be stopped. Once the arrhythmia reverts to normal, oral propranolol (1 to 4 mg per kg per day in four divided doses) should be started.

6. If the arrhythmia has not converted to normal and the infant deteriorates, DC cardioversion may be necessary. Since serious arrhythmias (for example, ventricular fibrillation) have been reported with electrical cardioversion in digitalized patients, these should be prevented by pretreatment with phenytoin (Dilantin). It should be administered in a dose of 5 mg per kg intravenously over a 10 minute period prior to DC cardioversion. This latter problem is not infrequently seen in pediatric patients, and many pediatric cardiologists are using DC cardioversion as a first step in therapy.

7. Once the arrhythmia is converted to sinus rhythm, antiarrhythmic drugs (usually digitalis and occasionally digitalis and propranolol) should be continued for 6 to 12 months for prevention of recurrences. In patients with the Wolff-Parkinson-White syndrome, it may be necessary to continue these drugs for a much longer time.

Older Children. PST in older children is not difficult to convert to normal, but it is usually more difficult to prevent recurrences. Vagal stimulating maneuvers are more likely to be effective in older children. The Valsalva maneuver or carotid massage is useful in the conversion of the arrhythmia. Digitalis is still the drug of choice in our experience. Methoxamine may be needed occasionally. Propranolol should be used, if the PST does not respond to digitalis. Once the conversion occurs, digoxin alone or along with propranolol should be administered for prevention of recurrences.

Ventricular Tachycardia (VT)

Treatment depends upon the clinical status of the patients. If the patient has short runs of VT (three or more consecutive PVCs) and is asymptomatic, propranolol, quinidine, or procainamide (see above for dosages) may be tried. Patients who are acutely ill need immediate treatment:

1. Sharp precordial thump (blow) may be delivered, which may convert the arrhythmia to normal.

2. Lidocaine, 1 mg per kg per dose, may be given intravenously while awaiting to have electrical cardioversion performed. If the rhythm reverts to normal with lidocaine, continue intravenous lidocaine infusion at a rate of 25 to 50 micrograms per kg per minute.

3. DC cardioversion should be undertaken as described above. Overdrive pacing may also be useful.

Caution: Digitalis is contraindicated in patients suspected of having VT. If digitalis was previously administered, pretreatment with phenytoin prior to DC conversion is necessary (see above).

4. Correct metabolic acidosis, hypoglycemia, and electrolyte abnormalities, if present.

5. Once the arrhythmia is converted, antiarrhythmic drugs to prevent recurrences should immediately be started. Propranolol, procainamide, or quinidine (see above for dosages) may be used. We prefer propranolol, 1 to 4 mg per kg per day in three to four divided doses.

Ventricular Fibrillation (VF)

Immediate treatment is indicated. DC cardioversion is the treatment of choice and should be performed as outlined above. While getting the instruments ready, the following should be done:

1. Establish an airway to provide mouth-to-mouth, Ambu bag, or endotracheal ventilation.

2. Circulatory assistance should be provided by closed-chest cardiac massage.

3. Correct metabolic acidosis with sodium bicarbonate or THAM.

Once cardioversion occurs, treat the cause if known. Antiarrhythmic drugs (propranolol, procainamide, or quinidine) may be needed to prevent recurrences of VF.

Atrial Flutter and Atrial Fibrillation

These are rare in children but, when present, are usually associated with longstanding underlying cardiac disease.

1. Digitalization should first be performed. This is useful not only because of the inotropic effect but also because it reduces conduction through the atrioventricular node and thus slows the ventricular response.

2. DC countershock can convert the rhythm to normal in 90 per cent of patients, but may revert to the original rhythm because of the chronic cardiac disease. Therefore, DC countershock is not usually helpful.

3. Quinidine (see Table 7 for dosage) may be administered to help convert the rhythm to normal. Procainamide or propranolol may be similarly used. When treating atrial flutter and fibrillation, always use digoxin prior to the use of these drugs; otherwise, rapid ventricular response and ventricular tachycardia may result.

4. In patients with longstanding atrial flutter and fibrillation, anticoagulants should be administered to prevent embolization.

5. If feasible, the underlying cardiac disease should be treated.

Sick Sinus Syndrome

This is rare in the pediatric patient; it may occur in patients with a repaired sinus venosus atrial septal defect or following the Mustard procedure for transposition of the great arteries, but may occur in patients with a structurally normal heart. Patients with severe bradyrhythmias, after adequate documentation, may need permanent pacemaker implantation. Patients with tachyrhythmias may need digitalis and quinidine.

Heart Block

First Degree Atrioventricular Block. This manifests as prolonged PR interval and does not usually require therapy. If any underlying cardiac disease is present, it should be treated.

Second Degree Atrioventricular Block. This is of two major types: Wenckebach phenomenon (Mobitz Type I) and fixed block (Mobitz Type II). Again, treat the underlying cause, if known. If it is related to digitalis excess, treat digitalis toxicity. If symptomatic, atropine (0.01 mg per kg per dose intravenously or subcutaneously), isoproterenol (1 microgram per kg per minute, intravenously), or pacemaker implantation may be necessary.

Third Degree or Complete Atrioventricular Block. Complete heart block (CHB) is most commonly seen with no other associated cardiac defects. Occasionally, it is seen in association with congenital heart defects or may be seen after intracardiac surgical repair.

1. Patients with congenital CHB do not ordinarily need a pacemaker throughout childhood and perhaps throughout adolescence. Pacemaker insertion may be indicated in the presence of the following: (a) Associated congenital cardiac defects producing significant hemodynamic abnormality. (b) Stokes-Adams attacks with dizziness, syncope, or loss of consciousness. (c) Congestive heart failure. (d) Significant cardiomegaly by

chest x-ray. (e) Resting (awake) ventricular rate less than 50 beats per minute in infants and less than 40 beats per minute in children. (f) Atrial (P wave) rate greater than 150 per minute. (g) Prolonged QRS duration (> 0.12 sec). (h) Lack of increase in ventricular rate with exercise (or atropine) when exercise tolerance is significantly reduced. (i) Electrophysiologically proved block within or distal to bundle of His.

2. Patients with surgically induced heart block need pacemaker therapy, since they usually do not tolerate CHB.

3. Patients seen with acute heart block or during a Stokes-Adams attack may be treated in the following manner: (a) Transvenous pacemaker insertion. (b) Treatment of hypoxia and acidosis, if present. (c) If acutely acquired, for example, secondary to myocarditis, steroids for their anti-inflammatory action. (d) Atropine, 0.01 to 0.02 mg per kg per dose, intravenously. (e) Isoproterenol, 0.5 to 1.0 microgram per kg per minute intravenously. (f) Digitalization if the patient is in heart failure.

4. Asymptomatic patients with CHB, not falling into categories 1 and 2 above, may need a temporary pacemaker during anesthesia or any other acute stressful situations.

CARDIAC CATHETERIZATION AND ANGIOGRAPHY

Cardiac catheterization is a specialized procedure which provides valuable anatomic and physiologic information which usually cannot be collected in any other manner and the data thus gathered confirm the diagnosis and allow for the intelligent planning of appropriate medical and/or surgical therapy. Selective angiography, i.e., the injection of radiopaque material into a specific chamber or vessel with simultaneous filming, is now an integral and inseparable part of cardiac catheterization. The indications for cardiac catheterization in a pediatric population are best discussed by making a sharp distinction between (1) the neonate and (2) the older infant or child with suspected heart disease.

The Neonate

There is general agreement concerning the necessity for early and aggressive management of the distressed neonate with cyanosis and/or congestive heart failure. The foremost indication for cardiac catheterization in the neonate is *cyanosis of cardiac origin.* The cyanotic infant often presents a diagnostic dilemma between cyanosis of pulmonary, metabolic, hematologic, or cardiac etiology. A brief discussion of the differential diagnosis of

cyanosis is given on page 000. Using these criteria, once cyanosis of cardiac origin is suspected, the infant becomes an urgent candidate for cardiac catheterization. Cyanosis of this type in the neonatal period does not improve with "careful observation." Despite lack of any other symptoms, these babies should be catheterized immediately and, indeed, catheterization prior to the development of distress may provide better anatomic and physiologic data, on the basis of which further surgical and/or medical therapy can be instituted safely.

The second major indication for cardiac catheterization in the neonate is *congestive heart failure.* Catheterization should be performed soon after starting the appropriate anticongestive measures, and one should not await complete improvement; indeed palliative or corrective surgery may be necessary prior to achievement of a stable state.

Balloon atrial septostomy may be considered a separate indication for catheterization, but by and large this follows hemodynamic and angiographic studies diagnostic of transposition of the great arteries or other lesions requiring septostomy.

Recently developed noninvasive methods such as echocardiography and radioisotope angiography may be of help in diagnosing some clinically suspected heart defects. These procedures, when conclusive, especially in relation to the hypoplastic left heart syndrome, may eliminate the need for catheterization in some babies. The decision with regard to catheterization should be largely based upon the expertise and experience of the pediatric cardiology staff in these noninvasive methods.

Not all patients with signs of cardiac disease need to be catheterized during the neonatal period. Specific examples include patients with an obvious murmur of a small ventricular septal defect or patent ductus arteriosus, or with abnormal pulses suggestive of coarctation of the aorta. These and the patients with an abnormal cardiac shadow on x-ray or an abnormal electrocardiogram are not candidates for cardiac catheterization in the neonatal period unless they show signs of impaired cardiac function.

In summary, all babies presenting with cyanosis which is probably of cardiac origin and/or congestive heart failure during the neonatal period are candidates for early evaluation by a pediatric cardiologist and cardiac catheterization with selective angiographic studies.

Infants and Older Children

The indications for catheterization of infants beyond the neonatal period, children, and adolescents are not as clearly defined as in the neonates. These indications may vary from institution to institution and depend in part upon the experience, confidence, and degree of aggressiveness of the pediatric cardiac and surgical teams. The following are generally considered the most acceptable indications for cardiac catheterization of children.

Prior to Planned Surgical Correction. Most patients having congenital or acquired cardiac defects should have a catheterization prior to surgery in order to (1) confirm the clinical diagnosis, (2) determine the severity, (3) exclude any associated lesions or complicating factors, and (4) provide the surgeon with as accurate an anatomic picture as possible. The data also serve as baseline information for patients requiring postoperative evaluation. However, exceptions to this general rule exist. Clinically typical cases of patent ductus arteriosus do not require catheterization prior to surgery. A similar approach may be used for children with classic findings of atrial septal defects (secundum type) and coarctation of the aorta. It is suggested that if the patient has any clinical, x-ray, or electrocardiographic findings which are not typical for and unaccounted for by the suspected lesion, the patient should be catheterized before surgery.

Obtaining Specific Physiologic and/or Anatomic Information. Under this heading are patients in whom specific physiologic or anatomic parameters are important in the patient management. These include pulmonary artery pressure or pulmonary vascular resistance in ventricular septal defect or transposition of the great arteries, the size of the pulmonary arteries and their relationships to the aorta in patients with complex cyanotic congenital heart disease with severe pulmonic stenosis, and the determination of aortic valve gradient (or aortic valve area) in patients with aortic stenosis. The last-named parameter can only be accurately assessed by catheterization, since the clinical data are not reliable.

Diagnostic Dilemmas. Pediatric patients with abnormal clinical or laboratory findings in whom a definite diagnosis cannot be made clinically may also need a cardiac study. Because of the large body of knowledge and experience acquired in the past few decades, children catheterized for this indication should now be very few.

Postoperative Evaluations. In most institutions where a large number of patients with congenital heart disease (CHD) are followed, routine catheterization is performed approximately 1 year after the corrective surgery for the more complex cardiac defects in order to evaluate the anatomic and physiologic results. Significant numbers of patients have been studied post-operatively at many institutions, and ideally, in the next few years, it will not be necessary to routinely catheterize as many patients after an operation. A postoperative catheterization will then be reserved for patients with residual defects or for those in whom a changing physiologic or anatomic variable has to be followed to intelligently manage the patient. The complex cardiac defects for which there have been only recent corrective (anatomic or physiologic) procedures would continue to need routine postoperative catheterization to evaluate adequacy of the surgery, to determine the need for additional medical and/or surgical therapy, and to advise the proper exercise and activity recommendations.

Determination of the Natural History. For certain types of congenital heart defects the natural history remains unknown. Therefore, it would be difficult to determine if the results of a given treatment are more favorable than the natural course of the disease. Natural history studies of this type may therefore be helpful in the management of patients with CHD. It should be noted, however, that studies of this type should be performed in an organized fashion.

Special Studies. Recent advances in His bundle electrocardiography have elucidated some of the electrophysiology of arrhythmias. In pediatric patients, arrhythmias, particularly those of the postoperative type, may require His bundle and other electrophysiologic studies to determine the exact abnormality, which may be helpful in clinical management.

Patients with heart block of any etiology can be paced temporarily by introducing a transvenous pacemaker catheter. This may be particularly helpful in digitalis intoxication.

Miscellaneous. Cardiac catheterization may be performed for research purposes to evaluate the effects of drugs or study a special type of physiologic measurement. Such catheterizations should be performed only after careful consideration of the risks of the procedure and possible benefits derived by the study. Of course, this should be done with clear parental understanding and consent. Increasing limitations (of recent times) placed on human experimentation and the legal implications would make this indication a rare one.

It has been suggested that the teenager with a murmur should be studied to confirm the innocent (functional) nature of the murmur so as to permit participation in competitive sports. In the opinion of the authors, innocent murmurs often can be distinguished from organic murmurs by careful examination and the usual laboratory studies, and cardiac catheterization should not be performed unless there are extremely unusual circumstances. Some may recommend catheterization for mild forms of CHD in patients ready to "graduate" from pediatric cardiac supervision; again, the authors do not see any reason to deviate from the criteria listed above.

In summary, the indications for elective catheterization in the older infants and children are multiple, but the most important are patients with correctable heart defects prior to operation and patients in whom there is need for special physiologic or anatomic parameters that cannot be obtained by noninvasive means.

Precatheterization Preparation. The preparation required may vary between the neonate and the remainder of pediatric patients. Upon arrival at the Regional Pediatric Cardiology Center, clinical as well as the usual laboratory data (chest x-ray, electrocardiogram, hemoglobin, hematocrit, and Dextrostix or blood sugar) are obtained immediately. No baby is too sick or too small to have the indicated cardiac study. Cardiac medications (digitalis and diuretics) are administered as indicated. Introduction of a catheter into the descending aorta via an umbilical artery for monitoring blood gases and blood pressure is highly recommended. Monitoring and maintenance of normal temperature, blood pH, blood sugar, and serum calcium cannot be overemphasized.

Older infants and children are usually admitted on an elective basis for any of the indications outlined above. Detailed explanation of (1) the need for the study, (2) description of the catheterization procedure, (3) risks involved, and (4) the length of the hospitalization is given to the parents at the time of scheduling for the study, and repeated at the time of admission. A booklet especially prepared for the parents, describing the catheterization, and a hospital coloring book for the older children are given. A pediatric play therapist presents a puppet show to the children above 4 years of age to possibly relieve some of the anxiety and bring out any questions and concerns the child and parents may have about the procedure. Catheterization is performed the day following the admission, and the child is usually ready for discharge within 24 hours after the study. Prior to discharge, the results of the catheterization and recommendations for further medical and/or surgical therapy are discussed with the parents.

In the newborn and younger infant, the procedure is performed without premedication, whereas older infants and children are premedicated with a mixture of meperidine (Demerol), 2 mg per kg of body weight (maximum 50 mg), chlorpromazine (Thorazine), 0.6 mg per kg (maximum 15 mg), and promethazine (Phenergan), 0.6 mg per kg (maximum 15 mg) given intramuscularly 30 minutes prior to catheterization.

CARDIOVASCULAR SURGERY

Surgical management of congenital heart disease may be discussed under two subheadings: (1) palliative surgery and (2) "corrective" surgery.

Palliative Surgery

The palliative surgical procedures are designed to improve a particular physiologic abnormality. These physiologic abnormalities are (1) decreased pulmonary blood flow, (2) increased pulmonary blood flow, and (3) inadequate interatrial mixing.

Decreased Pulmonary Blood Flow. Since the original description of subclavian artery–to–ipsilateral pulmonary artery anastomosis by Blalock and Taussig in 1945, several types of these shunt operations have been devised. These include other types of systemic artery–to–pulmonary artery shunt, namely Potts anastomosis (descending aorta–to–left pulmonary artery shunt), Waterston-Cooley shunt (ascending aorta–to–right pulmonary artery anastomosis), ascending aorta–to–main pulmonary artery anastomosis (creation of aortopulmonary window), and aorta–to–pulmonary artery Gore-Tex shunt and the Glenn procedure (superior vena cava–to–right pulmonary artery anastomosis). Maintenance of ductal patency by formalin infiltration of the ductus arteriosus and blind pulmonary valvotomy (Brock procedure) have also been used to palliate pulmonary oligemia. Systemic artery–to–pulmonary artery shunt operations are commonly used in surgical palliation. Because of the small size of the subclavian artery in the neonate and young infant, some surgeons have preferred central aortopulmonary (Potts and Waterston) shunts. Because of the complications associated with the latter shunts, most pediatric cardiologists recommend and most cardiovascular surgeons perform the Blalock-Taussig shunt as the procedure of choice. The recent modifications of the procedure and the use of microsurgical techniques make it feasible to perform the Blalock-Taussig shunt in very small infants and, indeed, at present we do not use any shunt other than the Blalock-Taussig anastomosis in infants with cyanotic heart disease and pulmonary oligemia. The cardiac defects in which this shunt is performed include pulmonary atresia with an intact ventricular septum, pulmonary atresia with ventricular septal defect, severe tetralogy of Fallot, tricuspid atresia, and complex congenital heart defects with severe pulmonary stenosis or atresia.

Increased Pulmonary Blood Flow. In infants with increased pulmonary blood flow and increased pulmonary arterial pressures (most of these infants will be in heart failure), surgical constriction or banding of the main pulmonary artery was recommended in the past. But because of improvements in open heart surgical techniques in younger infants, most of these infants, particularly those with large ventricular septal defects, will have primary surgical correction. Some defects, which cannot be completely corrected in small infants, may require pulmonary artery banding. The defects include muscular (Swiss cheese) type of ventricular septal defect, single ventricle, double outlet right ventricle, transposition of the great arteries with a large ventricular septal defect, and rare types of tricuspid atresia (all of the above without associated pulmonic stenosis).

Inadequate Interatrial Mixing. There are several congenital heart defects in which an interatrial septal defect with shunting across it is highly beneficial. Most important of these lesions is transposition of the great arteries with intact ventricular septum. In this cyanotic cardiac anomaly, the aorta arises from the right ventricle and the pulmonary artery from the left ventricle. Here the circulation is parallel instead of "in series." The systemic venous blood does not pass through the lungs to become oxygenated. Some intracardiac admixture is essential for patient survival. These infants will usually present in the first few days of life with severe cyanosis. In the past, the treatment of choice was surgical atrial septostomy, which carried a considerable risk in these sick cyanotic neonates. In 1966, Rashkind and Miller described a technique by which an atrial septostomy could be performed at cardiac catheterization. A deflated balloon catheter is advanced into the left atrium from the right atrium via a patent foramen ovale, and the balloon is inflated with diluted radiopaque liquid and rapidly pulled back across the patent foramen ovale, rupturing the lower margin of the atrial wall below the patent foramen ovale. Balloon septostomy renders palliation in most if not all infants until the age of 6 months to 1 year, when the defect can be corrected surgically with much less risk. Septostomy may also be performed in other cardiac defects in which a better mixing at the atrial level and/or relief of high right or left atrial pressure (as the case may be) are required. These defects include pulmonary atresia with intact ventricular septum, tricuspid atresia, mitral atresia, and total anomalous pulmonary venous connection.

TABLE 9. Lesions Which Can Be Primarily Repaired Without Prior Palliative Procedures

Acyanotic lesions
  Left to right shunt
    Atrial septal defect
    Ventricular septal defect
    Patent ductus arteriosus
    Endocardial cushion defect
    Partial anomalous pulmonary venous connection
  Obstructive lesions
    Aortic stenosis
    Coarctation of the aorta
    Interrupted aortic arch
    Pulmonic stenosis
Cyanotic lesions
  Tetralogy of Fallot
  Total anomalous pulmonary venous connection
  Single atrium
  Truncus arteriosus
  Double outlet right ventricle

Beyond the neonatal period, balloon atrial septostomy is technically difficult because the lower margin of the foramen ovale is thick and cannot be ruptured by balloon. Park and associates developed a catheter with a retractable knife which can be used to cut the septum, and then a balloon septostomy can be performed. If this technique is not successful or not readily available, atrial septostomy may be performed surgically either by the Blalock-Hanlon technique or by an open method.

"Corrective" Surgery

Since the introduction of cardiopulmonary bypass for open heart surgery by Gibson, Lillehei, and Kirklin in the 1950s and the introduction of these techniques in small infants in the 1960s and deep hypothermia technique in the early 1970s, there have been considerable advances in the surgical management of congenital heart disease. Almost every congenital heart defect can be "corrected," and the few that cannot be completely repaired can be effectively palliated. The term "corrective" surgery is used when defects of the heart or great vessels are anatomically repaired or the circulation is restored to a normal physiologic state. This does not necessarily mean that the cardiovascular system is restored to normal and that the patients are not without any residual cardiac defect. Corrective surgery in the purest form is possible in only a few defects, and therefore the term is used with quotation marks. Table 9 shows the lesions that can be completely repaired without prior palliative procedures, and Table 10 shows lesions which may require palliation before total correction several years later. Of course this classification is arbitrary and with considerable overlap.

TABLE 10. **Lesions Which May Require Prior Palliation**

Transposition of the great arteries
Pulmonary atresia
Tricuspid atresia
Single ventricle
Double outlet right ventricle

MISCELLANEOUS PROBLEMS ENCOUNTERED WITH CONGENITAL HEART DEFECTS

Anemia. Infants and children with acyanotic congenital heart defects but without cardiac failure can tolerate anemia similarly to normal children. Anemia is poorly tolerated by patients with impending or overt cardiac failure and therefore should be treated promptly. Packed red cell transfusions (10 ml per kg) over a few hours may be given if rapid correction is indicated. Evidence of volume overload should be scrutinized. Otherwise, oral iron therapy (6 mg of elemental iron per kg per day in three divided doses) may be given for iron deficiency anemia. Other types of anemia should be diagnosed by appropriate laboratory testing and treated accordingly.

In patients with cyanotic heart disease, there is usually polycythemia; this is a compensatory mechanism to increase O_2 carrying capacity in patients with a significant degree of arterial desaturation. Each patient, based on the level of arterial saturation, may have an optimal level of hemoglobin (or hematocrit) at which adequate oxygen is delivered to the tissues. In patients with cyanotic heart defects, the hemoglobin, hematocrit, and red blood cell indices should be periodically checked and at the first sign of iron deficiency anemia, it should be corrected by oral iron therapy (see above for dosage). Apart from providing adequate oxygen delivery to the tissues and near normal physical performance, optimal hemoglobin may help prevent cerebrovascular accidents. On occasion, correction of anemia may even result in reducing and preventing hypercyanotic spells.

Anemia secondary to the Waring Blender syndrome (intravascular hemolysis) will be discussed under Prosthetic Devices (p. 205).

Polycythemia. As described above, polycythemia is a compensatory mechanism in patients with cyanotic heart defects. In patients with severe and longstanding right-to-left shunting, progressive polycythemia develops, and as the central hematocrit reaches 65 to 70 per cent, it becomes counterproductive because the marked increase in blood viscosity elevates peripheral vascular resistance and decreases oxygen delivery to the tissues. At this point, symptoms of excessive polycythemia, namely headaches, chest pain, fatigue, muscle cramps, and irritability, develop. Furthermore, there is an increased risk of cerebrovascular accidents at these high levels of hematocrit. Although excessive polycythemia formerly was treated with phlebotomy, that practice is to be condemned. At present, the treatment of choice (in the absence of an appropriate palliative or corrective surgical procedure) is erythropheresis, i.e., removal of 20 to 30 ml aliquots of blood and replacement with an equal volume of Plasminate or fresh frozen plasma. The volume to be exchanged may be calculated as shown at the bottom of this page, where weight (L/kg) is body volume in liters, 0.11 is the blood volume as a fraction of body volume, and Hct_i and Hct_d are initial and desired hematocrits. We usually do not reduce the hematocrit by more than 10 per cent, nor do we recommend the desired hematocrit to be less than 55 per cent for fear of drastically reducing the oxygen delivery to the tissues.

The most frequent indication for erythropheresis is symptoms of excessive polycythemia along with a central hematocrit greater than 70 per cent. Other indications are coagulation abnormalities associated with polycythemia (see below), prior to cardiac catheterization, and preparatory to palliative or corrective surgery.

Coagulation Problems. Patients with cyanotic heart disease with a significant degree of polycythemia and arterial desaturation often have coagulation abnormalities. Although some of these abnormalities are artifacts related to inadequate amount of anticoagulant solution added to the blood sample, there are several types of well-documented coagulation problems in these patients. These include thrombocytopenia (thrombocytosis in patients with mild arterial desaturation), abnormal platelet function, decreased vitamin K dependent factors (prothrombin, factors VII, IX, and X), decreased consumable factors producing disseminated intravascular coagulation (fibrinogen, factors V and VIII), and increased fibrinolysis. Most if not all of these abnormalities can be corrected by erythropheresis. All patients with cyanotic heart disease (3 years and older) with a hematocrit greater than 50 per cent and O_2 saturation less than 60 to 70 per cent should be screened for prothrombin time, activated partial thromboplas-

$$\text{Volume to be exchanged} = \text{Weight (L/kg)} \times 0.11 \times \frac{Hct_i - Hct_d}{Hct_i}$$

tin time, and platelet count (after adding appropriate amount of anticoagulant) prior to any cardiac or noncardiac surgery or dental extraction. If abnormal, specific factor correction or preferably erythropheresis (see above) should be performed.

Hyperuricemia. Hyperuricemia, gout, and uric acid nephropathy may be seen in adolescents and adults with longstanding cyanotic heart disease with severe polycythemia. Serum uric acid levels should be measured periodically in adults and adolescents with cyanotic heart disease. Elevated uric acid levels (greater than 8 mg per 100 ml) should be treated with allopurinol (Zyloprim) in an attempt to prevent gout and uric acid nephropathy. If feasible, palliative or corrective surgery should be performed to relieve hypoxemia and thereby polycythemia and hyperuricemia.

Cerebrovascular Accidents. Cerebrovascular accidents (CVA) with resultant hemiplegia associated with cyanotic heart disease may be seen in two different situations: (1) infants (less than 2 years) with relative anemia and (2) older patients with severe polycythemia. Prevention of iron deficiency anemia by appropriate monitoring and prompt correction when present may prevent CVA of infancy. Similarly, prevention of severe polycythemia by performing appropriate palliative or corrective surgery or erythropheresis may reduce the incidence of CVA in the older age group. Once a CVA occurs, the treatment is supportive. This includes adequate hydration, correction of anemia or polycythemia if present, anticonvulsants (if seizures are present), and physiotherapy.

Brain Abscess. Patients with cyanotic heart defects are at risk for developing brain abscess because of the intracardiac right-to-left shunting bypassing the pulmonary filtering mechanism. The majority of the patients with brain abscess are beyond 2 years of age and usually have significant arterial hypoxemia and polycythemia. Any patient with cyanotic heart disease who has unexplained fever, headache, malaise, and neurologic signs is a suspect for brain abscess. Computerized tomographic scanning of the brain is very useful in detecting these lesions. Treatment include antibiotics and neurosurgical consultation for possible burr hole aspiration of the abscess.

Recurrent Respiratory Tract Infection. Children with congenital heart disease are not prone to develop upper respiratory tract infections. However, infants and young children with large left-to-right shunt lesions may have a higher incidence of lower respiratory tract infection; this is because of compression of the bronchi by the enlarged hypertensive pulmonary arteries and by compression caused by the enlarged heart. Infants with such problems should be promptly treated with antibiotics, physiotherapy, and postural drainage.

Prosthetic Devices. Prosthetic valves and conduits (with porcine valves) may be placed in many children during intracardiac repair. Many of these patients are then begun on sodium warfarin (Coumadin) to prevent thromboembolism. The dose of Coumadin should be adjusted to maintain the prothrombin time at 2 to 2½ times the control value; the prothrombin times should be monitored at monthly intervals.

These patients are in a high risk category for developing bacterial endocarditis, and therefore they should strictly adhere to the bacterial endocarditis prophylaxis regimen (to be discussed shortly) and should receive the prophylactic antibiotics parenterally.

Recent observations suggest that calcification of the porcine valves occurs with significant frequency in pediatric patients (and even in young adults). These valves may have to be replaced to alleviate the symptoms of porcine valve dysfunction.

Some patients with prosthetic valves may develop hemolytic anemia or intravascular hemolysis (Waring Blender syndrome). If this is severe, replacement of the prosthetic valve may be necessary. Mild forms can often be managed with oral iron and perhaps folic acid therapy.

Anesthesia. Acyanotic patients with minimal hemodynamic abnormalities can tolerate general anesthesia well. Patients with pulmonary vascular obstructive disease and severe cardiomegaly are at greatest risk from general anesthesia. Avoidance of hypoxia and hypotension is important because these are poorly tolerated by patients with significant heart disease. The blood pressure and the electrocardiogram should be monitored during the induction of anesthesia and during the operation. Adequate care should be taken in the cyanotic patients not to inadvertently inject any air intravenously because the air bubbles readily reach the systemic circuit.

In patients with tetralogy of Fallot, agents which reduce systemic vascular resistance (halothane and thiopental sodium [Pentothal]) or spinal anesthesia should not be used, because they may increase right-to-left shunting and thus hypoxemia. Cyclopropane and nitrous oxide are preferable because of their adrenergic effects. Cyclopropane should not be used in patients with pulmonary vascular obstructive disease because of its effects in increasing the pulmonary vascular resistance.

Prophylaxis in Asplenia Patients. Because of

a very high incidence of sepsis in asplenia patients, continuous antibiotic prophylaxis is recommended. After 3 months of age, amoxicillin by mouth is recommended; this is to prevent infection with pneumococcus and *Hemophilus influenzae*. Beyond 10 years of age, oral penicillin is adequate and should probably be continued indefinitely.

Prevention of Complications of Heart Disease. The prevention of the complications of congenital heart disease is an important and broad subject, and detailed discussion of these aspects is beyond the scope of this article. Pulmonary vascular obstructive disease is probably the most common cause of inoperability in children with otherwise technically operable congenital heart disease. Prevention of irreversible pulmonary vascular obstructive disease by early corrective or palliative surgery is an important aspect of management of patients with congenital heart disease. Such intervention should take place before 18 to 24 months of age in patients with large nonrestrictive ventricular septal defects. Much earlier intervention (6 months) may be necessary in patients with transposition of the great arteries with ventricular septal defect or common atrioventricular canal. Early referral by the family practitioner or the pediatrician and aggressive treatment by the pediatric cardiologists and cardiovascular surgeons are necessary to achieve this goal. Longstanding ventricular septal defect, mitral insufficiency, or aortic insufficiency (congenital or acquired) may cause deterioration of myocardial function. Appropriate surgery should be performed early enough to prevent myocardial damage. Late operation in coarctation of the aorta has been reported to produce residual cardiovascular effects, and this lesion should be operated upon early, i.e., before school age. Cerebrovascular accidents (secondary to anemia, hypoxemia, and polycythemia) and brain abscess should be prevented in cyanotic heart disease patients by timely and appropriate therapeutic measures. Bacterial endocarditis should be prevented in all patients with congenital heart disease.

Prophylaxis Against Bacterial Endocarditis. Patients with congenital or acquired heart disease tend to have hemodynamic trauma to the endocardium and vascular endothelium. These sites may form a nidus for circulating bacteria of either spontaneous origin or the result of any orodental, genitourinary, or other surgery or procedures. Therefore, antibiotics are indicated to reduce the degree and duration of bacteremia and thus prevent bacterial endocarditis. The following is a summary of preventive aspects of bacterial endocarditis:

1. All patients with congenital heart defects (as well as rheumatic heart disease or any other acquired cardiovascular malformation) should receive antibiotic prophylaxis prior to orodental, genitourinary, or gastrointestinal surgery or any other bacteremia-producing procedures, including labor and delivery. The recommended dosages and regimen of antibiotic prior to orodental procedures are listed in Table 11. Table 12 lists the recommendations prior to genitourinary or gastrointestinal surgery or procedures.

2. Prophylaxis for rheumatic fever should not be confused with prophylaxis for bacterial endocarditis. Rheumatic fever prophylaxis involves a low dose of penicillin (or sulfonamide) administered regularly in contrast to the episodic antibiotic prophylaxis prior to a bacteremia-producing procedure for prevention of bacterial endocarditis. Penicillin administered for prevention of recurrence of rheumatic fever cannot prevent bacterial endocarditis. In this group, because of the development of penicillin-resistant strains in the mouth flora, it is advisable to add an additional antibiotic (erythromycin or streptomycin) for bacterial endocarditis prophylaxis.

TABLE 11. **Summary of the Bacterial Endocarditis Prophylaxis Recommendations of the American Heart Association***

	ANTIBIOTICS AND DOSAGE	ROUTE AND FREQUENCY OF ADMINISTRATION
On the day of the procedure	Procaine penicillin G,† 600,000 units	Intramuscular, 30 minutes to 1 hour before the procedure
	plus Aqueous crystalline penicillin G, 30,000 units/kg *or*	
	Penicillin V, 1.0 gram‡	Oral, 30 minutes to 1 hour prior to the procedure
For 2 days after the procedure (start 6 hours after the procedure)	Penicillin V, 250 mg‡	Oral, every 6 hours§

*Reproduced, with permission of S. Karger, Basel, from Rao, P. S.: Paediatrician, *4*:320, 1975.

†For patients allergic to penicillin use erythromycin, 20 mg per kg orally 1½ to 2 hours prior to the procedure and 10 mg per kg orally every 6 hours for eight doses following the procedure.

‡For children weighing more than 60 lbs., the dosage of penicillin V should be doubled.

§The physician or dentist may choose to use the parenteral route of administration for these 2 days.

TABLE 12. **Bacterial Endocarditis Prophylaxis for Gastrointestinal and Genitourinary Tract Surgery or Procedures (Summary of the Recommendations of the American Heart Association)***

ANTIBIOTICS AND DOSAGE†	ROUTE AND FREQUENCY OF ADMINISTRATION
Aqueous crystalline penicillin G, 30,000 units/kg (not to exceed 2,000,000 units)	Intramuscular or intravenous, 30 minutes to 1 hour before the procedure and every 8 hours for two additional doses
or	
Ampicillin, 50 mg/kg (not to exceed 1.0 gram)	Same as above
plus	
Streptomycin, 20 mg/kg (not to exceed 1.0 gram)	Intramuscular, 30 minutes to 1 hour prior to the procedure and every 12 hours for two additional doses
or	
Gentamicin, 2.0 mg/kg (not to exceed 80 mg)	Intramuscular or intravenous, 30 minutes to 1 hour prior to the procedure and every 8 hours for two additional doses
or	
(For those patients who are allergic to penicillin) Streptomycin or gentamicin, as above	Same as above
plus	
Vancomycin, 20 mg/kg (not to exceed 1.0 gram per dose and 44 mg/kg/24 hours)	Intravenously given over 30 minutes to 1 hour; the administration of the dose should be begun 30 minutes to 1 hour prior to the procedure; repeat the same dose in 12 hours

*Reproduced, with permission of S. Karger, Basel, from Rao, P. S.: Paediatrician, *4*:320, 1975.

†In patients with significantly compromised renal function, it may be necessary to modify the dosage of antibiotics.

3. Attention to dental hygiene should be encouraged in children with cardiac defects.

4. A proper understanding of the reasons behind the prophylactic regimen is necessary for the patients to follow the recommendations. Therefore, the parents (and the patients) should be well educated as to the need for and the rationale of the prophylactic regimen.

5. No prophylactic treatment is necessary prior to cardiac catheterization.

6. Because of frequent endocarditis after open heart surgery, a combination of penicillin, streptomycin, and a penicillinase-resistant synthetic penicillin for 24 hours preoperatively and for 7 days postoperatively is recommended in all patients undergoing open-heart surgery.

7. There does not appear to be any need for antibiotic prophylaxis prior to closed-heart surgical procedures.

8. In many patients who have had corrective cardiac surgery, the risk of bacterial endocarditis does not change, and therefore they should receive prophylaxis as outlined above. The exceptions to this rule are patients with repaired atrial septal defect, patent ductus arteriosus, and ventricular septal defect without any residua; in this group, bacterial endocarditis prophylaxis may be discontinued 6 months after surgery.

9. Patients with prosthetic devices are at particular risk for bacterial endocarditis. Therefore, these patients should not only strictly adhere to the recommendations but also receive the antibiotic parenterally.

10. Patients undergoing open-heart surgery who have been on prolonged antibiotic therapy may be candidates for antifungal prophylaxis (oral nystatin, amphotericin B lozenges, and nystatin vaginal pessaries in women) for prevention of fungal endocarditis.

GENERAL PROBLEMS

Immunization. Patients with all types of congenital heart defects should receive routine immunizations on schedule. There is no contraindication for immunizations, nor should they be delayed. If intercurrent illness or hospitalization temporarily interrupts the immunization schedule, it should be resumed immediately thereafter. Children with large left-to-right shunt lesions, severe cardiomegaly, or severe cyanosis may be candidates for receiving polyvalent pneumococcal vaccine and trivalent influenza vaccine. Similarly, prompt immunization during epidemics is indicated.

Physical Activity and Exercise. The majority of the children with congenital heart disease will have only minimal hemodynamic impairment and should not be restricted in their physical activities.

Patients with moderate hemodynamic impairment should also be encouraged to participate in all normal activities. They should be allowed to determine their own level of activity; they usually learn to restrict their activity commensurate with their exercise tolerance. These children should be allowed to rest if they become fatigued.

Patients with moderate to severe aortic stenosis, severe pulmonic stenosis, pulmonary vascular obstructive disease, or severe cardiomegaly should refrain from participating in competitive sports. Patients with prosthetic valves also should not be allowed to participate in competitive sports.

Psychologic and Emotional Development. There are many adverse emotional effects on the children with heart disease and their parents. It has been suggested that poor psychologic adjustment and anxiety in the child with congenital heart disease is related to maternal anxiety and pampering, much of which can be greatly reduced by corrective operation. To prevent any adverse psychologic effects, one should recommend early corrective surgery for heart disease in children (if indicated and if it can be performed safely). Parents must be advised repeatedly to allow normal emotional and activity patterns in children not needing any surgery. Additional means that might be utilized to alleviate these problems are as follows:

1. Education of the child by providing information by simplified booklets, coloring books, tour of the catheterization laboratory or operating room, and puppet or play therapy when appropriate.

2. Counseling the parents at the time of diagnosis, cardiac catheterization, and cardiac surgery by nurse clinicians or social workers.

3. Encouraging parents' discussion with parents of other children with congenital heart disease.

4. The school age child should have his or her defect explained and drawn, and this should be repeated at the time of adolescence when some discussion of sex and the genetics of heart disease should also be undertaken. This education should be repeated to young adults, and we also insist they bring their spouses for an education session.

Prevention of Cardiac Nondisease. Findings that are either insignificant or very minor may be made to seem significant or major by the physician or perceived as such by the child or his parents and may cause "pseudodisease" or "nondisease" in the child and may lead to greater attention than deserved. Such a phenomenon associated with cardiac findings may be called cardiac nondisease. The common causes for this in the pediatric age group appear to be the functional (innocent, normal) heart murmur, congenital heart defects with minimal or no hemodynamic impairment, and "overdiagnosis" of acute rheumatic fever. Parents of patients with a functional murmur should be told that the child is entirely normal, and periodic follow-up is not necessary. Such follow-up of these patients will only accentuate the emotional problem and increase cardiac nondisease.

Many patients with congenital heart disease need only periodic follow-up and antibiotic prophylaxis prior to orodental or genitourinary surgery or procedures for prevention of bacterial endocarditis. There is no need for restriction of activity and exercise in children with congenital heart disease unless it is very severe. Therefore, it is important to impress on the parents the necessity for treating the child as "normal" with regard to both emotional needs and physical activity. Prevention of cardiac nondisease in children is the responsibility of the family physician, pediatrician, and pediatric cardiologists and should be kept in mind when dealing with functional heart murmurs and mild organic heart disease.

Genetic Counseling. Most parents have guilt feelings; they think that they are responsible for the congenital heart defect because of their heredity or something they have (or have not) done during pregnancy. These guilt feelings and anxieties should be relieved by making them understand that this is not the case with congenital heart disease.

In the majority of congenital heart defects, the causative factor or factors are not known; the defect is presumed to occur by multifactorial inheritance, i.e., genetic-environmental interaction. In the presence of congenital heart disease in only one member of the family, the recurrence risk in siblings (or offspring) is 2 to 5 per cent, which is only slightly higher than the general population incidence. Because of this low recurrence risk, we generally advise that the parents' decision to have future pregnancies be based on considerations other than the fact that the child under question has a congenital heart defect. Severity of the cardiac defect is another factor that must be taken into consideration. For example, recurrence of a defect such as patent ductus arteriosus, which can be easily operated in a sibling, is of far less concern than recurrence of a complex defect such as single ventricle or transposition of the great arteries.

A detailed genetic (family) history should be obtained prior to genetic counseling, and indeed, we, in our clinic, routinely record this information during the first visit for cardiac evaluation. The recurrence figures given above are valid if only one member of the family is involved. The risk of recurrence is considerably higher if more than one first degree relative is involved. Obviously, the risk is much increased if the given cardiac defect in the family is a mendelian dominant trait, as is the case with Marfan's syndrome.

Vocational Training and Rehabilitation. The majority of patients with congenital heart defects reaching adolescence and adulthood will have normal working capacity. These patients should not be denied jobs because of their defect without documentation by exercise testing. The primary physician and the pediatric cardiologist should assure the prospective employer of the lack of physical activity limitations of the congenital heart defect patient with minimal or no hemodynamic impairment.

Several patients will have limited physical working capacity, and in these patients vocational guidance is important. State rehabilitation agencies should be able to provide these services.

Sexuality, Contraception, and Pregnancy. The available data suggest that girls with congenital heart defects are as sexually active as their healthy peers. It is, therefore, mandatory to counsel the adolescent patients concerning their decision-making process. Since many will have made the decision to become sexually active, they should realize that they are responsible for making the next decision — to avoid pregnancy. The monograph "11 Million Teenagers" indicates that 35 to 45 per cent of 15- to 19-year-old girls have intercourse at some time. Therefore, at least 50 per cent do not, and the first alternative we have to offer these youngsters is abstinence or virginity. We can point out that not everyone is "doing it." This is obviously not a reasonable alternative to the adolescent who has decided to be active. The choices of contraception will then depend upon the individual. Table 13 lists the methods and their relative utility in adolescents who may have very few encounters with one individual or very frequent encounters with multiple partners.

At the time of counseling, the risk of pregnancy to the mother and to the infant should be discussed. Most women with mild to moderate acyanotic defects are at very low risk of complications of pregnancy, labor, and delivery. The exceptions are those with Marfan's syndrome and patients with uncorrected coarctation of the aorta. Some authorities think that Marfan's syndrome with aortic root dilatation (echographic) is an absolute contraindication to pregnancy because of the very high incidence of aortic dissection. Such a risk, plus the autosomal dominant nature of the defect, makes this a reasonable recommendation.

Individuals with cyanotic defects, especially those with Eisenmenger's syndrome, are at increased risk of deterioration and mortality during pregnancy, labor, and delivery. There is also a significant fetal wastage in some who are cyanotic.

Warfarin therapy in women with prosthetic valves causes a high incidence of a specific embryopathy (warfarin) and they should be informed of this high risk.

The risk of congenital heart disease (CHD) in the progeny of mothers with CHD is increased, and the data of Nora et al. are appropriate for this counseling.

Long-term Follow-up. The natural history of the patient who has had an operation or of the patient who did not have an operation is not clearly established, and long-term complications may occur. Therefore, long-term follow-up is necessary in all patients with congenital heart disease. Follow-up by the primary care physician, perhaps on a yearly basis, with visits to the pediatric cardiologists every 2 to 3 years is adequate. After reaching adulthood, follow-up of these patients by internist cardiologists or pediatric cardiologists once in 3 to 5 years is recommended.

TABLE 13.   **Contraception Methods and Comments**

Abstinence (virginity)	Reasonable in at least 50 per cent of 15 to 19 year olds; complications not reported
Birth control pills	Increased incidence of thromboembolic phenomena (less of a problem with mini pill); compliance is reduced in adolescent having infrequent encounters
Diaphragm and spermicidal	Effective when used appropriately; compliance is major detractor
Condom	Effective, can be carried by boy or girl; reduces incidence of venereal disease
Intrauterine device	Effective, but menorrhagia is common; pelvic inflammatory disease is frequent in females with multiple partners and increases the risk of bacterial endocarditis
Tubal ligation, vasectomy	An extreme measure which should be considered only after a great deal of discussion and counseling with clergy

ACKNOWLEDGMENT

The authors wish to thank Drs. Bruce Alpert, John Boineau, and Alex Robertson for reviewing this manuscript and for their constructive criticism.

CONGESTIVE HEART FAILURE

method of
RICHARD J. KATZ, M.D.,
and ALLAN M. ROSS, M.D.
Washington, D.C.

Definition

The sole function of the heart is to act as a pump. Heart failure exists (1) when there is inadequate blood provided to the pulmonary bed for oxygenation, (2) when there is excess pulmonary blood volume or pressure, or (3) when left heart forward cardiac output is inadequate to perfuse target organs.

Pathophysiologic Approach to Heart Failure

Understanding of the pathophysiologic basis of the types of "heart failure" is essential to the proper approach to the treatment of this group of disorders. The four major determinants of cardiac activity include (1) preload, (2) afterload, (3) contractility, and (4) heart rate. Abnormalities affecting one or more of these elements may disrupt pump function with resultant cardiac failure. *Preload* is defined as the initial stretch of the myocardial fiber (Frank-Starling mechanism). In man the strength of muscular contraction and the extent of myocardial fiber shortening are regulated by the length of the muscle at the onset of contraction (left ventricular end-diastolic volume). Excess preload will result in elevated pulmonary capillary pressure with subsequent pulmonary congestion and right heart failure. Common causes of elevated preload include cardiac dilatation from progressive myocardial damage of any etiology, overhydration from intravenous fluids, renal failure, transfusions, and contrast dye infusions. *Afterload* is the tension the heart must develop to empty the ventricle. The major determinant of afterload is peripheral vascular resistance, and the most common *extra*cardiac cause of increased afterload is systemic hypertension. The primary *intra*cardiac causes of elevated afterload include left ventricular outflow obstruction (aortic stenosis, idiopathic hypertrophic subaortic stenosis [IHSS]) and left ventricular dilatation of any etiology. In the failing heart the greater the outflow resistance facing the heart muscle, the less it will be able to empty. When outflow resistance is reduced (i.e., lowered blood pressure or surgical correction of aortic stenosis), cardiac function improves. *Myocardial contractility* is primarily dependent upon the number and size of myocardial fibers, the adequacy of their blood supply, and the quantity of calcium delivered to the heart's contractile proteins. These in turn influence the extent of myocardial fiber shortening. Common physiologic depressants of contractility are hypoxia, hypercapnia, acidosis, and hyperkalemia. These metabolic factors must be corrected to reverse cardiac pump dysfunction. Pharmacologic depressants of contractility include beta-adrenergic blockers, disopyramide phosphate, and possibly quinidine and procainamide. Pharmacologic stimulants of the contractile process include digitalis and sympathomimetic agents. *Heart rate* is normally determined by the rhythmicity of the sinus node. Both extreme tachycardia and bradycardia can result in congestive heart failure. Symptomatic tachycardia often requires treatment with antiarrhythmic drugs, whereas profound bradycardia must be treated with cardiac pacing.

One final category of causes of heart failure includes cardiac mechanical abnormalities. These include valvular stenosis (mitral, aortic), severe valvular regurgitation (mitral, aortic), acute ventricular septal rupture, and pericardial compression syndromes. In each of these situations operative correction (i.e., valve replacement, pericardiocentesis) of the mechanical lesion is the definitive mode of therapy, although pharmacologic treatment to improve preload, contractility, and afterload will be beneficial for interim therapy.

General Approach to Therapy of Heart Failure by Clinical Subsets

Heart failure commonly presents as one or two basic hemodynamic disturbances: (1) *Increased pulmonary capillary pressure*. This has been termed "backward failure," causing lung congestion with symptoms of dyspnea and orthopnea. (2) *Decreased cardiac output*. This has been called "forward failure," causing decreased oxygen supply to the peripheral tissues with resultant signs and symptoms of decreased organ function (fatigue, mental confusion, oliguria).

Therapy of heart failure should be selected based on the patient's clinical-hemodynamic subgroup (Fig. 1). *Subgroup A*, for comparison, is the asymptomatic patient with a normal Starling curve, requiring no treatment. *Subgroup B* represents patients with hypoperfusion alone (pure "forward failure"), in whom there is abnormally decreased preload (and thus no congestion). This group may have hypotension and reflex tachycardia owing to inadequate cardiac filling as caused by volume depletion (bleeding, overdiuresis), markedly decreased peripheral vascular resistance (anaphylaxis, septic shock), or profound bradycardia. Specific therapy should be directed at restoring preload by rehydration with intravenous fluids and colloid (blood, albumin), restoring peripheral vascular resistance with pressors, or maintaining adequate heart rate with cardiac pacing. *Subgroup C* includes patients with excessive preload but normal cardiac output and peripheral perfusion (pure "backward failure"). This clinical state often results from excess cardiac filling caused by overhydration or impaired diastolic ventricular function (pericardial effusion, mitral stenosis). The goal of treatment of this subgroup is to reduce lung congestion by reducing preload. The mainstay of therapy is diuresis either orally or intravenously. Other

CONGESTIVE HEART FAILURE: CLINICAL-HEMODYNAMIC SUBSETS

Figure 1.

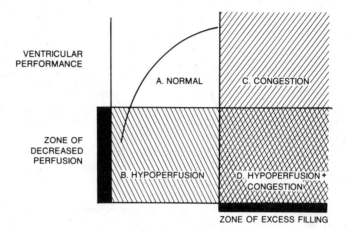

forms of preload reduction include venodilators (morphine, nitrates, or other vasodilators), venous pooling (upright position, tourniquets), or phlebotomy. As congestion is treated, however, it must be emphasized that *excessive* preload reduction will shift the patient from subgroup C to subgroup B, creating a *fall* in cardiac output and hypoperfusion. This complication is especially common when using potent diuretics. In addition, hypoperfusion may occur during diuresis of patients with impaired diastolic filling of the ventricles (pericardial effusion, mitral stenosis). In these cases effusion should be drained or stenosis surgically repaired. In *subgroup D*, patients present with combined symptoms and signs of pulmonary congestion and hypoperfusion (mixed "backward" and "forward" failure). Contractile function is reduced with decreased cardiac output and subsequent renal hypoperfusion, fluid retention, cardiac dilatation, and elevated pulmonary capillary pressure. Multiple drug therapy is usually required for this subgroup, and on occasion mechanical assist devices may be used. This extreme state with its attendant poor prognosis is often referred to as "pump failure," most commonly after a large myocardial infarction. In its extreme, subgroup D equates to "cardiogenic shock." Treatment of congestion should consist of diuretics and venodilators as discussed above for subgroup C patients; however, preload reduction will not augment cardiac output and hypoperfusion will persist. Further steps are needed to improve ventricular contractility; these may include digitalis orally or sympathomimetics intravenously (see Specific Pharmacologic Therapy, below). Additional improvement in ventricu-

lar systolic function may be achieved by adding an afterload reducing agent. Afterload therapy may be administered by either intravenous or oral routes, depending on the severity of the clinical setting. When congestive heart failure is severe and intravenous vasodilators are to be utilized, assessment should include invasive bedside hemodynamic monitoring with right-heart (pulmonary capillary wedge or Swan-Ganz) and intra-arterial catheters. Vasodilators are of particular benefit when blood pressure is elevated. When blood pressure is decreased (systolic <100 mm Hg), an intravenous inotropic agent with pressor activity such as dopamine may be required to be combined with a vasodilator. If congestive heart failure develops in the setting of ischemic heart disease, vasodilators are particularly preferable to inotropic agents, since the former usually reduce rather than raise myocardial oxygen demands.

Specific Pharmacologic Therapy

Diuretics. Thiazide diuretics are well tolerated orally administered agents with moderate potency. Their renal effects are primarily on the distal tubule and produce a notable kaliuresis. Most preparations in the thiazide group are relatively equipotent, with a half-life ranging from 12 to 48 hours, Hypokalemic metabolic acidosis is common, requiring supplementation with potassium chloride or combination with a potassium-sparing diuretic (see below). Serum uric acid elevation often develops but should not be treated with probenecid or allopurinol unless the patient has symptomatic gout. Since thiazide drugs are structurally related to sulfonamides, patients with known sulfa allergic reactions should avoid these medications.

Furosemide and ethacrynic acid are potent "loop diuretics" acting on the loop of Henle. They may be given orally, intramuscularly, or intravenously. Their diuretic effect may be preceded by systemic venodilatation within 5 to 10 minutes of administration, thus providing immediate preload reduction. The major advantages of this class of drugs are their rapid onset of action and marked diuretic effect, making them part of the first-line therapy of acute pulmonary edema. Oral and intravenous therapy with furosemide ranges from 40 to 200 mg and with ethacrynic acid from 50 to 250 mg once or twice a day. Hypokalemia must be monitored and treated as described with thiazides.

Potassium-sparing agents include spironolactone, an aldosterone antagonist (dose range 25 mg three or four times daily), and triamterene which acts on the distal tubule (dose range 50 to 100 mg one to two times daily). Both drugs are weak diuretics with slow onset of action and are best used in combination with either a thiazide or "loop" diuretic.

Occasionally severe congestive heart failure may be resistant to even a powerful intravenous "loop" diuretic. In such situations combination diuretic therapy with an oral thiazide approximately 30 to 45 minutes prior to an intravenous "loop" diuretic may help initiate diuresis by blocking the renal tubule at multiple sites. Another therapeutic maneuver for diuretic-resistant congestive heart failure is pretreatment of the patient with an oral, sublingual, topical, or intravenous afterload-reducing agent to improve renal perfusion and thus allow for effective diuretic action.

Inotropic Agents. DIGITALIS. For over 200 years digitalis has continued to be the only primary inotropic drug available for oral use. The digoxin preparation is absorbed approximately 80 per cent by the gastrointestinal tract and excreted primarily via the kidney. In the presence of normal renal function digoxin half-life is 36 hours and prolongs in proportion to increased creatinine. The daily maintenance dose must therefore be reduced with increased kidney failure. "Rapid digitalization" may be achieved by loading with digoxin, 0.5 to 1.0 mg intravenously or 1.0 to 1.5 mg orally. This is administered in divided doses (one half loading dose initially then the second half in two doses every 4 hours). "Slow digitalization" is attained by giving digoxin, 0.125 to 0.25 mg orally for 7 days. In the management of heart failure (as opposed to tachyrhythmia control) there is rarely or never a place for the

more rapid (and toxic) short-acting digitalis preparations such as ouabain.

Digitalis toxicity still occurs frequently (up to 30 per cent of cases). Digoxin serum levels are easily measured (therapeutic range 0.8 to 1.6 nanograms per ml) and can be helpful in assessing toxicity. Clinically this is usually manifest by cardiac arrhythmia (supraventricular or ventricular), particularly atrial tachycardia with block, accelerated junctional rhythm, or frequent ventricular ectopy. Specific therapy of digitalis toxicity is dependent upon the specific rhythm disturbance. In all cases digitalis should be discontinued and hypokalemia, if present, treated promptly with potassium supplements either orally or intravenously. Atrioventricular block is usually well tolerated unless it is of high degree, in which case temporary pacemaker insertion is required. Frequent ventricular ectopy should be treated initially with intravenous lidocaine. Phenytoin, procainamide, and propranolol also may be used (this use of phenytoin is not listed in the manufacturers' official directives).

CATECHOLAMINES. These intravenous drugs usually provide both increased contractility and a pressor effect. They are reserved for instances of severe refractory hypotension or as ancillary support during primary therapy with vasodilators (see below). The most commonly used agents include dopamine, isoproterenol, norepinephrine, and dobutamine. Each of these agents must be used with caution, since they often produce significant tachycardia and thus can aggravate myocardial ischemia. Dopamine (2 to 50 micrograms per kg per minute) has specific hemodynamic advantages compared to isoproterenol and norepinephrine in that at low doses (2 to 20 micrograms per kg per minute) it has predominant contractile (beta-adrenergic) effects without inducing hypertension or reducing renal blood flow. Dobutamine (2.5 to 15 micrograms per kg per minute) is a new inotropic agent with additional unique hemodynamic effects. This drug increases myocardial contractility without inducing marked tachycardia or greatly changing peripheral arterial resistance. Isoproterenol (1 to 10 micrograms per minute) and norepinephrine (4 to 8 mg in 1000 ml of 5 per cent dextrose in water [D5W] by infusion) possess powerful myocardial contractile properties; however, both are limited in use by marked tachycardia and by their actions to decrease (isoproterenol) or increase (norepinephrine) peripheral vascular resistance and thus lower or raise arterial pressure, respectively.

Vasodilators. This is a new class of drugs that has recently found widespread application for the treatment of congestive heart failure. The

TABLE 1.

DRUG	ROUTE OF ADMINISTRATION	VENODILATOR	ARTERIAL DILATOR	HALF-LIFE	DOSE
Isosorbide dinitrate	Oral	++	+	4–6h	10–40 mg q4–6h
Isosorbide dinitrate	Sublingual	++	+	1–2h	5–10 mg q4h
Nitroglycerine ointment	Topical	++	+	5–6h	½–2 inches q6h
Prazosin	Oral	++	++	6–8h	1–7 mg q6h
Hydralazine	Oral	0	++	6h	25–75 mg q6h
Morphine	IM, IV	++	++	2–4h	2–12 mg q4–6h
Nitroprusside	IV	++	+++	Minutes	15–400 micrograms/ min

vasodilators can be classified in Table 1 by their route of administration (intravenous, oral, topical, sublingual) and by their predominant site of effect — venodilatation (preload reduction) versus arterial dilatation (afterload reduction).

Nitrates provide effective preload reduction but must be combined with another drug, usually hydralazine, to provide significant afterload effects. They are further limited by short half-life and frequent headaches. Nitroglycerine ointment often may maintain a longer duration of action, but skin sensitization can limit its use. Prazosin has the advantage of a balanced preload and afterload lowering effect, but tachyphylaxis has been reported by some investigators and an increasing dose requirements can be anticipated. Also, significant hypotension may occur after the initial dose of prazosin or after increasing the dose. Hydralazine results in only afterload lowering and can cause further fluid retention. This can be treated by the addition of either diuretics or nitrates. A lupus-like syndrome may develop when dosage exceeds 200 mg per day. Morphine sulfate is a potent vasodilator drug. It has become a standard for treatment of pulmonary edema possessing both preload and afterload effects. Caution should be taken, however, since hypotension and respiratory depression may develop in some patients. Sodium nitroprusside is a powerful vasodilator that can be administered only intravenously and requires careful hemodynamic monitoring. Its rapid onset and short duration of action make it useful for acute severe congestive heart failure. Prolonged administration may result in neurologic signs of thiocyanate toxicity. It is imperative, when using any potent vasoactive drug, to recognize that rapid changes in a patient's hemodynamic status may result and that monitoring response is essential. Common examples of "oversuccessful" therapy include the conversion of a congestive failure patient to one who is functionally hypovolemic as a result of the administration of venodilators or diuretics. A patient requiring nitroprusside at one point could well require colloid infusion to sustain cardiac output an hour later.

INFECTIVE ENDOCARDITIS

method of
WALTER R. WILSON, M.D.,
and JOSEPH E. GERACI, M.D.
Rochester, Minnesota

Before the antibiotic era the mortality of patients with infective endocarditis (IE) was virtually 100 per cent. Today approximately 85 per cent of patients can be cured. In most other infectious diseases, host defenses play an important role. This is not the case with IE. Host defenses play little role in the control of IE. In no other infection does cure seem to be so dependent upon administration of appropriate bactericidal antibiotics. Advances in the technology of cardiac valve replacement have also reduced the mortality of patients with IE. Other factors influencing survival are the promptness of diagnosis and treatment, age and underlying conditions of the patient, and the microbiologic etiology.

General Principles of Therapy

Establish Bacterial Diagnosis. It is very important to establish the microbiologic etiology, if possible, before starting antimicrobial therapy. In the subacute form of IE, patients have often been ill for weeks or months and there is usually no great urgency to initiate antimicrobial therapy. Failure to establish the microbiologic cause in cases of suspected IE may result in prolonged hospitalization with increased cost to the patient and multiple iatrogenic complications related to the use of inappropriate therapy and possible relapse of infection.

The most important laboratory finding is the isolation of bacteria or fungi from at least two or more blood cultures obtained at intervals during a 48 hour period. Because bacteremias associated with IE are usually continuous, the timing of blood cultures is not critical, and if any blood cultures are positive, most of the other cultures drawn will also be positive. In patients who have not received prior antimicrobial therapy, streptococci may be isolated in 96 per cent of patients from the first blood culture and in 98 per cent from one of the first two blood cultures. Staphylococci may be isolated from the first blood culture in 90 per cent and from one of the first two cultures in 100 per cent of patients. It is rarely necessary to obtain more than three separate sets of blood cultures within a 24 hour period on 2 consecutive days in patients suspected of having IE. Blood culture bottles are inoculated so that a 1:10 ratio of bacteria to medium is achieved; this usually means an inoculum of 10 ml of blood. Each blood culture set should contain at least one bottle which is incubated anaerobically. Blood cultures should be incubated for at least 2 weeks before discarding as negative. If fastidious organisms are suspected, an even longer incubation period may be required. If after 48 to 72 hours of incubation the initial blood cultures remain negative, additional blood cultures should be obtained. These latter cultures are particularly helpful when patients have received antibiotics.

Use Bactericidal Therapy. Once the identification or Gram's stain and morphology of the organisms isolated from blood culture have been determined, bactericidal antibiotic therapy should be initiated promptly. The potential toxicity of the antimicrobial(s) chosen must be considered, and the least toxic, most effective regimen should be selected. The results of susceptibility tests may dictate changes in the antimicrobial regimen. The most widely used susceptibility test, and the simplest to perform, is the minimum inhibitory concentration (MIC) — the lowest concentration of antibiotics which will inhibit the growth of the causative bacteria. MIC may be measured by disc diffusion (Kirby-Bauer), agar dilution, or broth dilution methods. The minimum bactericidal concentration (MBC) — the lowest concentration of antimicrobial which will kill 99.9 to 100 per cent of the inoculum — is also helpful in determining optimal therapy. The MBC should be determined in all cases of IE to ensure that the antibiotic therapy is bactericidal. The peak serum concentration of the antibiotic administered should considerably exceed the MBC of the bacteria isolated from blood culture.

Use of Empiric Antimicrobial Therapy. In urgent cases or in the rare case of "culture-negative" IE in which empiric antimicrobial therapy must be initiated before the causative agent has been identified, the regimen should include a combination of antibiotics effective against enterococci and penicillinase-producing staphylococci.

Administer Antibiotics Parenterally. In general, antimicrobial therapy should be administered parenterally rather than orally. Absorption from the gastrointestinal tract of orally administered antimicrobial agents may be unpredictable.

Measure Serum Bactericidal Titer (SBT). The SBT measures the killing activity of the antimicrobial therapy in the patient's serum. Serial twofold dilutions are prepared of the patient's serum containing the antibiotic that has previously been administered to the patient. A standard inoculum of the patient's bacteria is transferred to each tube, and the tubes are incubated for 48 hours and subcultures performed. The results are expressed as the lowest dilution of patient serum which kills 99.9 to 100 per cent of the inoculum. Serum samples should be obtained at the anticipated peak serum antimicrobial concentration, usually 1 hour after administration of the antibiotic. Antibiotic therapy should be adjusted to achieve a peak serum concentration of antimicrobials which results in an SBT of 1:8 or more.

Consult with Cardiac Surgeon. It is preferable to treat patients with IE in facilities where emergency cardiac valve replacement may be performed if necessary. Patients with aortic valve IE may experience acute aortic insufficiency and severe congestive heart failure. Immediate cardiac valve replacement in these patients offers the only hope of survival.

Repeat Blood Cultures After Antimicrobial Therapy Started. Within 48 hours after institution of specific antimicrobial therapy, blood cultures should be obtained to assess the efficacy of treatment. Persistently positive blood cultures in spite of apparently appropriate therapy could indicate myocardial, aortic root, or distant abscesses, tolerance of bacteria to antimicrobial agents, or error in administration or dosage of antibiotics.

Perform Daily Physical Examinations During Treatment. Subtle changes in body weight, blood pressure, cardiac auscultatory findings, jugular venous distention, and so on may presage abrupt hemodynamic decompensation.

Identify and Eliminate Portal of Entry. Careful attention should be directed to eliminating the possible portal of entry, such as poor oral hygiene or urinary tract infections with or without stones. Dentulous patients with IE who are not critically ill should have dental x-ray films and an oral surgery consultation so that necessary dental work may be performed while the patient is receiving antimicrobial therapy for IE. Because of the association with inflammatory bowel disease and carcinoma of the colon, patients with IE caused by *Streptococcus bovis* should have a proctoscopic examination and colon x-ray studies while receiving antimicrobial therapy.

Instruct in IE Prophylaxis. Before dismissal from hospital, patients and their families should receive adequate instructions in prophylactic measures for IE.

Obtain Follow-up Blood Cultures. Follow-up blood cultures should be obtained at 1 and 2 months after completion of antimicrobial therapy. Relapses, if they occur, most often appear in the first two months after completion of therapy. Infections caused by fastidious microorganisms such as *Hemophilus* species may relapse later than 2 months.

Do Not Compromise with Therapy. Physicians should respect the seriousness of IE and should resist the temptation to compromise in the duration and means of administration of therapy or to switch to less effective antimicrobial agents. After initiation of therapy, some patients with IE, especially those with penicillin-sensitive streptococcal infections, will experience a dramatic improvement in general well-being and disappearance of fever. These improvements should not be interpreted as an indication that the antimicrobial may be switched to orally administered agents or that the length of treatment may be shortened. Symptomatic control of most hypersensitivity reactions should be attempted before changes are made to alternative therapy. If major hypersensitivity reactions or other complications occur which cannot be controlled by symptomatic measures, alternative therapy may be used. Clinicians should use only those accepted forms of alternative therapy outlined below or presented in standard texts and references.

Specific Antimicrobial Regimens

The antimicrobial therapy of choice and alternative regimens are given in Table 1. Additional information is provided below to assist in the selection of effective antimicrobial therapy.

Streptococcal IE. PENICILLIN-SUSCEPTIBLE STREPTOCOCCI (MIC < 0.2 MICROGRAM PER ML). The large majority of viridans streptococci and nonenterococcal group D streptococci (e.g., *S. bovis*) are exquisitely susceptible to penicillin.

Of the two regimens listed, the short-term (2 weeks) regimen is more cost effective than the 4 week regimen and is equally efficacious for the majority of patients. The 2 week regimen should not be administered to patients with symptoms of IE greater than 3 months in duration or to patients with suspected mycotic aneurysm, cerebritis, or shock, or with pre-existing renal insufficiency or vestibular abnormalities. In penicillin-allergic patients, the use of vancomycin is preferable to cephalothin. The in vitro susceptibility of streptococci to the cephalosporins is variable, and selection of a particular cephalosporin must be based on the results of susceptibility studies.

OTHER STREPTOCOCCI. Endocarditis caused by other groups of streptococci (e.g., groups B, C, G, H) and *Streptococcus pneumoniae* (pneumococci) should be treated with penicillin G, 20 million units intravenously, daily for 4 weeks. These microorganisms are highly susceptible to penicillin, and the addition of streptomycin to the therapeutic regimen in these patients does not increase the killing activity of penicillin.

RELATIVELY PENICILLIN-RESISTANT STREPTOCOCCI (MIC > 0.2 MICROGRAM PER ML). IE caused by relatively penicillin-resistant streptococci should be treated with aqueous penicillin G, 20 million units intravenously daily for 4 weeks, plus streptomycin, 500 mg intramuscularly every 12 hours, administered for the first 2 weeks of therapy.

ENTEROCOCCAL IE. Enterococci are inhibited but not killed in vitro by penicillin alone, and the successful treatment of patients with enterococcal IE requires the use of penicillin plus an aminoglycoside. The synergistic activities of the two antibiotics result in a bactericidal effect. The majority of cases should be treated with penicillin plus streptomycin. Recent studies have shown that approximately one third of enterococci are resistant to high concentrations of streptomycin (> 2000 micrograms per ml). Patients with infections caused by streptomycin-resistant enterococci should be treated with a combination of penicillin and gentamicin. The use of streptomycin may be associated with vestibular toxicity, and patients treated with gentamicin may develop renal insufficiency. Patients who are allergic to penicillin should be treated with vancomycin plus gentamicin. Cephalosporins *should not* be used to treat patients with enterococcal IE.

Staphylococcal IE. STAPHYLOCOCCUS AUREUS. A penicillinase-resistant penicillin (e.g., oxacillin or nafcillin) should be used initially in the treatment of *S. aureus* endocarditis. If the strain is shown not to produce penicillinase and to be susceptible to penicillin (MIC ≤ 0.1 microgram per ml), the oxacillin or nafcillin may be discontinued and therapy instituted with aqueous penicillin G. Vancomycin or the cephalosporins are suitable alternative agents for the treatment of *S. aureus* IE. In most instances, clindamycin is not bactericidal and not optimal therapy for these patients. Methicillin is not recommended because of the risk of methicillin-associated nephritis. The use of oxacillin or nafcillin may be associated with leukopenia and an elevation in hepatic enzymes. Periodic white blood cell count and liver function tests should be performed.

STAPHYLOCOCCUS EPIDERMIDIS. IE caused by *S. epidermidis* is usually associated with cardiac valve prosthesis or intracardiac foreign bodies. Most strains isolated from these patients are resistant to penicillin and methicillin, and most strains also contain subpopulations of organisms that are resistant to cephalosporins. Selection of antimicrobial therapy in these patients depends upon the results of in vitro susceptibility studies. The combination of vancomycin and rifampin is suggested for the treatment of methicillin-

TABLE 1.   **Treatment Regimens for Infective Endocarditis in Adults**

ORGANISM	REGIMENS OF CHOICE	DURATION (WEEKS)	ALTERNATIVE REGIMENS	DURATION (WEEKS)
Streptococci				
1. Penicillin-sensitive (MIC <0.2 microgram/ml) viridans and nonenterococcal group D; e.g., *S. bovis*	Aqueous penicillin G, 20 million units IV daily *or* Procaine penicillin, 1.2 million units IM q6h daily, or aqueous penicillin G, 10–20 million units IV daily *plus* Streptomycin,† 500 mg IM q12h daily	4 2 2	Vancomycin,* 7.5 mg/kg IV q6h daily *or* Cephalothin, 1.5 grams IV q4h daily	4 4
2. Other groups; e.g., A, B, C, F, H, *S. pneumoniae*	Aqueous penicillin G, 20 million units IV daily	4	Vancomycin* or cephalothin administered as above	4
3. Relative penicillin resistance (MIC >0.2 microgram/ml)	Aqueous penicillin G, 20 million units IV daily *plus* Streptomycin,† 500 mg IM q12h daily	4 2	Vancomycin,* 7.5 mg/kg IV q6h daily *plus* Streptomycin,† 500 milligrams IM q12h daily	4 2
4. Enterococcus	Aqueous penicillin G, 20 million units IV daily *plus* Streptomycin,† 500 mg q12h daily, or gentamicin,† 1 mg/kg IM or IV q8h daily	 4–6	Vancomycin,* 7.5 mg/kg IV q6h daily *plus* Gentamicin,† 1 mg/kg IM or IV q8h daily	 4–6
Staphylococci				
1. Penicillin-sensitive (MIC ≤0.1 microgram/ml) *S. aureus* or *S. epidermidis*	Aqueous penicillin G, 20 million units IV daily	4–6	Vancomycin,* 7.5 mg/kg IV q6h daily, or cephalothin, 2 grams IV q4h	4–6
2. Penicillin-resistant (MIC >0.1 microgram/ml), methicillin susceptible *S. aureus* or *S. epidermidis*	Oxacillin or nafcillin, 2 grams IV q4h daily	4–6	Vancomycin* or cephalothin administered as above	4–6
3. Methicillin-resistant *S. epidermidis*	Vancomycin,* 7.5 mg/kg q6h IV daily, plus rifampin,‡ 300 mg orally q8h daily	4–6	Cephalothin, 2 grams IV q4h daily, plus rifampin, ‡ 300 mg orally q8h daily	4–6
Gram-negative bacilli				
1. *Hemophilus* species, *Cardiobacterium hominis*, *Actinobacillus actinomycetemcomitans*	Ampicillin, 2 grams IV q4h daily	3	Penicillin allergy: desensitize patient and treat with ampicillin	
2. *Pseudomonas aeruginosa*	Carbenicillin, 35 grams IV daily, or ticarcillin 18 grams IV daily, in divided doses q4h *plus* Tobramycin,† 1.5 mg/kg IV q8h daily	6	Gentamicin,† 1.5 mg/kg, or amikacin,† 5 mg/kg, IV q8h daily (in lieu of tobramycin) if suggested by susceptibility tests	
3. Other gram-negative bacilli	See text	4–6		

TABLE 1.   **Treatment Regimens for Infective Endocarditis in Adults** (*Continued*)

ORGANISM	REGIMENS OF CHOICE	DURATION (WEEKS)	ALTERNATIVE REGIMENS	DURATION (WEEKS)
Miscellaneous bacteria				
1. *Neisseria* species	Aqueous penicillin G, 20 million units IV daily	4	Penicillin allergy: desensitize patient and treat with penicillin	
2. *Corynebacterium* species (diphtheroides) (MIC, gentamicin <4.0 micrograms/ml)	Aqueous penicillin G, 20 million units IV daily, plus gentamicin,† 1 mg/kg IM or IV q8h daily	4–6	Vancomycin,* 7.5 mg/kg IV q6h daily	4–6
(MIC, gentamicin ≥4.0 micrograms/ml)	Vancomycin,* 7.5 mg/kg IV q6h daily	4–6		
Fungi and yeast	Amphotericin B, 0.7–1.0 mg/kg IV daily, plus flucytosine, 150 mg/kg/day orally in divided doses q6h, plus cardiac valve replacement	6–8	None	
Culture-negative endocarditis	See text			

*Dosages of vancomycin must be adjusted in patients with renal insufficiency. Total daily dose of vancomycin is not to exceed 2 grams per day.

†Dosages of streptomycin, gentamicin, tobramycin, and amikacin must be adjusted in patients with renal insufficiency.

‡This use of this agent is not listed in the manufacturer's official directive.

resistant strains. Some authorities advocate the addition of gentamicin to vancomycin-rifampin therapy.

Gram-Negative Bacillary Endocarditis. HEMOPHILUS SPECIES, CARDIOBACTERIUM HOMINIS, ACTINOBACILLUS ACTINOMYCETEMCOMITANS. The great majority of these microorganisms are susceptible to ampicillin. *Hemophilus* strains should be tested for penicillinase production. In cases caused by susceptible strains, treatment with ampicillin alone is curative. Some authorities suggest the use of combined ampicillin-streptomycin therapy. In our experience, the use of streptomycin is not necessary. *Hemophilus* species endocarditis is frequently associated with the formation of large cardiac valve vegetations, and systemic embolization is not uncommon.

PSEUDOMONAS AERUGINOSA. Endocarditis caused by this organism usually occurs in addicts or patients with prosthetic heart valves. In addicts, the infection is frequently located on the tricuspid valve. These infections are highly resistant to antimicrobial therapy, and cardiac valve replacement or excision is frequently necessary.

OTHER GRAM-NEGATIVE BACILLI. The selection of antimicrobial therapeutic regimens for the treatment of endocarditis caused by other gram-negative bacilli is dependent upon the results of antimicrobial susceptibility testing. A combination of antimicrobial agents is often required. These combinations often consist of ampicillin, carbenicillin, or a cephalosporin plus an aminoglycoside administered parenterally for 4 to 6 weeks.

Miscellaneous Bacterial Causes of IE. NEISSERIA SPECIES.   IE caused by either the gonococcus or the meningococcus should be treated with aqueous penicillin G. *Neisseria gonorrhoeae* should be tested for penicillinase production.

CORYNEBACTERIUM SPECIES. These organisms are important causes of prosthetic valve endocarditis, especially that occurring during the initial months after cardiac surgery. The antibiotic susceptibility pattern of diphtheroids is unpredictable. The synergistic combination of penicillin plus gentamicin may be used when diphtheroids are susceptible to gentamicin (MIC < 4 micrograms per ml), regardless of the penicillin susceptibility. These bacteria are frequently susceptible to vancomycin, and this agent may be used to treat patients allergic to penicillin or those infected with a strain resistant to gentamicin.

Fungal or Yeast Endocarditis. Endocarditis caused by these microorganisms is rare and is usually associated with parenteral drug abuse or with recent cardiac valve replacement. Antifungal therapy should be administered with amphotericin B and 5-fluorocytosine (provided that the isolate is susceptible to 5-fluorocytosine in vitro). After 7 to 14 days' therapy the infected valve should be excised. Postoperative therapy with antifungal agents should be continued at least 4 weeks.

Culture-Negative Endocarditis. Improvement in microbiologic techniques has reduced the number of culture-negative cases to a small percentage of the total number of cases of IE. Prior use of antimicrobial agents is now the most common cause of "culture-negative" endocarditis. Rarely, culture-negative cases may be caused by Brucella species, *Coxiella burnetii,* fungi (especially Aspergillus), and fastidious gram-negative bacilli (e.g., Hemophilus species). Unless clinical epidemiologic or serologic data suggest otherwise, patients with culture-negative IE should be treated with regimens outlined for enterococcal endocarditis plus the addition of oxacillin or nafcillin. Noninfectious conditions which mimic culture-negative endocarditis include acute rheumatic fever, marantic endocarditis, atrial myxoma, carcinoid syndrome, and systemic lupus erythematosus.

Other Therapeutic Considerations

The Role of Cardiac Surgery in Patients with IE. During the antibiotic era, congestive heart failure has replaced sepsis as the leading cause of death among patients with IE, and most patients with IE who experience heart failure do so because of hemodynamic consequences of incompetent cardiac valves exacerbated by valvular infection. The operative mortality among patients who undergo cardiac valve replacement because of heart failure caused by IE is closely related to the degree of functional heart failure present at the time of operation, and patients with class IV heart failure have a significantly higher operative mortality than patients with class II heart failure. When compared with a similar group of patients without IE who undergo cardiac valve replacement, the operative mortality is remarkably similar to that of patients with IE when the degree of heart failure is the same at the time of surgery for both groups of patients. In patients with functional class IV heart failure or with sudden-onset severe aortic insufficiency associated with IE, urgent cardiac valve replacement probably offers the only hope for survival. Cardiac valve replacement may be successfully performed in these patients who have active infections even when blood cultures are positive in the immediate perioperative period. Procrastination in cardiac valve replacement in these patients in an attempt to stabilize heart failure by medical therapy or to complete a course of antimicrobial therapy preoperatively usually results in death from cardiac failure. We believe that the hemodynamic status of patients with IE should be the determining factor in timing of cardiac valve replacement rather than the activity of infection or the length of preoperative antimicrobial therapy.

Some authorities suggest that all patients with IE caused by *S. aureus* should undergo cardiac valve replacement. We do not believe that all patients with IE caused by *S. aureus* require cardiac valve replacement. In our experience, some patients with IE caused by this microorganism, especially those with tricuspid infection, can be treated successfully with medical management alone.

Cardiac valve infection may extend to adjacent myocardial tissue and result in myocardial abscess or sinus of Valsalva aneurysm, or the infection may involve the myocardial conduction system, resulting in dysrhythmia, variable heart block, and bradycardia. Physicians must be alert to these potential complications, especially those involving the conduction system. Urgent intervention with the use of transvenous or permanent cardiac pacemakers may be lifesaving in these patients.

The role of surgery in patients with recurrent systemic emboli is controversial. Emboli do not necessarily indicate antimicrobial failure. Recurrent major emboli may cause excess morbidity or may be fatal and are a possible indication for cardiac valve replacement.

Prosthetic Valve Endocarditis. Early surgical intervention in patients with prosthetic valve endocarditis is suggested in selected patients with one or more of the following complications: (1) most cases of endocarditis caused by staphylococci, (2) congestive heart failure caused by valve dysfunction, (3) valve dehiscence, and (4) recurrent relapse after appropriate antimicrobial therapy. Patients with prosthetic valve endocarditis who require the use of anticoagulants are cautiously maintained on warfarin sodium (Coumadin) with prothrombin times of one to one and a half times the control value. If central nervous system emboli occur in these patients, anticoagulants should be discontinued, the patient observed, and — if no additional emboli occur and there is no progression of central nervous system disease — anticoagulant therapy reinstituted cautiously.

Antibiotic Prophylaxis of Infective Endocarditis. The recommendations of the American Heart Association (Circulation 56:139A, 1977) are outlined in Table 2. The following cardiac abnormalities require prophylaxis: (1) congenital heart disease (except an uncomplicated secundum atrial septal defect and a ligated and divided ductus); (2) rheumatic or other acquired valvular heart disease; (3) idiopathic hypertrophic subaortic stenosis; (4) mitral valve prolapse with mitral regurgitation; (5) a prior episode of infective endocarditis; (6) all prosthetic cardiac valves; and (7) a calcified mitral annulus.

Prophylaxis is recommended during the following procedures: (1) all dental procedures likely to cause gingival bleeding, including professional cleaning; (2) surgery of the upper

TABLE 2. Antibiotic Prophylaxis to Prevent Endocarditis*

PROCEDURE	REGIMENS OF CHOICE	ALTERNATIVE REGIMENS
Dental procedures and surgery of the upper respiratory tract	Combined parenteral-oral program:† Aqueous penicillin G (1 million units IM) mixed with procaine penicillin G (600,000 units) given 30–60 minutes before procedure Follow with penicillin V (500 mg orally q6h for 8 doses)‡ Oral program: Penicillin V (2.0 grams orally) 30–60 minutes before procedure; thereafter 500 mg orally q6h for 8 doses† Combined parenteral-oral program:† Aqueous penicillin G (1 million units IM) mixed with procaine penicillin G (600,000 units IM) *plus* Streptomycin (1.0 gram IM) given 30–60 minutes prior to procedure; thereafter, penicillin V, 500 mg orally q6h for 8 doses‡	Program for patients allergic to penicillin: erythromycin (1.0 gram orally) 1.5–2 hours prior to procedure; thereafter, 500 mg orally q6h for 8 doses *or* Vancomycin (1.0 gram IV) over 30–60 minutes; vancomycin infusion started 30–60 minutes before procedure; thereafter, erythromycin, 500 mg orally q6h for 8 doses‡
Gastrointestinal and genitourinary tract surgery	Aqueous penicillin G (2 million units IM or IV) or ampicillin (1.0 gram IM or IV) *plus* Gentamicin (1.5 mg/kg IM, not over 80 mg total) Initial doses given 30–60 minute before procedure and repeated q8h for two additional doses‡	Program for patients allergic to penicillin: vancomycin (1.0 gram IV administered over 30–60 minutes) *plus* Streptomycin (1.0 gram IM) given 30–60 minutes prior to the procedure is probably sufficient, but the same dose may be repeated in 12 hours‡

*The interval between doses of aminoglycoside antibiotics must be modified if renal function is significantly reduced.
†The parenteral route of administration is preferred when practical, especially for patients considered to be at high risk.
‡In the case of delayed healing it may be wise to administer additional doses of antibiotics.

respiratory tract, e.g., tonsillectomy and adenoidectomy; (3) procedures of the upper respiratory tract, e.g., bronchoscopy, especially with a rigid bronchoscope; (4) surgery and instrumentation of the lower gastrointestinal tract and gallbladder; and (5) surgery or instrumentation of the genitourinary tract. Prophylaxis should also be used during obstetric infections and surgical procedures on infected tissues. In these latter situations, antibiotic regimens should be designed to be effective against the bacteria anticipated at the site of infection. Patients with prosthetic heart valves are at increased risk of developing endocarditis. Antibiotic prophylaxis in these patients is suggested, using the more vigorous parenteral regimens outlined in Table 2. In addition, in patients with prosthetic valves, prophylaxis is suggested for procedures that are not thought to require antibiotic coverage when performed on most patients with underlying heart disease. Such procedures include uncomplicated vaginal delivery, dilatation and curettage of the uterus, insertion and removal of intrauterine devices, liver biopsy, and upper gastrointestinal endoscopy.

The oral cavity of a patient receiving penicillin for rheumatic fever prophylaxis may harbor streptococci that are relatively resistant to penicillin. These patients should receive the penicillin-streptomycin regimen during dental or upper respiratory tract procedures.

HYPERTENSION

method of
JAMES W. WOODS, M.D.
Chapel Hill, North Carolina

Introduction

The benefits of blood pressure reduction and control are now well established. These benefits were evident for malignant hypertension in the late 1950s and were quickly demonstrated after hypotensive drugs became available, since most patients with this syndrome die within a year without treatment. It has also been shown that life can be prolonged by treatment in malignant hypertension even in the face of renal insufficiency. Establishment of the benefits of blood pressure reduction in patients with "benign" essential hypertension required a much longer period of study involving relatively large numbers of patients but had been accomplished by the Veterans Administration Cooperative Study by 1969 for patients with diastolic pressures above 105 mm Hg. The value of blood pressure reduction in mild hypertension (diastolic pressure 90 to 105 mm Hg) has just been shown by the large (10,500 patients), prospective, multicenter Hypertension Detection and Follow-up Program of the National Institutes of Health. These results were published in December 1979 and revealed a 20 per cent lower 5 year overall mortality for patients receiving aggressive stepped-care management when compared with patients referred back to their customary care (the control group). Further, there were 45 per cent fewer deaths attributed to cerebral vascular diseases and 46 per cent fewer deaths attributed to myocardial infarction in the aggressively treated group.

These results are of enormous potential significance for the nation's health, since 70 per cent of all hypertensives are in the stratum of diastolic pressures 90 to 105 mm Hg and approximately 60 per cent of the excess mortality attributable to high blood pressure overall occurs in this group. There is, therefore, a large potential for saving thousands of additional lives per year by identifying all persons with elevated diastolic blood pressure in the community and treating them effectively.

Management of the Hypertensive Patient

Initial Considerations. While the major thrust of this presentation will be on drug therapy, several important steps must precede the introduction of pharmacologic treatment.

1. A physician must question whether patients with mildly elevated routine blood pressure recordings are truly hypertensive, since anxiety, discomfort, physical activity, or other stress can acutely or transiently raise arterial pressure. It is therefore important to document significantly elevated pressure in the course of at least three examinations. This precaution is unnecessary in those with markedly elevated pressure or in those with evident target organ damage.

2. A carefully done diagnostic examination must be undertaken for the purposes of (a) detection of the severity of hypertension and the amount of end-organ damage (principally brain, eyes, heart, and kidneys), (b) detection of potentially curable causes, and (c) detection of other risk factors for cardiovascular disease.

3. Findings must be carefully explained to the patient. Understanding of the nature and risk of hypertension, the benefits of therapy, and the crucial importance of compliance with treatment are of greatest importance. Patients must be given the opportunity to ask questions and discuss points of concern. They must understand that this is a chronic disease which is often asymptomatic unless or until complications occur, that therapy is usually lifelong, and that benefits outweigh the nuisance value of drug therapy.

4. The patient's cooperation in adherence to a strict diet of about 85 mEq of sodium should be sought. The design of and instruction regarding such a diet by a therapeutic dietician facilitate this cooperation. Patients are told that adherence to the diet will enhance the response to diuretics, will reduce the chance of becoming hypokalemic, and may reduce the amount of pharmacologic treatment required. The latter is also true for reduction toward or to ideal weight if the patient is overweight. The diastolic pressure may be decreased about 4 mm of mercury for every 20 lb (9 kg) of weight loss.

Drug Therapy. A stepped-care approach to treatment has become popular and is quite rational. It calls for initiating therapy with a small dose of an antihypertensive drug, increasing the dose of that drug, and then adding, one after another, additional drugs as needed. The dose of each drug initially is low and subsequently is increased as needed to reach a predetermined therapeutic goal, usually below 140/90 mm Hg, while avoiding intolerable side effects. Any such plan should include periodic re-evaluation of blood pressure and regimen adjustment up and down as needed. Stepping down the drug dose, whenever possible, without compromising control, is obviously desirable. Such a stepped care plan might be as shown in Figure 1.

STEP 1: DIURETIC. Patients with mild hypertension (diastolic 90 to 105 mm Hg) will ordinarily be treated with a thiazide diuretic if blood pressure remains elevated after attempt at reduction to ideal weight and trial of a low sodium diet. The mechanism of hypertensive action is not certain, although chronic reduction of plasma volume, mobilization of sodium from arterial walls, a direct relaxing effect on smooth muscle, and production of decreased pressor responsiveness to endogenous pressors (catecholamines, angiotensin) are leading possibilities. Thiazide diuretics are the foundation of antihypertensive therapy, since they are often effective as single agents and are essential to multiple drug regimens by negating the sodium retention caused by each of the other drugs.

DRUG SELECTION (DOSE RANGE MG/DAY). Hydrochlorothiazide, 50–100. Chlorthalidone, 25–50. Furosemide, 40–120.

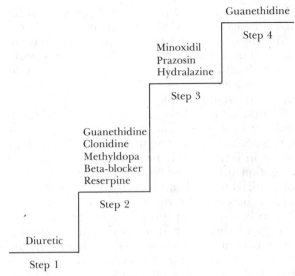

Guanethidine

Step 4

Minoxidil
Prazosin
Hydralazine

Step 3

Guanethidine
Clonidine
Methyldopa
Beta-blocker
Reserpine

Step 2

Diuretic

Step 1

Figure 1.

Hydrochlorothiazide and chlorthalidone are the most widely used diuretics. The thiazides, in contrast to furosemide, have relatively flat dose response curves, and doses larger than those shown above produce little additional hypotensive response but more hypokalemia and hyperuricemia. Furosemide is reserved for patients with renal insufficiency refractory to thiazide diuretics (serum creatinine above 3 to 4 mg per dl [100 ml]), hypertensive patients with intractable congestive heart failure, and hypertensive crises. When thiazides alone are inadequate, sodium intake is reviewed with the patient and a 24 hour urine sodium is measured. If excretion is greater than 100 mEq per day, the patient is given a choice of reducing sodium intake or having a second drug added to the regimen.

SIDE EFFECTS. 1. A decrease in serum potassium is frequent in thiazide-treated patients, but levels above 3.1 mEq per liter represent only mild total body depletion and do not require potassium supplement or addition of a potassium-sparing diuretic such as triamterene, spironolactone, or amiloride unless the patient is also receiving digitalis. Reductions of sodium intake and diuretic dosage are the simplest remedies. The cheapest potassium supplement is 10 per cent potassium chloride in water and is preferable if the patient can tolerate the disagreeable taste. Many flavored preparations and a slow release tablet are available. Foods rich in potassium are helpful, but their calories pose problems for the obese patient.

2. Asymptomatic hyperuricemia, unless very marked, does not require treatment or discontinuation of thiazide threatment. Acute gouty ar-

thritis obviously does require appropriate therapy.

3. Impaired carbohydrate tolerance is rarely a significant problem, is probably related to hypokalemia, and usually requires no more than a small increase in insulin dosage in insulin-dependent diabetics.

STEP 2: SYMPATHOLYTIC AGENTS. RESERPINE. Its mechanism of action is to prevent binding of norepinephrine and dopamine in the storage granules of postganglionic sympathetic fibers. This allows destruction of the unprotected catechols by the enzyme monamine oxidase. Neurotransmission is thus interfered with. Reserpine, in a dose of 0.1 to 0.25 mg daily, is an exceedingly useful drug in carefully selected patients. It should not be used in patients with chronic nasal obstruction, in patients inclined to mental depression, or in patients with active peptic ulcer disease. Although large doses of reserpine produce carcinoma of the breast in mice, there is no convincing evidence that this occurs in humans. It has the great advantage of once daily dosage and low cost. When combined with a diuretic, it may produce good blood pressure control in patients with moderate hypertension.

BETA-BLOCKING DRUGS. These agents are now widely used in hypertension. Propranolol has been the prototype drug in the United States, but several beta-blockers are now entering the market and they all differ from each other. They exert negative inotropic and chronotropic effects on the heart and appear to lower blood pressure principally by reducing cardiac output, although they also suppress plasma renin secretion and exert an effect on the central nervous system. A physician can now choose a beta-blocker which can be administered once daily (nadolol), which is relatively cardioselective (metoprolol, atenolol), and which is either largely metabolized by the liver or excreted by the kidney. If reserpine is contraindicated or not tolerated, these agents are our choice for a second drug to add to the diuretic. They should be used with caution in patients with asthma or congestive failure. Beta-blockers in adequate dosage will completely neutralize the reflex sympathetic stimulation produced by vasodilators such as hydralazine and minoxidil and serve an extremely useful role in such three drug regimens in patients with moderately severe or severe hypertension. Dosages of the currently Food and Drug Administration (FDA)–approved beta-blockers are as follows: propranolol, 10–160 mg every 12 hours; metoprolol, 25–200 mg every 12 hours; nadolol, 40–320 mg once daily.

GUANETHIDINE. This drug prevents uptake

of norepinephrine by postganglionic sympathetic fibers. It is customarily thought of as belonging in Step 4 but can serve a useful role in either Step 2 or Step 3 in low dosage (25 mg or less), with which the side effects of diarrhea, orthostatic hypotension, and retrograde ejaculation are rarely seen. At low dosage it has advantages of once daily administration and relatively low cost. The combination of thiazide, reserpine, and guanethidine is inexpensive, can be given once daily, and is quite potent. Oates demonstrated that 10 mg per day of guanethidine was as effective as reserpine. In severe hypertension up to 200 mg per day may be used. Its effect is blocked by tricyclics, phenothiazines, and ephedrine and may cause marked bradycardia in patients who are digitalized.

METHYLDOPA. This moderately potent drug is used when reserpine or beta-blockers are contraindicated and when a rapid effect is desired. An average dose is 250 mg every 8 hours, but up to 2 grams daily may be given and it is being used presently on a twice daily schedule. It exerts a direct alpha sympathomimetic inhibitory action on the vasomotor center and in this respect is similar to clonidine. Its adverse effects include drowsiness, fatigue, depression, hemolytic anemia, and hepatitis.

CLONIDINE. Its mechanism of action has been described previously. It may be used as a Step 2 drug when reserpine is not tolerated or when beta-blockers are contraindicated because of asthma or congestive heart failure. The dose is 0.1 to 1 mg every 12 hours. Drowsiness and dryness of the mouth are frequent side effects, but it produces little orthostatic hypotension or impotence. It should be used only in reliable patients, since sudden discontinuance may result in a rebound effect and even development of hypertensive encephalopathy. It may also be used as a Step 4 drug.

STEP 3: VASODILATORS. Three vasodilators are now available and are very useful when combined with a diuretic and a beta-blocker.

HYDRALAZINE. This is the oldest of this class, and it is effective in doses up to 150 mg twice daily. In larger doses a rheumatoid-like or lupus-like syndrome may be produced. Tolerance to it does not develop. It is being widely used now in cardiac patients for afterload reduction in low output syndromes.

PRAZOSIN. It dilates both arteries and veins and thus reduces both preload and afterload. In this respect, it is similar to nitroprusside and because of a more balanced effect does not produce as much reflex sympathetic stimulation as do hydralazine and minoxidil. Its mechanism of action is not well understood. The dose is up to 20 mg daily given in twice daily divided doses.

Tolerance may develop to this drug, but definitive studies are needed. The major side effect is "first dose syncope," marked postural hypotension occurring after the first dose and occasionally with an increase in dosage. The first dose or an increased dose is best given at bedtime in order to avoid this side effect.

MINOXIDIL. This very potent vasodilator is similar to hydralazine in action but perhaps ten times as potent. The dose is 5 to 20 mg daily given in one dose. It produces marked sodium retention unless used with furosemide (in place of a thiazide) and must be used in conjunction with a beta-blocker to prevent tachycardia and headache. It is very useful in severe hypertension, and this three drug regimen will control most patients with accelerated or malignant hypertension. Its most distressing side effect is increased facial hair. It is, therefore, tolerated better by males than females. Despite this side effect it may be lifesaving.

Preoperative withdrawal of antihypertensive drugs is usually unnecessary prior to surgery. Management of high blood pressure must be considered a lifelong endeavor, with the levels of blood pressure the criteria of its adequacy. After control has been demonstrated and the patient's blood pressure is stable, remeasurement every 3 to 6 months should be adequate for most patients. The need for repeat laboratory and baseline tests should be individualized according to the patient's age, initial severity of hypertension, and target organ damage.

Hypertensive Emergencies

Hypertensive patients with confusion, headache, somnolence, fleeting neurologic signs, papilledema, left ventricular failure, intracranial hemorrhage, and aortic dissection are in urgent need of rapid blood pressure reduction. Our first choice is sodium nitroprusside given by infusion pump in an intensive care unit with close blood pressure monitoring. The dose is 0.5 to 10 micrograms per kg per minute. Miniboluses of 50 to 100 mg of diazoxide given rapidly intravenously every 15 minutes until a desired level of blood pressure is reached may also be satisfactory. Its use must be accompanied by daily furosemide in order to prevent sodium retention. Oral regimens consisting of diuretic, beta-blocker, and either hydralazine or minoxidil may control pressure within 24 to 36 hours if an intensive care bed is not available and if the patient can take oral medication. Oral regimens should be started shortly after parenteral therapy is begun so that intravenous therapy and time in the intensive care unit may be as short as possible. Patients with malignant hypertension complicated by renal insufficiency should also be treated aggressively.

Summary

The means are now available for blood pressure control in most hypertensive patients, and the benefits of control, even in mild hypertension, have been demonstrated. Side effects and cost of drugs continue to be a problem but are not an unreasonable price to pay for health and life. Patient education and patient compliance with the regimen are of greatest importance. New understanding of etiologic mechanisms and continued development of new pharmacologic agents are anticipated.

ACUTE MYOCARDIAL INFARCTION

method of
L. DAVID HILLIS, M.D.,
and BRIAN G. FIRTH, M.D.
Dallas, Texas

Over the past 5 to 10 years the therapy of acute myocardial infarction has changed substantially. First, extensive evidence has accumulated in both experimental animals and man that the process of infarction following the cessation of blood flow to a portion of myocardium occurs over a period of at least several hours. As a result, therapeutic approaches have been devised which attempt to limit the extent of necrosis in patients with myocardial infarction. Second, preliminary studies suggest that coronary artery spasm may contribute to the occurrence and extent of acute myocardial infarction, at least in some patients. Therefore, therapeutic agents designed to alleviate spasm may be especially efficacious in patients with infarction. In short, as more information is gathered about the etiology and pathophysiology of myocardial infarction, the treatment of the patient with infarction is changing.

Care "in the Field" of the Patient with Acute Myocardial Infarction

About 50 per cent of the persons who die of acute myocardial infarction do so before the arrival of trained medical or paramedical personnel. Although some of these deaths are secondary to severe left ventricular dysfunction (with resul-

tant pulmonary venous congestion and inadequate cardiac output), most are due to either asystole or ventricular fibrillation occurring within seconds to minutes of infarction. Therapeutic efforts to reduce the incidence of dysrhythmic deaths have centered on programs designed to train the lay population in external cardiopulmonary resuscitation. If resuscitative maneuvers are initiated quickly and are continued until the victim reaches a hospital, many of these dysrhythmic deaths are preventable.

Ideally, a large portion of the lay population should be able to initiate external cardiopulmonary resuscitation. In turn, this widespread capability should be supported by a group of highly trained paramedical personnel who can continue the resuscitation, administer intravenous fluids and appropriate cardioactive medications, and transport the victim to a hospital. The rapidity with which these personnel reach the victim and accomplish his transfer is very important.

In some cities, the paramedical personnel attending the patient with an apparent myocardial infarction begin an intravenous infusion of a standard 5 per cent dextrose in water solution, after which they prophylactically administer atropine sulfate, 1.0 mg by intravenous bolus, and lidocaine, 50 to 100 mg by intravenous bolus, followed by a continuous infusion of 2 mg per minute. In addition, the patient is begun on oxygen at 4 liters per minute via nasal cannula or mask. The administration of atropine and lidocaine "in the field" to all patients with suspected myocardial infarction does not have proved utility.

Care in the Emergency Room of the Patient with Acute Myocardial Infarction

Once the patient with a myocardial infarction reaches the emergency room (ER), several therapeutic and diagnostic procedures are instituted immediately. The therapeutic maneuvers of greatest importance are as follows:

Intravenous Access. If the patient does not have a functioning intravenous line, one is established immediately, with 5 per cent dextrose in water as the standard solution.

Oxygen. The patient receives supplemental oxygen (4 liters per minute) by nasal cannula or mask.

Patient Comfort. The patient is allowed to assume whatever position is most comfortable (i.e., sitting upright rather than supine).

Analgesia. The patient is given sufficient analgesia to relieve pain completely. This is best accomplished with morphine sulfate (2 to 5 mg intravenously every 5 minutes) or meperidine (20 to 50 mg intravenously every 5 minutes), provided that systemic arterial pressure is well maintained.

Prophylactic Antiarrhythmic Agents. Although atropine and lidocaine are administered prophylactically at some institutions to all patients with suspected myocardial infarction, we do not administer these agents unless they are specifically indicated.

Avoidance of Intramuscular Injections. In the ER and coronary care unit (CCU), no intramuscular injections are performed, since they make it difficult to interpret subsequent elevations in cardiac enzymes.

In the ER, several diagnostic procedures are performed:

History and Physical Examination. When time permits, a brief history is obtained by the responsible physician, and a physical examination is performed.

Electrocardiogram (ECG). A 12 lead ECG is obtained and compared to previous tracings. In the early phase of myocardial infarction, the ECG may be completely normal. Therefore, the diagnosis of possible infarction is made on clinical grounds alone.

Continuous Electrocardiographic Monitoring. During the patient's brief stay in the ER, continuous electrocardiographic monitoring is performed.

Blood Tests. Blood samples are obtained for routine testing (i.e., complete blood count, serum electrolytes, blood urea nitrogen, serum glucose, serum creatinine, etc.) and for the quantitation of cardiac enzymes (creatine kinase [CK], serum glutamic oxaloacetic transaminase [SGOT], and lactic dehydrogenase [LDH]).

Chest Roentgenogram. A portable chest x-ray is performed.

As soon as the proper arrangements are made, the patient is transferred to the CCU with at least one physician in attendance and continuous electrocardiographic monitoring. The responsible physician has available a portable defibrillator; syringes of atropine sulfate, lidocaine, sodium bicarbonate, epinephrine, and calcium chloride; and a laryngoscope, an endotracheal tube of appropriate size, and an Ambu bag.

Care in the Coronary Care Unit of the Patient with Uncomplicated Acute Myocardial Infarction

Physical Activity. During the first 1 to 2 days after acute myocardial infarction, the patient's physical activities are limited as much as possible. Realistically, the patient is allowed to use a bed-side commode for urination and defecation, but his transfer from the bed to the commode and vice versa is accomplished with assistance. The amount of physical strain and exertion required of the patient is minimized during this 1 to 2 day period.

If the patient's initial course in the CCU is uncomplicated, he is allowed to sit in a chair for progressive periods on days 3 and 4 after infarction. Again, the transfer of the patient from bed to chair is performed with assistance. By day 4 after an uncomplicated infarction, the patient is allowed to sit in a chair for a total of 2 to 3 hours.

Diet. The diet served to the patient in the CCU is palatable and tasteful and yet does not contain an abundance of salt or rich, spicy foods that may cause indigestion. Salt intake is restricted to lessen the chance of the patient's developing venous congestion resulting from left ventricular dysfunction. In addition, the patient's meals are not unusually large or bulky, as a large meal may precipitate an episode of angina pectoris because of an increase in myocardial oxygen demands. Since unusually hot or cold foods may cause transient electrocardiographic ST and T wave alterations, they are avoided in this setting. Finally, in an attempt to encourage the patient on a long-term basis to minimize the ingestion of saturated fats, the diet in the CCU is low in such fatty foods.

Supplemental Oxygen. Humidified oxygen (at 4 liters per minute) is administered by nasal cannula or mask to all patients with myocardial infarction except those with severe chronic lung disease and resultant carbon dioxide retention.

Diagnostic Procedures. Several procedures are performed routinely to confirm the diagnosis of myocardial infarction. First, a 12-lead ECG is obtained at least once daily during the patient's stay in the CCU. Second, blood samples are obtained every 12 hours for cardiac enzyme quantitation. Third, a portable anteroposterior chest x-ray is obtained daily. Fourth, a 99m technetium stannous pyrophosphate scintigram is obtained 2 to 4 days after the clinical event in an effort to diagnose and to localize the new infarction. If the initial scintigram is negative in a patient in whom the clinical suspicion of myocardial infarction is strong, another scan is performed on the fifth or sixth day after admission.

Sedation. The patient receives enough sedation so that he is not anxious or emotionally distraught over his condition. In some CCUs nitrous oxide administered by mask is used for this purpose, but in our CCU oral diazepam, 5 to 15 mg every 6 to 8 hours, is preferred. In addition, a sleeping medication often is required. Flurazepam, 30 mg by mouth, or chloral hydrate, 500 mg orally, is employed commonly for this purpose.

Stool Softeners and Laxatives. Every attempt is made in the patient with myocardial infarction to reduce the necessity for vigorous physical exertion. Since straining at stool is undesirable, stool softeners and laxatives are administered to the patient in the CCU. We routinely give dioctyl sodium sulfosuccinate, 50 to 100 mg orally per day, and milk of magnesia, 15 to 30 ml by mouth per day, to all patients with myocardial infarction.

Analgesics. For the initial relief of the pain of myocardial infarction, morphine sulfate, 2 to 5 mg intravenously every 5 minutes, or meperidine, 20 to 50 mg intravenously every 5 minutes, is administered. The systemic arterial pressure is observed carefully, as these agents may cause hypotension.

Continuation of Maintenance Medications. Oftentimes the patient with a myocardial infarction has been taking cardioactive medications prior to infarction. Unless there is good reason to discontinue these medications, they are administered as usual.

DIGITALIS. If the patient has been on maintenance digitalis, it is continued at the usual dose unless there is evidence of intoxication. Patients with myocardial infarction develop digitalis intoxication more easily than patients without infarction.

PROPRANOLOL. If the patient has taken propranolol regularly prior to infarction, it is continued. However, if bradyrhythmias and/or left ventricular dysfunction appear, propranolol is tapered rapidly and eliminated over a 1 to 3 day period. If possible, propranolol is discontinued gradually, since sudden withdrawal may induce severe angina pectoris or even myocardial infarction.

NITRATES. If the patient has been maintained on long-acting nitrates prior to infarction, these are continued unless hypotension occurs, in which case they are discontinued.

ANTIARRHYTHMICS. If the patient has been on oral antiarrhythmic therapy prior to infarction, it is continued unless there is evidence of toxicity.

Prophylaxis Against Arrhythmias. Some physicians feel that all patients with myocardial infarction, even those who are totally without complications, should receive prophylactic intravenous lidocaine to suppress ventricular arrhythmias. At our institution, we do not administer lidocaine prophylactically, as it is not of proved utility when used this way.

Anticoagulation. Some physicians administer intravenous or subcutaneous heparin to all patients with myocardial infarction. At our institution, we initiate heparin therapy only if there is a specific and compelling clinical reason. For the patient with deep venous thrombosis, pulmonary embolism, or systemic embolism, heparin is given intravenously, either as 5000 to 7000 units every 4 hours by bolus or as 1000 to 1500 units per hour by continuous infusion. For the patient with peripheral venous congestion or the patient in whom prolonged bed rest is anticipated, heparin is administered subcutaneously in a dose of 5000 units every 12 hours in an attempt to prevent deep venous thrombosis and pulmonary embolism.

Care in the Coronary Care Unit of the Patient with a Complicated Myocardial Infarction

Abnormalities of Rate and Rhythm. ATRIAL ARRHYTHMIAS. *Sinus bradycardia* (sinus rhythm with a rate less than 60 beats per minute) is a relatively frequent accompaniment of myocardial infarction, especially when the inferior portion of the left ventricle is involved. Especially in this setting, it carries a good prognosis. If the sinus bradycardia is not severe (i.e., less than 40 beats per minute) and not associated with systemic arterial hypotension, angina pectoris, or ventricular irritability, it requires only careful observation. If treatment is necessary, atropine sulfate, 0.6 to 1.0 mg by intravenous bolus, is administered and can be repeated two to three times. If atropine is unsuccessful in abolishing the bradycardia, a temporary transvenous pacemaker is utilized. Isoproterenol, a positive chronotropic and inotropic agent, is avoided because of its marked augmentation of myocardial oxygen demands, which may aggravate myocardial ischemic injury, as well as its propensity to cause ventricular arrhythmias.

Sinus tachycardia (sinus rhythm with a rate greater than 100 beats per minute) in the setting of myocardial infarction can be caused by fever, fright or anxiety, persistent discomfort resulting from ongoing ischemia or pericarditis, or intravascular volume depletion. In addition, it may be a subtle manifestation of left ventricular dysfunction. A persistent tachycardia is deleterious in the setting of myocardial infarction because it increases myocardial oxygen demands; therefore, its underlying cause should be isolated and corrected as quickly as possible. Fever is controlled with an antipyretic agent such as acetylsalicylic acid, 650 mg by mouth every 4 to 6 hours. Fright or anxiety is treated with adequate reassurance and sedation. Persistent chest pain is relieved

TABLE 1. **Therapy of Dysrhythmic Complications of Acute Myocardial Infarction**

COMPLICATION	SPECIAL CIRCUMSTANCE	THERAPY (SEE TEXT FOR DETAILS)
Sinus bradycardia	Asymptomatic	Close observation
	Severe and/or symptomatic	IV atropine; if needed, temporary pacing
Sinus tachycardia		Correction of underlying cause
Atrial fibrillation with rapid ventricular response	Hemodynamically stable; no chest pain	IV digoxin or IV propranolol or IV verapamil*
	Hemodynamically unstable; chest pain	DC shock
Atrial flutter with rapid ventricular response		DC shock or IV verapamil*
Paroxysmal supraventricular tachycardia	Hemodynamically stable; no chest pain	Carotid sinus massage
		IV digoxin
		IV propranolol
		IV verapamil*
	Hemodynamically unstable; chest pain	DC shock
Ventricular premature beats	Infrequent, unifocal, far from preceding T wave	Close observation
	Frequent, multifocal, pairs or runs, close to preceding T wave	IV lidocaine; if needed, IV procainamide
Accelerated idioventricular rhythm	Hemodynamically stable	None
	Hemodynamically unstable	IV atropine
Ventricular tachycardia	Hemodynamically stable	IV lidocaine
	Hemodynamically unstable	DC shock
Ventricular fibrillation		DC shock

*Not available in the United States of America.

with intravenous morphine sulfate in the doses noted previously.

If sinus tachycardia persists despite these measures, a flow-directed, balloon-tipped catheter is introduced, and the pulmonary arterial and capillary wedge pressures are measured. In the absence of mitral valve disease, the pulmonary capillary wedge pressure is equal to left ventricular filling pressure. A wedge pressure less than 12 mm Hg indicates that the patient has inadequate intravascular volume. Therefore, the sinus tachycardia is a manifestation of hypovolemia and is corrected by amounts of normal saline or lactated Ringer's solution sufficient to increase the filling pressure to 16 to 20 mm Hg. In contrast, if left ventricular filling pressure is abnormally elevated (greater than 22 mm Hg), digoxin is initiated, 0.5 mg by intravenous bolus, followed by 0.25 mg intravenously 6 and 12 hours later, and then by a daily maintenance dose dependent on the patient's renal function. In addition, furosemide, 20 to 40 mg by intravenous bolus, is administered and can be repeated every 12 hours. The serum potassium is monitored to ensure that furosemide does not induce hypokalemia.

If the wedge pressure is between 12 and 22 mm Hg, the sinus tachycardia presumably is due to excessive catecholamine production and is best treated with small doses of intravenous propranolol, 1 mg every 3 minutes until either the sinus tachycardia subsides or a total dose of 5 to 7 mg is given. Both the systemic arterial and pulmonary

capillary wedge pressures are monitored as the propranolol is administered. Once the initial dosage of propranolol has been given intravenously, a small oral dose is instituted (i.e., 10 to 20 mg every 6 hours).

Atrial fibrillation occurs in about 10 per cent of patients with myocardial infarction. If the ventricular response is rapid, atrial fibrillation is especially deleterious in the setting of acute myocardial infarction, since any sustained tachycardia, regardless of its origin, increases myocardial oxygen demands and, consequently, infarct size. Therefore, in this clinical setting, the ventricular response is controlled as quickly as possible.

If atrial fibrillation with a rapid ventricular response causes *hemodynamic instability,* leading to pulmonary and/or peripheral venous congestion, systemic arterial hypotension, or cerebral or myocardial hypoperfusion, immediate therapeutic measures are instituted. After the patient has received diazepam to induce mild to moderate sedation (5 mg by intravenous bolus every 3 minutes until light anesthesia is produced), he is cardioverted with DC (direct current) countershock. The conversion of atrial fibrillation to sinus rhythm generally requires more than 100 watt-seconds. In contrast, if, despite a rapid ventricular response, the patient is *hemodynamically stable,* he is given digoxin or propranolol to slow the ventricular rate as quickly as possible. An initial dose of 0.50 to 0.75 mg of intravenous digoxin is followed every 3 to 4 hours by 0.25 mg until the ventricular response has fallen to 80 to

100 per minute. If the patient has no contraindication to propranolol (such as second or third degree atrioventricular block, left ventricular dysfunction, or severe pulmonary disease), it may be administered as a 1 mg intravenous bolus every 3 minutes up to a total dose of 5 to 7 mg.

Once the ventricular response is controlled with intravenous digoxin or propranolol, it is maintained with these same agents administered orally. Prior to the patient's hospital discharge, pharmacologic reversion to sinus rhythm may be attempted with oral quinidine or procainamide; if this is unsuccessful, DC countershock may be performed.

Verapamil has been used in Europe, Australia, and South Africa for the therapy of supraventricular tachyrhythmias, and it probably will be available in the United States in the near future. In the patient with atrial fibrillation and a rapid ventricular response, verapamil, 10 mg in 150 ml of 5 per cent dextrose in water, is infused intravenously at a rate sufficient to slow the ventricular response to 90 to 100 per minute. Once this ventricular response is achieved, the rate of infusion is adjusted appropriately. In the meantime, the patient is given digoxin. The verapamil infusion is continued long enough to allow the concomitantly administered digoxin to take effect. In a minority of patients, verapamil causes a reversion of atrial fibrillation to sinus rhythm.

Atrial flutter occurs occasionally in the setting of myocardial infarction. The resultant tachycardia may aggravate the extent of myocardial damage. DC countershock is the treatment of choice for the patient with mycardial infarction and atrial flutter. After initial dosages of digoxin and quinidine are administered, the patient undergoes DC countershock with light anesthesia provided by intravenous diazepam. Atrial flutter usually reverts to sinus rhythm with 10 to 50 watt-seconds of energy. Subsequent to reversion, the patient is maintained on digoxin and either quinidine or procainamide to prevent a recurrence of flutter.

Verapamil also may be used in the manner described previously. In the patient with atrial flutter, it increases the degree of atrioventricular block, thus slowing the ventricular response. Approximately 10 to 15 per cent of patients revert to sinus rhythm with verapamil.

Paroxysmal supraventricular tachycardia rarely occurs in the patient with myocardial infarction. Its deleterious effects in this setting are due to the resultant tachycardia and increased myocardial oxygen demands. Various maneuvers designed to stimulate the vagus nerve may revert this tachyrhythmia to sinus rhythm, such as carotid sinus massage. Pressor agents, edrophonium, and

the Valsalva maneuver should be avoided in the patient with a myocardial infarction. Intravenous propranolol, 1 mg every 3 minutes for a total of 5 to 7 mg, may be administered unless there is a contraindication. Alternatively, intravenous digoxin in the doses mentioned previously may be given to revert the tachycardia to sinus rhythm. If immediate reversion is necessary, DC countershock, 100 to 200 watt-seconds, is used after light anesthesia with intravenous diazepam.

When it becomes available, verapamil is the agent of choice for the treatment of paroxysmal supraventricular tachycardia. It is administered intravenously either as a bolus injection of 5 mg (which may be repeated once or twice at 5 minute intervals) or as a slow infusion as detailed previously. Verapamil induces a reversion to sinus rhythm in more than 90 per cent of patients with paroxysmal supraventricular tachycardia.

VENTRICULAR ARRHYTHMIAS. *Ventricular premature beats* (VPBs) occur commonly in the setting of myocardial infarction. During the first 24 to 48 hours after infarction, VPBs that are frequent (greater than 5 per minute), of more than one morphology, in pairs or runs, and/or in close proximity to the preceding T wave should be treated aggressively. The drug of choice for the treatment of VPBs is intravenous lidocaine. An initial bolus injection of 50 to 100 mg is followed by a continuous infusion of 1 to 4 mg per minute. The rate of infusion is reduced in the patient with venous congestion, cardiogenic shock, or hepatic dysfunction. Serious side effects of lidocaine include focal and grand mal seizures, psychosis, and rarely respiratory arrest. Paresthesias, muscle twitching, disorientation, drowsiness, and impaired hearing may necessitate a reduction in the rate of infusion.

If lidocaine cannot be given or is unsuccessful in the control of ventricular ectopy, procainamide may be effective. It is administered intravenously at 25 mg per minute to a total dose of 1 gram, after which a maintenance infusion of 2 mg per minute is employed. The systemic arterial pressure is monitored, since procainamide may cause hypotension. The effective plasma concentration is 4 to 8 micrograms per ml.

Disopyramide phosphate is an effective oral antiarrhythmic agent, especially for the management of ventricular ectopy. It is administered orally in a dose of 100 to 150 mg every 6 hours, which usually gives a plasma concentration of 2 to 4 micrograms per ml. Its untoward side effects are related to its anticholinergic properties and include dryness of the mouth, urinary retention, constipation, abdominal discomfort, blurred vision, and dizziness. In addition, it may adversely affect left ventricular function in the patient with poorly compensated congestive heart failure. Disopyramide is contraindicated in patients with acute pulmonary edema, uncontrolled congestive heart failure, cardiogenic shock, glaucoma, and urinary retention. In addition, it may be harmful to patients with sinus node dysfunction, sinus pauses, or sinoatrial exit block.

Quinidine sulfate may be used to suppress VPBs in the patient with myocardial infarction, although it is preferred more commonly for long-term suppression. Quinidine administered intravenously can cause severe hypotension, and at our institution intravenous administration is forbidden. Therefore, quinidine sulfate is given orally at a dose of 200 to 300 mg every 6 hours. Its mechanism of action is similar to that of procainamide. Nausea, vomiting, and diarrhea are the most frequent untoward effects.

When conventional doses of lidocaine, procainamide, disopyramide, and quinidine do not abolish ventricular ectopy, propranolol should be used in those patients in whom it is not contraindicated. The dosage of intravenous propranolol is the same as that employed to treat atrial fibrillation or flutter (1 mg every 3 minutes for a total of 5 to 7 mg). Once initial control of the ectopy is achieved with intravenous propranolol, the patient may be started on an oral maintenance dose of 10 to 40 mg every 6 hours.

Occasionally, phenytoin sodium (diphenylhydantoin) is useful for suppressing VPBs in the setting of myocardial infarction. (This use of phenytoin is not listed in the manufacturer's offical directive.) A loading dose of phenytoin is administered as 100 mg intravenously every 5 minutes to a total dose of 1 gram. Subsequently, the patient is given a maintenance dose of 100 mg every 8 hours either intravenously or orally. A therapeutic plasma concentration is 10 to 18 micrograms per ml. At our institution, phenytoin is used as an antiarrhythmic agent primarily when digitalis intoxication is of etiologic importance.

After the initial 48 hours of hospitalization, VPBs that continue to be frequent (greater than 5 per minute), multifocal, or in close proximity to the preceding T wave, as well as those occurring in pairs or runs, require long-term oral suppression. For this purpose, quinidine sulfate (200 to 300 mg every 6 to 8 hours), procainamide (250 to 750 mg every 4 to 6 hours), disopyramide phosphate (100 to 150 mg every 6 hours), and/or propranolol (10 to 40 mg every 6 hours) may be administered. Although chronic suppression of VPBs is recommended, its influence on survival has not been proved.

Accelerated idioventricular rhythm (AIVR, "slow ventricular tachycardia") appears transiently dur-

ing the first 48 hours after myocardial infarction in 30 to 50 per cent of patients. It generally occurs at a rate of 90 to 100 beats per minute. In most patients AIVR requires no therapy. If hypotension results, atropine sulfate, 0.6 to 1.0 mg by intravenous bolus, is administered.

Ventricular tachycardia is especially frequent in patients with large myocardial infarctions. If the patient with ventricular tachycardia maintains his systemic arterial pressure and peripheral perfusion, intravenous lidocaine, 50 to 100 mg by bolus injection followed by a continuous infusion of 1 to 4 mg per minute, is administered. If hemodynamic instability occurs with ventricular tachycardia, or if lidocaine is unsuccessful in reverting the hemodynamically stable patient to sinus rhythm, DC countershock is utilized. Most patients with ventricular tachycardia revert to sinus rhythm with very low energy DC shock (5 to 10 watt-seconds). Once sinus rhythm is achieved, a lidocaine or procainamide intravenous infusion is initiated to maintain sinus rhythm. Subsequently, the patient is placed on oral maintenance quinidine, procainamide, disopyramide, and/or propranolol in the doses mentioned previously.

Ventricular fibrillation is the underlying rhythm in 75 per cent of cardiac arrests in the setting of myocardial infarction. It is treated with 400 watt-seconds of DC countershock. Once sinus rhythm is restored, a lidocaine or procainamide infusion is initiated to prevent subsequent episodes.

CONDUCTION ABNORMALITIES AND ATRIOVENTRICULAR BLOCK. There is continuing uncertainty about the short- and long-term course of conduction disturbances and heart block in the patient with myocardial infarction. As a result, the specific conduction abnormalities that require insertion of a pacemaker, temporary or permanent, are ill defined. In the setting of myocardial infarction, a temporary transvenous pacemaker is indicated for the patient with (1) complete atrioventricular block with a slow ventricular rate and a wide QRS complex; (2) Mobitz type II second degree atrioventricular block with an associated slow ventricular rate and a wide QRS complex; (3) new right bundle branch block (RBBB) and left posterior or left anterior hemiblock; or (4) new left bundle branch block (LBBB).

The patient with old isolated RBBB, left anterior hemiblock, left posterior hemiblock, LBBB, or bifascicular block is observed closely, and a temporary pacemaker is inserted if more advanced conduction abnormalities appear. If there is no evidence that the conduction disturbance is old, it is regarded as new.

The long-term management of the patient with a conduction abnormality also is open to differences of opinion. Following myocardial infarction, a permanent pacemaker is indicated for the patient with (1) persistent complete atrioventricular block; (2) bifascicular block of any type in a patient in whom complete heart block was present, even though such complete block was transient, particularly if there is concomitant prolongation of the PR interval; or (3) persistent Mobitz II atrioventricular block, with an associated slow ventricular rate.

In general, atrioventricular block in association with an inferior infarction is transient and rarely requires a permanent pacemaker. In contrast, atrioventricular block in the presence of anterior infarction frequently does not resolve, reflects extensive ventricular damage, and, therefore, carries a poor long-term prognosis despite permanent ventricular pacing.

Abnormalities of Ventricular Function. LEFT VENTRICULAR FAILURE. The patient with a myocardial infarction is placed at complete bed rest and given a diet with a low salt content. If, despite this, the patient has symptoms and signs of *mild* failure without cardiomegaly, he is given furosemide, 20 to 40 mg intravenously every 12 hours. If the heart is *enlarged,* the patient also receives digoxin. There are numerous regimens whereby one can digitalize the patient. For example, digoxin may be given intravenously in doses of 0.50, 0.25, and 0.25 mg every 6 hours, followed by a maintenance dose of 0.25 mg per day.

If a patient with a myocardial infarction develops pulmonary edema, he is given, in addition to digoxin and furosemide, morphine sulfate, 2 to 5 mg intravenously every 5 minutes, and intermittent positive pressure breathing (IPPB) every 15 to 30 minutes. Rotating tourniquets may be of some benefit. If necessary, a phlebotomy

may be performed, although a substantial reduction of the hemoglobin and hematocrit is avoided, since anemia may worsen the extent of myocardial ischemic injury.

If, despite digitalis, diuretics, morphine sulfate, IPPB, rotating tourniquets, and phlebotomy, the patient continues to show evidence of left ventricular failure, he is considered for afterload reduction. In order to tolerate a reduction in afterload, the patient must not be hypotensive prior to its initiation. Long-acting nitrate preparations may be administered sublingually, orally, or topically: isosorbide dinitrate, as much as 20 to 30 mg every 3 hours either sublingually or orally, or nitroglycerin ointment, up to 2 inches topically every 6 hours, may be given. Intravenous nitroglycerin may be used both to reduce left ventricular filling pressure and to reduce afterload. Sodium nitroprusside in the setting of myocardial infarction remains controversial, since it may be deleterious to the ischemic myocardium. If arterial blood gases reflect ventilatory deterioration caused by left ventricular failure, the patient should be intubated and ventilated mechanically in order, first, to improve arterial oxygen saturation and, second, to relieve the heart of the work of breathing. Finally, if left ventricular failure is severe and unrelieved by all the aforementioned measures, intra-aortic balloon counterpulsation may bring about hemodynamic stability.

CARDIOGENIC SHOCK. If a myocardial infarction is extensive, it may compromise left ventricular function to the extent that cardiac output is inadequate, resulting in hypotension and hypoperfusion of vital organs (brain, heart, and kidneys). This condition is diagnosed with certainty only if several other conditions are excluded, including (1) spurious hypotension

TABLE 2. **Therapy of Mechanical Complications of Acute Myocardial Infarction**

COMPLICATION	SPECIAL CIRCUMSTANCE	THERAPY (SEE TEXT FOR DETAILS)
Left ventricular failure	Mild	IV furosemide
	Moderate	IV digoxin
		IV furosemide
	Severe	IV digoxin, furosemide; preload and afterload reduction with oral or sublingual nitrates
Cardiogenic shock		Pressors (dopamine, norepinephrine); intra-aortic balloon counterpulsation
Right ventricular failure	Mild	Close observation
	Moderate	IV digoxin
	Severe	IV digoxin
		Volume expansion
Acute, severe mitral regurgitation or ventricular septal rupture		IV nitroprusside and intra-aortic balloon counterpulsation
Myocardial rupture		Pericardiocentesis; emergent surgery

(that situation in which the arterial pressure cannot be determined satisfactorily with a cuff because of obesity or peripheral arterial disease), (2) hypovolemia, (3) right ventricular infarction (with resultant systemic venous congestion concomitant with a low left ventricular filling pressure), (4) a severe metabolic derangement (resulting in a transient depression of left ventricular performance), or (5) brady- or tachyrhythmias.

To confirm the clinical impression of cardiogenic shock, the following measures are undertaken: (1) Measurement of the pulmonary capillary wedge pressure with a flow-directed, balloon-tipped catheter. The patient with cardiogenic shock has a high wedge pressure (greater than 20 to 22 mm Hg). (2) Insertion of an intra-arterial cannula to confirm true hypotension and to allow one to monitor systemic arterial pressure accurately as therapy is initiated. (3) Insertion of a Foley catheter to allow the accurate quantitation of urine output. (4) Assessment of arterial oxygenation, acid-base status, serum electrolytes, and blood glucose.

If cardiogenic shock is present, the following measures are instituted:

1. The patient is digitalized as described previously.

2. A dopamine infusion is initiated at 2 to 5 micrograms per kg per minute. The rate of infusion should not exceed 10 to 12 micrograms per kg per minute, as above this rate dopamine's vasoconstrictive effects outweigh its positive inotropic effects.

3. If dopamine is unsuccessful in raising the systemic arterial pressure, an infusion of norepinephrine is instituted at 2 to 8 micrograms per minute (*not* 2 to 8 micrograms per kg. per minute).

4. If the patient does not respond to pressors, intra-aortic balloon counterpulsation is initiated.

At some institutions, patients with cardiogenic shock are stabilized by the aforementioned regimen and then undergo immediate coronary arteriography and, if technically possible, coronary artery bypass surgery. Even in the best of hands, the survival rate of patients with true cardiogenic shock is only about 25 per cent.

RIGHT VENTRICULAR FAILURE. An occasional patient develops extensive right ventricular infarction, generally in association with an inferior wall infarction, and, as a result, presents with a massive elevation of peripheral venous pressure and a reduced cardiac output. The lungs are not congested. The diagnosis of extensive right ventricular infarction and failure is confirmed by the insertion of a flow-directed, balloon-tipped catheter: the right atrial and right ventricular end-diastolic pressures are elevated, but the pulmonary artery and capillary wedge pressures are low or normal. The patient with right ventricular failure caused by myocardial infarction is treated as follows: (1) Colloid or saline solution is infused intravenously to increase right ventricular filling pressures sufficiently to increase left ventricular filling and, therefore, cardiac output. (2) Digitalis is administered to augment right ventricular contractility. (3) If necessary for the maintenance of systemic arterial pressure, dopamine or norepinephrine is infused in the doses described previously. (4) If systemic arterial pressure is not depressed substantially, afterload reduction with hydralazine, 25 mg orally three to four times daily, or prazosin, 1 to 5 mg by mouth three to four times per day, may be beneficial.

ACUTE MITRAL REGURGITATION AND VENTRICULAR SEPTAL RUPTURE. The patient with acute, severe mitral regurgitation (resulting from infarction and rupture of part or all of a papillary muscle) or an acute ventricular septal defect (resulting from infarction and rupture of the interventricular septum) typically develops sudden pulmonary venous congestion. A flow-directed, balloon-tipped catheter, through which pressures are measured and blood is sampled from the right-heart chambers, allows one to determine which of these complications has occurred. Once the diagnosis is made, therapy includes the following measures: (1) An intravenous infusion of sodium nitroprusside is given, beginning at 15 micrograms per minute and increasing gradually until the wedge pressure falls to 18 to 20 mm Hg and/or the systolic arterial pressure falls to 90 mm Hg. It is rarely necessary to infuse more than 200 micrograms per minute. (2) Along with nitroprusside, intra-aortic balloon counterpulsation is initiated unless there is a contraindication (i.e., severe peripheral vascular disease, severe thrombocytopenia, or aortic regurgitation). (3) If the patient does not stabilize hemodynamically within 24 hours, cardiac catheterization followed by surgical repair is performed.

MYOCARDIAL RUPTURE. An occasional patient with a transmural myocardial infarction acutely ruptures the free wall of the left ventricle. Most such ruptures are not recognized clinically and, therefore, are not treated appropriately; the patient dies suddenly of pericardial tamponade. If left ventricular rupture is recognized premortem, it is treated by immediate pericardiocentesis and emergency surgery to repair the rupture.

Miscellaneous Problems. ONGOING PAIN AFTER ACUTE MYOCARDIAL INFARCTION. After a myocardial infarction, some patients continue to have chest pain owing to continuing ischemia or infarction. Within 24 hours of the initial event, this is treated with morphine sulfate, 2 to 5 mg intravenously every 5 minutes. Subsequently, continuing pain is treated with the following measures: (1) Long- and short-acting nitrates, provided that they are not contraindicated (because of systemic arterial hypotension). Specifically, isosorbide dinitrate (long-acting), 10 to 30 mg orally or sublingually every 3 to 4 hours, or nitroglycerin ointment, up to 2 inches topically every 6 hours, may be administered, and sublingual nitroglycerin (0.6 mg) may be given when pain occurs. (2) Propranolol, unless it is contraindicated, at an initial dose of 10 to 40 mg orally every 6 hours. (3) Intravenous nitroglycerin for pain that continues despite good doses of nitrates and propranolol. It is begun at 5 to 10 micrograms per minute and is increased gradually until chest pain is relieved or systolic arterial pressure falls below 90 to 100 mm Hg. Both systemic arterial and left ventricular filling pressures are monitored during nitroglycerin infusion. (4) Intra-aortic balloon counterpulsation, for pain that continues despite intravenous nitroglycerin. (5) Emergency coronary arteriography and, if possible, coronary artery bypass surgery if, despite maximal medical therapy and the intra-aortic balloon, pain is still ongoing.

SEVERE SYSTEMIC ARTERIAL HYPERTENSION. In the setting of myocardial infarction, elevations of systemic arterial pressure are detrimental, first, because left ventricular wall tension is increased, causing an elevation of myocardial oxygen demands and an increase in infarct size and, second, because the chance of rupture of the intraventricular septum or the left ventricular free wall is increased. Therefore, the systemic arterial pressure is treated aggressively in the patient with a myocardial infarction.

MILD HYPERTENSION. Many patients with myocardial infarction have a mild elevation of systemic arterial pressure when they arrive in the ER or CCU, usually because of anxiety and/or persistent chest pain. Adequate sedation is administered to relieve anxiety (oral diazepam, 5 to 15 mg every 6 to 8 hours), and enough analgesia should be given to eliminate chest discomfort (morphine sulfate, 2 to 5 mg intravenously every 5 minutes, or meperidine, 20 to 50 mg intravenously every 5 minutes).

MODERATE HYPERTENSION. If the blood pressure remains elevated after adequate sedation and analgesia, long-acting nitrates are administered (isosorbide dinitrate, 10 to 30 mg orally or sublingually every 3 to 4 hours; nitroglycerin ointment, up to 2 inches topically every 6 hours).

SEVERE HYPERTENSION. If, despite sedation, analgesia, and nitrates, the patient remains hypertensive, a potent intravenous hypotensive agent is administered. Trimethaphan camsylate is administered by intravenous infusion at an initial dose of 3 to 4 mg per minute, after which the rate of infusion is adjusted according to the blood pressure response. Its onset of action is immediate, and its antihypertensive effect quickly disappears when it is discontinued. Since trimethaphan may produce severe hypotension, the systemic arterial pressure is monitored continually (via an intra-arterial cannula) during its infusion. Tachyphylaxis may develop to trimethaphan within 48 hours, at which time the dosage may have to be increased.

Alternatively, sodium nitroprusside may be given by intravenous infusion, beginning at 15 micrograms per minute and adjusting the rate of infusion until the systemic arterial pressure is controlled adequately. Since nitroprusside may worsen ischemic injury in the patient with myocardial infarction, we prefer not to utilize it in this clinical setting.

In addition to trimethaphan or nitroprusside to control systemic arterial pressure acutely, an oral antihypertensive medication is instituted, such as alpha methyldopa, 250 mg every 6 to 8 hours, hydralazine, 25 mg every 6 to 8 hours, or clonidine, 0.1 to 0.8 mg every 8 hours.

PERICARDITIS. Transient pericarditis is a fairly common accompaniment of transmural myocardial infarction. The patient may complain of pleuritic anterior chest pain that is worsened

TABLE 3. **Therapy of Miscellaneous Problems Accompanying Acute Myocardial Infarction**

PROBLEM	THERAPY (SEE TEXT FOR DETAILS)
Ongoing pain	(1) Long-acting and short-acting nitrates (oral, sublingual) (2) Propranolol (3) Nitroglycerin (intravenous) (4) Intra-aortic balloon counterpulsation (5) Emergency coronary arteriography and bypass surgery
Systemic arterial hypertension	
Mild	Sedation, pain relief
Moderate	Nitrates (oral, sublingual)
Severe	IV trimethaphan or IV nitroprusside; then oral antihypertensive agents
Pericarditis	Aspirin or indomethacin; avoid corticosteroids and anticoagulants
Pulmonary embolism	IV heparin
Arterial embolism	IV heparin (if CSF is not bloody)

by assuming the supine position and, alternatively, is improved by sitting up. On physical examination, a friction rub may be audible. The electrocardiogram (ECG) may demonstrate diffuse ST segment elevation.

The therapy of pericarditis associated with myocardial infarction includes acetylsalicylic acid, 650 mg orally every 4 to 6 hours, or indomethacin, 25 to 50 mg orally every 6 hours. (This specific use of indomethacin is not listed in the manufacturer's official directive.) These agents are equally efficacious in the therapy of this disorder. Corticosteroids are avoided, because they increase the chance of left ventricular rupture or aneurysm formation. Anticoagulants are avoided, as they may cause the accumulation of a bloody pericardial effusion with resultant tamponade.

PULMONARY EMBOLISM. In the setting of myocardial infarction, pulmonary embolism is uncommon but important to recognize, since it may cause hemodynamic instability and/or atrial tachyrhythmias. If a pulmonary embolus occurs, it is treated with heparin, administered intravenously by intermittent bolus injection, 5000 to 7000 units every 4 hours, or continuous infusion, 1000 to 1500 units per hour. The adequacy of heparin therapy is assessed by measuring the activated partial thromboplastin time (PTT); ideally, this should be 2 to 2½ times normal.

ARTERIAL EMBOLISM. Occasionally the patient with a myocardial infarction develops arterial embolization, manifested as a stroke, infarction of a specific organ, or acute arterial insufficiency of an extremity. If cerebral embolism occurs, anticoagulation is instituted if the cerebrospinal fluid does not show evidence of hemorrhage. If blood flow to an extremity is compromised, surgical embolectomy is performed.

Care Outside the Coronary Care Unit of the Patient with Acute Myocardial Infarction

The patient with a totally uncomplicated myocardial infarction remains in the CCU for 3 to 4 days, after which he is transferred to an intermediate facility, where he remains until hospital discharge. Similarly, the patient with a complicated myocardial infarction remains in the CCU until complications have resolved, at which time he, too, is transferred to an intermediate facility. Once the patient is moved from the CCU to this area, he remains in the hospital an average of 7 to 10 days. During this time period, therapy is designed as follows:

Physical Activity. Over the 7 to 10 days in the general hospital setting, the patient gradually increases his activities, so that by the last 2 to 3 days he is ambulating freely.

Diet. Upon transfer from the CCU, the patient is continued on a diet low in salt and saturated fats.

Antianginal Agents. As the patient increases his physical activity, he may develop angina pectoris, in which case he is placed on long- and short-acting nitrates (isosorbide dinitrate [long-acting], 10 to 30 mg orally every 3 to 6 hours, and sublingual nitroglycerin, 0.6 mg for episodes of pain) and, if necessary, oral propranolol, 20 to 80 mg every 6 hours. If anginal pain is severely limiting despite a good antianginal regimen, coronary arteriography and, if feasible, coronary artery bypass surgery are performed 4 to 6 weeks after infarction.

Patient and Family Education. During the period of convalescence following an acute myocardial infarction, the patient and his immediate family receive counseling about the rehabilitative process that will continue once the patient leaves the hospital. This includes specific recommendations about diet, physical activity, sexual activity, and return to work.

Protection of the Ischemic Myocardium

In the experimental animal, numerous pharmacologic, metabolic, and hemodynamic interventions have been shown to limit the severity and extent of myocardial ischemic injury following coronary artery occlusion, and in man several of these agents have been used, with generally encouraging results. Sublingual and intravenous nitroglycerin appears beneficial in the patient with acute myocardial infarction, as do hyaluronidase, propranolol, and a combination of hypertonic glucose, insulin, and potassium ("GIK"). Large doses of corticosteroids have been shown to limit infarct size, but they may increase the incidence of left ventricular rupture and aneurysm formation. Presently large clinical trials are assessing the abilities of propranolol, hyaluronidase, and GIK to protect the ischemic myocardium. The application of these agents to the patient with myocardial infarction awaits the results of these trials.

Abolition of Coronary Artery Spasm in the Setting of Acute Myocardial Infarction

Recent studies have demonstrated that coronary artery spasm may contribute to myocardial infarction in some patients. If this is true, antispasmodic agents may be efficacious in the setting of acute infarction. The relief of coronary artery spasm may be one way in which nitroglycerin minimizes the severity and extent of myocardial ischemic injury. In the setting of myocardial infarction, the calcium antagonists, such as nifedipine* and verapamil,* may diminish infarct size partly through their antispasmodic effects. As with the modification of infarct size, the use of potent antispasmodic agents in the patient with myocardial infarction awaits clinical trials to prove their efficacy.

---

*Not available in the United States of America.

REHABILITATION OF THE PATIENT AFTER MYOCARDIAL INFARCTION

method of
NANETTE K. WENGER, M.D.
Atlanta, Georgia

There are two major areas in rehabilitative programming for patients after myocardial infarction. The first involves activity: early ambulation during the hospitalization, and subsequent prescriptive exercise training on an ambulatory basis. A second and equally important component is patient and family education, beginning during the acute hospital stay and continuing on an ambulatory basis. Included in this component is the provision of a variety of counseling services as warranted — psychosocial, educational, and vocational.

Early Ambulation

Delineation of the deleterious effects of prolonged immobilization at bed rest provided the physiologic basis for recommending early ambulation. Immobilization is associated with a decrease in physical work capacity, with hypovolemia which results in orthostatic hypotension and tachycardia, with an increase in blood viscosity which predisposes to thromboembolism, with a decrease in lung volume and vital capacity, with a negative nitrogen and protein balance, and with a decrease in systemic muscle mass and muscular contractile strength; the last of these results in an increased oxygen demand compared with trained muscles to perform comparable work.

Early ambulation is appropriate for patients whose myocardial infarction is characterized by an uncomplicated clinical course — those without significant disturbances of cardiac rhythm, congestive heart failure, persistent or recurrent chest pain, or hypotension or clinical shock. Patients whose hospital course is characterized by complications of infarction become candidates for progressive ambulation once control or stabilization has been achieved.

Guidelines for suitable activities in the coronary or intensive care unit are that they be of low-level intensity, 1 to 2 mets (1 met = approximately 3.5 ml O_2 per kg of body weight per minute); be gradually progressive in work demand; and be supervised by an individual capable of assessing the patient's response to activity. These include self-care, with patients allowed to feed themselves, bathe, use a bedside commode, and sit in bed or in a bedside chair. Selected arm and leg exercises maintain muscle tone and joint mobility.

Activity surveillance is designed to identify disproportionate responses to the low-level activity: the development of chest pain, dyspnea, or palpitations; the occurrence of a heart rate greater than 120 beats per minute; the appearance of dysrhythmia; the occurrence of ST segment alterations on the electrocardiogram; and a fall of greater than 10 to 15 mm Hg in the systolic blood pressure, generally indicating inadequacy of the cardiac output to meet the demand.

An inappropriate response to low-level activity requires reduction of the activity and careful clinical reassessment of the patient. An appropriate response indicates that the patient can safely tolerate that workload and may be gradually progressed to a slightly greater intensity of activity.

After transfer out of the coronary care unit, rehabilitative physical activity for the remainder of the hospitalization is designed to achieve a functional level to permit the patient to perform usual homebound activities at the time of discharge from the hospital; this is currently typically at 7 to 14 days for the patient with an uncomplicated clinical course. Household tasks require a work intensity of 2 to 3 mets.

Patients continue to perform personal care, to sit in a chair for increasing periods of time, and to perform selected "warm-up" exercises. The major component of the activity program is walking, with both the pace and distance gradually increased. Patients who will have to climb steps at home should practice this in the hospital.

Ideally, prescribed daily exercises are associated with a parallel intensity of in-hospital daily activities, as well as recreational and educational activities. At Grady Memorial Hospital and the Emory University School of Medicine in Atlanta, Georgia, this format has been in use since the early 1960s. The current revision (Table 1) involves seven steps, the initial two performed in

TABLE 1.   **Inpatient Rehabilitation After Myocardial Infarction—Seven Step Program (as Revised 1980) at Grady Memorial Hospital and Emory University School of Medicine***

STEP	DATE	M.D. INITIALS	NURSE/PHYSICAL THERAPIST NOTES SUPERVISED EXERCISE	CCU/WARD ACTIVITY	EDUCATIONAL/RECREATIONAL ACTIVITY
Coronary care unit (CCU)					
1. ____			Active and passive range of motion (ROM) all extremities, in bed; Teach patient ankle plantar and dorsiflexion—repeat hourly when awake	Partial self-care; Feed self; Dangle legs on side of bed; Use bedside commode; Sit in chair 15 minutes 1–2 times a day	Orientation to CCU; Personal emergencies, social service aid as needed
2. ____			Active ROM all extremities, sitting on side of bed	Sit in chair 15–30 minutes 2–3 times a day; Complete self-care in bed	Orientation to rehabilitation team, program; Smoking cessation; Educational literature if requested; Planning transfer from CCU
Ward					
3. ____			Warm-up exercises, 2 mets; Stretching; Calisthenics; Walk 50 ft and back at slow pace	Sit in chair ad lib.; To ward class in wheelchair; Walk in room	Normal cardiac anatomy and function; Development of atherosclerosis; What happens with myocardial infarction; 1–2 met craft activity
4. ____			ROM and calisthenics, 2.5 mets; Walk length of hall (75 ft) and back, average pace; Teach pulse counting	Out of bed as tolerated; Walk to bathroom; Walk to ward class, with supervision	Coronary risk factors and their control
5. ____			ROM and calisthenics, 3 mets; Check pulse counting; Practice walking few stairsteps; Walk 300 ft b.i.d.	Walk to waiting room or telephone; Walk in ward corridor p.r.n.	Diet; Energy conservation; Work simplification techniques (as needed); 2–3 met craft activity
6. ____			Continue above activities; Walk down flight of steps (return by elevator); Walk 500 ft b.i.d.; Instruct on home exercise	Tepid shower or tub bath, with supervision; To occupational therapy, cardiac clinic teaching room, with supervision	Heart attack management; Medications; Exercise; Surgery; Response to symptoms; Family, community adjustments on return home; Craft activity p.r.n.
7. ____			Continue above activities; Walk up flight of steps; Walk 500 ft b.i.d.; Continue home exercise instructions—present information re outpatient exercise program	Continue all previous ward activities	Discharge planning; Medications, diet, activity; Return appointments; Scheduled tests; Return to work; Community resources; Educational literature; Medication cards; Craft activity p.r.n.

*From Wenger, N. K., *in* Hurst, J. W., et al. (eds.): The Heart. 5th ed. New York, McGraw-Hill Book Company, in press.

the coronary care unit and the subsequent five in a general medical care area.

In recent years there has been unequivocal documentation of the safety of this approach for appropriately selected patients. Advantages include the prevention of deconditioning, a decrease in pulmonary atelectasis and thromboembolic complications, and a decrease in anxiety and depression; the last point is particularly important in that most psychotropic drugs are contraindicated in acute infarction because of adverse effects on heart rate, blood pressure, and cardiac rhythm; hence, an added advantage to early ambulation. This approach tends to enable a shorter hospital stay with a saving in medical care costs and an improved use of hospital beds. Improved functional status of the patient at discharge is reflected by an earlier and more complete return to work.

Exercise Training: Cardiac Conditioning Physical Activities

The goal of physical activity during convalescence is to increase endurance to a level which will enable more rapid return to work and/or usual preinfarction activities. That this is appropriate is evidenced by the fact that of patients with uncomplicated infarction, over 85 per cent employed at the time of infarction typically return to work within 2 to 3 months, characteristically at their former job.

During the initial days at home, patients continue the activity level of the last days in the hospital. They perform usual household activities, are instructed in specific warm-up exercises, and gradually increase both the distance walked and the pace of walking. Recommendations are that sexual activity can be resumed when other components of daily life style are reinstituted.

Response to low-level convalescent activity can help guide the physician's recommendations regarding return to work. For example, walking at a speed of 3 to 3½ miles an hour entails 4 to 5 mets of work; when compared with the 3 or 4 met level of most sedentary desk and bench jobs, reassurance can be given to the patient who can walk at this pace without difficulty of the ability to perform these categories of work.

Individualized prescriptive physical activity is central to rehabilitation. Prescriptive components of exercise include its "dosage" — the frequency, duration, and intensity of exercise —and the specific type of exercise.

Multilevel exercise stress testing, typically done at 4 to 8 weeks postinfarction, is needed for accuracy and safety of exercise prescription. Recommendations are that the patient exercise two or three times weekly, with sessions of 30 to 45 minutes in duration, including warm-up and cool-down periods. The exercise intensity is such that patients should attain a heart rate between 70 and 85 per cent of the highest level safely achieved at exercise testing. Dynamic exercise is appropriate, i.e., activities involving the rhythmic repetitive movements of large muscle groups; these activities include walking, running, swimming, bicycling, selected calisthenics, rope jumping, and the like.

In general, individualized exercise is recommended at 70 to 75 per cent target heart rate intensity, with exercise in a supervised program at 80 or 85 per cent of the highest heart rate safely achieved at exercise testing. Typically, patients check the heart rate response by pulse counting; some supervised programs use intermittent or continuous electrocardiographic monitoring.

Program design should include activities which train both the arms and the legs, as the training effects are not interchangeable. In the course of an exercise program, serial exercise test assessment is recommended at 3 to 6 month intervals to document performance changes and permit revision of the exercise prescription.

The goal of prescriptive physical activity is an improvement in cardiovascular function, designated the "training effect." This includes a decrease in resting heart rate and systolic blood pressure, and a lesser increase in heart rate and systolic blood pressure for any level of submaximal work. Because these two components are major determinants of myocardial oxygen demand, the trained individual experiences less or no angina and demonstrates less or no ischemic electrocardiographic changes for any level of submaximal work. Peripheral oxygen extraction is also improved, as is the redistribution of exercise cardiac output. There is currently little evidence that exercise training improves myocardial performance, especially in the older individual with significant coronary disease, although this remains controversial.

Training can be accomplished in the patient receiving concomitant drug therapy, including vasodilator therapy, antihypertensive drugs, and beta-adrenergic blocking agents.

No evidence exists to date that exercise training alters coronary artery angiographic lesions or increases the coronary collateral circulation in man. The improvement in functional capacity is apparently primarily the peripheral effect described above. Equally important, there are no data as to whether exercise training alters the natural history of coronary atherosclerotic heart disease — longevity, recurrence of infarction, or coronary death. The effect of exercise training on arrhythmias is likewise controversial, although plasma catecholamine levels decrease with exercise. Serum triglyceride levels decrease, but the effect on total serum cholesterol is not predictable; high density lipoprotein cholesterol appears increased in physically active individuals. The effect on fibrinolysis is uncertain.

Additional beneficial effects of physical activity are psychosocial. Patients who exercise tend to feel better; have an improvement in self-confidence and self-esteem; show less anxiety, depression, denial, and dependency on standard psychometric tests; tend to participate increasingly in leisure time activities; and appear to have a better work attendance record. The importance of psychosocial features derives from the finding that more patients after myocardial infarction are disabled by psychologic than by physiologic features.

Patient and Family Education

Patient and family education is designed to provide enough information about the illness and its management to enable the involved individuals to assume some responsibility for health care. The physician must assume responsibility for the content of the educational program, but the actual teaching and development of teaching materials are often best accomplished by other health professionals who spend more time with the patient. The family life crisis of an episode of myocardial infarction creates motivation for learning; in the hospital, a variety of health professionals are available for teaching. In the coronary care unit, when fear, pain, anxiety, and fatigue impair the physical and mental readiness for learning, only very simple facts should be presented. These include a brief explanation of the diagnosis and the reasons for and safety features of regulations, procedures, and equipment.

During the remainder of the hospitalization, more detailed educational efforts are appropriate. They are designed to decrease the patient's feelings of helplessness and enhance the patient's ability to cope with the problems of illness.

A brief review is needed of normal cardiac function and of the atherosclerotic process causing coronary obstruction. The changes that occur with myocardial infarction should be described, with emphasis on healing. Prevalent myths regarding the precipitation of infarction must be dispelled, as many psychosocial outcomes relate to the patient's perception of illness, which may be favorably altered by education. The rationale for dietary changes should be presented, cessation of cigarette smoking recommended, and specific recommendations given for activity resumption and return to work. Discussion of resumption of sexual activity should include the guideline that it is appropriate and safe when other usual daily activities are reinstituted. Patients must be taught about medications they are to take and about the appropriate response to symptoms, particularly prolonged chest discomfort. Many hospitals teach cardiopulmonary resuscitation to families of myocardial infarction survivors. Community resources must be defined, including guidance and counseling serv-

ices, vocational rehabilitation facilities, home care agencies, and postcoronary educational groups or clubs.

Although specific patient concerns and problems necessitate individual teaching, the presentation of general information is best suited to a group format. This is economical of professional time and enables the patient to interact with a peer group confronting similar problems. Audiovisual materials facilitate learning, and take-home materials such as books, pamphlets, and instruction sheets are appropriate. Repetition is needed after the patient has returned home, as needs not perceived in the hospital become apparent when the patient must solve problems related to health care.

Patients who understand their disease and the rationale for its management appear to have an increased incentive and ability to cooperate in recommendations. An educational program helps define the patient's responsibility and role in the care of illness.

Summary

Effective rehabilitation can enable survivors of myocardial infarction to return rapidly to a relatively normal life style. The plan of care is designed to help the patient achieve realistically optimal physiologic improvement and attain an acceptable level of self-care and a useful activity level at home or at work. It is hoped that this approach will minimize the economic impact of the illness on the patient, family, and community through a shortened hospital stay for the acute event; de-emphasize invalidism; decrease the need for convalescent care; and promote an earlier and more complete return to work. The risk of recurrent coronary events and late complications may be decreased by implementation of a secondary prevention program. The responsibility for the initiation and coordination of rehabilitative efforts rests with the patient's primary physician; ideally rehabilitation is incorporated into the plan of care during the hospitalization, involves the patient's family and social environment as a support system, and continues in the office of the patient's physician and/or in a variety of community facilities. The ultimate goal is the improvement of the quality of life for the more than 600,000 patients who each year survive an episode of myocardial infarction.

Acknowledgment

With appreciation to Julia Wright for the typing of the manuscript.

PERICARDITIS

method of
CARL J. PEPINE, M.D.
Gainesville, Florida

Introduction

Rational management of the patient with pericarditis requires a thorough understanding of the pathophysiologic consequences of this disorder in addition to knowledge of the etiology. The consequences of pericarditis include pain, arrhythmias, effusion, constriction, and cardiac tamponade. Some of these consequences can be life threatening, while others often cause profound functional disability.

Management of Consequences of Pericarditis

Chest Pain. Pain is the cardinal symptom of acute pericarditis. Any etiologic type of pericarditis can produce pain arising through both direct and indirect effects of the actual inflammatory process. In general, pericardial pain is managed with analgesic and anti-inflammatory agents. Nonsteroidal anti-inflammatory agents (e.g., aspirin, indomethacin) are particularly useful. Occasionally more potent analgesic agents are required for a short period of time. If morphine or meperidine is required, one should remember that these narcotic agents will also directly relax vasoconstrictor tone. Resulting venodilation will reduce venous pressure, thereby decreasing both right and left heart filling pressures. Should some component of cardiac compression be present, because of pericardial constriction or tamponade, reduction in filling pressure could lead to marked reduction of cardiac output. If pain does not respond, corticosteroids may be used. Anti-inflammatory drug treatment should not be withdrawn abruptly, since recurrences can result. With chronic recurrent pericarditis, surgery, consisting of pericardial stripping, can be helpful to palliate pain.

Arrhythmias. Arrhythmias, both atrial and ventricular, are very common with acute and chronic pericarditis of any etiology. It is important to monitor patients with pericarditis electrocardiographically to detect, identify, and quantify these arrhythmias. I prefer propranolol for treatment of supraventricular tachycardia. This agent can be given orally (10 to 40 mg four times daily) if time permits (30 to 60 minutes) or intravenously (1 mg per 1 to 2 minutes) when more rapid control of the ventricular rate is required. On occasion, digitalis is used in combination with propranolol or alone to control supraventricular tachycardia. Once digitalis is used, however, it is difficult to differentiate subsequently occurring ventricular arrhythmias related to the inflammatory pericardial process from those related to sensitivity to digitalis. In addition, the risk of more serious rhythm disturbance becomes substantial should DC cardioversion be required. Therefore, I do not use digitalis as the initial agent for treatment of supraventricular tachyrhythmias.

Lidocaine is the agent reserved for treatment of ventricular arrhythmias occurring with pericarditis. For patients with ventricular arrhythmias not responding to lidocaine, propranolol is the drug that I use next by either intravenous or oral route. When ventricular dysrhythmias fail to respond or other problems (e.g., asthma, heart failure) limit use of propranolol, I recommend bretylium. This newly available drug does not depress myocardial function and has been very effective for resistant ventricular arrhythmias. Initial therapy should be 5 to 10 mg per kg intravenously. This dose may be repeated after 1 hour to a maximum total dose of 30 mg per kg. For maintenance, 5 to 10 mg per kg by intermittent intravenous infusion every 6 to 8 hours to a maximum of 30 mg per kg per day can be used. For oral use, quinidine and disopyramide have been helpful. I avoid procainamide in this situation because of the possibility of evoking a lupuslike syndrome with associated pericarditis which may obscure evaluation and/or response to therapy of the underlying pericardial disease process. Usually, once the etiologic type of pericarditis is identified and appropriately treated, these arrhythmias resolve.

Heart block, although not as frequent as tachyrhythmias, occurs occasionally in patients with pericarditis and is managed with a temporary transvenous pacemaker. The transthoracic route is to be avoided, except in life-threatening emergencies, until the possibility of an infectious cause of the pericarditis is definitely excluded. Even when this possibility is excluded, it is wise to avoid additional trauma to the pericardium with a transthoracic pacemaker. If heart block persists beyond 2 weeks, a permanent intravenous pacemaker is implanted.

Constrictive Pericarditis. Pericardial constriction usually occurs secondary to traumatic pericarditis or tuberculous pericarditis. Other types (i.e., viral, neoplastic, and pyogenic) of pericarditis, as a cause of constriction, are considered less common. Prompt management of these conditions is important to prevent subsequent constriction. The constrictive process is usually diffuse; however, on occasion it can be localized. Once evidence for constriction is established by either clinical examination or cardiac catheterization and the patient is limited by symptoms, pericardiectomy should be performed. Symptoms such as fatigue, dyspnea on exertion, edema, ascites (particularly out of proportion to edema), and elevated venous pressure should prompt early definitive evaluation to identify constriction. A protein-losing enteropathy and/or nephrotic syndrome can also occur. These findings will not resolve unless venous pressure is reduced. While restriction of salt and use of diuretics may be helpful in an occasional patient, delay of pericardiectomy only causes additional problems later. Furthermore, the risk from vigorous diuresis resulting in reduction in filling pressure and further reduction of cardiac output is substantial. If tuberculous pericarditis is encountered, antituberculous therapy should be used for 2 to 3 weeks prior to surgical intervention.

Cardiac Tamponade. The most serious life-threatening problem associated with pericarditis is cardiac tamponade. This finding is usually seen in patients with trauma to the chest or pericardium or patients with neoplastic disease. Occasionally, tamponade develops in patients with other forms of pericarditis who are treated with anticoagulants or who have abnormal blood coagulation. Tamponade is also seen in the patient with pericarditis caused by acute myocardial infarction when cardiac rupture occurs. Acute cardiac compression results when intrapericardial pressure exceeds right and left ventricular diastolic filling pressures. Thus, ventricular filling is abruptly reduced. Because diastolic fiber length is reduced, stroke volume declines and cardiac output is maintained only by the rise in heart rate. This rise in heart rate is, in itself, self-limiting because the duration of diastole is further shortened, thereby additionally decreasing diastolic filling. Consequences of acute cardiac compression are related to the rapidity of fluid accumulation, distensibility of the pericardium, and, to a small extent, the absolute quantity of pericardial fluid. For example, sudden accumulation of less than 100 ml of fluid can produce life-threatening tamponade in a patient with a stiff, fibrotic pericardium. In a patient with cholesterol pericarditis and a nearly normal pericardium, slow accumulation of more than 2 liters of fluid can be tolerated without evidence of cardiac compression. All patients hospitalized with a diagnosis of pericarditis should be localized in an area where emergency pericardial aspiration can be performed on very short notice. A pericardiocentesis tray with a blunt needle should be nearby with appropriate electrocardiographic and hemodynamic monitoring equipment. Pericardial aspiration is infre-

quently performed, but when done in the patient with acute tamponade the procedure is lifesaving. Before aspiration, one should use large amounts of intravenous fluids in an attempt to rapidly increase the ventricular filling pressure. Occasionally, infusion of catecholamines may increase contractility, allowing further use of systolic reserve mechanisms to promote more complete ventricular emptying to provide several additional minutes while the patient is prepared for pericardial aspiration. These measures should in no way delay appropriate aspiration and decompression.

Pericardial Effusion. Pericardial effusion can develop with any specific etiologic type of pericarditis. Asymptomatic effusions are usually very small and resolve spontaneously with treatment of the specific pericardial process. Larger effusions can cause symptoms attributable to cardiac compression as outlined above, in addition to vague types of chest discomfort. Effusion is usually manifest by cardiomegaly or change in cardiac silhouette on chest x-ray. In addition to classic electrocardiographic changes of pericarditis, however, in many cases of chronic effusion the electrocardiogram either is normal or shows only nonspecific changes. Echocardiography is extremely helpful in diagnosis and evaluation of therapy of patients with pericardial effusion. In general, pericardiocentesis with fluid analysis and culture is helpful in establishing the diagnosis and in further evaluation of patients not responding to therapy. Pericardiocentesis alone is limited in managing pericardial effusion recurring in pericarditis. After initial success, recurrences happen frequently, particularly when the underlying pericardial process is not treated appropriately.

Systemic anti-inflammatory agents, particularly nonsteroidal agents (e.g., indomethacin), have been advocated, but I have not been convinced of their long-term beneficial effect. Systemic corticosteroids may be helpful in selected etiologic types, as outlined below. Intrapericardial space infusion of corticosteroids combined with pericardiocentesis, have been advocated with certain types of pericardial effusions (e.g., uremic) with good results. Combining an indwelling pericardial catheter, to provide drainage, with periodic instillation of triamcinolone has been helpful. Surgical approaches include drainage procedures, such as pericardial window, pericardiostomy, and pericardiectomy. Such procedures are uniformly initially successful. However, the limited procedures (e.g., windows) are marred by recurrences, and in certain patient subsets the larger procedures have considerable morbidity. Complications include infection. However, pericardiectomy remains standard treatment for recurrent effusions in patients on medical therapy. In patients with cancer an alternative approach is usually attempted by obliteration of the pericardial space.

Management of Various Etiologic Types of Pericarditis

Acute Nonspecific Pericarditis. The major cause of this type of pericarditis is most probably viral. Echovirus 9, coxsackievirus, influenza, and other virus types have been isolated, and undoubtedly many other types also exist. The illness usually has an abrupt onset, lasts approximately 10 to 20 days, and is usually self-limited. The major treatment is symptomatic to control chest pain and other pathophysiologic consequences, as outlined above. Rest is probably helpful during the acute phase of illness. Analgesic and anti-inflammatory drug therapy is used to control pain, and no additional treatment is required in most patients. Recurrences, particularly when anti-inflammatory drugs are withdrawn, are not uncommon and may require use of corticosteroids or consideration of pericardial resection. Cardiac tamponade and significant pericardial effusion are infrequent and should be managed as outlined above.

Bacterial Pericarditis. Pneumococci, streptococci, staphylococci, or other gram-positive organisms may produce pyogenic pericarditis. This form of pericarditis usually results from hematogenous or direct spread of organisms from the lungs or pleural surface to the pericardial space. These types are not frequently observed today, possibly because of early widespread use of antibiotics for many infections before a causative organism is identified. Some unrecognized cases of pericarditis and some cases in which the specific etiologic agent cannot be identified may be a result of inadvertently treated pyogenic pericarditis. The patient with pyogenic pericarditis is very ill. Many appear toxic, with spiking fever, chills, and other symptoms. In such patients, pericardiocentesis should be performed early with Gram staining and cultures of aspirated fluid in addition to hematologic and chemical analysis. The initial antibiotic choice should be based upon the type of organism identified by Gram stain. Therapy, with the appropriate antibiotic, should be initiated *immediately* and in a dose sufficient to achieve adequate concentrations in the pericardial space. Antibiotic choice may be altered based on subsequent culture and sensitivity results. It is important to emphasize that delay in initiating antibiotic therapy not only causes considerable risk relative to life but also increases the possibility of subsequent pericardial

constriction. The role of pericardiocentesis alone as a drainage procedure is limited. Pericardiocentesis is useful to provide fluid for evaluation of patients with recurrence or patients who do not respond to initial antibiotic treatment. Surgical drainage of the pericardial space may be necessary along with continued antibiotic therapy. Tamponade and constriction are not uncommon.

Tuberculous Pericarditis. Tuberculous pericarditis is not common today. This type can be seen without pulmonary involvement, possibly the result of mediastinal lymph node or pleural tuberculosis. The onset is usually insidious, but occasionally an abrupt onset is observed. In addition to pain and arrhythmias, pericardial effusion is common. Cardiac tamponade or constriction may occur later in the course of illness. In almost all patients with tuberculous pericarditis, the skin test will be positive and negative tests are most likely limited to patients with anergy. An attempt should be made to identify the tuberculous organism in the pericardial aspirate by acid-fast stain or culture. In half or less of these patients, the tuberculous organism will not be positively identified by culture or acid-fast stain. Because of this fact and the 6 to 8 week period for culture, initial therapy with antituberculous drugs must be based upon clinical suspicion. Again, therapy must not be delayed. If the patient does not improve after 2 to 3 weeks of therapy, it is wise to reconsider the diagnosis, particularly if the tubercle bacillus has not been positively identified. Pericardial biopsy and pericardiectomy can be done at low risk to provide tissue diagnosis and lessen the probability of subsequent pericardial constriction. Therapy then can be altered accordingly. I recommend triple therapy with isoniazid, streptomycin, and ethambutol. Some recommend rifampin. After the initial phase of therapy (2 to 4 weeks) streptomycin may be discontinued. There is no place for "short-course" tuberculosis regimens in the patient with tuberculous pericarditis. At least two drugs must be continued for up to 2 years of therapy. One should remember that both isoniazid and rifampin are hepatotoxic. Isoniazid can cause peripheral neuropathy that can generally be prevented by prophylactic use of pyridoxine. Some believe that the simultaneous use of corticosteroid early in the course of tuberculous pericarditis reduces the possibility of subsequent constriction, and I employ this combination. Even with appropriate antituberculous therapy and corticosteroids, persistent or progressive elevation of central venous pressure, cardiomegaly, ascites, or other findings associated with pericardial constriction occur in a substantial proportion of patients. The earlier constriction is recognized, the easier it is to perform pericardiectomy. The possibility of complications relating to pericardiectomy is also lessened.

Fungal Pericarditis. Nontuberculous granulomatous types of pericarditis can be due to fungal organisms. Histoplasmosis, blastomycosis, nocardiosis, and coccidioidomycosis all can produce pericarditis. These problems are usually encountered in the immunologically compromised patient. Again, it is essential that the diagnosis be established by culture of pericardial fluid or culture of pericardial biopsy tissue prior to instituting therapy. Therapy consists of relatively toxic agents, such as amphotericin B. Direct instillation of this agent through an indwelling pericardial catheter may improve success of treatment and lessen toxicity.

Traumatic Pericarditis. Direct trauma to the pericardium usually occurs because of either penetrating chest injury or contiguous thoracic surgery and is the most frequent cause of traumatic pericarditis. If hemopericardium and signs of cardiac tamponade are present, prompt removal of fluid may be lifesaving and reduce the possibility of constriction. Usually, thoracotomy will be required and the lacerated myocardium in the region of the penetrating injury repaired or bleeding vessels sutured. Late problems, such as postpericardiotomy syndrome, are becoming very frequent. Even in situations such as coronary artery bypass surgery in which the pericardium is not closed, a postpericardiotomy-type syndrome is not uncommon. This complication usually presents with vague pain, which is blunted by use of analgesic agents for sternal discomfort related to the surgical procedure. In addition, fever and generalized malaise are not uncommon. This form of pericarditis may respond to nonsteroidal anti-inflammatory agents. However, some advocate a short course of corticosteroids. Constriction can also occur in these situations. Diagnosis is difficult in postoperative patients, but, once established, constriction can be managed as outlined above. However, in patients in whom adhesions and other mediastinal fibrotic reactions are extensive, pericardiocentesis can be difficult.

Another type of traumatic pericarditis arises after *blunt* chest trauma. Here, presumably veins or other small blood vessels are lacerated or traumatized. Hemopericardium can occur with usual signs of tamponade. Prompt removal of fluid can be lifesaving. Any patient with blunt chest trauma should be closely monitored for development of pericarditis.

Radiation Pericarditis. Acute pericarditis, clinically indistinguishable from other forms outlined above, associated with chronic effusion or even constriction, can occur after radiation therapy to the chest. This form of pericarditis is often difficult to distinguish from pericarditis more directly related to the disease for which radiation therapy was administered (i.e., neoplasm). Nonetheless, after evaluation and supportive care the patient should be monitored, as outlined, for other forms of pericarditis and consequences outlined above.

Pericarditis Associated with Connective Tissue Disorders. Patients with lupus erythematosus, rheumatoid arthritis, rheumatic fever, and other "collagen vascular disorders" (e.g., periarteritis nodosa, scleroderma) frequently develop pericarditis. Usually, therapy directed toward the underlying disease results in resolution of pericarditis. Systemic nonsteroidal anti-inflammatory agents or, if necessary, corticosteroids are usually beneficial. When questions arise as to differentiation of cardiac compression caused by constriction from right heart failure related to one of these disorders, appropriate catheterization studies are indicated to provide definitive diagnosis. Rarely tamponade or constriction occurs.

Pericarditis Related to Diseases of Contiguous Structures. MYOCARDIAL INFARCTION. Acute transmural myocardial infarction is often followed by some signs of pericarditis which can be detected if the patient is monitored closely. In general, these findings resolve within a few days and are of no consequence. Controversy continues as to use of or discontinuation of anticoagulants when findings of pericarditis are detected. I find this type of discussion irrelevant, since infarction involving the epicardial surface is associated with pericardial reaction in most if not all instances of transmural infarction. Only supportive therapy for management of pain is required. One must be careful to differentiate pain arising from associated pericarditis from pain caused by recurrent myocardial ischemia. In this instance, continuous electrocardiographic monitoring using multiple leads and pulmonary artery wedge pressure monitoring provide supportive evidence for or against transient myocardial ischemia. The clinical response to a trial of nitrate and propranolol treatment can be invaluable.

POSTMYOCARDIAL INFARCTION SYNDROME. In the later phase of acute myocardial infarction, usually after about 2 weeks, pericarditis can develop. This type of pericardial reaction may occur as late as 3 to 6 months after acute infarction. Recurrences are not uncommon. Effusion can result, but rarely constriction occurs. Treatment with nonsteroidal anti-inflammatory agents is usually successful. However, at times corticosteroids are needed.

DISSECTING AORTIC ANEURYSM. Dissection of the ascending aorta may produce a leak into the pericardial space. When this occurs, the patient develops severe pericardial pain and often aortic insufficiency. Such patients often require immediate surgery.

PLEURAL AND PULMONARY DISEASES. Pneumonia, pulmonary embolism, and various types of nonspecific pleuritis are frequently associated with signs of pericarditis. Other than differentiating these findings from that associated with acute myocardial ischemia, no specific treatment is required.

Pericarditis Associated with Disorders of Metabolism. RENAL FAILURE. Uremic pericarditis and dialysis-associated pericarditis are becoming common forms of pericarditis seen in large hospital referral centers that manage patients who have end-stage renal failure. Pericarditis can be subclinical with effusion detected only by echocardiography. Constriction is not uncommon and often occurs as a subacute process. Tamponade and secondary infection are also major problems. In general, this form of pericarditis can usually be managed by augmenting dialysis and supportive care with nonsteroidal anti-inflammatory agents given systemically. However, many patients have exacerbations of pericardial associated symptoms. In these patients, pericardiocentesis and instillation of nonabsorbable steroids through an indwelling catheter have been successful. I do not use systemic steroids. Fever (>38.5C [101F]) or a white count >15,000 suggests purulent pericarditis, which may be either contiguous or hematogenous in origin. This problem is managed as outlined under Bacterial Pericarditis, above. When constriction results or recurrences are frequent, surgical therapy should be considered.

HYPOTHYROIDISM. Effusion occurs in most patients with myxedema, resulting in a large cardiac silhouette on chest x-ray. This problem rarely produces chest pain, tamponade, or other consequences. Once appropriate thyroid replacement is instituted, effusion will begin to resolve over several weeks to months.

CHOLESTEROL PERICARDITIS. "Gold paint" pericarditis is associated with an effusion rich in cholesterol. This problem is infrequent but may be associated with antecedent trauma to the pericardium or with tuberculous pericarditis. In most instances the specific cause is untraceable. Yellowish or golden fluid containing cholesterol crystals without elevation of serum cholesterol and a biopsy revealing cholesterol plaques are diagnostic. This poorly understood condition is difficult to manage. Management consists of pericardial aspiration with analysis to establish the diagnosis. In general, because this form of pericarditis develops so slowly and the pericardium remains thin and normal in distensibility, the massive enlargement of the cardiac silhouette seen on chest x-ray does not cause hemodynamic compromise or chest pain.

PERICARDITIS ASSOCIATED WITH NEOPLASM. Secondary pericarditis resulting from metastatic hematogenous or direct extension of various malignancies, usually from lung or breast, occurs commonly. Appropriate treatment of the malignancy (i.e., radiation or chemotherapy) may control the pericardial effusion. If tamponade occurs, it is treated as outlined above. With recurrences, pericardiocentesis with intrapleural administration of chemotherapeutic agents may be necessary. Nitrogen mustard, thiotepa, quinacrine, and other agents have all been advocated and given by intrapericardial instillation with the goal of producing adhesions with fibrosis so that recurrent effusion is prevented. Tetracycline is much less toxic and irritating than these drugs. Administration is repeated every 48 to 72 hours, through an indwelling catheter, until no further fluid can be aspirated. It is important to differentiate reactions (e.g., fever) caused by this form of treatment from secondary pyogenic pericarditis.

Primary neoplasm of the pericardium causing pericarditis (e.g., mesothelioma) generally occurs in association with asbestosis. This condition is extremely difficult to manage because of the thickened pericardium and the very thick, almost gelatinous nature of the pericardial fluid associated with this condition. Asbestosis bodies, on pericardial biopsy, help establish the diagnosis. Instillation of tetracycline through an indwelling pericardial catheter might be helpful. In general, however, only primary management of the neoplastic process itself, i.e., chemotherapy or surgery, provides appropriate palliation.

DEGENERATIVE ARTERIAL DISEASE

method of
LARRY H. HOLLIER, M.D.
Rochester, Minnesota

Degenerative arterial disease is one of the few areas in medicine that lends itself readily to diagnosis based solely on a careful history and physical examination. Arteriosclerosis is a disease process which produces symptoms that are directly related to either acute or chronic reduction in blood flow and subsequent anoxia of peripheral nerves; the interruption or decrease in blood flow to an extremity deprives the muscles and nerves of the necessary oxygen required to maintain function and thus causes pain and restricted mobility. A gradual decrease in the amount of blood delivered to an extremity may produce symptoms only when the metabolic demands of the muscle are increased, as during exercise, while the sudden complete interruption of the blood supply may reduce oxygen and nutritional delivery to such a degree that the tissues are unable to maintain viability even at rest.

Acute Arterial Occlusion

Although the five "P's" of pain, pallor, paresthesia, pulselessness, and paralysis are well known, all are not invariably present with acute arterial occlusion. Many times the pain may not be that severe or the patient may not understand the significance of numbness that may occur and may ignore the occurrence. In general, however, the initial pain of an acute arterial occlusion is fairly characteristic, occurring as a sudden, severe, lancinating sensation that tends to make the extremity weak. If this occurs while a patient is standing, he is frequently forced to sit down immediately, or may even fall to the ground. Depending upon the degree of collateral circulation, the pain may decrease quickly after the initial episode of vasospasm subsides. However, if collateral circulation is inadequate to provide the needed nutrition to the lower extremity, the patient will develop progressive signs of acute ischemia.

If the diagnosis of acute embolism is fairly secure, the patient is treated with the immediate administration of 10,000 units of heparin given intravenously. Analgesics or narcotics are given as needed to ease the pain, but one must be cautious lest oversedation produce respiratory or cardiac compromise. The patient is prepared for immediate arterial embolectomy, utilizing embolectomy catheters; undue delay can only result in propagation of the clot with loss of more collateral vessels. The patient is brought to the operating theater and prepared and draped in sterile fashion to expose the involved extremity and adjacent vessels. Local anesthesia is generally satisfactory for simple embolectomies.

For an upper extremity embolus the entire arm and axilla are draped so that the brachial artery can be exposed and embolectomy catheters passed proximally and distally. Usually a small transverse incision in the brachial artery just above the antecubital fossa allows an adequate embolectomy to be performed.

For a lower extremity embolus with a good pulse in the opposite groin, the patient is prepared and draped, exposing both groins and the entire involved lower extremity. The involved groin is incised and the common femoral artery exposed. If the common femoral artery is free of atherosclerotic plaque, a transverse incision is made in the vessel after proximal and distal control is obtained. Embolectomy catheters are passed in antegrade and retrograde fashion, removing as much thrombus as possible. Both superficial and profunda femoris vessels should be freed of thrombus, after which heparin, 1000 units, is instilled in each vessel. If one is unable to obtain adequate removal of thrombus distally in the extremity, the distal popliteal artery or a pedal vessel may be opened to provide retrograde removal of thrombus. If good in-flow can be obtained from the iliac segment, heparin is instilled proximally and the transverse incision is closed with interrupted monofilament sutures. If adequate in-flow cannot be obtained despite repeated attempts at proximal embolectomy, then the opposite groin is opened and a cross-femoral graft is performed under local anesthesia. Adequacy of the peripheral revascularization may be ascertained by completion angiography prior to termination of the procedure.

If femoral pulses are not initially palpable in either groin, the patient must be prepared and draped in such a manner as to provide a sterile field wherein the procedure may be extended to include aortofemoral grafting or axillofemoral grafting if necessary. A saddle embolus such as this should initially be approached by bilateral groin incisions and bilateral proximal and distal embolectomy. If adequate flow can be obtained in this fashion, then each incision is simply closed after one is assured of the completeness of the embolectomy. If embolectomy of either iliac segment is unsatisfactory, then one should proceed with axillofemoral or cross-femoral grafting under local anesthesia. If the patient is in satisfactory condition, one may elect to place the patient under general anesthesia at this point and perform standard aortofemoral grafting.

Antibiotics (cephalothin [Keflin], 2 grams) are generally given preoperatively and continued postoperatively for 2 days. Intraoperative antibiotics are routinely used, both locally and systemically. Although reports in the literature suggest an increased incidence of wound complications with postoperative heparin, we routinely maintain the patient on heparin for 7 to 10 days postoperatively. This may be given intravenously (heparin, 1000 units per hour by constant infusion) or subcutaneously (heparin, 5000 units every 4 to 6 hours).

If one suspects by history and/or physical examination that the patient has an acute thrombosis superimposed on chronic atherosclerotic occlusive disease, one would prefer to have preoperative angiography performed if it can be obtained without undue delay. If angiography is unobtainable prior to surgery, then intraoperative angiography will help delineate the extent of the occlusive process and may indicate the need for endarterectomy or bypass grafting in addition to thrombectomy and embolectomy. If there is a large amount of atherosclerotic plaque present in the common femoral artery, we will frequently make a vertical incision in the common femoral artery, since femoral occlusion may require a femoropopliteal bypass if the patient has a secondary thrombosis superimposed on a highly stenotic plaque. If that proves to be the case, bypass is easily performed through the vertical incision for the proximal anastomosis. If, however, the patient proves to have a simple embolus with no significant distal occlusive disease that would require bypass, the vertical arteriotomy is closed with a small vein patch angioplasty to prevent narrowing.

In the case of superimposed thrombus the patient may have only the sudden onset of rest pain without extensive ischemia that immediately threatens the viability of the extremity. In this situation it is sometimes preferable to delay surgery until the patient can be adequately evaluated and prepared for more extensive bypass grafting under general anesthesia. We prefer to maintain such a patient on heparin until the time of his elective procedure, but would not continue heparin in the postoperative period.

After completion of successful embolectomy, it is important that the patient be thoroughly evaluated to determine the cause of the embolus. Repeat electrocardiograms, Holter monitoring, echocardiography, and angiography may be helpful in determining the precise source.

One must be constantly alert in these patients, as they will frequently have recurring emboli to the same extremity, to a different extremity, or to some other site such as cerebral or mesenteric vessels. If subsequent embolization occurs, prompt embolectomy may be lifesaving.

Some patients will present to the physician only after severe and extensive ischemic damage has occurred. If obvious gangrene is present, one must still consider embolectomy to reduce the level of amputation that may be needed. This may provide needed additional blood flow to assure healing of the amputation stump.

One must be very cautious whenever a delayed embolectomy is performed, since toxic metabolic byproducts which are released after reinstitution of flow may result in severe acidosis and hyperkalemia and may lead to lethal cardiac arrhythmias, even on the operating table. Intravenous sodium bicarbonate is generally indicated in any embolectomy in which treatment has been delayed for any extended period of time. The surgeon must also be aware of the possible need for fasciotomy if ischemia has been prolonged. Early fasciotomy may provide the necessary reduction in compartmental pressure to allow muscle to remain viable and the extremity to remain functional after embolectomy. Although the need for fasciotomy can generally be determined by clinical examination, techniques for measuring intracompartmental pressures are available and can provide helpful information in a questionable situation. Insertion of subfascial wicks or needles can be used to determine the pressure within the compartments of the leg and allow one to monitor this pressure in the early postembolectomy period. If the pressure within the compartment becomes significantly elevated, one is best advised to avoid delay and perform fasciotomy as soon as possible. Procrastination could lead to severe ischemic muscle and nerve damage with muscle necrosis, foot drop, and even gangrene.

Chronic Ischemia

Degenerative arterial disease of the lower extremities is a frequent phenomenon and is markedly increased in chronic cigarette smokers. The hallmark of chronic arterial insufficiency is *intermittent claudication*. The location of intermittent claudication is indicative of the site of arterial obstruction. Aortoiliac occlusive disease will generally result in buttock and thigh claudication and is frequently accompanied by impotence (Leriche's syndrome), while claudication that occurs in the calf is generally due to a superficial femoral artery occlusion. Rest pain and chronic skin changes are usually due to multiple lesions involving the iliac, femoral, and/or tibial arteries.

Any patient who has rest pain, ischemic ulcers, or gangrenous changes is a candidate for revascularization. If the primary occlusive process is in the aortoiliac segment, aortofemoral bypass is the treatment of choice. Presently, operative mortality approaches zero in elective cases, and the postoperative morbidity and mortality is in the range of 2 per cent. If the patient has rest pain as a result of superficial femoral artery occlusive disease, a femoropopliteal bypass utilizing the saphenous vein is the treatment of choice. If combined aortoiliac and superficial femoral disease is present, we generally find that aortofemoral bypass grafting with profunda-angioplasty is sufficient to relieve symptoms. We do not feel that routine use of sympathectomy in such patients is of any significant additional benefit. In patients with extensive occlusion of the superficial femoral and popliteal system, one may be forced to perform bypass grafting from the common femoral to the tibial vessel in the distal leg. In these situations it is important to perform this with a saphenous vein, even if this requires harvesting the vein from both extremities and/or the arms. Although synthetic grafts and composite grafts can be used in urgent situations, their patency rate is much lower than that of saphenous veins. Occasionally one finds patients with gangrene or severe rest pain who have such extensive disease that no direct arterial reconstruction can be performed. In the rare situation in which this is the case and the patient has only rest pain but still has some marginal flow to the lower extremity audible by a Doppler, lumbar sympathectomy will occasionally provide temporary relief from the rest pain. In most instances, however, amputation will eventually be required.

Since most patients with simple intermittent claudication will have adequate relief of their symptoms with cessation of smoking and an active exercise program, we prefer to treat these patients nonoperatively. Clinical studies indicate that only 4 to 7 per cent of patients with intermittent claudication of the calf secondary to superficial femoral artery occlusion will develop gangrenous changes. We will generally not perform femoropopliteal bypass unless the patient with intermittent claudication of the calf has a rapidly decreasing claudication distance, develops rest pain or skin changes, or requires a longer walking distance because of his type of employment or social obligations.

Inasmuch as aortoiliac disease is frequently seen in association with more peripheral occlusion, if the patient is in good condition, we will generally perform aortofemoral bypass for the treatment of aortoiliac occlusive disease, even though intermittent claudication is the only symptom. Aortofemoral bypass generally enjoys a very good patency rate, and complications are infrequently seen. Because of this we prefer to perform aortofemoral surgery soon if the patient is in good condition, as such surgery at a later date may become ill advised because of progressive cardiac, pulmonary, or renal diseases that are frequent concomitant occurrences.

Patients with chronic ischemia, but mild symptoms such as claudication, can frequently be effectively treated by the following nonoperative means:

1. They are advised to walk beyond the point of claudication several times daily and should be reassured that the discomfort which develops in the calf, although painful, is not something that is overtly dangerous to them. This will frequently allow them to extend their walking distance and stimulate collateral circulation.

2. It is mandatory that these patients stop cigarette smoking entirely. This must be emphasized to them repeatedly and reinforced by both the physician and family members.

3. As dietary habits are fairly difficult to change, we outline a nonatherogenic diet and suggest that the patient attempt to follow the guidelines as much as possible. However, as many of these patients are quite elderly, we do not feel that strict dietary restrictions serve the best purpose for these patients. Moderate alcoholic intake is not discouraged.

4. Patients who have atrophic changes of the feet are urged to pay particular attention to appropriate foot care. It is emphasized that they wear well-fitting shoes, bathe their feet daily, and, if necessary, use emollients such as lanolin to prevent drying and cracking of the skin.

5. Any evidence of cellulitis or trichophytosis must be vigorously treated. Calluses, corns, plantar warts, and ingrown toenails should be treated by a podiatrist.

6. We do not generally use vasodilators as part of the overall medical management of these patients. We have not been able to demonstrate clinically that they provide any measurable change in the patient's symptoms. However, some patients do benefit by at least a placebo effect, and we will occasionally prescribe vasodilators for that reason.

With increasing frequency, we are seeing patients who have severe ischemic disease of the lower extremities, but whose overall medical condition precludes general anesthesia. Patients with severe cardiac disease or debilitating lung disease, as well as patients with advanced renal disease, are frequently unsatisfactory risks for conventional anatomic reconstruction under general anesthesia. In situations such as this some physicians will delay surgical referral for these patients and decide without consultation that amputation is the appropriate treatment. However, extra-anatomic bypass, utilizing local anesthesia and possible supplemental intravenous sedation, is preferred over amputation if at all possible. Extra-anatomic bypass generally carries a mortality rate in the range of 2 to 6 per cent, whereas amputation has a mortality rate of 15 to 40 per cent. Axillofemoral, femorofemoral, and axillopopliteal bypasses can be satisfactorily accomplished under local anesthesia and, in many cases, can provide excellent revascularization of the extremity and prevention of progressive ischemic change that would otherwise lead to gangrene and loss of limb. In a situation such as this the patient is immensely benefited, not only by having a limb salvaged but also by having a reconstructive procedure that has a lower mortality rate than amputation.

Vasospastic Disease

Vasospastic arterial disease can affect upper and lower extremities and is seen in both sexes, with a female:male predominance of 5:1. In general terminology, *Raynaud's phenomenon* is used when the vasospasm is secondary to some underlying disease (e.g., collagen-vascular disease), while *Raynaud's disease* is a term reserved for those patients whose disorder has no apparent underlying cause.

Patients with Raynaud-type symptoms must have a thorough work-up for the possibility of an underlying cause such as chemicals (e.g., ergot alkaloids, arsenic, lead), occupational trauma ("pneumatic-hammer disease"), neurologic disorders, collagen-vascular disorders (e.g., periarteritis nodosa, systemic lupus erythematosus, dermatomyositis, rheumatoid arthritis, scleroderma), arteriosclerosis obliterans or thromboangiitis obliterans, and other disorders such as underlying lymphoma or malignancy, multiple myeloma, and sarcomas. It is also important to differentiate the relatively benign vasospastic disorders such as acrocyanosis and livedo reticularis from true Raynaud's disease.

We prefer to manage patients with Raynaud's phenomenon in the following manner:

1. Initial management should include protection of the extremities from cold. Mittens and woolen socks are especially helpful, as are various commercial handwarmers and electrically heated mittens and socks.

2. The involved digits must be protected from trauma, even if this means a change in the patient's occupation—e.g., typists, pneumatic drill operators, and pianists.

3. It is mandatory that the patients stop smoking entirely.

4. Vasodilators such as phenoxybenzamine (Dibenzaline), cyclandelate (Cyclospasmol), and dihydro-ergot alkaloids (Hydergine) may occasionally provide benefit in some patients. However, we find that prazosin, 1 mg orally once or twice daily, provides best relief of symptoms, although syncope is an undesirable side effect.

5. For any presence of ulceration or gangrene of the fingertips, Nitrol Ointment * (2 per cent nitroglycerin in a lanolin base) is sometimes efficacious.

6. The intra-arterial injection of 1 mg of reserpine* is reported to be of benefit. However, in our experience we have seen few significant longlasting effects from this treatment. Another technique that we have utilized occasionally with fair results for some patients has been the intravenous injection of 1 mg of reserpine* in 100 ml of isotonic saline solution while the extremity is occluded by a tourniquet. After maintaining tourniquet occlusion for 15 minutes, to allow "fixation" of the reserpine, the tourniquet is slowly released. Both intra-arterial and intravenous uses of reserpine in this disorder are fraught with many potential complications and should be reserved for refractory cases.

7. Any evidence of cellulitis of the involved digits must be vigorously treated with antibiotics and good local wound care. Because of the decreased circulation to these areas they are quite suceptible to any infection whatsoever. Both systemic and local antibiotics are used in these patients.

8. Some patients will progress to severe disabling conditions, despite all attempts at conservative medical management. When patients become incapacitated because of persistent painful vasospasm and/or redevelopment of digital ulceration and gangrene, we have found a signficant number to be benefited by appropriate sympathectomy. Many patients will have dramatic relief of symptoms for a period of several months, but most will eventually develop a recurrence of symptoms. In most cases in our experience recurrent symptoms have been of a lesser degree of severity than they were preoperatively. However, since the involved vessels can still elicit a definite response to local application of cold, patients should still continue good hand care and avoid cold stimuli.

Peripheral Arterial Aneurysms

Although peripheral arterial aneurysms can occur in virtually any vessel, over 90 per cent of them occur in either the popliteal or the femoral arteries. By far the most common cause is atherosclerotic occlusive disease with degeneration and weakening of the arterial wall. These patients will frequently have evidence of other manifestations of arteriosclerosis such as coronary artery disease, hypertension, transient ischemic attacks, or multiple aneurysms. Indeed, the presence of a peripheral aneurysm should be a warning signal to the evaluating physician because there is a very high incidence of multiple and bilateral aneurysms concomitant with a high incidence of

---

*This use of this agent is not listed in the manufacturer's official directive.

intra-abdominal aneurysms. The presence of a peripheral aneurysm carries a 50 to 75 per cent incidence of multiple aneurysms and a greater than 25 per cent incidence of a coexisting abdominal aortic aneurysm.

A common clinical manifestation of peripheral aneurysm is simply the presence of a mass. However, rupture and thrombosis can occur. Whereas abdominal aortic aneurysms have a propensity to rupture, popliteal aneurysms have a very high incidence of thrombosis. Symptoms of limb ischemia are common and either may present as chronic arterial insufficiency or may mimic acute arterial embolism owing to the sudden loss of blood flow in the distal leg. Occasionally a large aneurysm can result in neurologic compression symptoms with pain over the distribution of adjacent nerves. With popliteal aneurysms, phlebitis caused by pressure on the adjacent veins can be a presenting symptom.

Angiography is generally indicated in a patient with peripheral aneurysm and should include angiography of the abdominal aorta as well as the run-off vessels. Because of the high incidence of complications associated with peripheral aneurysms, surgical excision and interposition grafting should be performed whenever possible. One would prefer the use of the interposition saphenous vein to treat popliteal aneurysms, although sometimes femoral aneurysms, because of their involvement of adjacent branches, are treated as well with knitted Dacron grafts. In general, there is no good medical management for peripheral aneurysms. Attempts at early diagnosis and appropriate surgery prior to the development of complications provide the best means of treating this condition.

MASSIVE DEEP VEIN THROMBOSIS OF THE LOWER EXTREMITIES

method of
JOHN M. PORTER, M.D.
Portland, Oregon

Incidence

The magnitude of the clinical problem of deep vein thrombosis of the lower extremities is staggering. A careful review of annual mortality statistics suggests that about 150,00 deaths occur annually in the United States from pulmonary embolism, whereas another 700,000 to 1 million nonfatal pulmonary embolic episodes occur each year. It is clear that over 75 per cent of pulmonary emboli originate from thrombi in the deep veins of the lower extremities, and it appears that about one half of untreated episodes of deep vein thrombosis result in pulmonary embolism. This suggests that several million episodes of deep vein thrombosis of the lower extremities occur annually in the United States alone. The incidence of severe postphlebitic symptoms following deep vein thrombosis is not known, but the numbers must be massive. The treatment of patients with deep vein thrombosis must be directed at both the prevention of pulmonary embolism and the prevention of the long-term, disabling sequelae of the postphlebitic syndrome.

Definitions

Deep vein thrombosis of the lower extremities may occur in three variants: phlegmasia cerulea dolens, phlegmasia alba dolens, or tibial-soleal venous thrombosis. The first type, phlegmasia cerulea dolens, is the most severe and represents extensive deep vein thrombosis with massive obstruction of venous return from the limb. The extensive thrombosis involves the iliac, the femoral, and frequently the popliteal veins, and usually also the tibial and soleal veins. The internal iliac vein, the most important collateral venous drainage pathway of the lower extremity, is usually also thrombosed. The patient presents with severe swelling of the limb extending from the groin to the toes, a dusky cyanotic color of the limb, and dull, aching pain of variable severity. If leg elevation is not instituted early, venous hypertension may be so severe as to cause cutaneous bleb formation similar to that of a second degree burn. A most uncommon variant of phlegmasia cerulea dolens has been called venous gangrene. This rare condition, which results in gangrene of the distal extremities, is associated pathologically with extension of the venous thrombotic process into all the small veins and even the venules. The venous gangrene variant of phlegmasia cerulea dolens occurs almost exclusively in patients who are seriously ill with another disease process, frequently metastatic malignancy, and probably represents a variant of disseminated intravascular thrombosis.

Phlegmasia alba dolens denotes a less extensive venous thrombotic process, usually limited to the external iliac and common femoral veins with sparing of the internal iliac vein and other portions of the deep venous system. The clinical picture is that of limb swelling and discomfort, but massive swelling and cyanosis are absent.

Tibial-soleal venous thrombosis may be asymptomatic or present with only mild edema and discomfort of the lower leg, ankle, and foot.

Untreated venous thrombosis at or proximal to the popliteal vein carries a risk of pulmonary embolism of 50 per cent. Isolated tibial-soleal venous thrombosis carries a very low risk of pulmonary embolism if the popliteal vein is not involved. It is important to note, however, that initially isolated tibial-soleal venous thrombosis may spread to involve the popliteal vein, and for this reason I feel that this variant of venous thrombosis should be treated with the same anti-coagulant regimen as the other variants.

Treatment

The acute treatment of phlegmasia alba dolens and tibial-soleal venous thrombosis consists of leg elevation and heparin anticoagulation. The patient is placed at bed rest with the legs elevated 20 to 30 degrees, and this position must be constantly maintained. In the absence of any contraindications, heparin anticoagulation therapy is begun with the administration of 200 units per kg of body weight intravenously, followed by the continuous intravenous infusion of heparin sufficient to maintain the activated partial thromboplastin time two to three times normal. This is usually in the range of 800 to 1200 units of heparin per hour.

The treatment of phlegmasia cerulea dolens is identical, with the exception that early attention must be directed to replacement of the initially depleted intravascular volume that results from fluid sequestration in the massively edematous extremity. In these patients it appears prudent to use both central venous pressure and urinary output to guide appropriate intravascular volume replacement. I prefer equal volumes of plasma and saline for volume replacement.

Intravenous heparin anticoagulation is continued for 7 to 10 days and is followed by oral anticoagulation with warfarin. Warfarin is begun on day 3 or 4 of heparin therapy. The heparin is tapered gradually over a 24 hour period on about day 10 of therapy, at least 2 to 3 days after prolongation of prothrombin time to twice the control level has been achieved. It must be emphasized that the anticoagulant action of warfarin may lag several days behind the initial prolongation of prothrombin time.

The recognized contraindications to heparin use include known hemorrhagic diathesis, gastrointestinal bleeding, intracranial injury, gross hematuria, and immediate postoperative state. If the patient has one of these contraindications I prefer to use intravenous clinical dextran (average molecular weight 70,000), 500 ml per day of the 10 per cent solution for 5 to 6 days, with the simultaneous administration of warfarin. It must be noted that the efficacy of dextran used therapeutically for venous thrombosis is anecdotal only, and has never been documented by prospective randomized study. If the patient experiences a pulmonary embolus while on this regimen or has sufficient bleeding to require discontinuation of the dextran, I would recommend vena caval ligation as described below.

Warfarin anticoagulation should be continued for a minimum of 4 months, as several studies have shown that the first 4 months are the time of greatest likelihood of thrombus recurrence. If the patient has had previous venous thrombosis, oral anticoagulation should be maintained for 1 to 2 years. Although not proved, there is considerable evidence that patients taking oral contraceptives have a higher incidence of venous thromboembolism than matched patients not taking the drug. For this reason I recommend that all patients with a history of venous thrombosis not take oral contraceptives.

The clinician should remember that a number of frequently used drugs significantly alter the action of warfarin. Some of the drugs that potentiate the action of warfarin include quinidine, salicylates, phenylbutazone, chloramphenicol, and anabolic steroids. Barbiturates, glutethimide, and griseofulvin are among the more frequently used drugs that inhibit warfarin action. The physician should specifically ascertain the effect on warfarin of any other drug the patient may be taking.

The patient should not be allowed to ambulate until complete resolution of edema has occurred with bed rest and leg elevation, and then only while wearing firmly compressive elastic stockings. I prefer the 30 mm gradient below-knee Sigvaris elastic stockings, distributed in the United States by Camp International, Inc., Jackson, Michigan. The lightweight so-called "antiembolism" stockings are not sufficiently strong for use in this application.

Role of Surgery in Acute Deep Vein Thrombosis

The role of surgical thrombectomy in the acute treatment of deep vein thrombosis has evoked continuing controversy for years. At present it is clear that fewer and fewer surgeons favor thrombectomy despite the beguiling proposal of a "mechanical solution to a mechanical problem."

The two propositions brought forward in support of venous thrombectomy appear incorrect. One is the proposal that early thrombectomy in phlegmasia cerulea dolens may prevent the development of venous gangrene. It is important to emphasize that venous gangrene is clearly not the expected or normal evolutionary termination of untreated phlegmasia cerulea dolens. A large majority of patients with venous gangrene have metastatic malignancy, and the patients I have seen with this condition have all had clear hematologic evidence of disseminated intravascular coagulation. The reported use of thrombectomy for established venous gangrene has been strikingly unsuccessful. The other benefit claimed for early venous thrombectomy — namely, the avoidance of the postphlebitic syndrome — has not been supported by long-term critical follow-up of postoperative patients. Over 80 per cent of postoperative patients when followed for a period of years have developed typical postphlebitic symptoms. When this long-term functional failure is added to the reported operative mortality rate of 5 to 10 per cent, intraoperative pulmonary embolism rate of 5 to 20 per cent, and postoperative morbidity rate (primarily wound infection) of 20 to 30 per cent, one is forced to conclude that the procedure has little to recommend it. I have not performed venous thrombectomy in the past 10 years.

Fibrinolytic Therapy

Two fibrinolytic drugs, streptokinase and urokinase, have recently been marketed in the United States. Of these, only streptokinase has been approved for use in venous thrombosis. It appears likely that urokinase will be equally effective, but to date proof of efficacy has not been obtained.

The goal of therapy in patients with deep vein thrombosis, as previously stated, is the prevention of pulmonary embolism and the postphlebitic syndrome. Streptokinase, in selected patients, gives promise of achieving both these goals. Current reports suggest that patients experiencing their first episode of deep vein thrombosis and presenting less than 3 days after the onset of symptoms have a 50 per cent chance of complete thrombus resolution with restoration of normal venous valve function if treated with streptokinase.

If a patient meets these criteria and has no contraindication to the use of fibrinolytic therapy, I would begin treatment with a loading dose of 250,000 units of streptokinase, followed by 100,000 units per hour for 72 hours. The exact dose is usually regulated by maintaining the thrombin time at twice the normal value. After 72 hours treatment is switched to intravenous heparin, followed by warfarin as described above. The directions in the manufacturer's package insert describing contraindications to therapy, the recognition and treatment of allergic reactions, and drug dosage and monitoring should be carefully observed.

Postphlebitic Syndrome

This syndrome, caused by venous hypertension resulting from recanalization with destruction of valves in the previously thrombosed venous segment, consists in its fully developed form of malleolar ulceration, hyperpigmentation about the ankles, stasis dermatitis, and secondary varicose veins. This symptom complex can be completely incapacitating and constitutes the greatest cause of morbidity after deep vein thrombosis.

Clinical emphasis must be placed upon the prevention of the postphlebitic syndrome. It is clear that this syndrome may develop insidiously years after apparent total recovery from an episode of venous thrombosis. I feel it is most desirable that the physician follow a patient sequentially for life after an episode of venous thrombosis. The physician should impress upon the patient that his legs will never be normal and that his best chance of avoiding the postphlebitic syndrome lies in his careful adherence to the following regimen:

1. Wear fitted elastic stockings for life whenever out of bed. The patient should have at least two stockings so that he can wear one while the other is being laundered. Also, the stockings gradually lose their elasticity and require replacement about every 6 months. I prefer the 30 mm gradient below-knee Sigvaris brand stocking.

2. Elevate the foot of the bed 4 inches to promote venous drainage.

3. Carefully wash the leg, foot, and especially the intertriginous areas daily with soap and water.

4. Avoid leg trauma. Seek medical attention immediately even for such apparently trivial injuries as scratches or bruises. Several days of leg elevation and antibiotics, if indicated, should be prescribed until complete healing occurs.

5. Avoid long periods of leg dependency. If the patient must stand for long periods, he should develop the habit of frequent elevation onto the tips of the toes to promote venous return. Whenever sitting, the patient should elevate his leg on a second chair.

Various procedures have been described for the surgical treatment of refractory venous stasis ulcers. These consist of extra-or subfascial ligation of communicating veins, excision of regional varicose veins, and skin grafting. In my experience these procedures are rarely indicated. If the patient will wear elastic stockings and follow the instructions listed, venous stasis ulcers will heal without surgery. If surgery is performed with initial success, however, and the patient fails to wear stockings postoperatively, the ulcers will frequently recur. For these reasons I rarely recommend surgical treatment of venous stasis ulcers. Likewise, I find no merit in simple skin grafting of venous stasis ulcers.

Pulmonary Embolism

The most feared complication of venous thrombosis is pulmonary embolism. As noted earlier, untreated leg vein thrombosis is associated with an incidence of pulmonary embolism approaching 50 per cent, although many of these patients are not symptomatic. With adequate heparin anticoagulation, the incidence of pulmonary embolism is reduced to less than 10 per cent.

Vena Caval Interruption

Debate continues concerning the merits of vena caval interruption in the prevention of pulmonary embolism from leg vein thrombosis. Many have advocated the widespread use of this procedure even as a prophylactic measure while preforming abdominal operations upon patients who are believed to be at high risk for the development of venous thrombosis. Several recent reviews, however, have clearly pointed out the failure of vena caval interruption to achieve its stated goals. Recurrent embolization occurs in at least 5 to 10 per cent of patients, and possibly in many more. The operative mortality rate for the procedure is 5 per cent or higher, and the late incidence of the postphlebitic syndrome is at least 20 per cent.

Nevertheless, I do feel there is a definite, although limited, role for vena caval interruption. The only indications I regard as valid include (1) documented repeated small emboli, which may lead rapidly to the development of pulmonary hypertension and cor pulmonale; (2) septic emboli, usually from a septic pelvic focus; and (3) documented recurrent pulmonary embolism while on adequate heparin anticoagulation therapy. I feel it is absolutely essential to document the occurrence of embolism by pulmonary angiography; I personally do not accept the presence of an abnormal perfusion lung scan as diagnostic.

If vena caval interruption is indicated, I prefer transperitoneal caval ligation with two heavy ligatures placed just distal to the renal veins.

VARICOSE VEINS

method of
JOHN E. CONNOLLY, M.D.
Irvine, California

The treatment of varicose veins consists of external support, injection of sclerosing material, surgical excision, or a combination of these three methods of treatment. The patient is informed that although surgical treatment can be expected to markedly improve the situation, subsequent injections of sclerosing material or continued support with elastic stockings, or both these treatments, may also be necessary.

Elastic support or injection of sclerosing material alone is indicated only in the treatment of mild varices. For injection therapy, I prefer to use sodium tetradecyl (Sotradecol). The contents of the bottle are thoroughly agitated, and 0.5 ml of foam from the top is removed and injected into each varix with a 25 gauge needle.

Surgical Treatment

Although the classic high, middle, low ligation of the great and lesser saphenous veins has been very beneficial in the treatment of many patients with varicose veins, a much more satisfactory result in obtained by removal of the involved veins by stripping combined with additional ligation of incompetent communicating veins.

Technique

Immediately before the operation, with the patient standing, the sites of the communicating veins are located and scratched with a pin so that they can be easily identified after the leg has been prepared with antiseptics and the patient is in a horizontal position.

In our experience the deep veins are almost always competent unless the patient has had iliofemoral thrombosis in the past. If such a history is obtained or suspected, a preoperative venogram should be performed before embarking upon a stripping procedure.

Great Saphenous Vein Stripping Technique

1. A ½ to ¾ inch (1.25 to 2.0 cm) incision is made at the level of and just anterior to the medial malleolus. The saphenous vein is identified and ligated distally.

2. A small transverse incision is made in the saphenous vein. The small metal tip of a flexible internal vein stripper is introduced, and an effort is made to pass the internal stripper up the great saphenous vein as far as its junction with the femoral vein in the groin. This usually requires some bimanual manipulation with one of the operator's hands over the course of the ascending vein. I have found that it is easier to pass the stripper from below upward than from above downward.

3. Usually with proper manipulation the stripper is felt in the medial groin area.

4. A 2 to 3 inch (5 to 8 cm) transverse skin incision is made in the inguinal crease, centered over the palpable stripper. By this technique a smaller and more accurate groin incision is obtained than by employing a blind incision.

5. The great saphenous vein is then identified and divided close to its junction with the femoral vein after all tributaries have been ligated and divided. The stripper usually has to be pulled back a short distance before the vein can be transected. The proximal divided stump of the saphenous vein is both ligated and transfixed with nonabsorbable sutures.

6. After transection of the vein, the stripper is passed through the open end of the vein until the larger distal flanged end is caught by the small size of the vein at the malleolar level.

7. The malleolar end of the vein is then securely tied about the stripper flush with the large flanged end.

8. Prior to stripping of the greater saphenous vein, its upper transected end is grasped carefully with a clamp and elevated so that any residual tributaries into it near the saphenofemoral junction are clearly seen. They are then separated, ligated, and divided, taking care that no deep branches are missed.

9. Prior to stripping with the internal stripper in place, incisions are made over each previously marked perforator, and the perforating branches of the saphenous vein are ligated and divided. All incisions except the groin are then closed and dressed, and the leg is wrapped firmly from below with an Ace (elastic) bandage.

10. The great saphenous vein is then stripped by pulling the free end of the stripper out of the groin incision while the operator's other hand steadies the leg over the course of the stripper.

11. If the stripper cannot be passed the complete length of the vein initially, an incision is made over the vein at the level of obstruction and stripping is carried out as described, repeatedly if necessary, on up the leg.

12. The patient's legs are elevated in bed and he is encouraged to walk the same day with the supporting elastic bandages in place.

13. The patient is usually discharged from the hospital on the second or third day following surgery. Elastic bandages are worn for 2 weeks, after which they are generally replaced with elastic stockings which are worn for another several weeks.

Stripping of Lesser Saphenous Veins and Perforating Veins

If varices of the lesser system or perforators are diagnosed on the preoperative examination, they are handled as follows:

1. The short saphenous vein is located through a 1 inch (2.5 cm) transverse incision just lateral to the Achilles tendon.

2. An internal stripper is introduced into the vein at this point and passed upward to the popliteal crease, where a second transverse incision is made.

3. The lesser saphenous vein is then stripped from below upward in exactly the same manner as described for the greater saphenous vein.

4. Separate 1 inch (2.5 cm) transverse skin incisions are made over each perforating vein in the calf, and as much of the underlying vein as possible is excised. The final result of the operation depends in large part on the care and time devoted to ligating and excising the perforators.

Treatment of Stasis Ulcers

1. Elevation of the leg with strict bed rest is mandatory until healing of the ulcer occurs.

2. Cleansing of the ulcerated area by application of moist packs may be necessary if there is superimposed infection.

3. Large ulcers may require skin grafting.

4. In addition to stripping of the greater and lesser saphenous veins if not previously performed, subfascial division of perforating veins is necessary in the management of stasis ulcers. The perforators are most easily exposed by a longitudinal posterior incision from below the ulcer to well up on the calf, guided by a preoperative venogram to ascertain the location of all deep perforators.

5. Following subfascial ligation, the leg is kept elevated until wound healing has occurred.

SECTION 4

The Blood and Spleen

APLASTIC ANEMIA

method of
YVES NAJEAN, M.D.*
Paris, France

All the large series of aplastic anemia (AA) patients in the literature demonstrate the great severity of the disease (Williams et al., in a retrospective analysis in Salt Lake City; Camitta et al., reporting the results of a prospective American-British protocol; Sanchez-Medal in Mexico; Heimpel in West Germany; our group in France and Spain). When excluding very moderate pancytopenias (which do not require any therapy), the overall survival rate at the twentieth month is about 45 per cent. The treatments used, however, have their own risks: hepatic toxicity and growth arrest with androgens; anaphylactic shock and severe thrombocytopenia with antithymocytic serum; and severe infection and graft-vs.-host disease (GVH) in patients treated by allogenic bone marrow graft. So the choice of therapy is based upon a correct prognostic evaluation.

Prognostic Evaluation of Aplastic Anemias

Careful analysis of the prognostic factors in AA has been done. (For details see Lynch et al.: Blood 45:517, 1975, and Najean et al.: Am. J. Med. 67:564, 1979.)

Age is correlated with prognosis; AA in young patients (less than 30 years of age) is generally more severe than in older patients; on the other hand, the mortality rate in the oldest

*For the Cooperative Group for the Study of Aplastic and Refractory Anemias.

patients (over 70) is excessive because of excessive hemorrhagic and infectious risks. *Sex* is not clearly correlated with prognosis, even if slightly better survival is noted in females. *Secondary cases* do not appear different, in terms of severity, from primary cases. *Acute cases* are always more severe than those with a gradual onset.

The most important parameter is the degree of cytopenia. *Reticulocytopenia, thrombocytopenia,* and chiefly *granulocytopenia* are closely correlated to survival. Patients with less than 20×10^9 reticulocytes per liter, 0.5×10^9 granulocytes, and 20×10^9 platelets can be considered to have very severe disease with expected survival less than 25 per cent, and in such patients the risk of bone marrow graft appears fully justified.

Direct investigation of the bone marrow also helps evaluate prognosis. *Bone marrow slides* do not give valuable information on true marrow density, but the percentage of nonmyeloid cells is closely correlated with prognosis. *Bone marrow biopsy* gives useful information; qualitative abnormalities of the bone marrow (edema, hemorrhagic patches, disorganization of the reticulin network) are pejorative parameters. *Isotopic investigations* (^{59}Fe kinetics, bone marrow scintigraphy using Tc-colloids, ^{111}In or ^{52}Fe) give quantitative data on the remaining erythropoiesis, and may correct false interpretations of histologic data: rich bone marrow slides may be residual "hot pockets" in a globally poor bone marrow.

Unfortunately, *stem-cell quantification* does not bring useful prognostic information. Indeed, in all the cases the number of in vitro myeloid colonies is very low. This test, however, may be useful for investigating the mechanism of AA and for evaluating the myeloid repopulation.

From these parameters, which together are redundant, multivariate analysis allows the establishment of an "index of prognosis" closely cor-

251

related with short-term evolution, and so is very useful for the choice of therapy.

When considering the evolution of patients surviving the first 2 or 3 months of the disease, the most valuable prognostic parameter is the *evolutive tendency*. Those patients, even those whose disease was initially very severe, who have demonstrated an improvement, even slight, during the first 3 months have an excellent chance of survival compared to those who did not demonstrate any change. Such clinical information may be very useful when considering the use of a bone marrow graft.

Maintenance Therapy

Whatever the initial severity of the disease and the treatment chosen (androgen therapy, immunosuppression, bone marrow graft), adequate maintenance therapy is absolutely necessary. It has been noted that some bad results in a series of patients treated by androgen therapy alone could be due to insufficient maintenance and survey, and that no comparison of androgen-treated and grafted patients is valuable if the same maintenance therapy is not used in both groups.

Treatment of Anemia

As there is no possibility of stimulating bone marrow activity in these patients, the hemoglobin rate must be maintained at a level of 10 grams per 100 ml or more, chiefly in the oldest patients and in patients with vascular antecedents.

Before the first transfusion, a full study of the erythrocytic phenotype is necessary, in order to choose the best donors and to enable identification of subsequently developed alloantibodies. If possible, red packed blood cells compatible in the most immunogenic systems (Kell, Rhesus, Lewis, Duffy) are used. It is useful to use leukocyte-deprived transfusions to avoid alloimmunization in the HLA system (filtration on "leukopak," centrifugation, use of frozen blood).

In the management of these patients, regular surveys of possible alloantibodies and of material overloading are necessary. However, the risk of hemochromatosis in those patients who will be dead or cured at the twentieth month is not of consequence; not one patient in our large series (more than 100 patients living more than 2 years) died from hemochromatosis, so that the use of iron chelators (e.g., desferrioxamine) does not seem important.

Treatment of Granulocytopenia and Infectious Complications

When granulocytopenia is less than 0.5×10^9 per liter, the frequency of bacterial complications is very high. It is increased by the frequent and unjustified use of corticotherapy.

Preventive therapy is not easy. Isolation of the patient in a sterile enclosure for more than a few days is practically, financially, and psychologically difficult.

Most septicemias are caused by bacteria of endogenic origin, chiefly intestinal. This observation led to the use of systemic decontamination. However, even if such a treatment seems to be useful in the case of short aplastic phases, such as those induced by heavy chemotherapy in leukemia and cancer, its efficiency in chronic AA remains a matter of discussion. Its long-term use could induce local toxicity and development of resistant bacterial clones.

Conversely, antibiotic therapy is absolutely indicated as a curative therapy, should these patients develop a bacterial focus or only have a fever. Bacterial investigations for identification of the agent(s) and their sensitivity are needed, but polyvalent antibiotic therapy must be prescribed before the results are obtained with modification of therapy when results are known. Toxic shock in a patient with gram-negative bacteremia occurs frequently, and the prognosis of the cardiovascular collapse depends on the speed with which therapeutic measures are taken, i.e., perfusion, inotrope-positive drugs, diuretics. The use of granulocyte transfusions is reserved for such patients in the hope they can help cure the septicemia, although such therapy may be ineffective if a previous use had induced antibodies and reduced the survival of the transfused cells.

Granulocyte transfusions are effective only if the dose is sufficient and in the absence of alloimmunization. About 0.5×10^{11} granulocytes per square meter of body surface are needed to increase the granulocyte count to 1×10^9 per liter 1 hour after transfusion. The short life span of these cells (half-life of about 12 hours after ^{51}Cr labeling) implies a short-term repetition of these transfusions when fever does persist. From a technologic point of view, it is possible by continuous filtration or centrifugation to obtain enough granulocytes from a normal donor, chiefly for the treatment of children. In adults, the use of donors with chronic myeloid leukemia is convenient and efficient, but it raises two ethical problems: using blood of a patient with malignant disease for a patient with nonmalignant disease (which is theoretically forbidden), and delaying the treatment of a chronic leukemia by using the patient as a permanent donor. In any case, the donor selection should be done following HLA grouping.

Treatment of Thrombocytopenia and Hemorrhages

Only platelet transfusions are able to prevent and cure the hemorrhagic syndrome caused by thrombocytopenia. All other proposed therapeutic means are ineffective.

Platelets are obtained from a normal donor or donors, either as concentrates obtained from several units of blood by centrifugation and pooled or as a single concentrate obtained from a single donor by using continuous centrifugation technique. The dose, to obtain a platelet count high enough to stop hemorrhages, is generally 1 to 2 units per 10 kg of body weight, but a larger quantity may be required in previously transfused patients, in whom the platelet recovery and life span are lowered.

The use of platelet transfusion is not debatable in the case of life-threatening hemorrhage, but its use as a preventive measure can be criticized. Platelet transfusion can prevent sudden hemorrhages, cerebral hemorrhages in particular, which cannot be cured after they occur, and its use can be proposed in very severely thrombocytopenic patients, chiefly when headache, fundus hemorrhage, vascular antecedent, or associated infection makes the risk particularly high. In other cases, because of the risk of immunization and thus less efficacy of platelet transfusion, most authors prefer to delay its use.

Two general rules must be followed, whatever the blood fraction used (red cells, granulocytes, or platelets): (1) Close family relatives must be excluded as blood donors in order to avoid alloimmunization against a possible bone marrow donor. (2) In patients with a recent bone graft transplantation, irradiation of blood products at 1500 to 2000 rads is necessary to avoid the graft of potentially toxic lymphocytes in the immunodepressed recipient.

Androgen Therapy of Aplastic Anemia

Androgen therapy has been used for more than 15 years in primary and secondary AA, but with still poorly defined methods, with uncertain results, and on a poorly understood physiologic basis.

Experimental Data. Experimental data have shown the following effects of androgen on erythropoiesis: higher hemoglobin concentration in males compared to females, even when iron stores are identical; polycythemia caused by androgen-secreting tumors or by androgen therapy for breast cancer; and a drop of the red cell volume in animals and men after castration, which can be corrected by androgen therapy.

One of the ways androgens could act on erythropoiesis is by stimulation of erythropoietin secretion. It has been shown that the blood concentration and urinary excretion of erythropoietin increase after androgen infusion in animals and in human volunteers. This effect is abolished by bilateral nephrectomy. However, the erythropoietin rate in AA is always very high, and the androgen effect is probably not mediated in this way.

Another influence of androgens is direct inductive action on the stem cells. It has been proved that the number of erythroid colonies in vitro and the percentage of stem cells in cycle (i.e., in proliferative activity) increase with androgen added in vitro as well as after in vivo treatment. From the recent work of Singer and Adamson (Blood 48:855, 1976), it seems that the target cell of 5α-compounds (most usually used) and 5β-derivates could be different; the 5α-androstanes would modify the proliferation capacity of a very young cell (less differentiated, less erythropoietin-sensitive, larger, and less often in cycle than the target cell of the 5 α-derivatives).

Clinical Data. Numerous series of androgen-treated aplastic anemia patients have been published, from which the following conclusions can be drawn.

1. Actuarial survival curves of androgen-treated patients demonstrate better survival than that of controls with similar severity of disease. A comparison of several drugs in similarly followed patients has demonstrated significant differences between drugs in terms of survival and of hematologic recovery (Scand. J. Haemat. 22:343, 1979). Clear differences have been observed, in terms of survival, between patients treated with low (0.2 mg per kg) and high (1 mg per kg) doses of the same drug.

2. The prolongation of treatment at full dose for 10 to 20 months increases the percentage of complete remission and decreases the percentage of relapses and possible subsequent death.

3. After discontinuance of androgen therapy, even in the case of complete remission, relapse is observed in 40 per cent of patients. These relapses are androgen sensitive, with complete remission if the first remission was complete but with incomplete remission if it was previously incomplete.

4. Some patients demonstrate androgen dependency during a long-term survival (one of our patients for more than 10 years). In such cases

maintenance of a correct hematologic equilibrium requires permanent androgen supplementation.

The use of androgens given as soon as possible, at high doses, and for a long period is justified in AA from both a theoretical and a practical point of view.

Toxicity of Androgen Therapy. The most evident side effect and often the most difficult for the patient to accept is virilization (hirsutism, acne, hoarse voice, clitoris hypertrophy). It is important to inform the patient, chiefly young women or the parents of a child, that these side effects will regress after treatment is discontinued (to include return to normal menstruation, and possible pregnancies). Other minor side effects are weight increase, calf cramps, and hiccup. In elderly males, androgen therapy could favor prostatic tumors and acute urine retention.

In children, the risk of abnormal growth often has been emphasized by pediatricians. In our series, however, the children experienced an initial fast growth, and in long-term surviving patients adult height is normal or even superior to that of their parents.

In half the patients, hepatic abnormalities are observed when using C-17 alkylated as well as nonalkylated compounds. Icterus was observed in 30 per cent of our patients, and other biologic abnormalities in another 20 per cent; such a toxicity appears in the first 6 months in most cases. Icterus is not due to cellular hepatic toxicity, and may disappear even though the drug is not discontinued. None of our patients developed chronic hepatitis or cirrhosis in the absence of viral (blood-transmitted) hepatitis. A few patients did develop late hepatic tumor (generally benign hepatoma) or peliosis hepatis. In our series, four cases have been observed in 120 long-term survivors.

Limits of Androgen Efficacy. Improvement on androgen therapy is slow. Reticulocyte count (along with the need for transfusion) improves only after 3 to 6 months; granulocytes increase at the same time or even later, and platelets, if influenced, still later. This explains, at least partly, why there is failure in the most severe cases, the patients dying from infection or hemorrhages during the first weeks of the disease before any possible androgen-induced improvement could occur.

On the other hand, it has been said that androgen therapy acts only in less severe cases, i.e., in those patients who have preserved a pool of stem cells, the target cell of androgens. It is difficult to answer this objection, as patients with the most severe disease generally die or receive a bone graft during the first weeks of the illness; but in our few patients with severe disease who

survived for 3 months, it seems that androgen therapy could be effective in them as well as in less severely ill patients.

In genetic (Fanconi-type) anemia, androgen therapy is generally useful, but in most patients thrombocytopenia does not improve. All the published series, however, indicate that the improved patients remain androgen dependent for a long time and then relapse and die whatever the dose and type of androgen used during the terminal phase of the disease.

Assay of Lithium

Lithium salts–induced leukocytosis was reported in patients with psychiatric disorders as early as 1966 (Mayfield and Brown: J. Psych. Res.: 4:202, 1966). It has been proved that lithium stimulated the growth and number of granulocyte colony–forming cells and of colony-stimulating activity (Harker et al.: Blood, 49:263, 1977; Rohstein et al.: N. Engl. J. Med. 298:178, 1978).

Lithium is at present largely used in prospective protocols of chemotherapy in malignant disease, with the hope of reducing toxic granulocytopenia and its consequences. In primary AA, the results do not suggest any direct effect on stem cells and/or granulocytopoiesis (Barrett: Blut, 40:1, 1980).

Immunosuppression

Some investigations suggest that stem cell depression can be induced by an immunologic mechanism. An immune defect of bone marrow cells has been demonstrated in some acquired erythroblastopenias, but in these cases the maturing, already differentiated progenitor cells are targets of this immunologic process. Some patients with aplastic anemia have been cured after heavy immunosuppression without further bone marrow graft, or have experienced autologous repopulation after rejection of the allogeneic bone marrow cells. The efficacy of antithymocytic serum (Speck et al.: Lancet 2:1145, 1977) and of high-dose corticoids (Bacigapulo et al.: Fourth Congress of the French Society of Hematology, 1980), even if only temporary, is an argument favoring the immunologic basis of AA. In vitro inhibition of normal stem cell growth by the patient's lymphocytes, and its removal by antithymocytic serum (ATG), is another argument for a role of environmental factors in the pathogenesis of AA.

Antithymocytic Globulin (ATG)

This treatment, still under investigation, has already been used in a large number of patients, so some conclusions can be suggested. About 50 per cent of patients did demonstrate a clear increase of granulocyte and reticulocyte counts, but this was generally followed by a drop to initial levels. Further progressive improvement (with androgen therapy associated in most of the patients) was observed in responders and not in those who initially were nonresponders. There is a correlation between clinical response and in vitro effect of ATG on the granulocytic stem cell growth. Patients with the most severe cases (with multiparametric index of prognosis very low) do not respond to ATG assay, suggesting that the presence of some remaining stem cells is necessary for its efficacy.

At present, it seems that ATG infusion could be useful chiefly for discrimination of those patients susceptible of further response to androgens (or of spontaneous improvement). It is possible that this treatment could decrease, or suppress, the immunologic effect on the stem cells, and make them responsive to androgens or to spontaneous recovery.

ATG therapy is not easy to use. Severe platelet depression obliges one to use platelet transfusions. Anaphylactic reactions may be severe, even on corticoid preventive therapy, and prohibit sequential cures. At the least, a potential direct toxic effect on the stem cells, which are lymphocyte-like cells, has been suggested. It is our opinion that such assays must be reserved for specialized centers and within the framework of prospective protocols.

Corticoids

It has been largely proved that glucocorticoids used at the usual dosage (1 mg per kg or less) are ineffective in AA, and promote infectious complications; the possible effect of glucocorticoids as a preventive agent against hemorrhages is not clearly demonstrated. Glucocorticoid therapy is certainly not advisable.

Recently, Italian authors (Bacigapulo, Marmont et al.) observed surprising results in severe aplastic anemias after "bolus infusion" of a very high dose of glucocorticoids; they explain their clinical results as a consequence of immunosuppression. Their present results (not yet published) are 41 per cent (9 of 22 cases) autologous recovery at the thirtieth day following large dose corticosteroid therapy (100 mg per kg during the first week of treatment). However, the potential risk, the choice of patients, and the mechanism of the biologic effect still require further study, probably on a prospective, multicenter basis.

Bone Marrow Graft

Bone marrow graft has been tried in severe AA for a long time. But it is only recently that advances in choice of donors (better knowledge of transplantation antigens), in methods of immunosuppression of the recipient (chemo- and radiotherapy), in maintenance during the severe aplastic phase before repopulation (isolation, antibiotic therapy, platelet and granulocyte supplementation), and in treatment of graft versus host disease (GVH) have made this treatment available on a large scale. It should be noted, however, that the cost of such treatment is extraordinarily high (hospital facilities, medications, and chiefly the cost of the medical and biological staff — physicians, technicians, nurses), so that it must be limited to a few specialized institutions.

Technique of Bone Marrow Graft. The choice of the donor is the most important.

The least complex situation is the case (unfortunately rare) in which the patient has an identical twin. In such a circumstance no conditioning is necessary and no GVH or rejection is to be expected. (Recent British data, however, suggest that this is not always true.)

In most cases, we are obliged to use a brother or sister, of the same sex if possible, who is identical in the major system of histocompatibility (HLA-A, B, and C tested by serologic methods, and D by mixed lymphocyte culture). Statistically, the chance for a patient to have such a compatible brother or sister is only 25 per cent, which seriously limits bone marrow graft possibilities. The use of nonidentical donors still remains a matter for further developments.

The technique of bone marrow grafting is very simple. Under general anesthesia, bone marrow samples are taken from the pelvis and sternum of the donor, placed on a heparinized culture medium, filtrated, and infused intravenously after counting; at least 3×10^8 myeloid cells per kg are necessary.

Conditioning of the recipient is necessary to avoid bone marrow rejection. Several protocols have been proposed and are still being modified, so that no general directive can be given. All of them, however, use chemotherapy (cyclophosphamide) and/or radiotherapy (dose of 600 to 800 rads, with partial protection of the lungs) during the 5 days preceding the graft. Postgraft immunosuppression also seems necessary in order to avoid or reduce the frequency and severity of GVH disease; methotrexate is generally used for this purpose.

Bone Marrow Graft Complications. Two complications cause death in 50 to 60 per cent of the grafted patients: no-take or rejection, and graft-vs.-host disease and its infectious complications.

Rejection is observed in 30 to 50 per cent of patients and seems less frequent in the most recent series (better choice of the donor, better conditioning). It can be due to an insufficient number of transfused cells, but more often to

previous immunization of the recipient by transfusions; it is the reason why bone marrow grafting is proposed early in the course of the disease
in the severe cases.

Graft-vs.-host disease (GVH) remains the
most severe complication. Its most severe form,
leading to death (cachexia, diarrhea, cutaneous
rash, hepatic deficiency), is observed in about 30
per cent of patients. Less severe but chronic and
debilitating forms are at least as frequent. In
these patients infectious complications observed
during the second quarter after graft, favored by
immunosuppression, are frequent and severe;
they include bacterial diseases and pulmonary
infections or septicemias caused by cytomegalovirus and *Pneumocystis carinii*. Even in spite of
continuous progress in the control of GVH disease and its consequences, its occurrence limits
bone marrow graft to the most severe cases.

The long-term destiny of these chimeric patients remains unknown. We only know that
many of them survive, and remain chimeras for 3
to 6 years without relapse of AA or autologous
repopulation. In spite of the heavy hemo- and
radiotherapy used, at least one of the cured
female patients did experience normal pregnancy; but the males are azoospermic. The late
risk of carcinogenicity is not yet known.

Conclusion — Choice of Therapy

The choice of therapy is theoretically simple
from a statistical point of view but very difficult in
the presence of a·single patient. It must be
founded on a correct evaluation of the respective
risks of the disease and treatment. The more
severe the disease, the more risks of therapy that
can be accepted.

Every aplastic anemia patient should be hospitalized in a specialized institution in order to
make complete evaluation of the prognostic factors and to begin correct maintenance therapy.
When the expectancy of life is very low (i.e., when
our multiparametric evaluation is lower than 25
per cent of the normal value), bone marrow graft
should be proposed as soon as possible when a
potential donor is available, probably not excluding patients older than 35 to 40 even if their risk
appears excessive. When AA is severe but not
immediately life threatening (index 25 to 40),
androgen therapy should be initiated with assay
of immunosuppressive agents; secondary bone
marrow graft should be discussed at the second to
third month in the case of absence of any improvement or if worsening. Patients with the least
severe cases (index over 40) should be treated
with androgens alone, but would benefit from the
same maintenance therapy and survey as the
most severe, to avoid sudden infections or hemorrhagic accidents.

ANEMIA DUE TO IRON DEFICIENCY
method of
SEAN R. LYNCH, M.D.
Kansas City, Kansas

The diagnostic and therapeutic approach to iron
deficiency anemia should be governed by the clinical
setting in which it is suspected. In menstruating
women and young children it most often results from
an imbalance between a limited supply of available
iron in the diet and the increased physiologic requirements caused by child-bearing and menstruation
or rapid growth. The recorded prevalence of iron
deficiency among women and children in the United
States varies, depending upon the criteria used for
diagnosis as well as economic and other factors.
When iron deficiency has been identified clearly as
the cause, prevalence rates for anemia as high as 8
per cent in women and 5 per cent in children have
been reported in low income families. In contrast,
iron deficiency is rare in men and postmenopausal
women. Unless associated with gastric surgery, its
presence almost always implies blood loss.

Extensive investigation is often not warranted in
menstruating women and in children when the clinical features and peripheral blood smear support a
diagnosis of iron deficiency. A therapeutic trial of
iron is appropriate. On the other hand, failure to
respond to iron, anemia in a clinical situation in
which iron deficiency is uncommon, or the presence
of features not completely characteristic of iron lack
necessitates positive identification of iron deficiency
before an extensive search for a cause such as occult
blood loss is undertaken.

Chronic iron deficiency anemia is characterized
by the presence of microcytosis and hypochromia,
the mean cell volume (MCV) and mean cell hemoglobin (MCH) being the most reliable indices. However,
if the condition is of recent onset, the cells may still
be normocytic and normochromic. In addition a low
MCV is also characteristic of thalassemia minor, and
this possibility must be taken into consideration in
blacks and people from the Mèditerranean and
Southeast Asia, where thalassemia is common. Further evidence of iron deficient erythropoiesis is provided by the finding of a transferrin saturation of
less than 15 per cent and an increased free erythrocyte protoporphyrin concentration. It is important to
note that these results are indicative only of iron
deficient erythropoiesis and may be found in the
anemia of inflammatory disorders in which iron supply is curtailed but stores are normal or increased.
Confirmation of the presence of true iron deficiency
requires the demonstration of significantly diminished iron stores by the finding of a serum ferritin
level below 12 micrograms per liter or the absence of
stainable iron on a bone marrow aspirate. A low
serum ferritin is characteristic only of iron deficiency.
However, when inflammatory disease and iron defi-

ciency coexist, serum ferritin values may be in the normal range. The finding of particulate iron in the marrow excludes the diagnosis of uncomplicated iron deficiency unless parenteral iron has been administered in the preceding months. The interpretation of these laboratory investigations in infants and children should be based upon a comparison with age-specific reference standards, since there are marked developmental changes in the normal values for most of them.

Once the presence of iron deficiency has been established, the extent of further evaluation again depends upon the clinical assessment. Vigorous investigation may not be warranted with the first occurrence in menstruating women and young children, while a diligent search for the site of blood loss should always be instituted in men and older women or when the anemia fails to respond to iron. Occult bleeding from the gastrointestinal tract is the most common cause. Less frequently iron loss may result from hemosiderinuria in patients with prosthetic valves or paroxysmal nocturnal hemoglobinuria, idiopathic pulmonary hemosiderosis, or self-induced bleeding. Malabsorption of iron is rarely the sole cause of anemia but may be a contributing factor after gastric surgery or in patients with idiopathic steatorrhea.

Oral Iron Therapy

There are two objectives of iron therapy: repair of the anemia and restoration of the body iron reserve. Most patients will respond promptly to oral iron preparations. This occurs even in patients who have impaired food iron absorption following gastric surgery. Isotopic studies have demonstrated that ferrous salts in a dosage of 30 mg per day are absorbed approximately three times as well as ferric salts, and the difference increases with larger doses. Most ferrous salts are absorbed to about the same extent. Iron deficiency is therefore best treated with a simple ferrous salt such as the sulfate, gluconate, or fumarate. The quantity of elemental iron varies in different preparations. Ferrous sulfate is the last expensive, and most tablets contain about 65 mg elemental iron. Treatment should be initiated with 1 tablet of ferrous sulfate three times daily, taken between meals and the last dose taken just before going to bed. Iron taken with food is significantly less well absorbed, and some meals reduce absorption by 50 to 60 per cent. A dose of 3 mg per kg per day, which is comparable to the adult dose, usually in the form of an elixir, is recommended as adequate for infants and children. In the past, a dose of 6 mg per kg per day has been widely used, but this is probably unnecessarily high. An alternative and effective approach to the treatment of mild iron deficiency anemia in infants is the use of iron fortified formula. It has the advantages of not producing significant gastrointestinal side effects and removing the hazard of accidental ingestion of a large quantity of iron.

The side effects of oral iron therapy are largely confined to the gastrointestinal tract. Psychologic factors may be important in some instances, since 10 to 15 per cent of patients develop symptoms when taking a placebo which they believe contains iron. Nevertheless, physical intolerance undoubtedly does occur. Nausea, epigastric pain, constipation, diarrhea, and abdominal distention are the most common symptoms and are encountered in about 25 per cent of patients at a daily iron dose of 180 mg. An increase in dose causes a rise in the percentage of patients complaining of epigastric discomfort and nausea, but there is no increase in the frequency of other symptoms. Side effects appear to be uncommon in children, although iron solutions can produce temporary staining of the teeth. This may be minimized by placing the medication on the back of the tongue. A major concern in children is the serious toxicity which is a common consequence of accidental iron ingestion, and it is important to stress to parents the need to keep all iron preparations out of the reach of young children.

The rapid correction of iron deficiency is hardly ever important. Therefore when patients complain of untoward effects, particularly of upper gastrointestinal symptoms, the dose should be decreased or the patient advised to take the iron with meals. Iron administered with meals tends to be better tolerated but, as already mentioned, less well absorbed. Because of the important placebo effect, it is also helpful to change the preparation, although there is no evidence that different formulations containing the same quantity of available iron differ in the incidence of side effects.

Many iron preparations contain vitamins as well as other so-called hematinics. There is no evidence that any of these improve the therapeutic response to iron significantly, and the increased expense is not justified except perhaps during pregnancy, in which the use of a preparation containing both folic acid and iron may be convenient. Large quantities of ascorbic acid increase the absorption of ferrous sulfate by 30 to 40 per cent. However, there is a parallel rise in side effects and no therapeutic advantage over an equivalent increase in iron dosage.

Numerous attempts have been made to design iron preparations with fewer side effects. Enteric-coated tablets achieve this only by impairing the release of iron and reducing its availability for absorption. They should not be used. A number of slow-release preparations in which the solubilization of iron is purposely delayed are now on the market. Upper gastrointestinal tract side effects occur less frequently than with conventional oral iron therapy, and there is evidence that some of them are absorbed as well as or better than conventional formulas, particularly when both preparations are taken with food. Because of the high cost of slow-release preparations, their use cannot be advocated in all patients, but they should be considered as an alternative to parenteral iron in patients who develop epigastric discomfort or nausea on oral iron.

It is important to follow the therapeutic response after the institution of iron therapy. This is necessary both to confirm the diagnosis and to ensure that complete correction of the anemia occurs. Once the hemoglobin concentration is normal, therapy should be continued for 6 months to replete iron stores. Iron administration should then be discontinued because of the possible hazard of developing iron overload. A rise in the hemoglobin concentration of less than 2 grams per dl (100 ml) over a 3 week period or failure to correct the hemoglobin level within 2 months should be considered a therapeutic failure. In most cases this will result from poor compliance. Other causes are far less common. An incorrect diagnosis can be excluded by the demonstration of continued iron deficiency on the basis of the serum ferritin level or a bone marrow examination. Continued blood loss at a rate that matches the bone marrow's ability to produce new cells is easily detected, since this requires a loss of 20 ml of blood a day. Malabsorption of iron, although often considered, is very uncommon if a soluble ferrous salt is prescribed. It may occur in the presence of extensive small bowel disease. If suspected, the serum iron level should be measured before and 45, 90, and 120 minutes after the administration of 130 mg iron as ferrous sulfate. A rise of less than 150 micrograms per dl in the serum iron level suggests the possible existence of malabsorption and is an indication for more detailed investigation.

Parenteral Iron Therapy

Parenteral iron therapy is rarely justified, since most patients will respond rapidly to oral preparations. Moreover oral iron is usually well tolerated even by patients with gastrointestinal diseases such as peptic ulceration, regional ileitis, and ulcerative colitis, and the rate of rise in hemoglobin concentration is no faster after parenteral iron. The few definite indications for parenteral therapy include some patients with extensive small bowel disease and situations in which the rate of iron loss through bleeding exceeds the rate of absorption because of relative malabsorption or heavy blood loss. There are also occasional patients who cannot tolerate oral iron despite dosage reduction and the trial of different preparations and regimens. Parenteral iron should be recommended only after every attempt has been made to improve tolerance to oral iron.

Iron dextran (Imferon) is the best preparation available. It is a complex of ferric hydroxide with dextrans of molecular weight 5000 to 7000 daltons and is available as a colloidal solution containing 50 mg of iron per ml. The drug may be administered intramuscularly or intravenously after a 0.5 ml dose to test for anaphylaxis. Intravenous administration is preferable. The total dose given is based on the calculated iron deficit, as shown in the equation at the bottom of this page. Depending on body weight, an additional 500 to 1000 mg of elemental iron should be given to replenish stores. The approved method for intravenous use in adults in the United States is to give 0.5 ml on the first day to test for and minimize the chance of toxic reactions. Over the next 2 to 3 days, the dose may be raised to 2 ml (100 mg) per day given at a rate of less than 1 minute per ml or fraction thereof. Injections are repeated until the calculated dose of iron has been administered. An alternative method of administration which has gained wide acceptance elsewhere is that of "total dose infusion." The total quantity of iron required to replace the deficit is diluted in an isotonic saline solution (500 ml of saline for every 20 ml ampule of iron dextran [Imferon] containing 1000 mg of iron) and infused over several hours. Although "total dose infusion" is associated with some symptoms more frequently than is intermittent iron dextran administration, these symptoms tend to be relatively benign. (The total dose infusion method is not listed in the manufacturer's official directive.)

The most serious adverse reaction to iron dextran is anaphylaxis. Although rare, it may occur with both intramuscular and intravenous use and has been fatal on several occasions. The drug should therefore be administered only in situations in which full resuscitative measures are available. Other adverse reactions include fever, arthralgia and myalgia, pain and inflammation or

$$\text{Iron dose required to restore hemoglobin (mg)} = \frac{\text{Hemoglobin deficit (grams per dl)}}{100} \times \text{Estimated blood volume} \times 3.4$$

phlebitis at the injection site, and peripheral vascular "flushing" with intravenous infusion that is too rapid.

Blood Transfusion

Blood transfusion is very rarely necessary in iron deficiency anemia, because its gradual onset usually allows physiologic adaptations to occur. Occasionally, elderly patients present with severe congestive heart failure, angina, or cerebral vascular insufficiency. The cautious administration of 1 or 2 units of packed red cells together with a diuretic may then be justified.

IMMUNE HEMOLYTIC ANEMIA

method of
HARRY W. CARLOSS, M.D.,
and ROBERT McMILLAN, M.D.
La Jolla, California

Immune hemolytic anemia results from production by the patient of an antibody against either red cell (RBC) membrane antigens or extrinsic antigens which absorb to the RBC surface or result in the formation of immune complexes which bind to the RBC. The cell-bound antibody or immune complexes may also result in complement fixation. Destruction of the RBC occurs primarily by phagocytosis triggered by either cell-bound IgG antibody or the third component of complement (C'3).

Immune hemolytic anemia can be classified into two major groups on the basis of antibody characteristics: patients with warm-reacting IgG antibody (maximal activity at 37 C) and those with cold-reacting IgM antibody (maximal activity at 2 to 4 C). Each group can be further subdivided into primary (or idiopathic) and secondary types. Diseases commonly associated with secondary hemolytic anemias include lymphoproliferative diseases, collagen vascular diseases, infectious diseases, drugs, and other neoplasms.

General Treatment Measures

1. *Bedrest and oxygen,* to prevent or lessen symptoms of profound anemia.

2. *Folic acid (1 mg per day)* to prevent folate deficiency from rapid hemolysis.

3. *Transfusion.*

Warm Antibody Disease. It is usually impossible to find compatible blood for these patients, and for this reason transfusion should be given only when the anemia is life threatening. Symptoms such as angina, cardiac decompensation, and decreased sensorium in spite of bed rest and oxygen are indications for transfusion. It must be recognized that in some patients transfusion may be the sole measure available initially to support life and it *must* be used even if "most compatible" blood must be given. Techniques such as "warm autoadsorption" may be used by the blood bank to allow testing for alloantibodies. The aim of transfusion should be to alleviate life-threatening symptoms rather than achieving a certain level of hematocrit.

Cold Antibody Disease. Cross-matching must be performed at 37 C or the cold agglutinin removed by absorption prior to testing. Before transfusion, the RBCs must be washed and warmed to 37 C.

Specific Therapy

Warm Antibody Autoimmune Hemolytic Anemia. CORTICOSTEROIDS. Give prednisone, 1 to 2 mg per kg per day (usually 60 to 120 mg per day); equivalent doses of hydrocortisone sodium succinate (Solu-Cortef) or methylprednisolone sodium succinate (Solu-Medrol) may be substituted initially if oral therapy is not possible. The blood count should be monitored initially once or twice a week. Most patients respond within 3 weeks; no response after 3 weeks should be considered a steroid failure. A response is indicated by an increasing hematocrit and often initially an increasing reticulocyte count; the direct Coombs test frequently remains positive in spite of a response to steroids, although the titer may decrease. After normalization of the hematocrit or stabilization over 30 per cent, taper the prednisone 5 mg per week until the daily dose is 20 mg per day. Maintain this dose for 2 to 3 months. If the hematocrit remains stable, then taper more slowly over the next 4 to 6 months. Most patients require continued low doses of prednisone to maintain acceptable hematocrit levels. If more than 10 to 15 mg per day of prednisone is required to keep the hematocrit over 30 per cent, additional therapy is indicated. While on steroids, patients should receive antacids and potassium supplementation.

SPLENECTOMY. Splenectomy is indicated if (1) the patient's condition deteriorates rapidly; (2) no response to steroids occurs within 3 weeks; or (3) the patient cannot be maintained on acceptable long-term steroid dosage (<15 mg of prednisone per day). About 50 to 75 per cent of patients will undergo a complete remission or will markedly improve. If hemolysis continues after splenectomy, steroids should be reinstituted, since increased sensitivity to steroids often occurs after splenectomy. Organ sequestration studies using ^{51}Cr-labeled RBCs are not useful in individual patients in predicting their response to splenectomy. All patients who have undergone splenectomy have a small risk of severe infection, particularly pneumococcal septicemia, and should be immunized with pneumococcal vaccine (Pneumovax), 0.5 ml subcutaneously or intramuscularly at the time of surgery and approximately every 5 years thereafter.

IMMUNOSUPPRESSIVE DRUGS. These agents should be reserved for steroid- and splenectomy-resistant patients. They are more useful when given in conjunction with steroids. In rare patients, these drugs may be attempted as an alternative to splenectomy, but in general they are not effective unless the spleen has been removed. Cyclophosphamide and azathioprine are the most commonly used drugs. (This use of cyclophosphamide and azathioprine is not listed in the manufacturers' official directives.) Cyclophosphamide is a better immunosuppressant but has more side effects.

1. *Cyclophosphamide (Cytoxan)*, 1.5 to 2.0 mg per kg (100 to 200 mg per day) given daily. Dosage is monitored by weekly blood counts with the aim of maintaining the WBC >2500 per cu mm and the platelet counts >100,000 per cu mm. Responses usually occur in 6 to 8 weeks but may take up to 3 months. Side effects include marrow suppression, gastrointestinal intolerance, alopecia, and hemorrhagic cystitis. Patients should be instructed to drink at least 2 quarts of fluid daily to prevent bladder irritation. (This use of cyclophosphamide is not listed in the manufacturer's official directive.)

2. *Azathioprine (Imuran)*, 2.0 to 2.5 mg per kg per day (200 to 400 mg per day) given with dosage adjustments based on the blood counts as described above. Responses may take 3 to 4 months. Marrow suppression and gastrointestinal disturbances are the major side effects. (This use of azathioprine is not listed in manufacturer's official directive.)

If a response occurs with either of these drugs, they should be tapered with the aim of achieving the lowest possible dose that allows an acceptable hematocrit. Long-term administration of these agents carries the risk of developing a malignancy (e.g., acute leukemia) or serious infection.

INVESTIGATIONAL THERAPIES. (1) *Heparin* has known anticomplementary effects and may be useful in preventing thrombosis in the face of brisk intravascular hemolysis. (2) *Plasma exchange* may be useful in removing antibody under emergent circumstances until other forms of therapy become effective. (3) *Vinblastine-laden platelets* incorporate vinblastine and after sensitization with anti-platelet antibody theoretically deliver the drug to the reticuloendothelial system in high concentrations. These forms of therapy must be considered experimental and should be reserved for emergency situations when the aforementioned approaches are unsuccessful.

Cold Agglutinin Disease. Anemia is usually mild to moderate in these patients, and often no therapy is required. Patients should avoid exposure to cold. If they must go out in the cold, warm clothing to include earmuffs, mittens, and warm socks should be worn. Relocation to a warm climate may be necessary.

CHLORAMBUCIL (LEUKERAN). Patients with more severe anemia should be treated with chlorambucil, 4 mg per day. Increase the dose 2 mg per day at monthly intervals until improvement is noted or side effects occur, such as gastrointestinal symptoms or marrow suppression. (This use of chlorambucil is not listed in the manufacturer's official directive). Patients should be monitored initially with weekly blood counts until a maintenance dose is determined. At that point blood counts may be performed less frequently. Few patients are responsive to this therapy. Steroids and splenectomy are generally not useful.

Paroxysmal Cold Hemoglobinuria. This syndrome usually follows an acute infection and is self-limited. Patients require temporary protection from cold. Cold protection is also important in patients with the chronic form of the disease. If the diagnosis of syphilis is made, appropriate antibiotics should be given. Steroids and splenectomy are usually not useful.

Secondary Immune Hemolytic Anemia. Immune hemolytic anemia with serologic findings identical to idiopathic warm antibody autoimmune hemolytic anemia is frequently seen associated with other diseases, particularly lymphoproliferative disorders (Coombs' test — anti-γ, anti-C', or both) and collagen vascular diseases (Coombs' test — anti-C'). Cold agglutinins may also be seen in patients with lymphomas. Treatment of the primary disease will in some cases reduce the degree or alleviate the hemolysis, but by and large the approach to the hemolytic process is no different from that described above.

Hemolytic anemia seen with infectious mononucleosis and following mycoplasma pneumonia is due to cold-reactive antibodies and is self-limited and rarely symptomatic. Treatment is aimed at keeping the patient warm and giving transfusions if required.

Drug-Related Immune Hemolysis. Three major types are seen.

1. *Haptene mechanism* (e.g., penicillin). The drug combines with the RBC surface. An IgG antibody to the drug develops which reacts with the drug on the RBC surface, resulting in destruction. The Coombs test is positive (anti-γ type). The indirect Coombs test is positive only if drug-sensitized RBCs are used. *Treatment*: Discontinue the drug.

2. *Immune complex mechanism* (e.g., quinidine). The drug plus a possible carrier molecule forms immune complexes with circulating antibody. The complexes bind to the RBC, resulting in C' fixation and hemolysis. The Coombs test is positive for C' only (anti-C'), since the complexes elute off the RBC. *Treatment:* Discontinue the drug.

3. *Autoantibody mechanism* (e.g., methyldopa). Certain drugs induce antibody to be formed against RBC membrane antigens (Rh locus). A positive Coombs test (anti-γ, anti-C' or both) develops 3 to 6 months after beginning therapy with methyldopa in 10 to 36 per cent of patients; the effect is dose dependent. Only a small percentage of patients develop hemolysis. *Treatment:* Discontinue the drug. The hemolytic process may remain for 3 to 6 months, and on occasion corticosteroids and transfusion are needed.

HEMOLYTIC ANEMIA — NONIMMUNE

method of
RALPH ZALUSKY, M.D.
New York, New York

The normal life span of the adult red cell in the peripheral blood is 120 days. Reduction below this value, in the absence of hemorrhage, indicates a hemolytic state. When the rate of bone marrow erythropoiesis equals the rate of peripheral destruction, a compensated hemolytic state is present. However, if the rate of erythropoiesis, maximally six to eight times normal, fails in this compensation, anemia supervenes. In both circumstances, clinical and laboratory evidence for hemolysis is found. The former can include jaundice, often splenomegaly; and the latter, reticulocytosis, increased levels of serum unconjugated bilirubin, a variety of red cell morphologic abnormalities, and increased concentrations of red cell catabolic products.

Hemolytic disorders can be classified in a variety of ways, but the most convenient relies on an under-

standing of the basic pathophysiologic process involved. In this systematic approach, abnormalities extrinsic to the red cell (acquired) versus intrinsic red cell defects (generally inherited) are sought. A major category of hemolytic anemias includes those that are immune mediated, and these are considered in the article immediately preceding this one. It should be kept in mind that approximately 5 per cent of immune-mediated hemolytic anemias may be negative by direct antiglobulin testing, yet therapy is similar. In this article, the nonimmune causes of hemolysis will be considered.

Therapeutic Considerations

Red Blood Cell Transfusions. The whole blood volume is reasonably well maintained in chronic hemolytic states. Therefore, when the degree of anemia is sufficiently severe, packed red cell transfusions are given. Indications for transfusions depend upon the nature of the hemolytic process, age of the patient, cardiovascular status, and consideration for surgery. Especially in the elderly, volume overload can be avoided by monitoring central venous pressure and using judicious phlebotomy if necessary. A packed red cell volume of 30 per cent is generally sufficient to maintain normal tissue oxygenation.

Bone Marrow Decompensation. In the past, one of the complications of hemolytic anemia, characterized by sudden worsening of anemia and reticulocytopenia, was referred to as an "aplastic crisis." In fact, several factors can be causative. Most commonly, an intercurrent infection results in a failure of bone marrow compensation. Therapy is directed toward treatment of the infection. A second cause is a relative deficiency of folic acid, resulting in megaloblastic erythropoiesis and failure of effective red cell production. Because of this, folic acid, 1 mg orally twice a day, is generally prescribed for patients with chronic hemolytic anemia. Because of the long storage life of vitamin B_{12}, this vitamin deficiency is rarely a cause of this form of decompensation.

Cholelithiasis. All forms of chronic hemolytic anemia are associated with increased bilirubin turnover and its precipitation into gallstones, often at an especially early age. When surgical intervention is indicated, if the underlying hemolytic state requires splenectomy, then this procedure should be done first or simultaneously with the cholecystectomy.

Iron Overload. Since iron is reutilized in hemolytic anemia, unless hemoglobinuria with its iron loss is present and active erythropoiesis is associated with increased iron absorption, body iron stores are generally increased. When chronic transfusion therapy is necessary, significant iron overload and the complications of hemosiderosis may occur. Various programs have been designed to facilitate iron loss by the parenteral use of the iron-chelator desferoxamine. One such method now utilizes a portable infusion pump that delivers this drug subcutaneously over a 12 hour period. If the patient's hemoglobin level allows, judicious phlebotomy has also been utilized.

Extrinsic Causes of Nonimmune Hemolytic Anemias

Hypersplenism. Any disease process that causes splenic enlargement may result in the increased trapping function of that organ, with consequent lowering of one or more of the formed elements of the blood. Splenomegaly can be caused by congestion (portal hypertension), infection, inflammation, infiltration (lymphoma), or storage diseases (Gaucher's disease). The bone marrow is hyperplastic. Therapy is directed at the underlying disease, and, if not correctable, splenectomy is considered if the peripheral cytopenia is life threatening.

Fragmentation Hemolysis (Microangiopathic Hemolytic Anemia). There are several syndromes characterized by intravascular hemolysis and schistocytes in the peripheral blood smear. The underlying pathophysiology is an increased shear and stress on the circulating erythrocyte with fragmentation of the cell. In chronic forms of these syndromes, significant hemoglobinuria with attendant hemosiderinuria may lead to excessive iron loss and a superimposed iron deficiency state. When this occurs, iron supplementation in the form of oral ferrous sulfate, 0.3 gram twice daily, is indicated.

Perhaps the most common cause of fragmentation hemolysis is heart valve replacement, especially the aortic valve. A mild degree of hemolysis is usually acceptable, but when the syndrome is sufficiently severe to require frequent transfusions, then consideration for reoperation, in consultation with the cardiac surgeon, should be given. Thrombotic thrombocytopenic purpura is an acute, severe disorder usually associated with changing neurologic signs and, in the past, accompanied by a high mortality. Recently, plasma transfusion or exchange antiplatelet aggregating drugs, with or without splenectomy, have resulted in salutary clinical responses. When the syndrome is associated with severe hypertension or severe renal disease, as in the hemolytic-uremic syndrome, the underlying disorder requires active therapy. Disseminated intravascular coagulation, of diverse cause, may be associated with fragmentation hemolysis. Therapy is directed toward the

underlying cause, and in some instances this may include therapeutic doses of heparin. A rare disorder, March hemoglobinuria, is occasionally seen in runners (occasionally bongodrum players), in whom mechanical trauma appears to be transmitted to circulating red blood cells. Avoidance of such trauma, or appropriate padding, usually ameliorates the condition.

Drugs and Toxins. Even normal red blood cells are incapable of withstanding the onslaught of excessive exposure to oxidant drugs, especially such chemicals as aniline or its derivatives. Severe burns, heavy metals, and inadvertent use of hypotonic intravenous solutions can cause acute hemolysis. Certain bacterial toxins, especially from clostridial species, may induce significant hemolysis. Treatment includes removal of the causative agent and supportive measures such as hydration and vasopressor agents. On occasion, hemodialysis or exchange transfusion is utilized to remove the offending agent.

Intrinsic Causes of Nonimmune Hemolytic Anemia

Membrane Abnormalities. Hereditary spherocytosis is an autosomal dominant form of hemolytic anemia. Recent evidence suggests that this form of hemolysis may result from heritable alterations in the protein structure of the red cell membrane. Hemolysis begins early in life as a result of splenic trapping of poorly deformable spherocytes. The clinical picture may be punctuated by the complications of excessive hemolysis, such as gallstones, "aplastic crises," and, occasionally, chronic leg ulcers. Splenectomy is the therapy of choice, although the procedure is generally not performed before age 6 because of the vital role of the spleen in the prevention of certain bacterial infections, especially from encapsulated organisms. Currently, it is appropriate to immunize all splenectomized persons with pneumococcal vaccine (Pneumovax) against a large number of pneumococcal species. A much less common inherited membrane abnormality that occasionally causes clinically significant hemolytic anemia is hereditary elliptocytosis. Its mode of inheritance is similar to that of hereditary spherocytosis. Splenectomy is recommended when significant hemolysis is present. Rare inherited membrane disorders, whose mechanism is obscure, include Rh_{null} disease, hereditary stomatocytosis, acanthocytosis, and phospholipid abnormalities. Therapy for these disorders has not been established.

Acquired membrane disorders leading to hemolytic anemia by nonimmune mechanisms are relatively uncommon, and their therapy requires management of the underlying disease. Spur-cell anemia and stomatocytosis have been associated with severe liver disease. Hemolytic anemia, hyperlipidemia, and jaundice (Zieve's syndrome) is a self-limited disorder that may be seen in liver disease.

Paroxysmal nocturnal hemoglobinuria is an acquired clonal disorder of hematopoiesis giving rise to red cells that are peculiarly susceptible to complement-mediated hemolysis. The nature of the membrane defect remains obscure. Since this may be considered an immune-mediated form of hemolysis, this rare disorder is not discussed here.

Red Cell Enzyme Abnormalities. Deficiency or structural and functional abnormalities of erythrocyte enzymes may cause inherited, non-spherocytic hemolytic anemia. By far, the most common such disorder is glucose-6-phosphate dehydrogenase (Gd) deficiency. This X-chromosome–linked disorder includes over 110 variants of the enzyme. The two most common, Gd A⁻ ("primaquine-sensitive," found in black males) and Gd Mediterranean, are rarely associated with chronic hemolysis; however, upon exposure to a large variety of oxidant drugs, severe infections, and certain biologic agents (fava bean ingestion), an acute hemolytic anemia may ensue. Therapy consists of removal of the offending agent, vigorous treatment of infection or acidosis, and, when clinically indicated, judicious transfusion. Occasionally, chronic hemolysis, even in the absence of extrinsic factors, is observed with some Gd variants in which therapeutic interventions, including splenectomy, do not particularly affect the anemia. Over a dozen other red cell enzymopathies, of infrequent occurrence, may cause hemolytic anemia. In this group, pyruvate kinase deficiency is the most common, and marked shortening of the red cell life span with extreme reticulocytosis may be seen. In the severe form of the deficiency, splenectomy may be beneficial.

Hemoglobin Abnormalities. Inherited abnormalities of hemoglobin structure or synthesis account for a large number of cases of hemolytic anemia. The most common structural variant is hemoglobin S, and the homozygous state, sickle cell disease, causes an unremitting hemolytic disorder with episodic painful crises. Homozygosity for hemoglobins C, D, and E causes hemolytic disease of lesser severity. Double heterozygosity for hemoglobin S with other beta-chain variants or beta-thalassemia produces hemolytic disease of intermediate severity. Although active investigation is underway on drugs that might modify the structural abnor-

mality of hemoglobin S, therapy for these disorders is largely supportive at present. On occasion, when splenomegaly with secondary hypersplenism is present, removal of that organ may be beneficial.

Unstable hemoglobin hemolytic anemias are represented by over 40 structural variants. These are heterozygous codominant disorders in which the substituted hemoglobin is especially susceptible to denaturation and precipitation as Heinz bodies within the red cell. The clinical syndrome is characterized by hemolytic anemia, splenomegaly, and, frequently, the passage of mahogany-brown urine (dipyrroluria). Because of the inherent instability of these hemoglobins, ingestion of oxidant drugs may accelerate the degree of hemolysis and should be avoided. If hemolysis is clinically severe, splenectomy may partially ameliorate the anemia.

Unbalanced synthesis of alpha- or beta-polypeptide chains of hemoglobin underlies the thalassemia syndromes. In addition to impaired red cell production, the excess unbalanced chains form inclusions that lead to premature cell destruction. The more severe anemias are seen in homozygous beta-thalassemia and in hemoglobin H disease, in which three of the four alpha-chain genes are defective. The management of these disorders is considered on pages 265 to 269.

PERNICIOUS ANEMIA AND OTHER MEGALOBLASTIC ANEMIAS

method of
A. V. HOFFBRAND, D.M.
London, England

The megaloblastic anemias are a group of disorders characterized by an abnormal appearance of the erythroblasts in the bone marrow. This consists of delayed nuclear maturation with a fine, stippled chromatin pattern despite normal cytoplasmic development and hemoglobinization. Giant metamyelocytes and hypersegmented neutrophils are also present. There is an underlying defect of DNA synthesis in all cases, and this is usually due to deficiency of either vitamin B_{12} or folate. Vitamin B_{12} deficiency may also cause a severe neuropathy. Treatment consists largely of correcting whichever deficiency is present, treating the underlying cause, and preventing recurrence. It is important, therefore, to decide whether a patient with megaloblastic anemia is deficient of vitamin B_{12} or folate and then to pinpoint the exact cause of the deficiency in the individual patient.

Vitamin B_{12}

Adult daily requirements are about 2 micrograms and body stores 2 to 3 mg. Several years are needed to completely deplete the body stores whether from inadequate dietary intake (veganism) or malabsorption. Pernicious anemia (lack of gastric intrinsic factor caused by gastric atrophy) is the most common cause of vitamin B_{12} malabsorption in Western countries, but gastric resection and intestinal lesions, including ileal resection, the intestinal stagnant loop syndrome, tropical sprue, infestation with fish tapeworm, and rare congenital defects such as lack of intrinsic factor or abnormality of the ileal transport mechanism for vitamin B_{12}, may also cause deficiency. Deficiency of vitamin B_{12} caused by excess requirements or loss has not been described, but inactivation of vitamin B_{12} by nitrous oxide and rare plasma transport defects may cause megaloblastic anemia.

Folate

Requirements are relatively higher, 100 to 200 micrograms daily, and deficiency occurs readily, since body stores (8 to 12 mg) are sufficient for only about 4 months. Moreover, requirements for folate may be increased in conditions of increased cell turnover. Poor nutrition, malabsorption caused by gluten-induced enteropathy or tropical sprue, excess utilization in pregnacy or from diseases of increased cell proliferation (e.g., hemolytic anemias), and drugs (e.g., anticonvulsants and barbiturates) are among the more common causes of the deficiency.

Diagnosis

Peripheral blood and bone marrow examinations show the characteristic macrocytic and megaloblastic appearances, respectively. The results of serum B_{12} and folate and red cell folate measurements indicate which deficiency is present. In some patients both deficiencies occur, while in rare cases megaloblastosis is due to neither deficiency. In some laboratories, a deoxyuridine suppression of labeled thymidine uptake by bone marrow cells is used to diagnose deficiency of B_{12} or folate. Further tests are necessary to establish the underlying cause. For vitamin B_{12}, radioactive vitamin B_{12} absorption tests with and without added intrinsic factor, gastric secretion studies, tests for intrinsic factor and parietal cell antibodies in serum, barium studies, endoscopy, and gastric biopsy are most frequently carried out, whereas for folate, a detailed diet and drug history, tests of small intestinal function, including jejunal biopsy, and search for underlying disease are most often needed.

Initial Treatment

Vitamin B_{12} Deficiency. Patients with vitamin B_{12} deficiency from whatever cause are initially treated in the same way. Six intramuscular injections of hydroxocobalamin, each of 1000 micrograms, given over the first 2 to 3 weeks are adequate to replenish stores and give an optimal response. Hydroxocobalamin is the best therapeutic form, since it is retained in the body three times as well as cyanocobalamin, which, in my opinion, is now obsolete and should not be used. I continue with 1000 micrograms each week for 3 months or more in patients with vitamin B_{12} neuropathy, although there is no good evidence that this is more beneficial than the initial conventional loading of 6 injections described above.

Folate Deficiency. Folic acid, 5 mg, is given daily for 4 months. In cases of malabsorption 15 mg daily may be given. These doses completely replenish stores. There is no need for parenteral folic acid except in patients who are unable to swallow or who are receiving total parenteral nutrition. These doses of folic acid should be given only when vitamin B_{12} deficiency has been excluded or in severely ill patients in whom combined treatment with both vitamins is given before it is known which deficiency is present. Folic acid may precipitate neuropathy if given alone to a severely B_{12} deficient patient. Folinic acid (a reduced form of folate) is used only to reverse toxicity caused by antifolate drug therapy, e.g., methotrexate or pyrimethamine.

Assessment of Response

The patient feels better after 24 to 48 hours, with improvement in general well-being and appetite and relief of sore tongue. A reticulocyte response begins on the third day, with the peak on the sixth or seventh day, depending on the initial degree of anemia, reticulocytosis of over 30 per cent occurring in severely anemic patients. The white cell and platelet counts rise to normal after about 7 days and the hemoglobin rises by about 1 gram each week. A poor response suggests an associated disease, e.g., infection or malignancy; another deficiency, e.g., of iron, or an incorrect diagnosis.

Therapy Other Than Vitamin B_{12} or Folic Acid

1. In the severely anemic patient, transfusion may be essential. If so, only 1 or 2 units of blood should be given slowly as packed cells. If congestive heart failure is present, transfusion should be avoided or an equivalent or somewhat smaller volume of blood may be removed from the opposite arm.

2. Heart failure, if present, requires usual therapy with digoxin and diuretics.

3. Hypokalemia has been observed in patients with megaloblastic anemia during the initial response to treatment, as a result of potassium

entering developing hematopoietic cells from plasma. Although the definite indications for potassium therapy have not been determined, it seems advisable to give potassium orally during the first week or so of therapy to patients with heart failure and to patients in whom hypokalemia is found on initially testing serum potassium levels.

4. Occasionally, patients suffer an attack of gout at about the sixth day of therapy, owing to the sudden increase in uric acid excretion. The attack should be treated conventionally. In these patients there is usually a pre-existing tendency to gout, and long-term therapy with allopurinol or probenecid may be necessary.

Maintenance Therapy

Pernicious Anemia. 1. One thousand micrograms of hydroxocobalamin intramuscularly once every 3 months is satisfactory. On this, all our pernicious anemia patients maintain satisfactory blood counts and normal serum vitamin B_{12} levels immediately prior to the injection.

2. A physician should see the patient once every 6 to 12 months for a routine blood check and clinical examination.

3. A proportion of patients develop iron deficiency during the initial response to therapy. This should be treated with oral iron, e.g., anhydrous ferrous sulfate, 200 mg three times daily for 3 months or so, depending on the severity. Severe, recurring iron deficiency requires investigation.

4. There is a 2 to 3 per cent risk that carcinoma of the stomach will develop in patients with pernicious anemia. Routine x-rays and endoscopy are not necessary, but weight loss or other suggestive symptoms indicate the need for appropriate investigation.

5. Thyroid diseases, adrenal atrophy, and other autoimmune diseases are associated with pernicious anemia. The patient should be observed carefully for these.

Vitamin B_{12} Deficiency Other Than That Due to Pernicious Anemia. 1. Rarely, it may be possible to correct the cause of vitamin B_{12} deficiency so that long-term maintenance is unnecessary. Possible reversible causes include fish tapeworm, a stagnant loop of intestine, and tropical sprue. Vegans may change to a diet including vitamin B_{12}.

2. Prophylactic vitamin B_{12} therapy should be given for life from the time of operation to patients who undergo a total gastrectomy or an ileal resection.

3. There is no definite indication for vitamin B_{12} therapy in nonvitamin B_{12} deficiency states, except that massive amounts of vitamin B_{12} are needed in rare infants with transcobalamin II deficiency (defect of vitamin B_{12} transport). Hydroxocobalamin is indicated in nitrous oxide–induced megaloblastic anemia (inactivation of vitamin B_{12}). There are also suggestions that hydroxocobalamin is of benefit in Leber's optic atrophy and tobacco amblyopia.

Sensitivity to Vitamin B_{12}. This is extremely rare but, if suspected, may be confirmed by skin testing. It may be necessary to give vitamin B_{12} orally.

Oral Vitamin B_{12}. 1. Small amounts (about 1 per cent of an oral dose of vitamin B_{12}) can be absorbed by a nonintrinsic factor mechanism from the upper small intestine in normal subjects and in patients with pernicious anemia. It is possible, therefore, to maintain patients with pernicious anemia or other cause of vitamin B_{12} malabsorption with large (500 micrograms) oral doses each day. This may be done in patients who are sensitive to or refuse injections.

2. Vegans who develops vitamin B_{12} deficiency may be treated either by adding vitamin B_{12} to the daily diet or by regular injections (e.g., twice yearly).

Folate Deficiency. The need for maintenance therapy depends on whether or not the underlying condition is reversible (e.g., improved dietary intake of folate, a gluten-free diet) or is self-limiting (e.g., pregnancy). Patients who need long-term folic acid therapy include those with severe chronic hemolytic anemias (e.g., sickle cell anemia, thalassemia major), patients with chronic myelosclerosis or uncorrectable malabsorption syndrome, and patients receiving regular hemodialysis. In most of these conditions 5 mg of folic acid weekly is adequate to augment the diet and prevent recurrence of the deficiency.

Prophylactic folic acid is also given routinely in pregnancy and to premature babies (e.g., less than 1500 grams at birth).

THALASSEMIA

method of
JOSEPH H. GRAZIANO, Ph.D.,
and SERGIO PIOMELLI, M.D.
New York, New York

The thalassemia syndromes are a group of inherited disorders of hemoglobin synthesis which, in the United States, occur primarily in persons of Italian, Greek, or Oriental heritage, and to a lesser extent in blacks and Jews. The basic defect in thalassemia is an inability to synthesize one or more of the globin chains of hemoglobin. Whereas, under normal circumstances, alpha globin chain production is approximately equal to nonalpha ($\beta + \gamma + \delta$) globin chain production, the thalassemias are characterized by deficient synthesis of a particular globin, with a resultant excess of the complementary globin chain. For example, in beta-thalassemia, the form of the disease most common among people of Mediterranean origin, insufficient β-globin chain production leads to an excess of α-globin chains which aggregate and precipitate to form Heinz bodies in the red cell precursors. Such inclusion bodies lead to oxidation of membrane components and pitting of cells owing to removal of the inclusion bodies by the reticuloendothelial system. The end result is the production of poorly hemoglobinized cells with severely impaired survival.

There are two types of beta-thalassemia, one associated with decreased beta-chain synthesis (β^+) and the other with absent beta-chain synthesis (β^0). In the past few years, it has been established that each type in fact represents a heterogeneous group of diseases at the molecular level. Even with our present rudimentary knowledge of mammalian gene expression, it is obvious that numerous opportunities involving gene mutations and deletions could effect partial or complete reductions in globin mRNA transcription and translation. Numerous specific genotypes of beta-thalassemia will undoubtedly be described in the near future.

The heterozygous or carrier state of beta-thalassemia, referred to as thalassemia minor, is not a disease state, but may be associated with a mild asymptomatic, hypochromic, microcytic anemia, often more pronounced during pregnancy. The carrier state is often misdiagnosed as iron deficiency, but it can be distinguished from iron deficiency by hemoglobin electrophoresis, which reveals elevated hemoglobin A_2 ($\alpha_2\delta_2$) in beta-thalassemia trait, and by the erythrocyte protoporphyrin concentration, which is elevated in iron deficiency but is normal in beta-thalassemia trait. The homozygous state, referred to as thalassemia major, Cooley's anemia, or Mediterranean anemia, is usually first detected in the first year or two of life by the profound anemia which develops within a few months from birth, when the switch from fetal hemoglobin ($\alpha_2\gamma_2$) to adult hemoglobin ($\alpha_2\beta_2$) synthesis normally takes place. The measurement of globin chain syntheses by reticulocytes subsequently reveals insufficient (β^+) or absent (β^0) beta-globin production.

The genetics of the alpha-thalassemias are somewhat more complex. There are four alpha gene loci rather than two. The presence of one or two alpha-thalassemia genes does not produce any significant pathology. The double homozygous state produces hydrops fetalis because alpha-globin is necessary for the production of fetal hemoglobin ($\alpha_2\gamma_2$). The rare three-gene deletion produces hemoglobin H (γ_4) disease, a condition associated with a relatively mild hypochromic, microcytic anemia.

Pathophysiology of Thalassemia Major

During the past 15 years the pathophysiology of Cooley's anemia has changed as our approach to transfusion therapy becomes more aggressive. The basis of the pathophysiology is the unbalanced globin chain synthesis, which results in intramedullary red cell destruction and a tremendous rate of ineffective erythropoiesis. In response to the severe anemia, erythropoietin production becomes elevated, leading to extensive erythroid expansion of the bone marrow with concomitant increases in the delivery of iron to the marrow and plasma iron turnover. Thus, in the untransfused or inadequately transfused state, thalassemia major is characterized by the consequences of erythroid expansion and anemia: thinning of the bone cortices, resulting in frequent bone breaks, bone deformities, and the classic "chipmunk" facies; and markedly elevated iron absorption, which leads to hemosiderosis and eventually cardiac failure as a result of the combination of the massive cardiomegaly and high output state and myocardial iron deposition. Left untreated, patients with thalassemia major would maintain hematocrits of 10 or less, and would die of cardiac failure in the first few years of life.

Transfusion Therapy

The administration of red cell transfusions on a regular basis can prevent much of the pathophysiology associated with erythroid expansion and anemia. It is important to realize that the goal of transfusion therapy is not only to maintain life but also to shut down the erythroid marrow, decrease iron absorption, allow bone thickening, and improve the patient's sense of well-being and quality of life. Although blood transfusions lead to iron overload, which historically caused death near the age of 20, inadequately transfused patients fare no better because of elevated gastrointestinal iron absorption.

In order to inhibit intrinsic hematopoiesis, the pretransfusion hemoglobin concentration should not be allowed to fall below 10.5 to 11.0 grams per dl (100 ml). Some centers have suggested keeping patients above 12.0 grams per dl;

however, there is no evidence that this results in any improvement over the 10.5 to 11.0 grams per dl regimen. This can usually be accomplished by a transfusion schedule of 15 ml of packed red cells per kg of body weight every 3 to 4 weeks. Initially, blood may have to be administered more frequently in order to achieve the desired pre-transfusion hemoglobin concentration. Since packed red cells survive longer than washed, frozen cells, it is our practice to administer packed cells unless the development of antibodies requires the use of leukocyte-poor or eventually washed frozen cells. If begun very early in life, this transfusion program will completely prevent pathologic bony changes and cardiomegaly, will normalize cardiac work, and will permit a completely normal level of activity.

Current clinical research in Cooley's anemia is aimed at the development of young red cell transfusions in order to increase the time between transfusions, improve oxygen delivery to tissues, and ultimately decrease the amount of blood and iron administered each year. Because younger red cells are slightly larger and less dense than older red cells, the younger cells can now be isolated for transfusion by a number of techniques. Our laboratory is currently evaluating young cell transfusions by supporting a limited number of patients exclusively with young cells and quantitating red cell survival and the reduction in blood requirement. It seems reasonable to project that young cell transfusions may soon become routinely available at a reasonable cost at the major centers in the United States, and that such transfusions may decrease the annual frequency of transfusion, number of transfusions, and iron load by approximately 30 per cent.

Splenectomy

Persistent maintenance of the hemoglobin concentration above 10.5 to 11.0 grams per dl will generally prevent the acute onset of clinically overt hypersplenism. Nevertheless, if one carefully examines the annual transfusion requirement (ml per kg per year) of a large group of patients chronically transfused at the aforementioned 10.5 to 11.0 grams per dl regimen, it becomes obvious that the blood requirement increases with age even in the absence of overt hypersplenism. An analysis of the transfusion requirements of 37 patients with intact spleens revealed a requirement of 281 ml per kg per year for those over 5 years of age. In contrast, the mean blood requirement of 33 splenectomized patients over 5 years of age was only 190 ml per kg per year, with no increase as a function of age. Since the blood requirement must be kept to a

minimum if zero or negative iron balance is to be achieved through chelation therapy (see below), this data has led us to encourage splenectomy, even in the absence of overt hypersplenism, as soon as the blood requirement begins to rise by more than 20 per cent above the 190 ml per kg per year required by splenectomized patients. Typically, this occurs between 5 and 10 years of age. It is therefore essential to compute each patient's blood consumption in ml per kg per year at least once each year. Splenectomy invariably reduces the blood requirement to approximately 200 ml per kg per year or less and thereby facilitates the achievement of iron balance through chelation therapy.

Historically, there were problems with overwhelming pneumococcal, meningococcal, and *Hemophilus influenzae* infections in young splenectomized thalassemics. In recent times, with improved clinical management, these problems have become more manageable. After splenectomy, it is our practice to administer prophylactic penicillin indefinitely, and to administer the pneumococcal vaccine before surgery. It is also essential to educate patients and parents so that any instance of fever and possible infection may be treated aggressively until culture results are known.

Chelation Therapy

The pathology associated with iron overload, i.e., the cardiac, endocrine, and hepatic dysfunction, should be prevented by a chelation regimen which achieves iron balance. The achievement of iron balance is now possible in patients with thalassemia through the use of daily subcutaneous infusions of the iron-chelating drug deferoxamine B (Desferal). It is now standard, Food and Drug Administration–approved practice to administer daily subcutaneous infusions of Desferal on a home-care basis, using a small, portable, battery-operated infusion pump which can be attached to the patient's belt. Iron balance can be achieved with daily infusions of 20 to 40 mg per kg, administered as an 8-hour infusion. Most patients readily adapt to using the pump during sleep, with the needle placed under the skin in the abdomen or leg.

The quantity of iron excreted in response to an 8-hour subcutaneous infusion of Desferal increases as a function of the number of blood transfusions which the patient has received. The greater the iron load, the greater the response. Thus, while 20 mg per kg of Desferal is usually sufficient in patients older than 10 years of age, younger patients often require 40 mg per kg to achieve iron balance. The drug is usually mixed to a final concentration of 500 mg per 2 to 3 ml of sterile water and administered through a 25 or 27 gauge butterfly needle. The only adverse effects are occasional redness, pruritus, and swelling at the injection site, which appear to be due to mechanical irritation or poor needle placement. These problems usually diminish as the patient or parent gains experience.

Since preventing the tissue damage associated with iron overload is the goal of chelation therapy, the earlier that therapy is begun, the better the long-term prognosis will be; this is an assumption which is now being tested, since subcutaneous Desferal therapy has been in use only since 1976. In the absence of chelation therapy, myocardial thickening can be seen in the first years of life, and liver biopsies usually show marked fibrosis and occasionally cirrhosis by the age of 5 or 6 years. Thus, the age at which therapy is initiated depends more on the family than on anything else. Some families and patients adapt relatively easily by age 3, while others are still reluctant several years later. We have found it helpful initially to use the pump during transfusion visits so that the patient adjusts to it as he or she adjusts to venipuncture and blood transfusion.

Ascorbic acid, which is rapidly oxidized in patients with iron overload, is involved in the release of iron from the reticuloendothelial system. There is no question that ascorbate supplementation in ascorbate-depleted patients will increase the quantity of iron excreted with Desferal. But there is also no question that too much ascorbic acid is dangerous and cardiotoxic because too much iron is mobilized from the reticuloendothelial system. Based on our experience, we have reached two conclusions with regard to this issue. First, children under 10 years of age are usually not ascorbate deficient and do not require supplementation. Second, in children 10 years of age or older, 50 mg of ascorbate per day is enough to gradually replete the patient's reserves and improve the response to Desferal. In these cases, ascorbate is administered at the start of the Desferal infusion so that the released iron will be bound by the drug.

In discussing iron balance, one point should be re-emphasized. Chelation therapy will achieve iron balance only if the blood requirement is within reasonable limits. By 10 years of age, regardless of the prior transfusion history, the presence of an intact spleen makes the achievement of iron balance exceedingly difficult. For example, in one study of patients between 10 and 17 years of age who received 20 mg per kg of Desferal daily, 9 of 11 splenectomized patients were in negative iron balance, while only 2 of 11 with intact spleens achieved balance. Furthermore, the absolute quantity of iron excreted with Desferal does not diminish after splenectomy.

Thalassemia Intermedia

The thalassemia syndromes represent a spectrum of diseases varying widely in their severity, depending on the magnitude and type of globin chain deficiency. Although the spectrum of severity of the anemia is a continuous one, clinically patients are grouped into two groups: either they require transfusions to maintain life (thalassemia major) or they do not (thalassemia intermedia). The distinction between the two groups is one of clinical judgment. About 5 per cent of patients with thalassemia are able to maintain hemoglobin concentrations of 7 to 9 grams per dl without blood transfusions; these patients probably represent diverse genotypes, some of which are capable of compensating with fetal hemoglobin production. Although this group of patients demonstrates much of the typical pathology of thalassemia major such as bone deformities and hepatosplenomegaly, historically this group of untransfused patients usually survived longer and developed sexually better than transfused counterparts.

With the recent improvements in transfusion and chelation therapy, and improved but still ill-defined prognosis for patients with thalassemia major, the clinical decision of labeling a patient as an intermediate has become more difficult. The skeletal and facial deformities which occur early in life in untransfused patients are never completely reversed by blood transfusions later on. Thalassemia intermedia patients hyperabsorb and accumulate iron at an alarming rate and, when given Desferal, respond with as much iron excretion as age-matched patients with thalassemia major. Intermediate patients, therefore, should probably be placed on a low-iron diet and/or chelated. To our eyes the quality of life of patients with thalassemia major seems to be better than that of many of those who have been treated in the past as intermediates. Many patients treated as having thalassemia intermedia eventually require blood transfusions near the end of the second decade to alleviate the threat of vertebral relapse, for bone pain or cardiac arrhythmia. Often, the sense of well-being improves with transfusions to a level never before achieved.

The administration of folic acid (1 mg per day) is essential only for patients who are not transfused or who are, for whatever reason, only occasionally transfused. Folate, a vitamin which is not stored, is required for DNA synthesis. Massive bone marrow proliferation and ineffective erythropoiesis increase the daily requirement for folate. Likewise, massive DNA and purine degradation may require allopurinol administration to control hyperuricemia.

Antenatal Diagnosis

It is now possible to detect thalassemia major in utero by examining globin chain synthesis in fetal reticulocytes. Personnel at several major centers are capable of and adept at obtaining fetal blood samples during 18 to 20 weeks of gestation by fetoscopy. Although the risk of spontaneous abortion associated with this procedure was about 10 per cent for the first 500 cases, with experienced personnel the risk has fallen below 5 per cent. The procedure is almost routinely used by young families who already have a child with Cooley's anemia. Current research is aimed at the development of a simplified amniocentesis diagnostic technique.

SICKLE CELL DISEASE

method of
MARILYN H. GASTON, M.D.
Bethesda, Maryland

Introduction

Sickle cell disease is a major health concern throughout the world, occurring in Africa, the West Indies, the Mediterranean area, India, and the Middle East, as well as the United States. Inheritance of the gene for sickle hemoglobin results in the insertion of valine instead of glutamic acid in the sixth position of the β globin chains. When deoxygenated, sickle hemoglobin (HbS) gels and forms intermolecular aggregates which deform the erythrocytes (sickling) and cause rigidity. As a result of the sickle shape and loss of flexibility and deformability, these red cells are unable to transverse small vessels, and the resultant blockage with tissue anoxia accounts for most of the clinical manifestations of this illness.

Inheritance of the HbS gene from both parents results in homozygous S disease (SS) or sickle cell anemia. Inheritance of a sickle gene from one parent and a gene from the other parent for either β-thalassemia or another hemoglobin type, e.g., C, D, O_{Arab}, results in clinically significant disease. Therefore, these disorders or major genotypes (e.g., SS, SC, $S\beta^+$ thalassemia, $S\beta^0$ thalassemia, SD) in which the predominant hemoglobin is S produce clinical symptoms and constitute the syndrome of sickle cell disease.

Sickle cell trait (AS) is not classified as sickle cell disease because the predominant hemoglobin is adult hemoglobin, not sickle hemoglobin, and there is no associated anemia or painful crises. It is considered a benign carrier state with no clinical significance.

Sickle cell disease is characterized clinically by four different pathophysiologic mechanisms: (1) chronic hemolytic anemia from a shortened red cell survival; (2) acute and chronic organ damage from the vaso-occlusive phenomena; (3) the occurrence of secondary effects not related directly to the "sickled cell," e.g., gallstones, growth retardation, susceptibility to infection; and (4) psychosocial aspects resulting from an inherited chronic illness which is unpredictable in nature, requires frequent medical attention, is painful, and for which there is no available cure. These complications occur in all the major genotypes, but are usually most common and most severe in homozygous S sickle cell disease.

General Management

Management of patients with sickle cell disease not only includes treatment of specific complications but is directed toward helping patients reach their fullest potential and improving their overall quality of life. This is best accomplished with a comprehensive approach which utilizes and examplifies the team concept of health care management. This maintenance approach focuses on all the ramifications of the illness as it affects the total patient and the family. The "team" to provide medical care and support for the patient with sickle cell disease may be viewed as a primary team consisting of internist, pediatrician, hematologist, nurse, and social service components, which provides the continuity, stability, and coordination of all aspects of the patient's care. A secondary team consists of many medical subspecialties, as sickle cell disease may affect all major organ systems. The tertiary team includes other components within the life space of the patient and family, e.g., employers, visiting nurses, psychologists, and school officials.

This multifaceted, interdisciplinary approach and network of services should ensure (1) comprehensive care with close monitoring through routine visits and periodic measures of organ function; (2) ongoing continuous education to the patient, family, and outside individuals, e.g., school officials; and (3) recognition and support for the psychosocial aspects of this illness, focusing on the promotion of emotional well-being and assistance in the acquisition of educational and vocational goals.

Patients should be encouraged to lead as normal lives as possible and to realize that this illness has a broad spectrum of severity with considerable variability. Some patients have mild disease and few if any problems, while others manifest severe illness. At present, the etiology of the wide spectrum is unknown. The subsequent complications occur with variable frequency and severity from patient to patient.

Acute Complications

Painful Episode. This is the hallmark of sickle cell disease, with pain occurring anywhere but usually in the extremities, back, abdomen, or chest. The painful episodes vary in frequency, duration, and intensity for individual patients and from patient to patient; but for each patient the painful crises tend to be similar, which is helpful in distinguishing this pain from pain resulting from other causes.

Mild vaso-occlusive episodes can be managed at home with increased fluid intake, bed rest, and analgesics. Adult patients are encouraged to consume 2 to 3 liters of fluids daily and children 120 ml per kg daily. Analgesics include (1) acetaminophen (Tylenol) orally every 4 hours, 60 mg per year of age to age 5, 325 mg age 5 to 10 years, 600 mg over age 10 years; or (2) acetylsalicylic acid (aspirin or Empirin), 65 mg per kg divided into six doses; or (3) propoxyphene hydrochloride (Darvon), 3 mg per kg daily for patients over 12 years of age. Codeine phosphate, pentazocine (Talwin), and oxycodone hydrochloride (Percodan) are used on an individual basis and must be closely monitored. Patients with severe pain, atypical pain, infection, or other complicating aspects, e.g., vomiting, should be hospitalized.

Upon hospitalization, intravenous fluids should be administered and the patient's hydration *should not* depend on increased oral intake alone. Children receive 2000 to 3000 ml per square meter of body surface per 24 hours, and adults 4 liters per 24 hours. Alkali is indicated only if acidosis is present.

Pain severe enough to warrant hospitalization should be treated with intramuscular analgesics and *not* oral medication. The most important aspect of the entire regimen is to ease the pain and make patients as comfortable as possible. Therefore, the dosage is increased as necessary for relief and for the first 24 to 48 hours is administered every 3 to 4 hours on a regular schedule rather than on the usual as necessary basis. This single approach to pain management decreases the patient's anxiety and frustration in seeking pain relief, increases trust, and improves the doctor-patient communication. Meperidine (Demerol) is administered to children under 10 years of age, 1 mg per kg per dose every 3 to 4 hours intramuscularly; to adolescents, 25 to 75 mg every 3 to 4 hours intramuscularly; and to adults, 100 to 200 mg every 3 to 4 hours intramuscularly. The dosage is adjusted according to the severity of the pain and the response of the patient.

In addition, precipitating factors such as infection and acidosis should be sought and treated appropriately. Fever must be controlled around the clock, rather than as necessary, by antipyretics, especially in children to decrease further sickling. Routine management of the uncomplicated painful episode does not include oxygen, alkalis, blood transfusions, or antisickling agents.

Acute Anemic Episode. The chronic hemolytic anemia of sickle cell disease varies in severity among patients, but in the individual patient tends to be very steady. Patients tolerate their level of anemia quite well, and the anemia becomes a problem only if the hemoglobin drops significantly below the patient's usual level. An acute anemic episode may occur following an infection when the marrow production is diminished, resulting in an aplastic crisis with a rapid drop in hemoglobin and reticulocyte count. Transfusion to a hemoglobin level of 10 grams per cent with packed red blood cells is indicated (in children 10 ml per kg). Signs of congestive heart failure should be sought and treated appropriately.

A significant decrease in a child's hemoglobin level may be produced by acute splenic sequestration, which is a *medical emergency*. This results from the trapping of blood in the spleen and also liver, with a fulminant drop in hemoglobin and blood volume, producing shock and death. Immediate replacement of the blood volume is essential. While blood is being typed and cross-matched, volume expanders are given if the patient is in shock and are immediately followed by transfusions with packed cells or partial exchange transfusion (1½ volume exchange, 1.5 × 75 ml per kg = total ml whole blood). Subsequently, the child should be placed on a chronic transfusion program to maintain the hemoglobin S percentage below 30 per cent, and consideration should be given to splenectomy if the child is over the age of 2 years.

Acute Infectious Episode. Infection is the leading cause of death in young children, especially from pneumococcal septicemia. Therefore, management of patients with sickle cell disease includes a high index of suspicion for possible infections whenever medical attention is sought, thorough physical evaluation, frequent cultures, chest x-ray whenever fever is present, and lumbar puncture, as the incidence of meningitis is 600 times greater in patients with SS disease. Even though fever may occur with painful episodes, an unrelenting search must routinely be accomplished to rule out infection, since the risk for infection is great and the consequences severe. In addition, antibiotic therapy should be instituted early with dosages greater than those usually recommended. Septicemia, pneumonia, meningitis, osteomyelitis, and recurrent pyelonephritis occur with increased frequency in sickle cell disease. The most common bacterial pathogens are pneumococci, *Hemophilus influenzae*, meningococci, salmonellae, and streptococci. Therefore, the initial drugs of choice are penicillin G, 200,000 units per kg per 24 hours, and/or ampicillin, 200 mg per kg per 24 hours, intravenously in six divided doses. Other drugs are utilized as indicated by culture.

The pneumococcal vaccine is recommended for patients over the age of 2 years to prevent pneumococcal infections. Its efficacy in patients less than 2 years of age is being evaluated. In children under 2 years of age, penicillin VK, 250 ml daily, can be given prophylactically, but this approach is presently under investigation.

Acute Chest Syndrome. This is an acute illness characterized by chest pain, fever, tachypnea, and positive or negative x-rays. Differentiation between pneumonia and pulmonary infarct from in situ sickling is difficult. Pneumonia is the probable diagnosis in children under 10 years of age, with positive radiographic findings early and upper lobe infiltrates. Therapy includes parenteral penicillin or ampicillin, hydration, and oxygen. Transfusion is indicated with severe illness, hypoxemia, and/or multiple lobe involvement to decrease the hemoglobin S and also improve the oxygen carrying capacity.

Right Upper Quadrant Syndrome. Abdominal pain is common in sickle cell disease. Repeated episodes, especially in the right upper quadrant, require evaluation for gallstones and liver disease. Gallstones are also common, resulting from the chronic hemolysis and increased bilirubin, and have been reported in patients as young as 5 years of age. Cholecystectomy is indicated only if the patient is symptomatic. Acute right upper quadrant pain may indicate liver disease from hepatic infarction, or hepatitis. Treatment is supportive, but with severe liver damage partial exchange transfusions may benefit.

Cerebrovascular Accident. Partial or complete occlusion of small and large cerebral vessels occurs in sickle cell disease with significant resultant morbidity and mortality. Acute management includes exchange transfusion and supportive care. Long-term transfusion programs instituted immediately to keep the percentage of HbS below 30 have been shown to be effective in decreasing the stroke recurrence rate, which is considerably high. The length of time for continuation of the long-term transfusion program is uncertain but is over 2 to 3 years.

Priapism. This complication is frustrating and disconcerting for all involved, as present therapeutic modalities are inadequate, it can be recurrent, and impotence is a frequent and distressing sequela. Therapy ranges from exchange transfusions or aspiration of the corpora cavernosa to surgical shunting. The incidence of impotence is not affected by conservative or surgical treatment. It is essential that as much emotional support as possible be given during and following this difficult complication.

Chronic Complications

Repeated multiple blood vessel occlusions over a period of time result in chronic organ damage. The age of onset, rate of progression, and eventual outcome are essentially unknown but are presently being studied in a large 23 institution cooperative study. Every organ may be compromised by this process; however, the most commonly observed chronic complications are leg ulcers, aseptic necrosis of the femoral head, renal complications, and eye complications.

Leg Ulceration. This is an especially distressing feature of this illness, because ulcers recur, are often intractable to conservative and surgical management, and cause significant psychosocial morbidity, as time lost from school and work may be extensive.

Conservative management includes bed rest, debridement, and Burow's soaks followed by an antibiotic ointment. After an initial trial, the Unna boot with zinc oxide may be attempted. If the ulcer remains refractory, transfusions to decrease the HbS below 30 per cent and surgical skin grafts should be employed.

Ophthalmologic Complications. Patients with SC have the most severe fundus changes. The alterations in patients with S-thalassemia are less frequent and less pronounced, and patients with hemoglobin SS have the mildest changes for reasons which remain unclear. Nevertheless, all patients with sickle cell disease should be followed annually by an ophthalmologist beginning at age 6, as proliferative sickle retinopathy can lead to blindness resulting from vitreous hemorrhage or retinal detachment. Photocoagulation (xenon arc or argon laser) early appears to be effective in preventing visual loss.

Aseptic Necrosis. Aseptic necrosis of the hip is treated by standard orthopedic procedures, which in severe cases may include total hip replacement.

Renal Disease. Renal papillary necrosis occurs and may lead to hematuria. There is in addition an increased risk of urinary tract infection, proteinuria, and renal insufficiency. These complications are generally treated as with any other patient. Hematuria should be carefully evaluated to rule out other causes and treated conservatively with bed rest, hydration, and transfusions if necessary. Nephrectomy is contraindicated and the use of epsilon aminocaproic acid is not encouraged because of the risk of intrarenal clotting.

Health-Related Events

Surgery and Anesthesia. Prior to major surgery and general anesthesia, the patient should be transfused to increase the hemoglobin and hematocrit and decrease the percentage of hemoglobin S to 30 or below. This may be accomplished by simple transfusions with washed packed red blood cells or by partial exchange transfusion. Strict attention should be given to adequate fluid intake and oxygenation during the procedure and also during the postoperative period.

Pregnancy. There is increased risk for fetal and maternal morbidity with sickle cell disease, but this risk is significantly reduced with good prenatal and obstetric care. This includes monthly visits in the first trimester, biweekly in the second, and weekly in the third; multivitamins and iron; and folic acid, 1 mg per day.

The use of prophylactic transfusion during the third trimester, although reportedly beneficial, remains controversial at this point. Certainly with specific complications transfusions are employed. Normal vaginal delivery is the preferred route of delivery.

Transfusion. Blood transfusions, simple or exchange, should be employed only with specific indication in the management of patients with sickle cell disease. The risks of transfusion, including acute and delayed reactions, hepatitis, isoimmunization, and possible iron overload, must be weighed against the benefits. At present, specific indications include acute anemic episodes, splenic sequestration, cerebrovascular accidents, preparation for surgery with a general anesthetic, and acute chest syndrome with hypoxemia or life-threatening complications, e.g., septicemia. Chronic hypertransfusion programs to keep the hemoglobin S below 30 per cent over an extended period of time are recommended following cerebrovascular accidents and should be considered during pregnancy and with intractable leg ulcers.

NEUTROPENIA

method of
GERALD ROTHSTEIN, M.D.
Salt Lake City, Utah

Neutrophils are one essential part of a complex set of physiologic factors which prevent invasion by microorganisms. The neutrophils are produced in the bone marrow, stored there for 6 to 10 days, and then released into the blood. During their 10 hour sojourn in the blood, either neutrophils circulate freely and are accessible to the blood sampling needle or they are marginated along the walls of small vessels and escape detection by standard blood sampling techniques. Neutropenia or a decrease in the neutrophil count to less than 1600 cells per cu mm can come about because of a decrease in cell production, a decrease in the number of mature neutrophils stored in the marrow, or shortened neutrophil survival. When the neutrophil count is depressed because of increased cell margination, "pseudoneutropenia" exists because the total blood neutrophil content is normal. The finding of neutropenia demands answers to two questions: (1) What is the cause of the neutropenia? (2) Does this neutropenia signal a decrease in host resistance to infection?

The Detection of Neutropenia

In order to detect neutropenia, both a nucleated cell count (WBC) and differential count must be done. Then the absolute neutrophil count may be calculated by multiplying the WBC and the percentage of metamyelocytes + bands + polymorphonuclear leukocyes (PMN) in the differential. The normal range is 1600 to 7200 cells for Caucasians, with slightly lower limits for blacks.

Work-up of the Neutropenic Patient

The approach to the patient with neutropenia should be designed to determine the cause of the neutropenia and also to evaluate the patient's risk for infection. A history can be of great importance. Recurrent febrile illnesses, particularly those diagnosed as bacterial infection, should alert the physician to the possibility that neutropenia is so severe as to allow easy invasion by microorganisms. A history of progressive shortness of breath or petechiae should suggest that not only is there neutropenia but the red cell and platelet numbers are reduced as well. The presence of arthritis may suggest the diagnosis of lupus, rheumatoid arthritis, or other collagen vascular disease. A careful drug history should be obtained for chemotherapeutic agents such as cyclophosphamide or methotrexate. Some other drugs which may be associated with neutropenia are the antithyroid drugs, phenothiazines, colloidal gold, and some antimicrobial agents. Further examination of the blood should be used to determine whether not only the neutrophils but also other cell lines are involved, and the complete blood count should include hematocrit, WBC, platelet count, and differential count. Physical examination should be carefully performed to evaluate for pallor, petechiae, evidence of bacterial infection, lymphadenopathy, arthritis, or splenomegaly. A bone marrow aspirate and biopsy may also be helpful in evaluating marrow cell production and neutrophil stores. In the febrile patient, a thorough search for bacterial infection is indicated.

Causes of Neutropenia

Idiopathic Neutropenia. In this setting no underlying disease is found to account for the neutropenia, yet neutrophil counts of 250 to 1000 per cu mm are common. Splenomegaly is usually not present, and there is normal or increased marrow cellularity. During idiopathic neutropenia, reduced neutrophil counts may be sustained for years without supervening infection. If such infection does not occur, no therapy is indicated.

Neutropenia During Infection. Neutropenia may occur in a variety of viral and bacterial infections. When bacterial infection is associated with neutropenia a grave prognosis is suggested. Individuals with folate or B_{12} deficiency appear at unusually high risk for neutropenia during bacterial infection, dictating the use of folate or B_{12} treatment together with antibiotic therapy in such cases. Neonatal sepsis is frequently associated with depletion of the marrow storage pool of mature neutrophils, and when the marrow mature neutrophils constitute less than 10 per cent of the total nucleated cells in the bone marrow a fatal outcome is likely.

Chronic Neutropenia with Splenomegaly. When chronic neutropenia is associated with splenomegaly the diagnosis of inflammatory disease, lymphoma, or liver disease with portal hypertension should be considered. When associated with rheumatoid arthritis, the presence of neutropenia completes the features of Felty's syndrome. The neutropenia of Felty's syndrome is usually well tolerated by patients, even in the presence of very low blood neutrophil counts. Perhaps the explanation for this is that in many of these patients large proportions of circulating neutrophils are marginated, giving the impression of severe neutropenia when in fact the total blood content of neutrophils may be much more nearly normal. In most patients with splenomegaly and chronic neutropenia, the removal of the spleen does not produce a lasting increase in the blood neutrophil concentration. In fact splenectomy as a potential therapeutic maneuver for neutropenia should not be employed except as a treatment for patients with recurrent bacterial infections. Even in this setting splenectomy may fail to produce lasting improvement. Lithium carbonate treatment can elevate the neutrophil count of Felty's syndrome patients, but its effect upon the incidence of infection is unknown.

Neutropenia Due to Hypoproductive States. When neoplasms interfere with marrow cell production, neutropenia is a common sequel. For example, with acute leukemia the patient may present because of neutropenia and bacterial infection. Aplastic anemia is another hematologic disorder which may be associated with life-threatening infection. In this case survival of the patient depends upon obtaining a lasting remission from bone marrow hypoplasia. In addition, vitamin B_{12} or folate deficiency may interfere sufficiently with neutrophil production to result in neutropenia, and the administration of chemotherapeutic agents may induce neutropenia. Because neutrophils are stored in the bone marrow for 6 to 10 days before they are released into the blood, a drug-induced interference with marrow cell production may not be manifest in the peripheral blood until 1 to 2 weeks later. Suppression of the neutrophil count to as low as 500 per cu mm by therapeutic agents may be relatively well tolerated by patients, although support during bacterial infection may be needed. Usually ordinary treatment measures without neutrophil transfusions are sufficient, although severe neutropenia may require support with neutrophil transfusions for the period of 1 to 2 weeks before the marrow recovers.

Congenital Neutropenia. Neutropenia may appear as a congenital defect. Such neutropenia can be transiently mediated by maternal antibodies directly against the fetal neutrophils. On the other hand, neutropenia may be inherited as an autosomal dominant trait, but in this case the neutropenia is usually mild and does not affect survival. The Kostmann form of inherited neutropenia is transmitted by an autosomal recessive mechanism and usually results in death from infection within the first few years of life.

Neutropenia Due to Decreased Neutrophil Survival. In some cases, marrow cell production appears to be normal or even increased, but the survival of released neutrophils in the blood is short. Such a mechanism has been postulated as the cause of neutropenia in Felty's syndrome, and a number of cases of apparently immune-mediated neutropenia in adults have also been described. The response to this form of neutropenia is variable and may be associated with infection if neutropenia is sufficiently severe.

Cyclic Neutropenia. Cyclic neutropenia is an uncommon disorder, at least one variety of which appears to be due to a disorder of the stem cells that produce neutrophils in the bone marrow. There is some speculation that in other cases cyclic neutropenia occurs as a result of a deficiency in the hormone-like substances which simulate neutrophil production. Cyclic neutropenia is characterized by a fall in the neutrophil count at approximately 3 week intervals. Fortunately the infections are usually not severe and antibiotic therapy is usually reserved for the detection of a specific infection. Some patients have experienced improvement with corticosteroid treatment, and the use of lithium carbonate is also being explored.

General Principles in the Management of Neutropenia

The life-limiting consequence of neutropenia is infection. Therefore, neutropenic subjects at particular risk for infection must be identified and appropriately managed. Fortunately, most neutropenic patients do not experience an increased susceptibility to infection. However, when the neutrophil count falls below 500 cells per cu mm, life-threatening infections are most likely to occur. In such severely neutropenic patients, the presence of fever should always be considered a symptom of infection until proved otherwise. Thus in addition to the usual hematologic studies and diagnostic maneuvers to determine the etiology of neutropenia, a complete physical examination, x-ray of the chest, urinalysis, and culture of the urine, blood, and other body fluids should be performed. If evidence of a specific infection is obtained, antibiotic therapy should be directed against that particular infection. However, if no specific infectious site is identified, antibiotic therapy should be initiated in a hospital setting and should include a beta-lactamase–resistant antibiotic such as carbenicillin or ticarcillin, and an aminoglycoside antibiotic such as gentamicin or tobramycin. In some patients an antistaphylococcal agent such as nafcillin may be indicated. Any alterations in antibiotic therapy are dictated by the detection of a specific infectious agent. Neutrophil transfusions may be useful in severely neutropenic infected patients, particularly if the neutropenic period is believed to be of relatively finite and short duration. Neutrophils collected by the continuous flow centrifugation method appear to retain their functional properties better than those obtained by conventional fiber aggregation methods. In addition HLA-matched neutrophils have a higher survival rate when cross-transfused than do non-HLA-matched neutrophils.

Therapeutic Management of Chronic Neutropenia

A therapeutic approach to chronic neutropenia depends upon whether the neutropenia is severe enough to allow repeated bacterial infection. Such infection may be manifested by episodes of obvious localized disease such as pneumonia or cutaneous abscesses; on the other hand, it has been postulated that the frequent fevers these patients experience constitute a sign of limited systemic infection. In subjects without apparent infection, therapeutic maneuvers should be limited to specific treatment of the disease process. For example, B_{12} and folic acid therapy for megaloblastic anemia should be employed if this diagnosis is established. Occasional patients with cyclic neutropenia and infection benefit from alternate day prednisone therapy, and there is some indication that lithium carbonate therapy may be effective in selected cases of cyclic neutropenia. The question of splenectomy is a difficult one, since in some disorders such as myelofibrosis or chronic myelocytic leukemia the spleen may be a source of neutrophil production. Similarly, the effect of splenectomy in Felty's syndrome is transient in most cases. Occasional patients with aplastic anemia and neutropenia respond to androgen therapy. The neutropenia resulting from lupus erythematosus has sometimes been noted to respond to corticosteroid therapy.

HEMOLYTIC DISEASE OF THE NEWBORN

method of
JAMES W. KENDIG, M.D.,
and M. JEFFREY MAISELS, M.B., B.CH.
Hershey, Pennsylvania

Introduction

Hemolytic disease of the newborn refers to the hemolysis of fetal and newborn red blood cells which are coated with maternal IgG antibodies. In the past, the most important cause of this problem was Rhesus incompatibility (erythroblastosis fetalis), a disease which is rapidly becoming extinct with the decline in family size and the widespread use of $Rh_0(D)$ immune globulin. Hemolytic disease may also occur when the mother is Group O and the infant is Group A or B, and the most common cause of such hemolysis in the United States is OA incompatibility, although this disease is much less severe than that associated with Rh incompatibility. Hemolytic problems resulting from incompatibility of the minor blood types (e.g., Kell, Duffy, Kidd) also occur but are quite rare.

Obstetric Management of the Rh-Sensitized Mother

The obstetrician caring for the Rh-sensitized mother must periodically perform an amniocentesis to evaluate the severity of the Rh disease. The change in the amniotic fluid optical density at 450 millimicrons (ΔOD 450) is related to the bilirubin level, the degree of intrauterine hemolysis, and therefore the severity of fetal anemia. This information is correlated with measurements of lung maturity (amniotic fluid L/S ratios) to determine the optimal time for delivery.

Intrauterine death results from severe anemia. If the ΔOD 450 value suggests that significant anemia is present and the infant is too premature to permit delivery (with a reasonable prospect of intact survival), an intrauterine blood transfusion is indicated. Such patients should be referred to a high-risk perinatal center for continued antenatal care and subsequent delivery.

Prevention of Rh Disease

Rh$_o$(D) immune globulin (RhoGAM, Gamulin Rh, HypRho-D) should be given to all Rh negative unimmunized women who deliver Rh positive babies, abort, or undergo amniocentesis. Within 72 hours after delivery, Rh$_o$(D) immune globulin is administered intraumuscularly as a single dose. One vial is capable of neutralizing 15 ml of Rh positive red blood cells (packed cells, not whole blood). In the uncomplicated term delivery, a single dose (one vial) is adequate. In the case of a large fetomaternal hemorrhage, the acid elution test of Kleihauer-Betke should be used to determine the magnitude of the bleed and an appropriate dose of Rh$_o$(D) immune globulin administered to the mother.

Indications for Exchange Transfusion

There are two major indications for an exchange transfusion in the infant with erythroblastosis fetalis: (1) severe anemia and/or (2) hyperbilirubinemia or potential hyperbilirubinemia.

Severe Hemolytic Disease and Hydrops Fetalis. Hydropic infants and those that are obviously pale and asphyxiated require vigorous resuscitation and immediate treatment. They frequently need assisted ventilation and end-expiratory pressure. If the birth of a severely affected infant is anticipated, packed red blood cells from a Type O Rh negative donor, cross-matched with the serum of the mother in the last trimester, should be available at the time of delivery. In the presence of severe anemia (hematocrit 35 per cent or less), an exchange transfu-

sion of 25 to 80 ml per kg of packed red blood cells is done within 30 minutes of birth to raise the hematocrit to about 40 per cent. Phlebotomy should not be performed routinely on these infants, because they are usually normovolemic and may be hypovolemic. Acidosis, hypoglycemia, and hypothermia must be corrected.

Hemolytic Disease. Guidelines for the use of an exchange transfusion in the management of hyperbilirubinemia are given in Figure 1. These guidelines take into consideration the serum bilirubin level, the rate of rise of the bilirubin, the infant's age and birth weight, and other factors thought to affect the risk of developing kernicterus (acidosis, hypoxia, sepsis, hypothermia, and hypoalbuminemia).

In the past, various criteria for an early or immediate exchange transfusion were based on cord blood levels of hemoglobin and bilirubin. Recent studies suggest that these measurements do not predict the severity of hyperbilirubinemia with sufficient accuracy to warrant their use as therapeutic guidelines. Unless the infant is severely anemic or in shock, the timing of an exchange transfusion should be based on the rate of rise of the serum bilirubin, which must be determined from frequent measurements of serum levels.

A serum indirect bilirubin rising by more than 0.5 mg per dl (100 ml) per hour indicates that there is a relatively brisk hemolytic process which will require an exchange transfusion within the first 12 hours of life. An early exchange transfusion in this situation will also correct anemia and remove a significant proportion of the sensitized red blood cells.

Premature and severely ill newborn infants may develop kernicterus at bilirubin levels as low as 10 mg per dl, but it is impossible to define an absolutely "safe" level of bilirubin for an individual patient at this time. Multiple methods for determining albumin binding of bilirubin and free (unbound) bilirubin levels are currently under investigation. However, none of these tests have been evaluated in appropriate clinical trials, and no single test is sufficiently reliable to be recommended for routine clinical use.

Preparation of Blood for Exchange Transfusion

We use blood preserved in citrate-phosphate-dextrose (CPD) anticoagulant solution. Potassium levels in CPD blood increase rapidly with storage, and it is recommended that exchange transfusion blood be less than 4 days old.

Hospital blood banks have special procedures for the preparation of exchange transfusion blood. The donor's blood should not stimu-

Serum Bilirubin mg/100 ml	Birth weight	<24 hrs	24-48 hrs	49-72 hrs	>72 hrs
<5					
5-9	ALL	PHOTO-THERAPY IF HEMOLYSIS			
10-14	<2500g	EXCHANGE IF HEMOLYSIS	PHOTOTHERAPY		
	>2500g		INVESTIGATE IF BILIRUBIN >12 mg		
15-19	<2500g	EXCHANGE		CONSIDER EXCHANGE	
	>2500g		PHOTOTHERAPY		
20 and+	ALL	EXCHANGE			

☐ Observe   ▨ Investigate Jaundice

Use phototherapy after any exchange

In presence of:

1. Perinatal asphyxia
2. Respiratory distress
3. Metabolic acidosis (pH 7.25 or below)
4. Hypothermia (temp below 35° C)
5. Low serum protein (5g/100 ml or less)
6. Birth weight <1500 g
7. Signs of clinical or CNS deterioration

⎫ Treat as in next higher bilirubin category

Figure 1. (From Maisels, M. J., *in* Avery, G. B. [ed.]: Neonatology. Philadelphia, J. B. Lippincott Company, 1975, p. 349 [with permission].)

late the immunity of the baby to either ABO or $Rh_0(D)$ antigen, and the donor red cells must be compatible with the antibodies in the mother's (and therefore the baby's) serum. Our blood bank uses the following procedure: Babies with blood groups A, B, or AB are transfused with Group O packed cells reconstituted (to a final hematocrit of approximately 50 per cent) with Group AB Rh negative fresh frozen plasma (obtained from male donors who have no leukoagglutinins). Babies with Group O blood are transfused with Type O negative whole blood, and 65 ml of plasma is removed from the unit before use to raise the hematocrit of the adult donor blood, which has been diluted with 62 ml of anticoagulant. In order to carry out a 2 volume exchange transfusion one should order 170 to 200 ml of blood per kg of body weight.

Blood preserved with CPD anticoagulant has a number of advantages over that preserved with acid-citrate-dextrose (ACD) solution. The CPD solution permits longer maintenance of normal red cell 2,3-diphosphoglycerate (2,3-DPG) levels, enhancing oxygen delivery to tissues from the transfused red blood cells. CPD blood has less than half of the acid load of ACD blood at the time of drawing. At 7 days of age, CPD blood has a pH of 7.00, whereas ACD blood has a pH of about 6.7 at 3 days of age. However, the citric acid in CPD or ACD blood is readily metabolized by the liver to bicarbonate, and a metabolic alkalosis may occur and persist for up to 72 hours post-exchange. The blood is warmed to 37 C (98.6 F) in a commercial water bath (Hemokinetitherm, Dupaco Incorporated, San Marcos, California) before it is transfused into the infant.

The administration of intravenous albumin prior to an exchange transfusion has been advocated as a means of increasing the efficiency of the exchange. The value of this procedure has not been substantiated, and we do not currently advocate its use.

A few hospital blood banks prepare heparinized blood for exchange transfusions. This is the safest type of blood to use, since it produces no changes in ionized calcium, electrolytes, acid-base balance, and blood glucose levels. However, heparinized blood will affect the coagulation status of the infant, and it must be used within 24 hours of collection.

Technique of Exchange Transfusion

The umbilical vein is the safest route for conducting an exchange transfusion, even if an umbilical artery catheter is already in place for the monitoring of arterial blood gases. We have, on occasion, used the umbilical artery in sick, low birth weight infants over 1 week of age when an umbilical artery catheter was in place and the umbilical vein could not be cannulated. However, the umbilical artery route can lead to serious complications such as paraplegia and should not be used unless absolutely necessary.

Using sterile technique, the umbilical stump is scrubbed with povidone-iodine (Betadine), and the umbilical vein is catheterized with a No. 5.0 or 8.0 French exchange transfusion catheter (Pharmaseal Laboratories, Glendale, California 91201). A catheter in the umbilical vein should never be left open to the air, because a deep inspiration could draw air into the line, causing an air embolus. Unless the umbilical vein catheter can be passed through the ductus venosus into the inferior vena cava, we prefer to keep it low and therefore out of the portal system. The catheter is advanced only far enough to achieve a good blood return, which is usually 4 to 5 cm in the term newborn.

The blood is warmed in the water bath and passed through a filter to remove any small clots. The blood bag should be gently inverted periodically to prevent sedimentation of cells at the bottom of the bag. We conduct the exchange by the "push-pull" method, using a single syringe and a special four-way stopcock provided in a commercial exchange transfusion set (Pharmaseal Laboratories, Glendale, California 91201).

Blood is removed and added in increments of 5 ml in small premature infants and 10 ml in term newborns. The first aliquot removed is sent for determination of bilirubin, glucose, calcium, and electrolytes. If screening blood tests for phenylketonuria, T_4, and thyroid-stimulating hormone (TSH) have not been performed, they should also be sent from this first aliquot. For practical purposes, the size of the blood aliquots has no significant effect on the efficiency of the exchange. Therefore, exchanging in increments of 5 or 10 ml is just as efficient as using 20 ml. Withdrawing 20 ml of blood from a 3 kg infant represents an acute depletion of his total blood volume, causing a decrease in cardiac return, cardiac output, and blood pressure, particularly if done rapidly. The patient's heart rate is monitored electronically during the procedure.

There is no advantage and considerable risk in performing an exchange transfusion too rapidly. A rapid exchange aggravates the cardiovascular changes and may affect cerebral blood flow and intracranial pressure, and does not allow time for the liver to metabolize the infused citrate. A double-volume exchange should generally take about an hour in any baby.

The citrate in ACD and CPD blood will bind calcium and lower the total calcium level. In the past, it was common practice to administer calcium gluconate after every 100 ml of blood to counteract the citrate binding. We no longer administer calcium gluconate routinely, because measurements during exchange transfusions have not demonstrated any significant effect of calcium gluconate administration on the serum ionized calcium. It is also of interest to note that clinical signs such as jitteriness, crying, and irritability occurring during exchange transfusions cannot be correlated with levels of ionized calcium.

The final aliquot removed is sent for determinations of total and direct serum bilirubin, glucose, calcium, electrolytes, and hematocrit. Following a two volume exchange transfusion (170 ml per kg), the serum bilirubin will generally fall by about 50 per cent and rebound to 60 per cent of its pre-exchange value.

Following an exchange transfusion with CPD blood, the patient's blood glucose levels must be monitored carefully with periodic Dextrostix (Ames Company, Division of Miles Laboratories, Elkhart, Indiana 46514) determinations. Infants with erythroblastosis fetalis frequently have islet cell hyperplasia and high serum insulin levels. The CPD blood used for an exchange has a glucose content of 300 to 350 mg per 100 ml, which may further stimulate insulin secretion. Increased insulin levels at the conclusion of the exchange transfusion may cause rebound hypoglycemia. Dextrostix tests should be done every 15 minutes for the first hour post-exchange and then every 30 minutes for an additional hour. An intravenous glucose solution (10 per cent dextrose water in 0.25 isotonic saline) should be administered if hypoglycemia develops. Necrotizing enterocolitis and thrombocytopenia have also been reported as complications of exchange transfusions.

Phototherapy

Phototherapy should be used as an adjunct to exchange transfusion in the management of hyperbilirubinemia caused by hemolytic disease of the newborn. Mild hyperbilirubinemia caused by ABO incompatibility may be controlled by phototherapy alone. Infants who avoid an exchange transfusion because of the use of phototherapy are particularly likely to develop a late anemia at 4 to 8 weeks of age. This is due to the continued slow hemolysis of the sensitized red cells. These infants must be followed with serial hematocrits at 1 to 2 week intervals during the first 6 to 8 weeks of life. A transfusion of packed red blood cells (10 ml per kg) may be necessary to correct a severe anemia.

HEMOPHILIA AND RELATED CONDITIONS

method of
JEANNE M. LUSHER, M.D.
Detroit, Michigan

Definitions

Hemophilia A (factor VIII deficiency) and hemophilia B (factor IX deficiency) are hereditary bleeding disorders which are transmitted as X-linked recessive traits. Thus they affect males almost exclusively. Hemophilia A and hemophilia B are clinically indistinguishable but can easily be differentiated by factor VIII and factor IX activity assays. In hemophilia A the factor VIII procoagulant moiety is deficient or abnormal, while other components of the factor VIII system (factor VIII–related antigen and von Willebrand factor) are normal. In general the severity of clinical bleeding manifestations correlates well with the factor VIII activity value, assay values of less than 0.03 unit per ml (3 per cent) being associated with spontaneous hemorrhage into joints and soft tissues.

Hemophilia B (Christmas disease) is characterized by subnormal factor IX activity, which may reflect a quantitative or qualitative abnormality in the factor IX molecule. While the factor VIII complex has a molecular weight of about 1.5 million daltons, the human factor IX molecule is considerably smaller, having a molecular weight of 60,000 daltons. As in hemophilia A, a factor IX assay value of less than 3 per cent is generally associated with a clinically severe bleeding tendency (spontaneous bleeding into joints and soft tissues).

It is apparent that both hemophilia A and hemophilia B are heterogeneous conditions. At least six different subtypes of hemophilia B have been described. While all have low levels of factor IX activity, the degree of clotting factor deficiency varies and several of the subtypes have other laboratory evidence of abnormalities of the factor IX molecule. Within a given kindred, however, there does not appear to be heterogeneity.

While there are no accurate statistics at present, the estimated incidence of hemophilia in the United States is 1 in 10,000 individuals, or 1 in 5000 males. Hemophilia A is approximately four times as frequent as hemophilia B.

Von Willebrand's disease (vWD), another hereditary bleeding disorder, is characterized by mucous membrane bleeding. The disorder is inherited as an autosomal dominant trait with variable penetrance. In "classic" vWD all three components of the factor VIII system (factor VIII activity, factor VIII antigen, von Willebrand factor activity) are proportionately deficient. In addition, the bleeding time is prolonged as a result of the vW factor abnormality. In recent years it has become apparent that vWD is extremely heterogeneous. In addition to quantitative variants, qualitative variants also exist. The variant forms appear to be much more common than classic vWD.

Clinical severity varies considerably. Most affected individuals have only a mild or moderate bleeding tendency, and it is not uncommon to elicit a negative history for excessive bleeding. On the other hand some have epistaxis, menorrhagia, and other bleeding problems throughout life. *Severe* vWD is associated with a more extreme degree of deficiency of components of the factor VIII system (less than 10 per cent of normal values), and usually reflects homozygosity or a doubly heterozygous state. In addition to severe mucous membrane bleeding, such severely affected individuals may have acute hemarthroses and soft tissue bleeding as well.

It is thought that vWD is probably the most common of the hereditary coagulation disorders, although the majority of patients who have laboratory evidence of vWD have minimal bleeding symptoms and seldom if ever require treatment.

Although far less common than hemophilia A, hemophilia B, or vWD, hereditary deficiencies or abnormalities of other clotting factors also exist. While some of these (e.g., factor XII deficiency) are not associated with a bleeding tendency, congenital deficiencies or abnormalities of fibrinogen, prothrombin, and factors V, VII, X, and XIII (and sometimes XI) are associated with bleeding. The majority of these uncommon conditions are inherited in an autosomal recessive manner.

Treatment of Hemostatic Abnormalities in Hemophilia and Other Hereditary Coagulation Disorders

Blood Component Therapy. In general, if a person with a hereditary coagulation disorder is bleeding and treatment is judged to be indicated, he or she should receive an intravenous infusion of the clotting factor which is deficient. While through the mid-1960s one had only whole plasma to rely on, plasma components and clotting factor concentrates are now available, and these have become the mainstay of treatment for hemophilia A, hemophilia B, and vWD.

Fresh frozen plasma (FFP) is still useful in several situations, however. In the relatively rare hereditary deficiencies of prothrombin and factors V, VII, X, XI, and XIII, cessation of hemorrhage can generally be achieved with FFP in a dosage of 10 ml per kg. In addition, in mild hemophilia B with infrequent bleeding episodes, FFP may be preferable to commercially prepared factor IX concentrates. Although an estimated 15 per cent of activity is lost in the process of freezing and thawing plasma, an average unit of FFP of 230 ml will still contain approximately 200 units of activity for each of the clotting factors. (One unit of clotting factor activity is defined as the amount present in 1 ml of fresh plasma, e.g., 1 unit of factor VIII activity is the amount present in 1 ml of fresh plasma.)

Cryoprecipitates, prepared from single units of plasma, contain approximately 50 per cent of the factor VIII activity, von Willebrand factor activity, and fibrinogen which was present in the starting unit of plasma. Thus a single donor bag of cryoprecipitate should contain approximately 100 units of factor VIII activity and 0.25 to 0.30 gram of fibrinogen, in a volume of about 10 ml. Cryoprecipitates are generally regarded as the treatment of choice for vWD, as they contain the von Willebrand factor in addition to factor VIII activity. They can also be used for treatment of bleeding in hemophilia A, and in hypofibrinogenemia or afibrinogenemia. The main disadvantages of cryoprecipitates are that they must be stored in a deep freeze, they are somewhat difficult to reconstitute and administer, and bags of cryoprecipitates vary considerably in their factor VIII content.

Commercially prepared factor VIII concentrates are now produced by several different manufacturers in the United States and have become the mainstay of treatment of hemophilia A. Each lot of concentrate is produced from a large volume of starting plasma which has been obtained by plasmapheresis of as many as 5000 to 6000 donors. While these concentrates have considerable factor VIII activity, most do not contain enough vWF or fibrinogen to warrant their use in vWD or hypofibrinogenemia. Factor VIII concentrates are easy to store, reconstitute, and infuse, and each bottle is labeled with the number of factor VIII units contained.

Prothrombin complex concentrates (PCC), containing the four vitamin K dependent clotting factors, II, VII, IX and X, are currently produced by two manufacturers in the United States. In addition to nonactivated factors II, VII, IX, and X, the PCC contain some activated clotting factor in variable amounts as well. The main indication for use of PCC is in the treatment of severe hemophilia B. As is true of factor VIII concentrates, PCC offer several advantages over fresh frozen plasma. They provide factor IX replacement in a concentrated form, thus enabling achievement of high levels without danger of fluid overload. They can be stored for prolonged periods in an ordinary refrigerator and are easy to reconstitute and administer, thus making them ideal for home use. On the other hand, one must be aware of the thrombogenic potential of PCC, as described under Complications of Treatment, below. Over the last several years, PCC have also been widely used to treat bleeding episodes in patients with hemophilia A who have developed an inhibitor. In general, PCC are not recommended for use in patients with congenital deficiencies of factors II, VII, or X, as these can usually be successfully managed with FFP, which is associated with fewer potential complications than PCC.

Antifibrinolytic Therapy. *Epsilon aminocaproic acid (EACA)* is an antifibrinolytic agent which acts by inhibiting plasminogen activation. It is a useful adjunct in certain specific situations when one desires to prevent lysis of a clot which has already formed as a result of specific factor replacement therapy. Its greatest use in the hereditary clotting disorders has been in the management of bleeding in the oral cavity (e.g., extraction of permanent teeth or other oral surgical procedures, or tongue or mouth lacerations). One can usually decrease the amount of factor VIII replacement needed in such situations by the addition of EACA in a dosage of 75 mg per kg every 4 to 6 hours orally. It should be noted, however, that EACA may be hazardous if given in conjunction with PCC (which contain some activated clotting factors). The risk of thrombogenicity is enhanced when both these agents are used together.

Other Agents. In normal persons, and in those with only mild deficiencies, *estrogen preparations* raise the circulating levels of several coagulation factors (including factors VII, IX, and X and the factor VIII complex). Various estrogen-containing preparations have proved clinically useful in vWD women with extreme menorrhagia, and also in persons with vWD or mild hemophilia prior to dental extractions or other surgical procedures.

DDAVP, a synthetic analogue of the antidiuretic hormone 9-arginine vasopressin, has been used in Europe (as well as in some centers in the United States) as an alternative to plasma derivatives for patients with moderate (not severe) vWD. Infusion (or intranasal administration) of DDAVP produces a marked, transient increase in factor VIII activity, factor VIII antigen, and von Willebrand factor in normal persons and also in patients with vWD or mild hemophilia characterized by measurable baseline values. In those with measurable amounts to start with, there is a threefold increase over the starting value, with a disappearance time of several hours. This drug is thought to act via release of a second messenger, probably from the brain, which results in release of factor VIII from endothelial storage sites. Thus in patients with severe vWD there is none to be released, and in persons with a functionally abnormal form of factor VIII, the abnormal form will be released. However, it appears that in some vWD patients, correction of the bleeding time is possible with DDAVP.

Avoidance of Drugs Which Can Induce Platelet Dysfunction. Joint or soft tissue hemorrhage in hemophilia (or other hereditary coagulopathy) is often painful. If aspirin or an aspirin-containing compound is taken to relieve pain, the bleeding tendency may worsen as aspirin interferes with platelet function. A vicious cycle may ensue. (Aspirin inhibits platelet aggregation. This effect is mediated by inhibition of prostaglandin synthesis and is due to an irreversible inhibition of platelet cyclooxygenase.) Thus in persons with a coagulation disorder, aspirin-containing agents should be avoided. Acetaminophen is recommended for relief of mild pain or fever.

Among other drugs which interfere with platelet function are the antihistamines, phenothiazines, and nonsteroidal anti-inflammatory agents such as indomethacin.

Complications of Treatment. In using blood components and clotting factor concentrates, one must be aware of the potential complications of their use. While all these products undergo testing for hepatitis B surface antigen, such testing is by no means 100 per cent effective. Furthermore, it now appears that non-A, non-B hepatitis may be even more common than hepatitis B in persons receiving transfusions of blood or blood components. The risk of hepatitis is no doubt higher with the use of commercially prepared concentrates of factor VIII or factor IX, as each lot is prepared from plasma from hundreds or thousands of donors. Single units of fresh frozen plasma or single donor cryoprecipitates are generally associated with a lower hepatitis risk.

Thrombogenicity has been a concern in using large doses of prothrombin complex concentrates. Since these materials contain some activated clotting factors (principally factor IXa and Xa), disseminated intravascular coagulation and/or thromboembolic phenomena may occur in patients receiving repeated large doses over a period of several days, especially if they are immobile as after an orthopedic surgical procedure, major trauma, or extensive muscle hemorrhage. The risk of thrombogenicity is also increased in patients with active hepatitis, presumably as a result of (1) decreased levels of antithrombin III and (2) decreased ability to clear clotting factor intermediates from the circulation.

When used in hemophilia A patients with inhibitors, prothrombin complex concentrates may stimulate an anamnestic rise in factor VIII inhibitor concentration. This presumably results from small amounts of factor VIII procoagulant antigen present in these concentrates.

The anti-A and anti-B isoagglutinins present in the starting plasma will also be present in cryoprecipitates and in commercial factor VIII or factor IX concentrates made from them. Thus whenever possible, cryoprecipitates given to a patient should be ABO compatible in order to avoid hemolysis. While the relatively small amounts of anti-A and anti-B isoagglutinins present in most commercial concentrates will not often result in hemolytic anemia, significant hemolysis may occur if frequent repeated doses are given as in the postoperative period. If transfusion becomes necessary because of hemolytic anemia, type O cells should be used. Two manufacturers produce concentrate from A and AB donors, which can be obtained by special request for type A, B, or AB recipients who will be undergoing major surgery.

Another potential complication of prolonged intensive therapy with FFP, cryoprecipitate, or commercial factor VIII concentrates is that of an acquired platelet dysfunction. This may be associated with bleeding despite an adequate level of factor VIII, and is thought to result from an alteration of the fibrinogen molecule in these products.

Somewhat more common but less serious side effects of replacement therapy with plasma or cryoprecipitates include urticaria, headache, and low-grade fever. More severe immediate transfusion reactions such as anaphylaxis are rare. While urticaria or headache or both occasionally occur in association with infusion of commercial concentrates, such reactions are relatively uncommon.

Regional Comprehensive Care for Hemophilia. There are now a number of regional comprehensive hemophilia diagnostic and treatment centers in the United States which are partially subsidized by government grants. At each center a team of experts provides comprehensive periodic assessment of each individual seen, and makes recommendations to the patient and to his local health care providers. In addition to the internist and pediatric hematologist, comprehensive team members include an orthopedic surgeon, physiotherapist, dentist, dental hygienist, hemophilia project nurse, social worker, vocational counselor, psychologist, and genetic counselor. By such a multifaceted approach, the needs of the whole person and his family can ideally be met.

Patient education, vocational planning, and prophylaxis are stressed, including exercises and attention to dental hygiene. A booklet listing the federally funded hemophilia centers which provide such comprehensive evaluations can be obtained from the National Hemophilia Foundation, 19 West 34th St., New York, N.Y 10001.

Home Infusion Programs. During the past decade the concept of "home care" for hemophilia has steadily gained in popularity and acceptance. Most hemophilia centers now have programs for teaching the hemophiliac and his family not only the techniques of self-infusion but also when to treat, how to determine the proper dosage of concentrate, and when to call the center personnel. The advantages of home infusion include (1) promptness of treatment for an acute bleeding episode, (2) a greater feeling of independence, and (3) much less time lost from school or work. It is hoped that prompt home treatment of acute hemarthroses will prevent the development of chronic joint disease. In most states, those on home treatment must complete and return report forms which include the date, site of bleeding, lot number and dosage of concentrate used, perceived effectiveness, and any untoward side effects noted.

While a few centers prescribe cryoprecipitates for home infusion, most use commercially prepared concentrates of factor VIII and factor IX, as these are much easier to store, reconstitute, and administer at home. Children 11 or 12 years of age can usually learn to start their own intravenous infusions, while a parent of a child 3 years of age or older can generally be taught to start and administer the child's infusion.

Treatment of Hemophilia A

In general, clotting factor concentrates are used only for acute bleeding episodes. The most common indications for treatment are acute joint hemorrhage (hemarthrosis) and bleeding into a muscle mass. When such bleeding begins, it should be treated promptly, as early treatment will reduce complications (such as chronic joint disease) as well as the total amount of clotting factor needed for treatment of the episode. Treatment consists of factor VIII replacement and rest of the affected part. Factor VIII replacement can be achieved by infusion of either cryoprecipitate or commercial factor VIII concentrates. Because of their presumed lower hepatitis risk, single donor cryoprecipitates are preferred by some, especially in the management of patients with mild hemophilia A who require treatment infrequently. Most prefer commercial concentrates for the treatment of severe hemophilia A, mainly because of the ease of storing, reconstituting, and administering these lyophilized concentrates.

In calculating the dosage of factor VIII, it can be assumed that 1 unit of factor VIII per kg of body weight will raise the recipient's factor VIII level by 0.02 unit per ml (2 per cent). Thus if a severe hemophiliac with a baseline factor VIII level of less than 0.01 unit per ml received 20 units of factor VIII per kg, one would expect an immediate postinfusion factor VIII level of 0.40 unit per ml (40 per cent). The half-life of factor VIII is 8 to 12 hours; however, it may be less than this if the recipient is febrile or has had a major bleed (situations which may activate the coagulation system). While the label on each bottle of commercial concentrate indicates the amount of factor VIII present in that bottle, single donor cryoprecipitates have no such indication of their factor VIII content. For purpose of calculation one should assume that a bag of cryoprecipitate contains approximately 100 units of factor VIII. Since there is considerable variation in the factor VIII content of cryoprecipitates, however, it is recommended that one use at least three bags of cryoprecipitate even if calculations for a small child indicate that one or two bags would suffice.

Hemarthroses. Acute hemarthroses are the most common indication for treatment. Prompt treatment is of the utmost importance! If untreated or inadequately treated, acute hemarthroses eventually result in progressive, chronic joint disease which can be extremely disabling.

Each episode of acute hemarthrosis results in synovial inflammation. This synovitis may become chronic if repeated joint hemorrhages are not promptly treated. Chronic synovitis leads to (1) increased proliferation of the inflamed synovium, which is very vascular, thus making more frequent hemorrhages likely to occur; (2) destruction of cartilage and gradual resorption of bone, with cyst formation; (3) instability of the joint, resulting in more frequent bleeding into the joint and surrounding soft tissues; and (4) chronic joint pain, with subsequent disuse atro-

TABLE 1. **Hemophilia A—Recommended Dosages of Factor VIII**

TYPE OF BLEEDING	DOSAGE (FACTOR VIII UNITS/KG)	REPEAT DOSES (FACTOR VIII UNITS/KG)	ANCILLARY TREATMENT
Acute hemarthrosis			
Early	10	Seldom necessary	
Late (painful, with limitation of motion)	20	20 q12h	
Intramuscular hemorrhage	20–30	20 q12h (usually requires several days of treatment)	
Life-threatening situations*	50	25–30 q12h	
Intracranial hemorrhage			
Major trauma			
Major surgery			
Other serious bleeding*			
Tongue or neck bleeding with potential airway obstruction	40–50	20–25 q12h	
Severe abdominal pain	30–40	20–25 q12h	
Tongue and mouth lacerations*	20	20 q12h	EACA; sedation in small child
Extraction of permanent teeth	20	20 q12h	EACA, beginning day before extractions; continue 7–10 days
Painless spontaneous gross hematuria	None		Increased PO fluids

*These conditions should be treated in a comprehensive hemophilia center. If first seen in another hospital, the hemophilia center should be contacted and the patient transferred after initial treatment is given at the local hospital.

phy of surrounding muscles, and thus even greater instability of the joint.

Acute hemarthroses most frequently involve the knee, elbow, or ankle, although hemarthroses of the shoulder, hip, and wrist also occur. Joint bleeding may result from trauma or may be spontaneous. Recurrent bleeding without obvious trauma may occur in a particular joint, presumably because of the synovial irritation and increased vascularity which followed an earlier hemorrhage into the joint.

The early symptoms of joint bleeding can generally be recognized by the patient. Most describe a peculiar sensation or minimal discomfort or tingling in the joint before actual pain and swelling develop. *Treatment with clotting factor should be given at this time.* If joint bleeding is untreated, pain and joint swelling increase and there is progressive limitation of motion of the joint. By this time the joint hemorrhage is far advanced and synovial inflammation will begin.

Treatment consists of *clotting factor replacement* and immobilization or *rest* of the affected joint. The recommended dosage of factor VIII is shown in Table 1. In general, the earlier an acute hemarthrosis is treated, the less clotting factor is required. Thus, if a patient with hemophilia is on home treatment and treats himself at the earliest symptoms of bleeding into the joint, cessation of bleeding will generally result from half the dosage of concentrate that would be required for a hemorrhage of several hours' duration which has resulted in a very painful, distended joint. Rest of the affected joint during the acute phase of

bleeding is also important. For an elbow hemorrhage a sling is often helpful. In a small child with an extensive hemarthrosis of the knee, a lightweight splint may be helpful in protecting the joint from continued use. This is usually not necessary for early joint hemorrhages, however, as response to clotting factor concentrates is generally rapid. When immobilization is used, it should not be continued for more than a few days, because of the danger of muscle atrophy. Ice packs also may provide symptomatic relief from pain associated with an acute hemarthrosis.

Joint aspiration is seldom indicated, and should be reserved for acutely distended joints associated with severe pain. (Although this situation was commonly encountered prior to the 1970s, relatively few painfully distended joints are seen now, as most acute hemarthroses are being treated early.) When joint aspiration is judged to be indicated, it should be done with careful attention to aseptic technique and only after infusion of clotting factor concentrate.

As described above, frequent recurrent hemarthroses may result in disuse muscle atrophy. Thus *physiotherapy* is important. Isometric exercises are often quite useful in preventing atrophy of the quadriceps group, thus lessening the chance of reinjury to the knee. High top padded hiking boots will provide stability to the ankle and lessen the chances of ankle injury. Occasionally a long leg brace may be indicated for stabilizing and protecting a chronically swollen, severely affected knee.

In the case of frequent, recurrent episodes of bleeding into a single joint, a *prophylactic regimen* of every other day clotting factor concentrate may stop the cycle and allow healing of the inflamed synovium. Such prophylaxis, once begun, should be continued for at least a month and often considerably longer.

Muscle Hemorrhage. Intramuscular hemorrhage is the second most common indication for replacement therapy with clotting factor concentrates. As in the case of acute hemarthroses, pain and limitation of motion of the affected part usually occur. A longer course of replacement therapy is often necessary for a severe intramuscular hemorrhage than for joint hemorrhage. Clotting factor concentrates should be given every 12 hours until the affected muscle mass begins to soften and pain has disappeared. Several days of treatment are often required.

Whereas intramuscular bleeding in such areas as the calf or forearm is quite visible, with tense swelling and tenderness, the symptoms and signs of an iliopsoas hemorrhage are generally limited to ill-defined pain in the groin, flexion of the thigh, and pain on extension of the thigh. A large iliopsoas hemorrhage may result in displacement of the kidney and ureter, anemia from contained hemorrhage, and compression of the femoral nerve. Hospitalization with clotting factor concentrate given every 12 hours for a period of several days is indicated.

Oral Bleeding. Tongue and mouth lacerations occur most often in the toddler age group, but are occasionally seen in older children or adults. While clotting factor concentrate should be given to all, ancillary management depends on the age of the patient and the site and extent of intraoral injury. An infusion of clotting factor concentrate will result in local clot formation, but it is difficult to maintain an intact clot, particularly on the tongue. The mouth is a moist area where there is a great likelihood of dislodgement of the clot, especially in an infant or young child. In small children we have found that cessation of hemorrhage and healing of the wound can be achieved best by hospitalization, with (1) heavy sedation, (2) clotting factor concentrate every 12 hours, (3) no oral intake and maintenance with intravenous fluids, and (4) the use of epsilon aminocaproic acid (EACA), to prevent clot lysis. Three to 5 days of hospitalization are generally required for management of a tongue laceration in a small child. In an older child or adult with a similar lesion, outpatient management consists of clotting factor replacement, the local use of an orahesive gauze (such as Squibb's Stomahesive), EACA, and continued attention to preventing clot dislodgement. Cold, clear liquids followed by

a soft diet are recommended. (The orahesive gauze sheets can be cut to the desired size, and the cut piece is then placed firmly over the wound.) EACA should be continued for 7 to 10 days, until healing appears complete.

Hematuria. Gross hematuria may result from a blow or other injury to the kidney, in which case clotting factor concentrate is indicated. However, more commonly gross hematuria occurs spontaneously. Especially in children one should rule out other possible causes of painless, gross hematuria such as acute glomerulonephritis. If other underlying causes are excluded, it has been our practice to allow the patient to continue his usual activities and to drink extra fluids until hematuria stops. Most episodes of painless gross hematuria stop within 2 to 7 days. If it persists beyond that time, one may try one or two doses of clotting factor concentrate, but EACA should be avoided, as ureteropelvic obstruction by clots may occur with its use. While some recommend bed rest or the use of corticosteroids for the management of gross hematuria, these measures are not of proved benefit, and we have never used them.

Surgical Procedures. If the patient with hemophilia A does not have an inhibitor (see Inhibitors, below), surgery can generally be accomplished without undue risk as long as there is careful planning and cooperation betweeen surgical, medical, and laboratory personnel. Preoperative planning is essential and should include testing the patient for an inhibitor, as inhibitors can develop at any age and would make surgery hazardous. One should also ensure that an adequate supply of clotting factor concentrate is on hand for the entire postoperative period. If the patient has blood type A, B, or AB and a prolonged period of replacement therapy is anticipated, one should order a supply of concentrates specially prepared from A and AB donors which are available from two manufacturers in the United States. Clotting factor replacement should begin 45 minutes to 1 hour preoperatively, and continue every 12 hours for 7 to 10 days postoperatively for most major surgical procedures. A longer period of treatment (often 4 to 6 weeks) is required for extensive orthopedic procedures. Surgery should be undertaken only in a hospital where there is a hemophilia center, a reliable coagulation laboratory, a major blood bank, and an appropriate rehabilitation team for postoperative management. A notation taped on the front of the patient's chart should clearly indicate that no intramuscular injections should be given, and that all aspirin-containing compounds must be avoided.

For *oral surgical procedures,* EACA is begun 1

day preoperatively and continued for 10 days postoperatively in a dose of 75 mg per kg per dose every 6 hours. As for other surgical procedures, preoperative screening for inhibitors is mandatory. Clotting factor concentrate should be given 45 minutes to 1 hour preoperatively and continued every 12 hours for 1 or 2 days or longer depending on the extent of the procedure and the appearance of the local lesion.

Inhibitors. Inhibitors (antibodies) develop in an estimated 10 to 15 per cent of patients with hemophilia A and 2 to 3 per cent of those with hemophilia B. The inhibitor is an antibody which acts specifically against factor VIII (or factor IX) procoagulant activity. While some patients develop such inhibitors in only low titer (and can thus continue to be treated with factor VIII concentrates), the majority are high-titer antibody formers. At present, recommended management for bleeding episodes in those with high titer antibodies consists of prothrombin complex concentrates (PCC), in a dose of 75 factor IX units per kg of body weight. The precise mechanism of action of PCC in stopping bleeding in inhibitor patients is unknown, but it appears that one or more of the *activated* clotting factors present in PCC bypass the need for factor VIII (or factor IX) in the clotting sequence. Although both subjective and objective improvement occur following the use of large doses of PCC approximately 50 per cent of the time, the response is not nearly as good as is the response to factor VIII concentrates in a noninhibitor patient. However, for lack of a readily available, more effective form of treatment for inhibitor patients, most hemophilia centers use PCC at present.

An activated PCC (Hyland's Autoplex) was licensed for use in the United States in late 1979 and has been recommended for use in inhibitor patients. However, the clinical experience with this product has been limited, no controlled studies to determine its efficacy have been done, and it is currently quite costly and available in limited supply. However, this purposely activated PCC may prove to be superior to the standard, nonactivated PCCs in treating bleeding episodes in inhibitor patients.

Treatment of Hemophilia B

Hemophilia A and hemophilia B are clinically indistinguishable. Both are characterized by recurrent episodes of bleeding into joints and soft tissues, and in general the recommended management for hemophilia B is identical to that for hemophilia A. The major difference in treatment is in the type and dosage of clotting factor concentrate used. Since factor IX is a smaller molecule than factor VIII and diffuses from intravas-

cular to extravascular sites, a larger dose is needed in order to achieve the same factor level in the circulation. While a dosage of 1 unit per kg of factor VIII will raise the factor VIII level by 2 per cent, the same dosage of factor IX will raise the factor IX level by only 1 per cent. Although the factor IX level necessary to achieve hemostasis will depend on the severity and duration of bleeding, in general the hemostatic level appears to be less than for factor VIII. One should aim for a minimum factor IX level of 20 per cent for most hemorrhagic episodes, although larger amounts should be given for more serious situations (Table 2).

For persons with mild hemophilia B who require infrequent treatment, fresh frozen plasma (FFP) may be used. In such individuals hemostatic levels for factor IX can generally be achieved with FFP, and the risk of hepatitis is not as great as when PCC is used. For those with severe hemophilia B, however, acute bleeding episodes should be treated with PCC (see Table 2 for recommended dosages).

Surgery. Many hemophilia centers avoid elective surgical procedures in patients with hemophilia B because of the risk of thromboembolic complications following intensive use of PCC. The risk of disseminated intravascular coagulation, deep vein thromboses, and pulmonary embolism is accentuated in an adult who is relatively immobile following an orthopedic surgical procedure on a lower extremity. Such complications are far less common when the procedure involves an elbow or shoulder and the patient can be ambulated early. Nonetheless, if surgery is undertaken in a patient with hemophilia B, careful monitoring by the hematologist-coagulationist and other members of the medical team is essential. In view of the potential thrombogenicity it is recommended that heparin be added to the reconstituted PCC in a dosage of 5 units per ml of reconstituted material. In addition, it may be useful to infuse a unit of FFP (as a source of antithrombin III) prior to the administration of the initial dose of PCC for major surgical procedures when prolonged, intensive use of PCC is anticipated.

For *oral surgical procedures* when PCC is given preoperatively and postoperatively, EACA should be withheld until the day after the last dose of PCC in order to minimize the risk of thrombotic complications.

Hemophilia B patients with *inhibitors* are currently treated in similar fashion to hemophilia A patients with inhibitors. Bleeding episodes are treated with large doses (75 units per kg per dose) of PCC. In general, one or two doses will suffice for treatment of an acute hemarthrosis. However, response to treatment is generally suboptimal as compared to that in a noninhibitor patient.

Treatment of von Willebrand's Disease

Relatively few persons with vWD ever require treatment. Most have minimal bleeding problems which are self-limited or can be easily controlled by local measures. Those with moderately severe or severe bleeding, however, may require periodic treatment. Clotting factor replacement therapy is with cryoprecipitates. Cryoprecipitates contain the entire factor VIII complex, including von Willebrand factor, and are thus regarded as the treatment of choice for vWD. Recommended dosage is 1 bag of cryoprecipitate per 5 kg of body weight initially, followed by 1 bag per 10 kg every 6 to 8 hours until hemostasis is achieved (or, in the case of a tongue or mouth laceration in a small child, until healing occurs). If cryoprecipitates are not available, fresh frozen plasma can be used in a dosage of 10 to 15 ml per kg.

As shown in Figure 1, von Willebrand factor has a short half-life, and correction of the bleeding time is correspondingly short. Thus frequent infusions are necessary, especially in an individu-

al with severe vWD who has had a major hemorrhage or who has undergone a major surgical procedure.

For extractions of permanent teeth EACA should be used in addition to cryoprecipitates. As in hemophilia A, EACA should be started 1 day preoperatively and continued for 7 to 10 days. In patients with a moderate bleeding tendency a single dose of cryoprecipitate given an hour preoperatively will usually suffice, while in those with severe vWD, multiple doses may be required.

In the case of surgical procedures in patients with moderately severe or severe vWD, cryoprecipitate therapy should begin 18 to 24 hours preoperatively and can be monitored by the ristocetin cofactor assay or by bleeding times. Ristocetin cofactor values closely parallel the patient's hemorrhagic tendency, and this test is less traumatic than repeated bleeding times.

Estrogen-containing compounds will result in an increase in factor VIII activity, factor VIII antigen, and von Willebrand factor activity in persons who have some activity of these factors to begin with. Thus these compounds are often useful in controlling menorrhagia or other mucous membrane bleeding in patients with

TABLE 2.   **Hemophilia B — Recommended Dosage Schedules**

TYPE OF BLEEDING	INITIAL DOSAGE AND SOURCE OF FACTOR IX (FACTOR IX UNITS/KG)	REPEAT DOSE AND SOURCE OF FACTOR IX (FACTOR IX UNITS/KG)	ANCILLARY TREATMENT
Acute hemarthrosis			
In individual with mild hemophilia B who is treated infrequently	15 (FFP)	None	
Early, in severe hemophilia B	20 (PCC)	None	
Late (painful, with limitation of motion) in severe hemophilia B	30 (PCC)	20–25 (PCC) q12h	
Intramuscular hemorrhage			
In individual with mild hemophilia B	15 (FFP)	10 (FFP) q12h	
In severe hemophilia B	30–40 (PCC)	30 (PCC) q12h	
Life-threatening situations*	40–50 (PCC)	20–25 (PCC) q12h	A dose of FFP as a source of antithrombin III may be useful
Intracranial hemorrhage			
Major trauma			
Major surgery			
Other serious bleeding*			
Tongue or neck bleeding with potential for airway obstruction	40 (PCC)	20 (PCC) q12h	
Severe abdominal pain	40 (PCC) or 15 (FFP) for mild hemophilia	20 (PCC) q12h or 10 (FFP) q12h for mild hemophilia	
Tongue and mouth lacerations*	30 (PCC) or 15 (FFP) for mild hemophilia	20 (PCC) q12h or 10 (FFP) for mild hemophilia	EACA (if PCC is used, EACA is begun the day after PCC is stopped)
Extraction of permanent teeth	30 (PCC) or 15 (FFP) for mild hemophilia	20 (PCC) or 10 (FFP) for mild hemophilia	EACA (if PCC is used, EACA is begun the day after PCC is stopped)
Painless spontaneous gross hematuria	None		Increase PO fluids

*These conditions should be treated in a comprehensive hemophilia center. If first seen in another hospital, the hemophilia center should be contacted and the patient transferred after initial treatment is given at the local hospital. FFP = Fresh frozen plasma; PCC = prothrombin complex concentrates.

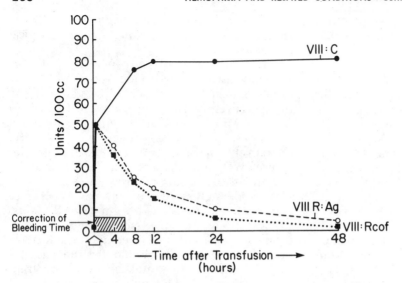

Figure 1. Transfusion response in vWD. Open arrow indicates infusion of 10 bags of cryoprecipitate. VIII:C = factor VIII procoagulant activity, VIII R:Ag = factor VIII–related antigen, and VIII:Rcof = ristocetin cofactor activity, which is an index of von Willebrand factor activity. Note that while factor VIII activity remains elevated for a prolonged period after infusion of cryoprecipitate, the ristocetin cofactor activity and bleeding time are only transiently corrected.

moderately severe vWD, but are generally ineffective in the occasional patient who has severe vWD with no factor VIII complex activity to start with.

As in normal women, in late pregnancy women with vWD have an increase in all three factor VIII components. If the hormonal changes during late pregnancy result in release of factor VIII from storage sites, it might be expected that those women who produce a functionally abnormal molecule will have no correction of bleeding time. Nonetheless, there are a number of well-documented cases of vWD women with extreme menorrhagia except while pregnant, who had no unusual bleeding during or immediately following delivery.

DDAVP has been used more widely in Europe than in the United States for vWD, but also appears to act by release of components of the factor VIII complex from storage sites. In some persons with mild or moderate vWD, correction of the bleeding time is possible with DDAVP. This agent can be used either parenterally or intranasally, and results in a transient threefold increase in all components of the factor VIII system. (This use of DDAVP is not listed in the manufacturer's official directive). European physicians report that DDAVP has proved to be a useful alternative to cryoprecipitates in patients with mild vWD undergoing dental extractions or other minor surgical procedures.

Epistaxis is a frequent problem in vWD. As in the case of any other hereditary coagulation disorder, aspirin-containing compounds should be avoided, as these drugs interfere with platelet function and thus aggravate the bleeding tendency. Other local measures which are useful in preventing epistaxis include the avoidance of drying mucous membranes by local application of petroleum jelly to the nostrils, or by the use of a humidifier. If epistaxis cannot be controlled with pressure alone, nasal packing with a greasy material (which can be readily removed without clot disruption) should be tried. If bleeding continues, cryoprecipitates should be given.

Recurrent epistaxis and/or menorrhagia often result in iron deficiency anemia. Thus supplemental iron is often a necessary part of treatment.

Treatment of Other Inherited Disorders of Coagulation

Hereditary deficiencies of all other known coagulation factors have been described, although they are far less common than hemophilia A and B and von Willebrand's disease. As is true of these three conditions, congenital deficiency states of the other clotting factors are heterogeneous, and thus not all families with a particular clotting factor deficiency have the same degree of deficiency or the same degree of bleeding. Nonetheless, the treatment of choice for hemorrhagic episodes in most of these rare disorders is fresh frozen plasma (FFP). FFP is generally effective, as the hemostatic level of most of these factors is relatively low and can thus be easily attained by infusion of FFP in a dosage of 10 ml per kg of body weight. Once hemostasis has been achieved, repetitive treatment for that episode is seldom required.

In those with congenital deficiency of factors II, VII, or X, FFP is preferable to PCC in view of the high incidence of hepatitis (and other complications) following its use. However, PCC should be used for such serious and life-threatening situations as intracranial hemorrhage.

Bleeding in patients with hypofibrinogenemia or afibrinogenemia should be treated with cryoprecipitates, as these are a rich source of fibrinogen. Often a single dose of cryoprecipitates will suffice. Recommended dosage is 4 bags of cryoprecipitate per 10 kg of body weight. If necessary, repeated doses of 2 bags per 10 kg are given every 48 hours.

Isolated deficiencies of the "contact factors" (factor XII, factor XI, Fletcher factor, and Fitzgerald factor) are seldom associated with a bleeding tendency and thus do not require treatment. If a patient with severe factor XI deficiency does bleed, FFP should be given.

BLEEDING DISORDERS SECONDARY TO PLATELET ABNORMALITIES

method of
SHERRILL J. SLICHTER, M.D.
Seattle, Washington

Abnormalities in either platelet number or function may be associated with hemorrhagic manifestations. Platelet-associated bleeding is usually mucocutaneous, and the patient presents with dependent lower extremity or posterior pharyngeal petechiae, ecchymosis after minimal trauma, epistaxis, or gum bleeding. There may be more serious forms of bleeding, such as hematemesis, melena, or hematuria. Management depends on categorizing the abnormalities (see Table 1) so that appropriate treatment can be provided.

THROMBOCYTOPENIA

Production Abnormalities

Aplasia

Idiopathic. Marked reduction in marrow megakaryocytes is associated with severe thrombocytopenia. The cause is often unknown but sometimes is related to drug exposure or hepatitis. Usually all cell lines are involved with associated depression of granulocyte and red cell production.

MARROW TRANSPLANTATION. Criteria for marrow transplantation are involvement of at least two cell lines (platelet count <20,000 per

microliter, granulocytes <500 per microliter, or reticulocytes <1 per cent) and a marrow biopsy showing pronounced aplasia with >65 per cent nonhematopoietic cells. If the marrow failure does not rapidly improve following discontinuation of possibly causative agents, the treatment of choice is bone marrow transplantation provided that a histocompatible sibling donor is available. In the event that a compatible marrow donor cannot be identified, some success has followed prolonged treatment with either antithymocyte globulin or androgens.

PLATELET TRANSFUSIONS. Until marrow recovery occurs, maintenance of platelet levels with transfusions of platelet concentrates is required.

INDICATIONS. Significant life-threatening bleeding usually does not occur until the platelet count falls below 5000 per microliter. Some individuals bleed at higher levels if they have associated platelet dysfunction. Aspirin, which is the most common drug causing platelet dysfunction, should never be given to thrombocytopenic patients. Acetaminophen is an appropriate substitute. If the patient has an infection, usually because of a low white count, the administration of a semisynthetic penicillin may cause platelet dysfunction, thus requiring more transfused platelets to prevent or control bleeding. Because of the high frequency of platelet alloimmunization with continued platelet transfusions, thrombocytopenic patients should be given platelets only with the onset of significant gastrointestinal (GI) or genitourinary (GU) bleeding. Prophylactic transfusions to prevent bleeding, often given for platelet counts of <20,000 per microliter, do not reduce morbidity and mortality as compared to transfusions given only for active bleeding. In fact, not only do prophylactic transfusions increase costs significantly but the subsequent alloimmunization may result in uncontrolled bleeding unless a compatible donor can be identified.

Mild bleeding expressed as petechiae or ecchymosis is not in itself an indication for platelet transfusion. Intermediate types of bleeding such as nasal or gingival may require platelet transfusions, depending on the severity. Central nervous system (CNS) bleeding rarely occurs with platelet counts above 5000 per microliter. The onset of severe headache with or without neurologic manifestations in a severely thrombocytopenic patient is the usual manifestation of CNS bleeding and is cause for immediate administration of platelets.

DOSAGE. One unit of platelet concentrate contains an average of 5.5×10^{10} platelets and in a 70 kg man should increase the peripheral platelet count by approximately 10,000 per microliter. Normally, about a third of the administered platelets are pooled in the spleen. In hy-

TABLE 1. **Classification of Platelet Abnormalities**

	PLATELET COUNT	MARROW MEGA-KARYOCYTES	BLEEDING TIME*	PLATELET SURVIVAL	OTHER
Disorders of platelet number					
Thrombocytopenia	Reduced				
Production					
Aplasia		Absent	Proportional	Normal	
Hypoproliferative		Reduced	Proportional	Normal	
Ineffective		Normal to increased	Proportional	Normal	
Distribution					
Hypersplenism		Normal	Proportional	Normal	Reduced platelet increment
Destruction					
Immunologically mediated		Increased	Shortened	Reduced	Antiplatelet antibodies
Consumption		Increased	Variable	Reduced	Abnormal coagulation screens
Dilutional		Normal	Proportional	Normal	
Thrombocytosis	Increased				
Secondary		Increased†	Proportional	Normal	
Malignant		Increased	Proportional or prolonged	Normal or reduced	
Disorders of platelet function	Normal	Normal	Prolonged	Normal	

*There is a direct inverse relationship between bleeding time and platelet count at levels between 100,000 and 10,000 per microliter, which is predicted by the following equation: bleeding time (minutes) $= 30.5 - \dfrac{\text{platelet count} \times 10^9/\text{L}}{3.85}$. Thus, the bleeding time may be either proportional to the platelet count, shortened, or prolonged.

†Megakaryocytes are increased in number but not in size.

persplenism, pooling is increased in proportion to the size of the spleen, and the number of platelet concentrates may have to be increased to achieve the desired increment. Conversely, in an asplenic recipient, the platelet increment per transfused unit is increased by about a third. The incremental response is best measured by a 1 hour post-transfusion platelet count.

The transfusion of a pool of platelet concentrates from 4 to 6 donors results in a post-transfusion increment sufficient to control bleeding in the majority of recipients. Survival of transfused platelets in nonimmunized thrombocytopenic recipients is approximately 5 days under optimal conditions, so a patient usually requires platelets twice a week. The actual survival of the transfused platelets is best determined by plotting a 1 hour, 4 hour, and 24 hour post-transfusion platelet count; this survival curve can then be used to determine transfusion frequency.

SOURCE OF PLATELETS. Random donor platelet concentrates prepared from units of routinely donated blood should be used initially. If the patient remains thrombocytopenic for extended periods of time and requires frequent transfusions, alloimmunization to random platelets results. Alloimmunization is documented by finding <5000 per microliter increase in the patient's 1 hour post-transfusion platelet count following a transfusion of at least 6 units of pooled concentrated platelets on two separate occasions. In the absence of significant hypersplenism or inadequately prepared platelets, alloimmunization is the only cause of a very poor 1 hour post-transfusion increment.

If immunization occurs, a compatible donor can be found within the patient's family about 50 per cent of the time. Enough platelets can be obtained from a single donor to provide an effective transfusion dose by use of pheresis procedures. Once the patient has become immunized to random platelets, approximately 80 per cent of HLA-matched siblings will still be compatible and 30 per cent of the HLA-haploidentical family members. HLA completely mismatched family members are not useful donors. Usually the patient is not immunized by the platelets of a compatible family member regardless of how many additional transfusions are required. If a compatible family member is not identified, then histocompatible random donors may be successful. Unfortunately, about a fourth of the time, HLA fully compatible random donors are incompatible, indicating that platelet antigens other than HLA are important for platelet transfusion compatibility. Therefore, platelet cross-match tests have been developed to select compatible platelet donors. Although these tests are highly predictive in individual laboratories, they are not widely available and have mainly been used on a research basis. Lymphocytotoxicity cross-match procedures are predictive about 60 per cent of the time. Usually, a positive cross-match test indicates an incompatible transfusion result, but there is a high percentage of false-negative results with this test.

Platelets should ideally be ABO compatible with the recipient because of the small number of contaminating red cells and the anti-A or anti-B antibodies in the plasma used to resuspend the platelet concentrate. However, if only ABO incompatible platelets are available, an incremental response about 80 per cent of that predicted will still be achieved and the platelets survive normally. The major concern is transfusion of platelets from a type O donor into an A recipient because of the high titer anti-A antibodies found in some O donors. However, the volume of donor plasma is low, and in most patients such transfusions have been well tolerated without significant red cell destruction.

COMPLICATIONS. 1. *Alloimmunization:* The major complication of platelet transfusion is alloimmunization to HLA or platelet-specific antigens. The frequency of immunization increases with each succeeding transfusion, reaching a peak of about 80 per cent of patients after 20 or more transfusions. If compatible donors cannot be identified, the patient is severely compromised because of uncontrolled bleeding. In addition to platelet and HLA antigen alloimmunization, Rh negative recipients can become immunized to the Rh antigen by platelet transfusions from Rh positive donors. This immunization is due to the contaminating red cells present in the platelet concentrate and should be of concern only for women before or during the childbearing period if the underlying disease process does not exclude subsequent pregnancies. For these individuals, platelets from Rh negative donors should be provided whenever possible.

2. *Infection:* Platelet concentrates as routinely prepared by most blood centers are stored at room temperature for up to 3 days. Although there was initial concern about bacterial contamination, this possible complication has rarely been documented. In fact, because of the extremely low incidence of contamination, the Bureau of Biologics no longer requires blood centers to perform periodic cultures on platelet concentrates. Viral infections such as hepatitis and cytomegalovirus can be transmitted with this blood product.

3. *Chills and fever:* After multiple transfusions, the platelet recipient may develop chills and fever approximately 30 to 60 minutes after a platelet transfusion. This finding usually heralds the onset of platelet alloimmunization, but the symptoms are actually due to the development of leukocyte antibodies which react with contaminating white cells in the platelet concentrate. The severity of the reaction can sometimes be lessened by administration of an antihistaminic prior to platelet transfusion. However, since there is usually associated platelet alloimmunization, definitive resolution of the problem is accomplished by finding a compatible platelet donor.

Disease-Related Marrow Failure. The most common cause of marked reductions in megakaryocytes is invasion of the bone marrow by malignant cells, particularly as leukemic infiltrates. The resultant thrombocytopenia may be as severe as that associated with idiopathic marrow aplasia. Again, marrow transplantation should be considered as the treatment of choice for patients with acute lymphoblastic leukemia in second remission and for patients with acute myeloblastic leukemia in first remission. Platelet supportive therapy should be provided for these patients along the same lines as those previously outlined under Idiopathic, above. The major difference in the leukemic patient is that the survival of transfused platelets may be significantly reduced because of a disease-related consumption of hemostatic factors. This process may reduce the transfused platelet survival to a day or less in severe leukemia. Therefore, the transfusion frequency may have to be substantially increased to accommodate the shortened platelet survival. In addition, leukemia-associated platelet dysfunction has been described, particularly in patients with acute myeloblastic leukemia, and larger numbers of transfused platelets may be required.

Any patient with a malignant disorder requiring treatment with chemo- or radiation therapy may be subjected to periods of transient marrow aplasia. The management of platelet transfusion therapy during these aplastic episodes should be as previously outlined for idiopathic marrow aplasia. The commonly prescribed chemo- or radiation therapies have not been shown to cause platelet dysfunction.

Hypoproliferative

Hypoproliferative marrow with decreased numbers of megakaryocytes is usually associated with modest reductions in platelet counts of between 20,000 and 100,000 per microliter. This is in a range in which the majority of patients do not have significant bleeding and therefore do not require either marrow transplantation or platelet transfusion therapy. The marrow can sometimes be stimulated by administration of androgens, but often there is progression to either complete aplasia or a leukemic transformation. Sometimes hypoplasia remains for long periods of time unresponsive to stimulating agents but not requiring any specific management.

Ineffective

B₁₂ or Folic Acid Deficiency. Deficiencies of either B_{12} or folic acid may be associated with ineffective production of platelets as well as red and white cells. The bone marrow in these situations shows megaloblastic hyperplasia in the red and white cell series and normal to increased numbers of megakaryocytes. Management consists of identifying and administering the deficient substrate.

Familial. Several families with autosomal dominant hereditary thrombocytopenia have been described. In these families the platelet count is usually in the range of 20,000 to 60,000 per microliter, with normal to increased numbers of bone marrow megakaryocytes and normal platelet survival. These patients are not known to be responsive to specific therapy, and because they are not severely thrombocytopenic they do not require platelet transfusions. In fact, every attempt should be made to prevent giving platelets to these individuals in order to avoid alloimmunization in case transfusions are required to control bleeding during operative procedures.

Distribution Abnormalities

Patients with splenic enlargement may have increased splenic pooling of platelets. Normally, about a third of the platelets produced by the bone marrow are pooled in the spleen, and this number is increased in proportion to the size of the spleen. However, even with severe hypersplenism, platelet counts are rarely below 30,000 per microliter, and platelet transfusion is not required. Since the platelet levels do not constitute a direct threat of bleeding, splenectomy should not be performed just to improve the platelet count. The procedure may be required for diagnosis of an underlying disease process or to manage associated deficiencies of white cells or red cells also pooled in a large spleen. Diagnosis of hypersplenic thrombocytopenia can be established by finding an enlarged spleen by physical examination or spleen scan or, if necessary, by actually transfusing platelets and documenting a substantially reduced platelet increment in the absence of alloimmunization.

Peripheral Destruction

Immunologically Mediated

Autoimmune. The highest incidence of autoimmune thrombocytopenia is found in young women, sometimes associated with systemic lupus erythematosus. Laboratory findings show an increased number and size of marrow megakaryocytes, indicating changes in platelet production in an attempt to compensate for removal of antibody-damaged platelets. Significantly, the bleeding time is usually shorter than that predicted from the platelet count, evidence that the platelets are hyperfunctional. Such hyperfunctional platelets are thought to represent early release from the bone marrow. The relationship between bleeding time and platelet count in this disorder is clearly different from that found in patients with marrow aplasia. This finding along with the marrow examination, serves as an important differential between the two disease states (Fig. 1). Because platelet function is better than normal, the patient's bleeding risk at any given platelet count is much less than that of an aplastic patient. Therefore, platelet transfusions are rarely required except for the very rare instances of CNS bleeding. Furthermore, transfused platelets, just as the patient's own platelets, circulate for only a few hours; thus it is not possible to raise the platelet count effectively. The primary treatment for immune-mediated thrombocytopenia is administration of corticosteroids in dosages of 1 to 2 mg per kg per day. An increase in the platelet count should occur within 2 weeks of starting high-dose therapy; as soon as the platelet count rises, the steroids should be rapidly tapered. In adults, cessation of steroids is usually associated with a fall in the platelet count, consistent with the autoimmune nature of the disorder. Because spontaneous remission rarely occurs in adult patients, the next step is to reinstitute the maximal dose of steroids and perform a splenectomy. In children, autoimmune thrombocytopenia is usually related to a viral illness, and treatment other than a short course of steroids is seldom required. If an individual has shown an increase in platelet count after steriod treatment, there is at least an 85 per cent chance that a remission will occur after splenectomy. However, if administration of high dose steroids did not improve the platelet count, then additional laboratory studies should be done to document the presence of autoantibodies to confirm the diagnosis. Those patients with autoimmune thrombocytopenia who have not responded to steriods have a splenectomy remission rate of little more than 20 per cent. However, because the next line of therapy involves chronic administration of immunosuppressive drugs, it is usually worthwhile to test the effect of splenectomy. If the patient does not respond to splenectomy or does so originally but subsequently relapses, then administration of immunosuppressive agents such as vincristine, azathioprine, 6-mercaptopurine, or cyclophosphamide is indicated. There is not enough information available to assess the relative efficacy of these immunosuppressive drugs; furthermore, individual patient improvement is quite variable. (This use of these agents is not listed in the manufacturers' official directives.) Some success has been achieved with a recently described form of treatment in which vinblastine-incubated platelets act as a conduit for localizing the therapeutic agent to the phagocytic cells, which remove antibody-coated platelets.

Drug Related. In some patients drug-related thrombocytopenia has been identified. The most common drugs associated with thrombocytopenia are the thiazide diuretics, some sulfur-containing compounds, quinine, quinidine, and heparin. Discontinuing the drug is associated with the return of a normal platelet count. However, in some people, the duration of the drug-related thrombocytopenia is much longer than expected on the basis of drug excretion rates. Particularly with quinidine-associated thrombocytopenia, the degree of platelet depression may be severe and the duration after stopping the drug as long as 2 to 3 weeks. Some of these patients require platelet support, with the recognition that the transfused platelets have a very short survival, necessitating infusion at least once a day. Transfusion therapy should be provided only for patients with significant bleeding resulting from severe platelet insufficiency. There is no evidence that steroid administration reduces the severity or duration of the thrombocytopenia. The other drug-related thrombocytopenias are more rapidly reversible and generally are less severe than that caused by quinidine.

Neonatal Isoimmune Thrombocytopenia. This disorder is related to a serologic incompatibility between the paternally inherited fetal antigens and the mother's platelet antibodies. During the course of pregnancy, fetal platelets may pass into the maternal circulation, resulting in the stimulation of antibodies against the paternally derived antigens of the fetal platelets. Since the antibody molecules are usually IgG, they can cross the placenta, causing thrombocytopenia in the baby. In contrast with most cases of red cell Rh incompatibility, the immunization process to platelets may occur during the first pregnancy. If the neonatal thrombocytopenia is severe, the mother's platelets should be transfused after washing to remove antibody-containing plasma. Platelet transfusions from the mother to the baby may be required for 3 to 4 weeks until the amount of maternal IgG in the infant's circulation falls sufficiently to allow autologous platelets to survive. Diagnosis of neonatal alloimmune thrombocytopenia is confirmed by demonstrating an antibody in the mother's plasma directed against the father's platelets or, after recovery, the baby's platelets.

Post-Transfusion Purpura. In this unusual syndrome, profound thrombocytopenia occurs approximately 5 to 10 days following a transfusion of blood or its cellular products. Usually, the affected individuals belong to the 2 per cent of people who lack the platelet-specific antigen PLA^1, and through prior pregnancies or transfusions they have been exposed to blood products from PLA^1-positive individuals. A subsequent transfusion of blood products containing PLA^1-positive platelets then results in an amnestic recall of an antibody which not only destroys the transfused donor platelets but, by a mechanism which is poorly understood, also destroys the patient's autologous PLA^1-negative platelets. The most likely explanation for this phenomenon is that during the process of alloantibody recall, an antibody which reacts with the patient's own platelets is produced. Because the thrombocytopenia is often profound with significant bleeding, plasma exchange may be required to clear the antibody from circulation. Transfused PLA^1 negative donor platelets are destroyed as rapidly as the patient's own PLA^1 negative platelets. In

Figure 1. Relationship between bleeding time and platelet count in production-related thrombocytopenia versus patients with autoimmune thrombocytopenia (ITP). The template bleeding time shows a direct inverse relationship to platelet count between 100,000 and 10,000 per microliter in patients with production-related thrombocytopenia (●). However, in patients with ITP (○) the bleeding time is disproportionately reduced, indicating the presence of hyperfunctioning platelets. Thus, patients with ITP have less tendency to bleed at any given platelet count than those with failure of marrow platelet production. (From Harker, L. A., and Slichter, S. J.: N. Engl. J. Med. 287:155, 1972.)

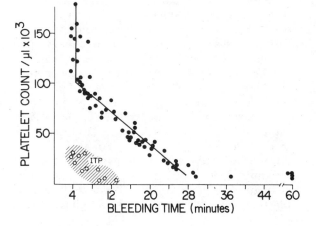

addition to plasma exchange, there is some evidence that high-dose steroid administration (2 mg per kg per day) may control the process or at least shorten the duration of the thrombocytopenia.

Thrombotic Thrombocytopenic Purpura. This syndrome is characterized by thrombocytopenia, microangiopathic hemolytic anemia, fever, and changing neurologic signs. Its exact etiology is unknown, but there is some evidence that the thrombocytopenia may have an immunologic origin or it may be caused entirely by the underlying vasculitis. The usual management consists of high dose steroids and other adjuvant therapy. It has recently been reported that a combination of daily plasmapheresis and administration of platelet function inhibitors (dipyridamole, 400 to 600 mg per day, and aspirin, 1200 to 2400 mg per day) is associated with a 90 per cent success rate. (This use of dipyridamole is not listed in the manufacturer's official directive.) Antiplatelet agents may have to be continued for 6 to 12 months. Plasmapheresis may either remove a toxic agent or provide a missing substance present in normal plasma. Another study demonstrated improvement with vincristine as a single agent. Splenectomy has been tried but is often not successful and may be associated with significant bleeding problems. The multiple treatment programs outlined indicate that optimal treatment has not been established.

Consumption

Increased peripheral utilization of platelets on a nonimmune basis and not related to vasculitis usually signifies a disorder associated with intravascular coagulation. These consumptive states are characterized by significant tissue destruction with release of thromboplastin into circulation and consumption of platelets and other clotting factors. The most common underlying events are severe trauma, surgery, burns, metastatic malignancies, bacteremia, or obstetrical complications such as abruptio placentae, retained dead fetus, or placenta previa. Consumption is diagnosed by demonstrating the underlying disease process in association with thrombocytopenia and abnormal coagulation tests such as prothrombin time, partial thromboplastin time, and fibrinogen level. Management of these patients consists of appropriate therapy to reverse the underlying disease process. If the disease cannot be readily controlled, then administration of platelet concentrates and plasma clotting factors is indicated for treatment of significant bleeding. Not only are the patients thrombocytopenic; they may also have dysfunctional platelets secondary to drugs being given to treat the underlying disease or to circulating fibrinogen/fibrin degradation products. The use of heparin in consumptive disorders prevents fibrin formation but does not interfere with platelet consumption. Thus, in the majority of patients bleeding is actually increased by heparin administration, since the patient remains severely thrombocytopenic.

Dilutional

Since platelets are not viable in stored blood, the administration of large volumes of transfused blood is associated with a progressive fall in the platelet count. After an average of 16 units of blood has been transfused, the platelet count may be less than 100,000 per microliter. Although in patients with marrow failure only 5000 platelets per microliter is required to prevent bleeding, in surgical or trauma patients with vascular injury platelet counts of at least 100,000 per microliter may be required to form a platelet plug. With severe trauma or extensive surgery, the platelet count may fall to levels <100,000 per microliter with fewer blood transfusions because platelets are also being consumed by tissue injury. In all patients, a platelet count should be obtained after the transfusion of 10 units of blood to anticipate the need for platelets.

THROMBOCYTOSIS

Secondary

Secondary thrombocytosis is characterized by an increase in the number but not in the size of marrow megakaryocytes. This type of platelet abnormality is usually a manifestation of iron deficiency, infection, or malignancy. Management consists of treating the underlying disease. Neither thrombotic nor bleeding complications associated wtih secondary thrombocytosis have been described.

Malignant

Autonomous thrombocytosis is characterized by an increase in both the number and the size of megakaryocytes. In blood films, the platelets are variably increased in size and irregularly shaped. These cells are often found to be dysfunctional by tests of platelet aggregation and bleeding time. In spite of thrombocytosis there is often bleeding or, conversely, thrombosis which in cerebral vessels results in significant neurologic sequelae. Management of these patients is related to administration of drugs that lower the platelet count; usually busulfan is the agent of choice. If the platelet count is >1 million per microliter, a level associated with the highest incidence of either bleeding or thrombosis, immediate reduction in platelet count may be achieved using plateletpheresis.

PLATELET DYSFUNCTION

The majority of these disorders are hereditary. Dysfunction is variable as measured by the bleeding time and in vitro response of platelets to aggregating agents. Almost all patients have a long bleeding time in proportion to their platelet counts, so this test serves as a good screening device. In addition to hereditary platelet dysfunction, there are some acquired types which are related to disease (von Willebrand's, uremia), drugs (acetylsalicylic acid), or antiplatelet antibodies. The majority of these patients do not have significant spontaneous bleeding, so no specific therapy is needed. Platelet transfusions may be indicated during surgical procedures in order to provide appropriate hemostasis. For the patients with lifelong hereditary disorders, the major concern is to avoid transfusing platelets because of the likelihood of alloimmunization.

DISSEMINATED INTRAVASCULAR COAGULATION (DIC)

method of
ERIC CHUN-YET LIAN, M.D.
Miami, Florida

Disseminated intravascular coagulation (DIC) is an intermediary reaction of disease which is initiated by the local or generalized activation of hemostatic systems, leading to the formation of systemic microthrombi associated with the consumption of platelets and plasma clotting factors and inhibitors. The process is usually accompanied by secondary fibrinolysis. DIC usually begins with subtle intravascular coagulation, presenting as a hypercoagulable state. When intravascular coagulation continues to increase, the equilibrium between hemostatic processes and homeostatic defense mechanisms (such as cellular clearance of activated clotting intermediates by liver and reticuloendothelial system, inactivation of activated clotting factors by antithrombin and other naturally occurring inhibitors, and fibrinolysis) becomes imbalanced. Depending on the local and circulatory conditions and the degree of hemostatic activation and consumption, the intravascular coagulation may become manifest as local thrombosis, chronic compensated DIC, and fulminant DIC with hemorrhage.

DIC is caused by excessive entrance of activating substances into the bloodstream. The process is enhanced or facilitated by excessive reactivity of platelets and clotting factors and defective control mechanisms. Triggering mechanisms can be divided into three types: (1) Contact activation of the intrinsic clotting pathway by agents which affect the contact phase of blood clotting, such as antigen-antibody complexes, particulate matter from amniotic fluid embolism, and collagen and basement membrane exposed after endothelial damage resulting from viremia, heat stroke, and septicemia. (2) Activation of the extrinsic clotting pathway by release of tissue thromboplastin into the circulating blood from leukocytes, cancer cells, brain, and endothelial cells. Tissue thromboplastin is also released in trauma, burn, surgery, and abruptio placentae to cause DIC. (3) Direct activation of factor X, prothrombin, and fibrinogen by proteolytic enzymes, such as trypsin, venoms, and extracts of mucin-producing adenocarcinoma.

The clinical picture depends upon the balance of opposing reactions of the coagulation processes and the limiting reactions. In some patients, thrombotic disease dominates, especially in the early stages. Clinical clues include oliguria, renal dysfunction, respiratory distress syndrome, liver dysfunction, mental confusion, and neurologic deficits. Bleeding may occur in the skin or mucous membrane (petechiae or ecchymosis); hematuria and gastrointestinal (GI) bleeding have been observed; and bleeding upon venipuncture sites or sites of surgical drainage tubes is common. In severe cases, shock frequently exists and microangiopathic hemolytic anemia may be observed.

In the early stages of DIC, clotting factors are still normal or even elevated; partial thromboplastin time is either normal or shortened. More sensitive tests are required for the detection of DIC. These include elevation of platelet factor 4, β-thromboglobulin, prothrombin fragment 1 or 2, fibrinopeptide A or B, circulating soluble fibrin, and thrombin-antithrombin complex and shortened half-life of platelets and fibrinogen. In the late stages of DIC, consumption of clotting factors, inhibitors, and platelets develops, along with the occurrence of secondary fibrinolysis. Laboratory studies may reveal a decreased platelet count; fragmented red cells; prolonged prothrombin time and partial thromboplastin time; abnormal clot formation and dissolution; decreased fibrinogen, factor II, factor V, factor VIII, and factor XIII; elevated fibrin-fibrinogen degradation products; prolonged thrombin time; positive protamine sulfate and ethanol gelation tests; and depressed plasminogen and antithrombin levels. Disseminated intravascular disorders should be differentiated from other acquired bleeding disorders such as vitamin K deficiency, liver disease, and acquired inhibitors. Many patients with DIC are debilitated and may not have eaten well for several days and are placed on antibiotics. Hence patients may have vitamin K deficiency as well.

Therapy of DIC

The aims of therapy for DIC are to prevent the further formation of microthrombi, to remove the microthrombi already formed, and to correct the hemostatic defects.

General Measures. Treatment should be started as early as possible once DIC is suspected or in disease states which are predisposing to DIC. The primary treatment should be directed toward the removal of underlying causes, such as evacuation of uterus for abruptio placentae and antibiotics for septicemia. Supportive treatment for the correction of hypoxia, shock, acidosis, and electrolyte imbalance is very important in order to slow down the intravascular coagulation process.

Anticoagulant Therapy. Heparin therapy of DIC is used on the basis that it interrupts the intravascular generation of thrombin and the further deposition of fibrin in the microvasculature. The choice of heparin dose should be individualized, depending on the underlying disease, vascular integrity, and hemostatic functions. A dose ranging from 5 to 25 units per kg per hour is usually sufficient. For acute DIC, continuous intravenous infusion is perhaps the safest way of attempting to treat DIC and prevent its complications. For subacute or chronic DIC, heparin can be given intravenously every 4 hours or subcutaneously every 8 to 12 hours. The prophylactic use of heparin in septic abortion, preeclampsia, and acute promyelocytic leukemia has been shown to be beneficial. For prophylactic use, low dose heparin, 10,000 to 20,000 units per day, is recommended and given by either intravenous infusion or subcutaneous injection. In addition, prophylactic use of heparin has also been recommended for patients with sepsis, severe burn, or other disease states predisposing to the development of DIC.

In heparin therapy for DIC, it is desirable to maintain a heparin level between 0.15 and 0.3 unit per ml based on antithrombin or protamine sulfate neutralization test. The effectiveness of heparin therapy is best monitored by fibrinogen level, fibrin degradation product, reptilase time, factor V assay, and fibrinopeptide A assay if available. Instead of heparin, warfarin (Coumadin) may be used in chronic DIC.

Activators and Inhibitors of the Fibrinolytic System. Secondary fibrinolytic activation is a protective mechanism against microthrombosis. During the intravascular coagulation process, plasminogen activator is decreased. The failure to activate fibrinolysis would favor persistence of microthrombi. Therefore, it is logical to use the plasminogen activators streptokinase or urokinase for DIC. Because of the high incidence of bleeding complications, their clinical application is limited. The use of streptokinase may be beneficial in hyaline membrane disease in premature infants and in the hemolytic-uremic syndrome.

Epsilon-aminocaproic acid (EACA, Amicar) is a potent antifibrinolytic agent. The administration of EACA alone in patients with DIC and secondary fibrinolysis is contraindicated. In those patients with massive hemorrhage caused by secondary hyperfibrinolysis and defibrination, low-dose EACA, 30 to 50 mg per kg every 6 hours, may be considered if heparin is given simultaneously.

Replacement of Hemostatic Elements with Blood and Plasma. Unless there is massive bleeding, hypovolemia, or a platelet count below 40,000 per cu mm, usually there is no need for blood transfusion or infusion of plasma or platelets. Replacement therapy for hemostatic components should be given after heparin therapy has been started. In obstetric complications, such as abruptio placentae, evacuation of conceptive product and massive transfusion with fresh blood and plasma without heparin have been proved to be of benefit.

THROMBOTIC THROMBOCYTOPENIC PURPURA

method of
ERIC CHUN-YET LIAN, M.D.
Miami, Florida

Thrombotic thrombocytopenic purpura (TTP) (Moschcowitz's syndrome) is a disorder characterized by thrombocytopenia, microangiopathic hemolytic anemia, neurologic signs, fever, and renal abnormalities. The disease is often accompanied by abdominal pain caused by pancreatitis or occlusion of visceral vessels, cardiac arrhythmia, and respiratory distress syndrome. Its etiology is not clear and has been reported to be associated with viral infection, rickettsial infection, vaccination, drug allergy, and various autoimmune disorders. Coombs' test is always negative, and coagulation tests are usually normal. Diagnosis can be confirmed by the demonstration of hyaline platelet thrombi in the arterioles and capillaries in the biopsied specimen from gingiva, skin, bone marrow, or lymph nodes, or by platelet aggregation induced by the patient's plasma and its inhibition by preincubation with normal plasma.

Therapy

Once the diagnosis of TTP is made, the patient should be treated immediately in an intensive care unit setting with constant cardiac and central venous pressure monitoring. Hematocrit should be raised to around 30 per cent. Exchange plasmapheresis should be performed as an emergency procedure. At least 1 plasma volume (2 to 3 liters) should be exchanged daily. In order to remove as much platelet-aggregating factor and its releasing substance as possible and, at the same time, to retain maximal amounts of normal plasma infused without volume overload, plasmapheresis can be performed with initial replacement with 0.5 to 1 liter of isotonic saline solution and 5 per cent dextrose in water and, later, with normal plasma. Plasma infusion can be continued even after plasmapheresis is completed so that a greater volume of plasma can be given and retained than has been removed. When lactic dehydrogenase (LDH) decreases to less than 600 units per dl (100 ml) or the platelet count rises, daily plasmapheresis can be discontinued and replaced by infusion with 600 to 1000 ml of normal plasma daily until the platelet count is normalized. After discontinuation of plasma infusion, the platelet count should be followed closely for several months. If there is a drop in the platelet count, plasma infusion should be reinstituted.

Platelet suppressants inhibit the platelet adhesion and aggregation caused by endothelial change and reduce the propagation of platelet aggregation caused by adenosine diphosphate (ADP), amines, and thromboxane A_2 released by aggregating platelets. Appropriate combinations and doses of various platelet suppressants (aspirin,* 200 mg once daily, dipyridamole,* 100 to 200 mg four times daily, and sulfinpyrazone,* 100 to 200 mg four times daily) would achieve some ancillary therapeutic effect. Cimetidine and antacid should be given concomitantly to protect gastrointestinal mucosa. Dextran 70 (Macrodex), which impairs platelet function and adherence to vascular surface, has also been used by some workers with some success in doses of 250 to 500 ml given intravenously over 30 to 60 minutes every 12 hours.

Platelets are the target of platelet aggregating substance. Infusion of platelet concentrates would increase the formation of circulation platelet aggregates and their deposition in the microcirculation, thus aggravating the clinical symptoms. Consequently, transfusion of platelet concentrates is contraindicated in TTP.

In those patients with an immunologic basis to their disease, it is reasonable to include corticosteroids in the treatment. Dosage up to 300 mg of hydrocortisone sodium succinate (Solu-Cortef) intravenously every 6 hours can be started from the beginning for 10 days and then replaced by prednisone 60 mg daily by mouth, which can be tapered off gradually depending on the course of disease.

From the literature and our experience, splenectomy appears to have no beneficial effect on the course of the disease.

---

*No drug is currently approved by the U.S. Food and Drug Administration as an antiplatelet agent. See manufacturers' official directives.

HEMOCHROMATOSIS AND HEMOSIDEROSIS

method of
DON M. SAMPLES, M.D.
New Orleans, Louisiana

Hemochromatosis is a disorder of iron overloading in which the excess iron is deposited in parenchymal tissues, causing cell damage, fibrosis, and impaired function, particularly of the liver, pancreas, and heart. There is a grayish bronze pigmentation of the skin owing primarily to the deposition of melanin, but there may be increased amounts of iron in 50 per cent of such patients.

Hemosiderosis indicates the deposition of iron in tissues without associated damage or impairment of function. Most of the iron is stored in the reticuloendothelial tissue rather than in the parenchymal cells.

In adults, total body iron is relatively constant at about 4 grams. Approximately two thirds of this is in hemoglobin and one fourth is stored as iron in the form of ferritin and hemosiderin. As there is no physiologic route for the excretion of iron, the avoidance of iron overloading depends upon the regulation of iron absorption. In normal nonanemic persons, absorption across the mucosa is inversely related to the total amount of storage iron. This serosal transfer of iron is probably part of an equilibrium between the plasma iron and the labile iron pool, which largely reflects the amount of storage iron. Daily absorption of approximately 1 mg of iron is needed to replace that lost by men and nonmenstruating women, and 1.5 mg by menstruating women.

In idiopathic hemochromatosis, excessive iron is absorbed irrespective of the need for iron. This may be as much as 3 to 5 mg per day, resulting in the accumulation of 25 to 60 grams of total body iron over 30 to 50 years.

Iron overloading resulting in secondary hemochromatosis may occur with ineffective erythropoiesis, particularly if accompanied by prolonged transfusion therapy, as in thalassemia major and less frequently in sideroblastic anemias. Prolonged excessive iron consumption and parenteral iron administration usually result in hemosiderosis, but secondary hemochromatosis has been observed.

In hemochromatosis serum iron levels are high and the iron binding capacity almost completely saturated. Serum ferritin levels reflect iron stores and are greatly elevated in patients, and they may detect approximately 90 per cent of the asymptomatic affected blood relatives. The diagnosis should be confirmed by iron stains on biopsies of the liver.

Treatment

Excess iron is pathogenic in hemochromatosis, and specific therapy is the removal of iron as rapidly as possible. Phlebotomy is the most effective way of doing this, as each 500 ml of blood removed contains 200 to 225 mg of iron. Initially, 1 unit of blood should be removed weekly and then the frequency increased depending upon the individual. Most will tolerate phlebotomy twice weekly. Phlebotomy should be continued at this rate until the patient is unable to maintain his hemoglobin level. At this point, the labile iron pool has been depleted, the serum ferritin level is normal, and the serum iron is normal or low. However, tissues may contain considerable amounts of more tightly bound iron, and phlebotomy should be continued at a slower rate until this has been removed. It may require 100 or more phlebotomies to exhaust the tissue iron accumulated over the years. Biopsies with iron stains of the liver and bone marrow should be done to confirm that all the iron has indeed been removed. In hemochromatosis excess iron absorption continues throughout life, and phlebotomies must be continued at 2 to 3 month intervals to prevent reaccumulation of excessive tissue iron. The role of chelating agents in promoting iron excretion in hemochromatosis has yet to be defined. Restriction of dietary iron is of no value.

The diabetes, cardiac problems, and cirrhosis of hemochromatosis are managed as in other patients. Removal of the excess iron may result in significant improvement of these conditions. However, there remains the high risk of hepatoma and there does seem to be a high rate of other cancers — namely, bronchial, pancreatic, gallbladder, and rectal. Family members who have large amounts of tissue iron but no evidence of injury should have this iron removed by phlebotomy and remain on a lifetime program of phlebotomies.

The iron overloading of patients with thalassemia major has shown dramatic benefit from continuous subcutaneous or intravenous chelating agents such as deferoxamine (Desferal) and is discussed elsewhere in this volume, as is the beneficial effect of phlebotomy in patients with prophyria cutanea tarda.

HODGKIN'S DISEASE: CHEMOTHERAPY

method of
HARVEY M. GOLOMB, M.D.,
and DONALD L. SWEET, M.D.
Chicago, Illinois

Introduction

Hodgkin's disease (HD) usually presents as asymptomatic lymphadenopathy. Diagnosis can be made only by biopsy and histologic evaluation. The extent or stage of disease at the time of diagnosis is the most important single guide to prognosis and treatment. Although there is unequivocal evidence that HD is curable at all stages of the disease, the frequency of cure is, indeed, stage dependent. During the past 20 years many centers have shown that patients with pathologic Stages I and II (about 50 per cent of all HD patients) have a 5 year survival rate of between 85 and 95 per cent. With the advent of combination chemotherapy with nitrogen mustard, vincristine sulfate (Oncovin), procarbazine, and prednisone (MOPP), it was shown that 80 per cent of patients with Stage IV disease could obtain a complete remission and approximately half of them would be surviving after 5 years. Treatment of patients with Stage III disease has recently been shown to be dependent on the distribution of the disease within the abdomen; there are probably substages of Stage III disease that require radiotherapy or combination chemotherapy.

It is obvious that the advances made in HD have required exacting histologic evaluation, careful staging, meticulous radiotherapy, and aggressive chemotherapy. The hematopathologist, surgeon, radiotherapist, and medical oncologist must cooperate initially and throughout the treatment course in order to allow each patient to be treated with intent to cure from the moment of diagnosis.

STAGING

The original histopathologic classification of Hodgkin's disease, suggested by Lukes and Butler and adopted after modifications at the Rye, New York, Symposium in 1965, is given in Table 1. The currently used staging classification was proposed by the Com-

TABLE 1. Histologic Classification of Hodgkin's Disease

LUKES AND BUTLER	RYE MODIFICATION

Lymphocytic and/or histiocytic
  a. Nodular
  b. Diffuse
	Lymphocytic predominance

Nodular sclerosis	Nodular sclerosis
Mixed cellularity	Mixed cellularity

Lymphocytic depletion
  a. Diffuse fibrosis
  b. Reticular
	Lymphocytic depletion

mittee on Hodgkin's Disease Staging Classification (Ann Arbor, Michigan, 1971) and is shown in Table 2. The Ann Arbor classification contained several new concepts. Musshoff proposed two forms of extranodal disease, one arising in contiguity with involved nodes ("E" extension), and the other associated with diffuse extranodal disease. The former had the same rate of cure as local or regional lymph node involvement when treated by radiotherapy; the latter had a less favorable prognosis requiring systemic therapy. A sharp distinction was made between the clinical stage (CS), based on data accumulated from the history, physical examination, radiographs, and radioisotope examinations, and the pathologic stage (PS), based on histologic material obtained from bone marrow biopsy, laparoscopy (peritoneoscopy), laparotomy, or other biopsied material.

TABLE 2. Hodgkin's Disease: Ann Arbor Modification of Rye Staging System (1971)

Stage I: Involvement of a single lymph node region (I) or of a single extralymphatic organ or site (I_E).

Stage II: Involvement of two or more lymph node regions on the same side of the diaphragm (II) or localized involvement of extralymphatic organ or site and of one or more lymph node regions on the same side of the diaphragm (II_E). Optional recommendation: number of node regions involved indicated by subscript—e.g., II_3.

Stage III: Involvement of lymph node regions on both sides of the diaphragm (III), which may be accompanied by localized involvement of extralymphatic organ or site (III_E), or by involvement of the spleen (III_S), or both (III_{SE}).

Stage IV: Diffuse or disseminated involvement of one or more extralymphatic organs or tissues with or without associated lymph node enlargement. The reason for classifying the involvement as Stage IV should be identified further by defining the site by symbols.

Note: Fever >38 C (100.5 F), night sweats, and/or weight loss >10 per cent of body weight in the 6 months preceding admission are defined as systemic symptoms and denoted by the suffix letter B. Asymptomatic patients are denoted by the suffix A.

Each patient received a CS and subsequently a PS designation.

The Ann Arbor classification has proved to be a workable schema and generally correlates with histopathology and prognosis. Lymphocyte predominance and nodular sclerosing types are typically associated with CS I or CS II disease; lymphocyte depletion type occurs infrequently and usually presents as CS III or CS IV disease. These stages correlate with prognosis: patients with PS I and PS II have a 5 year survival rate of greater than 86 per cent; patients with PS III and PS IV had survival rates of 81 per cent and 39 per cent, respectively.

Histopathology may not always correlate with prognosis. Fuller and coworkers observed no significant difference in disease-free survival for patients in PS I or PS II with lymphocyte predominance, nodular sclerosis, or mixed cellularity histologies when treated with radiotherapy alone.

The Ann Arbor classification refers only to patients at the time of presentation and prior to initial therapy. New designations were proposed at the International Symposium on Hodgkin's Disease in 1973 for patients in relapse, and are shown in Table 3. Restaging, including laparoscopy or laparotomy when indicated, may be necessary for patients who are suspected of being in relapse. This procedure permits determination of strategy for further therapy.

Staging Procedures

The recommendations of the Ann Arbor Committee on Hodgkin's Disease Staging Procedures (Ann Arbor, 1971) are shown in Table 4. The development of new techniques and greater appreciation of the sensitivity and specificity of older techniques may result in the obsolescence of certain of these recommendations.

Staging Laparotomy

The purpose of surgical staging is to determine accurately the presence or absence of intra-abdominal disease. Candidates for surgical staging include all patients who do not have a medical contraindication to elective abdominal surgery and in whom findings would modify therapy.

Surgical staging frequently detects abdominal dis-

TABLE 3. Staging Designation for Patients with Hodgkin's Disease in Relapse

Local recurrence (LR or TR): This is a recurrence in an area previously treated. Tumor dose of RT previously given should be specified.

Regional recurrence (MR, Adj R): This is a recurrence outside the previously treated area; however, it is confined to the same side of the diaphragm where disease was found initially.

Transdiaphragmatic recurrence (TDR): This signifies appearance of disease in lymph nodes (or spleen) but on the other side of the diaphragm than originally noted.

Extralymphatic recurrence (EL): This is the appearance of disease in extranodal or extrasplenic sites and may be designated as L^+, H^+, M^+, D^+, etc.

TABLE 4. **Recommendations on Staging Procedures**

A. Required evaluation procedures
  1. Adequate surgical biopsy, reviewed by a hematopathologist
  2. Detailed history of fever, sweating, pruritus, and weight loss
  3. Complete physical examination with attention to lymphadenopathy, Waldeyer's ring, liver, spleen, and bone tenderness
  4. Laboratory studies
     a. Complete blood count, platelet count, erythrocyte sedimentation rate, serum alkaline phosphatase level
     b. Evaluation of renal function and liver function
  5. Radiologic studies
     a. Chest roentgenogram (posteroanterior and lateral views)
     b. Intravenous pyelogram
     c. Bilateral lower extremity lymphogram
     d. Skeletal survey, especially thoracolumbar vertebrae, pelvis, proximal extremities, and areas of bone tenderness and/or pain
B. Required evaluation procedures under certain conditions
  1. Whole chest tomography, if abnormality on chest roentgenogram
  2. Inferior cavagraphy for equivocal lymphogram or pyelogram
  3. Bone marrow biopsy, by a needle or open surgical technique, if
     a. Serum alkaline phosphatase is elevated
     b. Unexplained anemia or other blood count depression
     c. Roentgenographic or scintigraphic evidence of osseous disease
     d. Generalized disease of Stage III category or greater
  4. Exploratory laparotomy and splenectomy, if management decisions will depend on the identification of abdominal disease
C. Useful ancillary procedures, not definitive for diagnosis
  1. Skeletal scintigrams
  2. Hepatic and splenic scintigrams
  3. Serum chemistries, including calcium and uric acid
  4. Estimate of patient's delayed hypersensitivity
D. Procedures and tests holding promise for clinical study at selected centers but experimental at this time
  1. Whole body gallium and selenium scintigrams
  2. Determinations of serum iron and iron binding capacity, copper and ceruloplasmin, zinc, haptoglobin, fibrinogen, alpha-2-globulin, as well as urinary hydroxyproline, leukocyte alkaline phosphatase, absolute lymphocyte count, antibodies to Epstein-Barr virus, human lymphocyte antibody typing

ease that was not anticipated by clinical evaluation. Intra-abdominal involvement has been found in 20 to 47 per cent of patients in whom other diagnostic methods, including lymphangiography (LAG), had not revealed disease below the diaphragm. Determination of splenic involvement has been a major function of surgical staging, since clinical evaluation of the spleen is inaccurate; the spleen may be the only site of infradiaphragmatic disease.

Additional advantages of surgical exploration with splenectomy are as follows: (1) decreased size of the radiation therapy port needed, with consequent reduced exposure of the left lung base and kidney, (2) application of clips to tumor masses and lymph node areas, which assist the radiotherapist in port design, (3) oophoropexy, and (4) possible increased tolerance to chemotherapy.

Detailed surgical staging has made it possible to subdivide patients with Stage III HD into two "anatomic substages," III_1 and III_2, which are defined as follows. In Stage III_1 patients, involvement is limited to those lymphatic structures in the "upper" abdomen that accompany the celiac axis group of arteries — spleen, splenic node, celiac node, or portal node. Stage III_2 includes patients with involvement of the "lower" abdominal nodes, that is, para-aortic, iliac, or mesenteric nodes with or without involvement of the spleen, splenic node, celiac node, or portal nodes.

Therapy

The accepted treatment for patients with pathologic Stage I and Stage IIA Hodgkin's disease is radiotherapy. Involved field (IF) radiotherapy has been compared to extended field (EF) radiotherapy in a national study. Although there were fewer complications with IF, there were more relapses. Conclusions as to survival differences have not been reached. Most centers recommend EF radiotherapy in all patients with Stages I and IIA HD who have undergone complete pathologic staging. For patients with Stages I_EA and II_EA disease, the use of radiotherapy alone, with adequate ports to encompass the extranodal sites effectively, is the treatment of choice. Even with careful pathologic staging, there is still a relapse rate of approximately 20 per cent of patients treated with EF radiotherapy. The majority of these patients can be re-treated with combination chemotherapy into a complete remission. Patients who have bulky mediastinal involvement that exceeds one third of the thoracic diameter have been postulated to be at high risk of developing extensions of their disease into extranodal sites in the lung, and adjuvant chemotherapy has been recommended. Whether these patients had pathologic Stage IV disease to begin with, or whether radiotherapy dosage and port design were less than adequate, or whether the patients are truly at increased risk to develop extensions remains to be determined.

Patients with systemic manifestations of HD ("B" symptoms; see note in Table 2) and local disease have not done well with radiotherapy alone, and many centers would recommend adjuvant chemotherapy. Our approach is to recommend extended field radiotherapy followed by combination chemotherapy if the disease is supradiaphragmatic in location. Staging laparotomy is still important to do in order to rule out PS IV or PS III_2 disease, since initial combination chemotherapy is the treatment of choice for PS IV and possibly for PS III_2.

Successful selection of therapy for patients with Stage III disease depends on the location of involved intra-abdominal sites. Patients with PS III_{S+N}-A or PS III_{N+}A, in which the upper abdominal nodes can be treated with the extended mantle, may be treated with radiation therapy alone. Patients with lower abdominal node disease probably require the early use of combination therapy alone, combination chemotherapy with supplemental radiotherapy, or alternating radiotherapy ports. This conclusion is of great importance because of the concern that aggressive multimodality therapy is associated with a striking incidence of induced second malignancies and leukemia. Recently, the Yale group has demonstrated the usefulness of combination chemotherapy and lowdose radiotherapy (1500 to 2000 rads). The incidence of leukemia in this study appears small, but a further period of observation is required. The point is that insufficient treatment leads to mortality from the primary malignancy; excessive therapy, especially combined modality therapy, leads to mortality from second malignancies, especially a refractory form of acute myeloblastic leukemia. The fear is that the percentage of patients salvaged by aggressive multimodality therapy (4000 rads total lymphoid irradiation plus MOPP) may be equal to the percentage of patients dying from induced second malignancies.

Patients with Stage IIIB or IVA or IVB HD are candidates for intensive combination chemotherapy. Approximately 75 per cent of all patients with advanced HD treated wtih combination chemotherapy can achieve a complete remission. In addition, over half of these remain disease free long enough to be considered cured. The challenge remains to increase the initial response rate as well as to decrease the significant relapse rate. This must be accomplished without increasing the initial treatment morbidity or the long-term morbidity and mortality of secondary malignancies.

Combination Chemotherapy

It has become a recognized fact that the standard and best combination chemotherapy treatment for patients with advanced HD consists of the four-drug MOPP combination (Table 5). The drugs are administered on a 28 day cycle, and dosage adjustments are made according to the schedule shown in Table 6. The scheduling of treatment is important, but dosage is equally important. If low blood counts persist at day 29, but have improved since day 22, then an extra week's delay is acceptable in order to administer as close to a maximal dosage as possible. Side effects are listed in Table 7. Use of antinausea medications such as prochlorperazine (Compazine), 25 mg per rectum 30 minutes prior to chemotherapy injection can be helpful in controlling this undesirable side effect. Procarbazine has monamine oxidase (MAO) inhibition activity, and the use of alcohol or other narcotics should be avoided during the treatment program. Dose modifications of vincristine sulfate (Oncovin) are necessary in patients who develop severe foot

TABLE 5. **MOPP Combination Chemotherapy—Every 28 Days**

DRUG	DOSAGE	ROUTE
Nitrogen mustard	6 mg/sq meter	days 1,8 IV
Vincristine (Oncovin)	1.4 mg/sq meter	days 1,8 IV
Procarbazine	100 mg/sq meter	days 1–14 PO
Prednisone*	40 mg/sq meter	days 1–14 PO

*Cycles 1 and 4 only.

TABLE 6. **MOPP Dosage Adjustments**

WBC COUNT ON PROPOSED DAY 1	ADJUSTMENT
>4000	100% of all drugs
3000–3999	100% vincristine (Oncovin), 50% nitrogen mustard and procarbazine
2000–2999	100% vincristine (Oncovin), 25% nitrogen mustard and procarbazine
1000–1999	50% vincristine (Oncovin), 25% nitrogen mustard and procarbazine
0–999	No drugs

PLATELET COUNT ON DAY 1	ADJUSTMENT
>100,000	100% of all drugs
50–100,000	100% vincristine (Oncovin), 25% nitrogen mustard and procarbazine
<50,000	No drugs

TABLE 7. **Chemotherapy Toxicities and Side Effects of Major Regimens**

REGIMEN	DRUG	MAJOR TOXICITY	SIDE EFFECT
MOPP	Nitrogen mustard	Myelosuppression	Nausea and vomiting
	Vincristine	Peripheral neuropathy	Alopecia, constipation
	Procarbazine	Myelosuppression	Nausea and vomiting
	Prednisone	—	Diabetes, hypertension, osteoporosis, peptic ulcer
ABVD	Doxorubicin (Adriamycin)	Myelosuppression	Nausea and vomiting, alopecia, mucositis, cardiac failure
	Bleomycin	Pulmonary fibrosis	Skin lesions, mucositis
	Vinblastine	Myelosuppression	Alopecia, neuropathy
	Dacarbazine (DTIC)	Myelosuppression	Nausea and vomiting
BVCPP	Carmustine (BCNU)	Myelosuppression (delayed)	Nausea and vomiting, flushing, local pain on administration

drop or other complications, such as unremitting constipation; they may necessitate discontinuation of the drug. The neuropathy can be so severe that patients can no longer ambulate; vincristine sulfate should be discontinued prior to this point. Hyperuricemia and attendant precipitation of urate crystals in the kidney can be prevented by the administration of allopurinol, 300 mg orally each day, which should be started 48 hours prior to initiation of chemotherapy.

A recent 10 year follow-up of 198 patients treated with MOPP at the National Cancer Institute (NCI) showed that all asymptomatic ("A") patients with Stage III or Stage IV disease achieved complete remission, and few relapsed. Overall, 80 per cent of the 198 patients achieved a complete remission. Two thirds of the complete remission group did not have a recurrence by 10 years. The 5 and 10 year survival rates of all treated patients were 65 and 58 per cent, respectively, whereas patients who achieved complete remissions had 5 and 10 year survival rates of 82 and 73 per cent, respectively. Further support for these results comes from the Southeastern Cancer Study Group, which recently reported on 324 patients with advanced or recurrent HD treated with a five-drug combination consisting of carmustine (BCNU), vinblastine sulfate (Velban), cyclophosphamide, procarbazine, and prednisone (BVCPP) (Table 8). Complete remission rates were 68 to 73 per cent for those patients who had not received prior chemotherapy; the rate was only 28 per cent for those who had.

The optimal number of cycles of MOPP chemotherapy remains to be determined and depends, in part, on the individual patient. Initially, 6 cycles were recommended, but more recently 10 cycles have been suggested. Most agree that patients should be treated until they have achieved a complete response, and then 2 additional cycles of drugs given as consolidation.

The completeness of the response should be determined prior to stopping therapy. The Southwest Oncology Group recently evaluated 82 patients with advanced HD who were in apparent complete remission after receiving 10 courses of combination chemotherapy. Occult HD was found in 10 (12 per cent) of these patients and was predominantly present in nodal sites (91 per cent) that were known to be involved at initial staging. Nine of the remaining 72 (13 per cent) thought to be free of disease after negative restaging subsequently relapsed within 8 months. Thus, the completeness of the response must be documented by performing all the clinical studies that were considered to be positive or abnormal at the initiation of treatment. It should also include a repeat bone core biopsy or liver biopsy if either was positive initially, but it may be necessary to resort to surgical biopsy or even laparotomy to define the completeness of the response.

If the response is complete, the therapy may be stopped. Studies from both the NCI and the Southwest Oncology Group have shown disease-free survival curves to be no different in the maintenance treated versus the untreated groups. There is no advantage in terms of survival, and because of the long-term morbidity associated with chemotherapy the use of maintenance therapy is not advisable.

TABLE 8. **BVCPP Regimen—Every 28 Days**

DRUG	DOSAGE	ROUTE
BCNU*	100 mg/sq meter	day 1 IV
Vinblastine	5 mg/sq meter	day 1 IV
Cyclophosphamide	600 mg/sq meter	day 1 IV
Procarbazine	100 mg/sq meter	days 1–10 PO
Prednisone	60 mg/sq meter	days 1–10 PO

*Bis-chloroethyl-nitrosourea or carmustine.

TABLE 9. **ABVD Regimen—Every 28 Days**

DRUG	DOSAGE	ROUTE
Doxorubicin (Adriamycin)	25 mg/sq meter	days 1, 15 IV
Bleomycin	10 units/sq meter	days 1, 15 IV
Vinblastine	6 mg/sq meter	days 1, 15 IV
Dacarbazine (DTIC)*	375 mg/sq meter	days 1, 15 IV

*Dimethyltriazeno-imidazole carboxamide.

Management of MOPP Failures

There are three failure groups to consider: (1) patients who progress through the initial induction therapy (20 per cent of MOPP induction failures), (2) those patients who relapse within 1 year of cessation of MOPP therapy, (3) and those patients whose treatment fails 1 year or more after cessation of MOPP therapy. The first two groups require treatment with another drug regimen that includes drugs that are non-cross-resistant. The combination ABVD (Table 9) has been shown to produce the equivalent percentage of complete remissions in previously untreated patients and also to produce complete responses in MOPP-resistant HD patients. Dose adjustments for ABVD are given in Table 10. Recently, a modification of the ABVD combination called B-DOPA, which includes bleomycin, DTIC, vincristine (Oncovin), prednisone, and doxorubicin (Adriamycin), has been used successfully in patients who failed MOPP treatment. The Stanford Group recently reported on the use of B-CAVe (bleomycin, 5 units per square meter body surface intravenously on days 1, 28, 35; CCNU, 100 mg per square meter orally on day 1; doxorubicin (Adriamycin), 60 mg per square meter intravenously on day 1; and vinblastine, 5 mg per square meter intravenously on day 1) in 22 patients who developed disease progression during or after MOPP therapy. Objective responses were achieved in 17 of 22 patients (77 per cent), and 11 of 22 responses (50 per cent) were complete.

For patients who relapse 1 year or longer after cessation of MOPP, it has been shown that 93 per cent of them can be reinduced to a complete remission with a second course of MOPP. These patients, however, require maintenance therapy in order to prevent relapse.

Radiotherapy plus Chemotherapy

The use of combined modality therapy in Hodgkin's disease needs careful scrutiny. The risk of a second malignancy is increased 29 times when both therapies are administerd, versus a threefold increase for either therapy alone, especially when total nodal irradiation is used. This increased risk of long-term complications with combined modality therapy requires careful attention to the exact stage of disease and to whether or not single modality therapy can be curative. The recent observations concerning Stage III anatomic substages (III_1 and III_2) may help to identify single modality therapy for Stage III patients (i.e., extended field radiotherapy for III_1 and combination chemotherapy for III_2). The ideal treatment for PS IB and IIB disease remains to be determined, but combination chemotherapy alone may be the advisable direction in attempting to cure the disease and decrease the long-term risk of a second malignancy.

Recently, the Yale group reported a treatment program for advanced HD emphasizing five-drug combination chemotherapy and low-dose radiation to sites of bulky disease. The chemotherapy program included nitrogen mustard, vincristine, vinblastine, prednisone, and procarbazine given in 8 week cycles for 5 cycles and radiotherapy of 1500 to 2500 rads given between cycles 3 and 4. Radiotherapy was given to the anatomic areas known to be involved with disease prior to the onset of chemotherapy. All involved areas were treated except the bone marrow. Of 80 patients treated, 60 obtained a complete remission. Most significantly, only 5 of the 60 complete responders relapsed, with follow-up from 1 to 6 years. The cumulative survival at 5 years of patients having complete remission was 92 per cent.

Re-treatment of Relapses After Radiation Therapy

Patients with PS I or PS IIA HD have a 20 per cent chance of relapsing within 5 years. Eighty-five per cent of these relapses occur within the first 2 years. Relapses are marginal or disseminated. The marginal relapses may be outside but contiguous to the original radiotherapy port, whereas others are true recurrences within the initial port. For the marginal relapses outside the original therapy port, the patient can be re-treated with radiotherapy alone for cure if no signs of dissemination are present. For true re-

TABLE 10. **ABVD Dose Adjustments**

WBC COUNT ON DAY 1	PLATE COUNT ON DAY 1	ADJUSTMENT
>4000	>130,000	100% of all drugs
3000–3999	90–129,000	100% of B, D; 50% of A, V
2000–2999	60–89,000	100% of B; 50% of D; 25% of A
1500–1999	40–59,000	100% of B; 25% of D
<1500	<40,000	100% of B

lapses, 2000 rads of radiotherapy can be given to partially control the local problem, but this must be followed by MOPP chemotherapy. Seventy-five per cent of relapsed patients can achieve a second complete remission utilizing these strategies. The chance for a complete response to MOPP combination chemotherapy is not reduced in patients who have received prior radiotherapy if adequate chemotherapy can be administered. One must adjust the chemotherapy dosages carefully in patients who have residual compromise of bone marrow function from previous chemotherapy.

Importance of Stage and Treatment Design to Prevent Long-Term Complications

Development of acute nonlymphocytic leukemia has been documented to occur in approximately 3 per cent of previously treated Hodgkin's disease patients. In most series it has been shown to occur approximately 5 years after the initial diagnosis and to be relatively refractory to treatment. Most patients show a preleukemic phase with a combination of cytopenias or pancytopenia. Chromosome studies have shown an abnormality in almost all patients as compared with only about 50 per cent of de novo acute leukemia patients. In fact, the chromosome abnormalities seem to be distinct in terms of both modal number and specifically affected chromosomes. This unusual syndrome suggests some relationship to the previous therapy, but an increased chance of a "second hit" because of increased longevity remains a possible explanation. However, because of this long-term complication, it is important to determine the exact stage of the disease and to use effective, curative single modality therapy, if possible, for each stage. As a result of these considerations and the data cited above, it is conceivable that the treatment programs such as that shown in Table 11 will be established for the next decade.

TABLE 11. **Future Treatment Programs to Maximize Staging Information and Therapy Regimens and Minimize Short- and Long-Term Morbidity**

STAGE	INITIAL THERAPY
I A and II A	Extended field RT
I B and II B	MOPP
III$_1$ A	Extended field RT
III$_2$ A	MOPP
III B	MOPP
IV A and IV B	MOPP

RT, radiotherapy.

HODGKIN'S DISEASE: RADIATION THERAPY

method of
STEPHEN L. SEAGREN, M.D.,
and JOHN E. BYFIELD, M.D.
San Diego, California

Great progress has been made in the therapy of Hodgkin's disease during the past 15 years. Several factors have contributed, including a better understanding of the natural history, more accurate clinical staging, widely accepted pathologic classification with important pathophysiologic correlations, effective combination chemotherapy, and more appropriate radiotherapeutic techniques.

The diagnosis is always made by biopsy, usually of supraclavicular, cervical, axillary, or mediastinal node. The histologic diagnosis is not always straightforward, and confirmation by an experienced hematopathologist is desirable. The pathologic classification of Lukes and Butler is employed (Table 1). It is generally agreed that lymphocyte predominant histology is prognostically favorable and lymphocyte depletion unfavorable. Whether there are significant prognostic differences between the two more common histologic types is less certain.

Once the diagnosis is established, staging must follow. Hodgkin's disease apparently begins in a single lymph node focus, and if it progresses, it does so in an orderly fashion to contiguous structures, usually nodes but also parenchyma. Only by assessing the extent of this progression can therapy be chosen and prognosis established. If the disease produces symptoms (unexplained fever, sweating, or weight loss), the tumor burden is presumably greater and the prognosis is adversely affected. Based on these concepts, a standard staging classification for Hodgkin's disease has been developed (Table 2). Many oncologists now believe that Stage III Hodgkin's disease is too broad a classification and that two subcategories are necessary, III$_1$ and III$_2$. III$_1$

TABLE 1.

TYPE	INCIDENCE
Lymphocytic predominant (LP)	10%
Nodular sclerosis (NS)	40%
Mixed cellularity (MC)	40%
Lymphocytic depletion (LD)	10%

TABLE 2. **Staging Classification**

Stage I	Involvement of a single lymph node region or single extralymphatic organ or site (I_E), excluding the liver or bone marrow
Stage II	Involvement of two or more lymph node regions on the same side of the diaphragm, or localized involvement of an extralymphatic organ or site (II_E)
Stage III	Involvement of lymph node regions on both sides of the diaphragm, or localized involvement of an extralymphatic organ or site (III_E) or spleen (III_S)
Stage IV	Diffuse or disseminated involvement of one or more extralymphatic organs with or without associated lymphatic involvement; the organ(s) should be identified by a symbol
A	Asymptomatic
B	Symptoms present, including fever, sweats, weight loss greater than 10 per cent of body weight

represents involvement of supradiaphragmatic nodes together with the high abdominal nodes, i.e., splenic, celiac, portal. III_2 represents similar involvement but including the lower para-aortic or pelvic nodes. This latter classification is controversial and not official, but we find that radiotherapy alone may be more beneficial to patients with III_1 disease than to those with III_2.

Some staging procedures are standard (Table 3), and others may be required under certain circumstances (Table 4). This standard staging approach may be modified as further experience is accumulated with newer imaging techniques. Exploratory laparotomy continues to be required when a therapeutic decision rests on the pathologic demonstration of the presence or absence of abdominal Hodgkin's disease. Since laparotomy has attendant morbidity (and mortality), patients for exploration should be highly selected. This is not a "routine" staging procedure. In general, patients whose disease already indicates chemotherapy as the initial therapy do not require laparotomy. In our opinion, these patients have Stages IB, IIB, III_B, and IV disease.

TABLE 3. **Staging Procedures**

1. Clinical history with special attention to fever, chills, and weight loss
2. Careful physical examination with special attention to all node-bearing areas and size of liver and spleen
3. Laboratory procedures
   a. Complete blood count
   b. Alkaline phosphatase
   c. Creatinine
4. Radiologic procedures
   a. Chest films, posteroanterior and lateral
   b. Bipedal lymphangiogram
5. Bone marrow needle biopsy

TABLE 4. **Procedures Sometimes Required**

1. Mediastinal or whole lung tomography if chest radiograph is abnormal
2. Gallium scan
3. Computed tomography of abdomen or pelvis
4. Liver and spleen scans (if abnormality is suspected)
5. Percutaneous hepatic needle biopsy (if abnormality is suspected)
6. Bone scan (if bony tenderness is present)
7. Skeletal radiographs of areas positive on bone scan
8. Exploratory laparotomy

Also, if lymphangiographic evidence of III_2 disease can be confirmed by gallium scan or computed abdominal tomography, this subset of patients may not require laparotomy. In addition, there are certain patients whose incidence of abdominal disease is sufficiently low not to warrant laparotomy, especially those with Stage I LP histology in the right neck and those with Stage I NS histology and a small mediastinal mass. In general, however, most patients selected for treatment by radiation will have had a laparotomy.

At laparotomy, selected nodes are removed and splenectomy is performed. Sites of nodes and splenic pedicle are identified by radiopaque clips, direct liver and bone marrow biopsies are done, and a preclosure abdominal roentgenograph is obtained in the operating room to be sure all nodes of interest (still opacified from the lymphangiogram) have been removed. Some surgeons will rotate the ovaries (marking them with clips) into the midline in female patients to shield them from radiation. However, we rarely radiate the pelvis in our patients as part of initial potentially curative radiotherapy.

Treatment

Much of the progress in Hodgkin's disease has been made because of randomized clinical trials. In general, when a trial we consider ethical and appropriate is open to us, we invite our patients to participate and treat them accordingly. When no trial is available or appropriate or the patient refuses entry, we treat him as follows.

The availability of effective chemotherapy and a recognition of the limitations of radiotherapy have led to an evolving therapeutic regimen based on pathologic stage. For Stages I_A, I_{EA}, II_A, II_{EA}, III_{SA}, and III_{1A}, extended field radiation (mantle, splenic pedicle, and para-aortic nodes) to curative dose levels is the treatment of choice.

For Stages I_B, II_B, and II_{EB}, the best treatment is not yet clear, but we treat patients with B symptoms with chemotherapy and usually recommend low dose radiotherapy to initially bulky (5 cm or larger) disease following chemotherapy.

For Stages III_{2A}, III_B, and IV, our treatment is primarily with chemotherapy. We recommend lower doses of consolidative radiotherapy to areas of initially bulky disease following 6 courses of MOPP. This is based on observations of failure patterns with chemotherapy alone, and some evidence of more lasting remissions with this approach. However, a clear survival advantage with a combined approach is not established.

Radiotherapy Technique

When radiation alone is used, the regions of involvement plus the next contiguous nodal chain are radiated. In almost all patients, this implies the mantle (axillary, clavicular, cervical, mediastinal, and hilar nodes), splenic pedicle, and para-aortic nodes. Unless very high cervical or pre-auricular nodes are involved, we do not treat Waldeyer's ring, thereby avoiding parotid radiation and a severely dry mouth. We prefer high energy x-rays from a linear accelerator (as opposed to Cobalt-60) because of better beam edge definition, which results in lower doses to normal tissue and fewer late complications. The dose to clinically involved areas must be at least 4000 rads in 4½ weeks, with an additional 500 rads to more bulky disease. The dose to clinically uninvolved regions may be lower (3000 to 3500 rads). We employ 180 rads per day, treating 5 days per week and two fields (parallel opposed) per day. We treat the mantle field first and the para-aortic field second. We have found the single extended field much too toxic and myelosuppressive. Overall treatment time is 2 to 2½ months.

Since most patients at risk for pelvic disease are treated with chemotherapy, we rarely treat the pelvic nodes. This, of course, means that patients at high risk for relapse will not have undergone prior pelvic radiotherapy with its attendant diminution of pelvic marrow reserve and limited tolerance for chemotherapy. Also, significant radiation to the gonads is virtually eliminated.

Patients are treated with arms overhead. Special divergent blocks are cut for each patient to block normal structures such as the lung, larynx, and cervical spinal cord. We treat the mantle first and then the splenic pedicle and para-aortic nodes (to the bifurcation) following the mantle. The fields are carefully matched and then 1 cm is added to the gap and a small (narrow 2 × 1 cm) midline cord block is added to the posterior field. All treatment is given by parallel opposed portals, and both fields are treated each day. Portal verification films are obtained at least weekly. The services of a radiation physicist, dosimetrist, and radiotherapy technologist in planning, administering, and monitoring this complicated therapy are indispensable.

When using radiation in combination with MOPP chemotherapy, we employ a lower dose (2000 to 2500 rads), treating only regions involved with bulky disease. Six full 28 day cycles of MOPP are given first. With smaller treatment volumes and lower doses, acute radiotoxicity is less.

Clinical Situations Requiring Special Approaches

Salvage Radiotherapy. A recurrence of Hodgkin's disease does not necessarily imply that the patient will die of his disease. In fact, at least half of the diminishing number of patients who relapse can be salvaged. Techniques vary with relapse pattern, and chemotherapy is normally the mainstay of salvage therapy. Nevertheless, we do use radiation therapy to bulky relapse regions in a similar fashion to the way we employ the modality in advanced primary disease. Occasionally relapse in untreated nodal regions can be salvaged by radiotherapy alone.

Large Mediastinal Mass. The patient with a large mediastinal mass (greater than one third chest diameter radiographically), but otherwise low stage (I_A, II_A, II_{AE}), presents a special therapeutic challenge. Radiotherapy alone in this subset of patients is apparently less effective in controlling the disease than in other low stage presentations, and the large volume of lung and heart requiring high dose radiation sets the stage for serious late sequelae in these organs. For these reasons we have recommended chemotherapy followed by 2000 to 2500 rads to the mediastinum in these cases.

Radiotherapeutic Emergencies. Occasionally a patient with known or suspected Hodgkin's disease will require immediate therapy.

TRACHEOBRONCHIAL COMPRESSION. When a patient presents with stridor, a mediastinal mass, and tracheal compression on chest film, we advise steroids, control of the airway with nasotracheal tube (if possible), and 400 rads to the mass; occasionally nitrogen mustard (10 mg per square meter) is used in addition. This normally widens the airway and allows subsequent diagnostic biopsy. Hodgkin's disease is usually found.

SUPERIOR VENA CAVA SYNDROME. In a previously untreated patient, we treat with oxygen, steroids, a sitting position, and sometimes diuret-

TABLE 5. **Five Year Survival**

	ABSOLUTE	DISEASE-FREE
Stage I	95–100%	90–95%
Stage II$_A$	85–95%	70–80%
Stage II$_B$	80–90%	70–80%
Stage III$_{A1}$	80–90%	60–80%
Stage III$_{A2}$	*	*
Stage IV	50–65%	40–50%

*Results with these methods are not yet clear.

ics (furosemide, 40 to 80 mg intravenously). Many patients respond and allow diagnostic evaluation. In nonresponding patients, we give a short course of radiotherapy (800 to 1200 rads in two to three fractions), which usually relieves the symptoms, and proceed with the work-up.

SPINAL CORD COMPRESSION. In a patient with known Hodgkin's disease (the usual situation) and a documented cord compression, we radiate a total of 3200 rads in 10 fractions over 12 days (400 rads per day for 2 days, then 300 rads for 8 fractions).

Results

Survival may be measured by either absolute or disease-free survival. Since many patients who relapse are salvaged, but since relapse represents a failure of primary therapy, both must be examined. The experience in most major centers is reflected in Table 5.

Consequences of Radiation to Normal Tissues

Early Effects. These are almost always self-limited and reversible.

OROINTESTINAL. A mild dry mouth and loss of taste result from radiating the submandibular and lower parotid salivary glands. In the presence of reasonable dental hygiene, radiation-induced caries are unusual. We encourage fluoride dental prophylaxis. Esophagopharyngitis results in a sore throat and dysphagia which may occasionally be severe. Nausea and vomiting may occur with the mantle, but are more common with abdominal radiation. Antiemetics used therapeutically and prophylactically are useful adjuncts, but sometimes the dose per fraction must be reduced to diminish this side effect. Mild diarrhea occasionally occurs with abdominal radiation.

SKIN AND HAIR. Skin erythema and even dry desquamation are not uncommon about the neck during mantle radiation, but rarely occur in the chest or abdomen. Occipital scalp epilation is common and usually reversible, but alarming to an uninformed patient.

FATIGUE. Most patients feel tired throughout the course of radiotherapy, but they are able to continue the majority of their normal activities.

MYELOSUPPRESSION. A generous portion of marrow is radiated when the mantle and para-aortic nodes are treated, even though the pelvis is excluded. A significant minority of patients will show a sufficiently severe neutropenia (segmented neutrophils plus bands less than 1700) to require interruption of therapy for marrow recovery. Significant thrombocytopenia (less than 75,000 platelets) similarly occurs, although less frequently. Lymphopenia with no known clinical significance is invariable. Weekly blood counts are routine.

Late Effects. Meticulous attention to detail in treatment planning and execution will minimize most clinically important late effects. Those which occur do so more commonly with higher doses or larger tissue volumes radiated. Many have no specific effective therapy.

PULMONARY. Two to 6 months following mantle therapy, some patients will experience dry cough and dyspnea and sometimes fever (which may imply a superinfection). Pulmonary fibrosis within the treatment portal is present. For the acute phase (if present), steroids and usually antibiotics are used; the chronic phase is usually asymptomatic, although mild persistence of symptoms sometimes occurs. The incidence is higher in patients with large mediastinal masses, who require a larger volume of normal lung in the portal.

CARDIAC. When, because of massive mediastinal adenopathy, a significant volume of the heart must be treated with more than 1500 rads, radiation pericarditis is possible. The clinical syndrome is similar to that of other pericardial disease and ranges from asymptomatic effusion to pericardial tamponade or to the clinical symptoms of acute pericarditis. Steroids may be useful for pericarditis; pericardiocentesis and often pericardiectomy are necessary for tamponade. If combined therapy for large mediastinal masses is employed with lower radiation dose, pulmonary and pericardial reactions may become less frequent. A rare patient will have radiation-induced damage to the coronary vascular supply, which can lead to lethal myocardial degeneration or infarction.

CENTRAL NERVOUS SYSTEM (CNS). Transient myelitis manifested as Lhermitte's sign (paresthesia of upper extremities with neck flexion) is said to be common if looked for, but is now rare within the inclusion of a posterior cervical spine block. The most devastating treatment complication, late transverse myelitis, is inevitably the consequence of field overlap; the tragedy is compounded in patients whose disease is controlled. By conservative field matching as discussed above, this complication should not ensue. We have not observed a relapse in this gap; but if it should occur, the patient still may well be salvaged. It is the efficacy of salvage chemotherapy which justifies this safeguard against radiation transverse myelitis.

ENDOCRINE. Among patients radiated for Hodgkin's disease, 20 to 30 per cent will develop biochemical evidence of hypothyroidism, although fewer will develop clinical symptoms or signs. Since the condition is easily treated, this complication must be remembered by a physician who undertakes the follow-up of Hodgkin's patients. Young females may be infertile as a secondary effect of this phenomenon.

SUBSEQUENT NEOPLASIA. Acute leukemia and malignant lymphoma occur more frequently than expected in patients whose Hodgkin's disease is controlled. Whether this is a consequence of therapy or an inherent tendency in the disease process is not clear. What is clear is that the incidence of these neoplasms increases sharply when aggressive chemotherapy and high dose radiation are used together, in which case incidence may be 7 per cent or higher. Whether a lower incidence will be observed when lower consolidative (1500 to 2500 rads) radiotherapy doses are used is not established, although this is suggested by some studies. In any case, this observation mandates that combined modality therapy be used judiciously and only with proper indication.

Follow-up

We see the patient 1 month following completion of radiotherapy. At this time we evaluate his or her recovery from the early effects. Then we see the patient every 3 months for 2 years, every 4 months for 2 years, every 6 months for 2 years, and annually thereafter. We do an interim history and physical examination, do a chest and abdominal x-ray (as long as dye remains in the nodes), and perform a complete blood count (CBC), sedimentation rate, and liver function tests, together with a test of thyroid function (T_4 and usually thyroid-stimulating hormone [TSH]). If we suspect recurrence, subsequent evaluation is guided by the symptoms and/or signs.

ACUTE LEUKEMIA IN ADULTS*

method of
HARVEY D. PREISLER, M.D.
Buffalo, New York

The last 10 years have brought significant advances in the treatment of acute leukemia. New drugs and therapeutic strategies have led to treatment regimens which induce complete remissions in the majority of patients ≤ 70 years old (65 to 75 per cent), with median durations of remission of 12 to 18 months and with 15 to 20 per cent of patients being long-term survivors (more than 2 years). The treatment of these diseases remains difficult, however, with the frequent occurrence of life-threatening complications produced by both the disease and the therapies employed.

Initial Evaluation of the Patient and General Approach to Supportive Care

The patient should be carefully and completely evaluated, since the results of the initial work-up will dictate the therapeutic approach. The initial evaluation should include a history, physical examination, complete blood count, bone marrow aspirate and biopsy (with at least Wright's-Giemsa, peroxidase, periodic acid–Schiff [PAS], and nonspecific esterase stains), coagulogram, renal function studies (serum electrolytes), liver function tests, and a posteroanterior and lateral x-ray of the chest. Particular attention should be paid to the temperature level, blood urea nitrogen (BUN), and serum uric acid and urine output, white blood cell count, coagulogram, chest x-ray, and rectal examination (looking for signs of perirectal abscess or cellulitis), since significant abnormalities in these areas mandate immediate therapeutic intervention.

Any febrile leukemic patient should be assumed to be infected unless proved otherwise. This includes all patients with a temperature of more than 38 C (100.5 F) not attributable to a recent transfusion of a blood product. Febrile patients should be immediately evaluated with a careful history, physical examination, and culture of the blood, urine, sputum, and any sites of suspected infection. Particular attention should

---

*Some agents mentioned in this article are considered investigational. Before using any of the drugs mentioned here, the physician should be well informed of their actions and of the information in the manufacturers' official directives.

be paid to the chest x-rays and rectal examination (looking for signs of a perirectal abscess or cellulitis), with the knowledge that a negative evaluation does not rule out infections in these areas, since the absence of infiltration of infected sites by normal granulocytes often precludes localizing signs of infection. Regardless of the physical findings, febrile patients with ≤500 circulating granulocytes per microliter of blood should be treated immediately with broad-spectrum antibiotics (do not wait for culture results), since in this setting infections can cause shock and death within hours. Antibiotic therapy should include an aminoglycoside antibiotic (gentamicin, tobramycin, or amikacin), a semisynthetic penicillin active against Pseudomonas sp. (carbenicillin or ticarcillin), with or without a member of the cephalosporin group. Antibiotic therapy should be continued (even in the absence of a documented infection) for 72 hours after the patient becomes afebrile — even if there is no documented source of infection. Serum aminoglycoside levels should be faithfully monitored to prevent renal toxicity. Patients who remain persistently febrile despite antibiotic therapy for more than 5 days should probably receive granulocyte transfusions containing at least 10^{10} granulocytes per transfusion. Patients with a rapidly progressing infection should receive granulocyte transfusions as soon as the rapid progression is recognized. At present it is clear that granulocyte transfusions are beneficial in those cases with documented infections. The benefit of granulocyte transfusions for patients with fevers of unknown origin is controversial. Superficial fungal infections are common in leukemic patients, but in my experience systemic fungal disease occurs primarily in patients who are in the later stages of remission induction therapy and who have been treated with broad-spectrum antibiotics for several weeks. Persistently febrile patients in this category should be treated with amphotericin B while continuing therapy with broad-spectrum antibiotics. It is uncommon for fever and infection to resolve completely until the leukemic patient enters complete remission.

Patients who present with evidence of disseminated intravascular coagulation (DIC) should be treated with 5000 units of heparin intravenously every 6 hours and replacement of any depleted plasma clotting factors. DIC should be especially suspected if there is persistent oozing of blood from venipuncture sites. Although this complication is most common in patients with acute promyelocytic leukemia and in some cases of acute monocytic leukemia, it may complicate the course of any acute leukemia. When considering the results of a coagulogram, special emphasis should be placed on quantitation of fibrin split products and on the thrombin time, since the disease itself, in the absence of a clotting disorder, can produce abnormally high levels of fibrinogen and factor VIII levels, making recognition of reduction in the levels of these factors difficult.

A blast cell count of more than 200,000 per microliter should be considered a medical emergency, since fatal intracranial bleeding may occur at any time. It should be emphasized that the likelihood of such bleeding is independent of the platelet count. Measures should be taken immediately to lower the white blood cell count. Leukapheresis may be employed, but it is probably safer to administer hydroxyurea, 3 grams per square meter orally, together with 400 to 500 R of whole brain radiation to rapidly lower the peripheral blood count and to destroy perivascular leukostatic nodules. Remission induction therapy for the leukemia should begin promptly. Since the rapid lysis of leukemic cells produces an outpouring of uric acid, measures must be taken to prevent urate nephropathy. These should include the administration of allopurinol, large amounts of fluids intravenously to ensure adequate urine flow, and alkalinization of the urine.

Who Should Be Treated?

Essentially all patients with acute lymphocytic leukemia should receive remission induction therapy. With respect to acute myelocytic leukemia, the outcome of remission induction therapy is often determined by the ability of the patient to survive the side effects of the disease and of intensive remission induction therapy. Hence, there are subpopulations of patients with acute myelocytic leukemia for whom the indications for intensive chemotherapy are unclear. Patients who are over 70 years of age generally do not survive intensive remission induction therapy unless they are physiologically younger than their chronological age. Patients with oligoblastic or smoldering leukemia represent a group for whom watchful waiting is better than the administration of intensive remission induction therapy. These patients have slowly progressing disease characterized at times by marrow hypocellularity, have less than 50 per cent leukemic cells in the bone marrow with relatively normal peripheral blood cell counts, and generally do poorly when treated aggressively. Therefore, it is probably advisable to withhold antileukemia therapy until the platelet count falls to less than 60,000 or the white blood cell count is less than 1000. Patients who develop acute myelocytic leukemia subsequent to radiation therapy and/or chemotherapy with al-kylating agents also respond poorly to therapy, primarily because of inadequate residual normal bone marrow reserve. These patients are best treated in a manner similar to that recommended for patients with smoldering leukemia. All other patients with acute myelocytic leukemia should receive remission induction therapy.

Therapeutic Regimens

Treatment should be directed at inducing a complete remission, defined as the absence of detectable leukemic cells in the bone marrow or peripheral blood with a normal bone marrow aspirate and peripheral blood cell count. All patients should be treated with allopurinol, 100 mg three or four times daily. Patients with acute lymphocytic leukemia or acute undifferentiated leukemia should receive remission induction therapy consisting of (1) daunorubicin, 45 mg per square meter intravenously on days 1, 2, and 3; (2) vincristine, 2 mg per square meter intra-venously (not to exceed 2 mg total dose) on days 1, 8, and 15; (3) prednisone, 40 mg per square meter per day orally on days 1 to 21, being tapered to zero on days 22 to 28; and (4) L-asparaginase, 500 IU per kg per day intra-venously for 10 days on days 22 to 31. Patients who fail to enter complete remission should receive a second cycle of daunorubicin, vin-cristine, and prednisone therapy. If they then do not enter remission, the patients should be-come candidates for new experimental regimens such as the "7 + 3" regimen used for the treat-ment of acute myelocytic leukemia. Once remis-sion is obtained, the patient should receive main-tenance chemotherapy, which should include prophylactic therapy of the central nervous sys-tem. The latter consists of cranial irradiation, 2400 rads administered over 18 days, together with weekly intrathecal methotrexate therapy for six doses (12 mg per square meter per week —not to exceed 10 mg per dose). Maintenance chemo-therapy should consist of 6-mercaptopurine, 200 mg per square meter per day orally for 5 days a week, and methotrexate, 7.5 mg per square meter per day orally for 5 days per week. During the period of intrathecal administration of meth-otrexate, the intrathecal administration of metho-trexate should be considered as day 1 therapy of the 5 day course of methotrexate. Every 3 months the course of mercaptopurine and methotrexate should be halted and the patient should receive two doses of vincristine (as above, with 1 week between doses) and prednisone, 40 mg per square meter per day orally for 2 weeks, with tapering to zero over 1 week's time.

Patients with acute myelocytic leukemia should receive remission induction therapy con-sisting of daunorubicin, 45 mg per square meter per day intravenously on days 1, 2, and 3, togeth-er with cytosine arabinoside, 100 mg per square meter per day by continuous infusion for 7 days (7 + 3 regimen). Seven days after the end of therapy a bone marrow aspirate and biopsy should be carried out. If persistent leukemia is detected, a second course of remission induction therapy (consisting of daunorubicin on days 1 and 2 and cytosine arabinoside on days 1 to 5 in dosages described above) should be adminis-tered. If the day 14 bone marrow is hypocellular without evidence of residual leukemia, no further therapy is administered until a decision can be made as to whether the cells which eventually repopulate the bone marrow are normal or leu-kemic. This often requires several bone marrow examinations separated by 3 or 4 days. It should be noted that the early appearance of blast cells may denote a regenerating normal bone marrow, so that unless the blast cells contain Auer rods it is usually necessary to continue to withhold therapy and repeat the bone marrow examination in 3 to 4 days to see if the myeloblasts have matured. Note that therapeutic decisions must be based upon examination of the bone marrow and not based on peripheral blood cell counts, which may be quite low despite the presence of a marrow packed with leukemia cells.

Remission maintenance therapy should con-sist of monthly 5 day courses of chemotherapy, all of which contain cytosine arabinoside, 100 mg per square meter twice daily for 5 days, together with each of the following in sequence: month 1 — daunorubicin, 45 mg per square meter intra-venously on days 1 and 2; month 2 — predni-sone, 40 mg per square meter orally for 5 days, and vincristine, 2 mg intravenously on day 1; month 3 — 6-thioguanine, 100 mg per square meter twice daily for 5 days. The sequence is re-peated.

Relapse in acute lymphocytic leukemia and acute myelocytic leukemia is defined as 5 per cent leukemic cells in the bone marrow. Marrow ex-aminations should be performed every 6 weeks. Remission maintenance therapy should be con-tinued for at least 3 years.

During maintenance therapy drug dosages should be adjusted so that the granulocyte count does not fall below 500 per microliter and the platelet count below 75,000 per microliter.

Complications During Remission Induction Therapy

Vital signs should be obtained every 4 hours on patients during remission induction therapy. Infection is the main complication. Since it is a life-threatening problem in granulocytopenic pa-tients, it should be handled as an emergency as described above. Since fever may be the only sign of infection, antipyretic agents should never be routinely administered to these patients, and the use of these drugs should be reserved for life-threatening temperature elevations.

Disseminated intravascular coagulation occasionally appears during remission induction therapy as a result of the massive lysis of leukemic cells and the resultant release of procoagulants. This complication should be treated as described above. Urine output should be kept at more than 50 ml per square meter per hour to decrease the likelihood of urate nephropathy.

Modifications of Drug Dosages

The presence of severe liver disease mandates avoidance of or reduction in dosages of the following chemotherapeutic agents: methotrexate, 6-mercaptopurine, 6-thioguanine, L-asparaginase, daunorubicin, and doxorubicin (Adriamycin). The following drugs may be administered at full doses but caution should be exercised: cytosine arabinoside, cyclophosphamide, vincristine, and prednisone.

For patients with severe renal disease, the following drugs should be avoided when possible: methotrexate, 6-mercaptopurine, 6-thioguanine, cyclophosphamide, and daunorubicin.

Daunorubicin or doxorubicin (Adriamycin) should not be administered to patients in congestive heart failure. Periodic measurement of the radionuclide cardiac ejection fraction should be carried out, since an ejection fraction of 50 per cent or less indicates compromised cardiac function and is an indication for withholding anthracycline antibiotic therapy.

Meningeal Leukemia

Meningeal leukemia is much more common in acute lymphocytic leukemia than in acute myelocytic leukemia in adults; hence, prophylactic central nervous system therapy should not be administered to the latter patients. The occurrence of meningeal leukemia necessitates intrathecal chemotherapy with methotrexate, 12 mg per square meter (total dose not to exceed 10 mg per administration) twice a week and continued for 2 weeks beyond the time that the cerebrospinal fluid (CSF) is cleared of leukemic cells. For meningeal leukemia refractory to methotrexate therapy, intrathecal cytosine arabinoside may be administered. Consideration should be given to inserting an Ommaya reservoir for ventricular perfusion.

Therapeutic Approaches Under Development

Several studies are underway evaluating more intensive therapy chemotherapy than that described above. Some intensive therapies under study are administered during remission induction therapy, shortly after complete remission is attained (early intensification), or after a patient has been in remission for 1 or more years (late intensification). While the initial results appear promising, it is too early to reach a conclusion regarding the efficacy of these approaches. The same can be said for allogeneic bone marrow transplantation for patients in complete remission. While interesting data have been presented, this approach also remains highly experimental. Studies of immunotherapy initially appeared promising, but at present this modality has fallen into disfavor because of the inability of many investigators to confirm the initial favorable results.

Conclusions

The treatment of acute leukemia remains difficult, with less than 20 per cent of all patients remaining alive 3 years after diagnosis. Intensive supportive care is required because of the complications resulting from the cytopenias produced by the disease and by remission induction therapy. Since many of these life-threatening complications are unique to these diseases, patients with acute leukemia should be treated by physicians who see many patients with these diseases in hospitals where the house staff are familiar with these problems and where intensive supportive care facilities are available.

The treatment of acute leukemia remains experimental, with the best regimens not yet discovered. For this reason, an effort should be made to gain knowledge from each leukemic patient who is treated. To this end, every effort should be made to treat leukemic patients within a Cancer Research Institution or on a Cooperative Group Study.

CHILDHOOD ACUTE LEUKEMIA*

method of
DENIS R. MILLER, M.D.
New York, New York

The improved outlook in childhood leukemia observed during the past 10 years has been the result of more accurate diagnosis, better

*Some agents mentioned in this article are considered investigational. Before using any of the drugs mentioned here, the physician should be well informed of their actions and of the information in the manufacturers' official directives.

supportive care, the use of multiple drugs to achieve and maintain remission, and the use of prophylactic therapy to prevent central nervous system leukemia.

Failure or success in disease control depends upon still ill-defined interactions between the host or patient, the leukemic cells, specific antileukemic therapy, and the responsible physician. Key factors include the growth and proliferative characteristics of the leukemic cell population, their sensitivity or resistance to chemotherapy, the presence of leukemic cells in protected sanctuaries unaffected by antileukemic therapy, variability in host response to therapy, underlying immunodeficiency states, and the competence and experience of the attending physician.

Designing a strategy for the treatment, control, and eradication of childhood acute leukemia requires an accurate diagnosis. Over 80 per cent of leukemic children under 15 years of age have acute lymphoblastic leukemia (ALL); the remaining 15 to 20 per cent of leukemias in children are acute nonlymphoblastic leukemia (ANLL) including acute myeloblastic leukemia (AML), acute promyelocytic leukemia (APML), acute myelomonoblastic leukemia (AMMoL), acute monoblastic leukemia (AMoL), erythroleukemia (EL), and chronic myelogenous leukemia (CML). It is essential that morphologic criteria, histochemical stains, and immunologic cell surface characterizations be utilized at the time of diagnosis in all patients to determine the exact type of leukemia and to plan appropriate therapy. Although the specific diagnostic and investigative studies are beyond the scope of this article, serious consideration should be given to referral of children with acute leukemia to centers with the laboratory and clinical resources to perform these studies and initiate therapy. Different therapeutic strategies are now employed for ALL and ANLL just as the prognosis of each group is markedly disparate. The appropriateness and effectiveness of initial therapy invariably determine the patient's eventual outcome. Patients who fail to achieve an initial successful complete remission seldom become long-term survivors.

In childhood ALL, over 50 per cent of children remain in complete continuous remission for 5 or more years after diagnosis, with the expectation that 85 per cent of this group will be long-term survivors with a good chance for cure. In contrast, the median duration of complete remission in childhood ANLL is only 12 to 14 months, and median survival only about 16 to 18 months. Approximately 20 per cent of children with ANLL are alive 36 months or more after diagnosis.

It is now recognized that prognosis in childhood ALL is determined by a number of clinical and biologic features of disease identifiable at the time of or shortly after diagnosis. Key significant factors recently identified by the Children's Cancer Study Group (CCSG) include (1) the leukemic cell burden, as measured by the initial white blood cell count (WBC) and the degree of adenopathy; (2) the age of the patient; (3) morphologic type of lymphoblast based upon a recent French-American-British classification; (4) the hemoglobin level; (5) the response of the bone marrow to initial antileukemic therapy; (6) immunoglobulin levels; (7) platelet count; (8) the presence or absence of central nervous system leukemia at diagnosis; (9) sex; (10) race; and (11) lymphoblast surface markers. Favorable and unfavorable prognostic factors (Table 1) are now being used in most centers to stratify patients at the time of diagnosis and to tailor therapy to the prognostic group of the patient. On the basis of initial WBC and age alone, which account for 75 per cent of the ability to predict remission and survival duration, three prognostic groups emerged in 700 children treated homogeneously in a recent study:

1. Good-prognosis patients, accounting for 27 per cent of the total, had an initial WBC of less than 10,000 per microliter and were between 3 and 7 years of age. Nearly 90 per cent of this group are in complete continuous remission 4 years after diagnosis.

2. An average- or intermediate-prognosis group, accounting for 55 per cent of the total, had initial WBC between 10,000 and 50,000 per microliter in all age groups or were less than 3 or greater than 7 years of age with an initial WBC of less than 10,000 per microliter. About 65 per cent are surviving 48 months after diagnosis.

3. A poor-prognosis group, comprising the remaining 18 per cent, had initial WBC greater than 50,000 per microliter and had a median survival of 2 years.

Interestingly, these factors, except for sex, lose their significance after 2 years and are no longer prognostic for remission duration or survival. Thus, these prognostic factors are most useful for identifying subsets of patients at high risk of induction failure, early relapse, or death. On the basis of these and other studies, children in the poor prognosis group are now receiving more intensive therapy than children in the good-risk and intermediate-risk groups. Still undetermined is whether more aggressive therapy will improve the outlook for patients in the unfavorable prognostic groups. On the other hand, less intensive but equally effective therapy for children in the favorable prognostic group is desirable if survival is prolonged and toxic side effects of treatment are obviated or reduced.

Morphologic subtypes in ANLL are not prognostic, but children with an initial WBC of less than 20,000 per microliter and who are in the age range of 5 to 10 years have a better rate of complete remission induction and a longer median remission duration and survival than do children who have a higher initial WBC or who are younger than 5 years or older than 10 years.

Supportive Care

General measures are required at diagnosis to restore physiologic homeostasis and are common to most varieties of childhood leukemia. Invariably, hospitalization at a center equipped with adequate resources and staff is required during the initial phase of therapy. Metabolic imbalances should be corrected or prevented, adequate hydration restored, deficits of hemoglobin and platelets corrected, and antibiotic treatment of possible infections instituted. Baseline cultures, renal and hepatic function, electrolytes, including calcium and phosphorus, and screening coagulation studies (PT and PTT) should be obtained before starting chemotherapy and should be followed carefully and frequently during the induction phase. Dietary manipulations, except for sodium restriction during steroid therapy and avoidance of pharmacologic doses of folic acid, are not necessary. Treatment in the protected environment of a laminar air flow room with gut sterilization and prophylactic nonabsorbable antibiotics and the use of prophylactic parenteral antibiotics is still experimental. In ANLL, this approach is associated with a lower incidence of septicemia but no improvement in remission rates or overall survival. Most children with ALL at diagnosis can be managed successfully without these special precautions or procedures, which often diminish access to the patient and compound the medical and nursing care without improving the remission rate. Gown-and-mask reverse isolation without specific infectious disease indications serves no useful purpose and is no substitute for meticulous handwashing and early diagnosis and treatment of infections. Psychosocial support is considered at the end of this article.

Anemia. Replacement of normal erythroid precursors by leukemic cells or loss of erythrocytes by hemorrhage invariably results in anemia, which should be treated when the hemoglobin level falls below 8 to 10 grams per dl (100 ml) and when severe infection, hemorrhage, or symptoms of anemia are present. If available, frozen erythrocytes are preferable to packed red cells to reduce the possibility of sensitization by white cell and HL antigens. Since every patient with acute leukemia is a potential recipient of a bone marrow transplant, HL-matched nonfamilial donors of all blood cell products are preferable to relatives and immediate family members.

The amount of red cells transfused depends on the patient's clinical status. A transfusion of 2 ml of red cells per kg of body weight will raise the hemoglobin concentration by 1 gram per dl. Generally, 10 to 15 ml per kg of packed red blood cells may be administered over a 2 to 4 hour

TABLE 1. **Prognostic Factors in Acute Lymphoblastic Leukemia of Childhood**

FACTOR	FAVORABLE	UNFAVORABLE
Demographic		
Age	2–10 years	<2, >10 years
Race	White	Black
Sex	Female	Male
Leukemic burden		
Initial WBC	<20,000 per microliter	>50,000 (>100,000 in girls) per microliter
Adenopathy	Absent	Present
CNS disease at diagnosis	Absent	Present
Hemoglobin	<10 grams per dl	>10 grams per dl
Platelet count	>100,000 per microliter	<100,000 per microliter
Mediastinal mass	Absent	Present
Morphology and histochemistry		
Lymphoblasts	L_1	L_2 or L_3
PAS stain	Positive	Negative
Philadelphia chromosome	Absent	Present
Immunologic factors		
Immunoglobulins	Normal IgG, IgA, IgM	Decreased IgG, IgA, IgM
Surface markers	Common ALL	T or B cell ALL
Response to induction therapy	M_1 marrow (<5% blasts) on day 14	M_3 marrow (>25% blasts) on day 14

period, but with half that volume over 4 to 6 hours if congestive heart failure exists.

Hemorrhage. The second most common cause of death in acute leukemia, after infection, is hemorrhage. Thrombocytopenic bleeding is preventable in the newly diagnosed child with histocompatible platelet concentrates prepared from ABO- and Rh-identical blood. Platelet transfusions should be given to any child with sepsis and active mucous membrane, central nervous system, pulmonary, gastrointestinal, or genitourinary tract bleeding, or such infusions should be given prophylactically if the platelet count falls below 20,000 per microliter, a level associated with an increased risk of life-threatening hemorrhage. Children with platelet counts below 50,000 per microliter who require invasive procedures (e.g., lumbar puncture, lymph node biopsy) should be given prior platelet transfusions as well. In the absence of alloimmunization by platelet or HL antigens, the transfusion of 1 unit of platelet concentrate per 6 kg of body weight will increase the platelet count by 80,000 to 100,000 per microliter, which is adequate for hemostasis. The frequency of platelet transfusions will depend upon the daily post-transfusion platelet count and the clinical condition of the patient. Bleeding, infection, and fever will increase platelet requirements. Salicylates, which impair platelet function by decreasing platelet aggregation, should not be used to treat fever and mild pain. Acetaminophen is the antipyretic of choice.

Severe bleeding may occur secondary to hepatic dysfunction or to disseminated intravascular coagulation (DIC) accompanying sepsis or APML. Fresh frozen plasma, 10 to 15 ml per kg per day, and platelet concentrates will replace most deficient coagulation factors. In APML, prophylactic heparinization with 10 units per kg per hour as a continuous infusion with increments to increase the partial thromboplastin time (PTT) and thrombin time to a value twice normal is beneficial. Endogenous and chemotherapeutically induced release of hydrolytic cytoplasmic granular enzymes triggers DIC, frequently associated with massive intracranial bleeding and death.

Infection. Infection is the primary cause of death in children with acute leukemia. Granulocytopenia caused by marrow replacement or later by therapy-induced bone marrow depression, immunosuppression (both cellular and humoral), damaged anatomic barriers secondary to gastrointestinal toxicity, and deranged granulocyte function induced by radiation or chemotherapy is responsible for the increased susceptibility of the leukemic child to bacterial, fungal, viral, and parasitic infections. About 25 per cent of patients are infected at diagnosis and 50 per cent may have documented infection during the first 6 weeks of therapy. Organisms causing sepsis during induction or remission include *Staphylococcus aureus, Escherichia coli, Pseudomonas aeruginosa, Hemophilus influenzae, Streptococcus pneumoniae,* Klebsiella species, *Proteus mirabilis,* the beta-hemolytic streptococci, and species of Candida.

The incidence of infection is related directly to the degree of granulocytopenia. Severe infection-sepsis (pneumonia, cellulitis, and meningitis) is associated with absolute neutrophil counts (total WBC × per cent neutrophils) below 200 per microliter. Any patient with fever and an absolute neutrophil count below 500 to 1000 per microliter should be suspected to be septic and admitted to the hospital. Chest radiograph and cultures of the blood, nasopharynx, gingiva, cerebrospinal fluid, urine, stool, and perineal area should be obtained and intravenous broad-spectrum antibiotic therapy started. The usual clinical and radiographic signs of infection are often absent in the granulocytopenic leukemic child. An effective initial regimen consists of gentamicin, 5 to 7 mg per kg per day; carbenicillin, 500 mg per kg per day; and a cephalosporin (Keflin), 200 mg per kg per day in divided doses every 4 hours. A semisynthetic penicillin, oxacillin, 200 mg per kg per day every 4 hours, can be used in place of a cephalosporin. Tobramycin, 5 to 7 mg per kg per day, or amikacin, 15 mg per kg per day every 6 hours, should be used in the presence of gentamicin-resistant organisms. If a specific organism is identified, antibiotic therapy should be altered according to in vitro sensitivities in each patient. If bacterial organisms are not isolated but the fever subsides, antibiotics should be continued for at least 7 to 10 days during periods of granulocytopenia. Antibiotics should be discontinued and a search made for opportunistic fungal or viral organisms such as Candida, Histoplasma, Aspergillus, Cryptococcus, cytomegalovirus, and herpes viruses if, after 2 weeks of antibacterial antibiotics, the patient remains febrile. With proved fungal infection, most often involving Candida species, amphotericin B should be started with an initial test dose of 0.1 mg per kg intravenously, and gradually increased to 1 mg per kg per day, infused slowly over a 6 hour period. Potassium levels and renal function chemistries must be followed closely, as hypokalemia, azotemia, and renal tubular acidosis are frequent complications of amphotericin therapy. Hydrocortisone, 25 mg intravenously, may be effective in decreasing severe chills and fever that accompany the amphotericin. The usual treatment course of a documented fungal infection is 4 to 6 weeks. Because of the sustained blood levels of the antibiotic, amphotericin can be given every other day during the latter half of treatment on an outpatient basis.

Suppression of cellular immunity reaches its nadir during the conclusion of central nervous system prophylaxis and the early part of maintenance therapy, particularly during or after tapering and discontinuation of corticosteroid therapy used to induce remission. Interstitial pneumonias caused by opportunistic and atypical infections are a particular problem and require open lung biopsy for diagnosis. Offending organisms include *Pneumocystis carinii*, cytomegalic inclusion virus, adenoviruses, herpes viruses, and fungi. No etiology is uncovered in over 50 per cent of children with interstitial pneumonia. Occasionally pulmonary leukemic infiltration, or cyclophosphamide or methotrexate toxicity, may produce a pneumonitis-like picture clinically and radiographically. The daily administration of prophylactic trimethoprim-sulfamethoxazole (Bactrim, Septra) as 5 mg per kg per day of trimethoprim is of proved benefit in preventing *Pneumocystis carinii* pneumonia. (This use of trimethoprim-sulfamethoxazole is not listed in the manufacturer's official directive.) Since late cases of Pneumocystis pneumonia may occur, prophylaxis should be continued throughout maintenance unless granulocytopenia compromises antileukemia therapy, in which case trimethoprim-sulfamethoxazole should be withheld.

Pneumocystis carinii pneumonia is treated effectively with either oral or intravenous trimethoprim-sulfamethoxazole (20 mg per kg per day and 100 mg per kg per day, respectively, for 10 to 14 days), or with pentamidine isethionate (available from the Center for Disease Control, Atlanta, Georgia), 4 mg per kg per day intramuscularly for 12 to 14 days. Trimethoprim-sulfamethoxazole is as effective as and less toxic than pentamidine and is preferred.

Administration of zoster immune globulin (ZIG) (obtained by contacting the ZIG Distribution Center, Boston, Massachusetts, 617–732–3121) within 3 to 4 days after direct exposure to varicella will modify or prevent clinical varicella in the susceptible child receiving chemotherapy for leukemia. Chemotherapy, especially prednisone, should be tapered or discontinued during the period of risk of developing varicella.

Because antileukemic therapy is associated with chronic immunosuppression and increased susceptibility to viral infections, live-virus vaccines, including measles, mumps, rubella, smallpox, and polio vaccines, should be avoided during treatment. Vaccination with killed-virus vaccines (e.g., influenza) may not be protective unless multiple doses are given.

Electrolyte Imbalance. Both hypercalcemia and hypocalcemia occur during the initial phases of treatment of childhood leukemia. Severe hypercalcemia (serum calcium level > 13 mg per dl), usually caused by ectopic hyperparathyroidism, is managed by vigorous hydration (at four times maintenance value) with 5 per cent dextrose in isotonic saline solution and furosemide, 40 to 80 mg every 4 to 6 hours, which induces a sodium (and calcium) diuresis. Magnesium and potassium depletion may occur as a side effect, and these electrolytes should be added to the intravenous hydration solution. In patients with hypercalcemia and severe renal disease (e.g., uric acid nephropathy) hemodialysis is used. Corticosteroids (hydrocortisone, 10 mg per kg every 12 hours) may be effective. In refractory cases, mithramycin, 25 micrograms per kg every 24 to 48 hours intravenously, reverses hypercalcemia in 48 hours.

Hypocalcemia occurs in patients with a large leukemic cell burden and arises as a complication of vigorous alkalinization of the urine. Initial antileukemic therapy results in hyperphosphatemia and secondary hypocalcemia. Calcium gluconate is used to treat this complication. Alkalinization should be discontinued until the deficiency is corrected.

Hyponatremia resulting from inappropriate antidiuretic hormone (ADH) secretion is a complication of vincristine or cyclophosphamide therapy and is treated with fluid restriction and withholding the offending drugs.

Hyperuricemia. Hyperuricemia characteristically is seen in children with a large leukemic cell burden (high initial WBC, massive organomegaly and adenopathy, leukemic conversion of non-Hodgkin's lymphoma) and reflects the increased degradation of purines, either from increased leukemic cell proliferation and death prior to the initiation of therapy or as a result of the therapy itself. A uric acid level greater than 10 mg per dl frequently results in precipitation of uric acid crystals in the renal tubules and renal failure. Regardless of the level of uric acid or the initial WBC, initial supportive therapy in newly diagnosed leukemic children should include adequate hydration, alkalinization of the urine, and allopurinol therapy. Allopurinol competitively inhibits xanthine oxidase. The catabolism of hypoxanthine to xanthine and xanthine to uric acid is blocked with subsequent increase in the urinary excretion of the more soluble oxypurine metabolites, hypoxanthine and xanthine. Allopurinol is given orally as 10 to 20 mg per kg per day in three divided doses. An intravenous preparation is available through the National Cancer Institute (NCI) as an experimental agent for patients unable to take the orally administered drug. Intravenous solutions with 5 per cent dextrose at a rate of 3000 ml per square meter per 24 hours should be administered to ensure an adequate urine flow. Alkalinization of the urine is achieved with intravenous sodium bicarbonate, 3 to 4 grams (36 to 48 mEq) per square meter per 24 hours to maintain urine pH values of 7.0 to 7.5. Alkalinization may cause hypokalemia and hypocalcemia, and appropriate replacement therapy will be required. This program should be initiated in hyperuricemic patients before chemotherapy is started and should be continued until the uric acid level has returned to normal, the WBC and organomegaly have returned to near normal, and renal function has been restored. The dosage of 6-mercaptopurine, which shares a common degradation pathway with purines, must be reduced by 75 per cent during allopurinol therapy.

If anuria or oliguria occurs, diuresis may be induced by intravenous mannitol infusions. Dialysis may be required in some patients. Diuretics, such as furosemide, which produces an acid urine, and thiazides, which increase serum urate levels and inhibit renal excretion of urate, are contraindicated, as are salicylates, which also inhibit uric acid secretion. Uricosuric agents (probenecid, colchicine, sulfinpyrazone) should be avoided as well because they transiently elevate urine uric acid levels and can exacerbate the nephropathy by increasing the precipitation of urate crystals in the kidneys.

Specific Therapy for ALL

Induction. About 95 per cent of children with ALL achieve an initial complete remission with currently employed multiple drug regimens. The objective of induction therapy is to destroy as many leukemic cells as rapidly as possible, to preserve normal hematopoietic cells, and to restore normal hematopoiesis quickly. Ideal combinations are selectively cytolytic for leukemic cells, are cell-cycle nonspecific in their mechanism of action, and have no significant suppressive effect upon normal marrow progenitor cells. Three agents fulfilling these criteria are prednisone, vincristine, and L-asparaginase (Table 2). Prednisone, 40 mg per square meter per day orally, is given in three divided doses for 28 days; vincristine, 1.5 mg per square meter (maximum 2.0 mg) per week, is given intravenously beginning on the first day of therapy, and then every 7 days thereafter for a total of five doses; and L-asparaginase (*E. coli* strain), 6000 units per square meter intramuscularly every other day of therapy, is given for a total of nine doses. Methotrexate is administered intrathecally on the first day of therapy and again 2 weeks later, if central ner-

vous system (CNS) leukemia is not present at diagnosis. The intrathecal dose of methotrexate is based upon the age-related volume of cerebrospinal fluid (CSF) rather than body surface area in order to decrease potential toxicity, using the following schedule:

Age (Years)	Intrathecal methotrexate dose (mg)
<1	6
1–2	8
2–3	10
>3	12

Patients with CNS leukemia at diagnosis should be given intrathecal methotrexate twice weekly until the CSF is clear, without interruption of induction therapy.

A bone marrow aspiration is performed on day 14 to determine the early response to therapy. If the day 28 bone marrow reveals complete remission (< 5 per cent lymphoblasts) CNS prophylaxis is begun. If the bone marrow is not in complete remission, prednisone and vincristine are continued for an additional 2 weeks (until day 42). The failure to achieve a complete remission after 6 weeks of induction with prednisone, vincristine, and L-asparaginase, or the early lapse of a poor-risk patient after successful induction, necessitates referral to a specialized pediatric cancer center and the use of more potent and investigational forms of therapy.

One of the single most important advances in the recent treatment of childhood ALL has been CNS prophylaxis, the objective of which is the eradication of microfoci of disease in the CNS. If unprotected, the CNS will become the eventual site of extramedullary relapse in 50 per cent of children. With CNS prophylaxis, 90 to 95 per cent of children never develop CNS leukemia. Standard CNS prophylaxis therapy consists of cranial irradiation (1800 rads) utilizing a supervoltage source (^{60}Co or 4 to 6 Mev) administered in a schedule of 180 rads per day, 5 days per week. Intrathecal methotrexate therapy is continued once weekly for four additional doses (total, six) using the same dosage schedule. During CNS prophylaxis, prednisone is tapered over a 2 week period, and 6-mercaptopurine, 75 mg per square meter per day orally, is given at the start of the CNS prophylaxis. Trimethoprim-sulfamethoxazole is also started at this time because the rate of *Pneumocystis carinii* pneumonia is highest during the first 2 months after complete remission is achieved. The bone marrow aspirate and lumbar puncture are repeated on day 56 at the end of CNS therapy. Maintenance therapy is started if the bone marrow remains in complete remission and the CSF is free of lymphoblasts.

The objective of maintenance or continuation therapy is to employ multiple drug combinations to control the disease and prevent bone marrow and extramedullary relapses without inducing severe myelo- or immunosuppression. An effective maintenance program for low-risk patients, and perhaps also for intermediate-risk patients, consists of 6-mercaptopurine, 75 mg per square meter per day orally; methotrexate, 20 mg per square meter per week orally; a monthly single dose of vincristine, 1.5 mg per square meter (maximum, 2.0 mg) intravenously; and prednisone, 40 mg per square meter per day orally in three divided doses for 5 days. During maintenance therapy, bone marrow and spinal fluid surveillance and blood chemistries should be performed every 2 months. Maintenance therapy is continued for 3 years from the completion of CNS prophylaxis. To date 3 years appears to be the optimal length of time of maintenance therapy for patients remaining in complete continuous remission. Males suffer a significantly higher rate of relapse (bone marrow and extramedullary) after discontinuation of maintenance therapy. Accordingly, all males should undergo bilateral open testicular biopsies as well as bone marrow and CNS surveillance prior to the discontinuation of therapy. Occult testicular leukemia has been detected in about 10 to 15 per cent of boys subjected to elective testicular biopsies. Obviously, therapy would be intensified and continued in males with occult testicular disease.

Unfortunately, more aggressive and intensive therapy for poor-risk patients has not improved their survival rates during the past 5 years. Subsets of patients with unfavorable prognostic characteristics (T and B cell leukemia, age under 1 year, initial WBC > 50,000 per microliter) are best referred to pediatric cancer centers for more experimental approaches to therapy. Standard therapy as outlined above is ineffective in this subset.

Physicians responsible for treating a child with ALL must be familiar with the mechanisms of action and side effects of the administered drugs (Table 3). Adequate laboratory and clinical supportive facilities are an obvious prerequisite before treatment can be initiated.

Extramedullary Leukemia. Isolated relapse in the central nervous system, testicles, or other extramedullary sites augurs ill for the patient and may precede bone marrow relapse. Central nervous system relapse can be treated in one of several ways. If the patient had received CNS radiation initially, an additional course of cranial radiation (1800 rads) plus spinal radiation (100 rads) can be given if high-dose methotrexate is not used. The combination of cranial irradiation (> 2400 rads), intrathecal methotrexate, and intravenous methotrexate (> 500 mg per square meter) has been associated with a progressive and sometimes fatal leukoencephalopathy, particularly evident in children with CNS leukemia. The addition of intrathecal or intraventricular methotrexate via an Ommaya shunt, per the dosage schedule described above, weekly for 6 weeks and then monthly is recommended for control of

TABLE 2.   **Chemotherapy of Childhood Acute Leukemia**

ALL	ANLL
Induction	Induction
Prednisone: 40 mg/sq meter/day PO, days 0 to 28 (divided doses tid)	Daunomycin: 30 mg/sq meter/day IV × 3 doses (maximum 540 mg/sq meter)
Vincristine: 1.5 mg/sq meter/week IV, days 0, 7, 14, 21, 28 (maximum 2.0 mg)	5-Azacytidine: 50 mg/sq meter IV, bid × 8 doses
L-Asparaginase: 6000 IU/sq meter IM, days 3, 5, 7, 10, 12, 14, 17, 19, 21	Cytosine arabinoside: 25 mg/sq meter IV q8h × 12 doses
Methotrexate intrathecally (see text for dosage; maximum 12 mg/dose), days 0, 14	Vincristine: 1.5 mg/sq meter/dose IV × 1 dose (maximum 2.0 mg) on first day of each course
Central nervous system prophylaxis	Prednisone: 40 mg/sq meter/day PO (divided doses tid) × 4 days
Cranial irradiation: 1800 rads (180 rads/day, 5 days/week)	Repeat each course every 14 days
Methotrexate intrathecally (see text for dosage; maximum 12 mg/dose), days 28, 35, 42, 49	Maximum 6 courses; minimum 4 courses
Prednisone: taper over 14 days	Maintenance
6-Mercaptopurine: 75 mg/sq meter/day PO	5-Azacytidine: 100 mg/sq meter/day IV × 4 days
Maintenance	Cytosine arabinoside: 75 mg/sq meter/day IV × 4 days
6-Mercaptopurine: 75 mg/sq meter/day PO	Cyclophosphamide: 75 mg/sq meter/day IV × 4 days
Methotrexate: 20 mg/sq meter/week PO	Vincristine: 1.5 mg/sq meter IV on first day of each course (maximum 2.0 mg)
Prednisone: 40 mg/sq meter/day PO (divided dose tid) × 5 days, every 28 days	6-Thioguanine: 75 mg/sq meter/day PO × 28 days
Vincristine: 1.5 mg/sq meter/dose IV, every 28 days (maximum 2.0 mg)	Repeat each course every 28 days
	Methotrexate intrathecally (see text for dosage; maximum 12 mg/dose) every 28 days × 6 courses

TABLE 3. **Side Effects and Toxicities of Drugs Used in Therapy of Childhood Acute Leukemia**

DRUGS	SIDE EFFECTS AND TOXICITIES
Vincristine sulfate	Neurotoxicity (paresthesias, jaw pain, loss of deep tendon reflexes, constipation, obstipation, ileus, hoarseness, sensory loss, ptosis, muscle weakness, slapping gait), local reactions with extravasation, alopecia, inappropriate ADH secretion, fever, and rare seizures.
Prednisone	Hypertension, increased appetite, weight gain, salt retention, cushingoid appearance, personality changes, myopathy, osteoporosis, diabetes mellitus, pancreatitis, increased susceptibility to infection, immunosuppression, and gastrointestinal ulceration
L-Asparaginase	Hypersensitivity reactions (urticaria and anaphylaxis), hepatotoxicity, fever, coagulation abnormalities, azotemia, weight loss, anorexia, nausea, vomiting, transient hyperglycemia, diabetes mellitus, pancreatitis, EEG changes, encephalopathy, and hyperammonemia
6-Mercaptopurine	Bone marrow suppression, hepatotoxicity, oral ulcerations, nausea, and vomiting (toxicity accentuated by allopurinol administration)
Methotrexate	Bone marrow suppression, megaloblastosis, gastrointestinal tract ulcerations, renal toxicity, hepatotoxicity, osteoporosis, pneumonitis, necrotizing enteropathy, anorexia, nausea, vomiting, skin rash, immunosuppression, cerebrospinal fluid pleocytosis, meningismus, arachnoiditis, and leukoencephalopathy
Cytosine arabinoside	Bone marrow suppression, megaloblastic marrow, oral ulcerations, anorexia, nausea, vomiting, fever, diarrhea and abdominal pain, hepatotoxicity, and alopecia
5-Azacytidine	Bone marrow suppression, nausea, vomiting, diarrhea, rash, fever, hepatotoxicity, phlebitis, and local reaction with injection site extravasation
Daunomycin, doxorubicin (Adriamycin)	Bone marrow suppression, gastrointestinal tract ulcerations, anorexia, nausea, vomiting, fever, alopecia, cardiac toxicity, abdominal pain, phlebitis, local reactions with injection site extravasation, and dark urine
Cyclophosphamide	Bone marrow suppression, alopecia, anorexia, nausea, vomiting, hemorrhagic cystitis, bladder fibrosis, sterility, immunosuppression, and inappropriate ADH secretion
6-Thioguanine	Bone marrow suppression, hepatotoxicity, and gastrointestinal abnormalities

CNS relapse, particularly if it occurs concomitantly with bone marrow relapse. Patients unresponsive to intrathecal methotrexate can be treated with cytosine arabinoside, 30 to 50 mg per square meter weekly for six injections, then monthly.

The treatment of choice for testicular relapse is bilateral testicular irradiation, 2000 rads, including the inguinal canal and iliac and para-aortic nodes, if the involvement of these areas is detected by lymphangiography, ultrasonography, computed tomography (CT) scan, or exploratory laparotomy. As with isolated extramedullary relapse, adequate management of testicular relapse requires that the patient be treated with an induction program as outlined above before continuing maintenance therapy.

Specific Therapy for ANLL

Obstacles to the successful treatment of ANLL in children include (1) the necessity of eradicating the malignant pluripotential stem cells to achieve a complete remission, (2) a significantly lower rate of induction of complete remission, (3) inadequate cytoreduction during maintenance, and (4) development of drug resistance.

Complete remissions are achieved in only 65 to 75 per cent of children with ANLL. Early deaths are caused by infection or hemorrhage, or both, often taxing even the most sophisticated support facilities. For these reasons, all children with ANLL should be referred to a pediatric cancer center with early consideration for bone marrow transplantation in selected patients with available HLA and mixed lymphocyte culture (MLC) compatible bone marrow donors.

Induction. To achieve complete remissions in ANLL, induction strategy employs different agents given in intensive courses, followed by rest periods designed to permit recovery of normal hematopoietic tissue. The Children's Cancer Study Group currently is using a five-drug induction regimen given as four to six courses every 14 days. The agents are daunomycin, 30 mg per square meter per day intravenously for three doses; 5-azacytidine, 50 mg per square meter intravenously twice daily for eight doses; cytosine arabinoside, 25 mg per square meter intravenously every 8 hours for 12 doses; vincristine, 1.5 mg per square meter (maximum, 2.0 mg) intravenously for one dose; and prednisone, 40 mg per square meter per day orally for 4 days (Table 2). Bone marrow aspirations are performed after each course, and the courses are repeated until remission is obtained or until a maximum of six courses is given. Daunomycin is discontinued when a total dose of 540 mg per square meter is reached to avoid cardiomyopathy and congestive heart failure. Because cardiomyopathy has been reported at lower total doses, patients must be monitored by serial EKG and cardiac ultrasonography. Maintenance therapy is begun on patients whose bone marrow aspirates contain less than 15 per cent abnormal blast cells and is given with the following drugs in 4 day courses every 28 days: vincristine, 1.5 mg per square meter (maximum 2.0 mg) intravenously on the first day of each course; cyclophosphamide, 75 mg per square meter intravenously per day for 4 days; and 5-azacytidine, 100 mg per square meter intravenously per day for 4 days. Thioguanine, 75 mg per square meter orally per day, is given continuously during maintenance.

An alternative approach to induction consists of daunomycin, 30 mg per square meter per day intravenously for three doses (or doxorubicin [Adriamycin], 30 mg per square meter per day intravenously for three doses), and cytosine arabinoside, 100 mg per square meter intravenously as a 24 hour infusion for 7 days. Repeat cycles are given every 14 days until the bone marrow contains 15 per cent or less blasts. Maintenance therapy is then started as outlined above. The optimal duration of maintenance therapy has yet to be established; conventionally, 3 years is given.

The role of CNS prophylaxis is not defined in ANLL primarily because the duration of remission is so short. The incidence of CNS leukemia in ANLL is about 7 per cent, but the attack rate is similar to that seen in ALL. Accordingly, intrathecal methotrexate, with or without cytosine arabinoside, is given intrathecally every 28 days for six doses during the maintenance phase of therapy.

Bone marrow aspirations should be performed every 2 months during maintenance. Blood chemistries and urinalysis to rule out cyclophosphamide-induced hemorrhagic cystitis should be done monthly. Generally, toxicity with maintenance regimens in ANLL are greater than in ALL, and alterations in drug dosage for hematologic or gastrointestinal toxicity are common (Table 3).

Psychosocial Support

Special competence is required for the medical management of the child with leukemia, but providing emotional support for the patient and the family is invariably more demanding of and challenging to the physician's skills. A team approach from the time of diagnosis is important. The enlistment of the combined resources of medical (attending pediatrician, hematologist-oncologist, house physician), nursing, medical social worker, and community personnel will improve the quality and continuity of care. The financial implications and burdens of the diagno-sis should be recognized early, and families should be referred to appropriate social agencies and societies for aid.

The initial interview with the parents and all subsequent discussions must be frank, open, and honest. These conferences should be held in an environment that minimizes distractions, interruptions, or lack of privacy, allowing ample time for questions. The diagnosis is explained and key aspects of supportive and specific therapy are outlined. Explanations should be simple, and jargon should be avoided. Emotionally distraught parents are unlikely to absorb the finer details of this initial interview. Misconceptions about the disease, parental guilt about delays in seeking medical attention, hereditary aspects, current knowledge about etiology, prognosis, and guidelines for psychosocial management of the patient, siblings, grandparents, and friends should be discussed as well. Considering the excellent remission rates and improved survival in ALL, a cautiously optimistic and hopeful approach is warranted, particularly for children in the good-risk group. Speculative, omniscient predictions of survival times and the creation of false hope should be avoided.

The physician must understand and deal with the initial reactions of shock, guilt, denial, hostility, and anger that frequently occur sequentially. Healthy patterns of adjustment and adaptive mechanisms developed by parents ("coping behavior") will protect them from overwhelming stress and permit them to function more effectively. Normal activities and discipline should be restored and overindulgence avoided.

Open communication between the physician, parents, and child is vital. Parents should be encouraged to contact members of the health care team whenever necessary. The willingness of the hospital staff to answer questions as they arise should be stressed. Follow-up conferences are invariably necessary to reinforce the points and progress made initially. Selected, informative printed materials are helpful.*

Most pediatric hematologists-oncologists agree that children should be told about their diagnosis. The diagnosis should be presented at a level commensurate with the child's age, maturity, and understanding. A child totally cut off from any meaningful discussion concerning his or her disease and its treatment may have anxieties and develop feelings of hopelessness and guilt. All children should be permitted to have an active role, ask questions, and maintain open and honest communication with their parents and

---

*You and Leukemia, A Day at a Time. Mayo Comprehensive Cancer Center, Rochester, Minnesota 55901.

physician. Children accept painful procedures, hospitalization, and changes in therapy or disease status much more readily if they are prepared for them and if they understand their rationale. The child must be allowed to retain hope of recovery, but inappropriate answers lead to increased fear and anxiety, decreased communication, depression, and feelings of abandonment. Fewer withdrawal and depressive reactions occur in patients who are aware of their diagnosis and who have access to honest discussion.

The physician must attend to the needs of the child and the family in a competent, conscientious manner and be available when needed. The family should be given his office and answering service telephone numbers to increase this availability. Competent and responsible medical coverage must always be provided in the absence of the primary physician. Sensitive, personalized, truly continuous care is better offered by one physician, although in many large centers or busy group practices this may be the ideal rather than the reality. The problems and reactions the physician himself may suffer should not be overlooked. Emotional overinvolvement may compromise medical management on the one hand, whereas repulsion by death and the impulse to retreat from medical failures, as exemplified by the relapsed or dying child on the other hand, may deny the child and his family vital emotional support. The physician who is responsible for providing optimal care to children with leukemia must find a compromise between these extremes.

When all reasonable therapeutic measures have failed and the death of a child is imminent, a frank and sympathetic discussion concerning the impending death should be held with the family. Preparing families for the death of a child ("anticipatory grieving") may decrease the sudden, overwhelming sense of loss that occurs in parents who were unwilling or unable to accept the implications of the diagnosis. Parents should be assured that the child's pain will be relieved and that needless procedures or heroic measures will not be entertained. The decision to withdraw life-prolonging care must be made by the responsible physician and discussed with the parents in terms of not prolonging the child's suffering. Frequently, parents will seek reassurance that artificial life support systems and attempts at resuscitation specifically will not be carried out. However, should the parents indicate a desire for prolongation of supportive care, the physician is obligated to continue these efforts. The physician must remain sensitive to the dying child's needs, with maintenance of personal attention, comfort, and adequate care. He must minimize his own tensions and anger, recognize and control his natural repulsion to death, and not reinvest his emotional and intellectual energies elsewhere until after the child dies.

Parents progress through mourning reactions that include sadness, anger, and finally reinvestment of their own energies into life, a process that may require several months. Recent studies have emphasized the high incidence of emotional disturbances and family discord occurring during the course of illness or following the death of a child with leukemia. A prolonged mourning reaction in a couple is an indication for psychiatric consultation. Parents of a deceased child should be encouraged to return for an interview to discuss autopsy findings if appropriate, to clarify unanswered questions, and to help ventilate and extinguish lingering feelings of guilt, anger, and anxiety.

THE CHRONIC LEUKEMIAS

method of
DAVID S. ROSENTHAL, M.D.,
and WILLIAM C. MOLONEY, M.D.
Boston, Massachusetts

Chronic Granulocytic Leukemia (CGL)

The median survival rate of patients with chronic granulocytic leukemia (CGL) has not changed appreciably in the last half century despite new technology and improved chemotherapy. Moreover, over 80 per cent of patients with CGL will develop and die of the "blast cell" transformation. For purposes of clinic research and therapy, we have divided the care of patients into three separate phases: (1) the early or preclinical stage, (2) the active stage, and (3) the blast crisis.

The patient in the *early or preclinical phase of CGL* is asymptomatic. The spleen is usually not palpable, but the diagnosis may be evident by the presence of relatively slight but significant changes in the peripheral blood. Further laboratory investigations reveal a marked decrease in alkaline phosphatase activity in segmented neutrophils and the presence of the Philadelphia (Ph^1) chromosome in the spontaneously dividing marrow cells. These patients may remain asymptomatic for many years. Unfortunately there is still no therapeutic advantage in detecting or treating these patients at an early stage. It has been our policy to withhold therapy for as long as possible, or until the white blood count rises significantly or the patient goes into the active stage. This group of patients, however, may furnish excellent opportunities to study leukemic granulocytes by new techniques.

The *active or symptomatic stage* features are the well recognized clinical and laboratory changes of CGL. As the leukocyte count rises, hypermetabolic symptoms, such as low-grade fever, fatigue, weight loss, and night sweats, may appear. The spleen becomes enlarged, and a low leukocyte alkaline phosphatase (LAP) score is universal. The Ph[1] chromosome is present in 80 to 90 per cent of cases. Specific therapeutic modalities employed in the active stage are listed in Table 1. Ancillary therapeutic modalities include hydration and allopurinol to prevent uric acid complications. Our usual treatment of this stage of disease is phenylalanine mustard (L-PAM, melphalan) given initially in doses of 8 to 10 mg orally per day with weekly follow-up blood counts and dose reduction. In some patients, after 1 month of therapy, the drug can be discontinued. Complete remission will be obtained in nearly all typical cases of CGL, but the drug may have to be intermittently restarted because of recurrent symptoms and a rising white blood cell count. Busulfan, which previously had been the drug of choice, has been used less frequently because with prolonged use cellular atypia occurs in various organs. Pulmonary fibrosis, cataracts, and a peculiar melanosis with addisonian-like syndrome may develop as late complications of busulfan therapy. To date these side effects have not been associated with prolonged L-PAM usage. In one trial, consecutive patients were successfully treated with low doses of splenic irradiation (less than 1000 rads over 14 to 21 days) with prompt fall in the white blood cell count and decrease in spleen size. However, patients all relapsed, and second courses were less successful. In our series of cases radiation to the spleen has been employed only with a very large or painful spleen resistant to chemotherapy. Hydroxyurea has also been used because the drug is thought to be nonmutagenic, unlike alkylating agents such as busulfan and L-PAM.

Hydroxyurea (HU) will cause immediate cytoreduction, occasionally within 1 week from the start of the treatment. Because it has such an immediate effect, blood counts have to be watched more closely, and when the drug is stopped the white blood count may rebound shortly thereafter. The starting dose of HU is 45 mg per kg orally daily, with a maintenance dose of about 20 mg per kg per day. Leukophoresis, originally employed for the emergency clinical situation of leukostasis, has also been used as a primary modality for therapy. This procedure, however, has proved too expensive and time consuming to be a practical method of long-term management.

It is generally conceded that little progress has been made in the treatment of CGL over the past several decades, despite the fact that nearly all typical cases will go into complete remission with the use of an alkylating agent or [32]P. Although it varies, the median survival time is only 40 months. Recently more aggressive measures have been advocated for the active phase, such as multiple drug therapy and splenectomy, in order to eliminate the Ph[1]-positive cells. To date, the results of this approach are unconvincing. More recently, patients who have an available HL-A and mixed lymphocyte culture compatible sibling have undergone bone marrow transplantation. This procedure, although performed in only a few patients at present, has been fairly successful, with complete replacement of the PH[1]-positive marrow cells by the transplanted marrow. Unfortunately, marrow cannot be transplanted in the majority of patients, and investigators are attempting to harvest white cells and marrow for freezing and storage. Since the ultimate cause of death in CGL is blast crisis, the hope would be to reinfuse the CGL cells after intensive chemotherapy for the blast crisis.

Blast crisis, the transition from a well-regulated chronic disorder to the calamitous acute form of leukemia, occurs in over 80 per cent of patients with CGL and is generally resistant to aggressive therapy. Although the median survival time for patients with the active phase of CGL is 40 months, that for patients with blast crisis is measured in weeks. Of 50 patients treated by us with aggressive therapy for blast crisis, only 2 achieved a complete remission and 15 a partial response. Recently, it has been recognized that the cells of some patients in blast crisis have surface properties, biochemical characteristics, and morphology that resemble those of lymphoblasts. Terminal deoxynucleotidyl transferase (TdT) present in almost all patients with acute lymphocytic leukemia (ALL) is found in 20 to 30 per cent of patients with blast crisis. It has become our policy to treat TdT-positive blast crisis pa-

TABLE 1. **Therapy of Chronic Granulocytic Leukemia (CGL)**

Busulfan	Splenic irradiation
Phenylalanine mustard	Leukophoresis
Hydroxyurea	Experimental: multiple drug programs ± splenectomy, marrow transplantation
[32]P	

TABLE 2. **Staging of Chronic Lymphocytic Leukemia (Rai Modification)**

STAGE	DESCRIPTION	AVERAGE SURVIVAL (MONTHS)
0	Lymphocytosis alone	Over 150
I	Lymphocytosis and adenopathy	101
II	Lymphocytosis and splenomegaly	71
III	Lymphocytosis with anemia (Hb < 11 grams/dl Hct < 33%) with or without adenopathy and splenomegaly	19
IV	Lymphocytosis with thrombocytopenia (platelets <100,000/cu mm), with or without anemia and organomegaly	19

tients similarly to those with ALL—i.e., with vincristine and prednisone first. In other patients, aggressive acute leukemic therapy is employed, including combination programs of cytosine arabinoside (Ara-C) and thioguanine, Ara-C and an anthracyclene, or a combination of cyclophosphamide, vincristine, methotrexate, and corticosteroids. However, blast crisis continues to be a form of acute leukemia most resistant to aggressive chemotherapy.

Chronic Lymphocytic Leukemia (CLL)

In CLL, therapy is not indicated solely because of an elevated white blood cell count. However, when anemia, thrombocytopenia, enlarged lymph nodes, splenomegaly, or invasion of the marrow or viscera occurs, therapy becomes necessary. Recent use of an Rai staging classification of CLL has clarified not only when to treat but also what the prognosis of this variable disease should be (Table 2). In Stages III and IV, the anemia and thrombocytopenia referred to are related to marrow infiltration and are not secondary to an immune mechanism. As with the preclinical phase of CGL, it may not be necessary to treat the patient with Stage 0, I, or II disease unless the enlargement of nodes or spleen is causing mechanical or aesthetic problems. If the nodes are quite large or the splenomegaly causes compressive symptoms, chemotherapy or local irradiation therapy may be employed. Alkylating agents, chlorambucil or cyclophosphamide, are used most commonly. Chlorambucil is administered in daily doses of 0.2 mg per kg of body weight orally. As the white blood cell count falls, the dose is reduced accordingly and the patient is maintained on 2 mg daily or every other day. Chlorambucil is quite effective, has relatively few toxic reactions, and is slow acting; however, long-term use has been associated with an increased incidence of acute nonlymphocytic leukemia. For

this reason, alkylating agents are now given in pulse oral form rather than as maintenance therapy: for example, for 7 consecutive days of every 4 weeks, an oral dose of chlorambucil at 0.2 mg per kg per day is given. When remission occurs, the drug may be stopped, and if symptoms or signs recur, therapy is restarted. Local radiation therapy in palliative doses (less than 2000 rads) may alleviate the symptoms of the enlarged nodes and spleen.

In the more aggressive stages, (Stages III and IV), intensive therapy similar to the treatment of non-Hodgkin's lymphoma may be necessary. If a simple alkylating agent is not beneficial, then addition of a corticosteroid, such as prednisone, 50 mg per day, may be helpful. Other combinations include weekly intravenous cyclophosphamide at 10 mg per kg and vincristine, 1 mg per sq meter, and oral prednisone at 50 mg daily. Relatively low doses of total body irradiation (TBI), 100 to 150 rads given over 4 to 5 weeks, has also been shown to produce good remissions. Comparative studies comparing TBI and chemotherapy are pending.

The immune complications of CLL, autoimmune hemolytic anemia and immune thrombocytopenia purpura, are best treated by prednisone and splenectomy if the immune process becomes refractory to corticosteroids.

It is somewhat discouraging to note that although chemical agents and ionizing radiation may induce remissions in both forms of chronic leukemia, little is known concerning either the cause or the pathogenesis of the disease. It seems unlikely that much progress will be made in the management of chronic leukemia until more is known about the basic biologic and metabolic activities of leukemic cells.

NON-HODGKIN'S LYMPHOMAS

method of
GIANNI BONADONNA, M.D.
Milan, Italy

The term non-Hodgkin's lymphomas (NHL) comprises a group of primary neoplasms of the lymphoreticular tissue involving stem cells and lymphocytes in varying degrees of differentiation. They occur essentially in a homogeneous population of single cell type. The term itself and the many classifications proposed reflect the difficulties encountered in the morphologic classification of these proliferative processes. During the past two decades important advances have been made, particularly in terms of histopathology, natural history, staging, and therapeutic approach. The diagnostic evaluation and the treatment of NHL demand considerable technical resource and skilled personnel. Consequently, before embarking on a staging work-up in a patient with malignant lymphoma, the physician should carefully and honestly evaluate the diagnostic and therapeutic facilities available to him. If these are inadequate, he should refer the patient to an established diagnostic treatment center. This recommendation particularly applies to patients with large cell lymphomas.

Histopathology

NHL comprise a broad spectrum of cell types and histopathologic patterns, and their accurate diagnosis and classification constitute one of the more difficult topics in morphologic pathology. An unequivocal diagnosis of malignant lymphoma can be made only by microscopic examination of one or more tissue specimens. Prerequisites include adequate biopsies and technical excellence in preparation of the tissue slides. Without benefit of the normal architecture of an intact lymph node, the pathologist frequently cannot differentiate a malignant lymphoma from a benign process. In primary extranodal lymphoma not associated with regional or distant lymphadenopathy, a tissue sample can often cause problems as to correct classification of the histologic subgroups. In recent years, the use of electron microscopy morphology and the study of immunologic membrane markers have greatly improved the classification of human lymphoid malignancies.

About a decade ago the histologic classification based on lymph node structure that Rappaport proposed in 1956 was in effect rediscovered and gradually applied to clinicopathologic as well as to treatment studies. The original as well as the revised Rappaport classification (Table 1), although not up to date with modern immunologic concepts, was found by clinicians to be an effective tool in identifying important distinctions in prognosis between the generally indolent nodular (or follicular) lymphomas and the more aggressive diffuse lymphomas. In addition to architectural patterns of growth, the Rappaport scheme describes the malignant cell population as lymphocytic, histiocytic, or mixed lymphocytic-histiocytic. Here, too, there is prognostic value, for in both the nodular and diffuse lymphomas a lymphocytic cytology is more favorable than a histiocytic one. The histiocytic lymphoma is the most common cell type, with poorly differentiated lymphocytic lymphoma the next most frequent. Most dissatisfaction with the Rappaport scheme resulted from the recognition that many lymphomas, termed histiocytic on morphologic grounds alone, have recently been shown by ultrastructural and immunologic techniques to be neoplasms of large transformed lymphocytes. Therefore, the term "histiocytic" is a misnomer and true histiocytic tumors are very rare. Thus, the Rappaport classification has become obsolete in concept, although it is still currently used by many hemopathologists. Another important objection to the continued use of the Rappaport classification is that it fails in some areas to distinguish certain entities of widely differing prognosis.

For the reasons mentioned above, in recent years there have been many attempts at providing new classification systems. With new immunologic and cytochemical techniques it is now widely acknowledged that all nodular lymphomas are composed of monoclonal neoplastic follicular B lymphocytes. Approximately 50 to 60 per cent of large cell lymphomas (Rappaport: histiocytic, mixed lymphocytic-histiocytic, and undifferentiated) have B cell features, while fewer (5 to 10 per cent) have T cell markers, and about one third lack detectable markers ("undefined" or "null"). In Burkitt's tumor "primitive" cells may be related to some B lymphocytes of normal germinal centers. In about 50 per cent of lymphoblastic lymphomas there are distinctive convoluted nuclear configurations (convoluted lymphoblastic lymphoma) and the immunologic features indicate that this new clinicopathologic entity is probably identical to acute lymphoblastic leukemia of T cell type. Other lymphoreticular neoplasms in which T cell markers have been detected in most cases are mycosis fungoides and Sézary's syndrome. The most widely debated and well founded classifications are those based on functional studies, such as the classification of Lukes and Collins and the Lennert classification, subsequently revised into the Kiel classification. Based on detailed morphologic studies of follicle center cells, together with cytochemical studies and some immunologic parameters, the Lukes and Collins and Kiel classifications are very similar in concepts but have an entirely distinct terminology.

In January 1980, at the conclusion of a large retrospective clinicopathologic study sponsored by the National Cancer Institute (NCI), a working formulation for clinical use was recommended in Palo

TABLE 1. Revised Rappaport Classification for Non-Hodgkin's Lymphomas

HISTOLOGIC SUBGROUPS	RELATIVE INCIDENCE (%)*	FIVE YEAR SURVIVAL (%)*
Nodular pattern		
Lymphocytic, well differentiated	1–2	75
Lymphocytic, poorly differentiated	15–20	70
Mixed lymphocytic-histiocytic	15–20	50
Histiocytic	4–7	70
Diffuse pattern		
Lymphocytic, well differentiated (with or without plasmacytoid features)	2–3	65
Lymphocytic, poorly differentiated (with or without plasmacytoid features)	8–15	40
Mixed lymphocytic-histiocytic	8–12	35
Histiocytic (with and without sclerosis)	28–35	40
Undifferentiated	1–2	< 10
Burkitt's tumor	1–2	< 5
Lymphoblastic (with or without convoluted cells)	2–3	30
Unclassified		

*In patients older than 15 years.

TABLE 2. **A Working Formulation of Non-Hodgkin's Lymphoma for Clinical Use—Recommendation of an Expert International Panel***

I. Low grade malignancy
   A. Malignant lymphoma
     Small lymphocytic
     Consistent with chronic lymphocytic leukemia
     Plasmacytoid
   B. Malignant lymphoma, follicular
     Predominantly small cleaved cell
     Diffuse areas
     Sclerosis
   C. Malignant lymphoma, follicular
     Mixed, small cleaved and large cell
     Diffuse areas
     Sclerosis

II. Intermediate grade malignancy
   D. Malignant lymphoma, follicular
     Predominantly large cell
     Diffuse areas
     Sclerosis
   E. Malignant lymphoma, diffuse
     Small cleaved cell
     Sclerosis
   F. Malignant lymphoma, diffuse
     Mixed, small and large cell
     Sclerosis
     Epithelioid cell component
   G. Malignant lymphoma, diffuse
     Large cell
     Cleaved cell
     Noncleaved cell
     Sclerosis

III. High grade malignancy
   H. Malignant lymphoma
     Large cell, immunoblastic
     Plasmacytoid
     Clear cell
     Polymorphous
     Epithelioid cell component
   I. Malignant lymphoma
     Lymphoblastic
     Convoluted cell
     Nonconvoluted cell
   J. Malignant lymphoma
     Small noncleaved cell
     Burkitt's tumor
     Follicular areas
   K. Miscellaneous
     Composite
     Mycoses fungoides
     Histiocytic
     Extramedullary plasmacytoma
     Unclassifiable
     Other

*Palo Alto, California, January 11, 1980.

Alto, California by an expert international panel (Table 2). In preparing the formulation, the experts have taken into consideration both the survival results of the aforementioned study and the different viewpoints, including terminology, concerning the appropriate morphologic classification of NHL. This formulation is currently being tested in many special-ized centers. Although its actual reproducibility and clinical relevance remain to be fully determined, the formulation represents, after innumerable controversies and debates, a step forward at least to exchange of information, utilizing a common, updated terminology.

Diagnostic Evaluation and Staging

The therapy prescribed for the patient with a lymphoma is dependent on the exact morphologic diagnosis as well as on the knowledge of the anatomic extent of that disorder. When lymphadenopathy is present, one or more intact lymph nodes must be excised. The most satisfactory nodes for the histopathologist are those from lower cervical or axillary regions. The pleomorphic presentation of NHL (e.g., pharynx, gastrointestinal tract, testicle, skeleton) requires different surgical approaches to establish the correct diagnosis. For certain anatomic sites (e.g., stomach, breast, uterus, testicle, thyroid) the diagnosis of carcinoma rather than that of lymphoma is frequently made on clinical grounds, and only histopathology reveals the presence of NHL once radical surgery is performed. When primary extranodal lymphoma presents with regional or distant adenopathy, biopsy from both lesions is highly recommended for a more precise histologic classification. Needle biopsy and frozen sections are contraindicated.

Accurate clinical (CS) and pathologic (PS) staging remain essential to the management of NHL, regardless of age and cell type. In general, once the diagnosis has been established, the principal aim of the staging work-up is to perform a sufficient number of procedures to determine whether or not the lymphoma is widely disseminated (Table 3). If involvement of the bone marrow is documented, the remainder of the work-up is concerned with collecting information necessary to properly assess the response to treatment (restaging). Ancillary procedures required in certain selected patients include mediastinal and chest tomograms, intravenous pyelogram (if bulky retroperitoneal nodes are present or if abdominal radiotherapy is planned); skeletal survey; roentgenogram of the base of skull; radioisotopic evaluation of liver, spleen, bone, and brain; abdominal sonography and/or computed tomography; and additional laboratory tests (e.g., Coombs' test, serum protein electrophoresis, quantitative immunoglobulin, cell membrane immunologic markers, labeling index). In children excessive staging procedures (e.g., laparoscopy) do not appear to be worthwhile in devising a therapeutic strategy. However, CS (whenever possible with lymphography) must be supplemented by marrow biopsy and cytologic examination of spinal fluid. If patients achieve apparent complete remission, pathologic restaging is indicated to establish whether further treatment is required. Repeat bone marrow and liver biopsies can in fact detect residual foci of disease in 5 to 25 per cent of patients.

Staging Classification

For the time being, the Ann Arbor international staging classification adopted for Hodgkin's disease (Table 4) remains the staging system to be utilized

TABLE 3. **Procedures Recommended
for Proper Staging**

Clinical staging
1. Detailed history with special attention to the presence or absence of systemic symptoms
2. Careful physical examination, emphasizing peripheral node chains, size of liver and spleen, Waldeyer ring, and bony tenderness
3. Adequate surgical biopsy reviewed by an experienced hemopathologist; in primary extranodal lymphomas biopsy should also include a lymph node when palpable
4. Routine laboratory tests: complete blood count, erythrocyte sedimentation rate, liver function tests, serum uric acid, serum copper
5. Chest roentgenogram (posteroanterior and lateral) and bilateral lower extremity lymphography
6. Roentgenologic examination of the gastrointestinal tract; gastroscopy should be added in the presence of Waldeyer's ring involvement

Pathologic staging
1. Core needle biopsy and aspirate of bone marrow from both posterior iliac crests
2. Laparoscopy with multiple liver biopsies (4 to 6) if bone marrow is normal and no other distant extranodal lesions are present
3. Staging laparotomy with splenectomy, needle and wedge biopsy of liver, and biopsies of paraaortic, mesenteric, portal, and splenic hilar lymph nodes—may be necessary as a final procedure for CS I diffuse "histiocytic" lymphoma
4. Lumbar puncture with cytologic examination of cerebrospinal fluid in all NHL of children
5. Cytologic examination of any effusion

also for NHL of adults and children. However, at the meeting held in Palo Alto in January 1980, a proposed modification of the staging system was considered in relation to the grade of malignancy. Thus, as illustrated in Table 4, patients with Stages I and II in the Ann Arbor classification may be grouped as Stage I if they have low grade malignant lymphoma, whereas those with Stage IV for only bone marrow invasion may be classified as Stage III, since the marrow involvement is a very common finding and does not represent per se a severe prognostic factor. In the other histologic subgroups, patients with Stages I to III and bulky disease could be classified as Stage IV according to the new staging proposal because of the prognostic relevance of massive disease. The definition of bulky disease in the thoracic cavity includes lymphoma occupying more than one third of the diameter of the chest; within the abdominal cavity, the lymphoma must be 10 cm in diameter or greater. As already mentioned for the histopathologic formation, the staging proposal must also be tested within research institutions in a large series of consecutive adults and children before being adopted as a new staging system.

Principles of Therapy

Modern treatment strategy for adults with NHL should first take into consideration the histologic subgroup and the disease extent. The underlying treatment principles are primarily based on the Rappaport and Ann Arbor classifications. High-energy radiotherapy (RT) still rep-

TABLE 4. **The Ann Arbor Classification and the New Staging Proposal**

		STAGING PROPOSAL	
ANN ARBOR SYSTEM	STAGE	Low Grade	Intermediate and High Grade
Involvement of a single lymph node region or of a single extranodal organ or site (I_E)	I	I	I
Involvement of two or more lymph node regions on the same side of the diaphragm, or localized involvement of an extranodal organ or site (II_E) and of one or more lymph node regions on the same side of the diaphragm	II		II
Involvement of lymph node regions on both sides of the diaphragm, which may also be accompanied by localized involvement of an extranodal organ or site (III_E) or spleen (III_S) or both (III_{SE})	III	II	III
Diffuse or disseminated involvement of one or more distant extranodal organs with or without associated lymph node involvement	IV Bone marrow only	III	A.A.*I-III Bulky IV
	IV Other	IV	

Fever >38 C (100.5 F), night sweats, and/or weight loss >10 per cent of body weight in the 6 months preceding admission are defined as systemic symptoms, and denoted by the suffix letter B. Asymptomatic patients are denoted by the suffix letter A. Biopsy-documented involvement of Stage IV sites is identified by the following symbols: marrow, M+; liver, H+; lung, L+; pleura, P+; bone, O+; skin, D+.

*A.A.: Ann Arbor system.

TABLE 5. **Single Agents Effective in Non-Hodgkin's Lymphomas***

DRUGS	USUAL DOSE, ROUTE, INTERVAL	CR PLUS PR (%)	MAJOR TOXICITY
Alkylating agents			
Chlorambucil	3–8 mg/m² PO daily	45–65	Bone marrow
Cyclophosphamide	1200 mg/m² IV q 3–4 weeks 300–500 mg/m² IV weekly 60–100 mg/m² PO daily	55–65	Bone marrow, cystitis, alopecia, nausea, vomiting
Vinca alkaloids			
Vincristine	1–2 mg/m² IV weekly	40–65	Neuropathy, constipation
Vinblastine	3–6 mg/m² IV weekly	20–35	Bone marrow, neuropathy
Vindesine	3–4 mg/m² IV q 7–10 days	30–40	Neuropathy, bone marrow
Antibiotics			
Doxorubicin (Adriamycin)	60 mg/m² IV q 3 weeks	45–65	Bone marrow, alopecia, vomiting, stomatitis, cardiomyopathy after 550 mg/m²
Bleomycin	5–10 units/m² IV weekly	35–45	Fever, stomatitis, hair loss, skin lesions, lung fibrosis after 200–250 mg/m²
Antimetabolites			
Methotrexate	20–30 mg/m² IM twice in a week 40–60 mg/m² IV weekly	25–30	Stomatitis, bone marrow
Cytosine arabinoside	150 mg/m² IV for 5 days q 2–3 weeks	25–30	Bone marrow
Nitrosourea derivatives			
Carmustine (BCNU)	150–250 mg/m² IV q 6–8 weeks	20–35	Bone marrow (delayed), local pain on administration
Lomustine (CCNU)	80–130 mg/m² PO q 6–8 weeks	15–25	Bone marrow (delayed)
Miscellaneous			
Procarbazine	75–150 mg/m² PO daily	30–50	Bone marrow
VP-16	250–300 mg/m² IV weekly	20–30	Bone marrow
L-Asparaginase	10,000–15,000 units/m² IV for 15 days q 2–3 weeks	40	Vomiting, allergic reaction, hepatic toxicity
Corticosteroids			
Prednisone	25–100 mg/m² PO daily	20–80	Diabetes, hypertension, osteoporosis, peptic ulcer

*Some agents mentioned in this table are considered investigational. Before using any of the drugs mentioned here, the physician should be well informed of their action, of their proper dose, and of the information in the manufacturers' official directives.

resents an important therapeutic tool for the large majority of adult patients with localized nodal or extranodal lymphoma regardless of the histologic subgroup. If such therapy is delivered in adequate doses (3500 to 4500 rads in about 4 weeks) and volumes, the cure rate can be maximized. At least the proximal adjacent clinical uninvolved nodal region(s) should always be included in the radiation field (regional extended RT). Since the main reason for treatment failure is not local recurrence but rather disease outside the irradiated area(s), namely extranodal sites, the question of whether RT should be supplemented with some form of systemic therapy has been considered in the past few years. As the result of prospective randomized studies carried out particularly in Milan and in other European centers, there is now evidence, in diffuse lymphomas treated with regional extended RT, that adjuvant combination chemotherapy can improve the 5 year relapse-free and total survival rates over use of RT alone. In selected patients with Stages III and IV follicular lymphomas, appreciable results can be obtained by utilizing total body irradiation (TBI) as primary treatment, since this type of irradiation offers a high probability of complete remission for an extended period of time with a minimum of attendant morbidity. TBI must be administered by use of conventional cobalt teletherapy unit or linear accelerator, and usually a 15 rad dose is given twice a week until the total dose of 150 rads is reached. A local boost irradiation of 1000 to 2000 rads is indicated in those with persistent disease after TBI.

NHL are notoriously responsive to chemotherapy. Table 5 lists the cytotoxic drugs most often utilized in clinical practice along with their conventional dose when administered as single agents and the major side effects. Today, single agent chemotherapy is seldom administered as first treatment and in but a few circumstances: (1) advanced lymphomas with low grade malignancy; (2) elderly patients with concomitant severe illnesses; (3) extremely low performance status; (4) patients living in isolated areas; and (5) patients with psychologic disturbances. In such instances, usually starting with one of the alkylating agents, chemotherapy is continued until the patient relapses or excessive toxicity occurs. Once the initial response is obtained, maintenance treatment is required to keep the patient in either complete or partial remission with minimal bone marrow toxicity. If and when the lymphoma becomes refractory to the alkylating agents, vincristine is tried next; when chemotherapy is still indicated because of further progression, one of the new effective antibiotics (doxorubicin [Adriamycin] or bleomycin) can be given.

The use of multiple drug combinations has revolutionized the chemotherapy of NHL. Today, several drug regimens are available, and Table 6 reports some of the most representative combinations utilized in NHL. Although none can specifically be recommended as the treatment of choice for given histopathologic subgroups, regimens containing doxorubicin (Adriamycin), bleomycin, and antimetabolites are considered particularly indicated in the management of lymphomas with high grade malignancy. The

difference in the reported incidence of complete response is primarily dependent upon the type of restaging (clinical vs. pathologic) carried out at the end of treatment. The principal aim of poly-drug chemotherapy is to achieve a prompt complete remission. There should not be a fixed period of induction therapy. Patients should receive, at a minimum, 6 cycles of therapy at maximally tolerated doses. If at the end of this period they are considered to be in pathologic complete remission, 2 more cycles of chemotherapy should be given as consolidation treatment. In some patients with nodular lymphomas or diffuse lymphocytic poorly differentiated lymphomas in the Rappaport classification, as many as 12 to 14 cycles are required before the patient can be considered in true complete remission. Once pathologic complete remission has been achieved, there seems to be no real advantage in prolonging treatment either with the same combination or with single agents in patients with diffuse histology. Re-treatment with the same combination at the time of relapse appears to be a

TABLE 6.   **Examples of Combination Chemotherapy Useful in Non-Hodgkin's Lymphomas***

ACRONYM	DRUGS	DOSE (MG/M^2)	DAYS OF TREATMENT	FREQUENCY
CVP†	Cyclophosphamide	400 PO	1 to 5	q 21 days
	Vincristine	1.4 IV	1	
	Prednisone	100 PO	1 to 5	
ABP	Doxorubicin (Adriamycin)	60–75 IV	1	q 21 days
	Bleomycin	10 units IV	1 and 8	
	Prednisone	100 PO, IM	1 to 5	
B-CHOP	Bleomycin	15 units IV	1 and 5	q 14–21 days
	Cyclophosphamide	750 IV	1	
	Doxorubicin (Adriamycin)	50 IV	1	
	Vincristine	2‡ IV	1 and 5	
	Prednisone	100‡ PO	1 to 5	
BACOP†	Bleomycin	5 units IV	15 and 22	q 28 weeks
	Doxorubicin (Adriamycin)	25 IV	1 and 8	
	Cyclophosphamide	650 IV	1 and 8	
	Vincristine	1.4 IV	1 and 8	
	Prednisone	60 PO	15 to 28	
M-BACOD	Methotrexate§	3000 IV	1	q 21 days
	Bleomycin	4 units IV	1	
	Doxorubicin (Adriamycin)	45 IV	1	
	Cyclophosphamide	600 IV	1	
	Vincristine	1 IV	1	
	Dexamethasone	6 PO	1 to 5	
COMLA	Cyclophosphamide	1500 IV	1	q 91 days
	Vincristine	1.4 IV	1, 8, 15	
	Methotrexate	120 IV	22, 29, 36, 43, 50, 57, 64, 71	
	Leucovorin	25 IM	q 6 hr × 4 doses; start 24 hrs after methotrexate	
	Cytosine arabinoside	300 IV	22, 29, 36, 43, 50, 57, 64, 71	

*Some agents mentioned in this table are considered investigational. Before using any of the drugs mentioned here, the physician should be well informed of their action, of their proper dose, and of the information in the manufacturers' official directives.

†NCI regimens.

‡Milligrams per day.

§Plus citrovorum factor.

much preferable therapeutic approach. We have observed in Milan that re-treatment with CVP alternated with ABP chemotherapy could induce a second complete remission in about half the patients with relapse, and the median duration of second response was in excess of 12 months. In patients not responding to re-treatment with the same regimen the prognosis is usually poor, particularly in the presence of large cell lymphomas. New drugs such as VP-16* or vindesine* can be tried, as well as L-asparaginase, vinblastine, procarbazine, cytosine arabinoside, or high dose methotrexate with citrovorum factor, either alone or in different combinations. Objective response, and occasionally complete remission, can be observed in not more than 20 to 30 per cent of patients and for a limited period of time (2 to 6 months).

Stages I and II, Nodular Histology. In this group of patients the suggested primary treatment is regional extended high energy radiotherapy (RT) to a tumor dose of about 4500 rads. The total 5 year survival is about 90 per cent. There is little evidence to support the use of total nodal RT in patients whose pathologic staging (PS) was carried out without exploratory laparotomy. Since occult mesenteric lymphadenopathy can be present in as many as 40 per cent of patients with negative lymphogram, if RT is to be administered with curative intent and surgical staging with laparotomy has not been performed, it would be advisable to encompass the entire abdominal contents (abdominal bath). In our experience, 6 cycles of adjuvant CVP (see Table 6) following regional extended RT have not significantly improved the 5 year relapse-free and total survival rates compared to RT alone. Therefore, unless one utilizes a more intensive and prolonged drug regimen, chemotherapy should be reserved for patients with relapse.

Stages I and II, Diffuse Histology. Regional extended RT must be supplemented with adjuvant chemotherapy. Our experience with 6 cycles of adjuvant CVP showed significantly improved 5 year relapse-free (76 per cent) and total survival rates (80 per cent), compared to irradiation alone (relapse-free 45 per cent, survival 52 per cent), both in lymphocytic and in histiocytic lymphomas. There was, however, marked distinction in the relapse-free survival between PS I (91 per cent) and PS II (53 per cent). Currently, we administer chemotherapy first (3 cycles) followed by regional extended radiotherapy, and treatment is completed with 3 more cycles of chemotherapy. In fact, if the rationale of employing chemotherapy is to eradicate tumor outside the irradiated volume, it seems illogical to delay

*May not be available or approved for use in the United States of America.

introduction of the systemic treatment. Furthermore, we utilize a combination containing doxorubicin (Adriamycin) and bleomycin (BACOP), and preliminary results appear more promising than with CVP, particularly in Stage II disease. Clinicians should be aware that in the presence of primary extranodal localizations or diffuse histiocytic lymphoma a tumor dose of at least 5000 rads must be delivered, as local (true) recurrence is not infrequent. Furthermore, RT for head and neck lymphomas, particularly those involving extranodal sites such as the orbital region or the paranasal sinuses, requires a very accurate technical approach to avoid severe postirradiation complications. Brilliant results were achieved by some investigators in diffuse histiocytic lymphoma either with total nodal RT alone in PS I after laparotomy or with intensive chemotherapy (CHOP) alone. Since, as outlined before, "histiocytic" lymphomas actually comprise different histologic subgroups, we do not presently recommend the routine use of the aforementioned forms of treatment.

Stages III and IV, Nodular Histology. There are no firm guidelines for routine primary treatment approach in all histopathologic subgroups. In the large majority of patients the disease can be easily controlled for prolonged periods of time with simple, relatively nontoxic regimens. Therefore, the patients should be started with single oral alkylating agent therapy, using a drug such as chlorambucil (see Table 5). Immediately prior to therapy patients are given allopurinol, 100 mg orally three times daily, to prevent urate nephropathy. Allopurinol may be discontinued after about 1 month of chemotherapy and serum uric acid monitored. Complete blood counts (CBC) and platelet counts are obtained weekly for the first 6 to 8 weeks and monthly thereafter. When the absolute granulocyte count falls below 2000 per cu mm or platelet count below 100,000 per cu mm, chemotherapy must be temporarily discontinued. When, after about 2 months of therapy, the disease is brought to good partial or complete remission, the drug dose is usually decreased by 50 per cent and treatment is continued until unequivocal signs of disease progression occur. There is a highly selective group of patients with nodular lymphomas who have limited extensive disease (small adenopathies, absence of large hepatosplenomegaly, no symptoms) and appear to have more indolent disease. They may be followed for prolonged periods of time without specific therapy. Treatment can be instituted when there is evidence of increasing adenopathy, hepatosplenomegaly, and systemic symptoms. Alternative treatments are represented by total body irradiation (TBI) or combination chemotherapy. They could be instituted in patients with particularly rapidly progressive lymphoma or bulky or symptomatic disease at the time of diagnosis or at relapse following the administration of chlorambucil. In nodular lymphocytic lymphomas TBI produces an overall 5 year survival ranging from 60 to 72 per cent.

TBI should not be considered a curative treatment, since all patients eventually relapse. At this point, they should be given combination chemotherapy. At times there are difficulties in repeating courses of TBI because of prolonged thrombocytopenia and the long-term bone marrow suppression resulting from this modality may prevent the effective use of subsequent combination chemotherapy. The polydrug regimen of choice is CVP or COP (see Table 6). Regardless of the schedule, response to therapy is usually prompt, and in more than 50 per cent of patients complete remission is achieved. Patients should receive allopurinol immediately prior to therapy. CBC and platelet counts are obtained weekly for the first two to three courses. If the nadir of absolute granulocyte counts is <1000 per cu mm or of platelets <75,000 per cu mm, the dose of cyclophosphamide should be decreased by 50 per cent in the subsequent course. The dose of this drug can be resumed to 100 per cent only if blood counts permit. Patients expected to have limited bone marrow reserve (age >65 years, prior TBI, prior chemotherapy) should be cautiously started at a 50 per cent dose, with subsequent escalation only if leukopenia or thrombocytopenia or both are moderate. CVP or COP also produce peripheral neuropathy, and severe paresthesias or foot drop is an indication to withhold vincristine temporarily.

Additional toxicities, including nausea and vomiting, hemorrhagic cystitis (discontinue cyclophosphamide and substitute another alkylating agent), alopecia, constipation, and loss of deep tendon reflexes, are fairly often observed. Gastric disturbances caused by corticosteroids and occasionally a bleeding gastric or duodenal ulcer may be encountered in patients treated for prolonged periods of time. The main problem with combination chemotherapy in nodular lymphomas is the duration of treatment. Since this type of lymphoma shows a high tendency to recur following treatment interruption, it is recommended in complete responders to administer maintenance therapy, utilizing a lower dose schedule. At relapse, other non-cross-resistant drug regimens, including doxorubicin (Adriamycin) or bleomycin, alone or in combination such as ABP, should be given. The expected response rate ranges from 30 to 50 per cent, and occasionally prolonged remissions are observed. In the presence of bulky adenopathy, palliative RT (2000 to 3000 rads) is indicated.

Stages III and IV, Diffuse Histology. Except for diffuse, well differentiated lymphocytic lymphoma, which is associated with a course and prognosis (low grade malignancy) similar to that of chronic lymphocytic leukemia, the diffuse lymphomas are definitely more aggressive tumors and they require prompt treatment of a more aggressive nature. In adult patients prognosis has definitely been improved only by the intensive application of various types of combination chemotherapy (Table 6). In this group relapse-free survival can be used as a measure of the efficacy of medical therapy. Currently, the most effective regimens are those including the new cytotoxic antibiotics (e.g., CHOP, BACOP, CVP alternated every 3 weeks with ABP) and/or the antimetabolites (e.g., M-BACOD, COMLA). High-dose methotrexate with citrovorum factor appears useful in decreasing or preventing lymphomatous meningeal infiltration because of methotrexate concentration in the cerebrospinal fluid. Since at present the combination of choice does not exist, it is difficult to suggest the optimal regimen to use in clinical practice. If the physician is not familiar with the use of high-dose methotrexate, he should not embark on the administration of M-BACOD or COMLA. Rather, he should properly utilize one of the regimens containing doxorubicin (Adriamycin) and bleomycin. Allopurinol should be administered as outlined for nodular lymphomas and CBC obtained weekly for the first 2 months and just before each course thereafter. Physicians should be aware that downward adjustments in the initial doses are required in patients with extensive prior irradiation, those over 65 years, or those with other evidence of impaired bone marrow reserve. Furthermore, the initial dose of doxorubicin (Adriamycin) should be reduced by 50 to 70 per cent in the presence of hepatic dysfunction. If the patients tolerate reduced doses well, gradual escalations toward full dosages should be attempted on subsequent courses of treatment. It is important to remember that the total cumulative dose of doxorubicin (Adriamycin) should be restricted to 550 mg per square meter of body surface area (450 mg per square meter in patients with prior mediastinal irradiation). Doxorubicin (Adriamycin) is probably contraindicated in patients with concomitant or past history of severe heart disease, congestive heart failure, or cardiomyopathy. Since pulmonary fibrosis is seen in 5 to 10 per cent of patients receiving bleomycin, the total cumulative dose should not exceed 250 units per square meter of body surface, and chest x-ray and pulmonary function tests should be utilized. Bleomycin is probably contraindicated in patients with severe pulmonary disease (e.g., emphysema, tuberculosis, prior lung irradiation).

Complete remission in pathologically restaged patients ranges from 55 to 65 per cent. The response rate is usually lower in patients with Stage IV (55 to 60 per cent) than with Stage III (68 to 72 per cent) disease, and is lower still in those with bulky lymphoma (35 to 38 per cent). Most patients with diffuse histiocytic lymphoma tend to enter prompt complete remission and either to relapse rapidly or not at all. Most patients who relapse are now known to have immunoblastic lymphoma. Seldom are relapses observed more than 1 year after cessation of treatment, and there is now substantial evidence that many of these patients are actually cured. The other types of diffuse lymphomas recur in patterns somewhat between those observed with nodular lymphomas and diffuse histiocytic lymphomas.

Childhood Lymphomas

In children with NHL chemotherapy is always indicated regardless of stage (often advanced) and histology (almost invariably of high grade malignancy). Treatment must be prompt and aggressive; it may include RT in patients with initially bulky disease, as well as central nervous system prophylaxis. Modern treatments are complex and difficult to summarize. In any case, once the histologic diagnosis is established, it is always advisable to refer the child immediately to a qualified pediatric oncologic team. Briefly, the approach to treatment can be divided into three phases. During Phase I (induction) the goal is to achieve the status of complete clinical remission within 4 to 6 weeks. This can be obtained in more than 85 per cent of patients with the effective use of combination chemotherapy, including known active agents such as cyclophosphamide, vincristine, doxorubicin (Adriamycin), and prednisone. After the second week of treatment some clinicians also irradiate the site(s) of initial massive disease with 2500 to 3000 rads to decrease the likelihood of early recurrence. Phase II then starts immediately and includes central nervous system prophylaxis (cranial irradiation with 2400 rads and intrathecal methotrexate at the dose of 10 mg per square meter of body surface for at least five doses). This treatment is mandatory in the presence of convoluted cell type lymphoblastic lymphoma, even if the disease is apparently localized, and in Burkitt's lymphoma with abdominal presentation, as well as in all children with initial bone marrow infiltration. Appropriate trials are in progress to establish the therapeutic value of high dose methotrexate plus citrovorum factor. Treatment continues with the third phase in complete responders, utilizing a cyclical maintenance treatment for about 2 years. The antimetabolites (6-mercaptopurine, 6-thioguanine,

methotrexate, cytosine arabinoside) are the drugs most often utilized. With an intensive treatment approach, 40 to 65 per cent of children are expected to be alive at the end of the second year. Stage III and IV patients as well as those with Burkitt's tumor have the worst prognosis, whereas most children with stage I and II disease can probably be cured.

Special Problems

Central Nervous System (CNS) Involvement. Leptomeningeal infiltration is a rather frequent event in diffuse lymphomas, particularly in children and in all patients with lymphoblastic convoluted cell (T cell) lymphomas. Epidural compression and intracerebral lymphoma are definitely more rare. This complication can occur when the patient otherwise appears in complete remission, since the CNS is a "drug sanctuary." Prompt diagnosis (e.g., myelography, examination of cytocentrifuge sample of cerebrospinal fluid) and appropriate treatment are essential to achieve remission and minimize permanent neurologic consequences. In the presence of leptomeningeal lymphoma, intrathecal medication (methotrexate, 10 mg per square meter of body surface, cytosine arabinoside, 25 to 30 mg per square meter, and hydrocortisone, 25 to 30 mg per square meter) should be administered every 4 days until complete remission. Treatment is usually supplemented by craniospinal irradiation (2000 to 2400 rads). In patients with slow epidural cord compression, RT (3500 to 4000 rads) eventually supplemented with systemic chemotherapy, represents the treatment of choice. The treatment for rapidly progressive extradural cord compression is represented by emergency laminectomy, followed within 1 to 3 days by local irradiation. When cranial nerves are involved or there are clinically documented cerebral masses, the approach of choice is RT as well as corticosteroids (e.g., dexamethasone, 8 to 12 mg per day orally). Subsequent therapy is that which is appropriate for the patient stage.

Superior Vena Cava (SVC) Syndrome. Rapid growth of lymphoma may cause compression of the major vessels. Childhood lymphomas and diffuse lymphomas in general, particularly the lymphoblastic convoluted cell type, are most likely to produce this syndrome. SVC obstruction constitutes a medical emergency. Therefore prompt diagnosis (usually with conventional roentgenograms) and treatment, even in the absence of tissue diagnosis, are required. If the patient is previously untreated, combination chemotherapy eventually combined with mediastinal irradiation (3500 to 4500 rads) represents the treatment of choice, and objective response is usually achieved within a few days. In patients previously treated with chemotherapy RT, corticosteroids, and diuretics should be given first, eventually followed by further cytotoxic drugs.

Pleural Effusions. Serous pleural effusions are common in lymphomas, complicating the course in about 20 per cent of patients who are not cured. This complication can be produced either by lymphatic obstruction in the mediastinum or by pleuropulmonary involvement of lymphoma. Treatment depends, in part, upon the cause. In the first case, appropriate RT to the mediastinum usually resolves the effusion. When cytology of the pleural fluid and/or pleural biopsy indicates the presence of visceral disease, combination chemotherapy provides the most successful treatment. In previously treated patients intrapleural instillation of mechlorethamine (8 to 12 mg per square meter of body surface in 20 to 30 ml of isotonic saline solution) or bleomycin (30 to 60 units per square meter) or doxorubicin (Adriamycin) (30 to 40 mg per square meter of body surface) should be administered after maximal removal of pleural fluid.

Acute Renal Failure. Renal failure resulting from bilateral replacement of kidneys by tumor is not infrequent in both adults and children with advanced disease. The most common signs are enlarged kidneys on radiograms with or without uremia, mild proteinuria, and arterial hypertension. Treatment of renal infiltration is best accomplished by systemic chemotherapy. RT to one or both kidneys is often utilized, particularly in patients resistant to first-line chemotherapy, but the dose should not exceed 1000 rads to avoid renal damage by irradiation. The strategic approach to be utilized in the presence of unilateral or bilateral ureteral obstruction is local RT combined with systemic treatment.

MYCOSIS FUNGOIDES AND THE SEZARY SYNDROME

method of
ERIC C. VONDERHEID, M.D.
Philadelphia, Pennsylvania

Mycosis fungoides (MF) is a distinctive lymphoma composed of atypical thymus-derived (T) lymphocytes with hyperchromatic convoluted nuclei, which has its initial manifestations in the skin. In typical cases, the cutaneous manifestations of the disease progress in a sequential fashion through premycotic, plaque, and tumor phases. Less commonly, MF

may develop rapidly as cutaneous tumors without antecedent skin lesions (tumor d'emblée) or as an extensive erythroderma with or without coexisting plaques and tumors (erythrodermic MF). The Sézary syndrome, characterized by generalized erythroderma and atypical mononuclear cells with cerebriform nuclei in the blood, is considered by most investigators to be a leukemic manifestation of MF.

Systemic involvement ultimately develops in most patients with MF and is almost always associated with extensive plaque, tumor, or erythrodermic skin manifestations. Although any organ system can eventually become involved, the peripheral lymph nodes seem to be infiltrated preferentially during the process of dissemination. The T lymphocyte membrane properties of the atypical cells may explain the "homing" of MF cells to epithelial structures in the skin and to thymus-dependent areas in lymph nodes and spleen.

The natural history of MF varies considerably from patient to patient, and the disease may last for decades with manifestations limited only to the skin. However, once the disease progresses to tumor phase or involves extracutaneous tissues, the median survival time of patients is less than 3 years. Infection is the most common immediate cause of death. It is incumbent on the physician to determine the extent of disease involvement in the patient in order that an adequate treatment program can be instituted.

Staging

The staging evaluation of the patient with MF begins with a complete history and physical examination (Table 1). The age and general health status of the patient and the rate of disease progression are important subjective considerations that may influence treatment planning. With slowly progressive

TABLE 1. **Recommended Staging Evaluation**

History and physical examination:
1. Age and general health status of patient
2. Duration and rate of progression of disease
3. Degree of lesion infiltration and extent of surface involvement
4. Status of peripheral lymph nodes and visceral organs

Laboratory and routine diagnostic studies:
1. Complete blood and platelet count
2. Smear to detect and quantitate circulating atypical lymphocytes
3. Serum chemistries for evidence of visceral abnormalities
4. Chest x-ray
5. Liver-spleen isotopic scan
6. Ultrasonic examination for intra-abdominal lymph node enlargement
7. Bipedal lymphangiography

Biopsy procedures:
1. Skin
2. Lymph node
3. Bone marrow
4. Others (as indicated by results of above studies)

Useful special studies:
1. Electron microscopy
2. Lymphocyte membrane properties of atypical cells
3. Cytogenetic analysis

disease, less intensive forms of treatment are usually favored for the patient with advanced age or in poor general health. Conversely, a relatively more intensive treatment program might be adopted in the otherwise healthy patient with rapidly progressive disease. The physical examination defines the magnitude of skin involvement in terms of the major prognostic parameters, i.e., degree of lesion infiltration and extent of surface involvement and the likelihood of coexisting extracutaneous involvement. Especially important is the search for palpable lymph nodes, since the disease seems to preferentially involve these structures during dissemination.

Skin biopsy specimens are next obtained from the most infiltrated lesions to confirm the diagnosis and to further characterize the status of cutaneous infiltration. In some patients with early MF, a definite histologic diagnosis can be made only after frequent biopsies and review of the histologic material by dermatopathologists experienced with this problem.

Additional staging procedures are also performed to detect involvement of extracutaneous tissues (Table 1). If abnormalities are found on routine tests, an effort should be made to confirm the involvement of visceral organs by histologic means. Detailed staging procedures, i.e., staging laparotomies, have been performed in MF patients, but their usefulness compared to less rigorous approaches is uncertain at present.

In staging the patient with MF, particular attention is given to the status of the peripheral lymph nodes, since experience indicates that involvement of other organ systems is unusual in the absence of lymph node involvement. A lymph node biopsy is mandatory in the patient with palpably enlarged lymph nodes, but its value in the patient with nonpalpable lymph nodes is less certain. Lymphangiography may have some usefulness in this regard, since positive correlations have been made between the degree of lymphangiographic abnormality and the probability of histologic detection of disease; however, this modality does not reliably distinguish between early involvement with MF and dermatopathic lymphadenitis or other reactive changes. A random biopsy of a nonpalpable lymph node seems indicated when advanced cutaneous manifestations are present, e.g., numerous plaques, tumors, or extensive erythroderma, or if suspect lymphangiographic changes are present.

Several special studies can help confirm whether tissues are involved with MF. The presence of clusters and sheets of lymphocytes with convoluted nuclei on electron micrographs is considered to be highly suggestive of MF and has been used to evaluate skin, lymph node, blood, and other specimens. Likewise, the demonstration that the abnormal cells have membrane markers of T lymphocytes is suggestive for MF. Cytogenetic analysis may reveal chromosomal abnormalities that help distinguish the disease from benign conditions.

Tables 2 and 3 present a staging classification based on the TNM System that has been recently adopted by the Mycosis Fungoides Cooperative Group.

TABLE 2. **TNM Classification of Cutaneous T Cell Lymphomas**

Magnitude of skin involvement (T):*
- T_0 Clinically or histopathologically suspicious lesions
- T_1 Premycotic lesions, papules, or plaques involving less than 10% of the skin
- T_2 Premycotic lesions, papules, or plaques involving more than 10% of the skin
- T_3 One or more tumors of skin
- T_4 Extensive, often generalized erythroderma

Status of peripheral lymph nodes (N):
- N_0 Clinically normal; pathologically not involved
- N_1 Clinically abnormal; pathologically not involved
- N_2 Clinically normal; pathologically involved
- N_3 Clinically abnormal; pathologically involved

Status of visceral organs (M):†
- M_0 Pathologically not involved
- M_1 Pathologically involved

*Stages T_1 to T_4 require pathologic confirmation. When more than one classification applies, indicate both ratings and use highest for staging—e.g., T_3 (T_2).

†The prognostic significance of atypical (Sézary) cells in the blood has not been determined.

Therapeutic Modalities

A number of well-established or investigative therapeutic modalities have a beneficial influence on MF, but their effectiveness may be of short duration or limited to earlier stages of disease. Furthermore, the capability of these modalities to modify the natural course of disease may not be established primarily because adequate numbers of patients have not been studied for long intervals. The recommended use, benefits, and adverse effects of available treatments are summarized briefly in the following paragraphs. The reader should refer to the key references provided for further details.

Corticosteroids

Topical and intralesional corticosteroids (Farber, E. M., Zackheim, H. S., McClintock, R. P., and Cox, A. J., Jr.: Arch Dermatol. *97*:165, 1968) are used for the temporary improvement of MF and occasionally may induce objective remissions. For patients with extensive MF, especially the Sézary syndrome, systemic corticoste-

TABLE 3. **Proposed Staging System for Cutaneous T Cell Lymphomas**

		T	N	M
Stage	I A	T_1	N_0	M_0
	B	T_2	N_0	M_0
	II A	T_{1-2}	N_1	M_0
	B	T_3	N_{0-1}	M_0
	III	T_4	N_{0-1}	M_0
	IV A	T_{1-4}	N_{2-3}	M_0
	B	T_{1-4}	N_{0-3}	M_1

roids may be administered to decrease pruritus and other manifestations of inflammation. However, the loss of therapeutic effectiveness (acquired unresponsiveness) and the potential adverse effects associated with long-term corticosteroid administration have limited the usefulness of these drugs.

Phototherapy

Conventional Ultraviolet Light. Intensive exposure to light from the sun or artificial light sources will often clear early manifestations of MF, but its overall influence on the natural course of disease is uncertain.

Methoxsalen Photochemotherapy. * (Gilchrest, B. Z., Parrish, J. A., Tanenbaum, L., Haynes, H. A., and Fitzpatrick, T. B.: Cancer *38*:683, 1976; Roenigk, H. H., Jr.: Arch. Dermatol., *113*:1047, 1977). Methoxsalen photochemotherapy, the oral administration of 8-methoxypsoralen (0.6 mg per kg), followed in 2 hours by exposure to titrated doses of long-wave (320 to 400 nm) ultraviolet light, is a recently introduced form of phototherapy whose long-term efficacy for MF has not yet been established. Preliminary results indicate that 90 to 95 per cent of patients with early MF will initially respond with treatment. However, maintenance therapy is necessary in most patients to discourage recurrence of disease, and supplemental treatment, e.g., local x-ray treatment, usually is required for thicker plaques or tumors because of the limited penetration by long-wave ultraviolet light. With careful supervision methoxsalen photochemotherapy is well tolerated by the patient, but there is a concern that long-term use may accelerate actinic damage and photocarcinogenesis in the skin.

Topical Chemotherapy

Topical Mechlorethamine (HN2) * (Vonderheid, E. C., VanScott, E. J., Johnson, W. C., Grekin, D. A., and Asbell, S. O.: Arch. Dermatol. *113*:454, 1977). The topical application of HN2 solutions has been found to induce complete remissions in 85 to 90 per cent of patients with early MF, and long-term disease-free intervals are achieved in a substantial proportion of these patients. The major advantage of topical NH2 is its availability and safety, but cost considerations and the development of contact allergic reactions in more than one third of patients limit its utility. Furthermore, there is concern that long intervals of HN2 use may induce epithelial neoplasms.

After a cleansing bath the patient applies a freshly prepared dilute aqueous solution of HN2 to the entire cutaneous surface once daily. An initial dose of 10 mg dissolved in 40 to 60 ml of tap water is usually well tolerated with minimal irritation. A therapeutic response usually becomes apparent during the first 6 weeks of treatment and complete clearing should occur by 6 months. If the response to treatment is slow or incomplete, the concentration of HN2 solution or frequency of applications, or both, may be increased as tolerated by the patient. Supplemental treatment, e.g., local x-ray therapy, is often necessary for patients with thick plaques, tumors, or erythrodermic disease. After a complete remission is achieved, maintenance therapy for several years is necessary to prevent recurrence of disease in most patients. For patients who develop allergic sensitization, both topical and systemic desensitization programs to circumvent this problem have been advocated.

Topical Carmustine (BiCNU) * (Zackheim, H. S., and Epstein, F. H., Jr.: Arch. Dermatol. *111*:1564, 1975). As with HN2, the topical application of an 0.1 per cent BiCNU solution may induce complete remissions, primarily in patients with clinically early MF. However, the potential for local and systemic toxicity is greater than for HN2, such that intermittent rather than sustained applications must be used. The long-term benefits have not been established because of the newness of the treatment.

Radiotherapy

Superficial X-Ray Radiation. Low-kilovoltage (80 to 140 kv) radiotherapy at a target-to-skin distance of 15 to 30 cm provides effective treatment for most localized infiltrates. Discrete, moderately infiltrated lesions almost always respond to doses of 150 to 300 R administered twice weekly to a total dose of 1000 to 2000 R. Markedly infiltrated lesions may require higher energy levels in the orthovoltage range (200 to 280 kv). However, only limited areas can be treated with orthovoltage radiation because of the risk of systemic toxicity.

Electron Beam Radiation (Hoppe, R., Fuks, Z., and Bagshaw, M.: Int. J. Radiat. Oncol. Biol. Phys. *2*:843, 1977). High-energy electrons (3 to 4 Mev) produced by linear accelerators or betatrons can be administered to extensive areas of the body without significant systemic toxicity. The entire body surface is usually treated in MF in order to avoid missing clinically inapparent lesions. The recommended total dosage, electron

---

*This use of this agent is not listed in the manufacturer's official directive.

* This use of this agent is not listed in the manufacturer's official directive.

energies, fractionation schedules, and treatment fields vary from institution to institution. Recent studies indicate that high-dosage schedules (3000 to 3600 rads) may be preferred over low-dosage schedules because of the high remission rates (over 90 per cent) and impressive 5 year disease-free survival rates that occur following aggressive treatment. However, treatment at higher dosages may also result in substantial acute (erythema, edema, blistering, hair loss) and chronic (atrophy, telangectasia, fibrosis) radiation sequelae. Other disadvantages include the expense and limited availability.

Single-Agent Systemic Chemotherapy

Multiple systemic drugs administered singly have been reported to produce beneficial, although temporary, responses in patients with MF. However, experience suggests that single-agent chemotherapy alone does not substantially improve the overall survival of patients. The most useful drugs for single agent chemotherapy are methotrexate and alkylating agents.

Methotrexate (MTX). This drug is particularly useful in MF because it can be safely administered with beneficial effects for long intervals. More than 50 per cent of patients treated with doses of 30 to 50 mg weekly show objective improvement, but complete remission occurs in less than 20 per cent. Serial monitoring of blood counts and liver function is required.

Mechlorethamine (HN2) (VanScott, E. J., Grekin, D. A., Kalmanson, J. D., Vonderheid, E. C., and Barry, W. E.: Cancer 36:1613, 1975). This drug is usually administered at a dose of 0.1 mg per kg intravenously daily for 4 days. Dramatic responses are sometimes achieved, but long-term remissions are unusual. Repeated courses may be administered but often result in prolonged bone marrow suppression. Recently systemic HN2 has been administered as daily 2 mg intravenous doses over a 2 to 3 week interval, with objective improvement in 70 per cent and complete remissions in about 25 per cent of patients treated. These responses were not compared to responses achieved by the conventional dosage schedule, but the "slow-dose" technique allows for improved control of side effects.

Cyclophosphamide (CTX) (VanScott, E. J., Auerbach, R., and Clendenning, W. E.: Arch. Dermatol. 85:499, 1962). Oral administration of CTX at a dose of 1 to 3 mg per kg daily produces objective improvements and occasionally complete remissions in over 50 per cent of patients. Bone marrow suppression, hair loss, and cystitis are troublesome adverse effects.

Chlorambucil (Campbell, E. W., and Fromer, J. L.: Surg. Clin. North Am. 39:585, 1959; Win-

kelmann, R. K., and Linman, J. W.: Mayo Clin. Proc. 49:590, 1974). Chlorambucil, at an oral dose of 0.1 to 0.2 mg per kg, has been used as adjunct therapy for patients treated with electron beam radiation. Low doses of chlorambucil (2 to 6 mg per day) administered in conjunction with prednisone have been reported to induce and maintain complete remissions in patients with Sézary syndrome. However, treatment often must be administered for 6 or more months before a therapeutic effect becomes apparent.

Multiple-Agent Systemic Chemotherapy

Combination chemotherapy is generally administered to patients with advanced MF, but limited information is available concerning the effectiveness of treatment because of the small numbers of patients so treated. Experience suggests that complete remissions occur more frequently than with single agents, but a beneficial influence on patient survival has not been demonstrated. Unfortunately, the undesired consequences of systemic chemotherapy further predispose the patient to serious infectious complications. The combinations of drugs that are used most frequently for MF are presented below.

MOPP

Mechlorethamine	6 mg/sq meter IV, days 1 and 8	
Vincristine	1.4 mg/sq meter IV, days 1 and 8	Repeated in 2 week cycles
Procarbazine	100 mg/sq meter PO, days 1 to 14	
Prednisone	40 mg/sq meter PO days 1 to 14 (cycles 1 and 4 only)	

COP or COP-Bleo

Cyclophosphamide	200 mg/sq meter PO, days 1 to 5	
Vincristine	1.4 mg/sq meter IV, day 1	Repeated in 3 week cycles
Prednisone	60 mg/sq meter PO, days 1 to 5	
± Bleomycin	10 units/sq meter, IV day 1	

CHOP

Cyclophosphamide	500 mg/sq meter IV, day 1	
Doxorubicin	40 mg/sq meter IV, day 1	Repeated in 3 week cycles
Vincristine	1.4 mg/sq meter IV, day 1	
Prednisone	60 mg/sq meter PO, days 1 to 5	

Of recent interest (Levi, J. A., Diggs, C. H., and Wiernik, P. H.: Cancer 39:1967, 1977) is the use of doxorubicin (60 mg per square meter body surface area intravenously once weekly for 3 weeks) to induce remissions in patients with advanced MF, followed by maintenance therapy with methotrexate (15 mg per square meter intramuscularly twice weekly) and cyclophosphamide (750 mg per square meter intravenously every 3 weeks).

Investigative Modalities

Topical Immunotherapy (Klein, E., Holtermann, O., Milgrom, H., Case, R. W., Klein, D., Rosner, D., and Djerassi, I.: Med. Clin. North Am. *60*:389, 1976). This provides application of various chemical antigens to the skin for immunologically mediated therapeutic benefits.

Transfer Factor (Zachariae, H., Grunnet, E., Ellegaard, J., and Thestrup-Pedersen, K.: Arch. Dermatol. *112*:1324, 1976). In this modality protein elaborated by sensitized normal lymphocytes is administered in order to enhance cell-mediated tumor resistance.

Leukapheresis (Edelson, R., Facktor, M., and Andrews, A.: N. Engl. J. Med. *291*:293, 1974). In leukapheresis there is mechanical removal of atypical cells from the blood of patients with the Sézary syndrome in order to reduce tumor burden.

Antithymocyte Globulin (Barrett, A. J., Brigden, D., Roberts, J. T., Staughton, R. C. D., Byrom, N., and Hobbs, J. R.: Lancet *1*:940, 1976; Edelson, R. L., Brown, J. A., Grossman, M. E., and Hardy, M. A.: Lancet *2*:249, 1977). Antithymocyte globulin is used to produce antibody-mediated destruction of abnormal (and normal) lymphocytes with thymus-derived membrane markers.

Methotrexate with Leukovorin Rescue (McDonald, C. J., and Bertino, J. R.: Cancer Treat. Rep., *62*:1009, 1978). Methotrexate, 60 to 240 mg per square meter, is given intravenously over 6 hours, followed by oral citrovorum factor (25 mg per square meter) every 4 hours for six doses.

Treatment Selection

Considering the number of therapeutic modalities currently available and the limited information regarding optimal use, it is difficult to make definitive statements regarding treatment selection at this time. Rather, our usual therapeutic approach will be indicated, followed by options that we frequently use depending on circumstances. The TNM Staging System (Table 3) will be used for the discussion.

Stage I A. Usual choice: topical HN2. Frequent options: ultraviolet light, photochemotherapy, topical immunotherapy. Infrequent options: electron beam radiation alone or followed by topical HN2; methotrexate.

Stage I B: Usual choice: topical HN2. Frequent options: electron beam followed by topical HN2; photochemotherapy; methotrexate. Infrequent options: slow-dose systemic NH2.

Stage II A. Treatment same as for Stage I B.

Stage II B. Usual choice: electron beam radiation followed by topical HN2 and methotrexate. Frequent options: slow-dose systemic HN2. Infrequent options: multiple-agent chemotherapy.

Stage III. Usual choice: topical HN2 and slow-dose systemic HN2 or methotrexate. Frequent options (particularly if there are more than 10 per cent atypical cells in blood): electron beam radiation followed by topical HN2; multiple-agent chemotherapy. Infrequent options: leukapheresis; antithymocyte globulin.

Stage IV A and B. Usual choice: multiple-agent chemotherapy alone. Frequent options: electron beam radiation or topical HN2 and multiple agent chemotherapy. Infrequent options: antithymocyte globulin, methotrexate.

MULTIPLE MYELOMA

method of
GIBBONS G. CORNWELL III, M.D.
Hanover, New Hampshire

Multiple myeloma is a disseminated malignancy of plasma cells which are located predominantly in the bone marrow. In a high proportion of patients, there is a monoclonal immunoglobulin present in the serum and/or urine and osteolytic lesions in marrow-containing bones. Specific supportive medical care remains the mainstay of managing patients with this disease, since reversible complications such as hypercalcemia, hyperuricemia, renal failure, infection, neurologic defects, and hyperviscosity pose life-threatening potential. Although chemotherapy increases the quality of life and prolongs survival in multiple myeloma, there has been little significant well-documented improvement in the chemotherapeutic approach to this disease in the past 20 years. However, several new developments on the horizon hold promise for prolonging survival in the foreseeable future.

Supportive Measures

The two most important goals for the patient with multiple myeloma are ambulation and adequate hydration. Since two thirds of patients present with osteolytic bone lesions and about 90 per cent have osteoporosis (in part related to the median age of 60 years), patients with this disease are highly prone to the development of bone pain and fractures. Bed rest accelerates the osteolytic process and increases the incidence of pathologic fractures. In patients with extensive localized lytic involvement of long bones (especially the femur), prophylactic surgical stabilization should be considered. Adequate hydration is essential in preventing renal disease and, in some patients, hyperviscosity secondary to high concentrations of certain monoclonal proteins. Patients with myeloma are at risk of potential renal failure as a result of dehydration, hypercalcemia, hyperuricemia, light chain proteinuria, and, in a small percentage of patients, amyloidosis. The prevention of hyperuricemia is thus a third important goal achieved by the prophylactic administration of allopurinol (Zyloprim) prior to initiation of specific therapy.

Management of Direct Complications

Hypercalcemia. Patients with serum calcium ≥12 grams per cent should be treated as medical emergencies. A normal or borderline elevation of serum calcium might be associated with a significant elevation in the ionized fraction if the serum albumin is low. Attempts to reduce the calcium level should be undertaken initially with corticosteroids (equivalent to prednisone, 40 mg per square meter per day), isotonic saline diuresis, and furosamide (Lasix), 40 mg two to four times per day. Treatment of the myeloma should commence as promptly as possible in conjunction with the measures outlined above. In patients who fail to respond within 24 to 48 hours, a single dose of mithramycin, 25 micrograms per kg administered over 4 to 6 hours in 1 liter of isotonic saline, may be given. This dose may be repeated after 3 days if necessary, but in view of potential hypocalcemia, renal toxicity, and myelosuppression, 5 day intervals are preferable.

Hyperuricemia. If hyperuricemia has developed, it should be treated promptly with allopurinol (Zyloprim), up to 600 mg per day. In addition, the urine should be alkalinized with sodium bicarbonate (1 to 2 grams orally every 4 to 6 hours), together with cautious hydration. Alternatively, acetazolamide (Diamox), up to 500 mg every 12 hours, may be used to maintain an alkaline urine.

Infection. Patients with myeloma are at increased risk of infection, predominantly as a result of decreased mobility and diminished normal B lymphocyte activity (and consequent diminished polyclonal immunoglobulins). Prophylactic gamma globulin has not been effective in preventing infections in one trial, and recent data indicate that myeloma patients show virtually no antibody response to pneumococcal antigens (Pneumovac). Patients suspected of infection should be cultured widely and treated aggressively with broad-spectrum antibiotics until culture results are available. Gram-negative organisms appear to have become an increasingly frequent cause of infection in myeloma patients.

Pain Associated with Bone Lesion. Prompt management of pain is essential in keeping patients ambulatory. Analgesics should be given on a fixed rather than on an as-necessary (PRN) schedule, and when possible they should include aspirin (which prevents the sensitization of pain receptors by the inhibition of prostaglandin synthesis). Local radiation therapy (1500 to 2000 rads over 5 to 10 days) results in symptomatic improvement in most patients within 3 or 4 days. Ambulation may be facilitated by corsets or back braces, provided that they are not too restrictive. A combination of sodium fluoride (50 mg orally twice a day) and calcium carbonate (1 gram four times a day) results in increased bone formation and should be considered in patients with significant bone involvement without hypercalcemia. (This use of sodium fluoride is not listed in the manufacturer's official directive.)

Renal Failure. In most patients with myeloma, acute renal failure is potentially reversible. Initial goals are to reverse renal effects caused by hypercalcemia, hyperuricemia, or dehydration. Recent studies have shown that aggressive plasmapheresis may be successful in reversing acute renal failure. Although short-term peritoneal dialysis has not been successful in a significant proportion of patients, long-term hemodialysis combined with chemotherapy has led to significant improvement in renal function in a high proportion of patients with chronic renal failure.

Pathologic Fractures. Since fracture sites invariably contain large amounts of tumor and associated lytic lesions, immobilization alone rarely results in satisfactory healing of weight-bearing bones. Consequently, surgical intervention with metal-supporting structures and methylmethacrylate may be required to assure early ambulation. Radiation therapy to the fracture site following fixation may facilitate bone healing.

Neurologic Deficits. Motor or sensory loss secondary to myelomatous tumor compression on the spinal cord or nerve roots represents an emergency. A myelogram should be performed when epidural compression is suspected and, when present, surgical decompression considered. In some patients, localized irradiation may be given as an alternative means of decompression or as an adjunct to surgery. A short course of high dose dexamethasone is indicated in most patients with neurologic deficits secondary to tumor compression.

Hyperviscosity. Hyperviscosity is most likely to occur in patients with multiple myeloma of the IgA and the IgG3 type and in those with high concentrations of serum monoclonal protein. Although the hyperviscosity syndrome occurs in only 5 to 15 per cent of patients, it should be suspected in any patient with mental changes, visual problems, thrombosis, or bleeding of unclear cause. When the relative viscosity exceeds 4, transfusion of packed red cells should be delayed until plasmapheresis has been instituted, so that significant increase in whole blood viscosity will be avoided. Since IgG and IgA are distributed throughout the extravascular compartment and re-enter the plasma following removal, plasmapheresis alone is only of temporary benefit in myeloma and must be combined with effective chemotherapy.

Amyloidosis. Amyloid of the immunoglobulin light chain type has been found in approximately 10 per cent of patients. When suspected on clinical grounds, a rectal biopsy (including the submucosa) will provide the diagnosis in approximately 90 per cent of patients. No chemotherapeutic program has yet been effective in reversing amyloid deposition.

Specific Therapy for Myeloma

Chemotherapy. SINGLE ALKYLATING AGENT. Melphalan or cyclophosphamide prolongs the survival of patients with myeloma, and direct comparisons have shown no advantage for either drug. The addition of prednisone to melphalan therapy appears to increase the response rate and survival in good risk patients, but improves only the response rate in poor risk patients. Continuous melphalan (150 micrograms per kg per day for 7 days, then 50 micrograms per kg per day when white count is rising) combined with prednisone (0.6 mg per kg per day tapered over 6 weeks) and intermittent melphalan (250 micrograms per kg per day for 4 days) combined with prednisone (2 mg per kg per day for 4 days) every 6 weeks result in equivalent median survival of approximately 2 years. However, these two programs have never been compared directly in a randomized trial. Patients who fail on melphalan may develop a significant response to cyclophosphamide given daily (0.5 to 1.0 mg per kg orally) or intermittently (0.6 to 1.0 gram per square meter intravenously every 3 to 6 weeks).

NITROSOUREAS. Intermittent carmustine (BiCNU) (150 mg per square meter intravenously every 6 weeks) or lomustine (CCNU) (100 mg per square meter orally every 6 weeks), combined with an initial 6 week tapering course of prednisone, is equally effective in previously untreated patients. A recent randomized trial indicates that both drugs are equivalent to melphalan in prolonging survival. Patients who have failed on melphalan may respond to a nitrosourea given alone or in combination with other drugs.

COMBINATION CHEMOTHERAPY. A variety of drug combinations have been studied in previously untreated patients and in patients who have become resistant to melphalan and prednisone. In most studies of untreated patients, combinations which have included doxorubicin (Adriamycin), carmustine (BCNU), or procarbazine have not been found superior to melphalan and prednisone alone. A four drug combination of melphalan, cyclophosphamide, carmustine (BCNU), and prednisone has shown a survival advantage in poor risk patients only. A five drug combination of vincristine, doxorubicin (Adriamycin), carmustine (BCNU), cyclophosphamide, and melphalan has been reported to result in significant objective remission in 87 per cent of untreated patients. As this trial contained a large proportion of good-risk patients (low blood urea nitrogen [BUN] and high performance status), confirmation of these results in a randomized trial would be of considerable interest. Other combinations containing vincristine have been shown to be somewhat superior to controls without vincristine, but the role of vincristine in myeloma is not yet clearly established. No large scale controlled trials have proved the superiority of any multidrug combinations (compared to single agents such as cyclophosphamide or CCNU) in prolonging survival in patients who have relapsed on melphalan therapy.

MAINTENANCE THERAPY. Several studies have attempted to determine whether continued treatment with melphalan and prednisone is indicated in patients who have shown a good response after 12 months of therapy. Results to date indicate that virtually all patients relapse after cessation of treatment, although the remission duration is longest in patients who had presented with a low tumor mass or had shown total disappearance of the serum monoclonal protein. Response to re-treatment has been smaller and of shorter duration than that following initial therapy. Further studies are required to resolve this issue.

Radiation Therapy. Total body irradiation, total bone marrow irradiation, and hemibody irradiation have all been studied in small numbers of patients with myeloma. None of these treatment modalities have yet proved effective in producing a significant number of good responses, but further trials are required in previously untreated patients.

New Developments

Interferon. A small number of patients have been treated with daily doses of human leukocyte interferon, and clear-cut responses have been observed in both previously untreated and treated patients. Further studies are presently underway in a small number of institutions to compare interferon with standard therapy.

Bone Marrow Cultures. Culture techniques have been applied to the study of various chemotherapeutic agents on myeloma cells in vitro. The successful development of methods for predicting in vivo response to chemotherapy would represent a significant development in the management of myeloma and other tumors.

POLYCYTHEMIA VERA, ERYTHROCYTOSIS, AND RELATIVE POLYCYTHEMIA

method of
HARRIET S. GILBERT, M. D.
New York, New York

Polycythemia vera is a clonal disorder of the pluripotential hematopoietic precursor cell in which cell proliferation is increased while differentiation and maturation of the hematic trilineage (erythroid and granulocyte precursors and megakaryocytes) are preserved. The intrinsic growth disturbance of the hematopoietic stem cell results in a chronic myeloproliferative disease with expansion of the bone marrow organ throughout the medullary cavity, as well as reactivation of hematopoiesis in extramedullary sites usually active only during fetal development, the most common involvement being splenic myeloid metaplasia. Myelofibrosis is a frequent epiphenomenon in myeloproliferative disease. The bone marrow fibroblasts are not derived from the abnormal hematopoietic clone, and the laying down of increased reticulin and collagen appears to be reactive to unknown stimuli. The clonal origin, autonomous growth pattern of the hematic populations, and tendency of the disease to undergo spontaneous transition to conditions characterized by greater degrees of stem cell dysplasia, such as post-polycythemic myeloid metaplasia with myelofibrosis, refractory anemia, or acute leukemia, support the classification of polycythemia vera as a malignant disease. On the other hand, the disease is chronic and one in which early diagnosis and appropriate management confer an average life expectancy that does not differ from that of an age-matched population without polycythemia vera. Because of the morbidity and life-threatening nature of the complications of uncontrolled disease and the potential myelotoxic and leukemogenic properties of some therapeutic agents used in their prevention, the management of polycythemia vera requires continual weighing of risk versus benefit. Disease manifestations vary widely from patient to patient as well as during the course of an individual patient, depending upon the type, location, and extent of cell proliferation. Stereotyped management is to be avoided in favor of an individualized and flexible approach in accordance with the general principles discussed below.

Establishing a Diagnosis

The need to satisfy rigorous criteria for a diagnosis of polycythemia vera cannot be overemphasized. A myriad of pathophysiologic alterations may produce an elevated hematocrit. In the majority of instances the increased hematocrit results from a reduction in circulating plasma volume rather than an absolute increase in the erythrocyte population. Acute dehydration is readily appreciated, but a chronic, low-grade state of dehydration may be overlooked. Because of its prevalence the reduction in plasma volume produced by tobacco smoking is of particular importance. The reversible nature of this form of relative polycythemia after 72 hours of abstention makes it readily detectable. The presence of a persistently elevated hematocrit without obvious explanation necessitates direct quantitation of the circulating red cell mass and plasma volume to distinguish true erythrocytosis from relative polycythemia caused by absolute reduction or shifts in circulating plasma. The volumes obtained for these two isotopically measured components of the total blood volume should be compared with predicted values based on the patient's weight, height, and sex, since red cell mass is closely correlated with lean body mass. A diagnosis of erythrocytosis should be accepted only when the observed red cell mass exceeds the predicted by 25 per cent. Erythrocyte indices should be assessed when there is a borderline elevation of hematocrit, and microcytosis resulting from iron deficiency should be corrected prior to a blood volume measurement to elicit a masked erythrocytosis. The red cell mass should be measured early in the evaluation of an elevated hematocrit and prior to any manipulation of the blood volume by phlebotomy. Blood removal is to be avoided, as it produces reactive changes in the peripheral blood that mimic myeloproliferative disease, a prime contender in the differential diagnosis of a polycythemic blood picture. Once this intervention is introduced, it becomes difficult to differentiate intrinsic features of the disease from iatrogenic phenomena.

Relative Polycythemia

Patients with a normal red cell mass in the presence of a polycythemic hematocrit level constitute an important group from the standpoint of prevalence, as they outnumber those who are truly erythrocytotic by a ratio of at least 5:1. The prototype is a young or middle-aged male smoker who is anxious and often engaged in a stressful occupation. He presents with multiple nonspecific complaints of headache, fatigue, dizziness, paresthesias, dyspnea, and epigastric distress, and is stocky or obese in habitus, plethoric, and hypertensive. Aside from a hematocrit level that is usually below 60 per cent, hematologic laboratory values are normal, but serum cholesterol, triglycerides, and uric acid may be elevated. These persons are prone to cardiovascular disease, and their management should be directed toward correction and prevention of coronary risk factors. Diuretic therapy should be avoided. Phlebotomy is contraindicated, as it further reduces a normal or already diminished plasma volume, confers no lasting correction of the blood volume abnormality, and produces a needless state of iron deficiency. Above all the patient must be protected from the inappropriate use of myelosuppressive therapy. This is best accomplished by a simple but adequate explanation of the nature and chronicity of the elevated hematocrit, emphasizing that it is not a hematoproliferative disorder.

Erythrocytosis

Once an absolute polycythemia with an observed red cell mass 25 per cent in excess of the predicted value has been documented, the diagnostic evaluation must proceed to differentiate between isolated erythrocytosis arising from exaggeration of normal erythropoiesis and erythrocytosis as an expression of a more generalized hematopoietic stem cell abnormality. Among the causes of erythrocytosis, polycythemia vera is unique for the presence of a panmyelosis with involvement of hematic populations other than the erythroid series and the occurrence of myeloid metaplasia. The initial screening for panmyelosis emphasizes the significance of splenomegaly, and if this organ is not readily palpable a spleen scan is recommended to detect subclinical splenomegaly. Other criteria of screening value for a diagnosis of polycythemia vera are leukocytosis greater than 12,000 per cu mm or neutrophilia above 7000 per cu mm, a platelet count above 400,000 per cu mm, direct basophil count above 65 per cu mm, increased leukocyte alkaline phosphatase activity, and unsaturated serum vitamin B_{12} binding capacity over 2200 picograms per ml. These criteria are invalid in the presence of infection, inflammation, or bleeding. If erythrocytosis and splenomegaly are present and there are no invalidating conditions, a diagnosis of polycythemia vera is satisfied when involvement of one other cell line is present. Erythrocytosis without splenomegaly requires documented involvement of two other cell lines to satisfy the diagnostic criteria. Patients with erythrocytosis who have minimal evidence of myeloproliferative disease or who have other conditions that invalidate the usual criteria require further studies to document myelodysplasia by means of marrow biopsy to detect megakaryocytosis and increased reticulin and fibrosis, bone marrow scan to seek expansion and peripheral extension of active marrow, bone marrow chromosome analysis to detect a karyotypically abnormal clone, and demonstration of erythropoietin-independent erythropoiesis as evidenced by low or absent circulating erythropoietin or autonomous erythroid colony formation in cultured bone marrow. The presence of erythrocytosis with two of the aforementioned criteria of abnormal growth properties of the hematic cell is sufficient for a diagnosis of polycythemia vera. Demonstration of isolated erythrocytosis without involvement of other hematic cell progeny should prompt a thorough investigation of key functions and organ systems involved in the regulation of erythropoiesis. The state of generalized tissue oxygenation should be assessed by measurements of arterial oxygen saturation and content as well as oxygen affinity of hemoglobin to detect causes of an appropriate compensatory erythrocytosis. Recognition of compensatory erythrocytosis is essential for proper management. Such patients require the extra oxygen carrying capacity conferred by the erythrocytosis and should not be phlebotomized to normal hematocrit levels. When the hematocrit reaches levels that compromise flow by reducing viscosity and offset the advantages of erythrocytosis, the patient may benefit from judicious phlebotomy. The therapeutic endpoint cannot be numerical and must be based on clinical criteria, such as increased exercise tolerance.

Causes of inappropriate erythrocytosis owing to increased erythropoietin elaboration from hypoxic renal tissue or from tumors or hyperplasias of extrarenal tissue that elaborate erythropoietin inappropriately should be sought. Patients with erythrocytosis in whom none of the aforementioned mechanisms can be invoked and who lack sufficient criteria for a diagnosis of polycythemia vera should be carried with a diagnosis of unclassified erythrocytosis. They should be observed carefully and restudied periodically for further clues to the nature of the erythrocytosis. Management should be restricted to manipulation of the circulating red cell mass with phlebotomy and to supportive measures discussed below. The use of myelosuppressive therapy is absolutely contraindicated on the basis that the patient does not have a hematologic malignancy that might otherwise justify the risk of using such agents.

Polycythemia Vera — Benefits and Risks

Disease-related complications that pose the most serious risks are thrombosis, hemorrhage, transition to acute leukemia, and development of marked myelofibrosis and myeloid metaplasia. Their incidence must be viewed with the realization that the median age at diagnosis is in the sixth decade, a time at which the incidence of vascular disease and malignancy is peaking in an age-matched population without polycythemia vera. Uncontrolled erythrocytosis with its attendant hypervolemia and hyperviscosity is the main contributory factor in the thrombotic and hemorrhagic complications. These risks are compounded further by thrombocythemia and qualitative platelet abnormalities. The presence of circulating platelet aggregates and degranulated platelets attest to intrinsic hyperfunction of the platelet population. Phlebotomy is the mainstay of therapy for polycythemia vera, in that it offers a simple and rapid means of correcting hypervolemia and hyperviscosity and has been shown to reduce the incidence of thrombosis and hemorrhage, although these complications still occur with greater frequency than in the general population. The normal stimulatory effect of phlebotomy on hematopoiesis is preserved and even exaggerated in polycythemia vera. The response includes a rise in the platelet count and the appearance of circulating platelets with increased hemostatic activity. The potential thrombogenic effect of this response can be mitigated by platelet deaggregating agents. These are useful adjuncts in management which should be introduced in conjunction with phlebotomy and continued for 1 week after the phlebotomy or series of phlebotomies is completed. They should also be used on a standing basis in patients with polycythemia vera who are high-risk candidates for thrombosis. This group includes patients with platelet counts greater than 500,000 per cu mm and those with a history of thrombosis or cardiovascular disease. Erythromelalgia and other symptoms of impaired small vessel circulation also respond dramatically and do not recur while this regimen is maintained. The long-term impact of platelet deaggregating therapy on thrombotic complications and survival has not been evaluated in a systematic way, but anecdotal experience suggests a substantial benefit.

Myelosuppressive therapy is a powerful tool in the management of polycythemia vera, and broad experience has accrued with the use of radioactive phosphorus and alkylating agents. Myelosuppression with normalization of the blood count and reduction or elimination of the need for phlebotomy can be induced in virtually all patients. Following induction with myelosuppressive therapy, the duration of unmaintained control of proliferative activity is highly variable, lasting from 2 months to several years. Since polycythemia vera is a chronic disorder, commitment to maintenance of a normal blood count and elimination of myeloid metaplasia using only myelosuppressive therapy requires a maintenance regimen in most patients. Median duration of disease is approximately 13 years, and such maintenance regimens entail extensive exposure to the risks of myelosuppressive therapy. Spontaneous transformation to acute leukemia does occur, but with low frequency, in patients who are managed without myelosuppression. There is documentation of an increased incidence of leukemic transformation in ^{32}P-treated patients, with a strong suggestion of a dose relationship. Alkylating agents have also proved to be leukemogenic in polycythemia vera, and the use of a vigorous induction and maintenance chemotherapy regimen may hasten the development of acute leukemia as compared with a ^{32}P regimen in which ceilings are observed for total dosage and for frequency of administration. Nonalkylating forms of chemotherapy are under investigation, but a standard regimen cannot be recommended at this time for lack of clinical experience. The reactive nature of the fibrosis raises the hope that appropriate therapy might abort the evolution of postpolycythemia myelofibrosis. However, the offending agent or process has not been discovered, and it is not clear to which aspect of disease activity it may be secondary and whether its development is retarded or stimulated by myelosuppression.

The physician who must select a treatment regimen for a newly diagnosed patient appears to be steering between Scylla and Charybdis when he faces the equally unacceptable risk of vascular complications versus leukemic transformation. The bleakness of this dilemma is mitigated by the fact that despite treatment-related differences in the types of complications that occur, there is no difference in survival among patients managed with phlebotomy alone, ^{32}P, or chemotherapy, and no overall difference in survival between the population with polycythemia vera and a contemporary, matched population. The presence of comparable survival in the face of the increased incidence of thrombosis and acute leukemia suggests that some benefit is conferred by having polycythemia vera. This may be the effect of improved general medical supervision, since the constantly changing clinical status of the patient requires close monitoring with frequent follow-up visits.

The aforementioned considerations suggest that an optimal regimen should incorporate the advantages of both approaches to therapy, while minimizing their potential disadvantages. This may be accomplished by employing phlebotomy and platelet deaggregating agents as the primary therapy to correct erythrocythemia and platelet hyperfunction and using minimal amounts of myelosuppressive therapy in short courses as a supplementary measure for specific high-risk indications. Prophylactic myelosuppression by means of maintenance therapy should be avoided in favor of periodic reinduction of control over myeloproliferative disease activity. There is no evidence that the patient with a normal hematocrit accompanied by low-grade thrombocytosis, leukocytosis, and splenomegaly fares any worse than one who has been myelosuppressed sufficiently to normalize these features of the disease.

Management with Phlebotomy and Adjunctive Therapy

Every patient with proved polycythemia vera should have an initial series of phlebotomies to restore the hematocrit to a level between 40 and 45 per cent. A phlebotomy of 500 ml should be performed every second or third day until this result is achieved. The number of phlebotomies required depends upon the degree of elevation of the red cell mass, and the amount of red cells removed can be estimated from volume of blood taken and the hematocrit at the time of each phlebotomy. Replacement of plasma or fluids is unnecessary, as the patient quickly reconstitutes his blood volume. Increased fluid intake should be encouraged. Little change in hematocrit may be observed after the first few phlebotomies; but as the red cell mass is decreased and the plasma

volume re-expands, the hematocrit begins to fall. In elderly patients or those with cardiovascular disease, smaller phlebotomies of 350 ml are preferable to avoid abrupt changes in blood volume. Simultaneously with correction of the hematocrit elevation, treatment of several other manifestations of proliferation should be initiated. Prior to or at the time of the first phlebotomy the patient should be placed on a regimen of acetylsalicylic acid at a dose of 500 mg twice a day and dipyridamole (Persantine) at a dose of 50 mg given three to four times a day. A buffered form of acetylsalicylic acid or concomitant administration of antacids is recommended. Allopurinol (Zyloprim) at a dose of 300 mg once each day should be prescribed regardless of the serum uric acid level to reduce the excessive load of uric acid presented by increased nucleoprotein turnover. Blocking the conversion of hypoxanthine to uric acid reduces the risk of developing secondary gout and urate stones or nephropathy. Pruritus, related to release of histamine from basophils, may be relieved by the antihistaminic cyproheptadine (Periactin) in doses of 4 to 16 mg, as needed. The severe itching that is induced by bathing, showering, or undressing can be attenuated by administration of 4 to 8 mg of cyproheptadine one half hour before exposure to the precipitating event.

After restoration of a normal hematocrit, the patient should be seen at 6 week intervals and the rate of rise in hematocrit should be assessed. Some patients display relatively indolent erythroid activity, and the hematocrit may be kept at normal levels with four to six phlebotomies a year. Management with phlebotomy alone should be employed in such patients, as well as in those with isolated erythrocytosis and patients with polycythemia vera in the childbearing age. Although most patiens with polycythemia have hypoferremia, depleted bone marrow iron stores, and a hypochromic, microcytic erythrocyte population, symptoms of iron deficiency are uncommon and iron replacement should not be given, since it produces an increase in hematocrit, requiring further phlebotomy. A normal diet is appropriate, and no attempt to limit iron-containing foods should be made. Reactive thrombocytosis may occur following the initial series of phlebotomies. This increase in platelet count will be superimposed upon any elevation present prior to phlebotomy but is transient, and the platelet count usually returns to the prephlebotomy level within several weeks.

Once the degree of erythroid and other proliferative activity and the need for control have been assessed, visits may be reduced to every

8 to 10 weeks and phlebotomies of 500 ml performed as needed to maintain the hematocrit between 40 and 45 per cent. If the platelet count is less than 500,000 per cu mm and the patient has no history of thrombosis or cardiovascular disease, platelet deaggregating therapy may be discontinued 2 weeks after the initial series of phlebotomies is completed and reintroduced for a 2 week period at the time of the next phlebotomy. If platelets remain at levels above 500,000 per cu mm or the patient is in a high-risk group for the development of thrombosis, deaggregating therapy should be continued with acetylsalicylic acid, 500 mg once daily, and dipyridamole, 100 to 200 mg daily in divided doses. Allopurinol should be administered continuously and antipruritic therapy given as needed.

Indications for and Management with Myelosuppressive Therapy

In some patients with polycythemia vera, erythroid activity may be so accelerated that the hematocrit cannot be maintained at normal levels by the aforementioned regimen. There are also occasional patients who do not tolerate the emotional or physical effects of phlebotomy. Myelosuppressive therapy should be employed when management with phlebotomy is unfeasible or when those features of the proliferative abnormality that cannot be controlled by phlebotomy are felt to be of clinical significance in the patient's disease. These include persistent thrombocytosis of greater than 1,000,000 per cu mm or modest thrombocytosis (500,000 per cu mm or greater) in patients with previous thrombotic episodes, or in elderly patients with compromised cardiovascular systems; patients with symptomatic splenomegaly manifested by early satiety, abdominal discomfort on a mechanical basis, or splenic infarcts; symptoms of "hypermetabolism" such as weight loss and excessive diaphoresis; significant symptoms attributable to iron deficiency; and intractable pruritus. Myelosuppression may be achieved with radioactive phosphorus or chemotherapy, administered as described below, and should be given only until the desired reduction in platelet count or spleen size or relief of symptoms occurs. The patient should be observed for the length of unmaintained remission and re-treated only when an indication for myelosuppression reappears. During unmaintained remission, phlebotomy should be employed to control the hematocrit level. If myelosuppression is used for one of the indications cited above, the patient's iron stores may be repleted during the period of suppression by administration of oral iron and treatment with allopurinol may be discontinued.

Radioactive Phosphorus. This agent is given intravenously in a dose of 2.3 millicuries per square meter of body surface area, the dose not to exceed 5 millicuries. Visits are made every 4 weeks and supplementary phlebotomy is used for control of the hematocrit. At 12 weeks the patient's response is evaluated to determine whether the desired endpoint for which myelosuppressive therapy was given has been attained. If not, a second treatment is given, using a 25 per cent increase in dose. If further suppression is required, a third dose at another 25 per cent increment, but not to exceed 7 millicuries, is given. Further treatment with ^{32}P should be administered only after a 6 month interval, and the total yearly dose should not exceed 15 millicuries. Control of proliferative activity is achieved in 85 to 90 per cent of patients, and a lengthy period of unmaintained remission may result. With repeated administration of ^{32}P there is a tendency toward a selective effect on megakaryopoiesis with a downward drift in platelet count while erythropoiesis remains accelerated. Heavy reliance on phlebotomy with the supplementary use of ^{32}P for myelosuppression should avoid the development of therapy-limiting thrombocytopenia later in the patient's course.

Chemotherapy. Of the several alkylating agents used in the treatment of polycythemia vera, chlorambucil (Leukeran) has been found to be one that provides the smoothest control with the least side effects. (This use of chlorambucil is not listed in the manufacturer's official directive.) Myelosuppression occurs gradually over 8 to 12 weeks, and counts may continue to fall during the lag period of 8 to 12 weeks after drug administration is discontinued. The duration of unmaintained myelosuppression after the first course of chlorambucil depends upon the degree of proliferative activity, but a course of therapy is usually required once or twice yearly. Induction of myelosuppression is begun with daily doses of 10 mg, taken in a single dose when the patient is in a fasting state. During induction a complete blood count is performed every 2 to 3 weeks and phlebotomy is employed for hematocrit control. If chemotherapy is being used for thrombocytosis, the drug should be discontinued when the platelet count reaches 500,000 per cu mm, as a further fall in count can be expected after its withdrawal. If it is being employed for control of other manifestations of proliferative activity, it may be continued until an effect is seen, provided that the platelet count remains above 150,000 per cu mm and the leukocyte count above 3000 per cu mm. During the induction phase, when the platelet or leukocyte count decreases by 25 per cent, the dose of chlorambucil should be adjusted downward to a daily dose of 4 to 6 mg. With a further decrease in count the drug should be discontinued. The thrombocytopenia and leukopenia that occur as a result of chlorambucil tend to be mild and short-lived. The desired control of proliferative activity is usually achieved in 3 to 4 months, and the response rate with chlorambucil is 85 to 90 per cent. The only side effect at the doses used is nausea, which usually subsides as the drug is continued. Once chemotherapy is discontinued, the patient returns to the 8 to 10 week visit cycle and management with phlebotomy. Chemotherapy is reintroduced for reappearance of specific indications for its use. Iron should be administered during the period of suppression and allopurinol discontinued.

Phenylalanine mustard (Alkeran) and busulfan (Myleran) have a more selective and profound effect on platelets than does chlorambucil and may be more appropriate for the patient with marked thrombocytosis and few other stigmata of myeloproliferative disease. Phenylalanine mustard or busulfan is given in doses of 4 to 6 mg daily in a single dose and fasting state. (This use of these two agents is not listed in the manufacturers' official directives.) Careful monitoring of the blood count is necessary at 2 week intervals, with downward reduction or cessation of drug to allow for the lag effect on platelets. An acceptable level of platelets is usually reached in 8 weeks, and no further drug need be administered until indications reappear. Drugs that produce selective platelet suppression are not suitable for control of proliferation in patients without thrombocytosis, as the attendant thrombocytopenia prohibits further treatment with chemotherapy that may be needed for control of other features of the disease.

The Young Patient with Polycythemia Vera

Polycythemia vera has a wide age distribution and may be encountered in young patients. In planning management several modifying factors should be considered: the optimal status of the cardiovascular system offers some protection against circulatory and thrombotic complications; a long survival and duration of disease are expected, making the need for myelosuppressive therapy at some time in the patient's course more likely; the patient is in the childbearing age and may wish to conceive; and myelosuppressive therapy may produce sterility or have a mutagenic effect on the germ cells. Myelosuppressive therapy should be avoided early in the patient's course and during the childbearing years unless there is a compelling indication for its use. In the case of male patients a semen analysis should be performed; if normal results are obtained, consider-

ation should be given to storage of sperm prior to introduction of myelosuppressive therapy. Any patient of childbearing age who must recieve myelosuppressive agents should be counseled against conception during and for at least 6 months after therapy.

Management of Complications

Thrombotic and hemorrhagic complications are managed in the same way as in the nonpolycythemic population. If medically indicated, anticoagulants may be employed. Patients with hemorrhagic manifestations should not be given platelet deaggregating agents. Surgical morbidity and mortality are increased in polycythemia vera, and elective surgery should be avoided. When surgery is indicated, the blood volume should be restored to normal with phlebotomy prior to surgery, and, if time permits, thrombocytosis should be controlled with myelosuppressive agents. Platelet deaggregating therapy should be introduced on the fourth or fifth postoperative day, if there is no postoperative bleeding, to prevent potential thrombotic complications from the reactive thrombocytosis that may follow surgery.

The erythrocytotic stage of polycythemia vera ranges in duration from 5 to 15 years. More than one third of patients eventually demonstrate a change in their proliferative disease and no longer manifest a polycythemic blood picture. The hematocrit may remain at normal levels without the need for phlebotomy for several years while myeloid metaplasia and myelofibrosis become more pronounced and the patient enters the spent phase of polycythemia vera. There is progressive enlargement of the spleen and liver and the hematocrit gradually falls. The anemia that results is usually refractory to hematinics, although iron or folate deficiency should be sought and corrected, if present. Splenomegaly is accompanied by an expansion of the plasma volume, and in some patients the anemia is primarily dilutional. Measurement of the red cell mass at this stage is useful, as it may reveal normal or even increased levels of circulating red cells and marked hydremia. The use of diuretics may partially correct this state and relieve any symptoms of circulatory overload that are present. An absolute reduction in red cell mass may result from decreased erythropoiesis or shortened red cell survival. In the latter case the patients may benefit from shrinkage of the spleen. This may be induced by the judicious use of myelosuppressive therapy or small doses of splenic irradiation. These therapies should not be administered to patients who have marked fibrosis of the marrow in the axial skeleton and little extension of hematopoietic activity to the distal skeleton. Bone marrow distribution should be examined by scanning to determine the total extent of the bone marrow "organ." In the case of anemia resulting from decreased erythropoiesis combined with a shortened red cell survival, the transfusion requirement may be reduced by administration of steroids. Androgens have also produced stimulation of erythropoiesis in some patients and are worthy of a trial. Response is slow to occur, and the therapeutic trial should be continued for 6 months before abandoning this form of treatment. Splenectomy may be of benefit in selected cases of postpolycythemia myeloid metaplasia in which there is evidence of hypersplenism. Although surgical morbidity and mortality are considerable, the diminution in transfusion requirement, rise in platelet count, and removal of physical discomfort produced by the enlarged spleen make splenectomy worthwhile in patients who are otherwise in good physical condition. Splenectomy is contraindicated in patients with thrombocytosis, since removal of the large storage pool results in marked thrombocytosis which may be difficult to control in the perioperative period and may lead to life-threatening complications. The patient with thrombocytosis should be prepared for splenectomy with a course of myelosuppressive therapy.

Acute leukemia terminates the course of 10 to 15 per cent of patients with polycythemia vera. Myeloblastic leukemia is the usual evolution, but in a small percentage the blasts bear properties usually seen in acute lymphoblastic leukemia. Management of the acute leukemic stage is complicated by the presence of a previously compromised bone marrow, and the remission rate is less than that of de novo acute leukemia. Nonetheless, successful remission induction has been attained with the standard regimens, and the patient should be given the benefit of this therapy. When this or other forms of malignancy arise in the patient with polycythemia vera the approach to treatment should not be altered, except to adjust medication doses according to the state of the proliferative activity. These patients have a favorable prognosis with respect to their myeloproliferative disease and should not be denied optimal therapy for any concomitant condition.

The patient with polycythemia vera presents a challenge in management, for the benefits conferred by proper treatment are dramatic in terms of improving survival and well-being. The multifaceted nature of the disease often taxes the physician's skill in manipulating the various forms of therapy that are available. Fortunately, these efforts are usually rewarded by the opportunity to participate in a prolonged and satisfying patient-doctor relationship.

THE PORPHYRIAS

method of
PETER V. TISHLER, M.D.
Boston, Massachusetts

The porphyrias are a group of inborn errors of heme biogenesis with clinical effects primarily on the nervous system, liver, and skin. Each porphyria is a genetically distinct entity with specific biochemical features. They have traditionally been classified according to their biochemical pathology into the hepatic and the erythropoietic porphyrias (Table 1 and Fig. 1). For purposes of this discussion of treatment, we shall depart from this classification to discuss the porphyrias according to their major clinical manifestations.

Porphyrias Presenting Primarily with Acute Symptomatology

The three acute porphyrias (or acute hepatic porphyrias) are intermittent acute porphyria (IAP), variegate porphyria (VP), and coproporphyria (CP). They are generally not distinguishable on clinical grounds. All three can present with acute attacks in which most signs and symptoms derive from autonomic, sensory, and motor neuropathy: severe pain, especially involving the abdomen or back; sensory and motor peripheral neuropathy, with paresthesias (pain in the extremities) and either indolent or rapidly progressive motor changes leading to a flaccid paralysis; constipation, tachycardia, and hypertension; acute psychosis; electrolyte abnormalities; and respiratory paralysis. Mortality and especially morbidity from the acute attack are high. Cutaneous manifestations are never seen in IAP, but may be found intermittently in some patients with either CP or VP. These cutaneous manifestations are similar to those of porphyria cutanea tarda (see below). IAP may also exist as a subacute or chronic syndrome notable only for severe psychiatric disease. Indeed, there is evidence to suggest that the prevalence of IAP in hospitalized psychiatric patient populations is significantly augmented.

All three acute porphyrias are inherited as strict autosomal dominants. However, there is considerable variability in clinical manifestations among those who have inherited a gene for one of these porphyrias, in large part because of the pharmacogenetic nature of these diseases (see below). Totally asymptomatic individuals are common, but they can have relatives with florid disease. Moreover, although the acute porphyrias rarely cause clinical problems before puberty, there is considerable intrafamily variability in the age at onset of any subsequent illness. Nonetheless, careful biochemical study will disclose the primary biochemical-genetic defect for these three porphyrias in most carriers of the gene, regardless of clinical status.

TABLE 1. The Porphyrias: Types, Manifestations, Means of Diagnosis*

BIOCHEMICAL TYPE	NAME	MAJOR MANIFESTATIONS	INHERITANCE	CRITERIA FOR DIAGNOSIS		
				Urine	Stool	Blood
Hepatic						
Acute	Intermittent acute porphyria (IAP)	Acute—attacks of pain, sensory loss, motor and respiratory paralysis, psychosis, hyponatremia; chronic—psychopathy	AD	↑↑ALA, PBG	nl	↓Uroporphyrinogen I synthetase (RBC)‡
	Variegate porphyria (VP)	Acute—as above; chronic—blistering, fissuring, scarring, hypertrichosis, hyperpigmentation, of sun-exposed skin	AD	↑↑ALA, PBG (intermittent)	↑Proto	↓Protoporphyrinogen oxidase (WBC)†
	Coproporphyria (CP)	Acute—as above; chronic—as above	AD	↑↑ALA, PBG (intermittent)	↑Copro	↓Coproporphyrinogen oxidase (WBC)†
Chronic	Porphyria cutanea tarda (PCT)	Blistering, friability, scarring, hypertrichosis, hyperpigmentation of sun-exposed skin	AD + ?sporadic	↑↑Uro (>Copro)	nl	↓Uroporphyrinogen decarboxylase (RBC)‡
Erythrohepatic	Protoporphyria (P)	Acute—skin photosensitivity, burning, erythema, swelling, itching, scarring; chronic—cirrhosis and hepatic failure	AD	nl	↑Proto	↓Proto (RBC) ↓Heme synthetase (WBC)†
Erythropoietic	Congenital erythropoietic porphyria (CEP)	Acute—skin photosensitivity as in protoporphyria, but bullous eruption predominates; chronic—serious scarring, mutilation	AR	↑↑Uro, ↑Copro	↑Copro	↓Uro (RBC) ↓Uroporphyrinogen III cosynthetase (RBC)‡

*Abbreviations: AD = autosomal dominant, AR = autosomal recessive; PBG = porphobilinogen, ALA = δ-aminolevulinic acid; Uro = uroporphyrin,
Copro = coproporphyrin, Proto = protoporphyrin; RBC = erythrocytes, WBC = leukocytes; nl = normal.
†These enzyme assays are not easily available for diagnostic purposes.
‡These enzyme assays are performed only at certain specialized laboratories.

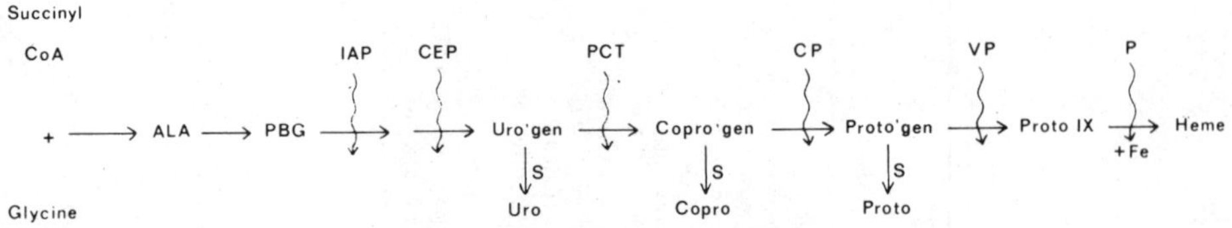

Succinyl

CoA

Glycine

Figure 1. Schema of porphyrin biosynthesis, including the genetically determined enzyme deficiencies of the porphyrias IAP, CEP, PCT, CP, VP, and P (see Table 1 for definitions of these abbreviations). The names of the enzymes deficient in the porphyrias are given in Table 1. In each case, excess quantities of metabolites proximal to the block may be demonstrated. Other abbreviations: CoA = coenzyme A; ALA = δ-aminolevulinic acid; PBG = porphobilinogen; Uro-, Copro-, Proto'gen = uro-, copro-, and protoporphyrinogen; Uro, Copro, Proto = uro-, copro-, and protoporphyrin.

Long-Term Treatment of the Acute Porphyrias

The cornerstones of treatment of the acute porphyrias are prevention and education. Prevention is a realistic goal because most acute attacks are precipitated by the ingestion of certain drugs, medications, or heavy metals, a dramatic change in diet, or an intercurrent illness. Concerning drugs or medications, a list of materials that are either safe or unsafe in the acute porphyrias is available from persons who specialize in these diseases. Unfortunately, this list is compiled from largely anecdotal reports and is incomplete for both old and new materials. Thus, patients should *avoid all medications unless they are absolutely indicated.* Specifically to be avoided are the barbiturates, sulfonamides, estrogen-containing preparations (including oral contraceptives), anticonvulsants, certain minor tranquilizers (chlordiazepoxide, meprobamate, possibly diazepam), alcohol, hypnotics (glutethimide), oral hypoglycemic agents, griseofulvin, and certain antihypertensive medications. Clearly, some major classes of medications are included in this list, and clinical indications for use of one of these may outweigh the contraindication. Seizures requiring treatment are a frequent accompaniment of the acute porphyrias. Certain affected individuals can take diphenylhydantoin (phenytoin) for seizure control without problem. In others, this will precipitate an acute attack, as will carbamazepine, methsuximide, and probably valproate. Clonazepam, diazepam, and even bromides have been used successfully as alternative forms of anticonvulsant therapy. Although certain antihypertensive medications (spironolactone, hydralazine, clonidine) appear to be potentially harmful in the acute porphyrias, others (reserpine, propranolol, thiazide diuretics, and possibly furosemide) have no deleterious effects. Anesthesia for surgery presents a real problem, since there is little experience with the newer inhalation agents. Ethyl ether is quite safe, but is rarely used nowadays. Isolated reports of acute attacks precipitated by halothane are contradicted by experimental evidence suggesting that it is not porphyrogenic,

while the converse is the case with enflurane. Other types of drugs that are safe for use in patients with an acute porphyria include salicylates, atropine, phenothiazines, narcotic analgesics, corticosteroids, penicillins, tetracyclines, antihistamines, digitalis preparations, and the aforementioned antihypertensive agents.

Preventive education of both patient and physician, particularly to the deleterious effects of drugs, is probably the major reason for the decline in mortality from the acute porphyrias in the past decade. Patients should also be educated to avoid all but modest alcohol intake, to maintain a constant reasonable caloric intake and specifically to avoid severe calorie restriction, and to keep their health care providers apprised of their medical problems. They should be urged to contact the physician early in the course of an apparently innocuous illness or at the time of undue emotional stress, and the physician must be alert to the possibility that acute attacks of porphyria can be precipitated by these events. Pregnancy constitutes an especially important period in which close observation and good rapport are essential, since acute attacks are relatively frequent. The primary emphasis in all these situations must be the prevention of the acute attack. The secondary emphasis must be on recognizing the acute attack before it becomes life threatening, removing the stimuli precipitating the attack, and/or offering expert treatment in a supportive environment. Patients must also carry some form of identification, such as a Medic Alert identification tag, in case they are unable to provide historical information.

Because the acute porphyrias may be life threatening, the study of family members to ascertain others with a gene for porphyria is prudent. These individuals, even if asymptomatic, should receive the same aforementioned education as their affected relatives. All carriers of a gene for an acute porphyria will profit from genetic counseling. Since all three diseases are autosomal dominant, the probability that each and every offspring will receive the gene for the porphyria is 0.5. However, the probability of frank disease, particularly with the simple precautions outlined above, is considerably less than this (perhaps one fifth to one half of those inheriting the gene will experience clinical manifestations at some time). Nonetheless, occasional patients will develop life-threatening complications. Prenatal diagnosis via amniocentesis is possible for IAP and probably for VP and CP. However, this would seem unnecessary under most circumstances.

Treatment of the Acute Attack

Removing the precipitating agent from the patient or from his or her environment is an essential first step in therapy. This may require diligent search, and is often ample justification for hospitalization and close observation, but the effort *must* be made. A second therapeutic measure is the institution of a high carbohydrate diet, of at least 300 grams daily by any route. This of itself will abort the acute attack in a significant proportion of affected individuals. Symptomatic treatment, such as phenothiazines or narcotic analgesics in moderate doses for pain, propranolol for autonomic dysfunction (tachycardia, hypertension), or anticonvulsants, may afford relief until the acute attack subsides. Acid-base, mineral, or electrolyte abnormalities, including those accompanying the inappropriate secretion of antidiuretic hormone, must be corrected by standard means.

The major pharmacologic treatment of the acute attack is the intravenous infusion of hematin (ferriheme hydroxide). This will dramatically interrupt the chemical pathology of the acute attack and abort the symptoms in most cases (Watson, C. J., et al.: Adv. Intern. Med. 23:265, 1978; Lamon, J. M., et al.: Medicine 58:252, 1979). Experience in the use of this material, although generally favorable, is still limited. Indeed, its availability is circumscribed by its investigational drug nature in the United States of America. Present indications for beginning hematin therapy would seem to be the following: (1) intractable symptoms unresponsive to other forms of therapy (see above) that are of themselves not a threat to life (e.g., persistent vomiting or obstipation, severe abdominal pain, acute psychosis); (2) a progression of manifestations, to include clear involvement of the peripheral nervous system (sensory or motor neuropathy); or (3) any acute, potentially life-threatening manifestations (respiratory paralysis). For any of these indications, early treatment maximizes the chances of a favorable therapeutic response. Hematin must be obtained from those few investigators who are permitted to dispense it for inves-

tigational use. It is given at a dosage of 2 to 4 mg per kg one or two times daily in saline solution in a large vein over 10 to 15 minutes. Treatment should probably be continued until the chemical manifestations (plasma or urinary ALA and PBG) demonstrate a reversion toward normal and the patient has experienced clear clinical improvement (including remission of life-threatening manifestations, if present), or there is no response to an adequate trial. Courses of hematin usually range from 3 to 13 days; at the dosage listed above, there have been remarkably few side effects. Multiple courses have also been given without adverse effect. Nonetheless, our knowledge concerning the indications, dosage, methods of termination of therapy, and other factors are so sketchy that the use of this material should be carried out only with the active collaboration of a clinician familiar with its use.

Throughout the acute attack, meticulous attention must be given to whatever mechanical supports are necessary to maintain life (e.g., assisted mechanical ventilation). Recovery from the neuropathy of an acute porphyria is often a very slow process, taxing the dedication of both the patient and the health care team. Very long term occupational and physical therapy will often result in total return of function, and thus should be pursued.

A Porphyria with Cutaneous and Hepatic Manifestations: Protoporphyria

Protoporphyria is an autosomal dominant inborn error characterized by cutaneous sensitivity to visible light (380 to 560 nm). Symptoms include burning, swelling, itching, and redness of the skin, and scarring may occur after repeated episodes. Its clinical onset is generally in the first decade of life, a fact that often differentiates it from the other cutaneous porphyrias. The diagnosis is made by the finding of increased concentrations of protoporphyrin IX in erythrocytes and plasma, or by demonstrating decreased activity of the mitochondrial enzyme heme synthetase (Table 1 and Fig. 1). These same studies are also useful in identifying asymptomatic affected relatives of index cases. Protoporphyria is a relatively newly described disease, and thus far the major manifestation seems to be these photosensitivity phenomena. The treatment of choice for this is oral beta-carotene (Solatene), starting at dosages of 15 to 180 mg per day according to age and increasing the dosage until the patient notes amelioration of photosensitivity. This usually correlates with a serum carotene of about 400 micrograms per dl. Treatment with beta-carotene produces a slight yellowish discoloration of the skin but seems to produce no side effects. In contrast, it produces a marked increase in tolerance for sunlight and a normalization of life style that otherwise may be limited to indoor activities during much of the year.

As experience with protoporphyria accumulates, there is increasing evidence to suggest that a severe, life-threatening liver disease may occur in certain patients. The prevalence in protoporphyria of liver disease in general, and fatal cirrhosis with hepatic failure in particular, is not known. Abnormalities of liver function may be minimal in patients in whom fatal hepatic failure is imminent, and there seems to be no good means for identifying these individuals before significant hepatic damage has ensued. Clearly, abnormal liver chemistries, particularly in association with markedly elevated plasma or erythrocyte protoporphyrin concentrations, are an indication for liver biopsy, both to quantitate the degree of hepatopathy and to search for the characteristic deposits of brown pigment that probably represent protoporphyrin. Early and prompt treatment of patients with liver disease with the ion exchange resin cholestyramine (Questran), in the usual dosages (12 to 15 grams per day in divided doses), with or without simultaneous vitamin E (100 units of Aquasol E daily) has reduced total body protoporphyrin concentrations and produced marked improvement of liver function in a limited number of patients.

Porphyrias with Cutaneous Manifestations

Of all of the porphyrias in this group, congenital porphyria (congenital erythropoietic porphyria, Günther's disease) is the most severe, with intense photosensitivity from infancy (Table 1). Repeated episodes of this photoeruption lead to severe scarring, with ultimate loss of the tips of the fingers, auricles, or nose in the extreme. Hemolysis, frequently with splenomegaly, is also the rule, but significant anemia is seen only rarely. Effective treatments of congenital porphyria have not been established with certainty. Dramatic reductions in photosensitivity have been observed in patients treated with betacarotene (orally, as outlined above), but only a few patients have received this treatment. Splenectomy may lessen the anemia and also the cutaneous manifestations in those patients with excessive hemolysis. Careful protection from sunlight is mandatory. Congenital porphyria is inherited as an autosomal recessive (it is the only porphyria that is not a dominant). Thus, parents (who may be consanguineous) may become aware of their heterozygosity for the gene for this disease only upon the birth of a clinically affected child. Such persons will benefit from referral to a geneticist for genetic counseling. The diagnosis of congenital porphyria can probably be made prenatally, since normal concentrations of uroporphyrinogen III cosynthetase have been demonstrated in cultured amniotic fluid cells in at least one at-risk fetus.

A more common porphyria is porphyria cutanea tarda (PCT or symptomatic porphyria), which in various small studies has a prevalence of about 2 per cent in patients with photosensitivity or with alcoholic cirrhosis. Cutaneous manifestations, involving primarily the light-exposed surfaces, include bullae, increased skin fragility, facial hypertrichosis, and hyperpigmentation. Scarring leads typically to skin that appears considerably older than expected by chronology. Certain phenomena are clearly associated with the development of these manifestations: the excessive use of alcohol, estrogen therapy, increased tissue iron stores, and exposure to halogenated hydrocarbons. The last appears to be an increasing problem as further industrial and environmental exposures to these common chemicals are documented. A decreased activity of the enzyme uroporphyrinogen decarboxylase has been demonstrated in liver and/or erythrocytes of many affected and some asymptomatic carrier individuals with PCT. However, controversy exists concerning the universality of this lesion in PCT, some authors claiming that only those individuals with clearly familial PCT have the enzyme deficiency as a primary gene defect. Furthermore, the relative roles of the aforementioned nongenetic precipitating agents and of this enzyme deficiency in the pathogenesis of this syndrome, while the subject of several critical studies in animals, have not been fully explained.

The primary treatment of PCT is, again, removal of the precipitating agents from the patient's environment. In some patients, the skin lesions will disappear and the liability for further sun-induced lesions will diminish solely with abstinence from alcohol or discontinuation of oral contraceptive agents. However, since most individuals with this syndrome have demonstrable iron overload that is not rectified by these maneuvers, further therapy by means of phlebotomy (removal of 500 ml every 2 to 4 weeks) is necessary for most patients. The efficacy and adequacy of phlebotomy are monitored carefully by frequent measurement of the hematocrit, serum ferritin, and urine uroporphyrin excretion. The aim is to reduce the urinary excretion of uroporphyrin to or toward normal, while also normalizing the ferritin and avoiding iron deficiency. With careful monitoring and conservatism in the rate at which blood is removed, particularly as treatment progresses and chemistries begin to normalize, this can be achieved without difficulty.

A return of the skin lesions or a significant increase in urinary uroporphyrin excretion (which should be monitored every 6 months) is an indication for resumption of therapy.

Both variegate porphyria and coproporphyria, the acute attacks of which were discussed above, may have cutaneous manifestations. These are generally indistinguishable from those of PCT, although the two acute porphyrias can be differentiated chemically from PCT by the pattern of fecal porphyrin excretion (Table 1). The cutaneous findings are not correlated with symptoms of the acute attack, or with exposure to the agents that precipitate the acute attack. Treatment should be aimed at minimizing the exposure to light. Beta-carotene might be helpful in preventing the photosensitivity, but has not been tried systematically. Sunscreens that have substantial absorption in the longwave untraviolet range (The Medical Letter *21*:46, 1979) may also be helpful, but again there are insufficient data to be predictive.

THERAPEUTIC USE OF BLOOD COMPONENTS

method of
JAMES W. LANGLEY, M.D.
San Antonio, Texas

Introduction

Maximal therapeutic effectiveness in the use of blood components requires development of a working knowledge of the characteristics and specific indications for use of the individual blood products, a full understanding of the transfusion risk involved, and objective assessment of the effectiveness of the transfused product. More widespread availability of sophisticated surgery as well as more aggressive medical treatment of all patients with diseases such as hemophilia, leukemia, lymphoma, and others has created a great demand for specific blood components.

One voluntary blood donation can be separated rapidly and efficiently into various components to meet the diverse needs of multiple patients. The careful selection of specific blood product(s) for treatment of individual blood component deficiencies allows for greater treatment effectiveness while reducing transfusion risks by decreasing additional exposure to cellular and plasma antigens.

With the increased demand for all blood components being placed on community blood centers, the use of whole blood transfusions can now only occasionally be justified.

Hypovolemia

Significant acute blood volume depletion can be clinically evaluated by a persistent increase in the pulse rate and a decrease in the systolic blood pressure to below 100 mm Hg. Most healthy adults can tolerate acute blood losses of 500 to 1000 ml with no or only minimal clinical effects. A blood loss of greater than 1000 ml may cause peripheral vasoconstriction, pallor, sweating, tachycardia, and postural hypotension. The loss of more than 2000 ml of blood will produce clinical shock which, unless reversed immediately, may cause irreversible organ and tissue damage. The immediate treatment of the acute blood loss must be directed primarily at restoration of adequate tissue perfusion by volume support and secondarily at replacing the red cell mass.

Crystalloid solutions such as isotonic saline and lactated Ringer's can be used to the immediate expansion of the intravascular volume when the acute blood loss is 1000 ml or less. Because of their loss from the intravascular space, these solutions must be infused rapidly and in quantities sufficient to maintain the vital signs.

Colloid solutions such as purified protein fraction and 5 per cent albumin remain longer in the intravascular space and are better able to maintain oncotic pressure. These solutions are effective when acute blood losses exceed 1000 ml. They should also be rapidly infused. These plasma-derived solutions are prepared with sophisticated fractionation and heat treatment processes which eliminate the risk of transmitting hepatitis. Some disadvantages of these solutions are the expense and their lack of coagulation factors. The purified plasma protein fractions have occasionally caused hypotensive episodes when administered rapidly during surgery. This is believed to be due to activated bradykinin contaminants.

When the acute blood loss is greater than 1500 ml, there is a significant decrease in red cell mass which must be corrected as well as the hypovolemia. This can be effectively done with either (1) packed red cell concentrates combined with colloid or electrolyte solutions or (2) whole blood. The use of stored whole blood in acute massive blood loss may require additional supplementation with platelets and occasionally labile clotting factors because of their poor preservation during storage at 4 to 6 C.

In rare emergency situations, in which the patient is in clinical shock with continuing hemorrhage and there is insufficient time to complete a routine crossmatch, uncrossmatched O $Rh_0(D)$ negative red blood cells can be given. However, this should seldom happen, since blood typing with an "emergency" crossmatch can be done usually within 10 minutes and group specific blood can be provided with some assurance of safety. The crossmatch can generally be fully completed within 1 hour while the patient is being transfused with electrolyte and protein solutions to maintain vital tissue perfusion.

Treatment to Improve Oxygen-Carrying Capacity

If medical assessment of the patient determines that there is a deficit in the red cell mass with impairment of oxygen delivery to peripheral tissues, the component which must be administered is an erythrocyte-containing preparation. These can be administered as whole blood, packed red cells, buffy poor packed red cells, saline-washed packed red cells, or frozen-washed packed red cells. Each of these products has its own characteristics and specific indications for use. All blood cell transfusions have the potential to produce fatal reactions, to transmit hepatitis, and to stimulate antibodies to various transfused antigens. Therefore the risks of the transfusion must be carefully evaluated in relation to the expected benefits. No patient whose oxygen-carrying deficit can be adequately restored without blood transfusion should be exposed to these additional risks. Patients with chronic anemia and megaloblastic anemia resulting from B_{12} or folate deficiency are usually best managed initially without transfusion. Patients with longstanding anemia, such as that seen in renal failure and collagen vascular diseases, usually have compensatory physiologic changes which allow increased oxygen delivery to tissues in spite of low hematocrit values. These patients, unless they have symptoms, should not be transfused merely to improve their abnormal laboratory values. Prior to the transfusion, it is absolutely essential that the blood product label be carefully examined to determine blood group and the unit number to verify that the unit of blood requested is actually going to be transfused to the correct patient. Clerical error and incorrect patient identification are the major causes of nearly all serious transfusion reactions.

Patients should normally receive group and type specific red blood cells. However, during periods of blood shortages, crossmatch compatible group O red blood cells can be safely given to patients of any group. Group AB patients can safely receive compatible red blood cells from group A, group B, or group O donors. When non-group-specific blood is transfused, the plasma should be removed to prevent a potential decrease in patient red cell survival caused by the transfused donor isohemagglutinins.

Red Blood Cells (Human). These packed red blood cell concentrates are prepared by centrifugation of whole blood and removal of most of the supernatant plasma. The unit volume is generally 250 ml and contains 250 mg of iron. It is equivalent in oxygen-carrying potential to a unit of whole blood. If stored in the anticoagulant CPD (citrate, phosphate, dextrose), it will have a maximal 21 day storage life. If stored in the new anticoagulant CPDA-1 (citrate, phosphate, dextrose with adenine supplement), the storage life is increased to 35 days. Removal of the plasma decreases the risk of circulatory overload in patients with a marginal cardiovascular status, and decreases the potential for citrate toxicity in massive transfusions. The hematocrit of 60 to 70 per cent may increase the viscosity of the packed cell concentrate. By adding at least 50 ml of isotonic saline solution to the blood unit by means of a Y tubing and applying a pressure cuff to the bag, the flow rate of the transfusion will be improved. Transfusion of 1 unit of packed red blood cells should elevate the hemoglobin 0.5 to 1 gram per dl and the hematocrit 2 to 4 percentage points in a 70 kg patient.

Red Blood Cells (Human), Leukocyte Poor. Whole blood or packed red cell concentrate may contain between 2 and 4×10^9 leukocytes. Seventy to 90 per cent of these leukocytes may be removed by centrifugation, nylon filtration, or saline washing techniques. Patients with a history of multiple pregnancies or exposure to multiple transfusions may develop febrile nonhemolytic transfusion reactions owing to antibodies to leukocyte antigens. These reactions may be decreased and even eliminated by the use of a red blood cell (human) leukocyte poor product. Some automated saline-washing procedures for red blood cells remove nearly 90 per cent of the leukocytes and nearly all plasma proteins. This product is indicated for patients with febrile nonhemolytic transfusion reactions, for patients with known reactions to plasma antigens (such as IgA deficient individuals), and for patients with a need for removal of plasma potassium, sodium, citrate, and ammonia (such as in pediatrics and in renal failure). Saline-washed red blood cells may have a 10 per cent loss of red cells during the procedure and a storage limitation of 24 hours to prevent potential bacterial growth.

Red Blood Cells (Human), Frozen, Deglycerolyzed. Blood may be stored frozen up to 3 years by adding the cryoprotective agent glycerol. After thawing and repeated washing to remove the glycerol, nearly all plasma and tissue antigens such as white cells are removed. The cost of frozen blood is high, and once thawed the units can be stored for only 24 hours. Patients with rare blood cell types can benefit most from receiving frozen red cells from a rare donor depot. Patients with rare blood should be strongly encouraged to store their own blood for potential future autotransfusion. Patients who continue to have febrile nonhemolytic transfusion reactions after receiving saline-washed or leuko-poor red cells will benefit from frozen deglycerolyzed red blood cells, because they essentially have few remaining white cell antigens. The use of frozen red cells can transmit hepatitis, but the risk is markedly decreased. The use of frozen blood in renal patients awaiting kidney transplantation may allow more patients to have an opportunity to receive transplants by preventing sensitization to leukocyte antigens, but may adversely affect the long-term kidney graft survival. There is current controversy about the benefits of this product for potential kidney transplant recipients.

Autologous Blood Donation. With the increased storage time of blood to 35 days in the CPDA-1 anticoagulant, any patient can easily donate at least 2 units of blood prior to any scheduled surgery. If additional units of blood are needed, supplemental oral iron can be given if necessary, and up to 6 to 8 units of blood can be collected and stored in the frozen state until needed. This therapeutic use of autologous blood is underutilized. There are no risks of transmission of hepatitis or sensitization to cellular or plasma antigens with the use of this product. With the additional blood storage time available with the new CPDA-1 anticoagulant, patient autologous blood donation is logistically simplified and should now be used to supply the blood needs of many scheduled surgical procedures.

Blood Components for Hemostasis

Patients may have disordered hemostasis because of congenital or acquired defects. These include quantitative or functional platelet or coagulation factor deficiencies.

Selection of the appropriate blood component to correct the hemostatic defect requires clinical evaluation of the patient history and the evaluation of the location and the nature of the bleeding. Laboratory evaluation, using the prothrombin time, partial thromboplastin time, fibrinogen level assay, and a platelet count, is usually helpful in documenting the deficiency. However, abnormal laboratory values alone are not justification for component therapy. Most clotting factors can be reduced to as low as 25 per cent of the normal levels before bleeding may actually occur. Platelet levels may also be reduced

to 10 to 15 per cent of normal (15,000 to 20,000 per cu mm) before spontaneous bleeding is seen. Normal hemostasis for surgical procedures may be provided with platelet counts of at least 50,000 per cu mm. Therefore, selection of components for hemostasis should be made only after evaluation of the clinical and laboratory information helps document and define the cause of the deficiency.

Platelet Concentrate (Human). Patients with thrombocytopenia resulting from decreased platelet production (e.g., aplastic anemia, leukemia, chemotherapy), dilutional effects from rapidly receiving 10 to 12 units of blood, or congenital or acquired platelet defects may show a beneficial response to platelet therapy. Thrombocytopenic patients with rapid platelet destruction and shortened platelet life spans (e.g., idiopathic thrombocytopenic purpura) generally receive no benefit from platelet therapy, and it should be reserved for life-threatening hemorrhage. After 48 hours, there are few hemostatically effective platelets in stored whole blood. Therefore, platelet concentrates are prepared by centrifugation from freshly drawn blood from random donors. These concentrates have a 30 to 50 ml volume and contain a minimum of 5.5×10^{10} platelets, 1 to 3×10^8 white cells, and approximately 0.5 ml red cells. Platelets do have ABO antigens. However, ABO incompatible platelets are effective when group specific platelets are unavailable. $Rh_0(D)$ negative children and $Rh_0(D)$ negative women of childbearing age should receive $Rh_0(D)$ negative platelets if possible. During blood shortages, $Rh_0(D)$ positive platelets may have to be given. $Rh_0(D)$ sensitization can be prevented by administering $Rh_0(D)$ immune globulin. Patients with fever, sepsis, splenomegaly, consumptive coagulopathy, and white cell sensitization may all have decreased response to platelet transfusions.

In a patient without fever and sepsis and who has not been sensitized by previous pregnancies or transfusions, 1 platelet concentrate should elevate the platelet count at 1 hour to at least 9000 per cu mm. A transfusion of at least 6 to 8 platelet concentrates normally produces effective hemostasis. For effective evaluation of platelet therapy, a pretransfusion platelet count and platelet counts at 1 and 24 hours should be done after each transfusion.

When the 1 hour post-transfusion platelet counts show either no or minimal increases in patients receiving repeated transfusions from random donors, new therapeutic approaches should be considered. These patients may respond to HLA-matched platelets from an HLA-typed random plateletpheresis donor provided from a regional blood center or from platelets from the immediate family. Plateletpheresis by automated blood cell separators are efficient in platelet collections. A plateletpheresis product from a single donor such as a family member or an HLA compatible random donor will provide from 3 to 6 × 10^{11} platelets in a 300 ml volume. This is equivalent to 6 to 10 conventional random donor platelet concentrates. The product should be transfused as soon as possible to get the maximal benefit. Plateletpheresis products should be reserved for patients with documented refractoriness to random donor platelet concentrates.

Single Donor Plasma (Human), Fresh Frozen. Fresh frozen plasma (FFP) contains all the plasma coagulation factors in a 250 ml volume and can be used to initially treat any of the acquired or hereditary clotting deficiencies. In a 70 kg adult 3 to 4 units of FFP can raise all the deficient clotting factors to at least 25 to 30 per cent. This may allow time for further clinical and laboratory documentation of a specific factor defect. Factor VIII and factor IX deficiencies in hemophiliacs usually require the use of factor concentrates because of the large volumes of FFP needed for effective hemostasis. FFP may provide short-term hemostasis effectiveness in patients with severe hepatic disorders. Vitamin K deficiency can often be adequately treated by oral or parenteral vitamin K alone. However, transfusion with FFP may occasionally be necessary.

Patients receiving massive quantities of blood usually greater than 10 to 12 units over a few hours may develop a dilutional thrombocytopenia. If the clinical and laboratory evaluations also indicate deficiency of clotting factor(s), then 3 to 5 units of FFP is usually sufficient to restore the levels to hemostatic effectiveness.

FFP takes 1 hour to thaw and should be administered promptly. It can cause nonhemolytic transfusion reactions and has the same risk of causing hepatitis as a single unit of red blood cells.

Cryoprecipitated Antihemophilic Factor (Human). One bag (10 to 20 ml) of this product is equivalent to 80 to 100 units of factor VIII coagulant activity and 200 to 300 mg of fibrinogen. This product is effective therapy for almost all patients with classic hemophilia A (factor VIII deficiency) and patients with fibrinogen deficiencies. Cryoprecipitate is also indicated in patients with von Willebrand's disease, in which the product corrects the factor VIII deficiency and improves platelet functions.

Factor VIII (AHF) Concentrates. These commercially prepared lyophilized concentrates are expensive. They are prepared from a large plasma pool and have a significant risk of transmitting hepatitis. However, the ease of storage and administration of known factor VIII dosage units makes this product very useful. Both cryoprecipitate and commercially prepared lyophilized factor VIII concentrates are effective for home therapy programs.

Factor IX Concentrates. These lyophilized preparations contain factors II, VII, IX, and X and have a very high risk of transmitting hepatitis. These concentrates should usually be used to treat patients with severe hemophilia B (less than 1 per cent factor IX coagulation activity). Because of volume limitations with fresh frozen plasma therapy, the use of factor IX concentrates is necessary for severe hemorrhages and home therapy programs.

Therapeutic Dosage Calculations. Prior to administration of either factor VIII or factor IX concentrates, an accurate diagnosis of the specific deficiency must be determined and the dose calculated based on the level of the deficient factor needed for hemostasis and the intravascular half-life of the product containing the clotting factor.

The metabolic intravascular half-life of factor VIII is 8 to 12 hours and of factor IX, 5 to 24 hours. Approximately 75 per cent of the transfused factor VIII concentrate and 30 to 50 per cent of the transfused factor IX concentrate remain in the intravascular space. Based on this information an adequate dose of clotting factor activity can be calculated depending on the patient's plasma volume and the clinical episode. The approximate plasma volume is calculated by the following formula:

$$\text{Weight (kg)} \times 70 \text{ ml blood per kg} = \text{blood volume}$$
$$(\text{Blood volume}) (1-\text{Hct}) = \text{plasma volume}$$

One ml of normal plasma contains 1 unit of factor VIII and 1 unit of factor IX activity. If a factor VIII level of 50 per cent is required in an adult with plasma volume of 3000 ml, at least 1500 units of factor VIII concentrate would be needed. Because of shortened intravascular half-life of factor IX the calculated dosage may have to be initially doubled. Laboratory assays of the deficient clotting factor levels should be done to effectively monitor the therapy.

Special Blood Component Products

Leukocyte Concentrate (Human). Granulocyte concentrates are prepared from single donors, usually family members, by the use of automated blood cell separators or nylon fiber filtration. The maximal granulocyte collection efficiency by a cell separator requires the use of hydroxyethyl starch and steroid premedication of the donor. The 3 hour procedure yields a 300 ml product which may contain from 2 to 5×10^{10} granulocytes, 1 to 4×10^9 lymphocytes, 2 to 3×10^{11} platelets, and 20 to 50 ml of red blood cells.

This special product has been shown to help reduce the mortality rates in infected leukopenic patients with severe marrow dysfunction not responsive to antibiotic therapy. Granulocytes should be administered to infected patients with absolute granulocyte counts (bands and segmented neutrophils of less than 500 per microliter). The granulocyte concentrates should be administered daily during the period of sepsis and severe granulocytopenia. They should be continued for a minimum of 4 days until the patient is afebrile or there is evidence of effective bone marrow recovery. The granulocytes should be ABO compatible with the patient. HLA compatibility and leukocyte crossmatch techniques have not been as effective in predicting transfusion response as ABO compatibility alone. The granulocytes should be transfused slowly through a blood filter over a period of 2 to 3 hours. Patient white cell counts and a differential prior to transfusion and at 1 hour post-transfusion are recommended. Granulocyte increments may be small owing to rapid mobilization to areas of infection. Granulocyte transfusions are frequently associated with chills, fever, and occasionally hypotension in a patient. It is generally recommended, because of the large doses of viable lymphocytes in each granulocyte concentrate, that they be irradiated prior to transfusion to patients with severe immune deficiency and patients who have received a bone marrow transplant and are severely immunosuppressed. This issue is controversial and is currently being evaluated.

The use of granulocyte concentrates is expensive, requires donor availability, and causes increased risk to the donor. This therapy should be reserved for severely ill patients who do not respond to antibiotic therapy and have a reasonable opportunity for bone marrow recovery and survival if their sepsis can be controlled.

Albumin. This is a purified product available as 5 and 25 per cent solutions. The 5 per cent solution is used most effectively for volume replacement in patients with acute hypovolemia. The concentrated 25 per cent albumin preparation can be used in patients with severe hypoproteinemia to temporarily increase the serum albumin level. However, hyperalimentation programs with oral or intravenous amino acid supplements are usually more effective to help increase protein synthesis in these patients. The

25 per cent albumin solution must be given cautiously to all patients with cardiac insufficiency because of its oncotic effect, which causes a marked increase in the intravascular blood volume.

Immune Globulins. Patients with agammaglobulinemia or hypogammaglobulinemia may be effectively treated by using plasma or commercial immune serum globulin, which is a 16.5 per cent solution of gamma globulin prepared from pooled human plasma. The initial dose is 0.5 to 2.0 ml per kg of body weight every 3 to 4 weeks. Further dose schedules will depend on the degree of the deficiency and amount needed to control symptoms and infections in each patient. Immune serum globulin is also used for prophylaxis or attenuation of hepatitis type A.

Hyperimmune gamma globulin preparations are commercially available. These include immune globulins for tetanus, pertussis, mumps, vaccinia, zoster, and hepatitis B. All gamma globulin preparations are given intramuscularly and are essentially free of hepatitis transmission.

$Rh_0(D)$ Immune Globulin. $Rh_0(D)$ immune globulin is a highly concentrated preparation of IgG antibody to the $Rh_0(D)$ antigen. It is administered intramuscularly. One vial (anti-$Rh_0(D)$, 300 micrograms) is usually sufficient to prevent sensitization of an $Rh_0(D)$ negative mother by 15 ml of red blood cells from a fetal-maternal hemorrhage from her $Rh_0(D)$ positive infant or abortus. The actual size of the fetal-maternal hemorrhage can be estimated by a laboratory procedure which can enumerate the number of fetal-maternal cells in the maternal circulation. If the estimated size of the fetal hemorrhage exceeds 15 ml, a second vial of $Rh_0(D)$ immune globulin is needed. This is usually rare. $Rh_0(D)$ negative children and women of childbearing age who may have been exposed to $Rh_0(D)$ positive red blood cells or blood products such as platelets should receive $Rh_0(D)$ immune globulin.

Filters

All blood and blood components should be administered through a blood filter. Red cells, plasma, and granulocytes should be transfused through the standard 170 micron blood filter. Platelet concentrates and cryoprecipitate should be administered through a special blood component filter. Microfilters (40 microns) were designed to prevent the build-up of cellular aggregates from stored blood in the patient's microvasculature. The indications for use of this filter are controversial. The routine use of this filter is not recommended, and it should not be used for platelet or granulocyte transfusions.

ADVERSE REACTIONS TO BLOOD TRANSFUSION

method of
THOMAS F. ZUCK, M.D., M.C.
Washington, D.C.

Despite the enhanced safety of transfusions of blood components which has been brought about by improved laboratory practice and intensified educational programs, transfusions are accompanied by significant risks of recipient mortality and morbidity. The more important risks are outlined in Table 1.

Before discussing the management of these complications, it should be noted that *prevention* remains the most effective, and for some complications the only, mode of management. Three general principles of prevention are important: First, transfusions should be used only in those clinical settings which defy practical management by any other means. Second, only those components necessary to correct a documented defi-

TABLE 1. **Risks of Blood Transfusions**

I. Immediate reactions
  A. Immune
    1. Hemolytic
    2. Febrile
    3. Allergic
    4. Anaphylactic
    5. Pulmonary hypersensitivity
  B. Nonimmune
    1. Circulatory overload
    2. Bacterial contamination
    3. Complications of massive transfusions
      a. Citrate toxicity
      b. Hyperkalemia
      c. Hypothermia
      d. Dilutional coagulopathy
    4. Hemolytic
    5. Air embolism
II. Delayed reactions
  A. Immune
    1. Hemolytic
    2. Post-transfusion purpura
    3. Graft-vs.-host reactions (GVH)
  B. Disease transmission
    1. Hepatitis
    2. Malaria
    3. Syphilis
    4. Postperfusion syndrome
    5. Other
  C. Microaggregates
  D. Transfusional hemosiderosis

ciency (or deficiencies) should be infused. In particular, other than replacing acute massive blood loss, infusions of whole blood rarely are indicated. Third, several of the most severe complications arise from administrative or clerical errors. All of the 22 preventable primary fatalities resulting from transfusion reactions in the operating suites and intensive care facilities reported to the Food and Drug Administration between 1976 and 1978 were due to clerical errors resulting in mismatch of ABO groups. These errors can be minimized only by meticulous adherence to proper identification procedures and administration techniques.

IMMEDIATE REACTIONS

These reactions occur during or within the first several hours following a transfusion.

Immune Immediate Reactions

Hemolytic. Because their occurrence can result in the death of the recipient through shock, through renal failure, or from a hemorrhagic diathesis, these reactions remain the most feared of all complications of transfusion practice. They most frequently are caused by clerical or administrative errors. Acute hemolysis of donor red blood cells results from reactions between preformed antibodies in the plasma of the recipient and corresponding antigenic determinants of the donor red blood cells. The ensuing red blood cell destruction usually results in hemoglobinemia and hemoglobinuria. Renal functional impairment following intravascular hemolysis is mediated by antigen-antibody-complement complexes leading to disseminated intravascular coagulation (DIC) and release of vasoactive compounds which decrease renal cortical blood flow. Severe complications are rarely seen in adults unless more than 100 ml of red blood cells has been destroyed.

No combination of signs and symptoms is reliable in establishing the diagnosis of an acute hemolytic transfusion reaction. Symptoms usually become manifest during the first 30 minutes of the transfusion and may include pain at the infusion site, tightness in the chest, lumbar or chest pain, chills, fever, and diaphoresis. The patient also may have tachycardia, tachypnea and hypotension, and, in massive reactions, vascular collapse. Indeed, in massive reactions uncontrollable hypotension may lead to death prior to the onset of bleeding or renal complications. In patients under general anesthesia, hypotension, hemoglobinuria, or generalized bleeding may be the first indication of an acute hemolytic reaction.

Management of a *suspected* acute hemolytic transfusion reaction should proceed using the following guidelines:

1. Since serious consequences are proportional to the amount of incompatible blood given, discontinue the transfusion immediately, but maintain a venous access with a slow infusion of isotonic saline solution. (If less than 100 ml has been infused into an adult, the outlet line from the unit may be clamped until the presence or absence of acute hemolysis has been determined.)

2. Notify the transfusion service or the blood bank. Reconfirm that the unit was administered to the right patient by rechecking clerical work. (If the patient has been administered the wrong blood, the transfusion service should be notified immediately; there is a likelihood that a second patient might also receive the wrong blood.)

3. Three samples of blood, one anticoagulated in citrate, one permitted to clot, and one anticoagulated with ethylene diaminotetraacetic acid (EDTA), should be drawn from a vein remote from the infusion site and submitted to the laboratory. Hemolysis should be avoided. If the unit of blood is disconnected, it also should be submitted, together with the transfusion set and attached intravenous solutions. Even emptied sets should be submitted.

4. Collect the first urine and monitor urinary output.

5. If the patient is in desperate need of oxygen-carrying capacity because of reduced hemoglobin concentration, another unit of packed red blood cells may be administered *if properly identified and tested for compatibility with a fresh blood sample.* If the reaction is due to an ABO incompatibility, it is best to give group O cells.

The laboratory should determine rapidly whether or not an acute hemolytic transfusion reaction is likely by the presence or absence of:

1. Clerical or administrative error.

2. Hemoglobinemia (plasma from the citrate sample compared with a pretransfusion compatibility sample of serum). Free hemoglobin is usually present in severe acute hemolytic transfusion reactions, especially if caused by ABO incompatibility.

3. Hemoglobinuria (presence of hemoglobin in a urine sample centrifuged to remove any intact red blood cells).

4. Positive direct antiglobulin (Coombs) test (EDTA sample).

5. Coagulation studies (on plasma from the citrated sample). Baseline studies should be performed only if there is evidence of acute hemolysis.

If the laboratory data *confirm* the likelihood of an acute hemolytic reaction, therapy should be directed toward prevention of renal failure by increasing renal blood flow and managing DIC. Baseline blood urea nitrogen, creatinine, and bilirubin also should be obtained.

Maintenance of renal blood flow should be attempted as follows:

1. Administer intravenously 1.25 mg per kg of the diuretic furosemide as an initial dose. This may be repeated in 2 hours if needed.

2. If there is no evidence of circulatory overload, concomitantly with diuretic therapy the patient should be provided some degree of water and sodium loading. Over 1 hour, infuse 1000 ml of either isotonic saline solution or 5 per cent dextrose in 0.45 per cent saline solution. An additional 500 ml may be given if within the first hour urine output has not reached 1 to 1.5 ml per kg per hour. *Caveat:* If a response in urinary output has not been observed within 3 or 4 hours, further fluid and diuretic therapy is unlikely to be effective, and may be harmful. In the presence of frank renal failure with oliguria, water and salt must be restricted, and the patient treated for acute tubular necrosis (see pp. 582 to 588).

The prevention and treatment of disseminated intravascular coagulation (DIC) is not without controversy. My approach is based on the estimate of the amount of red blood cells hemolyzed in a *confirmed* reaction. If less than 150 ml of incompatible red blood cells has been administered, DIC is unlikely to ensue, and anticoagulant therapy is instituted only if generalized bleeding occurs or the results of coagulation studies suggest DIC. The absence of fibrin degradation products in the patient's plasma makes the diagnosis of DIC highly improbable. If more than 300 ml of red blood cells has been destroyed, especially from ABO incompatibility, the onset of DIC is more likely, and prophylactic heparinization is considered. Heparin may be effective in preventing further DIC or lessening its intensification. Moreover, it may decrease destruction of incompatible red blood cells through its anticomplementary effect. Heparinization is accompanied by *considerable risk of bleeding,* especially in surgical patients, and should be undertaken only following confirmation that a severe acute hemolytic reaction has occurred.

If heparin is to be administered, the following regimen may be followed: (1) an intravenous loading dose of 60 units per kg, followed by (2) a continuous infusion of 20 units per kg per hour; (3) once instituted, heparin should be continued for 6 to 12 hours or until the likelihood of DIC has passed.

If DIC is confirmed, consumed procoagulants *must* be maintained at hemostatic levels. Cyroprecipitates should be used as a source of fibrinogen and factor VIII, and platelets replaced as necessary. If this is not done, bleeding may worsen, especially if the patient is heparinized.

Although most authorities have emphasized renal failure and DIC as complications of acute hemolytic transfusion reactions, a recent review of Food and Drug Administration records of reported fatalities suggested that in severe hemolytic transfusion reactions caused by ABO incompatibility, shock was the most common mode of death. There is some evidence that dopamine and maintenance of intravascular volume may be helpful in these patients; other vasopressures which decrease renal blood flow should be avoided. It is of the utmost importance that physicians expert in the therapy of shock, renal failure, and coagulation abnormalities be consulted early in the course of all confirmed severe acute hemolytic transfusion reactions. Their participation will assure the best available management.

Febrile Transfusion Reactions. Febrile transfusion reactions are common, and occur typically in patients who previously have been either transfused or pregnant. They are characterized by fever, chills, malaise, tachycardia, and increased blood pressure, and may be associated with frontal headache. Symptoms may occur almost immediately following the start of the transfusion (particularly when platelet concentrates have been given), but frequently the onset may be delayed for 1 or 2 hours. Although red blood cell lysis does not occur, the symptoms may mimic those of an acute hemolytic transfusion reaction. If the component administered contains red blood cells, the symptoms should be investigated to determine whether hemolysis has occurred.

Febrile reactions usually are caused by reactions of preformed recipient alloantibodies with leukocyte and platelet antigens of the donor.

Treatment is symptomatic through the use of antipyretics. Because of its inhibition on platelet function, aspirin should be avoided in patients with coagulation defects, especially thrombocytopenia. If the reaction is mild and the presence of hemolysis has been excluded, the transfusion may be resumed. Further transfusions following a severe nonhemolytic febrile reaction should be from another donor.

Patients who experience repeated febrile episodes associated with transfusions should be given either leukocyte-poor red blood cell preparations or frozen-thawed-deglycerolized red blood cells. These reactions are virtually impossible to prevent in patients who have repeated episodes and require platelet transfusions.

Allergic Transfusion Reactions. Immediate hypersensitivity dermal reactions occur in between 1 and 3 per cent of all transfusions, but are seldom serious. Symptoms include wheals, itching, urticaria, and very rarely fever. They may occur early in the course of the transfusion or within several hours. Rarely bronchospasms may occur. Although red blood cell lysis does not occur, these reactions may occur concomitantly with the more serious hemolytic reactions, the presence or absence of which must be determined if fever is present.

Allergic reactions are caused by preformed antibodies in the recipient plasma reacting with allergens in the donor plasma, usually foreign immunoglobulins, and may be observed during transfusions of plasma products as well as components containing cells.

The patient may be treated as follows:

1. An antihistamine (e.g., diphenhydramine in a dose of 50 to 100 mg) should be administered parenterally (intravenously if the patient has a bleeding diathesis).

2. If bronchospasms occur, 125 to 250 mg of aminophylline may be given intravenously over 5 minutes, together with oxygen.

3. In severe cases, it may be necessary to give hydrocortisone, 200 mg intravenously.

4. If hemolysis has been excluded, and the symptoms are not life threatening, the transfusion may be resumed.

Allergic reactions may be prevented in those patients who have repeated and severe episodes by administering red blood cells essentially free of plasma, either frozen-thawed-deglycerolized red cells or washed red cells. In such patients premedication with antihistamines parenterally or orally prior to the transfusion is usually effective in reducing the severity of the reactions.

Anaphylactic Transfusion Reactions. These reactions are the most hazardous form of allergic reactions, and are discussed separately because they are extremely dangerous. They usually occur almost immediately upon starting the transfusion, and are often dramatic. Symptoms include hypotension, flushing, cyanosis, wheezing, dyspnea, abdominal and/or back and chest pain, and nausea. These reactions can occur in patients with no previous history of transfusion or pregnancy.

Almost all severe anaphylactic reactions are due to anti-IgA antibodies in the recipient plasma reacting with IgA in the donor plasma. Although usually the recipient is IgA deficient, patients with normal levels of IgA may develop anti-IgA antibodies of limited specificity to an IgA subclass.

Anaphylactic reactions may be life threatening and must be treated vigorously:

1. Immediately stop the transfusion, but maintain an intravenous access with a saline infu-

sion; *give no other blood products until the cause of the reaction has been determined.*

2. Administer intravenously 0.5 ml of 1:1,000 epinephrine and 250 to 500 mg of hydrocortisone.

3. Support the patient with oxygen and fluids and, if necessary, vasopressors.

The most important aspect of prevention is to avoid any future infusion of plasma unless it is from an IgA deficient donor (about one in 700 donors). Transmembrane washed cell products (frozen-thawed-deglycerolized) may be relied upon cautiously, since even traces of IgA may initiate the reaction. A registry of IgA deficient donors is maintained by the University of California Medical Center in San Francisco. The rare donor files of the American Association of Blood Banks or the American Red Cross also may be able to find suitable donors. The patient *must* be told of the nature of the problem and should be issued medical alert identification.

Pulmonary Hypersensitivity. This is a relatively rare form of reaction seen with transfusions of granulocytes and is characterized by dyspnea, cough, and cyanosis associated with patchy pulmonary infiltrates on x-ray. These reactions have been said to be caused by preformed antileukocyte antibodies in either the donor or the recipient reacting with leukocytic antigens of the recipient or donor, respectively. The syndrome may begin very shortly after the transfusion is started. The treatment consists of epinephrine and steroids in addition to standard measures for pulmonary edema. These reactions may be avoided by administering HLA-matched granulocytes, and by avoiding donors previously responsible for passive transfer of antibody.

Nonimmune Immediate Reactions

Circulatory Overload. This is one of the more common untoward reactions to transfusion. It is usually encountered in pediatric and elderly patients with cardiac or pulmonary disease who have a normal or expanded total blood volume at the time the transfusion is started. The symptoms and treatment are as for other causes of pulmonary edema. It may be necessary to partially exchange the patient by withdrawing whole blood and replacing it with tightly packed (packed cell volume of 95 per cent) red blood cells.

This complication is prevented in patients at risk by slowly transfusing 1 ml per kg per hour of red blood cells tightly packed as above. In addition, if possible, these patients should be transfused sitting up in bed during daylight hours when their response can be monitored carefully by a full complement of nursing personnel.

Bacterial Contamination. Fortunately, this complication is rare with the availability of integrally connected sterile plastic blood drawing equipment. Accidental bacterial contamination and growth can occur, however, especially with psychrophilic (cold growing) gram-negative organisms. The reaction is due to endotoxin and can be seen with an infusion of as little as 50 ml of contaminated blood. The resulting hypotension, shock, fever, and chills can be dramatic, and can result in death. A bleeding diathesis caused by DIC may be seen.

The transfusion must be stopped *immediately* and steps taken as listed for the evaluation of a suspected acute hemolytic transfusion reaction (see p. 353). In addition, because it is quick and easy, the laboratory should perform an ordinary Wright's stain on smears of both the recipient's blood and the contents of the blood storage container. If bacteria are identified with Wright's stain, the organism then can be classified as gram-negative or gram-positive on additional Gram stained smears.

Treatment must be vigorous and consists of antibiotics and supportive therapy for shock caused by sepsis (see pp. 3 to 10). A physician expert in treating septic shock should be consulted.

Problems Associated with Massive Transfusions. The management of patients requiring massive blood replacement is a complex endeavor because the underlying disease leading to the need may greatly influence the patient's response to transfusions. It is highly desirable to enlist the services of a physician familiar with managing massive transfusions as soon as the need for them is apparent.

CITRATE TOXICITY. Anticoagulant-preservative solutions used to store blood and fresh frozen plasma contain an excess of citrate which will bind the plasma calcium of the recipient. The pathology of citrate toxicity is complex, however, and depends upon serum potassium concentrations and pH, as well as calcium concentrations. In general, a 70 kg man can tolerate 1 unit of whole blood every 5 minutes without manifesting hypocalcemia, which is heralded by electrocardiographic (EKG) changes and muscular tremors. The enthusiasm for giving calcium prophylactically in all massively transfused patients has waned because of the ventricular arrhythmias which may be produced by giving calcium to a patient who is not hypocalcemic. If the patient demonstrates EKG (prolonged electrical conductivity) or laboratory evidence of hypocalcemia, 5 ml of 10 per cent calcium gluconate (2.5 ml of 10 per cent calcium chloride) should be given intravenously and the response monitored.

The administration of packed red blood cells reduces the risks of citrate toxicity, but may have limited practicality in clinical settings requiring massive transfusions.

HYPERKALEMIA AND HYPOKALEMIA. The potassium level of the supernatant plasma of whole blood and packed red blood cells gradually rises during storage, primarily owing to the flux of potassium out of the red blood cells at 4 C. Following transfusion into the recipient, potassium re-enters the rewarmed red blood cells. Thus, except in newborns and patients in renal failure (for whom blood of less than 5 days old should be infused) hyperkalemia is more a theoretical than practical problem. Hypokalemia is observed more commonly following massive transfusions.

In patients who manifest hyperkalemia by laboratory test, units stored as whole blood for more than 2 weeks should be packed immediately prior to transfusion. Potassium from the recipient's plasma will enter the potassium-depleted transfused red blood cells as they are warmed. If hypokalemia is observed, potassium supplements may be administered intravenously.

HYPOTHERMIA. Patients receiving large amounts of blood stored at 4 C may become hypothermic. This is particularly common in infants. This reaction may be avoided by warming the blood with a device designed for this purpose and equipped with an alarm which will warn if the temperature of the blood has exceeded 38 C. Except in an emergency, the practice of passing the tubing of the administration set through a pan of "warm" water should be discouraged. Red blood cells will hemolyze at 45 C.

DILUTIONAL OR "WASHOUT" COAGULOPATHY. Abnormal bleeding may be manifest in patients who have received massive amounts of blood and other resuscitation fluids. This is usually attributed to the loss of labile procoagulants (platelets and factors V and VIII) during blood storage. In most massively transfused patients procoagulants do not fall below hemostatic levels even following replacement of their entire blood volume with transfused products. In my experience, in those patients exhibiting bleeding resulting from dilutional effect alone, platelets usually are the rate-limiting procoagulant. If a peripheral smear suggests a significant thrombocytopenia, 4 to 6 platelet concentrates should be administered.

If screening tests for deficiencies of soluble procoagulants (activated partial thromboplastin time *and* thrombin time) suggest a deficiency, an unsuspected acute hemolytic transfusion reaction, surreptitious heparin, or DIC must be excluded as causative. If it can be concluded that the cause of test abnormalities is purely dilutional, fresh frozen plasma and cryoprecipitates will be effective.

There does not appear to be any convincing evidence that the use of freshly shed blood is superior to the approach outlined above.

Hemolytic. Several events can cause in vitro hemolysis of donor red blood cells prior to the infusion. The results may be confused with immune hemolysis. Among the more common causes are warming of blood to more than 45 C (this is a particular hazard during cardiopulmonary bypass), freezing blood, storing blood heavily contaminated with bacteria, and mixing blood with incompatible intravenous solutions or drugs (such as 5 per cent dextrose and water). With the exception of transfusions of heavily contaminated hemolyzed blood, these misadventures are not associated with symptoms of an acute hemolytic reaction resulting from immune destruction, and the risk of renal failure or DIC is not great. Asymptomatic hemoglobinuria and hemoglobinemia should bring to mind the possibility of having transfused previously hemolyzed red cells. Treatment is supportive.

Air Embolism. Air embolisms are rare with the use of flexible plastic blood storage equipment. Nevertheless, they can occur, especially with the use of pressure, Y-administration sets, and glass bottles for other intravenous fluids. Their onset is suggested by the presence of cough, pain, and dyspnea not caused by circulatory overload or shock. The patient should be immediately placed on his or her left side with the head down in an effort to trap the injected air in the right side of the heart. Supportive measures to maintain blood pressure are indicated. If the patient continues to do poorly, and the cause is known to be an air embolism, cardiac aspiration may be required.

DELAYED TRANSFUSION REACTIONS

These untoward reactions occur days to months following the offending transfusion.

Immune

Delayed Hemolytic Transfusion Reactions. These reactions are suspected when a patient previously transfused with red blood cells develops an unexplained anemia. They may occur several days to weeks following the transfusion and, other than the manifestations of anemia, are usually asymptomatic. In rare patients, hemolysis may be brisk and resemble that of an acute hemolytic transfusion reaction with hemoglobinemia and hemoglobinuria. Death has been reported from these brisk delayed reactions.

Delayed hemolytic transfusion reactions occur through two similar mechanisms. In the more common form, the patient previously has been immunized, but the preformed antibody is of insufficient titer to be detected by routinely performed pretransfusion testing. Following transfusion, an anamnestic response to the incompatible red blood cells results in their lysis. The reaction usually becomes evident 5 to 10 days following transfusion. In the second, less common form the patient makes antibody de novo to incompatible red blood cells and lysis results. This second type of reaction occurs later and is almost invariably more mild.

Suspected delayed hemolytic transfusion reactions should be evaluated in a manner similar to that for a suspected acute hemolytic reaction, but the urgency is dependent upon clinical severity. A direct antiglobulin (Coombs) test is usually positve, and tests on an eluate usually will indicate the responsible incompatible red blood cell antigen(s).

In most patients these reactions do not require treatment; however, in the rare case in which red blood cell destruction is severe, treatment should proceed as for acute hemolytic transfusion reactions. If additional transfusions are required to augment oxygen-carrying capacity, red blood cells lacking the offending antigen and compatible with a *fresh* sample of recipient serum by pretransfusion testing should be used.

A positive direct antiglobulin (Coombs) test may occur owing to passive transfer of antibody in blood components and in vitro may mimic a delayed reaction. This usually results from transfusion of procoagulant concentrates, non-group-specific platelets, and group O universal donors. The transfused antibody reacts with the corresponding antigen on the recipient's red blood cells. Lysis occurs only rarely.

Patients who have experienced a delayed hemolytic transfusion reaction should be informed of its nature and implications, and issued an identification card so that the information is available should transfusion be required in the future.

Post-Transfusion Purpura. Post-transfusion purpura occurs approximately 1 week following transfusion and is characterized by severe thrombocytopenia with or without a bleeding diathesis. Reported cases indicate that antibody in the recipient's plasma reacts with platelet antigen(s) on the transfused platelets. Pl^{A1} is the antigenic determinant to which the antibody is formed, but, paradoxically, the recipient's own platelets lacking PL^{A1} antigen are also destroyed. This may result from the so-called "innocent bystander" phenomenon in which antigen-antibody complexes adsorb onto the recipient's own platelets, which are then destroyed. The resulting thrombocytopenia may be profound and life threatening and may last for several weeks.

Platelet destruction will not be resolved by corticosteroid therapy, and, since 98 per cent of the general population have the Pl^{A1} antigen on their platelets, bolus platelet transfusions from random donors are of little or no value. Transfusions of only Pl^{A1} negative platelets are generally impractical and not always effective.

If the thrombocytopenia is life threatening, intensive plasmapheresis or plasma exchange should be considered, since it has been successful in some patients. Until such a procedure can be performed, a *continuous uninterrupted* infusion of 1 platelet concentrate per hour obtained from random donors may be effective in stanching bleeding, although the rise in the recipient's peripheral venous platelet count may be minimal.

Graft-vs-Host Reaction (GVH). This syndrome consists of fever, skin rash, diarrhea, hepatitis, infections, and bone marrow suppression, and may be fatal. It occurs in patients who have either an acquired or hereditary immunodeficiency, and has been reported in newborns with extreme immaturity as well.

If immunocompetent lymphocytes from a donor are transfused with cellular blood components and the lymphocytes cannot be rejected by the immunoincompetent recipient, they may engraft in the recipient. The syndrome is an expression of these engrafted lymphocytes "rejecting" the recipient's foreign tissues.

Although there are no controlled clinical trials, it is generally accepted that GVH can be prevented by irradiating all blood components containing lymphocytes (whole blood, packed red blood cells, platelet concentrates, and granulocyte concentrates) with 1500 to 3000 rads prior to infusion. Although this dose is inadequate to prevent in vitro blastogenesis of lymphocytes, it appears effective in preventing GVH in susceptible recipients.

Disease Transmission

Under appropriate circumstances any pathogenic organism in the bloodstream of the donor at the time of blood collection may cause disease in the recipient. Fortunately, with the important exception of hepatitis, the fragility of most organisms at 4 C or in citrate and the effectiveness of the recipient's defenses make these complications infrequent. It is important that disease transmission by transfusion be considered in patients with unexplained symptoms days or even months following a transfusion.

Post-Transfusion Hepatitis. Hepatitis remains the most common complication of blood transfusion, and the magnitude of the problem cannot be overstated. Since most cases are subclinical and anicteric, the true incidence is not known. It is known that chronic active hepatitis can be a frequent sequela to nonicteric postinfusion hepatitis. It is clear that at least 90 per cent of post-transfusion hepatitis is so-called "non-A, non-B," or "C." The hepatitis A virus is rarely responsible, and pretransfusion screening tests of donors for HBsAg have largely eliminated the B virus as causative. There is currently no test available which will reliably detect the "non-A, non-B" agent(s) responsible for post-transfusion hepatitis.

Minimization of exposure to blood products is the only effective manner to manage this risk. The following guidelines should be followed:

1. Transfusions should be given only if absolutely necessary, and the benefits must be weighed against the hepatitis risks.

2. Blood products made from large pools of donor plasma (most commercial products) should never be given if several units of single-donor components would be effective.

3. Blood from volunteer donors is generally safer than that from paid donors.

4. Albumin, plasma protein fraction, and gamma globulin can be used without the risk of transmitting hepatitis.

Because most post-transfusion hepatitis is non-A, non-B, the routine prophylactic administration of hepatitis B immune globulin (HBIG) cannot be advocated at this time.

Malaria. Transmission of malaria is extremely rare, although occasional sporadic cases are reported. Its occurrence should be considered in any patient who develops unexplained fever 1 to 16 weeks following transfusion. The parasite can survive in liquid stored and in frozen blood components. Diagnosis and treatment should be as for malaria transmitted by other means.

The most effective prevention is careful screening of donors by blood banks according to the requirements of the American Association of Blood Banks and the American Red Cross.

Syphilis. The *Treponema pallidum* responsible for syphilis does not survive beyond 72 hours of 4 C storage in blood drawn into citrate, but transfusion of fresh and fresh frozen components can transmit the disease. The disease presents as secondary syphilis 1 to 4 months following the offending transfusion. A negative serologic test for syphilis performed on the donor's blood at the time of donation does not assure that the blood could not be contaminated with spirochetes.

Diagnosis and treatment are as for other cases of syphilis presenting in the secondary stage.

Postperfusion Syndrome. This syndrome refers to the development of fever, splenomegaly, and the presence of atypical lymphocytes in the peripheral blood of the recipient between 2 and 4 weeks after transfusion with blood stored at 4 C less than 48 hours. Less commonly, hepatomegaly, adenopathy, and a rash also may be observed.

Both the cytomegaloviruses and Epstein-Barr virus have been implicated as causative, the former much more frequently, probably because of the widespread immunity to the latter.

Treatment is symptomatic, as the disease is benign and self-limited to several weeks. It can be prevented by avoiding the transfusion of blood components less than 48 hours old.

Other Transmissible Diseases. There have been scattered and infrequent reports of several other diseases transmitted by blood transfusions. Among these are brucellosis, typhus, Rocky Mountain spotted fever, Chagas' disease, and salmonellosis. The principal danger is that their presence and cause may be overlooked and, as a result, they may not be treated appropriately.

Microaggregates

During the storage of whole blood and packed red blood cells in the liquid state, platelets, leukocytes, and fibrin form aggregates which will pass through the 170 μ mesh size of the standard blood administration filter. It has been postulated that these so-called microaggregates cause pulmonary pathology in heavily transfused patients; however, it appears that this complication is more theoretical than real. Extensive analysis of data from massively transfused battle casualties in Viet Nam has failed to confirm a relationship between the amount of stored blood transfused and the presence of clinical pulmonary insufficiency. The site of injury, i.e., thorax and abdomen, seems to be a more important variable. In neonatal patients with extreme immaturity, some increased risk of pulmonary damage from microaggregates has been suggested. This risk is probably minimized in these patients by use of blood less than 3 to 5 days old.

In patients who may have a particularly high susceptibility to pulmonary damage because of pre-existing lung disease, microaggregates larger than 20 to 40 μ may be removed by special infusion set filters designed for this purpose. It should be noted that these filters remove platelets, and their use is contraindicated in transfusions given to augment the recipient platelet count. These filters also retard flow rate, and for patients requiring rapid massive blood replacement prompt transfusion may be of greater importance than microaggregate removal.

Transfusional Hemosiderosis

Each unit of whole blood and packed red blood cells contains about 250 mg of iron. Since the body attempts to minimize iron loss, patients requiring chronic and numerous transfusions gradually will accumulate iron in their tissues. This transfusional hemosiderosis can result in parenchymal damage to many organs. Recently, some success in removing this iron has been reported using continuous subcutaneous infusions of the iron chelator deferoxamine. For patients who have long-term chronic transfusion needs (e.g., severe thalassemia, aplastic anemia) without a corresponding iron loss, this approach may be helpful. Its administration probably should be confined to physicians who are familiar with the technique.

The risks of transfusional hemosiderosis can be minimized, although not eliminated, by transfusing patients at risk as seldom as possible with the freshest available red blood cells. The use of frozen-thawed-deglycerolized red blood cells is suitable, and has the additional advantage of minimizing adverse reactions to foreign proteins, platelets, and leukocytes to which these patients also are prone.

SECTION 5

The Digestive System

BLEEDING ESOPHAGEAL VARICES

method of
JOHN T. GALAMBOS, M.D.
Atlanta, Georgia

The vigor and intensity of therapeutic or diagnostic interventions depend on the patient's clinical course. Although bleeding from varices can be life threatening and carries a high mortality rate, in a sizable proportion of patients bleeding stops spontaneously. Some patients will not even require blood transfusions, let alone other vigorous therapeutic procedures.

1. With a bleeding patient, hemodynamic stability is the primary concern. In those patients who require transfusions, a large intravenous access is established promptly and intravenous infusion of isotonic saline solution is started until blood becomes available, and 10 mg of phytonadione (Aquamephyton) is given intravenously.

2. Thereafter, other than blood or plasma, sodium-containing fluids are no longer administered intravenously. Depending on the estimated blood loss and the estimated rate of bleeding, a sufficient number of units of blood (usually 4 to 6) is typed and crossmatched. Transfusion begins if the patient is hemodynamically unstable (i.e., the blood pressure decreases in the sitting or upright position). The transfusions are to replace depleted intravascular volume and are independent of intragastric blood. It is preferable to transfuse a patient either with fresh blood or with packed cells and fresh frozen plasma rather than bank blood. If more than 4 transfusions are required, at least one half of the transfused blood should contain either fresh frozen plasma or fresh blood from recent donations.

3. If the bleeding is manifested only by melena, a nasogastric tube is placed in the stomach to confirm upper gastrointestinal bleeding. Once this diagnosis is made, and if the patient is conscious, 60 to 90 ml of milk of magnesia is injected in the stomach, and the nasogastric tube is removed.

4. Initial orders: Vital signs and urine output are recorded at least once hourly. Hematocrits are obtained immediately and at 4 hour intervals. The following laboratory tests are done: prothrombin time, bilirubin, albumin, total protein, serum glutamic oxaloacetic transaminase (SGOT), alkaline phosphatase, blood urea nitrogen (BUN), creatinine, electrolytes, and glucose. The complete blood count (CBC) should include reticulocytes and platelets. A urinalysis is obtained. Cimetidine, 300 mg every 6 hours, is given intravenously.

5. Once a patient is stable hemodynamically, the next step is to establish a specific diagnosis by endoscopy. The bleeding from gastric or esophageal varices is diagnosed by either (a) seeing blood issuing from a varix in the esophagus or stomach (this is the exception), or (b) seeing bleeding from the esophagus or from the fundus or body of the stomach but finding no specific lesion as the active bleeding site, such as esophagitis, Mallory-Weiss tear, erosive gastritis, or peptic ulcer, that would explain the bleeding of that vigor other than visible varices in the esophagus. (Gastric varices, although much bigger, are usually difficult to see during endoscopy.) If the endoscopy is done the morning after admission, commonly no blood, no active bleeding, and none of the lesions listed above are seen; only the varices are visualized.

6. Once a diagnosis of variceal bleeding is established and the bleeding is stopped, the patient can be evaluated for elective surgery (see below).

7. If urgent or emergency surgery is *not*

361

contemplated, a feeding schedule of 6 meals a day should be instituted. Remember that a patient who is not taking in a sufficient amount of calories is on a "high-protein" diet; i.e., gluconeogenesis can flood the urea cycle with ammonia from amino nitrogen. Probably, the maximal depression of gluconeogenesis, and therefore ammonia production from endogenous sources, is accomplished by an intake of 1600 calories per day. *Diet*: (a) If the patient has no ascites or other evidence of excessive salt and water retention, sodium restriction is not necessary. If the patient already had or develops ascites, sodium intake is restricted to 500 to 1000 mg per day, and spironolactone, 50 mg 4 times daily, is started. (The only sodium-containing fluid given intravenously is blood or plasma.) At this time more vigorous diuretic therapy should be undertaken with caution because prerenal azotemia may be overlooked. Even with normal creatinine concentration, the blood urea nitrogen is likely to be elevated owing to ingested blood accompanied by decreased renal perfusion as the result of gastrointestinal bleeding. However, as long as the BUN is decreasing and the creatinine clearances are well over 35 ml per minute, a potassium-wasting diuretic such as furosemide (Lasix) may be administered cautiously in addition to spironolactone if the patient is hemodynamically stable (see below for other complications). (b) If the patient shows no evidence of encephalopathy, protein restriction is unnecessary. However, it is advisable to avoid foods known to contain large amounts of preformed ammonia (Galambos, J. T.: *Cirrhosis.* Philadelphia, W. B. Saunders Company, 1979). If signs of encephalopathy develop, protein in the diet is reduced to 8 to 10 grams per day and purges with milk of magnesia or magnesium citrate or sulfate are administered. Neomycin, 1 gram every 4 hours, is given by mouth. In these patients lactulose is ill suited for control of encephalopathy. First, it is difficult to establish the optimal dose without inducing cramping abdominal pain and diarrhea. Neomycin is cheaper and is at least as effective as lactulose, if not more so. The nephro- or ototoxicity of neomycin, as a rule, is not an important consideration when it is administered for limited periods, such as for the treatment of encephalopathy precipitated by gastrointestinal bleeding.

8. If the bleeding continues, the next step is an intravenous infusion of vasopressin (Pitressin) (this use of vasopressin is not listed in the manufacturer's official directive). This can be administered either as a bolus (20 units in 15 to 20 minutes) or as a continuous infusion of 0.5 to 0.6 unit per minute. The former has the advantage of causing rapid evacuation of bloody intestinal

contents, but it also produces rather severe cramping abdominal pain and its effect may be short lived. The continuous infusion method is preferred. Monitor blood pressure and the electrocardiogram to recognize and to avoid excessive hypertension or myocardial ischemia. If the bleeding is controlled by this method, the infusion rate is gradually reduced by decrements of 0.1 unit per minute each 8 to 12 hours. If the bleeding recurs as the rate of infusion of vasopressin (Pitressin) is being reduced, the original effective dose of 0.5 to 0.6 unit per minute is reinstituted, and the rate of reduction is decreased.

9. If the bleeding continues despite high-dose intravenous vasopressin (Pitressin) infusion, angiograms* are obtained in preparation for possible urgent surgical intervention. When abdominal angiography is completed, the catheter is left in the superior mesenteric artery and vasopressin (Pitressin) is infused at 0.5 unit per minute. As bleeding is controlled, the infusion rate after 24 hours is reduced in 12 hour intervals by 0.1 unit per minute.

10. If the bleeding continues despite use of the intra-arterial vasopressin (Pitressin) infusion, the patient is considered for balloon tamponade with the use of the Sengstaken-Blakemore (S-B) tube. The major consideration is whether or not the patient is a candidate for urgent surgery if balloon tamponade does *not* control the bleeding. If the patient is not a candidate for surgery, it is preferable to use other means of control (if appropriate talent is available) than the balloon, because the bleeding in patients in whom balloon tamponade has failed will not stop short of surgery.

Care of the S-B balloon: Test the balloons before insertion to be sure that the gastric balloon does not leak. Determine the optimal inflation volume of the gastric balloon at the same time. Make sure that skilled personnel are available who can care for the patient with the balloon tamponade. Remember, the S-B balloon can cause life-threatening complications. Be sure that the gastric balloon is well in the stomach before it is inflated; inflate it fully, secure it with a strong clamp to avoid leakage of air, and pull it snugly against the gastric fundus. The balloon can be pulled against the nostril if the tube was passed through the nose, or it can be pulled against the face guard of a football helmet or some other

---

*Superior mesenteric, splenic, and hepatic arteriograms and hepatic and left renal venograms. At the same time, hepatic vein wedge pressure is measured and corrected sinusoidal pressure is calculated (wedge minus free hepatic vein pressure).

device. If the bleeding does not stop, inflate the esophageal balloon to a pressure just above portal pressure. When the esophageal balloon is inflated, it is imperative to put an additional small nasogastric suction tube above the balloon to aspirate secretions and prevent aspiration if you do not have a modified S-B tube equipped with a fourth channel for this purpose. The esophageal balloon is deflated in 6 to 10 hours. If bleeding has stopped, the gastric balloon is relaxed after 24 hours. *Note:* Beyond 36 to 48 hours of balloon compression of the fundus, the gastric mucosa undergoes hemorrhagic necrosis and can bleed vigorously in patients with portal hypertension. If the balloon tamponade does not control the bleeding, re-evaluate the diagnosis. If it is still variceal bleeding, the control of the bleeding requires surgery.

11. What type of operation is to be performed? If at all possible, surgery should be postponed and performed electively. If this is not possible because of continued bleeding, either despite the S-B balloon tamponade or as a result of recurrent bleeding after initial control with balloon tamponade in patients who are unresponsive to vasopressin (Pitressin) infusion, one of three types of operations may be considered: (1) the selective distal splenorenal (Warren) shunt, (2) one of the central or total shunts (such as a portacaval or mesorenal shunt), or (3) a nonshunting devascularization type of procedure.

The Warren shunt is performed if the abdominal angiography shows good portal venous flow (i.e., good opacification of the right and left portal veins during the venous phase of the superior mesenteric anteriogram and splenic arteriogram) and also shows appropriate anatomy for the splenic and left renal veins. In addition, if the patient does not have marked or refractory ascites, a Warren shunt should be performed. There are only a few but important technical differences in the performance of an elective versus an urgent or emergency Warren shunt. The most important difference is that during an urgent shunt the clamping of the splenic vein should be delayed as much as possible because during active or recent bleeding the clamping of the splenic vein may precipitate interoperative variceal bleeding.

If the patient does not have adequate visualization of the intrahepatic branches of the portal vein on the superior mesenteric angiogram —i.e., poor or no opacification of the portal vein —the patient should have one of the central or total shunts. The type of shunt is determined by the surgeon at the time of operation.

A nonshunting procedure is performed in those patients who have no vessels suitable for shunting. These are usually the ones who had previous shunts that clotted and usually had splenectomies as well, or ascitic patients who are at high risk of encephalopathy if a total shunt is performed. Remember that a nonshunting operation carries a mortality rate as high as or higher than a shunting operation. Furthermore, it does not provide the patient with long-term protection against recurrent variceal bleeding.

Postoperative encephalopathy after a total shunt is considerably more frequent than after the Warren shunt. There is a predictable impairment of hepatic function and intellectual function if the portal flow to the liver is diverted by a total shunt. The Warren shunt is just as effective in controlling bleeding as a total shunt is, although it may be more difficult technically when the patient is bleeding.

If the patient is not a candidate for surgery because of evidence of severe hepatocellular failure, unresponsive prolonged prothrombin time, high serum bilirubin levels, or low serum albumin concentrations, the therapy of choice is thrombosis of the varices. The procedures for variceal thrombosis fall into two categories: (1) transesophageal endoscopic sclerosis of the varices, and (2) angiographic thrombosis of these vessels.

Endoscopic sclerosis is performed by the injection of sclerosing solution (5 ml of a 5 per cent solution of sodium morrhuate) in each varix. As the needle is removed, the varix is compressed with a special sheet pushed over the flexible esophagoscope or with the use of a rigid esophagoscope. When bleeding stops, the next visible varix is injected, and so forth.

Angiographic thrombosis of varices is performed by percutaneously inserting a catheter into the portal vein and passing it into the left gastric vein. The varices can be thrombosed by injecting various substances. If the prothrombin time is prolonged and the anatomy is favorable, the portal vein is reached by the transjugular approach; otherwise the percutaneous puncture of the liver and direct catheterization of the portal vein is preferred. The gastroesophageal varices are identified by subselective venous angiography and may be thrombosed by the injection of a variety of substances, such as absorbable gelatin sponge (Gelfoam), thrombin, blood clots, metal clips, or a cyanoacrylate. Although variceal thrombosis is usually a temporizing measure, it may give long-term freedom from bleeding. Most importantly, it can give time for a patient with active parenchymal disease to improve from being an unacceptably high surgical risk to being a fair or even good surgical risk. After variceal thrombosis the patient can be treated in the bleeding-free interval and be sufficiently improved that an elective shunt operation can be performed with a much reduced mortality and postoperative morbidity rate. Bleeding recurs or the procedure is unsuccessful in the majority of patients. Because both endoscopic and angiographic thromboses of the varices are temporizing measures, repeated courses of injections may be required to reduce the risk of recurrent hemorrhage.

CHOLELITHIASIS AND CHOLECYSTITIS

method of
LARRY C. CAREY, M.D.,
and E. CHRISTOPHER ELLISON,
M.D.
Columbus, Ohio

Cholelithiasis is one of the most common health problems of adults in the United States, occurring in approximately 10 per cent of adults and in 20 per cent of persons over 40 years of age. The incidence of biliary calculi increases with age, so that one third of persons aged 70 or more will have gallstones. Cholelithiasis occurs four times more frequently in women than in men, although with increasing age the incidence among men approaches that in women. Other risk factors include hemolytic anemia (including sickle cell disease), pregnancy, and obesity.

In the United States, annual medical expenditures for the treatment of cholelithiasis approach $2 million. Approximately 600,000 cholecystectomies are performed yearly, making this the most frequent abdominal operation. When the procedure is performed electively, the operative mortality and morbidity are less than 0.5 per cent.

Natural History

Forty to 60 per cent of patients with gallstones are asymptomatic at the time of diagnosis. If they are followed for 5 to 20 years without operation, approximately 50 per cent of these patients will develop symptoms: biliary colic in 20 per cent, chronic cholecystitis in 10 per cent, and acute cholecystitis in 25 per cent. In addition, bile duct stones will occur in 10 to 15 per cent of patients. The natural history of cholelithiasis is the basis for early operative management of patients with this disease.

The Asymptomatic Patient

Since more than half the patients with gallstones will eventually have symptoms, the desirability of elective cholecystectomy in all patients younger than 65 years of age should be emphasized. Elective operation should be chosen particularly for patients with diabetes mellitus, who are predisposed to develop suppurative complications should acute cholecystitis occur, and for those with small gallstones, who are at increased risk to develop ductal calculi and pancreatitis. Patients with angina pectoris should undergo elective operation because myocardial infarction may occur during an episode of acute cholecystitis. In asymptomatic patients older than 65 years of age, or in younger patients with other major illnesses, including advanced cardiac disease, renal failure. or liver failure, cholecystectomy is delayed until symptoms make operation unavoidable.

Clinical Description

Therapeutic decisions concerning patients with symptomatic gallstone disease require differentiation of biliary colic and chronic cholecystitis from acute cholecystitis. Patients with biliary colic or chronic cholecystitis may be treated safely as outpatients and scheduled for elective cholecystectomy. Patients with acute cholecystitis should be hospitalized and, if not operated upon immediately, observed closely, so that the illness does not progress undetected.

Biliary colic is a self-limited disease, usually lasting less than 4 hours. The pain is of a "crampy" character, usually located in the right subcostal area with radiation to the tip of the right scapula. Its onset is often associated with the ingestion of a fat-rich meal. Dyspepsia associated with eating cabbage, Brussels sprouts, apples, and a variety of other foods has no relationship to biliary tract disease. Nausea and vomiting may occur. The patient is afebrile, appearing more uncomfortable than ill. Evidence of peritoneal irritation is uncommon.

Treatment of Chronic Cholecystitis

Once the diagnosis of chronic cholecystitis is confirmed, elective cholecystectomy with operative cholangiogram should be scheduled. The ideal time to perform cholecystectomy is when the symptoms are mild, not during an acute attack of cholecystitis.

Treatment of Acute Cholecystitis

The clinical diagnosis of acute cholecystitis justifies immediate hospitalization. The course of the disease is unpredictable, even though the patient may have had previous attacks that rapidly subsided. The uncertainties of diagnosis in an acutely ill patient who may have concurrent complicating disorders make early hospitalization a wise decision.

The initial treatment is nonoperative and supportive. Nasogastric intubation to decompress the stomach is accomplished early. Balanced electrolyte solutions are administered to correct predicted deficits and maintain urine output. Fluid requirements vary with the length and severity of preadmission illness and amount of vomiting. If gastric decompression does not give sufficient pain relief, merperidine (Demerol), 50 to 75 mg, is administered intramuscularly every 4 hours. Anticholinergics are of little benefit and should be avoided, particularly in the elderly patient.

Admission blood tests should include complete blood count (CBC) with differential, serum glutamic and pyruvic transaminase, alkaline phosphatase, bilirubin, amylase, glucose, blood urea nitrogen (BUN), and creatinine. Blood type and screen should be ordered to assure the availability of at least 4 units of packed red cells, should emergency operation become unavoidable.

Although the initial inflammatory process is the result of chemical irritation, bacterial infection may occur at any time. The benefit of antibiotics during the early course of acute cholecystitis is uncertain. They are not given if the onset of the attack is very recent, but are administered routinely if the patient has had symptoms for more than 48 hours, or if fever, leukocytosis, or jaundice indicates the presence of suppurative complications. Since enteric organisms are most common, antibiotics effective against these bacteria are selected. We prefer either ampicillin, 1 gram intravenously every 6 hours, or gentamicin, 60 to 80 mg intravenously every 8 hours, if empyema, perforation, gangrene, or emphysematous cholecystitis is suspected.

The most important aspect of early management is repeated and frequent examination of the patient by the same physician. This is the most reliable way to detect the development of complicated cholecystitis. White blood cell counts should be performed every 6 hours for the first 36 hours of hospitalization.

If gallstones have been demonstrated by previous roentgenographic studies, these need not be repeated during an acute attack. When the diagnosis is uncertain, ultrasonography is the best test to detect the presence of gallstones. Oral cholecystography may be performed within 24 to 48 hours after admission to the hospital, provided that the patient has had a regular diet for 24 hours. Intravenous cholangiography may be performed; however, this is rapidly being replaced by cholescintigraphy with 99^m technetium-labeled immunodiacetic acid (99^m Tc-HIDA). In either of these tests, the diagnosis of acute cholecystitis is made when the gallbladder is not seen with concurrent visualization of the common bile duct. Cholecystographic studies are useless if the bilirubin is greater than 3 mg per dl (100 ml). Radionuclide studies of the biliary tree are accurate when the patient has a bilirubin up to 7 mg per dl.

The timing of cholecystectomy should be individualized. Patients with evidence of complicated cholecystitis or whose condition worsens during medical treatment require immediate operation. The best time for operation on a patient with uncomplicated cholecystitis has been a point of debate in the past. However, most surgeons are convinced that cholecystectomy and operative cholangiography should be scheduled 24 to 72 hours after admission. This practice reduces the incidence of complications and length of hospitalization, and obviates the possibility of recurrent attacks requiring a second hospitalization. If the patient has another serious illness complicating cholecystitis, such as acute pancreatitis, myocardial infarction, congestive heart failure, renal failure, or severe pulmonary diseases, treatment should be expectant and cholecystectomy delayed for 6 weeks to 3 months.

Cholecystectomy with operative cholangiography is the preferred surgical treatment. Cholecystotomy performed under local anesthesia is indicated in patients with complicated cholecystitis if cholecystectomy is technically hazardous, or if the patient is elderly and has cardiovascular disease.

Choledocholithiasis

Approximately 15 to 20 per cent of patients undergoing cholecystectomy will have stones in the bile ducts. This should be suspected if the patient is jaundiced or has a history of jaundice, or has had previous episodes of pancreatitis. In the patient with hyperbilirubinemia, routine cholecystography is useless. Endoscopic retrograde cholangiopancreatography (ERCP) and transhepatic cholangiography are the best methods to study the biliary tract in these cases. Interestingly, half the patients with choledocholithiasis will have normal bilirubin levels.

Operative cholangiography is important in the identification of patients with unsuspected bile duct stones and prevents unwise and unnecessary exploration of the normal common bile duct.

After exploration of the bile ducts, a T-tube is placed and a second operative cholangiogram is made to ascertain the completeness of stone removal. If the cholangiogram is normal, the T-tube is allowed to drain by gravity. A final cholangiogram is taken 10 days after operation, and if the bile ducts are normal, the T-tube is removed 24 hours later. If retained stones are identified, the T-tube is left in place and clamped, and the patient is discharged. The patient returns in 6 to 8 weeks for stone extraction through the T-tube tract. Stone removal is performed under fluoroscopy with flexible probes and Dormia baskets. Irrigation of the ductal system with various agents to dissolve stone is costly, time consuming, and usually unsuccessful.

Postcholecystectomy Symptoms

The persistence or recurrence of symptoms following cholecystectomy is generally labeled the postcholecystectomy syndrome. There is no such syndrome. Rather, there are three sets of conditions which distress patients following removal of the gallbladder.

By far the most common is persistence of the symptoms for which the gallbladder was removed. In these cases, the patient frequently has dyspepsia, food intolerance, or other symptoms unrelated to cholelithiasis. It is likely that the majority of these cases can be prevented by the physician's adequately explaining the expectations of cholecystectomy to the patient and excluding peptic ulcer, diverticulitis, and other digestive diseases prior to operation.

In contrast to patients with persistent symptoms are those who are initially relieved of pain, but several months to years later experience symptoms identical to those for which cholecystectomy was performed. In the past, retained bile duct stones were estimated to account for 60 per cent of these cases, but increasing routine use of operative cholangiography will decrease the incidence of this complication. Other causes include partial cholecystectomy, long cystic duct remnant containing stones, cystic duct neuroma, and papillary stenosis. In addition to oral and intravenous cholangiography and ultrasonography, the evaluation of recurrent symptoms has been greatly facilitated by ERCP (endoscopic retrograde cholangiopancreatography). Using this technique, an exact preoperative diagnosis can be made in 95 per cent of patients and unnecessary surgery is avoided.

The third cause of distress following cholecystectomy is the development of new symptoms related to other organs of the digestive system. In these patients, hiatus hernia, duodenal ulcer, peptic ulcer, pancreatic, gastric, and colonic cancer, and a host of other possibilities must be considered and systematically excluded.

Medical Treatment of Cholelithiasis

Progress in the elucidation of the mechanism of gallstone formation has led to attempts to dissolve biliary calculi. Chenodeoxycholic acid is presently being studied in the National Gallstone Study to determine the safety and efficacy in humans of in vivo dissolution of gallstones. The treatment is still considered experimental.

Eighty per cent of patients are reported to respond to chenodeoxycholic acid, 15 mg per kg per day orally, with either a decrease in the size of the stones or complete dissolution. Only 40 per cent of patients will respond to less than this dose. The average time to dissolution or partial dissolution is about 15 months. Recurrence of gallstones occurs in 20 to 50 per cent of patients who stop treatment for 1 to 2 years. The efficacy of this drug is greatest in patients with radiolucent stones less than 2.5 cm in diameter and a functioning gallbladder. Chenodeoxycholic acid is not effective in the dissolution of radiopaque stones, in patients with a nonfunctioning gallbladder, or in patients with radiolucent stones greater than 2.5 cm in diameter. Adverse reactions are diarrhea and mild elevation in liver enzymes, which in humans studied to date are not associated with histologic injury. The question of hepatic toxicity of the drug in man has not been fully answered. Gallstone dissolution is at present experimental and imperfect. Cholecystectomy remains the preferred treatment of cholelithiasis.

CIRRHOSIS

method of
ROBERT H. RESNICK, M.D.
Brookline, Massachusetts

Cirrhosis may be defined as a chronic disorder of the liver characterized by two fundamentally different processes — the activation of mesenchymal elements to produce fibrosis and the proliferation of hepatocytes to form regenerative nodules. These pathologic alterations must coexist to allow the term cirrhosis to be applied. The microcirculation of the liver in cirrhosis is substantially reduced by the effects of fibrosis and nodule formation. An outflow or postsinusoidal block results in sinusoidal hypertension — the site of elevated portal venous pressure in cirrhosis. Intrahepatic shunts form, connecting the circulation of the portal triad to the central vein and bypassing adjacent hepatocytes. The anatomic derangement allowing intrahepatic as well as extrahepatic portal systemic shunting (e.g., esophageal varices, umbilical and perirectal veins) is a prerequisite for the major complication of encephalopathy in cirrhotic subjects. The pathologic picture of cirrhosis is thought to have its origin in hepatocellular necrosis.

This event appears to be responsible for inflammatory and fibrogenic sequelae. The micronodular and macronodular forms of gross pathology which are seen in Laennec's and postnecrotic cirrhosis, respectively, may indicate the intensity of the necrotizing injury.

Cirrhosis is the consequence of varied causes. The following may be identified: (1) Alcohol. (2) Virus (hepatitis B and non-A, non-B hepatitis). Note that hepatitis A is not a cause. (3) Drugs (methotrexate, alpha-methyldopa, isonicotinic acid hydrazide, oxyphenisatin). (4) "Autoimmune" type with evident serologic abnormalities (e.g., ANA, LE cells, smooth muscle antibody) and frequent extrahepatic involvement (arthritis, colitis, thyroiditis, Sjögren's syndrome, hemolytic anemia). Virus, drugs, and "autoimmune" liver injury may induce a chronic active hepatitis with bridging necrosis as a precirrhotic lesion. (5) Inborn errors of metabolism, including Wilson's disease, alpha-1-antitrypsin deficiency, and galactosemia. (6) Cystic fibrosis. (7) Cardiac cirrhosis. (8) Idiopathic or cryptogenic postnecrotic cirrhosis, which may be indistinguishable clinically and pathologically from the entities seen after ethanol, viral, or drug injury or in association with immunologic phenomena. (9) Primary and secondary biliary cirrhosis.

In every case the therapeutic goal should be to establish a possible etiologic diagnosis so that removal of the offending agent, if possible, might arrest progression of disease. Percutaneous liver biopsy is valuable in establishing cirrhosis and assessing the extent and activity of the process; it may be useful in determining etiology (e.g., alcoholic hyaline, copper content in Wilson's disease, iron content in hemochromatosis, and PAS-positive inclusions in hepatocytes of alpha-1-antitrypsin deficiency). It may also be useful in deciding on the potential benefits of corticosteroids in idiopathic postnecrotic cirrhosis or cirrhosis following chronic active liver disease. Since we are largely unable to reverse an established cirrhosis, our customary approach is generally concerned with treatment of complications. Certain aspects of management, however, are related to known etiologic factors.

Alcoholic Cirrhosis

There is reason to believe that current programs to encourage abstinence have not reduced the increasing evidence of cirrhosis in the alcoholic. While the early form of alcohol damage — fatty liver — is reversible in the absence of continued drinking, alcoholic hepatitis represents a clinical and morphologic entity of greater severity. In the latter case, progression to cirrhosis may develop in some patients even if abstinence is totally effective. The primary role of alcohol per se rather than malnutrition has been emphasized in pathogenesis by studies in apparently well-nourished baboons. The influence of malnutrition, nevertheless, is supported by noting that similar histologic abnormalities have been identified after jejunoileal bypass for morbid obesity in the complete absence of alcohol. Histopathologic findings of alcoholic hepatitis have also been observed in abstinent middle-aged women, often diabetic, with signs of chronic illness.

Treatment. What specific measures are needed? (1) Abstinence. Although it is clearly beneficial in early cirrhosis, debate rages concerning its efficacy in advanced portal hypertension. (2) Hospitalization — a requirement for accurate diagnosis (i.e., biopsy) and in the frankly jaundiced patient, particularly if ascites, encephalopathy, gastrointestinal bleeding, or fever is noted. (3) Caloric requirements. If hepatic encephalopathy is absent, protein intake should be at least 1 to 1.5 grams per kg of body weight; a 2000 calorie diet should be supplied. (4) Sodium restriction. The presence of ascites is a requirement for sodium reduction in the diet to 0.5 to 1.0 gram daily. I would not increase above 2 grams daily even in absence of demonstrable ascites. Fluid restriction is undesirable unless serum sodium is less than 120 mEq per liter or the inappropriate antidiuretic hormone (ADH) syndrome is present. (5) Nutritional deficits: folic acid, thiamine, and pyridoxal phosphate (vitamin B_6) have reduced serum concentrations in a majority of subjects with alcoholic liver disease. Associated features include macrocytic anemia, peripheral neuropathy, and other signs of malnutrition. Vitamin deficiency leads to impaired protein (vitamin B_6) and nucleic acid (folate, B_6, B_{12}) metabolism. The consequence is further tissue injury and inhibition of repair. Lack of micronutrient intake, reduced absorption, decreased storage, and impaired conversion to active metabolites (e.g., transketolase) as well as increased loss (e.g., zincuria) are underlying mechanisms. Replacement therapy should be based on identification of the nature and extent of nutrient loss.

Alcoholic hepatitis with or without cirrhosis may simulate acute biliary tract disorders with fever, leukocytosis, right upper quadrant pain, and elevated alkaline phosphatase. Ultrasound may be helpful in distinguishing the two entities based on the caliber of the bile ducts and observations of calculi. In equivocal cases, a percutaneous cholangiogram may provide diagnostic findings. It is vital to recognize that surgical exploration in clinically acute alcoholic hepatitis carries a prohibitive mortality. The evaluation of fever is another important aspect of care. Modest temperature elevations are common in decompensated alcoholic cirrhosis usually related to the inflammatory and necrotic hepatic lesions. Infections are frequent in these patients, however, and appropriate cultures of blood and body fluids (including ascites) are required for diagnosis.

The role of corticosteroids remains controversial in spite of nine controlled trials. Several groups, however, have been able to show benefit when alcoholic hepatitis has been complicated by encephalopathy. Review of all data in this field in my judgment fails to confirm these expectations. Similarly, favorable reports concerning colchicine, an inhibitor of collagen secretion by microbodies of fibroblasts, and propylthiouracil, an inhibitor of a presumed hepatic hypermetabolic state, require additional support in controlled trials. Initial enthusiasm for penicillamine, an inhibitor of collagen cross-linkage, has been challenged.

Postnecrotic Cirrhosis

This lesion represents a final common pathway for multiple etiologic states. The recognition of postnecrotic cirrhosis as a frequent pathologic entity in alcohol-related injury is comparatively recent.

Treatment. Whenever possible, the specific provoking agents should be removed — e.g., as in drug- or ethanol-induced disease. But it must be appreciated that in advanced cases, progressive injury and fatalities may not be reduced by removing the inciting agent. Termination of viral infection, correction of inborn metabolic errors, and comprehension of pathogenesis in cryptogenic cirrhosis remain for future investigation. In spite of these constraints certain measures are applicable to specific causes. In the case of postnecrotic cirrhosis following chronic active liver disease, corticosteroids may be useful in terms of reducing symptoms, suppressing hypertransaminasemia, and extending survival. This treatment should be utilized in the presence of an "active cirrhosis," defined by the Mayo Clinic Group in terms of clinical, biochemical, and histologic criteria. Some advantage may be obtained by the addition of azathioprine, 50 mg daily, to enable the maintenance dose of corticosteroid (prednisone) to be reduced to 10 mg daily. (This use of azathioprine is not listed in the manufacturer's official directive.)

Primary Biliary Cirrhosis

This disorder is a slowly progressive rare affliction, primarily of middle-aged women, marked by destruction of intralobular bile ducts. Increasing cholestasis noted clinically and biochemically leads to fibrosis, cirrhosis, and ultimately fatal hepatic failure. Multichannel analyzers frequently serve to detect the elevated alkaline phosphatase which may precede the onset of pruritus or jaundice by many years. With progression of illness, the patient experiences further hepatic dysfunction, hyperlipoproteinemia with xanthoma and xanthelasmas, and loss of fat-soluble vitamins caused by diminished intraluminal bile salts. Osteomalacia, osteoporosis, and hypoprothrombinemia may be important clinical consequences.

Treatment. Specific therapy for this poorly understood disorder is unavailable. Recent interest has been stimulated by the observation of high copper levels in liver of primary biliary cirrhosis. By analogy with Wilson's disease, investigators have proposed that D-penicillamine may effect copper chelation as well as possibly inhibit collagen deposition. Two of three controlled trials currently in progress have suggested both biochemical and possibly histologic benefit. Reduction in immune complexes which may have a pathogenetic role has been observed. A third trial of penicillamine, however, has shown no clear advantage to this therapy; moreover, serious and frequent adverse drug reactions, including Goodpasture's syndrome, a myasthenic reaction, and significant albuminuria, were noted. Steroid therapy is associated with an increased rate of pathologic bone fractures and is ineffectual.

Some reduction in pruritus may be obtained by use of cholestyramine, 4 grams with each meal; however, aggravation of steatorrhea and loss of fat-soluble vitamins may be anticipated. Management of steatorrhea with medium-chain triglycerides (in place of long-chain triglycerides) in doses of 50 ml is desirable. Vitamin D administration and supplemental calcium (1 gram daily) are employed to reduce the attendant osteomalacia.

Wilson's Disease

Wilson's disease is a recessively inherited defect resulting in excessive hepatic copper accumulation possibly related to enhanced intracellular binding processes.* Homozygous patients show a reduction in plasma ceruloplasmin, although some increase in Wilson's disease may follow hepatic inflammation or necrosis, or increased plasma estrogen levels. Hepatic copper usually exceeds 200 micrograms per gram dry weight; comparable concentrations have been noted in primary biliary cirrhosis, extrahepatic biliary obstruction, and occasionally chronic active hepatitis. The Kayser-Fleischer ring is seen in more than 90 per cent of patients and is reported only rarely in primary biliary cirrhosis. Wilson's disease should be suspected in a child or young

---

*An alternative view stresses the failure of biliary secretion of copper as a primary abnormality.

adult with subacute or chronic liver injury. Important diagnostic clues are the presence of hemolysis, a neurologic motor lesion, or family history of fatal liver disease in a sibling. Additional aid may be obtained by noting excess urinary copper excretion, a large cupruresis after a penicillimine test dose, or impaired incorporation of radiocopper into ceruloplasmin.

Treatment. Establishing a sustained negative copper balance is essential to improve hepatic, motor, and intellectual functions; regression of Kayser-Fleischer rings can be achieved. A poor clinical response indicates inadequate copper chelation or terminal disease. Penicillamine is the drug of choice; in most instances a 1 gram quantity in four divided doses will be well tolerated. Vitamin B_6 is also required in a dose of 50 mg twice weekly to prevent neurotoxicity. Toxic effects are not infrequent, however, and include bone marrow depression, albuminuria, and the nephrotic syndrome as well as the more common drug fever and skin rash. Occasionally the latter reactions have been overcome by restarting the drug in minimal quantities (e.g., 50 mg) with gradually increasing increments. Less common serious side effects include Goodpasture's syndrome and myasthenic reactions. An alternative chelating agent, triethylene tetramine, may be used when penicillamine toxicity is unacceptable. Substitution therapy, however, has a reduced decoppering effect.

Alpha-1-Antitrypsin Deficiency

This inborn error, which was initially described as a cause of chronic obstructive lung disease in adults, has been found to be a common cause of cirrhosis in infancy and childhood. Alpha-1-antitrypsin is a glycoprotein accounting for a major fraction of serum alpha-1-globulin and represents about 90 per cent of serum antitrypsin activity. The homozygous phenotype PiZZ (Pi protease inhibitor) results in cirrhosis in 15 per cent of affected patients. There appears to be a slight risk in the heterozygous state. Orthotopic liver transplants are the only means of preventing death in late-stage cirrhosis on the basis of recent experience. The phenotypes of the recipients become those of the donors after transplantation so that alpha-1-antitrypsin levels attain normal serum values.

Complications of Cirrhosis*

Portasystemic Encephalopathy (PSE). Portasystemic encephalopathy as it occurs in the context of chronic liver disease requires the following

---

*The problem of bleeding varices is discussed on pages 361 to 364.

elements for its presence: (1) Shunting of nitrogenous and possibly other toxic metabolites from the portal venous system to systemic channels; such anastomoses are created in the evolution of cirrhosis but are increased by the surgical formation of total (portasystemic) shunts. (2) Hepatic dysfunction as measured by conventional liver function tests or, more elaborately, by rates of maximal urea synthesis or aminopyrine clearance. (3) Biochemical activity by intestinal flora to generate neurotoxic substances.

Two differing theories underlie the pathophysiology. The first suggests that in the presence of hepatic damage the brain is rendered unusually susceptible to both endogenous and exogenous alterations. This concept helps explain the peculiar sensitivity of the central nervous system in cirrhotics to pharmacologic agents (e.g., tranquilizers), fever, and postoperative and other catabolic states. The second hypothesis deals with the significance of specific toxins which evade hepatic conjugation because of portasystemic shunting and impaired liver metabolism. These biologically active substances include ammonia, mercaptans, short-chain fatty acids, and certain aromatic amino acids (tryptophan, phenylalanine, tyrosine).

Patients affected by these metabolic disturbances show various degrees of neurotoxicity. In its simplest form PSE may appear as a subtle personality change detectable only by the most sophisticated observer. More profound effects can produce disorientation, confusion, psychotic behavior, sleep disorders, agitation, and excitement (Stage I). Still further aberrations may progressively lead to lethargy and stupor (Stage II) and loss of consciousness (Stages III and IV); decerebrate and decorticate states are particularly advanced changes. A flapping tremor (asterixis) is frequently present and represents a failure of maintenance of postural tone. The mild degrees of PSE may be monitored by use of psychometric examination and the Reitan trail-making test. Electroencephalograms can also be utilized for evaluation at any stage of illness. I have found the bedside performance of serial sevens, construction of a 5-pointed star, and a daily signature to be useful objective measures.

TREATMENT. The management of PSE is suggested in part by recognizing the specific precipitating factor in the patient's course. For example, attention to gastrointestinal hemorrhage should be promptly focused on diagnosing and terminating the source of bleeding; at the same time removal of intraluminal blood by cathartics and enemas is essential and must be promptly implemented. If encephalopathy makes aspiration possible, laxatives and other medications should be given by nasogastric tube.

If encephalopathy is considered to be related to exogenous agents (e.g., benzodiazepine), prompt recognition and cessation are urgent matters. Rapid correction of a hypokalemic alkalosis with intravenous potassium chloride needs prompt implementation. Treatment of hemorrhagic shock, antimicrobial control of sepsis, and avoidance of hypoxia are mandatory and self-evident. Hypovolemia producing azotemia must be promptly repaired.

In addition to these considerations, certain general therapeutic principles apply.

1. Restriction of dietary protein is essential. This is particularly vital in the patient who presents with no clear inducing event. At varying intervals after total shunts, many of these subjects are observed to present with an insidious chronic encephalopathic syndrome. Based upon the intensity of the clinical features, a daily intake of 20 to 40 grams of protein may be initiated, with increases to be determined by therapeutic response. Raising the level by 10 to 20 gram increments as tolerated every 5 days until a protein intake of 1.5 grams per kg is attained has been useful in my experience. If coma or gastrointestinal bleeding is the initial finding, a zero protein intake is required until clinical improvement is apparent and all blood has been removed from the gastrointestinal tract. Whenever possible, maximize protein intake while utilizing other therapeutic modalities to permit liver synthetic and reparative processes to function.

2. Pharmacologic treatment is of major benefit. Two drugs, neomycin and lactulose, have been shown independently to influence favorably the clinical effects of PSE. Regardless of the presence or absence of specific precipitating factors, these agents may be employed.

Neomycin, which historically preceded lactulose, results in a prompt and sustained reduction of intestinal flora based on its aminoglycoside action. Approximately 1 per cent of the drug is absorbed and undergoes renal excretion, providing an antimicrobial effect in the urine. Neomycin has been shown to have a similar efficacy to lactulose in a controlled trial but demonstrates significantly greater toxic potential (e.g., irreversible ototoxicity, mild intestinal injury resulting in malabsorption, bile salt precipitation, and possibly nephrotoxicity in azotemic patients). Therefore, use of neomycin should be limited to circumstances in which control of PSE is not obtainable by lactulose therapy alone. This use of neomycin is somewhat paradoxic, because lactulose is considered to require bacterial enzymatic action for its efficacy. Neomycin may be given initially in 8 gram oral dosage or via nasogastric tube in four divided doses; a maintenance level usually reached within a week consists of a 2 to 4 gram daily intake. When used as a 1 per cent colonic enema the drug may enhance the effect of oral administration. Ampicillin in 500 mg four times daily dosage may be used in those rare circumstances in which neomycin resistance has been observed.

Lactulose, a synthetic, nonabsorbable disaccharide, was considered to be of therapeutic advantage because of a presumed capacity to alter flora to enzymatically inactive forms (e.g., lactobacillus). Currently the mechanism of action is not believed to be related to changes in bacterial species. Several effects of lactulose appear to produce favorable responses in PSE. Colonic bacteria appear to degrade the lactulose into small acidic fragments such as lactic, formic, and acetic acids. A resulting osmotic effect shortens intestinal transit, and a low pH intraluminally inhibits ammonia absorption from the colon. Recent evidence also suggests that lactulose may shift bacterial metabolism away from nitrogenous substrates.

The practical use of lactulose may commence with 15 to 30 ml three times daily by mouth (or nasogastric tube), with rapid increments up to 150 ml daily if needed. The therapeutic goals should involve reduction of clinical encephalopathy without producing more than several soft stools daily. The lowest dose reversing PSE without significant diarrhea represents the desired effect. Lactulose may be utilized for both acute and chronic PSE and, like neomycin, may be used in enema form (300 ml added to 700 ml water). No unusual adverse reactions have been noted, but overzealous administration has led to severe diarrhea, hypovolemic shock, and electrolyte disorders (hypokalemia, hyponatremia).

Ascites.   Ascites represents a major complication of cirrhosis related to the development of portal hypertension. The importance of hepatic dysfunction in its genesis is implied by the observation that extrahepatic portal vein block alone is insufficient for the development of a significant permanent ascites. The prime factors for the occurrence of abdominal fluid are an elevated portal pressure and reduction of serum albumin concentration (colloid osmotic pressure). The presence or absence of ascites may be predicted by knowledge of these variables. Two conflicting theories describe the primary events leading to intra-abdominal fluid. The first hypothesis maintains that ascites forms from the hypertensive splanchnic and hepatic surface capillaries and lymphatics. An "ineffective" circulating plasma volume results and favors increased renal proximal tubular reabsorption of sodium and water. The alternative concept maintains that the renal events are primary and abdominal fluid forms caused by "overload" of the vasculature. Both theories are supported by experimental and clinical findings and may in fact be relevant at different times in a clinical setting. Regardless of mechanism the ascitic patient who is not diuresing avidly retains administered sodium and water by proximal tubular reabsorption.

TREATMENT. Debate concerning the necessity for treatment of ascites has evolved because of widespread clinical observations of complications following diuretic therapy. Hypovolemia with resultant azotemia, the hepatorenal syndrome, portasystemic encephalopathy, and electrolyte and acid-base disturbances after diuretic administration produce a sense of therapeutic wariness. However, ascites is often a harbinger of bleeding esophagogastric varices as well as the hepatorenal syndrome. Cardiorespiratory compromise, various sites of hernia formation, and the occurrence of infective ascites are additional factors favoring intervention. Finally, ascitic cirrhotics have a greater fatality rate than the nonascitic. These considerations weigh heavily for treatment when the fluid collection is sufficient to be detected by physical examination in the nonazotemic mentally alert cirrhotic without serum electrolyte disturbance. The following principles of management appear to be important: (1) Treatment should be undertaken under close surveillance in a hospital. The vagaries of response require observation at least until a satisfactory quantity of fluid has been mobilized without complication. (2) Dietary sodium restriction requires not more than 1 gram of sodium daily. Fluids should not exceed 1500 ml per day. Since many "virginal" cirrhotics will mobilize fluid on this regimen, a period of watchful waiting for 10 to 12 days is reasonable. Failure to respond calls for a pharmacologic approach. (3) Furosemide, 40 mg daily, is begun when weight reduction is inadequate. The drug may be increased by 40 mg increments every 5 to 7 days until diuresis is achieved up to a maximum of 160 mg daily. During this time the occurrence of potassium deficiency must be vigorously corrected if observed. (4) If diuresis has not ensued, aldosterone inhibition in the form of spironolactone should be instituted. The drug may be given at 100 mg daily for 5 days, increasing to 400 mg daily if necessary by 100 mg increments every 5 days. Furosemide at 160 mg daily is maintained throughout this period. (5) Body weight, intake and output, abdominal girth, and assessment of blood pressure for postural changes should be noted daily. Serum electrolytes, blood urea nitrogen, and creatinine should be obtained at intervals of 3 to 4 days after beginning treatment.

(6) Recognize that ascites cannot be mobilized at rates greater than 900 ml per day (approximately 2 lb [1 kg]). Substantially greater loss may be seen without hazard in those patients who demonstrate peripheral edema. In the absence of edema, however, losses exceeding this quantity reflect excretion of nonascitic extracellular fluid. Therapy with infused albumin in 25 gram units should be used to avert the dangers of azotemia, encephalopathy, and possibly the hepatorenal syndrome if oligemia occurs. (7) Successful therapy may be defined by loss of demonstrable ascites on examination. Failure is evident when mobilization of fluid according to the aforementioned protocol is not attained or when adverse reactions associated with treatment intervene. An additional group of treatment failures is composed of patients who are apparent therapeutic successes in hospital but relapse following discharge.

The management of treatment failures remains an unresolved issue. In the past, selected patients were treated by a side-to-side portacaval shunt if ascites was deemed "intractable." In view of a significant postoperative morbidity and mortality, use of this major surgical procedure has diminished. More recently interest has been generated by the LeVeen peritoneal-jugular shunt (PJS). This innovative concept allows the continuous direct transfer of ascitic fluid into the systemic circulation via a subcutaneously placed catheter introduced under local anesthesia. The patency of a one way valve situated in the central portion of the device is maintained by a pressure differential greater than 3 mm water between abdominal cavity and thoracic vein. When coupled with furosemide treatment, the PJS has resulted in very substantial diuresis in many ascitic cirrhotics. Claims have also been made that suggest possible benefit in the hepatorenal syndrome. Nevertheless, many potential pitfalls are apparent after PJS, including disseminated intravascular coagulation, bleeding varices, and congestive failure. At this time controlled trials have begun to evaluate the PJS both in the hepatorenal syndrome and in severe ascites.

Spontaneous Bacterial Peritonitis (SBP). This is a serious, frequently fatal feature of advanced cirrhotic portal hypertension that has been emphasized only during the past decade. The pathogenesis is usually obscure, since infection in a primary focus is found uncommonly. In some situations endoscopic or other invasive diagnostic maneuvers have been performed prior to detection; in other cases inflammation has been noted (e.g., cholecystitis) in an organ contiguous to the peritoneum. Since in most instances gram-negative organisms are responsible, it is possible that lumen-to-mucosal-to-serosal movement of bacteria occurs because of a gut compromised by portal hypertension.

TREATMENT.   From a clinical view, it is vital to recognize the possibility of SBP by performing a diagnostic paracentesis in all ascitic cirrhotics on admission to hospital. Because of the frequently dismal prognosis of this disorder, diagnostic taps should be repeated subsequently if unexplained fever or unanticipated clinical deterioration (e.g., encephalopathy without apparent cause) is observed. The fluid obtained should be studied for white blood cell count and differential, hematocrit, Gram stain of spun sediment, routine culture and sensitivities, acid-fast culture, and cytology. Anaerobic cultures are considered unnecessary routinely because of the rarity of SBP caused by these bacteria. A clearly positive Gram stain can be helpful but will be found in only a minority of instances. Antibiotic choice would still be empiric pending confirmation on cultures. The ultimate diagnosis depends on recovery of bacteria. The white blood cell (WBC) count and differential are important ancillary tests because of their rapid availability. A WBC count above 1000 organisms per cu mm is highly suggestive of SBP, particularly if greater than 75 per cent polymorphonuclear leukocytes are noted in the differential. On this basis it is reasonable to commence therapy awaiting definitive bacteriology. Between 500 and 1000 WBC per cu mm the data are equivocal, and the decision to begin immediate treatment may be made on the basis of associated findings, e.g., fever, positive peritoneal physical signs, per cent polymorphs, but it would be wise to await cultural information. If the WBC counts conflict with other clinical observations, it is reasonable to repeat the paracentesis for additional findings. If the analysis of all available information implies a high probability of SBP, antibiotic treatment should begin with gentamicin, 1.75 mg per kg every 8 hours if there is no azotemia, and cephalothin, 1 gram every 4 hours by the intravenous route, pending results of bacterial culture and sensitivities. Appropriate drug selection may then be made; or if the culture is negative, therapy may be stopped. In any case it is necessary to repeat the tap after a 3 to 5 day interval to assess progress. Effective management of SBP would be associated with some reduction of the WBC count and per cent polymorphs as well as sterilization of ascitic fluid. It is desirable to repeat the tap prior to terminating drug therapy after 12 to 14 days and again in the first week after cessation of treatment to confirm successful management. Failure to demonstrate sterile cultures may indicate an intra-abdominal septic focus requiring surgical drainage.

The Hepatorenal Syndrome (HRS).   The hepatorenal syndrome (HRS) is a poorly understood, almost invariably fatal late complication of cirrhosis. Its pathophysiology involves oliguria, rising blood urea nitrogen, and, terminally, hypotension. It is associated with renal cortical ischemia. Proper definition requires the absence of intrinsic renal disease, since it has been established that these kidneys function normally following transplantation to anephric patients. Furthermore in those unusual instances in which successful hepatic transplantation has been performed, the hepatorenal syndrome slowly reverts toward normality. There is speculation that prostaglandins and kinin peptides are influential in pathogenesis; the condition is aggravated by prostaglandin inhibition. Currently effective therapy is unavailable, although a few patients have benefited from hepatic transplants (as stated above) and reversal has followed portacaval shunts in a few selected patients. Unfortunately, portal decompression is inappropriate for the vast majority of patients in HRS because of poor operative risk. Recent enthusiasm for peritoneojugular shunts as proposed therapy requires confirmation.

Every effort should be made to differentiate between oligemia with potential for reversibility and HRS, which carries an ominous prognosis. The essential difference can be established by noting whether an infusion of osmotically active colloid such as serum albumin will result in reducing the significantly raised blood urea nitrogen and improvement in creatinine clearance. Azotemia may be corrected and diuresis established if hypovolemia is reversed. The differential diagnosis may be helped considerably by observing the response of central venous pressure before and after infusion of 2 units of serum albumin. Rarely if cardiac performance is suspect, a Swan-Ganz catheter may be required for differentiation. In many circumstances, however, because of a severe coexisting coagulopathy, invasive diagnostic aids may be contraindicated.

CONSTIPATION

method of
JOHN R. KELSEY, JR., M.D.
Houston, Texas

Probably the most misunderstood and mismanaged medical problem that the physician encounters is constipation. There still exists a large area of ignorance as to the cause and management of constipation, not only for the patient but also for the physician. There is a wide variation in the rate of passage of feces from the colon. Some healthy persons may have three stools daily, while others may go 3 or more days between stools. Because of this wide variation in pattern which is present among healthy persons, a precise definition of constipation is not possible, but may be considered to be dissatisfaction on the part of the patient as to the frequency, consistency, or ease in passage of digested waste from the gastrointestinal tract.

Although there are no specific measurements which one can use to define daily fecal output, the normal for 24 hours is less than 350 grams. The volume will depend upon the amount of fiber ingested and the content of fluid in the feces. Generally speaking the smaller the stool quantity, the less fluid and fiber, and the firmer the consistency. When the stool becomes extremely dry from the physiologic activity of the bowel extracting fluid and electrolytes, there results, in some people, difficulty in passage of fecal masses. The factors which lead to this are multiple and must be carefully analyzed before arriving at a helpful solution for the patient. Doctors are well advised to question the patient in detail to identify if the patient truly has a problem with elimination, and to try to identify specific causes and assist him in reaching a satisfactory solution to the problem.

Factors Responsible for Constipation

The following are the more common factors which must be considered:

First, dietary factors probably play the most important role. The American diet is typically low in fiber content. In our urban culture, fresh fruits and vegetables, which supply the major part of fiber content, are expensive, and over the years have progressively disappeared from the typical American diet. The low volume of fiber leads to low volume fecal output. Fiber may be obtained by the addition of breakfast cereals, or it may be added to bread, fruit, yogurt or other palatable or unpalatable concoctions to be included in the daily diet. These simple dietary measures will often correct constipation problems in a great majority of normal people.

Physical activity also encourages normal bowel functions, and, conversely, constipation is associated with inactivity, as experienced in traveling or in unusual sedentary periods such as hospitalization. Often dietary alterations or other measures may have to be taken as a preventive measure during sedentary periods.

Other factors which regulate bowel elimination are more complex and poorly understood, but relate to the digestive processes which take place in the proximal digestive tract. In most instances failure of proper digestion leads to diarrhea. It is not well understood why some people with normal anatomy and apparently normal physiologic function will have problems with eliminations while others do not. It is conceivable that the bowel may actually be more efficient in persons with constipation. It has been observed that although there is a wide variation in size and length of the colon among healthy persons, individuals with an unusually long bowel, so-called dolichocolon, or acquired megacolon, are more likely to have problems with fecal elimination.

Mechanical problems cause constipation in some patients. Anal fissuring and scarring may interfere with elimination. Higher bowel lumen pressure in patients with diverticular disease may result in bowel wall thickening and luminal narrowing, which may contribute to constipation. The correction of these basic disease problems may require medical or surgical treatment, which, when successfully accomplished, will eliminate the constipation. The possibility of bowel cancer looms prominently in the picture in an older patient who has had recent onset of constipation. This should serve as a stimulus to the physician to investigate properly, by appropriate diagnostic techniques, the possibility of a disease process.

In some patients, particularly the elderly and chronically disabled, bowel elimination becomes an increasing problem, and may even pose a serious life-threatening problem of fecal impaction. This is a unique group of patients for whom special care and attention are required to prevent impactions from occurring. If they occur, special nursing care and often hospitalization are required for management.

Finally, there is a very rare group of patients who appear to be refractory to any type of medical management. Some of these people have been found to have motor abnormalities of their bowel on the basis of toxic, neurogenic, or diffuse disease processes which damage the bowel musculature and affect its normal physiologic function. This has recently been given the name pseudo-obstruction. It is probably the most difficult problem relating to constipation, and in rare instances such patients may require surgical intervention or other heroic treatment measures.

Management of Constipation

After appropriate history, physical examination, and appropriate diagnostic studies, one is then prepared to approach the management of the patient's problem. By eradicating underlying causes, educating the patient, stopping the use of strong laxatives and enemas, establishing a regular living pattern, and improving the diet, most patients experience improvement. Cereals, particularly bran, may be added to the diet to supplement fiber usually obtained in fruits and vegetables.

Hydrophilic colloids from psyllium or tragacanth families are commonly employed agents which increase the bulk of the stool by holding water in the stool and thus creating a softer mass. Some of the common preparations used are Konsyl, Metamucil, Siblin, and Mucilose. One to 3 teaspoons of these preparations taken with fruit juice or other fluids on a daily basis will correct the problem without uncomfortable cramping. One side effect which is a problem to some patients, however, is increased gas formation, apparently from colonic bacteria. Rarely these agents have accounted for obstruction in the esophagus.

Stool softeners are substances which by decreasing surface tension are felt to account for mechanical softening of the stool. It is likely that they may stimulate some secretory function of the bowel as well. Common preparations in this category are dioctyl sodium sulfosuccinate (Colace, Doxinate) and calcium dioctyl sulfosuccinate (Surfak). These agents are particularly valuable in helping eliminate impactions. They may be ingested or given with enemas to help dissolve a large fecal mass.

Osmotic agents, such as Fleet's Phospho-Soda and lactulose, have the property of drawing fluid from the systemic circulation into the bowel lumen in large quantities, and are unsatisfactory agents to be used on a long-term basis. Laxatives such as cascara, senna, and phenolphthalein are common over-the-counter preparations which are irritating to the colon. Their use is commonly accompanied by abdominal cramping and discomfort. These agents are generally to be avoided in long-term use.

Bile salts, for many years, have been used as laxatives. They are obtained from animal sources and contain insoluble bile salts which are not absorbed by the intestinal tract. They cause secretory effects on the colonic mucosa, but when used in excessive amount they may also be irritating.

Finally, enemas, suppositories, and colonic irrigations are generally of limited value, and should not be used on a long-term basis except in the elderly or disabled, in the treatment of impactions.

DYSPHAGIA AND ESOPHAGEAL OBSTRUCTION

method of
LAWRENCE F. JOHNSON, M.D.,
and DAVID A. PEURA, M.D.
Washington, D.C.

Dysphagia is a cardinal symptom of esophageal disease and results from either lumen occlusion from a stricture or disordered esophageal motility. Mechanical obstruction of the esophagus produces dysphagia late in the disease process when lumen diameter is less than 13 mm or at least 50 per cent narrowed. In general, dysphagia resulting from mechanical obstruction occurs primarily with solid food, whereas dysphagia caused by disordered esophageal motility occurs with both solids and liquids. Dysphagia should be distinguished from odynophagia, pain with swallowing, an esophageal symptom resulting from mucosal diseases of different etiologies, most of which have specific therapy other than esophageal dilation. Dysphagia should never be considered functional, and all patients with this symptom should have a complete evaluation. Only when mechanical obstruction has been disproved should a diagnosis of a primary motor disorder of the esophagus be accepted as the cause of the patient's dysphagia.

Once the cause of the patient's symptoms has been determined, using history, physical examination and appropriate diagnostic studies, reestablishment and maintenance of an effective swallowing mechanism become the main goals of therapy. Peroral esophageal dilation can safely and effectively meet this goal in most patients with mechanical obstruction, as well as in some patients with motility disorders. Surgical therapy is rarely necessary for dysphagia.

Patients with dysphagia should be counseled to (1) chew their food carefully, (2) alter their diet as necessary to include such things as puréed foods, (3) drink sufficient fluid with their meals to facilitate passage, and (4) pay particular attention to their dentition. Adequate dentition is of primary importance to ensure thorough mastication of food with uniformity of bolus particle size prior to swallowing. Poorly fitted dentures should be corrected to prevent malocclusion. Patients with their hard palate covered by a dental bridge should be counseled that their awareness of bolus size prior to swallowing will be impaired and that they should thoroughly chew their food prior to swallowing. Patients should also be counseled to avoid drinking alcohol with their meals, since this may make them less aware of bolus size prior to swallowing. If a food impaction occurs, patients should be cautioned not to induce gagging or retching, both of which can potentially cause esophageal mucosal laceration or perforation. Patients should be instructed to seek immediate medical attention and be treated as outlined below.

Instruments for Dilation

Mercury-filled rubber dilators are commonly used in our clinical practice. The rounded tip (Hurst) and tapered tip (Maloney) dilators are supplied in sizes from 12 to 60 French units (Fr) (1 mm = 3 Fr.). Each subsequent dilator is 2 Fr larger than the preceding. Mercury-filled rubber dilators smaller than 30 Fr are so flexible that they prove ineffective in dilating most stenotic lesions. The tapered (Maloney) dilators are easier to pass and better tolerated by the patient; therefore, they are preferred in our clinical practice.

Metal olive dilators (Eder-Puestow) are supplied in sizes 21 to 45 Fr. The metal olive is attached to a flexible metal rod, and then passed over a flexible guide wire that has a distal spring tip (7 Fr.). Once the guide wire is passed and properly seated in the stomach, the metal olive dilators do not require patient swallowing effort for passage. The guide wire ensures a proper plane of passage through the hypopharyngeal-cricopharyngeal region and through the esophageal stricture. More force can be applied during the dilation effort because of added stiffness of the metal rod.

The pneumatic cardia dilator used for the treatment of achalasia comes in various sizes, shapes, and models. We use a modified Mosher pneumatic dilator that does not have a preformed waist. The indentation of the balloon by the lower esophageal sphincter ensures proper placement and is used as a monitor for insufflation pressure during the pneumatic dilation.

Patient Preparation for Esophageal Dilation

Patients should be fully informed of the indications, technique, and potential risks involved in their esophageal dilation. As with any peroral instrumentation there is a potential for complications. Bleeding, esophageal perforation, and pulmonary aspiration are all potential complications associated with this procedure. Esophageal dilation performed by experienced physicians can be done at low risk.

Patients should have no oral intake (NPO) for 6 hours prior to the procedure in order to prevent pulmonary aspiration of gastric or esophageal contents. Patients who have a dilated esophagus that empties incompletely, such as occurs in achalasia and some neoplasms of the gastric cardia, should have the esophagus aspirated with a large bore tube (Ewald, 34 Fr) prior to any dilation. Suction equipment to handle oropharyngeal secretions should also be available.

Most patients do not require a topical anesthetic agent applied to the hypopharynx prior to dilation; however, if desired, benzocaine (Cetacaine) gargles may be used. Sedation and general anesthesia should be avoided, since the patient must be monitored for pain both during and after the dilation procedure. Some chest pain may be associated with the dilation procedure; however, the intensity should promptly subside after the dilation. If this is not the case, the patient should be observed for a potential complication.

We use fluoroscopic control in all patients during the initial series of dilations. Subsequent dilations, using rubber dilators, may be conducted without fluoroscopy. However, fluoroscopy is mandatory when a metal or pneumatic dilator is used. Fluoroscopic control should also be used in patients with long tortuous strictures, or in those who have hypopharyngeal or esophageal diverticula.

Techniques for Dilation

All dilators should be thoroughly cleansed with a solution such as povidone-iodine (Betadine) prior to use. This prevents bacteremia from instrument contamination. During dilation patients may either sit or be in the lateral decubitus position, with the head elevated.

All dilators should be only lightly lubricated, because excess lubricant could wipe off in the hypopharynx and produce a foreign body sensation, occlude the airway, or be aspirated. Rubber dilators are passed into the midline of the hypopharynx much like a fiberoptic endoscope. The patient is asked to swallow in order to relax the upper esophageal sphincter, and the dilator is then gently advanced into the body of the esophagus. The degree of force used in advancing the dilator through the stricture is something that must be learned with experience. After the dilator passes through the strictured area, it is quickly withdrawn. It is important when using tapered dilators to document by measurement or fluoroscopy that the larger diameter of the dilator actually passed through the stricture.

Dilation with metal olives (Eder-Puestow) must always be done over a metal guide wire. This guide wire has a flexible spring tip that helps prevent an inadvertent perforation of the esophagus or stomach during passage, because the spring tip bends if any resistance is encountered. The guide wire is placed under fluoroscopic control through the strictured area and is positioned in the stomach. If the guide wire is difficult to pass, it can be inserted through the biopsy channel of a standard endoscope and, in turn, placed through the stricture orifice under direct vision. The appropriate sized metal olive is then attached to the dilator shaft, lightly lubricated, and passed over the guide wire through the strictured area. Since the metal shaft of the dilator assembly permits a forceful dilation, care must be taken that one's hand does not slip and injure the patient's face. Upon removal of the dilator, an assistant assures that the guide wire remains in position so that subsequent dilations may be performed. Once the series of dilations has been completed, the guide wire is pulled against the metal dilator shaft and the entire assembly is withdrawn.

The number of dilations done per session is dependent upon patient tolerance, the degree of resistance offered by the stricture, and resistance felt by the operator. Usually a maximum of three progressive size dilations can be safely accomplished during one session with minimal patient discomfort. If necessary, dilations may be performed daily. Usually the last dilator size passed at the previous session is passed first at the next session. The end point of dilation is determined mainly by the etiology of the stricture. Most peptic strictures can be dilated with minimal risk to a size 50 Fr. Other strictures with thick rigid fibrotic walls such as those caused by radiation or caustic injury should be dilated more cautiously and generally to size 40 Fr or less. Patients dilated to this size will be able to eat a regular diet if cautioned to chew their food well. We do not advocate dilation of strictures with an endoscope, because the tip was not designed for this purpose.

Specific Treatment Regimens

Dysphagia Due to Lumen Occlusion. BENIGN PEPTIC STRICTURES. These are generally short segment strictures located at the gastroesophageal junction, and result from gastroesophageal reflux. They are best treated with progressive dilation, using either Maloney or Hurst dilators. An estimate of the lumen size of the stricture can be obtained either radiographically or during the diagnostic endoscopy. These procedures aid in initial selection of the type and size of dilator to be used. Treatment of gastroesophageal reflux will retard the recurrence of these strictures and decrease future dilation requirement. A "benign peptic stricture" that requires dilation every week or two suggests the presence of an underlying malignancy.

LONG SEGMENTAL STRICTURES. These strictures may occur at various locations in the esophagus and are usually due to prior caustic ingestion or longstanding nasogastric intubation with reflux. Care must be taken that dilation of chronic strictures does not progress too rapidly and lead to a fracture and perforation of the fibrotic esophageal wall. These long strictures must often be managed with metal dilators.

ACUTE CORROSIVE INJURY. Esophagoscopy should be performed as soon as the patient is hospitalized and stable. This should be a limited examination, for once an injury to the mucosa is observed this implicates esophageal involvement resulting from the caustic agent. Therapeutic decisions can be made from this information, and the patient does not have to be exposed to added risk of a complete esophagoscopy. If an esophageal injury from the caustic agent is observed, we stop oral intake (NPO), and give intravenous fluids, broad-spectrum antibiotics, and corticosteroids. The efficacy of steroid therapy remains unproved. While esophageal edema can cause some dysphagia, stricture formation caused by fibrosis does not occur for at least 3 weeks. After several days, when the patient is no longer systemically ill and oral lesions and odynophagia have subsided, we institute dilation to ensure that the esophagus will not severely stricture over the next 3 to 4 weeks. The patient should have periodic esophageal dilation for the next several months to prevent a late stricture. The patient will be at risk of stricture formation up to 1 year following the injury. Patients with strictures resulting from corrosive injury of the esophagus have a higher incidence of squamous cell carcinoma and probably should have periodic surveillance.

RINGS AND WEBS. Dysphagia caused by esophageal webs and lower esophageal rings (Schatzki's) can be treated with peroral dilation, using a large rubber dilator (50 Fr). A single passage of a large dilator is usually effective in relieving symptoms.

FOOD IMPACTION. When a bolus of food impacts in the esophagus the major treatment depends upon the level of the impaction as well as the patient's ability to handle secretions. In order to demonstrate the level of an impacted bolus, plain films of the esophageal area are taken. Then a small amount of barium contrast may be either cautiously swallowed or instilled through a nasogastric tube. If the impaction is high in the esophagus and the patient is unable to handle secretions, immediate endoscopic removal of the bolus may be indicated. If the impaction is in the mid- or distal esophagus, attempts to dissolve the bolus may be undertaken, using a solution containing papain in the form of commercially available unseasoned meat tenderizer (Adolph's) mixed in a concentration of 1 rounded teaspoon dissolved in 4 ounces (120 ml) of water. If the patient is incompletely obstructed, this solution is slowly sipped. If the patient is completely obstructed, then 5 to 10 ml of solution is slowly infused above the area of the bolus through a nasogastric tube and aspirated after 5 minutes. Repeat instillation and aspiration is done every 30 to 60 minutes until the bolus passes. The attempt at dissolution may be continued for up to 48 hours.

If enzymatic dissolution of the bolus is unsuccessful and spontaneous passage does not occur, endoscopic removal may be attempted with biopsy forceps, a polyp remover, or snare. Occasionally, a rigid esophagoscope must be used so that the bolus can be grabbed with a larger biopsy forceps. Prior to endoscopic removal, plain films of the esophageal area should be reviewed to see if bone is present in the impacted bolus. Bones often preclude safe manipulation of the bolus, since they may cause esophageal perforation. One should not attempt to blindly push the bolus into the stomach. Once the bolus has been removed, a thorough evaluation of the esophagus must be undertaken to define the underlying pathology that caused the impaction.

FOREIGN BODIES.   Numerous foreign bodies have become impacted in the esophagus. We have removed an assortment of items such as a straight pin, coins, a thermometer, and dentures. The potential for removal of foreign bodies is limited only by the ingenuity of the endoscopist. Items may be grabbed with biopsy forceps, polyp snares, and retrievers. Caution should be taken in manipulating sharp objects within the esophagus, since perforation can occur. Occasionally it is helpful to attach a 2 to 3 inch Penrose drain rubber sheath hood over the tip of the endoscope into which sharp objects may be retrieved. When delivering foreign bodies through the cervical region, the patient's head should be extended in the position required for rigid esophagoscopy. This obviates a right angle turn and helps prevent loss of the foreign body in the cervical region or bronchial tree.

NEOPLASMS.   Squamous cell carcinoma is usually far advanced when the patient presents with dysphagia. We treat these patients with radiation therapy and esophageal dilation to relieve dysphagia, assure adequate nutrition, and prevent aspiration. Dilation should begin before radiation therapy and continue during radiation if necessary. It should extend thereafter to ensure esophageal lumen patency. We have published data to show that dilation in these patients can be done at low risk. Most malignant strictures will respond to rubber dilators; however, on occasion, some far advanced malignant strictures will require metal olive dilation. Dysphagia that occurs following radiotherapy and is refractory to periodic dilation may be treated with a nonoperatively placed polyvinyl prosthesis tube to ensure lumen patency. In a similar manner, these polyvinyl prosthetic tubes can palliate incessant coughing that results from aspiration caused by malignant tracheoesophageal fistula. While these prostheses may improve the patient's quality of remaining life, they do not prolong it, nor do they prevent known complications from the disease. Additionally, these tubes are not used without risk. Occasionally they may erode through the esophageal wall into a major vessel or organ. Therefore, we use them only in patients with the two previously stated indications.

Adenocarcinoma of the esophagus and cardia of the stomach is not a very radiosensitive tumor. It is our feeling that this tumor should be treated surgically with palliative resection. Recurrent dysphagia following surgery may be treated with dilation in combination with radiotherapy or chemotherapy.

Dysphagia Due to Disordered Motility. DIFFUSE ESOPHAGEAL SPASM (DES).   This entity is rare and requires specific manometric findings such as spontaneous, simultaneous, high amplitude esophageal contraction waves of long duration to confirm the diagnosis. Patients with retrosternal chest pain from DES occasionally do obtain symptomatic relief with periodic dilation with a large rubber dilator. Nitroglycerin and long-acting nitrates, such as isosorbide dinitrate (Isordil) may be helpful. In our experience, documented gastroesophageal reflux is rarely associated with DES; however, patients do occasionally obtain relief with vigorous antacid therapy. Patients with incapacitating symptoms associated with severe weight loss, characteristic manometric findings, and a thickened esophageal wall may derive some benefit from long surgical myotomy.

ACHALASIA.   Pneumatic dilation is our initial treatment modality for patients with achalasia. Once the diagnosis of achalasia has been firmly established by standard radiographic, manometric, and endoscopic criteria, the esophagus is aspirated clean and a large rubber dilator (58 Fr) is passed to ensure the absence of a stricture at the cardioesophageal junction that would compromise pneumatic dilation. A Mosher bag is then passed under fluoroscopic control so that the balloon is located in the cardioesophageal junction. In a patient with a dilated tortuous esophagus, it may be necessary to pass the pneumatic dilator over a guide wire. When the appropriate position of the bag has been fluoroscopically confirmed, the balloon is inflated to a pressure sufficient to straighten the waist indented by the lower esophageal sphincter. This pressure is maintained for 1 minute and then rapidly released. The balloon is reinflated to check the pressure needed to obliterate the balloon waist. This second pressure should be less than the original obliteration pressure if an effective dilation has occurred. Blood streaking on the balloon at the time of removal is also indicative of an effective dilation. Even though our patients complain of marked retrosternal pain during the dilation, we do not routinely give analgesic or sedative agents because we feel these drugs may have an adverse effect on the pneumatic dilation. After the balloon is deflated, the intensity of the patient's chest pain should markedly subside. We monitor the patient after the pneumatic dilation for any persistence of chest pain as well as for presence of fever, hypotension, tachycardia, or leukocytosis. If any of these signs occur, a small amount of water-soluble contrast material (Gastrografin) is given and esophageal x-rays are taken to rule out a perforation. Patients should be counseled that pneumatic dilation does not relieve all the dysphagia, for there is still a lack of primary peristalsis in the body of the esophagus. Should severe dysphagia return, a second attempt at pneumatic dilation may be performed prior to referring the patient for a surgical myotomy of the lower esophageal sphincter (Heller procedure). All patients require surveillance for carcinoma of the esophagus that reportedly occurs with increased frequency after many years with achalasia.

Odynophagia. Odynophagia, painful swallowing, usually indicates a disruption of the esophageal mucosa. It is caused by many conditions such as an acute infection with herpesvirus, Monilia, histoplasmosis, injury from a foreign body, corrosive agents, esophageal hematoma, or acute inflammation resulting from a pill maintaining prolonged esophageal mucosal contact (vitamin C, aspirin, tetracycline, quinidine, KCl). Patients presenting with odynophagia should have esophagoscopy done early to determine the cause, since the barium swallow is an insensitive detector of mucosal disease. At the time of esophagoscopy, biopsies and mucosal brushings, should be taken and examined for the presence of viral inclusion bodies, fungal and yeast elements, and malignancy. Symptomatic therapy for odynophagia should be instituted. This may include treatment with antacids or preparations such as lidocaine (Xylocaine viscous solution). We have found that a mixture of diphenhydramine (Benadryl elixir), 10 ml (25 mg), and 30 to 60 ml of antacid affords good symptomatic relief in most patients, regardless of the cause of the odynophagia. If the patient is found to have monilial esophagitis, vigorous therapy with oral nystatin suspension (500,000 units) four times a day is indicated. However, if the patient has evidence of deep esophageal fungal ulcers owing to immunosuppression, low dose amphotericin B (0.5 mg per kg per day) should be used to a total dose of 500 to 1000 mg. Patients with acute mucosal injury of the esophagus should be watched for evidence of stricturing; if this does occur, dilation should be instituted.

DIVERTICULA OF THE ALIMENTARY TRACT

method of
KENNETH ENG, M.D.,
and S. ARTHUR LOCALIO, M.D.
New York, New York

Diverticula of the alimentary tract may be congenital or acquired. The most common site by far is the colon. Colonic diverticular disease is also the most frequent cause of symptoms and complications.

Other sites involved, in order of decreasing frequency, are the duodenum, esophagus, stomach, jejunum, and ileum.

Zenker's (Pharyngoesophageal) Diverticulum

Zenker's diverticulum occurs as a posterior hernia between the oblique fibers of the inferior constrictor of the pharynx and the transverse fibers of the cricopharyngeus. Failure of relaxation of the cricopharyngeus during swallowing probably contributes to its pathogenesis.

Symptoms produced are the regurgitation of undigested food, splashing or gurgling noises in the neck, and a foul taste or odor in the mouth. A large diverticulum may cause dysphagia or obstruction. The diagnosis may be confirmed by an x-ray with contrast material. Perforation and hemorrhage are reported, but the most important complication is aspiration pneumonia.

These symptoms and the possibility of aspiration make early operation the treatment of choice for most patients. The operation may be accomplished under local anesthesia in poor risk patients. A liquid diet and postural drainage are instituted preoperatively to empty the sac. A broad-spectrum antibiotic such as cefazolin is administered in the preoperative and immediate postoperative periods. One-stage excision can be performed through an incision parallel to the left sternomastoid or a supraclavicular transverse incision. A large bore nasogastric tube is passed only after mobilization of the sac to avoid false passage and perforation. This tube is advanced beyond the diverticulum to serve as a stent during esophageal repair and is removed at the completion of the operation. The cricopharyngeus is divided. Cricopharyngeal myotomy alone has been suggested, but symptomatic diverticula are usually large enough to warrant excision. Fluids by mouth are permitted after 36 to 48 hours, and the patient is advanced to soft food by the fifth day. The mortality rate is less than 1 per cent. Complications — fistula, wound infection, and recurrent laryngeal nerve injury — occur in less than 2 per cent of patients.

Diverticula of the Esophagus

Diverticula of the thoracic esophagus occur most commonly in its mid-portion and in the epiphrenic area. Excision of these diverticula requires thoracotomy, and is reserved for patients with severe symptoms or complications. Carcinoma arising in an esophageal diverticulum has been reported.

Mid-esophageal diverticula are usually produced by contraction of adherent tracheobronchial lymph nodes. These traction diverticula are usually asymptomatic and require no treatment. Operation is reserved for the rare diverticulum which perforates into the trachea, lung, or mediastinum.

Pulsion diverticula are usually epiphrenic in location but may occur higher in the esophagus. These pulsion diverticula are often associated with achalasia, esophageal spasm, reflux esophagitis, or stricture. Asymptomatic epiphrenic diverticula may be managed nonoperatively. Surgical excision is indicated for patients with dysphagia, obstruction, or regurgitation, especially that occurring during sleep and associated with aspiration pneumonitis. Patients must be fully evaluated for motility disorders and reflux esophagitis. Transthoracic excision of the diverticulum should be accompanied by esophagomyotomy or antireflux procedure or both.

Diverticula of the Stomach

Gastric diverticula have been discovered as frequently as in 1 of 250 patients studied by upper gastrointestinal x-ray examination. They are usually single and typically occur in the cardia or the prepyloric region. Most gastric diverticula are asymptomatic and require no treatment. Postprandial dyspepsia, epigastric fullness, eructations, and substernal pain have all been ascribed to failure of these pouches to empty. Since these symptoms are nonspecific, other upper abdominal lesions must be excluded. Diverticulitis, perforation, and hemorrhage have also been reported. Operative treatment is indicated for the patient with severe symptoms or complications. The actual surgical procedure depends upon the location of the lesion. Proximal lesions are usually amenable to careful mobilization and excision. Prepyloric lesions are usually managed by distal gastrectomy.

Duodenal Diverticula

Duodenal diverticula are relatively common abnormalities and may be recognized in 1 per cent of upper gastrointestinal x-rays. They are usually solitary, arise in the descending duodenum near the ampulla of Vater, and project medially in proximity to the common bile duct and pancreas. Since these diverticula rarely produce definable symptoms and resection may be difficult, elective operation is rarely undertaken. Complications may be due to impingement upon the bile duct, pancreatic duct, or duodenum itself. Inflammation, hemorrhage, and perforation are also reported.

In patients presenting with obscure gastrointestinal bleeding, localization of the bleeder may be assisted by angiography or endoscopy. Treatment consists of suture of the offending vessel and excision of the diverticulum. The diverticulum is retroperitoneal, and adequate exposure requires full mobilization of the duodenum and head of the pancreas.

Perforated duodenal diverticulum is rarely recognized preoperatively. Treatment is excision and closure if possible, but defunctionalization by Billroth II gastrectomy may be necessary if inflammation is extensive or the ampulla is involved.

Obstruction of the common duct is most safely treated by biliary bypass.

Small Intestinal Diverticula

Acquired diverticula of the small intestine are found in 0.4 per cent of upper gastrointestinal x-ray examinations but may be demonstrated by inflation of the bowel in up to 1.2 per cent of autopsies. They occur most frequently in the jejunum but may occur in distal bowel. They are frequently multiple, occur on the mesenteric border in association with blood vessels, are deficient in muscle coat, and are seen with increasing frequency in older patients. These features held in common with colonic diverticula suggest a similar mechanism of disordered motility.

Although patients who present with complications often have a history of intermittent postprandial crampy pain and flatulence, most small bowel diverticula produce no recognizable pattern of symptoms.

Obstruction at the neck of a diverticulum may produce inflammation, perforation, hemorrhage, and intestinal obstruction. Small bowel diverticula should be included in the differential diagnosis of obscure gastrointestinal bleeding and the acute abdomen. Localization of a bleeding intestinal diverticulum may be aided by angiography. Diagnosis of peritonitis caused by a perforated diverticulum may be apparent only after careful exploration. Treatment is by segmental small bowel resection.

Bacterial overgrowth in the diverticulum may lead to malabsorption and megaloblastic anemia. Response of the diarrhea to a 7 to 10 day course of broad-spectrum antibiotics (tetracycline, 250 mg four times per day) confirms the diagnosis. This regimen may be repeated intermittently to prevent recurrence. Deficiencies of vitamin B_{12} and fat-soluble vitamins A, D, and K are treated by appropriate replacement.

Meckel's Diverticulum

Meckel's diverticulum, an embryologic remnant of the primitive yolk duct at its attachment to the distal ileum, is present in about 2 per cent of the population. It consists of all layers of bowel wall and arises on the antimesenteric border.

Complications occur in about 5 per cent, usually in childhood, but may occur at any age. Peptic ulceration resulting from aberrant gastric mucosa and intestinal obstruction by a variety of mechanisms are most commonly encountered. Diverticulitis, which may be indistinguishable from appendicitis, occurs less frequently.

The diverticulum rarely fills with contrast during a barium study, but a technetium scan may be diagnostic, since this isotope is concentrated by gastric mucosa. This study is particularly useful in patients with unexplained pain or bleeding.

Treatment is usually by excision, but segmental resection may be required in the presence of significant inflammation. Meckel's diverticulum found incidentally can be removed with minimal morbidity, but this is justified only if conditions are ideal and in young patients, since the incidence of complications is low.

Diverticular Disease of the Colon

The colon is the most common site for diverticular disease in the alimentary tract. One third of persons over 45 years of age and more than one half of those over 70 years of age are affected.

Colonic diverticula occur predominantly in the sigmoid, but the right side of the colon may be involved. Right-sided diverticular disease alone is infrequent. However, more than half of the cases of massively bleeding diverticula occur in the right colon. In addition, a cecal diverticulum has been recognized which is distinct from other colonic diverticula, in that it is solitary, contains all elements of the colon wall, and occurs in younger patients. Inflammation of solitary cecal diverticula may produce signs and symptoms which may be confused with acute appendicitis, appendiceal abscess, or carcinoma.

In the past, uncomplicated diverticular disease was thought to cause no symptoms. This view has been altered by several observations. Study of bowel resected for presumed sigmoid diverticulitis often showed no evidence of inflammation and sometimes few diverticula. The most consistent abnormality was hypertrophy of the muscular wall. Manometric studies revealed zones of elevated intraluminal pressure in the sigmoid colon with an exaggerated response to feeding and drugs which stimulate smooth muscle. Intraluminal pressure just a short distance away might be normal. Zones of elevated pressure have been correlated with segmentation of the lumen by adjacent rings of contraction. Diverticula are produced by herniation of mucosa where the muscular layers are penetrated by blood vessels. Symptoms such as crampy abdominal pain, flatulence, constipation, and occasionally diarrhea occur without inflammation and are due to this motility disorder.

Sigmoid diverticulitis represents a perforation of a mucosal sac and is distinguished from symptomatic diverticular disease by the presence of fever, leukocytosis and peritoneal signs or a tender mass. Such a perforation may result in peridiverticulitis, localized abscess, fistula, or, rarely, generalized peritonitis. Other complications of colonic diverticula are bleeding and obstruction.

Symptomatic Diverticular Disease

The treatment of diverticular disease by a high fiber diet is based upon the hypothesis that a moist bulky stool prevents segmentation and therefore reduces pathologic elevations of pressures. Although there is no evidence that a high fiber diet alters the natural history of diverticular disease or prevents complications, such a diet does lower intraluminal pressure and alleviates symptoms in most patients. Foods high in fiber content include whole wheat products, fruits, and vegetables. Indigestible particulate food such as nuts, corn, and seeds should probably be taken in moderation. If symptoms persist, additional bulk may be added in the form of unprocessed bran (2 teaspoonfuls added to foods, one to three times daily) or powdered psyllium seed (Metamucil, 1 teaspoonful twice daily). Severe episodes of pain may be alleviated by anticholinergics and nonopiate analgesics, but the patient must be warned of the significance of persistent pain, obstipation, and fever.

Acute Diverticulitis

Most patients with acute diverticulitis respond to supportive measures consisting of bed rest, parenteral fluids, and antibiotics. Early surgical consultation is advisable. Vital signs should be measured at least every 4 hours. Serial abdominal examination by the same observer will detect the earliest signs of spreading peritonitis. Abdominal masses should be outlined on the abdominal wall to follow changes in size.

If the patient is passing flatus, clear fluids by mouth are allowed. Nasogastric suction will be required for distention caused by ileus or obstruction. A broad-spectrum antibiotic such as ampicillin (2 grams every 6 hours) or cefoxitin (1 gram every 6 hours) is administered intravenously and altered as blood cultures and subsequent course dictate. Meperidine (75 to 100 mg every 4 hours) may be given to patients with severe pain. Morphine and other opiates which increase intraluminal pressure are contraindicated.

An objective response to treatment should be apparent within 48 to 72 hours. Fever and leukocytosis should diminish. Improvement in pain, tenderness, and abdominal distention and the passage of flatus or stool should ensue. Persistence or increase in abdominal signs or abdominal mass indicate failure to contain the perforation, and operation may be required.

The aforementioned measures are continued until all signs of inflammation have resolved, usually within 7 to 10 days. Oral intake is gradually advanced from liquids to a high fiber diet. Contrast studies are deferred as long as improvement continues, but should be obtained in several weeks to confirm the diagnosis and to rule out malignancy.

Diverticular Abscess

Failure of medical management as manifested by persistent fever, leukocytosis, mass, tenderness, or urinary symptoms is usually due to a walled-off abscess. The diagnosis may be aided by x-ray, using water-soluble contrast without cathartic preparation and without air insufflation. Extraluminal contrast or an eccentric filling defect is diagnostic, but often the study will demonstrate only diverticula, and the decision for operation is then based upon clinical findings.

If there is gastrointestinal function, the colon may be prepared with oral neomycin (8 grams in 24 hours) and erythromycin base (1 gram in 24 hours) and gentle rectal irrigations. At operation, if the colon is empty and the involved bowel and surrounding inflammatory process are removable en bloc, resection with primary anastomosis is possible. When the bowel preparation is inadequate or peritoneal inflammation or abscess wall remains after resection, anastomosis must be deferred. The proximal colon is brought out as an end colostomy, and the distal bowel exteriorized or oversewn. Intestinal continuity is restored after the inflammation has subsided.

Free Perforation and Generalized Peritonitis

In a few patients, a diverticulum will perforate directly into the peritoneal cavity or an enlarging abscess will perforate. Patients with spreading peritoneal signs should be prepared for emergency operation without delay. Vigorous intravenous fluid resuscitation to replace third space losses will be necessary. Clindamycin (300 to 600 mg every 6 hours) or cefoxitin (1 gram every 6 hours) and gentamicin (1 to 1.5 mg per kg every 8 hours, adjusting for serum creatinine) are given intravenously to provide broad coverage for intestinal microorganisms.

At operation, suture of the perforation, drainage, cecostomy, and proximal colostomy are all unreliable in controlling continued leakage of stool in patients with free perforation. Mortality rates of 30 per cent or more have been reported.

The continued contamination of the peritoneal cavity is most effectively eliminated by resection of the perforated segment without anastomosis. Colostomy and a mucous fistula or Hartmann's pouch are fashioned. The abdomen is irrigated thoroughly with saline solution, and drains are placed in the pelvis and left lumbar gutter. Definitive resection of diseased bowel and anastomosis are performed as a second stage.

Fistula

Patients with a well established fistula can usually be managed by one-stage resection with primary anastomosis of the colon and closure of the communicating viscus. Omentum or other normal tissue is interposed between the suture lines.

In cases in which a fistula appears acutely in association with a large abscess, the colonic anastomosis may have to be deferred.

Bleeding

Minor bleeding may occur in association with acute diverticulitis and is of no consequence. Treatment is directed at diverticulitis, but a coexisting carcinoma should be excluded.

Bleeding resulting from erosion of the artery at the neck of a diverticulum is characteristically massive and occurs without overt diverticulitis. Most will stop spontaneously. Monitoring of cardiovascular parameters, correction of coagulopathies, and prompt replacement of blood loss are vital, especially in elderly patients. The incidence of recurrent hemorrhage is approximately 30 per cent.

Nasogastric aspiration, upper endoscopy, and sigmoidoscopy should be performed to rule out other lesions. Angiography is the most useful study in massive lower intestinal bleeding. The site may be identified and the bleeding arrested at least temporarily by intraarterial vasopressin infusion (0.2 to 0.3 unit per minute by constant infusion).

Patients with continuing blood loss of 1500 to 2000 ml in 24 hours following replacement of the original deficit should undergo operation without delay.

If the bleeding site has been identified (more than 50 per cent are in the right colon), the appropriate segment is resected. If localization is unsuccessful, the procedure of choice is abdominal colectomy and ileoproctostomy.

Obstruction

Some degree of colonic obstruction is a feature of most patients with acute sigmoid diverticulitis. In most instances function returns with nasogastric decompression, parenteral fluids, and antibiotics. However, frequent abdominal x-rays must be obtained, and if progressive cecal distention develops, decompression by transverse colostomy will be necessary. Definitive resection and finally colostomy closure are performed in separate stages.

Small bowel obstruction resulting from entrapment by abscess or inflammatory mass should be suspected if nausea, vomiting, and intermittent crampy abdominal pain are prominent. Initial treatment consists of decompression by a mercury-weighted long intestinal tube which is placed at the pylorus by fluoroscopy and moni-

tored by frequent x-rays. Successful treatment, as evidenced by continued advancement of the tube, alleviation of pain and distention, decreased volume aspirated, and the passage of flatus should occur within 48 to 72 hours. Otherwise, this complication will necessitate lysis of adhesions as well as resection of the involved colon, usually with deferred anastomosis.

Elective Operation

A patient who recovers from a complication of diverticular disease may be a candidate for elective operation, particularly if he is 50 years old or younger. Primary resection and anastomosis can be accomplished with minimal morbidity and mortality under these conditions.

Among the accepted indications are previous episodes of documented acute diverticulitis, life-threatening hemorrhage, and partial colonic obstruction. Following a single episode of diverticulitis, resection is recommended for persistent tender mass, recurrent urinary symptoms, or x-ray findings of fixed narrowing or extraluminal barium. Resection is mandatory if carcinoma cannot be excluded after barium enema and colonoscopy.

CROHN'S DISEASE

method of
ROY G. SHORTER, M.D.
Rochester, Minnesota

As with the therapy of any other chronic condition, the management of Crohn's disease is best founded on a mutual trust between the patient and the physician. It is vital that such a relationship be established, starting with an understanding by the affected person that while no specific cure exists, with support and careful management he or she will be able to pursue a satisfying life style and that career goals can be achieved despite the disease.

Nutritional Therapy

General Principles. If the patient has no demonstrable nutritional deficits, the daily diet should be unrestricted, rich in protein (100 to 150 grams per day), high in calories (2500 to 3000), and well balanced. However, if the patient finds that any particular foodstuff causes unpleasant symptoms, it should be omitted from the diet. The nature of the offending item and its effects must be reported to the physician, as this may be of great significance to management. For example, such information is important in detecting intolerance of cow's milk because of lactase deficiency. If this is suspected, it should be evaluated further by lactose tolerance testing and by the trial of a lactose-free diet. As another illustration, when foods with a high fiber content cause abdominal cramping and distention in a patient with low-grade intestinal obstruction resulting from the disease process, these foods should be eliminated from the diet.

Dietary supplementation with a multiple vitamin preparation is advisable if the patient has even minimal signs of weight loss, and therapy with iron (ferrous sulfate, 300 mg three times daily) and folic acid (5 mg daily) also may be necessary. Calcium supplements are especially important if the patient is on a cow's milk–free diet. Monthly injections (100 micrograms) of vitamin B_{12} should be given if serum levels or a Schilling test indicates deficient absorption. Depletions of sodium, potassium, bicarbonate, or zinc require correction. If steatorrhea is significant, this should be treated by a low-fat diet (<70 grams) with replacement of the calories by protein, carbohydrate, and medium-chain triglycerides (MCT). A prepared liquid food containing MCT is available (Portagen). As a caveat, the quantity of MCT should not exceed 100 grams daily, because their high osmolality may result in worsening of the diarrhea, and their use is contraindicated in any patient with complicating cirrhosis. Calcium supplements are of particular import when steatorrhea is present, and magnesium deficiency also is a likely feature of severe malabsorption. The latter deficiency is best overcome by intramuscular injections of 1 to 2 ml of 50 per cent magnesium sulfate, with the use of a local anesthetic to reduce the discomfort.

Elemental Diets. To those patients who are unable to ingest or absorb adequate quantities of protein and calories in a regular diet, synthetic elemental diets can be given which are almost completely absorbable, even if only 100 cm of functionally absorptive intestine is present. These diets consist of a liquid containing amino acids, sugar, fats, and multivitamin supplements, including vitamin K, plus iron, magnesium, calcium, copper, zinc, and iodine. Numerous preparations are available commercially; in general all are similar in composition, and Vivonex and Flexical are two examples. Although some of the products are hyperosmolar compared to intestinal contents and thus may stimulate peristalsis and cause worsening of diarrhea, isotonic versions are available. They may be administered either through a small-bore (French No. 8) na-

sogastric tube directly into the stomach, using a variable speed pump, or as a drink. If given as a drink, although different flavors are available, none is particularly palatable for prolonged use, so a variety often are needed to persuade the patient to accept the diet. Chilling also may help make them palatable. As prepared for administration, they contain approximately 1 calorie per ml and thus permit a daily intake of up to 5000 calories per day. Initially small feedings (50 ml) every 1 to 2 hours are advisable, and the formulations should be in a concentration of 10 to 15 per cent weight per volume. Over 1 to 3 days, the concentration is increased to the usual level of 25 per cent. Additional water should be given to meet the patient's needs. The urinary output and its sugar content, the serum osmolality, electrolytes, and blood sugar all must be checked daily for the first few days, and then two to three times weekly. The management of these diets requires close collaboration with nutritionists familiar with their use, as problems may arise. These include nutritional deficiencies resulting from the use of a fixed dietary composition in the presence of variable needs.

Parenteral Venous Hyperalimentation. This form of nutritional therapy may be indicated in severely ill, malnourished patients who are unable to take sufficient food by mouth. In some of these patients it serves as part of the continuing medical treatment of their Crohn's disease, while in others it is used in their preparation for surgical therapy. Clearly, too, it has an important role for patients with Crohn's disease complicated by severe short bowel syndrome, in some of whom it has been used successfully as part of a home-treatment program.

Intravenous hyperalimentation provides an abundant quantity of nutrients and calories to promote positive nitrogen balance and weight gain. Positive nitrogen balance can be achieved by the infusion of either casein hydrolysates or amino acid solutions. The solutions also contain hypertonic glucose, and each liter provides 1000 calories as carbohydrate and 5 grams of nitrogen, plus all the necessary vitamins and trace minerals. A soya bean oil–egg lecithin fat emulsion also is available (Intralipid). Electrolytes, calcium, phosphorus, and magnesium are necessary supplements in quantities determined by the clinical situation and by the type of solution to be used. However, magnesium depletion may require correction by intramuscular injections of 50 per cent magnesium sulfate, as described above.

As a general rule, infusion rates of approximately 2000 ml per day are used initially, and then increased slowly. The maximal rate varies from patient to patient, and its control demands careful monitoring of the serum calcium, phosphorus, and magnesium and the urinary sugar. Careful attention also must be paid to detecting deficiencies of copper or zinc which may occur during the course of this nutritional therapy.

It cannot be emphasized too strongly that intravenous hyperalimentation should be used only in an environment in which careful control by physicians skilled in its management is readily available. The mechanical techniques involved require meticulous care, and its complications, which may be fatal, include those relating to the catheter, such as thrombosis and local and systemic infections, and also allergic reactions to the nutrients, metabolic acidosis, hyperosmolar coma, postinfusional hypoglycemia, severe hyperglycemia, fluid overload, electrolyte imbalance, hypophosphatemia, essential fatty acid deficiency, deficiencies of trace metals, hyperammonemia, and intrahepatic cholestasis.

Finally, while the use of this modality, with its important nutritional restorative capability, may be invaluable to some patients with Crohn's disease, there are no hard data to support the concept that it has any direct therapeutic action on the inflammatory process in the bowel, despite anecdotal suggestions to the contrary. However, it seems to be helpful in promoting the healing of fistulas, as does the use of elemental diets.

Therapy to Control Disease Activity

Prior to making recommendations for management in this therapeutic area, it is necessary to present certain important information:

Sulfasalazine (SAS) Therapy. The National Cooperative Crohn's Disease Study (NCCDS) has shown that the use of this drug alone in patients who had not been treated either with sulfasalazine, corticosteroids, or azathioprine or with surgical resection prior to their entry to the study was significantly superior to placebo for the treatment of active Crohn's colitis. This was true whether or not the ileum also was involved. However, sulfasalazine was ineffective when the disease was confined to the small intestine. Importantly, those patients who had been taking sulfasalazine prior to their entry to the trial seemed to be an especially drug-resistant group, and the continuation of its use in such patients was no better than a placebo. A similarly diminished effect was noted in those given corticosteroids before receiving treatment with SAS. The reasons for the selective effect of SAS in Crohn's colitis are obscure, although it is known that colonic bacteria metabolize the drug to form sulfapyridine and 5-aminosalicylate, and there is evidence to suggest that the latter is the active moiety in its beneficial action in chronic ulcerative colitis. Therefore, it has been speculated that this action of colonic bacteria also explains its effectiveness in Crohn's colitis and its inactivity when the small bowel alone is involved.

Finally, there is no evidence that SAS is effective in preventing relapse or recurrence of Crohn's disease.

Corticosteroid Therapy. In patients previously untreated with sulfasalazine, corticosteroids, or azathioprine or by surgical resection, the NCCDS found that prednisone was superior to placebo in the therapy of Crohn's disease when the ileum alone or the ileum and colon were involved, but was ineffective when the disease was confined to the colon. However, as the latter conclusion was based on a small number of patients, it must be accepted with caution. Again from observations in only a few patients, treatment with SAS, prednisone, or azathioprine prior to their entry to the study resulted in a reduced responsiveness to prednisone such that its effects were no better than those of placebo. Finally, the long-term use of prednisone has not reduced the incidence of recurrence or flare-ups of Crohn's disease.

Azathioprine Therapy. From the findings of the NCCDS, it can be concluded that azathioprine as a single agent in a daily dosage of 2.5 mg per kg is ineffective in the treatment of active Crohn's disease. In addition, there are no hard data to show that its use in combination with prednisone has a significant steroid-sparing effect. Finally, its long-term administration has not been shown to reduce the incidence of recurrence or flare-ups in patients with inactive disease.

Recommendations for the Treatment of Active Crohn's Disease, by Location. CROHN'S DISEASE OF THE STOMACH AND DUODENUM. Corticosteroids should be given, as for the treatment of small intestinal Crohn's disease.

SMALL INTESTINAL CROHN'S DISEASE. The drug of choice in the previously untreated patient with small intestinal disease is prednisone, provided that particular care is taken to monitor its catabolic effects when malabsorption coexists. We recommend initial doses of 40 to 60 mg daily in those with severely active disease and 20 to 40 mg daily if the activity is moderate. The use of azathioprine is not advised, but in those patients previously treated with any modality and in whom the initial response to steroids is poor, the addition of sulfasalazine (2 grams daily in divided doses) may be helpful. Unfortunately, the evidence on which this recommendation is based is anecdotal. The doses of steroids should be tapered subsequently in accordance with the clinical status of the disease in the hope, eventually, of total withdrawal. However, if two or more attempts to achieve this are unsuccessful, a maintenance dosage of 10 to 15 mg of prednisone daily is recommended, and careful consideration should be given to the need for surgical resection.

LARGE INTESTINAL CROHN'S DISEASE, WITH OR WITHOUT ILEAL INVOLVEMENT. The drug of choice for the therapy of Crohn's colitis in the previously untreated patient is sulfasalazine, initially in doses of 1 gram four times daily for 4 weeks, then reducing to 0.5 gram four times daily. If this initial dose is not tolerated, 0.5 gram four times daily can be tried, perhaps using enteric-coated preparations. In previously treated patients, or in those who do not respond to SAS alone, the addition of prednisone is suggested in the dosage schedules described above for the treatment of small intestinal Crohn's disease, but this advice is not based on hard data.

Antidiarrheal and Analgesic Therapy

The use of antidiarrheal medications often is of considerable symptomatic benefit, as some of these agents also relieve abdominal cramping. Diphenoxylate hydrochloride (2.5 mg three to four times daily), loperamide hydrochloride, codeine phophate or sulfate, or deodorized tincture of opium (10 drops, four to eight times daily) may achieve these goals. Anticholinergics (e.g., propantheline bromide, 15 mg four times daily) also may help. However, such drugs should not be given to patients with severe attacks of Crohn's colitis, as they may precipitate toxic dilatation of the bowel. In addition, hydrophilic mucilloids (e.g., psyllium or methylcellulose) may improve the consistency of the stools and relieve the urgency of defecation. In some patients with Crohn's disease of the ileum, and in some who have had ileal resections, the mechanisms of the diarrhea include an action of deconjugated bile salts. In these patients cholestyramine resin (Questran) may be helpful (4 grams one to three times daily). However, cholestyramine therapy is contraindicated in the presence of severe steatorrhea.

Mild analgesics, such as acetaminophen and propoxyphene, do not relieve pain of intestinal origin, and salicylates should be avoided if the patient is taking steroids.

Treatment of Emotional Problems

The most important factor in the control of these problems has been alluded to earlier — namely, the relationship between the patient and the physician. It is crucial for the patient to appreciate that the physician is interested in him or her as an individual, is sympathetic and supportive, is aware of the impact of the disease on the patient's life style, and is knowledgeable of its therapy. When necessary, sedatives or tranquilizers (e.g., diazepam, 2 to 10 mg, meprobamate, 400 mg) may be prescribed three or four times daily, plus a nightly sedative. Amitriptyline, 50 mg three times daily, can be helpful if depression is a problem.

Therapy of Certain Local Complications of Crohn's Disease

Treatment of Massive Hemorrhage. Although massive hemorrhage is rare, it requires immediate multiple blood transfusions, and usually the bleeding will stop. If not, emergency surgery is indicated, with consideration also being given to the possibility that a coagulation defect is involved, particularly that caused by deficiency of vitamin K.

Treatment of Toxic Megacolon in Crohn's Colitis. This must be considered as a medical and surgical emergency, and it demands close surgical collaboration starting at the time of the patient's admission to the hospital. The use of continuous suction applied to a Miller-Abbott or Cantor tube is recommended, with the tip of the tube in the ileum. Opiates or anticholinergics should not be given. Intravenous replacement and maintenance of water and electrolytes are necessary, and blood transfusions may be required. In some instances, intravenous injections of salt-free albumin are needed to correct hypoalbuminemia. After initial culturing of samples of blood and stool, antibiotics should be given parenterally to embrace a broad spectrum of aerobic and anaerobic bacteria. An example of such therapy is ampicillin, 1 gram intramuscularly 4 hourly, and kanamycin sulfate, 15 mg per kg per day in two doses either intravenously or intramuscularly. The intravenous use of ACTH or hydrocortisone, the latter if the patient previously has been receiving long-term steroid therapy, is recommended despite the lack of controlled trials to support this view. The regimen consists of 80 units of ACTH in the first 24 hours, followed by daily reductions of 10 units until either the patient requires surgery or, if a favorable response is achieved, the eighth day is reached. If surgery is necessary, the reduction in dosage is manipulated such that the drug is withdrawn on or about the twelfth postoperative day. A prompt beneficial response to medical therapy is mandatory; as a rough guide, if this is not achieved within 5 days, then surgical intervention is advisable.

Abscesses, Fistulas and Perianal Disease. If retroperitoneal or perienteric abscesses develop, these should be drained and cultured and the appropriate antibiotics given, with particular attention to anaerobic organisms. Fistulas, except for those involving the urinary bladder, ureters, or uterus, are not absolute indications for surgery, but their management involves surgical consultation. Treatment should be directed to the control of the primary disease, and elemental diets or parenteral nutrition, with supplementary vitamin C, may also be of help. Perianal disease, including abscesses and fistulas, requires therapy directed to the control of Crohn's disease, plus the use of warm sitz baths three or four times daily. Again, it is advisable to obtain surgical collaboration in management. The local application of topical steroids, either as a cream or as suppositories, may be helpful in some patients.

Intestinal Obstruction. Partial obstruction resulting from inflammation in the bowel wall is common in Crohn's enteritis and usually responds to nasogastric suction, intravenous fluids, and therapy with intravenous ACTH. More chronic or recurrent obstruction caused by scarring from the disease process requires surgical intervention.

Extraintestinal Manifestations

In general, the severity of the extraintestinal manifestations of Crohn's disease relates directly to the degree of activity of the intestinal lesions. As a result, successful treatment of the latter usually diminishes the intensity of the extraintestinal lesions.

Hepatobiliary Disease. Because fatty changes and pericholangitis most often are self-limited, their existence seldom directly influences management. For the attempted alleviation of some serious, progressive hepatic injury complicating Crohn's disease, it has been suggested that surgical resection of the diseased bowel may arrest or even cure the liver disease. However, the evidence for this was derived from uncontrolled, retrospective studies. Also from relatively slender data, T-tube drainage of the biliary tree has been recommended for the treatment of sclerosing cholangitis. Currently, in general it must be concluded that the best therapy for the complicating liver lesion is that which is best for the treatment of the bowel disease.

Musculoskeletal Disease. The severity of the acute arthritis which may complicate Crohn's disease parallels the degree of activity of the bowel disease. Corticosteroids are effective in the treatment of this arthritis and usually induce a rapid response, although in some cases doses of 25 mg daily, or more, for several weeks may be necessary.

Mucocutaneous Disease. Treatment with systemic corticosteroids, or by resection of the diseased bowel, is needed to control pyoderma gangrenosum. Erythema nodosum and aphthous stomatitis respond to effective treatment of the bowel disease.

Ocular Complications. These lesions usually respond well to successful therapy of the bowel disease. Nevertheless, local corticosteroids also are indicated for the treatment of uveitis or iritis, and the latter may require the use of systemic steroids. The management of patients with Crohn's disease, either with or without these ocular lesions, should involve ophthalmologic consultation, as any prolonged administration of steroids for the treatment of the bowel disease can result in the development of posterior subcapsular cataracts.

Urinary Tract Complications. Obstructive hydronephrosis complicating Crohn's disease requires surgical relief of the ureteral obstruction.

The risk of oxalate calculi formation is reduced by ensuring adequate fluid intake and by maintaining an alkaline urine with sodium bicarbonate. The treatment of hyperoxaluria and oxalate stones also includes certain dietary manipulations both to decrease the amount of oxalate and to reduce the intake of fats containing long-chain fatty acids. Medium-chain triglycerides can be used for caloric supplementation, with the caveat given earlier. Rich sources of oxalate include tomatoes, rhubarb, fruits, nuts, and cola drinks, so careful attention should be paid to their respective roles in the patient's diet if this is unrestricted. In addition, the oral administration of calcium or aluminum salts is helpful because it leads to the binding of free oxalate in the intestinal lumen, with the formation of insoluble oxalates, which then are excreted in the feces. Finally, because deoxycholic acid enhances the absorption of oxalate by the colon, the use of cholestyramine resin also may be of value in the treatment of hyperoxaluria, with the caveat mentioned earlier.

Surgical Treatment

The fact that approximately 70 per cent of patients require surgical intervention in the course of the disease emphasizes the need for close collaboration between the gastroenterologist, the surgeon, and the patient to achieve the best management. Resection should not be regarded as a "last ditch stand" but must be considered and timed to obtain optimal benefit to the patient. Lastly, it is emphasized that following total proctocolectomy for the treatment of Crohn's colitis, there is no role for Kock's (continent) ileostomy because of the risk of recurrent disease in the pouch.

HEMORRHOIDS, ANAL FISSURE, ANORECTAL ABSCESS, ANORECTAL FISTULA

method of
BERTRAM A. PORTIN, M.D.
Buffalo, New York

In all cases of the anorectal conditions to be considered, sigmoidoscopy (rigid or flexible fiberoptic) is a basic and necessary part of the diagnostic work-up. The presence of an obvious hemorrhoidal source for bleeding does not rule out more proximal pathology of a more serious nature. A short delay in performing sigmoidoscopy until acute and painful anorectal conditions subside, or until anesthesia is available, is acceptable. Similarly, barium enema and other appropriate studies, if indicated (e.g., family history of polyps or colonic cancer, suspicion of coexistent inflammatory bowel disease, passage of blood clots), should be carried out before completion of treatment.

Hemorrhoids

Hemorrhoids are grossly enlarged complexes of varicose veins of the anorectum. They may be external, internal, or mixed, depending on their location. Pure external hemorrhoids lie distal to the dentate line and are covered by anoderm. Internal hemorrhoids lie proximal to the dentate line and are entirely covered by mucosa. Mixed hemorrhoids are a combination of both.

External Hemorrhoids. The most common problem associated with external hemorrhoids is acute thrombosis. This often occurs following strain, especially from diarrhea or constipation. Thrombosis may result in a small painless mass and requires no therapy. Spontaneous absorption occurs in time. More often a larger, very tender thrombosis leads the patient to seek early medical care. These are well suited to office excision under local anesthesia. Simple incision and clot extraction are not recommended. After such extraction the skin edges may seal over and hematoma reaccumulate. More important, the clots are often multilocular and simple incision is not therapeutic. Finally, there is an indurated edematous tender mass present, and simple removal of the clot, if indeed possible, only adds a painful wound onto an already painful swelling. For these reasons, surgical excision is advisable.

TREATMENT OF THROMBOSED EXTERNAL HEMORRHOIDS. 1. All local anesthesia discussed in this article is either by bupivacaine (Marcaine) 0.25 or 0.5 per cent or lidocaine (Xylocaine) 0.5 per cent with 1:200,000 epinephrine. Each milliliter of anesthetic solution contains 5 to 10 units of hyaluronidase.

2. Infiltrate the area lateral to and beneath the thrombosis with 2 to 3 ml of anesthetic solution. Small needles (25 to 30 gauge) should be used, and adequate time allowed for the anesthetic to take effect. Gentle massage will help disperse edema.

3. An ellipse of overlying skin and the thrombosis is excised, preferably by a bipolar high frequency cutting current or, if not available, by a curved scissors. Do not extend the incision deep into the anal canal. An iatrogenic and painful chronic anal fissure may result.

4. Hemostasis, if a problem, may be assured by electrocoagulation or ligation with fine absorbable suture.

5. A plain cotton dressing is applied and the patient is advised to leave the dressing undisturbed for 6 to 8 hours. Thereafter, warm sitz baths for 10 to 15 minutes three times daily are advised. An oral analgesic is prescribed (acetaminophen, 300 mg, with codeine, 30 mg every 4 hours as needed). Topical anesthetic creams may enhance postoperative pain relief.

6. The routine use of laxatives is discouraged unless the patient had a constipation problem prior to the onset of the acute hemorrhoidal problem. The patient returns for examination in 1 week.

The circumferential rosette of large thrombosed external hemorrhoids which result from intrapartum straining does not lend itself to the foregoing plan of management. For these patients, continuous ice packs over glycerin and witch hazel pads (Tucks) will provide analgesia and help in the resolution of the painful and edematous process.

Internal Hemorrhoids. Internal hemorrhoids become of significance mainly because of bleeding and prolapse. They are almost uniquely a human ailment, most probably related to man's assumption of the upright position and to his heredity. Aggravating causes include pregnancy, constipation, diarrhea, portal hypertension, congestive heart failure, and occupation. A simple classification may help in determining the choice of therapy:

1. First degree — internal hemorrhoids with bleeding.

2. Second degree — internal hemorrhoids with bleeding and intermittent or self-reducing prolapse.

3. Third degree — internal hemorrhoids with bleeding and persistent prolapse.

TREATMENT OF FIRST DEGREE HEMOR-RHOIDS. Hemorrhoidectomy is rarely indicated for this stage of disease. There are other non-operative methods available, but two methods, injection and ligation therapy, are recommended. The objective of injection treatment is to promote a perivascular submucosal fibrosis with resultant shrinkage of the individual hemorrhoidal plexuses. Injections may be curative, but more often periodic reinjection series at 2 to 4 year intervals may be necessary. The solution used is a sterile 5 per cent quinine and urea hydrochloride mixture with 2 per cent benzyl alcohol. Five per cent phenol in cotton seed oil may also be used.

Technique of injection: 1. A 2 or 3 ml syringe is filled with 2 ml of solution. The use of a 2 or 3 inch extension or a long-angled Frankfeldt needle makes insertion technically easier. A 25 gauge needle is attached to the extension.

2. A beveled (Hirschman) or slotted ano-scope is gently inserted into the rectum. This allows the enlarged hemorrhoid to bulge into the lumen. With care taken to inject above the anorectal line and into the submucosa, approximately 1.5 ml of solution is injected directly into the plexus. The injection site should expand and blanch. It is not necessary to aspirate for blood prior to the injection.

3. The anoscope is then withdrawn and the injection site gently massaged to distribute the solution more widely. Repeat injections are done at 2 week intervals. Between three and five injections will usually control symptoms.

4. Nightly use of a bland emollient suppository (Calmol-4 or Anusol) is helpful in lubricating the rectum and providing a less traumatic passage of stool.

5. If constipation or diarrhea or frequent daily bowel movements are considered to be an etiologic factor, these should be corrected by proper dietary regimen and appropriate oral medications. Constipation may be treated by psyllium seed bulk agents (L. A. Formula, or Metamucil), stool softeners (Surfak 240, Kasof), or emulsified mineral oils (Kondremul, Petrogalar).

TREATMENT OF SECOND DEGREE AND SOME THIRD DEGREE HEMORRHOIDS. If prolapse of hemorrhoidal tissue occurs, sclerosing therapy usually is less effective. Occasionally, however, palliation for prolapsed hemorrhoids may be obtained, even with injections, if more effective methods are contraindicated. For example, the patient on anticoagulant therapy must not be treated with other than injection because of the possibility of massive hemorrhagic complications of ligation or excisional therapy.

Generally, for large redundant first degree and second degree hemorrhoids rubber band ligation treatment is most satisfactory. It is a more effective method than injection because hemorrhoidal tissue is actually destroyed rather than just sclerosed. Other contraindications to ligation are the coexistence of fistula, chronic fissure, or anal stricture. Since most sensory pain fibers are absent above the dentate line, the rubber bands may be applied at the base of excessive or redundant or prolapsing internal hemorrhoidal tissue, effectively strangulating the hemorrhoid. The devascularization leads to hemorrhoidal slough along with the release of the bands. In effect, the result is similar to a surgical internal hemorrhoidectomy.

Technique of ligation: 1. No anesthesia is required. With the patient in the Sims or knee-chest position, an anoscope (Hirschman) is inserted. While the anoscope is held by an assistant, the largest internal hemorrhoid is grasped by an alligator or Allis type forceps previously inserted through the barrel of the hemorrhoidal ligator (Barron or McGivney) loaded with two rubber bands. While exerting gentle traction on the hemorrhoid, the barrel is passed over the plexus and the trigger of the ligator compressed. This action deposits the bands at the base of the plexus. The compression of the bands immediately devascularizes the tissue.

2. The anoscope is withdrawn. There is usually a sensation of rectal fullness, sometimes discomfort, and rarely reflex lower abdominal cramping. These are usually transitory. It is best to ligate one plexus at a time and to perform subsequent ligations about every third week.

3. Postbanding instructions include prescribing acetaminophen with codeine, an emollient suppository at bedtime, warm sitz baths for discomfort, and a very clear warning to call the physician at any time should excessive bleeding occur. Such bleeding is unusual but does occur in 1 to 2 per cent of patients. The appearance of active hemorrhage following ligation occurs most often between the eighth and twentieth days. Treatment for this complication may be carried out in the office or emergency room. If known, the area of the plexus ligation should be anesthetized with 3 to 5 ml of local anesthetic. If, for example, the right anterior plexus has been ligated, the solution is injected into this quadrant from a site about 0.5 cm from the anal verge. A sigmoidoscope is inserted and all blood clots aspirated. When the bleeding site is identified, control may be by coagulation with an electrosurgical unit or by direct ligation, using an absorbable gastrointestinal suture.

TREATMENT OF THIRD DEGREE HEMORRHOIDS. Although injection and ligation therapy work best with first and second degree hemorrhoids, they may provide palliation for third degree hemorrhoids in patients who are not amenable to surgery (advanced or labile pregnancy, severe coexistent disease, and antipathy to surgery). In general, most third degree and some cases of very large first and second degree hemorrhoids are best treated by hemorrhoidectomy performed as an inpatient hospital procedure.

Technique of closed amputative hemorrhoidectomy: With the patient in a semi-jackknife prone position and with the buttocks strapped apart, 5 to 10 mg of diazepam (Valium) is given intravenously in 2.5 mg increments. The operation is then performed under local anesthesia. Using approximately 20 to 25 ml of one of the previously described mixtures, the injections are given subcutaneously and circumferentially. Then 4 ml is injected into the sphincter muscle and submucosally in each of the four quadrants. Gentle massage helps disperse the solution and provides anesthesia, tissue plane delineation, and hemostasis. Utilizing a large Hill-Ferguson retractor for exposure, the hemorrhoids are excised from approximately 1 cm lateral to the verge in a narrow oblong elliptical fashion up into the rectum, to and including the upper extent of the enlarged plexus. Wide radical excisions are to be avoided. Normal intervening mucosa must be left intact. Usually three quadrant excisions are necessary, and as a general rule more than four should be strictly avoided. The apex excisional site is ligated, and the mucosal defect is closed with a running lock suture of 3-0 chromic catgut. When the anoderm is reached, the suturing is continued with a simple running skin stitch to the outward or lateral end of the original incision and tied at this point. If there is evidence of internal sphincter fibrosis of the outlet, a partial internal sphincterotomy may be done to relieve this rigidity. At the conclusion of the procedure, there should be no question of adequate outlet if the anal retractor can still be inserted easily.

Postoperative recovery is rapid and patients are usually discharged on the second or third day, usually after passing a laxative-induced movement. Patients may return to work 1 to 2 weeks after surgery.

Anal Fissure

Fissures may be acute or chronic. The acute follow trauma such as that caused by passage of a foreign body or a hard or loose stool. These usually heal spontaneously. Chronic anal fissures cause pain and bleeding also, and usually require a higher level of treatment. The fissure is usually located posteriorly and less often anteriorly. Frequently, there is an associated fibrotic narrowed outlet secondary to hypertrophy and fibrosis of the internal sphincter. Consequently, examination is usually very painful. A gentle digital examination may not be possible without the injection of 1 to 2 ml of local anesthetic behind the fissure. A small anoscope can then be inserted to allow visual diagnosis. The classic triad of hypertrophied papilla, anal fissure, and posterior sentinel tag is often found. Lateral fissures, indolent-appearing fissures, and fissures without pain and sphincter spasm should make the examiner wary of an underlying diagnosis of Crohn's disease.

Chronic fissures which are not very tender or painful and do not show much sphincter spasm may be treated with stool softeners, bulk agents, or emollients, sitz baths, and a bland suppository. If there is much pain and sphincter spasm, lateral internal sphincterotomy should be performed. This can be done as an office procedure, but for the occasional operator a hospital setting and direct visualization of the internal sphincter make a better choice.

Technique of Internal Anal Sphincterotomy. With the patient either in the lateral Sims or modified jackknife position, local anesthesia infiltration is carried out as for hemorrhoidectomy. A left or right lateral radial incision about 1.5 cm long is made distal to the dentate line. The fibrotic sphincter is easily palpated and may be seen as a thickened whitish bundle lying transverse to the incision. With a Hill-Ferguson retractor in place, the muscle is stretched taut and is easily incised. There is immediate release of the stenosis. The anal skin is approximated with a short running fine absorbable suture. Healing occurs promptly, and the fissure is often healed by the fifth or seventh day. It is not necessary to remove the sentinel tag or hypertrophied papilla. If, however, these are large or are associated with large symptomatic hemorrhoids, appropriate excisions may than be carried out.

Anal Abscess and Fistula

An anal abscess presents as a tender, indurated, erythematous swelling in the para-anal area. It is usually the result of the spread of infection from an infected crypt and of the glands that lie in the crypt base. Less frequently an acute or chronic fissure may provide the source for the expanding infection. Severe throbbing pain without relief is the major symptom, along with a tender perianal swelling. Antibiotics and waiting for fluctuation provide an unnecessary period of prolonged suffering and progression of the infection. The proper treatment at the time of diagnosis is incision and drainage under local anesthesia. The relief is immediate and the disease process is aborted.

Technique for Incision and Drainage. 1. The indurated area is infiltrated with 1 to 2 ml of local anesthetic agent intradermally over the site chosen for incision. The incision site should lie close to the medial border of the swelling. If a subsequent fistula persists, the tract will then be shorter by this maneuver.

2. A 1 cm circle of overlying skin and subcutaneous tissue is excised. This is best done with an electrosurgical cutting current, but if that is unavailable, a scalpel is satisfactory.

3. Immediate drainage of pus occurs. Probing, packing, and antibiotics are not needed.

4. Warm sitz baths, two to three times daily, are prescribed. Re-examination is done at 1 week and again at 3 weeks. A fistula will persist in 35 to 50 per cent of patients. In some instances, the secondary opening at the drainage site may heal spontaneously, but recurrent abscesses in the same area indicate a persistent crypt infection and incomplete fistula. This will require further surgery.

Occasionally a patient will present with signs and symptoms of an ischiorectal abscess, lacking only external evidence of a swelling and external tenderness. Digital examination will reveal a tender submucosal mass. This is an intramuscular abscess, which, although cryptogenic, progressed upward into the space between the internal and external sphincters rather than downward into one of the subcutaneous spaces. Treatment requires hospitalization and surgery under caudal, spinal, or general anesthesia. The abscess is drained by incising from the crypt to the upper end of the cavity. Hemostasis is best accomplished by a whip stitch of running fine absorbable suture around the periphery of the incision. Fistulas do not follow proper incision and drainage.

Anorectal Fistulas

Complex fistulas such as supralevator fistulas do not fall within the scope of this discussion. Tracts which traverse deep to the entire sphincter mechanism, especially those lying anterior in the female patient, also require special techniques (staged fistulotomy with the use of a seton), and, again, these will not be discussed. Simple anorectal or cryptogenic fistulas are best treated by fistulotomy. Unless of a very short length and entirely subcutaneous, this should be performed in the operating room.

Technique of Fistulotomy. 1. Local anesthesia, as described earlier, is satisfactory.

2. Great care should be taken to find the primary or internal opening. If possible, a flexible probe is inserted gently from the external opening to the internal opening.

3. If the internal opening defies localization, 1 to 2 ml of a dilute peroxide–methylene blue mixture (peroxide 0.5 ml, methylene blue 0.5 ml, water 2 ml) may be gently injected into the external opening. As the oxygen gas is formed, a fine blue foam will emanate from the internal opening.

4. Direct incision through the overlying tissue to the probe lays open the entire tract. Packing is contraindicated.

5. Postoperative routine is identical to that of the posthemorrhoidectomy patient, except that diligent and more frequent examinations are necessary to ensure that early bridging of the skin edges does not occur and result in fistula recurrence.

Crohn's Disease

Commonly, granulomatous inflammatory bowel disease and atypical anorectal abscess with fistulas coexist. Indeed, the development of such a lesion may be the first indication or may even antedate the clinical onset of more proximal inflammatory bowel disease. Usually the abscesses are not acutely painful and, upon incision and drainage, do not result in the passage of much purulent matter. Furthermore, the abscess cavity appears chronic, indolent, and lined with a dull granulation tissue. Healing is poor. Chronic fistulas persist and are often multiple. Surgery, other than incision and drainage of abscess, is usually contraindicated. Simple fistulotomy may not heal, and incontinence may result. This is disastrous in a patient with unrelenting diarrhea.

GASTRITIS

method of
FRANCISCO VILARDELL, M.D.
Barcelona, Spain

The term gastritis implies an inflammation of the gastric mucosa; however, it is still usual for the clinician to use this term in connection with a variety of circumstances, some of which do not really presuppose detectable pathologic changes. In general, it may be said that gastritis as a disease entity does not display a specific symptomatology which may be correlated with physical, biologic, roentgenologic, or endoscopic diagnoses.

Gastritis is customarily divided into acute and chronic types.

Acute Gastritis

Exogenous Gastritis. Acute inflammation of the stomach may be caused by chemicals, drugs, alcohol, irradiation, and a variety of infectious agents. The gastric mucosa has a considerable capacity for regeneration, and it seems unlikely that chronic changes may develop as a consequence of acute gastritis.

Most often, acute gastritis is due to dietary indiscretion, alcohol, and the like. Symptoms will commonly last a few hours; malaise, epigastric fullness, nausea, and vomiting are prominent. Gastritis secondary to infectious agents may be accompanied by abdominal cramps and diarrhea. In the majority of cases, diagnosis can readily be made without ancillary procedures.

Treatment is supportive, since the process heals spontaneously. Bed rest is necessary. Nothing should be taken by mouth until nausea and vomiting have ceased. In mild cases nothing else is needed. For the relief of nausea, prochlorperazine (Compazine), 5 to 10 mg orally three times daily, or trimethobenzamide (Tigan), 250 mg three or four times daily, may be useful. If vomiting is present, a 25 mg rectal suppository of prochlorperazine (Compazine) may be effective.

In more severe cases adequate fluid and electrolytes (equal amounts of 5 per cent glucose and 0.45 per cent isotonic saline with 20 mEq K per liter) should be given intravenously. Prochlorperazine (Compazine), 5 to 10 mg, may be administered intramuscularly three to four times daily.

If nausea is persistent, gastric lavage with tepid water may be beneficial and alleviate symptoms. When heartburn is conspicuous, antacids should be prescribed; aluminum gels in liquid form (e.g., Amphojel, Maalox, Gelusil, Robalate) are preferred, 15 ml four to six times daily. Severe heartburn may respond more readily to aluminum gel associated with a local anesthetic, oxethazaine (Oxaine M), 1 to 2 teaspoonfuls three or four times daily.

Once the clinical picture has subsided, oral fluids are started such as plain water, tea with sugar, and bouillon with added salt, followed by strained soups and clear gelatin. From the second or third day a bland diet is instituted. After 4 or 5 days the patient can usually tolerate a normal diet.

Corrosive Gastritis. This type of gastritis follows ingestion of strong acids or, less often, alkalis. The patient should be immediately hospitalized and parenteral supportive and antiemetic therapy administered as outlined previously. For pain, meperidine (Demerol), 50 to 100 mg, may be necessary. In very early cases, immediate evacuation of the gastric contents and gentle lavage of the stomach with a soft wide-bore gastric tube, using weak acid or alkali solutions, may be of some benefit. In many cases, the patient is seen too late and these measures are useless, for the agent will be already fixed in the tissues. Until recently, a "wait and see" attitude was generally recommended, and in mild cases it is probably justified. However, in severe cases, in which there is a significant early mortality, endoscopic evaluation of the extent and intensity of the lesions have been increasingly recommended in order to detect signs of gastric wall gangrene, which may require emergency gastrectomy as a lifesaving procedure. Endoscopy should be carried out cautiously shortly after admission if an experienced endoscopist is available. Corticoids (15 to 30 mg of prednisone daily) and wide-spectrum antibiotics such as cefazolin (Kefzol), 1 gram every 6 hours intravenously, or ampicillin, 3 to 6 grams intramuscularly daily, may be given to prevent scarring, but their effectiveness has been questioned. Esophageal obstruction secondary to scarring may be treated later by bougienage. Pyloric stenosis often requires surgical intervention (gastrojejunostomy or gastrectomy).

Radiation Gastritis. Transient loss of appetite, mild aversion to food, and moderate nausea are symptoms associated with radiation of the stomach. No specific therapeutic approach is necessary, since gastritis usually subsides spontaneously after a few weeks. When symptoms are more prominent, patients should be treated as outlined for exogenous gastritis.

Erosive Gastritis. Gastric erosions are frequently seen during gastroscopy in symptomless patients and in many cases of acute gastritis. Although erosions can heal spontaneously in 48 hours, erosive gastritis, either diffuse or localized, may sometimes be the source of severe hemorrhage. This condition is seen after ingestion of salicylates and alcohol. It may be more prevalent in patients with chronic liver disease. Diagnosis can be made only by endoscopy.

The patient should be prepared for immediate gastroscopy by ice water lavage of the stomach. One or more liters of iced saline may be used. Gentle aspiration is of great importance, and a Toomey syringe is recommended for this purpose. After gastroscopy a gastric tube should be positioned in the stomach and intermittent aspiration applied to help in the evaluation of the clinical course. Blood transfusions should be prescribed in adequate amounts. Ice water lavage usually stops the bleeding. Afterward, intensive antacid therapy

(15 to 30 ml every 2 hours of magnesium–aluminum hydroxide preparations) should be prescribed to prevent further bleeding.

If the patient continues to bleed, lavage should be repeated. A series of measures has been recommended in these cases, such as irrigation of the stomach with levarterenol (Levophed, 8 mg in 200 ml of water) and the intravenous administration of cimetidine (Tagamet, 300 mg every 6 hours) (this use of these two agents is not listed in the manufacturers' official directives), but there is no convincing proof of their effectiveness, and in a minority of cases surgery may be unavoidable. The preferred operation is usually vagotomy associated with a drainage procedure. Unfortunately recurrent bleeding after this operation is not rare.

There is evidence that in patients suffering from severe infections or trauma or after major surgery, the occurrence of erosive gastritis can be prevented or reduced by intensive antacid therapy, as well as by cimetidine at the aforementioned dosage. It is therefore advisable to employ large doses either of antacids or cimetidine for preventive purposes in these cases. (This use of cimetidine is not listed in the manufacturer's official directive.)

Chronic Gastritis

Chronic gastritis should be diagnosed only on the histologic appearance of the biopsy material obtained at the time of endoscopy. A special form of gastritis which mainly affects the gastric fundus, producing gastric mucosal atrophy and achlorhydria, has been well documented. Other forms of chronic gastritis are more difficult to identify; antral gastritis may appear as an isolated lesion or in association with gastric or duodenal ulcer. The cause of these various forms of chronic gastritis is largely unknown, although autoimmune mechanisms as demonstrated by the finding of antibodies against parietal cells and intrinsic factor may play a role in the development of mucosal atrophy. The treatment of chronic gastritis is largely empirical, and no specific therapy is available.

Chronic Fundal Gastritis. Atrophy of the fundic glands along with chronic inflammation of the gastric mucosa may develop slowly through the years. In the final stages achlorhydria and the clinical picture of pernicious anemia may develop. There is no efficient therapy for achlorhydria, and the great majority of patients need no treatment at all except perhaps reassurance. Diluted hydrochloric acid used to be recommended, but it is probably of no use. Many patients seem to fare better on a soft,

bland diet. Large meals, hot beverages, greasy foods, and alcohol may cause abdominal discomfort and should then be avoided. Antacids are often useful to relieve dyspepsia and may be prescribed as aluminum gels alone or in combination with oxethazaine (Oxaine M) as outlined above.

Anemia, if present, should be correctly identified and treated. Most of the time it is secondary to iron deficiency and corrected accordingly. Although low vitamin B_{12} levels are common and intrinsic factor output may be almost undetectable in some patients, overt pernicious anemia is rare. Parenteral vitamin B_{12} therapy may be necessary in selected cases, but although the hematologic picture may improve, it has no effect on the gastric lesion.

Chronic Antral Gastritis. This condition is often associated with peptic ulcer, and treatment should include an ulcer regimen with antacids, as for acute gastritis. In severe cases, especially when intractable pain or bleeding occurs, gastrectomy may be considered. Surgical exploration may also be needed in rare instances of localized gastritis in which carcinoma cannot be definitely excluded by endoscopic biopsy.

GASEOUSNESS

method of
FRANZ GOLDSTEIN, M.D.
Philadelphia, Pennsylvania

The treatment of gaseousness is best approached by the realization that there is no effective medicinal therapy for this frequent and often disturbing complaint. Any treatment, in order to be effective, depends upon the physician's appreciation of existing knowledge of the underlying disturbances in gastrointestinal function and efforts to correct them.

Complaints about gaseousness can be divided into three broad categories: (1) excessive belching or gaseous eructations; (2) abdominal distention, bloating, and pains; and (3) excessive passage of flatus, together with associated odors.

Until relatively recently it was believed, on the basis of work done in the 1930s, that intestinal gas was predominantly nitrogen (N_2) and that its source was swallowed air. This belief was based on analyses of gas recovered through tubes placed in the small intestine of normal persons and of obstructed patients who were tested in the fasting state. Such studies ignored the composition of colonic gas and the influence of eating upon the volume and composition of intestinal gas. The work of Levitt, Bond, and others during the past decade has added greatly to our understanding of the mechanisms responsible for intestinal gaseousness and has led to more effective therapeutic approaches. Air swallowing is but one of several routes of gas entering the gastrointestinal tract. Diffusion of gases from blood into lumen is another source, albeit not a very important one, while intraluminal gas production is probably the most important source of colonic gaseousness.

While gas entering the gastrointestinal tract by swallowing has a composition approximating that of ambient air, and thus contains predominantly N_2, intraluminal gas production leads to important accumulations of hydrogen (H_2), carbon dioxide (CO_2), methane (CH_4), and trace amounts of other gases such as mercaptans. The oxygen (O_2) contained in swallowed air is rapidly diffused or utilized by bacteria, and hence O_2 is not a major constituent of intestinal gas. CO_2 can be produced in the stomach and duodenum through the interaction of hydrochloric acid (HCl) and bicarbonate (HCO_3) and thus may be a major constituent of gaseous eructations. Since it rapidly diffuses through biologic membranes, CO_2 produced in the duodenum does not readily reach the colon. Colonic CO_2, H_2, and CH_4 are the products of bacterial fermentation of undigested food residue. The concentration of the two last-named gases in flatus, as measured by Levitt and associates, may exceed 70 per cent, and mixtures of considerably lower concentrations of hydrogen and/or methane are potentially explosive. Indeed, explosions have occurred in the operating room or in endoscopy suites when high temperatures generated by electrosurgical instruments have ignited explosive gaseous mixtures in the intestine.

Since in the normal person most ingested nutrients are almost completely digested and absorbed in the small intestine, the amount of nutrients entering the colon and available for bacterial fermentation is relatively small. It follows that excessive colonic gas production is seen largely in patients with incomplete digestion and absorption of food (i.e., malabsorption) or in patients ingesting nutrients that are not digestible by the enzymes present in the normal small intestine. An outstanding example of the latter category of foods is the various types of beans which contain an oligosaccharide, stachyose, for which no human digestive enzyme exists. Hence, these oligosaccharides enter the colon, where they are fermented by bacteria with production of gas. The most important source of excessive gas production in the colon is undoubtedly lactose in lactase-deficient subjects. Primary lactase deficiency is present in about 70 per cent of the world's population and is closely related to ethnic and genetic background. In the United States, primary lactase deficiency not associated with small intestinal disease is found frequently in persons of Mediterranean (including Jewish), African, American Indian, South American, or Oriental origin and is encountered far less frequently in persons of Northern European origin. Since human populations are not racially pure, lactase deficiency should be kept in mind in dealing with all patients complaining of gaseousness, with the realization that the frequency of finding lactase deficiency is statistically greater in some populations than in others. As lactase deficiency appears to increase with age, its presence should be suspected particularly in older people, but the condition is also found in children and adolescents, though rarely in infants below age 2. Besides lactose, other unabsorbed nutrients can enter the colon and lead to fermentation and gas production. Studies of one particularly flatulent patient identified, besides milk and milk products, such foods as onions, beans, celery, carrots, raisins, bananas, apricots, prune juice, pretzels, bagels, wheat germ, and Brussels sprouts as particularly flatugenic foods. The withholding of lactose and wheat products proved especially effective in this patient. In some persons other sugars, including sucrose, have been the source of colonic gas production, but this is rare.

Since the fermentation of nonabsorbable foodstuffs leads to the production of both gas and short-chain fatty acids, affected subjects frequently complain of concurrent diarrhea produced by the osmotic effects of the fatty acids. In patients with small bowel stasis and bacterial overgrowth, excessive gas production can occur in the small intestine and occasionally in the stomach, as in diabetic gastroparesis or in the presence of large gastric diverticula.

The bowel normally contains relatively small quantities of gas, ranging from 30 to 200 ml, and patients complaining of excessive gaseousness often do not hold abnormally large volumes of gas in their intestines. However, some patients do have excessive gas volumes in their intestines, and this can be suspected from the physical findings of a distended abdomen and from the inspection of plain films of the abdomen, and can be proved by the washout technique introduced by Levitt. Since many patients who complain of gaseousness and accompanying abdominal pains do not have increased volumes of intraluminal gas, their symptoms presumably are caused by excessive contraction of their bowel and entrapment of gas between contracted segments, or by excessive sensitivity and pain perception to normal volumes of gas.

Part of the problem of gaseousness is the definition of what is normal, and patients should be advised that an occasional belch and passage of flatus are normal phenomena. Studies of normal young men indicate that such individuals have an average of 14 gas passages per day. Study of an extremely flatulent individual revealed as many as 20 passages per hour. This knowledge should aid physicians in differentiating flatulent from normal persons.

Many constipated patients complain of intestinal bloating and gaseousness. Such patients often have abdominal distention, and their colons probably contain excessive amounts of gas. It is further likely, although unproved, that with the prolonged intestinal transit such patients exhibit, prolonged fermentation of food residue leads to excessive accumulation of gas, often prevented from passage by fecal impaction. The ingestion of high fiber diets as treatment of constipation may lead to further gas production. Recent studies have shown that the cellulose of bran and other nondigestible carbohydrates contained in such diets are subject to fermentation by intestinal bacteria, largely obligate anaerobes, resembling ruminal bacteria of cattle. Hydrophilic mucilloid, consisting of hemicellulose or mucilages, also leads to gas production, but less than bran and related substances.

Therapeutic Approaches

With the foregoing explanations in mind, the physician can approach his gaseous patient in a more rational manner. Although no controlled clinical studies have been conducted in any of the subgroups of gaseous patients, the reported experience of others and one's own clinical experience will lead to successful management of most patients.

Management of Belching. Belching is a normal phenomenon, and patients should be reassured that an occasional eructation is not a sign of disease and does not require, or respond to, any specific medicinal therapy. What constitutes excessive belching is partly a matter of definition, but at times there can be no doubt. The most severe belchers tend to be severely neurotic individuals who draw in air with every inspiration and expel it with a loud noise on each expiration. Such patients have proved intractable to the ministrations of gastroenterologists, primary care internists, or family physicians and at times are best handled by psychiatrists. The more commonly encountered excessive belcher with less

dramatic sound effects can often be helped by being taught the elementary principles of normal eating. Patients should be taught to eat three meals a day, to chew carefully, to avoid gulping down food without chewing, and to avoid excessive imbibing of beverages with their meals. This applies particularly to carbonated beverages. Garlic and raw onions relax the lower esophageal sphincter and may cause belching. Excessive eating per se can lead to belching, and this should be avoided, particularly the ingestion of overly fatty meals. Perhaps the delayed emptying of the stomach caused by the ingestion of fatty meals leads to release of gas in the stomach or, more important, to the entrapment of swallowed air in the gastric air bubble (magenblase) and its eventual expulsion through belching. Patients of squatty build with a transverse stomach and a large gastric air bubble under the left diaphragm are particularly prone to air trapping that can produce severe pain radiating to the chest, at times mimicking coronary artery disease and myocardial infarction. This constellation has been called the "magenblase syndrome," and in acute phases can be relieved by the insertion of a nasogastric tube and the release of the trapped air. Patients predisposed to gas trapping in the stomach should be cautioned against ingesting such foods as soufflés, whipped desserts, and carbonated beverages. Reclining after meals appears to lead to belching in some persons, perhaps in part because of air trapping in the supine position and in part because of CO_2 production from contact of gastric acid and pancreatic HCO_3. Hence, patients should be cautioned not to recline after heavy meals. In rare instances belching is caused by gastric outlet obstruction, and, if so, the condition requires identification and correction of the underlying disease. Patients who purposely try to belch to relieve gastric distress should be cautioned against this habit, as it usually leads to more swallowing than expulsion of air and consequently offers no relief at all. Patients who belch primarily when nervous, and presumably swallow more air during periods of stress and anxiety, are occasionally helped by the use of tranquilizers.

Abdominal Distention and Pain. The aforementioned configuration of symptoms is usually caused by excessive gas accumulations in the colon and is likely caused by excessive gas production by bacterial fermentation. Where available, flatus analysis can be performed, and the composition of flatus would offer information as to the origin of colon gas. A predominance of N_2 indicates swallowed air, and the relative paucity of N_2 and abundance of H_2, CH_4, and CO_2

indicates colonic gas production by bacteria. Based on the explanations offered above, and on the relative frequencies encountered in clinical settings, we try to eliminate gas-producing foods from the diet.

In the vast majority of patients the offender is lactose. Lactose is present in all types of milk, and is present also in many cheeses, ice cream, milkshakes, chocolate, puddings, junkets, and many other food items. It should be kept in mind that the fermentation of 1 gram of the solid lactose can lead to the production of about 250 ml of gas, and that 1 glass of milk contains about 8 grams of lactose; thus the amount of gas produced from the ingestion of relatively small amounts of milk can be enormous. The amount of lactose in cheese varies greatly and no accurate data are or could be available on the thousands of varieties of cheese and their state of ripening. As a general rule, very ripe and smelly cheeses are virtually devoid of lactose, while most processed and pasteurized cheeses contain substantial amounts of lactose and hence can lead to substantial gas production. Regrettably, commercial food processors are apt to add milk solids, i.e., lactose, after the fermentation of cheese or yogurt, thus making them noxious to lactase-deficient patients. Homemade yogurt, permitted to ferment over 12 hours, usually is free of lactose, as is homemade or farm-produced cottage cheese. Much cottage cheese sold in food stores contains substantial amounts of skim milk or milk powder, as can be noted on the list of ingredients. *Lactase* is available commercially from a microbiological source in the form of Lact-Aid, a valuable product when used properly. Two packets of Lact-Aid or the appropriate number of drops of the liquid product should be added to a quart of milk, and the milk should then be kept in the refrigerator for 24 hours before use. Such pretreated milk contains minimal amounts of lactose and is tolerated by most lactase-deficient patients. So-called sweet acidophilus milk has not proved to be effective and cannot at present be recommended. Lactase deficiency can often be identified by simple dietary manipulation, i.e., by exclusion of all milk products for a week's time and rechallenge with a glass or two of milk between meals, comparing the effects of these dietary changes on gas production and its consequences. When the effects are not clear, a lactose tolerance test can be performed, or when available a hydrogen breath test can be carried out after ingestion of milk or lactose. However, it should be appreciated that even in patients with a normal lactose tolerance test, up to 8 per cent of lactose may not be absorbed and this amount can still lead to excessive gaseousness.

In patients who do not respond to elimination or reduction of lactose in the diet, other sources of gas production should be sought in the diet. The elimination of beans and other known gas-producing foods should be recommended. The search for lactose and other gas-producing sources can be quite intriguing. Thus, the continued use of lactose by the pharmaceutical industry as a filler should be noted; an example are some of the long-acting nitrates, marketed in lactose-containing capsules and hence potential sources of gaseousness. Diet soft drinks and diet gums should be interdicted, as they frequently contain lactose or the nonabsorbable alcohol sorbitol, another source of gas.

In patients who have gaseousness combined with constipation, efforts should be made to control the constipation. Our choice for this purpose rests on the use of bulking agents, such as psyllium hydrophilic mucilloid, even though they themselves may temporarily produce some gaseousness. The alternative use of bran leads to even more gaseousness. If psyllium mucilloid does not suffice to improve intestinal motor function and control constipation, stool softeners and senna alkaloid tablets or granules can be used in addition, at times with the further addition of milk of magnesia. For severe attacks of gas pains, an occasional enema may offer prompt relief. The use of antispasmodics has proved disappointing, even though segmental contractions and compression of gas in intestinal pockets may well be an important mechanism in the production of gas pains.

Excessive Passage of Flatus. The management of this distressing problem is similar to that described for the abdominal distention and pain and depends largely on the identification of the source of gas and its elimination. Thorough questioning of the patient regarding dietary habits and the ingestion of flatugenic foods is a prerequisite to proper management and the ultimate exclusion of gas-producing items from the diet. In instances of organic malabsorption syndromes, emphasis should be placed on specific therapy of the malabsorptive disorder, such as a gluten-free diet in celiac sprue, or the use of effective pancreatic enzyme preparations with each meal in patients with pancreatic insufficiency. Patients with bacterial overgrowth syndromes respond to antibiotics, preferably selected on the basis of the antibiotic sensitivities of recovered organisms obtained by intestinal intubation. The use of antibiotics for gaseousness of other causes has not been proved to be effective. Intestinal obstruction clearly requires specific measures directed at its relief, and is beyond the scope of this article.

In summary, most patients with intestinal gaseousness can be helped by inducing changes in habits and diets and by improving bowel function, rather than by using any pharmacologic agent.

ACUTE AND CHRONIC HEPATITIS

method of
J. SPALDING SCHRODER, M.D.
Atlanta, Georgia

The treatment of acute hepatitis has remained relatively unchanged over the past decade in spite of tremendous advances in understanding the nature of the causative organisms. The latter information has contributed to accuracy of diagnosis and prognosis, which may vary according to the type of hepatitis. Additional findings regarding the role of immune complexes in producing extrahepatic injury in association with viral hepatitis have also added to understanding of various related syndromes.

Acute hepatitis is usually recognized by demonstration of abnormal aminotransferase enzymes, with or without jaundice. From the standpoint of therapy it is important to establish whether a given case is due to viral hepatitis or to toxic hepatitis caused by drugs or alcohol. Extrahepatic obstructive causes may be confused with hepatitis in a significant number of patients. The subjective manifestations may vary from no symptoms at all even in the presence of abnormal laboratory tests to devastatingly prostrating illness in either viral or toxic hepatitis. The bilirubin elevation is just as variable but generally tends to parallel the degree of severity of the clinical manifestations. The laboratory tests are helpful in that the serum glutamic oxaloacetic transaminase (SGOT) and serum glutamic pyruvic transaminase (SGPT) levels are generally higher in viral hepatitis, usually over 500 in the early course of the illness, than in toxic hepatitis. Notable exceptions are those cases of toxic hepatitis causing extensive hepatocellular necrosis, such as may occur in halothane hepatitis.

The era of specific laboratory tests was ushered in by the development of methods to demonstrate hepatitis B surface antigen (HBsAg) and its corresponding antibody (anti-HBs). Other recent tests related to hepatitis B virus are antibodies to core antigen (anti-HBc) and "e" antigen (anti-HBe), the latter being associated with more progressive hepatitis B infection. Currently, the only specific test commercially available for hepatitis A is a test for antibody that reacts with hepatitis A virus (anti-HAV). The value of these antibody reactions in a given case is limited by the possibility that the antibody demonstrated may be due to passive prophylaxis from immune serum globulin or to active immunity acquired by previous exposure to the virus during an unrecognized bout of hepatitis. This dilemma may be resolved by demonstration of a significant increase in antibody titer in a convalescent specimen. Currently, there is no specific test to confirm the diagnosis of non-A, non-B hepatitis. In the presence of symptoms and signs of viral hepatitis, the demonstration of negative HBsAg, negative anti-HBs, and negative anti-HAV during the acute phase and 2 to 3 weeks later provides circumstantial evidence for this diagnosis. Non-A, non-B hepatitis is frequently transmitted by blood transfusions, needle contamination, and intimate physical contact. Its incubation period varies from 15 to 180 days.

Liver biopsy is especially useful in acute hepatitis when the etiology has not been established by serologic means and the clinical findings do not differentiate between viral and toxic hepatitis, drug-induced or alcohol-related. In addition to its usefulness in establishing the diagnosis of acute viral hepatitis, it is also helpful to estimate the prognosis of the individual patient with this diagnosis. Prognosis for complete recovery is excellent in the absence of "bridging necrosis," namely, zones of confluent hepatic cell necrosis that bridge adjacent portal triads and central veins. On the other hand, death or chronic hepatitis occurs in a significantly high percentage of patients with this lesion.

Treatment

The obvious management of toxic hepatitis is the removal of the toxin, whether drug or alcohol. Efforts to "reform" confirmed alcoholics are notoriously difficult, but many alcohol abusers are persuaded when confronted with a specimen of their own liver confirming the presence of alcoholic hepatitis, which is a reversible lesion prior to the development of cirrhosis. They may not have realized that the steady social or business-related alcohol consumption was damaging their livers, and the implications regarding future alcohol ingestion may prove to be the incentive needed to control their abuse.

Uncomplicated Viral Hepatitis. The majority of patients are treated successfully at home and may be followed on an outpatient basis by the physician. Twice weekly determinations of prothrombin time provide excellent prognostic information. In the uncomplicated typical case, jaundice and malaise will have subsided by the end of the second or third week of observation. Follow-up clinical evaluation with SGOT or SGPT evaluation at monthly intervals is recommended, with the realization that transaminase elevations may persist for a variable period of time following return to normal of other tests.

REST AND ACTIVITY. Complete bedrest need not be forced on the patient who does not feel too sick to walk to the bathroom or to sit in a comfortable chair where he may relax. On the other hand, the patient who feels too ill or too tired should not be forced out of bed or encouraged to ambulate. A generally satisfactory method is to advise the patient to remain in bed until he feels strong enough to prefer bathroom privileges and to gradually avail himself of the bedside chair as his returning strength dictates. As the days go by the average patient will gradually increase his ambulation without overexerting himself. He should be cautioned that fatigue must be avoided and that he must not exert himself beyond his limited endurance. Within 10 to 14 days of its appearance, the jaundice should have reached its peak in the average adult. A sense of well-being should begin to return with a return of strength at the same time. During the subsequent 1 to 4 weeks the level of bilirubin should decline to normal coincident with increasing ambulation. If the bilirubin reaches a plateau after 14 to 21 days and fails to decline, the possibility of complication should be considered and the patient's activity should be curtailed because of the possibility of progressive confluent necrosis, indicating need for more aggressive therapy as described below under Severe Acute Hepatitis.

DIET. The patients whose main complaints are anorexia and nausea have found a low fat, high carbohydrate diet more palatable than a general diet. As a result of such patient preference, not only have diets of this type been recommended by physicians in the past but fat has actually been forbidden in the diet of patients with hepatitis. This is unnecessary, and a general diet with normal distribution of carbohydrates, fat, and protein is now recommended. A forced high calorie or high protein diet is not beneficial. The general diet contains adequate vitamins, amino acids, and lipotropic agents, so that supplemental doses of these are unnecessary. Hard candy, carbonated drinks, and fruit juices are often well tolerated during this early period of anorexia and mild nausea. Parenteral feedings and vitamins are needed only when anorexia and nausea are severe enough to prevent the patient from retaining adequate caloric and fluid balance.

DRUGS. An antiemetic or antihistaminic medication taken before the principal meal helps overcome nausea. No other drugs are needed in uncomplicated acute hepatitis. As stated under dietary considerations, supplemental vitamins, amino acids, and lipotropic agents are unnecessary. The use of all drugs is avoided if possible, since drug metabolism is altered in the presence of significant liver dysfunction. Immunosuppressive therapy with corticosteroids or azathioprine has no place in therapy of acute uncomplicated hepatitis.

PROLONGED PROTHROMBIN TIME. Vitamin K_1 may be given intramuscularly (10 mg daily) in the presence of prolonged prothrombin time, because a cholestatic component in these patients may interfere with its absorption from the intestinal tract.

Severe Acute Hepatitis (Bridging Necrosis and Fulminant Hepatitis). The likelihood of progressive confluent hepatic cell necrosis (bridging necrosis) is to be considered in the patient whose symptoms and bilirubin and/or prothrombin levels fail to improve after 2 to 3 weeks. These are the rare patients (less than 1 per cent) who develop fulminant hepatitis with a very high mortality. Hepatic coma, gastrointestinal bleeding, and renal failure are the usual clinical manifestations of this complication. Treatment is best carried out in the intensive care unit with appropriate monitoring and immediate attention to each manifestation of system failure.

The protein intake should be discontinued and neomycin administered orally in doses of 4 to 6 grams daily. Neomycin enemas may be useful in reducing further ammonia absorption from the colon. Caloric intake is maintained through nasogastric tube feeding in addition to intravenous hypertonic glucose. Supplemental potassium is usually necessary, with daily monitoring of electrolytes to regulate dosage. Central blood volume monitoring may be needed to maintain adequate renal plasma flow with constant measurement of urinary output hour by hour, necessitating an indwelling catheter. Close monitoring of arterial blood gases is required, and appropriate appliances employed to assure adequate ventilation may become required to maintain adequate tissue oxygenation. Corticosteroid therapy has no proved efficacy in treatment of fulminant hepatitis, although the critical condition of the patient has led many physicians to employ very large doses in the desperate hope of maintaining stabilization of hepatocytes. The mainstay of treatment is to bide time while hoping for eventual regeneration of liver tissue.

Chronic Hepatitis. Chronic hepatitis may be recognized in a small percentage of patients, following a clinical bout of acute hepatitis B or hepatitis non-A, non-B, by the persistence of transaminase elevation beyond 3 to 6 months.

(Hepatitis A infection does not cause chronic hepatitis.) More often, the acute episode will have gone unrecognized, and the condition is suspected because of the finding of elevated transaminase levels on an automated screening procedure with persistence of the abnormality on repeated testing. The patient may have no symptoms or may experience nonspecific symptoms, including lassitude, fatigue, and anorexia. It is necessary to differentiate "chronic aggressive hepatitis" from "persistent hepatitis" in such patients, since immunosuppressive therapy may benefit the former but is undesirable in the latter, which is self-limited. The differential diagnosis is established by histologic findings of the needle liver biopsy specimen. These findings are infiltration of the portal zones with mononuclear cells and fibrosis and erosion of the limiting plate of liver cells by piecemeal necrosis. It is important to consider Wilson's disease and lupoid hepatitis as well as viral hepatitis as the cause of these histologic findings and to institute appropriate therapy with penicillamine in Wilson's disease and immunosuppressive therapy in lupoid hepatitis (which is continued for 2 years after apparent recovery).

Treatment with corticosteroids is recommended if the aforementioned histologic findings occur in the patient with nonspecific symptoms of lassitude, fatigue, and anorexia, associated with SGOT elevation over five times normal. If liver biopsy demonstrates multilobular (bridging) necrosis, with or without cirrhosis, treatment is begun immediately regardless of the presence or absence of symptoms. Prednisone is recommended in doses of 10 mg four times daily for 5 days, followed by 10 mg three times daily for 4 weeks, with weekly SGOT determinations. If improvement occurs, prednisone is reduced to 10 mg twice daily for another 4 weeks. If biochemical and symptomatic improvement is maintained, the dose can gradually be reduced to 10 to 15 mg per day. Clinical and laboratory evaluations are recommended every 2 to 4 months thereafter until remission is induced and maintained for 6 months. Liver biopsy should then be repeated, and if morphologic remission is seen, therapy may be gradually tapered and discontinued.

If the patient fails to respond to the regimen described above, then 50 mg of azathioprine a day may be added, and increased to 100 mg per day if necessary to induce remission. (This use of azathioprine is not listed in the manufacturer's official directive.) Higher doses of prednisone are not likely to be more effective and are likely to produce undesirable side effects.

Hepatitis Prophylaxis

The most effective protection known against hepatitis A and hepatitis B is meticulous personal hygiene and strict adherence to good techniques of "stool and needle isolation." Immune serum globulin is recommended for all persons having intimate contact with or living in the same house as the patient with hepatitis A. It should be administered early after exposure. The recommended dose is 0.5 ml for small children, 1 ml for children up to 100 pounds, and 2 ml for larger children and adults. In case of exposure to patients who have recognized hepatitis B infection through needle prick or through sexual or other intimate physical contact, it is recommended that 5 ml of immune serum globulin with high anti-HBs titer be given immediately and again in 30 days if the exposed person has negative HBsAg and anti-HBs titers. If these tests are not immediately available, sufficient serum should be obtained prior to administration of immune serum globulin to permit evaluation of results of this testing without interference from the administered immune serum globulin. Standard immune serum globulin is adequate for hepatitis A and hepatitis non-A, non-B until more precise information becomes available.

A vaccine to prevent type B hepatitis is now being developed, but further testing is required before it becomes available.

THE MALABSORPTION SYNDROME

method of
THOMAS W. SHEEHY, M.D.
Birmingham, Alabama

The malabsorption syndrome consists of many diseases, which, for the sake of simplicity, have been grouped into disorders of digestion and disorders of absorption.

Disorders of digestion occur whenever a disease interferes with the digestive process wherein nutrient molecules are reduced to immunologically inactive particles suitable for transfer across the intestinal epithelium. For example, in pancreatic insufficiency there is not enough pancreatic lipase to split dietary triglycerides into water-soluble fatty acids and beta-monoglycerides; in biliary tract disorders, there may be insufficient bile salts to solubilize amphiphatic molecules into macromolecules called micelles, which are necessary for fat absorption at the epithelial cell membrane. In these disorders, the intestinal mucosa is usually normal.

In disorders of absorption, mucosal lesions are prominent. These disorders include diseases that disrupt the transfer of digested nutrients across the intestinal mucosal cells into vascular and lymphatic channels. In celiac sprue, the mucosal epithelium is injured by the toxic action of gluten; in lymphoma and Whipple's disease the intestinal lymphatics are blocked; in abetalipoproteinemia, there is loss of lipoprotein lipase, a key intracellular enzyme required for intracellular re-esterification of fatty acid and monoglycerides into triglycerides.

Selective disorders of absorption result from failure to absorb or to digest specific substances; e.g., in pernicious anemia vitamin B_{12} cannot be absorbed owing to absence of intrinsic factor.

Table 1 lists over 40 diseases capable of causing maldigestion or malabsorption. As with any disease group, it is imperative that a specific cause be identified whenever possible. This is particularly so with this group of disorders, because diagnosis has both therapeutic and prognostic implications. Celiac disease is an eminently treatable disorder, whereas treatment for massive small bowel resection is far from satisfactory.

As always, a good history and physical examination are mandatory and often are all that is needed to indicate the disease process. A history of childhood diseases characterized by diarrhea or delayed growth suggests celiac disease or milk intolerance. Steatorrhea in the diabetic patient with neuropathy suggests diabetic enteropathy. Previous gastric or intestinal surgery can result in bacterial overgrowth and/or bile deficiency. Onset of malabsorption after return from the tropics suggests tropical sprue or

TABLE 1. **Diseases Causing Maldigestion or Malabsorption**

		MECHANISM
Disorders of digestion		
Stomach	Gastric resection	Surgery
	Gastrocolic-gastroileal fistula	
	Postvagotomy steatorrhea	
Pancreas	Pancreatic insufficiency	Insufficient pancreatic enzymes
	Pancreatic islet cell tumor	
	Carcinoma of head of pancreas	
	Cystic fibrosis	
	Protein deficiency states	
Hepatobiliary	Biliary tract obstruction	Insufficient bile salts
	Chronic parenchymal liver disease	
Endocrine	Thyrotoxicosis	?
	Hypoparathyroidism	
	Addison's disease	
	Sheehan's syndrome	
Other	Diverticulosis	Bacterial overgrowth–bile salt deconjugation
	Blind loop syndrome	Bacterial overgrowth–bile salt deconjugation
	Scleroderma	Stasis and bacterial–bile salt deconjugation
	Diabetes mellitus	Stasis and bacterial overgrowth–bile salt deconjugation
Disorders of absorption		
Mucosal defects	Tropical sprue	? Infection
	Celiac sprue	Gluten toxicity
	Lymphangiectasia	Congenital
	Short bowel syndrome	Surgery
Drugs	Neomycin	Toxic for epithelium
	Colchicine	Toxic for epithelium
	Para-aminosalicylic acid	Toxic for epithelium
	Methotrexate	Toxic for epithelium
Blockade	Whipple's disease	Infection
	Lymphoma – carcinoma	Infiltration
	Amyloidosis	Infiltration
	Carcinoid	Infiltration
Infections	Viral enteritis	?
	Giardiasis	?
	Strongyloidiasis	Inflammation
	Capillariasis	Inflammation
Inflammatory	Regional enteritis	?
	Radiation enteritis	X-ray
Selective disorders	Pernicious anemia	Lack of intrinsic factor
	Abetalipoproteinemia	Enzyme deficiency
	Disaccharidase deficiency	Enzyme deficiency
	Monosaccharide malabsorption	Transport failure
	Cystinuria, Hartnup disease	Transport failure

parasitic infection. Extensive pelvic radiation can cause enteritis, whereas recurrent pleuritis and arthritis with diarrhea suggest Whipple's disease.

Ordinarily, all dietary fat is digested and absorbed. The 5 to 6 grams excreted in feces comes from shed epithelium. With maldigestion or malabsorption, there is steatorrhea and large amounts of fat may be lost in feces. Indeed, steatorrhea is synonymous with the malabsorption syndrome, for it occurs in all the diseases listed in Table 1 except pernicious anemia, cystinuria, Hartnup disease, and primary glucose malabsorption. Malabsorption and maldigestion can also cause diarrhea, because unabsorbed long-chain fatty acids are broken down to short-chain fatty acids which act as bowel irritants. Since vitamins A, D, E, and K are dependent on fat transport for absorption, anything that interferes with the fat digestion or absorption may cause a deficiency of these vitamins.

Today, cost accountability demands that the clinician be able to readily establish the presence of steatorrhea. A simple microscopic examination of a fecal smear stained with Sudan III takes only minutes. If six or more fat globules per low power field are present, this is highly suggestive of steatorrhea. If one or more meat fibers per coverslip preparation are found, this is another indication that steatorrhea probably exists. Giardia and Strongyloides may cause steatorrhea, and stool examination may reveal their presence. A stool acid pH (<5) suggests bacterial overgrowth or a disaccharidase deficiency. An alkaline pH suggests shigellosis. A peripheral blood smear showing macro- or microcytosis has definite implications. Simple examination of gross stool may reveal the typical porridge-like foul-smelling feces so characteristic of steatorrhea.

While not diagnostic of any particular entity per se, when positive, these simple tests correlate well with the presence of steatorrhea. Then more definitive tests may be undertaken for diagnosis, e.g., a Schilling test, intestinal biopsy, tests of pancreatic function, a ^{14}C bile breath test, and even a therapeutic trial.

Disorders of Digestion

Pancreatic Exocrine Insufficiency. Pancreatic exocrine insufficiency may result from several diseases, e.g., alcoholism, cystic fibrosis, pancreatic neoplasm, and ductal obstruction caused by stones. The resultant inadequate production of lipase, amylase, and proteolytic enzymes disrupts the proper digestion of fat, carbohydrates, and proteins and leads to maldigestion with steatorrhea and often a deficiency of fat-soluble vitamins.

The objectives of therapy are to prevent recurrence, to control symptoms, and to improve digestion.

To prevent recurrent attacks of pancreatitis:

1. Encourage the patient to avoid alcohol.

2. Prescribe a bland, low fat diet, containing 75 to 150 grams of protein and 300 to 400 grams of carbohydrates; give anticholinergics before meals and at bedtime to reduce pancreatic stimulation.

3. Avoid thiazides and azathioprine, i.e., drugs capable of precipitating pancreatitis.

4. Recommend appropriate surgery when indicated for biliary or pancreatic stones or obstruction, pancreatic pseudocysts, or pancreatic ductal disease.

For pancreatic insufficiency:

1. Treat diabetes mellitus, if present.

2. Replace pancreatic enzyme (primarily lipase) with supplements, such as pancrelipase (Cotazym capsules) or pancreatin (Viokase) 0.3 gram (5 grain) tablets. For moderate steatorrhea, 2 to 4 tablets or capsules are given every 4 to 6 hours throughout the day; for severe diarrhea, 2 to 4 tablets every hour may be necessary. With improvement, dosage may be reduced to 2 to 4 tablets before meals and bedtime.

3. Concomitantly, use sodium bicarbonate, 1 to 3 grams per day, to prevent peptic acid inactivation of the enzyme supplements or to decrease acid inactivation of the patient's own lipase.

4. Use a low fat diet when the patient has severe symptoms and liberalize with clinical improvement.

5. Supplement the diet with medium-chain triglycerides in patients with severe diarrhea or weight loss. Medium-chain triglycerides (MCT) are rapidly hydrolyzed by both pancreatic and intestinal lipase. Depending on tolerance, 1 or 2 ounces can be given two or three times daily as salad dressing or medication. The oil can also be used for cooking purposes. Liquid formulas are available; however, one formula (Portagen) contains lactose. Unfortunately, MCT may cause diarrhea when given in excess of 300 calories per day.

6. Provide adequate fat-soluble vitamins and calcium, if necessary.

Postgastrectomy State. Malabsorption may occur after gastric operations for several reasons: bacterial overgrowth in an afferent loop; activation of latent celiac disease or disaccharidase insufficiency; intestinal hurry or chase, i.e., impaired delayed mixture of food with pancreatic juice and bile; and/or autodigestion of pancreatic enzymes. The objectives are to relieve symptoms, to improve nutrition, and to evaluate the patient for conditions amenable to surgery.

1. Increase caloric intake and give six small meals daily if weight loss occurs.

2. If the dumping syndrome is present, use

a diet high in fat and protein but low in carbohydrates; postpone beverages until 30 to 60 minutes after eating.

3. Treat iron deficiency or calcium depletion.

4. Give vitamin B_{12}, 100 micrograms monthly, after both total gastrectomy and partial gastrectomy.

5. Give paregoric (camphorated tincture of opium), 4 to 8 ml, or diphenozylate hydrochloride (Lomotil), 2.5 to 5.0 mg, if diarrhea is excessive. If milk increases symptoms, restrict the intake of milk and milk products and evaluate for lactose intolerance.

6. Evaluate the patient for celiac disease, pancreatic insufficiency, and afferent loop syndrome if steatorrhea is significant and difficult to control.

7. Consider the possibility of pulmonary tuberculosis in debilitated patients.

8. Try antibiotic therapy (tetracycline, 0.5 to 1 gram daily) if an afferent loop syndrome is suspected.

9. Consider surgical alteration of afferent loop syndromes.

Gastric Hypersecretion. In the Zollinger-Ellison syndrome, excessive amounts of hydrochloric acid pass into the proximal small intestine. This reduces the luminal pH to 2 or 3, which inactivates pancreatic enzymes, impairs micellar formation by precipitating conjugated bile salts, and injures the intestinal mucosa. Temporary relief may sometimes be obtained through use of antacids, cimetidine, or anticholinergic drugs. Total gastrectomy may be necessary if medical therapy is unsuccessful.

Gastric hypersecretion may also occur following massive intestinal resection. In this situation, antacids, anticholinergics, and pancreatic enzyme supplements should be tried.

Bile Salt Deficiency. All causes lead to impaired fat digestion and, with time, to deficiencies of fat-soluble vitamins and calcium.

BACTERIAL OVERGROWTH. Excessive bacterial overgrowth may occur in the proximal small bowel lumen of patients with diabetes mellitus, scleroderma, jejunal diverticula, or inflammatory diseases causing strictures, or with a blind loop or afferent loop. Anaerobic bacteria deconjugate bile salts and impair micellar formation of fat, a step essential to normal fat absorption; bacteria may also compete for vitamin B_{12} and cause a deficiency of that vitamin.

Effective treatment requires identification and eradication of the organism and relief of the stasis which permits bacterial overgrowth.

1. Culture the bowel contents for both aerobic and anaerobic organisms.

2. Treat with tetracycline, 250 mg four times a day, or ampicillin, 500 to 1000 mg four times daily. Indications of effectiveness are usually seen in 5 to 10 days, and include an increase in appetite, improved absorption of fat and/or vitamin B_{12}, and a decrease in stool frequency. Prolonged antibiotic therapy is often necessary in patients with scleroderma and diabetic steatorrhea. In these patients, reduce the daily dose of antibiotics to the lowest effective level and alternate use of tetracycline and ampicillin. This often permits control of gastrointestinal symptoms for years.

3. Treat vitamin B_{12} and fat-soluble vitamin deficiency and prescribe calcium, if necessary. Calcium requirements are 1 to 2 grams daily. Calcium carbonate (Titralac), 5 ml, contains 1.00 gram of calcium. Os-Cal tablets contain 250 mg per tablet; Titralac tablets contain 420 mg.

4. Supplement diet with medium-chain triglycerides.

5. Evaluate diabetics who have steatorrhea for gluten sensitivity or apathetic thyroid disease if effective control of their diabetes and treatment with antibiotics do not decrease the diarrhea or steatorrhea.

6. Correct lesions amenable to surgery.

BILIARY OBSTRUCTION. Biliary obstruction of prolonged duration may decrease intraluminal bile salt concentrations below the critical micellar level necessary for proper fat emusification and absorption. At present, oral bile salts cannot be used for replacement because of the large amounts necessary. Therefore the following measures should be undertaken:

1. Control the diarrhea by reduction of dietary fat intake. Limiting the intake of fat to 40 to 50 grams daily may decrease steatorrhea and reduce the loss of calcium and fat-soluble vitamins in the stools.

2. Supplement the diet with medium-chain triglycerides to maintain nutrition and weight.

3. Prescribe fat-soluble vitamins as needed. Give water-soluble vitamin A preparation (Aquasol) for better absorption if oral preparations are indicated. Vitamin D_2 (ergocalciferol), 25,000 units daily. Vitamin K (menadione), 4 mg daily.

4. Relieve surgically correctable lesions.

DECREASED HEPATIC SYNTHESIS. Bile acids are synthesized from cholesterol by the liver. With severe parenchymal liver disease, e.g., cirrhosis, viral or alcoholic hepatitis, chronic active hepatitis, there may be decreased production of bile acids. Fortunately, this type of bile deficiency is seldom encountered. When it is, treatment should be designed to (1) improve parenchymal liver cell function, e.g., use of steroids for chronic active hepatitis; (2) decrease diarrhea by prescribing a low fat diet, 40 to 50 grams daily; and (3) improve nutrition with medium-chain triglycerides and vitamins.

IMPAIRED BILE SALT ABSORPTION. Bile salts are absorbed in the distal ileum. With regional enteritis or extensive ileal resection, bile salt absorption may be impaired or eliminated. When bile salt loss exceeds hepatic production, maldigestion results.

1. Treat inflammatory bowel disease, e.g., Crohn's disease, as outlined on pages 382 to 386.

2. Use cholestyramine (a bile salt-binding resin), 5 grams three times daily in applesauce or with fruit juice, to decrease bile salt diarrhea. This resin binds bile salts and prevents their cathartic action.

3. Provide vitamin and calcium, as necessary.

Bile salt absorption is also impaired with extensive small bowel resection. This entity overlaps disorders of digestion and absorption because loss of bile salts may impair digestion, while extensive loss of gut area prevents absorption.

MASSIVE INTESTINAL RESECTION (SHORT BOWEL SYNDROME). Bile salt deficiency (excision of ileum) and cell surface area loss may both occur with this disorder.

Immediately following surgical shortening of the small bowel, there is little difference between problems presented by the patient with massive (more than 200 cm) resection and the patient with segmental resection. But once the patient with massive resection begins to eat, he usually presents a problem in management. Prognosis and management, after massive resection of the small bowel, are related to the preoperative condition, the amount and area of bowel resected, the state of remaining small intestine, the nutritional status of the patient, and the preservation of the ileocecal valve and right colon. Marked gastric hypersecretion of acid may also develop as a complication of massive resection. Patients without ileocecal valves have more diarrhea than those with an intact valve. Proximal resection of the small bowel is also tolerated better than distal resection. This is because the ileum is adapted to absorbing all nutrients in addition to being the sole site for bile salt reabsorption. Loss of all or most of the ileum may lead to severe diarrhea and sodium, calci-

um and magnesium loss. The cathartic action of bile salts increases colonic motility and impairs water and sodium absorption. Loss of 100 cm of distal ileum causes fecal bile salt loss to exceed hepatic synthesis with a resulting steatorrhea. Vitamin B_{12} deficiency also occurs. Medical management is designed as follows:

1. Maintain fluid and electrolyte balance and avoid hypokalemic acidosis. Supplemental calcium, magnesium, and vitamins are usually necessary.

2. Use intravenous hyperalimentation solutions via a central catheter in the vena cava to maintain nourishment as necessary. Most parenteral preparations contain approximately 1000 calories per liter. Infusion of 2 or 3 liters should be given over a 24 hour period at a slow rate. If glucosuria is prominent, check for diabetes and/or evidence of hyperosmolar hyperglycemia.

3. Assess the absorptive capacity of the remaining bowel.

4. Feed every 2 hours when oral feeding is started. Initially, a high protein, low fat diet should be tried. This provides 20 to 25 calories per pound of ideal body weight. As the patient becomes more tolerant of food, he can eat less frequently. Medium-chain triglycerides are often valuable, but they may induce diarrhea in some patients and they are not very palatable. The major portion of dietary fat should be given at breakfast when the bile salts reach their maximal intestinal concentration. Intake of lactose and milk should be restricted if they are tolerated poorly. Fortunately, many of these persons learn to adjust their food intake to their digestive tolerance.

5. Try antacids and anticholinergics if gastric hypersecretion develops; vagotomy may be necessary to help control secretion.

Lactase Deficiency. This deficiency is common in Asiatics (70 to 90 per cent) and in Blacks (10 to 15 per cent). Patients with this condition are unable to split milk sugar (lactose) into its component monosaccharides (glucose and galactose) because they lack the mucosal enzyme lactase. The unabsorbed lactose causes an osmotic diarrhea, and the sugar is degraded intestinally to short chain organic acids and to carbon dioxide. This leads to abdominal distention, cramping, and often diarrhea after drinking one or more glasses of milk.

Secondary lactase deficiency usually occurs in diseases involving the intestinal mucosa, e.g., celiac disease and tropical sprue. It may also occur in patients with ulcerative colitis, regional enteritis, and the irritable bowel syndrome.

1. Limit the intake of milk or milk products, such as powdered soft drinks, chocolates, cordials, instant coffee, and mashed potatoes.

2. Supplement the diet of children with calcium.

3. Treat primary conditions that may cause lactase deficiency.

Other Disaccharidase Deficiencies. Deficiencies of other disaccharidases may occur, e.g., sucrase, isomaltase, maltase, and trichalase deficiency. Of these, sucrase deficiency is usually the only clinically important deficiency. It may occur alone or in conjunction with lactase or other disaccharidase deficiencies or a congenital defect. Sucrase levels are often decreased significantly with severe mucosal disease, e.g., celiac or tropical sprue.

Glucose-galactose deficiency is another rare congenital condition. Here the transport mechanism responsible for conveying these sugars across the epithelial barrier is deficient. Treatment consists of eliminating these sugars and substituting foods or beverages containing fructose.

Disorders of Absorption

Malabsorption occurs in these disorders because of changes in the epithelium and damage of the subepithelial structures and/or the collecting channels.

Celiac Sprue. Gluten-sensitive enteropathy is also known as nontropical sprue and idiopathic steatorrhea. It is caused by the toxic effect of certain cereal grain protein fractions (gluten, gliadin) on the intestinal mucosa. The toxic effect of these agents results in loss of villi, a decreased absorbing surface, abnormal epithelial cells, and microscopic changes in the subepithelial structures.

About 20 per cent of patients with celiac disease have an associated nonspecific dermatitis. Dermatitis herpetiformis, however, is specifically related to the disease. Histocompatibility studies show that most patients with celiac disease and dermatitis herpetiformis have HLA-8 antigen. This suggests that the skin and gut lesions are manifestations of the same disease. Clinical observations support this concept, for adherence to a gluten-free diet leads to improvement in both the skin and the gut lesions.

Treatment is designed as follows:

1. Use a gluten-free diet — i.e., wheat, rye, oats, barley, buckwheat, and their byproducts must be removed from the diet. This means exclusion of bread, cakes, cookies, biscuits, pancakes, macaroni, ice cream cones, spaghetti, cold cuts, sausage, frankfurters, canned meats, gravies, certain commercial salad dressings, canned and creamed soups, sherbet, liqueurs, beer, ale, Ovaltine, and instant coffee containing the grains mentioned. Corn and rice are permitted.

2. Read all food labels carefully to avoid offending grains.

3. Continue the gluten-fee diet indefinitely. Clinical improvement in most patients should be evident within the first month of treatment, but an occasional patient requires several months for improvement. In such a case, make certain that the patient is adhering to the diet.

4. Investigate for other causes of malabsorption in those who fail to respond to the gluten-free diet or who respond partially, i.e., pancreatic insufficiency, thyroid disease, or diabetes.

5. Eliminate milk and milk products from persons with acquired intolerance to lactose.

6. Consider supplemental corticosteroid therapy for extremely ill patients. This is rarely indicated.

Tropical Sprue. The cause of this disease is not known; most likely it is a smoldering infection. The disease occurs in persons who reside or have resided in endemic tropical areas (Southeast Asia, the Caribbean). It may develop a few weeks after the patient arrives in an endemic area or years after departure from the tropics. Malabsorption is associated with partial villous atrophy, vitamin deficiencies, intestinal protein loss, and bacterial overgrowth. Therapy is designed to treat the associated vitamin deficiencies, anemia, and bowel lesion.

1. Give folic acid, 5 to 15 mg daily, for prolonged periods. This quickly corrects the anemia and the megaloblastic changes in other organs. It may cure sprue of short duration.

2. Administer tetracycline, 250 mg four times daily, for 1 month; then reduce the dosage to 500 mg daily for several months. In most patients, this regimen causes a remission. Tetracycline penetrates the intestinal epithelium rapidly and remains intracellularly for 1 to 2 hours. It is also phagocytized by macrophages and shed with them via the lamina propria into the lumen.

3. Correct vitamin B_{12} deficiency or iron deficiency if present.

4. Check for associated intestinal parasites and treat accordingly.

The value of prophylactic therapy with folic acid has not been established as a means of preventing the disease.

Whipple's Disease. Whipple (1907) considered this an infectious disease; today, most would agree with him. Although a specific organism has not been identified as causal, the periodic acid–Schiff (PAS) positive macrophages found in the lamina propria of the intestinal mucosa and in the peripheral blood contain bacillus-like organisms. These organisms are thought to be responsible for the arthritis, pleuritis, and other distant complications of this disease. In the intestine, lymphatic blockage leads to impaired nutrient transport and to malabsorption. The basis of treatment is long-term use of antibiotics.

1. Give penicillin, 1.2 million units, and streptomycin, 1 gram daily for 2 weeks.

2. Follow with tetracycline, 0.5 to 1.0 gram daily, for 6 to 12 months. The excretion of this drug in macrophages should enhance its activity against intracellular bacteria (personal observation).

3. If the patient is acutely ill, prednisolone, 10 to 20 mg daily, in combination with antibiotics, should be given initially and continued for 2 to 3 weeks.

Successful treatment leads to decrease of PAS-positive macrophages and to elimination of the bacillus-like organisms in the intestinal epithelium. The latter can be seen by light microscopy in sections of jejunal mucosa stained with toluidine blue or by electron microscopy. Relapses occur and patients should be followed closely so that early treatment can be reinstituted if necessary.

Immunoglobulin Deficiencies. Dysgammaglobulinemia may occur in association with celiac disease, lymphoma, intestinal protein loss, IgA sprue, and lymphoid nodular hyperplasia (LNH). In most of these diseases, IgA is the only deficient immunolgobulin, but in LNH there is a deficiency of two or more of the major serum immunoglobulins. Patients with LNH usually have recurrent pulmonary infections and associated *Giardia lamblia* infestation. After establishing a diagnosis; the following steps are taken:

1. Administer radiation or give chemotherapeutic agents if lymphoma is present.

2. Give a trial with gluten-free diet for IgA sprue, celiac disease, and LNH.

3. Try antibiotics for bacterial overgrowth, if (2) fails.

4. Treat giardiasis with quinacrine (Atabrine), 100 mg three times daily for 7 days, or with metronidazole (Flagyl), 250 mg four times daily for 10 days. (This use of metronidazole is not listed in the manufacturer's official directive.)

5. Try fresh frozen plasma or gamma globulin administration if other measures fail to reduce diarrhea or control infection.

Intestinal Lymphangiectasia. This defect may be congenital or acquired as a result of intestinal inflammatory lesions, infections, or neoplasm. Patients with primary intestinal lymphangiectasia usually present with edema, diarrhea, and/or mild steatorrhea.

1. Use a low fat diet supplemented with medium-chain triglycerides to reduce pressure in the lymphatics and improve fat absorption.

2. Restrict salt and use diuretics if helpful.

Other Conditions Associated with Malabsorption. These include pernicious anemia, Hartnup disease, cystinuria, and monosaccharide intolerance wherein specific substances cannot be absorbed. Most other entities have components of both maldigestion and malabsorption, e.g., radiation enteritis, Crohn's disease, hypoparathyroidism, giardiasis, tuberculous enteritis, abetalipoproteinemia, mesenteric artery insufficiency, kwashiorkor, lymphoma, and amyloidosis.

Nutritional Support

Nutritional supplements have improved steadily in the past decade and now provide a means of sustaining the seriously ill patient for considerable periods of time. Nutritional support can be supplied by enteral feeding, by parenteral supplemental feeding, i.e., Intralipid, or by total parenteral nutrition (hyperalimentation).

Enteral Feeding. The availability of small diameter tubes of polyethylene or Silastic and of numerous elemental diets have facilitated enteral feeding. Theoretically, supplemental feedings of this type are safer, cheaper, and more physiologic than total parenteral nutrition. For example, there is better maintenance of jejunal mucosal thickness and villus height. Enteral feedings are contraindicated with protracted nausea, vomiting, upper gastrointestinal bleeding, and intestinal obstruction.

Monomeric diets (Hy-Cal, Polycose, and medium-chain triglycerides) are supplements that usually contain one primary nutrient, e.g., fat or sugar. They are used when there is a minimal amount of marginally effective intestine, when a bulk-free diet is desired, when digestion is moderately impaired, and occasionally in chronic diarrheal states.

Polymeric mixtures, (e.g., Ensure, Vivonex, Compleat, Flexical, Isocal, Lonalac, Nutri-1000, Portagen, Sustacal, Precision) are used for oral ingestion in patients with short bowel syndromes, extensive regional enteritis, radiation enteritis, pancreatitis, and ulcerative colitis. They are readily assimilated from the bowel, and intraluminal digestion is not required. These preparations contain 1000 calories per liter and have osmolalities ranging from 350 to

1200 mOsm per kg of water. Their calorie-nitrogen ratio (150 to 300:1) is adequate to ensure a positive nitrogen balance. These agents contain varying percentages of predigested protein, amino acids, fats, carbohydrates, electrolytes, and minerals, such as calcium and phosphorus. Most contain lactose, but Ensure, Flexical, Isocal, and Precision do not. Some contain little fat — e.g., Vivonex and Precision have approximately 1 gram. If these are used as the sole source of nutrition, then 30 grams of safflower oil or 50 grams of corn oil must be added to the daily supplement. Some monomeric diets are isotonic (Portagen) and some are hypertonic (Vivonex-HN). Initially, the hypertonic preparations should be diluted to isotonicity and the concentrations increased over several days to avoid intestinal cramps and osmotic diarrhea.

MEDIUM-CHAIN TRIGLYCERIDES (MCT). These are fatty acids of 8 to 10 carbon chain length, whereas dietary fat consists predominantly of long chain fatty acids of 16 to 18 carbon length. MCT are hydrolyzed rapidly, even in conditions in which bile salts and pancreatic lipase are deficient. They are absorbed in disorders of absorption. Further, they require no resynthesis to chylomicrons within the intestinal epithelium, and they enter the portal system directly without the need for lymphatic transport. When they are used as a substitute for dietary fat, a low fat diet should be provided to avoid diarrhea or increased steatorrhea.

MCT are of considerable nutritional value (8.3 cal per gram) and help decrease steatorrhea in the conditions indicated previously, e.g., pancreatic insufficiency, massive small bowel resection. MCT oil is available for cooking purposes, and it can be used as a salad dressing. One teaspoon contains 125 calories.

Parenteral Nutrition. Parenteral nutrition is indicated when (1) the patient is unable to eat or absorb food adequately for over a week, (2) bowel rest is needed to aid in reducing secretion or allowing inflammation to subside, and (3) nutritional support is required.

Presently, two fat emulsions are available to the practitioner. Intralipid is a 10 per cent emulsion of soybean oil. Liposyn is a 10 per cent safflower oil emulsion. Both preparations have near normal osmolality. Their total calorie value, including fat, phospholipids, and glycerin, is 1.1 Kcal per ml. The major difference between these two products is their content of linoleic and linolenic acid. Soybean oil consists of 54 per cent linoleic acid, while safflower oil contains 75 per cent. Soybean oil contains 8 per cent linolenic acid; safflower oil preparation has none.

Linoleic acid is an essential fatty acid proved effective in correcting essential fatty acid deficiency (EFAD). To prevent EFAD, it is recommended that the daily calorie intake contain 1 to 4 per cent linoleic acid. This requirement can be met in poorly nourished patients by infusions of 500 ml of either fat emulsion, twice weekly. Both preparations are useful sources of calories for patients requiring parenteral nutrition.

INTRAVENOUS HYPEROSMOLAR SOLUTIONS OF GLUCOSE. Several preparations are currently available. Electrolytes and vitamins may be added as required. Hyperosmolar preparations are given through a central line to avoid sclerosis of peripheral veins. Their use also carries the risk of sepsis, hyperosmolar nonketotic coma, hypoglycemia, and hypophosphatemia. Other articles in this book describe hyeralimentation techniques in more detail.

INTESTINAL OBSTRUCTION

method of
ROBERT J. FREEARK, M.D.
Maywood, Illinois

The diagnosis of intestinal obstruction in adults is generally predicated on the demonstration of four characteristic findings: vomiting, obstipation, distention, and cramping abdominal pain (mnemonic VODCA). The diagnosis is usually confirmed by radiologic studies consisting of plain and upright films of the abdomen and contrast studies of the large intestine. Several variations of this classic pattern are noteworthy:

1. The degree of vomiting and abdominal distention varies inversely with the level of obstruction; e.g., patients with high small bowel obstructions vomit repeatedly but show minimal distention, whereas those with colonic obstructions are markedly distended but may not vomit.

2. Patients with closed loop and strangulation obstructions may have steady pain, local tenderness, atypical x-rays, and blood in the nasogastric or rectal drainage.

3. Neoplastic obstructions of the small bowel are often gradual in onset, with minimal vomiting, mild obstipation, and vague abdominal discomfort.

4. A clinical picture of mechanical intestinal obstruction may accompany a number of other acute and chronic abdominal conditions, e.g.,

acute appendicitis, inflammatory bowel disease, lymphoma. Under these circumstances, the symptomatology, diagnosis, and treatment may vary considerably from those outlined below.

The treatment of intestinal obstruction varies with the site, presumed etiology, risk of vascular compromise, and general condition of the patient. Four general categories of simple mechanical obstructions can be identified:

1. *Large bowel obstruction,* a disease of the elderly resulting from carcinoma of the colon (75 per cent), diverticular disease (10 per cent), or volvulus (10 per cent). *General approach:* Early surgical intervention to avoid cecal rupture. In most instances, a limited operation to provide decompression is advisable.

2. *Small bowel obstruction caused by incarcerated external hernia.* This occurs in all age groups and requires a search of all sites of abdominal wall herniation. *General approach:* Early surgical intervention to avoid strangulation of entrapped bowel. A limited incision over the site of external herniation may be carried out under local anesthesia if necessary.

3. *Small bowel obstruction resulting from intestinal adhesions.* This occurs in all age groups with a history of prior abdominal surgery or peritonitis. *General approach:* Initially nonoperative, with hope of spontaneous or therapuetic remission. Keen surgical judgment must be exercised here, and if a trial of nonoperative therapy is elected, the patient must be carefully observed to assure that the mechanism or progress of the obstruction does not result in gangrene or perforation of the involved bowel. Patients with a history of a sudden onset, localized tendernes, fever, leukocytosis, and so-called "sentinel loop" on x-ray should be operated upon promptly because of an increased risk of strangulation caused by an internal hernia or volvulus created by their peritoneal adhesions.

4. *Small bowel obstruction without external hernia or prior laparotomy.* A wide variety of uncommon conditions may be responsible, and assignment of this category should raise questions as to the diagnosis of intestinal obstruction, as well as the impact of a variety of etiologic conditions. *General approach:* Early surgical intervention. Formal laparotomy under general anesthesia is usually required.

Once the diagnosis of intestinal obstruction is entertained, the following therapeutic measures are advisable:

1. A No. 18 F nasogastric tube with air vent should be inserted and positioned so that the tip resides in the upper half of the stomach. Continuous suction with frequent irrigation of the lumen is advisable.

2. Intravenous fluids consisting of Ringer's lactate solution should be started and initially infused at a rate of at least 500 ml per hour. Following the infusion of 1500 ml, the rate of sodium and potassium concentration of the intravenous fluids should be adjusted on the basis of the urinary output and specific gravity, serum electrolytes, and clinical degree of dehydration.

3. Systemic antibiotics should be started, usually via the intravenous route. Our current preference is gentamicin (Garamycin), 3 mg per kg per day in three equal doses, or clindamycin (Cleocin), 300 mg every 8 hours.

4. Pain medication should be employed with extreme caution, particularly prior to surgical consultation or during a period of nonoperative treatment. When such medication is required, our preference is for meperidine (Demerol), 25 to 50 mg intravenously.

Immediate surgical consultation is advisable, and in most instances *operative intervention should be undertaken within the first 6 hours after the diagnosis is established.* In patients with chronic, partial (incomplete), or recurrent obstructions in which there is no evidence of vascular compromise (fever, tachycardia, elevated white blood cell [WBC] count, tenderness, gastrointestinal bleeding), a longer period of preparation and hydration may be advisable, and a long intestinal tube may prove useful. The use of long intestinal tubes (e.g., Miller-Abbott, Baker, Harris) as the principal treatment of intestinal obstruction is seldom advisable, and they should rarely be employed without surgical consultation and supervision.

ACUTE PANCREATITIS

method of
YNGVE EDLUND, M.D., PH.D.,
and TORE SCHERSTÉN, M.D.,
PH.D.
Göteborg, Sweden

The incidence of acute pancreatitis varies considerably between different countries. The same applies to the distribution of the most common etiologic factors. In most studies 60 to 80 per cent of the patients have either gallstones or a history of sustained alcohol abuse. Up to a decade ago, gallstone disease was commonly implicated. Recently, however, an increased incidence of pancreatitis associated with alcohol abuse has been reported from the United States of America and the Scandinavian countries. Hence, alcohol ingestion is now the major etiologic factor in patients with acute pancreatitis in these countries.

Pancreatitis associated with alcohol abuse tends to occur at a younger age than gallstone pancreatitis. The typical feature is recurring acute episodes. The first or second attack may be severe, including respiratory and cardiovascular failure, corresponding morphologically to necrotizing pancreatitis. The mortality rate during these primary attacks is significant, while it is negligible during later relapses. Patients with pancreatitis associated with gallstones are usually older and seldom have relapses. The mortality rate is relatively higher than in patients with alcoholic pancreatitis. The two most common types of pancreatitis, gallstone and alcoholic pancreatitis, can be considered as two different diseases with respect to pathogenesis and to some extent also as regards clinical features.

This presentation will be confined to a discussion of acute pancreatitis associated with alcohol abuse and biliary lithiasis. The treatment of acute pancreatitis associated with other etiologic factors, such as hyperlipoproteinemia, hypercalcemia, viral infection, corticosteroid and thiazide medications, and trauma, is primarily directed toward the cause but is otherwise similar to the treatment of alcoholic pancreatitis.

Clinical Course and Complications

Patients with acute pancreatitis show a wide spectrum of clinical illnesses. Many patients have a mild or moderate inflammatory reaction in the pancreas and recover uneventfully more or less independently of the conventional treatment consisting of nasogastric suction and intravenous fluid administration. Others rapidly develop a severe hemorrhagic pancreatic necrosis associated with serious respiratory, hypotensive, and septic complications which need intensive and specific treatment for patient survival. This means that early prognostic assessment to identify patients who have a high risk of developing serious or lethal complications is of the greatest importance.

Simple and accurate diagnostic criteria for pancreatitis do not exist today. However, there are some factors which may provide prognosis of the severity of the disease. At admission, the following variables suggest a severe attack: age above 50 years, history of no or only one previous episode, serum amylase values three times above normal levels, leukocytosis, and increased serum aminotransferases. The course during the first 24 to 48 hours after admission will give more positive evidence with respect to the severity of the episode. This is related to both the local abdominal sequelae and the general systemic manifestations of the disease. Proteolytic enzymes, trypsin, chymotrypsin, and elastase, as well as protease inhibitors, are released from the pancreas. Vasoactive polypeptides, such as bradykinin and histamine, and phospholipase are also released. It has been shown experimentally that an early and dramatic decrease in blood pressure occurs at the time when the protease inhibitors in the pancreatic exudate are fully saturated with enzymes. Saturation of the inhibitors is also followed by fibrinolysis and bleeding. Capillary damage may explain the tremendous losses of fluid and plasma proteins which occur in severe pancreatitis.

The circulatory shock in patients with severe pancreatitis is very complex and cannot be explained by hypovolemia alone. The finding of proteolytic enzyme and lipase activities in hemorrhagic peritoneal exudate indicates severe pancreatitis.

A pronounced decrease in the circulating blood volume and electrolyte losses may occur early in severe pancreatitis. Thus, hemoconcentration is initially a common feature. According to our experience, however, it is of minor prognostic significance. On the other hand, a rapid decrease in hematocrit during early treatment seems to correlate with the severity of the pancreatitis. Hypocalcemia during the initial 24 to 48 hours after diagnosis also seems to be related to the severity of the pancreatitis.

A decreased circulating blood volume results in hypotension, tachycardia, and decreased cardiac output. In some patients with acute pancreatitis, hypotension and hypoperfusion persist despite restoration of the intravascular volume. The mechanism of this cardiac failure is not known. It has been attributed to kinin formation by proteolytic enzymes or to a so-called myocardial depressant factor released from the pancreas or the intestines. Whatever the mechanism may be, this is a sign of a poor prognosis.

Respiratory complications in acute pancreatitis are common. The early occurrence of cyanosis, restlessness, tachypnea, and arterial hypoxemia, as well as an increased alveoloarterial oxygen gradient, indicates severe pancreatitis and a poor prognosis. Blood gas analyses often show an early mixed metabolic and respiratory alkalosis secondary to respiratory insufficiency and vomiting. This is not necessarily related to the severity of the pancreatitis. On the other hand, early metabolic acidosis, probably secondary to poor tissue perfusion, correlates significantly with the severity of the disease.

In severe acute pancreatitis, coagulation changes are often observed. There are correlations between the coagulation factor levels and respiratory, hepatic, and renal function impairment, suggesting that the clotting mechanism is involved in the pathogenesis of some systemic features of pancreatitis.

Hyperglycemia and hyperlipidemia are common in acute pancreatitis, especially when associated with alcohol abuse. The mechanism of these changes is probably a combination of islet cell dysfunction and peripheral insulin resistance. Insulin deficiency is associated with an increased lipolysis, which means a high flow of fatty acids from the periphery. This, in turn, causes increased blood viscosity, contributing to the impaired microcirculation. The fatty acid load on the liver is probably also the cause of the hepatic steatosis in acute pancreatitis. Hepatic dysfunction is clinically assessed by increased serum aminotransferases. These enzymes may be increased because of associated alcoholic hepatitis or biliary disease in patients with mild pancreatitis. However, in some groups of patients, the initial levels of these enzymes are correlated to the prognosis.

Medical Treatment

The principle that the patient should be treated initially with nonoperative measures is generally accepted. The primary objectives of treatment are: (1) to suppress the pancreatic inflammation, (2) to avoid complications by interrupting their pathogenesis, and (3) to treat complications as they arise.

To limit the severity of a pancreatic inflammation, it has been considered mandatory to reduce the metabolic and secretory activity of the pancreas, i.e., "put the pancreas to rest." This treatment includes complete fasting and also gastric suction medication with antacids, anticholinergics, aprotinin, glucagon, and calcitonin. The therapeutic efficacy of these measures has been questioned on the basis of controlled clinical studies. During recent years, we have not used medication with antibiotics, anticholinergics, aprotinin, and hormones such as glucagon, calcitonin, and somatostatin. Although the therapeutic role of nasogastric suction has been questioned, our clinical experience speaks in favor of this treatment. Our present practice, therefore, is to use nasogastric suction in all patients with acute pancreatitis and to maintain it until abdominal pain and tenderness have subsided and serum amylase levels are normalized. Antacid or cimetidine is given to decrease acid production and secretin release. In patients with mild acute pancreatitis, this treatment is usually enough. This means that in the vast majority of patients (70 to 80 per cent) the therapeutic problems are small.

So far no nonoperative therapeutic measure that is effective in reducing the severity of acute pancreatic inflammation has been described. In the absence of such specific measures to reduce or prevent complications of acute pancreatitis, the most important aspects of nonoperative treatment are supportive and symptomatic. It must be emphasized, however, that in this disease with its different causes and varied clinical manifestations, treatment must be individualized. Furthermore it should be kept in mind that surgery can be of importance in limiting the severity of pancreatitis or in interrupting the pathogenesis of complications (see below).

Supportive and symptomatic treatment involves measures to relieve pain, to restore and maintain respiratory and cardiovascular functions and electrolyte balance, and to prevent or limit metabolic host reactions.

The monitoring of circulating blood volume and cardiovascular function requires a central venous catheter and an indwelling urethral catheter for frequent measurements of central venous pressures, venous blood gases, and hourly urine output. Arterial blood gas values should be determined at least once a day. In patients with cardiac insufficiency, regardless of whether it is elicited by the pancreatitis or not, the monitoring of pulmonary arterial pressures by means of a Swan-Ganz catheter may be essential for the balance between fluid administration and medication with cardiac inotropic agents.

Intravascular volume and adequate urinary output usually can be satisfactorily restored and maintained by the administration of crystalloid and colloid solutions. Which colloid solution is the best in this situation has been debated. From a theoretical point of view, plasma may be better than other colloid solutions, since it contains protease inhibitors. Apart from determinations of central venous pressure and urinary output, serial measurements of the hematocrit are helpful to determine the amount of fluid to be given as well as the possible need of blood transfusions.

Sodium and potassium replacements are required. Replacements of calcium and magnesium are also recommended, although symptoms and complications directly related to hypocalcemia and hypomagnesemia are uncommon.

As mentioned above, enhanced lipolysis in adipose tissue resulting from insulin resistance or deficiency and release of catecholamines is common in acute pancreatitis. It has been suggested that fat necroses may be caused by factors activating the hormone-sensitive lipase in the adipose tissue. Insulin resistance and/or deficiency in combinations with catecholamines leads to hyperglycemia. These metabolic host reactions can be counteracted by the administration of insulin and glucose. The insulin dose can be regulated with close monitoring of blood glucose levels.

Respiratory failure is frequent in patients with acute pancreatitis. In the early phase, this respiratory failure can be subclinical. Therefore, it is essential that arterial blood gas values be determined regularly. Early hypoxemia may be lethal if it is untreated. Respiratory insufficiency can be enhanced by a fluid overload. In patients who are in progressive respiratory insufficiency, endotracheal intubation and respirator support should be instituted early. Indications for intubation and assisted respiration are a 50 per cent decrease in the arterial oxygen tension and a breathing rate of more than 30 per minute.

Surgical Treatment

The reason for surgical intervention in acute pancreatitis may be diagnostic or therapeutic. According to our view, early surgery is required only if it is clinically difficult to differentiate acute pancreatitis from other intra-abdominal catastrophes such as mesenteric infarction, perforated cholecystitis, or perforated ulcer.

It has been suggested that early biliary surgery may limit the severity of acute pancreatitis. Our experience does not support this view, and we recommend that biliary surgery be deferred until the signs of acute pancreatitis have subsided. The finding of pancreatitis with gallstones at early exploratory laparotomy does not necessarily mean that definitive biliary surgery should be performed. In patients with necrotizing pancreatitis, it is usually better to limit the operation to placement of drainage and lavage catheters.

Our own experience with early pancreatic resection or total pancreatectomy is very limited. However, we have no indications that these procedures lead to a reduced morbidity or mortality.

Patients with persistent or recurrent fever and leukocytosis after 10 to 20 days of treatment usually have an infected pancreatic abscess. Surgical exploration is necessary in these cases, and a wide drainage of the peripancreatic retroperitoneum should be instituted.

Concluding Remarks

The treatment results in patients with severe acute pancreatitis have improved in the last few years. This improvement, however, has nothing to do with specific treatment aimed at limiting the severity of the pancreatic inflammation. Instead, the improvement can be ascribed entirely to supportive and symptomatic treatment. It is due to the general improvement in the intensive care of severely ill patients.

The causative mechanisms of acute pancreatitis are not yet fully understood. This area presents a challenge not only to our understanding of the metabolic events in the early development of pancreatitis but also to our knowledge of factors controlling the severity of the disease. We will not have a basis for specific prophylaxis and therapy until the underlying mechanisms of pancreatitis have been clarified.

CHRONIC PANCREATITIS

method of
HENRY M. MIDDLETON, III,
M.D.
Augusta, Georgia

Chronic pancreatitis is characterized pathologically by loss of acinar and islet tissue, scarring, and ductular abnormalities with stricture, dilatation, and stone formation. Associated with these abnormalities is a loss of exocrine (acinar) and endocrine (islet) function. Clinically it may present as pain, malabsorption, diabetes, and pancreatic calcification. In the United States the majority of cases are related to alcohol abuse. Gallbladder disease is more associated with true acute pancreatitis and probably infrequently leads to the chronic form. Other causes of chronic pancreatitis, though of low incidence in the United States, include hyperparathyroidism, hemochromatosis, cystic fibrosis, trauma, malnutrition, and hereditary pancreatitis. In about 20 per cent of cases, the cause is not known. The management of chronic pancreatitis may be divided into four main areas: (1) diagnostic evaluation, (2) correction of malabsorption, (3) regulation of diabetes, and (4) control of pain.

Diagnostic Evaluation

On the initial evaluation other causes of chronic pancreatitis should be ruled out by appropriate clinical tests. Because a majority of cases will be due to chronic alcoholism, a careful history of alcohol ingestion should be obtained. Since it is often uncertain whether the first acute episode of pain represents true acute pancreatitis or simply the first clinical manifestation of an underlying chronic pancreatitis, evaluation of the biliary tract is mandatory to rule out cholelithiasis. The most useful tests include ultrasound and the oral cholecystogram (gallbladder series). Traditionally, nonvisualization of the gallbladder in the aftermath of a clinical exacerbation of pancreatitis has been said to be common. Therefore, conventional wisdom has dictated that nonvisualization should not be interpreted as demonstrating gallbladder disease for at least 6 weeks after the acute event. More recent data, however, suggest that this failure to visualize in the convalescent period is largely eliminated by making certain that the oral cholecystogram is done after the patient has resumed his regular diet.

Malabsorption

Malabsorption of fat and protein is due to inadequate secretion of digestive enzymes by the diseased pancreas and occurs after 90 per cent of acinar function is lost. Therapy consists of the oral administration of pancreatic preparations high in lipase and proteolytic enzyme activity. Examples include pancrelipase (Ilozyme, Ku-Zyme HP, Cotazym) and pancreatin (Viokase). Enteric-coated tablets are reported to have poorer bioavailability than the non-enteric-coated tablet preparations. In contrast, enteric-coated microspheres of pancrelipase (Pancrease) are reported to yield significantly better fat utilization and significantly decreased stool frequency when compared to conventional pancreatic enzyme preparations. Selection of one product over another will depend upon costs, local availability, and physician and/or patient preference. Initial therapy may reasonably consist of 2 or 3 tablets or capsules (or equivalent powders mixed with water or sprinkled over food) with each meal and snack. If response is inadequate, several options may be tried. First, the total dosage of the pancreatic preparation may be increased, with the higher doses given at mealtimes only or with the total amount divided into hourly doses while awake. In some patients, hourly enzyme replacement may be superior to administration only with meals. Second, an attempt may be made to raise the duodenal intraluminal pH in patients in whom it is low owing to inadequate pancreatic bicarbonate secretion. It is hoped that such an increase in pH will enhance replacement enzyme activity. Some patients will be helped; some will not. Agents which may be effective in this regard include sodium bicarbonate, antacids, and cimetidine (not a specifically approved indication for this drug). Third, the amount of fat in the diet may be decreased and isocalorically replaced with carbohydrate, protein, or medium-chain triglycerides.

Response to enzyme replacement may be measured both biochemically by 72 hour stool fat determinations and clinically by follow-up of changes in weight, character and frequency of bowel movements, and well-being of the patient. An optimal regimen from a practical point of view is one which corrects or adequately improves the biochemical and clinical parameters listed above with the simplest measures compatible with such a response.

Diabetes

If diabetes is present, it is treated similarly to the inherited disease. Although it may be reasonable to attempt initial control of mild hyperglycemia with oral hypoglycemic agents, insulin will usually be required for management. Some patients seem particularly sensitive to small changes in insulin doses and may demonstrate wide swings in serum glucose. Management may be complicated in part by changes in the efficiency of intestinal absorption related to the underlying malabsorptive process and to variations in the timing and/or dosage of pancreatic enzyme replacement. In such cases, hypoglycemia is a risk, and control of serum glucose may best be kept somewhat loose, permitting some degree of hyperglycemia. Control is not as good, but the risk of hypoglycemia should be correspondingly lessened.

Pain

Pain often is the most difficult problem of all. It may be severe and debilitating; often it is the complaint most frequently and emphatically expressed by the patient. Its relief may be elusive, and its persistence, in spite of multiple therapeutic trials, may try the patience and endurance of patient and physician alike. The cornerstone of therapy is total abstinence from alcohol; without such abstinence pain will probably continue, and little else is likely to give really satisfactory clinical resolution. Over time, the pain may decrease or even disappear in a significant percentage of patients in spite of continued alcohol consumption, probably because of a progressive destruction of remaining pancreatic tissue.

During clinical relapses associated with the acute onset of abdominal pain, nausea, and vomiting, with or without serum amylase elevations, therapy is that of acute pancreatitis with nasogastric suction, intravenous fluids, and analgesics. For more chronic complaints of pain, various non-narcotic preparations may be used. Since the risk of narcotic addiction is high in this population, the use of narcotics is best limited or avoided whenever possible. Pancreatic enzyme preparations also may be tried in a manner similar to their use for malabsorption. The object is to attempt to decrease endogenous pancreatic enzyme production and release. Such therapy appears to be of significant benefit in the relief of pain in certain patients.

The role of surgery in chronic pancreatitis (assuming that cholelithiasis has been ruled out) is primarily in the relief of intractable pain unresponsive to medical management. If the patient continues to drink, however, surgery is likely to be followed by persisting pain; continued alcohol consumption, therefore, is felt by many to preclude surgery. Thus, more specifically, the role of surgery in chronic pancreatitis is in the relief of intractable pain in the patient who has stopped drinking. The procedures advocated have included distal pancreatectomy for localized disease in that area, longitudinal Roux-Y pancreaticojejunostomy (Puestow procedure), and 95 per cent pancreatectomy. The 95 per cent pancreatectomy leads to an insulin-dependent diabetes which appears to have a high complication rate (hypoglycemia and hyperglycemia) in patients who continue to consume alcohol. Since disease is usually generalized rather than localized, and since it is desirable to use less radical procedures to accomplish an ideally similar end, the Puestow procedure is a reasonable choice for initial surgical management. Gastric surgery has been advocated in the past in an attempt to control pain by decreasing acid stimulation of the pancreas. There seems little value in such procedures, however. In a patient who already has pancreatic malabsorption, the malabsorptive tendencies that follow gastric surgery may only compound the problem. The result may be worse than the original problem.

PEPTIC ULCER

method of
FRANK J. BAUMEISTER, JR., M.D.
Portland, Oregon

A confirmed diagnosis of peptic ulcer disease generally heralds a lifetime diathesis with subsequent periodic flare-ups, and although an ulcer is usually only a minor disability, the potential exists for serious complications. The diagnosis should therefore be established with certainty prior to applying a diagnostic label and committing the patient to any therapeutic regimen. The pathophysiology of peptic ulcer is incompletely understood, but an imbalance between aggressive acid-peptic factors and intrinsic mucosal defenses has traditionally been implicated. Although mean acid secretory levels are higher in patients with peptic ulcer than in normal persons, there is considerable overlap, and sufficient numbers of patients develop an ulcer despite normal acid secretion to incriminate other mechanisms. The cause of peptic ulcer pain is similarly imperfectly explained, the simplistic explanation blaming the caustic effect of gastric acid on nerve endings in the ulcer crater, possibly with resultant local mural muscle spasm. Recent studies utilizing endoscopic surveillance have demonstrated poor correlation between the presence of an ulcer crater and the existence of ulcer pain, many patients continuing to experience typical ulcer distress despite ulcer healing, while many others become pain free despite persistence of a demonstrable crater. Nevertheless, the ulcer crater is a critical stage of chronic acid-peptic disease, during which symptoms may be severe and the complications of hemorrhage, perforation, or obstruction may occur.

Therapy therefore aims at healing the ulcer crater as quickly as possible and thereafter ideally preventing its recurrence. It is difficult to evaluate therapy in a disease with such an unpredictable course, in which symptoms wax and wane without rhyme or reason, even in the absence of any treatment. Lack of clear understanding of pathogenetic mechanisms is but one ingredient in the confusion. Another is the rather remarkable effect of placebo therapy both on pain relief and on healing time. Consequently, ulcer therapy historically has been empirical, founded upon traditional assumptions, some of which, with the passage of time, may become less tenable. With the recent development of the histamine H_2 receptor antagonists, ulcer therapy has come under scrutiny like never before, and endoscopic confirmation of diagnosis and response to treatment have been the common denominator of numerous controlled studies comparing various therapies, including placebo, antacids, and the H_2 receptor antagonist cimetidine. Plentiful data now appearing from such investigations are shedding new light on this old malady, and, ideally, further enlightenment will lead us to a rational, standardized therapeutic regimen based upon sound scientific principles.

Physician-Patient Relationship

A careful and thorough interview and physical examination by a concerned, compassionate physician initiate the therapeutic process. Judging by the profound placebo effect reported in all controlled studies to date, the doctor-patient interaction alone may be sufficient to relieve symptoms and promote healing in a significant number of patients with an ulcer. The diagnosis should be confirmed, utilizing endoscopy if radiology is not definitive, while excluding other, more sinister causes of upper abdominal misery. Once assured of the diagnosis, the physician can then proceed with therapy confidently and enthusiastically, educating the patient regarding the nature of the disease and the rationale of therapy while giving reassurance regarding the usual benign prognosis of an ulcer. The probability of expected recurrences can be discussed, and a plan of future action can be outlined, the goal of which should be to abort subsequent flare-ups and minimize the intrusion of the disease into the patient's life. The salutary effects of such a supportive relationship cannot be easily measured or objectively evaluated but undoubtedly play a beneficial role in management.

Reduction of Gastric Acid

Gastric acid reduction is the essential physiologic goal of current peptic ulcer management, and this end may be accomplished by either decreasing acid secretion (H_2 histamine receptor antagonists, anticholinergics, gastric surgery, gastric irradiation) or neutralizing intraluminal gastric acid (antacids).

H_2 Histamine Receptor Antagonists. The H_2 histamine receptor antagonist cimetidine (Tagamet) was approved for clinical use in the United States in 1977, with almost immediate enthusiastic acceptance and subsequent continued zealous use. Available in tablet form, cimetidine is preferred by patients to liquid antacid preparations, and the bowel disturbance so common with antacid regimens is not a problem with the drug. In all probability, the characteristic dramatic and rapid alleviation of symptoms makes believers of the patients themselves, thereby further encouraging adherence to a treatment plan. The beneficial effects of short-term treatment with cimetidine have been amply demonstrated by prompt pain relief and more rapid ulcer healing (70 to 80 per cent at 6 weeks) when compared with a placebo (40 to 60 per cent at 6 weeks). Prevention of ulcer recurrence has also been documented during maintenance therapy trials, the longest thus far reported extending to only 1 year. Only 15 to 25 per cent of patients with healed duodenal ulcers redevelop an ulcer while receiving cimetidine, 300 mg twice daily, whereas 75 to 100 per cent of such patients treated with a placebo suffer a recurrence during the same period of time (1 year). Unfortunately, the natural history and subsequent course of peptic ulcer disease appear to be unaltered by prolonged therapy, and recurrences are the rule following cessation of treatment. At least 50 per cent of patients will relapse within 1 year after discontinuing the drug.

The mechanism of action of cimetidine is blockage of the H_2 receptor sites for histamine on the gastric parietal cell. One theory considers histamine to be the final common path involved in acid secretion, regardless of the initiating stimulus. An alternate theory postulates individual receptors for each of the gastric secretagogues (gastrin, histamine, and acetylcholine), interaction of one with its receptor potentiating or increasing the affinity of the other sites for their respective secretagogue. Whatever the specific mechanism, cimetidine reduces basal acid secretion 90 per cent for 5 to 7 hours after a single dose and reduces meal-stimulated acid secretion 70 per cent over a 3 hour period.

Cimetidine is supplied as 200 and 300 mg tablets and in vials containing 300 mg per 2 ml for parenteral use. The drug is well absorbed from the small intestine, achieving peak blood levels within 60 to 90 minutes following an oral dose. Administration orally with meals delays absorption with resultant prolongation of action. The drug is rapidly excreted by the kidney, and with renal failure the normal serum half life of 1.5 to 2.0 hours is increased to 3.5 hours. The drug is dialyzable, and doses must be adjusted accordingly. The usual dose for peptic ulcer is 300 mg four times daily, with meals and at bedtime. In hypersecretory states (Zollinger-Ellison syndrome) doubling of the dose may be required. In renal impairment the dose is usually halved to 300 mg every 12 hours. The parenteral route may be utilized as needed.

Thus far, short-term therapy with cimetidine has been well tolerated. There may be mild, transient elevations of serum creatinine and amino transferase levels, and slight decreases in white blood count have been reported. There has been concern over reports of diminished libido and impotence, and raised serum gonadotropin levels have been seen and attributed to an antiandrogen effect. Gynecomastia is not rare, especially with larger doses and prolonged use, and an occasional skin rash is seen. Potentiation of warfarin is expected, and therapeutic doses of cimetidine can prolong the prothrombin time approximately 20 per cent. Central nervous system (CNS) disturbances have occurred in elderly patients and patients with renal impairment resulting in acute dementia or toxic psychosis. To date, all adverse effects have proved to be easily and rapidly reversible. Almost nothing is known about the consequences of long-term exposure to cimetidine. Suppression of gastric acidity alters gastric flora, and increased bacterial counts with a shift toward "fecal flora" have been documented during treatment. Theories projecting potential for increased risk of gastric malignancy in long-term treated patients would appear to be highly speculative at this time, and data from long-term, high dose animal experiments do not support such anxiety.

Anticholinergics. Anticholinergic drugs have been included in every suggested peptic ulcer regimen, even after Bachrach's thorough review in 1958 concluded that there was no convincing evidence to support their continued use. In recent years enthusiasm for anticholinergics has justifiably waned, but they are sometimes still used in combination with other agents or prescribed at bedtime for prevention of nocturnal pain.

Anticholinergics competitively inhibit the action of acetylcholine on structures innervated by postganglionic cholinergic nerves and on smooth muscles that respond to acetylcholine. The specific receptor site for acetylcholine on the parietal cell is presumably also competitively blocked, diminishing the synergistic interaction of acetylcholine with the other gastric secretagogues. Given before meals anticholinergics prolong and potentiate the effect of postprandial antacids, and small doses of anticholinergic potentiate the inhibitory effect of cimetidine on food-stimulated acid secretion. Anticholinergics alone can reduce basal acid secretion 50 per cent and meal-stimulated acid secretion 30 per cent. Unfortunately, generalized inhibition of parasympathetic function is inevitable, with resultant bothersome side effects which limit usefulness. Dry mouth, blurred vision, urinary retention, gastric retention, and intestinal atony with bloating are commonly noted, and precipitation of acute glaucoma is a risk. No endoscopically controlled studies have thus far addressed anticholinergic therapy, and previous data are unreliable.

When anticholinergics are used, the usual regimen employs one of innumerable available preparations, initially at low dosage, with subsequent incremental increases until minimal side effects are experienced. The dosage is then slightly lowered to maintain the maximal therapeutic dose without side effects.

At this time anticholinergic drugs should be assigned but a limited role in ulcer therapy. Used adjunctly with antacids or H_2 histamine receptor antagonists, they may occasionally be helpful, but there is no justification for their promotion as primary agents.

Gastric Irradiation. Gastric irradiation is a potentially useful, highly effective, relatively safe, and little appreciated method for treating peptic ulcer in poor risk patients. At least brief mention of the technique is warranted here, since considerable experience has now been gained by groups in Chicago and Baltimore with publication of impressive results. The rationale is that radiation injury of the parietal cells significantly reduces gastric acid secretion, and the method has proved to be very effective in accomplishing this goal. A single course of 2000 rads administered to the fundal, acid secreting portion of the stomach via anterior and posterior fields, 100 rads per field daily, effects a sustained, significant reduction of basal and stimulated acid secretion. Treatment is well tolerated and essentially without immediate side effects, and the incidence of ulcer recurrence is low (10 per cent). Although radiation nephritis has developed in a few patients after prolonged follow-up, restricting such therapy to the elderly minimizes the threat of this complication. In this "cimetidine era" of peptic ulcer therapy history, such treatment may be considered drastic and outmoded. However, in the occasional aged and infirm patient absolutely intolerant of cimetidine and unresponsive to conventional therapy, gastric irradiation may be a worthwhile alternative to surgery.

Antacids. Antacids traditionally have been the mainstay of therapy in peptic ulcer disease, but surprisingly few controlled investigations have objectively addressed the question of their efficacy. With the current interest generated by the arrival of H_2 histamine receptor antagonists on the scene and Food and Drug Administration (FDA) emphasis on controlled trials with endoscopic confirmation and surveillance, we are learning a great deal about antacid therapy as well. The rationale of antacid use is, of course, neutralization of secreted hydrochloric acid and prevention of pepsin activation. Effective therapy should relieve pain promptly, speed ulcer healing, and prevent recurrence. Several studies have failed to show superiority of antacids over placebos in relief of ulcer pain, and in the occasional study favoring antacids, the placebo success has generally been of such magnitude to minimize the benefit of medication. It does appear that antacids in full therapeutic doses do promote ulcer healing with about the same success as cimetidine (70 to 80 per cent healed at 6 weeks). Here again, however, as is the case with cimetidine, the race with placebo therapy is a close one. Chronic maintenance antacid therapy to prevent recurrence has not been well evaluated by current standards, and that issue remains unsettled.

Liquid preparations neutralize more acid than comparable doses in tablet form and are therefore preferred. Well absorbed antacids (calcium preparations and sodium bicarbonate) are superior neutralizing agents but should probably be avoided because of their adverse metabolic effects. Nonabsorbable products, usually aluminum-magnesium combinations, are therefore favored for long-term use, although they are not totally innocuous. Aluminum hydroxide binds phosphate in the small intestine and may induce phosphate depletion. Aluminum preparations are constipating, while magnesium commonly produces diarrhea. Aluminum-magnesium mixtures may avoid bowel disturbance, but they can interfere with the absorption of other drugs such as digoxin, tetracycline, and chlorpromazine. Problems of palatability and side effects notwithstanding, antacids do, however, effectively neutralize gastric acidity when administered in adequate, therapeutic doses. The recommended dose schedule consists of 30 ml of a standard, high potency antacid, given 1 and 3 hours after meals and at bedtime.

Mucosal Resistance

Mucosal resistance can be undermined by a number of commonly prescribed agents, particularly salicylates and the nonsteroidal antiinflammatory agents (e.g., indomethacin, ibuprofen, naproxen). Salicylates increase gastric mucosal permeability with resultant back-diffusion of acid, mucosal disruption, and local erosion or ulceration. Bleeding may ensue, facilitated by the anticoagulant effect (platelet dysfunction) of salicylates. Nonsteroidal anti-inflammatory drugs remove prostaglandin-supported "cytoprotective" defenses with similar mucosal injury. Corticosteroids, on the other hand, rarely produce endoscopically detectable mucosal injuries. The role of the aforementioned agents in chronic peptic ulcer disease is unknown, but all have been at least circumstantially incriminated in exacerbations and complications of chronic ulcer and should be avoided. Phenylbutazone has been similarly blamed without sufficient incriminating data, but it would seem prudent to avoid using the drug in patients with peptic ulcer until its safety is verified. Prostaglandins have been shown to protect the gastric mucosa by unknown mechanisms other than their known inhibition of acid secretion. This is certainly a fertile area for future research which offers great promise.

Behavior Modification

Behavior modification has traditionally been emphasized in the treatment of peptic ulcer, especially dietary restriction and the avoidance of unwholesome habits such as smoking and drinking. Diet is no longer regulated, since neither the quality nor the quantity of food ingested has been shown to have any bearing on the course of peptic ulcer disease. Current consensus recommends a liberal diet with avoidance of only those foods which are thought by the patient to consistently cause distress. There is no evidence to incriminate spices, "hot" or "rich" foods, coffee, or alcohol in the genesis, perpetuation, or exacerbation of peptic ulcer. Smoking remains a question mark. Tobacco smoking produces a number of gastrointestinal pathophysiologic effects, including delayed gastric emptying, decreased pyloric sphincter pressure, increased duodenogastric reflux, inhibition of secretin-stimulated pancreatic bicarbonate secretion, and lowered duodenal bulb pH. Peptic ulcer is more common in smokers than in nonsmokers. Whether the enumerated physiologic effects are responsible, or whether there are unknown factors responsible for both the ulcer diathesis and the tendency to smoke heavily, it would seem prudent to judge cigarette smoking harshly. As K. G. Wormsley concluded in a recent editorial, "We may dislike smoking by patients with duodenal ulcer, but we have no compelling reason for stopping them — yet!"

Gastric Ulcer

Gastric ulcer deserves special mention for several reasons. First is the potential for malignancy which demands endoscopy with biopsy and cytologic diagnosis. Second is the possible etiologic role of anti-inflammatory drugs, particularly aspirin. If aspirin ingestion is incriminated, mere abstinence thereafter might be sufficient to prevent further ulceration indefinitely, there being no true diathesis.

Recommended Regimen

The recommended regimen for peptic ulcer can be summarized as follows:

1. The concerned, compassionate physician is the essential ingredient in any regimen (recall the remarkable placebo effect), and treatment actually begins with the initial physician-patient interaction. Accurate diagnosis is absolutely critical. Reassurance and education of the patient are combined with exploration of emotional factors and conflicts. Provide ample ventilation of frustrations and support the patient in his coping attempts.

2. Prescribe cimetidine (Tagamet), 300 mg four times daily, with meals and at bedtime, or a standard, high potency antacid, 30 ml 1 and 3 hours after each meal and at bedtime, to hasten ulcer healing. Convenience and ease of administration, palatability and patient acceptance, effectiveness, and low incidence of side effects during short-term treatment all tend to favor cimetidine. Antacids, however, are time honored and may be preferred. Continue therapy for 6 to 8 weeks to assure total healing (around 90 per cent).

3. Caution the patient to avoid salicylate in any form, as well as all arthritis remedies. Encourage a liberal, balanced diet, moderation in alcohol consumption, and cessation of smoking if practicable.

4. At the conclusion of the first course of therapy all medication should be stopped. One should recall that peptic ulcer disease is, in general, a minor illness, and subsequent management must be tailored to the subsequent clinical course. Most ulcers recur, but many recurrences are asymptomatic, do not lead to complications, and are, therefore, of little consequence. However, should an ulcer soon recur symptomatic and again confirmed, then cimetidine or antacids should be again administered at full therapeutic doses and continued for sufficient duration to allow healing again (6 to 8 weeks). At this juncture a decision must be made whether to continue to treat expected periodic flare-ups with short-term (6 to 8 weeks) courses of therapy (either

cimetidine or antacids are acceptable), or whether to recommend maintenance cimetidine or possibly a definite surgical procedure. Maintenance cimetidine has not been studied for longer than 1 year, and although its effectiveness during such extended periods of observation seems proved, the natural history and subsequent course of peptic ulcer disease following cessation of therapy are unchanged, with subsequent recurrences the rule rather than the exception. Since little is known of the long-term side effects or potential toxicity of cimetidine, it would seem rational to recommend surgical intervention for the younger patient suffering from virulent ulcer disease punctuated by frequent, disabling flare-ups or complications. Continual cimetidine treatment at a dose of 300 mg twice daily might be justified in an aged, infirm patient considered a poor surgical risk or in a younger patient with other serious complicating or coexisting disease. The older patient could be offered the acceptable alternative of gastric irradiation. Perhaps someday in the near future indefinite maintenance therapy with either cimetidine or a safety-assured analogue will be feasible, but current data are insufficient to justify such a stance.

TUMORS OF THE STOMACH

method of
DAVID STATE, M.D.
Torrance, California

Benign Tumors

The most frequently occurring benign gastric neoplasms are (1) leiomyomas, (2) neurofibromas, and (3) polyps.

Leiomyoma and Neurofibroma. All extramucosal benign gastric tumors, i.e., leiomyomas and neurofibromas, should be excised because (1) a differential diagnosis from a malignant tumor can only be made when the neoplasm has been examined microscopically, and (2) malignant transformation occurs sufficiently frequently to warrant removal on this basis alone. When the tumor is small, local excision, including an inch of adjacent normal stomach wall, is sufficient. The tumor should be subjected to frozen section, and if malignant a subtotal gastric resection is indicated. Similarly, if the original lesion is large or if the lesion at laparotomy is very suspicious grossly, then extensive resection, even including total

gastrectomy, is indicated. The prognosis of these extramucosal lesions is very good, even when malignant transformation has occurred, and hence an aggressive surgical attack is indicated.

Polyp (Adenoma). The most common benign mucosal lesion is gastric polyp or adenoma. Usually this lesion is asymptomatic or at most produces ill-defined mild gastric disorder. On occasion, however, this tumor may produce clear-cut symptoms of obstruction and bleeding.

Considerable controversy surrounds appropriate therapy for this tumor. The essential problem relates to reported incidence of malignant transformation of this neoplasm. In a study conducted by the author and Dr. L. Hay at the University of Minnesota, it was found that in 54 patients having adenoma less than 1 cm in diameter, only one was malignant. In 29 patients with adenomatous tumors whose greatest diameter ranged from 1 to 2 cm, none was malignant. Of 13 polyps larger than 2 cm in diameter, seven were malignant.

NONOPERATIVE THERAPY. No surgery is recommended for (1) patients who are asymptomatic and whose polyps are less than 2.0 cm in diameter and appear benign to the gastroscopist and radiologist or (2) elderly patients who are poor surgical risks.

In these patients the tumors are observed roentgenologically every 4 months for the first year and then biannually. Any change in symptoms or size or shape of the neoplasms indicates the need for operative treatment.

OPERATIVE THERAPY. The following groups of patients are urged to have surgery: (1) patients with polyps larger than 2.0 cm; (2) patients with overt clinical symptoms; (3) patients with polyps smaller than 2.0 cm but whose radiologic and gastroscopic characteristics, including biopsy, suggest malignant transformation; and (4) patients who refuse or who are unable to accept adequate follow-up.

When surgery is decided upon, extensive gastric resection (75 to 85 per cent gastric resection) rather than polypectomy should be carried out. Removal of a polyp alone is insufficient, as it may be malignant; in addition, local removal is followed by a high recurrence rate. The one major exception to this policy is when the polyp is in the cardia of the stomach. Rather than proceed with a total gastrectomy, local removal of the polyp is recommended with immediate frozen section and histologic examination. If the polyp is benign and solitary, polypectomy with removal of 2.0 cm rim of normal mucosa is carried out. If the tumor is malignant, then a total gastrectomy must be performed.

Malignant Tumors of the Stomach

The two most frequently occurring primary malignant tumors of the stomach are carcinoma and lymphosarcoma.

Carcinoma. For reasons not understood, gastric carcinoma has shown a decreasing incidence over the last 20 years. The average physician thus will rarely see more than one or two such patients per year. Based on past experience and impression, the physician feels that gastric cancer is a hopeless condition and that little other than symptomatic palliative treatment is in order. If this article does nothing more than clear up this misunderstanding, it will have served an important purpose. Studies from a number of medical centers clearly show that appropriate surgery can bring about both significant survival and palliation. Of 100 patients, approximately 80 should be amenable to exploratory laparotomy. In this group the gastric neoplasm should be sufficiently well localized to permit resection in 60 patients. The mortality rate should not exceed 5 per cent. For those patients who have resection and survive, approximately 25 per cent will live 5 or more years free of the disease. If the tumor is confined to the stomach without regional lymph node metastases or direct invasion of adjacent organs, the 5 year survival is approximately 60 per cent.

It is apparent, therefore, that every effort should be made to arrive at a diagnosis of gastric cancer as quickly as possible. Patients with vague gastric symptoms, unexplained anemia, and occult blood in the stool, and those with a strong family history of gastric cancer, should have gastric roentgenograms. To this group should be added patients with pernicious anemia (even though under adequate therapy) and males over the age of 45 who are found on routine examination to have histamine-fast achlorhydria. These patients should be subjected to biannual x-ray studies of the stomach. Any suspicious gastric lesion should be aggressively investigated, and if gastric cancer cannot categorically be ruled out, then laparotomy should be recommended.

Primary Lymphosarcoma of the Stomach. These tumors make up approximately 3 per cent of all primary malignant tumors. Those that are of the round cell (lymphocytic) type are radiosensitive and can be cured either by surgical removal or by radiation. From the practical point of view, the diagnosis can be made only at operation, so that the decision as to which form of therapy should be employed is usually predicated on the extent of tumor at surgery. If it is well localized and in a position where a subtotal gastrectomy can be carried out, then this is to be preferred. If the tumor is more extensive or in a position (i.e., cardia) where a total gastrectomy would be necessary, then a biopsy is taken, the diagnosis is established, and x-ray radiation therapy is employed. With either form of therapy, the outlook is surprisingly good, with 30 to 40 per cent of the patients surviving 5 or more years.

The more radioresistant reticulum cell lymphosarcoma can be cured only by surgical extirpation. As in other types of malignant tumors, the success depends on the resectability of the tumor and whether there are lymph node or more distant metastases. All too often with this particular neoplasm, the outlook is grim indeed.

Palliation for Malignant Gastric Tumors. Despite exhortation for an aggressive attitude toward early diagnosis and treatment of gastric malignancies, all too frequently the role of the physician is one of providing worthwhile palliation to the patient. In this regard, the physician should know that the most effective form of palliation rests with surgical extirpation even though the extent of disease precludes a cure. When the main bulk of the tumor can be removed, periods of comfortable survival for as long as 12 to 15 months are the rule rather than the exception. What about the unfortunate patient whose disease is beyond surgical excision? The task is a most difficult one for the patient, his family, and the physician. First it should be remembered that external x-ray irradiation and chemotherapy have little to offer and may make the patient sicker and more uncomfortable. Judicious use of pain-relieving drugs and the clear exposition on the part of the physician that, even though he can do little, he is interested and cares will permit the patient to bear the trying terminal period of life with as much equanimity and dignity as possible.

TUMORS OF THE COLON AND RECTUM

method of
SIDNEY J. WINAWER, M.D.,
and PAUL SHERLOCK, M.D.
New York, New York

Management of colorectal tumors includes the following concepts: screening; diagnosis in symptomatic patients and in asymptomatic patients with positive screening tests; surgery; follow-up surveillance after surgery; chemotherapy; radiation therapy; and other supportive measures such as nutritional support.

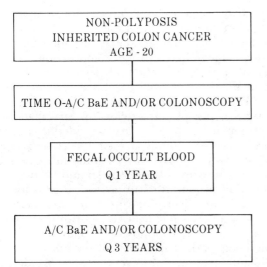

```
┌─────────────────────────────────┐
│         NON-POLYPOSIS            │
│     INHERITED COLON CANCER       │
│            AGE - 20              │
└─────────────────────────────────┘
                 │
┌─────────────────────────────────┐
│  TIME O-A/C BaE AND/OR COLONOSCOPY │
└─────────────────────────────────┘
                 │
┌─────────────────────────────────┐
│       FECAL OCCULT BLOOD         │
│            Q 1 YEAR              │
└─────────────────────────────────┘
                 │
┌─────────────────────────────────┐
│    A/C BaE AND/OR COLONOSCOPY     │
│            Q 3 YEARS             │
└─────────────────────────────────┘
```

Figure 1. Proposed algorithm for screening patients with a family history of non-polyposis inherited colonic cancer. Since fecal occult blood testing appears to have low sensitivity for detecting adenomas, the colon must be cleared of premalignant adenomas by direct visualization. The value of the barium enema has been questioned because of the young age at which screening begins, with possible periodic accumulative radiation exposure during repeated screening. The barium enema could be justified along with the colonoscopy initially on the basis that initially the screening is for cancers as well as adenomas. (Reprinted with the permission of the publishers of Harrison's Updates of Internal Medicine [in press].)

Inherited Colonic Cancer

In patients who have a family history of familial polyposis we prefer to do sigmoidoscopy once a year to see whether they are affected. Once patients with familial polyposis have had a diagnosis made that they are affected, they must be prepared psychologically for surgery and, at some time soon after the diagnosis is made, be subjected to a colectomy. There is great controversy as to whether this should be a total colectomy or a subtotal colectomy. A subtotal colectomy is appropriate, providing a small rectal segment with an end-to-end anastomosis of the ileum to the rectum. These patients, of course, must be kept under very close surveillance, with fulguration of additional polyps that develop. We continue to follow them by sigmoidoscopy every 6 months. It is interesting that in some patients who have had this procedure, some polyps remaining in the rectum after surgery have disappeared.

In patients who have had the nonpolyposis inherited colonic cancer family history, surveillance should be started at age 20 (Fig. 1). When we first start surveillance in this group of patients we usually do a double-contrast barium enema and colonoscopy to clear the colon of any adenomas and cancers. After this we like to get the patient back about every 3 years to check the colon once again, but at this time and for every 3 years thereafter we use only colonoscopy, since we are looking primarily for the adenomas that may appear after the colon has been initially cleared completely. The low sensitivity of the barium enema for adenomas, especially of the small type, makes it less desirable for use in periodic screening of these patients. In addition, since we begin screening these patients at a young age, we feel that the accumulative radiation exposure of periodic screening with the barium enema does not justify this approach. There is, of course, a potential complication rate of colonoscopy as well in these patients, but this has been shown to be extremely small, especially in well-type ambulatory people. We use Hemoccult (SmithKline Diagnostics, Sunnyvale, Calif.) slide testing annually in these patients as an interval examination along with the hemoglobin and an office visit.

Ulcerative Colitis

In patients with ulcerative colitis our approach is to begin surveillance after they have had universal colitis for 7 years, with annual colonoscopy. We perform the colonoscopy to the cecum, and on withdrawal of the colonoscope take multiple biopsies from the cecum and ascending colon, hepatic flexure, transverse colon, splenic flexure, descending colon, sigmoid, and rectum. We do this looking for dysplasia, and we mark the pathology slip to the attention of a single pathologist with whom we are working on this problem. If moderate or severe dysplasia is seen in the absence of significant inflammation, we perform another colonoscopy and obtain more specimens, and if this is documented once again, we recommend a total colectomy to the patient. The experience of most people, as well as our experience, is that only an occasional patient will have moderate to severe dysplasia. We like also to obtain lavage cytology from these patients, and, on withdrawal of the colonoscope, to lavage the colon segmentally, positioning the colonoscope first at the hepatic flexure, then the splenic flexure, then the sigmoid, and then the rectum. We also like to follow our ulcerative colitis patients with carcinoembryonic antigen looking for dramatic rises, since modest rises can be seen with active colitis without cancer. If there is a stricture present in the colon, we take multiple biopsies from the area of the stricture and insert a cytologic brush within the stricture for cytologic brushings. Pseudopolyps are not usually biopsied unless they are larger than 1 cm in size, are irregular in appearance, or look different from most other pseudopolyps. Under those circumstances we obtain brushings and biopsies from them to determine whether they are really pseudopolyps, or whether they are adenomas or polypoid carcinomas. We do not usually biopsy and brush benign-appearing polyps, but the pseudopolyp is one situation in which biopsy and brush will indicate the nature of the lesion that we are dealing with. We do not perform colonoscopy on patients who have active ulcerative colitis, and if we cannot obtain a quiescent colon by medical treatment, the patient will usually be a candidate for surgery for this reason. We use the same preparation for colonoscopy in patients with ulcerative colitis that we do in other patients, and if the patient's colon is not well enough to have this preparation performed, then the colonoscopy probably should not be performed either. We do not follow patients with barium enema who have ulcerative colitis unless there is some specific reason to obtain a barium enema, since this usually does not help in the diagnosis of early cancer.

Prior Colonic Neoplasia

Patients who have had a prior colorectal cancer or prior adenoma are patients who need follow-up surveillance (Fig. 2). In patients who

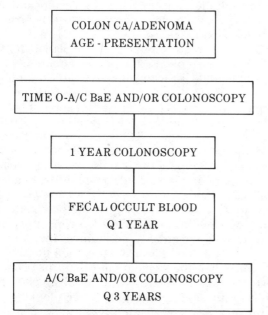

Figure 2. Proposed algorithm for screening patients who have had removal of a colonic cancer or adenoma. Follow-up surveillance should begin when their risk is identified regardless of age. The value of the barium enema in addition to the colonoscopy every 3 years has been questioned, since the lesion primarily being searched for is an adenoma, for which the barium enema has low sensitivity. The initial barium enema could be justified on the basis that initially the screening is for synchronous cancers as well as synchronous adenomas. (Reprinted with the permission of the publishers of Harrison's Updates of Internal Medicine [in press].)

have had a colonoscopic polypectomy in which the polyp has no cancer, a follow-up colonoscopy can be performed a year later, provided that the patients have had a total colonoscopy to the cecum at the time the polypectomy was performed and no residual adenomas remain. After the colon has been cleared a year later, these patients can be put on a follow-up surveillance of approximately every 3 years, provided that there were no lesions found at their last colonoscopy. In patients who have had a colonic cancer resection, a follow-up colonoscopy should be done at some point soon after surgery if a total colonoscopy had not been done prior to surgery. If a total colonoscopy had been done prior to surgery, then a follow-up colonoscopy could be done a year later, and, if normal, the patient can have follow-up examinations every 3 years. We do not routinely perform follow-up barium enemas in these patients every 3 years. However, patients who have had a colonic cancer resected should have barium enemas performed in the short term following their resection, perhaps a year after surgery and again 2 years after surgery to look for recurrences outside the bowel wall that could secondarily involve the bowel, which may be missed by colonoscopy. During colonoscopy performed in patients who have had a colonic cancer resection, we routinely brush the anastomosis within 3 years following their surgery to look for anastomotic recurrences. Anastomotic recurrences are usually infrequent unless the patients have had low anterior resections or have had their surgery performed under adverse circumstances, especially when they have presented with obstructing symptoms and the surgery may not have been as comprehensive as in more elective circumstances.

Colonoscopic Polypectomy

Polyps that we remove by colonoscopy include all pedunculated polyps of the colon regardless of size. We will remove sessile polyps by colonoscopy and electrocautery snare technique if they are up to approximately 2 cm in size. Although some people will remove polyps that are much larger than 2 cm in size, we are quite cautious about this, since they often harbor carcinoma, and it is questionable whether complete removal of these polyps can be performed consistently. This is especially hazardous on the right side of the colon where the wall is thinner. We will remove sessile polyps larger than 2 cm in size if the base is fairly narrow, that is, 2 cm in diameter or less. With a base such as this, large sessile adenomas can certainly be removed. Some people remove very large sessile adenomas with broad bases by segmental technique, but we do

TABLE 1. **Cancer in Adenomas—Surgery (?)**

Invasion through muscularis
Lymphatic invasion
Poorly differentiated
Invasion to resection line
Anatomic location
Patient
(These considerations are discussed in detail in the text)

not do this, since we feel that it is difficult to remove such a polyp completely and, in addition, much of the polyp is electrocoagulated in the process, rendering the diagnosis of carcinoma in the polyp very difficult. Smaller polyps of 7 or 8 mm in size or less, particularly if they are sessile, can be treated with hot biopsy technique, which consists of biopsy and fulguration of the remainder of the polyp at the same time. Polyps that are 1 or 2 mm in size are usually hyperplastic, and therefore we do not remove these. But polyps 3 mm in size or greater, above the rectum, are often true adenomas, and therefore we remove these by the hot biopsy technique. The risk for cancer in a polyp is higher if the polyp has a villous component than if it is merely adenomatous or tubular in type.

If there is carcinoma in situ or focal cancer in the tip of a polyp that has not penetrated the muscularis mucosae, no further surgery is necessary. If the carcinoma has penetrated the muscularis mucosae but is well clear of the margin of resection, we also do not advise surgical resection. We advise surgical resection if the polyp has had carcinoma that has invaded to the line of cautery or if there is lymphatic invasion observed or if the carcinoma is a poorly differentiated type. It is unusual to see the latter two factors (Table 1).

Surgery

Patients with colorectal cancer located anywhere in the colon, including the rectum, can have a primary resection and anastomosis. When the tumor is less than approximately 5 to 6 cm from the anal verge, an abdominal-perineal resection may be necessary with a colostomy, but this is necessary in only a very small percentage of patients. There is no improved survival following abdominal-perineal resection as compared to a low anterior resection for low-lying lesions in the upper rectum close to this 5 to 6 cm critical point. As a result of this, an attempt is usually made to avoid abdominal-perineal resection if at all possible. A colostomy may be necessary in patients who present with perforation or obstruction.

A subtotal resection is usually done in certain high-risk groups such as patients with inherited colonic cancer of either the polyposis or nonpolyposis type or in patients with multiple adenomas who are subjected to surgery for cancer. A total colectomy is performed in patients with ulcerative colitis of long standing who are suspected of having a superimposed cancer or who have moderately severe to severe dysplasia documented on multiple biopsies and have a recommendation made for surgery. There are usually no serious postoperative physiologic problems, except for some diarrhea and occasionally mild steatorrhea, in patients who have had a subtotal colectomy. This usually resolves within a few months of the time of surgery.

Following surgery for colorectal cancer, surveillance is initiated, including frequent examinations of the patient, carcinoembryonic antigen (CEA) assays, and colonoscopy at some point several months postoperatively to search for synchronous lesions if the patient has not had a total colonoscopy prior to surgery. Over a long period of time, there is a metachronous rate of 20 to 30 per cent for additional adenomas and 5 to 10 per cent for additional cancers. Periodic surveillance with colonoscopy in patients cured of their cancer is usually performed at intervals of 3 to 5 years.

Epidermoid cancers are handled with a different approach from that of adenocarcinomas of the colon. The epidermoid cancers that are resectable within the anal canal and higher than 6 cm from the anal verge are treated by low anterior resection. The epidermoid cancers in the rectum below 6 cm from the anal verge are usually handled by abdominal-perineal resection. Epidermoid cancers or junctional-type cancers below 6 cm from the anal verge that are deemed to be unresectable because of large, bulky size are usually treated by a combination of chemotherapy presently consisting of mitomycin C and 5-fluorouracil (5-FU), as well as radiation therapy for shrinkage of the tumor, and then when the tumor is felt to be resectable the patients are subjected to an abdominal-perineal resection. In patients who have had evidence of distant metastases and when the tumor has been controlled purely by chemotherapy and radiation therapy, in select circumstances surgery may be omitted.

We occasionally fulgurate tumors in the rectum if these are below the peritoneal reflection and if the patient has widespread metastases or for some other reason is considered not to be a surgical candidate. We do this primarily as a palliative procedure rather than a curative procedure and, if at all possible, prefer to operate on the patient for a primary resection. We can state as a general rule that we prefer to operate on the patient for resection of colonic cancer as primary management even if it is palliative, provided that the patient has a reasonable life expectancy. We feel this way because we find that if we do not operate on the patient, we may be faced in the near future with serious management problems of bleeding, perforation, or obstruction. As a result of this, even though there may be small liver metastases or lung metastases, we prefer still to operate on the patient for primary resection.

In patients who have solitary liver metastases at the time of surgery or at some later date, we like to work the patient up thoroughly for distant metastases elsewhere, and, if there are none, to remove these liver metastases. We have found, as others have, that there is a 20 to 30 per cent 5 year survival in these patients if these lesions are wedged out, and a 100 per cent mortality over a short period of time if they have not been removed.

Chemotherapy

Chemotherapy is usually reserved for those patients with known residual cancer or recurrent metastatic cancer. In former years, 5-fluorouracil (5-FU) was used as a single agent with approximately 15 per cent objective remission but no prolongation of life. At present, multiple agent combinations are being tested to determine whether they have increased efficacy over the single agent approach.

Protocols currently under trial are a combination of 5-FU and methyl-CCNU or 5-FU, methyl-CCNU, and streptozotocin. Although some of these protocols suggest some increased benefit, a longer period of time will be needed to determine whether this is indeed so. Chemotherapy is also being tried in an adjuvant approach in patients with Dukes' C cancers who are high risk for recurrence, to determine whether they will have a prolonged survival as compared to those patients with a similar stage who do not receive adjuvant chemotherapy. To date, there appears to be no benefit for adjuvant chemotherapy in colonic cancer, but studies have been too short in time to make a final assessment of this. There is a suggested benefit in rectal cancer. Patients often turn to us for recommendation for adjuvant chemotherapy, and in that setting we usually suggest that they be entered into a controlled trial of adjuvant chemotherapy, since we do not know the potential benefit or hazard of this.

Radiation

Radiation has been used in several ways in patients with colorectal cancer. It has been used for recurrent disease where there is a localized mass or pelvic recurrence, and occasionally in patients with metastatic disease to the liver with severe pain from distention of the liver capsule. Preoperative radiation therapy has also had trials in patients with rectal cancer. At present there is no uniform opinion as to its value in this situation. However, most colorectal surgeons make a determination of resectability preoperatively in patients with rectal cancer based on the digital examination and, if the patient appears to have a fixed lesion, administer preoperative radiation in an attempt to make the lesion more resectable. We individualize our approach to patients for preoperative radiation therapy who have rectal cancers and subject these patients to preoperative radiation therapy only if it is felt on digital examination that these are fixed lesions that may be unresectable.

We also use radiation therapy postoperatively in patients who have pelvic recurrences, since this is the most effective treatment for this type of recurrent disease. Occasionally we may use radiation therapy in patients who have extensive liver metastases, who have severe pain, and who have not been helped by chemotherapy. Under these circumstances a low-dose type of radiation to the liver, perhaps on the order of 2000 rads, has been helpful in some of our patients to alleviate this pain. It must be kept in mind that this could also provide further deterioration of liver function and hepatic coma, and therefore these patients must be watched very carefully and this potential problem weighed very carefully with the potential benefit. We use it only in select cases.

Follow-up Surveillance After Surgery

After surgery we like to follow patients very closely for the first year, seeing them on a monthly basis and each month obtaining a hemoglobin and a blood test for CEA, as well as performing a digital rectal examination and abdominal examination. For the first year we get liver function tests approximately every 3 months and a chest x-ray every 6 months. During the second and third years we perform the CEA, blood count, and liver function tests every 3 months and continue the chest x-ray every 6 months. We perform a colonoscopy soon postoperatively if the patient has not had a total colonoscopy preoperatively. If the patient had a colonoscopy preoperatively, we perform the colonoscopy at the end of the first year. At the end of the first year we also obtain a barium enema of the double-contrast type and repeat this after the second year. If the anastomosis is within reach of the sigmoidoscope, sigmoidoscopy is usually performed at 3 month intervals the first and second years and less often from the third year on. There is great variation in this kind of follow-up in patients. It is very important, especially in patients receiving adjuvant chemotherapy, to have a comprehensive approach. We may be doing abdominal examinations while the patient is developing a pelvic recurrence, which may be easy to detect by the examining finger. On the other hand, we may be doing frequent digital rectal examinations and sigmoidoscopies, but the patient may be having a rising CEA from intra-abdominal recurrences, and so the CEA is important to obtain as well. It is our approach now to operate on the patient for a second look if the CEA rises significantly and there is no evidence of metastases. Before we consider a second-look operation in a patient with rising CEA, we like to document the CEA several times over a short period and to obtain repeat liver function tests, chest x-ray, liver scan, and an abdominal computed tomography (CT) scan, as well as a physical examination, including a good rectal examination and a colonoscopy, to look for anastomotic recurrences. Usually the anastomotic recurrence is not the reason for the elevated CEA, since the anastomotic recurrence is usually very small unless it is secondary to growth outside the colon, invading inward toward the lumen. In patients who have borderline liver function tests or questionable liver scans, we try to do a laparoscopy prior to surgery to visualize the liver and see if there are recurrences prior to subjecting a patient to an exploration. However, laparoscopy is not available in many centers, and so this cannot be advised as a universal technique; in addition, it is often difficult to visualize the liver in a patient who has had extensive abdominal surgery because of the adhesions. We therefore do not do this routinely but only in select circumstances as indicated above.

Future

At present, colorectal cancer is a high-incidence cancer in this country, with a high mortality rate of close to 60 per cent of those patients who develop the tumor. Earlier diagnosis is possible by new screening techniques coupled with accurate diagnostic techniques. There are new concepts of high-risk groups and surveillance. It is very likely that dramatic changes will occur in survival from colorectal cancer and in the evolution of cancers in high-risk groups by rational application of these concepts and techniques.

ACUTE INFECTIOUS DIARRHEA

method of
FRANCIS J. TEDESCO, M.D.
Augusta, Georgia

Diarrhea is a common clinical problem. Infectious diarrhea is a major cause of morbidity and mortality in the general population of underdeveloped countries and in infants in the United States. In the adult population of the United States, acute diarrhea, although not a major cause of death, is a common problem which may result in a visit to a physician. It is one of the more common causes of absenteeism from work among healthy adults in this country.

Pathogenesis

Prior to 1980, infectious diarrhea was usually divided into two major groups according to its predominant type of pathogenesis: invasion of the mucosa or production of an enterotoxin. Recent investigation has improved and expanded our knowledge of the pathogenesis of infectious diarrhea.

Shigellosis is generally considered the prototype of invasive diarrhea. Although certain strains elaborate an enterotoxin, shigellae cause diarrhea principally by invasion of the epithelial cells initially in the small intestine and then the colonic mucosa. Microscopically, the mucosa and submucosa are infiltrated with polymorphonuclear leukocytes and gram-negative bacilli. Likewise, some strains of *Escherichia coli* have the capacity to adhere to gut epithelial cells and penetrate the intestinal mucosa as easily as virulent shigellae, producing a very similar type of invasive diarrhea. The diarrheal syndrome which may accompany the mucosal invasion by shigellae or *E. coli* is that of dysentery. Dysentery is characterized by the passage of frequent loose stools containing blood and mucus, frequently associated with abdominal cramps and tenesmus. Salmonellae likewise penetrate the mucosa, but the intestinal fluid loss may be in part the result of activation of a secretory enzyme system by bacterial toxins. Salmonella infection may cause fever, vomiting, and watery (occasionally bloody) diarrhea, but frank dysentery is unusual.

Other bacteria have been identified as causing invasive diarrhea. *Yersinia enterocolitica* may cause a variety of clinical syndromes ranging from acute enteritis to terminal ileitis with mesenteric lymphadenitis, the latter sometimes being clinically confused with acute appendicitis.

Vibrio parahaemolyticus, a halophilic, motile, curved bacillus ubiquitous in sea water, can be associated with a diarrheal disease following ingestion of contaminated seafood. Fish, oysters, clams, crabs, lobsters, and shrimp have been incriminated. The clinical syndrome is usually characterized by explosive watery diarrhea, abdominal cramps, nausea, and vomiting. Dysentery has also been reported. *Cam-*

pylobacter fetus has recently been recognized as a cause of infectious diarrhea in otherwise healthy individuals who are exposed to farm animals or their products. This organism is capable of producing a hemorrhagic necrosis of both the small and large bowel and causing a febrile diarrhea illness.

Several viruses can also be included as agents which cause diarrhea by mucosal invasion. The rotaviruses morphologically similar to reoviruses are responsible for 50 to 70 per cent of the wintertime diarrhea requiring hospitalization of children between the ages of 6 months and 2 years. The Norwalk agent, a parvovirus-like particle which primarily affects the upper jejunum, producing an inflammatory infiltrate in the lamina propria, has been implicated in smaller numbers of patients. Viral infections, though pathologically invasive types of diarrhea, are not usually associated with fecal leukocytes. Systemic signs such as fever, headache, and myalgias are commonly present.

Cholera is prototypic of toxin-induced diarrhea. The enterotoxin of *Vibrio cholerae* consists of two subunits: A (active) and B (binding). The B subunits combine with ganglioside components of principally small intestinal epithelial cells irreversibly and provide a channel in the cell through which the A component may diffuse. Subunit A activates adenyl cyclase, resulting in the breakdown of adenosine triphosphate (ATP) and accumulation of 3′,5′-cyclic adenosine monophosphate (AMP), with a resultant secretion of a protein-free isotonic fluid into the gut lumen. No histologic changes in the intestine are visible in cholera, and all manifestations of the disease can be attributed to the profound loss of fluid and electrolytes.

A similar type of toxigenic mechanism has been established for diarrhea caused by some *E. coli*, the so-called enterotoxigenic *E. coli*. Two types of enterotoxin have been described: heat-labile toxin, functionally similar to cholera toxin, and heat-stable toxin. While the mechanism of excessive intestinal secretion associated with the heat-stable toxin is unknown at present, adenyl cyclase is probably not involved. Moreover, the diarrhea caused by enterotoxigenic *E. coli* is rarely as massive as that found in cholera, and the illness usually lasts for 72 hours or less.

A third type of *E. coli* diarrhea has recently been reported. This diarrhea is associated with close adherence of the organism to the brush border of the small bowel with minimal or no invasion. Enterotoxin is apparently not involved.

Included in the toxigenic diarrheas are several "food poisonings." *Clostridium perfringens* is responsible for one third of the reported cases of food poisoning in the United States and Britain. The illness is associated with the ingestion of contaminated meat and poultry, is ordinarily mild, lasting less than 24 hours, and is unaccompanied by fever or systemic symptoms. Staphylococcal food poisoning is also mediated by an enterotoxin; in fact, five enterotoxins have been identified, designated A through E. The illness is associated with the eating of unrefrigerated foods such as eggs or cream-filled pastries, and 4 to 8 hours after ingestion of these foods an acute episode of vomiting, abdominal cramps, and diarrhea ensues. The disease is ordinarily short lived, subsiding within 8 hours, but symptoms may last for 24 hours.

Bacillus cereus has been linked to several foodborne disease outbreaks in Europe but is only infrequently recognized in this country. The mechanism of diarrhea production is unknown, but two types of syndromes, perhaps associated with two different enterotoxins, have been described. One, with an incubation time of 1 to 6 hours, mimics staphylococcal food poisoning; the second, with an incubation period of 6 to 24 hours, mimics *C. perfringens* food poisoning. Contaminated meat-containing foods, potatoes, vegetable sprouts, and fried rice have been suspected outbreak sources.

A final type of diarrhea, which has been shown to be enterotoxigenic in nature, is pseudomembranous colitis associated with antibiotic use. This diarrhea is usually a watery diarrhea, but may be bloody. Sigmoidoscopy usually demonstrates mucosal plaques composed of fibrin and cellular debris. It appears that antibiotics (particularly clindamycin, lincomycin, ampicillin, and cephalosporin) alter the intestinal microflora and allow *Clostridium difficile* to flourish and produce an enterotoxin.

Treatment

Enteric diarrhea is usually a self-limiting illness; however, in some cases specific therapy can shorten the illness. The major goal in treatment of acute diarrheal disease is the replacement of fluid and electrolytes. Frequent ingestion of small amounts of clear liquids is usually sufficient unless nausea and protracted emesis are present. Patients with diarrhea, profound systemic symptoms, hyperpyrexia, protracted emesis, or dehydration may be best managed in the hospital. For mild diarrhea, fruit juices, carbonated beverages, soups, Gatorade, or water will be adequate. Dairy products should be avoided because of the possibility of lactase deficiency associated with the diarrheal illness.

For more severe diarrhea and fluid loss, the United States Department of Public Health has recommended the following regimen: (1) fill one glass with 8 oz (240 ml) of any fruit juice (potassium content), and add one half teaspoon of honey or corn syrup (glucose facilitates absorption of sodium and chloride) and 1 pinch of table salt; (2) fill a second glass with 8 oz of water (boiled if contamination is likely) and add one half teaspoon of baking soda ($NaHCO_3$); (3) drink alternately from each glass. For moderate or severe dehydration, intravenous use of lactated Ringer's solution or isotonic saline solution with added potassium and/or bicarbonate may be used.

Symptomatic therapy in the approach to patients with diarrhea is not straightforward.

Kaolin-pectin preparations have been shown to alter the consistency of the stools but not to significantly ameliorate symptoms, number of bowel movements, or amount of fluid and electrolyte loss. Antimotility agents such as paregoric, 4 to 8 ml after each liquid stool up to four times a day, diphenoxylate hydrochloride with atropine sulfate (Lomotil), 5 mg (2 tablets) three or four times a day, or 30 mg of powdered opium and 15 mg of belladonna in capsule form three or four times a day seem to provide symptomatic relief of abdominal cramps and a decrease in the diarrhea. If shigellae or other invasive bacteria are the infecting agents, however, these antimotility drugs may delay the normalization of temperature and clearance of the pathogen from the stool. Thus, when prescribing an antimotility drug for an infectious diarrhea state, the need to control the diarrhea must be weighed against the possibility of altering the mechanism whereby the infecting organism is removed from the body.

Bismuth subsalicylate (Pepto-Bismol) has been used in some types of diarrhea. In a dosage of 240 ml (one bottle) given as 30 ml every one half hour for eight doses, this treatment effectively decreased the number of unformed stools as well as the subjective complaints of diarrhea, nausea, and abdominal cramps. Although bismuth may be the active antidiarrheal agent, there is growing evidence that the salicylate component, through its effect on prostaglandin metabolism, may be the active component. Its greatest effectiveness is in decreasing diarrhea caused by enterotoxigenic *E. coli.*

The use of antibiotics in diarrheal illnesses is based on the patient's systemic illness and an understanding of the natural history of the suspected infectious agent.

Shigellosis is treated primarily by correcting fluid and electrolyte deficits. In the patient who is clinically toxic or is having bloody mucoid stools, antibiotic therapy can be important. Because of plasmid-mediated resistance to a number of antibiotics, antimicrobials should ideally be withheld until susceptibilities are known. In significantly ill patients, therapy with ampicillin, 500 mg orally four times a day for adults, is appropriate. Amoxicillin has a spectrum of action similar to ampicillin, with the exception that ampicillin is more effective in the treatment of shigella infection. This exception negates the use of amoxicillin in shigellosis. Alternatives to ampicillin are trimethoprim-sulfamethoxazole, 1 tablet four times a day for 5 days, or tetracycline. Tetracycline can be given in a single dose of 2.5 grams orally with the same effectiveness as 500 mg four times a day for 5 days. Tetracycline should not be given to children or pregnant women, as it may stain developing teeth and has resulted in liver dysfunction.

Salmonella gastroenteritis is best treated by replacing fluids and electrolytes deficit. Antibiotics have no demonstrable beneficial effect on the clinical course and actually increase the duration of organism excretion; hence they are contraindicated in most forms of salmonella gastroenteritis. However, antibiotics should be employed in the treatment of salmonella enteric fever when there is profound illness or bacteremia.

Patients with cholera may be treated with tetracycline in a dosage of 30 to 40 mg per kg daily to eradicate the organism from the intestine and decrease the duration and volume of stool, but appropriate fluid and electrolyte replacement is the mainstay of treatment.

In summary, volume and electrolyte replenishment are crucial and the only treatment necessary in many patients with acute infectious diarrhea. Patients with dysentery or very ill patients with shigellosis or invasive or toxigenic *E. coli* may benefit from antibiotics. Patients with salmonellosis, except perhaps the very young or very old, ordinarily do not need to be treated with antibiotics. Bismuth subsalicylate and diphenoxylate with atropine may be effective, but in invasive bacterial diarrheas diphenoxylate with atropine sulfate is best avoided.

INTESTINAL PARASITES

method of
JAMES J. GIBSON, M.D.
Columbia, South Carolina

Certain populations living in the United States are at increased risk of infection with intestinal parasites, either through exposure overseas during travel to areas of high parasite prevalence or by infection in this country. Consequently, the clinician must maintain a high index of suspicion in recent returnees from foreign lands, and must remember that transmission of intestinal parasites still continues within the borders of the United States.

Correct diagnosis of the frequently subtle and nonspecific presenting symptoms of intestinal parasite infection thus requires taking a brief travel history; suspicion should be raised by recent return from a developing nation or other high-risk areas, e.g., Leningrad (giardiasis). Intestinal parasites and malaria have been among the most common medical problems in the recent immigrants from Southeast Asia.

Infection with the roundworms Ascaris and Trichuris is still common in children from impoverished families in local areas of the southeastern and south central United States; infection is associated with an environment of poverty and poor sanitation. Since these children are likely to become reinfected after treatment, repeated stool examinations and attempts at environmental improvement are indicated.

Several recent reports have appeared of intestinal protozoan infection (giardiasis, amebiasis) in male homosexuals, presumably after oral-anal contact.

Availability of Drugs

Many widely accepted antiparasitic drugs have never been approved by the Food and Drug Administration (FDA) for general use, or are not approved for use against a particular parasite. Several of these (Tables 1 and 2) can be obtained from the Parasitic Disease Division, Center for Disease Control, Atlanta, Georgia 30333 (telephone 404–329–3670 or 329–3644), along with consultation on therapy. When approved drugs are used for conditions other than those specified by the FDA, they are considered investigational, and informed consent should be obtained from the patient.

General Principles of Treatment

The availability of several new compounds with broad spectra of activity and/or fewer toxic effects has simplified the treatment of intestinal worm infections and schistosomiasis. Nonetheless, many antiparasitic drugs have significant toxicity, and in all infections the benefit of treatment must be compared with its potential toxicity. Asymptomatic or light infection may sometimes not justify treatment, particularly when the patient is unlikely to be re-exposed. Particularly for the helminths, which do not multiply in their host (with the exception of Strongyloides), the goal of therapy is reduction of parasitic load and symptoms, not cure. In cases of initial treatment failure in which the second-line drug is toxic, a second course of the initial drug may be indicated

TABLE 1. **Drug Therapy of Protozoan Infections***
(All Drugs Are Given Orally)

ORGANISM	DRUG	ADULT DOSE	PEDIATRIC DOSE	ADVERSE DRUG EFFECTS
Entamoeba histolytica	See Amebiasis (pp. 1 to 3)			
Giardia lamblia	1. Quinacrine HCl	100 mg tid × 5 days	2 mg/kg tid after meals × 5 days (maximum 300 mg/day)	Common: headache, nausea, dizziness, yellow skin Occasional: toxic psychosis, insomnia, blood dyscrasias, rash
	2. Furazolidone		1.25 mg/kg qid × 7 days	Occasional: nausea, headache Rare: antabuse-like reaction to alcohol, rash, arthralgia, hemolysis
	3. Metronidazole	250 mg tid × 5 days		Common: nausea, headache, metallic taste Occasional: vomiting, diarrhea, Antabuse-like reaction to alcohol, stomatitis, insomnia, rash, dark urine, paresthesias Rare: ataxia, depression
Dientamoeba fragilis	1. Tetracycline	500 mg qid × 10 days	10 mg/kg qid × 10 days (maximum 2 grams/day)	Common: nausea, diarrhea, tooth staining in children and fetus Occasional: liver damage, blood dyscrasias
	2. Diiodohydroxyquin	650 mg tid × 20 days	40 mg/kg/day in 3 doses × 20 days (maximum 2 grams/day)	Occasional: rash, thyroid enlargement, nausea, cramps Rare: optic atrophy after prolonged use
Balantidium coli	As for *Dientamoeba fragilis*			

*Certain drugs in this table may be investigational. See text and manufacturers' official directives before using, especially in children.

TABLE 2. Drug Therapy of Helminth Infections*
(All Given Orally Unless Otherwise Specified)

ORGANISM	DRUG	ADULT DOSE	PEDIATRIC DOSE	ADVERSE DRUG EFFECTS
Roundworms:				
Enterobius vermicularis	1. Mebendazole	100 mg once; repeat in 2 weeks	100 mg once (children >2 years); repeat in 2 weeks	Occasional: diarrhea, abdominal pain; contraindicated in pregnancy
	2. Pyrantel pamoate	11 mg/kg once (maximum 1 gram); repeat in 2 weeks	11 mg/kg once (maximum 1 gram); repeat in 2 weeks	Occasional: gastrointestinal disturbances, headaches, fever, rash
	1. Mebendazole	100 mg bid × 3 days	100 mg bid × 3 days (children >2 years)	See above
Ascaris lumbricoides	1. Pyrantel pamoate	11 mg/kg once (maximum 1 gram)	11 mg/kg once (maximum 1 gram)	See above
	2. Mebendazole	100 mg bid × 3 days	100 mg bid × 3 days (children >2 years)	See above
	3. Piperazine citrate	75 mg/kg/day × 2 days (maximum 3.5 grams/day)	75 mg/kg/day × 2 days (maximum 3.5 grams/day)	Occasional: gastrointestinal disturbances, dizziness, urticaria Rare: seizures, vision change, ataxia
Hookworm species	1. Pyrantel pamoate	11 mg/kg once (maximum 1 gram)	11 mg/kg once (maximum 1 gram)	See above
	2. Mebendazole	100 mg bid × 3 days	100 mg bid × 3 days (children >2 years)	See above
Strongyloides stercoralis	1. Thiabendazole	25 mg/kg bid × 2 days (maximum 3 grams/day)	25 mg/kg bid × 2 days (maximum 3 grams/day)	Common: dizziness, nausea Occasional: leukopenia, rash, hallucinations Rare: shock, tinnitus, Stevens-Johnson syndrome
Trichostrongylus species	1. Thiabendazole	25 mg/kg bid × 2 days (maximum 3 grams/day)	25 mg/kg bid × 2 days (maximum 3 grams/day)	See above
	2. Pyrantel pamoate	11 mg/kg once (maximum 1 gram)	11 mg/kg once (maximum 1 gram)	See above
Tapeworms:				
Taenia saginata Taenia solium Diphyllobothrium latum Dipylidium caninum	1. Niclosamide†	2 grams once chewed well	11–34 kg: 1 gram once >34 kg: 1.5 grams once	Occasional: nausea, abdominal pain
	2. Paromomycin	1 gram q 15 minutes × 4 doses	11 mg/kg q 15 minutes × 4 doses	Occasional: gastrointestinal disturbance Rare: eighth nerve damage, renal failure
Hymenolepis nana	1. Niclosamide†	2 grams daily chewed well × 5 days	11–34 kg: 1 gram daily × 5 days >34 kg: 1.5 grams daily × 5 days	See above
	2. Paromomycin	45 mg/kg daily × 6 days	45 mg/kg daily × 6 days	See above
Trematodes:				
Schistosoma haematobium	1. Metrifonate†	10 mg/kg every other week × 3	10 mg/kg every other week × 3	Occasional: nausea, bronchospasm, weakness, diarrhea, abdominal pain
	2. Niridazole†	25 mg/kg/day (maximum 1.5 grams) × 6 days	25 mg/kg/day (maximum 1.5 grams) × 6 days	Common: immunosuppression, vomiting, vertigo, headache Occasional: diarrhea, rash, paresthesias, EKG changes Rare: toxic psychosis, seizures, hemolysis in G6PD deficiency
Schistosoma mansoni	1. Niridazole†	25 mg/kg/day (maximum 1.5 grams) × 6 days	25 mg/kg/day (maximum 1.5 grams) × 6 days	See above
	2. Oxamniquine‡	15 mg/kg once	15 mg/kg once	Occasional: headache, dizziness, nausea, diarrhea, rash, change in hepatic enzymes or EKG Rare: seizures

*Certain drugs mentioned in this table may be investigational. See text and manufacturers' official directives before using, especially in children.

†See text for further information. These agents are available from the Center for Disease Control, Atlanta, Georgia.

‡For disease acquired in Africa, dose should be raised to 30 mg per kg per day for 2 days.

Table continued on following page.

TABLE 2. **Drug Therapy of Helminth Infections***
(All Given Orally Unless Otherwise Specified) (*Continued*)

ORGANISM	DRUG	ADULT DOSE	PEDIATRIC DOSE	ADVERSE DRUG EFFECTS
Schistosoma japonicum	1. Niridazole†	25 mg/kg/day (maximum 1.5 grams) × 10 days	25 mg/kg/day (maximum 1.5 grams) × 10 days	See above
	2. Sodium antimony dimercapto-succinate†	8 mg/kg IM once or twice/week × 5 doses	8 mg/kg IM once or twice/week × 5 doses	Common: muscle pain, bradycardia Occasional: colic, rash, pruritus, diarrhea, myocardial damage Rare: shock, sudden death, liver or renal damage, hemolysis
Fasciolopsis buski	1. Hexylresorcinol	1 gram once	1–7 years: 400 mg 8 years: 500 mg 9 years: 600 mg 10 years: 700 mg 11 years: 800 mg 12 years: 900 mg	Common: irritant to skin
	2. Tetrachloroethylene	0.1 ml/kg (maximum 5 ml) × 1 dose	0.1 ml/kg (maximum 5 ml) × 1 dose	Common: vomiting, abdominal pain Occasional: headache, vertigo, confusion in conjunction with alcohol
Liver flukes	1. Chloroquine phosphate	250 mg tid × 6 weeks		Occasional: nausea and vomiting, headache, rash, hemolysis, cataracts, retinal damage, alopecia, ocular palsies Rare: blood dyscrasia, nerve deafness, discoloration of nails and oral mucosa
Fasciola hepatica	1. Bithionol†	30–50 mg/kg every other day × 10–15 doses	30–50 mg/kg every other day × 10–15 doses	Common: photosensitive rash, vomiting, diarrhea, abdominal pain, urticaria

*Certain drugs mentioned in this table may be investigational. See text and manufacturers' official directives before using, especially in children.

†See text for further information. These agents are available from the Center for Disease Control, Atlanta, Georgia.

before trying the alternative therapy. In all cases, follow-up stool examination is necessary several weeks after therapy.

Data on safety in pregnancy is available on very few antiparasitic drugs. Treatment should usually be deferred until after delivery.

Mixed Infections

Patients are commonly infected with more than one intestinal parasite. Often a single broad-spectrum anthelmintic is effective for all species present, but if not, the organism causing symptoms or with potential for serious complications should be treated first.

Protozoan Infections (see Table 1)

Amebiasis. See pages 1 to 3 for *Entamoeba histolytica*.

Nonpathogenic Protozoa. *Entamoeba coli, Entamoeba hartmanni, Endolimax nana, Iodamoeba buetschlii,* and *Chilomastix mesnili* are not causes of disease and need no treatment. However, the presence of any of these commensal protozoa is evidence of recent oral ingestion of human fecal material, and mandates a careful search for intestinal pathogens and evaluation of the patient's food and water supply and fecal-oral contact.

Giardia Lamblia. This organism is endemic in all parts of the United States and many foreign countries, is spread by contaminated water supplies and also from person to person, and is associated with hypogammaglobulinemia. Stool examination is insensitive in diagnosing it, and examination of duodenal fluid may be necessary. Treatment of asymptomatic cases is indicated, to prevent future disease or transmission to others (Table 1). Quinacrine (Atabrine) is the primary treatment in adults; it is contraindicated in pregnancy. For children over 1 month of age, furazolidone (Furoxone) suspension is easily administered, causes less gastrointestinal toxicity, and is fairly effective. It causes mammary tumors in rats, but is approved for giardiasis with appropriate warnings to the patient or parents. It should not be given to patients receiving monoamine oxidase inhibitors or indirect-acting sympathomimetics. The alternative, metronidazole (Flagyl), is also less effective than quinacrine (Atabrine) and is not approved by the Food and Drug Administration for this indication. The package insert should be consulted for contraindications and toxicity, which include carcinogenicity and mutagenicity in other species.

Dientamoeba Fragilis. This organism can cause diarrheal disease in humans and should be treated. Either tetracycline (contraindicated in children under 14 years of age; see also manufacturers' official directives) or diiodohydroxyquin can be used. Diiodohydroxyquin dosage should not be exceeded, and the drug should not be given for multiple courses of therapy because of the possibility of optic neuritis; it is presently available under its generic name.

Balantidium Coli. This organism is rarely identified in the United States; it is treated as for *D. fragilis*.

Helminth Infections

Roundworms. ENTEROBIUS VERMICULARIS (PINWORM). This person-to-person–transmitted worm is extraordinarily common, particularly in temperate climate nations. Prevalence rates over 50 per cent can be seen in schoolchildren, and all social classes are affected. Many asymptomatic infections occur; unusual presentations include nocturnal enuresis and possibly urinary tract infection in girls. Principles of treatment include (1) simultaneous treatment of all family members when one is infected; (2) repeating therapy in 2 weeks; (3) discouragement of exceptional efforts at environmental or personal hygiene beyond laundering of bedclothes and personal clothing; and (4) counseling the family about the infection's benign nature and high prevalence. A single oral dose of mebendazole (Vermox) or pyrantel pamoate (Antiminth) is effective (see Table 2); however, mebendazole cannot be used in pregnancy and is available only in chewable tablets.

TRICHURIS TRICHIURA (WHIPWORM). Most infections are asymptomatic, but all should be treated, since the drug of choice, mebendazole (Vermox) (see Table 2), is effective and nontoxic. A few eggs on follow-up stool examination 4 weeks post-treatment are probably not an indication for retreatment.

ASCARIS LUMBRICOIDES. All infections with this worldwide soil-transmitted helminth should be treated because of the worm's potential for causing intestinal, biliary, or laryngeal obstruction. Heavy infections and occasional cases of intestinal obstruction are still seen in the southeastern United States. Uncomplicated infections are treated as in Table 2; all listed drugs are nontoxic and over 90 per cent effective, but mebendazole (Vermox) has the advantage of effectiveness in mixed infections with Ascaris, Trichuris, or hookworm. Treatment should be repeated if follow-up examination reveals any persistence of Ascaris eggs. Intestinal obstruction is treated with immediate duodenal intubation and suction, fluid and electrolyte replacement, and administration via tube of piperazine citrate, 150 mg per kg initially, then six doses of 65 mg per kg at 12 hour intervals to permit passage of the worms. Persistence of ileus requires surgery, which carries significant mortality.

HOOKWORMS. Both species of hookworm can be treated with mebendazole as for Ascaris; pyrantel pamoate* may be slightly more effective for *Necator americanus* (see Table 2). Oral iron supplements are indicated for the anemia accompanying heavy infections; asymptomatic light infections should be treated, with follow-up if the patient lives in an environment of continuing re-exposure.

STRONGYLOIDES STERCORALIS (STRONGYLOIDIASIS). This is the only helminth (along with certain tapeworms) with the ability to autoinfect and multiply in the host, and thus all infections should be treated, with follow-up examination. Diagnosis may require examination of duodenal fluid. Fatal hyperinfections have been reported in immunosuppressed patients (renal transplant, malnutrition), and persons undergoing immunosuppression should be carefully examined and, in high risk populations, perhaps treated prophylactically with thiabendazole (Mintezol). The only known effective drug is thiabendazole; side effects are frequent and can be life threatening (see Table 2). Caution is required in patients with liver or renal disease. Patients with disseminated infection should be treated longer, at least 5 days.

TRICHOSTRONGYLUS SPECIES. This infection is acquired only outside the United States, and there is no accepted standard treatment. Thiabendazole (Mintezol) is effective but toxic, so pyrantel pamoate (Antiminth) might be tried first; both are considered investigational drugs for this use by the Food and Drug Administration.

Tapeworms. Vague gastrointestinal symptoms have been associated with intestinal infection with adult tapeworms, but it is passage of tapeworm segments that usually prompts patients to seek treatment. *Diphyllobothrium latum* occasionally causes megaloblastic anemia requiring vitamin B_{12}. Therapy of adult forms of all the intestinal tapeworms (*Taenia saginata, Taenia solium, Diphyllobothrium latum, Hymenolepis nana, Dipylidium caninum*) is much simplified by the fact that all can be treated with the same drug, niclosamide (Yomesan), available from the Center for Disease Control (see Availability of Drugs, above). An alternative drug is paromomycin (Humatin); dosages and adverse effects are presented in Table 2. Neither drug is approved for this use in the United States. All the tapeworms are effectively treated with a single dose of niclosamide chewed thoroughly, except the dwarf tapeworm *Hymenolepis nana;* because its larval stages occur in intestinal villi and are resistant to the drug, the

---

*Considered an investigational drug for this purpose by the Food and Drug Administration.

treatment must be repeated for a total of 5 days. Follow-up for all should consist of warning patients to watch for proglottids and a stool examination 3 months after treatment.

In addition to intestinal infection by adult tapeworms, *Taenia solium* (pork tapeworm) and *Echinococcus granulosus* (dog tapeworm) can cause larval invasion of tissues (cysticercosis) and hydatid cysts, respectively. There is a theoretical possibility that treatment of an intestinal *T. solium* worm could cause larval tissue invasion and cysticercosis; this has never been reported. Oral mebendazole in massive doses may be effective for these larval infections; surgical resection is the accepted treatment.

Trematodes (Flukes). SCHISTOSOMIASIS. Adult worms of *Schistosoma mansoni* and *Schistosoma japonicum* inhabit the venules of the lower and mid-intestinal tract and lay eggs that are excreted in the feces. *Schistosoma haematobium* inhabits venules of the bladder and ureters, and its eggs appear in the urine. These infections are acquired only outside the United States.

All the drugs effective for schistosomiasis are experimental and/or significantly toxic; thus the benefits of treatment must be weighed against possible adverse effects. Consultation with a clinician experienced in parasitic diseases is recommended. *S. haematobium* is usually treated because of its potential carcinogenicity. Criteria for treatment of all three species include evidence that viable eggs are being passed (by egg hatching test or motility of flame cells), presence of heavy infection (egg count), symptomatic infection, and ability of the patient to withstand drug toxicity. Follow-up examination of stool or urine should be done every 3 months for 1 year.

The drug of choice for *S. haematobium* is metrifonate (Bilarcil), an acetylcholinesterase inhibitor; the alternative is niridazole (Ambilhar). Both are available from the Center for Disease Control (see Availability of Drugs, above). Niridazole has severe central nervous system side effects and is absolutely contraindicated in patients with hepatocellular disease, portal hypertension, or a history of psychiatric disease or seizures.

For *S. mansoni* and *S. japonicum* the drug of choice is niridazole (see contraindications above). There is some evidence that treating *S. mansoni* at half-standard dose (12.5 mg per kg) for 12 days may reduce toxicity without sacrificing efficacy. For *S. mansoni* the best alternative is oxamniquine (Mansil), but it was licensed in the spring of 1980 and may be difficult to obtain. For *S. japonicum*, the most severe infection and the hardest to treat, the alternative is an organic antimony compound, either sodium antimony dimercaptosuccinate (Astiban) or potassium antimony tartrate (tartar emetic). Astiban is available from the Center for Disease Control (see Availability of Drugs, above) and is contraindicated in patients with renal or cardiac disease, in liver disease not caused by schistosomiasis, and during other acute infections. Indications for stopping therapy include severe vomiting, albuminuria, severe joint pain, rash, infection, purpura, or progressive anemia. Contraindications for tartar emetic are the same, but toxic effects are more frequent and include spasms of cough and vomiting with rapid intravenous administration.

INTESTINAL FLUKES. *Fasciolopsis buski* is the most common of these; hexylresorcinol is the drug of choice (see Table 2). An alternative is tetrachloroethylene. This drug is safe and is approved, but is available only as Nema' worm capsules for veterinary use.

LIVER FLUKES. *Opisthorchis sinensis* and *Opisthorchis viverrini* often cause asymptomatic infection with minimal liver function abnormality, and should usually be left untreated. Chloroquine has been used, but it only suppresses egg production without killing the flukes and should not be used in children.

FASCIOLA HEPATICA. Bithionol is probably effective and is obtainable from the Center for Disease Control (see Availability of Drugs, above). Side effects of diarrhea and abdominal cramps are common, but subside in 2 to 3 days. It should not be used in young children.

ULCERATIVE COLITIS
(Chronic Ulcerative Colitis, Proctocolitis)

method of
HERMAN STEINBERG, M.D.
New York, New York

Definitions

Ulcerative colitis is a chronic, recurrent inflammatory condition of unknown etiology ("idiopathic" or "nonspecific" chronic ulcerative colitis) that *always* involves the rectum with or without variable extent of the remaining colon in *continuous* linear distribution. Thus the linear extent of the disease may vary from limited rectal disease ("proctitis") to involvement of the rectum and all the remaining colon ("universal colitis"). The disease *never* involves the small intestine except, rarely, as "backwash ileitis," which is a limited linear (no more than a few centimeters), insignificant radiologic abnormality of the terminal ileum. The constancy of rectal involvement and the anatomic restriction to the colon without small bowel extension render the term "proctocolitis" preferable to "ulcerative colitis."

Proctocolitis is to be distinguished from Crohn's colitis, which may or may not involve the rectum, and in which the linear distribution of the disease may or may not be segmental — that is, marked by skip areas of uninvolved colon. There are a number of other distinguishing features, including frequent small bowel involvement ("ileocolitis") and propensity for fistulization in Crohn's disease. However, perhaps 10 to 20 per cent of proctocolitis cannot be distinguished from Crohn's colitis.

Diagnostic Cautions and Screening

Proctocolitis must be distinguished from the "specific" colitides, such as amebiasis, shigellosis, Yersinia colitis, Campylobacter colitis, gonorrheal proctitis, and antibiotic-associated colitis, particularly amebiasis, since specific medications are available for these conditions, unlike proctocolitis. Furthermore, corticosteroid therapy, which is frequently employed in proctocolitis, is hazardous in the specific colitides.

All patients with an initial episode of suspected proctocolitis should be screened as follows:

1. At least three fresh stools for ova and parasites examined by an experienced technician, or examination of endoscopically collected exudate. Indirect hemagglutination tests for amebiasis in either rectal disease of greater than mild severity or more extensive linear disease of any severity. If a mucosal biopsy is performed, periodic acid–Schiff (PAS) stain for amebae may be helpful.

2. Stool cultures, properly and promptly plated, for the usual enteric pathogens, as well as Yersinia and Campylobacter.

3. When homosexuality and/or sexual promiscuity is suspected, rectal exudate promptly plated on Thayer-Martin medium for gonorrhea, if the linear distribution is limited to the rectum.

4. In a setting of recent antibiotic therapy, as well as in the deteriorating patient with proved proctocolitis who has been on antibiotics, cytopathic neutralization tests for *Clostridium difficile* if available, or a therapeutic trial of either vancomycin, 250 to 500 mg orally every 6 hours for 7 days, or metronidazole (Flagyl), 500 mg every eight hours for 7 to 10 days. (This use of metronidazole is not specifically mentioned in the manufacturer's official directive.)

Broad Principles of Therapy (Medical and Surgical)

Treatment is based on (1) linear extent of disease; (2) presence or absence of constitutional symptoms, colonic complications, and extragastrointestinal complications; (3) age of onset and duration of disease; and (4) psychologic tolerance by the patient of the vicissitudes of a chronic illness in his particular social, family, and financial setting.

Medical therapy is solely symptomatic and/or suppressive, but is preferred in the vast majority of patients. Surgery, which is the only curative therapy, is employed in (1) potentially lethal complications, such as uncontrolled bleeding, perforation, and malignant degeneration; (2) uncontrolled symptoms — either colonic or extragastrointestinal (intractable disease); or (3) the unequivocal presence of "severe dysplasia" on mucosal biopsy for cancer surveillance, particularly in the young or middle-aged patient.

Therapeutic Modalities (Principles and Dosage)

Dietotherapy. This is of relatively little benefit except in patients who have a coincidental lactose intolerance. All patients with proctocolitis should be evaluated for such intolerance early in their course. Those with moderate or severe symptoms should be carefully questioned as to whether milk and milk products cause increased diarrhea and/or flatulence, but a formal lactose tolerance test should be delayed until remission occurs. In the presence of suspected or proved lactose intolerance, a lactose restricted diet is indicated.

A low roughage and bland diet is not useful except during the phase of severe activity of the disease.

Psychiatric Therapy. Psychiatric therapy is of no benefit in altering the natural course of the disease, but may help the patient's ability to handle the psychologic ravages of the disease in a minority of cases. Avoid deep psychologic probing; supportive psychotherapy may be effective under these circumstances. Such support may be provided by the internist by means of sympathetic discussion of stress situations.

Sulfasalazine. This controversial drug is clearly not to be relied upon in the seriously ill patient and is probably not effective beyond placebo effect even in the mildly ill. A high incidence of innocuous, transitory initial side effects (headache, nausea) renders double blind studies suspect. Serious side effects (dermatitis, hemolytic anemia, hepatitis, agranulocytosis) may occasionally develop. The drug may have a role as a placebo for both the patient and the believer-physician in low-grade disease and as long-term prophylaxis. Initiate therapy with 0.5 gram twice daily and increase gradually over a 3 week period to a maintenance dosage of 4.0 grams daily in four divided doses. Daily folic acid (1.0 mg) will avoid the reported accompanying macrocytic anemia.

Antidiarrheal Agents. *Spasmogenic, nonperistaltic drugs,* such as the opiates and their derivatives, have *virtually no role in the moderately to seriously ill patient,* because they cause colonic distention and abdominal pain, occasionally of a serious nature (toxic megacolon). Under the best of circumstances, the diarrhea "catches up" in an even more distressing fashion before the next scheduled dose, or during the night. Nevertheless, an occasional dose is justified in this category of patient, given certain conditions — for example, urgent business or social engagement in the absence of convenient toilet facilities. This group of drugs may, however, offer reasonably symptomatic relief in those patients with extensive linear and mildly active disease, whose only symptom is diarrhea in the absence of significant bleeding and fever. Diphenoxylate (Lomotil), 2.5 to 5.0 mg, or loperamide (Imodium), 2 to 4 mg, up to four times daily; or codeine, 30 to 60 mg, paregoric, 5 to 10 ml, or tincture of deodorized opium, 6 to 12 drops, in order of increasing potency, once or twice daily, may be used.

Parasympatholytic drugs, including tincture of belladonna and the anticholinergics such as propantheline (Pro-Banthine), are not useful in the management of proctocolitis. They lead to abdominal distention without significant amelioration of the diarrhea, and predispose to toxic megacolon if abused in the seriously ill patient.

Antibiotics. This group of drugs has no role in the ongoing treatment of chronic symptoms, but is often indicated in the patient with "fulminant" proctocolitis, frequently a forerunner of toxic megacolon. The patient with abdominal distention, rebound tenderness, and high fever should be placed on intravenous antibiotics, particularly if on corticosteroids, for the possibility of walled-off perforation. Either cefoxitin, 1.5 to 3.0 grams every 6 hours, or triple antibiotic therapy (ampicillin, gentamicin, and clindamycin) may be employed. The course of therapy should be short — 5 to 10 days — for in this period of time either the fulminant status will have resolved itself or the patient will have been subjected to surgery. Triple antibiotic therapy is mandatory in toxic megacolon.

On *rare* occasions, exacerbations of disease of less than fulminant degree may be aborted by a short course of oral antibiotics, particularly me-

tronidazole, 500 mg every 8 hours. (This use of metronidazole is not listed in the manufacturer's official directive.)

Corticosteroids (Steroids). GENERAL. These drugs are the only clearly effective agents in the therapy of proctocolitis. Although not curative, they are dependably suppressive when properly employed, particularly on initial use. Steroids are indicated when the disease prevents adequate functioning of the patient. In general, moderate to severe disease requires steroids. Since proctocolitis is often a cyclic disease, the course of therapy should be limited to periods of activity. However, long-term maintenance therapy is justified in unremittent disease.

Prior to the *initial* use of steroids in mild and in selected cases of moderately severe disease, a limited course of sympathetic observation should be attempted. On occasion, the natural course of the disease will produce a spontaneous remission during this period of time without the necessity for resorting to these potent drugs.

The key to the use of corticosteroids is "start high and wean slowly." The oral route of administration should be employed except if the patient is vomiting, in fulminant disease, or in toxic megacolon. Intravenous therapy should be reserved for these situations. Retention steroid enemas are indicated in symptomatic proctitis or proctosigmoiditis, whether as a solitary lesion or as part of more extensive linear disease.

DURATION OF THERAPY. The usual course of oral therapy is a minimum of 3 to 6 months, but not infrequently a long-term, low-dose, once daily, or alternate day regimen, is indicated. It cannot be emphasized too strongly that continual attempts to taper corticosteroids to zero dosage should always be made. Intravenous (or intramuscular) therapy may be required up to 10 days before oral medication can be substituted. Steroid retention enemas are always given at bedtime and occasionally also on arising after the morning bowel movement, until the symptoms of proctitis subside (a few days to 2 weeks), whereupon the patient is slowly weaned by decreasing the frequency of the enemas to zero over a period of 2 to 6 weeks.

Oral therapy is initiated with 40 to 100 mg of prednisone (or equivalent) daily in three or four divided doses. The beneficial effect, if it is to occur, will be apparent in from a few days to 3 weeks. The patient is then weaned to zero dosage, or to a low maintenance dose, over a period of 3 to 6 months. If a "safe" maintenance dose, that is, either no more than 7.5 mg in one morning dose or 20 to 25 mg on alternate mornings, is ineffective after a limited number of weaning attempts over perhaps a year or two, consideration should be given to surgery, depending upon individual circumstances. Such circumstances include age of patient; social and financial considerations; associated medical conditions; psychologic tolerance of chronic symptoms, including steroid side effects; and fear of surgery.

Parenteral therapy, usually intravenous, is initiated with 100 or 120 mg of prednisolone (or equivalent) daily in three or four bolus injections, but may be given intramuscularly. There is absolutely no advantage to ACTH therapy over corticosteroids.

Rectal retention enemas usually contain 100 mg of hydrocortisone in solution (Cortenema), of which perhaps 30 to 40 per cent is absorbed. This significant amount of absorbed steroids should be taken into consideration in any long-term maintenance program, particularly if combined with oral steroids.

Corticosteroid failure occurs (1) if there is no beneficial response, (2) if steroid disease develops, or (3) if the proctocolitis persists in an unacceptably smoldering form.

Sedatives. Sedation is not ordinarily effective in proctocolitis, but may occasionally be useful when episodes of activity are precipitated by, or coincide with, periods of emotional stress. These drugs (phenobarbital, diazepam) may be useful as a delaying action before committing the patient to a course of corticosteroids if the patient's condition permits.

Total Parenteral Nutrition (TPN). TPN is indicated in the following circumstances: (1) The child with growth retardation, provided that the epiphyses have not closed; on rare occasions, 4 to 8 weeks of such therapy will produce a growth spurt. (2) The markedly depleted preoperative patient, in whom colectomy may be relatively hazardous because of long-term, high-dose steroid therapy. Healing of the perineal wound particularly may be enhanced by a course of preoperative TPN. (3) The markedly depleted postoperative patient, in whom surgery was urgent or of an emergency nature, in an attempt to promote wound healing.

Enteric Hyperalimentation. Enteric hyperalimentation is of no benefit and is never indicated in proctocolitis.

Azathioprine (Imuran). Use of azathioprine in proctocolitis is of no benefit and hazardous.

Psychotropic Drugs. Psychotropic drugs are of no benefit except in the severely depressed patient. The hazards of anticholinergic therapy must be considered when using these drugs.

Colitis Clubs. In general, the "stoma" clubs (United Ostomy Associations) prove helpful either if the patient does not have access to a good stomal therapist (usually a specially trained nurse) or as a social avenue for young, unmarried ileostomy patients. The "colitis" clubs (National Foundation for Ileitis and Colitis), on the other hand, cater to the fears and anxieties of the patient and his family. The latter foundation tends to provide the patient with overoptimistic reports of "significant advances" and other misinformation, leading to a deterioration of the relationship between the patient and his physician. Such unfortunate situations can be avoided if the patient's physician is knowledgeable in the disease and allows the time to discuss the confusion surrounding the cause and therapy of proctocolitis.

A Scheme of Therapy Based on Linear Extent and Complications

Proctitis (Proctosigmoiditis). Many patients with low grade disease, limited to the rectum, have only one or two daily movements containing small amounts of blood. The bleeding is almost never severe enough to produce anemia, but the patient reacts to the sight of blood with fright. These patients should be reassured by emphasizing the minimal degree of blood loss and dealt with sympathetically, but not otherwise treated. On the other hand, symptoms of tenesmus, associated with multiple, urgent passages of bloody exudate with the passage of an occasional hard stool, require the use of local corticosteroids. Steroid retention enemas (Cortenema) are usually effective, but on occasion the tenesmus prevents retention of the liquid hydrocortisone solution. Under these circumstances, a foam preparation of hydrocortisone acetate (Cortifoam) is usually better tolerated, although the surface area of effective application is less. In minimal disease, limited to the distal few centimeters of rectum, a suppository containing 25 mg of hydrocortisone may be all that is required.

Distal (Left-Sided) Disease. Active disease extending into the splenic flexure produces a pattern of frequent, often bloody, loose stools (bloody diarrhea) and usually requires suppressive therapy with systemic steroids. If the diarrhea is not bloody and in the absence of both significant anemia and constitutional symptoms, cautious use of the spasmogenic antidiarrheal agents may suffice.

Extensive Linear Disease (Universal Colitis). When active, such disease distribution requires systemic steroids. Not infrequently, however, as in distal disease, the activity may be minimal, the diarrhea, if present, free of gross blood, and the patient free of both anemia and constitutional symptoms. Under these circumstances, judicious use of spasmogenic antidiarrheal agents may be adequate. As with disease of any linear distribution, a significant element of tenesmus should be treated with rectal steroids, with or without systemic corticosteroids.

Toxic Megacolon. If the patient has had no previous steroid therapy, a strictly limited trial of high-dose parenteral corticosteroid therapy should be initiated. If toxic megacolon develops while the patient is on low to moderate steroid dosage, increase to high-dose range. If this very serious complication of proctocolitis develops while the patient is on high-dose steroids, prompt colectomy is indicated after adequate blood, fluid, and electrolyte replacement, under triple antibiotic coverage. The trial period of high-dose steroids (medical therapy) should rarely extend beyond 1 to 3 or 4 days, by which time either the toxic megacolon should show clear improvement or colectomy should be undertaken. The patient must be observed compulsively from the moment of initiation of the medical trial; any evidence of deterioration demands prompt colectomy. All patients with toxic megacolon require triple antibiotic coverage, nasogastric suction, and appropriate blood, fluid, and electrolyte replacement.

Massive Bleeding. A trial of high-dose steroids is indicated. If unsuccessful, total colectomy is preferred to subtotal colectomy, provided that the patient's condition permits, since the bleeding is usually from an extensive area of the colon, including the rectum and sigmoid. On rare occasions, significant bleeding, although not massive, may originate in one or two large pseudopolyps, which may be removed endoscopically.

Perianal Fistula, Rectovaginal Fistula. These are rare in proctocolitis. Suspect Crohn's colitis, particularly if multiple perianal fistulas are present. Patients may respond (usually temporarily) to metronidazole, 250 mg every 6 to 8 hours for a period of 4 weeks, although local conservative surgical therapy may be necessary. (This use of metronidazole is not listed in the manufacturer's official directive.)

Pyoderma Gangrenosum. Oral steroids are used, or occasionally local infiltration with steroids; skin grafts may be necessary.

Erythema Nodosum. Salicylates usually are adequate therapy, since the lesions tend to resolve spontaneously. On rare occasions, systemic steroids are necessary if the lesions are disabling.

Arthritis. Large joints are generally attacked, with a lower extremity distribution. Salicylates or nonsteroidal anti-inflammatory agents, naproxen (Naprosyn), 250 mg twice daily, usually suffice. On rare occasions, systemic steroids are required. The arthritis tends to be cyclic, not necessarily coinciding with colonic activity, and usually subsides spontaneously over a reasonable period of time.

Ankylosing Spondylitis and Sacroiliitis. This is a genetically determined accompaniment of proctocolitis (and Crohn's disease), and not, strictly speaking, a complication. It should be treated on its own merits. Salicylates, nonsteroidal anti-inflammatory agents (indomethacin [Indocin], 25 mg twice daily, or phenylbutazone [Butazolidin], 100 mg daily), or, rarely, low-dose steroids are indicated.

Iritis-Episcleritis. Steroids are indicated. Iritis may require both the local (topical drops and local infiltration) and systemic routes, together with cycloplegics. For episcleritis, topical application of steroids suffices. Iritis is a potentially serious complication and requires the attendance of an ophthalmologist.

Liver Disease (Pericholangitis, Sclerosing Cholangitis/Choledochitis). These three types of liver disease probably represent the spectrum of the same underlying process. Low-grade liver disease, as manifested by minor cholestatic chemical abnormalities in the young person with proctocolitis, is more of a threat than in the older patient, because progression to bile duct cancer and/or biliary cirrhosis may take place over the many remaining decades of life. Once the diagnosis of sclerosing cholangitis/choledochitis is established, the decision as to total colectomy must be made. There is only tenuous evidence that such prophylactic surgery prevents the progression of the liver disease. However, in the relatively young person, serious consideration should be given to such surgery.

Thromboembolic Disease. This is a very serious, potentially fatal complication, requiring active therapy and *not* a wait-and-see attitude. If the rectal bleeding is mild to moderate, anticoagulants — heparin to be followed by maintenance warfarin (Coumadin) — are indicated. In the presence of more severe colonic bleeding, ligation of the inferior vena cava or placement of an umbrella device in the inferior vena cava should be performed with or without colectomy.

Special Problems

Growth Retardation. Although not so common a problem in proctocolitis as with small bowel involvement in Crohn's disease, this distressing complication deserves special attention in the youngster prior to epiphyseal closure. Both the attendant malnutrition and corticosteroid therapy are contributory, probably predominantly the former, except in the face of long-duration, high-dose steroid therapy. Elemental and semielemental diets are ineffective. Total parenteral nutrition (TPN) over a period of 4 to 8 weeks may be followed·by a growth spurt. If the growth retardation is severe, total colectomy is indicated before epiphyseal closure.

Pregnancy. Proctocolitis may either develop for the first time or exacerbate during pregnancy, as well as in the immediate postpartum period, although it is not unusual for remissions to occur when a patient becomes pregnant. Moreover, available statistics suggest that the incidence of active disease is no greater during pregnancy than otherwise. The postpartum period is the time when the disease is most likely to exacerbate, followed in frequency by the first trimester.

The principles of therapy during pregnancy are not altered by the fact of pregnancy, except that possibly extended periods of high-dose steroid therapy should be avoided if at all possible during the first trimester, in order to avoid the theoretical teratogenic sequelae. It should be emphasized that such sequelae are exceedingly rare. Thus, attention should be directed to the treatment of the mother, rather than to concern for the effects of therapy on the fetus. Therapeutic abortions are not indicated. The relative resistance of the fetus to deleterious effects of maternal corticosteroid administration is explained by placental inactivation. The general health of the mother is far more important in maintaining the integrity of the fetus than is the therapy directed to the mother's proctocolitis.

Cancer Surveillance. The incidence of colonic cancer in the patient with longstanding proctocolitis is clearly significantly increased. The greater the linear extent of the disease, the higher the incidence over a set period of time. Although controversial, it seems that the onset of the disease prior to or during puberty may further predispose to malignant degeneration. Since there is no relationship between duration of activity and the incidence of malignant degeneration, patients with longstanding inactive disease require cancer surveillance with the same diligence as do those with ongoing active disease.

Surveillance should begin 8 to 10 years after the onset of universal or extensive linear disease, and 15 to 20 years after the onset of left-sided disease. The exact form of surveillance will depend on the facilities available. If both a competent colonoscopist and either an experienced and interested pathologist or a "reference center" are available, colonoscopy should be performed yearly with multiple proximal and distal biopsies. Histologic cancer and unequivocally "severe" dysplasia are indications for total colectomy. If colonoscopy is not available, careful air contrast barium enema should be performed every year, together with yearly rigid tube sigmoidoscopy on an alternate 6 month schedule. At the time of sigmoidoscopy, at least three rectal-sigmoidodal biopsies should be collected. Biopsies for cancer surveillance should be taken from "inactive" flat or velvety (villous) areas of mucosa and *not* from sites of active inflammation; the latter often contain "inflammatory dysplasia," which is of no cancer significance.

Metabolic Disorders

BERIBERI
(Thiamine [Vitamin B$_1$] Deficiency)

method of
CHUICHI KAWAI, M.D.
Kyoto, Japan

Beriberi, "I cannot," in Singhalese, signifying that the person is too ill to do anything, is a spectrum of disease states characterized by multiple neuritis, cardiovascular changes, and, frequently, edema, attributable to thiamine deficiency. Thiamine pyrophosphate, vitamin B$_1$, has two independent roles: (1) a coenzyme function in intermediary carbohydrate metabolism and (2) a significant role in the nerve excitation process.

Clinical beriberi is seen among populations whose chief source of calories is carbohydrates with lack of thiamine, such as polished rice in the Orient. It has been reported recently that relative thiamine deficiency is commonly induced by the current tendency for teenagers in Japan to take excessive sweet carbonated soft drinks, instant noodles, and powermill-polished rice without thiamine supplementation. The sudden increase in thiamine requirements caused by strenuous exercise in summer results in overt beriberi heart disease. The sporadic case of beriberi in the Western world is common in alcoholics because of the displacement of thiamine-containing food by alcohol. Relative thiamine deficiency may also be induced by a hypermetabolic state or increased urinary excretion of thiamine secondary to prolonged use of diuretics.

Clinically, beriberi can be divided into three types: (1) wet beriberi, (2) dry beriberi, and (3) shoshin beriberi (acute pernicious beriberi heart disease).

The state in which the beriberi patient develops acute sudden onset of severe biventricular failure associated with cardiovascular shock is called "shoshin"; in Japanese "sho" means acute damage and "shin" heart. Shoshin beriberi is occasionally seen in infants or pregnant or lactating women, but more frequently in young healthy individuals with only minimal prodromal symptoms. Death may ensue within hours unless properly treated. Typical "shoshin" beriberi is rare now in developed countries.

Prevention

Adequate dietary intake of thiamine is the key to the prevention of beriberi. The minimal daily requirement of thiamine ranges from 0.23 mg to 0.45 mg per 1000 calories, according to previous investigations. In rice-eating countries, intake of germ-retaining polished rice, under-milled rice (for example, 70 per cent milled rice), or rice enriched with thiamine is highly recommended. A daily supplement of 1 mg of thiamine is enough to prevent beriberi in adults who are known to have a decreased intake or an increased utilization or excretion of thiamine. Excessive intake of sweet carbonated drinks should be avoided by those who perform strenuous exercise during the hot summer and who eat well-milled white rice or instant foods without thiamine supplementation.

Thiaminase, which is contained in clams, raw fish, or ferns, may sometimes cause beriberi. Cooking such as baking or broiling inactivates thiaminase.

Treatment

In mild beriberi, especially in young patients, a favorable therapeutic effect can be obtained with rest alone, but a well balanced diet, consisting of appropriate protein, lipids, and carbohydrate fortified with thiamine, is recommended. A prompt therapeutic effect is achieved by parenteral administration of thiamine hydrochloride or thiamine propyldisulfide (TPD, Alinamin),* 50 to 100 mg, followed by 10 to 50 mg three times daily for 1 week, and then the same dose orally as

---

*May not be available in the United States of America.

maintenance therapy. Through its action of rapid conversion to thiamine intracellularly, TPD, a lipotropic thiamine derivative, is said to be effective in patients with chronic thiamine deficiency who fail to show an increase in blood thiamine level or to improve clinically in spite of prolonged administration of thiamine hydrochloride. Therapy for "shoshin" beriberi consists of prompt parenteral administration of thiamine, 100 mg, and a maintenance dose of 10 to 50 mg three times daily for several days, followed by oral administration. At the same time digitalis may be given very carefully. Sometimes diuretics are indicated to remove volume overload.

Polyneuropathy tends to respond slowly to therapy; therefore, large amounts (50 to 100 mg) of thiamine should be given for a prolonged period. Physiotherapy is also recommended to prevent muscular atrophy and contractures.

HYPO- AND HYPER-VITAMINOSIS A

method of
DONALD S. McLAREN, M.D.
Edinburgh, Scotland

Vitamin A (retinol) is essential for life, reproduction, normal growth, retinal rod and cone function, and integrity of most epithelia, especially the conjunctiva and cornea, and the immune response. The vitamin is derived from several of the many carotenoid pigments of plants, notably β-carotene, by central fission of the molecule. Excessive ingestion of carotene, frequently as a result of food faddism, produces hypercarotenosis with staining of body tissues. This does not lead to hypervitaminosis, and treatment consists of withdrawal of the source of the carotenes.

Hypovitaminosis A

Most adult human dietaries have about one third of their vitamin A activity as preformed vitamin A from animal sources and the remaining two thirds in the form of carotene. Much of the carotene is not absorbed, and the rest is either absorbed unchanged or converted to vitamin A in the lumen of the small intestine. The liver is capable of storing vitamin A, mainly as retinyl palmitate, in high concentrations and releases it coupled to retinol-binding protein and prealbumin for transport to the tissues. Vitamin A deficiency caused by dietary lack is endemic among young children in many parts of Southeast Asia, the Middle East, Africa, and Latin America and is the most common cause of blindness in this age group. Recent estimates suggest that 250,000 go blind annually. Hypovitaminosis A occurs sporadically secondary to impaired absorption (any cause of malabsorption such as celiac disease, sprue, cystic fibrosis), transport (abetalipoproteinemia), or storage (cirrhosis). Clinical signs in the order of increasing severity of deficiency consist of impairment of dark adaptation and night blindness, xerosis of the conjunctiva and the type of Bitot's spots that accompany this xerosis, xerosis of the cornea, and, finally, keratomalacia. They appear only after liver stores have been depleted and serum levels have fallen below about 10 micrograms per 100 ml.

Prophylaxis. The recommended daily dietary allowance is 1000 micrograms of retinol, increasing to 1200 micrograms in pregnancy and about 1400 micrograms in lactation (1 microgram = 3.33 units). Most adult dietaries provide sufficient vitamin A from green leafy vegetables and animal sources to meet daily needs and to maintain considerable liver reserves. In states of impaired physiology or inadequate intake, daily aqueous supplements of 2000 micrograms (6666 units) are indicated. The requirement of the young child is relatively great, about 750 micrograms (2500 units), and this is the age group in which the stress of infections and a poor dietary intake are especially prone to produce deficiency. Puréed green leaves should be incorporated early into the supplementary dietary. In several countries preventive programs are under way, using either a 4 to 6 monthly capsule (66,000 micrograms) of retinyl palmitate in oil (half this dose for children under 1 year) or fortification of sugar or monosodium glutamate.

Treatment. The deficiency is seldom isolated, and the general nutrition must be improved by a balanced diet and precipitating factors and underlying disorders corrected.

Because of the threat of corneal damage and blindness, all patients should receive prompt and full treatment; thus also building up liver reserves and guarding against future relapse. The 66,000 microgram retinyl palmitate capsule is given on diagnosis, again on the second day, and once more before discharge. If there is persistent vomiting or diarrhea, 33,000 micrograms of water-miscible retinyl palmitate is given in the same regimen by intramuscular injection. Oil injection must never be used, as it is not absorbed from the injection site. Maintenance therapy is continued with 10 ml of cod liver oil two or three times daily.

Hypervitaminosis A

Excess intake of vitamin A may be acute or chronic. Acute toxicity in children from a dose of ' several hundred thousand micrograms produces symptoms of raised intracranial pressure. Spontaneous recovery occurs with no residual damage when administration of the vitamin is stopped; fatalities have not been reported. Most children tolerate a large single dose, but a very few appear to be hypersensitive. In adults ingestion by Arctic explorers of several hundred thousand micrograms of vitamin A in a single meal of polar bear or bearded seal liver has produced headache, vomiting, and subsequent peeling of the skin with ultimate recovery.

Chronic poisoning develops after daily doses of tens of thousands of micrograms of vitamin A for many months in adults and smaller doses over a few weeks in infants. Symptoms include anorexia, weight loss, headache, pruritus, liver enlargement, anemia, and pain in the limbs, with periosteal thickening of long bones. Symptoms and signs disappear in from 1 to 4 weeks after cessation of vitamin A intake.

DIABETES MELLITUS IN ADULTS

method of
E. A. HAUNZ, M.D.,
and MARY BLAINE, B.Sc.
Grand Forks, North Dakota

The newly revised classification and diagnostic criteria of diabetes mellitus have significantly altered our previous concepts of this ubiquitous disease to the extent that a brief review of the National Diabetes Data Group (NDDG) recommendations (Harris, Cahill, et al.: Diabetes *28*:1039, 1979) should appropriately precede current therapeutic considerations. Heretofore the classification has been a hodgepodge of ambiguous terminology wherein even the "experts" have differed on acceptable ground rules in defining variants of this disease.

The glucose tolerance test (despite its rejection as a diagnostic parameter by certain clinicians and investigators) is endorsed by the NDDG, but *with decided limitations on its significance and interpretation.* Medicolegally, the practicing physician should be aware that these recommendations are now approved by the American, British, European, and Australian Dia-

betes Associations as well as by the expert committee of the World Health Organization. Indeed, it represents the first worldwide effort to establish consistent, revised criteria for glucose tolerance and screening test values to diagnose diabetes mellitus with *minimal* chance of error.

The most significant conclusion of the immense study is that previously accepted "positive" criteria (blood glucose levels) have been generally too low, explaining in part the high prevalence of false-positive diagnoses heretofore made by well-intentioned clinicians. The NDDG concedes that "this classification is based on contemporary knowledge of diabetes and also represents compromises of different points of view," and that amended revisions will be necessary as continuing research reveals new facets of understanding.

The following brief outline of revised classification and diagnosis should be utilized to afford some medicolegal protection against pitfalls in clinical recognition of adult diabetes, especially in early stages of this heterogenous syndrome.

Classification

1. The term "juvenile diabetes" is no longer appropriate. This insulin-dependent, ketosis-prone type of diabetes (with variable frequency of certain HLA antigens on chromosome 6 and islet cell antibodies) is now designated as *Type I diabetes,* because it may manifest itself initially at any age.

2. Non-insulin-dependent diabetes is now designated *Type II diabetes,* which frequently presents with minimal or no symptoms (as opposed to the usual abrupt onset of symptoms, insulinopenia, and dependence on injected insulin to sustain life which characterizes Type I diabetes). Here insulin levels may be normal, moderately depressed, or excessive. Many of these patients do not have fasting hyperglycemia, may be asymptomatic for years with slow progression of the disease, but are not exempt from vasculopathy. While the onset is typically beyond age 40, it may occur in young subjects, invalidating the previous terms "adult or maturity-onset" diabetes. A more frequent familial pattern of occurrence suggests a stronger genetic basis, including children, adolescents, and adults in whom an autosomal dominant inheritance is well established. Type II diabetes also includes what was previously termed "maturity-onset diabetes of the young" (MODY) — another designation to be abandoned. From 80 to 90 per cent of Type II diabetics are obese subjects in whom hyperglycemia and glucose intolerance are usually improved by adequate weight reduction (and occasionally totally reversed) (Fig. 1) and aggregation of HLA types and islet cell antibodies are absent.

3. The remaining types of diabetes are "lumped" into a subclass of certain other conditions and syndromes with clinical features not generally associated with the "diabetic state." Included are pancreatic disease, acromegaly, Cushing's syndrome, pheochromocytoma, glucagonoma, primary aldosteronism, somatostatinoma, and exposure to exogenous hormones and drugs. Here we see varying degrees of hyperglycemia and glucose intolerance,

"REVERSIBLE DIABETES"
45 YR. OLD FEMALE LOST 98 LBS. IN 9 MOS. WITH STRICT DIET. (MOTHER DIABETIC)

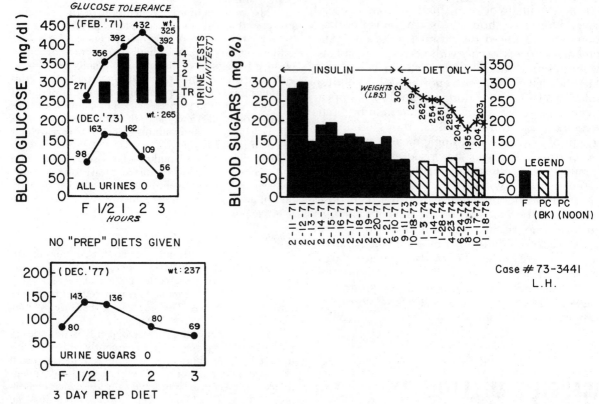

Figure 1. Dramatic illustration of "total reversal" of florid diabetes effected by weight loss of 98 pounds (initial weight, 302 pounds). Referring physician had performed an obviously unnecessary glucose tolerance test (the severe fasting hyperglycemia was unequivocally diagnostic). Insulin was stopped after 3 weeks on a diet of 1000 calories when hyperglycemia disappeared. Follow-up glucose tolerance tests have remained normal to date. Such patients need regular follow-up visits to ensure continued motivation in a reducing program.

which may be induced in part by abnormalities in numbers or affinity of insulin receptors or antibodies, compromising the receptor mechanism.

The practicing physician should utilize the new classification as a "frame of reference" *with decided limitations in applicability to the individual patient.* Because diabetes is more commonly a "dynamic" than a "static" syndrome, a given patient may shift from one classification to another at unpredictable intervals as evidenced by remissions often encountered in early stages of the disease. It is obvious, therefore, that the real purpose of the new classification is to establish more uniform, definitive terminology, eliminating previous overlapping or ambiguous nomenclature which has been so confusing to date. To repeat, it is not an attempt to provide definitive guidelines for therapy of the individual patient.

Recommended Diagnostic Criteria for Adult Diabetes

The diagnosis of so-called "florid" diabetes in a noncomatose patient is nearly always immediately dis-

cernible by its classic triad (polydipsia, polyuria, and polyphagia) and frequent concomitant features of weight loss, drowsiness, dehydration (e.g., soft eyeballs, dry skin), blurred vision, and, not uncommonly, abdominal pain with nausea and vomiting. When such patients are seen in the emergency room or physician's office, the diagnosis (even in a previously known diabetic) should include "stat" procedures as follows: (1) blood (or plasma) glucose determination; (2) plasma sodium, chlorides, blood urea nitrogen, potassium, and ketones; (3) blood gases and pH; (4) routine urinalysis; and (5) complete blood count (CBC) and hematocrit.

Hyperosmolar nonketotic coma (HNKC) must always be considered and recognized promptly, the cardinal features including very high blood glucose levels (often over 1500 mg per dl [100 ml]) and absence (or only a trace) of plasma ketones, together with hyperosmolarity.

The diagnosis of early asymptomatic diabetes in adults, on the other hand, can be a hazardous pursuit because of pitfalls in analysis of laboratory values (Haunz: Geriatrics, Oct. 1979). Indeed, a former Chairman of ,the Committee on Professional Education of the American Diabetes Association has been quoted in a nationwide news release as stating that "one-third of the patients being labeled 'diabetic' don't have the disease." Although this number of "false-positive" diagnoses appears overdrawn, many diabetologists are voicing increased concern over the frequency of such diagnostic errors.

In general, most of these errors are incurred by a physician's naive acceptance of one (or even two) elevated blood glucose levels as unequivocally diagnostic, when in fact more meticulous reappraisal would have negated the diagnosis. Until very recently this whole problem was further compounded by an inclination to "overread" the clinical significance of borderline to mildly positive glucose tolerance tests. The medicolegal implications of "diagnosing" diabetes (which is nonexistent) are self-evident in such a mislabeled patient who thus incurs lifelong stigmata which may erode into every facet of his future life style, with the imposition of insurance riders, restricted driving privileges, limited employability, heightened anxieties over future well-being, and unwelcome self-discipline of diet and daily routine. When reasonable doubt exists, the error of commission (false-positive diagnosis) renders the physician far more vulnerable than the error of omission. Our collection of over 100 patients who presented with an erroneous diagnosis of "diabetes" and were previously subjected to long-term management with diet, oral agents, or insulin attests to the urgency of preceding any discussion of therapy with the following brief review of currently revised techniques as recommended by the NDDG (with minor modifications predicated on our own extensive experience):

Current opinion still supports the a priori assumption that estimation of plasma glucose levels is the sole criterion for early clinical recognition of the diabetic state. (Glycosylated hemoglobin [A_{1C}] is gaining stature in "reinforcing" the significance of hyperglycemia, but remains controversial in its reliability as a single diagnostic test. Indeed, hemoglobin A_{1C} tends to rise with blood glucose levels during the glucose tolerance test, presumably owing to a loosely attached fraction of glucose to hemoglobin.)

"Positive diagnostic criteria" are currently subdivided into the following groups:

Group 1. "Diabetes mellitus (in nonpregnant adults)." *In this group the diagnosis of diabetes is justified if any one of the three following factors is present:* (1) Classic symptoms with gross or unequivocal elevation of plasma glucose. (2) Elevated fasting plasma glucose on more than one occasion. (Oral glucose tolerance test is not required if fasting plasma glucose is 140 mg per dl or more on repeated venous samples.) (3) Fasting plasma glucose less than (2), but sustained elevation of glucose seen during oral glucose tolerance test (OGTT) occurs on more than one occasion. Both the 2 hour venous sample and one other sample taken between a 75 gram oral glucose load and 2 hours later must be 200 mg per dl or more.

Group 2. "Impaired glucose tolerance in non-

pregnant adults." (The diagnosis of "diabetes mellitus" is deferred.) *In this group, three criteria must be met:* (1) The fasting venous plasma glucose must be *below* the diagnostic value for diabetes (viz., less than 140 mg per dl). (2) The plasma venous glucose at 2 hours after a 75 gram oral glucose load must be between normal and diabetic values (viz., less than 200 mg per dl but more than 140 mg per dl). (3) A venous plasma glucose value between ½ hour, 1 hour or 1½ hours after a 75 gram oral glucose load must be less than 200 mg per dl but more than 140 mg per dl.

Summary of normal plasma glucose levels in nonpregnant adults (new NDDG criteria): Fasting value: below 115 mg per dl. Two hour OGTT value: Below 140 mg per dl. OGTT value between ½ hour, 1 hour, or 1½ hours: below 200 mg per dl.

It must be remembered that values for plasma are 15 per cent (not 15 mg per dl) higher than equivalent whole blood values (to extrapolate from plasma to whole blood equivalent, simply multiply the former by 0.86). In our experience capillary (arterial) blood should not be used for precise diagnostic evaluation. Likewise, the Eyetone or Dextrometer (Ames Co., Elkhart, Indiana), Sta-Tek (Biodynamics, Indianapolis, Indiana), and similar devices should not be used for these purposes.

The clinician must be aware of the methodology utilized in his laboratory source. For example, do not use fluoride as a preservative of blood if the glucose oxidase reaction is used, because fluoride interferes with this reaction. Instead, heparin or ethylenediamine tetra-acetic acid (EDTA) should be the anticoagulant of choice.

It should be noted that the time-honored 3 hour value (post 75 gram glucose load) has been deleted by the NDDG. We still prefer inclusion of this in the OGTT since so-called "reactive hypoglycemia" is most apt to appear at this time and may be the first sign of early or impending diabetes, although not diagnostic in itself.

The author's modifications in accepting the new NDDG recommendations are basically three-fold:

1. We believe the 3 hour plasma glucose level should be retained because of its value in detecting reactive hypoglycemia, frequently signaling possible "early" diabetes.

2. We perform a glucose tolerance test (after a 3 day "preparatory diet" of at least 150 grams of carbohydrate daily) whenever the fasting plasma glucose ranges from 125 mg per dl to 150 mg per dl (on two determinations) and/or the 2 hour postprandial plasma glucose ranges from 150 mg per dl to 200 mg per dl on two determinations after a "loading meal" of at least 100 grams of carbohydrate. In nonketotic asymptomatic patients exhibiting values in this range, a glucose tolerance test is entirely innocuous and serves to *quantify* more precisely the severity of the disease as a guide to therapy. (Indeed, a positive afternoon glucose tolerance test, repeated in the morning, has sometimes been normal, disproving the validity of fasting and postprandial determinations.) The prevailing opinion that this test is time consuming, expensive, and unnecessary is an unjustified aversion to the procedure when viewed in the context of avoid-

ing the erroneous diagnosis of a lifelong, incurable disease with its attendant psychologic and socioeconomic stigmata.

3. We utilize "age-dependency criteria" in interpreting the oral glucose tolerance test in subjects over age 50 (viz., add 10 mg per dl per decade beyond age 50 years to all values except the *fasting* * level). While this is controversial, it obviously encourages conservatism in diagnosis and therapy in this group.

As already delineated for the glucose tolerance test, postprandial screening tests should be performed in the forenoon (after breakfast), since studies in diurnal variations in response to glucose loading have been repeatedly shown to exhibit higher "normal" blood glucose levels in the afternoon than after breakfast. Indeed, we have found this to be a common cause for the erroneous diagnosis of diabetes.

In summary, it is imperative that the practicing physician have practical insight into the revised classification and diagnostic criteria of diabetes mellitus before implementing therapy, at least for his medicolegal protection. In essence, the term diabetes mellitus should now be restricted to those persons who have (1) overt diabetic symptoms and unequivocal hyperglycemia, (2) fasting plasma glucose levels exceeding 140 mg per dl on more than one occasion, or (3) if fasting plasma glucose is not elevated, plasma glucose levels during the OGTT that exceed 200 mg per dl at 2 hours post-glucose loading and at some other point between fasting and 2 hours on more than one occasion.†

Childhood and gestational diabetes are omitted from this discussion because of space limitation. (Classification and diagnostic criteria for these groups are available on request from Maureen Harris, Ph.D., M.P.H., Westwood Building, Room 607, National Institutes of Health, Bethesda, Md. 20205.)

Therapeutic Considerations

Once the diagnosis of diabetes is *unequivocally established*, appropriate therapy, including thorough indoctrination of the patient in self-management, must be *carefully tailored to that individual's need*. For many years we have utilized a simple technique of therapeutic classification as "categories of response." Thus, whether treatment is initiated in a newly discovered diabetic or a previously established case, each patient should fit into one of four groups:

Group 1: Control requires only simple restriction of free sugar ("qualitative diet"). The patient's weight is optimal, the urine remains essentially sugar free, and fasting and post-

---

*Most authorities concur that fasting levels remain essentially constant throughout life in nondiabetics.

†It has long been the author's opinion that the glucose tolerance test, properly executed with adequate preparatory diet, attains its greatest reliability in *excluding* the diagnosis of diabetes when it is *normal*.

prandial plasma glucose levels do not exceed 125 mg per dl and 170 mg per dl, respectively, without use of insulin or sulfonylureas.

Group 2: Control requires a carefully measured ("quantitative") diet to achieve optimal weight, minimize glycosuria, and maintain fasting and postprandial plasma glucose levels below 140 mg per dl and 180 mg per dl, respectively, without use of insulin or sulfonylureas. (These patients are usually obese and may revert to Group 1 with adequate weight reduction.) (*It is recommended that an "official" diagnosis of diabetes in Groups 1 and 2 be held in abeyance, pending reappraisal after 6 to 8 weeks of diet therapy.*)

Group 3: Control requires, in addition to a quantitative diet, up to 40 units of exogenous insulin (or a sulfonylurea compound) to minimize glycosuria and maintain fasting and postprandial sugars equivalent to those achieved in Group 2. In the asymptomatic, uncomplicated patient, insulin (or a sulfonylurea compound) should not be started until the obese subject has attained ideal weight via strict dietary supervision. If all attempts fail, it becomes a highly objectionable "therapy of concession."

Group 4: Control requires in excess of 40 units of exogenous insulin with appropriate diet to achieve minimal glycosuria and blood sugar levels equivalent to Group 2. A sulfonylurea compound may be a successful substitute for insulin, but *should not be tried until control has initially been established with insulin*. (If the patient is ketosis-prone, sulfonylureas are contraindicated.) Here, again, in the obese subject the physician may temporize on the use of insulin during strict dietary supervision but at considerable risk of morbidity (e.g., infection, dehydration, active triad, weakness, neuropathy). Close follow-up is imperative.

Plasma sugar values proposed herein as indices of "control" are obviously arbitrary and as such cannot be the sine qua non for therapeutic grouping. Hypoglycemic episodes, insulin-sensitive metabolic instability, and poor compliance in those who require insulin may invalidate attempts at precise grouping. Furthermore, ketosis-prone patients who exhibit inordinately high glucose levels with ketonuria, frank ketoacidosis, or diabetic coma constitute medical emergencies, often requiring immediate hospitalization with skilled nursing care. The management of diabetic ketoacidosis with or without coma will be considered separately.

In summary, the categories of response described above are designed solely as a guide to institute immediate therapy for the *chemical severity* of the disease. Above all considerations, significant ketonemia or ketonuria (with or without impending acidosis), or both, in an established case of diabetes *always requires appropriate insulinization promptly.*

The American Diabetes Association has recently officially endorsed the concept that optimized control of the blood sugar on a long-term basis does indeed significantly reduce the evolutionary tempo, severity, and prevalence rates of ultimate dreaded complications, especially as they relate to microvasculopathy (Cahill, Etzwiler, and Freinkel: N. Engl. J. Med. *294*:1004, 1976). It follows, therefore, that all difficult cases should have the benefit of expert consultation, since "diabetology" is now a recognized specialty. Likewise, the physician who lacks adequate facilities for thorough, detailed education of the patient in self-management should refer his patient to a diabetes teaching center (available in most larger hospitals). Because about 25 per cent of the diabetic population have some form of diabetic retinopathy, every patient deserves funduscopic examination by an ophthalmologist at regular intervals to avoid delay in early treatment.

Diet

All diabetologists concur that "diet is the keystone in the arch of all therapy," especially in the case of obese Type I and II diabetics. But more specifically, enlisting the patient's full cooperation in adhering to a prescribed diet (preferably by a dietitian) and *achieving ideal weight on a permanent basis represents the greatest challenge in the entire therapeutic spectrum of adult diabetes.*

In 1970 the Food and Drug Administration (FDA) stated: "The initial and essential foundation for the management of diabetes is diet and weight control. When symptoms of the disease (and hyperglycemia) are adequately controlled by these measures, no other therapy is indicated." Thirty years' experience with over 5000 private diabetic patients has convinced this author that to achieve any degree of success in all patients (exclusive of Group 1) a qualified dietitian is indispensable as part of the health care team. The physician who lacks such facilities can usually obtain outpatient instruction from a hospital dietitian, and cases of intractable obesity require frequent follow-up visits with weight checks. In such cases it has been repeatedly shown that "single encounters between a dietitian and the patient are useless. Lifelong habits cannot be altered in one session" (Arky). It is far too complicated and time consuming for the busy clinician to achieve an in-depth analysis of a patient's ethnic preferences, timing of meals, diet composition and energy content thereof, and level of physical activity peculiar to that subject's lifestyle. Yet it is his responsibility to prescribe the appropriate caloric intake and percentages of carbohydrate, protein, and fat, together with features to correct lipid disturbances, coexistent hypertension, and the like.

The author has utilized full-time dietitians for 30 years and repeatedly reaffirmed that *the greatest single therapeutic deficit in adult diabetes is proper dietary instruction and supervision.* While the "Exchange System" of the American Diabetes Association can be taught by competent nurses and "diabetes educators," the efforts of these participants usually lack the motivation, respect, and compliance engendered by the dietary career-nutritionist. It cannot be overemphasized that under these most ideal conditions the success rate in effecting weight loss among the obese remains relatively poor! A cavalier approach to diet by the physician is certain to be reflected in the poorest adherence by the patient. Only after intensive efforts to achieve weight loss can the clinician justify the use of insulin (or oral agents in particular) to control severe degrees of hyperglycemia as a "therapy of concession."

The Food Exchange System* of the American Diabetes and Dietetic Associations is the most workable diet for the average patient. The exchange lists for meal planning were revised in 1977. Foods have been divided into six lists (Table 1). Exchanges are units of equality. Food portions within an exchange group are equal to one another in kilocalories, carbohydrate, protein, fat, and more important, available glucose. Adherence to prescribed exchange meal plan enhances day-to-day consistency in caloric intake, thereby reducing variations in glucose peaks.

The appropriate calorie level for a diabetic is one which achieves and maintains ideal weight. This level can be determined in several ways:

1. Based on weight history (fluctuations) and diet inventories as evaluated by the dietitian.

2. Estimated basal caloric requirements, which can be approximated by multiplying the ideal body weight in pounds (from height-weight tables) by 10. Add approximately 25 per cent for the sedentary person, 50 per cent for the moder-

Text continued on page 445

---

*For information on the Food Exchange System, write the American Diabetes Association, Inc., 600 Fifth Avenue, New York, New York 10020. The exchange lists are based on material in the Exchange Lists for Meal Planning prepared by Committees of the American Diabetes Association, Inc., and the American Dietetic Association in cooperation with the National Institute of Arthritis, Metabolism, and Digestive Diseases and the National Heart and Lung Institute, National Institutes of Health.

TABLE 1. ADA Exchange Lists

List 1. Milk Exchanges
12 grams of carbohydrate, 8 grams of protein, a trace of fat, and 80 calories

Nonfat fortified milk	
Skim or nonfat milk	1 cup
Powdered (nonfat dry, before adding liquid)	1/3 cup
Canned, evaporated—skim milk	1/2 cup
Buttermilk made from skim milk	1 cup
Yogurt made from skim milk (plain, unflavored)	1 cup
Low-fat fortified milk	
1% fat fortified milk (omit 1/2 Fat Exchange)	1 cup
2% fat fortified milk (omit 1 Fat Exchange)	1 cup
Yogurt made from 2% fortified milk (plain, unflavored) (omit 1 Fat Exchange)	1 cup
Whole milk (omit 2 Fat Exchanges)	
Whole milk	1 cup
Canned, evaporated whole milk	1/2 cup
Buttermilk made from whole milk	1 cup
Yogurt made from whole milk (plain, unflavored)	1 cup

List 2. Vegetable Exchanges
5 grams of carbohydrate, 2 grams of protein, and 25 calories; one Exchange is 1/2 cup

Asparagus	Greens:	Onions
Bean sprouts	Beet	Rhubarb
Beets	Chards	Rutabaga
Broccoli	Collards	Sauerkraut
Brussels sprouts	Dandelion	String beans, green or yellow
Cabbage	Kale	Summer squash
Carrots	Mustard	Tomatoes
Cauliflower	Spinach	Tomato juice
Celery	Turnip	Turnips
Eggplant	Mushrooms	Vegetable juice cocktail
Green pepper	Okra	Zucchini

The following raw vegetables may be used as desired:

Chicory	Escarole	Radishes
Chinese cabbage	Lettuce	Watercress
Cucumbers	Parsley	
Endive	Pickles, dill	

Starchy vegetables are found in the Bread Exchange list

List 3. Fruit Exchanges
10 grams of carbohydrate and 40 calories

Apple	1 small	Mango	1/2 small
Apple juice	1/3 cup	Melon	
Applesauce (unsweetened)	1/2 cup	Cantaloupe	1/4 small
Apricots, fresh	2 medium	Honeydew	1/8 medium
Apricots, dried	4 halves	Watermelon	1 cup
Banana	1/2 small	Nectarine	1 small
Berries		Orange	1 small
Blackberries	1/2 cup	Orange juice	1/2 cup
Blueberries	1/2 cup	Papaya	3/4 cup
Raspberries	1/2 cup	Peach	1 medium
Strawberries	3/4 cup	Pear	1 small
Cherries	10 large	Persimmon, native	1 medium
Cider	1/3 cup	Pineapple	1/2 cup
Dates	2	Pineapple juice	1/3 cup
Figs, fresh	1	Plums	2 medium
Figs, dried	1	Prunes	2 medium
Grapefruit	1/2	Prune juice	1/4 cup
Grapefruit juice	1/2 cup	Raisins	2 tablespoons
Grapes	12	Tangerine	1 medium
Grape juice	1/4 cup		

Cranberries may be used as desired if no sugar is added

TABLE 1. **ADA Exchange Lists** (*Continued*)

List 4. Bread Exchanges
15 grams of carbohydrate, 2 grams of protein, and 70 calories

Bread			Dried beans, peas, and lentils	
White (including French and Italian)	1 slice		Beans, peas, lentils (dried and cooked)	1/2 cup
Whole wheat	1 slice		Baked beans, no pork (canned)	1/4 cup
Rye or pumpernickel	1 slice		Starchy vegetables	
Raisin	1 slice		Corn	1/3 cup
Bagel, small	1/2		Corn on cob	1 small
English muffin, small	1/2		Lima beans	1/2 cup
Plain roll, bread	1		Parsnips	2/3 cup
Frankfurter roll	1/2		Peas, green (canned or frozen)	1/2 cup
Hamburger bun	1/2		Potato, white	1 small
Dried bread crumbs	3 tbs		Potato (mashed)	1/2 cup
Tortilla, 6"	1		Pumpkin	3/4 cup
Cereal			Winter squash, acorn, or butternut	1/2 cup
Bran flakes	1/2 cup		Yam or sweet potato	1/4 cup
Other ready-to-eat unsweetened cereal	3/4 cup		Prepared foods	
Puffed cereal (unfrosted)	1 cup		Biscuit 2" dia (omit 1 Fat Exchange)	1
Cereal (cooked)	1/2 cup		Corn bread, 2" × 2" × 1" (omit 1 Fat Exchange)	1
Grits (cooked)	1/2 cup		Corn muffin, 2" dia (omit 1 Fat Exchange)	1
Rice or barley (cooked)	1/2 cup		Crackers, round butter type (omit 1 Fat Exchange)	5
Pasta (cooked), spaghetti, noodles, macaroni	1/2 cup		Muffin, plain small (omit 1 Fat Exchange)	1
Popcorn (popped, no fat added, large kernel)	3 cups		Potatoes, French fried, length 2" to 3-1/2" (omit 1 Fat Exchange)	8
Cornmeal (dry)	2 tbs		Potato or corn chips (omit 2 Fat Exchanges)	15
Flour	2-1/2 tbs		Pancake, 5" × 1/2" (omit 1 Fat Exchange)	1
Wheat germ	1/4 cup		Waffle, 5" × 1/2" (omit 1 Fat Exchange)	1
Crackers				
Arrowroot	3			
Graham, 2-1/2" sq	2			
Matzoth, 4" × 6"	1/2			
Oyster	20			
Pretzels 3-1/8" long × 1/8" dia	25			
Rye Wafers, 2" × 3-1/2"	3			
Saltines	6			
Soda, 2-1/2" sq	4			

List 5. Meat Exchanges:
Lean Meat
One Exchange of lean meat (1 oz) contains 7 grams of protein, 3 grams of fat, and 55 calories

Beef:	Baby beef (very lean), chipped beef, chuck, flank steak, tenderloin, plate ribs, plate skirt steak, round (bottom, top), all cuts rump, spare ribs, tripe	1 oz
Lamb:	Leg, rib, sirloin, loin (roast and chops), shank, shoulder	1 oz
Pork:	Leg (whole rump, center shank), ham, smoked (center slices)	1 oz
Veal:	Leg, loin, rib, shank, shoulder, cutlets	1 oz
Poultry:	Meat *without skin* of chicken, turkey, cornish hen, guinea hen, pheasant	1 oz
Fish:	Any fresh or frozen	1 oz
	Canned salmon, tuna, mackerel, crab, lobster	1/4 cup
	Clams, oysters, scallops, shrimp	5 or 1 oz
	Sardines, drained	3
Cheeses containing less than 5% butterfat		1 oz.
Cottage cheese, dry and 2% butterfat		1/4 cup
Dried beans and peas (omit 1 Bread Exchange)		1/2 cup

Table continued on following page

TABLE 1. **ADA Exchange Lists** (*Continued*)

List 5. Meat Exchanges:
Medium-Fat Meat
One Exchange of medium-fat meat (1 oz.) contains 7 grams of protein, 5 grams of fat, and 75 calories

Beef	Ground (15% fat), corned beef (canned), rib eye, round (ground commercial)	1 oz
Pork:	Loin (all cuts tenderloin), shoulder arm (picnic), shoulder blade, Boston butt, Canadian bacon, boiled ham	1 oz
Liver, heart, kidney, and sweetbreads (these are high in cholesterol)		1 oz
Cottage cheese, creamed		1/4 cup
Cheese:	Mozarella, ricotta, farmer's cheese, neufchatel	1 oz
	Parmesan	3 tbs
Egg (high in cholesterol)		1
Peanut butter (omit 2 additional Fat Exchanges)		2 tbs

List 5. Meat Exchanges:
High-Fat Meat
One Exchange of high-fat meat (1 oz) contains 7 grams of protein, 8 grams of fat, and 100 calories

Beef:	Brisket, corned beef (brisket), ground beef (more than 20% fat), hamburger (commercial), chuck (ground commercial), roasts (rib), steaks (club and rib)	1 oz
Lamb:	Breast	1 oz
Pork:	Spare ribs, loin (back ribs), pork (ground), country style ham, deviled ham	1 oz
Veal:	Breast	1 oz
Poultry:	Capon, duck (domestic), goose	1 oz
Cheese:	Cheddar types	1 oz
Cold cuts		4-1/2″ × 1/8″ slice
Frankfurter		1 small

List 6. Fat Exchanges
One Exchange of fat contains 5 grams of fat and 45 calories

Margarine, soft, tub or stick*	1 teaspoon
Avocado (4″ in diameter)†	1/8
Oil, corn, cottonseed, safflower, soy, sunflower	1 teaspoon
Oil, olive†	1 teaspoon
Oil, peanut†	1 teaspoon
Olives†	5 small
Almonds†	10 whole
Pecans†	2 large whole
Peanuts†	
Spanish	20 whole
Virginia	10 whole
Walnuts	6 small
Nuts, other†	6 small
Margarine, regular stick	1 teaspoon
Butter	1 teaspoon
Bacon fat	1 teaspoon
Bacon, crisp	1 strip
Cream, light	2 tablespoons
Cream, sour	2 tablespoons
Cream, heavy	1 tablespoon
Cream cheese	1 tablespoon
French dressing‡	1 tablespoon
Italian dressing‡	1 tablespoon
Lard	1 teaspoon
Mayonnaise‡	1 teaspoon
Salad dressing, mayonnaise type‡	2 teaspoons
Salt pork	3/4 inch cube

*Made with corn, cottonseed, safflower, soy or sunflower oil only.
†Fat content is primarily monounsaturated.
‡If made with corn, cottonseed, safflower, soy, or sunflower oil, can be used on fat modified diet.

ately active, and up to 75 per cent for the strenuously hard worker.

3. "Maintenance diet": multiply the person's weight in kg by 30. "Reducing diet": multiply weight in kg by 20. "Gaining diet": multiply weight in kg by 40.

The recommended distribution of these kilocalories has now been revised upward to 50 to 60 per cent from carbohydrate, while protein and fat have been correspondingly lowered to 12 to 20 per cent and 30 to 35 per cent respectively. (See Table 2 for exemplary diabetic meal plan.) (We have observed exceptions to this; occasionally glucose tolerance is *not* improved by upgrading the complexed carbohydrate.) The value of dietary fiber in improving glucose tolerance among certain diabetics remains controversial, as results are often conflicting or statistically insignificant. Whenever acceptable to the patient, natural foods containing unrefined carbohydrate with fiber should be substituted for highly refined carbohydrates, which are lower in fiber and which usually result in hyperglycemic "spikes."

The revision in the Exchange Lists for Meal Planning makes it possible to distinguish between saturated and polyunsaturated fat. The level of saturated fatty acids in the diet should be decreased to less than 10 per cent of the total kilocalories. Polyunsaturated fatty acids should supply up to 10 per cent of the total kilocalories, and the remainder of ingested fat is derived from monosaturated sources (Principles of Nutrition and Dietary Recommendations for Individuals with Diabetes Mellitus, American Diabetes Association, 1979). Control of body weight is likely to be more rewarding than change of dietary lipids in decreasing the risk of coronary heart disease in adult men.

The dietary program is carefully planned by the dietitian with the patient. The first step is a detailed analysis of the foods eaten, quantities, and frequency. Meal plans are adapted as nearly as possible to the individual within the principles of optimal diabetic control. Consistency is the watchword of a newly established diet plan. Hypoglycemia is minimized in the Type I diabetic by an orderly routine of prompt mealtimes and using supplementary snacks commensurate with increased physical activity.

Except for refined carbohydrate restriction, the diet differs little from that of the nondiabetic, since both are premised on sound principles of nutrition. The major change for most new diabetics is loss of "random" eating. The only "side effect" of the exchange diet is boredom. Thought and ingenuity by the dietitian in diet planning with proper food selection is the best way to offset this. Foods included in the list are only as dull and

TABLE 2. Diabetic Meal Plan

Carbohydrate, 220 grams; Protein, 90 grams; Fat, 60 grams; Kilocalories, 1800

Food for the Day

2 1/2 cups	Milk (List 1)
1 cup	Vegetable exchanges (List 2)
3	Fruit exchanges (List 3)
10	Bread exchanges (List 4)
7	Meat exchanges (List 5)
5	Fat exchanges (List 6)

Menu Suggestions

Exchanges	
Breakfast	
1 fruit (List 3)	1/2 cup orange juice
2 bread (List 4)	2 slices toast
1 meat (List 5)	1 poached egg
2 fat (List 6)	2 pats margarine
1/2 milk (List 1)	1/2 cup skim milk
Any amount	Coffee or tea
Morning lunch	
1 bread (List 4)	6 Saltines
Lunch or supper	
2 meat (List 5)	1/2 cup cottage cheese
2 bread (List 4)	2 slices rye bread
1 vegetable (List 2)	Lettuce
1 fruit (List 3)	1 small apple
1 fat (List 6)	1 pat margarine
1 milk (List 1)	1 cup skim milk
Afternoon lunch	
1 bread (List 4)	2 graham crackers
1 milk (List 1)	1 cup skim milk
Dinner	
3 meat (List 5)	1 baked pork chop
2 bread (List 4)	1 slice bread, 1/2 cup mashed potatoes
1 vegetable (List 2)	1/2 cup carrots
1 fruit (List 3)	3/4 cup strawberries
2 fat (List 6)	2 pats margarine
Any amount	Coffee or tea
Bedtime lunch	
2 bread (List 4)	2 slices bread
1 meat (List 5)	1 slice cheese
Any amount	Lettuce
	Coffee or tea

monotonous as the preparer wants them to be, because variations within the exchange system are almost unlimited. Frequent follow-up visits with the dietitian are vital to ensure continued patient compliance.

The standardized exchange diets facilitate selection of foods which are familiar, desirable, and economically feasible for the individual patient. Special dietary foods are not necessary and, in fact, often contain excessive calories. *Foods that are sugar-free are not necessarily calorie-free.* Many labels on dietetic foods are misleading. It is necessary, however, to use only water-packed, unsweetened, or artificially sweetened canned fruits, carbonated beverages, dietetic gums, candies, gelatin desserts, and the like. Non-nutritive sweeteners are allowed. With regard to saccharin, the American Diabetes Association's policy statement implies that the perceived need and benefit of saccharin to the public generally, and especially to the individuals afflicted with diabetes mellitus and/or obesity, are too great to warrant a ban, particularly since no substitute is available. More recently the Food and Drug Administration has taken a less stringent posture against saccharin as a possible carcinogen.

The purpose of patient education is to enhance the insight of the patient in diagnosis and treatment and to inspire compliance and self-responsibility. The merits and psychologic value in convincing obese individuals that they can change their long-established and deeply ingrained eating habits are self-evident. The best motivation is the total thrust of the physician and the health care team, who should actively protect patients from massive exploitation by the news media, including "diet pills," and diet schemes.

Exercise

Extensive research has unequivocally demonstrated that adequate physical activity enhances affinity of receptor sites for insulin action, usually lowering requirements for exogenous insulin in linear relationship to the degree of exercise. It is postulated that exercise reduces excess platelet adhesiveness typical of the diabetic state and thus may delay or prevent retinopathy. It is thus imperative that diabetics receiving insulin or oral agents maintain a strategic equilibrium through proper timing of meals and uniform physical energy, carefully reconciled with the temporal action of the hypoglycemic modality. Intermeal and bedtime snacks are usually essential to avoidance of hypoglycemic episodes. In Type II diabetes (not requiring insulin or oral agents) snack feedings are not necessary.

Oral Antidiabetic Agents

The University Group Diabetes Program (UGDP), first reported in 1970, sparked one of the most heated controversies in the history of modern therapeutics in concluding that the use of tolbutamide (Orinase) and phenformin (DBI) more than doubled the cardiovascular mortality among diabetics so treated. Clinicians and researchers still remain divided on the merits of this

study. However, all physicians are in accord with the fact that the major favorable impact of this report was to discourage the indiscriminate use of insulin and especially oral agents as a substitute for an optimized diet to effect weight reduction in the obese diabetic. For medicolegal reasons, in particular, more physicians have become motivated to implement proper dietary control before resorting to these agents. Another "spinoff" has been more cautious dosage calibration among subjects so treated.

Table 3 should be memorized by all physicians utilizing the four agents still in use. *Far more important than which of the four agents should be used is a thorough knowledge of dosage, time action, pharmacology, and side effects inherent in utilizing the one chosen.* Package inserts contain adequate clinical information and should be carefully read before prescribing. Space limitation permits only a brief résumé of basic differences of these compounds:

Tolbutamide (Orinase) is a butyl compound, carboxylated in the liver into inactive substances, which are then excreted by the kidneys. Its brief half-life requires divided dosage (i.e., two or three doses daily). Oxidation end-products may produce spurious albuminuria.

Acetohexamide (Dymelor) and *tolazamide* (Tolinase) are intermediate-acting compounds, metabolized by the liver. The bulk of acetohexamide is converted to hydroxyacetohexamide, which accounts for about 75 per cent of its hypoglycemic effect, while tolazamide is metabolized to at least three active "daughter compounds" in the liver as hypoglycemic end-products. Divided dosage (twice daily) is usually necessary.

Chlorpropamide (Diabinese): Recent studies suggest that about 20 per cent of this compound is excreted unchanged by the kidneys, the remainder being metabolized. (It should be realized that all sulfonylureas are relatively contraindicated in the presence of significant impairment of renal function.) It is the only sulfonylurea which can and should be given in single daily dosage because of its extended half-life (35 to 72 hours). Gastrointestinal intolerance occasionally requires divided (twice daily) dosage, but we rarely see this.

TABLE 3. **Action Times and Dosages of Current Oral Antidiabetic Agents**

DRUG	TIME (HOURS)	DOSAGES	FREQUENCY OF ADMINISTRATION	TABLET OR CAPSULE SIZE
Tolbutamide (Orinase)	8	1000 to 3000 mg	b.i.d. or t.i.d.	500 mg
Acetohexamide (Dymelor)	12–24	500 to 1500 mg	Once daily to b.i.d.	250 and 500 mg
Tolazamide (Tolinase)	16–24	100 to 1000 mg	Once daily to b.i.d.	100 and 250 mg
Chlorpropamide (Diabinese)	24–36	125 to 500 mg	Once daily	100 and 250 mg

TABLE 4. **Efficacy of Chlorpropamide**

1. Reduces hyperglycemia and improves insulin binding to mononuclear cells (Olefsky and Reaven, 1976)
2. Inhibits glucagon-stimulated glucose production by augmenting endogenous insulin action (thus potentiating hepatic action of insulin) (Blumenthal, 1976)
3. Significantly improves HbA_{1C} levels, denoting improved control of diabetes (Peterson and Jones, 1978)
4. Can improve hyperglycemia even after maximal stimulation of endogenous insulin is attained (extrapancreatic pharmacokinetics)
5. Hypoglycemia is rare in *properly managed* patients
6. SIADH syndrome* is rare and usually due to excessive dosage

*Syndrome of inappropriate antidiuretic hormone secretion.

The author's preference for chlorpropamide is based on over 20 years' observation of its clinical utility among more than 700 patients. Until a superior compound is forthcoming, this appears to be the drug of choice because: (1) dosage is most cost effective, (2) compliance is enhanced by its uniform effectiveness in once daily dosage, and (3) side effects (especially cumulative hypoglycemia) are indeed rare *when the drug is used properly with adequate follow-up, in minimally effective dosage, and when "refills" coincide with follow-up visits.*

To date there are approximately 2500 publications on chlorpropamide, many of which attest to its overall clinical superiority. Current research suggests that *in properly selected cases* sulfonylureas in general (and chlorpropamide in particular) may be superior to insulin in metabolically stable, nonketotic diabetics (Table 4).

Following is a summary of therapy with sulfonylureas, along with caveats on their use:

1. Do not use in patients under 30 years of age, in pregnancy, or in ketosis-prone subjects.

2. Use *minimal effective dose* and prescribe only enough for the interim between office visits. (Label prescription "no refill without permission.")

3. Inform the patient of all potential hazards, including primary and secondary failures, disulfiram reactions with alcohol, cumulative hypoglycemia and skin rash. ("Primary failure," by definition, occurs within the first month; "secondary failure" occurs at any time thereafter.)

4. Patients who prefer insulin should be encouraged to take it, in view of the UGDP controversy.

5. Do not give sulfonylurea compounds or insulin if blood sugar levels are within the limits of Group 1 or 2 in "categories of response" (see p. 440).

6. Do not combine insulin with sulfonylurea therapy.

7. Do not permit patients to defer follow-up visits longer than 3 months, at which time both fasting and postprandial plasma glucose determinations protect both physician and patient. (Obviously, certain patients require more frequent office visits, and patients with very mild cases, less frequent visits.)

8. When transfer from chlorpropamide to insulin is indicated, proceed cautiously because the hypoglycemic effects of chlorpropamide may persist as long as 5 or 6 days after the drug is discontinued. Conversely, the author agrees with Shuman (Medical Times, 1980) that some patients with rather severe (nonketotic) hyperglycemia may become sulfonylurea responsive from pretreatment with insulin, which "permits regranulation of beta cells depleted of secretory granules and reduces plasma concentration of competing substrate fatty acids." This requires close supervision.

9. *Remember:* The medicolegal risk of cumulative hypoglycemia or undetected primary or secondary failure from sulfonylurea therapy in a "neglected" patient is much greater than that which obtains with insulin-taking diabetics. (The aged are more vulnerable to unpredictable cumulative hypoglycemia. They can and should be protected by less puristic control of hyperglycemia.)

10. As this article goes to press, a final ruling of the FDA to insert a warning on the use of sulfonylurea agents in the context of UGDP study results is still in limbo. If the warning of a possible two-and-one-half-fold increase in cardiovascular mortality, occurring from sulfonylurea therapy, is incorporated in package inserts, patients should sign an "informed consent," including a refusal to take insulin. While this does not provide immunity from a malpractice suit, it does provide documentary evidence of a properly informed patient.

The biguanide phenformin (DBI) is purposely omitted from the discussion of oral agents, since its use has been virtually totally banned by the FDA because of burgeoning case reports of lactic acidosis incident to its use. (The medical community is also divided on this issue, however.)

In summary, sulfonylureas are not and never have been a substitute for strict dietary adherence. In properly selected cases they may be superior to insulin by (1) augmenting endogenous insulin release by reducing hepatic glucose output, (2) increasing insulin secretion via beta-cytotropic action, and (3) enhancing receptor sites.

So-called "second generation" sulfonylureas at present await FDA approval, viz., glyburide

TABLE 5. **Currently Available Insulins**

TYPES	FORM	ACTION	PEAK ACTIVITY (HOURS)	DURATION (HOURS)
Regular (crystalline)*	Clear solution	Rapid	2–4	5–7
NPH	Crystalline	Intermediate	6–12	24–28
Protamine zinc (PZI)	Amorphous	Prolonged	14–24	36+
Semilente	Amorphous	Rapid	2–4	12–16
Lente†	30% amorphous 70% crystalline	Intermediate	6–12	24–28
Ultralente	Crystalline	Prolonged	18–24	36+

*Clinicians should be aware that "the time of maximum effect and total duration of action of regular insulin are significantly longer than current textbook data indicate," the peak effect persisting for several hours and the total duration up to 17 hours in many patients (Field et al.: Clin. Endocrinol. Nutr. 1980). This is why two injections of regular insulin are often successful in achieving 24 hour glycemic control.

†Recent studies suggest that in some diabetics Lente falls short of 24 hour time action.

and glipizide. Many authorities question the wisdom of introducing these compounds, since they possess no real advantages over those in current use, until the UGDP controversy might be resolved.

The Insulins

Insulin preparations in current use with corresponding durations of action are illustrated in Table 5. The indications for use of insulin are self-evident from the above, viz., all Type 1 diabetics in Groups 3 and 4 of categories of response. But again it must be remembered that patients may "shift" from one type or category to another. Early insulin therapy in newly discovered Type 1 cases may induce remissions for weeks, months, and rarely *years,* after which the diabetes invariably reasserts itself, insidiously or abruptly. (Globin insulin is omitted because it is rarely used.)

The "New" Insulins. Physicians should be aware of recent progress in purification of beef-pork preparations via ion exchange chromatography, known as *chromatographic refinement,* by Lilly Research Laboratories. The major advance in their new purification process is the reduction of undesirable proinsulin from 1 to 5 per cent (in the conventional insulin preparations) to less than 0.005 per cent in the newest product. This new "advance" should not be confused with the initial development of single peak insulin in 1972, when the proinsulin content was reduced to less than 0.3 per cent via gel filtration chromatography. The practical clinical implications for the physicians are two-fold:

1. Close supervision is essential when converting a patient from "old" to "new" insulin, because in occasional cases hypoglycemic episodes might result from its relatively higher potency.* The physician can avoid embarrassment by discussing this before the patient reads the "patient information leaflet" now included when purchase is made.

2. Insulin lipoatrophy has been virtually eliminated (Galloway, Wentworth, Haunz, et al.: in press) by these new preparations, while lipohypertrophy and insulin allergy are now less common. Do not resort to the pure pork preparation (now known as Iletin II) in cases of allergy or lipoatrophy until a thorough trial with the new insulin has proved unsuccessful. Iletin II (pork) is more expensive and may be needed on a temporary basis only. Because the risk is minimal, it has been our policy to rechallenge the patient with the standard preparation (beef-pork) again in 2 to 4 weeks and, if the allergy persists, every 2 months thereafter. Persistent insulin lipoatrophy will nearly always disappear if Iletin II (pork) is injected directly (hypodermically) into atrophic areas. This should be a "last resort" and the usual beef-pork insulins reinstituted when the lipoatrophy disappears.

How to "Insulinize" the New Patient in an Office Setting. 1. First establish indication for insulin via criteria already mentioned. (The initial visit is of crucial significance to the patient. It must be an unhurried, skillful, compassionate exercise by the physician who should, himself, give that historic "first shot" before referring the apprehensive patient to the "diabetes educator" and dietitian.)

2. The patient should be on sick leave from employment but remain physically active to a degree commensurate with energy expenditure

*At present it is not possible to identify which patients need a reduction in dosage and, if so, whether it occurs abruptly or gradually.

of his or her usual daily routine. In difficult-to-control cases, driving and other potentially hazardous pursuits should be interdicted until optimal control is established.

3. Patient education and dietary supervision should be concomitants of the "regulating" process, but must be highly individualized to avoid teaching faster than the patient can "learn" and vice versa.

4. In the "average" case, experience has taught us that from 3 to 6 days are usually necessary to achieve optimal response to appropriate insulin dosage and complete basic instruction in diet, self-management, insulin self-injections, and recognition and treatment of insulin reactions. Plasma glucose is measured three times daily (fasting, postprandially, and 4:00 P.M.) and reconciled with urine diaries recording premeal and bedtime glycosuria. ("Second voidings" are tested when considered necessary.) Not many patients object to this extensive routine when reminded that expensive hospitalization is being circumvented and that they are investing a few days' time to ensure maximum longevity and minimize the potential of ultimate serious complications of a lifelong incurable disease.

These same principles of management are utilized in previously known diabetics who present themselves "out of control" or with complications not requiring hospitalization. Refresher courses are nearly always necessary.

Split-Dose Insulinization. The split-dose principle of insulin therapy consists of giving approximately two thirds of a dose of modified insulin (Lente or NPH) with or without regular insulin admixture before breakfast and the remaining one third of the same insulin (again with or without regular admixture) before supper or at bedtime. Several publications emphasize that better overall control can be achieved around the clock with this approach, especially in childhood Type 1 diabetes. However, this author believes that every patient being "regulated" deserves, a priori, a carefully executed initial trial of single daily dosage of a modified insulin, mixed with regular insulin (if the latter appears indicated), with a scrupulous, painstaking analytic distillation of his or her life style, dietary formulation (and adherence thereto), uniformity of physical activity, proclivity to hypoglycemic episodes, emotional stance, and compliance with principles of optimal diabetes self-management, before resorting to a divided dosage schedule. All too often we have found the split dose technique unjustified if there is enhanced motivation of both physician and patient in careful restructuring of these critical factors. Much time, patience, and serial plasma sugar determinations (including a baseline Hb

A_{1C}) over several days of ambulatory observation that as closely as possible simulate patient's daily routine will not infrequently result in adequate control of the diabetes on single daily insulin dosage. (If it proves satisfactory, you have spared that patient 3650 injections of insulin over the next decade! Several days of outpatient visits and close supervision are a small price to pay for a decision so vital to the patient.) It is incumbent upon the physician to exercise circumspection and reasoned judgment and not succumb to what, in some cases, may be exposed as whimsical faddism.*

Following are four "guidelines" in selecting patients who may unequivocally benefit from a split-dose regimen:

1. When fasting hyperglycemia cannot be adequately reduced without inducing nocturnal hypoglycemic episodes by simply increasing the single morning dose of modified insulins.

2. When "brittle" diabetes becomes *unequivocally* more stable by initiating a second injection before supper or sometimes at bedtime.

3. When single-dose modified insulin (with or without regular insulin) induces hypoglycemic episodes during the day despite ideal structuring of meals, intermeal feedings, and energy output. (This is uncommon in our experience.)

4. When Hb A_{1C} and 24 hour urinary glucose determinations are significantly improved over several weeks of observation.

In so-called true "brittle diabetics" whose control is still inadequate on split dosage, we resort to multiple injections of regular insulin. Initially the patient is given only two doses daily, viz., one before breakfast and the second before supper. If the fasting plasma glucose is not adequately controlled thereby, we add a third (smaller) dose at bedtime.

A dose preceding the noon meal is usually avoided, if possible, because: (1) with careful diet planning it is usually unnecessary, the plasma glucose rising just before supper (when this occurs, we omit the midafternoon snack); and (2) for most working patients this is an inconvenient time to prepare and inject a dose.

Experience has shown considerable variation in time-action curves incident to regular insulin at the individual patient level. Indeed we have seen

---

*At a recent symposium the author reported four exemplary Type 1 diabetics who had taken but one dose of insulin daily for 25 to 40 years' duration of the disease. While control was considered "fair to good" throughout their diabetic careers, all four patients were totally devoid of any complications. By avoiding a second injection daily, these patients were spared a total of 48,545 injections. Thus to state that "split dosage" is necessary to prevent or reduce complications is an oversimplification.

three patients in whom a single morning dose of regular insulin maintained good control for 24 hours for reasons unknown. (See footnote, Table 5.)

When is Hospitalization of Diabetic Patients Necessary?

Diabetes should be regarded as essentially an outpatient disease, unless serious complications such as gangrene, advanced nephropathy, cardiovascular accidents, systemic or serious localized infection, or severe ketoacidosis with threatening coma are in evidence. Extremely brittle cases may require hospitalization to rule out extraneous contributory factors such as noncompliance (dietary or otherwise) or emotional disturbances, which can be disclosed only by removing the patient from his usual environment for a few days.

Unnecessary hospitalization of diabetics for so-called "regulation" continues to be a widespread practice nationally. A carefully controlled study revealed that as much as $2 billion may be wasted annually, which could otherwise have been saved by good office (or outpatient) management of these cases (Miller and Goldstein: N. Engl. J. Med. *236*:1388, 1972). Indeed, there is no valid reason why mild, uncomplicated cases of ketoacidosis cannot be treated on an outpatient basis if the physician has access to competent laboratory facilities to carry out frequent measurements of plasma glucose, pH, bicarbonate, and basic electrolyte panels, together with equipment for simple intravenous replacement of insulin, potassium, in saline infusions, all carefully monitored by a competent office nurse under physician supervision. In clear-cut cases without other serious concomitant medical infirmities, the costly intensive care unit is certainly unnecessary.

Self-Monitoring for Glycemic Control

Recently several publications have reported favorable results with self-monitoring rapid testing devices such as the Dextrometer (Ames Co., Elkhart, Indiana) and Sta-Tek (Biodynamics, Indianapolis, Indiana). These instruments are expensive (from $350 to $675 each). When skillfully used they are surprisingly accurate (within 5 to 10 mg per dl), but results are in capillary (arterial) whole blood values. However, in our experience successful application of this do-it-yourself therapeutic method has decided limitations:

1. The technique for reliable results is too difficult for many patients.

2. Those patients who do master the technique are often tempted to treat themselves and may fail to return to their physician frequently enough for adequate supervision.

3. They are often unable to test themselves for hypoglycemia before premonitory symptoms impair their capacity to do so.

The greatest value of home monitoring is among brittle diabetics, to expose spurious symptoms of hypoglycemia.

This approach is hardly beyond the investigative stage, and simple, less expensive machines may render it more feasible in the future.

Surgery and Diabetes

The pre- and postoperative medical management of uncomplicated, maturity-onset, stable diabetes is relatively simple, and when properly executed the surgical risk is nearly equal to that of the nondiabetic. Criteria to be fulfilled are as follows:

1. Thorough preoperative examination, including routine laboratory tests such as blood urea nitrogen, fasting and postprandial plasma sugars, chest x-ray, electrocardiogram, a review of recent urine tests, and description of time, frequency, and severity of recent insulin reactions. A so-called "metabolic panel" should be included. Optimal control must be established unless the patient is a surgical emergency.

2. *Never permit the patient to enter the operating room until a plasma sugar determination is made and reported within 1 hour prior to surgery.*

3. *Always insist on early morning scheduling on the surgeon's list.* (This is a vital measure to prevent deterioration in control.)

4. If the patient is "stable," requiring 30 units or less of insulin daily, and the preoperative plasma sugar is less than 150 mg per dl, there is no harm in omitting insulin entirely until the patient returns from the operating room, at which time another plasma sugar test will reveal whether a small dose of insulin is required. Thereafter, supplements of crystalline insulin are given as indicated by serial plasma sugar tests.

In more complicated, unstable or "brittle" cases, the same principles are implemented except that closer monitoring is necessary, including plasma sugar determinations about every 2 to 3 hours until the diabetes is restabilized. Plasma ketones may be estimated, but this is not as reliable as plasma sugar tests, which are still the most definitive yardstick of insulin action, especially if the plasma is negative for ketones. When the patient is taking more than 20 units of insulin and the preoperative plasma sugar ranges between 150 to 200 mg per dl, the total daily dose may be halved on the day of surgery, and divided doses of crystalline insulin are given for the first 24 to 48 hours.

The chief objective of the preoperative plasma

sugar determination is to guard against any risk of hypoglycemic shock on the operating table, because ketoacidosis virtually never occurs in a matter of a few hours in the previously well-controlled patient. If the plasma sugar is "close to the line," 5 per cent glucose infusion should be started before anesthesia is induced, and insulin should be omitted from this first bottle. The importance of listing the diabetic as the first case on the surgeon's list at 8 A.M. cannot be overemphasized.

In acute surgical emergencies the clinician must carefully weigh the risk of further operative delay against the urgency of establishing better preoperative control, and this may be a very difficult decision. Since the abdominal pain and rigidity of the diabetic can mimic the acute surgical abdomen, distinction of one from the other poses a genuine clinical challenge. A careful history usually reveals whether the abdominal symptoms preceded the onset of acidosis or vice versa.

Postoperative plasma sugar levels should be estimated at least three times daily until control is re-established and the patient is taking adequate food. Allowance must be made for some distortion of plasma sugar levels owing to intravenous glucose infusions. Urine tests for sugar and acetone are made four to six times daily as an ancillary guide to therapy. Catheterization should be avoided insofar as possible, and when it is necessary concomitant prophylactic chemotherapy should be given.

The choice of anesthetic should be left to an experienced anesthesiologist so long as the diabetes is in good control, but the patient's physician must assume primacy in ordering all doses of insulin.

Diabetic Ketoacidosis and Coma

Full-blown severe diabetic ketoacidosis with marked depression of serum bicarbonate and pH and inordinately high plasma glucose remains a serious medical emergency and requires immediate hospitalization in the intensive care unit. Authorities disagree on when the term "coma" is appropriate, but in this author's opinion it should be restricted to the total absence of conscious perception and lack of response to auditory, tactile, or visual stimuli. In such cases the prognosis is much more guarded. Ketoacidosis with or without coma should never occur in a previously known diabetic who is cooperative and properly schooled in self-management of the disease.

Total Management of the Acute Case. It is imperative to prepare or have available a diabetic ketoacidosis and coma chart to ensure continuous, orderly analysis of laboratory data and clinical course of the patient, as illustrated in Table 6.

1. Treatment objectives include correcting acidosis, dehydration, and electrolyte depletion and eliminating any concomitant infection simultaneously.

2. "Constant bedside vigil is the hallmark of therapy" (Ann Lawrence, M.D., Ph.D.). A major criticism is that physicians too often fail to repeat plasma glucose at least hourly for the first 6 to 8 hours and repeat serum pH, potassium, hematocrit, and blood gases at least every 2 hours for the first 10 hours.

3. As soon as "baseline" plasma glucose and acetoacetate, electrolytes, pH, hematocrit, and blood gases are obtained, start an intravenous drip with regular insulin in isotonic saline, preferably with Abbott pump, delivering approximately

TABLE 6. **Diabetic Ketoacidosis and Coma Chart**

DATE AND HOUR	TIME SINCE ADMISSION	URINE			BLOOD								INSULIN— KIND AND DOSE	FLUID		BLOOD PRESSURE	REMARKS AND HYPOGLYCEMIA
		Volume (ml)	Glucose	Acetest or Ketostix	Glucose	Ketones	HCO₃	pH	BUN	K	Cl	Na		Intake IV and Orally	Output Urine Emesis		

10 units per hour, after a "priming" dose of 16 units. (Insulin delivery is critical, requiring *constant vigilance* of nursing personnel!)

4. Monitor urine sugar and acetoacetate every hour as obtainable (no catheter unless acute retention occurs).

5. Be prepared to give a total of 7 to 12 liters of isotonic saline in the first 24 hours, constantly assessing degree of rehydration with clinical judgment and serial hematocrits.

6. Sodium bicarbonate is usually not required, as insulin and saline therapy will correct the acidosis. However, if blood gases disclose HCO_3 at 10 mEq per liter or less and pH is 6.9 or less, add two ampules of $NaHCO_3$ (44.6 mEq per 50 ml ampule) to each liter of saline. (*Warning:* Indiscriminate use of $NaHCO_3$ may induce cerebrospinal fluid acidosis!)

7. Start potassium replacement 3 to 4 hours after treatment is begun (40 to 60 mEq per liter of intravenous fluid). Monitor additionally with serum potassium levels and serial electrocardiograms (ECG). Urine output must be adequate.

8. *Warning:* Despite claims in literature that "low-dose" insulin therapy is the treatment of choice and insulin resistance is not seen, we have encountered two patients who failed to respond and required 50 to 100 unit boluses of insulin to overwhelm apparent insulin antagonism. If hyperglycemia does not respond adequately within 2 hours, resort to 50 unit boluses intravenously.

9. Do not use fructose, but 5 per cent dextrose infusions may be started when blood sugar falls to 200 mg per dl or less. (Excessive glucose infusions may render it difficult to calibrate insulin dosage.)

10. Phosphorus deficiency is a well-known concomitant of diabetic ketoacidosis, but the necessity of corrective replacement is controversial. However, since it is a simple matter to replenish any deficiency concomitant with potassium replacement, we would recommend its use. The rationale of this is basically to replete erythrocyte 2,3-diphosphoglycerate and improve oxygen delivery to tissues (Kreisberg R. A., 1978).

Treatment of Hyperosmolar Nonketotic Coma.
1. First be certain of diagnosis. Basic features are striking hemoconcentration with hyperosmolarity as high as 462 mOsm/per liter H_2O (normal 280 to 310). Plasma sugars may be 600 to 3000 mg per dl! Hyperosmolarity has been promptly identified by utilizing the following formula:

$$\text{Serum osmolality (mOsm/L)} = 2\,[\text{Na (mEq/L)} + \text{K (mEq/L)}\,] + \frac{\text{plasma glucose (mg/dl)}}{18} + \frac{\text{BUN (mg/dl)}}{2.8}$$

The pH usually is normal and serum acetoacetate trace to negative. However, the course may be complicated by lactic acidosis if the patient goes into shock.

2. Give *hypotonic* saline infusions intravenously and also orally if tolerated.

3. Monitor venous pressures.

4. Insulin requirement may be much lower than in ketoacidosis despite the extreme hyperglycemia. (Hourly blood glucose levels are advised!)

5. Be alert for hypokalemia, which can be more severe than in diabetic ketoacidosis.

6. *Warning:* Too rapid correction of hyperosmolarity may contribute to fatal cerebral edema!

For an excellent exhaustive review of current opinion regarding hyperosmolar nonketotic coma, the reader is referred to the section entitled Hyperosmolar Non-Ketotic Coma: Underdiagnosed and Undertreated, in *Clinical Diabetes: Modern Management*, by Stephen Podolsky (ed.), New York, Appleton-Century-Crofts, 1980.

Acknowledgment

We wish to express our deep appreciation to Miss Eleanor Tveit, medical secretary, for her untiring efforts in preparing this manuscript.

DIABETES MELLITUS IN CHILDHOOD AND ADOLESCENCE

method of
MICHAEL B. AINSLIE, M.D.,
and DONNELL D. ETZWILER, M.D.
Minneapolis, Minnesota

Introduction

The child or adolescent who develops insulin-dependent diabetes mellitus presents many problems to the physician. It is a serious disease for which there is adequate treatment, but no cure. Perhaps in no other disease state do we ask so much participation of patients in their own care. It is estimated that of the 2.5 million people with diabetes in this country, approximately 100,000 have juvenile-onset diabetes.

Because of confusion over the various terminologies used for diabetes mellitus, it has been recommended that juvenile-onset diabetes mellitus, or insulin-dependent, ketosis-prone diabetes be referred to as Type I diabetes. We will use that terminology throughout this article.

At present the cause of Type I diabetes is unknown. Numerous theories have been proposed in the past. Usually there is a family history of diabetes in the immediate family. Although it was believed that diabetes was an autosomal recessive, autosomal dominant, or sex-linked disorder, it is now known that this is false. If diabetes is inherited, it must be on a complex, multifactorial basis. We know that the risk for a child's developing diabetes is fairly slight, even if one parent has the disease (10 to 15 per cent). Several viruses have been implicated in the past, especially because of Type I diabetes' peak incidence in fall and winter of the year when viral illnesses are more prevalent, but no virus has been consistently shown to produce diabetes. Certainly no single virus will be found to cause all Type I diabetes. Finally, autoimmune mechanisms have been implicated. Anti-islet antibodies are demonstrable early in many patients with Type I diabetes. They are not consistently found, nor does the sudden onset of symptoms suggest an autoimmune mechanism in all patients. Environmental factors may play a role also.

In summary, the cause of Type I diabetes is unknown. The child probably inherits the genetic susceptibility to the disease; then later in life a viral infection may directly cause or trigger an autoimmune process to cause development of diabetes.

Initial Management

The onset of Type I diabetes is sudden. Frequently the patient or the parents can pinpoint the exact day when the symptoms began. Usually the child will present with the classic 3P's of diabetes — polyuria, polydipsia, and polyphagia. Weight loss, lethargy, and frank diabetic ketoacidosis may become manifest if these early symptoms are ignored. The physician must maintain a high index of suspicion. The diagnosis of Type I diabetes is quite easy once considered. All that is necessary is a blood test for glucose. Then a simple confirmatory test is a fasting blood sugar. This does not have to be done in the morning. A simple 4 to 6 hour fast during the day is sufficient. Indeed, delaying the diagnosis by obtaining an overnight fast or a glucose tolerance test will be extremely dangerous to the child. A child with diabetes and not on insulin therapy is at great risk to develop ketoacidosis. This deterioration can occur over a matter of a few hours. *The importance of prompt diagnosis and equally prompt institution of insulin therapy cannot be overstressed.*

If the child and family have had no experience with diabetes, the child should be immediately hospitalized. In a few communities an outpatient diabetes program and service are available to these children and hospitalization is not necessary. However, because of variance in susceptibility to insulin, the risk of insulin therapy (hypoglycemia), and the need for education about diabetes, hospitalization is usually the method of choice for their initial care.

Ketoacidosis

If the child presents in ketoacidosis, its care must be instituted without delay. A few important points must be considered in the care of diabetic ketoacidosis.

Fluids. Over the last several years, it has become clear that fluid therapy is the most important aspect of ketoacidosis care. Meticulous recording of fluid balance and body weight and estimation of stage of dehydration will usually allow successful reversal of ketoacidosis. The patients in ketoacidosis are usually moderately to quite severely dehydrated. Because of the high osmotic load induced by hyperglycemia, the dehydration is of the hypertonic type. Clinical estimation of the degree of dehydration is at best tenuous with hypertonic dehydration. Therefore, it is wise to consider every patient in ketoacidosis to be at least 10 per cent dehydrated; many may be more so. Patients with 15 to 20 per cent dehydration will be in shock, and many are quite hypothermic. Immediate expansion of blood volume with 20 to 40 ml per kg of isotonic saline (0.9 NaCl) solution or 1 ml per kg of salt-poor albumin may be used. Fresh whole blood may also be used and has the theoretic advantage of providing more oxygen-carrying capacity than the patient's blood owing to higher 2,3-DPG levels.

After the initial volume expansion or if the patient is not in shock, fluid correction is begun, using a balanced electrolyte solution. Glucose is usually not necessary in the initial fluids, but will become necessary later in therapy. A solution containing approximately 50 mEq of sodium and chloride per liter, with addition of potassium (see below) and bicarbonate (see below), is then instituted. The fluid calculation should be the sum of the following factors:

1. Simple maintenance fluids: 100 ml/kg for each of the first 10 kilograms of body weight; 50 ml/kg for the next 10 kilograms; 20 ml/kg for each kilogram over 20; e.g., 40 kg adolescent maintenance = 1900 ml = 1000 (100 × 10) + 500 (50 × 10) + 400 (20 × 20).

2. Replacement fluids: ½ × maintenance for 5 per cent dehydration; 1 × maintenance for 10 per cent dehydration; 1½ × maintenance for 15 per cent dehydration.

3. Ongoing losses: (a) hyperventilation (an additional 10 per cent of maintenance); (b) os-

motic urinary loss (an additional 25 to 50 per cent to maintenance fluids).

Obviously, the total amount of fluids may be enormous. Frequently, three to four times the normal maintenance fluids must be given. At least half of the correction of the fluid deficit should occur in the first 8 hours of therapy. The remainder can be corrected over the next 16 hours. The importance of frequent recalculation of fluid cannot be overemphasized.

When the blood glucose reaches the 200 to 300 mg per 100 ml level, 5 per cent dextrose is added to the repair solution. If the blood glucose falls below 200 mg per 100 ml, then 10 per cent dextrose may be necessary to prevent hypoglycemia.

Potassium.   When children with diabetes develop ketoacidosis, they experience a large whole body potassium loss. This is primarily an intracellular potassium loss, so that serum potassium is usually in the normal range or slightly elevated when initially obtained. The physician, however, must anticipate this potassium loss and begin replacing large amounts of potassium even though serum potassium may be normal.

Anuria is rarely a problem in pediatric diabetes; therefore potassium may be started soon after the initiation of therapy (1 to 2 hours). Potassium may be replaced safely at 4 to 6 mEq per 100 ml of fluid. A larger amount of 6 to 8 mEq per 100 ml may be necessary if the child has severe ketoacidosis, but these large doses are recommended only when constant cardiac monitoring is available to avoid cardiac toxicity of hyperkalemia.

Most of the replacement potassium is the chloride salt (KCl). We usually replace 1 mEq per 100 ml as the phosphate salt (K_2HPO_4, KH_2PO_4). This replaces some of the phosphate deficiency recently shown to accompany ketoacidosis. Phosphate should not be given in a higher dose, as the solution is quite acid and hypocalcemia may be caused by a large influx of phosphate.

Bicarbonate.   The use of bicarbonate in all patients with ketoacidosis can be dangerous. Rapid correction of acidosis with bicarbonate is necessary only when the pH is less than 7.00 to 7.10. Because of a more rapid diffusion of CO_2 than bicarbonate across the blood-brain barrier, a paradoxical fall in cerebrospinal fluid pH may take place with deterioration of the patient's status.

If bicarbonate is necessary, it should be infused slowly, over 1 to 2 hours. Also, the amount given should correct the pH only to the 7.10 to 7.20 range. The patient's own buffer will correct the rest of the deficit. Too much correction will lead to alkalosis after the ketoacidosis is corrected.

Only 10 to 20 mEq of bicarbonate is used in most cases. A larger amount may be necessary in severe acidosis, or in a large adolescent.

Insulin.   It is clear from recent studies that only a small amount of insulin is necessary to correct most cases of ketoacidosis. A dose of 0.1 unit per kg as a continuous intravenous drip, or every hour intramuscularly, is usually sufficient to lower the blood glucose at a constant rate (100 mg per 100 ml per hour). There have been claims for fewer problems with hypoglycemia and hypokalemia with this therapy. However, we feel that this may be an artifact and that the patients continue to need constant observation. If the ketoacidosis and hyperglycemia do not respond to low dose infusion, or if the patient's condition deteriorates at all, the low dose infusion should be abandoned in favor of the high dose intermittent therapy. If the low dose therapy is unsuccessful, or if the physician is more comfortable with high dose therapy, a dosage of 1 to 4 units per kg of regular insulin is used. The dose is given subcutaneously in a mildly ill child. In severe ketoacidosis half or all of the dose can be given intravenously. Subsequent regular insulin is given in 2 to 4 hours, pending the patient's blood glucose response. A higher dose is given if the blood glucose rises, a smaller dose if it falls.

Through careful consideration of the four points enumerated above, most patients with ketoacidosis should respond. Hypothermia and shock remain significant problems and account for most of the mortality still present with ketoacidosis.

Most children and adolescents do not usually present in ketoacidosis, so that the initial dose of regular insulin will be instituted when the child is admitted to the hospital. This initial dose of insulin is usually 0.25 to 0.5 unit per kg subcutaneously. Blood glucoses are obtained in 4 to 6 hours to assess the response to this insulin, and subsequent regular insulin given at 6 hour intervals for the first 24 hours. A sliding scale of insulin is not recommended, because it measures only what the patient's blood glucose has done, not any future considerations. For example, a 2 per cent urine glucose at noon may require a different insulin dose than the same test at bedtime. On the second day of therapy, a combination of a dose of regular and an intermediate insulin (Lente or NPH) is given in the morning. Some diabetologists are routinely placing all their patients on a split dosage of insulin (A.M. and before dinner). While most adolescents require such a schedule, only rarely does a child need a split dose initially. The dose of insulin is approximately 0.25 to 0.5 unit per kg of body weight. This amount is divided into one third regular and the rest as NPH or Lente insulin. The dose of insulin is adjusted on subsequent days, depending upon the patient's response. Blood glucose is obtained before each meal, at bedtime, and whenever necessary. Urine tests are done before each meal and at bedtime. It is not our policy to try to obtain close control of the blood glucose in this initial hospitalization. This can be attempted upon discharge, when the patient is back in the usual environment.

Urine tests are taught, using the percentage system. The old plus system is being phased out, and the physician should be familiar with percentage urinary glucose. Two types of tests are taught, dipstick (Diastix, Ketodiastix) and tablet (Clinitest). Paper tape testing (Testape) is not recommended because of very subtle color changes with this test.

We find that the dipstick test is the easiest, and therefore more likely to be actually done by the patient. Also, the Clinitest tablets are quite toxic if ingested, and therefore should not be used in a household with small children.

Urine testing should be done using the second voided urine (urine obtained 30 to 60 minutes after voiding) before each meal if possible and at bedtime. A child under age 5 to 6 may be able to obtain only a first voided specimen. Ketones are measured if the urine has a large amount of glucose (1 to 2 per cent) or if the child is ill.

The child is started on a diet regimen that should be nutritious and sufficient for growth. Dietary therapy is still one of the mainstays of controlling the glucose level. Calories should be distributed among three meals and two to three snacks. The exact quantity at each meal depends upon personal preferences. We have found that the exchange system is the easiest quantitative dietary system to use. The "free system" is really not such, and the child must avoid concentrated forms of sugar regardless of the diet chosen. The weighed diet is difficult to follow. So the exchange system provides enough flexibility to be easily applied to all situations, and yet provides a framework for a fairly consistent food pattern. The total calorie intake is usually never limited in the child and should allow sufficient calories for normal growth and development.

The hospitalization then becomes a time of education about diabetes. Its care with insulin and diet, urine testing, and insulin administration are covered in depth. Recognition and care of acute complications of hypoglycemia and ketoacidosis are taught.

The educational process in diabetes can be divided into three goals, as shown in Table 1. The initial education should be accomplished during the initial hospitalization period. Unfortunately, in many communities there are no resources for an in-depth educational experience, so that this will have to be provided initially. We have found that patients rarely remember the important con-

TABLE 1. **Educational Process in Type I Diabetes**

I. Initial education
Goal:
To inform the patient that he or she has diabetes and to provide the information necessary for the immediate management of the disease
Objectives:
1. Assess the patient's knowledge of diabetes and explain the diagnosis and basic nature of the disease
2. Explain the necessity of the patient's participation and knowledge of the disease
3. Jointly plan an immediate education and management program
4. Teach the necessary skills of urine testing, diet selection, and insulin administration
5. Inform the patient of the nature of the acute complications of diabetes, their prevention, recognition, and treatment

II. In-depth education
Goal:
To increase the patient's knowledge of diabetes once the newness of the disease has subsided and the patient's personal experiences permit acceptance
Objectives:
1. Provide an in-depth educational experience covering all facets of the disease, its management, and its complications
2. Inform the patient on how to control the disease under unusual and adverse circumstances
3. Motivate the patient to carry out his or her responsibilities
4. Develop a long-term program of management and education

III. Continuing education
Goal:
To meet the current and changing needs of the patient's knowledge base as well as to review and update information taught previously
Objectives:
1. Answer all immediate questions patients have regarding management
2. Continually assess patient knowledge and understanding of the disease and review previous essential information which requires updating
3. Inform the patient of any new knowledge in the field or add information which becomes pertinent to the individual's changing needs; e.g., pregnancy
4. Provide continuing rapport and communications which can increase patient motivation and cooperation

siderations covered in the in-depth experience if they have not lived with diabetes for a few weeks or months. Therefore, we recommend this in-depth course 4 to 6 weeks after the onset. Continuing education, of course, occurs throughout the patient's lifetime. We have found that review of a certain topic, such as illness or injection technique, should be done at least every two years.

Immediate Post-Hospitalization Management

Usually 4 to 5 days of hospitalization are required for the child and family to learn the critical items of care of Type I diabetes. The child is then discharged to the usual environment. Usual activities are resumed as soon as possible. We routinely keep in phone contact with the family at least daily for the first week. Insulin needs usually decline because of increased activity. Our goal is to reduce glycosuria to a minimum without hypoglycemia. This phone contact provides support and continuity for the family. Also, a specially trained group of experienced parents of children with diabetes is useful at this time, because the parents and child will thus find people who have experienced the same feelings and frustrations that they now have.

After a few weeks at home, the child may enter the period called the "honeymoon phase" of diabetes. For unknown reasons, the child may reacquire the ability to make insulin. The physician must warn the family that this may occur; otherwise, they may think that the diabetes is disappearing. This is only a transient phase, and permanent diabetes soon ensues. Insulin requirements may fall dramatically at this time. About 10 per cent of the patients may require only a small amount of insulin (1 to 2 units per day). Usually the children are kept on insulin to emphasize the fact that they still have diabetes, and for the theoretical reason of insulin antibody–induced insulin resistance when insulin is reinstated. Insulin requirement usually rises as the "honeymoon phase" ends. Approximately 1 unit per kg of insulin is necessary for permanent diabetes.

The family and patient are seen in the office approximately 3 weeks after discharge and every 3 months thereafter. A team of a physician, dietician, and nurse educator sees them at each visit. The physician is primarily concerned with insulin adjustment, adjustment caused by dietary changes, or changes resulting from growth or exercise pattern changes. All intercurrent illnesses are assessed and appropriately treated. Overall control, as measured by growth and development, urine testing, 24 urinary glucose loss, and Hgb A_{1c} if appropriate, is estimated. Particular attention is paid to the areas of long-term complications, such as the eye, kidney, and nerves. Discussion of ways the patient may attain better blood glucose control are discussed, and recommendations for insulin changes are made.

The dietitian is the member of the team who assesses the patient's dietary needs and instructs the patient and family how to handle the dietary changes that occur in that season of the year. Usually the diet will need some reduction after the first 3 weeks, because the patient has usually reattained his or her previous weight. Special ways of buying and preparing food are discussed. School lunches and needs for special occasions are covered.

The nurse educator deals with the continuing education of the patient. Subjects such as hypoglycemia, ketoacidosis, insulin injection, urine testing, exercise, and illness are regularly discussed.

The team then confers about each patient. If a special problem such as a psychologic problem, surfaces, referral to appropriate care may be made. Many clinics have a clinical psychologist working as a member of the team. Through this team approach an in-depth assessment of the patient's present status may be made, and appropriate changes suggested.

Long-Term Management

The long-term management of any chronic disease is at best difficult, and perhaps nowhere is this more true than in the care of insulin-dependent diabetes mellitus. The data from animal experimentation and a few human experiments seem to demonstrate that long-term control of blood glucose can delay or prevent the long-term complications of diabetes.

Four aims of long-term care should be kept in mind:

1. *Monitor growth and development.* We are very careful to plot the height and weight of all our patients on a growth grid at each visit. Through this careful attention to growth we can recognize potential problems early and make appropriate adjustments. For example, a child's weight may be accelerating from the fiftieth percentile into the ninetieth percentile, while his height stays at the fiftieth percentile. This may be due either to the child's overeating, or to overinsulinization of that child. Excessive insulin dosage may manifest itself as excessive weight gain.

We recommend that the child pursue any sports, activities, and career choice desired. There is still much discrimination against people with diabetes in various fields and only through diligent effort by diabetic children and their families will these barriers be broken.

2. *Minimize episodes of hypoglycemia and ketoacidosis.* The prevention of hypoglycemic episodes

is important, as these episodes are uncomfortable and dangerous for the child and the family. Sometimes the fear of a severe hypoglycemic episode overwhelms the family and the child is allowed to be quite hyperglycemic. While this may be an aim in a very young infant who can have a severe reaction without warning, hyperglycemia should never be allowed in an older child or adolescent. Most episodes of hypoglycemia are quite mild and can be handled easily by the child and family. If they become persistent and repetitive, then adjustments in insulin or diet must be made.

The prevention of ketoacidosis is discussed below. A few children truly have "brittle" diabetes, that is, frequent episodes of severe ketoacidosis without warning. These children are most difficult to treat. Frequently a strong emotional reason may be found for these episodes. Through proper care and patience these children usually lose this propensity after 1 to 2 years.

3. *Prevent or delay the long-term complications.* The long-term complications of Type I diabetes can be divided into three main groups: microvascular, macrovascular, and neuropathic complications. The microvascular complications are frequently seen in Type I diabetes (56 per cent in 20 years). This small blood vessel disease affects two major organ systems — the eye and the kidney. The eye changes can lead to proliferative retinopathy and blindness. Indeed, diabetes is the leading cause of acquired blindness in the United States in persons over age 20. The small blood vessel nephropathy leads to renal failure and the need for chronic dialysis.

The macrovascular or large blood vessel disease affects the coronary arteries, carotids, and leg vessels. This process seems to be an accelerated atherosclerosis. It leads to occlusion of larger leg vessels and, coupled with the neuropathy of that leg, may lead to gangrene and loss of that limb. Heart attacks and strokes are frequent causes of death in adults with diabetes.

The neuropathy usually affects the longest nerves of the body, i.e., the legs and may affect both sensory and motor components. The autonomic nervous system may also be affected. These complications are rare before 10 years after onset, but increase rapidly so that 50 to 75 per cent of patients with Type I diabetes have one or more of these complications within 20 years after onset.

It is most difficult to convince a child, adolescent, or even adult that what he or she is doing now in the care of diabetes will make any difference in prevention or delay of these complications. In addition there is disagreement in the medical literature as to the value of long-term control.

4. *Keep the loss of carbohydrate calories to less than 5 per cent in the urine.* This is one of the few objective measures of control. It is preferable to obtaining occasional blood glucoses. The usual diabetic diet contains approximately 50 per cent carbohydrates. A 24 hour urine is collected by the patient in four time periods:

Corresponding Insulin

I.	Breakfast-lunch	A.M. Regular
II.	Lunch-dinner	A.M. NPH (Lente)
III.	Dinner-bedtime	P.M. Regular
IV.	Bedtime-breakfast	P.M. NPH (Lente)

If the patient is receiving only one injection of insulin daily, then the A.M. NPH would cover the rest of the day. By dividing the collection times in this manner, the appropriate corresponding insulin can be adjusted. An example of this calculation is for a child who is on a 2000 calorie diet. Approximately 1000 calories are carbohydrate. Our aim is to lose less than 5 per cent of these calories, or 50 calories. Since there are 4 calories in every gram of carbohydrate, this calculates to 12.5 grams. So the total spill should be less than 12.5 grams. Now if the spill is over 12.5 grams and one time period accounts for this loss, then the corresponding insulin should be adjusted. This urine collection and testing can be done at home, using the two drop Clinitest method and a metric volume measure. The percentage of glucose spill (e.g., 2 per cent) means there are 2 grams of glucose per 100 ml of solution. So simple multiplication by the number of milliliters will give the total gram amount.

Special Problems

Illness — Ketoacidosis. The key to the management of ketoacidosis is its early recognition and treatment. Indeed, many children can avert full ketoacidosis by following a few simple measures. Two important measures should be followed on an ill day. First, the child needs insulin, at least in the usual amount and in most cases additional regular insulin. Second, the child needs a source of glucose, such as sugar-containing soft drinks. Frequent small sips of these soft drinks may alleviate the nausea and forestall any vomiting. Several doses of regular insulin (4 to 10 units) at 2 to 6 hourly intervals may be necessary. As the urinary glucose, acetone, and symptoms begin to clear, then less insulin may be used. Frequent phone contact is made with the physician. Through a regimen such as this, hospitalization for acute ketoacidosis can be minimized. Of course, it is equally important to diagnose and appropriately treat the precipitating illness.

Hypoglycemia. The acute complication of hypoglycemia sometimes hangs like the sword of Damocles over the heads of the child and family. Because of its sudden onset and fairly rapid progression of symptoms, the family may become overly protective. It is seen more frequently as control increases. The child and family should always be prepared to treat hypoglycemia. Sugar cubes and hard candy are the easiest to carry. Regular candy or soft drinks are unfortunately often consumed long before the child needs them, and frequently small children may use a reaction to obtain candy. These substances should be used only in the conscious child. Reactose, a gel substance containing glucose, is useful in that it can be carried by the patient. Its gel nature helps prevent aspiration in the event of its use in the unconscious patient. It is not absorbed through the buccal mucosa, and must enter the stomach to effect a rise in blood glucose.

Finally, glucagon may be used by the patient to treat a severe reaction. The dose is 0.5 unit to children less than 10 years of age and 1.0 unit for those over 10 years of age. Glucagon requires 15 to 20 minutes to act. Our studies showed a 70 mg per 100 ml glucose rise in 20 minutes. Also it requires mixing when used, so the family should be familiar with this procedure, because during the stress of a severe reaction one cannot take time to read directions. Preparations should be made for the patient to receive intravenous dextrose if glucagon is not successful. This must be done by a qualified rescue squad or in an emergency room. Glucagon should be used only in an unconscious patient. Vomiting after its use is a frequent side effect. Intravenous dextrose should be given only in 10 gram (20 ml of D_{50}) increments. Monitoring of the blood glucose rise must be done. Remember that this solution is quite hyperosmotic. Many deaths have been caused by overzealous attempts to treat hypoglycemia.

In a very young child control may have to be relaxed to prevent frequent and serious hypoglycemia. Usually by age 5 the child can recognize the early symptoms of hypoglycemia, and tighter control can be achieved.

Adolescence. This is a time of great emotional turmoil, both for the child and for the family. A child who develops diabetes at a younger age (less than 10 years) is usually fairly well adjusted to the disease. The young adolescent who develops the disease is at a great disadvantage. During this age (10 to 14) the child's self-image is just being formulated, and here is one more thing to tell him or her that something is wrong. Also, the parents naturally tend to try to protect their child with diabetes. Frequently this leads to excessive concern and later rebellion on the part of the child. A psychologist or psychiatrist must be consulted frequently.

By allowing the child to take over as much control as early as possible in the disease, many problems may be alleviated. Frequently, interaction with peers with diabetes is useful. Threats and discussions about the dire consequences of poor control are of no use. All too often the only parameter of control in an adolescent is whether the patient is in the hospital or not.

Adolescent girls with diabetes present numerous problems. Menstrual periods may be quite irregular, especially in poorly controlled girls. Birth control in those girls who are sexually active is another problem. Birth control pills have many potential dangers in a diabetic girl. However, pregnancy does also, so that this is a frequently used method of contraception.

Surgery. Any child or adolescent with diabetes who undergoes general anesthesia must be in an institution where close monitoring of the blood glucose is available. Elective surgery, even tooth extraction, should be scheduled early in the day. The child should enter the hospital the night prior to surgery so as to be in reasonable control prior to surgery (no acetonuria). Blood glucose should be done early on the day of surgery. Insulin should be given on that day. Dosage is variable. We usually give one third to one half of the usual regular insulin and the usual intermediate (NPH or Lente) insulin if the surgery will be short. We may give frequent injections of regular insulin with decreased intermediate if a prolonged procedure is expected. An intravenous infusion of 10 per cent dextrose is started and should run throughout the surgery. If the procedure is over 4 hours in length, a blood glucose should be obtained in the operating room. Blood glucose should be done in the recovery room regardless of the length of the surgery. The major aim during surgery is to prevent hypoglycemia.

Somogyi Phenomenon. This problem is not uncommon. It is frequently seen when the child, family, or doctor tries to be overly aggressive with insulin therapy. The phenomenon itself is reactive hyperglycemia following asymptomatic hypoglycemia. It is frequently present when the child is receiving more than 1 unit per kg of insulin and is in poor control. All too often excessive doses of insulin (100 to 200 units per day) are given in an overzealous attempt to clear all glycosuria. The treatment of this phenomenon is a simple reduction of insulin. This may have to be done in small decrements.

The Somogyi phenomenon may be seen in an adolescent who takes one large dose of insulin in the morning. Frequently, by late afternoon the patient has a voracious appetite and consumes large quantities of food. Later when the insulin effect wears off, nocturia ensues. Many show excessive weight gain during this period. Treatment is a reduction of insulin and splitting the dose into a morning and evening injection.

Hgb A$_{IC}$. When normal adult hemoglobin (Hgb A) is present in a glucose solution, it will bind glucose at a constant rate proportional to the concentration of glucose. Since this occurs over a long time interval, it has been applied to diabetes as a measure of long-term control of the blood glucose. Normally a person has approximately 5 per cent of hemoglobin as Hgb A$_{IC}$. With diabetes this increases to 7 to 20 per cent. We have studied Hgb A$_{IC}$ in our patients, and in general those with higher Hgb A$_{IC}$ percentages tended to be those in poorer control. However, there was a wide overlap in the groups. So Hgb A$_{IC}$ at best is only one index of control and must be coupled with urine tests, 24 hour urines, compliance, and other measures to get an overall index of control.

Future and Summary

Recent changes in insulin delivery systems such as the constant insulin infusion pump and home glucose monitoring may soon make this entire article obsolete. These systems return the blood glucose to normal and allow the patient to lead a normal life. Through their use we may obtain the answer as to whether close control of the blood glucose will prevent the long-term complications.

The care of Type I diabetes must be individualized to each patient. There is no one right or wrong way to treat a child. Only through diligent effort by the family and patient will adequate control be obtained. We feel that this is best obtained in patients who are highly informed and educated about their diabetes and who cooperate with a knowledgeable and concerned health care team in a planned system of care.

HYPERURICEMIA AND GOUT

method of
THOMAS D. PALELLA, M.D.
Ann Arbor, Michigan

The gouty diatheses represent a spectrum of diseases related to the persistent elevation of the serum urate concentration above 7.5 to 8.0 mg per dl (100 ml). At this concentration, serum may be considered saturated with urate. Statistically hyperuricemia is associated with an increased risk of development of the clinical manifestations of gout. Gout should be considered to include gouty arthritis (monosodium urate monohydrate crystal–induced synovitis), tophaceous gout (the deposition of monosodium urate crystal aggregates in soft tissues), uric acid nephrolithiasis, and sustained asymptomatic hyperuricemia. Additionally, in the presence of systemic hypertension, hyperuricemia predisposes to urate nephropathy.

Uric acid is the final degradative product of purine catabolism in humans. Although purines are ingested in significant amounts in an average diet, the contribution of exogenous purines to the production of uric acid is probably less than 20 per cent. The remainder of uric acid production derives primarily from the de novo synthesis of purines for nucleic acid synthesis.

The disposition of uric acid occurs via renal and extrarenal routes. The latter is the least significant, accounting for one fourth to one third of daily uric acid excretion. The extrarenal metabolism of uric acid occurs primarily in the gut, where the intestinal flora hydrolyzes it to allantoin. The renal handling of uric acid is somewhat more complex. Uric acid is freely filtered by the glomeruli. Greater than 90 per cent of the filtered uric acid is subsequently reabsorbed by an active mechanism in the proximal tubule. Virtually all the uric acid finally excreted in the urine is thus actively secreted into the tubular lumen at a more distal site.

Hyperuricemia can result from the overproduction of uric acid, insufficient excretion of uric acid, or both. The overproduction of uric acid often results from increased de novo synthesis of purines. Overproduction of uric acid is reflected by hyperuricosuria, that is, urinary acid excretion in excess of 800 mg per 24 hours. Conversely, the finding of a normal 24 hour urinary uric acid in the presence of hyperuricemia suggests underexcretion of uric acid and usually indicates an abnormality in renal clearance. These two mechanisms may be operative simultaneously. A note of caution should be added here. The recognition of excessive urinary excretion of uric acid as an abnormality is predicated upon the total excretion of uric acid in 24 hours. Attempts at approximating the "24 hour urine uric acid" by extrapolation from spot urine specimens are likely to be inaccurate, since they ignore the sizable diurnal variation of the renal excretion of uric acid.

The distinction of primary versus secondary hyperuricemia is an important one. Secondary hyperuricemia is the result of overproduction or underexcretion of uric acid as a manifestation of an underlying disease state or drug ingestion. Examples of conditions leading to overproduction of uric acid include myeloproliferative disorders, radio- or chemotherapy, and psoriasis. Abnormalities in the renal handling of uric acid leading to hyperuricemia on the basis of underexcretion include renal failure, low dose aspirin therapy, diuretics, and acidosis. Primary hyperuricemia, on the other hand, is the elevation of serum urate levels in the absence of a precipitating disorder. The cornerstone of the treatment of secondary hyperuricemia rests with the treatment of the disorder from which it arises, as well as treatment of the biochemical abnormality. In contrast, therapy of primary hyperuricemia, which is presumably genetic in origin, relies on the treatment of the biochemical anomaly itself. Statistically the risk of development of gouty arthritis increases both with the level of hyperuricemia and with the length of time over which the elevated level is sustained. However, factors such as cost and the potential toxicity of therapy mitigate against treatment of the serum abnormality itself. Because of the rather significant risk of the development of renal stones, hyperuricemia coexistent with hyperuricosuria constitutes an indication for antihyperuricemic therapy. Therefore, when biochemical screening identifies hyperuricemia which is subsequently confirmed, a search for causes of secondary hyperuricemia should be made. Such a search should include a history with special reference to medication and alcohol use, physical examination, and laboratory evaluation of renal and hematologic status. Additionally, a measurement of urinary uric acid over a 24 hour period should be obtained. There is no reason to collect such a specimen routinely on a purine-free diet. The outcome of such an evaluation should then direct the therapy of hyperuricemia. Certainly, patients with hyperuricemia about to undergo chemotherapy of malignancies should receive prophylactic antihyperuricemic therapy. Allopurinol, 300 mg, should be administered by mouth 12 to 24 hours prior to the institution of chemotherapy. The demonstration of hyperuricosuria on a 24 hour urine specimen is thought by many, but by no means all, to represent an indication for antihyperuricemic therapy. Hyperuricemia as an isolated finding does not constitute an indication for antihyperuricemic therapy.

Acute Gouty Arthritis

The clinical manifestations of acute gouty arthritis are those of a crystal-induced synovitis. Typically, the patient is a middle-aged male with the acute onset of pain and marked inflammatory signs in a single distal joint. A single attack usually lasts on the order of 3 to 4 days, with the peak of discomfort occurring within the first 36 hours. Although strongly suggestive of gouty arthritis, the classic presentation is by no means specific, and atypical presentations occur as well. Consequently, physical evidence to support the diagnosis of gout should be sought in the form of monosodium urate crystals aspirated from either an involved joint or a tophus. In synovial aspirates, characteristically needle-shaped negatively birefringent crystals should be demonstrated within the cytoplasm of neutrophils. The time-honored therapeutic response to colchicine is hardly as reliable, since a similar response is sometimes seen in other crystal-induced arthritides. Conversely, a lack of response to colchicine does not exclude gout. Attempts at therapy are then directed initially at the acute attack and subsequently at the long-term management of hyperuricemia to forestall recurrent episodes.

The management of the acute gouty attack depends on anti-inflammatory therapy. The persistent popularity of colchicine is testimony to its effectiveness when given by either the oral or intravenous route. Orally, 0.6 mg of colchicine is given hourly. Hourly administration is continued until (1) the attack improves, (2) gastrointestinal toxicity ensues (primarily vomiting and diarrhea), or (3) 7.2 mg (12 doses) has been administered without benefit. Intravenous administration requires the dilution of cholchicine (1 or 2 mg in 25 to 50 ml of isotonic saline) and slow infusion through a well-running intravenous catheter. A recommended dosage schedule employs an initial 1 or 2 mg dose followed by one or two subsequent 1 mg doses at 4 hour intervals. Intravenous colchicine therapy is not limited by gastrointestinal side effects. Therapy may be complicated by painful extravasation and resultant soft tissue necrosis if care is not taken when infusing the drug. Arrhythmias and respiratory arrest have rarely been associated with intravenous colchicine therapy. Regardless of the presence or absence of a therapeutic effect, the maximal intravenous dose of colchicine in 24 hours is 4 mg.

With the advent of nonsteroidal anti-inflammatory drugs (NSAID), it has become possible to adequately treat the patient who is intolerant of colchicine or for whom contraindications to colchicine exist. Indeed, since these agents nonspecifically suppress inflammation with a minimum of side effects, they have for many become the treatment of choice for acute gouty attacks. Indomethacin should be the first NSAID considered because of its demonstrated efficacy in the acute gouty attack and the large experience to date with its use. A tapering schedule is usually employed with an initial single oral dose of 150 mg. Therapy should be continued with 50 mg three times daily for 2 to 3 days, and then reduced to 50 mg twice daily until symptoms abate. Patients should be instructed to take indomethacin with meals or antacids to minimize gastrointestinal side effects. Headache, dizziness, and rarely psychosis have been demonstrated as dose-related side effects of indomethacin. Bone marrow suppression, elevation of liver enzymes, and fluid retention are complications of long-term therapy only.

Less experience has been garnered in the treatment of the acute gouty attack with the variety of other NSAID, and there are no specific advantages to indicate that any are preferred over indomethacin. Both sulindac and naproxen have long enough half-lives to permit two or three doses daily. Sulindac should be given orally in a dose of 200 mg twice daily; naproxen may also be given orally in doses of 250 mg two or three times daily. (This use of naproxen is not listed in the manufacturer's official directive.) The propionic acid derivatives ibuprofen and fenoprofen calcium require more frequent administrations. The manufacturers' maximal recommended daily dose has been 600 mg four times daily, although doses as high as 900 mg four times daily may be necessary acutely to alleviate symptoms. (This use of ibuprofen and fenoprofen is not listed in the manufacturers' official directives.) After improvement has been obtained, returning to the lower dose seems advisable. Gastrointestinal side effects predominate with the use of all these agents except perhaps sulindac; administration with meals or antacids may minimize these effects. The more serious side effects of these agents, particularly fluid retention, are related to duration of therapy in most instances. The wide spectrum of NSAID available currently has virtually precluded the necessity to employ phenylbutazone or its derivatives, which have a higher potential for serious side effects. The decision to continue prophylactic anti-inflammatory therapy hinges on both the frequency of recurrent attacks and the choice and success of antihyperuricemic employed.

Antihyperuricemic Therapy

Documentation of clinical manifestations of gout in association with hyperuricemia constitutes indication for antihyperuricemic therapy. The decision to institute antihyperuricemic therapy should be delayed at least 14 days after the resolution of an acute attack. Normalization of the serum uric acid level is the goal of such therapy. The rationale for this objective is to promote the resolubilization of urate crystals de-

posited in the joints and other soft tissues. Approaches to antihyperuricemic therapy are aimed at promoting the excretion of uric acid or decreasing its production by inhibiting its formation from its biochemical precursors, xanthine and hypoxanthine. Inhibition of reabsorption of uric acid in the renal tubules results in uricosuria and lowering of the serum urate level. Such agents are designated uricosurics and are indicated in those patients in whom hyperuricosuria has been excluded. Probenecid and sulfinpyrazone are the most commonly employed agents. Their relatively long history of safety and efficacy makes them the agents of choice in hyperuricemia on the basis of underexcretion of uric acid. (Indeed, these agents are contraindicated in overproductive states, since they enhance the hyperuricosuria that is the hallmark of overproduction. Obviously, patients with uric acid nephrolithiasis should not take uricosurics.) Additionally, renal function must be such that enhanced uric acid excretion can result from inhibition of reabsorption. Concomitant salicylate therapy promotes reabsorption and obliterates the effect of uricosuric therapy. Therefore, patients should be advised against the use of aspirin while taking probenecid or sulfinpyrazone.

Probenecid at high doses competes with uric acid for reabsorptive sites in the proximal tubule. Initial therapy should be 250 or 500 mg daily, preferably in the morning. The dose may be escalated at 2 to 4 week intervals by increments of 250 mg to a total morning dose of 1 gram. Further increases in therapy should be directed by serum urate levels which should normalize in the dose range of 1.0 to 2.0 grams daily. Doses larger than 1.0 gram should be divided throughout the day for maximal benefit. Renal dysfunction is a side effect of probenecid therapy, and use of this drug should be avoided in patients with established renal disease. While taking probenecid, patients should be advised to maintain a daily urinary output in excess of 2 liters to avoid the promotion of uric acid stone formation. Alkalinization of the urine in the early stages of therapy with probenecid may further reduce the likelihood of the development of uricolithiasis secondary to the enhanced solubility of uric acid at alkaline pH values. Nausea and vomiting, skin rash, and drug fever occur in a small percentage of patients taking probenecid.

Sulfinpyrazone also inhibits the tubular reabsorption of uric acid, consequently increasing urinary uric acid excretion. Therefore, like probenecid, sulfinpyrazone predisposes to uricolithiasis, and the same precautions to minimize this predisposition should be taken. Therapy should begin with a dose of 50 mg twice daily. At monthly intervals, the dose may be advanced by 100 mg until as much as 400 mg daily is given. Total daily doses above 100 mg should be administered in 100 mg single doses two, three, and four times daily. Both hepatic and renal toxicity are side effects of sulfinpyrazone. Sulfinpyrazone is structurally related to phenylbutazone, and bone marrow suppression has been described. Sulfinpyrazone also decreases platelet adhesiveness and capacity to aggregate. This effect does not seem to predispose to bleeding, but care must be exercised in administering sulfinpyrazone to patients with coagulopathies or on anticoagulant therapy.

The agent of choice in the treatment of hyperuricemia on the basis of overproduction in the setting of chronic renal failure or in patients intolerant to uricosurics is allopurinol. Allopurinol and its metabolite oxypurinol inhibit xanthine oxidase, the enzyme responsible for the oxidation of hypoxanthine to xanthine and xanthine to uric acid. Oxypurinol (alloxanthine) is the principal metabolically active form of the drug. Greater than 90 per cent of an orally administered dose of allopurinol is excreted as oxypurinol with a half-life of approximately 20 hours. Probenecid promotes the excretion of oxypurinol and hence reduces its effectiveness. The long half-life of the metabolically active form of the drug makes single daily dosing practical. The usual initial dose is 300 mg (or 4 mg per kg per day) orally as a single daily dose. The onset of lowering of serum urate levels is apparent in 72 to 96 hours with the maximal effect occurring within 2 weeks of the institution of therapy. When renal insufficiency is present, the antihyperuricemic effect may be delayed owing to delayed elimination of uric acid formed prior to xanthine oxidase inhibition. Gastrointestinal side effects are relatively common, as is genuine toxicity (primarily rash, drug fever, leukopenia, and elevated liver enzyme studies). More serious side effects have been encountered, particularly toxic epidermal necrolysis and, rarely, xanthine stones. The former is seen more frequently in patients with chronic renal failure.

In summary, allopurinol should be used in the following settings: gouty arthritis associated with a 24 hour urinary uric acid in excess of 800 mg (overproduction of uric acid); gouty arthritis secondary to chronic renal insufficiency; tophaceous gout; gouty arthritis in patients intolerant of uricosuric therapy; prophylactically in patients undergoing chemotherapy for malignant neoplasms; and in patients with uric acid stones or who are at high risk for stone formation by virtue of massive hyperuricosuria (24 hour urinary uric acid in excess of 1000 to 1100 mg).

The relationship between the onset of antihyperuricemic therapy and precipitation of acute gouty arthritis apparently derives from sudden shifts in uric acid levels in the various compartments in equilibrium with the intravascular pool of uric acid. The likelihood of precipitating attacks may be minimized by the prophylactic administration of anti-inflammatory medication during the first 6 months of antihyperuricemic therapy. Either colchicine (0.6 mg twice daily) or indomethacin (50 mg twice daily) is effective. In the setting of chronic tophaceous gout, discontinuation of such prophylaxis should await the dissolution of tophi.

Chronic Tophaceous Gout

The therapy of chronic tophaceous gout is identical to the two phase management outlined above, namely, anti-inflammatory therapy for acute attacks and long-term antihyperuricemic therapy. Chronic tophaceous gout is destructive to varying degrees, depending on the sites of deposition of monosodium urate crystal aggregates. When deposited in the articular cartilage of synovial membranes, resultant bony damage may lead to both deformity and degenerative joint diseases. The principles of management of these sequelae are identical to the comprehensive care of patients with degenerative and erosive joint diseases on other bases. Since tophaceous deposits are most common in the first metatarsophalangeal joints, the distal interphalangeal joints, and the knees, these are the most common sites of secondary degenerative changes.

Tophi can be expected to reduce in size and eventually disappear with effective antihyperuricemic therapy. During the course of their resorption, it is not uncommon for tophi to become cystic in nature and occasionally drain a thick suspension of monosodium urate ("milk of urate"). Local inflammation and secondary infection of resorbing tophi are treated with anti-inflammatory drugs and appropriate antibiotics, respectively. Aspiration of cystic lesions may lead to more rapid resolution of such inflammatory episodes.

Associated Conditions

The identification of gouty diatheses prompts the physician to look for associated metabolic abnormalities in an effort to facilitate antihyperuricemic therapy as well as identify remediable causes of morbidity in such a population. The constellation of obesity, abnormalities in lipid and carbohydrate metabolism, and hypertension is encountered in sum or in various combinations of its parts in patients with hyperuricemia. Attempts at weight reduction, control of hypertension, and appropriate dietary and medical management of lipid and carbohydrate metabolism abnormalities will have salutary effects on antihyperuricemic therapy. Control of hypertension and the resultant reduction of the risks of cardiac and renal consequences of elevated blood pressure should receive primary attention. Diuretic therapy for hypertension is not contraindicated in the hyperuricemic patient despite the fact that it may worsen the degree of hyperuricemia. Effective antihyperuricemic therapy is usually obtainable after the blood pressure is satisfactorily controlled. Excessive alcohol consumption in patients with hyperuricemia and gout should be discouraged as well.

HYPERLIPOPROTEINEMIA

method of
BASIL M. RIFKIND, M.D.
Bethesda, Maryland

The major plasma lipids are cholesterol, triglyceride, and phospholipids. Lipids, by definition, are insoluble in aqueous media; however, when they are complexed with various apolipoproteins in the form of lipoproteins, they can be transported through the plasma.

Four families of lipoproteins are normally observed in the postabsorptive state. The *chylomicrons* are formed in the intestinal epithelium, composed predominantly of dietary (exogenous) triglyceride, and travel thence to the systemic circulation via the intestinal lacteals and the thoracic duct. Their removal from the plasma depends on the integrity of several enzymes collectively named lipoprotein lipase. The *very low density lipoproteins* (VLDL) are formed primarily in the liver and are rich in endogenous triglycerides assembled from precursors such as free fatty acids or carbohydrate. After their release into the plasma, their fate is incompletely understood but involves the transformation into a transient intermediate lipoprotein form, which, in turn, is converted into *low density lipoprotein* (LDL). (Current views hold that LDL is wholly or largely derived from the catabolism of VLDL through the formation of *intermediate density lipoprotein* [IDL].) LDL is cholesterol rich, normally accounting for 60 to 70 per cent of the total plasma cholesterol, but triglyceride poor. The fourth lipoprotein class, *high density lipoprotein* (HDL), has a complex origin, its components being derived through chylomicron and VLDL catabolism, and by hepatic synthesis. All the lipoprotein fractions contain cholesterol, triglyceride, and phospholipid in more or less characteristic amounts.

Hyperlipidemia; Hyperlipoproteinemia

Hyperlipidemia refers to an abnormal concentration of one or more of the plasma lipids, usually cholesterol or triglyceride. "Normal" limits are usually based on the ninetieth or ninety-fifth age- and sex-specific percentiles for these lipids. It must be emphasized that this is somewhat arbitrary. Lipid concentrations are distributed continuously in populations. Cholesterol levels are directly related to the risk of coronary heart disease (CHD), the main clinical consequence of hyperlipidemia, and within the range of cholesterol levels encountered in industrialized societies such as the United States of America there is no level below which the risk disappears. The clinical custom of focusing on subjects at the upper end of the distribution is based on identification of those subjects at greatest risk and, through them, members of their kindreds, with specific forms of genetically determined hyperlipidemia. Although these are important goals, it should be understood that only a small part of all CHD is attributable to the high risk subjects at the top 5 or 10 per cent of the cholesterol distribution. There is a growing awareness that physicians have a role to play in reducing CHD risk factors such as cholesterol levels in the whole community, and not merely in those of subjects with unusually high levels.

Since, as indicated, it is as lipoproteins that the plasma lipids circulate, hyperlipidemia is best translated into hyperlipoproteinemia. One reason for doing this is to distinguish between different patterns of lipoprotein increase that can result in similar degrees of hypercholesterolemia or hypertriglyceridemia. Also, it is becoming increasingly apparent that lipoproteins differ in their role in atherogenesis. LDL, which normally carries approximately 70 per cent of the total plasma cholesterol, is atherogenic, depositing cholesterol in the artery. HDL, however, appears to exert a protective role, since its concentrations are inversely related to CHD risk.

Analogous to hyperlipidemia and subject to the same limitations, hyperlipoproteinemia is usually defined on the basis of lipoprotein concentrations exceeding the age- and sex-specific ninetieth or ninety-fifth percentiles.

The hyperlipoproteinemias are a heterogeneous group of disorders characterized by abnormal concentrations of the plasma lipoproteins. The most common classification in use distinguishes five major patterns of lipoprotein increase (Table 1). Each pattern may occur as a consequence of other diseases, including common ones such as hypothyroidism, the nephrotic syndrome, or obstructive liver disease.

TABLE 1. **Main Types of Hyperlipoproteinemia**

TYPE	
I	Chylomicrons in fasting plasma
II	Increased LDL concentration without (IIa) or with (IIb) a VLDL increase
III	Presence of intermediate lipoprotein form ("floating" beta: d <1.006 grams/ml)
IV	VLDL increase only
V	Chylomicrons and VLDL increase in fasting plasma

Each may also occur as a primary, often familial and genetically determined abnormality. Each of these five lipoprotein patterns is often associated with characteristic clinical and genetic features. This approach to classification also emphasizes the need to design therapy to reduce abnormally high lipoprotein levels and to explain the mode of action of therapeutic agents in terms of whether they reduce lipoprotein synthesis or increase lipoprotein catabolism.

The main clinical consequences of hyperlipoproteinemia are as follows:

1. Recurrent abdominal pain, pancreatitis, hepatosplenomegaly, lipemia retinalis, and eruptive xanthomas, which are characteristic of hyperlipoproteinemias Types I and V, in which marked chylomicronemia is a feature.

2. Atherosclerotic vascular disease, especially coronary heart and peripheral vascular disease, which often occurs in Types II, III, and IV hyperlipoproteinemia and is, by far, the main clinical problem related to hyperlipoproteinemia.

3. Hyperglycemia, hyperuricemia, and obesity, common associations of Types IIb, III, IV, and V hyperlipoproteinemia, all of which share endogenous hypertriglyceridemia as a feature.

4. Tendinous, tuberous, tuboeruptive, and planar xanthomas, which variously occur in Types II and III and are mainly of cosmetic significance.

Therapeutic Objectives

The main aim of treating hyperlipoproteinemia is to prevent its vascular consequences. An undoubted association exists between certain forms of hyperlipoproteinemia and CHD. Evidence relating total plasma and LDL cholesterol levels to CHD is especially strong. Total and LDL-cholesterol have been identified as powerful independent risk factors for CHD in many prospective studies. Additional evidence comes from other epidemiologic approaches, animal experimentation, clinical observation, and detailed biochemical studies. The relationship is much less clear between triglyceride (and VLDL) levels and CHD. Prospective studies suggest that although triglyceride levels are directly related to CHD, this is not independent but reflects a relationship of triglyceride to other CHD risk factors.

The evidence for cholesterol strongly suggests that its reduction would prevent CHD. Animal experiments, especially studies on non-human primates, suggest that lowering cholesterol can decrease the rate of the progression of atherosclerosis, or even lead to some regression of lesions. There is little evidence in man, as yet, to confirm this. Despite many clinical trials of cholesterol lowering by diet or drugs, some encouraging, it remains to be conclusively demonstrated that primary or secondary prevention of coronary heart disease can be effected by such treatment. For triglyceride there is much less

circumstantial information, and virtually no clinical trial experience, to sustain the view that decreasing triglyceride is of benefit, though the possibility exists. These considerations have led the Food and Drug Administration to require pharmaceutical firms that market lipid-lowering drugs to caution that correction of hyperlipidemia cannot be equated with proved benefit for coronary heart disease.

Long-Term Toxicity Considerations

In contemplating lipid lowering (especially drug therapy), it is important to consider that such a course, once embarked upon, is lifelong. Under these circumstances problems with drug toxicity assume additional dimensions. Toxic effects have been described for all lipid-lowering drugs in use and are probably inevitable for those that will be developed. Toxic effects of low frequency that can often be tolerated in therapeutic interventions of short duration may be of considerable importance during the long-term administration of a hypolipidemic drug. Some attempt must be made to balance the increased toxicity rate against the possible (and as yet unproved) benefits of reducing CHD rates through cholesterol lowering. Thus, as long as definitive evidence of benefit is lacking, caution should be exercised in embarking on long-term therapeutic regimens with possible toxicity. A certain arbitrariness is involved in selecting patients for treatment, and it is not possible to make categorical recommendations for all varieties of hyperlipoproteinemic patients. Nevertheless, in certain subjects, the risk of CHD seems sufficiently strong to justify aggressive measures, and for the many more who are at lesser risk, effective, apparently safe dietary treatment may be used.

Certain benefits undoubtedly accrue from treatment of certain forms of hyperlipidemia, such as resolution of the clinical features associated with chylomicronemia, including prevention of recurrent attacks of abdominal pain and sometimes fatal pancreatitis, and the partial or complete disappearance of the different types of superficial xanthomas.

Correction of endogenous hypertriglyceridemia by dietary means also frequently improves the concomitant abnormal glucose tolerance, hyperuricemia, and hypertension.

High Density Lipoprotein

HDL is emerging as a protective factor for CHD. Considerable attention is presently being paid to factors that raise or lower plasma HDL levels. So far, however, no systematic, reliable, and safe means of substantially raising HDL levels has been developed. Furthermore, much more evidence is required to decide whether or not raising HDL appears to be a suitable means of preventing GHD. Accordingly, it is not presently recommended that therapy should be directed to raising low HDL levels. Nevertheless, subjects under treatment for hyperlipidemia should be observed to ensure that it is also not resulting in a significant fall in their HDL levels.

Therapy

In attempting to prevent CHD through lipid lowering, it should be remembered that other risk factors, such as cigarette smoking and hypertension, should be simultaneously corrected. The treatment of secondary hyperlipoproteinemia is primarily through the correction, when possible, of the primary disorder.

Diet

Diet, the cornerstone of primary hyperlipoproteinemia therapy appears to be safe, and many hyperlipoproteinemias adequately respond to it alone (Table 2). It is only for those subjects in whom an unacceptable degree of hyperlipidemia persists that diet should be supplemented by drugs. The main lipid-lowering diets are (1) low cholesterol, high polyunsaturated:saturated fatty acid (P:S) ratio — to reduce elevated LDL; (2) low fat — to correct chylomicronemia; (3) weight reduction — to reduce elevated VLDL or IDL; and (4) maintenance diet — to maintain previously reduced VLDL or IDL levels. Combinations and modifications of these diets may be used under certain circumstances to be described.

Diet manuals embodying these principles and tailored for adults and children with the different types of primary hyperlipoproteinemia are available from the National Heart, Lung, and Blood Institute, Bethesda, Maryland 20205. The diet outlines described below are based on these manuals, which should be consulted for detailed prescription. Ideally a nutritionist should instruct the patient and whoever is responsible for the patient's meals in the diet. The patient should be subsequently seen by the nutritionist to deal with any problems in adherence.

Low Cholesterol, High P:S Diet. This diet reduces the daily cholesterol intake from its usual level of over 600 mg to less than 300 mg and increases the P:S ratio almost tenfold from about 0.2 to 2.0. Cholesterol restriction is achieved mainly by avoidance of egg yolk in any guise and all organ meats such as liver and kidney, and restriction of most other dairy products. Beef, lamb, and ham or pork are limited, and fish and lean meats such as chicken, turkey, and veal are used instead. Skimmed milk and skimmed milk products are used in preference to whole milk,

ice cream, cream, and cheese. These changes and the use of polyunsaturated fat substitutes and supplements provide the increased P:S ratio. Carbohydrate and protein intakes are not limited. Revised figures for the cholesterol content of shellfish indicate that, with the exception of shrimp, they may now be included in such a diet. Alcohol restriction is unnecessary. Children receive an essentially similar diet.

Weight reduction is not a feature of the low cholesterol, high P:S diet, simplifying adherence to it. The present and predicted growth of low cholesterol commercial food substitutes also facilitates adherence. The low cholesterol, high P:S diet usually reduces the total plasma cholesterol by 15 to 25 per cent, apparently by increasing LDL removal. Although such a reduction is substantial, it is, in many Type II subjects, insufficient to achieve normal lipid levels.

Low Fat Diet. The low fat diet reduces abnormal chylomicron concentrations by decreasing production of this lipoprotein class from dietary triglyceride. Highly effective in principle, its use is complicated by the difficulty in constructing a palatable diet in the face of severe fat restriction. It is necessary to provide some fat in the diet, and although the chylomicronemia may not be completely corrected, the plasma lipids are usually maintained at a low enough value that the patient is free of abdominal symptoms.

For the adult, the fat intake is restricted to 25 to 35 grams per day; the P:S ratio is unimportant, and the cholesterol, carbohydrate, and protein intakes are not limited.

Such a diet is constructed by (1) eliminating all separated fats, e.g., butter, margarine, shortening, oils, (2) eliminating nuts, (3) using lean meats, (4) avoiding many baked goods, and (5) restricting the use of many dairy products containing fat.

Medium-chain triglycerides (MCT), in the form of MCT oil, can be used as an alternative source of fat, because they do not require chylomicron formation for their absorption.

In children, fat is restricted to 10 to 15 grams per day, using the same principles as for the adult. Formula feeding is available for treatment of the infant with chylomicronemia. An MCT preparation, Portagen, is useful.

Weight Reduction. Subjects with endogenous hypertriglyceridemia (Types IIb, III, IV, V) are often obese, and reduction to ideal weight frequently results by substantial or total correction of hypertriglyceridemia, presumably by decreasing VLDL production.

Balanced Diet. Having restored ideal weight and improved hyperlipidemia, it is necessary to prescribe a diet with a calorie content to maintain

TABLE 2. **Dietary Treatment of Hyperlipoproteinemia***

FACTOR	TYPE I	TYPE II	TYPE III	TYPE IV	TYPE V
Dietary prescription	Low fat, 25 to 35 grams	Low cholesterol, polyunsaturated fat increased	Low cholesterol approximately 20% cal. protein, 40% cal. fat, 40% cal. CHO	Controlled CHO (approximately 40 to 45% calories); moderately restricted cholesterol	Restricted fat (30% calories), controlled CHO (50% calories), moderately restricted cholesterol
Calories	Not restricted	Not restricted, except in Type IIb, in which weight reduction is often indicated	Achieve and maintain "ideal" weight—reduction diet if necessary	Achieve and maintain "ideal" weight—reduction diet if necessary	Achieve and maintain "ideal" weight—reduction diet if necessary
Protein	Total protein intake not limited	Total protein intake not limited	High protein	Not limited, other than control of patient's weight	High protein
Fat	Restricted to 25 to 35 grams in adults and 10 to 15 grams in children; kind of fat not important	Saturated fat intake limited; polyunsaturated intake increased	Controlled to 40 to 45% calories (polyunsaturated fats recommended in preference to saturated fats)	Not limited, other than control of patient's weight (polyunsaturated fats recommended in preference to saturated fats)	Restricted to 30% calories (polyunsaturated fats recommended in preference to saturated fats)
Cholesterol	Not restricted	Less than 300 mg or as low as possible; only source of cholesterol is meat	Less than 300 mg; only source of cholesterol is meat	Moderately restricted to 300 to 500 mg	Moderately restricted to 300 to 500 mg
Carbohydrates	Not restricted	Not restricted (may be controlled in Type IIb)	Controlled; most concentrated sweets eliminated	Controlled; most concentrated sweets eliminated	Controlled; most concentrated sweets eliminated
Alcohol	Not recommended	May be used with discretion	Limited to two servings (substituted for carbohydrate)	Limited to two servings (substituted for carbohydrate)	Not recommended

*After Levy et al.: Ann. Intern. Med. 77:267, 1972.

CHO = carbohydrate; cal. = calories.

both weight and lipids. Carbohydrate foods are limited to about 40 to 45 per cent of total calories, because excessive carbohydrate consumption often elevates triglyceride concentrations in these patients. Concentrated sweets are especially restricted by an intake not exceeding 4 to 5 grams per kg of body weight. The amount of protein and fat is dictated only by its contribution to the overall caloric intake. Polyunsaturated rather than saturated fat is used when possible. The cholesterol intake is restricted to 300 to 500 mg for Type IV and to less than 300 mg for Types III and IIb subjects. A limited amount of alcohol may be used but should be taken into account in calorie calculations.

Drug Therapy

Hypolipidemic Drugs. Various drugs often result in further substantial falls in plasma lipid levels. However, recent toxicity problems with several of them, coupled with a relatively limited evaluation of others, have severely restricted the number of effective, apparently safe drugs that can be considered for use.

Drug therapy reduces lipid concentrations either through decreasing lipoprotein production or increasing lipoprotein removal rates. With the exception of neomycin, all have been approved by the Food and Drug Administration for use as hypolipidemic agents. It should be emphasized that the use of these drugs in pregnancy and childhood has not been approved.

Nicotinic Acid. Nicotinic acid therapy causes VLDL to fall within several days, and reduced synthesis of LDL occurs. The ability of nicotinic acid to reduce both lipoprotein classes makes it an especially useful drug and potentially of value for treatment of Types IIa and IIb, III, IV, and V hyperlipoproteinemia. Several forms of the drug exist, but plain nicotinic acid is preferable, being less toxic than sustained action preparations, no

more prone to produce side effects, and inexpensive.

Both flushing and pruritus are prominent side effects, but these usually occur only in the initial weeks of therapy. Gastrointestinal disturbances such as nausea, vomiting, and diarrhea are common but also often subside during treatment. Liver function tests (SGOT, SGPT, LDH, and alkaline phosphatase levels) frequently become abnormal but also quickly improve if therapy is discontinued and significant hepatotoxicity is not a problem. Nicotinic acid can aggravate the hyperuricemia that often accompanies Types IV and V hyperlipoproteinemia, and may precipitate acute gout. Reduced glucose tolerance, glycosuria, and symptomatic diabetes may result from its use but disappear on discontinuation of the drug. Nicotinic acid probably should not be used in known diabetics. General or local skin hyperpigmentation and dry skin may occur. The vasodilating and postural hypotensive effects of ganglioplegic antihypertensive agents may be enhanced by nicotinic acid.

In adults the maintenance dose is 1 to 2 grams three times daily. To reduce the likelihood of gastrointestinal irritation it should be taken with meals, commencing with a dose of 100 mg three times daily, which is built up over a 1 to 2 week period until the maintenance dose is reached. In children a dose of 25 to 75 mg per kg per day is used (Table 3).

Clofibrate (CPIB). The main effect of clofibrate is to decrease the triglyceride-rich VLDL, apparently by both decreasing VLDL synthesis and increasing VLDL catabolism. Often, when used for this purpose in subjects with Type IV hyperlipoproteinemia, this is accompanied by an increase in LDL, an effect which may be undesirable. HDL levels, however, may be increased. Its effect on lowering LDL levels of Type II subjects is usually modest, reducing it by less than 10 per

TABLE 3. **Treatment of Primary Hyperlipoproteinemia in Childhood***

TYPE	DIET	DRUG	EFFECT OF TREATMENT
I	Low fat (10 to 15 grams/day), medium-chain triglyceride	—	Normalizes lipids; prevents bouts of recurrent abdominal pain and pancreatitis
II Heterozygote	Low cholesterol (100–150 mg/day), high P:S ratio (2:1)	Cholestyramine (250–800 mg/kg per day)	Normalizes lipids; ? decreases cardiovascular risk
II Homozygote	Low cholesterol (100–150 mg/day), high P:S ratio (2:1)	Cholestyramine (0.5–1.5 grams/kg per day); nicotinic acid (25–75 mg/kg per day); ? clofibrate; ? D-thyroxine	Usually substantial lowering of lipids; tuberous xanthomas decrease; ? decreases cardiovascular risk

*See manufacturer's official directives before using these agents in children.
P = Polyunsaturated fat; S = saturated fat.

cent or not at all and making it unsuitable for most Type IIa subjects. However, it may occasionally produce a more marked fall. The widespread use of clofibrate for the treatment of "hypercholesterolemia" is to be deprecated, because in most such subjects a Type II pattern is responsible. It is of little or no use in Type I and is only of occasional value in Type V.

Clofibrate has been in use for many years and has been found to produce a variety of usually mild side effects, including gastrointestinal disturbances, weight gain, drowsiness, weakness, giddiness, skin rashes, and alopecia. Moderate and transient serum transaminase rises occur but do not indicate hepatic injury. Uncommon but serious side effects are acute myositis, especially likely to occur in nephrotic patients, and cardiac ventricular irritability.

Subjects on coumarin anticoagulants show decreased dosage requirements when clofibrate is introduced; it is recommended that the anticoagulant maintenance dose be halved when clofibrate is added and thereafter adjusted according to the results of monitoring. The dose of clofibrate is 1.0 gram twice daily.

Two clinical trials, the Coronary Drug Project and the World Health Organization (WHO) Clofibrate Study, have considerably extended the experience with clofibrate. Both failed to show any improvement with respect to fatal heart attacks. Nonfatal heart attack was reduced only in the WHO study but was offset by a rise in total deaths. This excess of deaths was contributed to by hepatic, biliary, and gastrointestinal diseases. In addition, both studies reported an increased incidence of gallstone disease. These findings suggest that use of clofibrate should be restricted to (1) subjects with Type III hyperlipoproteinemia, in addition to their standard diet, (2) subjects with severe Type II, in whom a combination of appropriate diet and biliary sequestrant therapy has insufficiently lowered LDL levels and (3) subjects with severe Type IV hyperlipoproteinemia unresponsive to diet therapy. Clearly it should continue to be used only in such circumstances when it produces a marked degree of lipid lowering.

The Biliary Sequestrants — Cholestyramine and Colestipol. The introduction of the biliary sequestrants cholestyramine and colestipol constitutes a major advance in the treatment of Type IIa hyperlipoproteinemia. There is more experience with cholestyramine than colestipol, although both drugs appear to be similar in most respects. After ingestion, cholestyramine resin binds intestinal bile acids, interferes with their enterohepatic circulation, and increases their fecal excretion. An increased rate of conversion of cholesterol to bile acid results, and despite increased cholesterogenesis, the net effect is a reduction in the total plasma and LDL cholesterol. An increased LDL removal rate has been noted. The sequestrants do not reduce VLDL (and triglyceride) levels and may actually increase them, and therefore they should be cautiously employed in subjects with Type IIb hyperlipoproteinemia. They may result in a slight rise in HDL.

The effect of cholestyramine on cholesterol levels is dose related. Normally 16 to 24 grams per day (or 12 to 15 grams per day of colestipol) is used to produce falls in the total plasma cholesterol of 20 to 25 per cent through its effect on LDL cholesterol. Higher doses (up to 36 grams per day) are occasionally employed in severe Type II heterozygotes and in Type II homozygotes. (This dose is higher than that stated in the manufacturer's official directive.) In homozygous children a dose of 0.5 to 1.5 grams per kg of body weight per day is used. The drug is taken in powder form, a 9 gram packet containing 4 grams of the active preparation. Earlier preparations, which were unpleasant to take (Cuemid), have been replaced by an orange-flavored, palatable form (Questran). It is always taken suspended in water, another liquid, or a fruit purée with a high fluid content. Cholestyramine is usually taken in divided doses four times a day, after each meal and at bedtime.

It has recently been demonstrated that administration of the total dose in two equal doses with breakfast and supper is as effective as a four times daily regimen, eliminating the need for a lunchtime dose, a considerable convenience for persons such as school children or business people who do not regularly eat lunch at home. The nonabsorption of cholestyramine explains its freedom from direct systemic toxicity. Gastrointestinal side effects are quite common and include nausea, vomiting, abdominal cramps, distention, and constipation. Constipation is most prone to occur in the elderly, in whom the need for the drug can be doubted. It is especially to be avoided in patients with angina and can be readily countered by the use of stool softeners such as dioctyl sodium succinate (Colace) up to a dose of 300 mg or a mild aperient. It is best avoided in patients with chronic intestinal disease such as ulcerative colitis or diverticulitis. Constipation often spontaneously improves despite continued treatment with sequestrants. Hyperchloremic acidosis occasionally occurs in small children on high dosage.

Despite its effect on bile acids, cholestyramine does not induce steatorrhea unless a very high dose (more than 32 grams per day) is used or pre-existing asymptomatic malabsorption is present. The risk of producing fat-soluble vitamin deficiency is more theoretical than real. Nevertheless patients, especially children, should be periodically evaluated for this.

Cholestyramine can bind other drugs, including digoxin and related compounds, coumarin anticoagulants, thyroxine and triiodothyronine, phenylbutazone and thiazides, and possibly oral iron. These and probably all other drugs should be taken at least 1 hour before the cholestyramine dose.

The main problem with the biliary sequestrants is difficulty in compliance related to their bulk and gastrointestinal side effects.

Probucol. This drug was recently approved by the Food and Drug Administration (FDA) for cholesterol lowering. It reduces total and LDL cholesterol levels by 10 to 15 per cent but does not reduce triglyceride (or VLDL). A disquieting feature is a substantial reduction of HDL. Its mode of action is unclear. It has a half-life of several weeks. Worrisome but apparently specific fatal cardiotoxicity was originally reported for dogs; recently cardiotoxic deaths have been reported in monkeys. Although the problem has not been apparently observed in man, it would seem prudent to restrict the use of this drug to severe Type II subjects who fail to respond to appropriate diet and sequestrant therapy, and who show a substantial fall in cholesterol levels with probucol.

D-Thyroxine. Sodium dextrothyroxine (Choloxin) appears to be most effective in Type II subjects in whom it decreases cholesterol, possibly by increasing LDL catabolism. It is also sometimes effective in Type III. Although without significant hypermetabolic effects, D-thyroxine is unfortunately cardiotoxic, as was recently confirmed in the Coronary Drug Project, in which an increased coronary and other cardiovascular mortality and a high rate of nonfatal myocardial infarction were noted in certain categories of men with a history of previous myocardial infarction. These findings suggest that D-thyroxine should not be used in subjects with coronary heart disease and is not the drug of choice in hyperlipoproteinemic subjects free of, but at risk for, coronary heart disease.

The drug is used in doses of 4 to 8 mg per day, commencing with 1 mg per day and increasing this by 1 mg per month. Subjects previously on warfarin therapy may show decreased anticoagulant dosage requirements.

Drug and Dietary Treatment of Primary Hyperlipoproteinemias

Type I. The treatment of Type I hyperlipoproteinemia is entirely dietary. No drug is known to be effective. A low fat diet, appropriate to the age of the patient and supplemented by medium-chain triglycerides (MCT), is employed and results in reduction of chylomicronemia within several days and resolution of all clinical features. Triglyceride levels of 500 to 800 mg per 100 ml are usually achieved, sufficiently low to avoid the complications. During severe attacks of acute abdominal pain, with or without pancreatitis, oral intake should be suspended and parenteral fluids employed.

Type II. A strict low cholesterol, high P:S diet is employed in all subjects with Type IIa hyperlipoproteinemia. No adverse effects of such diets have been observed to date. In Type IIb the combination diet to be described for Type III is often effective in controlling the hypercholesterolemia and hypertriglyceridemia.

In the uncommon Type II homozygote, aggressive drug therapy is added to the diet. The drug of choice is cholestyramine, using the high dosage described earlier. Combined diet and cholestyramine therapy is still usually insufficient, and a further addition of nicotinic acid is then necessary. The rationale in combining nicotinic acid and cholestyramine is their complementary action, the former decreasing LDL synthesis, the latter increasing LDL removal. The addition of clofibrate to cholestyramine or colestipol and diet treatment is occasionally effective. Some subjects remain resistant to all therapy.

In the much more common heterozygote adults and children, diet is sometimes sufficient to normalize lipids, but more often LDL cholesterol levels still remain too high. Whether or not to administer drug therapy in the absence of categorical information regarding the effect of therapy on vascular disease is an individual decision. One must take into account the age of the patient, the severity of the hyperlipoproteinemia, the presence or absence of CHD in the patient, and whether there is a history of premature vascular disease in near relatives. In heterozygous children with mild to moderate hyperlipoproteinemia, especially if the family history is not striking, it is prudent to rely on diet alone. In those with a more severe degree of hyperlipoproteinemia not totally corrected by diet, and especially if the family history is adverse, cholestyramine or colestipol is the drug of choice. In severely hyperlipoproteinemic adults, combined nicotinic acid and sequestrant therapy may be used as for homozygotes. In subjects with Type IIb, if sequestrants aggravate the hypertriglyceridemia, it may be necessary to try the effect of nicotinic acid or clofibrate, although only after diet has been found inadequate.

I do not favor the use of ileal bypass procedures for the treatment of Type II hyperlipoproteinemia, because the majority of subjects can be successfully managed by the diet and drug regimens and especially because the means by which sequestrants reduce cholesterol levels is not far removed from that of the surgical procedure. Procedures such as portacaval shunting or plasmapheresis are restricted to a few centers and must be regarded as experimental.

Type III. Primary Type III consistently responds to a combination regimen consisting of (1) clofibrate, 1 gram twice daily (nicotinic acid is also effective but clofibrate is much less likely to produce troublesome side effects); (2) low cholesterol diet (less than 300 mg per day); and (3) weight reduction, followed by a balanced diet.

Patients on such treatment show a prompt fall in their lipid levels and gradual resolution of superficial xanthomas.

Type IV. The relationship of Type IV and endogenous hypertriglyceridemia to coronary heart disease is much less securely established than that of Type II and hypercholesterolemia, making advice about treatment even more difficult.

Reduction to ideal weight followed by a balanced diet with moderate cholesterol restriction (300 to 500 mg per day) nearly always improves hypertriglyceridemia in Type IV subjects and often normalizes lipids. In those in whom significant hypertriglyceridemia (more than 500 mg per 100 ml) persists, clofibrate is the drug of choice of many physicians, although I favor nicotinic acid. Alcohol use should be restricted.

Type V. It is important to reduce lipids and prevent the potentially dangerous symptomatology characteristic of this disorder. Initial treatment consists of reduction of body weight to ideal and usually makes a substantial contribution to lowering lipid levels. Diet therapy is aimed at reducing both chylomicronemia and VLDL concentrations, and combines fat and carbohydrate restriction. It involves the following measures: (1) Restriction and modification of fat intake to 25 to 30 per cent of total calories or 50 to 85 grams of fat. The fat intake must not exceed 0.9 to 1.3 grams per kg of body weight per day. Polyunsaturated fat should be substituted for saturated fat. (2) Control of carbohydrate to approximately 50 per cent of total calories and not exceeding 5 grams per kg of body weight. (3) Moderate restriction of cholesterol to 300 to 500 mg a day.

The protein intake is high as a result of measures 1 and 2. Alcohol must be avoided, because its use may precipitate hypertriglyceridemia and severe abdominal pain. During an acute abdominal attack, treatment consists of suspension of oral intake and administration of intravenous fluids.

Diet therapy is often sufficient to maintain the Type V patient, but in some it is necessary to use additional drugs. Nicotinic acid in a dose of 3 to 6 grams per day is often quite effective. However, coexisting hyperuricemia and hyperglycemia may preclude its use. Clofibrate is occasionally helpful, but care must be exercised on withdrawal of the drug, because a troublesome aggravation of hypertriglyceridemia can occur. Norethisterone acetate (investigational) has been found to be effective in female patients, but less so in males, at a dose of 2.5 to 5.0 mg per day.

REACTIVE HYPOGLYCEMIAS*

method of
BOYD E. METZGER, M.D.,
and NORBERT FREINKEL, M.D.
Chicago, Illinois

Diagnosis

Hypoglycemias which occur during the period of metabolic disposition of dietary carbohydrates are designated reactive hypoglycemias or hypoglycemias of the fed state. Thus, symptoms are characteristically elicited within 2 to 5 hours after eating and do not occur after overnight fasting or when meals are omitted.

Reactive hypoglycemia should be suspected in anyone complaining of episodic weakness, "dizziness," "jitteriness," palpitations, or hunger in the postprandial period. When such symptoms are present chronically or are sustained and unrelated temporally to meals, hypoglycemia rarely can be demonstrated as the cause of the symptoms. Hypoglycemia can best be documented by reproducing the fed state with a 5 hour oral glucose tolerance test performed after the patient has received a 300 gram carbohydrate diet for at least 3 days. Blood specimens should be drawn every 30 minutes for analysis of plasma glucose and insulin. If symptoms develop, blood should be drawn immediately, since a transient hypoglycemic dip can be missed by strict adherence to a 30 minute sampling interval. Furthermore, subjects may experience other phenomena which produce symptoms that are similar to those experienced during reactive hypoglycemia (e.g., hyperventilation or anxiety reaction). For these reasons, a physician, nurse, or technician should be

*Supported in part by AM-10699, AM-07169, HD 11021, and RR-48 from the National Institutes of Health, Bethesda, Maryland, and by grants from the National Foundation March of Dimes and the Kroc Foundation.

available for observation of the patient, immediate sampling of blood, and measurement of blood pressure, pulse, and respirations at any time symptoms are experienced.

Many factors contribute to the oral glucose tolerance curve, and failure to elicit a hypoglycemic reaction during a single 5 hour oral glucose tolerance test (OGTT) does not entirely exclude the presence of reactive hypoglycemia. If such a disorder is strongly suspected from the history, repeated testing is warranted.

Alimentary Hypoglycemia. Under ordinary circumstances, pyloric outflow is modulated so that ingested foodstuffs are presented to the absorptive sites in the small intestine at a finite rate. Blood insulin rises quickly in response to gastrointestinal absorption of glucose and release of gastrointestinal hormones or "gut factors," but the effects of insulin upon blood sugar are buffered by the reservoir of carbohydrate which slowly leaves the stomach for continuing absorption.

Both these aspects of normal absorption are modified as a consequence of gastrectomy or pyloric bypass. Alimentary carbohydrate is quickly poured into the small intestine. The ensuing rapid and excessive rise in blood sugar and perhaps the increased release of "gut factors" elicit secretion of insulin that is greater than normal, although appropriate to the hyperglycemia. Prompt utilization of glucose follows, but since the stomach is soon empty, absorptive input of glucose quickly diminishes and hypoglycemia frequently supervenes, usually about 2 hours after eating. In the postgastrectomy patient, postprandial hypoglycemia must be differentiated from the "dumping syndrome," although the two may be present concurrently. The osmotic phenomena of "dumping" develop within a few minutes to a half hour after eating, while hypoglycemia is rarely seen earlier than 1½ hours postprandially. When "dumping" is suspected, blood pressure, pulse, and hematocrit as well as blood sugar should be monitored carefully during an oral glucose tolerance test.

Rapid gastric emptying with accelerated absorption of glucose and increased release of "gut factors", e.g., gastric inhibitory polypeptide (GIP), is also the probable mechanism mediating the hypoglycemia which may be found in a significant number of patients with active peptic ulcers. Alimentary mechanisms may also play a major role in some subjects who have reactive hypoglycemia without demonstrable gastrointestinal disease, as well as in some patients with hyperthyroidism.

Hypoglycemia in Early Non-Insulin-Dependent Diabetes Mellitus (NIDDM). When glucose absorption is normal, but release of insulin to alimentary challenge is sluggish (as in most subjects with NIDDM), the immediate restraint to hepatic glucose output and deposition of glycogen may be subnormal. Thus, more of the ingested carbohydrate escapes the liver and enters the systemic circulation. The resultant hyperglycemia provides a continuing stimulus to insulin secretion and evokes a delayed peak in plasma insulin concentration. Hence, influx of glucose from the gastrointestinal tract may have ceased while plasma insulin is still relatively elevated. Characteristically, the glucose tolerance curve is elevated during the first 2 or 3 hours, with a fall to hypoglycemic levels in the fourth or fifth hour. Postprandial hypoglycemia in mild NIDDM is more common than generally appreciated and can be recognized with increased frequency by extending routine oral glucose tolerance tests beyond the conventional 2 or 3 hour period. It is not seen in patients with sustained fasting hyperglycemia, in whom acute insulin secretory response is markedly obtunded.

Functional Hypoglycemia. Symptomatic hypoglycemia may occur 2 to 5 hours after eating in subjects in whom no abnormalities in glucose tolerance are demonstrable during the first 2 hours — functional hypoglycemia. Inappropriately high plasma insulin levels following oral glucose can be demonstrated in some but not all of these patients.

It is still not certain whether functional hypoglycemia exists as a distinct entity. We have observed several subjects in whom the patterns of glucose and insulin during OGTT have fulfilled the criteria of "functional hypoglycemia" on some occasions and on others have shown impaired glucose tolerance and sluggish insulin release as in early NIDDM. Likewise, alimentary hypoglycemia cannot be excluded solely by the shape of a single oral glucose tolerance curve.

Treatment

Although the episodes of reactive hypoglycemia are usually transient and self-limited, a prolonged fall in blood sugar can be encountered in patients who are also receiving drugs which can compromise counter-regulation to hypoglycemia. Thus such drugs should be avoided in any subjects with a propensity toward reactive hypoglycemia. In particular, adrenergic blocking agents such as propranolol, or agents which deplete catecholamine, e.g., reserpine, should not be administered to these patients. Ingestion of alcohol prior to or concurrently with carbohydrates may also precipitate symptoms in some cases and should be avoided whenever historical information suggests such a response.

Not infrequently, patients with reactive hypoglycemia have learned by experience that they can avoid symptoms by repeatedly nibbling food. Consequently, they are often overweight when first seen by a physician. Restriction of calories should in such cases be instituted within the framework of the various specific dietary regimens (see below).

Alimentary Hypoglycemia. The objective of therapy is to reduce the wide excursions of blood sugar which characterize the alimentary hypoglycemias. Dietary carbohydrate ingestion should be restricted to less than 150 grams daily and protein intake increased from the normal 14 to 15 per cent to 25 to 30 per cent of total dietary calories. The remainder of the necessary calories is made up of fat. The food intake should be divided into six small meals to minimize the total load at any one time. In those patients with hypoglycemia associated with prior gastric surgery, some additional benefit may be achieved if food is taken dry, i.e., omitting water and other liquids at mealtime.

When hypoglycemia is associated with active peptic ulcer, treatment of the ulcer with diet and anticholinergic medications usually results in abatement of symptoms. By reducing the rate of discharge of food from the stomach, anticholinergic drugs may also be of benefit to those subjects who display alimentary hypoglycemia without demonstrable gastrointestinal disease, and should be employed if dietary manipulation alone does not eliminate the episodes of hypoglycemia.

Hypoglycemia in Early NIDDM. If symptoms persist after institution of a diabetic diet restricted in sucrose and monosaccharide or after weight reduction in the 60 to 80 per cent of subjects who are obese, rectification of postprandial hypoglycemia in mild NIDDM can frequently be achieved by treatment with oral sulfonylureas. If these measures are not entirely successful, the diet should be split into multiple feedings, keeping total caloric intake constant.

Functional Hypoglycemia. Dietary manipulation has proved to be the most successful form of therapy in "functional" hypoglycemia. Feedings of a diet high in protein and low in carbohydrate on a regular three meal schedule should be tried initially. If hypoglycemic episodes are not completely eliminated, small between-meal feedings should be added, keeping the total daily caloric intake constant. Weight control may be necessary and is especially desirable in view of the suggestive evidence that "functional" hypoglycemia may be a "prediabetic" abnormality in some persons.

OBESITY

method of
SAUL GENUTH, M.D.,
and VICTOR VERTES, M.D.
Cleveland, Ohio

General Considerations

Obesity is a distressing problem for the patient, a frustrating problem for the physician, and a vexing problem for the public health professional. For all three, however, recent progress — albeit slow — is perceptible.

A precise definition of obesity is not possible, because adipose tissue mass does not follow a bimodal population distribution and not all "excess weight" is fat. Therefore, the most reasonable way to define obesity is by its effect on mortality experience. At 130 per cent of desirable body weight (Metropolitan Life Insurance Company tables, 1959), an increase in mortality experience is already evident. Above 160 per cent of desirable body weight, the increase in mortality rates is exponential rather than linear. Hence, even in the absence of other complicating medical disease, obesity may be *conservatively* defined as a morbid condition at 150 per cent of ideal body weight. In the presence of concomitant hypertension, cardiac disease, or diabetes mellitus, a body weight in excess of 120 per cent of desirable weight constitutes morbid obesity.

In a very minute fraction of patients, obesity results from specifically diagnosable disorders such as hypothalamic tumors or infiltration, Prader-Willi syndrome, insulinoma, glucocorticoid excess, and hypothyroidism. In the overwhelming majority, the cause is unknown and the primary cause cannot be removed. That obesity is a heterogeneous disorder is suggested by differences in familial incidence, in age of onset, in adipose tissue hyperplasia versus hypertrophy, in rapidity of weight loss and weight regain, and in vulnerability to the development of diabetes mellitus. This conclusion is further supported by significant variations in hormone profiles and/or enzyme capacities in animal models of obesity. The one common denominator in the development of obesity, regardless of its penultimate cause, must be a period of time during which energy input as food exceeds energy expenditure. Therefore, all present forms of nonspecific treatment consist of reversing this imbalance until a lower, healthier weight is achieved.

The therapy of obesity today may be characterized, in general, as follows. Palliation, defined as temporary reduction to desirable body weight followed by inexorable weight regain, can be achieved in 70 to 80 per cent of patients. Control, defined as reduction to desirable body weight, followed by long-term maintenance of that weight through constant or intermittent regulation of energy intake and expenditure, may be achieved in up to 20 per cent of patients. Cure, defined as reduction to desirable body weight followed by maintenance of that weight on an entirely ad lib basis, is rarely achieved. Palliation, with the additional hope of long-term control, should be offered to all patients with morbid obesity. No matter what method is employed, it is a sine qua non for success that the physician be sincerely committed to the effort. A skeptical attitude and/or perfunctory performance will inevitably communicate itself to the patient and sabotage the therapeutic program. Medical practices based solely on the treatment of obesity run the risk of self-delusion by the physician and unrealistic expectations by the patient. Hence, obesity is probably best treated by physicians with a serious interest in the disorder who are willing to use various therapeutic modalities in a systematic fashion but who have sufficient other medical responsibilities so as to maintain their perspective. Reputable community group programs may appropriately serve patients with nonmorbid obesity, primarily desiring cosmetic relief, who do not respond readily to simple dietary prescription by the physician. A small fraction of patients with morbid obesity who have previously exhibited psychiatric disturbance or social pathology when their weight was drastically reduced are probably best left untreated as the lesser of two evils.

Methods

We endorse a logical hierarchy of treatment which begins with conventional, minimally intrusive dieting, proceeds to supplemented fasting, and reserves surgical procedures as a last resort.

Conventional Dieting. The basic approach used is a diet containing 800 to 1500 kcal per day. No particular distribution of carbohydrate, protein, and fat is of advantage so long as protein deficiency is avoided. The greater the degree of obesity, the greater should be the degree of caloric restriction. More energy expenditure in everyday life should be encouraged, e.g., walking instead of riding short distances, climbing stairs instead of taking elevators. Simple instruction in behavior modification techniques such as eating more slowly, more formally, more regularly, with others rather than alone, more purposefully, and without entertainment distractions may increase success and instill better long-term habits. This approach should be offered all patients less than

150 per cent of desirable weight who are seeking medical help for the first time. It may also be appropriate for a small number of patients who repeatedly fail on more drastic regimens but who have a strong psychologic need to feel that they are still trying to deal medically with their obesity. At the least, it maintains physician surveillance for the development or worsening of medical complications of obesity.

We do not recommend adjunctive use of drugs. There is no reasonable justification for human chorionic gonadotropin injections. Amphetamines may increase rates of weight loss by 0.25 to 0.5 kg per week, but resistance often develops by 12 weeks, while side effects such as irritability and palpitations may continue. Observations that overeating may accompany life tensions, relieve frustration, or be used to sublimate or ward off sexual activity have fostered the notion that in many patients obesity is the result of emotional disturbances. Nonetheless, formal psychotherapy aimed specifically at weight reduction is almost never successful. It may occasionally be indicated during dietary treatment for management of associated psychiatric disorders, of which depression is the most common. Psychotherapy is mandatory when depression or sexual panic results from weight reduction.

Supplemented Fasting. The high failure rate of conventional diet therapy has led to the development of "supplemented fasting" or "protein-sparing modified fasting." These techniques guarantee a high initial rate of success on which to base long-term maintenance programs. They are designed to exploit the anorexic effect and rapid weight loss of fasting in outpatient safety. By administration of sufficient protein and a small amount of carbohydrate, the clinical debilitation, chemical derangements, and attrition of lean body mass which characterize total fasting are minimized. Some authors recommend the use of 1.2 to 1.4 grams of protein per kg of body weight supplied as lean meat, fowl, and fish. We employ a daily ration of 70 grams of egg albumin and 30 grams of carbohydrate — the latter to further limit ketosis and hyperuricemia. This formulated supplement of 400 calories is given in five equal doses and also supplies 1000 mg of calcium, 550 mg of phosphorus, 400 mg of magnesium, 18 mg of iron, 40 mEq of sodium, 20 mEq of potassium, and 100 per cent recommended dietary allowances of copper, zinc, manganese, iodine, and all vitamins. An additional 20 mEq of potassium is routinely prescribed to maintain normokalemia.

Most patients are begun ambulatory on this program of complete food withdrawal. Hypertensive and diabetic patients, however, are usually admitted to the hospital for the initial week of therapy. Diuretics, antihypertensive drugs, sulfonylureas, and insulin are withdrawn. In diabetics taking more than 50 units of insulin daily, the dose is tapered over several days as food calories are simultaneously reduced. Diabetics with a previous history of ketoacidosis are excluded. Other previously prescribed medications may be continued; extra potassium may be needed for patients maintained on digitalis preparations.

After discharge, the vast majority of patients carry on their usual occupational, social, and family activities. They are monitored weekly in the clinic by symptom review and weight and blood pressure measurement; routine blood chemistries with emphasis on serum potassium, uric acid, blood urea nitrogen (BUN), and glucose are measured every 2 weeks and hematocrit every 4 weeks. Seventy to 80 per cent of patients lose more than 18 kg. The average rates of loss are 1.4 kg per week for women and 2.0 kg per week for men. This regimen has been maintained for a full year in patients with starting weights above 180 kg. Customarily, however, food is reintroduced in slowly increasing amounts after weight losses of 25 to 35 kg. Sodium and carbohydrate intake must be carefully regulated during this time to avoid refeeding edema.

This program often succeeds in patients with morbid obesity who have failed on conventional dieting. It is especially useful for patients urgently requiring weight reduction for medical reasons. This includes patients with the pickwickian syndrome, uncontrolled diabetes, hypertension, or severe pulmonary disease; patients needing coronary arteriography and, if indicated, bypass surgery; patients needing semi-elective surgery as colectomy for ulcerative colitis, hysterectomy for chronic menorrhagia, or aneurysectomy; and patients needing elective surgery such as hip replacement, laminectomy, or herniorrhaphy. In diabetics hyperglycemia may be expected to abate within 3 weeks, and 80 to 90 per cent of hypertensives normalize their blood pressure, usually without drug therapy. Needed surgery can usually be carried out after 3 to 6 months of weight reduction. Improvements in agility, social life, self-image, and employment status are other benefits of significance.

In the initial week of supplemented fasting, diarrhea, fatigue, headache, and hunger pains are common but transient symptoms. Orthostatic dizziness, cold intolerance, skin dryness, hair loss, muscle cramps, decreased libido, amenorrhea, and euphoria are seen later and may persist for several months after cessation of supplemented fasting. These seldom cause premature termination of the program, however. Unilateral and reversible peroneal nerve palsy occasionally occurs after very large losses of weight. Rarely, cholecystitis or pancreatitis has complicated the reinstitution of food if the patient did not follow the recommended diet. A very widespread and largely unsupervised use of so-called "liquid protein diets" during the 1970s resulted in reports of 16 unexplained sudden deaths in obese women aged 23 to 51, thought to be otherwise healthy. In relation to the estimated use, this death rate significantly exceeded that expected for nonobese women in the same age range. In an experience of 2500 patients treated by supplemented fasting, we have observed seven deaths. Five occurred in patients with evidence of preexisting heart disease, one was accidental, and one, in a hypertensive male, remains unexplained. The risk of death unrelated to known heart disease appears very low (and far less than that associated with intestinal bypass surgery) if patients are given high-quality protein and adequate potassium, are carefully monitored, and are not extended to heroic lengths of weight reduction.

A high rate of recidivism plagues all nonsurgical treatment programs for obesity. Without follow-up, complete weight regain can be expected in 90 per cent of patients within several years of successful weight reduction. This dismal prognosis obligates the conscientious therapist to continue an organized program of assistance with weight maintenance. We currently employ two tools in concert.

Regular exercise is best conducted in a formal structured group program with a trained supervisor. Physical fitness is first estimated in simple fashion with a 5 minute walk at 3 miles per hour. Resultant pulse rates of 120 and 100 are graded "poor" and "fair." Stress testing may also be indicated if there is a question of coronary disease. For poor and fair categories, exercise may be initially prescribed at 60 per cent or 70 per cent of maximal allowable heart rate (220 minus age in years), respectively. For example, a patient may begin by walking 5 to 15 minutes three times a week with speed and duration limited by the aforementioned heart rates and by avoidance of dyspnea. Gradually, as fitness improves, patients may achieve optimal walking or jogging periods of 45 minutes five times per week. Group sessions help maintain compliance; patients who exercise alone should be asked to keep activity logs. Although exercise does not materially accelerate the rate of weight reduction, it may still be usefully started during supplemented fasting. This helps preserve lean body mass, improves the patient's sense of well-being, and emphasizes, at the outset, the importance of behavior change.

A second tool used is systematic modification

of life style as it affects eating behavior. Irrespective of the ultimate reason for overeating, some patients are· definitely benefited by a careful, guided *self-analysis* of the circumstances and proximate cause for individual instances of unrestrained and unphysiologic eating. The patient must first be taught to record all eating — its quantity, quality, time, place, purpose, mood, and associated companions and activities. As patterns of consistent antecedents or stimuli to unnecessary or unwise eating are identified (e.g., eating alone while watching television), tactics are devised to remove or replace them. As the new behaviors are learned, they must be positively reinforced; success comes when these behaviors become habit and the weight control automatic. While the responsibility for change of behavior rests with the patient, family help may be enlisted in both the observational and corrective stages. The patient's efforts at weight control, however, often become a part of interpersonal family dynamics, and ways must be found to mitigate this as a source of family conflict. Life style change can be taught through individual counseling or more economically in groups of six to ten. Groups offer the advantages of peer empathy and support as well as surprising flashes of insight. Group leaders require considerable skills (different from those of individual counseling) to teach group dynamics, to distribute time and attention equitably, to defuse conflict, and to prevent victimization of individual patients.

The use of these tools should not detract from traditional, ongoing dietary education. Patients must still be taught caloric contents and nutritional values of food. However, dietary counseling does not succeed if it is totally rigid. Patients can be taught to arrange their caloric affairs so as to eat more freely and enjoyably at certain times of the week, making up for the excess at other times when restriction of calories is more socially acceptable.

It must be admitted by the realistic therapist that even intensive programs, such as those described above, produce only limited success. In the flush of successful weight reduction, a large fraction of patients forsake the physician or clinic immediately, certain that this time "they have learned their lesson." Another group disengages more slowly because of guilt, shame, or fear of chastisement if their weight begins to increase. This self-defeating maneuver is especially frustrating to the physician. Some patients are also unwilling or unable to bear the cost of continuing the professional attention from physician, nutritionist, exercise physiologist, or psychologist. For these reasons, reliable long-term follow-up data are frustratingly difficult to obtain. Of those patients who choose to remain in our regular maintenance program, about half control their weight successfully for at least the first 2 years as defined by a weight regain of less than 25 per cent. Therapeutic nihilists may view this salvage rate as too low to justify their or the patients' efforts. Others who have achieved splendid individual results with solid medical and social benefits will continue to offer current therapy in a responsible and patient-informed manner while seeking better solutions to the problem.

Surgery. Refractory morbid obesity in psychiatrically suitable patients can, as a last resort, be treated by either ileal or· gastric bypass. In the former procedure, all but approximately 50 cm of jejunum and ileum is functionally bypassed. Weight loss occurs both because of the reduced absorptive surface and because of an anorexogenic effect of the shunt. An average of one third of body weight is gradually lost, and in most patients weight remains stable thereafter. The undeniable medical benefits of this procedure must be balanced against its disadvantages. Almost all patients suffer from chronic diarrhea, and many exhibit intermittent, dangerous electrolyte depletion. Arthritis, osteomalacia, renal lithiasis, and hepatic dysfunction are complications of formidable magnitude and frequency. Perioperative mortality rates have averaged 4 per cent. Gastric bypass, or stapling, is designed to reduce the functional capacity of the stomach and thereby greatly limit the amount of food which can be comfortably ingested at any one time. Rates of weight loss and weight maintenance are similar to those of ileal bypass. However, perioperative mortality appears to be lower and subsequent medical complications are much less frequent and hazardous. A longer period of experience is needed before the final role and indications for this operation can be judged.

PELLAGRA

method of
RICHARD W. VILTER, M.D.
Cincinnati, Ohio

Pellagra was endemic in the southern United States until the practice of enriching flour and improvement in the standard of living occurred after World War II. Now pellagra is recognized principally in alcoholic addicts who replace vitamin-rich calories with "empty" ones, food faddists, neglected or depressed elderly persons, drug addicts, persons with malabsorption syndromes of various types, and those with illnesses such as thyrotoxicosis that increase the requirement for essential nutrients. An interesting association is the occurrence of pellagrous dermatitis in persons with malignant carcinoid tumor. This tumor can convert tremendous amounts of tryptophan to serotonin rather than to coenzymes containing niacinamide. In developing countries where corn and millet are dietary staples, the deficiency state is apt to occur because these two grains are severely deficient in tryptophan and niacin.

Niacinamide is an essential component of respiratory coenzymes NAD and NADP. The enzyme systems activated by these coenzymes are involved in glycolysis, synthesis of fat, and production of energy.

Niacin deficiency never occurs as an isolated entity under natural circumstances. Other vitamins, particularly the water-soluble ones, are lacking also. Anemia may be due to folic acid deficiency; peripheral neuritis may be due to thiamine deficiency; seborrheic scrotal dermatitis may result from riboflavin deficiency; and vitamin B_6 deficiency may cause any of the symptoms just mentioned.

Prevention

The most important aspect of prevention is provision of an adequate diet sufficient in calories to meet the energy requirements of the patient and including fish, poultry, legumes, cereals, dairy products, and fruits. Such a diet, providing 2400 calories, 70 grams of protein of good biologic quality, and 20 niacin equivalents,* will prevent pellagra. If a sick patient is unable to eat such a diet, a complete multivitamin capsule or vitamin-enriched protein supplement should be prescribed that provides one, two, or three times the recommended dietary allowances of the Food and Nutrition Board of the National Academy of Sciences. According to the recommendations, healthy infants and children under 4 years should receive 6 to 9 niacin equivalents. Adults and children over 4 years of age should receive 11 to 19 niacin equivalents, and pregnant or lactating women should receive an additional 2 to 5 niacin equivalents.

Treatment

Acute manifestations of pellagra should be treated with niacinamide orally, intramuscularly, or intravenously, as most easily meets the needs of the patient. For children the dose would be 25 to 50 mg three times a day for 14 days and for

---

*One niacin equivalent is 1 mg niacin or 60 mg tryptophan.

adults 100 mg three times a day for the same period. Electrolyte imbalances should be rectified by intravenous fluids according to the patient's needs. Other associated vitamin deficiencies should be treated with a mixed vitamin capsule two or three times a day as described under Prevention. As quickly as possible, the patient should receive a diet of 2500 to 3000 calories similar to that described under Prevention. Until the patient's mouth has healed, a liquid or puréed diet may be needed, offered to the patient in multiple feedings. The patient must be encouraged constantly by the personnel of the hospital to eat the food, and this aspect of treatment must be most carefully monitored. If therapy is properly provided, improvement in the oral mucous membranes and in emotional disturbances may be anticipated within 6 to 12 hours. Diarrhea may abate within 24 hours, and gradual return to good health will usually require 10 to 14 days.

RICKETS AND OSTEOMALACIA

method of
SUDHAKER D. RAO, M.B., B.S.,
and BOY FRAME, M.D.
Detroit, Michigan

Rickets is a disease in which there is impaired mineralization of cartilage, leading to a defect in enchondral bone formation, and which, by definition, can no longer be manifested after epiphyseal fusion. Osteomalacia, on the other hand, is characterized by excessive accumulation of osteoid (the poorly mineralized bone matrix) as a result of slowing or arrest in the initial phases of mineralization. Thus, osteomalacia can manifest itself as soon as significant amounts of lamellar bone have been formed in replacement of woven bone. Adults, therefore, have only osteomalacia, but in children rickets and osteomalacia usually coexist. Despite this difference, the pathogenesis of rickets and osteomalacia is similar, and therapy of the two conditions can conveniently be considered together.

Recent major advances in our knowledge of vitamin D (calciferol) metabolism have led to the realization that this compound is the precursor of a well-regulated hormonal system. Through a series of successive hydroxylation reactions, more active metabolites of the parent vitamin are formed in the liver and kidney (Fig. 1). The

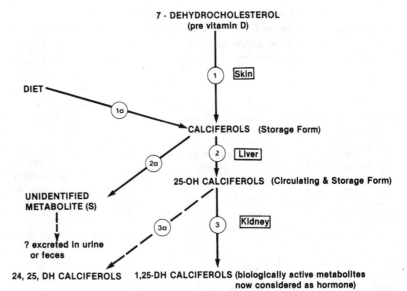

Figure 1. Schematic representation of vitamin D metabolism.

7 · DEHYDROCHOLESTEROL
(pre vitamin D)

① Skin

DIET

1a

CALCIFEROLS (Storage Form)

② Liver

2a

25-OH CALCIFEROLS (Circulating & Storage Form)

UNIDENTIFIED
METABOLITE (S)

3a   ③ Kidney

? excreted in urine
or feces

24, 25, DH CALCIFEROLS   1,25-DH CALCIFEROLS (biologically active metabolites
                          now considered as hormone)

Legend: (1) photochemical conversion by UV light
         (1a) affected by malabsorption, ? genetic
         (2) CALCIFEROL 25-hydroxylase
         (2a) enzyme (s) induction
         (3) 25-hydroxy CALCIFEROL · 1α hydroxylase
         (3a) 25-hydroxy CALCIFEROL, 24 hydroxylase

terminology used in this article will reflect the hormonal nature of the vitamin D system (Table 1).

Availability of newer metabolites for treatment of rickets and osteomalacia necessitates the understanding of metabolic derangements in various forms of these two conditions. A classification based on mechanisms involved in the pathogenesis of rickets and osteomalacia provides a rational approach to therapy (Table 2 and Fig. 1). In most instances the underlying metabolic defect can be pinpointed such that response to adequate treatment is usually most gratifying in alleviating the skeletal disability.

Ergocalciferol, the only compound available for general use in the United States, remains the mainstay of current therapy for rickets and osteomalacia. However, newer metabolites of calciferol currently under extensive clinical trials are likely to become available in the foreseeable future. One such metabolite, 1,25-dihydroxycholecalciferol (1,25-DHCC, calcitriol) has been approved by the Food and Drug Administration for limited use in renal osteodystrophy. When appropriate, we will indicate the form and dose of these newer metabolites in the treatment of rickets and osteomalacia. The metabolites of calciferol offer several advantages over conventional ergocalciferol therapy: lower and more physiologic doses, more rapid onset of action, shorter half-life (this becomes important if hypercalcemia develops during treatment), and greater specifici-

TABLE 1. **Nomenclature of Vitamin D and Its Metabolites**

AS A VITAMIN	AS A HORMONE
Vitamin D (parent compound)	Calciferol
Vitamin D_2*	Ergocalciferol (EC)
Vitamin D_3*	Cholecalciferol (CC)
25-Hydroxyvitamin D_3 (D_2)†	25-Hydroxychole(ergo)calciferol (25-HCC,25-HEC)
1,25-Dihydroxyvitamin D_3 (D_2)‡	1,25-Dihydroxychole(ergo)calciferol (1,25-DHCC;1,25-DHEC)
24,25-Dihydroxyvitamin D_3 (D_2)†	24,25-Dihydroxychole(ergo)calciferol (24,25-DHCC;24,25-DHEC)

*Available for general use.
†Available for investigational use only.
‡Available for use only in patients on dialysis.

TABLE 2. **Common Causes of Rickets or Osteomalacia or Both (A Classification Based on Mechanisms)**

Vitamin D deficiency (1)*
  1. ? Skin pigment
  2. Inadequate exposure to sunlight
Vitamin D malabsorption or malnutrition (1a)
  1. Inadequate intake
  2. Gastrectomy
  3. Small intestinal disease, resection, or bypass
  4. Sprue syndrome ± gluten enteropathy
  5. Pancreatic insufficiency
  6. Laxative abuse
  7. Cholestyramine
Impaired vitamin D-25 hydroxylation (2)
  1. Chronic liver disease ± alcoholism
  2. Biliary cirrhosis
  3. Neonatal hepatitis
  4. Immaturity
  5. ? Genetic enzyme defect
Increased catabolism and/or excretion (2a)
  1. Increased catabolism
    a. Phenytoin (Dilantin)
    b. Barbiturates
    c. Glutethimide
  2. Increased excretion
    a. Primary biliary cirrhosis
    b. Nephrotic syndrome
Impaired 25-hydroxy vitamin D–1α-hydroxylase (3)
  1. Chronic renal failure
  2. Genetically ineffective enzyme (vitamin D dependency)
  3. Parathyroid hormone deficiency or "resistance"
Substrate deficiency (1a, in some instances)
  1. Hypophosphatemia
    a. Vitamin D refractory rickets or osteomalacia
    b. Oncogenic osteomalacia (associated with tumors)
    c. Inadequate intake
    d. Excessive or prolonged use of antacids
  2. Hypocalcemia (uncommon)
  3. Hypomagnesemia (uncommon)
Miscellaneous
  1. Renal tubular acidosis (all forms)
  2. Ureterosigmoidostomy
  3. ? End organ (bone or intestine) resistance to 1,25-DHCC

*Numbers in parenthesis represent site of metabolic abnormality. See Figure 1 for explanation.

ty for certain rachitic or osteomalacic conditions.

Since calciferol and its various metabolites are now available in pure chemical forms, units of weight rather than the obsolete terminology of International Units (IU) will be used. Forty thousand IU of calciferol is equal to 1 mg, and 10 micrograms is equal to 400 IU.

General Principles and Precautions of Therapy

When dealing with simple nutritional deficiency rickets or osteomalacia, it is our invariable practice to begin therapy with a higher dose than the expected maintenance dose (EMD). In this way, onset of healing is expedited and the risk of hypercalcemia is negligible. However, when using pharmacologic doses of ergocalciferol, an initial high-dose regimen may be extremely hazardous. In this situation use of ergocalciferol is analogous to the use of digitalis. During the initial phase of treatment, body stores of calciferol and its metabolites must be repleted or filled to a given level; this level varies between diseases, between different patients with the same disease, and in the same patient at different times. Injudicious use, as with digitalis, will increase the risk of intoxication. It is therefore best to initiate therapy with somewhat less than the EMD, and only then to increase the dose by small amounts, depending upon the biochemical and roentgenologic response.

An erroneous belief still exists in the general population that "bone meal" (a combination of calcium carbonate and small amounts of ergocalciferol) improves the strength of the bones. Quite regrettably, many physicians also believe that large doses of ergocalciferol and calcium are helpful in preventing osteoporosis. Current evidence and our own experience do not support this contention except in a small number of patients. Pharmacologic use of ergocalciferol and calcium has deleterious effects on the bone cell function when these agents are used over a long period of time. Therefore, routine use of ergocalciferol as a supplement is strongly discouraged.

Therapy of Specific Categories of Rickets and Osteomalacia

Because of their frequent use, the time-honored terms for various forms of rickets and osteomalacia will be used in the following discussion. When appropriate, we will indicate the alternative (and probably more suitable) terms.

Vitamin D Deficiency. The widespread use of vitamin supplements and fortification of foods has largely eliminated vitamin D deficiency in the Western Hemisphere. Not infrequently, however, poverty, ignorance, and unusual dietary habits have resulted in the re-emergence of such cases within small segments of the population. Dark-skinned persons with little exposure to sunlight are particularly susceptible, since the synthesis of cholecalciferol that normally occurs in the skin is reduced under these circumstances (Fig. 1). Rickets is more apt to occur in premature infants and in infants receiving unenriched cow's milk.

PROPHYLAXIS. The minimal daily requirement (MDR) of calciferol in children to prevent rickets is about 10 micrograms per day. In adults, 2.5 micrograms per day is considered adequate to prevent osteomalacia. Some enthusiastic mothers may give additional calciferol supplements to infants who are already receiving the MDR of the vitamin in fortified milk and other foods. This should be discouraged, as some infants are unduly sensitive to the effects of calciferol and may develop hypercalcemia with its attendant risks.

TREATMENT. Although smaller doses may occasionally be effective, it is advisable to administer at least 100 micrograms of erogocalciferol daily for children and 50 to 100 micrograms daily for adults until a response is obtained. This is measured by a return of the plasma calcium and phosphorus levels to near normal in 7 to 10 days. Radiologic improvement of rachitic changes or pseudofractures is apparent in about 2 to 4 weeks, but it may be several months before the elevated alkaline phosphatase level returns to normal.

Not infrequently, symptomatic hypocalcemia may be present either before or immediately after initiation of treatment with ergocalciferol, especially in infants. Under these circumstances intravenous calcium gluconate should be given initially, to be followed by oral calcium supplements until normal plasma calcium levels are attained. A poor response or a delay in response may suggest the possibility of vitamin D dependent rickets or osteomalacia.

Vitamin D Dependent Rickets (1α-Hydroxylase Enzyme Deficiency). Because of its resemblance clinically, biochemically and roentgenologically to vitamin D deficiency, this disorder is sometimes referred to as "pseudo-calciferol deficiency rickets." Response to treatment is usually complete as in the case of vitamin D deficiency rickets, but lifelong pharmacologic doses (0.5 to 1.5 mg per day) of ergocalciferol are required for correction of mineral and skeletal defects.

Recent studies have demonstrated that there is a defective synthesis of 1,25-DHCC in this disease. It appears to be a genetically (autosomal recessive) determined 25-HCC 1α-hydroxylase enzyme deficiency. Biochemical and skeletal response occurs with as little as 1 to 2 micrograms (or 0.04 microgram per kg of body weight per day) of 1,25-DHCC (see Table 1 for use). Whether this metabolite will become the drug of choice in the treatment of vitamin D dependent rickets remains to be seen.

Sporadic cases of vitamin D dependent osteomalacia have been reported in adults. There is no familial occurrence, but the incidence seems to be high in certain parts of the world. Therapy of this condition is similar to that of vitamin D dependent rickets.

Vitamin D Refractory Rickets (Primary Hypophosphatemia, Rickets, and Osteomalacia). This term is applied to all forms of hypophosphatemic rickets and osteomalacia. There is no identifiable defect in vitamin D metabolism in this disease,

and plasma calcium (unlike vitamin D deficiency and vitamin D dependent rickets) is almost always normal prior to therapy. Pathogenesis of this disorder has not yet been clearly defined, and treatment, therefore, cannot be based on rational correction of a specific metabolic error. Proper therapy requires a long-term close cooperation between the patient, the family, and the physician.

It is important to realize that the main objectives of therapy are to alleviate symptoms and promote normal activity, to avoid hypercalcemia, to achieve normal linear growth, and to prevent deformity. The optimal dose of ergocalciferol to achieve these goals is often most difficult to determine. A deliberate undertreatment is probably better than prolonged moderate overdose.

Therapy with 1 to 2 mg of ergocalciferol daily is initiated, and 0.25 to 0.50 mg increments in the dose are considered every 3 to 4 months. Rarely if ever are higher doses required. Improvement is gauged by radiologic signs of healing and prevention of deformities, and toxicity is measured by the appearance of hypercalciuria and hypercalcemia. Hypophosphatemia and elevated plasma serum alkaline phosphatase levels may not return to normal even in the presence of radiologic healing. After closure of growth cartilage, the dose of ergocalciferol can often be reduced to 0.5 to 1.0 mg per day. Lifelong treatment, however, is required to prevent reactivation of the disease, which may occur during later life.

Corrective osteotomies are best delayed, if possible, until after cessation of growth. Either the dose of ergocalciferol should be markedly reduced or the therapy discontinued altogether during the period of bed rest, before and several months after corrective surgery. If this is not done, the added factor of immobilization may be sufficient to cause hypercalcemia.

Although phosphate supplements alone do not initiate healing of rickets, their use will reduce the daily requirement of ergocalciferol by 0.5 to 1.0 mg. One to 2 grams of elemental phosphorus given orally in frequent small doses is better tolerated, and a more persistent elevation of plasma phosphorus level is achieved. Troublesome diarrhea (a frequent side effect) and the nonpalatable nature of these supplements can be circumvented by the use of powdered forms of phosphorus in the cooking of stews, hamburgers, and so on.

Rarely, sporadic and vitamin D resistant hypophosphatemic osteomalacia occurs for the first time during adolescence or in adulthood. The biochemical findings are similar to the X-linked forms of vitamin D resistant rickets but are different in that severe skeletal pain and muscle weakness are invariably present. The principles of ergocalciferol administration are similar in both instances, but phosphate supplements are more efficacious in the adult-onset variety. In fact, a number of such patients have shown improvement in both muscle weakness and osteomalacia with 2 to 3 grams of oral phosphate supplements as the only form of therapy. Excessive phosphate may lead to hypocalcemia and secondary hyperparathyroidism with its deleterious effect on the skeleton.

An acquired form of sporadic hypophosphatemic osteomalacia has been reported in association with certain vascular and giant cell tumors. This form of the disease will respond to phosphate supplements and ergocalciferol therapy. However, if the tumor is resectable, the osteomalacia is usually cured or greatly improved once the tumor is removed.

The general principles of therapy for primary hypophosphatemic rickets and osteomalacia also apply when there are associated findings of renal glycosuria and aminoaciduria, as in some of the complex renal tubular disorders.

Vitamin D Malabsorption. In a number of gastrointestinal and hepatobiliary disorders there is, for different reasons, an impaired absorption of ergocalciferol and its metabolites. In some there is increased urinary and fecal loss of 25-HCC. Symptoms of malabsorption in these patients may not be obvious, and careful history-taking and thorough evaluation are needed to uncover any underlying malabsorption. Both rickets and osteomalacia can result purely as a consequence of malabsorption of ergocalciferol, calcium, or phosphorus. Osteoporosis frequently accompanies the osteomalacia in malabsorption states and does not respond to treatment with ergocalciferol.

Postgastrectomy osteomalacia results from a combination of poor dietary intake of ergocalciferol and calcium, impaired absorption of calciferol, and possibly phosphate depletion as a result of excessive use of phosphate binding antacids. Parenteral administration of 2.5 micrograms per day of ergocalciferol results in a complete cure of osteomalacia. Since the degree of malabsorption in this disease is only mild, the oral dose of ergocalciferol should not be very much greater than the parenteral dose, unless there is associated pancreatic disease. There is no established correct oral dose of ergocalciferol, since most patients are given large pharmacologic doses. An approximate dose would be no more than 100 to 150 micrograms per day (i.e., twice the suggested dose for simple dietary deficiency rickets or osteomalacia).

In *intestinal mucosal disease* (with or without signs of overt malabsorption) there is both impaired absorption of ergocalciferol and increased endogenous fecal calcium excretion. In some patients dietary calcium absorption may be normal or increased. In gluten enteropathy, despite marked depression of absorption of ergocalciferol, complete cure of rickets and osteomalacia is possible with a gluten-free diet alone. If more rapid treatment of the bone disease is required, 1 to 2 mg of ergocalciferol may be administered daily until the radiologic improvement is noted and the elevated alkaline phosphatase levels return to normal. In other forms of intestinal malabsorption that do not respond to treatment of the primary intestinal disorder, lifelong administration of as much as 1 to 10 mg of ergocalciferol per day may be required, along with dietary calcium supplementation.

25-Hydroxycholecalciferol may be the drug of choice for treatment of rickets and osteomalacia occurring in patients with *hepatobiliary disease*. It is the increased excretion of 25-HCC (or its catabolic products), rather than impaired absorption, that is a major contributing factor to the development of bone disease. Until 25-HCC is available for general use, administration of large doses of ergocalciferol (1 to 5 mg per day) are probably sufficient for treatment of osteomalacia and rickets.

In the absence of associated intestinal mucosal disease, both rickets and osteomalacia are less common in *pancreatic disease*. The therapeutic requirement of ergocalciferol is approximately the same as that in hepatobiliary disease.

Parenteral administration of ergocalciferol might usually be recommended in treatment of rickets or osteomalacia caused by various gastrointestinal disorders, except that unfortunately a reliable preparation of ergocalciferol for parenteral use is not readily available. Magnesium supplements may also be required before symptomatic hypocalcemia is corrected in some instances of intestinal malabsorption.

Hyperchloremic Acidosis. Rickets and osteomalacia may be associated with hyperchloremic metabolic acidosis. Both developmental (distal) and acquired (ureterosigmoidostomy and paraproteinemias) forms of renal tubular acidoses may result in defective mineralization of osteoid. Metabolic acidosis, renal phosphate leak, and hypophosphatemia all contribute to the development of rickets and osteomalacia. Disabling skeletal symptoms are often incapacitating. Therapy with both ergocalciferol and alkali is often required. In general, 1 to 2 mg per day of ergocalciferol over a period of 6 to 8 months is adequate to restore normal mineralization of the osteoid tissue. In addition, sufficient alkali in the form of sodium bicarbonate or sodium citrate is given to correct the metabolic acidosis. Up to 10 to 15 grams of sodium bicarbonate may be required each day, which might present problems in patients with underlying cardiac disease. After the healing of bone disease, therapy with alkali alone will prevent recurrence. Hypophosphatemia, when present, should be corrected with oral phosphate supplements to expedite the healing of rickets and osteomalacia.

Renal Osteodystrophy. Progressive renal insufficiency results in two important metabolic abnormalities: decreased phosphate clearance leading to hyperphosphatemia, and reduced functioning renal tissue with the consequent impairment of 1α-hydroxylation of 25-HCC. The resultant hypocalcemia (caused by decreased synthesis of 1,25-DHCC and decreased intestinal absorption of calcium) and hyperphosphatemia invariably lead to the development of moderate to severe secondary hyperparathyroidism with its attendant skeletal effects.

Renal osteodystrophy is a complex metabolic disorder that includes osteomalacia (or rickets), osteitis fibrosa, osteoporosis, and osteosclerosis. A detailed account of pathogenesis of various components of renal osteodystrophy is beyond the scope of this discussion. The course of bone disease is quite variable. Although the biochemical evidence of secondary hyperparathyroidism is demonstrable when creatinine clearance falls below 70 ml per minute, osteomalacia is uncommon before the creatinine clearance falls to 30 ml per minute or less. Some patients (i.e., those on anticonvulsant therapy) are more prone to develop osteomalacia earlier in the course of renal failure.

Major goals of therapy are (1) prevention of phosphate retention, (2) correction of hypocalcemia, (3) suppression of secondary hyperparathyroidism, and (4) healing of bone disease.

Adequate attention to diet is probably more important in the treatment of renal osteodystrophy than in any other skeletal disease, with the exception of nutritional osteomalacia. Restriction of dietary phosphate intake, as renal function declines, prevents the development of both secondary hyperparathyroidism and soft tissue calcification. Daily calcium intake should be maintained at 1 gram and is best accomplished by supplementing the diet with calcium carbonate. This form of calcium supplement has an advantage over other forms of calcium salts (e.g., calcium lactate or gluconate), since it provides more elemental calcium per gram of salt (thus reducing the number of tablets per day) and binds phosphate in the intestine, thereby helping maintain a more normal plasma phosphate. Calcium carbonate is not, however, an effective phosphate binding agent, and most patients require aluminum hydroxide in addition to dietary phosphate restriction and calcium carbonate supplementation.

If the primary objectives of treatment are correction of symptomatic hypocalcemia and suppression of secondary hyperparathyroidism, the aforementioned maneuvers alone may be quite effective. Symptomatic bone disease such as osteomalacia, on the other hand, often requires therapy with ergocalciferol or its analogues or metabolites. In large doses (usually 2.5 mg per day or higher), ergocalciferol causes significant healing of osteomalacia in most patients. It is usual to start with 0.5 mg daily and increase the dose until there is a symptomatic improvement. Plasma calcium increases as ergocalciferol begins to take effect, and plasma alkaline phosphatase level usually rises (the alkaline phosphatase flare) as bone healing occurs. The dose of ergocalciferol should be titrated according to the biochemical response to avoid hypercalcemia.

Crystalline dihydrotachysterol (DHT), an analogue of ergocalciferol, offers some theoretic advantages. First, it does not require renal 1-hydroxylation to be effective; second, onset and offset of action are shorter than those of ergocalciferol; and third, if hypercalcemia develops during therapy, discontinuation of DHT is quickly followed by return of plasma calcium to normal level. The usual dose of DHT is 0.25 to 0.75 mg per day.

The newer metabolites of calciferol, 25-HCC, 1,25-DHCC, and 1α-HCC, have been somewhat disappointing in clinical trials with respect to treatment of the osteomalacic component of renal osteodystrophy. They have, however, been shown to be of great benefit in suppressing secondary hyperparathyroidism. 1,25-DHCC (calcitriol, Rocaltrol) has been approved specifically for use in patients on maintenance hemodialysis who have persistent hypocalcemia. (In all other circumstances this compound must still be considered an experimental drug.) The recommended starting dose is 0.5 to 1 microgram per day, reducing to a maintenance dose of 0.25 microgram as the plasma calcium level rises to normal and the plasma alkaline phosphatase level falls (see also dosage in the manufacturer's package insert). It has not yet been determined how long patients should be maintained on this dose of 0.25 microgram per day, but current evidence indicates that there are no long-term deleterious effects from this drug provided that hypercalcemia is avoided. The doses of 25-HCC that have been used in most clinical trials have been from

50 to 100 micrograms per day, but an occasional patient has required 150 micrograms per day before a significant rise in plasma calcium is observed. The dose of 1-hydroxycholecalciferol used in clinical trials has been 1 to 2 micrograms per day, but there is no convincing evidence that this compound has any advantages over 1,25-DHCC.

The ideal and probably the best treatment for renal osteodystrophy is unquestionably renal transplantation, which restores normal renal function. There are, however, certain skeletal complications peculiar to the post-transplant state. Immediately following renal transplantation, plasma calcium rises, occasionally to hypercalcemic levels. This is usually a transient phenomenon that reverts spontaneously over a period of a few weeks or months. Persistence of hypercalcemia beyond 6 to 8 months may necessitate subtotal parathyroidectomy. Hypophosphatemic osteomalacia may be an occasional skeletal complication of renal transplantation. This is due to an acquired renal tubular defect in phosphate reabsorption in the transplanted kidney. Supplemental phosphate is all that is required to correct the skeletal lesion.

SCURVY AND VITAMIN C DEFICIENCY

method of
WILLIAM B. BEAN, M.D.
Iowa City, Iowa

Clinical scurvy follows prolonged reduction in the intake of vitamin C and the depletion of body stores. In experimental scurvy, blood levels of vitamin C decline rapidly. Nucleated cells, particularly platelets, retain it longer than plasma, but ultimately it disappears. Chemical depletion exists for some time before clinical scurvy appears. Symptoms and signs come unpredictably and sometimes with explosive violence.

Prevention. Citrus fruits and tomatoes are the best source of vitamin C, but there is enough in many foods to provide ample safety. Ripe uncooked fruits and vegetables have more than stored or cooked items. Vegetables are not very rich but because they are used in bulk are a significant source of ascorbic acid.

Occurrence. Although scurvy may develop whenever the diet is low in vitamin C, it had become rare in North America well before the megavitamin C Goliaths went out to do battle ineffectually with the clinically more experienced Davids. Scurvy occurs sporadically, particularly in elderly bachelors, widows, or widowers usually living alone, in food faddists, and in those who abuse drugs or alcohol, as well as in the very poor, the rejected and neglected. Many forms of malnutrition occur in such persons.

Requirements. Plasma ascorbic acid levels below 0.2 mg per 100 ml suggest at least recent ascorbic acid deprivation. In patients with such levels any intercurrent disease or conditions requiring an operation have a much worse outlook than in those with normal vitamin C levels, unless the depletion is promptly corrected. Recommended daily allowances of vitamin C are 35 mg for infants, 40 mg for children up to 4 years of age, 45 mg for adults, 60 mg for pregnant women, and 80 mg for women during lactation. Water-soluble vitamins are needed in increased amounts when their loss is increased, their absorption is diminished, or there are excess metabolic needs.

Decreased Absorption. Severe or chronic diarrheas may result in reduced absorption of ascorbic acid because of the rapid transit; and sometimes it falls after jejunoileal bypass operations or those which eliminate much of the small intestine.

Peptic Ulcer. When large amounts of antacids are taken, the ascorbic acid in food may be destroyed. Those troubled with hyperacidity are likely to avoid citrus fruits and juices, tomatoes, and other good sources of vitamin C. When pernicious anemia or other forms of anacidity exist, alkaline digestive juices from small bowel, pancreas, or liver may destroy most of the ingested ascorbic acid. Smokers may have chronically low levels, perhaps because the bioavailability is diminished when that in the gut is pre-empted for the biosynthesis of serotonin, which is stimulated by nicotine.

Increased Utilization. Thyroid overactivity, pregnancy and lactation, sustained fevers, and exposure to extremes of heat and cold may be associated with increased metabolic needs. Infection, inflammation, and injury are associated with an increased requirement of vitamin C, which is particularly important in wound healing and repair.

Hemodialysis. Since vitamin C is lost in hemodialysis, its replacement is mandatory.

Drugs. Long-term use of aspirin is followed by reduction of ascorbic acid in plasma and buffy coat. Indomethacin and related agents may have similar effects. Phenytoin-like drugs lower plasma vitamin C levels.

Poisonings. Large doses of ascorbic acid have been used with apparent success in carbon monoxide poisoning, in cadmium poisoning, and in the nephrotoxic state produced by tetracyclines, although controlled studies are rare. It has also been claimed to increase the tolerance of arsenicals, inhalation anesthetics, muscle relaxants, and mercurial diuretics. All currently available parenteral tetracyclines contain significant amounts of ascorbic acid.

Stress. It is not yet clear whether stress is a regular stimulus to increase vitamin C requirements, but occasional examples have been reported.

Toxicity. Large doses of ascorbic acid may reduce the prothrombin time of patients being treated with warfarin sodium. In dogs and rats heparin and ascorbic acid are reported to be antagonistic. Ascorbic acid itself is one of the most bland and least toxic of chemicals. Doses of several grams a day have been used to acidify the urine.

Colds. There is no increase in the frequency of colds or viral infections in victims of scurvy. Megadoses of vitamin C have been claimed to reduce some of the symptoms of colds but not to shorten their duration or prevent their occurrence.

Bleeding Gums. Most gums which bleed do so from irritation of food or trauma, perhaps through overaggressive cleaning. In scurvy the gums are spongy and bleed around the teeth. If the mouth is edentulous, the gums do not bleed even in advanced scurvy. In anyone whose bleeding persists, gingivitis should be attended to, and a trial of 200 mg of vitamin C a day might be used for a few days or a week. Any other vitamin deficiency should be treated appropriately.

Treatment of Scurvy. When scurvy is diagnosed, 1 gram of ascorbic acid should be given quickly by intravenous injection. One gram a day should be given orally as soon as the patient can swallow comfortably and continued for several days. Strict bed rest is needed until the deficiency has been corrected. There is usually a remarkable improvement and a surge of returning health, although patients must be warned not to overdo. Any patient who has had severe malnutrition is a poor risk for operations; if an elective operation is planned, the patient should be built up with all the necessary food elements and vitamins.

Maintenance Therapy. Unless there is some form of obligatory malabsorption, oral therapy is necessary when one is dealing with a state that requires increased amounts. An effort should be made to keep the plasma ascorbic

TABLE 1.

	DAILY DOSE
Increased metabolism or work	
Hyperthyroidism	100–200 mg
Pregnancy or lactation	100 mg
Exposure to extreme temperatures	100 mg
Decrease absorption	
Chronic peptic ulcer	100 mg
Pernicious anemia or other gastric anacidity	100 mg
Diarrheas, severe	100–200 mg
Acute and chronic inflammation and infection	
Tuberculosis	100–200 mg
Burns, severe	200–500 mg
Ulcerative colitis	200–400 mg
Urinary infection, severe	200 mg
Wounds, granulating, chronic	100–200 mg
Postoperative convalescence, uncomplicated	100 mg

acid at a level of at least 0.4 mg per 100 ml. A rough rule of thumb for oral therapy in several disorders is given in Table 1.

Diet. The ultimate objective is to have the patient eat adequate amounts of ascorbic acid in the diet. This is provided by approximately 5 oz (150 ml) of orange juice or grapefruit juice, either fresh or canned, since synthetic vitamin C has been added to many canned juices. Foods with high vitamin C content include oranges, lemons, limes, peppers, grapefruit, tomatoes, strawberries, cranberries, currants, potatoes, and many green vegetables. Heat and alkalis destroy ascorbic acid.

VITAMIN K DEFICIENCY

method of
ROBERT CHILCOTE, M.D.
Chicago, Illinois

Vitamin K (from Danish word Koagulation) is a fat-soluble vitamin that has no appreciable storage pool in the body. A constant supply is required for the synthesis of the coagulation factors II (prothrombin), VII, IX, and X. Alterations in gastrointestinal fat absorption, motility, and bacterial flora may have significant effects on vitamin K absorption. Leafy green vegetables supply the principal dietary source of vitamin K (vitamin K_1). A supply of vitamin K_2 is also available from the metabolism of bacterial flora within the large bowel. The vitamin K-dependent coagulation factors are all trace proteins in the plasma. They achieve high local concentrations near damaged vessels by becoming bound at calcium-dependent membrane binding sites. So anchored, they participate in the cascade of coagulation reactions that result in a firm fibrin clot. Vitamin K helps carboxylate the terminal glutamic acid residues in the precursors of factors II, VII, IX, and X. The resulting gamma carboxyglutamic acid residues determine the binding sites and convert the precursors into their physiologically active counterparts. In vitamin K deficiency, precursors to factors II, VII, IX, and X are present in adequate concentrations but are physiologically inactive. These nonfunctional precursors are rapidly converted to their normal configurations by the administration of vitamin K, and correction of the hemorrhagic tendency is dramatic. There are no other known clinical effects from vitamin K deficiency.

When vitamin K deficiency is suspected, blood for determinations of prothrombin time and partial thromboplastin time is drawn and vitamin K_1 (AquaMephyton, Konakion), 10 mg, is administered intramuscularly or subcutaneously with a 25-gauge needle. In patients with poor tissue perfusion owing to shock, the intravenous route may be preferred. Vitamin K_1 does not cause hemolysis in glucose-6-phosphate dehydrogenase (G6PD) deficiency. Aspirin, or products that contain aspirin, should not be given to any patient with a hemorrhagic tendency. In vitamin K deficiency, aspirin may exacerbate the bleeding tendency by competitive inhibition of available vitamin K and decreasing platelet function. Four to 8 hours after administration, repeat prothrombin time and partial thromboplastin time are determined. If hemorrhage persists, the dose is not repeated and other causes for bleeding are sought. However, in those patients with vitamin K deficiency, oral prophylaxis with 1 mg daily or parenteral administration every 4 days in hospitalized patients is indicated. In many clinical situations, increased consumption of coagulation factors caused by the various categories of disseminated intravascular coagulation may coexist with decreased synthesis. This may result in a complicated laboratory coagulation profile. In these situations, it is useful to determine factors V (synthesized by the liver but not vitamin K dependent), VII, and VIII, fibrinogen, fibrin split products, and platelet levels. These determinations are repeated several hours after vitamin K is administered and adequate tissue perfusion is restored. Changes in the levels can help assess the relative contributions of vitamin K deficiency, liver disease, and disseminated intravascular coagulation to persisting hemorrhagic phenomena.

There is no faster way to correct a vitamin K deficiency coagulation problem than by parenteral administration of vitamin K. It takes less time for the vitamin K-deficient patient to synthesize coagulation factors after the administration of vitamin K than it takes to obtain and infuse type-specific fresh frozen plasma.

Vitamin K in Neonates

The normal neonate receives vitamin K from transplacental passage. Hepatic immaturity, particularly in premature infants, can lower the levels of factors II, VII, IX, and X. In general, however, at birth the levels are adequate to assure hemostasis.

Vitamin K-dependent factor levels normally fall in the first few days of neonatal life until vitamin K is obtained from endogenous flora and the diet becomes adequate to assure continuing synthesis. Formulas are supplemented with vitamin K_1, but the breast-fed infant has less endogenous bacterial production of vitamin K_2 as well as a decreased dietary intake.

Vitamin K_1, 0.5 to 1.0 mg (AquaMephyton, Konakion) should be administered to all newborns. The traditional dose of 1 mg (1000 micrograms) far exceeds the physiologic requirement but is safe. The omission of vitamin K can result in catastrophic hemorrhage.

Infants who are exclusively breast fed or poorly nourished patients of any age with, for example, severe congenital heart disease, neoplasia, or chronic diarrhea should receive 1 mg of vitamin K_1 before any surgical procedure.

Coagulation Disturbances in Infants of Mothers Who Take Medicines with Anticoagulant Properties

Severe hemorrhagic tendency resulting from vitamin K deficiency is seen in infants born to mothers with seizure disorders who have taken hydantoins or barbiturates. In contrast to the usual hemorrhagic disease of the newborn seen on the second or third day of life, hemorrhage in these infants may take place at birth. Although the mothers of these infants have normal coagulation values, fetal vitamin K-dependent factors are depressed. Hydantoins and barbiturates cross the placenta and competitively inhibit vitamin K action similarly to the action of warfarin. Since the drugs are metabolized more slowly by the immature fetal liver than by the maternal liver, higher levels are attained within the fetus.

These mothers should be instructed not to take aspirin during pregnancy and should receive 10 mg of vitamin K_1 intramuscularly during early labor. The infant should receive vitamin K_1 immediately after birth (1 mg). If severe hemorrhage is present, administer 10 ml per kg of fresh frozen plasma. Alternatively, prothrombin complex concentrates (Konyne or Proplex) may be administered. Currently available preparations may cause hepatitis.

Coagulation Disturbances in Liver Disease

Hepatic cell dysfunction causes decreased synthesis of vitamin K-dependent coagulation factors. Intrahepatic cholestasis may lessen fat absorption and decrease absorption of vitamin K. In uncomplicated hepatitis, administration of vitamin K is not required. In patients with severe hepatitis and hemorrhage, coexistent thrombocytopenia may complicate the picture; vitamin K_1 and platelets should be given. Fresh frozen plasma (10 ml per kg) may supply sufficient coagulation factors to bring the levels above the usual 20 or 25 per cent of normal seen in patients who have a clinical hemorrhagic tendency. The prothrombin complex concentrates have been noted to cause sudden death from pulmonary emboli in patients with severe liver disease. Apparently, some preparations of prothrombin complex contain activated factors that are ordinarily cleared by a healthy reticuloendothelial system. In severe liver disease, however, these activated coagulation factors may precipitate intravascular thrombosis.

Malabsorption Syndromes

Short bowel syndrome, pancreatic cancer, biliary atresia, idiopathic cholestasis, cystic fibrosis, gluten enteropathy, and sprue may cause vitamin K deficiency. Patients with these conditions should receive oral prophylactic water-soluble vitamin K_3, as either a sodium disulfate or a sodium diphosphate salt (Hykinone, Synkayvite). An adequate prophylactic dose is 5 mg by mouth once a day. For hemorrhagic symptoms, intramuscular vitamin K_1 (1 mg for an infant to 10 mg for an adult) should be administered.

Infants with severe and protracted diarrhea may develop malabsorption and coagulation abnormalities. Bacterial flora is suppressed by antibiotic therapy, and endogenous vitamin K_2 synthesis may also decrease. Although these coagulation abnormalities remit as the diarrhea clears, severe hemorrhagic phenomena have developed in a few of these children. Therefore, it is prudent to administer vitamin K_1 (1 mg) every 4 to 7 days after the first week of illness. Most special formulas now contain vitamin K_1. Infants who are on intravenous hyperalimentation programs may develop hemorrhagic disease if vitamin K_1 supplementation is not given (1 mg every 7 days). Alternatively, 0.1 mg of vitamin K per 100 ml of intravenous fluid can be administered.

Marginal Vitamin K Deficiency

Dietary deficiency may be present but a relative hemorrhagic tendency may not appear until after a major surgical procedure has been done. In older patients, in patients with chronic renal failure, in patients chronically taking antibiotics, and in patients with cancer it is reasonable to give 10 mg of vitamin K preoperatively. This appears to be a more reasonable procedure than performing diagnostic factor assays preoperatively or waiting for a postoperative hemorrhagic event.

OSTEOPOROSIS

method of
CHARLES H. CHESNUT III, M.D.,
Seattle, Washington
and HELEN E. GRUBER, Ph.D.
Tacoma, Washington

Definition

The underlying clinical problem in osteoporosis is a deficiency of bone mass, or skeletal osteopenia, resulting in fractures of the spine, distal radius and ulna, and femoral neck. While bone mass is reduced in osteoporosis, current research data suggest that the bone that is present is essentially normal.

Pathogenesis

Significant osteopenia may be associated with numerous diseases (e.g., Cushing's disease, rheumatoid arthritis, thyrotoxicosis) and medications (e.g., adrenocorticosteroids, heparin), but it presents most frequently as postmenopausal osteoporosis in the elderly female; perhaps 25 to 30 per cent of all Caucasian females will experience an osteoporosis-related fracture by age 65. Although numerous factors contribute to the development of osteoporosis (e.g., age, estrogen deficiency, diet, racial factors in postmenopausal osteoporosis; steroid excess in Cushing's disease), the basic abnormality in all forms of osteopenia is some disturbance of the normal bone remodeling sequence.

Therefore, to understand the pathogenesis of osteoporosis (and also to understand its treatment), some knowledge of bone remodeling is necessary. Bone is constantly turning over, with the initial event an increase in bone resorption mediated by the osteoclast and (to a lesser extent) the osteocyte. This event is generally followed by an increase in bone formation mediated by the osteoblast. The processes of bone resorption and bone formation are normally (perhaps homeostatically) "coupled": an increase or decrease in bone resorption produces a corresponding increase or decrease in bone formation, such that the net change in bone mass is zero. In postmenopausal osteoporosis, however, bone resorption is thought to be increased over normal bone remodeling levels, without a corresponding increase in bone formation, leading to a net loss in bone mass. Bone remodeling is "negatively uncoupled." In other forms of osteoporosis an increase in bone resorption is usually the principal bone remodeling abnormality, although a primary decrease in bone formation may occur (such as in the glucocorticoid excess of Cushing's disease).

Rationale for Therapy

While osteoporosis associated with other disease processes may be improved by treatment of the underlying disease (i.e., alleviation of the hyperthyroid state in the thyrotoxic individual), the ideal goal of treatment in any form of osteopenia should be either preventive or restorative, depending upon the patient's bone mass and history of fracture. (1) For instance, in menopausal and postmenopausal females with relatively normal bone mass and no previous fractures, the goal of therapy should be the prevention of an osteopenic state sufficient to cause fracture. Attainment of the goal involves a slowing of the bone loss that normally occurs in the aging per-

son. (2) On the other hand, in menopausal and postmenopausal females with a relatively low bone mass and previous fractures, treatment should be directed at restoration of bone mass to a level at which fracture risk is substantially reduced. Achieving this goal involves a slowing of age-related bone loss as well as replacement of bone previously lost.

In terms of bone remodeling, prevention and restoration may obviously be accomplished by two therapeutic maneuvers: (1) a decrease in bone resorption and/or (2) an increase in bone formation. To prevent osteopenia, a decrease in bone resorption may suffice if bone formation is maintained at a normal level. However, the restoration of bone mass ideally requires a decrease in bone resorption as well as an increase in bone formation; an increase in bone resorption with a greater increase in bone formation, or a decrease in bone resorption with a lesser decrease in bone formation, also results in the desired net positive bone mass change. In other words, these therapeutic maneuvers attempt to "uncouple" ("positive uncoupling") the normal coupling mechanism of bone remodeling.

As will be seen, a number of therapeutic agents can slow the loss of bone mass, probably by decreasing bone resorption. To date, however, few agents appear capable of restoring previously lost bone mass and preventing further fractures. In addition, little definitive information is available confirming the efficacy of various therapies in preventing significant osteopenia development in the pre-, peri-, or postmenopausal female.

Specific Therapy

In our laboratory a program of combination therapy for the osteoporotic individual is utilized, as noted in Table 1 (items 1 to 4).

TABLE 1. **Therapeutic Agents for the Treatment of Postmenopausal Osteoporosis**

AGENT	DOSAGE	COMPLICATIONS
1. Calcium carbonate	600 mg PO b.i.d.	Increased urinary calcium
2. Vitamin D_2 (in multivitamin form)	400 IU PO q.d.	—
3. Anabolic steroid:		
Methandrostenolone (Dianabol) or	2.5–5.0 mg PO q.d. cycled 3–4 weeks ⎫	Abnormal liver function tests, fluid
Stanozolol (Winstrol)	2–6 mg PO q.d. cycled 3–4 weeks ⎬	retention, masculinizing effects
4. Exercise		Tiredness
Other:		
5. Estrogen (Premarin)	0.3 mg PO q.d. cycled 3–4 weeks	Endometrial carcinoma, uterine bleeding, ? gallbladder disease
		Fluid retention
6. Sodium fluoride*	22–44 mg PO q.d.	Gastric irritation, tendinitis
7. Synthetic salmon calcitonin* (Calcimar)	100 MRC units SC or IM q.d.	Allergic skin reaction at site of injection
8. Dichloro-MDP (clodronate disodium)*	Exact dosage not yet defined	Possible diarrhea

*Experimental; usage in osteoporosis not currently approved by the Food and Drug Administration.

Calcium. The pre-, peri-, and postmenopausal female should probably consume at least 1000 mg of elemental calcium daily in the form of dietary calcium and/or oral calcium supplements (the latter particularly in those persons with milk intolerance). We usually administer 600 mg of calcium carbonate twice daily to supplement our patients' dietary calcium. Excessive calcium intake can be monitored with 24 hour urinary calcium determinations; in our experience urinary calcium excretion of up to 250 mg per 24 hours is acceptable (without risk of renal lithiasis).

Calcium appears to be of short-term benefit (probably by decreasing bone mass loss by decreasing bone resorption), but its potential long-term value is unproved. It appears unlikely that oral calcium alone can restore previously lost bone mass; its value in preventing the development of significant osteopenia is currently under investigation. In our opinion, however, adequate calcium intake should be mandatory in any osteoporosis combination treatment program.

Vitamin D. A multivitamin with 400 IU of vitamin D appears to be a quite reasonable program inclusion, primarily in treating a mild D deficiency that may exist in many elderly osteoporotic females. There is little evidence at this time to indicate a beneficial effect of vitamin D and its various congeners (25-hydroxycholecalciferol, 1,25-dihydroxycholecalciferol, and 24,25-dihydroxycholecalciferol) in the treatment of postmenopausal osteoporosis, although it may be of value in the treatment of steroid-induced osteopenia (see below).

Anabolic Steroids. In our laboratory the anabolic steroids are the cornerstone of our osteoporosis combination therapy; these modified male hormones are administered in a dosage of 2 to 6 mg daily of stanozolol (Winstrol), or 2.5 to 5 mg daily of methandrostenolone (Dianabol), for 21 of every 28 days. Methandrostenolone produces fewer side effects than does stanozolol, although it also appears somewhat less potent than stanozolol in its beneficial effect upon bone. Elevations of hepatic enzymes, fluid retention, and androgenic effects (hirsutism, acne, hoarseness) appear to be dose related; most side effects appear transient and are improved with reduction or discontinuation of dosage. A serum glutamic-oxaloacetic transaminase (SGOT) value should be obtained at 6 month intervals, and dosage manipulated accordingly.

The anabolic steroids exhibit definite long-term (27 months in our experience) benefit in slowing the loss of bone (probably by decreasing both bone resorption and urinary calcium) and in increasing bone mass above pretreatment levels (a 4.2 per cent increase in total bone mass was noted in our studies with stanozolol, as well as a decrease in spinal compression fracture occurrence). It appears quite likely that the anabolic steroids can prevent bone mass loss and (to a limited extent) replace bone previously lost. However, the clinician using these agents in osteoporosis should be fully cognizant of their potential side effects, and should balance the need for an apparently effective agent against the possibility of less desirous drug actions.

Exercise. A reasonable exercise program (walking and swimming are of particular value and safety in the elderly female) should be an integral part of any osteoporosis treatment protocol; exercise is done up to and slightly beyond the point of bone pain, although it is frequently important to reduce exercise in the patient with an acute fracture. Exercise may decrease bone mass loss by increasing bone formation to a greater extent than it increases bone resorption.

Our designation of individual patients for components of our treatment protocol is as follows: In patients with essentially normal bone mass (as established by radial bone mass measurements by photon absorptiometry techniques) and/or without fractures, but at high risk for the development of significant osteopenia (familial, racial, dietary, or medical predispositions) — calcium supplements, vitamin D in multivitamin form, exercise, and close follow-up (clinical evaluation and bone mass measurements if available) at 6 to 12 month intervals. In patients with low bone mass and fractures — calcium supplements, vitamin D, anabolic steroids, and exercise.

Should the aforementioned therapeutic regimen prove not to be of benefit (as determined by decreasing bone mass and the occurrence of new fractures) within a reasonable period of time (6 to 12 months), additional agents as noted in Table 1 (items 5 to 8) may be added to the program.

Estrogens. Estrogen preparations may be utilized in combination therapy. Owing to the potential development of endometrial carcinoma, 0.3 mg per day of conjugated estrogen (Premarin) should be prescribed as the minimal replacement dose in unhysterectomized individuals.

Estrogens appear to act by decreasing bone resorption (perhaps by decreasing bone responsiveness to parathyroid hormone), and consequently by slowing (and possibly preventing) bone mass loss; there is essentially no evidence that estrogens can significantly replace bone mass previously lost. Indeed, despite the widespread use of these preparations in the past for the treatment of postmenopausal osteoporosis, few controlled studies exist definitively establishing their efficacy.

Fluoride. Sodium fluoride in a dosage of 22 to 44 mg per day may also be utilized in multiple drug regimens; calcium supplements are usually administered concomitantly. As noted in Table 1, certain side effects may be noted with fluoride ingestion. Also, it should be noted that use of fluoride in osteoporosis is experimental; fluoride is not currently approved by the Food and Drug Administration for osteoporosis therapy.

Of the various therapeutic modalities available for osteoporosis, fluoride alone appears to directly increase bone formation; theoretically, it would therefore not only slow bone mass loss but also restore bone mass previously lost. However, concern has arisen regarding the structural integrity of the bone produced by the patient while on fluoride therapy; recent data have suggested an increased fracture incidence following long-term fluoride treatment, possibly because of the formation of fluorapatite (rather than hydroxy-apatite) bone crystal. Whether inclusion of fluoride in a combination therapy protocol circumvents this difficulty is unproved; its use in such programs remains empirical.

Calcitonin. Synthetic salmon calcitonin, one of the experimental modalities for osteoporosis currently under evaluation in our own and other laboratories, is one of the few agents that has been shown to increase total body calcium, and it is the least noxious. It is an anti-bone resorber with proved efficacy in Paget's disease and potential benefit in osteoporosis. Apart from the disadvantage of injection and the possibility of allergic skin reaction at the injection site, calcitonin is a safe medication with few side effects, and may prove extremely efficacious in preventing the development of an osteopenic state.

Diphosphonates. The diphosphonate dichloro-MDP (clodronate disodium) is another experimental modality which we are currently evaluating. Although not yet well tested, diphosphonates have proved value in Paget's disease; they also act by decreasing bone resorption (although probably by a mechanism different from that of calcitonin) and thereby slow bone mass loss. Prolonged clinical use studies are still in preliminary stages but offer promise that, aside from the possible side effect of diarrhea, diphosphonates may prove an effective clinical way to block bone resorption.

Secondary Osteoporoses

Unfortunately, few studies are available assessing the value of these and other therapies in preventing and treating the osteopenia associated with other disease processes; ostensibly such combination treatment programs would be of value. As noted previously, the primary aim in such situations remains discontinuation of the osteopenia-producing agents (e.g., corticosteroids, heparin) or treatment of the underlying pathologic process (e.g., hyperthyroidism). In corticosteroid-induced osteopenia there are data suggesting a decrease in bone mass loss with a regimen of 50,000 IU of vitamin D (available in capsule form as Drisdol) orally weekly for 12 weeks, plus calcium carbonate supplements, 600 mg orally twice daily; 24 hour urinary calcium should be monitored at 1 to 2 month intervals for significant hypercalciuria. Fluoride, 22 to 44 mg orally daily, may also be added to the regimen, although definitive data establishing its efficacy in this clinical situation are lacking.

In conclusion, it would appear that the major beneficial effect of most of the currently available therapeutic agents is in decreasing loss of bone mass. Furthermore, even with those agents that may increase bone mass, the observed increase may be insufficient to improve bone strength substantially or, in the elderly osteoporotic female, to replete skeletal mass fully within the expected life span. Nevertheless, osteoporosis may be an extremely morbid and incapacitating disease; any decrease in bone mass loss or increase in total bone mass will be of benefit. In addition, it should be noted that the prophylactic potential of these medications (either singly or in combination) has not been defined, but may be quite substantial. Overall, it would appear that osteoporosis is now a treatable disease, and in the future it may be a preventable disease as well.

PARENTERAL FLUID AND ELECTROLYTE THERAPY IN ADULTS

method of
HARRY F. WEISBERG, M.D.
Milwaukee, Wisconsin

Parenteral fluid therapy requires some knowledge of the physiology and pathology of body water, electrolyte, and acid-base balance. Parenteral fluid therapy must be directed to the administration of the daily *basic* requirements for water, electrolytes, calories, vitamins, and protein (nitrogen). In addition, *continued* losses and prior *deficits* must be replaced. The patient receiving parenteral fluid therapy must be re-evaluated as often as necessary and changes made in the prescribed fluids as indicated by his condition.

GENERAL CONSIDERATIONS

Body Water

The total body water was described by Gamble to be 70 per cent of the body weight expressed in kilograms* (50 per cent intracellular and 20 per cent extracellular). Present values (and ranges) for total body water in adult males and females, respectively, are 60 (50 to 71) and 50 (40 to 60) per cent of the body weight. Body water content is inversely related to body fat content. Values (and ranges) for fat content in adult men are 18 (4 to 32) per cent and 32 (18 to 42) per cent of the body weight in adult women. The plasma volume (intravascular fluid) is the same in adults — about 4.5 per cent (total blood volume differs because of the difference in red cell mass) — and the interstitial and lymphatic fluid compartment (12 per cent) is similar in men and women. From these values, the average intracellular water would be 43 and 33 per cent of body weight for man and woman, respectively. More recent studies (on males) have revealed three additional components of the extracellular fluid — connective tissue–cartilage (4.5 per cent), bone (4.5 per cent), and transcellular (1.5 per cent) fluid compartments. Thus, the "correct" average values for the intra- and extra-cellular fluid compartments, respectively, are 33 and 27 per cent for men and 23 and 27 per cent for women.

Administration of Parenteral Solutions

The *enteral* administration of water and electrolytes is preferred. In many instances, a patient with mild dehydration can be encouraged to drink a water or electrolyte prescription (e.g., meat broth). Elemental diets consisting of solutions of carbohydrates, electrolytes (and trace minerals), pure amino acids, and vitamins (but no fat) are readily absorbed from the gastrointestinal

---

*The weight in pounds can be converted to kilograms by a simple mental calculation. Divide pounds by 2; 10 per cent of this quotient is subtracted from the quotient to obtain the weight in kilograms. For example, a 180 pound patient weighs 81 kg; 180 divided by 2 equals 90, and 10 per cent of 90 is 9, which is subtracted from the 90 to give 81 kg.

tract and may be taken *orally* or via a transnasal gastric tube. *Rectal* administration may also be utilized (especially in nursing home situations where intravenous fluids are not easily administered); a slow drip of 5 per cent dextrose in isotonic saline may obviate the admission of a patient to a hospital.

Parenteral fluids are usually administered subcutaneously or intravenously. The use of hyaluronidase preparations has been advocated to alleviate the problems associated with *subcutaneous* fluid therapy. Hyaluronidase will hasten the absorption of subcutaneously injected *isotonic saline* only. Hyaluronidase will cause the spreading out of other solutions but *does not hasten their absorption*. Hypertonic solutions should *not* be administered by hypodermoclysis because of the danger of sloughing and infection. Oliguria, anuria, and circulatory collapse may result from the subcutaneous administration of nonelectrolyte solutions, especially in patients with incipient shock, dehydration, or salt deficiency. It is best *not* to utilize the subcutaneous route.

The *intravenous* route should be reserved for the patient with severe dehydration, acid-base imbalance, and so forth. The rate of administration of the fluids should vary with the patient's condition; a slower rate can adequately combat moderate dehydration, but rapid intravenous administration may be necessary in severe depletion, especially if peripheral circulatory failure is present. Water and electrolytes are retained better when given over long periods in contrast to short intervals. This will avoid a sudden loading of the cardiovascular system and subsequent long periods without any intake of water and electrolytes. Fluids are best started in the morning so that the administration can be maintained during the day and their effect on the patient observed. The use of an indwelling polyethylene catheter, or plastic needle, will permit prolonged intravenous therapy for several days (with proper aseptic technique and precautions) without the necessity for repeated venipunctures.

The use of Y tube infusion sets available commercially is of benefit in allowing the physician to administer two "compatible" solutions at the same time (or at alternate intervals, e.g., fat emulsions should not be mixed with other solutions) and thus to be able to "mix" them without actually mixing the contents of the two bottles. For TPN or "total parenteral nutrition" (a better term than "hyperalimentation"), in-line filters have been used to screen out bacteria and particulate matter. Filters with pore size less than 0.22 micron require the use of a peristaltic pump.

Calculation of Rate of Administration of Parenteral Fluids. The physician must prescribe the *rate* at which the parenteral fluids should be administered to the patient. Administration sets vary in size of drop issuing into the drop chamber (the "size" of the needle inserted into the vein is not relevant). Administration sets from various manufacturers do not necessarily conform to the US Pharmacopaeia definition of 20 drops to the milliliter (for aqueous solutions) but vary from 10 to 20 and 50 to 60 drops for regular and "pediatric" sets, respectively. Sets supplied for the administration of blood or plasma products range from 10 to 15 drops per ml. If the physician knows the number of drops contained in 1 ml (usually printed on the container), the use of Formula 1 allows the calculation of the *number of drops per minute* to be written on the order sheet (see bottom of this page). I have therefore devised a simple pocket calculator which requires only one setting for this "difficult" calculation.*

Many hospitals have special peristaltic pumps to regulate the rate of flow of parenteral solutions (or enteral feedings); these are usually set at ml per minute or ml per hour. However, most patients receiving parenteral fluids do not have a pump available; thus the ability to "calculate" the proper rate of administration is very valuable.

Types of Intravenous Solutions

Carbohydrate and Water Solutions. *Isotonic* solutions have the same osmotic pressure as the body fluids and will neither increase nor decrease the size of the red blood cells in a test tube. Carbohydrates added to water serve to make the solution isotonic and, by providing calories, to institute a series of measures that overcome abnormal metabolic reactions.

The administration of carbohydrate solutions serves several purposes: (1) It spares the loss of extracellular electrolytes, e.g., sodium. (2) It conserves the intracellular electrolytes, e.g., potassium. (3) It spares the excess loss of nitrogen caused by breakdown of tissue protoplasm. Maximal nitrogen sparing requires about 750 (nonprotein) kcal per day, equivalent to 200 grams of invert sugar or fructose or to 220 grams of dextrose ("hydrated"). (4) It provides a source of calories (although not sufficient for the daily total) required for the daily metabolic needs,

*Distributed free of charge through the courtesy of Travenol Laboratories, Inc., Morton Grove, Illinois 60053, as MINISLIDE.

especially for protein synthesis. (5) It prevents or stops the production by the liver of excess ketone bodies owing to depletion of the liver glycogen. Our studies in animals reveal that invert sugar (dextrose plus fructose) is best for repletion of liver glycogen. (6) Water per se and water from the oxidation of the carbohydrate supply the body needs for insensible perspiration and urine output. (7) It spares the loss of intracellular water. (8) It decreases the amount of water necessary for kidney excretion by presenting a decreased load of ketone bodies, nitrogenous products, electrolytes, and other solutes that must be excreted by the kidneys.

Plasma osmolality ranges from 270 to 300 mosmol per kg of plasma water.* The average isotonic glucose (dextrose) solution is 5.5 per cent (range 4.8 to 5.9), and the average isotonic saline solution is 0.9 per cent (range 0.79 to 0.96). The US Pharmacopaeia requires a parenteral solution with dextrose as the only carbohydrate to be in the form of the monohydrate ($C_6H_{12}O_6 \cdot H_2O$), so that the 5 per cent solution really contains only 4.5 per cent sugar (equivalent to about 250 mosmol per liter). However, sugar solutions containing dextrose and fructose (invert sugar) do not contain the hydrated form of dextrose. A 5.5 per cent dextrose (anhydrous, USP) solution has the same "tonicity" as the 0.9 per cent saline solution (about 310 mosmol per liter).

Many physicians are fearful of using 10 per cent carbohydrate solution as a medium for the administration of water and calories because it is "hypertonic" and therefore may result in diuresis. Many of these same physicians usually do not consider "5 per cent glucose in isotonic saline" to be hypertonic or to have any diuretic effect; yet this solution has more osmotic pull (588 mosmol per liter) than the 10 per cent dextrose solution (500 mosmol per liter). Hexoses do have an "osmotic diuretic" effect when administered as the 1 molar solution (1000 mosmol per liter) equal to 18 per cent, or greater concentrations.

Actually, hypotonic and hypertonic solutions *may* be administered intravenously provided that the infusion rate is *slow* enough to allow for

*The correct terminology for expressing the "osmotic" concentration of a solution is *"osmols per kilogram of solvent."* In medicine the solute concentration is so dilute (milliosmols) and body temperature so relatively constant that the terms mosmol per liter of solution (plasma or urine) ("osmolar") and mosmol per kg of solvent (water)("osmolal") can be used interchangeably without any significant "error."

$$\text{Drops/minute} = \frac{\text{Drops/ml} \times \text{total volume to be infused (ml)}}{60 \text{ minutes/hour} \times \text{duration of infusion (hours)}} \qquad (1)$$

adequate mixing of the infused solution with the blood (in a relatively large vessel with relative fast flow of blood) so that no major changes occur in the volume of blood cells. In addition, the carbohydrate is oxidized, leaving the "water" intermixed with the body fluids.

Toward the end of long-continued intravenous carbohydrate administration, the rate of administration should be *decreased slowly* to prevent the onset of hypoglycemic reactions. The use of carbohydrates in water does *not* supply electrolytes needed for the daily body needs.

Electrolyte and Water Solutions. The electrolytes may be added to distilled water, various carbohydrates, amino acids, or alcohol combinations. Although many solutions are available commercially, it is unfortunate that the majority used consist of the "oldest" three — 5 per cent glucose (dextrose) in distilled water, isotonic saline, and 5 per cent dextrose in isotonic saline. Some of the electrolyte solutions available commercially are shown in Table 1, in comparison to normal plasma. Normal plasma also contains 1 mEq of sulfate and 16 mEq of proteinate per liter of plasma; when these anions are added to those shown in the table, the sum of the cations and of the anions will balance, each total being 154 mEq per liter.

Isotonic saline is erroneously called "normal saline" or "physiologic saline." It is *not physiologic*, because it contains more chloride than is normally found in the blood. The blood level of chloride is 103 mEq per liter, and the concentration of sodium is 142 mEq per liter. Isotonic saline solution, however, contains 154 mEq of sodium and 154 mEq of chloride per liter. Isotonic saline is *not normal,* in the chemical sense of the term; chemically speaking, a normal (or molar, because it is monovalent) saline solution is a 5.85 per cent solution of sodium chloride — the closest commercial solution is the 5 per cent saline. The so-called physiologic or normal saline solution should be referred to as *isotonic saline.*

For routine use, Ringer's-lactate solution is more beneficial than isotonic saline. In addition to the sodium and chloride, Ringer's-lactate contains potassium and calcium; even though the additional cations are present in small quantities, the use of this solution serves to prevent a *dilution* of these electrolytes in the blood and thereby to prevent the appearance of a latent tetany or a dilutional hypopotassemia. The sodium concentration is 130 mEq per liter and the chloride 109 mEq per liter; these concentrations are closer to those existing in normal blood plasma. The plasma "bicarbonate" is supplied by the presence of lactate ion, which under normal circumstances is oxidized or built up into glucose or glycogen. Ringer's-lactate has been the solution of choice in treating diabetic acidosis.

TABLE 1. **Composition of Typical Electrolyte Repair Solutions**

SOLUTION	CATIONS (mEq PER LITER)					ANIONS (mEq PER LITER)			
	Na	K	Ca	Mg	NH_4	Cl	HCO_3	*Lactate*	PO_4
Plasma, normal	142	5	5	2		103	27	5*	2
Duodenal, modified (or No. 1)	80	36	5	3		63		60	
Gastric (Cooke and Crowley or No. 3)	63	17			70	150			
Multiple electrolyte solution (Butler or No. 2)	57	25		6		50		25	13
Potassium chloride (0.3%) and sodium chloride (0.45%)	77	40				117			
Ringer's	147	4	4			155			
Ringer's-lactate (mod. Hartmann)	130	4	3			109		28	
Saline, hypertonic (5%)	855					855			
Saline, hypertonic (3%)	513					513			
Saline, hypotonic (0.45%)	77					77			
Saline, isotonic 1/6M (0.9%)	154					154			
Sodium bicarbonate 1/6M (1.4%)	167						167		
Sodium bicarbonate (5%)	595						595		
Sodium bicarbonate (7.5%)	892						892		
Sodium bicarbonate (8.4%)	1000						1000		
Sodium r-lactate, 1/6M (1.9%)	167							167	
Manufacture proscribed by FDA:									
Ammonium chloride, 1/6M (0.9%)					169	169			
Ammonium chloride (2.14%)					400	400			
Darrow's	121	35				103		53	

*Total organic acids in plasma; lactate concentration about 1 to 2.

Solutions with *high* concentrations of potassium should be administered intravenously only after the kidneys excrete an adequate urine volume. The concentration should *never exceed 80 mEq of potassium per liter,* and preferably not more than 60 mEq per liter; it is best to administer a maximum of 30 mEq of potassium *per hour.* Potassium may be administered orally in the form of meat broth or meat extract.

Ammonium chloride solutions (0.9 and 2.14 per cent) have been proscribed by the FDA from manufacture; they are available until present stocks are depleted. Yet the gastric solution which contains 70 mEq of ammonium can be manufactured!

Darrow's solution will also not be manufactured. A substitute for this solution can be prescribed by adding 50 mEq of sodium lactate (e.g., 20 ml of Abbott Ion-O-Trate Sodium lactate or 12.5 ml of Cutter Quadrate Sodium lactate) to 1 liter of potassium chloride (0.3 per cent) and sodium chloride (0.45 per cent) solution. An alternative substitute solution can be prepared by adding 40 mEq of potassium chloride and 50 mEq of sodium lactate to 1 liter of hypotonic saline (0.45 per cent) solution.

Amino Acid Solutions. Commercial preparations of digested proteins ("amino acids") are available for parenteral use: "protein hydrolysates," "enzyme digests," and so forth. They contain about 80 per cent "utilizable protein" (amino acids) and 20 per cent short-chain peptides. On the basis of total "solids," each gram yields 3.4 kcal, whereas "amino acids" yield 4.2 kcal (see Table 2). These solutions are available in various combinations with electrolytes, carbohydrates, alcohol, and so forth. "Protein" solutions serve to furnish the body with a supply of nitrogen (and phosphorus) essential for growth, cellular repair,

and wound healing. The presence of potassium, magnesium, and phosphate is necessary for the assimilation of parenteral amino acids; these are present in commercial protein solutions. Average American diets contain 1 gram of protein per kg per day; for minimal maintenance 0.5 gram is sufficient in the presence of adequate calories.

The term "hyperalimentation" has been applied to the administration of about 5 per cent protein hydrolysate or synthetic amino acid solutions with about 25 per cent carbohydrate via a large central vein. More accurate descriptive terms are "total parenteral nutrition" (TPN) or "intravenous alimentation" (IVA). This type of therapy is best used for sustaining and saving lives of patients with severe disease of the intestine or severe catabolic states such as burns. Some of the possible complications are systemic infection, metabolic acidosis, hyperosmolar nonketotic coma, hyperammonemia, and hypophosphatemia. If insulin is prescribed for the high concentration of dextrose (to avoid hyperglycemia), it is best to administer it subcutaneously, for the insulin (protein) can be and is absorbed onto the glass or plastic container and plastic tubing. (If insulin is mixed with the contents of the container, 25 to 40 units of regular insulin should be used.)

Fat Emulsions. Fat emulsions are of special importance in supplying extra calories for utilization of protein nitrogen and in supplying essential fatty acids essential in prolonged intravenous alimentation (TPN). A weekly infusion of 500 ml of 10 per cent Intralipid will satisfy the needs for fatty acids. Since this fat solution is isotonic, it may be administered via a peripheral vein.

Colloids. Examples of colloid solutions are whole blood, human serum albumin, and plasma expanders such as dextran, polyvinylpyrrolidone

TABLE 2.   **Caloric Equivalents of Foodstuffs Based on USP "Parenteral" versus Usual "Dietary" Calculations***

FOODSTUFF	USP "PARENTERAL" KCAL	USUAL "DIETARY" KCAL
1 gram dextrose (monohydrate)†	3.4	4 (1 gram CHO)‡
1 gram dextrose (anhydrous)	3.75	4 (1 gram CHO)
1 gram fructose	3.75	4 (1 gram CHO)
1 gram invert sugar (dextrose and fructose)	3.75	4 (1 gram CHO)
1 gram "solids" of protein hydrolysates	3.4	4 (1 gram protein)
1 gram "crystalline" amino acids	4.2	4 (1 gram protein)
1 ml ethyl alcohol (absolute)	5.6	5.6 (1 ml ethanol)
1 gram lecithin	6.5	9 (1 gram fat)
1 gram cottonseed oil	9	9 (1 gram fat)

*Modified from Weisberg, H. F.: Water, Electrolyte and Acid-Base Balance, 2nd ed. Baltimore, Williams & Wilkins Company, 1962.

†USP requirement when used as sole carbohydrate in the parenteral solution.

‡CHO = carbohydrate.

(PVP), and gelatin. (Human plasma is no longer available.) Colloid solutions are used to prevent shock, to support the circulatory system in the presence of shock, and to supply additional proteins or large molecules to support the plasma osmotic pressure. Sodium chloride is present in whole blood, plasma, and some colloid preparations. Whole blood (preferably washed packed cells) is best for the replacement of red blood cells.

The potassium present in the plasma of aged bank blood may reach 25 mEq per liter. Solutions with high concentrations of potassium are contraindicated for patients with oliguria or anuria, adrenal insufficiency, or chronic renal disease, or for those who require massive, multiple transfusions; the freshest blood available should be used.

Daily Requirements

Water. A simple formula for the calculation of the total daily water needs for insensible water loss and excretion of urine is

$$\text{Total water (ml/kg/day)} = 125 - (5 \times \text{years}) \quad (2)$$

Formula 2 is satisfactory for the ages from 1 year to adulthood; the *minimal* need for the adult *male* is 30 ml per kg per day, and the *minimal* need for the adult *female* is 25 ml per kg per day.

Formula 3 gives the amount of water lost per day via insensible perspiration:

$$\text{Insensible perspiration (ml/kg/day)} = 30 - \text{years} \quad (3)$$

Formula 3 is used for ages up to 15 years, since the adult requires a *minimum* of 15 ml per kg per day for the water of insensible perspiration. The remainder of the daily water loss is excreted via the urine. Thus a normal man with normal fluid intake should excrete 15 ml per kg per day of urine, whereas a normal woman will excrete only 10 ml per kg per day. If the intake of water is decreased, the insensible perspiration water loss takes precedence over the urine excretion and thus oliguria results.

Electrolytes. The exact *minimal* requirements of the various electrolytes are not known; the supposed average intake of different salts varies according to various authorities. The following daily requirements apply to the average *normal* adult. The need for *sodium* will be satisfied by about 100 mEq, contained in approximately 6 grams of sodium chloride (range from 4 to 7 grams). The *chloride* requirement of about 120 mEq is contained in 7 grams of sodium chloride

(range from 5 to 8 grams). The *potassium* requirement will be satisfied by the daily intake of 60 mEq, equivalent to about 4.5 grams, of potassium chloride (range 4 to 6 grams).

These three electrolytes are the most important in therapy. Other electrolytes are *also necessary;* even though the exact minimal requirements are not known, *magnesium* and *phosphate* are being used more extensively. A normal person who is *eating a normal balanced diet* will satisfy his needs for the various electrolytes.

Other Requirements. Formula 4 (by Wallace) gives a scheme for the calculation of calories needed under normal circumstances.

$$\text{kcal/kg/day} = 100 - (3 \times \text{years}) \quad (4)$$

This formula is good for all ages but must not fall below the *minimum* for an individual in bed — 25 kcal per kg per day. Light physical work or a patient with a fever requires 30 to 35 kcal per kg per day, moderate physical work or a septic patient requires 35 to 40 kcal per kg per day, and heavy physical work or a patient with extensive burns requires 40 to more than 50 kcal per kg per day.

Table 2 gives the caloric equivalents of "foodstuffs" used parenterally and their equivalents as calculated for the usual "dietary" calories. The caloric needs of a patient cannot be satisfied by the infusion of 2 to 3 liters of water containing hexoses. The kilocalories derived from 1 liter of solution are 170 for 5 per cent dextrose, 340 for 10 per cent dextrose, and 375 for 10 per cent invert sugar. One liter of 5 per cent amino acids, 12.5 per cent fructose, and 2.4 per cent alcohol will yield 780 kcal. A typical TPN solution of 4.2 per cent crystalline amino acids in 25 per cent dextrose solution supplies 1000 kcal per liter. Some fat emulsions (10 per cent dextrose and 40 per cent fat) have been used for *oral* feedings; such solutions furnish 4000 kcal per liter.

If the patient is to be treated with parenteral fluids for more than 3 days, he should be supplied with proteins in the form of an amino acid solution. Nitrogen balance can be achieved with a *minimum* of 0.5 grams of protein (approximately 0.1 gram of nitrogen) per kg per day; this can be supplied by 1 liter of a 5 per cent amino acid solution. In order to utilize the 0.5 gram protein regimen, one must supply the *basal* caloric requirement of 25 kcal per kg per day. In addition to calories, the deposition of nitrogen as protein requires potassium, magnesium, and phosphate. Some articles have been published advocating the infusion of 3 per cent crystalline L-amino acids (*without* 5 per cent dextrose) to replace the usual volume of dextrose usually administered. The reasoning is that without dextrose there is less stimulation of insulin secretion which thus allows for lipolysis and facilitates anabolism of the amino acids.

Vitamins. The B complex and C vitamins are necessary for the intermediary metabolism of carbohydrates. They should be administered to patients who will be maintained on parenteral fluid therapy for more than 4 days by adding to the infusion fluid or, *preferably*, by separate intramuscular injection. For patients on TPN the water-soluble and fat-soluble vitamins are indicated.

THE B-C-D OF PARENTERAL THERAPY

Parenteral fluid therapy should be a three-pronged program: (1) administration of the *Basic* requirements, (2) replacement of *Continued* losses, and (3) replacement of the prior *Deficit*. Optimal treatment should supply water, calories, nitrogen, electrolytes, and vitamins.

Basic Requirements

Short-Term. Butler's multiple electrolyte solution (No. 2) will supply the basal maintenance needs for the major electrolytes in addition to the daily basal water needs when Formulas 5 and 6 are used as a guide to therapy.

$$\text{ml/day for males} = 30 \times \text{kg} \qquad (5)$$

$$\text{ml/day for females} = 25 \times \text{kg} \qquad (6)$$

Thus a 60 kg woman will require 60×25 or 1.5 liters of Butler's solution; this will provide the basal 90 mEq of sodium, 37.8 mEq of potassium, and 75 mEq of chloride, as well as some lactate, magnesium, and phosphate (Table 3). If 10 per cent dextrose were included, the 1.5 liters (135 grams of anhydrous dextrose) would provide 506 kcal, whereas with 10 per cent invert sugar 562 kcal would be supplied; in both cases the basal caloric needs of the patient would *not* be satisfied.

Long-Term. The daily prescription for an 80 kg male is calculated as 80×30 or about 2.5 liters. This quantity of Butler's solution will provide the basal 144 mEq of sodium, 60 mEq of potassium, and 120 mEq of chloride as well as lactate, magnesium, and phosphate. If administered with 10 per cent dextrose, 850 kcal would be provided; with 10 per cent invert sugar 937 kcal would be supplied.

TABLE 3. **Electrolytes Provided by Butler's Multiple Electrolyte Solution (No. 2)**

ELECTROLYTE	CONCENTRATION (mEq/LITER)	ELECTROLYTES PROVIDED BY FORMULAS* Males (mEq/kg)	Females (mEq/kg)
Sodium	57	1.8	1.5
Potassium	25	0.75	0.63
Chloride	50	1.5	1.25
Lactate	25	0.75	0.63
Magnesium	6	0.18	0.15
Phosphate	13	0.39	0.33

*Using basal maintenance formulas:
Males: ml/day = 30 × kg.
Females: ml/day = 25 × kg.

For "long-term" maintenance (*over 4 days*) of a patient *without* dehydration, the prescription should include 1 liter of a "protein" solution (and multivitamins).

1000 ml 10 per cent carbohydrate in Electrolyte No. 2.

1000 ml 5 per cent protein in 12.4 per cent fructose and 2.4 per cent alcohol solution.

500 ml 10 per cent carbohydrate in Electrolyte No. 2.

This prescription will supply 121.4 mEq of sodium, 55 mEq of potassium, and 92 mEq of chloride (plus lactate, magnesium, and phosphate) and 40 grams of utilizable protein (satisfying the minimal 0.5 gram per kilogram). The kcal would be 1342 (87 per cent nonprotein), close to the basal, "resting" caloric needs of the average individual.

Replacement of Continued Losses

A patient may still be losing extra water and electrolytes even after therapy has been started. The use of a water and electrolyte balance sheet, recording fluid *intake* and *output* and the types of solutions administered, will aid the physician in adjusting the quantity and composition of the repair solutions to be administered. Water and solutes may be lost via the urine as a result of the polyuria of *diabetes mellitus* or the protein catabolism resulting from *surgery*, whereas only water will be lost in patients with fixed low specific gravity urine, in seriously ill elderly patients, or in those with intrinsic renal disease (Table 4).

A febrile patient will be losing more water via hyperventilation and insensible perspiration; electrolytes *and* water will be lost via the sensible

TABLE 4. **Clinical Estimation of Continuing Water and Electrolyte Needs***†

CONDITIONS CAUSING LOSS	REPLACEMENT SOLUTION INDICATED	
	Quantity ml/kg/day	*Type*
Via urine		
Increased loss of solutes	5	Multiple electrolyte solution (Butler or No. 2)
Isosthenuria (fixed low specific gravity)	5–10	Water (with CHO‡)
Via insensible perspiration		
Prolonged temperature elevation		
(temperate zone)		
Fever *Room*		
>38 C (100 F) >26 C (79 F)	5	Water (with CHO)
>39 C (102 F) >29 C (84 F)	10	Water (with CHO)
>40 C (104 F) >32 C (90 F)	15	Water (with CHO)
>41 C (106 F) >35 C (95 F)	20	Water (with CHO)
>42 C (108 F) >38 C (100 F)	25	Water (with CHO)
>41 C (106 F)	30	Water (with CHO)
Ventilator or endotracheal tube	15	Water (with CHO)
During surgery (ml/kg for each *hour*)	7	Water (with CHO)
Via sweating		
Moderate	5	Multiple electrolyte solution (Butler or No. 2)
Severe	10	Multiple electrolyte solution (Butler or No. 2)

*Modified from Weisberg, H. F.: Water, Electrolyte and Acid-Base Balance. 2nd ed. Baltimore, Williams & Wilkins Company, 1962.

†In *addition* to daily basal maintenance needs.

‡CHO = carbohydrate.

perspiration (sweat). Such unseen abnormal losses must be considered and included in the therapeutic regimen. It is best to record the losses and prescribe their replacement as part of the fluids ordered on the succeeding morning.

For a 50 kg female adult with fixed specific gravity of the urine, sweating moderately in a hospital room with ambient temperature of 30 C (86 F), the prescription for fluids can be calculated as 50 × 25 (Formula 6) to give 1250 ml of 10 per cent carbohydrate in Electrolyte No. 2 to satisfy the basal water and electrolyte needs. From Table 4 one calculates the extra No. 2 solution as 50 × 5 = 250 ml for the moderate sweating (which occurred the previous day). Extra water needs for the fixed specific gravity are 50 × 5 = 250 ml. Insensible perspiration water losses are equal to 50 × 10 = 500 ml for the elevated room temperature. The total fluid prescription for the day therefore would consist of:

1500 ml 10 per cent carbohydrate in Electrolyte No. 2.

750 ml 10 per cent carbohydrate in water.

Surgery. At the time of operation a *slow* infusion of *hypotonic* saline solution can or should be started to facilitate the job of the anesthetist and to allow a ready inlet for any needed blood transfusion. The danger of clumping of red cells which may occur when blood is mixed with an infusion of carbohydrate in water is avoided if the carbohydrate solution contains *electrolytes*. Many surgeons abhor the administration of saline solution on the day of surgery. This has resulted from the old type of therapy in which only saline solutions were administered, resulting in overtreatment and pulmonary edema, and so forth. Despite the extra secretion of adrenocortical steroids as a reaction to the general stress of surgery, the administration of the *minimal* requirements of sodium, potassium, and chloride will not result in edema and other complications. This is important, because the daily maintenance of a surgical patient, even without abnormal losses, is complicated by the reaction to surgical trauma; there is an *increased loss of potassium via the kidneys*.

With the over-enthusiastic use of Ringer's lactate solution *during* the surgical procedure to increase the volume of the interstitial (and intravascular) fluid compartment, patients may be overtreated with electrolytes! It is wiser to start such infusions the night before surgery, resulting in a saving of time in the operating room and in the patient's being slowly rehydrated before surgery.

Assume that an adult male weighing 90 kg is to undergo surgery. His normal minimal water and electrolyte requirements would be 90 × 30 = 2700 ml of multiple electrolyte solution. The surgery lasts 2 hours, requiring an additional 90

× 2 × 7 = "1250" ml of 10 per cent carbohydrate in water (Table 4). Practically, the fluid prescription for the day of surgery may be:

250 ml hypotonic saline (slow drip for possible transfusion in operating room).
3000 ml 10 per cent carbohydrate in Electrolyte No. 2.
1000 ml 10 per cent carbohydrate in water.

Since surgery usually results in negative nitrogen balance and loss of potassium, the water and electrolytes for *subsequent* days, provided that there are no abnormal losses, may be scheduled as:

2000 ml 10 per cent carbohydrate in Electrolyte No. 2.
1000 ml 5 per cent amino acids in 12.5 per cent fructose and 2.4 per cent alcohol.
Vitamins.

Replacement of Prior Deficits

Dehydration. The history is essential in ascertaining the type and approximate amount of water and electrolytes lost. Accurate knowledge of the patient's usual body weight is very important. For example, a male patient whose weight has been 65 kg (143 pounds) may present himself to the physician after having had a bout of diarrhea for the preceding few days, during which time the weight loss has amounted to approximately 3 kg (6 to 7 pounds). Since his body is approximately 60 per cent water, the loss of total body weight is equivalent to a loss of about 2 kg (2 liters) of body fluid (water and electrolytes). The lost fluid is approximately 3 per cent of the patient's body weight, a loss which the body can tolerate with little evidence of functional impairment. The patient will be thirsty and will show evidence of lassitude, with possible giddiness on suddenly assuming the upright position.

Therapy for this patient should include 2 liters (65 × 30 = 1950 ml) of water and electrolytes for daily maintenance (10 per cent carbohydrate in Electrolyte No. 2), plus the estimated previous losses — 2 liters (which can be supplied as Ringer's-lactate solution.) This *theoretical* plan of therapy should be altered, depending on the clinical evaluation of the patient and on the determinations performed in the laboratory. If the diarrhea ceases owing to adjuvant and antibiotic therapy, the second day of parenteral fluid therapy will repair the calculated deficit. However, if the diarrhea continues, an estimate must be made of the amount of fluids lost; this quantity must be added to the original projected plan of therapy.

Clinical dehydration will be quite apparent when approximately 6 per cent of the body weight has been lost; thirst is severe, eyeballs are sunken, mucous membranes are dry, skin and muscle have lost turgor, oliguria develops, peripheral circulation begins to fail, pulse rate increases, blood pressure falls, and renal function becomes impaired. Such a dehydrated patient requires active supportive therapy with colloid solutions for the *incipient shock* as part of his maintenance and replacement needs; such therapy will require about 2 to 3 days for complete replacement. The proportions of water and electrolyte may be changed, depending upon the laboratory results; more water (with carbohydrate), for instance, being needed if the hematocrit, plasma protein, and electrolyte concentrations are elevated. A normal or low electrolyte concentration in the blood in the presence of a low hematocrit would indicate the need for relatively more electrolyte solution than water (with carbohydrate).

If 10 to 20 per cent of the body weight is lost, shock is well established and requires vigorous therapy with colloid and electrolyte solutions. Losses greater than 20 per cent of the body weight (equivalent to *body fluid* losses greater than 14 per cent of the body weight) result in irreversible circulatory failure.

Gastrointestinal Tract Losses. The prolonged use of a tube within the gastrointestinal tract is irritating and causes further secretion of the various juices. *The tube should be removed as soon as feasible.* Water is not satisfactory as an irrigant for such tubes; isotonic saline solution is much better. Allowing a patient to have "sips of water" or to eat ice chips results in removal of electrolytes from the blood via the gastrointestinal tract wall. It would be much better if the ice chips were made from electrolyte solutions so that the *"ice"* given to the patient is *"Ice-Chip-Electrolytes."*

Dehydration is very often present as the result of losses of water and electrolytes from the gastrointestinal tract by vomiting, suction drainage, fistula, diarrhea, and other causes. The type of parenteral fluid to be administered will vary with the source of the fluid loss. Table 5 illustrates the types of solutions available commercially which can be used for volume-for-volume replacement to make up the losses from the gastrointestinal tract; accurate collections must be made!

Gastric juice which has a pH of 3 or less (normal gastric acidity) has high concentrations of chloride and potassium and a low concentration of sodium; replacement is accomplished by use of the commercial "gastric" solution (Table 5). If, however, the pH of the gastric contents is

TABLE 5. **Volume-for-Volume Replacement for Losses of Gastrointestinal Secretions***

SOURCE OF FLUID LOSS	REPLACEMENT SOLUTION INDICATED
Gastric	
pH 3 or less	Gastric (Cooke and Crowley or No. 3)
pH 5 or less	Potassium chloride (0.3%) and sodium chloride (0.45%)
Bile	Ringer's-lactate
Pancreatic	Duodenal, modified (or No. 1)
Small intestine	Ringer's-lactate
With obstruction and/ or excess losses	Darrow's or substitute†
Large intestine	Multiple electrolyte solution (Butler or No. 2)
With excess losses, e.g., diarrhea, severe	Darrow's or substitute†

*Modified from Weisberg, H. F.: Water, Electrolyte and Acid-Base Balance. 2nd ed. Baltimore, Williams & Wilkins Company, 1962.

†To 1 liter of potassium chloride (0.3 per cent) and sodium chloride (0.45 per cent), add 50 mEq of sodium lactate (e.g., 20 ml of Abbott Ion-O-Trate sodium lactate *or* 12.5 ml of Cutter Quadrate sodium lactate).

high (over 5), such as is seen in infants, patients with gastric carcinoma or pernicious anemia, and the elderly (increased incidence of hypochlorhydria), the "gastric" solution should *not* be used but the potassium chloride (0.3 per cent) plus sodium chloride (0.45 per cent) solution should be used. In addition, the potassium chloride plus sodium chloride solution should be used to replace gastric secretion whenever a patient has liver disease, because such patients do not tolerate the ammonium ion present in the "gastric" solution. *Bile* has a composition approximating that of the extracellular fluid; replacement is accomplished by using Ringer's-lactate solution. *Pancreatic* fluid has a high sodium and potassium concentration and a relatively low chloride concentration; this should be replaced with the modified duodenal type of solution (Table 5).

Losses from the *small intestine*, if moderate in quantity, can be replaced with Ringer's-lactate solution; however, if the quantity lost is excessive, as in obstruction, great amounts of potassium are lost and replacement is accomplished with Darrow's solution or its substitute (Table 5). The losses of juices from the *large intestine* are replaced with a hypotonic solution, e.g., multiple electrolyte solution; however, as for the small intestine, if the losses are excessive (e.g., *diarrhea*),

Darrow's solution or its substitute is indicated. These volume-for-volume replacement fluids are administered in addition to the daily maintenance needs!

Treatment of Complications

The patient with dehydration may also present other complicating factors which require additional therapy. A burned patient requires colloid solutions, alterations of acid-base balance need extra vigilance and treatment, and so on.

Hypertonicity and Hypotonicity. The blood is considered hypertonic (or hyperosmotic) if the plasma sodium is elevated above 155 mEq per liter; it is hypotonic (or hypo-osmotic) if the sodium value is below 130. The normal "osmotic pressure" of the plasma is 270 to 300 mosmol per kilogram (or per liter) of plasma water. A simple formula to calculate osmolality (and correcting for the water content of plasma) is shown at the bottom of this page (Formula 7). If a patient has an elevation of the blood glucose or urea nitrogen or both, the total osmolality (tonicity) of the blood is increased and will "displace" some of the sodium (which enters the cells or is excreted via the urine). An 80 kg male adult has a blood sugar of 450 mg per 100 ml and a serum urea nitrogen of 65 mg per 100 ml in the presence of a sodium of 115 mEq per liter. Substituting in Formula 7 results in $(2 \times 115) + 450/20 + 65/3 = 230 + 22 + 22 = 274$ mosmol per kg of plasma water, indicating that despite the very low sodium concentration, therapy for the hyponatremia is *not* indicated at this time.

Use of Formula 7 is valuable to determine the "osmolal discriminate" by substracting the calculated osmolality from the actual value determined with an osmometer. Normally, the difference is about 10 mosmol. Increased values of the osmolal discriminate may signify the presence of alcohol or drugs, and a value of more than 40 mosmol per kg denotes a grave prognosis (usually seen in patients in shock with "idiogenic" osmoles).

Hypotonicity (low concentration of sodium) may result from a depletion of salt ("low salt syndrome") as seen in acute severe diarrhea, or from dilution caused by the overzealous administration of carbohydrates in water without electrolytes, or by inappropriate secretion of antidiuretic hormone (symptomless hyponatremia) as seen in pulmonary tuberculosis or bronchogenic carcinoma. If therapy with hypertonic sa-

$$\text{mosmol per kg of plasma water} = (2 \times \text{Na mEq/L}) + \frac{\text{Sugar mg/100 ml}}{20} + \frac{\text{Urea N mg/100 ml}}{3} \quad (7)$$

line is indicated, it must be remembered that the *oral intake of fluids is restricted* and the administration of nonelectrolyte-containing parenteral fluids should be delayed. The calculated amount of hypertonic saline solution should be given in *divided doses,* because many patients will have a normal concentration of sodium when less than the calculated dose is administered. It is best to give *one half* of the calculated dose on the first day of therapy; the sodium determination should be repeated on the following day and the deficit recalculated. Some authorities administer diuretics to a patient with hyponatremia and replace the volume of urine excreted with a similar volume infusion of isotonic saline.

Formula 8 is used to calculate the volume of repair solution needed to treat hyponatremia or hypernatremia.

$$\text{ml of solution} = F \times kg \times mEq \text{ change desired in Na} \quad (8)$$

The various factors are listed in Table 6. Before treating a hyponatremic patient with a hypertonic saline solution, the physician should be sure that the *blood glucose and blood urea nitrogen values are normal.* A 60 kg female patient has normal glucose and urea nitrogen values and the sodium concentration is 122. From Formula 8 and Table 6, assuming that we wish to raise the sodium concentration to the normal 142,

$$\text{ml 5 per cent saline solution needed} = 0.6 \times 60 \times 20 = 720 \text{ ml}$$

If 3 per cent saline were used, the volume required would be 1200 ml.

Hypertonicity is usually seen in pure water dehydration or in a mixed dehydration in which more water than salt is lost; in such cases the hematocrit, hemoglobin, serum protein, and so forth will also be increased. A male patient weighing 80 kg has a sodium concentration of 162 mEq per liter, a value which is 20 mEq above the

TABLE 6. **Factors (F) in Formula* for Therapy of Hyponatremia or Hypernatremia**

SOLUTION	FACTORS	
	Males	*Females*
For hyponatremia:		
3% NaCl	1.2	1.0
5% NaCl	0.7	0.6
For hypernatremia:		
Carbohydrate in water	4	3

*Ml of solution = F × kg × mEq change desired in Na.

normal 142. Instead of attempting to bring the sodium concentration back to the "normal," it is desired to reduce the concentration to 147 mEq per liter. Substituting in Formula 8 (factors in Table 6),

$$\text{ml water needed} = 4 \times 80 \times 15 = 4800 \text{ ml}$$

It should be realized that this quantity is in *addition* to the daily maintenance needs for water and electrolytes already discussed (80× 30 = 2400); the total quantity of 7200 ml of fluid should be administered over the entire 24 hour period. Even without additional losses, the patient may not be "normal" after being treated and should be re-evaluated; further fluids should be prescribed if necessary.

Acid-Base Imbalance. The terms "acid" and "base" are sometimes used erroneously in physiology and medicine. An *acid* is a substance that can furnish a proton in the form of the hydrogen ion (H^+), e.g., H_2CO_3, HCl, H_2SO_4; a *base* is a substance that can accept or unite with a proton (H^+). The symbol pH is an index of the hydrogen ion concentration in blood (plasma); the normal average (and range) is 7.40 (7.35 to 7.45) for arterial blood and 7.37 (7.32 to 7.42) for venous blood; the extremes compatible with life are 6.80 to 7.80. The pH is controlled by *blood buffers* — bicarbonate and carbonic acid, hemoglobin, protein, and phosphate. *Acidosis* or *acidemia* is present if the ratio of bicarbonate to carbonic acid is *decreased* and the blood pH is *decreased. Alkalosis* or *alkalemia* is present if the ratio of bicarbonate to carbonic acid is *increased* and the blood pH is *increased.* The normal ratio of bicarbonate to carbonic acid in the Henderson-Hasselbalch equation is 20 to 1 for arterial blood (pH 7.40) and 18.6 to 1 for venous blood (pH 7.37).

A pH value alone can tell the physician if acidosis or alkalosis is present; however, he will not know what type (metabolic or respiratory or mixed) is present and how much, if any, compensation has occurred. A full picture of the state of acid-base is achieved by also having the P_{CO_2} value. The normal average values and ranges for P_{CO_2} are 40 (35 to 45) and 46 (42 to 55) mm Hg, respectively, for arterial and venous blood. A modification of the Hastings pH–carbon dioxide content diagram is shown in Figure 1, with the major diagnostic areas. Knowing the pH and P_{CO_2} is sufficient to diagnose most of the acid-base abnormalities; this can be done on venous or arterial blood, arterial blood being needed for the evaluation of P_{O_2}. In patients with pulmonary disease (hypoxia) and shock, it is best to know the values for both arterial and venous blood.

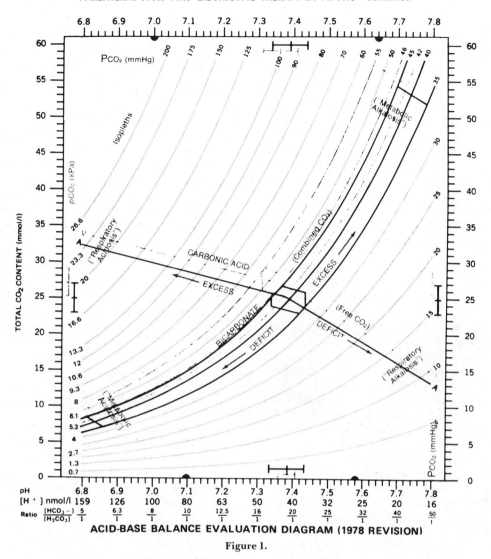

ACID-BASE BALANCE EVALUATION DIAGRAM (1978 REVISION)

Figure 1.

A patient may have a normal carbon dioxide content of 25 mmol per liter; without a knowledge of the pH one could misconstrue the actual condition of the patient. Thus with a content of 25 mmol per liter the pH may be 6.90, as seen in a mixed carbonic acid excess (respiratory acidosis) and bicarbonate deficit (metabolic acidosis); with a pure carbonic acid excess at this pH the carbon dioxide content should be 31 mmol per liter (Fig. 1). This value of 31 mmol per liter is the "theoretical" CO_2 content (CO_2CT) for arterial blood at pH 6.90 and can be found by inspection of Figure 1 (intersection of the carbon dioxide buffer line — from northwest to southeast) with the actual pH or from the TRI-SLIDE/CO_2rrec°t-O_2-slide calculator* designed by the author, or from Formulas 9 to 12.

Formulas 9 and 10 are for arterial blood; Formula 9 is used when the arterial pH is less than 7.40 (acidosis) and Formula 10 when the arterial pH is more than 7.40 (alkalosis).

$$\text{Arterial theoretical } CO_2CT_{(acid)} = \qquad (9)$$
$$25 + 12 \,(7.40 - pH)$$

$$\text{Arterial theoretical } CO_2CT_{(alk)} = \qquad (10)$$
$$25 + 28 \,(7.40 - pH)$$

Formulas 11 and 12 are for venous blood; Formula 11 is used when the venous pH is less than 7.37 (acidosis) and Formula 12 when the pH is more than 7.37 (alkalosis).

$$\text{Venous theoretical } CO_2CT_{(acid)} = \qquad (11)$$
$$27 + 12 \,(7.37 - pH)$$

$$\text{Venous theoretical } CO_2CT_{(alk)} = \qquad (12)$$
$$27 + 28 \,(7.37 - pH)$$

*Obtainable from the author, 2574 N. Terrace Avenue, Milwaukee, Wisconsin 53211.

The "delta content" (ΔCT) is obtained by subtracting the theoretical CO_2 content from the proper corresponding value determined in the laboratory.

$$\Delta CT \text{ ("BE/D")} =$$
$$\text{Actual } CO_2CT - \text{theoretical } CO_2CT \qquad (13)$$

A "negative" delta content signifies a bicarbonate deficit and is equivalent to "base deficit" (old "base excess negative") of Astrup and Siggaard-Andersen. A "positive" delta content signifies a bicarbonate excess and is equivalent to "base excess" (old "base excess positive") of Astrup and Siggaard-Andersen. The normal ΔCT ranges from -2 to $+2$.

Formula 14 gives the milliliters of 1/6 molar sodium lactate (or bicarbonate, acetate, citrate, gluconate) needed to correct a bicarbonate deficit or the amount of 1/6 molar ammonium chloride to correct a bicarbonate excess; it is better to use such calculated values *as a guide*, administering a *portion* at a time and *re-evaluating* the patient subsequent to therapy. The factor 1.5 applies to 1/6 molar repair solutions (about 167 mEq of cations and of anions). (See bottom of this page.) Table 7 gives various factors for various solutions used in the therapy of metabolic alterations of acid-base balance.

Knowledge of the pH and P_{CO_2} will help the physician diagnose most acid-base imbalances. Compensated acid-base imbalance is present when the pH is in the normal range, even though the P_{CO_2} is abnormal. Examples are normal pH with high P_{CO_2} with compensated respiratory acidosis (compensated metabolic alkalosis is less likely) and normal pH with low P_{CO_2} with compensated respiratory alkalosis (compensated metabolic acidosis is less likely). The physician should be cautious in treating such conditions, since the pH is already normal.

In the therapy of *bicarbonate deficit* (metabolic acidosis), exemplified by low pH and normal (uncompensated) or decreased (partially compensated) P_{CO_2}, Ringer's-lactate has been used. For the very serious case of acidosis with extreme hyperpnea (Kussmaul respiration), 1/6 molar sodium *r*-lactate can be used. Sodium lactate is not completely metabolized in the presence of poor liver function or extreme congestive heart failure with passive congestion of the liver; in such cases sodium bicarbonate may be used with caution. The slower the infusion of sodium bicarbonate, the more effective it is. Use of sodium bicarbonate implies good pulmonary function to get rid of the extra carbon dioxide which is produced. In cases of cardiac arrest, haste in therapy is extremely important, without waiting for laboratory data.

For the therapy of *bicarbonate excess* or metabolic alkalosis exemplified by high pH and normal (uncompensated) or increased (partially compensated) P_{CO_2}, Ringer's solution has been used. In very severe cases, ammonium chloride solutions may be administered at a rate of 1 liter in 4 hours; this slow rate of administration is necessary because of the tendency of ammonium chloride solution to cause hemolysis of the red blood cells. Ammonium chloride releases hydrochloric acid when ammonia is split off to form urea or glutamine. (In infants and special cases as discussed earlier, the 0.3 per cent potassium chloride–0.45 per cent saline solution is used.) In the future, the only "ammonium chloride" solution produced will be the gastric (No. 3) solution. The infusion of 0.1 molar hydrochloric acid has also been used.

In a patient with *carbonic acid excess* or respiratory acidosis (low pH and elevated P_{CO_2}), the *dehydration* is treated by the administration of hypotonic electrolytes and carbohydrates. If the respiratory acidosis is severe, Ringer's-lactate should be administered; sodium bicarbonate or 1/6 molar sodium lactate should be administered with caution. Such measures will further *increase* the carbon dioxide content but will bring the pH back toward the normal range. The intravenous administration of sodium bicarbonate should be preceded by the intravenous administration of 10 ml of 10 per cent calcium gluconate or calcium levulinate, to prevent the onset of tetany. Tris buffer (an organic amine) has also been used to treat carbonic acid excess.

In treating *carbonic acid deficit* or respiratory alkalosis (high pH and decreased P_{CO_2}), the solution of choice is Ringer's solution which contains calcium ion, replenishing the depleted ionized calcium. A low ionized calcium level will not result in manifest tetany if the potassium level is

---

Condition	Therapy with	Quantity (ml)
Bicarbonate deficit (−) ("base deficit")	1/6 molar sodium lactate (−)	
=		$= 1.5 \times kg \times \Delta CT$
Bicarbonate excess (+) ("base excess")	1/6 molar ammonium chloride (+)	

$$(14)$$

TABLE 7. **Factors in Formula* for Therapy of Metabolic Acid-Base Abnormalities†**

MOLARITY (OR NORMALITY FOR MONOVALENT IONS)	TOTAL CATIONS OR TOTAL ANIONS (mEq PER LITER)	FACTOR (F) FOR THERAPY EQUATION*	EXAMPLES OF SOLUTIONS
0.070	70	3.5	Gastric (No. 3) solution (for ammonium chloride)
0.100	100	2.5	0.1 molar hydrochloric acid
0.167	167	1.5	All 1/6 molar solutions
0.400	400	0.6	2.14% ammonium chloride
0.500	500	0.5	4.2% sodium bicarbonate
0.600	600	0.4	5.0% sodium bicarbonate
0.892	892	0.28	7.5% sodium bicarbonate ("ampules")
1.000	1000	0.25	8.4% sodium bicarbonate ("ampules")

*Ml/kg = F × kg × ΔCT.
†Based on 25 per cent extracellular fluid compartment.

low; the administration of potassium to such a patient may cause the onset of tetany. The amount of potassium present in Ringer's solution is not sufficient to do this. If tetany does occur, it should be treated with calcium chloride or calcium gluconate intravenously. In very severe carbonic acid deficit it may be necessary to administer ammonium chloride (or hydrochloric acid) intravenously to bring the pH back toward normal, but the carbon dioxide content may be *depressed* still further, the result being a compensated alkalosis.

The delta content (ΔCT) or "base excess/deficit" is needed to distinguish acute and chronic respiratory, and "mixed" imbalances for proper therapy to be instituted. The pH is low and P_{CO_2} high in acute and chronic carbonic acid excess (respiratory acidosis) and in a mixed metabolic acidosis and respiratory acidosis. However, the delta content (BE/D) is normal in acute and increased in chronic carbonic acid excess; it is decreased in the mixed acidosis. The pH is high and P_{CO_2} low in acute and chronic carbonic acid deficit (respiratory alkalosis) and in a mixed metabolic alkalosis and respiratory alkalosis. However, the delta content (BE/D) is normal in acute and decreased in chronic carbonic acid deficit; it is increased in the mixed alkalosis.

FLUID THERAPY IN CHILDREN

method of
SOLOMON A. KAPLAN, M.D.
Los Angeles, California

Expenditure of water and electrolytes in children is considerably greater per unit of body weight than in adults for the following reasons: (1) The ratio between surface area and volume of the body is inversely proportional to the size of the body. Therefore the surface area of children per unit of body weight is larger than that of adults. Thus in infants and children there is a relatively larger surface from which evaporative or insensible losses can occur. (2) Renal powers of water conservation are diminished in the first few weeks of life, leading to a relatively large turnover of water. (3) Water expenditure is related to basal metabolic rate, which governs in part the amount of heat production and waste solute excretion by the kidney. Basal metabolic rate and caloric requirements are related to surface area and are considerably greater per kg in infants than in adults. (4) Infants generally react to infections with higher temperatures than do adults, and higher body temperature results in excessive evaporative water loss.

In adults the water requirements per 24 hours per kg are between 30 and 40 ml. Infants require 150 to 200 ml per kg per 24 hours. The larger volumes of water (and also sodium and potassium) continuously turned over by infants and children predispose to the rapid development of precarious situations if intake is not adequately maintained. Therefore, infants and children who are unable to ingest required amounts of electolytes and water or those who lose excessive quantities through vomiting or diarrhea must be treated promptly.

The amounts of water, sodium, and other electrolytes required per unit of body weight vary through life. There is a gradual decline of water requirement, for example, from about 200 ml per kg in infancy to 35 ml per kg in adult life. While it is possible to memorize the requirements of water and electrolytes at different ages per unit of body weight, it is a simpler mnemonic device to remember the requirements per unit of surface area. Fluid expenditure is related to surface area, as has been previously pointed out, and it is not unexpected that requirements of fluid and electrolytes are related to body surface area.

TABLE 1. **Percentage of Body Surface Area of Sections of the Body at Different Ages**

	NEW-BORN	3 YEARS	6 YEARS	12–20 YEARS
Lower extremity (each)	13	15	16	18
Front of torso	21	20	20	18
Back of torso	21	20	20	18
Upper extremity (each)	6	7	8	9
Head and face	17	15	11	9
Neck	1	1	1	1

Principles

The fluids used to treat dehydration and electrolyte loss consist of two parts:

1. *Maintenance*: This refers to the intake required by a well infant of the same age and size.

2. *Replacement*: This refers to abnormal fluid losses which have occurred and which must be replaced.

Maintenance Therapy. It is convenient to relate the quantities of fluid and electrolyte normally required to body surface area. Once the amount per unit surface area is known, the calculation may be applied to an individual of any age from 1 week of life to adult life. (Special considerations apply to the first week of life; these will be discussed subsequently.) The surface area may be read off standard nomograms, but, except for small infants, a close approximation can be reached by remembering that the average surface area of a 10 kg infant is 0.5 square meter, of a 30 kg child 1.0 square meter, and of a 60 kg person 1.5 square meters. The average requirements of average-sized adults may be calculated on the assumption of a surface area of 1.7 square meters.

The normal requirements per square meter are water 1500 to 2000 ml, sodium 35 to 50 mEq, and potassium 30 to 40 mEq. The minimal amount of fluid compatible with homeostasis is 900 ml and the maximum 2700 ml. Minimal needs under conditions of health for sodium and potassium are 10 mEq and the maximal tolerance for both electrolytes is 250 mEq. In infants and children we generally administer 2000 ml per square meter per day. In teenagers and adults we generally use the figure of 1500 ml. On the first day of life the requirements are about two fifths of the aforementioned amounts (800 ml water, 20 mEq sodium and 15 mEq potassium per square meter). The amounts are increased gradually over the first week so that at the end of the first week the requirements are as for older children.

Replacement Therapy. AMOUNT OF FLUID. This is best based on the patient's weight. Use of surface area as a basis for calculating deficits may lead to inaccuracies. The amount of fluid lost is estimated from the following considerations. A loss of 5 per cent of the body weight in fluid is the smallest amount that is clinically detectable, and a loss of 20 per cent is about the maximum compatible with life. Children moribund from dehydration are, therefore, estimated to have lost about 20 per cent of their body weight, those with severe dehydration about 15 per cent, and those with moderate dehydration about 10 per cent of the body weight. In cases of mild dehydration, the weight loss is assumed to be about 5 per cent of the body weight.

Attempts to replace all the lost fluid in 24 hours may result in water intoxication. As a rule, therefore, *one half* of the estimated fluid loss is given in the first 24 hours. This is equal to 7.5 per cent of the body weight in severe dehydration, 5 per cent in moderate, and 2.5 per cent in mild dehydration. For example, on the first day a child weighing 10 kg will receive 750 ml if he is severely dehydrated and 500 ml if moderately dehydrated. In all instances the fluid is calculated on the basis of the admission weight rather than the predehydration weight.

Since it is difficult to make an accurate assessment of the amount of dehydration, and since there are variables such as rate of loss of fluid from the skin, kidneys, and lungs, the patient must be examined frequently and the rate of fluid administration adjusted according to the physical findings. Periorbital edema is usually the first indication that the amount of fluids being administered is excessive. Peripheral or pulmonary edema is a late sign that too much fluid has been administered.

TYPE OF FLUID. In nearly all cases in which abnormal losses are to be replaced, the replacement solution should be 0.9 per cent saline, modified to include potassium if there is potassium deficiency, and bicarbonate (or lactate) if there is acidosis. Lactate is rapidly metabolized and is equivalent, therefore, to bicarbonate (except possibly in diabetic acidosis and salicylate poisoning). Alkali should be administered if the serum bicarbonate level is less than 15 mEq per liter and should be given in doses calculated to raise the level by about 10 mEq per liter per 24 hours. The dose of 7.5 per cent bicarbonate (which contains 0.9 mEq sodium bicarbonate per ml) is 6.6 ml (6 mEq) per kg per 24 hours. After calculating the amount of saline to be given as replacement, the figure is adjusted by subtracting the amount of bicarbonate. For example, in the case of the child weighing 10 kg to whom 500 ml of saline is given for moderate dehydration over 24 hours, the dose of bicarbonate calculated is 10 × 6.6 or 66 ml. This contains 60 mEq of Na. The original figure of 500 ml saline (75 mEq) is then adjusted to 100 ml saline (15 mEq) plus 66 ml of 7.5 per cent bicarbonate (60 mEq) plus 140 ml of water or 5 per cent dextrose in water. If the serum bicarbonate concentration increases at a rate faster than 5 mEq per liter over 12 hours, the volume of bicarbonate administered should be reduced.

Potassium Deficiency

The diagnosis of potassium deficiency in a patient with acute dehydration depends almost entirely on the history. If the cause of the dehydration is abnormal loss from the gastrointestinal tract (vomiting, diarrhea, surgical fistula, or diabetic acidosis), it may be safely assumed that some degree of potassium deficiency exists. The serum potassium concentration, the electrocardiogram, and certain physical signs such as hypotonia, abdominal distention, or lethargy are of little value in a patient with moderate or severe dehydration. Potassium deficiency in the absence of dehydration is usually characterized by low serum potassium, high serum bicarbonate, low serum chloride, and normal serum sodium concentration. In spite of the alkalosis, the urine is acid. These abnormalities are corrected only by administration of potassium.

In cases of potassium deficiency, the actual deficit may amount to 8 or 9 mEq per kg. However, it is usually unwise to administer more than 5 mEq per kg per 24 hours as the total dose of potassium. If this amount of potassium is given, the "maintenance" potassium (40 mEq per sq meter) is omitted. KCl is available in several concentrations. A form frequently used contains 3 mEq K per ml. Calculations in this article refer to this solution. If the patient has oliguria, it is advisable to wait for the development of adequate urine flow before administering potassium. Generally, potassium should not be administered during the first 6 hours of therapy to such patients. In diabetic ketoacidosis in children, on the other hand, the patient usually has polyuria, and potassium should be included in the administered fluids from the outset or profound hypokalemia may occur.

Calcium Deficiency

Calcium may be given if increased irritability or convulsive seizures are noted. It may be given only by the oral or intravenous routes. It must not be given intramuscularly, and when given intravenously scrupulous care must be taken to prevent its escape into the perivascular tissues. The oral dose of elemental calcium is 2 grams of calcium per sq meter given in two or three divided doses per 24 hours. One gram of calcium chloride is equivalent to 360 mg of calcium, 1 gram of calcium gluconate is equivalent to 110 mg of calcium, and 1 gram of calcium lactate is equivalent to 180 mg of calcium. Calcium chloride may be given orally as a very dilute solution only (preferably never exceeding 1 per cent), since more concentrated solutions are irritating to the gastric mucosa. The intravenous dose is variable, but as a rough approximation 10 ml of a 10 per cent solution of calcium gluconate per square meter may be given intravenously slowly over a 20 minute period to a patient with hypocalcemia and convulsions. If there is no immediate response, the dose may be repeated twice or three times in the first hour. In newborn full-term infants with hypocalcemic tetany it is sometimes necessary to give as much as 10 ml of 10 per cent calcium gluconate over a period of 30 minutes. For premature infants 5 ml will usually be adequate. Once the convulsions are controlled, medication with oral calcium should be started. It should be remembered that calcium chloride is an "acidifying" salt, and serum pH or bicarbonate concentration should be carefully checked if this agent is administered over more than 24 hours. Because calcium, given by rapid injection, may cause cardiac arrest, it must be administered very slowly intravenously (10 ml over 5 minutes), and during its injection the heart rates should be checked and the injection stopped if the heart rate slows by more than 10 beats per minute. Most patients who suffer convulsions during intravenous therapy for diarrhea are not helped by administration of intravenous calcium. In many patients the cause of the convulsions is never determined. Water intoxication with cerebral edema may possibly be the most frequent cause. "Maintenance" quantities of calcium may be added to the fluids administered over 12 or 24 hours (300 mg elemental calcium per square meter of body surface per day).

Magnesium Deficiency

Magnesium deficiency of sufficient degree to require therapy is rarely encountered in pediatric practice. Excessive loss of magnesium occurs in chronic diarrhea, treatment of heart failure with diuretics, certain types of chronic renal disease, diabetic acidosis, primary aldosteronism, and hyperparathyroidism. The symptoms include tremor, incoordination, tetany, convulsions, and stupor. The diagnosis may be made if the level is below 1 mEq per liter in the serum. Treatment consists in administration of 1 to 2 mEq of magnesium per kg of body weight per 24 hours.

Phosphorus Deficiency

Phosphorus deficiency may occur in diabetic acidosis, diarrhea, and other conditions. If phosphorus deficiency is severe, replacement of 1 to 2 mmol of phosphate per kg per day may be undertaken.

Rate of Administration

In case the patient is moribund and in a state of unresponsive collapse, the initial fluid should be composed of isotonic saline, plasma, albumin solution, or blood. The primary objective here is to restore circulating blood volume. This can be done only with saline, blood, or plasma; dextrose solution is relatively inefficient.

If saline or plasma is used, 20 to 30 ml per kg is injected over the first hour. At the end of this time, the rate of administration is changed to the usual rate previously described. (Blood, 10 to 20 ml per kg, should be reserved for patients with anemia and collapse, or surgical shock.)

If the patient is not in imminent danger of collapse or shock, the daily dose of intravenous fluids is divided into 4 aliquots and each of these is administered over 6 hours. Others prefer to give half the day's dose of fluids in the first 8 hours.

Diagnosis of Dehydration

Clinical Diagnosis. Loss of skin turgor, sunken eyes, and depressed fontanelle are signs of dehydration. The skin is sometimes doughy in hypernatremic dehydration. Dryness of the mucous membranes is an unreliable sign.

Laboratory Aid. The blood urea nitrogen (BUN) or nonprotein nitrogen (NPN) content of the plasma may be a rough index of the degree of dehydration. An increase in concentration occurs in renal disease, in dehydration (prerenal azotemia), and in massive gastrointestinal hemorrhage. If increased concentration is due to dehydration, the level will fall to normal when fluid loss is replaced (usually within 48 hours). In the first year of life, the upper limit of normal of BUN is 24 mg per 100 ml and of NPN 40 mg per 100 ml. Elevation of the concentration of plasma protein and red cell count are unreliable signs of dehydration in the first years of life because the "normal" levels of hemoglobin or protein concentration undergo fluctuation during this period. The plasma sodium may be increased, normal, or low, depending on the relative losses of sodium and water from the body. The majority of patients with dehydration, however, have normal levels of serum sodium (134 to 148 mEq per liter). In the presence of metabolic acidosis, the plasma bicarbonate level falls and the chloride level rises (this also occurs in respiratory alkalosis, a rare syndrome in pediatric practice.)

Examples of Fluid Therapy

The following examples of application of these principles will be discussed. The examples are illustrations of typical problems occurring in pediatric practice.

1. A newborn with a tracheoesophageal fistula.
2. A 4-week-old child with pyloric stenosis.
3. An infant aged 5 months with diarrheal disease.
4. A child aged 5 years with acute renal failure.
5. A child aged 8 years with diabetic ketoacidosis.

EXAMPLE 1: A NEWBORN INFANT WITH TRACHEOESOPHAGEAL FISTULA (weight 2.5 kg., surface area (SA) 0.2 sq meter). The infant will be fed entirely by vein until feedings by gastrostomy are begun (or until oral feeding is possible). The infant's requirements per sq meter are 20 mEq Na (130 ml saline), 15 mEq K, and 800 ml water. The daily fluids are:

26 ml	0.9 per cent saline
1 ml	3 mEq per ml KCl
133 ml	5 per cent dextrose in water
160 ml	per 24 hours

i.e., 6.0 ml per hour.

When gastric feedings are begun, their volume is subtracted from this amount. For example, if half an ounce (15 ml) of milk formula is given every 6 hours (60 ml per day), then only 100 ml should be given by vein. This rate is usually too slow to be maintained for continuous flow, but at the end of the first week the total fluid requirement is increased to 300 ml per 24 hours.

EXAMPLE 2: A 3-WEEK-OLD INFANT WITH PYLORIC STENOSIS (weight 5 kg, SA 0.3 sq meter) in a state of moderate dehydration. Because there are abnormal losses from the gastrointestinal tract, potassium deficiency is assumed to exist.

Replacement
5 per cent body weight	250 ml saline
Potassium (5 mEq per kg)	8 ml KCl solution (24 mEq)

Maintenance:
330 ml saline per sq meter	100 ml saline
Total water (2000 ml per sq meter)	500 ml 5 per cent dextrose (600 to 100 ml)
Total	860 ml

One quarter (90 ml saline, 120 ml dextrose, no potassium) is administered over the first 6 hours at 36 ml per hour. The rest (including potassium) is given over the next 18 hours. Surgical intervention is usually possible after 24 hours or less of such therapy but may be delayed longer if the infant's condition is not considered satisfactory for surgery.

On the second day, if hydration is adequate, only maintenance amounts need be given (100 ml saline, 4 ml KCl, and 500 ml 5 per cent dextrose). If there still is evidence of dehydration, additional saline equivalent to 2.5 to 5 per cent of the body weight is given, depending on whether the dehydration is mild or moderate.

Alkalosis is usually present in these patients, partly because of the loss of acid in the vomitus and partly because of the potassium deficiency. However, it is not necessary to give "acid producing salts" such as ammonium chloride. When oral feedings are begun, intravenous therapy is reduced by an equal amount; e.g., if daily requirement is estimated at 600 ml and 6 ounces (180 ml) of milk is ingested, only 420 ml need be given by vein.

EXAMPLE 3: AN INFANT AGED 3 MONTHS WITH ACUTE DIARRHEAL DISEASE (weight 7.5 kg, SA 0.4 sq meter) with severe dehydration. Loss of fluid is assumed to be 15 per cent. In first 24 hours plan to replace 7.5 per cent body weight plus maintenance.

First 24 hours: *Replacement* 7.5 per cent body weight or 560 ml saline.

Bicarbonate replacement	$7.5 \times 6.6 =$	50 ml
	7.5 per cent bicarbonate	
Adjusted saline figure		260 ml
5 per cent dextrose in water		
to make up volume		250 ml
Potassium (5 mEq/kg)		5 ml
		565 ml

One fourth of this is given every 6 hours. Potassium is omitted from the intravenous fluids until urine flow is established. This usually happens after 6 hours. The entire dose of potassium is administered over the last 18 hours.

Note: It must be emphasized that in this example, as in all fluid therapy, the initial calculations described above represent only the initial estimate of the days' fluid orders. The patient is to be examined frequently and samples of blood obtained at appropriate times to measure serum electrolytes. The fluid orders must be changed if too much or too little of any of the constituents of intravenous fluids are being administered.

Second 24 hours: If the diarrhea ends and the patient is adequately hydrated, he may require only "maintenance" amounts. If the diarrhea continues unabated, fluid therapy on the second day will resemble that on the first day. Between these two extremes will fall the majority of patients who will need 2.5 to 5 per cent of body weight as saline, and potassium in addition to "maintenance" water and sodium. When fluids are given by mouth their volume is subtracted from the total amount and the rest given by vein. If there is no diarrhea or vomiting, fluids given by mouth or vein have equal value at this time. An estimate of the volume of stool loss can be obtained by weighing the diapers first dry and then containing the stool.

EXAMPLE 4: A CHILD AGED 5 YEARS WITH ACUTE RENAL FAILURE (weight 20 kg, SA 0.75 sq meter). The approach to treatment is governed by the cardinal principles that (1) nothing can be done to hasten healing of the necrotic renal tissue and (2) death is hastened by administering too much fluid, thus overloading the circulation and inducing circulatory failure.

The normal urine output is equal to about half the water requirement; i.e., 1000 ml per sq meter per 24 hours. Oliguria is arbitrarily defined as a urine output of less than 200 ml per square meter per 24 hours. When the patient is admitted, however, it may not be clear whether the anuria is due to dehydration or renal failure. Under these conditions, it may be necessary to administer fluid intravenously to determine if the oliguria is caused by acute renal failure. One third of the daily requirement (550 ml made up of 1 part saline to 4 parts dextrose) is given intravenously over 4 hours. At the end of this time if oliguria persists, no more fluids are given for the rest of the first day. If this test does not provide a clear-cut answer as to whether the oliguria is caused by acute renal failure, mannitol (1.0 gram per kg of a 20 per cent solution) may be infused intravenously over a 20 minute interval. If urine flow is not established (10 to 15 ml per gram of mannitol over the next 4 hours) after injection of the volume of fluid previously mentioned, it is advisable to treat the patient as suffering from acute renal failure.

The daily fluid therapy is limited to replacement of insensible losses (500 ml per sq meter). Ten mEq of sodium bicarbonate is included as part of this total. Bicarbonate should be given from the beginning in order to anticipate the invariably developing acidosis. The remaining fluids (440 ml) may be given as 5 or 10 per cent dextrose.

A quantity equal to the urine flow is added to the previously mentioned solution. One third of this volume is given as lactate and the rest as dextrose in water. Potassium administration is contraindicated. Calcium gluconate may be given intravenously if hypocalcemia develops.

Peritoneal dialysis or hemodialysis may be necessary if urine flow is not established and if the clinical condition deteriorates.

When urine flow increases during recovery it will be necessary to increase intake to keep pace with output. The urine volume for the previous day is added to calculated insensible loss. The total amount administered in 1 day generally should not exceed 2500 ml per sq meter. The amount of sodium given should be determined by the amounts excreted in the urine over the previous day. It should be given as sodium bicarbonate until the plasma CO_2 exceeds 20 mEq per liter.

EXAMPLE 5: DIABETIC ACIDOSIS AND MODERATE DEHYDRATION in a child weighing 30 kg (SA 1 sq meter). *Insulin*: This may be given as regular insulin immediately in the amount of *2 units per kg* of body weight. It may also be given as a constant infusion. After a loading dose of 0.1 to 0.25 unit per kg, 0.1 unit per kg per hour is infused intravenously. The subsequent dosage of insulin varies with the clinical response of the patient.

Replacement fluid therapy:

5 per cent body weight	1500 ml saline
Sodium bicarbonate 6.6 ml/kg	200 ml
	7.5 per cent bicarbonate
Adjusted saline figure	
(0.9 per cent)	900 ml
Water to make up volume	400 ml
Potassium (5 mEq/kg)	50 ml

(Potassium solution is made up of 4 parts potassium chloride, 1 part potassium phosphate)

Maintenance fluid therapy:

Saline (0.9 per cent),	
330 ml per sq meter	330 ml
5 per cent dextrose to final volume of	
2000 ml,	1670 ml

The intravenous fluids may be divided into two portions, one containing bicarbonate, saline, water, potassium chloride, and potassium phosphate. The other contains all the 5 per cent dextrose mixed with saline to a concentration of 75 mEq per liter. Administration of bicarbonate to patients in diabetic ketosis is considered undesirable by many because of untoward responses, including induction of paradoxical acidosis in the cerebrospinal fluid. It is my practice to administer bicarbonate if the serum bicarbonate level is less than 15 mEq per liter at the time the patient is first seen. The total calculated for the day is about 3500 ml. Half of this is given over the first 12 hours. Potassium is given from the beginning because severe potassium deficiency develops rapidly in children who generally do not yet have evidence of renal disease. Because hyperglycemia is present, glucose solutions should not be administered at the beginning. Blood glucose and serum electrolytes should be measured every 2 to 4 hours, and when the blood sugar falls below 250 mg per dl (100 ml) the rate of insulin infusion is slowed down and glucose solutions are administered until the blood glucose concentration is stabilized.

NOTES

Premature Infants

The fluid requirements of premature and full-term infants are the same per sq meter. Until the premature weighs more than 5 pounds, however, his sodium requirement is best considered as only 30 mEq per sq meter. This is because hypoproteinemia is frequent in prematures, and there is therefore a greater tendency for edema formation with sodium retention. It appears that prematures can handle injected potassium with reasonable facility.

Body Temperature Changes

For every degree (centigrade) of temperature lowering, the body requires about 10 per cent less fluid, and in patients for whom extreme hypothermia is being used the fluid requirements should be lowered accordingly. In prolonged hyperthermia, fluid requirements should be increased by the same amount. In general, fluctuations of temperature of less than ±2 C need not be taken into account in calculating the fluid replacement.

In experimental animals hypothermia induces a sodium diuresis. In human subjects, diuresis may occur without increased excretion of water. Because there is considerable individual variation from patient to patient, the amount of sodium which could be administered must be determined by measurement of its loss in the urine over 12 or 24 hours. The amount of sodium lost in the urine should be replaced over the next period.

Hypernatremia

Hypernatremia is found in approximately 25 per cent of all patients with acute diarrhea in infancy. It may also occur in chronic renal disease and primary aldosteronism. In acute diarrheal disease, hypernatremia may be suspected if the skin is warm and dry, rather than cold and moist as frequently occurs when the serum sodium is normal or reduced. The skin is often doughy. In addition, nuchal rigidity and a positive Kernig sign are frequently present. The spinal fluid is usually under increased pressure and often contains increased amounts of protein. The cell count is often normal. Extreme irritability, restlessness, and convulsions are frequent in this type of dehydration.

When dehydration is accompanied by hypernatremia, it is usually unnecessary to change the previously outlined scheme of therapy. These patients usually have some deficit in total body sodium, and it has been shown that administration of sodium-free solutions to these patients may aggravate their condition by lowering the serum sodium too rapidly. The scheme of therapy suggested here recommends the administration of hypotonic solutions with respect to sodium. With mild dehydration the concentration of sodium in administered solutions is usually about 30 mEq per liter. In moderate dehydration it is usually about 50 mEq per liter. It is recommended, however, that the concentration of sodium in the fluids used for subjects with hypernatremic dehydration should never exceed 50 mEq per liter.

Hyponatremia

If the serum sodium is below 125 mEq per liter, rapid correction of the concentration is sometimes required. In acute diarrhea this is usually not necessary, because the serum sodium concentration will increase gradually with usual therapy. In certain acute dilutional syndromes in the absence of dehydration, it may be necessary to correct the sodium concentration more rapidly. Under these circumstances the following calculations are made. It is assumed that the volume of distribution of freely exchangeable sodium is equivalent to the total body water because of osmotic movement of water from within the cells following injection of sodium. It is also considered unwise to correct the serum sodium by more than 10 mEq per liter in one dose. Thus, if the serum sodium is 115 mEq per liter, it is preferable to attempt to correct to 125 mEq per liter over 6 hours. Subsequently, the rest of the correction may be made. In the case of an infant weighing 10 kg whose serum sodium is 115 mEq per liter, the volume of the total body water is 60 per cent or 6 liters. The amount of sodium injected will be $10 \times 6 = 60$ mEq. This is given in a hypertonic solution, e.g., 5 per cent sodium chloride, which contains 900 mEq sodium per liter or approximately 1 mEq per ml. This can be run in over 6 hours in addition to the other fluids being given.

Additional Notes on Surgical Applications

Fluid therapy in surgical patients is generally governed by the same principles applicable to nonsurgical patients. Preoperative and postoperative fluid therapy will depend on an estimate of the deficits incurred and anticipated. The management of an infant with tracheoesophageal fistula (example No. 1) will afford an example of how most surgical conditions can be treated in the first week of life. In older children (example No. 2) treatment of pyloric stenosis may be used as a model for the preoperative treatment of dehydration. Notes on the requirements of premature infants for fluid are given above, and the use of various types of solutions are covered in various parts of the scheme presented.

Because there is evidence that the stress of surgical procedures results in antidiuresis and retention of sodium, it is recommended that the amount of sodium administered to the patient be half that recommended in other situations, i.e., in the first 24 hours postoperatively, 25 mEq per sq meter per 24 hours. Although urine losses of water are diminished, losses by other routes such as the skin may be exaggerated during the surgical procedure, and it is, therefore, advisable not to reduce the total amount of water administered in the postoperative period. The amount of potassium administered should also be reduced by half. In the second 24 hours postoperatively, the usual amounts of sodium, potassium, and water should be administered.

The concentration of sodium and chloride in fluid from nasogastric decompression varies markedly, but is generally approximately half that in the serum, i.e., approximately 70 mEq of sodium and 70 mEq of chloride per liter. The concentrations of sodium and chloride in small bowel fluid are approximately 125 mEq per liter each. The concentration of potassium in practically all gastrointestinal secretions is between 3 and 20 mEq per liter, and an average value of 10 mEq per liter may be taken as a working guide. It is preferable, wherever possible, to measure concentrations of electrolytes in gastrointestinal secretions.

Burns

The amount of fluid given depends on the percentage of the body surface having a third degree burn. The percentages of surface of the body which each part makes up are shown in Table 1. In the treatment of burns, the surface area rule is applicable to children, i.e., 1 ml each of electrolyte solution per per cent burn per kg per 24 hours. In addition to this, it is important that maintenance fluids as recommended be administered. These can conveniently be calculated as 2000 ml of water and 50 mEq of sodium per sq meter per 24 hours. Because of tissue destruction and liberation of potassium, it is advisable that potassium not be given in the first 3 days of treatment of a burn. On the second day, it is advisable to give approximately half the volume of the electrolyte solutions but not to change the quantity of maintenance fluids being infused. On the third day the maintenance fluids remain the same in volume and quantity, but the electrolyte solutions should be reduced to one third. This is only a general rule, and the clinical condition of the patient must serve as a guide for the therapy used. One of the most satisfactory measurements which may be used as a guide is the volume of urine excreted. A simple rule for estimating the normal volume of urine excreted is that approximately 50 to 70 per cent of the ingested fluid is excreted as urine. An average volume of 1000 ml per sq meter per 24 hours may be used as the normal rate of urine excretion; thus, an attempt should be made to keep the urine volume at a level at least half of this.

Treatment must be geared to the patient's response, however, and adjusted according to the degree of shock, hematocrit, and reduction in urine volume. One of the dangers not to be overlooked is overtreatment. In any case, no more fluid should ever be given than that calculated for a 50 per cent burn. For example, if a patient has a 60 per cent or 70 per cent burn, he would still receive only the amount of fluid calculated for a 50 per cent burn.

SECTION 7

The Endocrine System

ACROMEGALY*

method of
JOHN A. LINFOOT, M.D.
Berkeley, California

Acromegaly and gigantism represent multisystem diseases resulting from either a primary pituitary tumor or an ill-defined hypothalamohypophyseal dysfunction causing somatotropic cell hyperplasia and tumor formation. Clinical manifestations of the disease result from three major processes: (1) excessive growth hormone (HGH) secretion, (2) deficiencies of other pituitary tropic hormones, and (3) local invasion of parasellar neural and vascular structures.

Treatment Evaluation of Acromegaly

Immunoreactive HGH level is elevated and tumors can be demonstrated in a majority of the patients. Recent studies suggest that abnormalities of the hypothalamohypophyseal axis exist in many acromegalic patients and the overproduction of HGH could be due to excessive hypothalamic stimulation or a deficiency of HGH release inhibiting factor(s), such as somatostatin. Although somatostatin has been characterized and synthesized, neither this tetradecapeptide nor an HGH releasing factor has been clearly implicated as a causal factor in acromegaly or gigantism.

In the typical pathologic literature, acromegaly and gigantism have been classified as diseases resulting from tumors that have eosinophilic or chromophobic staining properties with standard hematoxylin and eosin stains. It is only recently that more complex histologic charac-

*This work was supported by the Biology and Medicine Division of the United States Department of Energy.

teristics of pituitary tumors have been recognized. The availability of the electron microscope and specific immunohistologic staining with immunoperoxidase and related techniques have provided a more precise characterization and classification of pituitary tumors. Using these techniques, Kovacs, Horvath, and Ezrin have classified pituitary tumors associated with acromegaly into eosinophilic stem cell, somatotropin cell, and mixed somatotropin–prolactin cell adenomas. Since most so-called chromophobic cells can be demonstrated to contain specific hormone-containing granules, the traditional light microscopic classification of eosinophilic, basophilic, and chromophobic tumors should be abandoned.

It is noteworthy that in approximately 40 per cent of our acromegalic patients, coexisting hyperprolactinemia and hypersomatotropinism have been demonstrated. The significance of this hyperprolactinemia in acromegaly is complex. Hyperprolactinemia may result from the presence of mixed adenomas, from a separate adenoma, or from suppression of the prolactin inhibiting factor (PIF) by an invasive pituitary adenoma. The recognition of the coexistence of separate HGH and prolactin secretion in patients with acromegaly is important, since removal of two separate adenomas may be required to achieve the optimal treatment.

Acromegaly and gigantism are associated with a variety of complications. The disease is not only disfiguring but ultimately may cause physical impairment because of joint and other musculoskeletal abnormalities. It has also been estimated to shorten life by approximately 10 years.

Treatment

Surgical Treatment. Frontal transcranial hypophysectomy, which at one time was the common surgical approach to pituitary tumors, is

509

now limited primarily to those rare tumors with large suprasellar extensions that cannot be decompressed by the transsphenoidal route. Transsphenoidal microsurgery, developed by Guiot in Paris and revolutionized by Jules Hardy in Montreal with the operating microscope, has largely replaced craniotomy. This delicate procedure provides better visualization of the pituitary and facilitates selective tumor removal (microadenectomy). The reduced morbidity and low mortality rates have established it as the procedure of choice for the surgical treatment of pituitary tumors.

Cryogenic hypophysectomy, developed by Rand, has been used effectively in the control of acromegaly. The limitations of this procedure are (1) difficulty in adequate cryogenic destruction in the large invasive tumors, and (2) technical problems, which include the necessity of conducting the procedure in the sedated but conscious patient. Its primary role now appears to be in conjunction with translabial transsphenoidal operation for recurrent tumor and cryogenic destruction of residual tumor tissue under direct vision with the binocular operating microscope.

Radiofrequency thermal coagulation, developed by Zervas, has a similar role in acromegaly. The thermal probe is more easily controlled than the cryogenic probe, and the thermal lesion is more evenly distributed throughout a large pituitary fossa.

Both procedures are highly effective for total therapeutic hypophysectomy in metastatic mammary carcinoma and diabetic retinopathy. Their use in acromegaly should be limited to patients selected for total pituitary ablation and performed by operators who have extensive experience with these procedures.

The indications, limitations, and complications of translabial transsphenoidal microsurgery require additional amplification. Surgical exposure of tumor tissue and its physical separation from the normal pituitary gland is a direct, selective, and specific form of therapy. Pressure on adjacent tissues is promptly relieved, and within minutes blood levels of HGH drop to the normal range. However, total effectiveness of this operative approach is determined by the tumor size and extension into the surrounding intrasellar and parasellar structures. Anatomic classification as suggested by Hardy is essential in predicting the outcome of surgery. Microadenomas that measure 10 mm or less in diameter (Grade I tumors) and larger, enclosed, noninvasive (Grade II) tumors without suprasellar extension can be treated with high degrees of success by an experienced neurosurgeon. Total operative removal of these tumors is the treatment of choice when

prompt lowering of HGH is desired. Because delayed fall in circulating blood levels occurs after irradiation therapy, selective microsurgical adenectomy may also have a particular advantage in younger patients. The incidence of hypopituitarism is generally low, although there are insufficient long-term data on the incidence of post-treatment hypopituitarism following transsphenoidal microsurgery. Transient diabetes insipidus does occur in a significant number of patients, but permanent diabetes insipidus is uncommon. Minor local complications of surgery include perforation of the nasal septum, numbness of the upper lip, and, rarely, dental disturbances.

Contraindications for the transsphenoidal procedure include the presence of the empty sella syndrome (because of potential difficulty with cerebrospinal fluid rhinorrhea), anomalous dural venous sinuses (which could lead to uncontrollable hemorrhage), coexistent intrasellar aneurysms, and, rarely, buckling or other anomalies of the carotid arteries.

Patients with high HGH levels (greater than 100 nanograms per ml) and those patients with large invasive tumors (Grades III and IV of Hardy) are infrequently cured by surgical procedures. These tumors often extend suprasellarly (may or may not involve the optic chiasm), inferiorly into the sphenoid sinus, laterally into the cavernous sinus, and, rarely, posteriorly into the clivus. In our experience, a combined surgical and irradiation approach improves the results of treatment in these difficult conditions. Combined therapy should include extensive surgical reduction of tumor mass, placement of clips on the diaphragma sellae as a landmark, and definition of the residual tumor in a detailed descriptive operative note. A postoperative pneumoencephalogram (PEG) using hypocycloidal polytomography to localize the optic chiasm and to define an empty sella and other unsuspected landmarks will assist in the accurate and effective delivery of alpha particle or proton beam irradiation. If the residual tumor lesion is massive, photon therapy should be employed.

Use of yttrium (^{90}Y) or gold (^{198}Au) radioactive implantation has been used successfully at several centers in Europe. The experience at Hammersmith Hospital in London by Joplin and his coworkers demonstrate this to be an effective procedure in the majority of cases of acromegaly. Similar experience has been reported in France and Italy. In the United States, these procedures were never widely used, and as a result of less experience, complications (e.g., cerebrospinal fluid rhinorrhea, extraocular palsy) occurred. These procedures were replaced by cryogenic and thermocautery techniques before introduction of the transsphenoidal microsurgery procedure.

Radiation Therapy. PHOTON THERAPY. Photon therapy with high-kilovolt (kv) x-rays have been used in the treatment of acromegaly with varying degrees of success for many years. More recently, radiation therapy with photon (x-rays and gamma rays) from ^{60}cobalt or linear accelerators has been used in the treatment of pituitary tumors. Early photon therapy studies frequently showed persistently elevated HGH in most patients; permanent control of HGH secretion, however, was uncommon.

Currently, photon therapy appears to control tumor growth with reasonable effectiveness in acromegaly. A fall in HGH has been observed in patients treated with photon therapy, although the rate of fall is delayed. Five to 10 years after photon therapy, a substantial number of patients have HGH ≤10 nanograms per ml. Levels <5 nanograms per ml are unusual in our experience. It should be emphasized, however, that clinical improvement such as disappearance of headaches, decreased sweating, and improved energy may occur before HGH levels are substantially lowered. Although the data are less clear in acromegaly, tumor recurrence with combined surgical and photon therapy is probably reduced, much as it has been reported for nonfunctioning (chromophobe) tumors.

Complications of radiation therapy (Table 1) are infrequent and are related to the type and size of the radiation field (isodose curve), total

TABLE 1. **Complications of Treatment for Acromegaly**

A. Surgery
  1. Anesthesia and surgical
  2. Hemorrhage
  3. CSF leak
  4. Meningitis
  5. Diabetes insipidus
  6. Hypopituitarism
  7. Cranial nerve damage
  8. Empty sella syndrome
B. Radiation
  1. Epilation (photon therapy only)
  2. Postirradiation necrosis
    a. Extraocular motor nerve
    b. Optic chiasm
    c. Temporal lobe
    d. Empty sella syndrome
    e. Hypopituitarism
C. Pharmacologic
  1. Variable and often incomplete HGH suppression
  2. Failure to have a consistent and clear-cut effect on tumor growth
  3. Rapid rise of HGH to pretreatment levels after discontinuation of medication
  4. Drug reaction

dose, duration of therapy, and dose delivered per fraction. During the mid-1960s and early 1970s, there was a trend toward increasing the total dose and the rate per fraction with the idea that therapy could be improved. With doses of 5000 to 6000 rads the effect on tumor growth and hypersecretion was apparently improved; however, there was a slight but significant increase in complications of radiation, e.g., postirradiation necrosis of the parasellar structures. Minor complications of photon therapy include epilation of the scalp and occasionally mild headache. Acute tumor swelling caused by infarction and hemorrhage into the tumor rarely occurs.

In the past few years there has been a trend to reduce the total radiation dose as well as the dose per fraction. The effects of these modifications are uncertain, but we might anticipate that the results of treatment may be substantially different from those observed with higher doses. Several years of follow-up will be required to observe the effects of these changes. A knowledge of the experience and the current treatment program employed by the radiotherapist is essential, since photon therapy is not conducted in the same fashion in all centers.

HEAVY PARTICLE THERAPY. Currently, 910 Mev alpha particles (helium ions) from the 184 inch synchrocyclotron are used in the treatment of acromegaly, Cushing's disease, and prolactin-secreting and nonfunctioning pituitary tumors at the Lawrence Berkeley Laboratory in California. The Berkeley facility has employed a multiplane rotational technique using the plateau portion of the helium ion beam. This dosimetry provides an isodose curve that fits the contour of the pituitary gland and significantly lowers the radiation dose in the coronal plane, sparing the optic chiasm, hypothalamus, and other parasellar structures. The patient's head is immobilized with a clear plastic mask, and doses of 3500 to 7500 rads are delivered in 4 fractions on consecutive days. Bragg peak therapy, with alpha particles has been limited to a few patients with massive tumors.

In 1963 the Neurosurgical Department at the Massachusetts General Hospital, under the leadership of Dr. Raymond Kjellberg, initiated a heavy particle procedure employing protons. Because of the lower particle energy from the Harvard cyclotron, this treatment exclusively employes the Bragg peak. A stereotaxic headholder is employed, and treatment with doses from 3000 to 12,000 rads is delivered in a single sitting using 6 to 12 radiation ports. The higher energy, greater biologic effect, and precision of localization, as well as the stopping properties and dense ionization, of the Bragg peak provide advantages of heavy ions over conventional photon therapy.

Over 800 patients with acromegaly or gigantism have been treated with heavy particles at these two institutions.

Three hundered and five patients with acromegaly have been treated with alpha particle pituitary irradiation (APPI). This treatment program provides abundant clinical data and can now serve as a treatment model for the management of acromegaly by other modalities. A large number of patients have had consistent follow-up over an extended period of time (>20 years), so that both acute and long-term effects of treatment have been determined. The selection criteria developed for patients treated with APPI are shown in Table 2. Ninety per cent of patients achieve normal fasting HGH levels within 5 to 6 years after treatment. A fall of 50 to 60 per cent typically occurs in the first year, which is often associated with striking clinical and metabolic improvement (see Table 3), such as improved glucose tolerance, loss of insulin resistance, and a fall in elevated serum phosphorus levels. These metabolic improvements are usually seen before the HGH levels fall to less than 10 nanograms per ml. More striking improvement is observed when HGH falls to ≤5 nanograms per ml. Ultimately, in most patients, there is normalization of the paradoxic responses to thyrotropin-releasing hormone (TRH) and other stimuli and in many, return of normal suppressibility of glucose stimulation.

Soft tissue changes occur in essentially all patients, the degree of which depends on the duration and the severity of acromegaly. The bony changes regress much more subtly and are generally appreciated by careful examination of x-rays for remineralization of the sella and widening of the thickened metacarpal spaces on x-rays of the hand. The rapidity and ultimate result of treatment is related to the size of the tumor. Patients with microadenomas (Grade I tumors) have rapid normalization of HGH levels

TABLE 2. **Selection Criteria for Alpha Particle Pituitary Irradiation**

1. Presence of a confirmed functioning or nonfunctioning pituitary tumor
2. No prior therapeutic irradiation to the pituitary or parasellar lesions
3. Total tumor mass ≤2.0 cm in maximal diameter
4. Suprasellar extension <4 mm
5. Adequate definition of tumor in large sphenoidal extensions
6. Adequate definition of tumor and normal anatomic landmarks in postsurgical patients

TABLE 3. **Desired End Points of Treatment for Acromegaly**

A. Physical findings
 1. Cessation of acral growth
 2. Cessation of hyperhidrosis and skin tag (fibroma) formation
 3. Soft tissue regression
 4. Improvement in fatigue and lethargy
 5. Stable visual fields and neuro-ophthalmologic examination
B. X-ray findings
 1. Lack of erosion or expansion of sella
 2. Remineralization of sella
 3. Remineralization of metacarpal medullary space
 4. Stabilization and variable regression of heel pad and other soft tissue thickening
C. Metabolic
 1. Improvement of diabetic state and/or glucose tolerance
 2. Loss of insulin resistance
 3. Fall in elevated serum phosphorus level
D. Growth hormone
 1. Fasting HGH ≤10 nanograms/ml, preferably ≤5 nanograms/ml
 2. Absent paradoxic rise to thyroid releasing hormone (TRH) stimulation
 3. Partial return of suppressibility to glucose stimulation
 4. Normal serum somatomedin levels

after APPI within 12 to 24 months. Relapse is extremely unusual in these patients. The HGH response in Grade II tumor patients after APPI parallels the microadenoma response, but tends to be delayed. The invasive tumors, which usually have higher HGH levels, represent difficult therapeutic geometry and have a less favorable prognosis for cure. If the lesion is incompletely defined radiographically, inadequate HGH response or therapeutic failure will result. APPI appears to be the more effective treatment of invasive lesions if the tumor mass can be accurately defined. Combined surgery and irradiation often is the optimal treatment in many of these difficult cases. A review of 65 patients with invasive lesions who have had previous transfrontal, transsphenoidal, and/or cryogenic surgery showed a slower but parallel fall in HGH levels compared to patients treated de novo with APPI. Patients with massive invasive lesions are probably better treated with photon therapy or proton or alpha particle Bragg peak therapy, since the biplanar rotational technique is less satisfactory when large radiation fields are required.

Analysis of endocrine side effects in the acromegalic patients reveals that about 34 per cent of the patients required adrenal or thyroid replacement 6 to 10 years after APPI. Lesser numbers of patients required gonadal steroid hormone replacement. These figures appear comparable to or less than those observed with photon therapy and greater than those reported for transsphenoidal microsurgery.

The complications of therapy are given in Table 1. Neural complications of APPI were limited to six patients who were treated prior to 1961 after unsuccessful photon therapy (large Grade III and Grade IV tumors). These complications included partial third nerve lesions and temporal lobe epilepsy, which was controlled easily with anticonvulsant therapy. Because of these early complications, patients who have received prior photon therapy have not been accepted since 1961. Patients who have received ≥4000 rads of photon therapy within 2 years likewise are not accepted for proton beam therapy.

Pharmacologic Therapy. Logically somatostatin should hold great promise as a therapeutic agent in acromegaly. Control of HGH secretion with somatostatin has been limited by the lack of a sufficiently long-acting derivative of somatostatin and the transient HGH suppressive action following somatostatin injections. Potential side effects from the suppression of other hormones (e.g., insulin, glucagon, gastrin) as well as a possible effect on hemostatic processes have also limited the ultimate pharmacologic usefulness of this potent peptide.

Although a number of pharmacologic agents have been shown to lower HGH in acromegaly, most of these agents have only transient and unpredictable effects. Glucocorticoids (C-21 steroids) are potent suppressors of HGH, but the doses required produce significant side effects. The importance in recognizing the effects of pharmacologic doses of glucocorticoids lies in the interpretation of a serum HGH level in the postoperative (hypoxic) patient who is still receiving large doses of steroid following surgery. Measurements of HGH levels should be deferred until the patient's therapy has been tapered to physiologic maintenance doses of glucocorticoids. Medroxyprogesterone is the C-21 steroid that has been most widely used. Unfortunately, extensive use of medroxyprogesterone has shown that in many patients HGH secretion is not consistently suppressed, and most patients either fail to respond or ultimately escape control by the drug. Estrogens antagonize the peripheral effects of HGH, including the generation of somatomedin. They have a limited role for short-term management in some patients because of menorrhagia and endometrial hyperplasia. Chlorpromazine (Thorazine) has even less value in the treatment of acromegaly. None of these agents has an important pharmacologic role at the present time.

Currently, the only medication for acromegaly that offers any promise is bromocriptine. Bromocriptine is a long-acting dopamine agonist that causes a paradoxic fall of growth hormone level in most acromegalic patients, whereas in normal subjects either a rise in basal plasma growth hormone levels or an augmented HGH release during stimulation tests is observed. Long-term studies with bromocriptine have been limited, but in general responses to bromocriptine can be predicted if a 55 per cent or greater fall in basal HGH level occurs after a single 2.5 mg oral dose. Since the effect of a single dose lasts 6 to 8 hours, daily treatment with three to four divided doses is usually required. The total dose normally ranges between 7.5 and a maximum of 30 mg per day. Intolerance to bromocriptine develops in some patients, and rapid rebound to pretreatment levels occurs upon discontinuation of medication. Side effects include nausea, postural hypotension, blanching of the fingers, and mild constipation. Since there is no certain effect on tumor growth, current use should be restricted to elderly, symptomatic patients who are not suitable candidates for surgery or as adjunctive therapy in patients who have undergone unsuccessful surgical hypophysectomy or radiation therapy. Its most important role probably will be a temporary measure in patients subjected to alpha particle or proton beam therapy while awaiting the full effects of the treatment. It should be emphasized that bromocriptine has not been released for the treatment of acromegaly in the United States; the data cited were based on studies from Europe and Asia.

Summary

In order to select a therapy for the patient (see Table 4), the physician must be aware of the therapeutic goals (see Table 5) and weigh the side effects and complications against the ultimate success in achieving hormonal as well as tumor control. It is clear that patients with microadenomas can be satisfactorily managed with either surgery or radiation therapy. Invasive lesions will reduce the likelihood of cure with transsphenoidal surgery, and primary heavy ion therapy or combined therapy, or both, will probably be required in more of these patients. With massive tumors, photon therapy may be used equally effectively. With better localization techniques of microadenomas within the sella, it is conceivable that complete tumor removal will be even more

TABLE 4. **Treatment of Acromegaly**

A. Surgical
   1. Transfrontal craniotomy
   2. Transsphenoidal microsurgery
   3. Cryogenic surgery
   4. Radiofrequency thermocoagulation
   5. Intrasellar implantation (^{90}Y, ^{198}Au)
B. Radiation
   1. Photon radiation, "conventional radiation"
     a. High voltage x-ray
     b. ^{60}Co
     c. Linear accelerator
   2. Heavy particle (Cyclotron)
     a. Alpha particle (Berkeley)
     b. Proton beam, Bragg peak (Boston)
   3. Stereotaxic radiosurgery (Stockholm)
C. Pharmacologic
   1. Bromocriptine
   2. Glucocorticoids
   3. Medroxyprogesterone
   4. Estrogens
   5. Chlorpromazine
D. Combined therapy
   1. Radiation and pharmacologic
   2. Multiple surgeries
   3. Surgery plus irradiation
     Heavy particle
     Photon
   4. Surgery and pharmacologic

expeditiously achieved and treatment failures limited to patients with pituitary hyperplasia or multiple (or mixed) adenomas. Better tumor localization by computed tomography (CT) scanning or heavy ion radiography will also facilitate the use of stereotaxic heavy ion radiation adenectomy, sparing the surrounding normal gland. Finally, neuroendocrine research should provide more potent and effective pharmacologic agents for the control of growth hormone secretion.

Because of the slow rate of tumor growth and the subtle endocrine symptoms of patients with partial or total hypopituitarism, all patients require annual evaluation of their current hormonal and tumor status for an indefinite period of time.

TABLE 5. **Therapeutic Goals in the Treatment of Acromegaly**

1. Permanent control of tumor growth
2. Permanent normalization of hormone hypersecretion
3. Minimal tropic hormonal side effects
4. Minimal CNS side effects
5. Minimal surgical and/or anesthetic morbidity and mortality

ADRENOCORTICAL INSUFFICIENCY

method of
ALFRED M. BONGIOVANNI, M.D.
Philadelphia, Pennsylvania

Adrenocortical insufficiency is usually the result of a gradual destruction of functioning tissue caused by granulomatous, autoimmune, or other poorly understood processes. Therefore the clinical manifestations often develop gradually, and the diagnosis should be established before hormonal insufficiency is complete. In most forms both the glucocorticoids and mineralocorticoids are deficient.

Chronic Insufficiency

The treatment is relatively simple and the results gratifying. Cortisone acetate by mouth, 20 mg in the morning and 10 mg in the evening, affords good control. Alternatively prednisone, 7.5 mg and 5 mg, may be used. The latter has the advantage of a longer biologic half-life. Dexamethasone (Decadron) should not be used because of its unusually long half-life and its natriuretic action. In addition a mineralocorticoid is indicated. For this purpose 9-alpha-fluorocortisol acetate by mouth, 0.05 to 0.1 mg once daily, is adequate. The dosage of the latter may require individual adjustment and should be lowered if excessive salt and water retention or hypertension occurs.

In the face of intercurrent disease, such as severe respiratory infection, the dosage of cortisone acetate should be doubled. With illnesses such as severe gastroenteritis, or in any condition which precludes oral medication, intramuscular cortisone acetate, 50 mg daily, should be administered. The patient should be instructed in selfmanagement for such events. Sterile syringes and a small supply of parenteral cortisone acetate should be on hand. This last approach is also advisable in preparation for surgery, using 100 mg of cortisone acetate, and in the postsurgical management until the crisis has passed and oral medication is once more possible. In addition, intravenous hydrocortisone phosphate or hemisuccinate should be on hand in the operating room, but its use is not often required provided that a sufficient preoperative intramuscular dosage has been administered and provided that administration is continued daily until recovery. During the time that the patient is unable to accept oral fluids, 5 per cent dextrose in isotonic saline solution, 30 ml per kg of body weight daily, should be continuously administered and the serum electrolytes and blood glucose monitored. More fluid and/or plasma may be required if there is dehydration or unusual blood loss.

As a rule supplemental sodium chloride is not needed in the management of chronic insufficiency provided that the patient ingests a normal amount of salt according to his taste. It is advisable for the patient to wear a suitable identification tag with a notation such as "I have Addison's disease" or "I take cortisone — notify a physician." Appropriate therapy for concomitant disease such as tuberculosis or multiglandular deficiency should be employed.

Acute Insufficiency

Precipitous cardiovascular collapse may occur in unrecognized cases of chronic insufficiency (sometimes precipitated by stress), sudden withdrawal of steroid therapy employed for other conditions, adrenal hemorrhage (as in the Waterhouse-Friderichsen syndrome), or surgical removal of a functioning unilateral adrenocortical tumor. Rapid suitable treatment is most urgent.

Intravenous 5 per cent dextrose in isotonic saline solution should be started as soon as possible. Concomitantly 100 mg of hydrocortisone phosphate or hydrocortisone hemisuccinate should be injected intravenously over 3 minutes and 100 mg of cortisone acetate given intramuscularly. Within the first 24 hours approximately 65 ml per kg of body weight of the intravenous fluid should be given, half of this rapidly within the first 4 hours. After the first day, the intravenous fluid requirement is approximately 30 ml per kg. Usually by the second or third day the patient is able to take fluids by mouth. Cortisone acetate, 100 mg daily intramuscularly, should be continued daily until the patient is able to take the steroid by mouth, as discussed previously for chronic insufficiency. If there is intercurrent disease, such as pneumonia, the oral dosage should be double the maintenance amount until recovery has occurred. Although in the first day or two of treatment the large amounts of parenteral cortisone acetate have sufficient mineralocorticoid action, I employ intramuscular desoxycorticosterone acetate in oil, 2 to 3 mg intramuscularly for 3 days. Recovery is usually rapid and gratifying.

In extremely severe shock it may be necessary to give a vasopressor substance such as epinephrine intravenously, 0.2 mg every 6 to 12 hours. It should be remembered, however, that the rapid administration of cortisone or other glucocorticoids is essential for a permissive action of the vasopressor agent. Under these circumstances it is also rarely necessary to administer plasma, 5.0 ml per kg (or other expander in equivalent volume), during the first day. Following recovery from the acute stage, the long-term management is as outlined for chronic insufficiency.

CUSHING'S SYNDROME

method of
ADRIAN M. SCHNALL, M.D.
Cleveland, Ohio

Effective treatment of Cushing's syndrome is possible only when the underlying cause has been correctly identified. In order of frequency, the causes of the clinical syndrome and the source of the excessive glucocorticoid are (1) iatrogenic, (2) pituitary-dependent, (3) ectopic ACTH production, (4) adrenal adenoma, (5) adrenal carcinoma, and (6) nodular adrenocortical hyperplasia. Measurement of cortisol and its metabolites in blood and urine under conditions of suppression and stimulation is the cornerstone of differential diagnosis of these entities, and various radiologic techniques may help in differentiating them.

Iatrogenic Cushing's Syndrome

This form of Cushing's syndrome usually occurs in patients receiving large doses of glucocorticoid or ACTH as treatment for a serious underlying disease, but may also result from the surreptitious use of these substances by psychologically disturbed persons. Excessive serum corticosteroid levels may result from absorption of skin creams and nasal sprays as well as from oral and intramuscular medications. If the glucocorticoid taken is not cortisone or hydrocortisone, the plasma cortisol level will be low despite the clinical picture of Cushing's syndrome. The physician must choose one of three treatment methods.

1. The most effective treatment is to discontinue the glucocorticoid medication. If a satisfactory alternative treatment is available for the disease for which glucocorticoid was prescribed, the physician must balance the risks of the alternative therapy against the dangers of Cushing's syndrome. If no effective alternative is available, one must balance the risks of the underlying

disease against those of glucocorticoid excess. Glucocorticoids should never be discontinued abruptly in iatrogenic Cushing's syndrome, because patients invariably have abnormal endogenous ACTH and cortisol secretion, a condition which may persist for 6 to 9 months after the glucocorticoid dose is reduced below 30 mg per day of hydrocortisone equivalent. To avoid "steroid withdrawal" symptoms of malaise, arthralgias, and fever, it is wise to halve the dose repeatedly at weekly intervals until reaching 30 mg per day hydrocortisone equivalent, and then to gradually reduce from this level to zero over a 6 to 9 month period. Such a gradual reduction in dosage allows the patient's pituitary and adrenal glands to escape from the chronic suppressive effect of higher doses and to gradually resume normal secretory function. It is sometimes necessary to reduce the initial dose more slowly in order to avoid a sudden exacerbation of the underlying disease.

2. One may sometimes lessen the intensity of iatrogenic Cushing's syndrome by carefully reducing the dose of glucocorticoid to the lowest level which maintains acceptable suppression of the disease under treatment. To help prevent recrudescence of the underlying disease, a satisfactory alternative therapy may be instituted, if available, before the dose of glucocorticoid is reduced.

3. Converting from daily administration of glucocorticoid to an alternate day schedule often results in dramatic improvement in iatrogenic Cushing's syndrome. Patients who receive one morning dose each 48 hours frequently experience regression of the clinical features of hypercortisolism even though the total dose of medication remains the same. Such alternate day treatment is not effective for *initial control* of diseases which respond to glucocorticoids and is successful in treating iatrogenic Cushing's syndrome only when a short-acting agent such as prednisone is used. Once the underlying disease is under control with daily doses of such an agent, the patient begins to take *twice* the established daily dose as a single morning dose on alternate days. On the "off" days, he progressively reduces the dose to zero, the individual clinical situation dictating the pace of the tapering process. In the case of prednisone, the following protocol is often successful: reduce by 10 mg every 2 cycles for doses of 40 mg or more, by 5 mg every 2 cycles for doses between 40 and 20 mg, and by 2.5 mg every 2 cycles for doses below 20 mg.

When the physician decides that continuation of glucocorticoid medication is the wisest alternative, he should encourage a diet high in protein (at least 1 gram per kg of body weight), encourage regular exercise to minimize muscle wasting and osteoporosis, and treat hyperglycemia and hypertension appropriately if they occur. Because of patients' impaired wound healing and reduced resistance to infection, surgical procedures should be avoided if possible.

Pituitary-Dependent Cushing's Syndrome

Autopsy studies and recent reports of patients undergoing pituitary surgery have shown that 60 to 90 per cent of patients with pituitary-dependent hypercortisolism ("Cushing's disease") have pituitary tumors. Most such tumors are small (less than 10 mm in diameter) and not invasive, only 15 to 20 per cent producing abnormalities on routine x-ray studies of the sella turcica, and another 30 to 40 per cent causing minor abnormalities visible on thin section polytomography of the sella. Computed tomography (CT) brain scanning may visualize microadenomas in a few more patients, but a significant number of patients reported have had all available radiographic techniques demonstrating no abnormality, and have been found at surgery to have small adenomas. Rare cases of diffuse ACTH-cell hyperplasia have been reported, but a primary hypothalamic abnormality is postulated as causing overproduction of ACTH in the other 20 to 30 per cent of cases of pituitary Cushing's disease.

Patients over 20 years of age with abnormalities of the sella turcica consistent with a microadenoma should have a microsurgical exploration of the sella by the transsphenoidal approach, but it is essential that referral be made to a neurosurgeon experienced in this technique. In experienced hands, mortality is nil and morbidity minimal. If the tumor is small, normal pituitary tissue can usually be preserved, and replacement glucocorticoids can be tapered and discontinued 3 to 6 months after surgery. In the few patients in whom the tumor is large and cannot be removed completely, persistent hypercortisolism usually can be treated effectively by pituitary radiation. It is important to measure morning blood cortisol levels in the few days postoperatively to document complete removal of the tumor. The remaining (normal) ACTH-producing cells will be suppressed for several weeks to months, requiring temporary glucocorticoid replacement (30 mg per day hydrocortisone equivalent).

In adult patients with pituitary dependent Cushing's disease who have no radiographic abnormality of the sella turcica, physician and patient should recognize that a pituitary microadenoma may be present, and should weigh the alternatives of pituitary microsurgery, pituitary radiation, bilateral adrenalectomy, and pharmacologic treatment.

Transsphenoidal microsurgery frequently offers an uncomplicated cure if a tumor is found (over 50 per cent of cases), but the patient must decide before surgery whether to consent to a complete adenohypophysectomy in case the surgeon finds no tumor. This procedure will lead to cure of Cushing's disease in virtually all cases, but will also necessitate lifelong treatment with thyroid hormones and cortisone, and with gonadotropins as well in patients who desire an active reproductive life. When the patient chooses not to accept such lifelong hormone treatment and no tumor is found at surgery, the alternative modalities of treatment are available.

Conventional external pituitary irradiation delivering 4000 to 5000 rads to the pituitary leads to improvement in 50 per cent of adults but to remission in only 20 per cent. In critically ill patients such treatment is not satisfactory by itself because of the 6 to 18 month lag time between dose and maximal effect. Proton beam or alpha particle radiation can deliver 8000 to 12,000 rads to the pituitary fossa and leads to a higher remission rate, but also to a higher incidence of cranial nerve damage and hypopituitarism. Children are more sensitive to conventional radiotherapy than adults, and achieve an 80 per cent remission rate with the doses noted above. Growth rates return to normal, and sexual development and reproductive function are usually not impaired by such therapy. Since experience with transsphenoidal surgery in children is limited, conventional radiotherapy is the treatment of choice for pituitary Cushing's disease in this age group.

Total bilateral adrenalectomy usually causes total remission of pituitary-dependent Cushing's syndrome, but even in experienced hands perioperative mortality approximates 10 per cent. After successful surgery, patients require lifelong cortisone replacement. Remnants of adrenocortical tissue lead to recurrence of the disease in 5 to 10 per cent of patients. The major disadvantage of this modality of treatment, however, is the occurrence, years after adrenalectomy, of Nelson's syndrome — a generalized hyperpigmentation of the skin which is mediated by high plasma levels of ACTH and β-MSH (melanocyte-stimulating hormone), occurring in association with a large and sometimes invasive pituitary tumor. The incidence of this complication has been 10 to 15 per cent in older series but as high as 50 per cent in some recent reports. Transsphenoidal surgery is less successful in removing these large tumors than the small ones associated with pituitary-based Cushing's disease, and radia-

tion therapy is often necessary to prevent optic nerve compression by the tumor. Some authorities recommend prophylactic pituitary radiation for patients in whom bilateral adrenalectomy is planned, but Nelson's syndrome has been reported in a few patients who had received such prior radiation therapy. Certainly all patients with pituitary dependent Cushing's disease who have had total adrenalectomies should be followed with annual radiographic studies of the sella turcica and visual field examinations. Progressive rises in serum ACTH levels in such patients may portend the development of a pituitary tumor.

Pharmacologic treatment of Cushing's disease involves the use of drugs which either interfere with pituitary ACTH production or impair the synthesis of cortisol in adrenal cells. Drugs of the former group available for general use are cyproheptadine hydrochloride (Periactin)* and bromocriptine mesylate (Parlodel).*

Cyproheptadine, a drug with antiserotonin, antihistamine, and anticholinergic effects, has been reported to induce remission of the clinical syndrome and to lower corticosteroid levels to the normal range in many patients with pituitary-dependent Cushing's disease. Since serotonin is known to have a major influence on ACTH production, we presume that the drug's effectiveness depends on its serotonin antagonism. The drug used alone induces remission in less than 50 per cent of patients, however, and must be used in relatively large doses (24 to 32 mg per day), which frequently cause drowsiness and increased appetite. Maximal effectiveness sometimes does not occur until 4 or 5 months of continuous treatment, and the disease recurs when cyproheptadine is discontinued. Bromocriptine, a dopamine-receptor agonist, has been reported to reduce ACTH and corticosteroid levels in several patients with Cushing's disease, usually in conjunction with other forms of treatment. The doses used have been low (2.5 to 7.5 mg per day), but nausea, headache, and dizziness are common adverse effects. Both cyproheptadine and bromocriptine are most effective when used in conjunction with a more definitive mode of treatment (e.g., to control the disease while waiting for radiotherapy to exert its maximal effect).

Pharmacologic agents which impair production of cortisol include metyrapone, aminoglutethimide, and mitotane (o,p'-DDD). The two former drugs reduce cortisol levels by inhibiting its synthesis in adrenocortical cells. Their effectiveness is limited by the fact that reduction of cortisol levels stimulates increased ACTH pro-

---

*Use of these drugs for the treatment of Cushing's disease is not listed in the manufacturers' directives.

duction in patients with otherwise untreated pituitary-dependent hypercortisolism, thereby driving the cortisol biosynthetic pathways and counteracting the blocking action of the drug. If pituitary ACTH cell function has been altered by partial hypophysectomy or radiation therapy, however, both drugs are very effective in reducing cortisol levels.

Aminoglutethimide is an investigational drug not available for general use in the United States. Metyrapone (Metopirone) blocks the biosynthesis of both cortisol and aldosterone, but does not produce mineralocorticoid deficiency because it increases production of the immediate precursor of aldosterone, 11-desoxycorticosterone, which is itself a potent mineralocorticoid. Metyrapone is given in divided doses up to 4 grams per day and frequently produces nausea, an effect which can be avoided in most cases by administering the drug with meals or a snack. (This use of metyrapone is not listed in the manufacturer's official directive.) Another disadvantage of this drug is its high cost.

Mitotane (o,p'-DDD), a much more potent and toxic drug, exerts its effect by a direct toxic action on adrenocortical cells, specifically those in the zona fasciculata. Mineralocorticoid production is relatively spared. The slow onset of action and lack of predictable response make it advisable to add glucocorticoids in replacement doses when plasma cortisol levels approach normal. Mitotane alters the metabolism of cortisol as well as its production, and urinary 17-hydroxycorticosteroid levels may be deceptively low for weeks after its discontinuation. Divided doses of 2 to 12 grams per day are usually effective in bringing plasma cortisol levels down to normal, and permanent remission of Cushing's disease has been reported in 75 to 80 per cent of patients so treated. (This use of mitotane is not listed in the manufacturer's official directive.) Unfortunately, the majority of such "cured" patients require permanent cortisone replacement, and at least half the patients taking the drug have severe nausea or vomiting.

Spironolactone, a competitive inhibitor of aldosterone, is useful in patients with Cushing's disease who have severe hypertension or hypokalemia, especially those who cannot tolerate oral potassium preparations. The usual dose is 100 to 150 mg per day in divided doses, but up to 400 mg per day may be given.

Ectopic ACTH Production

Neoplasms which originate outside the pituitary gland may secrete ACTH autonomously, producing adrenocortical hyperplasia and hypercortisolism. The most common tumor type is small cell carcinoma of the lung, but tumors in many other organs may produce the same syndrome. Plasma ACTH levels are frequently elevated to astronomical levels, perhaps because the abnormal tumor cells may produce large amounts of immunoassay-detectable but biologically inactive ACTH-like peptides. Presumably for the same reason, patients with ectopic ACTH hypercortisolism may have only minimal clinical features of Cushing's syndrome despite high plasma ACTH concentrations. Such patients often demonstrate a clinical picture dominated by hypokalemic alkalosis and hypertension. Ratios in plasma of β-lipotropin/ACTH greater than 1.0 are characteristic and helpful in diagnosis.

Surgical removal of the ACTH-producing tumor is the treatment of choice but can rarely be accomplished because such tumors tend to be rapidly growing and are usually widely disseminated by the time they are discovered.

Primary debulking of tumors readily accessible to surgery may help lower ACTH production, and chemotherapy or radiation directed at the underlying malignancy may achieve the same results. The mainstays of treatment of the hypercortisolism are the adrenal blocking drugs aminoglutethimide, metyrapone, or mitotane (see above), alone or in combination. Spironolactone and potassium replacement are often important in controlling the often prominent mineralocorticoid features.

Adrenal Adenoma

Surgical excision is the primary treatment and is usually curative if perioperative complications are avoided. Adrenal angiography, CT body scanning, and iodocholesterol isotopic scanning are helpful in localizing the lesion, and these studies as well as endocrinologic testing provide clues as to its nature, but *both* adrenal glands must be examined carefully by the surgeon. The following unexpected occurrences may be encountered: (1) a lesion thought before surgery to be benign may be malignant, and spread to the opposite adrenal may have occurred; (2) bilateral benign adenomas may occur, one side larger than the other; or (3) nodular adrenocortical hyperplasia may be present.

Intraoperative and postoperative complications are common, and the experience and skill of the surgical team are of utmost importance. The physician should be alert for poorly controlled bleeding at the operative site, rapid changes in blood pressure, thromboembolism postoperatively, poor wound healing, and infection. All are commonplace in patients with Cushing's syndrome.

Because the unaffected adrenal gland is frequently chronically suppressed and atrophic, moderately large doses of glucocorticoids must be administered in the perioperative period. The following measures are offered as a guide to glucocorticoid treatment: (1) Give hydrocortisone sodium succinate, 50 mg intramuscularly, 4 hours before surgery. (2) Begin an intravenous infusion of hydrocortisone sodium succinate when surgery begins and infuse at a continuous rate of 300 mg per day (or give "push" doses of 50 mg every 4 hours) for the first 48 hours. (3) If no fever, hypotension, electrolyte imbalance, or other complications develop, reduce the dose by 50 mg per day beginning on the third day after surgery until reaching 50 mg per day. (4) When the patient can take oral medications, discontinue intravenous administration and give the same dose orally, two thirds in the morning and one third in the afternoon. (5) After 1 week, when the dose should be 50 mg per day, reduce to 30 mg per day. If unilateral adrenalectomy has been done, taper gradually and discontinue hydrocortisone in 6 to 9 months; if bilateral adrenalectomy has been performed, maintain the patient permanently on hydrocortisone, 20 mg each morning and 10 mg each afternoon.

Adrenocortical Carcinoma

These tumors frequently attain a large size before diagnosis, tend to be highly malignant, and often have spread to liver, lung, bone, or the contralateral adrenal gland before the patient seeks medical attention. Although the tumor often cannot be removed completely, extensive excision is sometimes justified for the purpose of minimizing the cellular mass secreting cortisol, thereby facilitating control of hypercortisolism. The surgeon must choose the operative approach and technique of tumor removal and will necessarily be guided by the location and degree of metastasis in each individual case as well as by his own experience.

Mitotane (o,p'-DDD) is used almost universally as the palliative drug of choice for adrenocortical carcinoma which cannot be totally excised. Its cytotoxic effect on adrenocortical cells makes it a useful chemotherapeutic agent as well as an effective inhibitor of cortisol production. Use in combination with metyrapone or glutethimide may allow the physician to reduce the dosage and thereby minimize nausea and anorexia.

Nodular Adrenocortical Hyperplasia

The clinical and endocrinologic features of this rare disorder are similar to those in adrenal adenomas, but both adrenal glands contain multiple cortical nodules of various sizes with frequently a grossly visible dark brown pigmentation. Occasionally the involved adrenal glands appear normal grossly, and microscopic examination reveals the nodules. Total bilateral adrenalectomy is the preferred treatment and is curative, but rare cases of Nelson's syndrome following adrenalectomy for this disorder have been reported. Patients require lifelong glucocorticoid replacement therapy.

DIABETES INSIPIDUS

method of
RICHARD H. STERNS, M.D.
Rochester, New York

Diabetes insipidus (DI) is a disorder of water conservation manifest clinically by polyuria, polydipsia, and inappropriately dilute urine. DI results either from a deficiency of the antidiuretic hormone arginine vasopressin (central DI) or from a failure of the kidney to respond to the hormone (nephrogenic DI).

Diabetes insipidus must be distinguished from other causes of polyuria. A large urine volume may result either from the excretion of large amounts of solute (usually glucose, sodium, or urea) in an isotonic urine (*osmotic diuresis*) or from the excretion of a normal amount of solute in a dilute urine (*water diuresis*). In conditions causing *osmotic diuresis*, such as poorly controlled diabetes mellitus, the recovery phase of acute renal failure, or postobstructive diuresis, the urine osmolality tends to equal or exceed the plasma osmolality and urine specific gravity equals or exceeds 1.010. During polyuria caused by a *water diuresis*, the urine is considerably more dilute than plasma and the urine specific gravity is less than 1.005.

A water diuresis may be either a physiologic response to a large water intake (such as occurs in patients with psychogenic polydipsia) or a pathologic abnormality in water conservation (nephrogenic or central DI). Since polyuria caused by excessive water intake is a consequence of mild water overload, a water diuresis in a patient with dehydration and hypernatremia is diagnostic of diabetes insipidus; in this case the response to vasopressin can be assessed without further evaluation. In patients who are *not hypernatremic*, a water deprivation test is necessary to distinguish between pathologic and physiologic water diuresis. It is important to monitor urine volume and body weight during the test to ensure that the patient does not continue to drink or does not become rapidly dehydrated. If after 18 hours or the loss of 3 to 5 per cent of body weight, urine osmolality remains lower than plasma osmolality, a diagnosis of DI can be made; the response to exogenous vasopressin is then assessed to distinguish between nephrogenic DI (no response) and central DI (greater than 50 per cent increase in urine osmolality). Some patients with DI have only partial vasopressin deficiency (incomplete DI) and may be difficult to distinguish from patients with psychogenic polydipsia, since in both disorders the urine osmolality exceeds plasma osmolality after water deprivation. The administration of exogenous vasopressin to patients with incomplete DI results in a further increase in urine osmolality, while in patients with psychogenic polydipsia urine osmolality does not change.

Central Diabetes Insipidus

Once the diagnosis of central DI has been established, a careful search should be made for potentially remediable causes. Although the majority of cases of central DI are idiopathic or secondary to trauma, approximately 25 per cent are caused by surgically correctable lesions such as pituitary tumors and craniopharyngiomas or by granulomatous processes which are amenable to specific medical therapy.

Patients with DI do well, except for the nuisance of polyuria and polydipsia, as long as they drink sufficient amounts of water to prevent dehydration. In fact, patients with minimal DI need not be treated as long as they have a normal thirst mechanism. In rare patients, both DI and hypodipsia may be present concomitantly, resulting in severe (although usually asymptomatic) hypernatremia. It is important to provide all patients with DI with appropriate medical identification to alert medical personnel of the need for fluid and/or hormonal therapy in case of emergency.

In unconscious patients with DI, the physician's control of intravenous fluid therapy must substitute for normal thirst mechanisms. In patients who have become dehydrated and hypernatremic before DI is recognized and treated, sufficient hypotonic fluid must be administered to correct the hypernatremia over the course of 1 to 2 days. Once the water deficit has been corrected and the serum sodium concentration has returned to normal, fluid administration should be adjusted to match urine and other losses with periodic adjustment based on the serum sodium concentration.

In the patient with symptomatic polyuria, specific therapy is justified. Although a variety of nonhormonal medications are available, administration of some form of vasopressin remains the mainstay of treatment for central DI. It should be remembered that DI following head injury or intracranial surgery is often temporary; attempts should be made to withdraw therapy periodically.

1. *Aqueous vasopressin* (Pitressin) is a water-soluble pituitary extract containing a variable mixture of arginine and lysine vasopressin in a concentration of 20 units per ml. The usual dose is 5 to 10 units administered subcutaneously or intramuscularly; antidiuresis usually begins within 30 to 60 minutes and continues for 4 to 6 hours. Since absorption after subcutaneous or intramuscular injection may be unpredictable, the drug may be diluted and administered as a slow intravenous drip (5 milliunits per minute for at least 1 hour); onset of action is immediate and lasts 30 to 60 minutes (this route of administration is not mentioned in the manufacturer's official directive).

Since vasopressin is a potent vasoconstrictor, patients suffering from vascular disease, especially coronary artery disease, should be treated with caution. Hypertension and coronary insufficiency are unusual at the recommended doses, however. Vasopressin may cause abdominal cramps and nausea resulting from stimulation of intestinal smooth muscle contractility. Women may also experience menstrual-like cramps owing to stimulation of uterine contractility. Aqueous vasopressin is used in the diagnosis of DI (see above) and in the treatment of acute (and often transient) central DI. It has little use in the long-term treatment of DI.

2. *Desmopressin acetate (1-desamino-8-D-arginine vasopressin)* (DDAVP) is a new synthetic analogue of arginine vasopressin which is now the drug of choice in the treatment of chronic central DI. It has several advantages over other forms of vasopressin therapy: (1) it is administered intranasally, freeing the patient from painful intramuscular injections of vasopressin tannate in oil (see below); (2) it has a longer antidiuretic action than lysine vasopressin nasal spray (see below), freeing the patient from nocturnal polyuria; and (3) it has very little pressor or vascular activity, freeing the patient from many of the adverse systemic and local reactions associated with other forms of vasopressin therapy. Intranasal desmopressin acetate (DDAVP) may also be preferable to parenteral aqueous vasopressin in the diagnosis of DI.

The drug is currently available in 2.5 ml vials containing 0.1 mg per ml of solution for intranasal use. (A parenteral preparation of the drug is currently available for investigational use only.) A small calibrated catheter comes with each ampule so that exact amounts can be measured and inhaled intranasally. The usual dose is 5 to 20 micrograms. Antidiuresis begins within 1 hour, and, since the drug is slowly absorbed from the nasal mucosa and has a longer plasma half-life than other agents, antidiuresis may last for 6 to

20 hours. One or two doses daily are usually sufficient. Although dose-related headaches, nasal congestion, and abdominal cramps have occurred in some patients, side effects have been few. Most patients have preferred desmopressin acetate (DDAVP) to other forms of therapy. The cost of therapy with this agent (about $10 to $35 per week) is, however, two to four times the cost of therapy with vasopressin tannate in oil (see below).

3. *Vasopressin tannate in oil* (Pitressin Tannate in Oil) is a mixture of arginine and lysine vasopressin in a long-acting preparation. It is supplied in a concentration of 5 units per ml and can be administered subcutaneously or intramuscularly. The usual dose is 2 to 5 units; antidiuresis begins within 2 to 4 hours and continues for 24 to 72 hours. This preparation should never be used intravenously. Before use, the ampule must be vigorously shaken and warmed for several minutes in order to suspend the hormone (the brown precipitate) in the form of an emulsion. The preparation is highly viscous and requires a large needle for injection.

Adverse reactions include the pressor effects associated with aqueous vasopressin, allergic reactions, and the usual problems associated with long-term injections (e.g., pain, abscesses). Too frequent use of the medication may result in dilutional hyponatremia. This agent, like aqueous vasopressin and desmopressin acetate (DDAVP), can also be employed in the diagnosis of DI, but its long duration of action may be a disadvantage in this setting.

4. *Synthetic lysine vasopressin* (Diapid) is available as a nasal spray containing 50 units per ml. Local nasal irritation and systemic side effects are frequent. Its other major disadvantage is the short duration of action; it must be administered every 4 to 6 hours. This preparation completely replaced the use of posterior pituitary powder ("pituitary snuff"), which is more irritating to the nasal mucosa and has also been associated with allergic pulmonary complications. More recently, the use of lysine vasopressin nasal spray has been largely superseded by the development of desmopressin acetate (DDAVP) (see above).

5. *Nonhormonal therapy* of central DI includes such agents as the thiazide diuretics, chlorpropamide, clofibrate, and carbamazepine (the use of these agents is not mentioned in the manufacturers' official directives). The use of one or more of these agents, especially when combined with dietary restriction of protein and salt (to reduce urinary solute and hence obligatory water excretion), can markedly reduce the degree of polyuria and can therefore be a useful adjunct to hormone replacement therapy. The thiazide diuretics can be employed in patients with complete or incomplete central DI, whereas the other agents are effective only in patients who have some residual capacity to secrete vasopressin (incomplete central DI).

The *thiazide diuretics** cause mild volume depletion. This results in increased isotonic resorption of glomerular filtrate in the proximal convoluted tubule and decreased delivery of fluid to the distal portions of the nephron where dilute urine is formed. Since this effect is dependent on maintaining a state of sodium depletion, an excessive intake of sodium will reduce the effectiveness of thiazide therapy. Conventional doses of hydrochlorothiazide (50 to 100 mg daily) or its equivalent are effective, and side effects other than hypokalemia are uncommon.

Chlorpropamide,* an oral hypoglycemic agent, is capable of reducing the degree of polyuria in one third to one half of patients with incomplete central DI. It acts by enhancing secretion of vasopressin and by potentiating the action of circulating vasopressin on the collecting tubules; hence, it is ineffective in complete central DI and nephrogenic DI. The initial dose should be 125 to 250 mg daily; this can then be increased in increments of 250 mg every 3 to 4 days to a maximum of 750 mg daily until a satisfactory antidiuretic response is achieved. Doses in excess of 500 to 750 mg daily are associated with a significant incidence of hypoglycemia. Since the mechanism of action of chlorpropamide differs from that of the thiazides, the action of the two drugs is additive.

Clofibrate* is an oral hypolipemic agent which in conventional doses (1 to 2 grams daily) enhances secretion of vasopressin, resulting in an antidiuretic action in patients with incomplete central DI. It is somewhat less potent than chlorpropamide and since it has a short duration of action (6 to 8 hours), it must be given four times daily. Clofibrate is associated with a variety of side effects, including gastrointestinal symptoms, myositis, and abnormalities of liver function. Since its only advantage over chlorpropamide is freedom from hypoglycemic reactions, it should not be used as the initial agent in the treatment of incomplete central DI.

Carbamazepine* is used as an anticonvulsant and in the treatment of tic douloureux; it is also effective in reducing polyuria in patients with partial central DI. Since it has few advantages over chlorpropamide or clofibrate, it is not rec-

---

*This use of this drug is not mentioned in the manufacturer's official directive.

ommended for the routine therapy of incomplete central DI.

Nephrogenic Diabetes Insipidus

A variety of disorders of the renal medulla (e.g., sickle cell disease, interstitial nephritis, or advanced renal failure of any cause) commonly impair the ability to maximally concentrate the urine. However, since the urine is not dilute, but rather isotonic or submaximally concentrated, patients with these disorders do not usually suffer from polyuria and polydipsia. Severe hypercalcemia or hypokalemia causes a similar concentrating defect, but does result in polyuria and polydipsia, possibly because of an effect of these metabolic disorders on thirst centers. Excessive volumes of dilute urine despite water deprivation and exogenous vasopressin (nephrogenic or vasopressin-resistant DI) are seen more rarely: as a sex-linked inherited disorder presenting shortly after birth; in medullary cystic disease (nephronophthisis); in partial urinary tract obstruction; in infiltrative diseases affecting the collecting duct (e.g., amyloidosis, myelomatosis); and as a consequence of certain drugs (methoxyflurane anesthesia, amphotericin B, demeclocycline, or lithium).

Patients with nephrogenic DI do not respond to exogenous vasopressin or to therapies which enhance the effects of endogenous vasopressin. Some reduction in polyuria can be achieved by restriction of dietary protein and salt, which limits urinary solute content. In some instances, this is sufficient therapy, since the polyuria of nephrogenic DI tends to be less severe than that seen with central DI. If necessary, thiazide diuretics can be added as described for central DI. In patients with nephrogenic DI as a consequence of chronic lithium therapy, however, thiazide diuretics will increase the risk of lithium toxicity and should be avoided.

Psychogenic Polydipsia

Inappropriate treatment of these patients with antidiuretic agents can lead to life-threatening water intoxication. However, since it is sometimes difficult to distinguish this disorder from incomplete DI, a *closely supervised* therapeutic trial may be necessary in some cases. Compulsive water drinkers usually continue to drink excessively even after the urinary volume has been reduced and maintain that the hormonal therapy is of no benefit to them.

SIMPLE GOITER

method of
MORELLY L. MAAYAN, M.D.
Brooklyn, New York

The term simple goiter applies to any non-malignant thyroid growth present in a euthyroid individual. While this definition would appear to embrace both diffuse and nodular goiters, it usually refers to the diffuse anterocervical, nonsubsternal form of the disease.

The treatment of simple goiter may be medical or surgical.

Medical Treatment

For a better understanding of medical therapy, the causes and forms of simple goiter will be reviewed.

The pathophysiology of goiter involves the feedback mechanism of the adenohypophyseal-thyroid axis. When thyroid hormone secretion decreases, its plasma concentration falls and the hypophyseal secretion of thyroid-stimulating hormone (TSH) increases; speaking teleologically, this is an attempt (almost always inadequate) to re-establish normal thyroidal function. In goiter the feedback mechanism responds to stimuli that impair normal thyroid hormone biosynthesis and release. Hence, hyperplasia occurs as a response to increased TSH secretion.

Thyroid function is impaired in goiter by the following factors:

1. Dietary iodine deficiency in a specific geographic area (leading to endemic goiter).

2. Dietary presence of substances that prevent trapping of iodine, such as thiocyanate or perchlorate.

3. Dietary presence of thiourea compounds that prevent iodide oxidation and hence its incorporation into tyrosine (organification).

4. Inability of the thyroid to "trap" and further utilize the iodine even if available (enzymatic deficiencies affecting thyroid hormone biosynthesis).

5. Familial factors, as yet poorly defined, leading to cases of sporadic goiter, in which the enzymatic deficiencies in the process of thyroid hormone biosynthesis are below the threshold of detection by current methods.

6. Unusual causes, i.e., increased urinary loss of iodide induced by high sodium chloride

intake, pregnancy, or increased fecal loss of thyroxine in soybean diet.

Although all the enumerated causes lead to the same outlined pathophysiologic mechanism, identification of the specific cause is necessary to design an appropriate therapy. It is improbable that supplementation with iodide will have any positive effect when there are iodide-depleting or organification-inhibiting factors or both in the diet. It is also unlikely that "suppressive" or "replacement" therapy with L-thyroxine (see below) will be efficient if there is loss of thyroxine through the intestinal tract.

The most common medical treatment of goiter consists in administration of suppressive doses of thyroid hormone (L-thyroxine or L-triiodothyronine). The term "suppressive" refers to the thyroid hormone–induced inhibition of the hypophyseal TSH secretion responsible, as outlined above, for the thyroidal hypertrophy leading to goiter. As a result of TSH "suppression" the enlarged thyroid will shrink. This therapeutic effect is most dramatic in children or juveniles. Large goiters may disappear completely if the treatment is vigorous and prolonged enough. In older patients the therapeutic effects are less impressive. Presently, almost all patients given suppressive therapy receive thyroid hormone in the form of L-thyroxine. However, until only a few years ago in the United States of America, thyroid hormones were given as desiccated thyroid extract (DTE); this is still the practice in many overseas countries. DTE is a purified, desiccated thyroid powder, whose potency was standardized by its iodine content. The suppressive dose of DTE was equated to that necessary to bring a hypothyroid patient to laboratory values (PBI, serum T_4) diagnostic for a euthyroid state. The average dose varied between 150 and 200 mg (2½ to 3 grains) of DTE per day. Much has been said and written about the advantage of taking the given dose of thyroid hormone around the clock, but for the desiccated thyroid powder this is not essential. On many occasions the practical advantage of taking the entire dose once a day has prevailed over any theoretical advantages of having a constant serum level of thyroid hormone. As mentioned above, DTE has been replaced in the last several years by L-thyroxine, a pure and scientifically standardized preparation. It is available under several brand names (Synthroid, Letter, and others) or its generic name of L-thyroxine. Initial assessments equated 1 grain of thyroid extract with 100 micrograms of L-thyroxine, but subsequent clinical evaluations indicate that 200 micrograms of L-thyroxine has biological effects closer to those of 3 grains of DTE per day.

The obvious advantages of changing from DTE to L-thyroxine are standardization, purity of preparation, and ability to follow the therapeutic effect by simple and appropriate laboratory tests. Thus, a dose of 200 micrograms of L-thyroxine per day will usually be reflected by a serum T_4 titer of 9 micrograms per 100 ml (for a laboratory indicating normal values between 5 and 10 micrograms per 100 ml). In determining the dose, whether the patient is euthyroid or hypothyroid, the eventual excess given for suppressive reasons will induce a feedback effect, diminishing TSH, and will put the thyroid gland to rest (which in simple goiter is the desired effect). This treatment will be efficient in all patients with goiters except those, mentioned above, who lose thyroxine because of dietary factors. Obviously, in such rare cases, these patients will lose not only the endogenously produced thyroxine but also that ingested. In such patients administration of the suppressive doses of L-thyroxine (T_4) should be preceded by removal of the agent(s) or cause(s) inducing the L-thyroxine escape.

An alternative to L-thyroxine is administration of L-triiodothyronine. For treatment of simple goiter this is seldom used, since the preparation is expensive and short acting. The suppressive dose of L-triiodothyronine would be 50 to 75 micrograms per day. If it is used, the medication should be given in divided doses around the clock, usually at no more than 8 hour intervals. Another disadvantage of L-triiodothyronine administration is the difficulty in following the therapeutic effects by laboratory tests (with the exception of T_3 determination by radioimmunoassay, which is unnecessarily elaborate and expensive). While administration of L-thyroxine leads to a normal plasma L-triiodothyronine (T_3) titer by its conversion to T_3, administration of L-triiodothyronine (T_3) greatly diminishes the measurable T_4 owing to its TSH suppressive effect. The laboratory values for T_4 in the serum may thus be in the myxedematous range in a euthyroid person. This can cause needless difficulties if the patient comes under the care of a physician who is unaware of this situation, as may happen in an emergency.

Despite the therapeutic effectiveness of thyroid hormone preparations which makes them the preferred treatment in cases of sporadic goiter, in most endemic areas simple goiter is treated with iodide salts. There are several reasons for this, more pertinent perhaps in overseas countries than in the United States:

1. The cost of iodized salt is much less than that of L-thyroxine or triiodothyronine.

2. Endemic goiter areas are widespread in parts of the world where medical facilities and medications are scarce and the population to be treated is relatively uneducated. While intake of a prescribed, standardized medication represents a disciplined and costly action that can probably not be properly followed by a large portion of the population, the mass treatment with iodized salt in endemic goiter involves administration of this compound in forms easy to take and difficult to avoid. Although this aspect does not concern the individual practitioner but rather a public health organization, the treating physician should be aware of the public measures taken in a given area to avoid misinterpretation of laboratory or clinical findings related to excess iodide administration.

In endemic goiter areas, iodide may be distributed as daily tablets of 1 mg of iodide salts (KI) given primarily to children and pregnant women under the supervision of ancillary health personnel in schools, nurseries, hospitals, or other organizations. The effect in simple goiter is preventive and sometimes also curative. Where these facilities are unavailable, iodide is administered as a supplement in kitchen salt (20 mg per 1000 grams) and even in cattle fodder. In the latter, the iodide will prevent goiter in animals and will reach the human population in animal products such as milk. The excess of iodide is apparently sufficient to overcome the lack of iodide substrate; the amount necessary for normal biosynthesis of thyroid hormone is thus supplied and eradicates goiter. This effect has been repeatedly demonstrated by the disappearance of large endemic goiter areas so common in the past.

Another form of iodide administration, this time involuntary, has been achieved by using iodide salts in the process of baking bread in the United States. The result is a supplementation of the iodide ingestion in all individuals, an elevation of the level of iodide in serum, and an alteration of the normal values of uptake of radioactive iodide. However, the overall effect is presumably beneficial.

In infrequently encountered forms of goiter, representing impaired thyroid hormone biosynthesis resulting from a trapping defect of iodide, the small doses of iodide, as mentioned above, are insufficient as therapeutic agents. Larger amounts should be given to promote diffusion into the gland so as to overcome the impaired biosynthesis of thyroid hormones. This must be administered under physician observation, since 60 to 180 mg per day of iodide may be required and reactions to iodide (iodism) may occur.

Surgical Treatment

Unfortunately there are still a large number of goiters for which medical treatment is given too late. Again, in regions of endemic goiter there is a very high incidence of old, lobulated goiters palpable and visible, of large size, inducing mechanical compression effects. These old goiters are by and large fibrotic, and hormonal treatment aimed at inducing a diminution in size of the thyroid parenchyma has no effect on the patches of connective tissue. The differential diagnosis of such goiters is made by clinical examination and thyroid scans with either radioactive iodine (^{131}I or ^{123}I) or ^{99m}technetium–pertechnetate. While there are some discrepancies in scans obtained after the administration of the 2 radionuclides, existence of large "cold" patches within an enlarged mass of thyroid parenchyma suggests that the normal thyroid tissue has been displaced by, or replaced with, fibrotic tissue. The differential diagnosis should include malignant formations, which are also "cold" by scanning. The definitive diagnosis is obtained by biopsy performed during thyroid surgery. Occasionally, needle biopsy is used in some departments, presenting the advantage of avoiding surgery but the disadvantage of a less positive diagnosis than in "open" biopsy.

Mere presence of cold areas within a thyroid gland is not an absolute indication for thyroidectomy. This procedure should be done either for cosmetic reasons or when compressive signs such as tracheal deviation or esophageal obstruction are present, as shown by dyspnea or dysphagia and corroborated by x-ray procedures. Then thyroidectomy becomes mandatory and, although still elective, the procedure should be performed at the first opportunity.

It is essential to have the surgery performed by an expert surgeon with extensive experience. Even then the patient should be informed of the potential risks of thyroidectomy. The most common are injury of the recurrent laryngeal nerve and subsequent hoarseness; an unesthetic, sometimes keloidal scar; post-thyroidectomy myxedema that should be properly evaluated and treated by administration of thyroid hormones; and post-thyroidectomy compensatory hypertrophy of the thyroid remnant. A rare risk is hypoparathyroidism through inadvertent removal of or injury to the parathyroids. The treatment of compensatory hypertrophy is either administration of suppressive doses of thyroid hormone or repeated thyroidectomy. In general, the latter is to be avoided, since the operative risks are much higher during a second thyroid procedure. To prevent post-thyroidectomy hypertrophy, the patient, after surgery, is given a less than suppressive therapeutic dose of L-thyroxine (100 micrograms) or desiccated thyroid extract (65 mg [1 grain] per day), with the expectation of continuing or discontinuing at his physician's orders. Usually patients undergoing thyroidectomy should be followed with monthly visits the first 3 months; bimonthly visits during the following 4 to 6 months; quarterly visits for the remainder of the first year; biannual visits the next 2 years; and annual visits for up to 5 years. Complications, or lack of them, may change this schedule, but most often it should be faithfully followed during the first postoperative year.

HYPER- AND HYPOPARATHYROIDISM

method of
PETER GREENBERG, M.D.
Melbourne, Australia

HYPERPARATHYROIDISM

The object of treatment is to relieve symptoms and prevent complications resulting from excessive secretion of parathyroid hormone. Choice of treatment depends on the particular clinical situation and on whether the hyperparathyroidism is due to disease of the parathyroid glands (primary) or the result of longstanding hypocalcemia associated with chronic renal failure, malabsorption, or, rarely, vitamin D–resistant rickets and osteomalacia (secondary).

Primary Hyperparathyroidism with Symptomatic Hypercalcemia

Moderate or severe hypercalcemia leads to polyuria because the kidneys are unable to form a urine of high specific gravity. Nausea, anorexia, and vomiting may also occur, and hypercalcemic patients tend to become dehydrated and uremic.

Oral fluids may be adequate for rehydration, but intravenous fluids are usually required. Isotonic saline solution should be infused to correct extracellular fluid losses, and potassium should be given unless renal failure has developed. With very severe hypercalcemia, a forced diuresis can be attained by combining saline infusion with diuretics (e.g., initially furosemide, 20 to 40 mg every 8 hours), but severe sodium, potassium, and magnesium depletion may occur, and hypovolemia can result. Careful clinical and laboratory monitoring is therefore required.

In most patients, restoration of plasma and extracellular fluid volume produces diuresis and reduction of serum calcium concentration. In patients who remain markedly hypercalcemic, the following additional treatments should be considered:

Phosphate. Buffered sodium or potassium phosphate can be infused intravenously at a rate not exceeding 1 gram of elemental phosphorus per 24 hours. This treatment is contraindicated in patients who are already hyperphosphatemic or uremic. In severe hypercalcemia, calcium phosphate deposits may occur in the veins at the site of the infusion. Oral phosphate can be administered in daily doses containing 1 to 2 grams of elemental phosphorus, but doses exceeding 3 grams usually produce diarrhea.

Calcitonin. The administration of calcitonin may help control the condition in patients with refractory hypercalcemia by inhibiting bone resorption. Calcitonin is given in a dose of 50 to 100 MRC (Medical Research Council) units 12 hourly by intramuscular or subcutaneous injection. The hypocalcemic effect is apparent within several hours, but as it is seldom sustained for more than several days, parathyroidectomy should not be unduly delayed.

Dialysis. Dialysis against a fluid of low calcium concentration can result in prompt resolution of hypercalcemia and should be considered in refractory patients, particularly those with uremia and cardiac failure.

Primary Hyperparathyroidism with Bone Disease

Hyperparathyroidism is rarely associated with bone disease (osteitis fibrosa cystica). In such patients, however, severe hypocalcemia may occur following parathyroidectomy and may continue for several months, until the bones are healed.

It is useful to administer vitamin D (e.g., ergocalciferol [vitamin D_2], 50,000 units [1.25 mg] daily for several weeks) prior to parathyroidectomy. Serum calcium and creatinine levels should be measured weekly to detect worsening hypercalcemia or the development of uremia. Most patients with bone disease will require vitamin D postoperatively and, because it takes several weeks to effect the full biologic action of ergocalciferol, it is best to begin this before surgery.

Primary Hyperparathyroidism with Renal Calculi

In patients with hyperparathyroidism and renal calculi, parathyroidectomy is indicated.

Primary Hyperparathyroidism with Uremia

Parathyroidectomy is recommended. A transient deterioration in renal function may occur in the early postoperative period.

Biochemical Hyperparathyroidism

An increasing number of patients are found to have hyperparathyroidism as a result of biochemical screening. In elderly patients with mild hypercalcemia (e.g., less than 3 mmol per liter) no particular treatment may be required, but the patient and his medical advisers should be aware of the need to avoid dehydration, which may accentuate the degree of hypercalcemia. In patients with moderate or severe hypercalcemia, and in those patients with mild hypercalcemia and hyperparathyroidism complicated by renal stones, bone disease, or uremia, parathyroidectomy is advisable.

Although the serum calcium level can be reduced with oral phosphate therapy, the safety and efficacy of this treatment has not been confirmed and it should not be given to asymptomatic patients with mild, uncomplicated hyperparathyroidism.

Secondary Hyperparathyroidism

Prevention. Secondary hyperparathyroidism in patients with uremia can be prevented by prescribing antacids, e.g., aluminum hydroxide (Amphojel), in divided doses sufficient to keep the serum phosphate level within normal limits. Patients find it difficult to comply with this treatment over long periods.

Treatment. Treatment of asymptomatic bone disease should be attempted in the first instance with ergocalciferol (Calciferol) in a dose sufficient to effect healing without producing hypercalcemia or deterioration in renal function. Fifty thousand to 100,000 units (1.25 to 2.5 mg) daily usually suffices, but careful clinical and laboratory control is required in order to prevent complications. The serum concentration should be kept normal by the concomitant administration of antacids. If hypercalcemia results, subtotal parathyroidectomy is recommended.

Parathyroidectomy may also be indicated in patients with bone pain refractory to medical treatment and in those with metastatic calcification.

In patients with secondary hyperparathyroidism and severe bone disease, profound hypocalcemia is common after parathyroidectomy, and it is best to commence ergocalciferol treatment several weeks before parathyroidectomy.

Tertiary Hyperparathyroidism

In this condition, hypercalcemia occurs in patients who develop hyperparathyroidism because of previous longstanding hypocalcemia. Subtotal parathyroidectomy is indicated. If possible, bone disease should be treated preoperatively.

Parathyroidectomy

Localization of Abnormal Parathyroid Tissue. Although the measurement of immunoreactive parathyroid hormone in samples obtained during selective catheterization of the neck and upper thoracic veins sometimes permits preoperative localization of abnormal parathyroid tissue, this procedure is not recommended routinely. When the parathyroid surgeon and pathologist are experienced, the additional information obtained seldom contributes to management.

Primary hyperparathyroidism is most commonly associated with a single parathyroid adenoma and, if this is confirmed, the adenoma should be removed and the other parathyroid glands identified.

In patients with four enlarged parathyroid glands, subtotal parathyroidectomy should be performed, the surgeon removing three glands and half of the remaining gland. Patients with a family history of hyperparathyroidism or other endocrine adenomas are most likely to have enlargement of several glands.

If one enlarged gland and one normal or atrophic gland are identified, it is unlikely that the remaining parathyroid glands will be enlarged, and removal of the enlarged gland is appropriate. If two or more enlarged glands are found, a particularly careful search should be made for the remaining glands, as these are also likely to be abnormal.

Metabolic Complications of Parathyroidectomy. Following parathyroidectomy there is often transient impairment of renal function and hypocalcemia and hypomagnesemia may occur, particularly in patients with preexisting bone disease. Severe metabolic problems can be prevented by preoperative treatment of these patients (see Primary Hyperparathyroidism with Bone Disease, above). Patients should be examined for latent tetany (Trousseau's sign and Chvostek's sign) twice daily in the early postoperative period, and levels of serum calcium, albumin, and magnesium should be monitored daily. As latent tetany may sometimes occur with normal serum calcium and magnesium levels, pretreatment levels should always be obtained.

Symptomatic hypocalcemia is treated by injecting 10 ml of 10 per cent calcium gluconate over 5 minutes. For severe hypocalcemia, 100 to 200 ml of 10 per cent calcium gluconate should be infused over 12 to 24 hours in 1 liter of isotonic saline solution with appropriate clinical and laboratory controls. If hypomagnesemia occurs, this can be treated by giving magnesium sulfate, 50 per cent, 1 to 2 ml intramuscularly each 12 to 24 hours. Hypomagnesemia may itself produce hypocalcemia, and the need for calcium supplements becomes less when serum magnesium concentration becomes normal.

If hypocalcemia persists, the patient should be given a high-calcium diet (e.g., 1 to 2 pints of cow's milk containing 0.5 to 1 gram of calcium) or supplementary calcium containing 1 to 4 grams of elemental calcium daily, in divided doses, or both. Effervescent calcium in doses exceeding 4 to 6 grams daily is seldom tolerated because of diarrhea.

In patients with hyperparathyroid bone disease, calcium supplements should be given until the tissues are healed as shown by clinical and laboratory (e.g., serum alkaline phosphatase) values. If normocalcemia cannot be maintained by calcium supplements alone, ergocalciferol should be added in doses of about 50,000 to 100,000 units daily (1.25 to 2.50 mg), with serum calcium measurements done at least each 4 weeks to avoid producing hypercalcemia.

Recurrent Hyperparathyroidism

When hypercalcemia occurs after apparent surgical cure of primary hyperparathyroidism, the possibility of missed parathyroid adenoma, parathyroid hyperplasia, and parathyroid carcinoma should be considered.

The estimation of parathyroid hormone in samples obtained during selective catheterization is particularly helpful in these patients because of the technical difficulties associated with reexploration.

If the mass of residual parathyroid tissue cannot be reduced and hypercalcemia persists, the plan for treatment will depend upon the severity of the hypercalcemia and the symptoms and complications produced by this. In patients with severe symptomatic hypercalcemia caused by parathyroid carcinoma, treatment with phosphate (see p. 525), calcitonin (see p. 525), mithramycin (e.g., 15 to 25 micrograms per kg intrave-

nously over 4 hours on 2 to 3 consecutive days with appropriate regard to hematologic, renal, and hepatic toxicity), or estrogen (e.g., ethinyl estradiol, 50 micrograms daily) should be considered (this use of ethinyl estradiol is not listed in the manufacturer's official directive). As increased absorption of calcium occurs in hyperparathyroidism, a low calcium diet (no milk or cheese) is prescribed.

HYPOPARATHYROIDISM

Acute Postoperative Tetany

Hypoparathyroidism may complicate thyroidectomy, parathyroidectomy, and radical neck dissection. In thyrotoxic patients with bone disease, hypocalcemia sometimes associated with tetany may follow thyroidectomy. This is particularly common in young patients in whom prior drug treatment has only partially controlled the disease. The hypocalcemia probably reflects rapid uptake of mineral into bone, and similar responses are sometimes seen in patients with hyperparathyroid bone disease following parathyroidectomy (see p. 526).

Hypomagnesemia

Functional hypoparathyroidism occurs in hypomagnesemic patients as a result of impaired release of parathyroid hormone and inhibition of the peripheral action of the hormone. This may be seen after parathyroidectomy in patients with hyperparathyroid bone disease (see p. 526). Hypomagnesemia should be considered as a cause of hypocalcemia or tetany in alcoholics, patients receiving parenteral nutrition, or those with a malabsorption syndrome, and also in the diuretic phase of acute tubular necrosis (for treatment, see Parathyroidectomy, above).

Chronic Hypoparathyroidism

This is usually seen following parathyroidectomy but may also be due to agenesis of the parathyroid glands, secretion of biologically inert parathyroid hormone, or impaired peripheral responses to parathyroid hormone. Postoperative hypoparathyroidism may be associated with hypothyroidism and idiopathic hypoparathyroidism with Addison's disease.

The main object of treatment is to prevent tetany and seizures from hypocalcemia. It is also desirable to maintain serum calcium levels within normal limits in order to possibly prevent long-term complications, e.g., cataract. Few patients respond to a high-calcium diet or calcium supplementation (see p. 526), and most require vitamin D supplementation.

Vitamin D_2 (ergocalciferol), is usually required in doses of 50,000 to 100,000 units (1.25 to 2.50 mg) daily. It takes 1 to 2 weeks before ergocalciferol has its biologic effects and so there is a considerable latent period before serum calcium level changes after an increase or reduction in dose.

Clinical response is determined by symptoms and by monitoring the signs of latent tetany (Trousseau's sign, Chvostek's sign). Hypoparathyroid patients should have serum calcium levels measured at 4 monthly intervals, at least, because (1) some patients continue to have latent tetany when normocalcemic, (2) mild or moderate hypercalcemia can be asymptomatic, and (3) the dose of ergocalciferol needed to maintain normocalcemia tends to vary from time to time. Hypoparathyroidism, once established, is usually permanent, but because of the risk of hypercalcemia and its complications, the smallest dose of ergocalciferol needed to keep serum calcium in the low to midnormal range should be given. In patients whose conditions are not controlled by supplementary calcium alone, it is simplest to control serum calcium level with ergocalciferol alone.

Pregnancy and lactation seldom present problems for hypoparathyroid mothers, but serum calcium levels should be measured more frequently in order to ensure that the patient remains normocalcemic.

HYPOPITUITARISM

method of
BARRY M. SHERMAN, M.D.
Iowa City, Iowa

The anterior lobe of the pituitary secretes at least six hormones: growth hormone (GH), adrenal corticotropin (ACTH), thyroid-stimulating hormone (TSH), follicle-stimulating hormone (FSH), luteinizing hormone (LH), and prolactin (PRL). ACTH is synthesized as part of a peptide of substantially greater molecular weight, beta lipotropin. Another portion of this same precursor peptide is beta endorphin, an endogenous opiate. The existence and exact nature of the hormone responsible for regulating skin pigmentation are at present in doubt. The hypothalamus regulates the release of these hormones from the pituitary through secretion of both stimulatory and inhibitory factors. The concentration of circulating hormones from the target glands (such as thyroid, adrenal, or gonad) exerts a negative feed-

back control on secretion of its corresponding tropic hormone. High concentrations of thyroid hormones or of cortisol, for example, diminish pituitary TSH and ACTH secretion, respectively. These effects are mediated at the level of the hypothalamus, the pituitary, or both. For prolactin a hypothalamic inhibiting factor predominates, while for growth hormone both a releasing hormone and a release-inhibiting hormone (somatostatin) have been demonstrated.

Pituitary hormone deficiency may involve one or more hormones. Panhypopituitarism is a relatively rare occurrence. The causes of hypopituitarism are listed in Table 1. Pituitary adenomas, craniopharyngiomas, and idiopathic hypopituitarism of childhood are by far the most common causes. A pituitary tumor may be recognized because of excess hormone production, hormone deficiencies, or mechanical consequences such as headache and visual field abnormalities.

In some patients, especially those with pituitary tumors, there may be progressive loss of pituitary function. The pituitary hormones usually become deficient in the following order: (1) GH, (2) LH and FSH, (3) ACTH, and (4) TSH. Prolactin deficiency is very unusual. Because of these considerations, periodic reassessment of pituitary function is important. The initiation of hormone replacement usually commits the patient to lifelong therapy. For that reason, a diagnosis of pituitary hormone deficiency should be carefully documented, using appropriate testing procedures.

Patients with hypopituitarism should be instructed to register with the Medic Alert Foundation, P. O. Box 1009, Turlock, California 95380, and to obtain an identification tag that lists their hormone treatment.

Growth Hormone

The adult patient experiences few symptoms directly referrable to growth hormone deficiency. Insulin-requiring diabetics may have a dramatic increase in insulin sensitivity, with a decrease in requirement for insulin therapy. Growth hormone–deficient children will have greatly retarded growth with the history of normal birth weight. This type of dwarfism is characterized by normal body proportions and may be associated with other endocrine deficiencies.

The treatment of growth hormone deficiency in children is dependent upon the availability of growth hormone purified from human cadaver pituitary glands. That material is made available for investigational use from the National Pituitary Agency and now is available commercially from Calbio or Kaby Pharmaceuticals. The response is dose related. The usual dose is 1 or 2 IU given intramuscularly on alternate days or three times weekly. Continuous treatment is more effective than intermediate dosing. Growth hormone administration results in linear growth, weight gain, and bone maturation. Growth is

TABLE 1. **Causes of Hypopituitarism**

CLASSIFICATIONS	CAUSES
Neoplasms	Primary intrasellar tumors
	Craniopharyngioma
	Metastatic carcinoma
	Histiocytosis
Granulomas	Sarcoidosis
Infection	Fungal diseases
	Tuberculosis
	Syphilis (gumma)
	Pyogenic infections
	Meningitis (sequel)
Vascular	Infarction—intrapartum or postpartum
	Ischemic vascular disease
	Aneurysm of internal carotid artery
Idiopathic	Hypopituitarism of childhood
	Isolated hormone deficiency
Surgical Trauma	Hypophysectomy or stalk section

generally better when treatment is started at an early age and is almost always greatest during the first year of treatment. About 35 per cent of patients will develop circulating antibodies to growth hormone, but this does not seem to impair the growth response.

In children with multiple pituitary hormone deficiencies, treatment with other hormones requires careful consideration. Adequate thyroid hormone is necessary for optimal growth. Excessive glucocorticoid hormone therapy can reduce the response to growth hormone, and for that reason patients should receive the smallest steroid dose consistent with alleviation of symptoms. Sex hormone replacement speeds epiphyseal closure and should be delayed until the maximal growth hormone effect is attained. This often conflicts with the patient's emotional and social needs and requires careful counseling.

Gonadotropin Deficiency

Gonadotropin deficiency results in loss of libido in both men and women, impotence in men, and amenorrhea. In women, this secondary estrogen deficiency causes atrophy of breast tissue and vaginal epithelium and development of fine wrinkles around the eyes and mouth. In men the testes may become smaller and softer, and the rate of beard growth is often reduced. Preadolescent gonadotropin deficiency results in failure to develop secondary sex characteristics.

A functional form of gonadotropin deficiency that results in amenorrhea and infertility occurs in patients with hyperprolactinemia. Lowering the prolactin concentration to normal, either surgically or medically, results in resumption of menstrual cycles and return of fertility in premenopausal women.

In patients who have gonadotropin deficiency because of defect in the secretion of the hypothalamic-releasing hormone for LH and FSH, treatment of gonadotropin deficiency is theoretically possible by administration of the synthetic releasing hormone. This material is available only for investigational use, and those studies have not resulted in an effective or practical treatment schedule.

In men, androgen replacement is carried out using the parenteral preparations testosterone enanthate (Delatestryl) or testosterone cypionate (Depo-Testosterone). These are more effective in maintaining secondary sex characteristics than are oral preparations such as fluoxymesterone. In adults, the usual dose is 200 mg intramuscularly every 3 to 4 weeks. We measure the serum testosterone concentration before the next dose and adjust the dosing interval to maintain the serum testosterone level in the normal range of 3 to 10 nanograms per ml. The dose can be halved in older men to reduce the likelihood of prostatic hyperplasia and obstructive uropathy.

There are other considerations in the initiation of treatment in adolescents. Sex hormone therapy results in epiphyseal closure. Ideally, treatment of androgen deficiency should be delayed to provide an opportunity for maximal linear growth, and when started is begun in a lower dose, 75 to 100 mg monthly. This consideration often has to be balanced against the emotional needs of the patient for normal adolescent changes.

In the adolescent male, it is often difficult to distinguish physiologic delayed puberty from permanent hypothalamic-pituitary gonadotropin deficiency. Normal puberty may follow a 4 to 6 month trial of androgen replacement in some patients with physiologic delay. Such a therapeutic trial should be followed by a reassessment of pituitary-gonadal function. In these circumstances, some physicians prefer to use human chorionic gonadotropin (HCG), 2000 IU three times a week, to stimulate Leydig cell testosterone production. This is usually effective but is expensive and requires frequent injections.

Side effects of androgen replacement include the development of acne and transient gynecomastia in adolescents. Adults may be troubled by mild fluid retention.

The treatment of the infertility that accompanies pituitary dysfunction in men is unsatisfactory. This has been attempted in a variety of ways with HCG, purified LH and FSH, gonadotropin-releasing hormone (GnRH), or one of its long-acting analogues. Research with each of these methods continues, but none has yet been shown to be consistently effective.

Gonadotropin deficiency in women is treated by cyclic replacement of both estrogen and progesterone. This is done conveniently with a combination oral contraceptive containing 20 to 50 micrograms of ethinyl estradiol. Alternatively, we use 20 or 50 microgram tablets of ethinyl estradiol or 0.625 mg tablets of conjugated estrogens (Premarin) for 25 days and add 5 to 10 mg of medroxyprogesterone (Provera) for the last 5 days. These programs provide for cyclic sloughing of the endometrium and avoid the potential consequences of persistent estrogen stimulation.

Induction of fertility in women with LH and FSH deficiency can be accomplished by administration of gonadotropins. Purified LH and FSH are now available for experimental use. However, ovulation induction is carried out with human menopausal gonadotropin (HMG) menotropins (Pergonal). This material is recovered from the urine of menopausal women and is rich in both LH and FSH. Each ampule contains 75 IU of FSH and 75 IU of LH.

Induction of ovulation requires the qualitative, quantitative, and temporal replication of the events of the normal ovulatory cycle, resulting in follicular maturation, ovulation, and corpus luteum function.

Follicular maturation is promoted by daily administration of 1 or more ampules of HMG for 9 to 12 days. Serum and/or urinary estrogen concentrations are measured daily to assess the adequacy of follicular maturation and to judge the appropriate timing of a single dose of HCG, 5000 or 10,000 units. The bolus of HCG mimics the midcycle LH surge and causes follicular rupture and ovulation.

The success rate of ovulation induction is approximately 35 per cent. This treatment is complex, expensive, and fraught with potential complications. It should be done only by physicians experienced in the use of these drugs and with adequate laboratory support. Complications include ovarian enlargement, multiple pregnancies, and the hyperstimulation syndrome characterized by abdominal pain, nausea, vomiting, ruptured ovarian cysts, and ascites.

ACTH

Loss of ACTH secretory capacity usually results in decreased stamina, exhaustion, hypopigmentation, and loss of axillary and pubic hair. In general, symptoms referable to mineralocorticoid deficiency such as postural hypotension and vascular collapse are not prominent in the absence of unusual stress.

Most of our patients do well on a program of cortisone acetate, 25 mg orally in the morning and 12.5 mg in the late afternoon. An alternative is hydrocortisone, 10 mg in the morning, 10 mg at noon, and 5 mg in the late afternoon. Individual dose adjustment is necessary, depending upon the patient's response. Some will experience an increase in appetite and weight gain, even on standard doses. Laboratory tests are not helpful in determining the precise dose for an individual patient.

Postural hypotension and hyponatremia, while uncommon, will occur in some patients with hypopituitarism and indicate the need for mineralocorticoid replacement. Fludrocortisone acetate (Florinef) is used in a dose as small as 0.05 mg on alternate days and rarely more than 0.1 mg daily. If ankle edema or hypertension develops, the dose should be reduced.

Patients taking glucocorticoid replacement should receive special instructions. They should register with and obtain an appropriate identification tag from the Medic Alert Foundation. During intercurrent illnesses or gastroenteritis they should double their usual steroid dose. They should have available a parenteral dose of glucocorticoid hormone in a prefilled syringe, either 4 mg of dexamethasone phosphate or 100 mg of hydrocortisone sodium succinate (Solu-Cortef). The patient and a family member should be instructed on how to use it in the event of an acute catastrophic illness or when nausea and vomiting preclude oral medications.

Patients with pituitary disease require special hormone treatment before and during surgery. Our routine is to give cortisone acetate, 100 mg intramuscularly, on the morning of surgery. During surgery hydrocortisone sodium succinate (Solu-Cortef) is given intravenously in a dose of 10 mg per hour. Another 100 mg dose of cortisone acetate is given after surgery and is continued in a dose of 100 mg twice daily during the immediate postoperative period. Thereafter the dose can be reduced commensurate with the clinical course.

Patients with hypopituitarism and ACTH deficiency can develop the syndrome of acute adrenal insufficiency just as patients with primary adrenal disease. Treatment is as for acute primary adrenal insufficiency, including immediate intravenous administration of hydrocortisone sodium succinate (Solu-Cortef), 100 mg, and intravenous saline.

Thyroid

The entire spectrum of symptoms and signs of thyroid deficiency can be observed in hypopituitarism and is indistinguishable from, though often milder than, primary hypothyroidism. The same therapeutic considerations apply as in the treatment of primary hypothyroidism.

L-Thyroxine is the standard therapy for hypothyroidism. The usual adult dose is 0.1 to 0.2 mg in a single daily dose. Treatment can usually be started with a 0.1 or 0.15 mg dose. In children, a thyroxine dose of 3 to 5 micrograms per kg per day is used. Desiccated thyroid hormone is a suitable alternative, but triiodothyronine or combinations of thyroxine and triiodothyronine have no place in the management of hypothyroidism.

The adequacy of therapy is assessed by the patient's clinical response and by measurement of the serum thyroxine concentration in patients taking L-thyroxine or desiccated thyroid.

It is prudent to begin treatment with low doses of thyroxine (0.025 or 0.05 mg daily) in the elderly, in patients with known ischemic heart disease, and in patients with longstanding, severe hypothyroidism. That dose is doubled at 3 to 4 week intervals, depending on the patient's response and the serum thyroxine concentration.

Most patients with secondary hypothyroidism will have other pituitary hormone deficits, including ACTH. Treatment with replacement doses of glucocorticoid hormone should be started when thyroid hormone treatment is begun.

HYPERPROLACTINEMIA

method of
BARRY M. SHERMAN
Iowa City, Iowa

An elevated serum prolactin concentration is a marker for the presence of a prolactin-secreting tumor in both men and women. Prolactin-secreting tumors make up 60 per cent or more of all pituitary tumors, including most of those previously thought to be chromophobic or nonfunctioning. During the past decade advances in endocrinologic, radiologic, and neurosurgical methods have changed the amenorrhea-galactorrhea syndrome from a relative medical curiosity to a well-recognized and frequently diagnosed disorder. The spectrum of women with hyperprolactinemia and prolactin-secreting tumors includes postpartum amenorrhea-galactorrhea described by Chiari and Frommel, spontaneous amenorrhea-galactorrhea described by Argonz and Del Castillo, and the amenorrhea-galactorrhea syndrome with evidence of a pituitary tumor on conventional skull x-rays described by Forbes and Albright. In our own experience, the majority of patients with this disorder (60 per cent) developed amenorrhea following discontinuation of oral contraceptive therapy.

Hyperprolactinemia is found in about 30 to 40 per cent of women with secondary amenorrhea and in more than 75 per cent of those in whom galac-

torrhea accompanies amenorrhea. The patient's clinical presentation, whether related to sustained hyperestrogenemia, as in postpill or postpartum amenorrhea-galactorrhea, or apparently unrelated to estrogen action, as in those with primary amenorrhea or the spontaneous onset of secondary amenorrhea, may be an important factor in the choice of therapy.

Radiographic changes suggestive of a pituitary tumor are found in about half the patients with hyperprolactinemia and amenorrhea. However, it is possible that all patients with amenorrhea and hyperprolactinemia have pituitary tumors, some of which are so small or are in such a location that they do not cause erosive change in the sella turcica. In our series, six patients without x-ray abnormalities on polytomography had tumors verified by immunocytochemical study of tissue removed at surgery.

Other causes of hyperprolactinemia are listed in Table 1. Particular attention should be given to exclude hypothyroidism and the use of neuroleptic drugs.

The management of the amenorrhea-galactorrhea syndrome caused by prolactin-secreting tumors is unsettled. Considerations in the management of these patients include (1) restoration of fertility, (2) resolution of galactorrhea, and (3) prevention of tumor growth. In premenopausal women normalization of the serum prolactin concentration usually results in resumption of regular ovulatory menstrual cycles and cessation of galactorrhea.

Two forms of therapy are available for women desirous of pregnancy, but only transsphenoidal surgery has been widely used in the United States because of federal regulations restricting the use of dopamine agonists for treatment of infertility. A dopamine agonist, bromocriptine, has been reported to result in normalization of serum prolactin and the resumption of menses in 80 to 85 per cent of patients with hyperprolactinemia. The therapeutic success of transsphenoidal surgery approaches that of bromocriptine, with minimal morbidity or compromise of pituitary function.

Bromocriptine is a polypeptoid alkaloid derivative of the ergotoxine group. It is a dopamine receptor agonist in that it activates postsynaptic dopaminergic receptors. Dopaminergic neurons of the thalamic or hypothalamic areas modulate the secretion of prolactin from the anterior pitu-

TABLE 1.   **Causes of Abnormal Prolactin Secretion**

Pituitary adenoma
Pituitary stalk section
Neuroleptic drugs
Estrogen therapy
Hyperthyroidism
Chest wall lesions
Renal failure

itary gland either directly or by stimulating the release of prolactin inhibitory factor. Pharmacologic· experiments and clinical evidence have demonstrated the selective activity of bromocriptine in suppressing prolactin secretion in animals and humans with hyperprolactinemia from a variety of causes.

Data on the efficacy of bromocriptine in women with amenorrhea and hyperprolactinemia are based upon a review of 22 separate studies involving a total of 226 patients. Eighty per cent of the patients resumed menses during treatment. The average time to resumption of menses was 6 weeks. Forty-seven per cent of the patients had complete resolution of galactorrhea as well as resumption of menses, while 63 per cent had resumption of menses accompanied by a marked reduction in galactorrhea. After 4 weeks of therapy, 66 per cent of the patients had a serum prolactin concentration less than 25 nanograms per ml. There were 31 pregnancies, resulting in 25 normal children.

Acute toxicity of bromocriptine is largely confined to the consequences of postural hypotension. This often accompanies the initiation of treatment. For that reason, therapy is begun with a single 2.5 mg dose daily for 3 to 5 days and then increased to a total dose of 5 to 7.5 mg daily in divided doses. During that time, tolerance develops to the hypotensive action of the drug. Common side effects of chronic treatment include nausea, headache, dizziness, fatigue, and lightheadedness. Chronic treatment with large doses results in digital vasospasm in a small number of subjects. No consistent hematologic or biochemical changes resulting from bromocriptine treatment in low or high doses have been reported. The drug is not curative. Amenorrhea and galactorrhea generally recur when the drug is discontinued, with recurrence rates ranging from 70 to 80 per cent.

The growth of prolactin-secreting pituitary tumors and development of visual field defects have been reported during pregnancies that followed bromocriptine treatment. If patients become pregnant while taking bromocriptine, the drug should be stopped and they should be followed carefully with serial visual field evaluations during the course of pregnancy.

The overall success rate of transsphenoidal surgery for prolactin-secreting tumors ranges from 46 to 83 per cent and was 58 per cent in our series of 73 patients. The resumption of regular menses and normalization of serum prolactin after transsphenoidal surgery is inversely related to the preoperative serum prolactin concentration and the surgeon's estimate of tumor size. However, it is not possible to generalize from these results to determine whether transsphen-oidal surgery will be successful in an individual patient. In our surgically treated patients, treatment success, defined as resumption of regular menses and/or normalization of the serum prolactin concentration, was achieved in 72 per cent of those women with postpartum or post–oral contraceptive amenorrhea-galactorrhea, compared with 33 per cent in women with primary amenorrhea or spontaneous onset of secondary amenorrhea. I believe that the clinical presentation may be the most important factor in predicting a successful response to transsphenoidal surgery and should be a prime consideration in selection of therapy for prolactin-secreting adenomas.

The reason for the differences in surgical success in these groups is not readily apparent. Women with "non-estrogen-related" amenorrhea may have larger tumors as reflected by more prominent changes on polytomography, by higher prolactin levels, and by longer duration of symptoms. These large tumors may be technically more difficult to remove.

Transsphenoidal surgery for pituitary adenomas is a safe procedure, not accompanied by significant morbidity or complication. Selective removal of the tumor can be accomplished without compromise of pituitary function. Mild diabetes insipidus occurs occasionally, but is usually transient. The procedure can be recommended as effective therapy, particularly for patients with postpartum and post–oral contraceptive hyperprolactinemia who are desirous of pregnancy.

Transsphenoidal surgery remains the accepted procedure for those patients with large tumors who present with visual impairment. Preliminary studies suggest that bromocriptine may reduce the size of prolactin-secreting tumors and relieve visual loss caused by suprasellar extension.

Treatment with a dopamine agonist may have a special place in the treatment of prolactin-secreting tumors in women with primary amenorrhea or those whose secondary amenorrhea is unrelated to estrogen use. There are several considerations that add to the complexity of this therapeutic recommendation. Those tumors that express themselves in the absence of exogenous estrogen use or pregnancy appear to have a greater spontaneous growth potential. These patients may therefore be at greater risk for progressive tumor growth if not treated surgically. A case could be made that these women should receive bromocriptine for treatment of infertility and perhaps on a long-term basis to reduce the risk of tumor growth. While recent reports suggest that complications associated with bromocriptine-induced pregnancies are rare, it is possible that women whose amenorrhea-galactorrhea and hyperprolactinemia develop unrelated to estrogens might be at a higher risk for tumor growth during bromocriptine-induced pregnancies.

A specific recommendation regarding treatment of women in whom fertility is not an issue requires more information about the natural history of prolactin-secreting tumors. The proportion of these tumors that enlarge progressively, causing headache, visual loss, and hypopituitarism, is not known but is probably small. Neither surgery nor chronic bromocriptine can be recommended as routine treatment. The efficacy of external pituitary irradiation is not known. These women should be followed closely with yearly measurements of serum prolactin concentration and biannual tomography of the sella turcica.

The diagnosis of prolactin-secreting tumors in men is often delayed, and the lesions are usually quite large when finally discovered. Normalization of the serum prolactin concentration after surgery or bromocriptine has been reported to result in restoration of both normal spermatogenesis and testosterone secretion.

HYPERTHYROIDISM

method of
ROBERT VOLPÉ, M.D.
Toronto, Ontario, Canada

Introduction

Hyperthyroidism may be defined as the excessive production of thyroid hormones. The most common cause is Graves' disease (Basedow's disease, Parry's disease, autoimmune hyperthyroidism), which appears in 1 to 2 per cent of the population. Less common causes include toxic nodular goiter, the hyperthyroid phase of thyroiditis, and hyperthyroidism resulting from hydatidiform moles or choriocarcinoma. Rare causes include pituitary thyroid stimulating hormone (TSH) excess, widespread functioning metastatic thyroid carcinoma, and excessive ingestion of iodide or thyroid hormone. We shall concern ourselves here primarily with the treatment directed to counteract the thyroid activity.

Graves' disease is currently considered to be an autoimmune disorder. The most likely possibility is that it results from a defect in immune regulation, quite possibly a defect in a population of suppressor T lymphocytes. This permits a normally randomly mutating "forbidden" clone of thyroid-directed "helper" T lymphocytes (which normally would be suppressed) to survive, interact with an antigen on the thyroid cell membrane, and then direct groups of already present appropriate B lymphocytes to produce an immunoglobulin (thyroid stimulating immunoglobulin) against the TSH receptor. This immunoglobulin has the peculiar (if not unique) capacity to be able to attach to the TSH receptor or a closely contiguous site on the cell membrane (presumably by an antigen-antibody union) and then to stimulate the thyroid cells in a manner indistinguishable from that of TSH. The disorder is often associated with ophthalmopathy, and less commonly with dermopathy (pretibial myxedema). The ophthalmopathy seems clearly to be due to autoimmune processes as well, although this is not directly related to the hyperthyroidism. The cause of the dermopathy is yet unclarified. The disorder is most common in women, and the predisposition is genetically transmitted. Remissions of the condition are not uncommon. Since Graves' disease thus appears to be an autoimmune process, rational therapy would be to interfere with the specific autoimmune condition. This, however, is not yet practicable, and thus therapy continues to be directed at the control of excessive thyroid hormone production, either by suppression (antithyroid drugs) or by the destruction of tissue (radioactive iodine or subtotal thyroidectomy). Nonspecific forms of therapy, such as rest, sedation, and beta-adrenergic blockers, are also quite useful.

Toxic nodular goiter, the second most common form of hyperthyroidism, is not of autoimmune origin. It may occur in an evolutionary fashion from preexisting nontoxic goiter. Presumably such nontoxic goiters, having undergone periods of involution and hyperplasia, have developed foci of tissue which are no longer under TSH control. This evolutionary metaplasia may not result in hyperthyroidism, despite the autonomous foci, at least until the focus or foci are large enough and active enough to produce excessive amounts of thyroid hormone. Remissions are virtually unknown in this condition.

Other forms of hyperthyroidism will be mentioned briefly below.

Antithyroid Drugs

Antithyroid drugs can be employed as long-term therapy for Graves' disease, or as interim therapy prior to thyroid destructive therapy (surgery or radioactive iodine). While antithyroid drug therapy can be employed in forms of hyperthyroidism other than Graves' disease, there are special considerations in the latter which must be taken into account. The antithyroid drugs are structurally classified as thionamides. They fall into two main groups, the thiourea group (e.g., propylthiouracil) and the imidazole group (e.g., methimazole). Propylthiouracil is available in 50 and 100 mg tablets and methimazole in 5 and 10 mg tablets. Propylthiouracil has three known actions: it inhibits the peroxidase enzyme system, thus preventing oxidation of trapped iodide and subsequent incorporation into iodotyrosines and ultimately iodothyronine; it inhibits coupling of the iodotyrosines; and finally it inhibits the conversion of L-thyroxine to L-triiodothyronine (T_3)

in peripheral tissues. The imidazole group appears to act only on the peroxidase enzyme system. There is, however, little to distinguish the two groups in terms of clinical response. Propylthiouracil (PTU) is often prescribed in doses of 100 to 200 mg every 8 hours, and methimazole in doses of 10 to 20 mg every 8 hours. While the duration of these drugs is considered to be approximately 8 hours, there is now evidence that they will inhibit synthesis of thyroid hormone for 24 hours or longer. Thus, after the initial treatment period of the first few weeks, the drug can be given at longer intervals and in smaller doses, titrating the dosage against the response. Once patients are under control, PTU in single doses of 50 or 100 mg per day will often maintain a patient in a euthyroid state. Similarly, single doses of 5 mg of methimazole once daily may be equally effective. The timing of clinical improvement will depend upon the amount of thyroid hormone stored within the thyroid gland, because the drugs do not interfere with the secretion of preformed hormone. Improvement is usually evident within 3 weeks, and a euthyroid state may be achieved within 6 to 12 weeks. The dosage is then gradually reduced, although it is necessary to monitor the patient's response continually, and it may be necessary to titrate dosage even after some months. Estimations of serum thyroxine and triiodothyronine are very useful for this purpose.

Only rarely is it necessary to use larger doses than those mentioned above at the commencement of therapy. Under such circumstances the goiter is often found to be extremely large, and ablative therapy generally proves to be the ultimate manner of controlling such patients.

Enlargement of the goiter during therapy may be due either to progression of the basic underlying disease or to development of PTU-induced hypothyroidism. If the serum thyroxine declines below normal and plasma thyrotropin rises, it is important to reduce the dosage of PTU rather than add thyroxine. Also, there is recent evidence that the antithyroid drugs in addition have a mild immunosuppressive effect, although it is doubtful that this reaches clinical significance. In any event, it is generally felt that patients should be on antithyroid drug therapy for at least 1 year, and in some centers for a few years, so as to enhance the incidence of long-term remissions. Evidence suggests that the longer the treatment period, the more remissions will ultimately occur, at least to the point of 2 to 3 years of treatment. However, there are now means at hand to determine whether or not patients are likely to go into remission after several months' (rather than several weeks') therapy.

Patients who are clinically most likely to remain in remission following antithyroid drug therapy are those with moderate or mild hyperthyroidism and relatively small goiters.

Patients with Graves' disease who have been shown to have thyroid stimulating antibody will often show a decline in this abnormal stimulator during antithyroid drug therapy. In those patients who do *not* show a decline, hyperthyroidism will recur once the antithyroid drug therapy is discontinued. Moreover, if patients are found to have the histocompatibility gene HLA-Dw3 (in Caucasians), then the chances of recurrence are greater. These considerations hold only for Graves' disease, and do not hold for any other forms of hyperthyroidism such as toxic nodular goiter.

It is generally our view that all patients with Graves' disease, except perhaps those with very large goiters, should be given at least one course of antithyroid drug therapy prior to embarking on destructive therapy. About 30 per cent of patients will go into long-term remission and thus be able to avoid destructive treatment. However, should one recurrence develop, then I recommend ablative therapy, rather than a second course of antithyroid drug therapy, although views differ in this respect. Moreover, it should be remembered that even if patients do remain in remission for years after antithyroid drug therapy, late recurrences are still possible, and late, spontaneous hypothyroidism may also develop, possibly a result of Hashimoto's thyroiditis.

Although patients with toxic nodular goiter can also be treated with antithyroid drug therapy, remissions will *not* occur. Thus the reason for treating such a patient with these agents is generally to render the patient euthyroid before other forms of therapy are undertaken.

Complications of Drug Therapy

The most serious side effect is agranulocytosis, which is observed in 0.4 to 0.7 per cent of patients. This complication develops precipitously, and there is thus no point in performing frequent or routine leukocyte counts. However, the harbingers of agranulocytosis include severe aphthous stomatitis and pharyngitis, and/or fever, and/or rashes. If the patient develops any of these symptoms, the medication must be discontinued and an immediate leukocyte count performed. The patient should be warned about these symptoms and advised to discontinue the medication and report to the physician immediately. Fortunately, the agranulocytosis is usually reversible. Common, but less severe, side effects include dermatitis, arthralgia, myalgia, jaundice, hepatitis, fever, and lymphadenopathy. Rarely aplastic anemia has been reported. Under such conditions, it is considered wise not to use another antithyroid drug, but to revert to a form of ablative therapy.

Thyroidectomy

Historically, thyroidectomy was the first effective treatment for hyperthyroidism. However, it did not really become feasible until Plummer in 1923 demonstrated the value of iodine in the preparation of patients for surgery. Iodide was shown to reduce the vascularity of the gland and produce a temporary involution. It did this by interfering acutely with the release of thyroid hormone and with the biosynthesis of thyroxine; the latter effect was prolonged in some patients and persisted almost indefinitely when the iodide therapy was continued in at least a small number of patients. This form of preoperative preparation with iodide made it possible to operate on patients who were no longer severely hyperthyroid, and this reduced the incidence of complications considerably. Later the introduction of antithyroid drugs made it possible to have an even more effective preoperative preparation. At present, with advances in anesthetic techniques, surgical procedures, and postoperative care, the mortality of thyroidectomy is virtually nil.

Many centers in the world continue to prefer subtotal thyroidectomy as the optimal form of definitive therapy for Graves' disease, although in Toronto most endocrinologists regard thyroidectomy as the treatment of choice only in selected patients, particularly children or adolescents who cannot be controlled with antithyroid drug therapy. It is, of course, accepted that the patient must be rendered euthyroid before surgery by the administration of antithyroid drug therapy for some weeks, often with the addition of iodide in the last few days. Associated disorders must be treated accordingly; e.g., a patient with cardiac disease should be digitalized and arrhythmias must be corrected or controlled before surgery. Diabetes mellitus, if present, should also be properly controlled.

Although it is generally a safe procedure, subtotal thyroidectomy is still attended by a variety of complications. It is noted that from 3.6 to 42.8 per cent of patients develop hypothyroidism postoperatively, either shortly after the procedure or many years later. The higher incidence was detected by follow-up studies many years after surgery, so it would appear that the thyroid remnant is incapable of continued secretion after a limited period in many patients. The onset of hypothyroidism may be subtle, and often may go undetected for many years while the patient's health gradually deteriorates. The cause of this late postoperative deterioration may be due, at least in some patients, to autoimmune destruction. Consequently, it is clear that annual follow-up is essential, even in those patients who do exceedingly well. Patients who have transient hypothyroidism after operation are particularly prone to develop permanent myxedema later. The presence of thyroid autoantibodies in moderate or high titers at the time of surgery may also be a harbinger of hypothyroidism.

Postoperative hypoparathyroidism will develop in about 1 per cent of patients following subtotal thyroidectomy and indeed in occult form may occur in up to 10 per cent. Patients with the overt form of this condition must be treated with lifelong calcium and vitamin D therapy. Untreated hypoparathyroidism is associated with a high incidence of cataracts, convulsions, and metastatic calcification. Vocal cord palsy resulting from trauma of the recurrent laryngeal nerve is usually unilateral and occurs in 0 to 5.6 per cent. At the very least this complication alters the voice, particularly for singing, and usually results in chronic hoarseness. Paralysis of both cords produces spastic airway obstruction and may require tracheostomy.

The persistence or recurrence of hyperthyroidism has been observed in 0.6 to 17.9 per cent of patients, and is more common in children. A variety of other complications have been described, such as bleeding, scars, keloid formation, wound infections, and phlebitis. It should be emphasized, however, that, in general, subtotal thyroidectomy is an extremely effective form of therapy which controls the disease quickly and well in 90 per cent of patients.

In toxic nodular goiter, removal of the nodule surgically is an effective form of therapy, although generally radioactive iodine may be very effectively employed in older patients with this disorder. In younger persons with toxic adenomas, however, surgery is to be preferred, for reasons which will be discussed under the heading Radioactive Iodine Therapy.

Radioactive Iodine Therapy

Since the thyroid gland is the only tissue to retain iodide for any prolonged interval, it is an ideal organ for the use of therapeutic radioactive iodine. ^{131}I with a half-life of 8 days has been the isotope of choice since it became available. Actually, ^{131}I was first used to treat hyperthyroidism in the late 1930s, but only in the 1950s when it become widely available was this radioisotope established as an effective agent to control hyperthyroidism. This isotope is largely a beta-emitter; only about 10 per cent of its effect is derived from gamma-emission. Because the beta rays travel only about 2 mm, the ^{131}I within the thyroid gland will not damage surrounding structures, and therefore considerable radiation can be applied to the gland. The radiation destroys some cells, leaves other intact, and in some effectively reduces the synthesis of hormone. In many centers it has become the treatment of choice for adult hyperthyroidism. It has many advantages: the treatment is usually definitive; it is convenient and can generally be administered without admitting the patient to hospital; it avoids the morbidity and complications of surgical treatment; and only rarely is ^{131}I administration followed by radiation thyroiditis with tenderness in the neck and an increase in hyperthyroid symptoms.

The first clinical effects of radioactive iodine become evident no earlier than 1 month, with gradual improvement following treatment in most patients. The goiter usually disappears after one dose, while most of the remainder require only a second dose. Only a very small percentage of patients require three or more treatments.

Dosimetry formulations have been proposed, utilizing the units of absorbed radiation, i.e., rads. Thus one formula is as follows:

$$\text{Dose (rads)} = \frac{90 \times \text{microcuries administered} \times 24 \text{ hour uptake}}{\text{Gland weight (in grams)} \times 100}$$

General experience suggests that a dose between 5000 and 7000 rads is appropriate for the diffusely enlarged gland of Graves' disease. In terms of microcuries per gram delivered to the thyroid, the equivalent of this rad dose is 56 to 78 microcuries per gram of thyroid tissue.

Once a dose of microcuries per gram has been determined, the following simplified expression may be used:

$$\text{Administered dose (microcuries)} = \frac{\text{Microcuries/gram desired} \times \text{gland weight} \times 100}{\text{Per cent uptake at 24 hours}}$$

With some experience, the weight of the thyroid gland can be estimated. Such estimates are within 10 to 20 per cent of actual gland weight if the gland is 50 grams or less in size. This simplified system has been termed a "guesstimate."

There is a very considerable variation in turnover rate in the thyroid gland, making sophisticated dosage formulations of less value than heretofore expected. Most simply, 80 microcuries per estimated gram of thyroid tissue may be administered when the 24 hour radioactive iodine uptake is approximately 50 per cent. If the radioactive iodine uptake is considerably higher than this, then the dosage is reduced somewhat. If the uptake is lower than 50 per cent, the dosage is increased slightly. Generally, physicians have tended to overtreat small goiters and thus increase the incidence of hypothyroidism. On the other hand, large goiters are often undertreated. While this "guesstimate" technique seems primitive, it seems to provide results which do not differ greatly from those obtained with more sophisticated formulations. Moreover, there does not appear to be any great advantage in reducing the dosage, since this merely increases the number of patients who are still hyperthyroid 3 months after the initial dose and yet does not prevent the late onset of hypothyroidism once the hyperthyroidism has been controlled (although it may delay that onset for several years).

There are several variables which have been shown to influence the outcome of radioactive iodine therapy. Men are less likely to have hypothyroidism than women, and blacks appear to be more resistant to the ^{131}I. Large thyroid glands appear to be more resistant, but also there is a tendency to underestimate their weight. Patients who are most severely hyperthyroid also seem to be more resistant.

Hypothyroidism is the only significant adverse effect of radioactive iodine therapy. In our hands, about 20 per cent of patients become hypothyroid within 1 year. Thereafter the incidence gradually increases, so that about 50 per cent are hypothyroid within a decade. Follow-up must be continued not only in the early months following radioactive iodine therapy but also on an annual basis for life. Since the onset of hypothyroidism may be subtle, the patients must be exhorted to return for annual examinations to check their thyroid status. However, once patients have become hypothyroid and are taking thyroxine therapy, the chief point of follow-up is to ensure that they continue to take their medication.

The aforementioned considerations relate only to Graves' disease, as much larger doses are required to treat toxic nodular goiter. Doses in the order of 35 millicuries are necessary for this purpose. However, with such large doses, it is usually possible to ablate the offending autonomous nodule, while not damaging the surrounding, resting parenchyma (which has been suppressed by the action of the elevated thyroid hormone concentrations on pituitary TSH secretion and thus does not pick up ^{131}I). Thus the incidence of late hypothyroidism in toxic nodular goiters treated with ^{131}I is much lower than that in Graves' disease. However, although radioactive iodine is very useful in the treatment of toxic nodular goiter, and in our view is the agent of choice in older patients with this disorder, it should not be employed in younger patients with this condition. The autonomous nodule will receive an adequate number of rads to destroy the autonomous area, but the marginal regions just beyond the nodule may receive low dose radiation in the range that might produce thyroid neoplasia years later. This is not the case in Graves' disease, in which all cells are irradiated with high dose radiation (see below).

The late incidence of hypothyroidism in Graves' disease treated with ^{131}I may only partially be due to the radioactive iodine. Radioiodine seems to prevent replication of thyroid cells, and thus late hypothyroidism may be a consequence of the body's failure to replace cells that wear out. This failure may also be due to autoimmune destruction stimulated by irradiation applied to an already susceptible gland.

The other possible hazards of radioactive iodine are largely hypothetical. Abnormalities of leukocyte chromosomes have been reported after ^{131}I therapy, but the increased incidence of leukemia predicted following the use of radioactive iodine in hyperthyroidism has not materialized. There is, however, a slightly increased incidence of leukemia in patients with Graves' disease generally, no matter what form of treatment is prescribed, and it seems to be unrelated to the treatment.

There has been no increased incidence of mutations secondary to gonadal radiation by radioactive iodine. The radiation to each ovary is approximately 0.12 rad per millicurie. The conventional dose of radioactive iodine delivers approximately the same dose of radiation to the ovaries as does roentgenologic examination of the colon or kidneys. The dose of radioactive iodine usually employed in hyperthyroidism would thus produce only a small amount of gonadal radiation, and as a "genetically significant gonadal dose" this source does not contribute nearly as much to the whole of the North American population as does diagnostic radiology.

Concern has been expressed that radioactive iodine might produce carcinoma of the thyroid, because it is well known that radiation to the neck in childhood or adolescence is one of the major causes of thyroid carcinoma. However, the doses of radiation that induce thyroid carcinoma must be low — in the order of 50 to 1500 rads. As the doses of radiation become higher, the incidence of carcinoma of the thyroid declines sharply. It would appear, therefore, that our concern can readily be allayed, because the dosages used for the treatment of Graves' disease are much greater than those referred to previously, and are in the order of 5000 to 10,000 rads. Indeed, the incidence of thyroid carcinoma in patients who have received radioactive iodine for hyperthyroidism appears to be lower than that found in patients subjected to subtotal thyroidectomy, i.e., the incidence of spontaneous thyroid carcinoma in Graves' disease. The low incidence of thyroid carcinoma after ^{131}I may have the same explanation as the fact that so many patients become hypothyroid following such therapy: the radiation in the doses used impairs the ability of the cells to replicate. Once again, however, it should be emphasized that such considerations apply when all the cells within the thyroid gland are receiving high dose irradiation, and thus would not apply when the irradiation is delivered in a spotty manner, such as in toxic nodular goiter.

It is our view that radioactive iodine constitutes the best form of destructive therapy of the thyroid gland, and should be employed as definitive therapy for adult hyperthyroid patients with Graves' disease. Our own youngest age for such therapy is 20 years old. In many European centers, radioactive iodine treatment is not utilized until age 40, whereas in some American centers even children receive this form of therapy.

Other Drugs

Iodide is not an ideal agent for the long-term treatment of hyperthyroidism, because its therapeutic response is frequently incomplete or transient. It is used in the last few days of preoperative preparation, along with an antithyroid drug (primarily to reduce vascularity of the thyroid), or in the treatment of thyroid storm, again in combination with an antithyroid drug.

Lithium carbonate has effects similar to those of iodide. However, the place of lithium in the treatment of hyperthyroidism remains to be defined, and this agent should be considered experimental.

Drugs that deplete catecholamines may also be useful as adjuncts in the treatment of hyperthyroidism. Both reserpine and guanethidine suppress the clinical symptoms of hyperthyroidism caused by the increased action of sympathetic amines, although they do not appear to affect tissue hypermetabolism. (This use of these agents is not listed in the manufacturers' official directives.) Propranolol, a potent beta-adrenergic blocking agent, has a prominent position in the treatment of hyperthyroidism. It generally has no effect on the fundamental disease, although it does cause some reduction in the monodeiodination of thyroxine to triiodothyronine. However, it ameliorates many of the signs and symptoms of hyperthyroidism through its beta-adrenergic blocking; rapid heart beat is controlled, nervousness declines, and sweating and tremor are reduced. The patient generally feels much improved. Improvement has also been noted in myocardial efficiency, and the exaggerated myocardial oxygen consumption has been reduced. Propranolol has been useful as symptomatic therapy while awaiting the improvement from antithyroid drugs or radioactive iodine. Some patients have even gone into remission on propranolol therapy alone. These drugs should be used cautiously when there is evidence of myocardial insufficiency, although control of tachycardia in Graves' disease often permits improved circulatory efficiency. Propranolol is usually given orally in doses of 20 to 40 mg every 6 hours. In thyroid storm it may be given intravenously, 1 to 3 mg over 3 to 10 minutes.

Special Considerations

Treatment of Children. Hyperthyroidism is comparatively rare in young children. Generally antithyroid drug therapy is preferred in children and adolescents, and treatment for 2 years or longer is recommended. If remissions do not occur and if the disorder cannot be controlled with antithyroid drugs, most conservative clinicians recommend subtotal thyroidectomy, at least until age 20, although the complications of thyroidectomy appear to be more frequent in children (perhaps because the structures are smaller). Radioactive iodine has been advocated by some groups for use in children and adolescents, although it has not yet received wide approval. Although the fear of carcinogenesis appears unfounded, a longer period of follow-up is still required before radioactive iodine is approved for wider application in children.

Pregnancy. Radioactive iodine is contraindicated in pregnancy because the fetal thyroid concentrates iodine after the twelfth week of gestation. However, radioactive iodine therapy has been prescribed inadvertently to some gravid women in the first and second trimesters without apparent injury to the fetus. Nevertheless, such risks should not be taken knowingly, and it is wise to be certain that women are not pregnant before radioactive iodine is administered. Surgery is to be avoided in the first trimester because it results in a high incidence of spontaneous abortion, although it seems reasonably safe in the second trimester.

Generally, the hyperthyroid state during pregnancy is treated with antithyroid drug therapy. It is our practice to continue antithyroid drugs throughout the period of gestation. In the early part of pregnancy, the usual doses of antithyroid drugs are used, as has been discussed previously. However, the drugs cross the placenta and, if the

dosage is excessive, may produce goiter and hypothyroidism in the fetus. Such goiters may be of a size that may interfere with vaginal delivery. Thus, particularly in the last part of the second trimester and throughout the third trimester, dosages must be reduced considerably; doses of PTU below 200 mg per day have not been reported to cause goiter in the newborn. The dose of PTU during pregnancy must be titrated to ensure that the mother does not become hypothyroid because this state is associated with an increased incidence of spontaneous abortion. Aside from maternal hypothyroidism, there is no point in adding thyroxine to the mother's treatment during this stage of pregnancy because thyroxine does not traverse the placenta. In the latter part of gestation it is therefore important to reduce the dose of antithyroid drug to low levels, even if this results in a slight return of hyperthyroidism. Following delivery the mother should not nurse her infant, because the antithyroid drug (which should be continued following delivery) is secreted in the mother's milk. On the other hand, it may be possible to discontinue therapy at that time if there is evidence that the mother is in a state of remission.

Since thyroid stimulating immunoglobulin (TSI) crosses the placenta, the infant should be carefully examined for neonatal Graves' disease. This will be present only if large amounts of thyroid stimulating immunoglobulin were present in the mother. The early advent of this condition in the newborn infant will not be seen when the mother has been on antithyroid drug treatment throughout pregnancy, since the fetal TSI-induced goiter will have been suppressed as this agent crosses the placenta. Thus, several days may elapse after delivery before neonatal Graves' disease makes its appearance. It must then be treated with antithyroid drug therapy once again, and will subside as the thyroid stimulating immunoglobulin disappears from the infant's bloodstream.

Thyroid Storm. Thyroid storm (thyroid crisis) is a life-threatening condition that is characterized by the greatly heightened signs and symptoms of hyperthyroidism and by hyperpyrexia. The elevation in body temperature may reach 106 F (41.2 C) and be associated with marked restlessness, agitation, severe tachycardia, heart failure, profound prostration, nausea, vomiting, diarrhea, delirium, psychosis, jaundice, and subsequent dehydration. The disorder is now rare. Factors that precipitate this crisis include infections, trauma, surgery, and withdrawal from antithyroid drugs. Treatment is usually commenced with iodide because this drug reduces the secretion of thyroid hormone very quickly. Doses of

500 mg every 6 hours orally or 0.5 gram of sodium iodide in a constant intravenous drip every 8 hours should be used. It is important to give propylthiouracil in doses of 300 to 600 mg per day *before* giving the iodine, so that synthesis of thyroxine will also be quickly blocked. If iodine is prescribed first, there may be a considerable delay in response to the antithyroid agent. Propranolol, intravenous fluid therapy, the mechanical treatment of hyperthermia, and corticosteroids, may also be used during this emergency.

Ophthalmopathy. There is no truly rational or satisfactory treatment for severe ophthalmopathy of Graves' disease. Fortunately, the ophthalmopathy is often mild and does not require stringent methods of treatment. In such cases, methylcellulose drops can be employed for comfort. In severe cases of infiltrative ophthalmopathy or even malignant exophthalmos, systemic corticosteroids in very large dosages (e.g., prednisone, 120 mg per day) are necessary. Similar dosage schedules are necessary if vision is in danger, particularly if there is papilledema or visual field scotomas. This therapy can sometimes be augmented by immunosuppressive therapy in the form of cyclophosphamide, but this agent is of little value alone. (This use of cyclophosphamide is not listed in the manufacturer's official directive.) In any event, very large dose corticosteroid therapy will generally result in a considerable decrease in the acute inflammatory manifestations and an objective reduction in proptosis. Some ophthalmologists favor retrobulbar steroid injections, but patients dislike this modality, and there is no great advantage in this method over systemic steroid administration.

In oculopathies of this severity, consideration should be given to supervoltage radiotherapy to the orbits, particularly while the patients are still receiving corticosteroids. This may result in some degree of permanent reduction in the infiltrative inflammatory reaction.

The treatment of ophthalmoplegia is less satisfactory. While on occasion ophthalmoplegias will respond to the aforementioned measures, more frequently by the time they are observed the muscle shortening is already permanent.

In any event, it is clear that large dosage corticosteroid therapy cannot be maintained for more than a few weeks, and must be gradually reduced and then discontinued. Often, however, the most severe manifestations of the oculopathy will not return. Nevertheless, one is often left with very severely proptotic eyes, and one still may have severe infiltrative ophthalmopathy. In such instances, surgical correction should be considered. Transantral decompression is probably the most favored operative procedure, although it can make diplopia more marked. About one third of patients who did not have diplopia before surgery will have it following this surgical procedure, and this may require a second surgical procedure. For ophthalmoplegias, if mild, prismatic lenses may sometimes be appropriate, but often muscle recessive surgery is required. Such surgery should be performed only when the oculopathy has been stable for at least several months. Other surgical techniques that have been employed to improve oculopathies include tarsorrhaphy, or lowering of the lids.

Other Types of Hyperthyroidism

Thyrotoxicosis associated with subacute thyroiditis or silent (painless) thyroiditis is frequently associated with a hyperthyroid phase in the initial stage of the disease. This is a result of the release of massive amounts of thyroid hormones through destruction of the thyroid gland. While painful (de Quervain's) thyroiditis has been a well-known entity for decades, recently the entity of painless thyroiditis has gained increasing attention. Painless thyroiditis differs from the painful form in a number of different ways. First, the thyroid gland may be minimally enlarged or not enlarged at all; moreover, the sedimentation rate is only slightly elevated or not at all. Finally, the pathologic picture in the painless variety is that of a lymphocytic infiltration which resembles Hashimoto's thyroiditis (although Askanazy cells are usually lacking). However, it does not truly represent Hashimoto's thyroiditis, as thyroid autoantibodies are in low titer or lacking altogether, and the gland goes on to full recovery with the pathologic picture returning to normal. The painful variety is generally treated with corticosteroids when severe, or with analgesics when mild. The painless variety requires only propranolol therapy for the control of the hyperthyroid symptoms. Antithyroid therapy on the one hand and destructive therapy on the other are completely contraindicated.

Hyperthyroidism resulting from hydatidiform mole or choriocarcinoma is due to the very high levels of human chorionic gonadotropin elaborated by these lesions. Thus the treatment of the hyperthyroidism primarily consists of removing the source, although it may be necessary to treat the hyperthyroidism with antithyroid drugs and iodide during the interim period.

Hyperthyroidism resulting from excess intake of iodide (jodbasedow syndrome) may require propranolol therapy and sedation until the disease abates when the iodine intake is reduced. Hyperthyroidism resulting from excess production of TSH will, of course, be cured if the TSH-secreting pituitary microadenoma is removed. In some of these patients, a definite microadenoma is not demonstrable, although it is possible that all such patients do have tiny pituitary microadenomas. In hyperthyroidism caused by widespread functioning metastases of follicular carcinoma of the thyroid, clearly the therapy is to destroy those functioning metastases. Finally, in hyperthyroidism caused by the excessive ingestion of thyroid hormones, the treatment is obvious.

HYPOTHYROIDISM

method of
PAUL J. DAVIS, M.D.,
and FAITH B. DAVIS, M.D.
Buffalo, New York

Appropriate treatment of hypothyroidism depends upon knowledge of (1) the cause of thyroid hypofunction, (2) its severity, (3) the clinical context in which hypothyroidism has been detected (e.g., patient age, presence of coronary artery disease), and (4) patient compliance. Implicit in the responsibility for therapy is measurement of the effectiveness of instituted therapy ("end point"). In acute clinical settings in which the question of the diagnosis of profound hypothyroidism has been raised, it is appropriate to institute replacement therapy before results of thyroid function tests are available. The risks of temporarily treating eumetabolic patients with replacement thyroid hormone are negligible. It is also important to recognize the effect of nonthyroidal illness on serum thyroid function tests so that hypothyroidism is not overdiagnosed.

Causes of Hypothyroidism

More than 95 per cent of patients with hypothyroidism have primary thyroidal failure ("thyroidal hypothyroidism") resulting from spontaneous chronic lymphocytic thyroiditis or ablation of a previously thyrotoxic thyroid gland by radioiodine administration or surgery. Nonetheless, the possibility of pituitary hypothyroidism must be considered in all patients who present with signs and symptoms of thyroid hypofunction. Treatment of pituitary hypothyroidism with thyroid replacement therapy alone may precipitate adrenocortical insufficiency. An occasional patient with longstanding thyroidal hypothyroidism may experience relative adrenocortical insufficiency when thyroid replacement therapy is started. Relative adrenocortical insuffi-

ciency must be distinguished from irreversible adrenocortical failure (Addison's disease), which occasionally coexists with chronic lymphocytic thyroiditis. Pituitary hypothyroidism is either idiopathic or due to a locally destructive process, such as primary or metastatic tumor involvement of the pituitary, intrapituitary hemorrhage, or granulomatous disease of the hypothalamus and pituitary. It should also be kept in mind that administration of several nonendocrine medications may precipitate hypothyroidism. For example, cholestyramine and colestipol are bile salt chelators which also bind thyroid hormone in the gastrointestinal tract; the use of these resins in hypothyroid patients reduces the effectiveness of replacement therapy. Administration of iodide as a putative mucolytic agent to patients with chronic obstructive lung disease who are euthyroid but have chronic lymphocytic thyroiditis (Hashimoto's thyroiditis) can induce reversible hypothyroidism; the damaged thyroid is unable to escape the inhibitory effects of iodide on thyroid hormone biosynthesis. Finally, the use of aminoglutethimide as an antiadrenal agent in patients with ectopic ACTH syndrome or with Cushing's syndrome may also lead to hypothyroidism, since aminoglutethimide is also an antithyroid agent.

Severity of Hypothyroidism

Myxedema stupor and coma are far-advanced thyroprival states occurring in patients over the age of 50 years and require high dose thyroid hormone replacement intravenously as well as other measures as described below. In contrast, the majority of patients with hypothyroidism are 40 to 70 years of age, present with longstanding, mild to moderate hypometabolism, and may develop significant adverse cardiovascular and nervous system effects from thyroid hormone administration unless such therapy is initiated in low dosage and only gradually increased to full replacement levels. Patients under the age of 40 years with recent-onset, mild hypothyroidism — for example, after thyroidectomy or because of chronic lymphocytic thyroiditis — may be candidates for full-dose oral replacement thyroid hormone therapy at the time of diagnosis of thyroid hypofunction.

Nonthyroidal Disease Which Is Concomitant with Hypothyroidism

Concurrence of hypothyroidism and coronary arteriosclerosis or cerebrovascular disease can influence the approach to management and prognosis of hypothyroidism. Worsening of angina pectoris or congestive heart failure is a well-known complication of thyroid hormone replacement therapy, and, although the contrary may be hoped, dementia may become more apparent as thyroid hormone replacement therapy is instituted in certain elderly patients. It should also be recalled that the pharmacokinetics and dose requirements of a variety of nonthyroidal drugs may be changed as hypothyroid patients are returned to the euthyroid state.

Patient Compliance

The possibility that a hypothyroid patient is failing to take replacement thyroid hormone appropriately must always be considered in outpatients whose course does not conform to conventional expectations. It should first be determined that adverse effects of thyroid hormone replacement have not caused the hypothyroid patient to discontinue replacement therapy. Patients who chronically omit replacement therapy may be given at one time a week's dose of thyroid hormone (hebdomadal therapy) either in the physician's office or in the course of house calls by visiting nurses. In those instances in which the hypothyroid patient knowingly takes excessive doses of thyroid hormone, prescriptions for limited amounts of thyroid hormone, pill counts at the time of office visits, or once per week administration of thyroid hormone may be utilized.

Indications for Initiating Thyroid Hormone Replacement Therapy Prior to Laboratory Confirmation of the Diagnosis

Before the laboratory diagnosis of hypothyroidism is secure, it is appropriate to consider administration of thyroid hormone in the following settings:

1. Hypothermia (body temperature less than 93 F [33.9 C]) in the context of a history of any form of "thyroid disease."
2. Conventional clinical findings of hypothyroidism associated with impaired sensorium or hypotension.
3. Suspected neonatal hypothyroidism.

Clinical Settings in Which the Presumptive Diagnosis of Hypothyroidism Does Not Warrant Thyroid Replacement Therapy

Obesity or infertility in the presence of normal serum thyroid function tests should not be construed as subtle indicators of the presence of hypothyroidism. Drug-induced depressions of serum T_4 and T_3—as may be attributed to the administration of diphenylhydantoin (phenytoin) or androgens—do not mandate thyroid hormone replacement therapy. The finding of normal serum thyroid stimulating hormone (TSH) levels in this setting is assurance that thyroidal hypothyroidism is not present.

The term "premyxedema" has been applied to the concurrence of hyperlipidemia and circulating antibodies to thyroid gland antigens; serum thyroid function tests such as T_4 RIA, free T_4, and resin T_3 uptake are normal. No case can currently be made for instituting thyroid hormone in this setting. Impaired peripheral (i.e., extrathyroidal) conversion of T_4 to T_3 occurs in a variety of nonthyroidal illnesses, such as hepatic disease, chronic renal failure, and diabetes mellitus. Caloric deprivation may in part underlie the inability to generate normal quantities of T_3 from T_4 in tissues such as the liver, kidney, and muscle. Current evidence is insufficient, however, to confirm that such patients are in fact hypometabolic if their serum free T_4 levels remain within the normal range.

Forms of Thyroid Hormone Available for Replacement Therapy

The following forms of thyroid hormone are commercially available:

L-Thyroxine (Levothroid; Synthroid). In virtually all clinical presentations of hypothyroidism, L-thyroxine (T_4) is the preferred form of thyroid hormone to be employed. The preparation contains no significant quantity of other active or inactive analogues of thyroid hormone and is not contaminated with nonhormonal iodide. It is of synthetic origin, and therefore no thyroid gland proteins or other proteins are present in its formulation. Absorption from the gastrointestinal tract depends upon the time relationship of drug administration to the fasting and fed states. Up to 80 per cent of L-thyroxine may be absorbed when patients are in the fasted state, and 50 per cent is absorbed by patients in the fed state. An intravenous preparation of L-thyroxine is available for use in emergent settings when myxedema stupor or coma is present (see below). It is thought that most of the metabolic activity of L-thyroxine is expressed as a result of its conversion to L-triiodothyronine (T_3) following its administration. In virtually all patients with hypothyroidism, this conversion of T_4 to T_3 is believed to occur at a rate consonant with the patient's metabolic needs. Circulating levels of T_3 in hypothyroid patients treated with T_4 rise smoothly toward the euthyroid range as the dosage of T_4 is increased progressively to full replacement levels. The cost of L-thyroxine is competitive with all other commercially available forms of thyroid hormone replacement. It is supplied in strengths ranging from 0.025 to 0.300 mg per tablet.

L-Triiodothyronine (Cytomel). Administration of this form of thyroid hormone—which is two to five times as metabolically potent as L-thyroxine—results in brief periods of high levels of blood T_3 after each oral dose. Because of the metabolic activity of T_3, such elevations are theoretically, if not clinically, undesirable. The half-life of T_3 is about 1 day, roughly one seventh that of T_4, and occasionally we consider using this short-lived form of thyroid hormone replacement in situations in which thyroid hormone toxicity may be anticipated and particularly detrimental. For example, patients with previously untreated hypothyroidism and stable angina pectoris may be started on small doses of T_3 as replacement. If angina accelerates, lowering of the dose of T_3 or its withdrawal will usually result in a prompt improvement in cardiac symptoms. We have used propranolol and small doses of T_3 in this clinical situation in order to control symptoms of hypothyroidism and of coronary artery insufficiency. Another undesirable aspect of T_3 administration is that full replacement dosage results in a lowering of the serum T_4 level into the profoundly hypothyroid range. Thus the commonly available and reasonably priced serum T_4 RIA is of no value in assessing metabolic state in patients whose thyroid hormone replacement has been carried out with T_3. L-T_3 is not commercially available for parenteral use.

Desiccated Thyroid. Of either beef or porcine origin, desiccated thyroid gland tablets are not recommended for replacement therapy in patients with hypothyroidism. These preparations have been standardized on the basis of iodine rather than thyroid hormone content. Included in their formulation are a variety of iodinated analogues of thyroid hormone of low or high potency, as well as undisclosed amounts of thyroid gland proteins.

Thyroglobulin (Proloid) and Combination Tablets of Synthetic T_4 and T_3 (Euthroid, Thyrolar). A standardized preparation of porcine thyroid gland–source thyroglobulin is commercially available and contains a fixed proportion of L-thyroxine and L-triiodothyronine (about 2.5:1). Combination tablets containing synthetic T_4 and T_3 in a 4:1 ratio are also available. No therapeutic advantage is gained with the administration of these generally more expensive forms of thyroid hormone.

Thyroid Hormone Replacement Regimens

The conventional goal of treatment of hypothyroidism is obviously reestablishment of the eumetabolic state. Recent evidence suggests that administration of a single dose of L-T_4 in the amount of 2.2 micrograms per kg body weight per day achieves eumetabolism in the vast majority of hypothyroid subjects. "Full replacement" is inferred from suppression by thyroid hormone administration of previously elevated serum thyrotropin (TSH) levels into the normal range.

In most patients, then, the total daily replacement dose of T_4 is 0.15 to 0.175 mg (150 to 175 micrograms). Data from our laboratory suggest that in patients with hypothyroidism who are over the age of 60 years, a lower replacement dose (e.g., 1.6 micrograms per kg per day) may suffice.

Mild Hypothyroidism, Recent Onset, Patients of Age 40 Years or Younger. In most of these patients, full replacement therapy can be initiated at the time of confirmation of diagnosis of hypothyroidism.

Mild to Moderately Severe Hypothyroidism, Patients Over the Age of 40 Years. In the absence of clinical, electrocardiographic, echocardiographic, and radiologic evidence of heart disease, initiation of full replacement dosage of thyroid hormone can be considered at the time of diagnosis of thyroid hypofunction. Ordinarily, however, it is difficult to exclude the possibility of concomitant heart disease, and it is appropriate to begin thyroid hormone replacement in this group of patients with a low dose of T_4 and progressively increase the replacement dose with time until eumetabolism is obtained. The initial dose of T_4 is 0.025 or 0.050 mg per day (25 to 50 micrograms per day) in these patients. At 2 to 6 week intervals, the daily dose is increased by steps of 0.025 or 0.050 mg (25 or 50 micrograms). If congestive heart failure, tachyrhythmia, or a change in anginal pattern occurs, the dose is adjusted downward by 1 step and maintained for 1 to 2 months, at which time the patient is again challenged with an increase in dose.

Occasionally we encounter patients who cannot tolerate thyroid hormone replacement dosages needed to achieve full replacement. Worsening angina pectoris or arrhythmia may be the factors limiting thyroid hormone replacement. Such patients may be maintained indefinitely on suboptimal doses of T_4, e.g., 0.025 or 0.050 mg per day (25 or 50 micrograms per day). These patients will be symptomatically hypothyroid and usually require propranolol or other antianginal therapy. They are at risk for myxedema stupor or coma when subjected to the stress of major nonthyroidal illness.

Some patients with mild to moderately severe hypothyroidism may require corticosteroid replacement, because of relative adrenocortical insufficiency, during the initiation of thyroid hormone replacement. We do not introduce steroid therapy unless the patient (1) has clinical evidence of volume depletion during thyroid hormone replacement, (2) develops new, or worsens already present, hyponatremia, or (3) has documented pituitary insufficiency. Because hyponatremia is frequently seen in hypothyroidism and accounted for by the latter through several mechanisms, the presence of low serum sodium concentrations is not itself a mandate for corticosteroid replacement. When they are required for management of relative adrenocortical insufficiency, glucocorticoids should be administered at a dosage of 100 to 150 mg of hydrocortisone (or its equivalent in corticosteroid analogues) per day in divided dosage. Higher doses of glucocorticoids (e.g., 300 mg per 24 hours) are frequently recommended but represent twice maximum ("stress") endogenous corticoid production.

Myxedema Stupor or Coma. These states are medical emergencies with extraordinary mortality when left untreated. Despite the clinical presence of heart disease in many patients who present with myxedema stupor or coma, high-dose intravenous thyroid hormone replacement therapy is indicated and is lifesaving. The dose of parenteral T_4 (Synthroid) is 250 to 500 micrograms as a bolus injection; the dose is repeated in 12 to 24 hours if no significant change in sensorium or improvement in hypothermia is noted. Full replacement corticosteroid, as detailed above, is also supplied via the intravenous route. Additional supportive measures include treatment of concomitant nonthyroid illness which may have triggered myxedema coma, such as superimposed infection. The patient may then be maintained on 50 to 75 micrograms of T_4 intravenously daily until he is able to take thyroid hormone replacement by mouth, after which time stepwise upward progressions in replacement dosages to the full replacement range may be made. Stress-level corticosteroid replacement need be continued only through the hypothermic phase of the patient's illness and may be tapered thereafter, unless the suspicion of a hypopituitary basis for the patient's hypothyroidism remains.

Hypothyroidism in Children. It is important to initiate thyroid hormone replacement in the neonate as soon as thyroid hypofunction is suspected and serum for determinations of T_4 and TSH has been sent to the laboratory. The dose is 10 to 12 micrograms of T_4 per kg of body weight; after 3 months the T_4 dose is reduced to 8 to 10 micrograms per kg. In the age group 1 to 5 years, 6 micrograms of T_4 per kg is recommended, and 4 to 6 micrograms per kg is sufficient between the ages of 5 and 15 years. Therapy is monitored clinically (normal growth pattern, remission of symptoms of hypothyroidism) and by normalization of serum T_4 and TSH content. By midadolescence, the "adult replacement dose" of 2.2 micrograms per kg is recommended.

Assessment of End Points of Thyroid Hormone Replacement Therapy

The criteria by which hypothyroid patients may be evaluated to determine the appropriateness of a given replacement dose of thyroid hormone include (1) subjective impressions provided by the patients, (2) objective assessments by the physician of certain physical findings of hypothyroidism, and (3) the use of several laboratory tests. Because neither patient nor physician may have adequate insight into the premyxedematous state of patients, the weighting of improvement in symptoms and signs of hypothyroidism during replacement therapy may be difficult. Remission of periorbital edema, voice hoarseness, and abnormal deep tendon reflexes is an obvious end point. Unfortunately, this end point may be reached either with too much thyroid hormone and the risk of thyroid hormone toxicity or with relatively low levels of hormone replacement which do not achieve normality of any of a variety of biochemical parameters. The goal we recommend is a mid-normal range serum T_4 concentration in patients receiving T_4 replacement and a return into the normal range of the previously elevated serum TSH concentration. In elderly patients, in whom it becomes increasingly important to establish that nontoxic thyroid hormone replacement is instituted, we occasionally will carry out a thyrotropin-releasing hormone (TRH) test during thyroid hormone replacement and define full replacement as that daily dose of T_4 which normalizes, but does not suppress, the TSH response to the administration of TRH.

THYROID MALIGNANCY

method of
ANTHONY J. EDIS, M.D.,
and OLIVER H. BEAHRS, M.D.
Rochester, Minnesota

Introduction

Until recently, malignancies of the thyroid gland were considered uncommon. However, in a study conducted at the University of Michigan in 1976, thin-section and meticulous histologic examination of thyroid glands removed at routine autopsy revealed tiny cancers in fully 13 per cent. Similar studies in Japan have shown an even higher prevalence of thyroid cancer in the Japanese population (approaching 30 per cent). The question is whether these tumors, which look like typical papillary cancers under the microscope, share the same biologic potential for growth and metastasis as their counterparts encountered clinically. Apparently they do not, otherwise we would expect to see many more patients with clinically evident disease than we do. Thyroid cancer in its clinically overt form remains uncommon, and it is still a very rare cause of death in the United States (about 1100 annually).

There is renewed interest in thyroid cancer as a result of recent recognition of the fact that persons exposed to x-ray treatment of the head and neck are at increased risk of developing thyroid malignancy. It is estimated that before the 1950s, more than 1 million people in the United States received x-irradiation of the head and neck as treatment for conditions such as tonsillitis, acne, cervical lymphadenopathy, thymic enlargement, keloid scars, and hemangiomas of the skin. We now know that thyroid cancer may develop in these persons even as long as 20 or 30 years after the initial x-ray exposure. If a thyroid nodule is palpable in such persons, surgery is indicated; according to several authorities, the chances of finding a thyroid malignancy approach 30 to 40 per cent. Concern about this problem has prompted many clinics and hospitals throughout the United States to institute recall programs aimed at identifying and treating patients at risk.

Hopes for early diagnosis and, hence, prompt and more effective treatment have been realized recently for at least one form of thyroid malignancy — namely, the rare, inheritable type known as medullary thyroid carcinoma (MTC). This has been facilitated by the development of a reliable radioimmunoassay for the hormone calcitonin. Calcitonin is the unique secretory product of MTC, and it therefore serves as a specific tumor marker. To screen familial MTC suspects for the disease, one has only to measure their circulating plasma calcitonin levels. An increased basal level of plasma calcitonin or an exaggerated increase in concentration in response to a challenge with intravenous calcium or pentagastrin provides definite evidence of MTC or its precursor, C-cell hyperplasia.

Thyroid malignancies can be categorized into three broad groups according to the cell of origin (Table 1). Treatment differs for each group, and there are also special therapeutic considerations that apply to the various subgroups listed.

Tumors of Follicular Cell Origin

Papillary Carcinoma. Papillary carcinoma is by far the most common malignant tumor of the thyroid gland. Papillary carcinoma is generally regarded as relatively indolent in its behavior. It is characteristically a slow-growing lesion, and although spread to regional lymph nodes is not uncommon, more distant metastasis via the bloodstream is rarely encountered. If the primary tumor has not breached the capsule of the thyroid to invade adjacent structures in the neck (extrathyroid type), it is usually amenable to cure.

In our practice, the primary treatment is total lobectomy on the side of the lesion and, because of the significant incidence of multicentric lesions, a near-total lobectomy on the opposite side. If a remnant of 1 to 2 grams of thyroid tissue is left, at least one parathyroid gland can be preserved consistently, and the risk of postoperative hypoparathyroid tetany is thereby minimized. If parathyroid glands are devascularized in the course of thyroidectomy, salvage is possible by dicing the glands into small pieces and autotransplanting them into the sternocleidomastoid muscle. Lymph nodes from the tracheoesophageal groove on each side (middle compartment of the neck and upper anterior mediastinum) are routinely dissected and removed in continuity with the thyroid specimen, but clearance of the lateral region of the neck is indicated only if enlarged nodes are palpable either on clinical examination or at the time of operation. Involved nodes, together with adjacent node-bearing fascia and fat, are dissected en bloc; the internal jugular vein and the cosmetically important sternocleidomastoid muscle are preserved. A classic radical neck dissection is required only in the rare patient in whom lymph node involvement is truly massive. Although it seems paradoxic, a number of clinical studies attest to the fact that the presence or absence of nodal metastasis has no bearing on the curability of a given tumor. This is an unusual, if not unique, situation in tumor biology.

As a matter of routine, we prescribe lifelong thyroid hormone therapy in fully suppressive doses after surgery for papillary thyroid cancer,

TABLE 1.   **Classification of Thyroid Cancers**

CELLULAR ORIGIN	HISTOLOGIC TYPE		PATHOLOGIC STATE	
Follicular	Papillary	62%*	Occult (<1.5 cm diam)	35%
			Intrathyroid	50%
			Extrathyroid (thyroid capsule breached)	15%
	Follicular	18%	Angioinvasion	
			Minimal	50%
			Moderate or marked	50%
	Anaplastic	14%		
Parafollicular (C cell)	Medullary	6%		
Lymphoreticular		<1%		

*Percentages are relative incidence among 1181 cases at the Mayo Clinic, Rochester, Minnesota, 1926 through 1960.

because there is at least suggestive evidence that thyroid cancers of follicular cell origin are thyroid-stimulating hormone growth-dependent. We have also been influenced by the results of a recent United States Armed Forces Institute of Pathology study highlighting the importance of follow-up radioiodine therapy after surgery for papillary cancer. Our indications for postoperative radioiodine ablation of the thyroid remnant have been liberalized to include all cases of papillary cancer except occult tumors (those less than 1.5 cm in diameter) without nodal metastasis. A radioiodine uptake study and scan are performed 6 to 8 weeks postoperatively. All thyroid medication is discontinued several weeks before the scan (3 weeks if triiodothyronine is used; 6 weeks for thyroxine) to induce hypothyroidism and to encourage avid uptake of the administered tracer dose of ^{131}I. If the only uptake is from residual thyroid tissue in the neck, the remnant is ablated by giving an appropriate dose (usually less than 29 millicuries [mCi]) of ^{131}I. If distant metastatic foci are revealed by the scan, a therapeutic dose (50 to 200 mCi) of radioiodine is administered. The results of therapy are monitored by subsequent scans at judicious intervals. In the interim between scans, thyroid hormone is given in full suppressive doses. Regular follow-up of these patients is, of course, mandatory. This conservative surgical approach to papillary adenocarcinoma of the thyroid gland has resulted in a very low surgical mortality rate (0.1 per cent) and minimal morbidity. If the primary lesion has not breached the thyroid capsule to invade surrounding structures in the neck, the survival rate is excellent; only with the extrathyroidal type of tumor is long-term survival significantly decreased.

Follicular Carcinoma. In contrast to papillary cancer, follicular carcinoma of the thyroid gland rarely spreads to regional lymph nodes. Instead, it shows a pronounced predilection to invade adjacent blood vessels and then to spread to distant sites, such as bone and lungs. It is the degree of vascular invasion seen on microscopic examination of the tumor capsule that determines the prognosis. A 40 year follow-up study carried out at the Mayo Clinic revealed that when there was no angioinvasion or only slight angioinvasion of the capsule, survival did not differ from that of normal persons of comparable age and sex. When angioinvasion was moderate or severe, however, survival decreased to only half that of the normal population.

Treatment of follicular carcinoma of the thyroid follows exactly those guidelines discussed above for papillary cancer.

Anaplastic Carcinoma. Anaplastic cancer of the thyroid gland is a rapidly growing lesion that spreads early into adjacent neck structures and also to distant sites via the bloodstream. It is uniformly fatal, regardless of treatment; most patients die within 36 months after diagnosis.

Occasionally, it is possible to relieve obstructive airway symptoms for a time by a palliative debulking of tumor, but most often the surgeon can do no more than simply biopsy the lesion.

Tumors of Parafollicular Cell Origin

Medullary Thyroid Carcinoma (MTC). The parafollicular or C (for calcitonin-secreting) cells of the thyroid gland are derived embryologically from the neural ectoderm in common with a number of different cells that are subsequently found dispersed throughout the endocrine system of the adult. It is, therefore, not altogether surprising to find MTC associated with tumors of the adrenal medulla and parathyroid glands. This particular clinical conglomerate is referred to as multiple endocrine neoplasia syndrome, Type 2a. Patients with Type 2b syndrome differ from those with Type 2a only in that they also have a peculiar marfanoid habitus and distinctive lumpy ganglioneuromas of the lips, mouth, conjunctiva, and bowel. These syndromes, like familial MTC itself, are transmissible from one generation to another by autosomal dominant inheritance. Thus, in patients with proved MTC, it is important not only to look for associated endocrine disease before planning therapeutic priorities (pheochromocytoma first, thyroid and parathyroid disease second) but also to make a careful appraisal of family members in a search for clinical or subclinical disease. It is here that plasma calcitonin screening has such great utility (see above).

Sporadic MTC usually involves only one lobe of the thyroid gland, but the familial form of the disease, in our experience, is invariably bilateral. Lymph nodes are involved with metastatic disease in about 50 per cent of patients overall. However, in patients in whom the diagnosis has been made by calcitonin screening, only 35 per cent have positive nodes. It is to be hoped that this will translate into a higher cure rate for this group of patients, because in MTC, unlike papillary cancer, the presence or absence of lymph node involvement is a most important determinant of prognosis. The 10 year survival rate for patients without nodal metastasis closely approximates that of normal persons of comparable age and sex; for patients with positive involvement of nodes, it is only 40 per cent. Other factors are important in determining survival; for example, the familial form of MTC appears to have an intrinsically better prognosis than the sporadic form — unless the patient also has the neuroma phenotype, in which case the disease appears to be particularly lethal. One has to be impressed also with the great variability in the biologic behavior of MTC. Some tumors may cause death within a year of diagnosis, whereas others enjoy an almost symbiotic relationship with their host for many years.

Because of the high incidence of bilaterality, we believe that MTC is best treated by total thyroidectomy. Biopsy of lymph nodes of the midline compartment of the neck and of the internal jugular chains should be performed routinely, and if metastases are found, thorough en bloc neck dissection should be carried out.

Tumors of Lymphoreticular Cell Origin – Lymphosarcoma

Previously, most small-cell tumors of the thyroid gland were regarded as anaplastic carcinoma; but during the past 20 to 25 years or so, they have been recognized increasingly as malignant lymphomas. Typically, these tumors present as large, rapidly growing goiters in older women. The diagnosis can be confirmed by percutaneous core needle biopsy of the thyroid. If thyroidectomy is feasible, this should be carried out, and the neck is subsequently irradiated. If thyroid lymphoma is locally unresectable or is part of a disseminated process, external irradiation to the neck after biopsy is the recommended treatment. The prognosis is good for lymphoma confined to the thyroid; if it is part of a generalized lymphoma, the prognosis is a function of the generalized disease.

Conclusion

The differing biologic behaviors of the various types of thyroid malignancy must be recognized so that the proper therapy can be selected. When favorable prognostic factors are present, the chances of cure are excellent for all tumors except anaplastic carcinoma.

PHEOCHROMOCYTOMA

method of
NORMAN H. ERTEL, M.D.,
and ROBERT S. MODLINGER,
M.D.
East Orange, New Jersey

Pheochromocytomas are chromaffin cell tumors, derived from neuroectoderm. Eighty-five per cent or more occur in the adrenal medulla. Most extra-adrenal tumors are found within the abdomen, oc-curring either in the superior para-aortic area or in the organ of Zuckerkandl at the bifurcation of the aorta. They are rarely seen in the posterior mediastinum, urinary bladder, neck, and brain. Pheochromocytomas are most likely to present in the fourth to sixth decades, but they are an important source of hypertension in children under 15 years of age. About 10 per cent of pheochromocytomas are familial, bilateral, multiple, malignant, or extra-adrenal.

This uncommon disease is important because it is one of the curable causes of severe hypertension. Hypertension-screening programs reveal an incidence of 0.1 to 0.7 per cent, and 1000 deaths per year have been attributed to pheochromocytoma in the United States alone. Most cases of pheochromocytoma are suspected because of sustained hypertension or a history of paroxysms or both.

Preoperative Medical Management

The treatment of choice for pheochromocytoma is surgical removal of the neoplasm. In those patients with no contraindications to surgery (see below), it is advisable to operate within the shortest time compatible with preoperative preparation. As a general rule, it is best that such patients undergo no unnecessary tests or manipulations, as seemingly innocuous procedures have occasionally been associated with sudden death.

In the past, surgery for pheochromocytoma was associated with a mortality rate greater than 50 per cent, mainly because of hypertensive crisis, shock, and cardiac arrhythmia occuring during induction of anesthesia or surgery. Such complications have largely been eliminated by the development of potent alpha- and beta-sympathetic blocking agents.

Most physicians, including those in our group, prefer to use the long-acting alpha-blocking agent phenoxybenzamine (Dibenzyline) in all patients with norepinephrine-secreting pheochromocytomas. However, at least one prominent group reserves preoperative alpha-adrenergic blockade for high risk patients or for patients with accurately localized tumors. When the location of a pheochromocytoma is uncertain or the likelihood of encountering more than one tumor is anticipated, those workers do not advocate complete alpha-blockade. We do not agree with that approach and have been successful in locating single or multiple tumors intraoperatively in over 200 cases, despite clinically complete blockade.

The noncompetitive blockade produced by phenoxybenzamine has a half-life of approximately 24 hours in intact man. The effects of daily oral administration are cumulative for nearly a week. Therefore, it is advisable to treat the patient for not less than 1 week before proceeding to invasive radiologic studies or emergency surgery. The usual starting dose is 10 mg given every 12 hours, with an increase of 10 to 20 mg every 2 to 3 days until the hypertension and paroxysms are controlled. (This dose may be higher than that advised in the manufacturer's official directive.) It is unwise to give a large dose initially, because this drug inhibits the uptake and reuptake of catecholamines into adrenergic nerve terminals and therefore can theoretically cause a hypertensive crisis. We have not had to administer more than 80 mg per day to our patients, but doses greater than 150 mg per day have been reported in the literature. Although generally well tolerated, this agent may cause nasal stuffiness, gastrointestinal distress, and orthostatic hypotension. Metyrosine (alpha-methyl-L-tyrosine) (Demser) has recently been approved for the preoperative preparation of patients with pheochromocytoma. This agent, when given orally in a dose of 250 to 1000 mg four times daily, blocks the initial and rate-limiting step of catecholamine synthesis and decreases urinary excretion of catecholamines and metabolites by up to 80 per cent within 2 to 3 days of administering the effective dose. This is accompanied by improvement in the clinical status of the patient and by decreases in blood pressure, pulse rate, sweating, palpitations, and headache. Side effects are prominent, particularly diarrhea, which is attributable both to a direct effect on the bowel and to diminished sympathetic input. Other side effects include sedation, anorexia, anxiety, tremor, and galactorrhea. It is probably best reserved for patients not adequately controlled by phenoxybenzamine or in patients with metastatic or inoperable pheochromocytoma. Prazosin (Minipress), a postsynaptic alpha-adrenergic blocker, and Labetalol, an agent with both alpha- and beta-adrenergic blocking activity, have been successfully used in the treatment of pheochromocytoma. However, the status of these newer agents will not be clearly defined until comparative studies with phenoxybenzamine are published.

Phentolamine (Regitine), a short-acting alpha-adrenergic blocking agent, is useful as both a therapeutic and diagnostic agent during pheochromocytoma crisis. Although it has been used as preoperative therapy when given orally, we do not recommend its use, since it must be given every 4 to 6 hours, even at night. It produces significant gastrointestinal side effects, and gives uneven control of blood pressure. In addition, it can cause tachycardia and arrhythmias, which are more than just a reflex response to peripheral vasodilation.

We do not customarily start beta-blockade unless the patient develops persistent tachycardia with a pulse rate greater than 130 per minute or there is a history or objective evidence of recurrent ventricular arrhythmias. These cardiovascular abnormalities may be present initially, particularly in epinephrine-secreting tumors, or may emerge as a result of alpha-blockade. Propranolol (Inderal) is currently the beta blocker of choice. Patients with pheochromocytoma may be extremely sensitive to propranolol, and the starting dose should not exceed 30 mg (10 mg three times daily). This may be increased cautiously every 3 to 4 days until there is control of the tachycardia and arrhythmia. It must be emphasized that propranolol should not be begun before adequate alpha-blockade is achieved and never used prior to starting alpha-blocking agents. Resulting unopposed alpha effects with generalized severe vasoconstriction and hypertensive crisis could result in death. There are, however, patients with predominantly epinephrine-secreting tumors in whom propranolol may be the only indicated treatment. Indeed, some physicians routinely wait for fractionation of epinephrine excretion before instituting definitive therapy. We do not routinely do this unless there are clinical clues to an epinephrine-secreting tumor, such as hypotensive episodes, persistent or recurring arrhythmias, unusual weight loss, or raised basal metabolic rate. Patients on preoperative propranolol therapy should continue this drug until the time of surgery. Sudden cessation can lead to paroxysmal tachycardia and arrhythmias, and has been implicated in myocardial infarction in patients with ischemic heart disease.

Patients with pheochromocytoma are occasionally blood volume depleted at the time of presentation, although this is seen in less than 30 per cent of patients. Adequate sympathetic blockade, however, usually corrects the depleted blood volume, since it is caused by peripheral vasoconstriction and contraction of the vascular space. If this has not been accomplished by the time of surgery, it should be corrected with either colloid or blood. Although some centers substitute phentolamine for phenoxybenzamine in the days preceding surgery, experience has shown that the latter drug can be continued until the morning of surgery without causing hypotension refractory to therapy during surgery or making operative localization of the tumor more difficult. Hypercalcemia, if present either because of concomitant hyperparathyroidism or because of ectopic parathormone secretion by the pheochromocytoma, should be treated with fluids and loop diuretic agents, as hypercalcemia can stimulate catecholamine secretion. Hypokalemia, present in some patients with pheochromocytoma, should be corrected by oral administration of potassium. Digitalis should be administered cautiously in patients with congestive heart failure, because it may lead to arrhythmias in hearts sensitized by excess levels of catecholamines. It is preferable for patients to be well controlled for at least 10 to 14 days preceding surgery.

Localization of the Tumor

Since greater than 95 per cent of pheochromocytomas are located beneath the diaphragm and are either multiple or bilateral in more than 10 per cent of patients, a thorough exploration is required even when location has been suggested by a variety of invasive and noninvasive radiographic techniques. When selective adrenal arteriography was the major technique to be considered, differences of opinion concerning routine preoperative use were common, with surgeons usually exerting pressure to obtain as much preoperative information as possible. However, the introduction of computerized axial tomography (CAT) scans has revolutionized localization techniques and should now be considered a routine part of the preoperative workup. CAT scans are noninvasive and without risk even to unblocked patients. Tumors as small as 1 cm in diameter have been detected by this technique. It should be emphasized, however, that the diagnosis of pheochromocytoma should be established by biochemical testing, not by radiologic techniques more appropriately reserved for localization of the tumor already proved to exist.

Intraoperative Management

The management of the patient is a combined effort by an anesthesiologist, surgeon, endocrinologist, and cardiologist who have experience and knowledge of the specialized problems concerned with this type of surgery. Before intubation or induction of anesthesia, an intra-arterial catheter should be placed to allow constant monitoring of blood pressure. A central venous or Swan-Ganz catheter and electrocardiographic leads should be positioned and ready for use. In several centers an infusion of blood or intravascular volume expander is begun routinely at the commencement of surgery in anticipation of the hypotension which frequently follows tumor removal. Several dozen ampules of phentolamine should be available, and lidocaine, propranolol, norepinephrine, angiotensin, phenylephrine, hydrocortisone, and sodium nitroprusside delivery systems should be prepared for immediate use. Muscle relaxants will usually be required for intubation and sustained skeletal muscle relaxation in order to provide the surgeon with a broad operative field, thus allowing easy exploration of both suprarenal areas and the entire paravertebral area. Pancuronium (Pavulon) has been considered the competitive neuromuscular blocking agent of choice, as it does not release histamine after ordinary doses. Although rapid injection of curare can result in histamine release with symptoms in man, it should be noted that phenoxybenzamine is a potent antihistaminic agent and that the use of d-tubocurarine has not been associated with hypertensive crises in patients adequately prepared with phenoxybenzamine. Succinylcholine seems to be widely recommended, but it, too, can cause histamine release and has been reported to produce recurrent ventricular bigeminy when administered to a patient with pheochromocytoma. Gallamine (Flaxedil) should never be used in these patients, because it is vagolytic and produces undesirable tachycardia and arrhythmia.

Much of the controversy concerning preoperative medication and the anesthetic of choice was generated before the routine use of adrenergic blocking agents. Short-acting barbiturates, such as secobarbital, and scopolamine are commonly used preanesthetic medications. Atropine is generally considered to be contraindicated because of the hypothetical side effects of tachycardia and potentiation of the vasopressor activity of catecholamines. Our anesthesiologists have, on occasion, used atropine in the adequately prepared patient without untoward effects. Diethyl ether and cyclopropane are contraindicated because they are explosive and stimulate release of catecholamines during surgery; the latter markedly sensitizes the myocardium to these catecholamines. Halothane has been widely used because it induces little or no sympathoadrenal release during anesthesia in man, as measured by changes in plasma norepinephrine levels. However, since many patients develop significant ventricular arrhythmias, we no longer consider it an acceptable anesthetic agent. Innovar, a combination of the neuroleptic compound droperidol and the narcotic analgesic fentanyl citrate, has been widely used in combination with nitrous oxide with success in patients with pheochromocytoma. Although Innovar has resulted in increased urinary epinephrine and norepinephrine excretion in other conditions, electrocardiographic abnormalities are rare, and this agent may actually protect against ventricular arrhythmias caused by epinephrine. Methoxyflurane (Penthrane) and enflurane (Ethrane), usually used along with nitrous oxide, have been recommended for use in pheochromocytoma, as they do not appreciably lower the arrhythmia threshold of the myocardium to catecholamines at currently used anesthetic doses. Enflurane, in particular, would seem to be an excellent agent because it is nonexplosive, produces excellent muscular relaxation, and does not produce the renal toxicity reported with methoxyflurane.

The surgeon should make an anterior abdominal incision through which the entire abdominopelvic area can be explored. If the tumor has been localized by radiologic means prior to surgery, the surgeon should proceed to this area and attempt to ligate the venous drainage. No attempt should be made to separate the tumor from surrounding normal adrenal tissue, as the capsule should be kept intact in order to prevent seeding by benign or malignant tumor. In the event that the tumor is adherent to the adjacent kidney, the kidney and adrenal may have to be removed en bloc.

The major intraoperative and postoperative complications are cardiac arrhythmia, hypertensive crisis, and shock.

Arrhythmias occur most frequently during induction, intubation, and tumor manipulation. Most common are extrasystoles, bigeminy, and ventricular tachycardia. Premature contractions usually accompany rises in blood pressure and may often be adequately treated by pressure reduction. Lidocaine (50 to 100 mg bolus) or propranolol (1 mg) may be required to reverse significant ventricular arrhythmias. Equipment for electric cardioversion should be available at all times.

The treatment of hypertensive crisis during induction of anesthesia or tumor manipulation is the rapid intravenous injection of phentolamine. It should be given as 1 to 5 mg injections. Its action is usually evident within 30 seconds, with a peak effect within 5 minutes. Repeated boluses may be used as needed. Alternatively, nitroprusside by continuous infusion is equally effective, in addition to being useful in the occasional patient found to be refractory to phentolamine.

Ligation of tumor venous drainage usually results in hypotension, often to shock levels in the unblocked patient. This is caused by a sudden decline in alpha-adrenergic–induced vasoconstriction with resultant disproportion between vascular capacity and blood volume. The therapy of choice is rapid replacement of estimated blood loss plus as much blood as is needed to maintain adequate blood pressure without causing a hazardous increase in central venous pressure. Should this be unsuccessful, the depth of surgical anesthesia may be raised. Infusion of norepinephrine (Levophed) or phenylephrine (Neo-Synephrine) is sometimes necessary to maintain blood pressure levels. In the event that these measures are not effective, angiotensin (Hypertensin), a vasoconstrictor which does not act through alpha receptors, can be lifesaving. This drug must be obtained directly from Ciba Pharmaceutical Company. In patients subjected to bilateral adrenalectomy, intravenous hydrocortisone should be begun at the time of surgical attack on the second gland and the patient thereafter managed as an addisonian undergoing surgery.

Postoperative Management

The patient should be closely monitored, with intra-arterial and central venous catheters left in place for at least 24 to 48 hours after surgery. It is rarely necessary to continue pressor agents if blood volume has been adequately repleted. Persistent hypotension may indicate bleeding at the postoperative site or inadequate steroid replacement in the bilaterally adrenalectomized patient. Failure of the blood pressure to fall significantly by the third postoperative day suggests a second tumor, metastatic disease, irreversible small vessel disease, or renal artery stenosis secondary to the surgical procedure (poor suture placement). Immediate aortography may be indicated. Raised tissue stores of catecholamines may remain for up to 10 days after successful surgery as reflected in urinary catecholamine or metabolite excretion. During this time, it is hazardous to treat the patient with drugs that release stored catecholamines, such as guanethidine or reserpine. Very recent work has demonstrated the usefulness of serial plasma catecholamine determinations after surgery in establishing completeness of tumor removal and return to normal levels.

After surgery, patients must be watched carefully for an indefinite period of time. Plasma and urinary catecholamine determinations should be obtained every 6 months or with a return of clinical symptoms to ensure the early diagnosis of multiple or recurrent pheochromocytomas. It is advisable that all relatives of patients with bilateral pheochromocytomas be screened for the presence of such a tumor. In addition, the patient with multiple tumors and all close relatives should be screened for medullary carcinoma of the thyroid and hyperparathyroidism.

Medical Therapy

Long-term medical therapy is always required in patients with functioning metastatic pheochromocytoma in whom complete removal is not possible. In such patients, it is important to remove as much of the tumor as possible, as these tumors generally do not respond to radiotherapy or to the currently available cytotoxic agents. They are slow growing, and survival beyond 5 years is not unusual, although half die within 2 years despite adrenolytic management. Nonoperative therapy is also frequently necessary in patients bearing multiple tumors or with medical contraindications to definitive surgery, such as severe cardiomyopathy or recent cardiac infarction.

Chronic medical therapy with alpha- and beta-blocking agents differs little from the regimen described under Preoperative Medical Management. Phenoxybenzamine has been the agent of choice for long-term administration, but metyrosine may also prove to be an effective agent for long-term use.

Special Problems

Pheochromocytoma in Pregnancy. Pheochromocytoma during pregnancy is a rare but extremely serious disorder. In the undiagnosed case, maternal mortality approaches 50 per cent, whereas fetal wastage is approximately 33 per cent. Mortality, however, is significantly less if the pheochromocytoma is detected prior to term. Management does not differ significantly from that outlined under Medical Therapy. If the tumor is detected during the second trimester, it is probably best to attempt removal, after appropriate preoperative preparation. For patients whose pheochromocytoma is diagnosed during the third trimester, management depends upon both the degree of success obtained with medical therapy and the maturity of the fetus. If near term, cesarean section with subsequent search for the tumor appears indicated. If the fetus is judged nonviable and the patient is adequately controlled by medical management, careful observation with operative delivery at a later date appears indicated. Patients who are poorly controlled should be subject to surgery for pheochromocytoma removal, despite the risk of spontaneous premature delivery.

Pheochromocytoma of the Bladder. Pheochromocytoma of the urinary bladder is relatively uncommon. It is usually easily identified by the typical postmicturition symptomatology. The majority of such tumors may be identified during cystoscopy. Since cystoscopy can induce an attack of paroxysmal hypertension, it is important that the patient be adequately blocked with phenoxybenzamine therapy prior to any manipulation. Surgery should include exploration of the entire abdominopelvic area in order to search for multiple tumors.

THYROIDITIS

method of
MERRILL W. EDMONDS, M.D.
London, Ontario, Canada

Acute (Suppurative) Thyroiditis

This rare condition is usually due to bacteria such as *Staphylococcus aureus, Streptococcus hemolyticus,* or the *pneumococcus,* or more rarely other bacteria or fungi such as Actinomyces. The clinical presentation is sudden, with severe neck pain, malaise, fever, chills, and tachycardia. Extreme tenderness, swelling, redness, and increased warmth in the region of the thyroid mark the physical examination. Normal circulating thyroid hormone levels and a normal 24 hour radioactive iodine uptake (RAIU) help distinguish this condition from subacute thyroiditis. The scintiscan may show a cold area in the region of the thyroiditis. A fine needle aspiration biopsy for both cytology and culture can also be helpful in making the diagnosis. Treatment includes the use of aspirin, stronger analgesics as necessary, and appropriate antibiotics (penicillin is the initial drug of choice unless the identity of the microorganism is known), followed by surgical excision of the affected area or incision and drainage if excision is impossible.

Subacute Thyroiditis

This not uncommon inflammation of the thyroid is probably a viral disease. As a result, it is more common in fall and spring and is often preceded by an upper respiratory infection. There are three main types of clinical presentation:

1. Severe pain and tenderness with marked systemic symptoms (temperature up to 40 C [104 F]) and clinical and biochemical features of hyperthyroidism (common).

2. A painless enlarged thyroid with a few systemic symptoms and clinical euthyroidism.

3. Hyperthyroidism alone with no local symptoms (rare).

In addition to the increased circulating thyroid hormone levels, the RAIU is very low (often 0 per cent). The erythrocyte sedimentation rate is elevated (often above 80 mm per hour). Thyroid antibodies are usually negative but may be present in low titer during recovery. Fine needle aspiration biopsy may again help confirm the diagnosis.

No treatment may be necessary for the milder cases. Symptoms of hyperthyroidism can be controlled by propranolol, 10 to 80 mg four times daily. Analgesics can be used for the pain if necessary, but when the pain is severe only prednisone, 10 mg four times daily, results in immediate relief. The prednisone dose should be gradually reduced over 1 month. If the pain recurs, the prednisone is restarted at a higher dose. L-Thyroxine, 0.1 to 0.2 mg daily, may help prevent any further recurrences when the patient is euthyroid or hypothyroid. The L-thyroxine can be stopped after 6 to 12 months. Spontaneous recovery usually occurs within 2 to 5 months. Recurrence is seen in 20 per cent of patients, and 25 per cent develop transient hypothyroidism during recovery.

Lymphocytic (Autoimmune) Thyroiditis

This common thyroid disorder is thought to be an autoimmune disease. Both cell-mediated immunity (T cells) and antibody-mediated immunity (B cells) are involved. This disease appears to be very closely associated with Graves' disease. In Graves' disease, however, the antibodies appear to be directed against the thyrotropin receptor area of the cell membrane and produce stimulation of the thyroid cell. The four subtypes include the classic type of Hashimoto's thyroiditis, (commonly occurring in the 30- to 50-year-old female), juvenile thyroiditis, chronic thyroiditis, and atrophic thyroiditis (idiopathic myxedema of the elderly).

The clinical presentation of lymphocytic thyroiditis is quite varied and may include (1) asymptomatic diffuse rubbery firm goiter (most common cause of goiter in patients over the age of 11); (2) hypothyroidism with or without a diffuse rubbery firm goiter; (3) hyperthyroidism resulting from the presence of stimulating as well as destructive antibodies (hashitoxicosis); (4) firm solitary thyroid nodule; or (5) spontaneously resolving hyperthyroidism (SRH) (10 per cent postpartum period), in which the gland may or may not be tender.

A family history of autoimmune thyroid disease can be found in at least 30 per cent of cases if looked for. Circulating thyroid hormone levels may be normal, low, or high. Serum thyroid-stimulating hormone (TSH) may be normal or high. Thyroid antibodies are usually positive except in the juvenile type. The radioactive iodine uptake (RAIU) may be low (SRH), normal, or high, and the scan may show a patchy uptake. The fine needle aspiration biopsy may be quite helpful in confirming the diagnosis.

Suppression or replacement with L-thyroxine, 0.1 to 0.2 mg daily, is the treatment of choice. This will result in some decrease in the size of the gland, depending on the amount of fibrosis, and amelioration of any hypothyroid symptoms or signs. This should be started cautiously in the hypothyroid subject who is elderly or has any cardiovascular disease (0.0125 to 0.025 mg daily, with gradual increases at 2 to 4 week intervals as tolerated). Some patients may, in addition, have stimulating antibodies present and their own thyroid function will, therefore, not completely suppress. Thus peripheral thyroid hormone levels must be checked after 4 weeks to be sure the patient is not taking too much thyroxine. Surgery is rarely necessary to relieve local symptoms of obstruction or to rule out associated malignancy. Corticosteroids are not recommended, since they have only a temporary effect. Lithium and excess iodide may induce frank hypothyroidism. Propranolol in a dose of 10 to 40 mg four times daily can be quite useful in controlling the symptoms of thyrotoxicosis.

Fibrous (Riedel's) Thyroiditis

The fibrosis of this very rare type of thyroiditis does not have a known cause but often involves retroperitoneal and mediastinal areas as well. A patient with this condition presents with a very firm goiter or nodule and may develop pressure symptoms involving the trachea and esophagus, making it difficult to distinguish it from carcinoma. Peripheral thyroid hormone levels are usually normal. The RAIU is normal, but thyroid scintiscans usually show the area to be cold. Thyroid autoantibodies are usually negative. Surgery is sometimes necessary to rule out malignancy or to relieve pressure symptoms by resection of the isthmus.

MALIGNANT CARCINOID SYNDROME

method of
HAROLD BROWN, M.D.
Houston, Texas

The dramatic symptomatology of the classic malignant carcinoid syndrome is usually a late manifestation of the disease, and the physician will be confronted with a long-term management problem. The syndrome is characterized by episodes of flushing, particularly of the upper part of the body, with cyanosis and venous telangiectasia; intestinal hyperperistalsis with abdominal cramps, borborygmi, and diarrhea; a peculiar valvular heart disease with collagenous deposits on the endocardium, particularly of the right side of the heart, resulting in pulmonic stenosis and tricuspid regurgitation and stenosis; and bronchial constriction, which is the least frequent component of the syndrome.

In most subjects with the syndrome the tumor arises from the ileum and there are extensive deposits in the liver, but the origin may be from any portion of the gastrointestinal tract, including the pancreas and gallbladder, lung, ovary, testis, thyroid, and thymus.

At first the symptomatology was attributed to the elaboration of serotonin, but it is now appreciated that these tumors may secrete other substances, including 5-hydroxytryptophan, histamine, prostaglandins, kallikreins — which form bradykinin — catecholamines, ACTH, melanocyte-stimulating hormone (MSH), insulin, calcitonin, gastrin, antidiuretic hormone (ADH), glucagon, and vasoactive intestinal peptide.

Since patients with the syndrome are usually not surgical candidates, except in specific instances to be detailed, symptomatic therapy is usually employed.

Surgery

Occasionally, the syndrome may arise from carcinoids in the lung, ovary, or testis, and resection may be curative. In most patients there will be extensive hepatic metastases that preclude surgery. Rarely some palliation may be achieved by resection of a large mass of tumor in the liver or omentum. The anesthesiologist should be aware of the tendency of these subjects to develop hypotension, particularly with the administration of sympathomimetic compounds.

Flushing

In some patients the attacks may be precipitated by specific foods, alcohol, or large meals, and avoidance of these factors will diminish attacks. The bouts of flushing may be brought on by emotional upsets, and sedation with tranquilizers such as chlorpromazine (Thorazine) may be effective. The phenothiazines are also mild alpha-adrenergic blocking agents that tend to inhibit kinin formation. Phenoxybenzamine (Dibenzyline), an alpha-receptor blocker, may also be tried, beginning with a dose of 10 to 20 mg per day and increasing to 60 mg if necessary. (This use of phenoxybenzamine is not listed in the manufacturer's official directive.)

A number of carcinoid syndrome patients with severe flushing attacks have responded to a combination of H_1 and H_2 blocker therapy — namely, diphenhydramine and cimetidine — even when there was no evidence of excess histamine production.

Gastrointestinal Symptoms

There is considerable evidence that serotonin is involved in the gastrointestinal manifestations, and antiserotonin agents usually give relief. Methysergide (Sansert), a potent antiserotonin agent, can be tried in doses of 2 to 4 mg as often as every 4 hours, with most of the medication being taken during the period when symptoms are maximal. (This use of methysergide is not listed in the manufacturer's official directive.) One should omit therapy for several weeks every 6 months after gradually decreasing the dose to reduce risk of producing retroperitoneal or other organ fibrosis, which is, however, reversible. Cyproheptadine (Periactin) has also been effective in doses of 4 to 8 mg two or three times per day. The diarrhea will also respond to traditional antidiarrhea medication such as paregoric or diphenoxylate with atropine (Lomotil).

Heart Disease

The manifestations of heart disease are treated in the usual fashion. Patients with valvular heart disease and intractable failure should be considered for a valvular prosthesis.

Antitumor Therapy

Response to radiation and chemotherapy leaves much to be desired, although radiation is useful to treat local deposits in skin or bone.

Various chemotherapeutic agents have been tried with little success and should be employed only on an investigational basis in desperate situations. It is hoped that new and more effective agents or combinations will be forthcoming.

Asthma

Attacks of bronchoconstriction can be relieved by administration of epinephrine or similar agents via nebulizer. The small amount of drug delivered locally to the lung does not appear to cause exacerbation of the flushing attack or to provoke hypotension.

General

The life span of these patients may be decades, and they must be encouraged to tolerate minor discomforts. Their symptoms may vary in intensity from time to time for unknown reasons. Some of the attacks are accompanied by hypotension, which usually resolves without specific treatment. If a vasoconstrictive agent is required, the usual sympathomimetic agents — norepinephrine (Levophed), metaraminol (Aramine), or mephentermine (Wyamine) — are avoided, and only the direct acting α-receptor agents, such as phenylephrine (Neo-Synephrine) or methoxamine (Vasoxyl), should be employed after volume replacement if the patient remains symptomatic.

Patients with marginal food intake and those with high 5-HIAA excretion should receive supplements of 50 to 100 mg of niacin per day as part of their daily multivitamin supplement.

SECTION
8

The Urogenital Tract

BACTERIAL INFECTIONS OF THE URINARY TRACT (MALE)

method of
C. LOWELL PARSONS, M.D.
San Diego, California

Bacterial infections of the male genital tract (excluding urethritis) are often associated with definable abnormalities such as urethral stricture, benign prostatic hyperplasia, or vesicoureteral reflux. In the male patient with a bacterial genitourinary tract infection, a search for an underlying cause with intravenous pyelography (IVP), voiding cystourethrography (VCUG), and cystoscopy is usually indicated. The object of therapy is twofold: resolution of the primary disorder, if one is present, and treatment of the bacterial infection with the antimicrobial agent that is best fit in terms of effectiveness, toxicity, and cost.

Urethritis

Gonococcal Urethritis. Acute gonococcal urethritis may be treated with several different compounds. If aqueous penicillin is to be used, the standard dose is 4.8 million units given intramuscularly, preceded by administration of 1.0 gram of oral probenecid 30 to 60 minutes before the injection. Ampicillin, 3.5 grams orally following 1.0 gram of oral probenecid, may also be used. Spectinomycin, 2.0 grams intramuscularly, may be employed in relapsing patients or in those who cannot tolerate penicillin. Tetracycline in a dose of 500 mg four times a day for 10 days is also effective but has the disadvantage of depending on patient compliance.

Nonspecific Urethritis. It is currently felt that chlamydial organisms are the cause of most cases of nonspecific urethritis. Initial therapy should consist of tetracycline, 250 mg four times a day

for 10 days. Minocycline or doxycycline (Vibramycin) may be used in doses of 100 mg two times a day, but these agents are far more expensive. Another alternative is erythromycin in doses of 250 to 500 mg three times a day. If possible, the consort should also be treated. In the event of relapse even with therapy of the consort, medication should be continued for 1 to 3 months.

Prostatitis

The symptom complex of dysuria, perineal ache, and painful ejaculation accompanies prostatic inflammatory disease of both bacterial and nonbacterial origin. The former condition is rare; the latter is common. The patient with a nonbacterial inflammation often shows no objective signs of disease, such as white blood cells in the prostatic fluid, and will probably respond no better with antimicrobial therapy than without it.

If true bacterial prostatitis is present, effective antibiotics include tetracycline, 500 mg four times a day for 2 weeks; trimethoprim-sulfamethoxazole (Septra, Bactrim), one double-strength tablet two times a day for 2 weeks; carbenicillin (Geocillin), 1 tablet four times a day for 2 weeks; or nitrofurantoin (Macrodantin), 50 mg four times a day for 2 weeks. Relapse is common; when it occurs, full-dose therapy for 3 months will help many patients.

Recurrent cystitis is often the cause of the major symptoms in patients with true bacterial prostatitis that is not controlled by the modes of therapy described above. The pathogen in these cases is usually *Escherichia coli*. After acute therapy of cystitis for 1 week, the infection may be suppressed with nitrofurantoin (Macrodantin), 50 mg per day at bedtime; penicillin V-potassium, 250 mg per day at bedtime; sulfisoxazole (Gantrisin), 0.5 gram per day at bedtime; or trimethoprim-sulfamethoxazole (Bactrim, Septra), 1 single-strength tablet per day at bedtime. If no breakthrough infections occur, the suppres-

555

sive dosages may be reduced to 1 tablet every other day at bedtime. In addition to the antibiotic therapy, increased sexual activity to drain the prostatic acini is encouraged.

Epididymitis

Acute epididymitis requires strict bed rest until pain is greatly reduced. The scrotum should be elevated — for example, by placement of a rolled towel beneath it. Younger males tend to have a high incidence of chlamydial epididymitis; in older males, *Escherichia coli* is the principal cause of infection. For both younger and older males, tetracycline in a dosage of 500 mg four times a day is suggested as the first-line antibiotic. If *Escherichia coli* is the causative agent, ampicillin, 500 mg four times a day, may be used; cephalexin (Keflex), cephradine (Velosef), or cephadroxil monohydrate (Duricef) in doses of 500 mg four times a day or trimethoprim-sulfamethoxazole (Septra, Bactrim) may be substituted but are more expensive alternatives.

Cystitis

Cystitis in the male is usually associated with a definable underlying cause such as bladder outlet obstruction (secondary to benign prostatic hyperplasia or strictures), bacterial prostatitis, neuropathic bladder, vesicoureteral reflux, or even chronic pyelonephritis. Such a cause should be sought and, if possible, corrected.

Escherichia coli is usually the infecting microbe in acute cystitis. Effective therapy may include one of several drugs. Inexpensive and nontoxic compounds should be tried first: penicillin V-potassium 250 mg four times a day (for *Escherichia coli,* Proteus, and enterococci), sulfisoxazole (Gantrisin), 0.5 gram four times a day, nitrofurantoin (Macrodantin), 50 mg orally four times a day, ampicillin, 250 mg orally four times a day, and nalidixic acid (NegGram), 1 gram four times a day. A 7 day course of therapy is usually more than adequate to clear the infection. If relapse occurs owing to an uncontrollable cause of infection, e.g., prostatitis, suppressive therapy with any of the aforementioned drugs in a dosage of 1 tablet per day at bedtime is recommended.

If the patient is unable to tolerate any of the less expensive drugs, trimethoprim-sulfamethoxazole (Septra, Bactrim), cephalexin (Keflex), cephadroxil (Duricef), cephradine (Velosef), carbenicillin (Geocillin), or amoxicillin may be used.

Pyelonephritis

Acute Pyelonephritis. Severe acute pyelonephritis is a significant life-threatening disease that should be treated vigorously with parenteral medication. Two populations of patients with pyelonephritis are seen.

The first type is the patient with a community-acquired infection; microorganisms of concern that should be included in initial broad-spectrum coverage are *Escherichia coli,* enterococci, Klebsiella, Proteus, and Enterobacter species (not Pseudomonas, Serratia, or Providencia). Consequently, an aminoglycoside is required: either kanamycin, 7.5 mg per kg of body weight every 12 hours, or gentamicin, 1.5 to 2.0 mg per kg body weight every 8 hours. For enterococcal coverage 2 grams of ampicillin every 6 hours should be employed. It must be emphasized that the acute swelling and inflammation in the pyelonephritic kidney reduces the blood flow and diminishes function so that attainment of adequate serum levels of drug is important. Once the results of urine culture and sensitivity are obtained, the single best agent should be administered parenterally in doses adequate to prevent recurrence of infection or development of perinephric abscesses, e.g., ampicillin 2 grams intravenously every 6 hours.

In cases of non-community-acquired (complicated) pyelonephritis, e.g., in patients with neuropathic bladder, indwelling catheters, or infectious stone disease, protection must also be provided against additional bacterial species, including Pseudomonas, Serratia, and Providencia. The broad-spectrum coverage should also include any problem organisms that a specific hospital may have. The drugs initially should be gentamicin or tobramycin, 1.5 to 2.0 mg per kg of body weight every 8 hours, plus carbenicillin (Geocillin), 2 grams every 4 hours. Once the results of urine culture and sensitivity testing are available, the best single drug should be used. If Pseudomonas is involved, however, both carbenicillin and an aminoglycoside should be administered. In cases in which the hospital has a problem species that is susceptible only to amikacin (Amikin), this compound should be the aminoglycoside of choice. The dosage is 7.5 to 10.0 mg per kg of body weight every 12 hours. (This dose may be higher than that listed in the manufacturer's official directive.)

Chronic Pyelonephritis. Chronic pyelonephritis may be treated with the same regimen of oral drugs that is described above for cystitis. Should relapse persist, high dose intravenous therapy with the single safest, cheapest drug will often control the infection. As always, one must use the aforementioned antibiotics with caution in patients with compromised renal function, reducing dosages and frequency of doses when appropriate.

BACTERIAL INFECTIONS OF THE URINARY TRACT (FEMALE ADULTS)

method of
ANTHONY J. SCHAEFFER, M.D.
Chicago, Illinois

Urinary tract infections are a common and often frustrating problem for patients and physicians alike. Most episodes of bacteriuria are accompanied by considerable discomfort, anxiety, and expense; fortunately only a few patients are at risk of significant renal function impairment and death, and these sequelae can usually be prevented by judicious management.

The approach detailed below is based on documentation of urinary infections and the effect of therapy by urine culture. Reliance on symptoms or urinalysis alone to diagnose and treat "urinary tract infections" is scientifically unsound and potentially dangerous. The major objections to performing urine cultures (i.e., patient inconvenience and excessive cost) can now be overcome by the use of dip slide (e.g., Uricult) or other such devices which provide accurate, quantitative urine cultures for approximately $1 each.

Our assessment and management of culture-documented urinary tract infections is based on the classification of different infection patterns as outlined by Stamey:

1. First infection (symptomatic)
2. Unresolved bacteriuria during therapy
3. Recurrent urinary tract infections
   a. Reinfections
   b. Bacterial persistence

First infections are generally caused by common gram-negative organisms (*Escherichia coli* in approximately 85 per cent of cases), although gram-positive staphylococci and streptococci are not uncommon. The source of the pathogen is usually the patient's bowel flora. A variety of antimicrobials are effective, and recurrent infections are rare. Approximately 5 to 10 per cent of patients will have unresolved bacteriuria during therapy because the pathogen was naturally resistant or acquired resistance to the first drug selected. Antimicrobial sensitivity testing is necessary in these patients to delineate effective alternative drug therapy. The vast majority of recurrent infections are reinfections caused by the reintroduction of organisms into the urinary tract. The increased susceptibility to infections appears to be predisposed by a biologic defect which permits frequent colonization of the vaginal vestibule by bacteria from the rectal flora. These women characteristically have clusters of symptomatic infections (two thirds will have reinfections within 6 months), followed by 6 to 12 month infection-free intervals. A much smaller group of women have true "chronic" infections owing to bacterial persistence within the urinary tract, usually in a stone or anatomic abnormality. These recurrences are always caused by the same organism and usually occur within several days of stopping antimicrobial therapy. Identification of the structural or functional cause is mandatory for effective management of these women.

Thus, this classification can be used to characterize groups of patients with different infectious etiology and patterns, to identify those who may be at risk or require further urologic evaluation, and to plan appropriate therapy based on a predictable course of infection.

Before discussing individual treatment regimens, three general therapeutic principles deserve emphasis. First, the fecal flora is the ultimate reservoir for most urinary tract pathogens. Antimicrobial therapy, whether for urinary tract or other infections, can rapidly and significantly alter bacterial susceptibility either to the original drug (chromosomal resistance) or to other antimicrobials (R-factor resistances). Considerable care should therefore be exercised in selecting drugs for treatment of urinary tract infections when patients have recently been exposed to or are likely to require future antimicrobial therapy. Second, the cure of urinary tract infection depends upon whether or not the infecting strain can be killed by the antimicrobial concentration in the urine rather than the serum. Achievable urine levels of antimicrobials are generally 50 to 100 times those in the serum unless renal failure impedes concentrating ability. It is important therefore to note whether in vitro antimicrobial sensitivities reflect urine concentrations achievable in vivo. Finally, in vitro sensitivity testing is based on the assumption that the organisms tested are representative of those causing the infection. In fact, the population is not entirely homogeneous; some organisms are more or less sensitive to the reported minimal inhibitory concentration. The therapeutic implication is clear; in order to minimize selection of resistant mutants, one should choose the drug that can achieve urinary concentrations which exceed the minimal inhibitory concentration by the widest margin.

First Infection

First infections are almost always responsive to a variety of oral antimicrobial agents. I manage these patients in the following way, unless the

557

infection may be complicated by an underlying functional or structural urinary tract abnormality (see High-Risk Patients, below). Although a pretherapy culture is not essential, I usually obtain one to document the infection. Antimicrobial sensitivity testing is not ordered unless I suspect that the pathogen is resistant (owing to a history of previous antimicrobial therapy) or that the patient has pyelonephritis.

Generally, I use one of the following drugs:

1. Penicillin G, 250 mg (400,000 units) orally four times daily for 5 days. Ampicillin, 250 mg orally four times a day, is slightly more potent, but the difference is small and in my opinion not worth the extra cost. Other penicillin derivatives, such as penicillin V and methicillin, are substantially inferior. Penicillin G achieves high urinary levels (100 micrograms per ml) that are remarkably effective against most strains of *Escherichia coli, Proteus mirabilis, Streptococcus faecalis, Staphylococcus aureus,* and about 25 per cent of Klebsiella. The drug should be taken on an empty stomach so that complete absorption and full therapeutic urinary levels are achieved. It should be noted that cephalexin is not effective against most strains of *S. faecalis,* but is quite effective against Klebsiella.

2. Nitrofurantoin, 100 mg orally four times daily for 5 days. This drug is almost completely absorbed from the upper gastrointestinal tract, and therefore does not lead to the development of resistant bacteria in the fecal flora. Bacteria thus remain sensitive if future therapy is required. Nitrofurantoin is usually active against *E. coli, S. faecalis,* and *Staphylococcus aureus.* Some strains of Enterobacter species and Klebsiella species are resistant, and it is not active against most strains of Proteus. Gastrointestinal side effects are said to be reduced by the use of nitrofurantoin in macrocrystals (Macrodantin) or when the drug is taken with food or milk.

3. Sulfonamides. Sulfamethoxazole (Gantanol), 1 gram orally twice daily, may be preferable to sulfamethizole (Thiosulfil Forte), 500 mg four times daily, because increased patient compliance should be expected with the twice daily dosage. In addition, less protein binding may make more of the active drug available in the urine. Sulfisoxazole (Gantrisin), 500 mg four times daily, produces about half the urinary concentration of biologically active drug as the same dose of sulfamethizole. *E. coli* is the most susceptible species, followed by Klebsiella sp., *P. mirabilis,* Pseudomonas sp., and *S. aureus; S. faecalis* is resistant.

4. Trimethoprim-sulfamethoxazole (Bactrim or Septra), 2 tablets (regular strength) or 1 tablet (double strength) orally twice daily.

5. Cinoxacin (Cinobac), 250 to 500 mg orally twice daily. Trimethoprim-sulfamethoxazole and cinoxacin are both very effective against common gram-negative urinary pathogens and usually ineffective against gram-positive organisms. The dosage schedule probably increases patient compliance. They are particularly attractive choices in patients with recurrent urinary tract infections because they do not favor development of resistant strains (see below). Cinoxacin is not associated with multiple drug (R-factor) resistance, so I use it when a patient is likely to be infected with a resistant strain owing to recent exposure to sulfonamides, tetracycline, or penicillin.

Other drugs such as oxytetracycline or tetracycline, 250 to 500 mg orally four times daily, and cephalexin (Keflex), 250 to 500 mg four times daily, are usually reserved for therapy based on antimicrobial sensitivity testing.

I rarely obtain a culture during therapy, unless persistent symptoms suggest unresolved bacteriuria. I believe a follow-up culture 3 to 5 days after stopping therapy is mandatory. If the culture is positive, further therapy is based on antimicrobial sensitivity testing and repeat cultures are obtained during therapy. If the culture is negative and either the patient is still symptomatic or if the urinalysis continues to show pyuria, the patient is re-evaluated several weeks later. Persistent symptoms or findings of inflammation warrant consideration of urologic evaluation for other lesions such as stones, tumors, or tuberculosis.

Recurrent Infection

Reinfection. Recurrences at long intervals (usually greater than 2 weeks) and with different bacterial strains are characteristic of reinfection. It should be noted, however, that reinfections at shorter intervals and with the same species and even serotype of *E. coli* are not uncommon.

Urologic evaluation has a limited role in the evaluation of women with reinfection. Excretory urography appears to be of little benefit and carries a significant risk. I limit its use to patients with other risk factors — i.e., a history of unexplained hematuria, obstructive symptoms, neurogenic bladder dysfunction, renal calculi, analgesic abuse, or severe diabetes mellitus.

Cystoscopy, on the other hand, has essentially no risk under local anesthesia and occasionally yields information helpful in future management, such as enterovesical or vesicovaginal fistula, patulous or ectopic orifices, ureterocele, or findings suggestive of neurogenic bladder dysfunction.

Whether urethral stenosis contributes to reinfection remains controversial. It is apparent that without vaginal colonization with fecal organisms, reinfection is unlikely to occur no matter how stenotic the urethra. On the other hand, it is possible that urethral stenosis in susceptible women can contribute to reinfections. Dilatation of the stenotic urethra may be appropriate in these patients. There is little evidence, however, that urethral dilatation or reconstruction is useful in the routine management of the vast majority of patients with reinfections.

The primary goal of antimicrobial therapy should be to eliminate or reduce the rate of reinfections in the most convenient and inexpensive way. We usually institute low dose preventive therapy with one of the following drugs after we have documented that the urine culture shows no growth (most commonly as the patient is completing a full-dose course of antimicrobial therapy for an antecedent infection).

1. Trimethoprim-sulfamethoxazole (Bactrim or Septra), half a tablet orally at bedtime. The effectiveness of this drug is due to the diffusion and concentration of trimethoprim into vaginal fluid at therapeutic concentrations which prevent vaginal colonization with potential urinary pathogens. Reinfections occur rarely and are usually due to susceptible strains.

2. Cinoxacin (Cinobac), 250 to 500 mg orally at bedtime. This is a new synthetic antibacterial agent which is chemically similar to nalidixic acid and shares its activity against gram-negative bacteria most frequently isolated from the urinary tract. It has distinct advantages over nalidixic acid, including the fact that it achieves a many-fold higher urinary concentration with equivalent dosage, is less neurotoxic, and is less prone to induce resistant mutants. Breakthroughs occur rarely and are usually due to gram-positive organisms.

3. Nitrofurantoin, 50 mg orally at bedtime. As noted above, this drug is an ideal agent for preventive therapy because it is almost completely absorbed from the upper gastrointestinal tract, has a minimal impact on selection of resistant strains, and is excreted in high concentration in the urine.

I usually continue preventive therapy for 6 months, and then obtain frequent cultures off therapy. It is often helpful to give the patient a dip slide so that she can conveniently perform a culture at the first symptoms of infection. An infection is treated with full dose therapy, and cultures are obtained during and off therapy. Many patients prefer to use the dip slide technique and intermittent therapy for infrequent reinfections. Otherwise, a 6 month course of preventive therapy is reinstituted.

Bacterial Persistence. Infections in these patients are repeatedly caused by the same species and tend to recur rapidly. Thus the first infection is usually followed by a second within days of stopping therapy. It is obviously important to establish that the first infection was actually eradicated by antimicrobial therapy (i.e., negative culture on therapy). A thorough urologic evaluation is mandatory to identify within the urinary tract the focus of bacterial persistence which antimicrobials cannot reach and/or eradicate. The most common cause of bacterial persistence is infection stones resulting from urea-splitting organisms such as *Proteus mirabilis*. A congenital or acquired anomaly (such as calyceal diverticulum, nonfunctioning renal segment, or nonrefluxing ureteral stump) which has become secondarily infected represents a less common cause.

Surgical therapy plays a pivotal role in the management of these patients. When the focus of bacterial persistence has been localized, it should be removed or the responsible defect corrected. Although surgery can cure these patients of recurrent infections temporarily, the susceptibility for reinfection frequently remains and can lead to further episodes of bacteriuria. In some cases, long-term suppressive antimicrobial therapy may be required to control infection in lieu of definitive surgery.

High-Risk Patients

Any situation which predisposes to bacterial contamination of the urinary tract (e.g., catheterization) or diminishes the capacity to transport and void urine or concentrate antimicrobial agents increases the risk of infection. Patients at increased risk include those with renal failure, obstructive uropathy, or nephropathy caused by diabetes, analgesic abuse, or sickle cell disease, in whom there is a tendency toward papillary necrosis and secondary ureteral obstruction. Additional patients at increased risk from infection include those with neurogenic disorders of the urinary tract, patients with urea-splitting bacterial infections (e.g., *Proteus mirabilis* — see above) that can lead to formation of struvite infection stones, and patients with indwelling catheters. Finally, women who are pregnant require careful monitoring for and treatment of bacteriuric episodes. I generally treat infections during pregnancy with a short course of penicillin G or nitrofurantoin. If recurrences are frequent, I may institute preventive therapy with nitrofurantoin, 50 mg daily at bedtime, for the remainder of the pregnancy. I avoid tetracyclines, sulfonamides, and cinoxacin because of their potential effects on the fetus.

BACTERIAL INFECTIONS OF THE URINARY TRACT (FEMALE CHILDREN)

method of
LOWELL R. KING, M.D.
Chicago, Illinois

Bacterial urinary infections (UTI) occur frequently in girls, particularly after age 3, when toilet training has been begun or has been completed. Thus, there is empiric evidence that holding urine, or voiding infrequently, is a predisposing cause in some patients who later prove to have no other specific abnormality after thorough evaluation. At any given time, slightly more than 1 per cent of schoolage girls have urinary infections; about half of these are asymptomatic, or, more accurately, the symptoms are not severe enough to bring the child to the doctor. It is estimated that 5 to 10 per cent of girls have at least one UTI during their growing years. The diagnosis is best made by looking at a fresh, spun urine sediment under the microscope. Therapy can be started while the culture and sensitivities are pending. Most non-hospital-acquired infections are caused by *Escherichia coli,* and can be effectively treated by an antibacterial, such as nitrofurantoin, nalidixic acid, trimethoprim and sulfamethoxazole combinations, or a sulfonamide alone, as well as the relatively safe antibiotics such as ampicillin, given in weight-related doses. The antibiotics are more apt to cause diarrhea by altering bowel flora, and should usually be reserved for resistant cases and prescribed on the basis of the bacterial sensitivity tests. Therapy of an acute infection is usually continued for 10 to 14 days, although evidence is accumulating that suggests 3 to 5 days of therapy are usually adequate. A single dose of amikacin or amoxicillin given in the office at the time the diagnosis is made is adequate in about 90 per cent of instances, again excluding the hospital-acquired infections, which tend to be caused by more sophisticated antibiotic-resistant bacteria. A fresh urine should again be examined microscopically at least 3 days after the cessation of therapy to ascertain that the infection has been eradicated. A clear urine with 0 to 3 white blood cells per high power field and no visible bacteria (spun sediment) is reliable. Reculture should be done if the urinalysis is equivocal. Commercially available home or office culture kits, such as Uricult, are inexpensive and useful in this regard, as well as in follow-up.

What tests are pertinent in the evaluation of girls with urinary infection, and when should they be done? These include x-ray evaluation of the urinary tract by cystogram and intravenous pyelography (IVP), urethral calibration and dilatation with cystoscopy, and urodynamic testing. Deciding which child needs which test is one of the many arts of medicine, but some general guidelines can be used. First, urine infections occurring in infant girls are much more apt to be associated with anatomic anomalies which result in the presence of residual urine, most commonly vesicoureteral reflux, than those found in older girls. For instance, in one sample, 45 per cent of infants under 2 years of age presenting with infection exhibited reflux, while in the older girls in our clinic the rate was 22 per cent. About 4 per cent of each group had ureteropelvic or ureterovesical junction obstruction. We feel, therefore, that infants of either sex should be screened by voiding cystourethrogram and IVP after a first infection. It is desirable that the infection be eradicated before the cystogram is performed, because acute cystitis may cause transient mild reflux, but if the infection is resistant to therapy, the x-rays should be obtained without delay. Anatomic abnormalities which are detected are, of course, then evaluated and corrected surgically when necessary. The same is true in older girls, except that radiographic investigation is generally deferred unless the infection persists in the face of therapy or recurs within a year. Follow-up is, therefore, very important; urinalyses are recommended every 2 months for the first year plus whenever the child becomes ill from any apparent cause. Primary reflux, particularly when mild in degree and not associated with hydronephrosis on IVP, is often corrected with growth of the intravesical ureter, but surgical correction to protect the kidney is safest when infections recur. Cystoscopic evaluation is often helpful in prognosticating whether the reflux will stop. Children with known reflux are usually maintained on an antibacterial at about half the therapeutic dose, i.e., trimethoprim-sulfamethoxazole once a day or nitrofurantoin twice a day, until the reflux is known to have stopped on follow-up cystogram.

The majority of girls have normal x-ray studies, and for them the next step in evaluation or treatment is currently the subject of considerable debate. Urethral dilatation is an old, some would say time-tested, empiric treatment for urine infection in females. Girls have two narrow places in the urethra — the meatus and the distal urethral ring — which can each be permanently enlarged by a single overdilatation to No. 28 or

30 French. This is easily accomplished, but is painful and requires a general anesthetic in children. There is no scientific evidence that concomitant dilatation works any better than antibacterial medication alone in preventing reinfections, and there is considerable evidence that the urethral caliber in girls with a history of urine infection is not statistically different from that in urologically normal girls. Thus, the rationale for routine urethral dilatation, at least in girls with urine infection, is weak, and the procedure is not likely to be effective in preventing reinfection, except perhaps in a small minority with a very narrow urethral ring or meatus.

However, cystoscopy is of value. Girls with recurrent infection but without anatomic abnormalities on x-ray tend to fall into two groups: those who become reinfected as soon as suppressive medications are stopped, and those in whom infections are sporadic but occur at greater intervals. If infection recurs within 10 to 14 days after cessation of therapy or sooner, chronic cystitis, cystitis cystica, or cystitis glandularis is apt to be present. This can be confirmed cystoscopically, and means that long-term — at least 6 months (mean, 3½ years) — antibacterial therapy will be needed before the child stays well without medication. In order to get maximal information, cystoscopy should usually be performed while the child is infected and before treatment is begun. Cultures can be taken from the kidneys via urethral catheters after the bladder has been washed. Localization of infection is important, because common clinical signs, such as the presence or absence of high fever or the site of pain, do not permit the physician to distinguish pyelitis or pyelonephritis from cystitis with accuracy. Even without reflux and with a normal IVP, about 7 per cent of girls will prove to have renal infections as well as cystitis and longer-term therapy is then again considered. While the girl is asleep for the cystoscopy, the urethra is calibrated and usually overdilated (one time) to enlarge the caliber at the narrow points. This does not increase the morbidity from cytoscopy, which is generally dysuria with some hematuria for 1 to 3 days.

Girls with recurrent UTI also require further evaluation even when the infections are relatively infrequent — more than two or three a year. A urodynamic evaluation is needed when the cystogram and IVP are normal in such patients. In general, even though sphincter dyssynergia can cause intermittent incomplete emptying, residual urine, and even hydronephrosis, a relatively small proportion of such girls, perhaps 25 per cent, are shown to have a urodynamic abnormality. Nonetheless, sphincter dyssynergia can easily be tested for on an outpatient basis, and can usually be successfully treated, if detected, with appropriate medication or biofeedback. If undetected and if infections continue to recur, (1) cystoscopy during an episode to localize the infection and to check for rare causes such as a foreign body or enteric fistula and (2) a urethral dilatation are next performed. If no cause is found and infections are frequent, long-term therapy with a safe antibacterial agent may be the only maneuver effective in preventing most recurrences. If the kidneys are uninfected, it is equally appropriate to treat each infection as it occurs with a short course of medication. Given a negative workup, there is about a 20 per cent chance that each episode of reinfection will be the last. Since not all patients are symptomatic, parents should usually be instructed in home cultural techniques, but the urine should also be examined by the physician on a periodic basis.

CHILDHOOD ENURESIS

method of
MELVIN E. JENKINS, M.D.
Washington, D.C.

Nocturnal enuresis is a common complaint which accounts for a significant number of difficult-to-manage problems confronting the physician who treats children. Actually, its prevalence is probably much higher than office visits indicate because many parents have come to accept nocturnal enuresis as a "fact of life" and do not see the necessity to seek help. Under these circumstances, it is probably correct to estimate that at least 15 per cent of all 5- to 6-year olds are nocturnally enuretic. This frequency decreases progressively and significantly to almost 4 per cent in the early adolescent age group.

In this article, I shall outline the management approach to a child with enuresis in stepwise fashion, briefly justifying the rationale for each modality recommended.

Step I — History

A careful medical history of the child, including a family history, can prove most helpful. In this connection, it is well to remember that the diagnosis of enuresis should be limited to girls beyond the age of 5 years and to boys beyond the age of 6 years — this sex difference in age being related to developmental variation. The male counterpart age appears to exceed the female in all age groups observed.

The toilet training history bears relative significance to the problem. The age at which this was introduced, the response of the child during the time period, and the attitudes and approaches of the parents toward this aspect are important indicators in determining the mode of treatment. The effect of current environmental influences on the severity of the symptoms should be noted. Approximately 10 per cent of enuretics are also encopretic, which may reflect either organic pathology or deficiencies in toilet training. It is also necessary that the family history be considered, since a *positive* correlation has been found in 18 to 79 per cent of patients.

Step II — Physical Examination

A full physical examination is mandatory in these situations. The patient's urination process should be carefully observed for signs of straining, a small stream, emission, or dribbling. Any minor or major anomalies of the genitourinary tract should be assessed, e.g., undersized testes and/or meatal stenosis. A neurologic examination is needed to assess any lower spinal cord dysfunction. Obviously the child's blood pressure must be taken and growth rate evaluated and followed by 3 to 6 month visits to the pediatrician. Both these parameters may be useful in detecting reflections of chronic renal disease.

Step III — Urinalysis

A urinalysis is crucial to evaluate the possibility of diabetes mellitus, diabetes insipidus, urinary tract infections, psychogenic water drinking, and renal anomalies. Intravenous pyelography and voiding cystourethrography are done only if an organic disease is suspected, based on the results of the history, the physical examination, and/or the urine studies.

Step IV — Bladder Control Training

There is no specific therapy for enuresis, and yet this complaint can be responsive to methods which include positive reassurances for both the younger and the older child who bedwet because of environmental stresses. Other measures which have proved useful involve limiting fluid intake, emptying the bladder at bedtime, or taking the child to the bathroom during the night. These may temporarily decrease the symptoms but do not hasten a full remission.

A method utilizing progressive earlier waking has been introduced for the treatment of enuresis. This program involves waking the child 2 hours after he or she falls asleep and then progressively allowing the child to retain urine for longer periods before consecutive voidings. During daytime training, gradually increased periods of daytime retention of urine are reported to be followed by better nighttime control. This training is based on the fact that many enuretic children have a decreased functional bladder capacity, and this therapy attempts to transform an infantile bladder into one of a more adult volume capacity.

There are also mechanical conditioning techniques involving a mattress with a moisture-sensitive device which triggers an alarm to awaken the child upon initiation of wetting. Primary enuretics respond much better to this technique, but response bears no relation to the severity of the enuresis. Treatment failures may be due to patient resistance, sound sleep, or mechanical difficulty with a device.

Step V — Medication

Anticholinergic or sympathomimetic drugs have been used successfully in the treatment of enuresis. The mechanism of action is either a direct relaxation effect on the detrusor muscle or an antidepressant effect on the central nervous system.

Imipramine is the most commonly used agent in this disorder. It is generally given ½ to 1 hour before bedtime, with the initial dose 25 mg for children under 12 years and 50 mg for older children. (It is not recommended for use in children younger than 6 years of age.) Once a successful therapeutic response is achieved, the child is maintained on the medication for 2 or 3 months. The drug is then tapered to one dose every other night, then to every third night, and finally discontinued 4 to 6 weeks after tapering commenced.

Common side effects of the drug are nervousness, sleep disorders, and mild gastrointestinal complaints or even withdrawal symptoms. Imipramine poisoning when it occurs can be fatal in young children. This means that careful instructions must be given parents regarding storage of this medication to prevent access to small children.

Step VI — Supportive Counseling

Supportive counseling can prove to be curative therapy but must also be used as an adjunct to other specific regimens. Counseling is able to accomplish the following goals: (1) an understanding by the child that he or she can have some control over the enuresis; (2) acceptance by the child of the symptoms; (3) full acceptance of the child by the parents; and (4) good understanding by the parents of the multiple causes and effects of enuresis.

Genuine love and understanding by the parent may be the most important factor in resolving functional childhood enuresis. This common problem must be approached in an orderly fashion, with treatment carefully individualized and made appropriate for each patient.

EPIDIDYMITIS

method of
FRAY F. MARSHALL, M.D.
Baltimore, Maryland

Acute epididymitis is an inflammatory process affecting men of any age except prepubertal males. There are generally two groups of patients. In the first group, patients tend to be older with urinary tract infections and an obstructive uropathy. They generally have an easily identified bacterial epididymitis. The second group consists of younger males, often without evidence of bacterial infection. Many of these patients may have a chlamydial infection. Reflux of sterile urine up the ductus deferens to the epididymis is also a possible pathogenic mechanism. In prepubertal males epididymitis is rare but, if present, congenital anomalies of the urinary tract, especially ectopic ureters inserting into the vas deferens or seminal vesicle, must be suspected.

Treatment

Bed Rest. Continued activity will often delay resolution of symptoms and physical findings.

Scrotal Support. In the severe acute phase a towel between the thighs may aid in elevation. At a later stage an athletic supporter is often very helpful.

Antibiotics. A urine culture should be obtained before instituting any antibiotic therapy. If there is any question of tuberculosis, an acid-fast bacteria (AFB) culture should also be obtained. In patients with apparent urinary tract sepsis, aggressive early management with aminoglycosides may be required. In other patients with obvious infection, bacterial sensitivities from the culture should be used to direct therapy. In the younger patient, tetracycline (7 to 10 days) is indicated, because chlamydial organisms do not grow on ordinary urine cultures but the infection responds to tetracycline.

Pain Medication. Pain is often severe and may require narcotics. However, immobilization usually eases the pain dramatically. Infiltration of the spermatic cord with 1 per cent lidocaine (Xylocaine) has been advocated, but bleeding and injury to the spermatic vessels are possible complications.

Supportive Measures. Decrease in fever and lesser degrees of analgesia can be achieved with the use of aspirin or acetaminophen (Tylenol). Ambulation is restricted until the pain or tenderness is minimal.

Surgical Therapy. Surgical therapy is generally not indicated unless there is a question of torsion of the testes or a testicular tumor. The use of the Doppler or a testicular scan within the first few hours of symptoms can be helpful, but surgical exploration may still be required. If on exploration an abscess is found, it should be drained. In an elderly person with a large abscess, an orchiectomy may speed convalescence. If the epididymitis or mass does not appear to respond to management and there appears to be a possible testicular mass, a high inguinal exploration with possible orchiectomy should be considered.

Complications

Errors in diagnosis can create worse complications. Torsion of the testis or a testicular tumor clearly requires entirely different therapy. Chronic epididymitis is another complication. The pain can sometimes be a symptomatic problem. The inflammatory response can also lead to fibrosis and subsequent ductal obstruction, with sterility as a possible result. Fortunately, most cases respond to treatment.

BALANITIS AND BALANOPOSTHITIS

method of
ROBERT T. PLUMB, M.D.
San Diego, California

Balanitis is inflammation of the glans penis and posthitis is inflammation of the prepuce. These inflammations usually occur in uncircumcised men.

Etiology

Phimosis, with its associated desquamating epithelial cells, glandular secretions, bacteria,

Candida, and *Mycobacterium smegmatis,* provides an ideal culture medium for resulting balanoposthitis. Also, uncontrolled diabetes mellitus must be included as a cause. The specific venereal diseases and precancerous and cancerous lesions must be considered in the differential diagnosis.

Management

Management consists of clearing the nonspecific inflammation, using *vinegar compresses* (dilute 1 to 2 ounces [60 ml] of vinegar to 1 pint [470 ml] of room temperature water) and resoaking the compresses at 2 to 3 hour intervals. This should give good results within 24 hours.

Topical antibacterial or antimycotic agents such as polymyxin B, neomycin, and gramicidin (Neosporin); nystatin (Mycostatin); or neomycin sulfate and triamcinolone acetonide (Mycolog) may be applied three to four times daily. Correction of glycosuria is essential. If these methods do not produce results, a dorsal slit of the prepuce or circumcision should be performed.

GLOMERULAR DISORDERS

method of
ROBERT C. GOLDSZER, M.D.,
and J. MICHAEL LAZARUS, M.D.
Boston, Massachusetts

Introduction

The signs and symptoms of diseases affecting the glomerulus should be well known to physicians. Diseases may primarily affect the glomerulus or may be systemic with prominent glomerular involvement. Exclusion of diseases of other sites in the urinary tract such as cystitis, nephrolithiasis, interstitial nephritis, tumor, or obstruction is obviously important. Edema, hypertension, hematuria (gross or microscopic), or proteinuria, alone or in combination, strongly suggests glomerular involvement. Red cell casts are considered pathognomonic for parenchymal disease. In many patients therapeutic decisions will depend upon interpretation of renal biopsy material.

There are five major clinical syndromes produced by glomerular disorders: (1) *Nephrotic syndrome* is defined as proteinuria in excess of 3.5 grams per day, hypoalbuminemia, edema, and hyperlipidemia. Most cases of nephrotic syndrome are due to glomerulonephritis, primarily membranous nephritis, focal glomerulosclerosis, and minimal change disease. Other common causes include diabetes mellitus, drug nephropathy, systemic lupus erythematosus, and amyloidosis. (2) Patients with *chronic glomerulonephritis* may or may not have had a history of glomerular disorder, including any of the other four clinical syndromes. Small kidneys, urinary abnormalities, and varying degrees of azotemia characterize this syndrome. (3) *Rapidly progressive glomerulonephritis* causes urinary abnormalities, hypertension, and rapid deterioration of renal function, that is, azotemia occurring in less than 2 to 3 months' time. The most common pathologic finding in this clinical syndrome is crescentic glomerulonephritis. (4) Patients with *acute glomerulonephritis* present with edema, hypertension and hematuria or red blood cell casts, and proteinuria of acute onset, commonly following streptococcal infection. The disorder is common in children, may manifest mild azotemia, but usually remits. (5) Patients with *asymptomatic urinary abnormalities* may present with hematuria and mild proteinuria but without other signs and symptoms such as hypertension, edema, or azotemia. On renal biopsy many of these patients will demonstrate some form of glomerulonephritis, most often focal proliferative or mesangial proliferative glomerulonephritis.

Patients with glomerulonephritis may have problems with fluid retention, hypoproteinemia, hyperlipidemia, increased risk of thrombogenicity, renal failure, hyperuricemia, and hyperphosphatemia. We will discuss the approach to each of these problems before proceeding to therapy of glomerulonephritis.

Increased proximal tubular reabsorption of sodium leads to excessive retention of salt and water, causing periorbital and pretibial edema, ascites, and pleural effusion, and contributes to hypertension and possibly pulmonary edema. Hypoalbuminemia and hyperaldosteronism may contribute to this excessive sodium and water retention. Sodium restriction should be the first phase in management of these patients. A diet with 2 grams of sodium per day (88 mEq of sodium per day) is a reasonable starting point, although a few patients may require their sodium intake reduced to 0.5 gram per day. Some patients may prefer or require diuretic therapy rather than undergo extreme sodium restriction. Those with normal renal function will usually respond to thiazide diuretics. In patients with impaired renal function (serum creatinine greater than 3 to 4 mEq per dl (100 ml) or creatinine clearance less than 10 to 20 ml per minute), more potent diuretics, e.g., loopblocking diuretics such as furosemide or ethacrynic acid, will be required. Dosage should be titrated to reach a diuretic threshold (varying from 40 to 800 mg per day). (This dose may be higher than that listed in the manufacturer's official directive.) Deafness has been reported with both furosemide and ethacrynic acid, especially in patients with compromised renal function. The effect of ethacrynic acid is the more serious of the two, as irreversible deafness has been recorded with this agent. Fluid overload should be treated with the knowledge that prerenal azotemia may result if there is excessive loss of intravascular volume. Pulmonary edema, hypertension, and symptomatic pleural effusions require vigorous diuretic therapy. Peripheral edema, however, should be treated only if it is debilitating the patient. Pulmonary edema can frequently be managed with diuretics and blood pressure control; however, a digitalis preparation may be required in those patients in whom depressed myocardial function is a contributing factor. With impaired renal function, the dosage of digoxin must be modified.

Hypoproteinemia occurs because of excessive urinary protein losses and the inability of the liver to maintain synthesis. In addition to albumin loss, these patients lose globulins, causing significantly low serum levels of IgG, thyroxine-binding globulin, cortisol-binding globulin, and calciferol-binding globulin. Hypoalbuminemia and protein malnutrition can be minimized with dietary protein supplement of up to 1.5 to 2.0 grams of protein per kg per day. Because of difficulties in diuresis in patients with hypoalbuminemia, intravenous administration of albumin followed by furosemide may be transiently effective. Bed rest and elastic support hose may be helpful in mobilizing interstitial fluid to potentiate diuresis.

Hyperlipidemia is due to excessive production associated with hepatic compensation of protein losses. Hypercholesterolemia may lead to accelerated atherosclerosis. Dietary restriction of cholesterol and high fat foods is advisable; however, if one is to be vigorous in cholesterol control, drug therapy utilizing agents such as clofibrate is advisable. In patients with a compromised renal function this agent must be significantly reduced in dosage.

Thromboembolic complications such as renal vein thrombosis and pulmonary embolism may be seen in patients with nephrotic syndrome. Urinary losses of antithrombin III and increased hepatic synthesis of coagulation factors II, V, VII, and X lead to increased thrombogenicity. Patients should be monitored closely for this complication and, if it is present, treated with anticoagulation, initially continuous heparin infusion, followed by warfarin sodium therapy.

Hypertension associated with glomerular disorders may be due to excessive fluid retention and expansion of intravascular volume or stimulation of the renin-angiotensin system. Elevation of blood pressure to levels greater than 150/90 requires treatment. Initial management of mild hypertension is the same as that described above for edema. If blood pressure is not controlled with diet and diuretics, a second drug should be added, such as one of the sympatholytic agents — e.g., propranolol (40 to 200 mg two to four times

per day),* alpha-methyldopa (250 to 500 mg two to four times per day), or clonidine (0.1 to 0.6 mg two to four times per day). If blood pressure is still not controlled despite maximal dosages of one of these drugs, a third group, e.g., a vasodilator, should be added. These include hydralazine (25 to 100 mg two to four times per day),* prazosin (1 to 4 mg two to four times per day), or one of the newer antihypertensive agents such as minoxidil (2 to 5 mg per day) or, if available, the oral angiotensin converting enzyme inhibitor (Captopril). Malignant hypertension may be associated with glomerular disease and should be treated promptly and vigorously regardless of the state of renal function. A slight and transient decrease in glomerular filtration may occur because of decreased renal blood flow as blood pressure is lowered. Despite this, evidence suggests that control of pressure is essential to avoid more significant renal injury. Treatment should include intravenous furosemide and either diazoxide (100 to 300 mg) or nitroprusside infusion (0.5 to 10 micrograms per kg per minute), with close monitoring in an intensive care setting.

Glomerulopathy may lead to renal failure with varying degrees of rapidity. Patients developing renal failure must be evaluated for a reversible component and treated vigorously to avoid progressive azotemia and its complications. Therapy of this manifestation includes maintenance or correction of acid-base and electrolyte status, maintenance of calcium, phosphorus, and magnesium balance, correction of fluid status, proper nutrition, and prevention and treatment of infection, as well as correction of specific complications of uremia. Hyperuricemia often occurs in patients with impaired renal function caused by decreased excretion. Those patients who have a history of gout or urate renal stones should be treated with allopurinol, 100 mg two to three times per day. Acute gouty attacks require colchicine, 0.5 mg per hour, until relief is obtained. In the absence of gouty arthritis or nephrolithiasis, the treatment of hyperuricemia caused by renal insufficiency is debatable. Hyperphosphatemia is important in the development of secondary hyperparathyroidism, and some have suggested that this is important in the progression of renal disease. Serum phosphorus is controlled by administration of aluminum hydroxide–containing antacids that reduce phosphate absorption from the diet. Treatment of hypertension and of hyperphosphatemia are two important considerations in slowing the progression of renal insufficiency.

---

*This dose of this agent may be higher than that listed in the manufacturer's official directive.

Specific Treatment of Disorders Affecting the Glomerulus

Etiology of glomerulonephritis is unknown except for a few types, e.g., poststreptococcal infection, drug nephrotoxicity, bacterial endocarditis, heavy metal poisoning, bee sting, and hepatitis B virus. Most glomerulonephritides are thought to be due to an immune disorder related to antigen-antibody complexes, which in turn activates complement and white blood cell enzymes, causing injury to glomerular basement membranes. The glomerular basement membrane is typically associated with a granular pattern on immunofluorescent studies. A second major immune mechanism which may cause glomerulonephritis is the production and deposition of antibody directed against the glomerular basement membrane itself. This antibody deposition is responsible for the linear or smooth immunofluorescent staining of glomerular basement membrane such as that seen in Goodpasture's syndrome. The treatment of these various conditions is currently evolving. Few controlled prospective trials evaluating the efficacy of potentially toxic therapies have been performed. Therapy is determined by the clinical status of the patient, laboratory and immunologic parameters, and pathologic identification on renal biopsy.

Minimal Change Disease (Nil Disease, Lipid Nephrosis). This form of glomerulonephritis may have five possible courses: (1) spontaneously remittent, (2) responsive to therapy and not recurrent, (3) responsive to therapy and recurrent, (4) treatment dependent, and (5) progressive and unresponsive to treatment. Unless spontaneous remission occurs very early (within several weeks), patients should be treated for approximately 8 weeks with corticosteroids (prednisone, 1 mg per kg per day). Alternate-day steroid therapy has been shown to be effective as well (2 mg per kg every other day) and is associated with fewer side effects. Response is judged by excretion of protein and renal function studies. Many patients who respond do so within 4 weeks and should have the steroid dosage tapered. Repeated courses of therapy should be administered with each recurrence of the nephrotic syndrome. If there is no decrease in urinary protein excretion, the biopsy should be reviewed. In the past, focal glomerulosclerosis, which sometimes involves only deep, juxtamedullary glomeruli, has been missed and the diagnosis of minimal change disease mistakenly made. If the diagnosis is indeed minimal change disease and the patient is unresponsive to prednisone, a short course of either cyclophosphamide (1 to 1.5 mg per kg per day) or chlorambucil (0.2 mg per kg per day) may be considered. (This use of cyclophosphamide and chlorambucil is not listed in the manufacturers' official directives.) If there is no response after this time, patients will likely not respond and therapy should be discontinued.

Membranous Glomerulonephritis. Approximately 30 to 50 per cent of adults with nephrotic syndrome will demonstrate membranous glomerulonephritis on renal biopsy. Spontaneous remissions have been reported to occur in 15 to 20 per cent of these patients. This pathologic entity is usually idiopathic but may be seen in patients with solid tumors, drug nephropathy, heavy metal poisoning, and viral infections. Treatment includes reversal of any underlying disorder if possible. Prospective studies of prednisone in patients with idiopathic membranous glomerulonephritis suggest that those treated are less likely to progress to renal failure than those not treated. This finding is independent of the effect on proteinuria. Corticosteroids (prednisone, 2 mg per kg every other day) should be given for 2 months and then tapered for 1 month. If patients relapse, therapy should be repeated with each episode, provided that the patient has suffered no side effects of therapy. If renal function has severely deteriorated (serum creatinine greater than 4 to 6 mg per 100 ml or creatinine clearance less than 5 to 10 ml per minute), therapy is not likely to be beneficial. Studies with cytotoxic agents have not clearly demonstrated effectiveness in this disorder.

Focal Glomerulosclerosis. Focal glomerulosclerosis accounts for approximately 10 per cent of adults with nephrotic syndrome. Generally, deeper glomeruli are affected earlier with sparing of those in peripheral tissue. Progression to renal failure is common, but the time course may vary. No form of therapy has been proved effective.

Membranoproliferative (Mesangiocapillary) Glomerulonephritis. This histopathologic form of glomerulonephritis is the cause in approximately 5 to 10 per cent of adults with nephrotic syndrome. Patients commonly present with urinary abnormalities, hypertension, and variable degrees of renal insufficiency. At present there are few data on efficacy of therapy. Treatment modalities such as corticosteroids, immunosuppressive agents, and anticoagulants have been tried and reported with varying degrees of success, but none are of proved value. Approximately 50 to 60 per cent of these patients may be expected to develop end-stage renal disease.

Focal Proliferative Glomerulonephritis. The variable pathologic presentation, the variable course, and the association with systemic disease have made the role of therapy difficult to evaluate. The patient with focal proliferation may present with nephrotic syndrome or with asymptomatic urinary abnormalities. If renal function begins to decline, a 2 month course of alternate day corticosteroids as described above might be tried on an empirical basis early in the course. There is insufficient evidence to support continued treatment if there is no response or if there is contraindication to corticosteroid therapy.

Mesangioproliferative Glomerulonephritis. A diffuse increase in mesangial cells without capillary wall thickening or extracapillary proliferation is occasionally encountered in cases of idiopathic nephrotic syndrome. Patients will follow a variable course with most having a favorable prognosis. This lesion has not been shown to respond to therapy.

Crescentic Glomerulonephritis — Rapidly Progressive Glomerulonephritis. This disorder may be idiopathic or associated with systemic disease (Goodpasture's syndrome, systemic lupus erythematosus, or vasculitis) or may occur after streptococcal infection. The characteristic finding on biopsy is extracapillary crescents involving greater than 70 per cent of the glomeruli. Patients have hypertension, hematuria, and rapid deterioration of renal function and often become oliguric. Those patients who have developed oliguria and uremia have a poorer response to therapy. Treatment is most beneficial when initiated early in the disease process, ideally before renal function deteriorates and when urinary output is adequate. Various treatment regimens have been proposed and include pulse-dose methylprednisone (1 gram intravenously per day for 3 days) followed by high dose corticosteroids (prednisone, 1 to 1.5 mg per kg per day) along with an immunosuppressive agent (cyclophosphamide, 1 to 1.5 mg per kg per day) for 1 month and then tapered. (This use of cyclophosphamide is not listed in the manufacturer's official directive.) Plasmapheresis is a new mode of therapy which may have a role, especially in patients with demonstrable circulating antiglomerular basement membrane antibodies. Plasmapheresis is usually used in conjunction with corticosteroid and cytotoxic therapy. Anticoagulants, antiplatelet agents, and antifibrinolytic agents have been suggested but have not been proved effective to date. Because of the poor prognosis of patients with oliguria and renal failure, toxicities of these therapies may warrant a more conservative approach to such patients.

Acute Glomerulonephritis (Diffuse Proliferative Glomerulonephritis). These patients may have mild degrees of azotemia, but renal failure and nephrotic syndrome are rare. Therapy for this condition is supportive and includes treatment of edema, hypertension, and congestive heart failure, as noted above, and eradication of streptococcal infection. Corticosteroids and/or immunosuppressive agents are not indicated. Prolonged bed rest, advocated in the past, is probably not necessary. Most patients have a good prognosis; however, a rare patient with persistent proteinuria or early azotemia may have progressive loss of renal function.

Asymptomatic Urinary Abnormalities. Patients with microscopic hematuria, alone or in combination with mild proteinuria, but no other signs or symptoms usually have some type of glomerulonephritis when histopathology is obtained on renal biopsy. Examples are IgA nephropathy (Berger's disease), IgM nephropathy, hereditary nephritis, or some systemic diseases. Prognosis is variable for these entities, and therapeutic programs have been difficult to evaluate. Some patients may have spontaneous remission, but a few will progress to renal failure. A search should be undertaken for systemic disease which might be amenable to treatment.

Management of Systemic Disorders with Prominent Glomerular Involvement

Diabetes Mellitus. Tight control of blood glucose has been a generally accepted treatment to minimize progression of renal disease. There is little evidence, however, that therapy can delay the progression of diabetic glomerulonephritis once proteinuria is present. Many of these patients will develop nephrotic syndrome and progress to renal failure. Drug therapy for renal disease resulting from diabetes mellitus is not indicated.

Drug Nephrotoxicity. Many agents have been reported to cause glomerulonephritis. A partial list includes D-pencillamine, gold, heroin, and sulfa drugs. The drug nephrotoxicity may present as nephrotic syndrome or renal insufficiency. The renal disease in most of these patients will remit upon withdrawing the medication.

Systemic Lupus Erythematosus. Renal involvement is common, and the exact type can be identified only by histopathology with kidney biopsy. Patients with mesangial or focal proliferative glomerulonephritis whose renal function has not deteriorated probably require no therapy from the renal standpoint. Diffuse proliferative, membranous, or membranous with proliferative glomerulonephritis has been reported by some investigators to respond to corticosteroid therapy (1 to 1.5 mg per kg per day initially, with taper to the lowest dose that maintains remission). Rapid deterioration of renal function, when it occurs, is most commonly associated with the diffuse proliferative form. A trial of high dose pulse methylprednisolone has been suggested, but its benefit has not been proved. In some series, those patients who fail to respond to corticosteroid therapy are treated with cytotoxic agents (cyclophosphamide* or azathioprine*). Some have shown these agents to be effective; however, there is no agreement as to their indication. Plasmapheresis has also been suggested for the management of rapidly deteriorating renal function and SLE, but again it is not of proved benefit.

Vasculitides. These patients present with active urine sediment, hypertension, and varying degrees of renal function impairment. A partial list of these diseases includes hypersensitivity angiitis, polyarteritis nodosa, Wegener's granulomatosis, and Goodpasture's syndrome. These patients should probably be treated with a trial of corticosteroids (1 to 1.5 mg per kg per day) and an immunosuppressive agent, e.g., cyclophosphamide (1.5 mg per kg per day) if there are no major contraindications. (This use of cyclophosphamide is not listed in the manufacturer's official directive.) Cyclophosphamide is shown to be particularly beneficial in patients with Wegener's granulomatosis. Many of these patients present with rapidly progressive glomerulonephritis. Plasmapheresis has been suggested, but again has not been systematically studied to date.

Glomerulonephritis Associated with Systemic Infection. Such varied diseases as hepatitis B, toxoplasmosis, syphilis, and malaria have been associated with glomerulonephritis. In most cases, glomerular involvement will respond to successful treatment of the underlying disorder.

Complications of Treatment

The several drugs suggested as possible therapy for glomerular disorders have many potential and serious side effects. These are listed below:

Diuretics — hypovolemia, hypokalemia, hyponatremia, hyperuricemia, mild hyperglycemia, deafness, and interstitial nephritis.

Corticosteroids — cosmetic changes (acne, moon facies, hump back, striae), glucose intolerance, hypertension, cataracts, osteoporosis, aseptic necrosis of the femoral head, psychiatric disorder, and increased propensity to infection.

Immunosuppressive agents: Cyclophosphamide — bone marrow suppression, leukopenia with an increased susceptibility to infection, gonadal failure, alopecia, and hemorrhagic cystitis. Azathioprine — bone marrow suppression, leukopenia, hepatocellular dysfunction, and oncogenicity. Chlorambucil — gonadal failure and bone marrow depression.

Allopurinol — vasculitis, bone marrow suppression, and interstitial nephritis.

---

*This use of this agent is not listed in the manufacturer's official directive.

PYELONEPHRITIS

method of
HOWARD E. FAUVER, JR., M.D.
Aurora, Colorado

Evaluation

In addition to a detailed history and physical examination the following studies are indicated:

Laboratory Data

Urinalysis. A high urine pH may suggest infection with a urea splitter such as Proteus. Microscopic examination routinely demonstrates large numbers of white blood cells (WBC), at times associated with WBC casts and variable amounts of hematuria. Bacteria in a drop of unspun urine is virtually diagnostic of significant bacilluria.

Urine Culture. This generally will show greater than 100,000 colonies per ml of the causative organism in the properly collected, preserved, and cultured specimen. In the male a midstream specimen is acceptable. In the female a clean catch specimen monitored by a nurse or aide is often all that is necessary. However, if any question of the adequacy of collection exists, a simple in-and-out catheterization using aseptic technique is usually without significant risk and will be diagnostic. A suprapubic tap is extremely useful in children and represents a reasonable alternative in adults. Uncommonly, more than one type of organism will be present, or the colony count even with known infection will be less than 10^5. The laboratory should therefore be admonished to identify all organisms regardless of colony count if your index of suspicion is high.

Blood Count. Leukocytosis is routinely present in the acutely ill patient and provides an additional parameter by which to follow response to therapy.

Chemistries. Creatinine and blood urea nitrogen should be determined at the outset and periodically therafter if potentially nephrotoxic drugs are employed.

X-Ray

Radiographic changes on excretory urography in acute uncomplicated pyelonephritis are evanescent and equivocal at best. Despite this an intravenous pyelogram (IVP) is indicated immediately to rule out obstruction in certain patients, e.g., those in sepsis, those with known prior urinary obstructive or calculous disease, or those with pain mimicking renal colic. Those patients who fail to respond to therapy within 48 to 72 hours should also be studied.

Cystoscopy

Endoscopy is avoided in the presence of acute infection unless necessary to relieve obstruction.

Treatment

The first critical therapeutic decision is whether the patient should be hospitalized for treatment. As a rule, only those patients with minimal or moderate constitutional symptoms are candidates for outpatient therapy. Marked fever and/or pain, inability to maintain adequate oral hydration as a result of vomiting or inanition, and the presence of significant underlying disease such as diabetes mellitus all mandate admission.

General. 1. Bed rest initially.

2. A minimal fluid intake of 2000 to 2500 ml per day is necessary. Fever greater than 101 F (38.4 C) may increase the requirement by 500 ml or more. The oral route is preferred if tolerated, but intravenous use of appropriate balanced electrolyte solutions may be necessary.

3. Moderate or severe pain may be managed by codeine sulfate 30 to 60 mg orally every 4 to 6 hours. If oral medications are inappropriate, meperidine, 50 to 100 mg intramuscularly every 4 hours, may be needed.

4. For fever greater than 101 F (38.4 C), acetylsalicylic acid should be administered in dosage of 600 mg orally every 4 hours or, alternatively, 600 mg in suppository form.

Specific Antibiotics. A staggering number of antimicrobial agents are available, varying in their spectra, their potential toxicity, and, also to be considered, their expense. Initial choice of drug is influenced by the patient's condition, the likelihood of a resistant organism (e.g., community- versus hospital-acquired), the feasibility of the oral route of administration, and an awareness of the usual sensitivity pattern in an individual hospital. Evidence of clinical improvement is normally present by 48 to 72 hours and coincides with the reporting of sensitivity testing. Appropriate changes in medication or dosage can then be made.

In the individual patient, the following drugs may be suitable according to sensitivities:

WHEN PARENTERAL MEDICATION IS APPROPRIATE. 1. Aminoglycosides. These have in common the widest available spectrum for organisms usually involved in acute pyelonephritis, although displaying some variations in predictability of serum levels, potential for oto- or nephrotoxicity, and frequency with which resistant strains are seen. They are not active against enterococci.

In hospital-acquired infections, in the septic patient, or in pyelonephritis complicated by urinary obstruction or stasis, these should be considered first-line drugs.

Amikacin may be administered in dosage of 15 mg per kg per day either intravenously or intramuscularly, not to exceed 1.5 grams daily, in divided doses of 7.5 mg per kg every 12 hours or 5 mg per kg at 8 hour intervals. Serum levels for this drug appear to be more predictable at pre-scribed dosages than with the other aminoglycosides, and this may represent an advantage.

Gentamicin may be used in a range of 3 to 5 mg per kg per day in divided doses every 8 hours. If long-term therapy is indicated or if a sensitive organism is slow to respond, serum levels should be monitored, since interpatient variation in serum levels at normal dosages may be considerable even in the presence of normal renal function.

Tobramycin may be used in the same dosages as gentamicin.

The aminoglycosides should not be mixed with other drugs in the same container. Blood urea nitrogen and serum creatinine should be determined frequently during administration of these agents and the dose adjusted if evidence of renal impairment is present. Courses of treatment extending beyond 7 to 10 days, if felt to be imperative, should also be an indication for audiometric tresting. These drugs as a class are concentrated in the kidney, so downward adjustment of dosage may be appropriate once clinical response is apparent.

2. Penicillins. Ampicillin, 1 gram intravenously every 6 hours, is often effective as a single agent. In the septic patient, however, we prefer to use it together with an aminoglycoside to protect against the significant but uncommon pathogen enterococcus until sensitivities are known.

Carbenicillin is also effective against enterococcus as well as a variety of gram-negative organisms, including Pseudomonas, in dosages of 200 mg per kg per day intravenously in divided doses. Synergism with gentamicin against Pseudomonas has been reported. Use of this combination discourages the emergence of resistant strains, which is sometimes seen when carbenicillin is used as a single agent.

3. Cephalosporins. A variety of these antibiotics with comparable spectra are available. These drugs do not routinely cover enterococci, Pseudomonas, or indole-positive Proteus, although some of the newer agents such as cefamandole are effective against some strains of the latter organism. Cross-allergenicity with penicillin has been documented.

Cefazolin, cephapirin, or cephradine, 500 mg to 1 gram every 6 hours either intravenously or intramuscularly, may be given.

Cefamandole may be used in a dosage of 500 mg every 8 hours by the same routes.

WHEN ORAL TREATMENT IS APPROPRIATE. 1. Penicillins. Ampicillin, 500 mg every 6 hours, or indanyl carbenicillin, 1 to 2 tablets four times a day, may be used.

2. Cephalosporins. Cephradine or cefadroxil, 1 gram twice daily, may be appropriate.

3. Tetracyclines. These are contraindicated

in pregnancy and childhood. If used at other times, my preference is for doxycycline, 200 mg in divided doses on the first day, followed by 100 to 200 mg per day.

4. Miscellaneous agents. Numerous other drugs are available and may be appropriate in a given patient. These include the long-acting tri-methoprim-sulfamethoxazole (TMP/SMX) combinations, 1 tablet twice daily; nitrofurantoin macrocrystals, 50 to 100 mg four times a day; nalidixic acid, 1 gram four times daily; or the generically similar oxolinic acid, 750 mg twice a day.

In general, the patient is changed from parenteral medications to an appropriate oral agent 24 to 48 hours after clinical resolution of symptoms has occurred. Total course of treatment in an uncomplicated first episode of pyelonephritis is 10 days.

Follow-up

Urine sterility at the end of the course of treatment must be confirmed. Additional cultures are performed monthly for 3 months, then every 3 months thereafter for 1 year, to detect those patients with asymptomatic bacilluria. Recurrence of infection even without symptoms during this period is an indication for a second course of treatment for 7 to 10 days with full therapeutic dosages, followed by 6 weeks of treatment with maintenance dosages, e.g., nitrofurantoin, 50 mg twice daily, or ½ tablet of a long-acting trimethoprim-sulfamethoxazole (TMP/SMX) combination twice a day.

If excretory urogram (IVP) was not performed previously, it should be accomplished. Because of a high association with vesicoureteral reflux, a retrograde cystogram should also be done after 8 to 12 weeks. Abnormal findings on either study should occasion urologic consultation.

GENITOURINARY TRACT TRAUMA

method of
IRVING M. BUSH, M.D.,
PATRICK GUINAN, M.D.,
and SALVADOR ZAMORA, M.D.
Chicago, Illinois

Introduction

All patients with traumatic disease have to be evaluated individually. This is particularly true in patients with genitourinary trauma, since they more often have concomitant injuries of several organ systems. One cannot be dogmatic in these situations but must mentally balance the life-threatening injuries with the less serious ones.

As in all trauma, treatment begins simultaneously with diagnosis. Whether in the ambulance or in the emergency room, as soon as the patient is determined to be suffering from trauma, the following measures are taken:

1. An airway is obtained or maintained.
2. Gross bleeding is stopped.
3. Vital signs are obtained.
4. Intravenous fluids are started.
5. Any burns or open wounds are covered with sterile dressings. Dismembered organs or appendages are wrapped with sterile, cold, saline-soaked dressings.

The patient should, on arrival at the hospital or after initial care in the emergency room, be moved to a specially designated area or portion of the emergency room which has enough room so that all clothes can be removed (cut off) and all parts of the body reached with ease. Next:

1. Blood is obtained for complete blood count (CBC), electrolyte concentrations (blood gases), typing and cross matching (2 to 4 units).
2. A central venous pressure catheter is inserted, if deemed necessary.
3. Vital signs are confirmed.
4. A urine specimen is obtained for urinalysis, microscopic examination, and culture (except if a urethral injury is suspected).
5. A history is obtained. It is important to verify the following: (a) When did the accident or incident occur? (b) Where was the patient struck? (c) Where is the pain? (d) Is it increasing? (e) Was any tissue lost and recovered? (f) Was the injury caused by an auto accident, a fall, machinery, a blunt blow, a stab, or a low- or high-velocity bullet? (g) Was there loss of consciousness? (h) Is there a history of previous urologic disease or surgery (nephrectomy, calculi, congenital problems, urinary tract infection)? (i) Did the patient urinate a short time before the accident? (j) Did the patient void after the accident? Was it bloody? Was it a full amount?
6. A physical examination should then be performed, including the following: (a) Inspection for ecchymosis in the flank, over the abdomen, or in the perineum. (b) Percussion of the bladder. (c) Rectal examination for position of the prostate. (d) Estimation of flank, chest, or abdominal tenderness. (e) Measurement of the abdominal circumference.
7. Appropriate x-rays can then be ordered.

A working diagnosis of the extent of injury is then made and the need for the following is assessed:

1. Fluid and blood replacement.

2. A Foley catheter (see Urethral Trauma) to monitor urine output.

3. Peritoneal lavage, which has replaced four-quadrant abdominal tap in many institutions. A No. 14 Intracath can be inserted just below the umbilicus. Hematocrit and amylase determinations should be performed on the fluid return. A technetium scan for residual abdominal radionuclide can also be obtained or substituted for peritoneal lavage. Remember that a negative lavage does not prove the absence of injury.

Urologic Trauma

If it is suspected that the patient has genitourinary injury, the urologic work-up continues parallel to the management of other injuries. This is essential because 60 per cent of patients with penetrating renal trauma have associated abdominal injuries, and 15 per cent of these same patients will have an associated chest injury. Blunt injuries also may involve multiple organs, especially with significant pelvic fractures. The most serious injury takes precedence in the management of the patient. Patients with isolated urologic injuries whose conditions are stable are generally treated more conservatively, whereas patients whose conditions are unstable are managed surgically. Often the presence of associated injuries dictates surgical exploration. This aids in the assessment of a urologic injury, since the abdomen and retroperitoneum can be examined directly during laparotomy.

Renal Injury

When the initial evaluation points to a renal injury from either a gunshot or stab wound or blunt trauma, an infusion intravenous pyelogram with nephrotomograms, if feasible, should be obtained. Indications for selective renal angiography when available include the following:

1. Absence of function on either side or both sides.

2. Evidence of a collecting system leak.

3. Significant renal fractures.

Angiography also delineates the number of renal arteries and segmental artery damage and occlusion. Specific indications for operative intervention include the following:

1. Any major injury of the renal substance or collecting system.

2. A gunshot wound.

3. Evidence of an injured major vessel.

4. A dropping hematocrit level (the need for 2 units of blood).

5. One helpful sign indicative of an unstable vascular system is the inability of a patient to maintain his systolic blood pressure if moved from the recumbent to sitting position.

Absence of the aforementioned signs suggests the need for observation. It is well known that the presence or absence of gross hematuria does not correlate with the need for exploration or extent of injury, since a significant injury to the renal parenchyma or vascular pedicle does not necessarily communicate with the collecting system.

When renal exploration is indicated, the pedicle is isolated first and control of the artery and vein is obtained. This is best performed by a long midline transabdominal incision. If there is complete disruption of the renal pedicle or a shattered kidney (especially with high-velocity bullet wounds), a nephrectomy is usually performed. Always ascertain that there is a viable kidney on the opposite side by intravenous urography, palpation, or indigo carmine injection with the ipsilateral ureter isolated and occluded. Bench surgery with autotransplantation is rarely available or indicated except in associated pancreatic or duodenal injuries. If the renal vein or artery is injured but the remainder of the kidney is intact, the vessels can be repaired.

In arterial injuries, renal ischemic time, associated renal damage, the extent of intimal damage, the length of time necessary to obtain a vein segment for a patch or replacement graft or the advisability of using an artificial graft, and the ease of repair all play a role in whether arterial repair or nephrectomy should be performed. All arterial contusions should be evaluated for intimal arterial damage. Review of the arteriogram should be followed by intraoperative Doppler studies after the use of procaine to relieve the spasm, or by arteriotomy and direct observation. In injuries of arterial branches, ligation should be considered if the distal end cannot be freed from the renal parenchyma or renal pelvis. Thrombectomy in all arteries, if performed, should include intimal repair.

Right-sided vascular injuries are usually more difficult to repair because of the shorter veins. Small veins can be ligated most of the time. If the kidney seems swollen at initial inspection, translocation of the renal vein lower on the vena cava is indicated. If the venous injury is close to the left kidney, proximal to the ovarian/spermatic and adrenal veins, major branches can be ligated following diagnostic clamping (the kidney should not swell).

In upper pole and lateral parenchymal injuries, the significant devitalized tissue should be debrided. Minimal devitalized tissue does not have to be resected. Partial nephrectomy is in many instances a simple procedure. All bleeding vessels are ligated carefully with figure-eight sutures of 3-0 absorbable material. The collecting system is then sutured closed. Attempts to close or fill every defect with perirenal fat or omentum may not be necessary. The capsule (if available) is then closed. A free peritoneal graft can be used for this purpose. Perirenal fat can also be used as bolsters or to cover raw surfaces. Extraperitoneal drainage with Penrose drains is then performed.

Conservative Approach to Renal Injuries

If there is no evidence of significant injury on an intravenous pyelogram (IVP) or angiography, the following "delayed treatment" protocol can be undertaken in blunt and stab wound injuries. Since most of these patients will be treated conservatively, an organized plan is important and should include these elements:

1. Repeat hematocrit readings every 2 hours for the first 3 to 6 hours and then every 4 hours for the next 6 to 12 hours, twice daily for the next 2 days, and then daily for at least 3 days after ambulation.

2. Give nothing by mouth (NPO) during evaluation and until exploration is no longer considered.

3. Bed rest is mandatory until gross hematuria stops and hematocrit level stabilizes.

4. Technetium arteriography and renal scan, renogram, and sonograms (and rarely CT scans) may be helpful in delineating extent of injury.

5. Follow-up IVPs in 10 days to 2 weeks and in 3 to 6 months should be done.

If there is a limited renal injury and the abdomen is to be explored for some other reason, a conservative approach, which includes possible use of partial nephrectomy, can be employed. The retroperitoneum is examined prior to the repair of the nonurologic injuries, and the extent of the peritoneal hematoma is evaluated. After repair of the other injuries, Gerota's fascia is opened only if the hematoma has progressed. If there is a question about the extent of the renal injury, an intraoperative arteriogram can be performed.

Recurrence of Hematuria

Recurrence of hematuria or a drop in hematocrit upon ambulation usually indicates nonhealing of the injury. Persistent or recurrent fever indicates continued extravasation or infection. Infusion pyelography, arteriography, retrograde pyelography, and occasionally ureterorenoscopy will identify the bleeding site. The presence of an arteriovenous fistula must always be considered. Recurrent bleeding necessitates exploration, the use of partial nephrectomy, or nephrectomy, which is determined best by correlation of radiographic and operative findings.

Remember:

1. Do not be alarmed at superficial gaping wounds of the flank, since many times they do not involve the kidney substance or collecting system. This is a common situation seen in shotgun wounds.

2. Evaluate the contralateral kidney and ureter whenever possible by palpation and use of indigo carmine.

3. While observing the patient, repeatedly measure the abdomen and examine the patient for flank and abdominal masses.

4. Placing serial urine specimens in a bedside rack permits all personnel to observe the progress of hematuria.

5. In case of massive injury, an infusion pyelogram can be started on the way to the operating room table.

6. Always suspect splenic injury in left renal injury and liver damage in right renal trauma.

7. If a bleeding segmental renal artery is discovered during selective angiography, blockade by autologous clot or gelatin sponge (Gelfoam) has been successful.

8. Always suspect congenital abnormality or tumor in a child who develops hematuria from simple cases (e.g., hitting the side of a table, falling off a swing).

9. If the renal fossa is explored, mobilize the kidney so that the entire renal surface can be examined.

10. Follow-up for hypertension should be performed for at least several years. Although the incidence of hypertension following renal injury in both conservatively and surgically treated cases has seemingly decreased over the past 20 years, it is still between 1 and 5 per cent.

Ureteral and Renal Pelvic Injury

Ureteral and renal pelvic injuries are evaluated, much like renal injuries, with an infusion pyelogram. A prone film and a delayed film are especially important. Oftentimes retrograde pyelography is of benefit, particularly in iatrogenic injuries, which usually occur in the lower third of the ureter. A retrograde pyelogram is performed as the last test in the work-up or if a management change is contemplated. Tears in the renal pelvis are best handled by suture placement, stenting, and drainage. In upper ureteral disruption, a dismembered pyeloplasty yields the best results. If there is a massive injury or underlying congenital defect, a nephrostomy tube may be substituted or added to the stenting.

Loss of less than one third of the ureteral diameter requires only debridement and stenting with or without repair. Loss of more than one third of the diameter requires end-to-end spatulated or Z-plasty watertight anastomosis with 4-0 or 5-0 chromic or Dexon suture. Proximal stenting through a high linear ureterotomy may be used. Loss of over 3 to 4 cm of length in the upper third of the ureter is best managed by inferior nephropexy or bowel interposition. With significant middle third ureteral loss, end-to-side transureteroureterostomy is the technique of choice. Lower third ureteral injuries are managed by reimplantation (antireflux) psoas hitch or the Boari flap technique. In unusual cases, cutaneous ureterostomy or nephrectomy may be necessary to save the patient's life.

Remember:

1. The diagnosis of ureteral or renal pelvic injuries is made when the physician has a high index of suspicion.

2. Stab wounds of the duodenum, lateral abdominal gunshot wounds, and trigonal injuries should be especially investigated for renal pelvis and ureteral injury.

3. Use of intravenous indigo carmine is helpful in these injuries.

4. A prior cystogram with extravasation may obscure a concomitant injury to the lower ureter.

5. If there is no tension on the ureteral repair, ureteral stents may be eliminated.

6. In these injuries, adequate drainage, careful observation, and long-term follow-up are always necessary.

7. Delayed recognition of a ureteral injury may require local drainage and diversion by nephrostomy for several weeks before actual repair can be performed.

8. Immediate identification of ureteral ligation can be treated by *disligation* and stenting in urgent situations. A clamped or securely tied ureter probably should be treated by resection and repair except in the presence of abscess or tumor.

9. Use of renal capsular flaps to repair the upper ureter and ureteropelvic junction should be considered when a nondilated intrarenal pelvis is present.

10. In exposing the renal vessels, the incision in the posterior peritoneum should be made over the aorta just medial to the inferior mesenteric vein.

11. In using a bladder flap technique, make sure that the base of the flap is broad and has an adequate blood supply and that the ureteral implantation, if possible, is through a submucosal tunnel.

12. In autotransplantation of the kidney to the ipsilateral iliac fossa, a ureteroneocystostomy is not usually necessary.

13. If pressed, a ureter can be quickly reimplanted by triangulating the end with three sutures (serosa to mucosa) inserting each suture through a hole in the bladder (mucosa to serosa), and tying the sutures outside the bladder wall.

14. In performing any reimplantation or flap procedure, try to make the bladder entrance as close to the trigone as possible.

15. If the pancreas and the renal pelvis or ureter are injured, nephrectomy may be the wisest course. On the other hand, if individual drainage of each injury is used, a separation can be achieved by interposing significant tissue between the two injured organs, employing adequate proximal urinary diversion, and obtaining a tension-free watertight closure in an attempt to avoid nephrectomy. Secondary nephrectomy can always be performed.

Bladder Injury

Bladder injuries are diagnosed accurately and rapidly by a cystogram with an emptying film. Although the use of an infusion pyelogram first will better demonstrate lower ureteral injuries, the cystogram should be performed initially, if no urethral injury is suspected. Although an emptying film may miss 5 per cent of perforations, it is especially helpful in identifying small leaks and in distinguishing between extraperitoneal and intraperitoneal injuries. Again, a high index of suspicion will often locate an inapparent perforation. All perforations of the bladder are best managed with cystotomy, although extraperitoneal perforations may be treated by a large urethral catheter and suprapubic drainage in a healthy female. In closing penetrating lesions of the bladder, it is best to close the peritoneal defect first and then the bladder in two layers with absorbable suture. Also, look for and close the second hole in the bladder, which is often seen in penetrating wounds. More recently, the use of a disposable illuminating catheter has been a help in demonstrating low ureteral defects.

Remember:

1. In pelvic fractures, remove all visible bony fragments before bladder closure.

2. Gynecologic and obstetric injuries to the bladder can be best diagnosed by suspicion and the use of milk (boiled?), which is nonstaining and can be used before and after repair. A two-layered closure with interposing peritoneum or omentum is to be recommended.

Urethral Trauma

As the trauma patient is evaluated initially, it is important to consider the possibility of urethral injury by carefully obtaining the following information:

1. History taking (straddle injuries, pelvic fractures).

2. Visual inspection (perineal ecchymosis, blood at meatus).

3. Physical examination (high-riding prostate).

A urethrogram taken before insertion of the Foley catheter, using intravenous contrast material and instilled initially under gravity, will usually delineate most urethral trauma and distinguish anterior from posterior (prostatomembranous) and partial from complete urethral injuries.

If there is only a partial urethral injury, a No. 14 or No. 16 Foley catheter can be gently passed. In partial anterior injuries, a pressure dressing should be applied after the Foley catheter is inserted. If a catheter cannot be passed, the following method for complete anterior injuries should be carried out.

In complete anterior urethral injuries, a catheter should not be passed and the patient should not be encouraged to void. If the patient's condition is stable and there are no associated bladder injuries, exploration and end-to-end anastomosis can be performed primarily. Otherwise, a cystotomy can be performed initially with end-to-end anastomosis delayed for 6 weeks to 4 months.

In a complete posterior urethral tear, in which a small Foley catheter or catheter coudé cannot be passed, or in massive or contaminated urethral injuries, a suprapubic cystotomy should be performed initially and a gentle attempt at restoration of continuity can be tried. We attempt a single retrograde passage of a flexible fiberoptic catheter, and if this is not successful, a soft red rubber catheter is passed antegradely. If this is successful, we attach a heavy No. 1 silk suture to the distal end and pull a Foley catheter in place. Lateral transperineal fixation sutures (Mersaline strips over dental rolls or nylon sling sutures, sutures attached to an elastic band strapped to each thigh) are inserted from the inside out to bring the bladder and prostate back down onto the perineum. The catheter is not placed under any tension. A very long, heavy silk strand is tied to the end of the Foley catheter and brought out alongside the cystotomy tube. The space of Retzius is well drained. If urethral continuity cannot be re-established immediately, do not repeatedly attempt to pass a catheter or use interlocking sounds (which are useful in later procedures).

Since it is difficult to estimate the effect of the initial injury on later potency and continence, it is wise not to induce more damage, which will cause subsequent fibrosis or scarring, by vigorous or prolonged manipulations. Patients and relatives should immediately be made aware that urethral injuries, even with the best management, may take months to years to finally correct.

If perineal fullness is detected several days after the injury, the treating physician should suspect persistent urine leakage around Colles' fascia. In this situation the following are done:

1. Repeat the urethrogram with minimal to moderate pressure.

2. Perform suprapubic cystotomy.

3. Do not explore for urethral defects.

4. Insert multiple perineal drains and suprapubic drains.

5. Perform extensive debridement of all necrotic or gangrenous areas.

6. Examine for crepitation.

7. Culture and treat with large doses of appropriate antibiotics as if gas-producing or anaerobic infection were present.

Foreign bodies in the urethra and bladder should always be considered when the history is not straightforward and sexual dysfunction is a concern. Bobby pins, pencils, parts of knitting needles, and so forth, are not uncommonly found in the female urethra and bladder. Clothespins, nail files, parts of candles, cut Foley catheters, "superglue," and similar objects can be seen in the male urethra. Plain x-ray films may not be of value without contrast material. Dilute contrast urethrography is necessary, since many of the objects found in recent years are of plastic, wood, or wax. Cystopanendoscopy is confirmatory and can be used to remove most small urethral and bladder foreign bodies. Cystostomy is necessary for larger objects in the bladder. Every now and then variously shaped objects (vibrators, soda bottles) are "lost" by the same persons in their rectums.

Remember:

1. The most common form of urethral trauma causing stricture formation is poor catheter insertion, placement, and care.

2. In partial posterior urethral injury, a finger in the rectum will help guide the catheter and immediately determine if the catheter is outside of the urethra.

3. In all types of trauma, a Foley catheter in males should be taped up on the abdomen to prevent stricture formation.

4. Use of a multi-hole catheter to drain the entire urethra, especially the posterior prostatic urethra, is at times helpful.

5. Primary urethral repair should always be performed by a surgeon with prior experience. Indications for primary repair are the following: (a) The hematoma is not extensive. (b) There is no continuous bleeding. (c) The torn edges are

easily identified. (d) The edges are not edematous or severely traumatized (this will prevent breakdown of the wound).

6. In end-to-end anastomosis, illuminating catheters passed retrogradely and antegradely (through the cystotomy) may help to identify the torn ends with ease and minimize trauma.

7. In dilating urethral strictures, following total posterior disruption, it should be remembered that fibrosis may cause an S-shaped deformity.

8. A delayed scrotal flap technique for urethral disruption repair after cystotomy alone as an initial treatment has been very successful in several centers.

9. Delayed transpubic approach to traumatic strictures of the posterior membranous urethra affords direct observation and decreased sexual complications.

Scrotum and Testes

Small hematomas of the scrotum, especially from blunt trauma, that do not expand should be treated conservatively by observation, bed rest, icebag, and antibiotics. Large or expanding scrotal hematomas (especially caused by penetrating injury) should always be explored. Specific efforts should be made to conserve all genital tissue, especially skin, whenever possible. In scrotal avulsion injuries all clothing should be carefully removed in a sterile manner. In clean avulsions, it is best to bury the exposed testicles in the thigh. In potentially infected or necrotic scrotal wounds, it is important to debride the area widely and let the testicles remain exposed but covered with sterile dressings. A method that can be followed in injury to the scrotum includes the following:

1. Measure the size of the testicles and scrotum with a tape measure or calipers in several directions.

2. Obtain permission for possible removal of testicle or ligation of the spermatic vein.

3. Prepare for surgical exploration.

4. Doppler readings of both spermatic cords and testes to evaluate blood flow are helpful, if available.

5. Observe scrotum within ½ to 1 hour.

6. If the hematoma is small and not expanding, continue to observe.

7. If the hematoma is expanding or if it was caused by significant penetrating injury, explore the scrotum through a wide incision and express the clot, taking care not to traumatize scrotal skin.

8. In penetrating injury, look for a specific vessel and ligate it, if small.

9. If the spermatic artery is damaged, repair if at all possible with 6-0 arterial suture.

10. In blunt injuries or postvasectomy hematomas, the specific vessel is hard to find. Before establishing dependent drainage, quiet observation of the open scrotum for 5 minutes (Feldman technique) often leads to discovery of the bleeding vessel.

11. Use compression dressing, elevation, and icepacks for at least 24 to 48 hours.

Because of testicular mobility and the thick tunica albuginea, rupture of the testicle is somewhat unusual. If the tunica albuginea is ruptured, protruding tubules should be snipped off flush with the tunica and the tunica closed with a tight running 3-0 catgut suture. When there has been attempted self-castration with spermatic cord injury, extend the incisions high into the inguinal regions, since the spermatic arteries immediately retract. In massive injuries, retain as much testicular tissue as possible to preserve hormonal function.

Remember:

1. Urethrograms should always be performed in penile and scrotal injuries to detect inapparent urethral injuries.

2. If a vas or ductus is injured, immediate repair with 6-0 nylon, avoiding the mucosa over an intraluminal chromic catgut suture or over a No. 28 or No. 30 wire stent, brought out 2 to 3 cm proximal and distal to the repair should be performed. The wire can be removed in 7 to 10 days. The catgut suture will be absorbed.

3. Many patients will have delayed psychologic reactions to scrotal and testicular injuries.

Penis

The most common penile injuries seen in the emergency room are zipper injuries. Instead of retracting the zipper down, cut off the fasteners with shears on the movable head and part the zipper. Rings and other circular objects that mimic paraphimosis usually have to be cut off because the edema is too advanced. Placing a protective shield between the circular ring and the skin is always a good idea. When the penis is entrapped in a metal carafe or closed cylinder, insert a lubricated red rubber catheter along the side of the shaft of the penis to break the suction, instill some mineral oil, and suspend the object above the body. This may prevent having to blindly cut the thick metal with heavy equipment. Strings, shoelaces, or hair are sometimes tied around the penis. As with vacuum cleaner injuries, it is important to ascertain if the injury is superficial or if there is a thrombosis of the deep dorsal artery. Superficial injuries (e.g., suction devices, electric brooms) are treated by catheterization, antibiotics, and delayed debridement. Lack of a dorsal blood supply by Doppler studies suggests use of immediate revascularization procedure (bilateral superficial epigastric artery to corpora cavernosa anastomoses). Significant venous occlusion with resultant priapism can be treated with multiple corpora cavernosa to corpora spongiosa shunting by formal surgical windows or by the use of a biopsy needle inserted through the head of the penis into each corpus cavernosum.

Cases of thrombosis of the superficial veins of the penis are being recently seen owing to an increased use of constricting leather bands, rubber bands, and metal rings to prolong erection. These patients usually present in the progressing phase of the thrombosis and need rest, aspirin, or a regimen of heparin or warfarin therapy. At times, a very swollen penis will be seen with a brawny edema. A high index of suspicion and a few pointed questions will elicit a history of the use of a suction "penis enlarger" advertised in certain magazines. Stopping the use of the device will "cure" the edema. However, subsequent fibrosis of the corpora may occur.

In cases of penile self-mutilation (now seen less often with the availability of transsexual surgery), perineal urethrostomy, ligation of bleeding vessels, and psychiatric consultation are usually proper. Any reconstruction should be delayed until a later date. In penile transections or avulsions caused by machine injuries or knife wounds, the patient and the severed organ (wrapped in cold, sterile, saline-soaked dressings) should be brought to a facility having microsurgical equipment for possible reanastomosis, within 6 to 8 hours, before infection becomes significant. In gunshot wounds of the penis, microsurgical repair of the deep dorsal artery may be necessary although extensive injury precludes immediate arterial repair.

Remember:

1. Human bites must be vigorously debrided but should not be sutured.

2. In penile degloving injuries, it is mandatory to save all viable skin.

3. Penile fractures can be diagnosed by corpus cavernography using 10 ml of contrast material through a No. 19 gauge butterfly needle and treated by immediate suture of the fractured tunica albuginea with 2-0 chromic catgut sutures of Dexon.

4. Buttonhole pieces of foreskin or scrotum can be used as a good cover for large penile defect.

5. Superficial penile hematomas should be treated with bed rest, ice packs, urethral catheterization, and moderate wraparound gauze dressing.

BENIGN PROSTATIC HYPERPLASIA

method of
HUGH P. ROBINSON, M.D.
Portland, Maine

Treatment of prostatic hyperplasia preserves renal function and restores normal voiding. An effective plan requires assessment of symptoms, objective findings, and appreciation of the pathophysiology of urinary obstruction. Individual therapy is further modified by the patient's general health, expected survival, and particular concerns.

Definition

Benign prostatic hyperplasia, or enlargement of the prostate gland, is a natural phenomenon in the elderly male. Many patients have some degree of hypertrophy, but most will be asymptomatic with negative urine sediments, normal renal function, and stable urinary tracts as shown by intravenous pyelography. Nevertheless, many will require treatment for dysuria, frequency, stranguria, nocturia, and progressive decompensation of the bladder and upper tracts. Occasionally, complications such as acute urinary retention, suprapubic pain, and uncontrolled bleeding will precipitate urgent attention, but usually treatment is elective.

Pathophysiology

Prostatic hypertrophy and bladder neck obstruction develop from hyperplasia of glandular and fibromuscular tissue in the central luminal or periurethral area of the normal prostate, resulting in a "doughnut-shaped" adenoma which, by continued growth, compresses the normal prostatic tissue in an external shell called the surgical capsule. The fibroelastic capsule in turn resists peripheral expansion and compresses the internal urinary channel, making the "hole in the doughnut" smaller and increasing voiding resistance. There is some element of obstruction with all hypertrophy, and the ability of the bladder detrusor to compensate to the increased voiding restriction determines the clinical symptoms and secondary obstructive changes in the urinary tract. Initially, the bladder adapts by hypertrophy of individual detrusor muscle bundles, resulting in trabeculation and cellule formation, but later may decompensate with increasing residual urine, diverticula, infection, vesical calculi, and ultimately hydronephrosis and impaired renal function. These changes in the bladder as well as the size of the adenoma are important in the selection of the type of surgery, and also serve as a guide in anticipating early postoperative results. Marked detrusor irritability dictates avoidance of a transvesical incision and may require antispasmodics to control discomfort from bladder spasms and to reduce troublesome postoperative urgency incontinence. On the other hand, a large atonic bladder may require both preoperative and postoperative catheter drainage for detrusor recovery. The clinical enigma of a large prostatic hypertrophy, urgency incontinence with no residual urine, and the antithesis of no palpable prostatic enlargement yet overflow incontinence can be appreciated only with an awareness of the pathophysiology of obstruction.

Conservative Treatment Options

Moderate prostatic obstruction may be aggravated by infection, calculi, and distal urethral stricture. Correction of these complications may obviate specific treatment to the prostate. Digital rectal massage for recurrent prostatic congestion may give considerable symptomatic relief, but should be considered a temporary measure. Timed voiding and double voiding may reduce residual urine, but the general condition of the patient may dictate indefinite conservative management by urethral catheter diversion. In the ambulatory patient who is no longer sexually active, catheter drainage is well tolerated. Normal bathing, forced fluids to include 1000 ml of water daily, and careful observation of urethral irritation are routine. Cranberry juice is popular to acidify the urine and discourage encrustation of the catheter tip. Prophylactic suppressive low dose drug therapy with nitrofurantoin, 25 mg twice a day, or combination drug therapy with sulfamethoxazole, 400 mg, and trimethoprim, 80 mg, one-half tablet twice a day, is optional. Bedridden or nursing home patients require closer supervision, including frequent meatal hygiene to remove urethral secretions and fecal contamination. Small caliber catheters such as 14 to 16 F 5 ml Foley cause less urethral irritation and may be safely inflated to 15 ml to prevent displacement into the urethra. Catheters are carefully changed monthly to observe for encrustation and possible retained fragments of a ruptured retention bag. Demineralization of the bones by disuse may make encrustation and stone formation inevitable; this will require instillation in the bladder of half strength solution "G" (citrate solution) for dissolution of calculi. Sixty to 120 ml is instilled and the catheter is clamped, followed by vigorous irrigation with isotonic saline solution until returns are free of sediment. Periodic clamping of the catheter for "bladder training" is ill advised because of the hazard of pyelonephritis from reflux of infected urine. Patients should be warned of serious septic complications from long-term drainage, as well as increased risk of bladder cancer from chronic infection and irritation. Specific antibiotic therapy is used only with complications such as periurethral abscess or epididymitis. If a trial of voiding without a catheter is contemplated, appropriate urine cultures should be obtained and indicated antibiotic therapy begun 24 hours prior to catheter removal. A determination to replace the catheter should be made within 4 to 6 hours, and should not await obvious retention with the associated high incidence of bacteremia.

Surgical Options

In spite of encouraging progress in the investigative treatment of prostatic obstruction by hormonal or chemical manipulation, surgical removal of the obstructing adenoma remains the method of choice. The surgical approach can be either endoscopic resection through the urethra or enucleation through an incision in the lower abdominal wall or through the perineum. Each has its advantages and limitations; each is considered with regard to the pathophysiology of obstruction.

Suprapubic Prostatectomy. The transvesical approach allows easy access to the bladder neck and prostate for removal of moderate or large adenomas — particularly the intravesical type — and for the coincidental treatment of bladder calculi, diverticula, and large atonic bladders. Hemostasis is secured with stick ties of the major prostatic vessels in the posterior quadrants of the vesical neck and supplemented with light traction on the Foley bag balloon. Secondary bladder neck contracture can be avoided by suture of mucosa in the midpoint of the trigone into the depth of the prostatic fossa. The bladder neck may be further revised by the interposition of an anterior bladder flap. Direct visualization of the trigone also assures protection of the ureteral orifices from inadvertent suture obstruction. Suprapubic prostatectomy remains the most adaptable procedure and is ideally suited for removal of huge adenomas when blood loss might be excessive. Immediate placement of a hemostatic bag avoids procrastination and frustrating delay in securing active bleeding points in an obscured fossa. Also, the routine use of the suprapubic catheter is advantageous if prolonged drainage is expected for recovery of the detrusor. Early removal of the urethral catheter may prevent strictures and disappointing recurrence of obstructive symptoms.

Intermittent trials at voiding are facilitated by clamping with periodic release of the suprapubic tube for evaluation of residual urine. The major intraoperative limitation of the procedure is the inability to remove an unsuspected infiltrating carcinoma or fibrous contracture. Postoperative bladder spasms may be increased, particularly if there is marked detrusor irritability. Occasionally, opening the prevesical space may result in abscess formation with delayed healing of the suprapubic fistula and pelvic phlebitis with increased risk of pulmonary embolism.

Retropubic Prostatectomy. The transcapsular approach allows direct vision of the prostatic fossa, precise ligature of bleeding points, and, with modification, optional extension of the incision into the vesical neck for limited exposure of the bladder cavity. There is no need for a secondary suprapubic catheter, less detrusor irritation, prompt healing, and earlier voiding. Exposure may be compromised in the obese patient, and extreme caution must be used to avoid laceration of periprostatic veins. Small or fibrous adenomas can be removed advantageously by sharp dissection. The procedure is particularly suited for large intraurethral adenomas. A rare complication of pubic pain from osteitis pubis is self-limited and may be due to the necessary use of retractors for exposure.

Perineal Prostatectomy. The perineal approach is seldom used for benign adenomas, although it has a decided advantage of fewer pulmonary complications, dependent tissue drainage, rapid wound healing, and the option of precise biopsy of suspicious prostatic nodules. Limitations include intraoperative ventilatory problems and distressing postoperative low back pain associated with the exaggerated lithotomy position. If bleeding requires replacement of the catheter, there is some hazard, with improper instrumentation, of disruption of the posterior capsular repair and injury to the rectum. Finally, a competent internal sphincter or vesical neck may compensate for an undetected injury to the external sphincter, with normal urinary control preserved. Accidental injury to the rectum must be promptly recognized and repaired to avoid a rectourethral fistula.

Transurethral Resection (TUR). Improved fiberoptic illumination with the electrotome and Thompson resectoscope has extended the premier position of transurethral resection. With low morbidity, low mortality, accurate hemostasis with pinpoint fulguration, and short hospital stay, TUR gives results comparable to those of any other approach. In the absence of a painful surgical incision, there is less ileus, less respiratory depression from narcotics, early ambulation with rapid return to independent self care, and patient optimism for early recovery. Mortality is reduced primarily by the avoidance of surgical trauma to the deep pelvic veins and possibly delayed pulmonary embolism. A decided advantage is the rapidity with which the procedure can be modified or terminated in the event of intraoperative complications. Although complete resection of all adenomatous tissue is the optimal goal, circumstances may dictate compromise, but an incomplete resection leaves the patient with reasonable options. The incompletely resected patient may be returned to the operating room for a planned secondary resection which carries no increased risk, or he may be given a trial at voiding, and if this is successful, surgery can be indefinitely postponed. Careful attention to urethral calibration with appropriate internal urethrotomy and avoidance of unnecessary resection of the vesical neck can minimize postoperative anterior urethral stricture and vesical neck contracture.

Specific Patient Concerns

Specific patient concerns often delay proper treatment and deserve special consideration. The four most common fears concern cancer, loss of sexual potency, loss of bladder control, and the misunderstanding that transurethral resection removes only a portion of the adenoma whereas an open surgical incision removes the entire prostate. Routine pathologic examination of the resected tissue may fail to identify carcinoma in the peripheral or capsular portion, and areas of induration may require biopsy either before or during definitive surgery. The ability to have satisfactory sexual intercourse should not be altered, but retrograde ejaculation of seminal fluid into the bladder is common. Some degree of urgency and stress incontinence can be anticipated during early recovery, but this is seldom permanent. Finally, all surgical procedures for removal of prostatic adenomas are designed to be complete, but some regrowth can be expected following any procedure, particularly in younger patients.

Patient Selection for Treatment

Almost any patient suffering from prostatism, who has a reasonable life expectancy and whose associated infirmities are under good medical control, can be considered for surgery. Initial evaluation excludes illness or treatment which aggravates mild or subclinical prostatic obstruction, such as congestive failure, patient noncompliance with diuretic treatment schedules, anticholinergic drugs used as antispasmodics or cold remedies, cerebral vascular accidents, diabetic neuropathy, and specific central nervous system disease. The voiding history of hesitancy, frequency, stranguria, nocturia, and terminal dribbling is obtained with special evaluation of incontinence from urgency or overflow. Urologic examination includes palpation of vesical distention and prostatic enlargement, with attention to suspicious areas of induration or nodularity suggesting chronic prostatitis or malignancy. Urinalysis is obtained to exclude glycosuria, infection, or hematuria. Finally, personal observation of the voided stream confirms the clinical diagnosis. If initial findings are significant, further preoperative studies, including renal function, excretory urography, urine cultures, and general medical consultation, are obtained. Vesical detrusor instability with urgency incontinence deserves cystometric and neurologic evaluation. The findings are reviewed with the patient and his spouse or family. Indication for surgery may be conveniently classified into urgent, optional, and deferrable. Findings of upper tract dilatation with secondary impaired renal function, calculi with uncontrolled infection, massive residual urine, or large diverticula are all urgent indications for treatment, whereas modest retention, trabeculation, stable upper tracts, and negative urine sediment are optional indications for surgery primarily for relief of symptoms. Most patients even with large adenomas void normally and will not need treatment, but should be re-evaluated periodically.

Preparation for Surgery

With increasing recognition by the public of early prostatic obstructive symptoms, most patients present with moderate and uncomplicated prostatism and are best treated by transurethral resection. However, unusually large adenomas or those with associated calculi, diverticula, or huge atonic bladders may require open surgery. Occasionally, severe limitation of hip mobility by osteoarthritis may preclude TUR. Acute urinary retention precipitates immediate treatment by catheter drainage. The bladder is drained rapidly, and the volume of urine measured. Retention greater than 1000 ml requires investigation for chronic detrusor decompensation, and the patient is continued on constant drainage. A cystogram is obtained to exclude large diverticula, and initial cystometrograms are performed to predict detrusor recovery. A few days' drainage may produce marked improvement with decreasing capacity and improved urge to void. Drainage also reduces prostatic congestion and lessens intraoperative blood loss. Cystoscopy is deferred until operation to avoid infection or retention,

and pyelograms are obtained before the day of surgery to prevent dehydration, disturbed preoperative sleep, and rectal discomfort. Spinal anesthesia is preferable, as it allows prompt recognition of intraoperative complications and reduces postoperative discomfort and restlessness, but general anesthesia is equally acceptable, and the decision is made by the patient in consultation with the anesthesiologist. Type and screening is routine, but in cases in which blood loss greater than 500 ml is possible, cross-matched blood should be available. Electrolytes are obtained on patients with severe retention, or who are on diuretic therapy. Preoperative hydration by intravenous fluids is given to ensure diuresis during surgery.

Complications

Most complications are avoided by simple preparation. Indeed, the risk of complication should determine the choice of operative technique. Patients at risk of septic reactions, such as those with significant preoperative infection, bladder calculi, long-term catheter drainage, or valvular heart disease, are treated prophylactically with antibiotics such as cephalothin, 2 grams intravenously, and gentamicin, 80 mg intramuscularly. Intravenous fluids are continued liberally to ensure diuresis, prevent postoperative oliguria, and lower nephron nephrosis.

With spinal anesthesia, time is allowed for stabilization of the vascular system. If there is limitation of hip mobility, the patient is personally, by the surgeon, placed in the lithotomy position with care taken to prevent excessive abduction of the legs. Those at risk of thrombophlebitis require special padding and tensor bandages in severe cases. The bladder is drained, a culture obtained to aid in treatment of possible postoperative infection, and a final rectal examination of the prostate performed under anesthesia, as preoperative findings are occasionally misleading as to size or consistency. Suspicious areas of induration indicative of malignancy are identified, and a biopsy with the Hutchins modification of the Silverman needle is obtained through the perineum, or tissue is recovered by deep capsular biopsy at the conclusion of the procedure. Selection of specific prostatic chips for examination by the pathologist avoids embarrassment of delayed revision of the postoperative diagnosis. Calibration is done to identify and treat pre-existing strictures by urethrotomy. Cystoscopy confirms clinical findings and excludes unsuspected bladder pathology such as neoplasm and interstitial cystitis. A nonhemolytic irrigating solution such as aminoacetic acid (glycine 1.5 per cent) is used to prevent intravascular hemolysis; nevertheless, undetected intravascular infusion can occur through the periprostatic venous plexus. Nausea, vomiting, disorientation, and hypertension may indicate fluid overload, which is promptly treated by rapid conclusion of the procedure, a diuretic such as furosemide, 40 to 80 mg intravenously, concentrated 3 to 5 per cent saline infusion, electrolytes and serum hemoglobin determination, and antihypertensive medication in extreme instances. Response to treatment may be followed by a sudden fall in blood pressure, and cross-matched blood should be available.

Occasionally, operative blood loss may become alarming, particularly from large capsular veins, and if not easily controlled by fulguration and traction on the inflated standard 24 F 75 ml Foley bag catheter, immediate cystotomy for control of bleeding points is necessary. Fulguration, suture ligation, or packing may be unsatisfactory, with continued bleeding from the prostatic fossa. Such seeming disasters respond promptly to the use of a specially designed hemostatic device called the Brake bag. This extra large balloon, which unfortunately has been all but forgotten in urologic artifacts, is threaded over a 20 F 30 ml Foley catheter in the bladder, inflated with 200 ml, and pulled against the bladder neck and pelvic diaphragm with immediate hemostasis. The suprapubic wound is only partially closed, allowing urine to drain into the dressing. No routine irrigation is done, and the bladder remains undistended at rest. Within 24 hours the balloon is deflated and removed through the cystotomy incision under sterile conditions at the bedside, the wound closed with previously placed sutures, and drainage continued through the urethral catheter. Wound healing is prompt and convalescence normal.

Another complication is perforation of the bladder signaled by abdominal rigidity, diaphragmatic or shoulder pain, reduced irrigating returns, and hypotension. Extravasation requires immediate cystogram for evaluation and appropriate drainage.

Immediate Postoperative Complications. Recognition of many operative complications may be delayed until the immediate postoperative recovery period. With stable blood pressure and normal electrolytes, the routine use of intravenous diuretic such as a single dose of furosemide, 20 mg intravenously, assures continued diuresis. The use of traction on the Foley catheter to discourage venous bleeding results in moderate bladder discomfort, spasms, and rectal tenesmus with occasional uncontrolled desire to defecate,

and must be promptly relieved by the judicious use of intravenous narcotics and tranquilizers such as meperidine, 25 mg, and diazepam, 2.5 mg, with careful attention to blood pressure. If the patient continues to strain, there will be overwhelming bleeding from the prostatic fossa by increased venous pressure. Initial hemostasis from accurate fulguration of bleeding points is re-enforced by a generalized spasm of the prostatic capsule, but early returns of clear irrigating fluid may rapidly change to bleeding and clot retention with relaxation of the prostate. Continued periodic irrigation in spite of clear returns is essential to identify this change of events. Finally, the proper position of the inflated bag of the Foley catheter, whether in the prostatic fossa or in the bladder cavity resting on the vesical neck, may be unnecessarily controversial. In general, if the catheter becomes occluded by clot and requires replacement, the optimal position is intravesical. A 24 F 75 ml bag catheter is passed into the bladder cavity, inflated with as much as 150 ml, and then withdrawn against the bladder neck with light traction.

Early Postoperative Complications. The most serious and fortunately the most infrequent complications are coronary occlusion and pulmonary embolus. Cardiac patients who are stable for 6 months preoperatively return to normal risk, but transient hypotensive episodes call for careful review of silent infarct. Prophylactic use of anticoagulants for those at risk for embolus must be carefully weighed against the inevitable increased blood loss attendant with its use. In general, anticoagulant therapy should be discontinued or avoided for 1 month unless there is an acute embolus. Coronary occlusion may occur during hospitalization, but embolus usually occurs after discharge.

Less serious complications include continued bleeding and must be evaluated by personal irrigation of the catheter and estimated blood loss. Oliguria is excluded by careful measurement of the first hour's output the day after surgery; also, a hemoglobin, hematocrit, and blood urea nitrogen (BUN) are obtained. Early fever may indicate undetected extravasation, and a broad-spectrum antibiotic such as ampicillin, 250 mg orally four times a day, is given empirically in spite of a negative operative culture. Bladder discomfort is lessened with release of the traction, partial deflation of the Foley bag, and antispasmodics such as propantheline, 15 mg orally every 4 hours. The patient is discouraged from moving his bowels the first day, as straining may cause delayed bleeding. However, a mild laxative such as milk of magnesia, 30 ml, is given daily thereafter. A light diet is given the first day to avoid ileus, liberal fluids are encouraged, and the patient is ambulated. The genitalia are examined daily for urethritis, which is treated with replacement of the catheter by one of smaller size and local hygiene. Epididymitis is rare and most likely associated with preoperative infection. Routine vasectomy is not done, as morbidity appears to outweigh its advantages. The catheter is removed when the urine is clear, and the patient observed for bleeding or retention. Some stress and urgency incontinence can be expected for 24 to 48 hours and should not be treated with condom or sheath drainage. Continued forced fluids and hot sitz baths encourage resolution. Persistent retention or unsatisfactory voiding does not require immediate cystoscopy, but usually responds to continued drainage on an outpatient basis. On discharge the patient and his spouse are instructed on limitation of physical activity, sexual abstinence, and continued liberal fluid intake. The patient is provided with low dose suppressive chemotherapy such as nitrofurantoin or sulfamethoxazole and trimethoprim. Delayed bleeding, which can occur within 2 weeks, is usually precipitated by strenuous activity and responds to complete bed rest and forced fluids to 3000 ml daily. Any feeling of bladder fullness or incomplete emptying requires catheterization for removal of clots. Return to surgery is seldom necessary.

Late Complications. Initial office recheck is done at 1 month. The patient's voided stream is observed, and the sediment examined. Sterile pyuria may persist for 3 months during normal healing and requires no further antibiotic therapy. If bacilluria or urethral discomfort persists, suppressive therapy is continued or changed. Rectal examination of the prostate is deferred, as this may precipitate bleeding or epididymitis. Persistent infection can also indicate incomplete resection or retained prostatic chips, and recurrent obstructive symptoms may occur with stricture in the anterior urethra or at the bladder neck. Those at risk of stricture should be identified preoperatively by calibration of subclinical stricture, or by cystoscopy, to identify unusual prostatic configuration which predisposes to postoperative contracture of the vesical neck. Most respond to early dilatation, and few will require operative repair. The patient returns for a final check at 3 months. Digital examination of the prostate is done, normal voiding assured, and the patient discharged to his referring physician, with encouragement to obtain periodic examination of the prostatic remnant at 6 month intervals to exclude latent carcinoma.

PROSTATITIS

method of
LESTER A. KLEIN, M.D.
Boston, Massachusetts

Prostatitis — inflammation of the prostate — causes urinary frequency, dysuria, stranguria, reduced force of stream, and urgency sometimes associated with incontinence. Urethritis and cystitis cause similar symptoms and may coexist with prostatitis. Both factors make it difficult to determine which problem or problems the patient has. Table 1 lists the major symptoms and their occurrence in these three diseases and is included to help the reader make the correct diagnosis.

Prostatitis takes one of three forms: acute bacterial, chronic bacterial, and nonbacterial. Acute prostatitis is often a fulminating disorder. It is essentially cellulitis of the prostate, and thus manipulation of the tissue is to be avoided. Thus vigorous or frequent rectal examinations and especially prostate massage are contraindicated. If bladder drainage is required, a suprapubic tube is preferred over a urethral (Foley) catheter. Treatment includes bed rest, hydration, and antibiotics. Initial drug therapy is gentamicin or tobramycin, 3 to 5 mg per kg per day intramuscularly, plus ampicillin, 2 grams intravenously per day, all in divided doses. When the results of culture and sensitivity testing are available, treatment should be altered accordingly. After a week, treatment may be converted to an oral preparation and should be continued for at least a month. Chronic bacterial prostatitis produces the same symptoms as acute prostatitis, but the patient has fewer systemic signs (fever, leukocytosis); the condition is characterized by relapsing urinary tract infection with the same pathogen. Trimethoprim-sulfamethoxazole, 1 regular strength

TABLE 1.

	PROSTATITIS	URETHRITIS	CYSTITIS
Frequency	++	0	++++
Urgency	++	0	++++
Dysuria	++	+++	+
Discharge	0	+++	0
Hematuria	0	0	+++
Bacteruria			
First glass	0	+++	+
Third glass	+++	0	+
Total	±	±	+
Tender prostate	±	0	0

In using Table 1, you must remember the lesions often coexist!

tablet twice a day, or nitrofurantoin, 100 mg by mouth three times per day, is used during exacerbations, and the same drugs, once per day, may be used for long-term suppression. Treatment should continue for 1 to 4 months in order to achieve cure rates approaching 40 to 70 per cent. Patients who fail to respond within that time may be helped by longer treatment, but other causes should be sought. Prostatic calculi may cause irremediable chronic prostatitis, and their removal by operation may be required before cure can be effected. Occasionally, the resistant problem is solved by total prostatectomy. Unfortunately, partial prostatectomy (e.g., transurethral resection [TUR]) may exacerbate the problem.

Nonbacterial prostatitis is the most common form of the disease seen today, but because the cause is obscure the treatment remains unsatisfactory. Ureaplasma (T-mycoplasma) and chlamydia have been suggested as causative agents (the latter clearly is a cause of nonspecific urethritis), although the evidence supporting their role is debatable. Tetracycline or erythromycin, 500 mg four times per day for prolonged periods, may be helpful. Often the symptoms will resolve during this time of treatment (? spontaneously), but if they do not, further treatment should be symptomatic. Such measures as hot sitz baths, alteration of sexual activity, and aspirin may be helpful. Clearly not helpful is prostatic massage or dietary restriction.

Most men with symptomatic benign prostatic hypertrophy have prostatitis and are helped by treating that component of the problem; the rest must be considered for prostatectomy.

Urethritis may be bacterial or nonspecific. Gonococcal urethritis should be treated with procaine penicillin G, 4.8 million units intramuscularly on the first visit, along with 1.0 gram of probenecid orally. If the patient is allergic to penicillin, use spectinomycin, 2.0 grams as a single dose intramuscularly, or tetracycline, 30 mg per kg per day for 4 days. A repeat culture should be made in 1 week. Nonspecific urethritis probably runs a course unrelated to treatment, but most authorities suggest using tetracycline or erythromycin, 500 mg orally four times per day for 1, 2, or 4 weeks. Usually, within that time period the patient will improve; if not, antibiotics may be continued up to 3 months. Recurrences are common.

Finally, a word about cystitis. The diagnosis of pure cystitis in the male should be made with extreme caution and then only rarely. It is usually associated with prostatitis, but if the latter is lacking, the diagnosis is more likely bladder cancer. Urine cytology and cystoscopy are required in all cases diagnosed as pure cystitis in the male.

ACUTE RENAL FAILURE

method of
CHRISTOPHER R. BLAGG, M.D.
Seattle, Washington

Acute renal failure (ARF) is an abrupt, frequently reversible reduction in renal glomerular and tubular function associated with biochemical changes and acute uremia. Acute tubular necrosis (ATN) is a pathologic diagnosis, often used synonymously with ARF, confirmed on renal biopsy by finding appropriate anatomic renal tubular changes, and most commonly associated with either administration of a nephrotoxin or the occurrence of prolonged renal ischemia. Patients with ARF usually become clinically and biochemically uremic within a few days of the renal insult, developing acidosis, anemia, hyperphosphatemia, and hyperkalemia. The rate of development of uremia is dependent on the rate of protein catabolism, and is more rapid in patients developing ARF following trauma or surgery.

Early management of ARF requires establishment of the diagnosis. Urinary tract obstruction of the urethra, bladder, or ureters — *postrenal failure* — may produce a clinical picture resembling ARF. Anuria (< 50 ml urine output in 24 hours) or alternating polyuria and oliguria are suggestive of obstruction.

Reduced renal perfusion from any cause can result in an appreciable elevation of the blood urea nitrogen (BUN) concentration, but with a less marked increase in the serum creatinine level to 2 to 4 mg per dl (100 ml) — *prerenal azotemia*. Unless appropriate measures are taken, this frequently proceeds to development of ARF.

The usual first sign of ARF is a decrease in volume of urine output. Anuria (urine output < 50 ml per day) is not common with ARF, and suggests the possibility of postrenal failure, vascular obstruction, acute cortical necrosis, or acute glomerulonephritis. More commonly, ARF presents with oliguria (urine output 50 to 400 ml per day), with a "normal" urine volume, or with polyuria (urine output > 2.5 liters per day) — so-called *nonoliguric ARF*. Polyuria is more frequent following exposure to a nephrotoxin (especially aminoglycoside antibiotics), while oliguria is more frequent after prolonged hypotension, after traumatic rhabdomyolysis, and with some other nephrotoxins.

Etiology of Acute Renal Failure

In 50 to 60 per cent of patients, ARF follows surgery or an episode of severe trauma. Cardiac and aortic surgery and surgery of large vessels and of the biliary tract are particularly common causes of postsurgical ARF. These patients have a high mortality, on the order of 50 per cent.

Other patients develop ARF subsequent to receiving radiographic contrast media, antibiotics, or other nephrotoxic agents, and have a much better prognosis, with a survival rate of about 85 per cent. ARF following radiographic procedures is particularly common in patients who have had multiple injections of contrast media over a short period of time. This has become much more frequent as a cause of ARF over the last 10 years, presumably because of increased use of radiographic tests. Characteristically, patients at greatest risk of ARF from radiographic contrast media are those with multiple myeloma or diabetes, although the aged, patients with hypertension, and others are also subject to this risk. The incidence of ARF after receiving contrast media probably is greater than realized, because many patients may develop transient, nonoliguric ARF which may recover with or without recognition. The overall incidence of ARF induced by contrast media in high risk patients may be as great as 5 to 10 per cent. All iodinated contrast compounds are potentially dangerous, including those used for oral cholecystography, and the nephrotoxic effect can be additive. Consequently, it may be preferable to delay repeated studies, particularly in high risk patients. Prevention depends on prior identification of patients at risk, avoidance of contrast studies when ultrasound or radioisotopes can give the same information, avoidance of frequent or multiple contrast studies, judicious use of dehydration before pyelography, and consideration as to whether a further contrast study can provide information sufficient to outweigh the potential morbidity or mortality associated with ARF (Carvallo et al.: Am. J. Med. 65:38, 1978).

The last 10 years have also seen development of new aminoglycoside antibiotics which are potential nephrotoxins. As a result, antibiotic-induced ARF is now a frequent cause of ARF. Nephrotoxicity can result from inappropriate or overprolonged administration of such an antibiotic; failure to follow blood levels and to monitor renal function closely during treatment; combination of an aminoglycoside with another potentially nephrotoxic drug such as another aminoglycoside, a cephalosporin, or, perhaps, some diuretics; lack of knowledge of the effects of such agents; and lack of recognition of potential risk factors such as age, pre-existing renal disease, recent surgery, sepsis, and trauma.

The most widely used aminoglycoside antibiotics are gentamicin, tobramycin, amikacin, kanamycin, and streptomycin. Oliguria is less frequent and may be less marked in ARF caused by aminoglycosides, and often develops 1 to 2 weeks after initial therapy. Consequently, ARF may occur after treatment is discontinued, perhaps as a result of slow release of antibiotic from tissue sites. At least in rats, tobramycin appears to be less nephrotoxic than an equivalent dose of gentamicin. Cephalosporins can potentiate aminoglycoside nephrotoxicity and may be potentially nephrotoxic themselves; thus, a combination of cephalosporin and aminoglycoside is more nephrotoxic than a combination of methicillin and aminoglycoside. Furosemide may potentiate the nephrotoxicity of aminoglycosides and of aminoglycosides plus cephalosporins. Other nephrotoxic drugs include methotrexate and cis-dichloroammineplatinum used in cancer chemotherapy; the latter is nephrotoxic because of its heavy metal content. Again, use of these compounds in combination with other nephrotoxic drugs such as aminoglycosides is likely to increase the incidence of ARF.

Other common causes of ARF include sepsis, pancreatitis, mismatched blood transfusion, and obstetrical problems such as septic abortion, and accidental hemorrhage.

Complications of ARF (McMurray et al.: Arch. Intern. Med. 138:950, 1978)

Complications, which occur in 90 per cent of patients, are the usual cause of death in patients with ARF, because uremia itself can be well controlled with dialysis. Among frequent complications of ARF are infection, cardiovascular problems such as arrhythmias and pulmonary edema, gastrointestinal bleeding, disseminated intravascular coagulation, wound dehiscence, and metabolic encephalopathy.

Infection occurs in the majority of patients, more frequently in postsurgical and post-traumatic ARF, and accounts for approximately half the deaths. Almost all postsurgical patients become infected, frequently with peritonitis, and usually with the common pathogens. Opportunistic organisms tend to be infrequent, except in patients receiving immunosuppressive or prolonged broad-spectrum antibiotic therapy. The physical signs of infection are similar to those in patients without ARF, including fever, leukocytosis, abdominal pain, and guarding. Since uremia frequently is associated with a falling basal body temperature, occurrence of fever in a patient with ARF must be viewed with suspicion.

Mortality in Acute Renal Failure

Death in ARF is usually due to the underlying cause of the ARF or its complications, rather than uremia. Apart from infection, death is most commonly associated with arrhythmias, pulmonary edema, or acute myocardial infarction. In postsurgical and post-traumatic ARF the mortality is 50 per cent or more, the most common causes including pulmonary insufficiency, wound dehiscence, systemic sepsis, or gastrointestinal bleeding. The mortality in postobstetric and nephrotoxin-induced ARF is 15 per cent or less.

Because common causes of death include hyperkalemia, intravascular fluid overload, and sepsis, the aim of treatment in ARF is to minimize these complications by dialysis and other measures, while paying attention to other complicating surgical and medical problems.

Diagnosis of Acute Renal Failure

Diagnostic measures should be instituted as soon as the possibility of ARF is considered, with the aim of excluding treatable causes of oliguria such as postrenal obstruction and prerenal azotemia. Such measures include the following:

Exclude Urinary Tract Obstruction. Lower urinary tract obstruction may be obvious from the history and, on physical examination, by finding a distended bladder, but other causes of obstruction, such as bilateral urinary calculi, retroperitoneal fibrosis or tumor, and papillary necrosis with obstructed ureters, may be difficult to detect without further investigation. Whenever the possibility of obstruction exists, urologic consultation should be obtained to confirm or exclude this diagnosis, as early relief of obstruction is necessary. Investigations include (1) measurement of renal size and check for presence or absence of hydronephrosis by sonography, (2) unilateral ureteral catheterization if obstruction above the bladder is suspected, and (3) measurement of residual urine by bladder catheterization in elderly males.

Exclude Prerenal Azotemia. Shock, hypotension, and extracellular volume depletion associated with hemorrhage, burns, or other severe fluid losses may reduce renal perfusion, thus depressing urinary output. Consequently, the diagnosis of ARF should not be made until normal blood pressure and extracellular fluid volume are restored. Some characteristics of prerenal azotemia and ARF are contrasted in Table 1 (Miller et al.: Ann. Intern. Med. 89:47, 1978). Nevertheless, whether or not the results of such tests are available, the first step is to treat shock, if present,

and to check the effect of volume expansion. Provided that the patient does not have obvious volume overload, the possibility of reduced effective plasma volume should be evaluated by the following means:

1. Infusion of appropriate fluid (blood, plasma, or 0.9 per cent saline solution) to treat shock and to restore volume while observing urine output, neck vein filling, and blood pressure. In critically ill patients a Swan-Ganz catheter should be placed to evaluate and monitor volume status. If infusion is well tolerated, resulting in increased urine flow > 50 ml per hour, vigorous fluid replacement should be maintained, as the patient has prerenal azotemia rather than ARF.

2. If there is no response to volume restoration, a bolus of 25 grams of mannitol together with 80 mg of furosemide should be given intravenously. These diuretics will restore urine output to > 50 ml per hour in many oliguric patients who do not yet have ARF. Should urine output improve, additional doses of these diuretics can be given, together with continuing volume restoration with saline or other appropriate fluid in order to maintain urine output.

3. If there is no response after 1 hour, a further bolus of 25 grams of mannitol and 500 mg of furosemide should be given, together with an infusion of dopamine at a rate of 1 to 2 micrograms per kg of body weight per minute. Again, a response in terms of increased urine output is a sign to continue fluid replacement, diuretics, and possibly dopamine infusion. Failure of response indicates ARF. Use of these measures may prevent progression of prerenal azotemia to ARF, or may result in development of nonoliguric ARF rather than oliguric ARF.

Identify Any Specific Disease Causing ARF. 1. History and physical examination may suggest acute glomerulonephritis, renal artery obstruction, or other renal parenchymal disease.

2. If renal artery obstruction is suspected, especially in association with abdominal aneurysm, immediate surgical relief is necessary.

3. Give tests for antiglomerular basement membrane antibody (Goodpasture's syndrome and rapidly progressive glomerulonephritis).

4. Give serologic tests for systemic lupus erythematosus.

5. Consider percutaneous renal biopsy, pro-

TABLE 1. **Differential Characteristics of Prerenal Azotemia and ARF**

	PRERENAL AZOTEMIA	ARF
Urine osmolality	>500 mosm/Kg H_2O	<350 mosm/Kg H_2O
BUN: creatinine concentrations	>10:1	10:1
Urine Na concentration	<20 mEq/liter	>40 mEq/liter
Fractional excretion of filtered sodium	<1	<1

vided that the patient has two normal-sized kidneys and an intact coagulation mechanism.

Immediate Therapy

The most important requirement on first seeing a patient with ARF is to decide whether a medical emergency exists. In the comatose, uremic patient, prompt dialysis is essential. Equally dangerous, and usually not apparent on physical examination, is the presence of severe hyperkalemia.

The following should be considered when first seeing a patient with ARF:

Hyperkalemia and Its Treatment. No elevated serum potassium level is safe in the patient with ARF, as the myocardial effects of hyperkalemia are potentiated by hyponatremia and acidosis. If the serum potassium level exceeds 5.5 mEq per liter in an oliguric patient, especially a catabolic patient with traumatic or postsurgical ARF, potentially fatal cardiac arrhythmias may develop without warning. Consequently, an electrocardiogram (ECG) should be taken and an immediate serum potassium level should be estimated. Monitoring of existing hyperkalemia is best done by continuous or frequent ECGs, comparing the lead showing the greatest abnormality, usually precordial lead V_3 or V_4. In usual order of appearance, the common ECG signs of hyperkalemia are (1) symmetrical, peaked or "tented" T waves greater than 6 mm in height; (2) flattening and disappearance of the P wave; (3) prolongation of the PR interval; (4) widening of the QRS complex; and (5) fusion of the QRS complex and T wave to form a sine wave; this heralds imminent cardiac arrest. With appropriate therapy all these changes are reversible in minutes.

In a patient with ARF, the presence of hyperkalemia with ECG changes that do not respond promptly to conservative therapy is an indication for immediate dialysis. Peritoneal dialysis may usually be rapidly instituted, especially if facilities for hemodialysis are not available.

The following measures should also be taken:

1. If the serum potassium is greater than 6.5 mEq per liter and there are major ECG abnormalities (absent P waves, wide QRS complexes, or ventricular arrhythmias), 10 ml of 10 per cent calcium gluconate solution should be injected intravenously over 5 minutes, with continuous ECG monitoring. Calcium opposes the adverse effect of hyperkalemia on myocardial muscle, and can immediately revert the sine wave ECG of severe hyperkalemia to normal. Because this effect of calcium is transitory, it is essential to institute other measures to control the hyperkalemia (see below), and to make plans for early

dialysis, while continuing ECG monitoring and a rate of intravenous calcium infusion sufficient to maintain a reasonably normal ECG.

2. With a serum potassium level of greater than 6.5 mEq per liter, but without such marked ECG changes, rapid lowering of the serum potassium level still is essential. This may be accomplished within 15 to 30 minutes by intravenous infusion of 100 ml of 50 per cent glucose, with or without 25 units of regular insulin. Alternatively, 2 ampules (44 mEq per ampule) of sodium bicarbonate or 1 liter of isotonic sodium bicarbonate may be given intravenously to partially correct the acidosis. Both glucose and bicarbonate cause intracellular movement of potassium ions. Generally, glucose is preferable to bicarbonate, because the latter expands extracellular fluid volume, possibly inducing cardiac failure. The possibility of reactive hypoglycemia following intravenous infusion of glucose should be considered, particularly if insulin is given, the danger of this being greatest about 3 hours after insulin administration.

3. If the serum potassium level is between 5.5 and 6.5 mEq per liter, administration of sodium polystyrene sulfonate resin (Kayexalate) should be started, either orally or as a retention enema. Orally, the dose is 15 to 20 grams of resin, with 20 ml of 70 per cent sorbitol, three or four times daily. (Sorbitol increases the rate of passage of resin through the gastrointestinal tract.) For retention enema, 50 grams of resin is mixed with 50 ml of 70 per cent sorbitol and 100 ml tap water, administered, retained for 30 to 45 minutes, and then expelled. Resin results in reduction of the serum potassium level over several hours. The rectal route may be preferred because of the lesser risk of vomiting. Because the resin exchanges sodium for potassium ions in the gastrointestinal tract, repeated use of exchange resin may result in sodium overload.

4. Prepare for immediate dialysis.

Assessment of Cardiovascular Status. Cardiovascular complications of ARF include hypertension, pulmonary edema, arrhythmias, and pericarditis. It is unusual for a previously normal heart to develop congestive heart failure during ARF, and heart failure most often results from circulatory overload. Cardiac output usually is increased in response to anemia, even when pulmonary edema is not present. Hypoxemia in ARF may result from anemia, fluid overload, or pneumonia.

Dyspnea, hypoxemia, and volume overload in ARF are managed as follows:

1. Administer oxygen (4 liters per minute) by nasal catheter.

2. If the patient is hypertensive, reduce the

blood pressure to no more than 150/100 mm Hg by giving clonidine, 0.1 mg orally every 2 to 4 hours. In patients unable to take oral medication, use a sodium nitroprusside drip of 50 mg in 500 ml of 5 per cent dextrose in water (100 micrograms per ml) at a rate of 0.5 to 8.0 micrograms per kg of body weight per minute.

3. Transfusion of packed red cells should be considered for patients with post-traumatic and postsurgical ARF and for elderly patients whose hematocrit is below 30 per cent. Younger, otherwise healthy patients usually tolerate hematocrit levels as low as 15 per cent, and should not be transfused because of the risk of fluid overload.

4. Weigh the patient. Intake and output records should be maintained, but usually are inaccurate. Patients with ARF may receive large volumes of parenteral fluid in association with prescribed medications, and volume overload usually is iatrogenic. A constant or falling body weight is the only sure evidence that volume overload is being avoided. Fluid intake should be restricted to no more than 500 ml per day (50 per cent glucose and water), in addition to other measured fluid losses, preferably given orally.

5. If pulmonary edema is clearly attributable to overadministration of parental fluid, phlebotomy of 500 ml of blood should be considered if the hematocrit is 35 per cent or greater.

6. Digitalis should be used only in patients with cardiac failure caused by primary cardiac disease, generally the elderly and some diabetic patients. Digoxin, 0.25 mg every 6 hours to a total of 1 mg, should be prescribed, and continued at the appropriate maintenance dosage if clinical improvement is apparent. The hazardous effect of lowering the serum potassium level by dialysis in a digitalized patient must be remembered.

7. Distended neck veins and pulsus paradoxus should suggest the possibility of cardiac tamponade, and this should be checked by echocardiography. Should significant pericardial effusion be detected, a diagnostic (and therapeutic) pericardial tap should be performed. (Cardiac tamponade is uncommon in ARF and more frequent in patients with chronic renal failure.)

8. Hemodialysis with ultrafiltration, or peritoneal dialysis with hyperosmolar dialysate, will remove large volumes of fluid from the patient. Early dialysis also solves most of the uremic problems of ARF, and is the treatment of choice for severe fluid overload.

Treatment of Hemorrhage. Hemorrhage is associated with 35 per cent of deaths in patients with ARF, and should always be controlled by a combination of dialysis and surgery. Bleeding may occur as a complication of severe uremia, but this will cease within 24 hours of starting dialysis.

Treatment of hemorrhage must never be delayed because of the presence of ARF, as a combination of vigorous dialysis and urgent surgery has proved lifesaving both under battle conditions and with ARF in civilian life.

Management of Sepsis. Septicemia occurs in up to 30 per cent of patients with ARF. Pulmonary, wound, genitourinary, and peritoneal infections are common. Mortality is reduced by early and vigorous dialysis. Additional steps of value in the control and treatment of sepsis include the following:

1. Removal of a bladder catheter. There is no value in knowing the severity of oliguria in a patient with ARF, and there is substantial risk that an indwelling bladder catheter will result in infection.

2. Avoidance of parenteral fluids in a patient who can tolerate oral feeding.

3. Adjustment of antibiotic and other drug dosages to compensate for impaired renal excretion. Excellent guidelines for drug dosage in uremia are available (Bennett et al.: Ann. Intern. Med. 93:62, 286, 1980). Potentially nephrotoxic antibiotics should be discontinued if effective alternatives exist. Serum levels of all potentially toxic agents should be monitored.

Maintenance Therapy

Oliguria in ARF usually persists for 2 to 3 weeks, although protracted oliguria has been recorded for as long as 60 to 90 days. During the period of oliguria, treatment is directed to maintaining nutrition and to preventing complications.

Maintenance of Nutrition. Previously, when dialysis was not readily available, patients with ARF were treated with an unpalatable diet of fat, carbohydrate, and minimal water. Today, assuming that the cause of ARF does not involve the gastrointestinal tract, properly managed patients with ARF may be ambulatory, free of intravenous lines, and able to eat reasonably appetizing meals. Guidelines for nutrition include the following:

1. If the patient can eat, use as normal a diet as possible, including food containing protein of high biologic value. No specific limitations of protein or sodium intake are necessary if dialysis is available, and every effort should be made to provide protein and calories in an appetizing form.

2. Give fluids as desired to control thirst. Avoid citrus juices, which have a high potassium content.

3. Avoid magnesium-containing antacids, as uremic patients are already hypermagnesemic.

4. Bind phosphorus in the gut, using alu-

minum hydroxide gel (Amphojel), 30 ml with each meal.

5. Sodium bicarbonate may be given in the event of development of respiratory symptoms from severe acidosis, with a serum bicarbonate level of 13 mEq per liter or less. All ARF patients are acidotic because of retention of organic acids and reduced renal acid secretion. However, sodium bicarbonate is best avoided unless symptomatic acidosis develops, because of the risk of volume overload. Rather, development of severe acidosis is an indication for dialysis.

6. Give a multiple vitamin capsule twice daily, as deficiencies of water-soluble vitamins are common in patients with ARF and aggravated by dialysis.

7. Calcium supplementation usually is not needed, as severe hypocalcemia is unusual in ARF.

8. Provided that the patient can be fed orally, hyperalimentation is unnecessary. Parenteral administration of hypertonic glucose solution with a mixture of essential amino acids has been reported to decrease mortality and lessen catabolic rate and consequent rate of increase of blood urea nitrogen (BUN) and serum creatinine levels in patients with ARF, and should be considered in all patients unable to eat (Abel et al.: N. Engl. J. Med. *288*:695, 1973).

Prevention of Complications. Dialysis in ARF should be used to maintain the BUN level below 70 to 100 mg per dl and the serum creatinine level below 5 mg per dl. This has been shown to lower the mortality rate and to lessen the frequency of complications (Conger: J. Trauma *15*:1056, 1975). Hypercatabolic patients may require daily dialysis, whereas for less catabolic patients with ARF caused by nephrotoxins, less frequent dialysis may be sufficient.

The choice between hemodialysis and peritoneal dialysis for the individual patient requires nephrologic consultation. Both treatments are effective. Factors affecting this choice are shown in Table 2.

Neurologic, hematologic, gastroenterologic, and cardiovascular complications of ARF are all managed by dialysis, and most uremic complications are entirely preventable by frequent (daily if necessary) prophylactic dialysis. In the absence of extrarenal disease, a well-dialyzed patient with ARF may appear to be as well as a patient with chronic renal failure on maintenance dialysis.

To minimize iatrogenic complications, the effect of reduced renal function should be reviewed before prescribing any medication. Most antibiotics, analgesics, and digitalis preparations require reduced dosage because of impaired drug clearance in ARF.

Diuretic Phase

The diuretic or recovery phase follows the oliguric phase of ARF and is commonly marked by an increase in urine output of several hundred ml per day over several days. The magnitude of diuresis is largely determined by the quantity of excess fluid accumulated during the oliguric phase. The massive diureses reported in the past occurred in inadequately dialyzed, fluid-overloaded patients, and, too often, diuresis was sustained by inappropriate volume-for-volume repletion.

Death from electrolyte abnormalities or sepsis still may occur during the diuretic phase. Consequently, daily electrolyte estimation should be continued, and continuation of dialysis may be necessary, even in a patient voiding large volumes of urine. A patient recovering from ARF with a daily urine output of 2 to 4 liters may have a glomerular filtration rate of only 10 ml per minute.

Treatment in the diuretic phase consists of the following measures:

1. Fluid replacement equivalent to urine output up to 2 liters daily. For outputs exceeding 2 liters per day, replace with 2 liters plus two thirds of fluid losses over 2 liters.

2. Administration of sodium-containing fluids and foods to replace urinary losses. Conscious patients, able to feed by mouth, can be given a normal diet. Unconscious patients should be infused with 0.9 per cent saline and 5 per cent glucose solutions as required, based on electrolyte estimations, and hyperalimentation should be continued.

TABLE 2. **Factors Influencing Choices Between Hemodialysis and Peritoneal Dialysis in ARF**

	PERITONEAL DIALYSIS	HEMODIALYSIS
Delay in starting	None	May be hours
Usual urea clearance rate	20–35 ml/min	120–180 ml/min
Special indications	Peritonitis, severe CVS insufficiency	Extensive abdominal surgery, hypercatabolism
Common complications	Peritonitis, punctured viscus	Hypotension
Fluid removal	Slow, 1 liter q6h	Fast, 1 liter q1h
Stress to cardiovascular system	Mild	Mild to severe, depending on rate of fluid removal

3. Potassium replacement may be necessary, especially in patients receiving digitalis. In patients with a massive diuresis, measurement of serum potassium concentration offers guidance to the need for parenteral replacement by slow infusion. For patients with a mild to moderate diuresis, addition of fruit juice to the diet may be sufficient.

4. An otherwise free diet, as desired.

Acute-on-Chronic Renal Failure

Hypotension and volume depletion are particularly hazardous conditions for the elderly and for patients with nephrosclerosis, diabetes, or plasma cell dyscrasias, and radiographic procedures using contrast media should be limited to essential examinations in such patients. Treatment of acute-on-chronic renal failure is no different from that of ARF, except that recovery of renal function may be less marked or nonexistent.

Nonoliguric Acute Renal Failure (Anderson et al.: N. Engl. J. Med. *296*:1134, 1977)

As many as 30 per cent of patients with ARF do not develop oliguria and have nonoliguric ARF. Rhabdomyolysis, surgery, and burns are the most common causes of this condition. Characteristically, nonoliguric ARF results in a urine output of 1 to 2 liters daily, and as a result such patients have reduced dialysis requirements and a lower mortality. Diagnosis may be difficult because the usual criteria for identifying oliguric ARF (high urinary sodium concentration and urine/plasma osmolality approaching 1) may not occur. Rising serum creatinine and BUN levels in the absence of other causes of renal disease, particularly when following an appropriate insult, are presumptive evidence for a diagnosis of nonoliguric ARF. Management is identical to that of oliguric ARF, although severe acidosis, hyperkalemia, and fluid overload are infrequent because of continuing urine output. A 40 gram protein, 2 gram salt diet may be tolerated without need for dialysis. On occasion the distinction between prerenal azotemia and nonoliguric ARF may be blurred.

Post-Transplant Acute Renal Failure

Approximately 20 per cent of transplanted kidneys obtained from cadavers develop reversible ARF. Diagnosis of post-transplant ARF is complicated by the possibility of acute or hyperacute allograft rejection or transplant renal artery obstruction. Management of the post-transplant oliguric patient includes the following measures:

1. Obtain radionuclide studies of renal perfusion and function. If arterial flow is interrupted, surgical exploration is indicated.

2. If transplant perfusion is normal but function is reduced, monitor clinical status for systemic signs of allograft rejection (fever, lymphocyturia, tenderness over transplant). Rejection and ARF may be indistinguishable clinically.

3. Perform percutaneous transplant biopsy if the diagnosis remains in doubt.

4. Continue pretransplant treatment of renal failure by dialysis until graft function develops or nephrectomy is done. Early and repeated dialysis is appropriate.

5. Increased steroid dosage if rejection is suspected. More than 90 per cent of post-transplant kidneys with ARF will function, the mean oliguric interval being 5 days. Rejection occurring during oliguric ARF may be difficult to recognize, despite careful diagnostic studies. Management of the immediate post-transplant period necessitates a team approach by nephrologist, transplant surgeon, urologist, and radiologist.

Residual Renal Damage

Studies of patients following ARF have shown that glomerular filtration rate and renal plasma flow may remain somewhat impaired, as compared with matched control subjects, for as long as 1 year following recovery from oliguria.

CHRONIC RENAL FAILURE

method of
ELI A. FRIEDMAN, M.D.
Brooklyn, New York

A precise definition of chronic renal failure is lacking, although the term is understood to imply azotemia resulting from irreversible kidney disease. The clinical onset of chronic uremia may be abrupt, as in diffuse bilateral renal cortical necrosis associated with abruptio placentae, or gradual, over a decade, as in bilateral polycystic kidney disease. Formulation of a strategy for patients suffering chronic uremia requires establishing a renal diagnosis and recognition and treatment, when possible, of coincident systemic extrarenal disease which might limit rehabilitation, such as retinopathy in diabetes and cardiomyopathy in systemic sclerosis.

Management

Not every azotemic patient has intrinsic renal disease. Just as an initial step in the management of acute renal failure involves exclusion of prerenal and postrenal (obstructive) failure, the first concern in assessment of an azotemic patient is identification of remedial causes of renal failure. Dehydration and administration of potent diuretics, especially furosemide and ethacrynic acid, with inadequate fluid replacement can induce elevation of the blood urea nitrogen level. Any cause of reduction in effective plasma volume may reduce renal perfusion, leading to diminished excretion of urea and, to a lesser extent, creatinine. A volume-depleted patient generally has a high urine to plasma urea concentration ratio (> 4) and a low urinary sodium content (< 15 mEq per liter). If dehydration is suspected as the cause of azotemia, cautious fluid repletion with up to 2 liters of 0.45 per cent saline solution may be administered while monitoring venous pressure. Congestive heart failure, by reducing renal perfusion, can simulate uremia and should be treated by a combination of diuretics such as furosemide, 80 mg orally or intravenously twice daily (provided that the creatinine clearance exceeds 10 ml per minute), and digoxin in reduced dose because of lower renal excretion (0.125 mg orally daily) while periodically checking blood digoxin levels for toxicity. Distinction between salt and water overload in uremia and azotemia resulting from congestive heart failure may be difficult on physical examination, although the first few hours of therapy usually provide clarification.

Obstructive uropathy must be excluded in every uremic patient because its early discovery and correction is often rewarded by reversibility of renal insufficiency. While postrenal (obstructive) failure is an obvious diagnostic thought in an 80-year-old man with a recent history of difficulty in starting and ending micturition, prostatic hypertrophy in a 50-year-old man, or bilateral ureteral obstruction by cystine calculi in a 20-year-old woman, will be recognized only if an orderly approach to renal diagnosis is pursued. Unless the patient complains of frequency, urinary incontinence, or an inability to empty the bladder, or examination discloses a palpably distended bladder, urethral catheterization is unwarranted.

Quantitation of Renal Status

Once it is clear that irreversible renal failure is the correct diagnosis, the next step in management of the azotemic patient is to quantify the severity of renal malfunction. Calculation of the patient's endogenous creatinine clearance is a simple and noninvasive means of approximating the glomerular filtration rate. Creatinine is excreted in the urine in proportion to muscle mass (greater in men than women), and age (less in children and the elderly). At very high plasma concentrations (> 15 mg per dl [100 ml]) creatinine is excreted by the renal tubule, causing an overestimate (5 to 20 per cent) of true glomerular filtration rate as defined by inulin clearance. For clinical use, however, the creatinine clearance is reliable, reproducible to within 10 per cent, and relatively inexpensive. To perform a creatinine clearance a timed urine collection of from 6 to 24 hours is obtained and the plasma (serum) creatinine level is measured once during the collection period. Clearance is calculated using the formula

$$C_{ml/min} = \frac{U mg/dl \; V ml/min}{P mg/dl}$$

where C = creatinine clearance in ml per minute, U = urinary creatinine concentration, V = rate of urine flow which is calculated by dividing the total urine volume by the number of minutes in the collection interval (1440 minutes in a day), and P = the plasma (or serum) creatinine concentration. A satisfactory approximation of creatinine clearance can be predicted from the patient's serum creatinine concentration, age, and weight as follows (Dialysis and Transplantation 9:251, 1980):

$$C_{cr\,ml/min} = \frac{(140 - age) \; wt \; (kg)}{72 \times P_{cr} \; mg/dl}$$

Healthy adults younger than 40 years of age have a creatinine clearance of at least 100 ml per minute. Thereafter, each decade of aging reduces creatinine clearance by about 10 ml per minute; a 90-year-old woman with a creatinine clearance of 46 ml per minute thus has normal renal function.

As part of the initial renal assessment, the 24 hour urinary protein excretion should be determined if a screening (dipstick) test has detected more than + proteinuria. Subsequent urinary protein measurements may indicate response to therapy, as in allergic vasculitis, or multiple myeloma. A carefully collected urine specimen for bacterial culture should also be obtained, as persistent renal infection can accelerate loss of kidney function, especially in polycystic disease or diabetic nephropathy. The 24 hour excretion of sodium should be measured in patients with less than 20 ml per minute of creatinine clearance to provide a guide to dietary salt allocation (see diet below).

Initiation of Surveillance

Management of a diagnosed patient with progressive renal insufficiency is mainly a matter of preventive medicine until renal clearance falls below the level essential to continue active life (usually 5 to 10 ml per minute). There is good correlation between the creatinine clearance and the signs and symptoms of renal failure (Table 1). Outpatient "checkups" every 2 to 4 months are sufficient when the creatinine clearance is above 30 ml per minute. More frequent visits are required as the clearance falls; unstable patients with clearances < 10 ml per minute often need weekly adjustment of medication and diet.

Dietary Prescription

Before the ubiquitous availability of dialytic therapy, manipulation of the content of an unpalatable, severely protein restricted (< 20 grams) diet was the keystone of conservative care for advanced uremia. Neither protein nor salt restriction is necessary so long as the creatinine clearance is over 15 ml per minute. For clearances below 15 ml per minute, metabolic balance studies have shown that a 40 gram protein diet, about 0.5 gram per kg of body weight, when fed with sufficient calories (30 calories per kg of body weight) prevents negative nitrogen balance. Nephrotic patients will need an extra protein allotment to replace urinary losses, at about the rate of 6 grams per gram of urinary protein. If the creatinine clearance is below 3 ml per minute, muscle catabolism and nitrogen wasting are inevitable no matter what diet is consumed.

Dietary salt need not be curtailed until the creatinine clearance declines to 15 ml per minute or less. Daily weight measurements serve as an excellent guide to salt intake. The usual patient in advanced renal failure (creatinine clearance of 5 to 10 ml per minute) excretes 2 to 6 grams of salt daily. Several renal tubular disorders, such as medullary cystic disease and interstitial nephritis, may induce the loss (salt wasting) of 10 to 30 grams of urinary salt daily. By starting with a 4 gram salt prescription the patient's daily weights can be followed as a guide to increased salt content (for falling weight) or further restriction (if edema worsens). Hypoproteinemic uremic patients, particularly diabetics, may retain edema even on a 2 gram restricted salt diet. Diuresis with furosemide, 40 to 120 mg one to three times daily, or metolazone, 5 to 20 mg once or twice daily, is often effective so long as the creatinine clearance is at least 5 ml per minute. To counteract excessive salt loss while correcting acidosis, which is characteristic of renal failure, sodium bicarbonate tablets totaling 1.2 to 12 grams per day may be given in gradual daily increments, using the daily weight as a sign of under- or overcorrection.

Limitation of dietary potassium is, like protein and salt restriction, of increasing importance as the creatinine clearance falls below 15 ml per minute. Patients should be advised to avoid foods high in potassium content such as citrus fruits and potatoes. It is seldom necessary to include a potassium-depleting drug such as sodium polystyrene sulfonate (Kayexalate) resin in the regimen for chronic uremia. Should hyperkalemia develop, if more than a transient episode caused by dietary indiscretion, the end of conservative management has been signaled. The risk of sudden death caused by otherwise silent hyperkalemia makes continuation of conservative therapy an avoidable danger.

Bone Preservation

Renal osteodystrophy is the term applied to the combination of osteomalacia, osteosclerosis, osteoporosis, and osteofibrosis which is found in the bones of uremic patients. In chronic renal failure, the diagnosis of a diseased skeletal system may be made after a pathologic fracture occurs, or from the finding of bone cysts or subperiosteal resorption (easily detected in the phalanges). The mechanism of uremic bone disease is complex. Enlargement with hypersecretion of parathyroid hormone (PTH) by the four parathyroid glands develops because of phosphate retention which causes hypocalcemia. Diseased kidneys further contribute to hypocalcemia by reduced synthesis of active vitamin D (1,25-$[OH]_2D_3$) from its liver-synthesized precursor (25-[OH] D_3) which is essential to normal intestinal absorption of calcium. PTH levels are elevated early and constantly in

TABLE 1. **Correlation of Clinical and Laboratory Signs in Renal Failure**

CREATININE CLEARANCE (ML/MM)	SIGNS AND SYMPTOMS
60 to 120	None (PTH ↑)
30 to 59	Mild anemia, decreased work tolerance, mild hypertension
15 to 29	Hypertension, decreased cerebration, salt retention, fatigue, nausea, anemia, acidosis, azotemia
5 to 14	Anorexia, weight loss, emesis, edema, urochrome pigmentation, restless legs, insomnia, fetid breath, overtly uremic but functional
2 to 4	Obviously sick, cachexia, pericarditis, neuropathy, bleeding diathesis, asterixis, seizures, hypothermia
< 2	Coma

progressive kidney disease. Preservation of bone integrity can be effected by binding dietary phosphate in the gut with aluminum hydroxide or aluminum carbonate liquid gels (1 tablespoonful before meals or 2 tablets four times daily). Phosphate binders induce constipation and nausea in some patients, who require constant encouragement to continue their use. In conjunction with phosphate binders, for patients who are not hypercalcemic, Rocaltrol, an active vitamin D preparation (1,25-$[OH]_2D_3$), is now available. Starting at a dose of 0.25 microgram per day, the dose can be increased by 0.25 microgram per day every 2 weeks until a total dose of 1.0 microgram per day is reached. Should hypercalcemia develop during treatment, the drug must be discontinued temporarily to avoid metastatic calcification. Uncontrolled renal osteodystrophy is an indication for subtotal parathyroidectomy, although sufficient dialysis or renal transplantation may facilitate a reduction in PTH level. Clinical trials in progress suggest that cimetidine treatment may prevent synthesis or release of PTH, serving as a "medical parathyroidectomy."

Hypertension

Sustained hypertension, present in 85 per cent of patients with severe renal insufficiency (creatinine clearance <15 ml per minute), increases mortality and morbidity, and can be treated. Control of hypertension, as shown in diabetic nephropathy by Mogenson, will also retard the rate of decline of renal function. No specific drug regimen has been found clearly superior, and most depend on a combination of a diuretic such as furosemide, 40 to 120 mg once or twice daily, and a central or peripheral vasodilator. The goal of treatment is a diastolic blood pressure of 90 mm Hg or less. Switching of drugs because of severe side effects, especially somnolence and impotence, may prove necessary until an acceptable regimen is devised. Relatively effective drugs include clonidine (Catapres), 0.1 to 0.4 mg two to four times daily; methyldopa (Aldomet), 250 to 500 mg two to four times daily; hydralazine (Apresoline), 10 to 150 mg two times daily; prazosin (Minipress), 1 to 5 mg two to three times daily (after a test dose of 1 mg to exclude sensitivity manifested by syncope); and propranolol (Inderal), 40 to 120 mg two to four times daily. For initial control of malignant hypertension, intravenous sodium nitroprusside (Nipride) may be employed at a dose of 0.5 to 6 micrograms per kg per minute. Bilateral nephrectomy as a means of controlling virulent hypertension resistant to drug therapy is no longer necessary. Minoxidil (Loniten) in a dose of 10 to 40 mg twice daily will reduce diastolic pressure to normal in nearly every instance. Minoxidil should be reserved for patients in whom other drugs have failed, because of its potency and side effects of fluid retention (use furosemide) and angina-tachycardia (use propranolol). Excessive facial and chest hair growth makes minoxidil objectionable to women. Nearly all hypertensive uremic patients can respond to a regimen of blood pressure reduction. During dialysis, normalization of blood pressure is the rule (Fig. 1).

Anemia

Once creatinine clearance has dropped below 10 ml per minute, anemia becomes a universal finding. A hematocrit of 20 to 25 per cent is usual, and is not in itself an indication for therapy. Unless coronary insufficiency or reduced tolerance for activity limits rehabilitation, the anemia of uremia requires no treatment. Iron or folate deficiency, when identified, should be corrected. The benefit of androgenic steroids such as testosterone enanthate (Delatestryl) is still to be proved. Transfusion before surgery has not been needed, as safety during general anesthesia has been observed provided that fluid overload does not compromise pulmonary function.

Drug Choice

To minimize adverse drug reactions in patients with renal failure, a good guideline is to

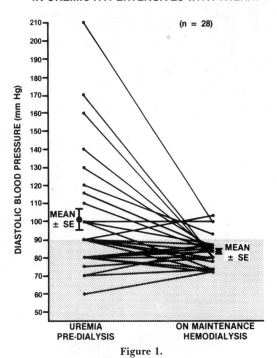

NORMALIZATION OF DIASTOLIC PRESSURE IN UREMIC HYPERTENSIVES WITH THERAPY

Figure 1.

avoid administration of any drug in the absence of a strong indication. Modification of dosage for drugs excreted by the kidney can be effected by either a reduction in dose or an increase in the interval between doses. A detailed reference (Ann Intern. Med. *86*:754, 1977) has been prepared to assist in drug choice and dose selection. Aminoglycoside drugs (amikacin, gentamicin, kanamycin, and tobramycin) require careful dose decrease, with a standard dose given at 18 to 25 hour intervals for clearances < 10 ml per minute. No modification of commonly used analgesics (opiates, meperidine, acetaminophen, or propoxyphene), sedative-hypnotic drugs (benzodiazepines, chloral hydrate, and most barbiturates), or tranquilizers is required, although the central nervous system effects of uremia may be enhanced by these drugs. Cardiac glycosides may be risky in uremia; the dose of digoxin must be reduced to half the normal amount (0.125 mg per day) and followed with blood concentration measurements. Lidocaine, propranolol, and phenytoin are preferred over procainamide and quinidine, which must be administered in lower doses. Nitrofurantoin (Furadantin) may cause peripheral neuropathy, and tetracyclines, which impede hepatic protein metabolism, should not be prescribed in renal failure.

Symptomatic Treatment

Progressive debility, fatigue, lassitude, nausea, and dyspepsia accompany the decline in creatinine clearance below 10 ml per minute. A reduced protein intake and the use of phenothiazines such as prochlorperazine maleate (Compazine), 10 mg orally twice per day, may produce temporary relief of the gastrointestinal complaints. Uremic pruritus is responsive to treatment of secondary hyperparathyroidism, and is thought to be a manifestation of increased circulating PTH. Starch baths, ultraviolet phototherapy, and trimeprazine (Temaril), 5 mg four times a day, have all proved helpful to some but not all patients with persistent itching.

Pericarditis, colitis, motor neuropathy, convulsions, and a reversed diurnal sleep pattern are signs that the interval of conservative therapy has ended.

Life Plan

As shown in Figure 2, the uremic patient has a choice of treatments, including an option of no therapy. For a patient with uncontrolled extensive metastatic cancer causing uremia by ureteral obstruction, the decision not to accept a dialysis regimen is understandable. Similarly, an institutionalized, demented, psychotic patient, who neither understands nor communicates with his medical team, may not be treated because of the absence of staff capable of devoting sufficient time to the struggle to effect therapy.

For most uremic adults, however, prior knowledge of the benefits and limitations of each treatment option allows for selection of the best (for that individual) alternative. In the months preceding final deterioration in renal function, a surgically created internal arteriovenous fistula should have been formed in the nondominant arm, and tissue typing of potential intrafamilial donors should have been completed if renal transplantation is contemplated. Each of the steps in the management of progressive azotemia through formulation of a life plan is reviewed in Figure 3.

Uremia Therapy

Hemodialysis. Maintenance hemodialysis, consisting of thrice weekly 4 to 6 hour treatments performed in a hospital, outpatient ambulatory facility, or the patient's home, is the uremia

MANAGING THE AZOTEMIC PATIENT

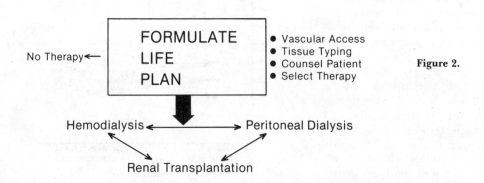

Figure 2.

MANAGING THE AZOTEMIC PATIENT

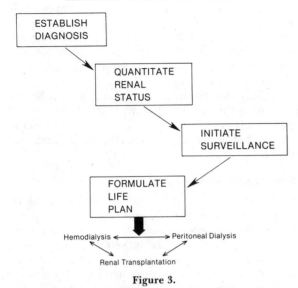

Figure 3.

therapy most commonly utilized in the United States. In mid-1980, approximately 54,000 Americans were undergoing maintenance hemodialysis under federal support, representing about 85 per cent of all treated patients. The hemodialysis regimen is dependent on a vascular access, most commonly enlarged forearm veins resulting from creation of an internal arteriovenous fistula months earlier. Vein to vein hemodialysis at a blood flow rate of 200 to 400 ml per minute through a disposable coil, parallel plate, or hollow fiber cellulose membrane device of about 1 square meter surface area extracts urea at about a clearance of 175 ml per minute and creatinine at approximately a clearance of 125 ml per minute. Water is removed from the patient's blood at a rate of up to 1500 ml per hour by maintaining a pressure differential across the cellulose membrane which is higher in the blood than in the dialysate compartment.

Hemodialysis patients have only partially corrected uremia and remain azotemic, anemic (hematocrit of 20 to 30 per cent), and acidotic (predialysis blood pH of 7.2 to 7.35). All uremic complications which occur in undialyzed patients may develop at some point during dialytic therapy. Uremic bone disease, cardiovascular disease, and postdialysis muscle cramps and fatigue are the most troublesome indicators of persistent renal insufficiency. As a component of the treatment regimen, dialysis patients adhere to water, protein, and potassium-restricted diets. Depression, subnormal sexual performance, and persistent urochrome skin pigmentation are common. Nevertheless, return to work, home, or school responsibilities is usual, particularly for those who perform self-dialysis at home. Long-term

survival is increasingly reported for hemodialysis patients free of systemic diseases such as diabetes. A newly treated home hemodialysis patient between the ages of 18 and 45 years has at least an 80 per cent chance of living 5 years. Survival of Delano's initial series of patients in Brooklyn is shown in Figure 4. Overall mortality, including elderly, diabetic, and cancerous patients on institutional hemodialysis, is 12 per cent per year. Surgical procedures and medical diseases during hemodialysis are handled as in an azotemic patient with a creatinine clearance of about 10 ml per minute without a noticeably increased complication rate.

Peritoneal Dialysis.   Until about 3 years ago, very few patients were sustained by intermittent peritoneal dialysis because of its poor efficiency and high rate of peritonitis. Introduction of continuous ambulatory peritoneal dialysis (CAPD) prompted a resurgence of interest in its potential. Now in wide clinical trial, CAPD machine-free treatment requires that the patient have a permanent plastic intraperitoneal catheter inserted surgically. In CAPD, dialysate, 2 to 3 liters, flows into the peritoneal cavity by gravity and is drained 6 hours later. Recycling of dialysate is performed four times daily 7 days per week by the trained patient or an assistant. Advantages of CAPD include a short training period, which may be as brief as 2 weeks, and its minimal negative psychologic implications, absence of a machine, and a feeling of well-being presumably resulting from a relatively steady level of nitrogenous solutes in the blood. Free of the post-dialysis swings which typify hemodialysis, the CAPD patient apparently has more energy and experiences enhanced reha-

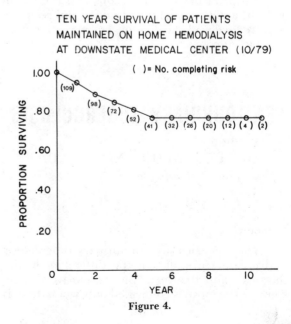

Figure 4.

bilitation. Disadvantages of CAPD include a high rate of peritonitis and a tendency to hyperlipidemia and weight gain caused by dialysate glucose levels of 1500 mg per dl or higher. The relative importance of CAPD as a uremia therapy is under study. Enthusiastic reports by nephrologists and their patients indicate the need for serious attention to this novel and simple therapy.

Renal Transplantation. A functioning renal transplant will totally reverse all aspects of uremia, maximizing rehabilitation in uremia therapy. As yet, few transplant recipients have a perfect course, and most are affected with either graft rejection, in days to years, or toxic or infectious consequences of antirejection drugs. Combined immunosuppressive therapy with azathioprine (Imuran), 0.5 to 3 mg per kg, and prednisone, 0.25 to 2.0 mg per kg, will retard graft rejection in well-matched recipients. Intrafamilial living donor kidney recipients have about a 90 per cent chance of living 2 years and an 80 per cent probability of graft function for 2 years. Recipients of cadaveric renal grafts have a 2 year survival of about 80 to 85 per cent and a functional 2 year graft survival of about 50 per cent. The young uremic patient free of systemic disease lacking a living donor must choose between the higher mortality and better rehabilitation of cadaveric transplantation and the safety and morbidity of dialytic therapy. Uremia therapies should not be viewed as competitive or exclusive. A dialysis patient may at any time opt for a transplant. Transplant recipients with failed grafts become dialysis patients until they once again request a new kidney. Improved results of cadaveric kidney transplantation are now being reported in Western Europe. Beneficial effects of pretransplant blood transfusions and the use of HLA-D antigen matching of donor and recipient are credited with facilitating an increasingly favorable outcome.

GENITOURINARY TUBERCULOSIS

method of
DUDLEY SETH DANOFF, M.D.
Los Angeles, California

Introduction

The incidence of genitourinary tuberculosis is decreasing overall, but the difficulties in the diagnosis and treatment of this elusive disease remain. Diagnosis is confirmed only when there is a minimum of three positive urine cultures for *Mycobacterium tuberculosis* taken from three early morning first voided (concentrated) urine specimens, collected on 3 separate days. Direct aspiration of the renal lesions or cultures taken directly from the surgical specimen are occasionally necessary to confirm the diagnosis.

Once the diagnosis of genitourinary tuberculosis is confirmed by appropriate cultures, treatment falls generally into two categories: specific chemotherapy and urologic (surgical) management.

Specific Chemotherapy

There are at present 12 antituberculotic drugs available throughout the world, some being more effective than others. After the start of appropriate antituberculotic chemotherapy, the patient is rapidly rendered noninfectious, and almost all of the genitourinary tuberculous lesions can be cured by chemotherapeutic regimens alone.

The general rule that we follow is the rule of "2 and 2", that is, two drugs for a duration of 2 years. The older literature emphasizes the importance of using three drugs, but that was at a time when para-aminosalicylic acid (PAS) was considered the first-line drug. By today's standard, this drug is not very effective, and its replacement by isoniazid (INH) has mitigated the necessity of using three troublesome drugs. Our personal preference is the *combination of isoniazid (INH) and rifampin.* Both these drugs are bactericidal; their combination is highly effective, with an extremely low incidence of the development of resistant forms. It is the most cost-effective combination, and the combination with the least unfavorable side effects. The combination of *isoniazid and ethambutol* is also quite an acceptable first-line therapy regimen, although it is somewhat less effective, because ethambutol is bacteriostatic and there is greater possibility of the emergence of resistant strains.

After the culture diagnosis is confirmed, brief hospitalization, usually less than 2 weeks, is advisable. It is best to do the initial urologic workup in the hospital at a time when the greatest degree of infectivity exists, prior to the initiation of chemotherapy. Hospitalization permits baseline studies to be completed, including intravenous pyelogram; retrograde pyelography if the lower ureter is not well visualized; cystoscopic examination and appropriate bladder biopsies if bladder lesions are seen; skeletal bone survey; and full chest tomograms. In addition, the hospital setting allows the clinician the opportunity to educate the patient with particular emphasis on the importance of meticulously adhering to the drug regimen outlined. After the start of anti-tuberculotic chemotherapy, the patient is rapidly rendered noninfectious.

First-Line Drugs. First-line drugs should be administered as follows:

1. Isoniazid (INH), given in doses of 8 mg per kg per day (in combination with rifampin or ethambutol). The usual dose of isoniazid is 300 mg per day, and it is best given in divided doses. INH should be continued for a minimum of 18 to 24 months after the cultures have become negative. INH is the least toxic of all of the drugs currently used. It has infrequent side effects. A mild peripheral neuropathy may be seen, for which pyridoxine is given along with the isoniazid. This combination results in good protection against the neuropathy. Some unusual side effects to be aware of with the use of isoniazid include occasional psychosis, dizziness, rare optic neuritis, and rare convulsions. Although mild changes in liver function may occur with INH, these changes are unusual, unpredictable, and *not* dose related. It is suggested that stimulants such as caffeine or amphetamine derivatives not be used when the patient is taking INH, as there is often a cumulative irritative effect on the central nervous system.

2. Pyridoxine (vitamin B_6), 100 mg daily by mouth. This is always used in combination with isoniazid to protect against the peripheral neuropathy.

3. Rifampin, 300 mg orally twice daily. This is always taken in combination with isoniazid. Rifampin is the single most effective antimycobacterial drug and the combination of INH-rifampin is the most effective by today's standards. Rifampin is bactericidal. It is excreted by the liver and is therefore unaffected by any renal impairment caused by the primary genitourinary tuberculosis lesion. It is relatively nontoxic, but because it is excreted by the liver, it may alter liver function test results slightly. Rarely thrombocytopenia has been reported. A mild skin rash may develop and on occasion the urine may be colored a bright orange, which has no clinical consequence, but may surprise or alarm the patient.

4. Ethambutol, 25 mg per kg per day for 2 months initially, then 15 mg per kg per day by mouth, taken in combination with INH. Because ethambutol is bacteriostatic, it is a less effective drug to be used in combination with isoniazid than is rifampin. However, the combination of isoniazid-ethambutol is a good one and of relatively low toxicity. It is still widely used, although not our first choice. The main side effect of ethambutol is retrobulbar neuritis with decreased visual acuity. All patients on ethambutol therefore should have visual acuity testing before treatment is instituted (baseline) and then at periodic intervals while they are taking ethambutol. Visual acuity is often reduced, sometimes unilaterally. The earliest effect is manifested by the inability to perceive the color green. Visual acuity returns to normal when the drug is stopped. Tests of renal function should also be done periodically while the patient is on ethambutol, since the drug is excreted primarily by the kidney and will often cause a minor renal impairment.

With the combination of isoniazid-rifampin *or* isoniazid-ethambutol, the cultures from the vast majority of patients will be converted to negative within 6 weeks. It is wise to check other signs, including the presence of pyuria or microscopic hematuria, as a rough guideline to the effectiveness of the drugs. Within the first 6 to 8 weeks after starting treatment, repeat cultures for *Mycobacterium tuberculosis* are obtained, and sensitivity studies should be performed to be certain that the correct and most effective combination of drugs is being used.

Second-Line Drugs. It is rarely necessary to introduce a third drug when the two-drug combination of INH-rifampin or INH-ethambutol is used. Occasionally there is a failure of the urinary culture to become negative. Severe cavitary infections may infrequently result in treatment failure. More commonly, however, treatment failures are due to underlying problems, such as malnutrition, diabetes, the use of immunosuppressive agents in renal transplantation, or alcoholism. Failure resulting from chemotherapeutic resistance is unusual, and therefore these second-line drugs are almost never used as initial therapy because of their relatively high toxicity or their decreased acceptability to both the patient and the physician. The second-line drugs are used in cases of re-treatment or treatment failure caused by the emergence of resistant organisms after the first-line therapy has proved to be ineffective. The rule of thumb is that when additional drugs are required after the standard two-drug start, it is best to introduce a drug with a different mode of action than the drug that was primarily being used. Therefore, for example, it would be well to introduce injectable streptomycin along with INH if one is substituting or adding to rifampin or ethambutol.

Second-line drugs include the following:

1. Streptomycin. Of all the second-line drugs, this is the most common drug added to our primary two-drug regimen. It is often given initially, particularly in severe infections or in infections that seem at least to be unresponsive to the standard two-drug starting combination. It is

given intramuscularly, 1 gram daily for 8 to 12 weeks, and then is usually discontinued. It may cause eighth nerve toxicity with auditory and vestibular impairment and this must be watched very closely. Renal function must be monitored as well, and if impairment of renal function is reported, the drug is discontinued.

2. Para-aminosalicylic acid (PAS). This was formerly regarded as a first-line drug but has been almost universally abandoned because of its intolerable gastrointestinal side effects and its relatively low effectiveness compared to INH. However, it is occasionally used when the patient cannot take INH and then is given 5 grams three times daily by mouth. The sodium form of PAS can decrease the effects of nausea and diarrhea, but there is the added problem of a large sodium load. PAS is most commonly used today in pregnant women and small children but is not considered an important drug.

3. Pyrazinamide. To be used in doses of 25 mg per kg per day with a maximal dose of 3 grams per day. It can cause hepatotoxicity, elevation of the serum uric acid level, and minor aberrations in renal function. It is not an important drug but can be used when either rifampin or ethambutol cannot be used with isoniazid.

4. Cycloserine. Usually given in doses of 250 mg orally twice daily. Its major side effect is central nervous system stimulation, which mimics toxicity from amphetamines and caffeine. When used in combination with isoniazid and pyridoxine, the pyridoxine may decrease the central nervous system's stimulant side effects of cycloserine, as it does with isoniazid alone.

Many recent studies have advocated the use of "intermittent" chemotherapy, particularly with the unreliable or uncooperative patient. Instead of the daily dose schedule usually used with the combination of INH-rifampin, a combination of INH given in the dose of 14 mg per kg and intramuscular streptomycin at 27 mg per kg, administered *twice weekly* by a visiting nurse in the patient's home, can also be effective. Some reports have indicated that the combination of INH-ethambutol *or* INH-rifampin, administered in this twice-weekly regimen, is equally effective. However, we do not recommend intermittent chemotherapy in the treatment of genitourinary tuberculosis, nor do we recommend the short-course chemotherapy, i.e., less than 18 to 24 months, because the long-term bacteriologic relapse rate for this group has been significant.

Chemoprophylaxis. A brief word must be said about chemoprophylaxis. This should not be considered chemotherapy, but should be reserved for those patients who are at high risk of contracting the disease.

The dose in this group is INH, 300 mg daily for 1 year. The group to receive chemoprophylaxis in this dose regimen should include these persons:

1. A household contact.

2. A skin test converter, particularly a young adult.

3. A patient who had a previous history of tuberculosis and who is now inactive but exposed to active tuberculosis.

4. A recent transplant recipient with a positive purified protein derivative (PPD) test result or a positive contact history.

Urologic (Surgical) Management

Urologic and surgical management usually have no place in the *cure* of genitourinary tuberculosis. However, the *prevention* of permanent damage to the urinary tract from the scarring, ureteral stenosis, and narrowing of all drainage structures, often with disastrous renal consequences, depends on meticulous urologic care.

The role of nephrectomy in the management of renal tuberculosis has sharply declined with the advancement of adequate chemotherapy over the past several years. Today urologic management is aimed at the treatment of the complications of genitourinary tuberculosis. All the complications are related to the results of *retractile sclerosis*, and the key to urologic treatment is directed toward management of the following:

1. Narrowing and stenosis of the distal ureter.

2. Contraction of the urinary bladder, resulting in small bladder capacity and intractable urinary frequency.

3. Vesicoureteral reflux secondary to bladder contracture and trigonal fibrosis.

4. Renal infundibular stenosis producing calyceal diverticula, often with pyocalix, microabscess formation, chronic infection, papillary necrosis, calculus formation, and eventual renal destruction.

Urologic therapy is therefore directed against these sequelae and involves radiographic evaluation with the following:

1. An initial intravenous pyelogram and cystogram at the time chemotherapy is instituted to obtain a baseline study and assess any significant ureteral or bladder damage.

2. Repeat intravenous pyelogram done 6 to 8 weeks after chemotherapy is begun. If ureteral stenosis is noted, prompt retrograde pyelography and ureteral dilatation must be done.

3. Intravenous urography or retrograde pyelography, or both, should then be repeated every 8 to 10 weeks if there is any evidence of progressing ureteral stenosis. *Complete* ureteral

obstruction and cessation of unilateral renal function (autonephrectomy) may occur quite silently.

4. In the absence of any evidence of significant renal damage after the first 8 to 12 weeks following the start of chemotherapy, intravenous pyelography (IVP) or retrograde pyelography should be repeated at 6-monthly intervals while the patient is under treatment, and at yearly intervals for 5 years after treatment has been completed.

Urologic Treatment and Evaluation. 1. Initial cystoscopy, retrograde pyelography, and calibration of the ureters at the start of chemotherapy should be done. If there is evidence of ureteral narrowing or stenosis, the ureters should be dilated to a size No. 6 French ureteral catheter. At the time of the initial cystoscopic examination, retrograde studies are made and urine specimens are obtained from each kidney separately in order to lateralize the disease, if possible. Bladder biopsy may also be taken for both pathologic and bacteriologic confirmation.

2. During treatment, if there is any evidence of ureteral stenosis, ureteral calibration and dilatation can be repeated as often as every 6 weeks, since ureteral strictures are the major single cause of autonephrectomy. If there is persistent ureteral stenosis, it is often wise to add corticosteroids to the regimen along with mechanical ureteral dilatation.

Steroids, i.e., prednisone (15 to 20 mg per day), may be beneficial in minimizing strictures and may be started when urine cultures are sterile and continued until x-ray evidence of ureteral narrowing is gone. Chemotherapy must be continued for 6 months after steroid treatment is stopped.

3. It may be necessary to place an indwelling *stenting* ureteral catheter (Silastic type) during treatment if ureteral narrowing persists.

4. If contraction of the bladder appears to be a problem early in treatment, consideration should be given to hydraulic overdistention of the bladder at the time of cystoscopy, even though the results of this are usually not long lasting.

5. If a small contracted bladder results in vesicoureteral reflux, it may become necessary to perform ureterovesical reimplantation. One of the various distal ureteral remodeling or bladder-flap procedures may be indicated if the degree of distal ureteral stenosis is severe.

6. With marked and persistent bladder contracture (with or without vesicoureteral reflux), it may be necessary to perform either (a) an enterocystoplasty (augmentation cystoplasty), utilizing an isolated loop of small or large intestine, to increase bladder size, or (b) if the bladder is badly damaged, a complete urinary diversion using an ileal loop (conduit, as described by Bricker) or a colonic conduit.

The use of augmentation cystoplasty or urinary diversion must be considered when the resultant contracted bladder is associated with renal insufficiency.

7. Calcified renal tuberculin lesions have been mistakenly treated as for primary stone disease. Surgical removal of these calcifications (partial nephrectomy) may be necessary to ensure adequate chemotherapy and eradication of the organisms.

8. Nephrectomy is to be reserved only for these conditions: (a) intractable pyonephrosis with pain; (b) uncontrollable fever secondary to distal ureteral stricture and obstruction, unresponsive to chemotherapeutic manipulation; (c) troublesome calcification or inability to distinguish the tuberculous renal lesion from possible neoplasm; or (d) organisms unresponsive and resistant to *all* chemotherapy.

9. Tuberculosis is often manifested in the epididymis, presenting with so-called "beading" of the ductus epididymidis and terminal epididymis. Local abscess formation and draining scrotal fistulas are seen and epididymectomy or orchiectomy, or both, may be necessary if these troublesome lesions do not respond to chemotherapy.

10. A draining perineal fistula from tuberculous prostatitis may be encountered and will usually respond to chemotherapy.

GENITOURINARY TUMORS

method of
E. DAVID CRAWFORD, M.D.,
and THOMAS A. BORDEN, M.D.
Albuquerque, New Mexico

Introduction

Physicians dealing with genitourinary tumors have witnessed a number of changes in both the diagnosis and treatment of these tumors during the last decade. These changes stem from the development of new and innovative surgical techniques, in addition to advancements in the field of irradiation and chemotherapy, which in some diseases have modified the timing of the surgical approach. Nonetheless, the primary therapy for localized genitourinary tumors remains complete surgical excision. It has become very clear that many patients who succumb to disease after successful definitive surgery do so because of unrecognized distant metastases at the time of the procedure. It would appear that surgery and irradiation have achieved about as much as they are going to achieve in terms of curability and control of local disease, and future advances will depend upon the development and use of other adjuvants in the form of chemotherapy and/or immunotherapy. Therefore, the use of systemic chemotherapeutic adjuvants has become increasingly important. Institutional studies are currently underway to define which patients might benefit from such systemic adjuvant chemotherapy.

Aldosteronoma

Aldosteronomas are benign tumors of the adrenal cortex which secrete an excess amount of aldosterone. The tumor is often discovered during an evaluation for hypertension, and rarely does the patient present with complaints related to electrolyte abnormalities (hypokalemic alkalosis).

Treatment. The treatment of an aldosteronoma is straightforward if the presence and location of the tumor have been established preoperatively. Total adrenalectomy is the treatment of choice. If surgery is exploratory, it should be performed through an anterior incision which provides access to both adrenal glands. Under these circumstances, if no definite tumor is identified, a left adrenalectomy is performed, since most tumors are located within the left adrenal gland. If no tumor is found on multiple step sections of the left adrenal, a partial right adrenalectomy is performed. We feel that total bilateral adrenalectomy should not be done because of the risks associated with chronic steroid replacement therapy. Patients whose hypertension is well controlled with antihypertensives are not subjected to exploration when the presence of a tumor cannot be verified preoperatively.

Pheochromocytoma

Complete surgical excision is the treatment of choice for pheochromocytoma. Prior to the surgical procedure, we employ preoperative preparation with alpha-adrenergic blockade. Since most patients with pheochromocytoma have a diminished blood volume, 2 units of whole blood and plasma expanders are administered preoperatively. The assistance of a knowledgeable anesthesiologist is mandatory.

The tumor should be approached through an anterior transperitoneal incision. A total adrenalectomy (or complete excision of the tumor when not arising from the adrenal) is performed. Occasionally these tumors are malignant; thus, if the tumor seems unusually adherent or invasive, the kidney and surrounding tissue are also removed. Under these circumstances, or if the lymph nodes are palpably enlarged, we also perform a regional lymphadenectomy. The contralateral adrenal gland, para-aortic tissues, and pelvic structures should then be carefully and systematically palpated to rule out a second, unsuspected tumor. The blood pressure should be continuously monitored during this exploration, and sudden increases in systolic pressure while palpating along the great vessels may indicate the presence of a small extra-adrenal tumor. Since histologic criteria for the diagnosis of malignant pheochromocytoma have not yet been established, the patient should be monitored postoperatively for the development of recurrent hypertension or other signs of metastases.

Treatment of metastatic or unresectable pheochromocytoma with ortho-para-DDD (mitotane) has been disappointing, but it is the only chemotherapeutic agent currently available.

Neuroblastoma

Neuroblastoma is the most common solid malignant tumor of infancy and childhood. While most frequently arising from the adrenal medulla, it may develop in any cells of neural crest origin. The majority of patients with neuroblastoma have metastatic disease at the time of diagnosis.

Treatment. The treatment of neuroblastoma remains highly controversial. The frequency of spontaneous regression, the markedly better prognosis in children under 1 year of age, and the frequency of metastatic disease at the time of diagnosis have made the efficacy of treatment difficult to assess. Treatment must be individualized, and is predominantly based on the age of the patient and the stage of the disease. The importance of a multidisciplinary approach cannot be overemphasized. We employ the staging system of Evans:

Stage 1:   Tumor limited to organ of origin
Stage 2:   Regional spread that does not cross the midline
Stage 3:   Tumors extending across the midline
Stage 4:   Patients with distant metastases
Stage 4-S: Patients with a small primary and metastases limited to liver, skin, or bone marrow, without radiographic evidence of bony metastases

Patients with Stage 1 and Stage 2 tumors are treated by surgical extirpation. Radiation is generally reserved for selected patients over 1 year of age with Stage 3 disease. Irradiation may also be extremely helpful in treating patients with isolated metastatic lesions. Other patients with increased stage disease are treated with chemotherapy. In infants, chemotherapy is reserved for those with disseminated disease. Cyclophosphamide alone, or in combination with vincristine or doxorubicin (Adriamycin), remains the regimen of choice. Initial experience with the use of cisplatin seems encouraging. Chemotherapy or localized radiation therapy may also be indicated in infants with severe liver involvement, and can be instrumental in the management of severe pain secondary to widespread bony metastases. Surgery may be important in establishing the diagnosis of neuroblastoma and in both defining and marking the extent of the disease, in addition to treating localized lesions. At times, surgery is indicated for the relief of acute processes as well, such as ureteral obstruction. Although the role of tumor debulking and second-look procedures remains controversial, in some instances large tumors respond to chemotherapy or irradiation and may in turn become resectable.

Benign Renal Tumors

Benign tumors of the kidney may arise from the renal capsule, renal parenchyma, or renal pelvis, and may be cystic or solid. The most common benign renal tumors of importance are the cystic lesions. The solid varieties include adenoma, fibroma, lipoma, leiomyoma, angioma, rhabdomyoma, dermoid, and angiomyolipoma. Renal cortical adenoma is the most common of the benign solid parenchymal tumors, and considerable debate exists as to the natural history of this lesion. Most pathologists classify adenomas as lesions smaller than 3 cm, whereas larger lesions are classified as true renal carcinomas. We find it difficult to distinguish renal adenoma from adenocarcinoma in most cases, and recommend surgical excision. Small lesions may be treated by partial resection of the kidney.

Angiomyolipomas (hamartomas) occur most commonly in patients with tuberous sclerosis. However, approximately 50 per cent of the patients we see with angiomyolipomas have no stigmata of tuberous sclerosis. These tumors may reach a very large size and produce flank pain, hematuria, obstruction, and marked distortion of the collecting system. Computed tomography is often helpful in diagnosing this disease because the attentuation coefficient is that of adipose tissue. We treat large tumors restricted to one renal unit with nephrectomy. Bilateral tumors are best treated conservatively.

Renal Pelvic Tumors

Cancer of the renal pelvis accounts for approximately 5 per cent of renal cancers. The peak incidence occurs in the sixth to seventh decades of life, and males predominate by a 3:1 ratio. Eighty-five per cent of these malignant tumors are transitional cell, 14 per cent squamous cell, and 1 per cent adenocarcinomas. Papillomas of the renal pelvis are relatively rare, and are connected to the renal pelvis by a narrow stalk a few millimeters in diameter. Pathologically, these papillomas never show invasion; however, approximately 25 per cent of patients will develop frank carcinoma somewhere else in the urinary tract. Chronic noxious stimulation of the uroepithelium may produce a variety of proliferative changes, including squamous metaplasia. Of paramount importance in the management of upper tract tumors is the synchronous or metachronous association with bladder cancer in approximately 30 to 50 per cent of patients.

Staging. We employ the following pathologic staging system in these tumors:

Stage 1: Benign papilloma with no evidence of invasion
Stage 2: Low stage, noninvasive tumors which have not extended into the muscularis of the ureter
Stage 3: High stage, papillary lesions extending to the level of the muscularis, which may extend beyond the muscularis into intrarenal portions of the renal pelvis if confined to the kidney
Stage 4: Extension beyond the renal parenchyma

Treatment. Since the majority of the lesions encountered are invasive and have the propensity for lymphatic permeation, vascular invasion, and multicentricity, we use nephroureterectomy as the preferred surgical procedure. The surgical specimen should include an excision of a cuff of bladder surrounding the ureteral orifice, as there is a 30 per cent incidence of recurrent tumor in the ureteral stump in those patients in whom a stump remains. We employ a thoracoabdominal approach, thus necessitating only one incision. Some urologists recommend an upper excision for the nephrectomy portion, followed by a lower abdominal incision to complete the nephroureterectomy. An occasional patient may have a low stage lesion in an upper or lower pole calyx, which may be treated by partial nephrectomy encompassing the involved collecting system. Nephroscopy should be used to locate the tumors within the collecting system of the kidney, and the remaining intrarenal collecting systems should be inspected carefully before they are considered for a partial nephrectomy. Patients with a solitary kidney may best be treated by a conservative approach. With this approach, patients must be followed carefully to detect the presence of tumor elsewhere in the urinary tract.

Squamous cell carcinoma and adenocarcinoma of the renal pelvis are rare tumors that tend to be associated with chronic infection and stone formation. These diseases are usually discovered at a more advanced stage, accompanied by a poor prognosis. They are not always multifocal, as is the transitional cell variety; however, they are best treated by radical nephroureterectomy.

Patients with positive lymph node involvement are best managed with postoperative irradiation therapy to the renal bed and major lymph node areas. In addition, we have employed cisplatin (see Bladder Cancer) for patients with advanced or metastatic disease. Several patients have survived for extended periods of time with this combined treatment adjunct.

Ureteral Carcinoma

Cancers of the ureter are relatively rare lesions, and account for only 1 per cent of carcinomas of the upper urinary tract. Eighty per cent of these lesions are transitional, 11 per cent squamous, and less than 1 per cent adenocarcinomas.

Stage 0: Disease limited to the mucosa
Stage A: Tumors with submucosal infiltration
Stage B: Lesions having muscular invasion
Stage C: Lesions extending through the ureteric wall into the surrounding adipose tissue
Stage D: Metastases by direct extension to adjacent organs or distant hematogenous or lymphatic metastases

Treatment. Solitary, low grade, low stage distal ureteral tumors can be treated by distal ureterectomy coupled with ureteral reimplantation. Lesions in the proximal ureter, high grade invasive lesions, or multifocal lesions are best handled with a nephroureterectomy and bladder cuff procedure (see Renal Pelvic Tumors). In all instances, excision of the regional lymph nodes provides a valuable staging adjunct. We treat patients who have high grade invasive lesions or distant metastases with adjuvant irradiation and cisplatin as outlined under Bladder Cancer. We have treated one patient who had a low grade, low stage proximal lesion with excision and autotransplantation of the kidney. An ileoureter is also a consideration.

The diagnosis of in situ carcinoma of the ureter is generally made at the time of cystectomy, when one has the opportunity to examine the distal ureter by frozen section. The question arises as to what to do for such a patient and the natural history of such lesions. These tend to occur in from 8 to 30 per cent of patients who undergo cystectomy. There is no current documentation as to the natural history of the disease; however, our preference is to remove as much distal ureter as is compatible with the performance of a standard and uncomplicated ileal conduit diversion.

Renal Cancer

Renal tubular carcinoma is the most common malignant tumor of the adult kidney, and accounts for approximately 3 per cent of all adult malignancies. There are approximately 15,000 new cases of renal cell carcinoma per year, and about 30 per cent of these present with distant metastases. It is often called the "internists' tumor" because of the diagnostic dilemma it presents. We employ the staging system shown below:

Stage 1: Tumor confined to the kidney
Stage 2: Tumor involving the perinephric fat, but confined within Gerota's fascia
Stage 3: Tumor involving the renal vein or regional nodes, with or without involvement of the vena cava or perinephric fat
Stage 4: Distant metastases secondary to renal cell carcinoma present on admission, or histologic involvement by tumor of contiguous visceral structures

Treatment. The mainstay of treatment for localized renal cell carcinoma is surgical excision. We feel the surgical specimen should include a complete excision of Gerota's fascia and its contents, including the adrenal gland and kidney. We have routinely removed the regional nodes for staging purposes; however, there is little evidence, once the nodes are involved with tumor, that removal would improve patient survival.

We do not routinely employ percutaneous catheter occlusion of the renal artery prior to the nephrectomy. But it has been advocated by some to decrease hemorrhage during surgery and to facilitate radical nephrectomy, and may be of some value in extremely large tumors. When infarction is employed, nephrectomy should be done at some time within the ensuing 24 to 48 hours, since there is an associated toxicity (fever, pain, and vomiting).

Patients who present with disseminated disease have an extremely poor prognosis. In the past, many urologists have performed a palliative nephrectomy in this situation, but it does little to increase the survival of patients with metastatic disease. Those who perform nephrectomy in the setting of metastatic disease should be aware that spontaneous regression of metastases occurs in less than 1 per cent of cases. The operative mortality is much higher. However, we perform nephrectomy in the face of metastatic disease for one of three reasons: (1) when the primary lesion is causing severe pain or uncontrolled hemorrhage; (2) in patients who have one or two distant metastases amenable to primary resection; and (3) in patients who have demonstrated response to a trial of systemic chemotherapy.

Hormonal therapy has been employed in patients with metastatic disease; however, true objective responses are rare, and probably occur in only 10 per cent of patients. The standard dose is 100 mg of medroxyprogesterone (Provera) by mouth three times daily, or 500 mg of medroxyprogesterone acetate (Depo-Provera) intramuscularly twice a week. Most of the chemotherapeutic drugs employed in the treatment of metastatic renal cell carcinoma have given disappointing results. The most effective agent appears to be vinblastine (Velban), which produces responses in the range of 15 to 25 per cent. Five to 8 mg per square meter is given intravenously every week. The dosage should be titrated to the patient's white blood cell count. The use of radiotherapy in the treatment of renal cell carcinoma does not appear to have a definite role, as there is no improvement in survival with irradiation to the renal bed, either preoperatively or postoperatively. However, very large tumors can sometimes be decreased to resectable size by radiotherapy. We do employ irradiation therapy for the treatment of symptomatic metastatic lesions.

Wilms' Tumor

Wilms' tumor (nephroblastoma) is the most common renal malignancy occurring in infants and children, with an incidence of one per 200,000 per year in children under age 14. The potential benefit of collaborative and multidisciplinary protocol management has been dramatically demonstrated by the National Wilms' Tumor Study (NWTS) group. As a result of this combined effort, the prognosis for this tumor has greatly improved, and currently the majority of children afflicted with the neoplasm are cured. NWTS-1 and NWTS-2 have been completed. The optimal treatment and surgical principles for managing most patients have been very clearly defined, and we strongly recommend that protocol. NWTS-3 has also been initiated, and its major objectives are aimed at minimizing treatment side effects and improving therapy for those children who can be identified as having a poor prognosis. Physicians involved in the care of patients with Wilms' tumor should be familiar with these protocols and should avail themselves of the benefit of multidisciplinary management. It is extremely important that treatment be started promptly; if a patient is to be entered into NWTS-3, he must be registered within 72 hours of the time of diagnosis.

The NWTS-3 requires the following minimal evaluation: complete blood count, urinalysis, blood urea nitrogen (BUN), creatinine, liver function profile, electrocardiogram, chest x-ray, and an excretory urogram. A skeletal survey and liver scan are desirable in most patients. Inferior vena cavography, angiography, sonography, and computerized axial tomography are elective and are employed as indicated in selected cases. We employ the staging system below:

Stage 1: Tumor limited to the kidney and completely excised

Stage 2: Tumor extending beyond the kidney but completely excised

Stage 3: Residual nonhematogenous tumor confined to the abdomen

Stage 4: Patients with hematogenous metastases and all patients with unfavorable histology

Treatment. Surgery plays a vital role in both the treatment and staging of patients. If possible, the primary tumor is removed in all patients regardless of stage, and if a patient is to be entered into the NWTS-3, a specific protocol should be followed and a checklist (available from the NWTS group) should be completed at the end of the surgical procedure. The tumor is generally approached through a wide transperitoneal incision. The diagnosis must be made with certainty. The entire abdomen, including the lymph nodes, opposite kidney, and liver, is explored, and suspicious lesions and lymph nodes are biopsied and marked with clips, as are representative lymph nodes. In the unusual case in which the tumor cannot be removed, its extent is marked with clips. If the tumor can be removed, a radical nephrectomy and regional lymphadenectomy are performed, with early control of the renal vessels. The procedure should be performed with a minimum of manipulation of the tumor, and every attempt is made to avoid tumor spillage. If residual tumor is present following the procedure, these margins are marked with silver clips.

Staging is based on the clinical evaluation, surgical findings, and the histologic examination of the surgical specimen. An important conclusion of the NWTS-2 was recognition of the fact that patients with unfavorable histology have a poor prognosis regardless of their stage. Unfavorable histology is defined as those tumors which are sarcomatous or which are diffusely anaplastic. In the third study, all patients with unfavorable histology are treated as Stage 4. NWTS-1 and NWTS-2 demonstrated that Wilms' tumors are sensitive to irradiation and also respond to chemotherapeutic agents, specifically actinomycin D, vincristine, and doxorubicin (Adriamycin). Treatment complications were predominantly related to the long-term use of actinomycin D and vincristine, the cardiotoxic effects of doxorubicin (Adriamycin), and the irradiation effects on the growing child. As a result, NWTS-3 is designed to ensure that each patient receives the maximum therapeutic benefit found in the earlier study and at the same time be randomized to see if the treatment can be refined in order to diminish side effects. Infants under 11 months of age receive age adjusted x-ray and chemotherapeutic dosage. The basic treatment protocol for NWTS-3 and the variables which are randomized are listed in Table 1.

Bladder Cancer

Cancer of the urinary bladder represents a formidable cause of cancer-related deaths each year. Of the 30,000 new cases diagnosed annually, 70 per cent are localized to the bladder at the time of diagnosis, yet 10,000 people will succumb to the disease this year. The high mortality stems from many factors, including the physician's confusion about the natural history of the disease, resulting in postponement of aggressive management until metastases have rendered salvage impossible. Bladder carcinoma represents one of the few tumors in which carcinogenic agents have been identified. It is estimated that up to one-third of the cases of bladder cancer in the United States may be related to industrial exposure to one or more compounds: β-naph-

thylamine, 4-aminobiphenyl, 4-nitrobiphenyl, and benzidine. Tobacco abuse has been incriminated as producing increased amounts of known carcinogens in the urine—beta-naphthylamine and tryptophan. Artificial sweeteners in the form of cyclamates and saccharin have been implicated as bladder carcinogens.

Staging. The current preferred method of staging is Marshall's modification of the Jewett-Strong system; the TNM system is not widely employed in this country.

Stage 0: Superficial tumor of bladder epithelium

Stage A: Superficial tumor through the lamina propria but not into muscle

Stage B: Tumor invading the muscularis

Stage C: Tumor through the bladder wall and into the perivesical fat

Stage D_1: Metastases limited to the pelvis, usually in the form of lymph nodes

Stage D_2: Distant metastases

The accuracy of preoperative staging is somewhere between 50 and 70 per cent. In addition to staging, treatment is also based upon the degree of cellular differentiation of the tumor. In general, the more high grade tumors are treated with aggressive therapy.

Treatment. Commonly accepted treatment modalities include transurethral resection, irradiation therapy, partial cystectomy, total cystectomy with urinary diversion, intracavitary chemotherapy, systemic chemotherapy, immunotherapy, and various combinations of the above. Patient survival is dependent upon the time employment and proper selection among these regimens.

CARCINOMA IN SITU. The subject of carcinoma in situ (severe epithelial atypia) needs special emphasis. It is considered to represent the uroepithelium's reaction to a diffuse, neoplastic stimulus. It may be associated with high grade, high stage malignancies, occasionally occurs as the sole finding in patients with crippling, irritative bladder symptoms, or can accompany low grade, low

TABLE 1. **Basic Treatment Protocol NWTS-3***

STAGE	TREATMENT	RANDOMIZED VARIABLE
1	AMD; VCR	Duration of treatment
2	AMD; VCR	ADR; RT (2000 rads)
3	AMD; VCR; RT	ADR; RT (2000 rads), RT (1000 rads)
4 (favorable histology)	AMD; VCR; ADR; RT (2000 rads)	CPM
4 (unfavorable histology)	AMD; VCR; ADR; RT (age adjusted)	CPM

*AMD = actinomycin-D; VCR = vincristine; ADR = doxorubicin (Adriamycin); CPM = cyclophosphamide; RT = radiation therapy.

stage lesions. Inasmuch as the prognosis for patients with this finding is poor, aggressive treatment (radical cystectomy) seems imperative. Carcinoma in situ is not a radiosensitive tumor.

STAGES 0 AND A. Transurethral resection is the preferred treatment for low grade, low stage malignancies (0 and A, well to moderately well differentiated). Transurethral resection is accompanied by low morbidity and low mortality, requires a short period of hospitalization, and preserves bladder and sexual function. Patients treated with this modality should be followed cystoscopically, and have appropriate bladder biopsies to detect recurrence every 3 months the first year, every 6 months the second year, and then yearly. The cycle is repeated with each recurrence, and changes in grade, stage, or frequency of recurrence signal the need for more aggressive therapy (radical cystectomy). Urinary cytology is a helpful adjunct, but does not replace the necessity of repeat cystoscopic examination. Superficial bladder tumors are commonly treated by the instillation of the radiomimetic drug triethylenethiophosphoramide (Thiotepa). Patients with recurrent superficial tumors should have a trial of 30 to 60 mg doses in 60 ml of water instilled intravesically every week for 6 weeks, followed by monthly instillations. Recent evidence suggests that Thiotepa instilled immediately after a transurethral resection reduces the chance of recurrence. Several critical points concerning the use of Thiotepa must be emphasized: (1) the bone marrow must be monitored for toxic effects (leukopenia and thrombocytopenia); (2) previous radiotherapy tends to accentuate toxicity, therefore requiring selective treatment; and (3) the effect of Thiotepa is confined to the surface epithelium and may mask deeper penetration, thus delaying diagnosis of an infiltrating lesion. Intravesical insulation of other agents such as bleomycin, triethylene glycol diglyceridyl ether (Epodyl), and 5-fluorouracil also appear to benefit patients with superficial tumors. We employ 5-fluorouracil (5-FU) because it seems to have fewer side effects than Thiotepa. One gram of 5-FU undiluted is administered intravesically as outlined for Thiotepa. (This use of 5-fluorouracil is not listed in the manufacturer's official directive.)

STAGES B AND C. Radiation therapy alone for invasive bladder cancer achieves a 5 year survival of 16 to 20 per cent; therefore, this form of treatment is reserved for the poor risk patients, those with advanced pelvic disease, or as an adjunct to another form of therapy. Recent evidence suggests that cystectomy coupled with preoperative irradiation has achieved survival rates at 5 years approximately twice that of irradiation alone. In these patients, no increase in the operative morbidity and mortality has been observed, other than a slight increase in the incidence of wound infection. We recommend that patients receive 2000 rads of preoperative irradiation to the bladder in 5 days, followed by radical cystectomy within 7 days of completion of the radiotherapy. We employ the ileal conduit as our standard form of diversion and, in select patients, either a transverse colon conduit or ureterosigmoidostomy. A total urethrectomy is performed in those patients with overt tumor or carcinoma in situ near the bladder neck. Those not undergoing urethrectomy at the time of cystectomy should be followed with saline washes of the urethra for cytology every 3 months. Urethrectomy is then performed if positive cytology exists. We recommend partial cystectomy only in those patients who have a solitary infiltrating tumor in an accessible portion of the bladder, with no evidence of surrounding carcinoma in situ. Few patients meet these rigid criteria.

STAGE D_1. Patients with positive lymph nodes below the aortic bifurcation are treated with lymphadenectomy and radical cystectomy. Inasmuch as the prognosis is poor, we administer adjuvant chemotherapy (see below). This mode of treatment has not been proved to be effective. Those patients with gross tumor remaining in the pelvis after cystectomy, or who are felt to be locally unresectable, may benefit from postoperative radiation. Adjuvant chemotherapy may also be given in this setting.

STAGE D_2. Systemic chemotherapy is generally administered for the treatment of advanced bladder cancer, Stage D_2. Those drugs known to produce objective responses include cisplatin, doxorubicin, 5-fluorouracil, methotrexate, mitomycin C, and cyclophosphamide. The response rate varies from 20 to 40 per cent, but few complete responses occur and most patients relapse within 10 months, regardless of therapy. In patients with normal renal function, we administer cisplatin, 80 mg per square meter, in 500 ml of saline over a 4 to 6 hour period, with mannitol and hydration every 3 weeks. (This use of cisplatin is not specifically listed in the manufacturer's official directive.) Cyclophosphamide is given in those with compromised renal function (1 gram per square meter intravenously every 3 weeks).

The primary goal of palliation for the treatment of advanced bladder carcinoma is the relief of symptoms (severe gross hematuria and localized pain), while preserving bladder function. Numerous procedures are now available, including instillation of formalin, hydrostatic pressure balloons, intravesical hyperthermia, cryotherapy, radiation therapy, DMSO (dimethyl sulfoxide), arterial infusions of chemotherapeutic agents, and palliative surgical procedures. We reserve the more aggressive surgical techniques (cystectomy) for the patient in whom other measures have failed to relieve symptoms.

Carcinoma of the Female Urethra

Carcinoma of the female urethra is an uncommon tumor that accounts for less than 0.03 per cent of all malignant diseases occurring in women. We employ the staging system of Grabstald, as follows:

Stage 0:   In situ (limited to mucosa)
Stage A: Submucosal (not beyond submucosa)
Stage B: Muscular (infiltrating periurethral muscle)
Stage C: Periurethral: (1) infiltrating muscular wall of vagina; (2) infiltrating muscular wall of vagina with invasion of vaginal mucosa; (3) infiltrating other adjacent structures such as bladder, labia, and clitoris
Stage D: Metastasis: (1) inguinal lymph nodes; (2) pelvic lymph nodes below aortic bifurcation; (3) lymph nodes above aortic bifurcation; (4) distant

Treatment.   Distal urethral lesions are treated by local excision; however, there is a risk of incontinence. We have recently employed interstitial radiation implantation for the treatment of low stage distal urethral carcinoma, with or without local excision. Anterior lesions and most distal lesions are best managed by anterior exenteration, with excision of the urethra and part of the vagina. These tumors will frequently involve the vagina, cervix, and vulva. With involvement of the labia or vulva, a radical vulvectomy is included as part of the surgical procedure. Since these lesions metastasize to the inguinal lymph nodes, inguinal lymphadenectomy is indicated when palpable adenopathy exists. Inguinal lymphadenectomy is employed only in those patients with demonstrable metastasis because of the potential morbidity of the procedure. With the more advanced lesions, we employ preoperative external irradiation followed by anterior exenteration and, if necessary, vulvectomy and inguinal lymphadenectomy. There is a high incidence of local recurrence (in the range of 50 to 60 per cent) following single modality therapy. Patients who have proved pelvic lymph node involvement undergo palliative irradiation and chemotherapy. We employ cisplatin as outlined under Bladder Cancer. (This use of cisplatin is not specifically listed in the manufacturer's official directive.)

Carcinoma of the Male Urethra

Secondary involvement of the urethra by direct extension of bladder or prostatic cancer is not unusual; however, primary malignancies of the male urethra are distinctly uncommon. These tumors most frequently occur in the fifth and sixth decades of life. Epidermoid carcinoma accounts for three fourths of all lesions, and predominantly involves the bulbomembranous urethra. Transitional cell carcinomas and adenocarcinomas constitute the remainder. Adenocarcinoma originating in the urethra is rare, and most often appears secondary to extension of prostatic adenocarcinoma. Urethral carcinoma generally presents as symptomatic outflow obstruction, and approximately 40 per cent of patients may have an antecedent history of urethral stricture requiring dilatation. Other symptoms include urethral discharage, initial hematuria, dysuria, palpable urethral mass, or cutaneous fistulization. Treatment and prognosis depend upon the stage of the tumor and its position in the urethra. We employ the following staging system:

Stage 0:   In situ carcinoma
Stage A: Invasion of basement membrane, but not into the corpus spongiosum or prostate
Stage B: Invasion of the corpus spongiosum or prostate
Stage C: Invasion outside the corpus spongiosum or prostate
Stage D: Metastatic disease

Treatment.   We treat superficial tumors of the anterior urethra with partial urethrectomy and inguinal lymphadenectomy when palpable lymph nodes persist. The more advanced Stage B and C lesions invade the corpus spongiosum, and require partial or total penectomy. Biopsy-proved inguinal adenopathy, when present, will require a superficial node dissection.

Lesions of the posterior urethra tend to be invasive and are best treated with a radical cystoprostatectomy, en bloc urethrectomy, and bilateral pelvic lymph node dissection. In most posterior urethral tumors, partial or total penectomy is not required. Invasive tumors in and around the membranous urethra require more aggressive surgery in the form of radical cystoprostatectomy, en bloc urethrectomy, and excision of the symphysis pubis. The routine employment of preoperative or postoperative irradiation has not been proved beneficial, but we continue to administer preoperative irradiation in deep, invasive epidermal, and transitional cell carcinomas.

Carcinoma of the Penis

Carcinoma of the penis accounts for less than 1 per cent of all male cancers. This neoplasm, associated with chronic irritation and smegma, occurs almost exclusively in uncircumcised male patients. In some Far Eastern countries, it accounts for approximately 18 to 20 per cent of cancers in men. We employ the following staging system of Jackson:

Stage 1: Tumor limited to the glans penis and/or prepuce

Stage 2: Invasion into the shaft or corpora, but without nodal or distant metastases

Stage 3: Tumor confined to the shaft, with proved regional node metastases

Stage 4: Invasion from the shaft, with inoperable regional node involvement or distant metastases

Treatment. STAGE 1. Circumcision alone is used for small lesions confined to the foreskin. Superficial lesions on the penile shaft should be excised with an adequate margin of normal tissue. In either case, careful follow-up is required to rule out any local recurrence. Radiation therapy has been proposed as a method of preserving the phallus, and presents an alternative to local excision for superficial lesions.

STAGE 2. For this stage of the disease, partial penile amputation is employed 2 cm proximal to the area of cancer involvement. Total penectomy is required in those cases in which the lesion is near the penile base. Large lesions involving the base of the penis or abdominal wall are best treated by penectomy with en bloc peniculectomy and bilateral node dissection. External beam irradiation is not preferred in Stage 2 lesions, since necrosis and stricture often result. Also, approximately 50 per cent of these lesions will be refractory to treatment, or will recur.

STAGE 3. Patients with palpable nodes at the time of penectomy are followed for 4 weeks before they are considered to be true clinical Stage 3. During this time, a course of antimicrobials is given to distinguish an inflammatory reaction from actual nodal involvement with tumor. Those patients with positive inguinal nodes remaining 4 weeks after removal of the primary tumor are classified as Stage 3, and undergo lymphadenectomy. Routine sentinel node biopsy may also be of value. We feel that bilateral dissection is indicated because of the desiccation of lymphatics at the base of the penis. We avoid incision into the groin crease, and employ a skin bridge technique of node dissection, making a pair of curved incisions above and below the groin crease. If the lymph nodes appear negative at the level of the bifurcation of the iliac vessels, the lymphadenectomy is begun at this area and continued downward to include the superficial and deep iliac nodes, in addition to the obturator nodes. The specimen is passed en bloc under the skin bridge and dissection of the superficial and deep groin lymphatics, as well as muscle fascial coverings, is carried out through the lower part of the incision. We treat the more involved site first, followed by a 6 week rest period, and then proceed with the opposite groin dissection.

STAGE 4. Patients with disease extending beyond the regional lymph nodes have a dismal prognosis. Although responses with the use of bleomycin have been reported, its value in the chemotherapeutic treatment of metastatic epidermoid carcinoma of the penis has been limited. Some studies show that the combination of bleomycin and methotrexate may be effective in the treatment of this metastatic disease. We employ high dose methotrexate followed by citrovorum factor rescue in patients with Stage 4 disease.

Sarcoma

Pelvic sarcomas are relatively uncommon, and the site of the primary tumor may be obscure. They are consequently considered collectively. In children, sarcomas of the bladder have a somewhat more favorable prognosis than rhabdomyosarcoma of the prostate. However, the prognosis for either is poor. Surgical excision often requires radical pelvic exenteration, since involvement of contiguous organs is typical. Preoperative irradiation and chemotherapy (vincristine, actinomycin D, cyclophosphamide) have improved the results of treatment and may dramatically decrease the size of a tumor, rendering it resectable. Leiomyosarcoma of the prostate is more commonly seen in the older adult, often a circumscribed lesion, and tends to be less aggressive than those seen in children. Limited procedures, such as transurethral resection of obstructing lesions, and chemotherapy may provide dramatic symptomatic relief in patients who are not candidates for radical extirpation.

Malignant Tumors of the Prostate

Adenocarcinoma. Prostate cancer is the second most common malignancy in men, ranking third in cancer-related deaths for those 55 years of age and older. An estimated 60,000 new cases of prostate cancer will be diagnosed this year, along with 20,000 deaths attributable to the disease. Adenocarcinoma is the most common malignant tumor of the prostate gland; occurrence is higher in blacks than in whites.

The staging system which we have adopted is as follows:

Stage A: Tumor not suspected clinically

Stage A_1:   One or several microscopic foci of tumor in transurethral resection (TUR) or open prostatectomy specimen

Stage A_2:   Multiple foci of tumor in TUR or open prostatectomy specimen, usually higher grade

Stage B: Clinically detectable tumor confined to the gland

Stage B_1:   Tumor involves one lobe and is less than 2 cm in size

Stage B_2:   Tumor involves more than one lobe

Stage C: Tumor extending through the prostatic capsule or into the seminal vesicle

Stage D_1:   Tumor invading local structures or metastasizing to pelvic lymph nodes

Stage D_2:   Distant metastases

In addition to clinical staging, the tumor should be graded pathologically. Evidence exists that survival correlates not only with clinical stage but also with initial pathologic grade of the tumor. Prostatic neoplasms spread by local extension, lymphatics, and hematogenous dissemination. Thus, tests to determine the spread of prostatic cancer should evaluate the primary roots of metastases to lymph nodes, bones, liver, and lungs. Radiologic staging should include chest x-ray, intravenous pyelogram, radionucleotide bone scan, and radiographic skeletal roentgenograms of suspicious areas. Ultrasound and computed tomography scanning, although new, seem to offer assistance in tumor staging. The value of lymphangiography in staging remains uncertain. Serum acid phosphatase is elevated in extracapsular and metastatic disease, and is elevated in two thirds of patients with Stage D lesions. An abnormal high value is seen in only 5 per cent of patients with disease limited to the prostate; thus, the acid phosphatase is not a screening test for prostatic cancer, since it shows elevated levels only late in the disease process. A number of nonprostatic diseases will elevate acid phosphatase, including multiple myeloma, osteogenic sarcoma, thrombocytopenia, Gaucher's disease, nonprostatic malignant tumors with bone metastases, Paget's disease, hyperparathyroidism, osteoporosis, and hematologic neoplasms. The newer methods of acid phosphatase determination, including radioimmunoassay and counterimmunoelectrophoresis, have been proved more sensitive and may improve our ability to detect occult metastases and perhaps even lesions confined to the prostate.

Treatment. Few diseases generate more controversy concerning treatment than prostatic cancer. The following staging categories and their definitions incorporate our approach to treatment modalities for this disease.

STAGE A_1. This stage is defined as being unsuspected clinically and found in the course of transurethral resection or open prostatectomy for "benign disease." The patient's pathology report will usually show one to several microfoci of well differentiated adenocarcinoma. We believe that this patient should be restudied in 3 months, with transurethral resection and biopsies, either transperineally or transrectally. If tumor is then detected, either radical prostatectomy or definitive irradiation is recommended.

STAGE A_2. This patient's pathologic report demonstrates more than 25 per cent of the gland involved with adenocarcinoma. The grade is usually moderately to poorly differentiated. These patients are offered staging pelvic lymphadenectomy along with radical retropubic prostatectomy or definitive irradiation therapy.

STAGE B. The incidence of positive pelvic lymph nodes with a Stage B neoplasm approaches 20 per cent. The propensity for lymph node involvement tends to increase with the size and grade of the tumor. We therefore recommend a staging pelvic lymphadenectomy followed by radical prostatectomy. The radical prostatectomy may be via either the perineal or the retropubic approach; however, most urologists favor the retropubic approach. Both approaches, in our experience, have been followed by an almost 100 per cent incidence of impotence. Varying degrees of urinary stress incontinence may be expected with each procedure as well (6 to 25 per cent).

Radiation therapy offers some distinct advantages over radical surgery; these include avoidance of extensive surgery and preservation of potency in about 50 per cent of cases. However, complications do occur, and include posttherapeutic enteritis, prostatitis, lymphedema, impotence, and urethral stricture. Our radiotherapists treat the pelvis with 5000 rads, and an additional boost of 2000 rads to the prostate is given over a 7 to 8 week period. Radiotherapy has become a definite alternative to surgery in the treatment of Stage B disease, but external beam irradiation therapy does not achieve results comparable to those obtained with radical prostatectomy for Stage B carcinoma. We therefore favor radical prostatectomy over irradiation for Stage B_1 disease, as well as for Stage B_2, although there is no current information supporting surgery for true Stage B_2. Regardless, patients should be advised as to this alternative mode of therapy. Those patients refusing radical prostatectomy are offered staging pelvic lymphadenectomy coupled with either radioactive ^{125}I seeds into the prostate or definitive postoperative irradiation therapy. It should be emphasized that pelvic lymphadenectomy is only a staging procedure, and there is no evidence that it is curative with lymph nodal involvement.

STAGE C. This neoplasm has extended beyond the confines of the prostatic capsule, acid phosphatase level is normal, and radiologic bone survey is negative for tumor spread. Approximately 60 per cent of patients with Stage C will have positive lymph nodes, and therefore are reclassified as Stage D. We recommend that most Stage C patients have a staging lymphadenectomy and either external beam radiotherapy postoperatively or implantation of radioactive material at the time of the lymphadenectomy. We do not recommend interstitial irradiation in bulky Stage C lesions, since the tumor borders are indistinct and accurate placing of needles or seeds is difficult, resulting in an uneven and often inadequate dose. Occasionally, a patient with a fairly small, well to moderately differentiated tumor may be treated by radical prostatectomy. Some surgeons have given such patients preoperative estrogens in an attempt to shrink the primary neoplasm prior to radical prostatectomy; endocrine manipulation alone, however, has no effect on the survival rates in Stage C disease.

STAGE D_1. The concept of dividing the D categories into D_1 and D_2 is relatively new, resulting from the recent introduction and use of pelvic lymphadenectomy in the detection of lymph node involvement. The chance for cure for patients with even minimal metastatic carcinoma is slight, although there are a few reports of cure after radical treatment of Stage D_1 prostatic carcinoma. Upon finding positive lymph nodes at the time of staging lymphadenectomy, we complete the lymphadenectomy and implant radioactive seeds into the prostate, following this with external beam irradiation to the pelvis. An alternative management plan is definitive postoperative photon therapy alone. Because errors occur in the evaluation of lymph nodes at the time of frozen section, some urologists recommend staging lymphadenectomy alone, followed in 3 to 4 days by perineal prostatectomy if permanent sections are pathologically negative. We do not routinely employ this form of treatment unless there is a reasonable question of the status of the lymph nodes on frozen section. Patients who are found to have numerous positive lymph nodes above the bifurcation of the internal and external iliac vessels are not candidates for local therapy; recommendation is made for an orchiectomy or diethylstilbestrol therapy.

STAGE D_2. The point at which hormonal manipulation is instituted remains controversial. At present, hormonal therapy is the treatment of choice for metastatic carcinoma of the prostate, and 70 to 80 per cent of patients will experience improvement with this treatment. Patients receive endocrine manipulation, in the form of either orchiectomy or diethylstilbestrol (DES), 1 mg three times daily. It is often helpful to obtain a serum testosterone evaluation on patients taking DES to confirm complete suppression. We occasionally see a patient who has relapse of the disease because the prescribed or adequate doses of DES are not administered. Orchiectomy or adequate estrogen therapy is equally effective in controlling the symptoms of metastatic carcinoma of the prostate. In relapse or tumor escape following initial therapy with either estrogens or orchiectomy, the tumor is frequently hormonally unresponsive to other agents. Further treatment with hypophysectomy, bilateral adrenalectomy, or antiandrogens rarely improves symptoms or survival rates.

We currently reserve chemotherapy for patients who fail to respond to hormonal manipulation; in the future, we may find that earlier institution of chemotherapy will prolong the survival. For patients unresponsive to hormonal therapy, we employ cyclophosphamide, 1 gram per square meter intravenously every 3 weeks. An alternative form of treatment is as follows: methotrexate, 15 mg per square meter intravenously weekly for 8 weeks, total dose not to exceed 25 mg weekly; 5-fluorouracil, 300 mg per square meter weekly intravenously for 8 weeks, total dose not to exceed 500 mg per week; and cyclophosphamide, 100 mg orally daily. Prednisone is administered daily with dose reductions at 2 week intervals, 30 mg, 15 mg, 5 mg, and then discontinued. Vincristine, 1 mg intravenously weekly, is administered until neurotoxicity develops and is then discontinued. At the end of 8 weeks 5-fluorouracil and methotrexate are continued orally at the same dose.

Dose reductions for both of the aforementioned regimens are necessary in patients with previous irradiation therapy. Localized bone pain can be successfully treated with cobalt irradiation therapy in some instances. Analgesics have been used to control pain secondary to metastatic disease with varying results. Simple aspirin-containing compounds have relieved pain in about 70 per cent of patients, and Brompton's cocktail has also been proved useful in treating severe pain.

Carcinoma of the Testis

Roughly 2 per cent of cancers in the male occur in the testis. Nearly 60 per cent of these tumors, occurring in a young age group, are found in men between the ages of 25 and 44, and represent the most common malignancy in men between 29 and 35 years of age. There are an estimated 2500 new cases annually; the overall incidence has been reported to be 2.2 per 100,000 male subjects per year.

Testicular tumors begin as small intratesticular lesions contained within the tunica albuginea. Seminoma, teratoma, and embryonal cell carcinoma usually spread by the lymphatic route, but choriocarcinoma is disseminated not only by the lymphatic group, but also by the venous system. Thirty-five per cent of patients with testicular tumors will have either lymphatic or distant metastases when first diagnosed. The etiology of these tumors remains elusive; however, there may be an association with cryptorchidism.

During the last decade, we have witnessed marked changes both in the modes of therapy and the survival rates in patients with testicular tumors. These changes stem from progress in three areas: chemotherapy, employment of meticulous retroperitoneal lymphadenectomy, and the use of serum markers. The timely employment of these three advances has dramatically improved the poor prognosis formerly associated with nonseminomatous tumors; thus at present, these tumors carry the best prognosis of any genitourinary malignant tumor, and of any solid tumor encountered in the adult male.

Staging. Testicular tumors are divided into two major groups: seminomas and nonseminomas. We stage testicular tumors clinically or pathologically as follows:

Stage A: Tumor confined to the testis with no metastasis
Stage B: Metastases to retroperitoneal lymph nodes
Stage B_1:   Retroperitoneal metastases, in fewer than six lymph nodes
Stage B_2:   Retroperitoneal metastases, more than six positive lymph nodes
Stage B_3:   Massive retroperitoneal disease
Stage C: Metastases to lymph nodes above the diaphragm or other viscera (most commonly pulmonary metastases)

The pretreatment diagnostic evaluation of patients with testicular tumors will depend upon the cell type. In general, tests should include chest x-ray with full lung tomography, intravenous pyelography, and liver function tests. Ultrasound and computed tomography of the retroperitoneum are also helpful in defining the stage of the disease. Lymphangiography is employed only in patients with seminoma. We do not routinely employ scalene lymph node biopsy. One of

the more dramatic advances during the last 5 years in the management of testicular tumor has been the development of tumor markers, which are helpful in the early detection, staging, and follow-up of such tumors. Two proteins that have been isolated in the serum of patients with germ cell tumors of the testis are the beta subunit of human chorionic gonadotropin (beta HCG), and alpha-fetoprotein. While the presence of elevated markers indicates nonseminomatous germinal cell tumors with great accuracy, negative studies do not rule out their presence. Therefore, patients with suspicious testicular masses should undergo appropriate surgical evaluation. Patients with the histologic diagnosis of seminoma accompanied by elevated alpha-fetoprotein will have nonseminomatous elements present, since pure seminoma does not produce an elevated alpha-fetoprotein. In addition, some seminomas can cause elevation of serum beta HCG. We feel this portends a poor prognosis, and thus patients who have persistently elevated beta HCG after orchiectomy for seminoma should be included in the treatment plan for nonseminomas (see below).

Pretreatment elevation of serum markers returns to normal with effective therapy. If there remains a persistently elevated level after appropriate therapy, recurrent tumor is invariably present. In addition to alpha-fetoprotein and beta HCG, a number of other markers are currently being investigated for their use in tumor detection.

Treatment. SEMINOMA, STAGES A, B, AND B_2. The diagnosis of seminoma of the testis, as with nonseminoma, is made by a radical inguinal orchiectomy with excision of the cord and testis. Scrotal orchiectomy carries the risk of contaminating the scrotum and providing other means of metastasis, particularly to the inguinal lymph nodes. The radiologic procedures previously outlined are performed in an attempt to stage the disease accurately. Primary treatment for these low stage seminomas is definitive irradiation therapy; patients with Stage A disease receive a total of 2500 rads over a 3 week period to the ipsilateral inguinal, iliac, and bilateral para-aortic caval nodes to the level of the diaphragm. Those patients with Stage B_1 and B_2 tumors should receive an additional boost of 1000 rads to the involved retroperitoneal areas, as well as 2500 rads to the mediastinum and supraclavicular regions. The ipsilateral hemiscrotum should also be irradiated if a scrotal orchiectomy has been performed.

SEMINOMA, STAGES B_3 AND C. The survival rate for patients with Stages B_3 and C tumors treated with irradiation therapy alone has been poor (22 per cent). Because of the dismal prognosis associated with advanced disease, routine irradiation is not felt to be adequate for these patients, even when whole abdominal irradiation and boosts are given to areas of known tumor. For this reason, we feel that aggressive preirradiation chemotherapy is indicated. Currently, our treatment plan for advanced seminoma consists of an induction course of intensive systemic chemotherapy followed by irradiation. The dosage schedule for such chemotherapeutic agents, if given subsequent to x-ray therapy, would almost certainly have to be reduced. The drugs consist of actinomycin D, vincristine, and cyclophosphamide: 0.5 mg of actinomycin D is given on days 1 through 5 of the 8 day cycle; vincristine in a dose of 1.8 mg is administered intravenously on days 1 and 8; 600 mg of cyclophosphamide is given intravenously on days 1, 3, and 8 on the cycle. The patient is admitted on day 1 and discharged on day 3. The rest of this cycle is carried out on an outpatient basis. In elderly patients, or in patients who have received previous irradiation therapy, it is necessary to decrease the dosages of the chemotherapeutic agents. We have found good patient tolerance and minimal side effects when employing this regimen. The cycle is repeated in 3 weeks, and the disease process reassessed. Those patients demonstrating a complete response to the program undergo irradiation therapy as outlined for Stage B lesions. In those patients not demonstrating a complete response, another course of chemotherapy is given, followed by irradiation. Upon completion of the irradiation, we commence with adjuvant chemotherapy for 6 months, consisting of 1 gram of cyclophosphamide per square meter every 4 weeks. Any residual retroperitoneal tumor mass would necessitate a radical retroperitoneal lymphadenectomy. During the last 2 years, we have managed 5 patients with this regimen, and all remain alive and well.

NONSEMINOMATOUS GERMINAL CELL TUMORS. Our treatment plan for all stages is based on a radical retroperitoneal lymphadenectomy. Bilateral lymphadenectomy is performed, including both renal lymphatics, aortic, caval, ipsilateral iliac, and obturator lymphatics. We classify nonseminomatous lesions into two groups: those with no or minimal disease (Stages A, B_1 and B_2), and those with advanced disease (Stages B_3 and C).

STAGE A. If after the appropriate radiologic evaluation no disease is detected in the retroperitoneum, the patient undergoes a radical retroperitoneal lymphadenectomy. When the retroperitoneal nodes are negative and there is no evidence of other distant metastases, we recommend close follow-up in the form of chest x-ray and serum markers every 3 months for 2 years, and every 6 months thereafter.

STAGE B_1. These patients are found to have fewer than six positive nodes at the time of radical retroperitoneal lymphadenectomy. It is felt that these patients are at high risk for tumor recurrence; postoperative chemotherapy is therefore employed in the form of vinblastine (Velban) and bleomycin. Bleomycin is given in doses of 30 units intravenously twice weekly for 5 weeks. Vinblastine is used in a dose of 10 mg intravenously on day 1, 15 mg on day 8, and 20 mg on day 22. We then continue adjuvant chemotherapy with cyclic actinomycin D, given every 2 months for the remainder of the first year, and every 3 months for the second year (10 micrograms per kg per day, each day for 5 days).

STAGE B_2. Treatment is as outlined for Stage B_1.

STAGES B_3 AND C. Because of the difficulty in excising large retroperitoneal tumor masses, these patients should undergo prior chemotherapy. Our preference is a combination of vinblastine (Velban), bleomycin, and cisplatin. The dosages are as follows: cisplatin, 20 mg per square meter intravenously daily for 5 days every 3 weeks for three to four courses; bleomycin, 30 units intravenously weekly (day 2 of each week) for 12 consecutive doses; and vinblastine, 0.15 to 0.2 mg per kg intravenously (days 1 and 2) every 3 weeks for three to four courses. This chemotherapeutic regimen can be very toxic, and at times fatal; it should be used only by clinicians well qualified in the administration of chemotherapeutic drugs. Upon completion of the course outlined above, the patient then undergoes a radical retroperitoneal lymphadenectomy. Those patients found to have no tumor or mature teratomatous elements at lymphadenectomy then receive another course of vinblastine, bleomycin, and cisplatin, followed by cyclic actinomycin D for 2 years. Patients showing persistent primitive elements receive two further courses of vinblastine, cisplatin, and bleomycin, followed by cyclic actinomycin D for 2 years. The total dose of bleomycin in any of these regimens should not exceed 400 units.

Patients with Stage C disease are treated similarly. Persistence of radiographically detectable tumor, especially in the lungs after chemotherapy, indicates the need for excision of the residual lesions. Such patients should be followed with chest x-ray and serum markers every 2 months for 2 years, and every 6 months thereafter.

We have recently seen three patients with persistence of pulmonary metastases and abdominal disease after three to seven courses of vinblastine, bleomycin, and cisplatin. They were approached surgically through a median sternotomy coupled with a midline abdominal incision. In this fashion we have resected multiple pulmonary nodules, enlarged supraclavicular masses, and abdominal disease.

URETHRAL STRICTURE

method of
CECIL MORGAN, Jr., M.D.
Birmingham, Alabama

Treatment of urethral stricture is so intertwined with diagnosis that the two must be considered simultaneously. Stricture is suspected when a patient complains of narrow urinary stream with straining to void and postvoiding dribbling, perhaps accompanied by discomfort on urination. Recurrent urinary tract infection which either does not clear on appropriate antimicrobials as indicated by urine culture or immediately recurs after adequate treatment is also an indication to search for urethral stricture. Other symptoms are urinary urge and stress incontinence and persistent urethral discharge. When there has been pelvic trauma and difficulty voiding, recent urethral or prostatic surgery, or even catheterization, there may be stricture.

Diagnosis is based on radiographic and direct visualization of the stricture, and/or calibration with either sounds or bougies à boule. Should Foley catheter or sounds encounter resistance on passage, they must not be forced, because if stricture is present, injury to the mucosa or a false urethral passage may occur. This causes bleeding, making further diagnosis and treatment much more difficult. Gentleness is the byword! Diagnosis should include an accurate evaluation of properly collected urine by microscopic examination of the centrifuged sediment, and urine culture. If infection is present and emergency relief of urinary retention is not necessary, appropriate antimicrobial treatment is given for 5 to 7 days. The standard procedure demonstrating urethral stricture is retrograde instillation of contrast material into the urethra for radiographic study. Fifty per cent sodium diatrizoate (Hypaque) is quite satisfactory for all urethral strictures. The voiding cystourethrogram is the best method for determining presence and location of obstruction by posterior urethral valves and other strictures. The usual technique requires catheter passage. If this is impossible, a voiding film taken during intravenous urogram may show stricture. Van Buren sounds rarely localize stricture adequately and may miss multiple lesions. Bougie à boule in progressive sizes can give exact location as related to external anatomy. To further delineate composition, length, and multiplicity, direct vision urethroscopy completes the diagnostic regimen.

Treatment varies with location. Urethral meatal stenosis in males is often revealed by chronic irritation and, in small boys, by frequent pulling of genitalia. Urethral meatotomy is easily done on infants by clamping the meatus ventrally with a mosquito hemostat without anesthesia, and then cutting the clamped tissue. This is too painful in older boys, but can be done in the office using local anesthesia. More often it is done on an outpatient basis, using general anesthesia. Sutures are not used, as they may cause small scars which may deviate the urinary stream. It is simple and totally effective to instruct parents to daily open the meatus by separating the little incision, usually after a bath, for 7 days and then every other day for 7 more. Close inspection and follow-up are necessary to ensure that the meatus heals open. Results are usually dramatic and quite pleasing.

Urethral meatal stenosis in female children is best found by bougie à boule calibration under anesthesia. A normal size for the meatus is not recognized by me as it relates to symptoms, for some may be of small size and the children have no voiding problems. Others with marked dysuria or recurrent urinary infections and small meatus benefit greatly from meatotomy. It is done by incising the ring-like fibrous band at the meatus over Walther sounds ventrally at the 6 o'clock position so that a bougie à boule of the caliber of the rest of the urethra will pass easily. Lateral and apical areas of the incision are sutured mucosa to mucosa with three 5–0 Dexon sutures. Meatotomy in adult females may be done in the office, using local anesthesia. A single urethral dilatation may be effective in some female children, but recurrence of the stenosis occurs and repeated dilatation should be avoided, as it is quite traumatic to the child. A theoretical problem of creating hypospadias in females with accompanying infection and incontinence has not been encountered as the children grow up. In older females, mild urethral stenosis dilatation may be entirely satisfactory.

After diagnosis and control or suppression of infection with nitrofurantoin or trimethoprim-sulfamethoxazole, if there is urinary retention and gentle catheterization fails, a more direct approach is needed. It is quite difficult to do an adequate urethral instrumentation while the patient is lying in bed. A stricture is much easier to negotiate with the patient in lithotomy position in either a treatment room or cystoscopy suite. Genitalia are prepared with povidone-iodine (Betadine) and parenteral or intravenous sedation is given, using narcotics or diazepam (Valium). Local urethral analgesia is achieved by low pressure instillation of 5 to 10 ml of 1 or 2 per cent lidocaine by small Asepto syringe into the urethra. The urethra should be gently compressed distally (penile clamp) for 5 to 10 minutes. Using sterile technique with draping and handling of instruments, filiforms can then be placed into the urethra. A pigtail or spiral tip is usually most effective, although straight tips may function well. Often there are several blind-ending pockets, and if filled with multiple filiforms, usually another one will be free to pass into the true urethra.

The injection of lubricating jellies in the urethra is to be avoided for two reasons: (1) By urethrogram, contrast material injected under pressure can be seen in the venous system of the penis and pelvis. Therefore, lubricating jellies can be injected into the general circulation. The increased risk of sepsis is obvious. (2) Pulmonary emboli of these materials have been reported.

Some patients have great intolerance for stricture negotiation, even under adequate sedation. General or spinal anesthesia is then waranted, and often the stricture can be passed with much greater ease because of total perineal relaxation.

For ease of passage in males, the penis should be extended by stretch. In difficult cases, using a gloved finger in the rectum as a proprioceptive guide, Van Buren sounds can be passed without forming a false passage. Once a filiform has been passed through the stricture into the bladder, it can be followed by progressive sizes of Philips woven bougies or catheters, or by Le Fort metal sounds, using their screw-on tips. Depending on the density of stricture, the size of final dilatation is variable, but usually 24 French is adequate. If filiforms cannot be placed in this manner, the urologist may be able to place one by direct visualization of the lumen in stricture by cystoscopy. Whenever stricture dilatation occurs, scar tissue is torn and must heal by new scar formation, which will again contract to reform a stricture.

In emergency situations, suprapubic catheter placement can be done, using a trochar passed into the distended bladder at bedside. Specialized kits are available for small temporary plastic catheter (Bardic Desert Supracath, C. R. Bard Co.), and instructions must be followed carefully to avoid injury. Suprapubic cystostomy is done if other methods fail, and placement of the catheter obliquely through the abdominal wall exiting high above the pubic symphysis prevents fistula formation. Catheters of size 26 to 30 French should be used for best drainage. Later, with bladder decompression and reduction of edema, urethral calibration will be easier. If a filiform can be passed, catheter drainage may be established by using the specialized Councill Foley and obturator with a screw tip which passes through the end of the Councill catheter. Once the device follows the filiform into the bladder and the Foley balloon is inflated, the obturator attached to the filiform is removed, leaving the Foley catheter in place. A less traumatic method is dilating the stricture over catheters by changing to a larger size every 36 to 48 hours until 24 French is reached. Using a metal catheter guide can be dangerous, possibly causing bladder perforations and false passages, and should be attempted only by the most experienced.

Once an adequate channel has been established, periodic dilatation, from weeks to months, may be required. Each time, complications such as sepsis, bleeding, and false passages can occur. Slight bleeding will be self-limiting, and the patient can use a gauze sponge held over the meatus by a small rubber band after office dilatation to prevent soilage. For patient comfort, phenazopyridine HCl (Pyridium), 100 to 200 mg orally every 6 to 8 hours as needed, may be prescribed. Antibiotic use is optional.

Definitive surgical repair can be attempted by endoscopic or transurethral means. For bladder neck contracture, deep incisions at 5 and 7 o'clock from the bladder neck to the veru can be done with Collins knife electrode, often resulting in permanent relief. If bladder neck contracture is recurrent, a suprapubic approach and YV-plasty of the bladder neck is satisfactory.

The Otis urethrotome has long been used for incision of urethral strictures, but an alternative approach is the newly developed direct vision, cystoscopic cold knife incision. Injection of the treated stricture with steroids has been advocated to reduce the inflammatory response and gain more lasting results. Posterior urethral valves in children are managed by transurethral incision, electroresection, or mechanical rupture for definitive treatment.

Choice of open surgical procedures depends on location and extent of the stricture. If it is quite short in the pendulous or bulbous urethra, simple excision with reanastomosis, using beveling of the ends, is effective. The most extensively used is the method of Johanson, a two-stage procedure. First, the stricture is opened and marsupialized, sewn to surrounding skin. This fistula is allowed to heal for 4 to 6 months, and if the proximal and distal urethral openings are adequate, secondary closure is done, using the principle of Denis Browne (buried intact epithelium). When the stricture is deep in the perineal urethra, at or near the urethral sphincter, a two-stage technique (Turner-Warwick), using scrotal skin inlay may be used. Pelvic fracture and disruption of urethra require either immediate suprapubic cystostomy or an attempt at repair by the urologist. If only cystostomy is done and the urethra is scarred and the ends widely separated, the transpubic approach of Waterhouse is used.

In those unfortunate individuals who have severe stricture and infection resulting in numerous urethrocutaneous fistulas (watering-pot perineum), the initial treatment is suprapubic cystostomy and control of infection. After 6 or more months definitive repair may be attempted.

The most important recent surgical development is the single stage repair by Horton and Devine. The stricture is incised to normal urethra, and the defect is closed by a non-hair-bearing, full thickness free skin patchgraft, usually taken from the foreskin. It is sewn with the epithelial surface in the urethral lumen. Strictures of any length, including those going through the membranous urethra, can be repaired. Recurrent strictures and those partially treated by first stage operations can likewise be treated with the skin patchgraft. Although it is not 100 per cent successful, even failures can be repaired with this same technique, which is my method of choice.

RENAL CALCULI

method of
WILLIAM H. BOYCE, M.D.
Winston-Salem, North Carolina

Modern medical management of renal calculi is capable of preventing new stone formation in the majority of patients; of slowing or stabilizing growth of existing stones; and of effecting dissolution of certain types of calculi. From the clinician's point of view the presence of a renal calculus is a sign of a vast array of metabolic, endocrinologic, infectious, malignant, degenerative, and other diseases or disturbances of function, especially in the urinary, gastrointestinal, and skeletal systems. Categorically, some 16 per cent of patients with stones have "infectious calculi," and approximately 12 per cent have an endocrinologic, malignant, myeloproliferative,

metabolic, or other recognizable syndrome. The remaining 72 per cent are generally labeled "idiopathic." This article will be limited to consideration of the idiopathic category, since the recognition and treatment of other categories are generally well known and exceed the scope of this review. It is important that every patient with a renal calculus have an adequate diagnostic evaluation. This is especially true of patients with infectious stones since the infection is most frequently, if not always, a secondary phenomenon. In this situation there is no satisfactory simplistic classification which ipso facto can direct treatment. The time-honored classification based on chemical or crystalline analysis of the stone is a case in point. The stone should be analyzed, but composition of the stone should not be the sole determinant for therapy, since a diversity of factors may result in formation of stones of similar composition. The vagaries of so diverse a system are largely related to the complex interplay of the mechanisms by which crystalline substances develop in the urinary passages. Nucleation, aggregation, crystal growth, and possibly induction are all aspects of stone formation. The initiation or nucleation of crystals may be due to simple supersaturation of urine, but this is never the sole factor, since heterotopic nucleation, epitaxy, and a host of other factors are always operational. Growth of urinary crystals is influenced by time, retention, relative concentrations of crystalloids, inhibitors, and many other influences. Our knowledge of crystal nucleation and growth in urine is relatively meager, yet it greatly exceeds our knowledge of crystal aggregation and true induction of crystal deposition on certain substrates. This should not lead the patient or the physician to despair of effective treatment but rather to understand such apparent contradictions as why gouty patients may form calcium oxalate stones, why most uric acid stones occur in nongouty patients, and why relative concentrations of urinary crystalloids are more important indices for treatment than are absolute excretion rates. In stone-forming patients there is no absolute numerical description for hypercalciuria, since the term is relative to concentrations of other ions, especially oxalates, urates, cystine, and phosphates. The important guide for treatment is a complete biochemical profile of the individual plus his or her response to deprivation or loading of selected crystallites.

The essentials for successful management of the stone former require:

1. A proper metabolic and urologic evaluation of each patient.

2. A complete program designed for each patient.

3. Adequate explanation to the patient in such manner as to enlist his or her full understanding and cooperation.

4. A system to monitor the effects of the program and to make adjustments until the desired results have been achieved.

The Detailed Evaluation of Stone-Formers

A minimum of 5 days' continuous observation is required for even the most elementary work-up. There are many published "protocols," any of which is satisfactory if the results are interpreted in light of the history, physical examination, and related data available for each patient. The anatomic and physiologic function of the urinary system is important in all patients with stones but especially so when infection coexists.

This basic screening protocol will identify hypercalciuria as defined by the specific conditions of the study. It will determine if the hypercalciuria is simply alimentative or tractable, that is, relatively responsive to reduced intake; or intractable, that is, continues even with prolonged starvation. Pak has referred to the latter as "renal leak" hypercalciuria. The presence of persistently low urinary phosphate levels or high oxalate, cystine, or urate excretion may be significant factors in developing a program for the individual patient. "High" in this terminology is not above a theoretic "normal range" but rather reflects concentrations persistently above one standard deviation for the protocol in force. This is modified by ratios with other crystalloids; a high calcium level is "higher" if oxalate level is also increased.

It is virtually impossible to develop a satisfactory diagnostic evaluation of the stone-forming patient within the environs of a hospital geared to general patient care without a protocol-like program to control the variables of diet, sample collections, and testing.

Design of a Therapeutic Program for Each Patient

In their most elementary form, the current concepts of therapy are directed toward achieving a urine dilute in all potentially crystallizable substances. To this end there are general measures applicable to all patients and specific measures designed to reduce absolute or relative concentrations of individual crystalloids.

General Measures

Fluid Intake. Fluid intake should include water in maximal tolerable quantities. The majority of the common beverages, especially tea and citrus juices, contain undesirable amounts of oxalate, sodium, sugars, and other substances.

There is no substitute for water, although the need for distilled as opposed to tap water is debatable.

Diet. Diet should be designed to provide an adequate nutrition with avoidance of excess of calories and stone-forming crystalloids, especially calcium, oxalate, and urate. Highly specialized diets are poorly tolerated, and their efficacy in "idiopathic" stone disease is questionable. Since the majority of calculi are calcigerous, the most commonly used diet attempts to reduce calcium absorption by limiting calcium content to 400 mg per day and sodium intake to 100 mEq per day, and reducing caloric intake to achieve a minimal functional body weight. This diet is also relatively low in acid ash, purine, and oxalate content.

Specific Measures

The need to consider all aspects of the patient's metabolic profile and to undertake correction of *all* rather than a single aberration cannot be overemphasized. The key to success is continued monitoring of the patient after the program is established.

Hypercalciuric Patients. Hypercalciuric patients exhibit a wide range of responses to restrictive measures. Seventy-three per cent of sterile calcium oxalate stone-formers are demonstrably hypercalciuric; the remaining 27 per cent are normocalciuric. The alimentative or simple absorptive hypercalciuric (47 per cent of oxalate stone formers) responds promptly to reduced oral intake of calcium, a response that is accentuated by a low-sodium diet. Indeed, for the patient who has formed only an occasional stone, adjustment of diet and water intake may be the only required therapy.

At the other extreme of hypercalciuria are the "renal leak" patients (12 per cent of oxalate stone formers) whose response to oral restriction is neither prompt nor dramatic. In addition to all the aforementioned measures, these patients require hydrochlorothiazide. The average maintenance dose of 50 mg every 12 hours is reached by increasing the dosage gradually over a period of 4 weeks.

Approximately 14 per cent of oxalate stone formers occupy a position intermediate between the tractable and the intractable hypercalciuric patients. Since they exhibit many of the traits of both groups, they probably represent varying combinations of hyperabsorption and renal loss of calcium. Treatment of these patients is usually begun with the aforementioned general measures plus administration of neutral potassium phosphate. The indications for phosphate supplementation may include either a persistently low urinary phosphate excretion, or a relatively intractable hypercalciuria. The dosage is adjusted to maintain a urinary phosphorus excretion above 1200 mg per 24 hours. This usually requires 4 to 6 tablets of neutral K-Phos, each containing 250 mg of phosphorus. Larger amounts of 8 to 12 tablets (2 to 3 grams of phosphorus per day) usually require gradual increase in dosage to prevent gastrointestinal irritation. The neutral buffered salt is preferable, since it eliminates the danger of systemic acidosis and does not add significant sodium to the diet.

The usual precautions regarding administration of potassium are observed. Fortunately, virtually all oxalate stone formers for whom phosphates are indicated retain excellent renal function.

Uric Acid Metabolism. Metabolism of uric acid is abnormal in a surprisingly large number of stone formers regardless of the crystalline composition of their stones. This is apparent in the metabolic profiles, in which mean values for serum or urinary urate concentrations are persistently above the normal. These patients may respond well to simple dietary restriction of purines. Many of these patients are habitual aspirin users and should be advised to discontinue taking aspirin. The other uricosuric drugs are to be avoided for obvious reasons. The most effective medication in this situation is xanthine oxidase inhibition with allopurinol (Zyloprim). Relatively low dosage of 200 to 300 mg daily is effective in reducing urinary urate levels and is generally well tolerated. The drug should not be administered with ampicillin (which causes increased incidence of dermatitis).

Combinations of Drug Therapy

The three drugs mentioned previously — phosphate, hydrochlorothiazide, and allopurinol — may be administered in various combinations. These decisions are based not only upon the initial metabolic survey but more importantly upon the response during the follow-up period and the severity of the disease, that is, the rate and number of oxalate stones formed.

Fortunately, these three drugs tend to supplement one another. The potassium in the phosphates is generally adequate to replace that lost by thiazide administration. The nitrogen retention associated with thiazides is reduced by allopurinol. There are well-known side effects to administration of each of these, and such double or triple drug therapy should not be employed indiscriminately.

The Homozygous Cystinuric Patient. Treatment of the homozygous cystinuric patient who forms stones containing cystine is well established. This includes the maximal intake of water, alkalinization of the urine to pH 8, reduction of cystine and acid ash in the diet, and, in special circumstances, administration of the disulfide D-penicillamine. The complications of penicillamine administration are well known, and the drug should be reserved for dissolution of existing stones or for intractable stone formation when urinary cystine excretion exceeds 1200 mg per day.

The Heterozygous Cystinuric Patient. The metabolic evaluation of all stone formers should include a scanning test for cystine. Heterozygous cystinuric patients excrete mean quantities of cystine intermediate between those of normal persons and those of homozygous cystinurics. The incidence of such individuals in the general population is estimated at 1 in 200, but we have found an incidence in oxalate stone formers of 1 in 7. The oxalate stone former who persistently shows rapid rates of stone formation and growth in spite of a favorable biochemical response to the aforementioned measures for treating oxalate stone formation should have definitive quantitative analyses for urinary cystine, lysine, arginine, and ornithine concentrations. The demonstrable presence of heterozygous cystinuria should invoke the general measures for treatment of cystinuria. If the rate of oxalate stone formation is sufficient to warrant additional therapy, D-penicillamine has resulted in dramatic reduction of stone formation in a small number of such patients. This therapy is ineffectual in oxalate stone formers who do not also have cystinuria.

Explanation, Evaluation, and Adjustment of Therapeutic Programs

The enlistment of patient cooperation is best achieved by his enlightenment as to the rationale and objectives as well as possible complications of the program.

The periodic monitoring and adjustment of such programs is of even greater importance than the initial decisions as to structure of the program itself. A single uncontrolled biochemical profile of blood or urine may have little value as an initial diagnostic test, but when viewed against the background of the initial metabolic evaluation and as a measure of response of the individual to treatment, it becomes invaluable. In addition to the established guidelines for monitoring patients on thiazide, allopurinol, and phosphate therapy, the follow-up should include the following pertinent observations:

1. Patients who continue to pass stones should be informed whether these antedated treatment, or whether they are new stones.

2. Long-term thiazide therapy may unmask a latent hyperparathyroidism, as indeed may any other long-term period of observation.

3. Patients with infectious stones, who are usually normocalciuric when first seen, may demonstrate their latent hypercalciuria when the infection and obstruction have been relieved.

4. Patients on phosphate therapy who develop urinary infection, azotemia, or hyperphosphatemia should have their drug regimen discontinued.

The list is much longer, but these are some of the common checkpoints.

Summary

The guidelines for therapy are defined by the relative and absolute concentrations of crystallizable substances in the urine.

The specific therapeutic measures are based upon the individual patient's response to a controlled metabolic evaluation of how the crystalloids in question are transported and excreted.

The simplistic objective is to create a urine as selectively dilute in all these crystalloids as is consistent with good nutrition.

The program must be explained to the patient, monitored, and periodically adjusted. Programs of therapy not included in this article have proved to be ineffectual in our experience or have such highly specialized application as to be utilizable only in patients with diseases other than "idiopathic" stones, which are the sole consideration here.

The Venereal Diseases

CHANCROID

method of
RICHARD B. ODOM, M.D.
San Francisco, California

Chancroid is a specific sexually transmitted disease characterized by multiple, painful, foul-smelling, necrotic, nonindurated genital ulcerations caused by *Hemophilus ducreyi*, a small gram-negative bacillus. The incubation period averages 4 to 5 days. Individual lesions may vary in diameter from 1 mm to 2 cm and are usually two to five in number. Approximately 50 per cent of patients develop usually unilateral, painful, tender, inflammatory, or suppurative inguinal adenopathy 1 to 2 weeks following the appearance of the genital ulcers. If early treatment is not instituted, the lymph nodes may become fluctuant, rupture spontaneously, and drain sanguinopurulent material. Other complications include phimosis, paraphimosis, urethral fistulas, rupture of the frenulum, and scarring and deformity of the inguinal regions and tissues of the penis. Coexistent infections with other sexually transmitted diseases, especially primary syphilis, must be ruled out by darkfield examinations and serial serologic tests for syphilis. Genital herpes simplex infections may become secondarily infected with bacteria, producing a clinical picture simulating chancroid.

Treatment

Local hygiene is important and can be accomplished through use of cleansing tepid soaks or compresses of isotonic saline solution for 15 minutes four times a day. Obviously, sexual contacts should be avoided until definitive therapy has been completed and all signs and symptoms of disease activity have disappeared.

The drugs of choice in the treatment of chancroid are the sulfonamides. Sulfonamides do not mask coexistent syphilis. Sulfisoxazole (Gantrisin), 1.0 gram orally four times a day, is the preferred treatment schedule. Sulfamethoxazole, 800 mg, in combination with trimethoprim, 160 mg, is an effective alternative drug and has the advantage of a 12 hour dosage interval. (This specific use of this combination of drugs is not listed in the manufacturer's official directive.) If there is no improvement within 5 days, tetracycline, 500 mg orally four times a day, may be initiated as the sole therapeutic agent or added to the sulfonamide drug. Sulfonamides and/or tetracycline are given for a minimum of 14 days or until there is complete healing of all lesions, including any lymphadenitis.

I have consulted on several patients with chancroid who have failed to respond to sulfonamide drugs, tetracycline, or a combination of both. To date, all such patients have responded to minocycline (Minocin), 100 mg orally twice a day for 2 weeks. As a result of therapeutic efficacy and the twice daily dosage schedule, I currently prescribe minocycline routinely. I do perform darkfield examinations and serologic tests for syphilis in all such cases. The only disadvantages to minocycline are the side effects of vertigo and lightheadedness and the expense versus the sulfonamides and tetracycline. Also, intramuscular kanamycin, 0.5 gram twice a day for 5 to 14 days, can be used in those patients with chancroid resistant to treatment with the sulfonamides and tetracycline. Erythromycin, streptomycin, and cephalothin have also proved effective.

Fluctuant lymph nodes should be aspirated to avoid spontaneous rupture. Aspiration may be accomplished by entering with a large gauge needle through normal skin superior to the bubo or directly overlying the fluctuant node. Incision should not be performed.

In patients with paraphimosis or phimosis, a dorsal slit and/or circumcision may be required. Such procedures should be delayed until infection has subsided.

GONOCOCCAL INFECTION

method of
RICHARD R. HOOPER, M.D.
Oakland, California

Over the last few years, effective treatment regimens for infections caused by *Neisseria gonorrhoeae* have come into widespread use, and the proportion of gonococcal organisms resistant to various antibiotics has declined. There has also been a concomitant increase in the complexity of treatment for gonococcal infections. Factors which must be considered in the selection of an appropriate course of therapy include the following:

1. *The certainty of diagnosis.* If *N. gonorrhoeae* has not clearly been identified, a regimen effective against more than one etiologic agent should be chosen. For example, tetracycline would be a reasonable choice of drugs to treat epididymitis in a male with a Gram stain–negative urethral discharge.

2. *The resistance of the organism.* Rational therapy of gonococcal infection requires a knowledge of the resistance patterns in a given geographic area. For example, *N. gonorrhoeae* acquired in the western Pacific, particularly the Philippines, is likely to be resistant both to penicillin and to tetracycline. The prevalence of penicillinase-producing *N. gonorrhoeae* (PPNG) in this area of the world has been estimated to be 20 to 40 per cent of infected persons. Even within the United States the resistance patterns vary considerably.

3. *The anatomic site of infection.* Pharyngeal infection with *N. gonorrhoeae* is more difficult to treat. Spectinomycin is not effective in treating infection at this site.

4. *The likelihood of adverse host reaction to the antibiotic.* About 5 per cent of the population are allergic to penicillin and its analogues. Reactions to the procaine vehicle can also occur. Ampicillin is associated with rashes, and tetracycline is contraindicated in pregnant women and in children less than 8 years old.

5. *The reliability of the patient.* Single dose regimens are more likely to be effective, since patient compliance is not a factor. The difficulty in adhering to the four times daily between meal, low calcium regimen advocated in the use of tetracycline is an illustration of a difficult-to-follow regimen. The recommended test of cure culture 3 to 7 days after cessation of therapy is difficult to obtain on an unreliable patient, especially those on multiple dose oral regimens.

6. *The effectiveness of the regimen against coincident diseases.* For example, tetracycline, penicillin, and amoxicillin regimens abort incubating syphilis, whereas the spectinomycin regimen probably does not. Similarly, tetracycline is effective against chlamydial infection, but penicillin, amoxicillin, and spectinomycin are not.

7. *The severity of disease.* Generally speaking, the treatment of gonococcal infection with local extension or systemic involvement requires higher dosages of medication over longer periods of time, despite evidence that the gonococcal organisms in these cases are usually sensitive to the recommended antimicrobials. Aggressive therapy is indicated because of the increase in morbidity and mortality associated with inadequate treatment of disseminated disease.

8. *The cost of treatment.* While the cost of gonococcal treatment regimens may vary tenfold, the choice of the antibiotic should be based primarily on the effectiveness of the regimen. An ill-advised regimen will cost physician and patient additional time for re-treatment, may result in more adverse reactions, and may lead to continued spread of the disease.

9. *Legal consideration.* Regimens which follow the approved standards for medical practice should be chosen. Ineffective regimens include benzathine penicillin, oral penicillin V, and tetracycline or its analogues in *single dose* therapy.

The regimens outlined in this article are based primarily on the recommendations of the Center for Disease Control. However, I do not recommend ampicillin for the treatment of uncomplicated gonorrhea. It is less effective than penicillin, less reliably absorbed than amoxicillin, associated with the selection of resistant strains of *N. gonorrhoeae*, and responsible for idiosyncratic rashes in approximately 10 per cent of patients. Also, ampicillin is not effective in the treatment of nongonococcal urethritis (NGU). Not all the regimens available for the treatment of gonococcal infections will be mentioned. For example, the long-acting tetracyclines are probably as effective as tetracycline and less dependent on patient reliability. However, there have been insufficient widely based studies to document their effectiveness as clearly as the recommended agents.

Localized Gonococcal Infection

Table 1 lists the recommended antimicrobial regimens for the treatment of localized gonococcal infections, such as urethritis, cervicitis, pharyngitis, and proctitis. In addition to these medications, I would suggest the following:

1. Perform a serologic test for syphilis at the time of diagnosis, and, if using spectinomycin, repeat this test one or more times at 4 week intervals. When a patient has findings compatible with primary or secondary syphilis, the regimens advocated for treatment of gonococcal infections are inadequate.

2. Report the case to local health authorities so that sexual partners can be identified and treated. In the case of pediatric gonococcal infections, child abuse should be considered.

3. Have the patient return for a test of cure 3 to 7 days after treatment.

4. Urge the patient to refrain from sexual intercourse until the follow-up culture has been taken.

Gonococcal Conjunctivitis — Ophthalmia

While gonococcal conjunctivitis usually remains a localized infection, the sometimes rapid progression of the disease with resultant blindness makes aggressive therapy with close monitoring advisable. Management includes the following measures:

1. Hospitalization with isolation for the first 24 hours.

2. Antibiotics. (a) *Adult:* Give aqueous penicillin G, 10 million units per day intravenously, until active infection is arrested, followed by amoxicillin, 500 mg orally four times daily for 10 days. (b) *Pediatric:* Aqueous penicillin is the drug of choice. In the neonate, give 50,000 units per kg per day, divided into two or three doses, for 7 days. For a child over 1 year of age but weighing less than 45 kg, give 100,000 units per kg per day intravenously, divided into four doses, for 7 days. (c) The child less than 8 years of age with penicillin allergy should receive cephalothin, 60 to 80 mg per kg per day intravenously, divided into four doses, for at least 7 days.

3. Saline irrigation of the eye, followed by antibiotic drops (penicillin or tetracycline every 15 minutes initially, then less frequently as a response is noted).

Gonococcal Infection with Regional Spread — Epididymitis and Pelvic Inflammatory Disease (PID)

The antimicrobial regimens recommended for the treatment of epididymitis and PID caused

TABLE 1. **The Treatment of Uncomplicated Gonococcal Infection (Urethritis, Pharyngitis, Proctitis, Cervicitis, Vaginitis; for Conjunctivitis See Text)**

PRIORITY		DOSE	ADVANTAGES	DISADVANTAGES
1	Procaine penicillin	*Adult:* 4.8 million units intramuscularly divided into 2 doses, with 1 gram probenecid PO given simultaneously	Widespread effectiveness; works well at all anatomic sites; aborts incubating syphilis; single dose regimen	Risk of allergic or idiosyncratic reaction; not effective against NGU,* PPNG,† or other penicillin-resistant strains
		Pediatric (less than 45 kg): 100,000 units/kg intramuscularly and 25 mg/kg of probenecid PO		
2	Tetracycline	*Adult:* 500 mg PO q6h, taken 1 hour before meals for a total of 10 grams—i.e., for 5 days	Effective against NGU; aborts incubating syphilis; effective for pharyngitis	Usually not effective against Asian-acquired strains; contraindicated in pregnancy and in children less than 8 years old; patient compliance important
		Pediatric: Over 8 years old, 40 mg/kg/day, not to exceed 2 grams, in four divided doses, for 5 days PO		
3	Spectinomycin	*Adult:* Two grams intramuscularly	Particularly effective against Asian-acquired strains and PPNG; single dose regimen	Not effective against NGU and syphilis; not effective against pharyngeal infection
		Pediatric (less than 45 kg): 40 mg/kg in two divided doses		
4	Amoxicillin and probenicid	*Adult:* 3 grams PO + 1 gram probenecid PO given simultaneously	Single dose regimen; orally administered	Generally less effective than penicillin; contraindicated in penicillin allergy; not effective for NGU
		Pediatric (less than 45 kg): 50 mg/kg amoxicillin + 25 mg/kg probenecid PO		

*NGU = Nongonococcal urethritis.
†PPNG = Penicillinase-producing *N. gonorrhoeae.*

TABLE 2. **The Treatment of Gonococcal Infection with Regional Spread (Epididymitis, Pelvic Inflammatory Disease [PID])**

Hospitalized
Drug of choice:
    Aqueous crystalline penicillin G, 20 million units intravenously daily divided into four doses, until improvement, followed by amoxicillin, 500 mg PO qid to complete 10 days of therapy
Alternative:
    Tetracycline, 250 mg intravenously qid until improvement, then 500 mg PO qid to complete 10 days of therapy*

Nonhospitalized
Drug of choice:
    Aqueous procaine penicillin G, 4.8 million units intramuscularly in two sites, with 1 gram probenecid PO simultaneously, followed by amoxicillin, 500 mg PO qid for 10 days
Alternatives:
    Tetracycline, 0.5 gram PO qid for 10 days*
    Amoxicillin, 3.0 grams PO with 1 gram probenecid simultaneously, followed by amoxicillin, 0.5 gram PO for 10 days
    Spectinomycin, 2 grams intramuscularly every 12 hours for 3 days

*Preferable if chlamydial infection suspected.

by gonococcal infection are outlined in Table 2. Other management considerations include the following:

1. Indications for hospitalization: (a) Uncertain diagnosis (e.g., surgical emergencies such as appendicitis, ectopic pregnancy, or testicular torsion). (b) Severe illness (e.g., generalized peritonitis, heart murmur, or arthritis). See Disseminated Gonococcal Infection, below. (c) Pregnancy. (d) Inability of the patient to follow or tolerate an outpatient regimen. (e) Failure to respond to outpatient therapy.

2. Identification and treatment of sexual partners.

3. For epididymitis, scrotal support with bed rest.

4. For PID, removal of an intrauterine device, if present, and bed rest, preferably in semi-Fowler's position.

5. Follow-up with culture following completion of therapy.

6. Surgical drainage of abscesses that develop as a consequence of regional spread.

Disseminated Gonococcal Infection (Arthritis, Dermatitis, Meningitis, Endocarditis)

The antimicrobial regimens appropriate for the management of these severe forms of gonococcal infection are outlined in Table 3. Hospitalization is advisable because of the potential complications associated with disseminated disease and because the etiologic diagnosis is often uncertain in these cases.

As with localized disease, identification of sexual partners and follow-up test of cure are indicated.

Since the gonococcal organisms responsible for disseminated disease are usually sensitive to penicillin analogues, ampicillin is an appropriate alternative drug. Erythromycin can also be used.

Other Considerations

Persons exposed to known gonococcal infections should be regarded as having local disease and treated as soon as cultures have been obtained, regardless of the results. Neonates born to mothers with gonococcal infection should receive procaine penicillin, 50,000 units intramuscularly if term, or 20,000 units if of low birth weight.

TABLE 3. **The Treatment of Disseminated Gonococcal Infection (Arthritis-Dermatitis, Meningitis, Endocarditis)**

Treatment of choice:
    Aqueous penicillin G, 10 million units per day intravenously until patient improves, followed by amoxicillin or ampicillin, 500 mg PO qid to complete 7 days of therapy
Alternatives:
    Ampicillin, 3.5 grams, or amoxicillin, 3.0 grams, PO, plus probenecid, 1 gram PO, followed by ampicillin or amoxicillin, 500 mg PO qid for 7 days
    Tetracycline, 0.5 gram PO qid for 7 days
    Spectinomycin, 2 grams intramuscularly every 12 hours for 3 days*
    Erythromycin, 0.5 gram intravenously every 6 hours until patient improves, followed by 0.5 gram PO qid to complete 7 days of therapy
For endocarditis: Aqueous penicillin, 20 million units intravenously daily for 4 to 6 weeks, with bactericidal blood level determinations for the isolated organism; no acceptable alternate regimen has been established
For meningitis: Aqueous penicillin G regimen same as for endocarditis; alternative regimen is chloramphenicol, 1 gram intravenously qid daily for 14 days

*Treatment of choice for disseminated infection with PPNG.

GRANULOMA INGUINALE

method of
HUBERTO BOGAERT, M.D.,
Santo Domingo, Dominican Republic

Granuloma inguinale or granuloma venereum is a chronic infectious granulomatous disease of the genitalia and the surrounding skin caused by *Donovania granulomatis*. The incubation period is approximately 3 or 4 weeks. The first lesion is a soft, elevated nodule which breaks out to form a beefy red ulcer with a sharply defined edge. These lesions are painless and enlarge very slowly. There is no inguinal adenopathy. The course is chronic with no tendency to spontaneous cure. The laboratory diagnosis is based on finding the Donovan body. Adequate deep tissue should be removed with a curette or a punch biopsy and spreads made with the undersurface of the tissue. The preparations are stained with Wright's or Giemsa stain.

Therapy

Tetracyclines are effective in doses of 500 mg orally every 6 hours for 3 to 4 weeks. Erythromycin may be administered at the same dosage. Occasional recurrences may require a second course for a longer period.

Streptomycin, 1 gram intramuscularly every 24 hours for 2 to 3 weeks, is effective.

Trimethoprim-sulfamethoxazole (Septra, Bactrim) is also effective in doses of 2 tablets twice daily for 2 weeks (this use is not listed in the manufacturer's official directive).

Ampicillin, chloramphenicol, gentamicin, and minocycline have been used with varying degrees of success.

Local treatment is useful to control secondary infection and as a deodorant.

Potassium permanganate (1:20,000) or hydrogen perioxide soaks are useful.

Follow-up

Periodic examination every 2 to 3 months should be continued for a year. Successive serologic tests for syphilis should be performed; it should be kept in mind that broad-spectrum antibiotic therapy may mask concomitant syphilitic infection. Plastic surgical repair may be indicated.

LYMPHOGRANULOMA VENEREUM

method of
HUBERTO BOGAERT, M.D.
Santo Domingo, Dominican Republic

Lymphogranuloma venereum or lymphogranuloma inguinale is a systemic disease, usually sexually transmitted, caused by an organism of the genus Chlamydia, manifested by constitutional signs and symptoms and acute or chronic tissue changes affecting primarily the lymphatics and other tissues of the inguinal, genital, and anorectal regions. The incubation period is approximately 10 to 15 days. The first lesion is a small papule on the genitals; this heals within a few days and may pass unnoticed. There are two main varieties: the inguinal and the late anorectal-genital syndrome.

The inguinal syndrome is more common in men. Within 2 to 4 weeks after exposure, enlargement of the inguinal lymph nodes begins, usually on one side. The nodes are matted; the overlying skin is reddish purple, edematous, thickened, and attached to underlying tissue. The nodes subsequently suppurate and show multiple draining sinuses.

The anorectal-genital syndrome is found mainly in women and is a late chronic manifestation. It may be manifested by proctitis, rectal stricture, elephantiasis of the penis or vulva, and ulcerations.

The suspected diagnosis should be confirmed by skin testing with Frei antigen.

Therapy

Sulfisoxazole (Gantrisin), sulfadiazine, or sulfathiazole* is effective in doses of 4 grams initially, followed by 1 gram orally every 6 hours for 3 to 4 weeks.

Trimethoprim-sulfamethoxazole (Bactrim, Septra) is effective in doses of 2 tablets twice daily for 2 to 3 weeks (this use is not listed in the manufacturer's official directive).

Also effective are tetracycline hydrochloride, 500 mg orally every 6 hours for 3 to 4 weeks, and minocycline, 200 mg initially, followed by 100 mg every 12 hours for 3 to 4 weeks. Longer and repeated courses are necessary in the anorectal-genital syndrome. Other tetracyclines and erythromycin may also be effective. Local treatment for buboes includes bed rest, application of ice bags, and aspiration of fluctuant lesions. Incision is contraindicated.

Follow-up

Continued surveillance of the patient is important; remissions and exacerbations are frequent. A persistent high titer of lymphogranuloma venereum–complement fixation test (LGV-CFT) is an indication for re-treatment.

---

*May not be available in the United States of America.

SYPHILIS

method of
EDMUND C. TRAMONT, M.D.
Washington, D.C.

General Considerations

An appreciation of the pathogenesis of syphilis, the doubling time of *Treponema pallidum*, and the pharmacokinetics of penicillin forms the basis of the rationale for the treatment regimens of syphilis.

Soon after the host becomes infected but before the appearance of a primary chancre, a *spirochetemia* develops, which can potentially infect any organ in the body, most notably for therapeutic considerations the central nervous system.

Treponema pallidum divides every 30 to 36 hours, which necessitates the maintenance of an adequate antibiotic level for more than 1 week. Single dose, short-acting antibiotic regimens cannot be relied upon to cure established syphilis.

Penicillin G is the treatment of choice for all forms of syphilis unless the patient is allergic to the drug. There is no evidence that *T. pallidum* has developed increased resistance to penicillin or to any other antibiotic. Benzathine penicillin G is the principal preparation recommended for the treatment of syphilis because it maintains adequate blood levels for up to 3 weeks. As will be discussed later, its principal drawback is that one cannot rely upon it to attain adequate levels in the central nervous system.

Early Syphilis

Early syphilis is the arbitrarily designated terminology to denote the first year of disease. In most patients, it encompasses the primary chancre, the florid secondary stage (when the number of live spirochetes infecting the host reach their greatest concentration), and the early latent period when there is a positive serologic test but an absence of clinical symptoms.

Benzathine penicillin G, 2.4 million units, by intramuscular injection in the buttock is the treatment of choice. Half can be given in each buttock to reduce the after-soreness.

Patients allergic to penicillin may be given tetracycline, 500 mg orally four times a day for 15 days, or erythromycin enteric-coated base, 500 mg four times a day for 15 days. Patients should be advised to take the drugs on an empty stomach (30 minutes before or 2 hours after a meal), and cautioned not to take tetracycline with milk or antacids. Erythromycin stearate or ethylsuccinate may be substituted for erythromycin base.

Although never adequately studied, other theoretical regimens would be a cephalosporin

TABLE 1.   **Quick Guide for the Treatment of Syphilis (See Text for Details and Other Alternative Schedules)**

STAGE	PENICILLIN THERAPY	ALLERGIC TO PENICILLIN
Early syphilis (primary, secondary, latent syphilis of less than 1 year's duration)	Benzathine penicillin G, 2.4 million units total by intramuscular injection at a single session; half may be given in each buttock	Tetracycline hydrochloride, 500 mg four times a day orally for 15 days *or* Erythromycin enteric-coated base, 500 mg four times a day orally for 15 days
Syphilis of more than 1 year's duration (latent syphilis of indeterminate or more than 1 year's duration, cardiovascular, late benign)	Benzathine penicillin G, 7.2 million units total: 2.4 million units by intramuscular injection weekly for 3 successive weeks *or* Aqueous procaine penicillin G, 9.0 million units total: 600,000 units by intramuscular injection daily for 15 days	Tetracycline hydrochloride, 500 mg four times a day by mouth for 28 days *or* Erythromycin (stearate, ethylsuccinate, or base), 500 mg four times a day by mouth for 28 days
Neurosyphilis	Aqueous crystalline penicillin G, 2.4 million units every 4 hours for 8–10 days	Chloramphenicol, 2 grams/day for 15 days

Congenital syphilis	Infants with normal CSF:
	  Benzathine penicillin G, 50,000 units/kg intramuscularly in a single dose
	Infants with abnormal CSF:
	  Aqueous crystalline penicillin G, 50,000 units/kg intravenously daily in two divided doses for a minimum of 10 days
	or
	  Aqueous procaine penicillin G, 50,000 units/kg intramuscularly daily for a minimum of 10 days	

Pregnant women should be treated in dosage schedules appropriate for the stage of syphilis as recommended for nonpregnant women. Pregnant women allergic to penicillin should be treated with erythromycin in dosage schedules appropriate for the stage of syphilis as recommended for nonpregnant patients.

antibiotic, doxycycline, or minocycline for 15 days.

Early incubating syphilis is probably aborted when gonorrhea or nongonococcal urethritis is treated with penicillin or tetracycline, but in some patients this treatment may modify the clinical presentation. Spectinomycin has no effect on syphilis.

Latent Syphilis of Indeterminate Duration or More Than 1 Year's Duration, Cardiovascular Syphilis, or Late Benign Syphilis

It is generally felt that syphilis of longer duration requires prolonged therapy. The regimen of choice is benzathine penicillin G, 7.2 million units total, given in 2.4 million unit doses by intramuscular injection for 3 successive weeks. A far less acceptable regimen to most patients and one that is more painful is to administer procaine penicillin G, 600,000 units intramuscularly daily for 15 days.

The adequacy of other drug regimens for syphilis of more than 1 year's duration has never been adequately studied. Thus, a history of penicillin allergy should be carefully documented before embarking on alternative treatment regimens. However, by extrapolation, penicillin-allergic patients may be treated with 500 mg four times a day of tetracycline hydrochloride (on an empty stomach with water or fruit juice), doxycycline, 200 mg, or erythromycin enteric-coated base, 500 mg, four times a day, by mouth for 30 days.

Neurosyphilis

Since the central nervous system (CNS) is invaded in a small but significant number of patients who suffer a spirochetemia, and since a spirochetemia develops soon after the infection is established, all patients should be considered to have neurosyphilis. A careful neurologic examination and a cerebrospinal fluid (CSF) examination are mandatory. Any patient with an abnormal physical examination (particular attention should be paid to second and eighth cranial nerves and posterior spinal cord column functions) or an abnormal nontreponemal test (VDRL, PRP, ART) or FTA unabsorbed test on the cerebrospinal fluid (CSF) should be considered to have possible neurosyphilis.

The treatment of neurosyphilis is controversial. Since benzathine penicillin G rarely produces detectable levels of penicillin G in the cerebrospinal fluid, this form of penicillin is theoretically inadequate for the treatment of neurosyphilis. On the other hand, there is evidence to suggest that when 6,000,000 units or more of any form of penicillin is given, the cure rates reach acceptable levels. However, treatment failures have been documented, and since the potential damage of neurosyphilis to the patient years later can be so devastating, many clinicians prefer to treat with 12 to 24 million units of aqueous crystalline penicillin G intravenously every 24 hours for 8 to 10 days to assure that adequate levels are attained in the central nervous system for a sufficient period of time. On the other hand, the United States Public Health Service currently accepts as adequate therapy the same penicillin treatment regimens that are recommended for the treatment of syphilis of greater than 1 year's duration. Recent evidence suggests that amoxicillin, 3 grams per day, plus probenicid (1 gram) orally for 15 days may also be adequate. (This use of amoxicillin is not listed in the manufacturer's official directive.)

Chloramphenicol (2 grams per day for 14 days) would theoretically be a good alternative choice in patients allergic to penicillin, because it achieves adequate levels in the central nervous system and the aqueous humor of the eye and has been shown to be effective in the treatment of early syphilis. Other alternatives would be doxycycline or minocycline, 200 mg orally, or tetracycline or erythromycin enteric-coated base, 500 mg, four times daily for 28 days.

Prednisone, 80 mg orally every other day for 1 to 3 months, plus penicillin may be efficacious in patients with syphilitic hearing loss. The response to treatment should be documented with audiograms and the prednisone discontinued if there is no improvement after 1 month. Treatment is continued until the audiogram stabilizes.

Syphilis in Pregnancy

Pregnant patients should receive penicillin in dosage schedules appropriate for the stage of syphilis. The choice is more difficult in penicillin-allergic patients because the efficacy of such treatment regimens for effecting a cure in the fetus are not well established. Erythromycin enteric-coated base is the drug of first choice. Tetracycline, erythromycin estolate, and chloramphenicol are contraindicated because of adverse effects on the mother or fetus.

Congenital Syphilis

Since immediate hypersensitivity to penicillin is not a problem in neonates, it is common practice to treat all infants born to mothers with gestational syphilis regardless of maternal treatment, but especially for those who were treated with an antibiotic other than penicillin. All infants should have a CSF examination. If the CSF is normal, a single dose of benzathine penicillin, 50,000 units per kg intramuscularly, may be given. If the CSF is abnormal, they should receive aqueous crystalline penicillin G in two divided doses intramuscularly, or aqueous procaine penicillin G intravenously at 50,000 units per kg for 10 days.

Treatment of Contacts

Because of the high communicability of syphilis (up to 50 per cent of contacts become infected) and the contagion of the infection before the serology becomes reactive, it is wise to treat all contacts of patients with early syphilis based on epidemiologic considerations. Adequate early treatment will often prevent the development of seroreactivity.

Follow-up and Re-treatment

It is absolutely essential that all patients with syphilis have a follow-up evaluation. All patients with early syphilis and congenital syphilis should have repeat quantitative nontreponemal tests (VDRL, RPR, ART) at 3, 6, and 12 months or until they become negative in two tests. All patients with secondary syphilis or syphilis of more than 1 year's duration should have a repeat nontreponemal serologic test up to 24 months or until they become negative in two tests. Examination of the CSF is also warranted in all patients with syphilis. All patients with neurosyphilis must be carefully followed with repeat CSF examinations for at least 3 years.

Treatment should be reinstituted whenever there is a sustained or an increase in titer of a nontreponemal test or when a titer persists beyond 12 months in primary syphilis (chancre) or 24 months in secondary syphilis. Re-treatment should also be considered whenever clinical signs and symptoms of syphilis persist, even in late syphilis when pathologic changes may have taken place and reversal is unlikely, i.e., the patient should be given the benefit of the doubt.

Jarisch-Herxheimer Reaction

The Jarisch-Herxheimer reaction is a systemic reaction occurring 1 to 2 hours after the initial treatment of syphilis with antibiotics, especially penicillin, and is felt to be due at least in part to the release of endotoxin from the lysed spirochetes. It consists of the abrupt onset of fever, chills, myalgias, headache, tachycardia, hyperventilation, flushing, and mild hypotension. It is particularly prone to occur in the secondary stage of the disease. It is usually self-limited and can be treated symptomatically with aspirin and bed rest. It can be aborted with 10 mg of prednisone given orally every 4 hours and may require up to six doses in severe cases. Pretreatment with 10 mg of prednisone may be given to all patients before the treatment of neurosyphilis to abort any adverse effects of this reaction on the central nervous system.

SECTION 10

Diseases of Allergy

ANAPHYLAXIS AND SERUM SICKNESS

method of
PHIL LIEBERMAN, M.D.
Memphis, Tennessee

ANAPHYLAXIS

Definition

Anaphylaxis is a systemic, immediate hypersensitivity reaction caused by the immunologic release of chemical mediators from mast cells and basophils. These mediators exert effects on smooth muscle and the vasculature resulting in increased capillary permeability, vasodilatation, and bronchoconstriction. Immunoglobulin E (IgE) is responsible for most if not all anaphylactic attacks in man.

Anaphylactoid reactions are clinically similar or identical to anaphylaxis but are not mediated by IgE.

The most common cause of anaphylaxis is drugs. Penicillin, radiographic contrast material, plasma expanders, and aspirin are probably the most frequent drugs producing anaphylaxis and anaphylactoid reactions. Hymenoptera stings and foods are also frequent causes.

Prevention of Anaphylaxis and Anaphylactoid Reactions

Although anaphylaxis is an unavoidable aspect of the practice of modern medicine, its incidence can be decreased by employing certain preventive measures. These are noted below:

1. A thorough drug allergy history should be obtained prior to the administration of any drug. When a history of an allergic reaction to a drug is present, a substitute, structurally unrelated drug should be administered whenever possible.

2. Anaphylaxis is usually more severe when the route of administration of the drug is parenteral. Therefore, whenever possible, a drug should be administered orally in terms of the prevention of severe anaphylactic attacks.

3. A patient receiving a drug in an office setting should remain in the office for 30 minutes after the administration. The more severe episodes of anaphylaxis usually occur shortly after the administration of a drug. Anaphylactic morbidity and mortality can be reduced by rapid institution of therapy.

4. Patients predisposed to anaphylactic attacks should carry appropriate identification. For example, patients allergic to drugs or Hymenoptera stings should carry an identification card in their wallet or purse. Identification jewelry is also available for this purpose.

5. Predisposed patients should also be taught the self-injection of epinephrine and should keep an anaphylactic treatment kit consisting of a loaded syringe with epinephrine with them at all times. Inhaled epinephrine is a poor substitute for the injected variety, since it is not absorbed in large quantities and therefore is beneficial only for bronchospasm. It should also be noted that sublingual isoproterenol might be contraindicated, since it produces peripheral vasodilatation and could thereby worsen hypotension.

6. If it is absolutely essential to administer a drug to a patient who has demonstrated hypersensitivity to it, the patient should be desensitized. This is true for drugs producing immediate hypersensitivity reactions in sensitive patients. These patients may be skin tested to document such hypersensitivity. The drug should be administered only by employing a carefully monitored desensitization procedure. Examples of drugs lending themselves to this form of administration are penicillin, animal antisera, and insulin. It should be noted that drugs that produce anaphylactoid reactions do not lend themselves to skin testing and administration by desensitization.

625

Examples of such drugs are radiographic contrast material, gamma globulin, aspirin and other nonsteroidal anti-inflammatory drugs, and sulfobromophthalein.

In addition to the general principles of prevention of anaphylaxis and anaphylactoid reactions as noted above, certain drugs bear special mention in regard to prevention because of the frequency with which they present clinical problems. These drugs are dealt with separately below.

Penicillin. Penicillin is probably the most frequent cause of anaphylaxis in the United States today. It has been estimated that it causes 400 to 800 deaths per year in the United States alone. Whenever possible, patients who give a history of immediate hypersensitivity to penicillin should be treated with an alternative drug. If there is no suitable alternative, the patient should be skin tested, using both aqueous penicillin G and benzylpenicilloyl polylysine (Pre-Pen). In the face of a positive history and a positive skin test the drug should be administered using a standard desensitization regimen with anaphylactic precautions available and the physician at the bedside at all times.

Immediate hypersensitivity reactions to penicillin are produced by allergic responses to metabolic products of the betalactam and thiazolidine rings. Since cephalothin sodium (Keflin) contains an identical betalactam ring and a very similar dihydralathiazolidine ring, metabolic products are structurally related to those of penicillin. For this reason cephalosporins cannot be given with impunity to patients truly allergic to penicillin. In addition most patients allergic to one form of penicillin are at risk of experiencing a similar reaction to related penicillins.

Radiographic Contrast Material. Reactions to radiographic contrast material are anaphylactoid in nature. That is they are not mediated by IgE. For this reason skin testing is of no predictive value. The incidence of anaphylactoid reactions to radiographic contrast material probably approximates 1 per cent. Based on this figure and the number of procedures employing this material performed annually, reactions to radiographic contrast material rival those to penicillin in terms of frequency.

The most frequently encountered problem regarding reactions to radiographic contrast material involves patients who have had previous such reactions. Approximately one third of such patients will develop another reaction upon readministration of the drug. Therefore these patients should not receive radiographic contrast material unless the diagnostic study is essential. If the study is deemed essential, most such reactions can be prevented by pretreatment of the patient with corticosteroids and diphenhydramine (Benadryl). The pretreatment schedule consists of the administration of prednisone, 50 mg orally every 6 hours beginning 18 hours prior to the procedure, and 50 mg of diphenhydramine (Benadryl) administered by intramuscular injection 1 hour prior to the procedure. It should be noted that this pretreatment protocol is not universally effective in preventing reactions. Therefore, if the previous reaction was life threatening, an additional precautionary measure should probably be employed. This measure consists of the administration of weak concentrations of radiographic contrast material in gradually increasing amounts while observing the patient for symptoms. Over a period of approximately 1½ hours the full strength and amount can be given. This procedure is time consuming and requires a physician at the bedside. Most patients will not require such measures, since the pretreatment protocol noted above is effective in the vast majority of instances.

Heterologous Serum. The importance of heterologous serum as a cause of anaphylaxis has been greatly reduced with the development of human antisera. However, animal antisera are still used for prophylaxis against snakebites, rabies, gas gangrene, and botulism, and for immunosuppression in the form of antilymphocyte or antithymocyte globulin. Anaphylactic shock occurs with significant frequency in patients receiving animal antisera. The incidence can be as high as 2 per cent. Whenever possible, human antiserum should be administered. If there is no available human antiserum, the administration of animal antiserum should be performed only after cutaneous testing. Prick testing should be performed initially with a 1:100 concentration. If the test is negative, a 1:10 concentration should be employed. If prick tests are negative, intradermal tests are done. Testing is done first with a 1:100 and then a 1:10 concentration. If the test to a 1:10 concentration is negative, anaphylaxis is unlikely. If the test is positive, administration is hazardous. It should be done only with anaphylactic precautions available and using a careful desensitization procedure. This procedure is outlined in the package insert supplied with the antiserum.

Hymenoptera Stings. As noted above, patients who have immediate hypersensitivity to stinging insects should carry warning identification with them and should be taught the self-injection of epinephrine and supplied with an emergency epinephrine injection kit. Patients with previous anaphylactic sensitivity to Hymenoptera should also receive immunotherapy to the appropriate Hymenoptera venom. Finally, they should be instructed in avoidance procedures.

Aspirin and Related Nonsteroidal and Anti-inflammatory Drugs. Aspirin and other non-steroidal, anti-inflammatory drugs produce anaphylactoid events. The mechanism of production of these reactions has not been clarified but is believed to involve the production of prostaglandins and possibly slow reacting substance of anaphylaxis. There is no predictive test to identify patients at risk.

Most patients who exhibit reactions to aspirin are also sensitive to all nonsteroidal anti-inflammatory drugs. They must therefore be instructed to avoid not only aspirin and all aspirin-containing products but also all nonsteroidal anti-inflammatory agents such as indomethacin, naproxen, tolmetin sodium, and others. Most such patients will also suffer from asthma, nasal polyposis, and chronic hyperplastic sinusitis.

Local Anesthetics. Local anesthetics may be divided into those containing a highly antigenic para-amino phenyl group (benzocaine, butacaine, procaine, tetracaine, and others) and those not containing this group (lidocaine, mepivacaine, dibucaine, and others). True anaphylactic reactions to local anesthetics have decreased radically in frequency as there has been a shift away from the use of those containing the para-amino phenyl group to those without this group. In most instances, even patients who have had a questionable reaction to local anesthetics can take an anesthetic lacking the para-amino phenyl group without difficulty. However, if there is any question, the drug should be administered in a carefully monitored, graded fashion. Administration is initiated with dilute concentrations. The concentration should be increased gradually and carefully in a fashion similar to that noted above for radiographic contrast material. In most instances, over a period of 2 hours, the full therapeutic dose can be given. Large series of patients treated in this manner have now been reported.

Therapy of the Acute Attack

The therapy of anaphylaxis and anaphylactoid reactions is subdivided into those procedures which are to be performed immediately and those which require a more detailed evaluation of the patient prior to their institution. The steps of therapy are summarized in Table 1. Procedures which should be instituted immediately are noted below:

1. The administration of epinephrine is the most important single therapeutic measure. Epinephrine should be administered at the first

TABLE 1. **Therapy of Anaphylaxis and Anaphylactoid Reactions**

A. Immediate therapy
   1. Epinephrine
   2. Check of airways
   3. Tourniquet proximal to injection site
   4. Patient in recumbent position, feet elevated
   5. Administration of oxygen
   6. Vital signs
B. Therapy instituted after further evaluation
   1. Corticosteroids
   2. Diphenhydramine (Benadryl)
   3. Fluids
   4. Plasma expanders
   5. Vasopressors
   6. Aminophylline

appearance of symptoms. Early administration can prevent more serious manifestations. The route of administration should be intramuscular or subcutaneous. Intravenous administration should be avoided if possible, being reserved only for those rare instances in which there is loss of consciousness and obvious severe cardiovascular collapse.

The dose of intramuscular or subcutaneous epinephrine is 0.3 to 0.5 ml of a 1:1000 concentration. Injections may be administered every 10 to 15 minutes until an effect is achieved or until tachycardia or other side effects supervene. If epinephrine must be given intravenously, the recommended dose varies between 0.1 to 0.5 ml of a 1:10,000 or a 1:100,000 solution. This solution can be made from the 1:1000 concentration by dilution with saline solution. Intravenous administration should be done cautiously over a period of approximately 5 minutes.

The aforementioned subcutaneous and intramuscular dose is for adults. Children should receive a dose of 0.01 ml per kg, to a maximum of 0.3 ml.

2. The airways should be checked immediately. Laryngeal edema and angioedema of the tissue surrounding the airway is the most rapid cause of death.

3. A tourniquet should be placed above the injection site if the agent producing the anaphylaxis was administered by injection. This tourniquet should be removed every 10 to 15 minutes for a 2 to 3 minute period. It has also been suggested that epinephrine be injected into the site of the original injection of antigen. This may slow the absorption of antigen. The dose of epinephrine placed into this injection site is 0.1 to 0.3 ml.

4. The patient should be placed in a recumbent position and his feet elevated.

5. Nasal oxygen should be started.

6. Vital signs should be obtained and monitored every 10 to 15 minutes for the duration of the attack.

After the procedures noted above have been done, a more extensive evaluation can be performed. Oftentimes the injection of epinephrine is sufficient to prevent further symptoms. If, however, the patient continues to have difficulty, other measures are instituted as deemed appropriate according to patient evaluation. These are noted below:

7. In any protracted attack not relieved immediately by epinephrine, the institution of corticosteroids is indicated. It should be emphasized that corticosteroids do not exert an immediate effect. They are therefore not lifesaving. However, the duration of any given attack of anaphylaxis cannot be predicted. It is clear that corticosteroids can exert biologic effects in vivo within 1 hour. Therefore for any attack not relieved by the measures noted above, corticosteroids should be given in the form of hydrocortisone (Solu-Cortef), 300 to 500 mg initially and every 4 hours as needed.

8. Diphenhydramine (Benadryl) should also be given for any attack which is not relieved by epinephrine alone. As in the case of corticosteroids, diphenhydramine is not lifesaving. Antihistamines act as competitive inhibitors of histamine. They therefore will not reduce symptoms which have already been produced by the action of histamine on receptor sites. However, they are indicated in protracted cases of anaphylaxis to prevent further binding. The dose of diphenhydramine is 25 to 50 mg given intramuscularly or intravenously according to the severity of the situation.

9. Shock with protracted hypotension is one of the major causes of death during episodes which persist after the administration of epinephrine. The treatment of choice in such instances is fluids and plasma expanders. Isotonic saline solution should be employed initially. If hypotension has not responded to the injection of epinephrine and the administration of 1000 ml of isotonic saline solution, the use of plasma volume expanders should be considered. Hydroxyethyl starch is probably the volume expander of choice. Human serum plasma or albumin can also be administered. Rapid infusion of the expander to a volume of 500 ml followed by slow infusion thereafter is recommended. The blood pressure can be monitored as a means of titrating the infusion rate. The aforementioned recommendations are for an adult of approximately 75 kg weight. Appropriate dosage adjustments in fluid administration and volume expanders should be made for children.

The use of vasopressors in the treatment of hypotension during anaphylaxis and anaphylactoid reactions has become somewhat controversial. This is because of the observation that hypotension and shock can occur in the face of an increase in peripheral resistance. In such instances shock is presumably due to a decreased cardiac output and extravascular leakage of plasma. However, vasopressors are still felt by many to be useful agents. Levarterenol or metaraminol can be employed. The dose of levarterenol in an adult is 8 to 16 mg diluted in 500 ml dextrose and water and administered by slow drip. Metaraminol can be administered in a dose of 100 to 200 mg in 500 ml dextrose and water, again given by slow drip. Vasopressor drugs may be "piggybacked" into the saline intravenous set. The rate of infusion is titrated according to the blood pressure response.

10. Persistent bronchospasm should be treated with intravenous aminophylline. Caution should be taken when aminophylline is given to a hypotensive patient. Administration should be performed by slow intravenous infusion. The dose is 4 to 7 mg per kg given at a rate of 10 mg per minute. If prompt resolution is not obtained, consideration should be given to the initiation of an intravenous drip administered at a rate of 0.5 to 0.7 mg per kg per hour. The drip should employ aminophylline, 500 mg in 1000 ml of 5 per cent dextrose in water.

11. Further measures may be needed according to the clinical response. Laryngeal edema may require intubation or tracheostomy. Intractable wheeze may require intubation and assisted ventilation. Arrhythmias and prolonged cardiovascular shock will require appropriate agents. Under these circumstances therapy is of course continued in an intensive care unit with appropriate careful monitoring of cardiovascular status and blood gases.

SERUM SICKNESS

Serum sickness is a form of immune complex disease. Antibody (IgG, IgM) and antigen complexes result in the activation of complement and the subsequent release of inflammatory mediators and chemotactic attraction of polymorphonuclear leukocytes. The end result of these series of events is the release of lysosomal contents and tissue damage. The name is derived from the observation that a large percentage of patients receiving heterologous serum will develop the syndrome. The symptoms consist of fever, lymphadenopathy, hepatosplenomegaly, arthralgias, arthritis, and rashes, the most frequent of which is urticaria. Other manifestations such as mononeuritis multiplex, Guillain-Barré syndrome, and glomerulonephritis can also occur.

Treatment

1. Antihistamines, corticosteroids, and salicylates may all be employed. Diphenhydramine (Benadryl), 50 to 100 mg every 6 hours, or hydroxyzine (Atarax), 25 to 50 mg every 4 to 6 hours, can be employed. There is some evidence that initiation of antihistamines during the course of therapy with heterologous serum may prevent the occurrence of serum sickness.

2. Aspirin is used to control joint pain and fever.

3. Severe cases can be treated with a tapering course of prednisone, beginning with an initial dose of 40 to 60 mg daily.

Classic serum sickness is a self-limited illness, usually subsiding in 1 to 3 weeks.

ASTHMA IN ADULTS

method of
RICHARD R. ROSENTHAL, M.D.
Fairfax, Virginia

Characteristics

Asthma may be described as a condition resulting primarily from narrowing of the bronchi, which characteristically has some reversibility. Although bronchospasm is the primary abnormality, mucosal edema and bronchorrhea often play an important role in the pathogenesis of the illness. Clinically, chest tightness and dyspnea are the hallmark symptoms, and wheezing, cough, and rhonchi are included among the signs. Laboratory findings may include an elevated total eosinophil count, regardless of the cause of the asthma, and an obstructive pattern on pulmonary function testing (decreased flow rates, such as FEV_1). Both show some reversal after treatment with a bronchodilator. Total and antigen specific IgE levels may or may not be elevated, depending upon the patient's state of atopy (allergy). The white blood count and differential may be helpful if bronchiolitis or pneumonia is suspected as well. Other illnesses which cause wheezing, such as congestive heart failure, pneumonia, endobronchial tumors, and foreign bodies, should always be kept in mind.

Causes

Allergy. Atopic asthma is often called "extrinsic," or coming from without. Bronchospasm in response to allergens follows the inhalation of antigens such as animal dander, pollen fragments, mold spores, or dust particles. Alternatively patients may have asthma after ingestion of certain foods, such as shellfish, or medications, such as aspirin, penicillin, and radio-contrast media. Stinging insect hypersensitivity may also cause bronchospasm. The mechanisms are immunologic and, in some cases of drug sensitivity, idiosyncratic. Reactions may be immediate or delayed by 8 to 12 hours.

Irritant. Bronchial hyperreactivity, either acquired, such as after influenzal infection, or "intrinsic," a constitutional predilection of sorts, may result in bronchospasm following the inhalation of fumes, smoke, chemical odors, dust as an irritant, various pollutants, and cold air. Even mild cooking odors can trigger bronchospasm in a sensitive individual. The primary mechanism is thought to be cholinergic, and is modulated by parasympathetic vagal irritant receptors in the upper airways and the efferent vagus nerve to the bronchi.

Infections. Sinusitis, bronchitis, and bronchiolitis as well as pneumonia can all cause bronchospasm. The majority of these infections are viral but may be bacterial.

Exercise. Almost all asthmatics are sensitive to the bronchospastic effects of exercise. The mechanism is not well understood but is linked directly to the inhalation of cold air.

Emotions. Happily, asthma is no longer stigmatized as an "emotional illness." Intense emotional states, including laughter, can, however, trigger or exacerbate an attack of asthma. Patient suggestibility can play a role in the intensification or amelioration of symptoms, and there is no doubt that the illness can be manipulated for secondary gain.

Treatment of Mild Asthma

Mild asthma is characterized by intermittent bronchospasm in otherwise asymptomatic patients. Such patients will have little or no physical limitations resulting from the illness, and mild but not disabling exercise intolerance may occur. Many patients can participate in competitive sports. Pulmonary function tests are normal or near normal between episodes. Acute disabling attacks, while uncommon, may occur, especially in association with respiratory infections or exposure to particular inhalants to which the patient is unusually sensitive. This category is used to describe patients who require only intermittent therapy.

A theophylline preparation that gives rapid blood levels, such as Elixophyllin capsules, may be given for a short course of therapy. The recommended loading dose is 6 mg per kg, followed by 3 mg per kg at the sixth and twelfth hour, with maintenance of 3 mg per kg every 8 hours. Depending on the size of the patient and his sensitivity to the drug, a single 100 or 200 mg capsule is often all that is needed on an as necessary (PRN) basis. Alternatively, beta agonists such as terbutaline or metaproterenol may be given as necessary (PRN) or four times daily until symptoms are under control, and then withdrawn. Terbutaline may cause some tremor and jitteriness, which can be modified by starting with a dose of 2.5 mg for several days and then graduating to 5 mg four times daily if the patient can tolerate this. The side effects often diminish with prolonged use. Metaproterenol is usually given in the dose of 20 mg four times daily, but some prefer 10 mg four times daily because of jitteriness. There has been a movement away from fixed combinations such as theophylline and ephedrine, and there is some evidence that such combinations offer no therapeutic advantage over theophylline alone but may in fact be synergistically toxic. Others believe that they are useful, and there are a number of such combinations available. Tedral contains theophylline, 130 mg, ephedrine, 24 mg, and phenobarbital, 8 mg, added to decrease the stimulatory effects of the combined ephedrine. Although less relevant in the mild asthmatic, it is important to remember that barbiturates can increase the metabolism of steroids because of liver microsomal enzyme induction, thereby potentially increasing steroid requirements in patients who might need them. The Marax formulation is similar to Tedral, except that hydroxyzine is used instead of phenobarbital. Exercise-sensitive asthmatics who are otherwise well may benefit from the inhalation of a single capsule of cromolyn (Intal) before exercise or an athletic event as this drug seems to have specific inhibitory activity in exercise-induced bronchospasm. Metered dose inhalers of beta agonists such as isoproterenol or metaproterenol may also be particularly useful for the relief of mild acute symptoms, provided that the patient is properly educated regarding the potential for abuse. The effects of metaproterenol may be longer lasting than those of isoproterenol when inhaled.

Treatment of Moderate Asthma

Patients with moderate asthma usually experience mild wheezing which is persistent and have some physical limitations resulting from exercise intolerance. Exacerbations may be frequent and are characterized by excessive coughing and wheezing as well as dyspnea. There may be some hyperinflation at all times. Pulmonary function tests taken at any time usually reveal some airways obstruction, which is usually reversible to some extent following administration of an inhaled bronchodilator. Moderate asthma requires around-the-clock medication with occasional augmentation needed for exacerbations.

Patients are usually started on continuous theophylline therapy, which may be expedited by the use of long-acting theophylline preparations. Theo-Dur is one such preparation which has zero order kinetics, that is, a constant rate of drug dissolution. This feature implements the achievement of a steady state with minimal peaks and valleys in the theophylline serum level. New patients may be started on 200 mg twice daily and graduated to 300 mg twice daily within 3 days if there are no side effects. After an additional 3 days the dose is raised to 400 mg twice daily. It is advisable to draw a serum sample for theophylline determination between 3 and 8 hours after a dose in order to establish that the proper maintenance level has been reached. The desired therapeutic level is between 10 and 20 micrograms per ml. The chart below will give some guidance regarding theophylline dosage adjustments. Patients who are on theophylline maintenance should have serum theophylline determinations repeated after every dosage adjustment and routinely every 6 months. Beta-adrenergic agents such as metaproterenol or terbutaline are often added as discussed above, if treatment is still not optimum. Doing so, at least theoretically, is therapeutically synergistic, although some hold that only the toxic effects cumulate. It is common practice, however, to add the beta agonists, but it is important to stress that patients be followed closely. A subset of patients may respond to cromolyn, and a therapeutic trial of 1 month is in order, especially if it appears as if the patient may require steroids, as cromolyn may be steroid sparing. Outside the United States it is common to start mildly asthmatic patients on cromolyn before initiating theophylline therapy. Often the cromolyn responders are improved symptomatically but show little measurable change in pulmonary function. Acute exacerbations may require short bursts of steroid therapy. A methylprednisolone (Medrol) dose pack is a convenient preparation to use and is easily understood by the patient, thereby augmenting compliance. The initial day's dose of Medrol is 24 mg, which is tapered to 4 mg on the sixth day. A higher initial dose with a longer taper may be desirable in order to treat more aggressively and minimize the chances for rebound.

TABLE 1.

THEOPHYLLINE LEVEL, MICROGRAMS/ML	ADJUSTMENT IN DAILY DOSE*	COMMENT
Under 5	100%	If patient is asymptomatic, consider discontinuation of drug
5–10	25%	Even if patient is asymptomatic, an increase into the therapeutic range may be desirable in order to help ameliorate the exacerbation of symptoms which occur after respiratory tract infections or inhalant exposures
11–13	10% only if clinically indicated	Increase cautiously only if symptoms supervene despite maintenance in this range
14–20	None	Consider change to long-acting preparation if a short-acting preparation is being used and there seem to be "breakthrough" symptoms
	10% decrease if intolerant	Side effects of gastric distress, nausea, vomiting, or diarrhea may occur in sensitive patients or slow metabolizers
21–25	10% decrease	Reduce dose even if side effects are absent
26–34	25–33% decrease	Omit next dose and reduce subsequent doses even if side effects are absent
Over 35	50% decrease	Omit next two doses and decrease subsequent doses

*A dosage increase of 0.5 mg per kg per hour will increase the serum level by 1 microgram per ml. Generally patients should be maintained between 10 and 20 micrograms per ml. Always check serum theophylline after dosage adjustments 2 to 3 hours after short-acting preparations and 3 to 8 hours after long-acting preparations.

Treatment of Severe Asthma

Severe asthma is characterized by persistent symptoms with more frequent and often severe exacerbations. There is greatly diminished exercise tolerance to the point that even normal activities are often intolerable. Sleep is often interrupted. Symptoms are usually moderate to severe, often exacerbated, and patients may require frequent hospitalizations. These patients run an increased risk of respiratory failure and frequently need augmented therapy. At best they require around-the-clock medication in order to maintain stability and are usually steroid dependent.

Initial therapy should be conducted as outlined above with the contingency of steroid therapy to be added when control is yet inadequate. It is usually more appropriate to initiate steroid treatment with "burst therapy," utilizing a high initial dose, followed by a gradual tapering. Initial doses may range from 30 to 60 mg of prednisone or the equivalent and taper over 5 days or more. Prednisone may be given twice daily and the total dose decreased by 5 mg every other day until a dose of 15 mg is reached. If the patient is doing well, you may start every other day dosing at 15 mg, or, if there is still some instability, double the dose and administer every other day. Taper the every other day dose to 10 or 15 mg every morning if possible. Exacerbations may require readministration of every day dosing. Many patients can be taught to titrate their own prednisone doses *within limits* which should be set by the physician. Many patients who were previously on oral steroids may now be maintained on inhaled beclomethasone. I find it helpful to initiate beclomethasone therapy (Vanceril) as oral steroids are being withdrawn. The usual dosage is one or two inhalations (42 to 84 micrograms) given three or four times a day. In patients with severe asthma it may be appropriate to start with up to 20 inhalations a day (no more) and taper to the usual dosage. Patients using inhaled bronchodilators routinely should inhale them first in order to maximize the deposition of the beclomethasone in the pulmonary tree. Patients who require more than 15 mg of prednisone a day should have the beclomethasone started when they are stable. After 1 week systemic steroids may be tapered slowly. It has been emphasized that the steroid taper must be quite gradual in order to avoid the symptoms of steroid withdrawal, joint and muscle pain, lassitude, and depression, as well as adrenal insufficiency caused by steroid suppression of the adrenal axis. An early morning resting serum cortisol will help determine if there is endogenous production of steroid or if there is still suppression of the adrenal glands. In steroid-dependent patients, smaller decrements of 2.5 mg of prednisone should be made only every week or two. Stress or severe asthma will require a boost of systemic steroids, and patients must be monitored for signs of adrenal insufficiency such as weight loss or hypotension. Alternatively, moderately ill asthmatics may be started on inhaled beclomethasone initially rather than systemic steroids if they are relatively stable and not in need of burst therapy. Beclomethasone may be started at the usual maintenance dose or higher as suggested above and then tapered to maintenance. Allow from 1 to 4 weeks for a response. Complications include oral candidiasis and hoarseness, as well as oral aspergillosis. If this occurs, patients may be treated with nystatin mouthwash and will usually respond quickly when the beclomethasone is withdrawn. Long-term effects are not yet fully appreciated, but there seems to be no particular suppression of the adrenal axis in doses under 1000 micrograms per day.

Treatment of Acute Asthma and Status Asthmaticus

Acute asthma is an exacerbation of pre-existing asthma or the rapid onset of broncho-spasm in relatively asymptomatic patients who have this predilection. Status asthmaticus is usually an intense crisis owing to refractoriness to medication, necessitating emergency treatment and aggressive intervention. Patients in this predicament are most often taking various drugs such as theophylline and inhaled bronchodila-tors, and the possibility of drug toxicity must be taken into account when treating patients in this state. The modalities of treatment are as follows:

1. Epinephrine 1:1000, 0.15 to 0.3 ml, may be given subcutaneously and repeated in 20 minutes if necessary. Blood pressure should be monitored and the drug used with caution if the diastolic pressure is over 95 to 100 mm Hg. Alternatively terbutaline, which is less cardio-selective, may be used in the dose of 0.25 mg, and is also given subcutaneously. It may be repeated in 20 to 30 minutes, but preferably only once.

2. Intravenous aminophylline is often the next drug of choice. It is ideal to have a serum theophylline level before determining the dose to be given. When this information is not available, the loading dose of aminophylline is 2.5 mg per kg, diluted in Volutrol to 50 ml, and given over 30 minutes. When the patient has not been on theophylline, the loading dose is 5 to 6 mg per kg administered in the same way. A continuous infusion of aminophylline, 0.5 to 1.0 mg per kg per hour, is recommended thereafter. A Harvard pump or IMed volumetric infusion pump is particularly convenient for dosing accurately. Serum theophylline determinations must be done routinely in order to accurately titrate the patient to the desired range of 10 to 20 micrograms per ml. Remember that a 2 mg per kg elevation in dose will raise the serum level by 4 micrograms per ml.

3. Aerosolized bronchodilators are often used in addition to intravenous drugs. Isoetharine (Bronkosol) 1 per cent may be given in the dose of 0.5 ml in 1.5 ml of saline solution and delivered from any convenient nebulizer. Slow deep inspirations favor bronchial penetration. It should not be used if the heart rate is above 180 beats per minute. Atropine sulfate or hydrochloride may also be used as a bronchodilator, especially if there is refractoriness toward beta agonists. One ml of a 1 mg per ml solution may be given by inhalation for relief of bronchospasm caused by increased vagal tone. Vagal reflexes play an important role in the bronchospasm associated with irritant inhalation and may be increased after coughing excessively, IPPB, or inhalation of aerosols.

4. Steroids are often given intravenously during an acute attack, especially if the patient has been refractory to treatment and is in status. Hydrocortisone (Solu-Cortef) may be given in the dose of 4 to 10 mg per kg and repeated in 6 hours. Methylprednisolone (Solu-Medrol) has less salt retention and can be substituted when available. The dose is one fourth that of hydrocortisone. Alternatively the patient may be started on prednisone, 60 to 80 mg, and the dose tapered over the next several days according to the patient's clinical status.

5. Oxygen is clearly indicated if the patient is hypoxic. This is usually due to ventilation-perfusion mismatching. Arterial blood gas determinations should be considered a requirement for the management of an acutely ill asthma patient and will serve as a guide for both oxygen and ventilatory needs as well as treatment of acidosis. The Pa_{O_2} should be kept above 50 mm Hg and ideally between 65 to 100. Venturi masks may be used to deliver from 24 to 40 per cent inspired oxygen. Nasal cannulas, especially the short prongs that fit only into the nares, are less desirable, as patients are usually mouth breathing.

6. The presence of acidosis with a pH of less than 7.2 and a base deficit of more than 7 mEq per liter may require treatment with sodium bicarbonate. The amount required in mEq may be calculated by multiplying the base deficit (mEq) by 0.3 by the patient's weight in kg (base deficit $\times$ 0.3 $\times$ kg). Give half the calculated dose slowly and then recalculate in 1 hour after repeating electrolytes and arterial blood gases. Generally ventilation is a better way to treat respiratory acidosis, but try not to lower the P_{CO_2} by more than 10 mm Hg per hour.

7. Antibiotics may be indicated for treatment of supervening infection. The sputum should be examined for color and consistency and Gram stained. A broad-spectrum antibiotic such as tetracycline, 250 to 500 mg four times daily, or ampicillin, 250 mg four times daily, may be selected pending the return of sputum culture. Always ascertain any history of penicillin or other drug allergy first.

8. Expectorants are of dubious value but are used in hopes of helping to liquefy secretions. Saturated solution of potassium iodide (SSKI), 10 drops in a glass of water, or guaifenesin may be useful. Hydration by intravenous fluids or encouragement to take oral fluids may be just as useful. Oxygen should be humidified in order to prevent drying of mucous membranes, and a Maximist or other humidifier may be used to deliver humidified air to the tracheobronchial tree in hopes of liquefying viscous secretions.

9. Hypokalemia may occur, especially if steroids and bicarbonate are used. Potassium may be added to the intravenous infusion at the rate of 2 to 3 mEq per kg per day. Intravenous solutions should not contain more than 40 mEq per liter of potassium.

10. Once the acute stage has passed, chest physiotherapy and postural drainage may be of benefit. Patients should be encouraged to cough in order to help raise mucous plugs, especially in areas of atelectasis. Antihistamines are generally avoided because of their drying effect on mucous secretions. Tranquilizers and sedatives are also relatively contraindicated.

Respiratory Failure

A $Paco_2$ of 65 mm Hg or higher, especially if the rise has been progressive, accompanied by decreased or absent breath sounds, cyanosis on 40 per cent ambient oxygen, depressed consciousness, poor muscle tone, severe inspiratory retractions, and use of accessory muscles of respiration, indicates respiratory failure and the need for assisted ventilation. Although not all these signs may occur, the appearance of any of them is cause for concern and dictates increased surveillance. Controlled ventilation must be done with endotracheal intubation, preferably orotracheal intubation, which is easier to suction. Muscle relaxants such as succinylcholine, 2 mg per kg every 2 hours, will facilitate intubation and control of ventilation. Pancuronium (Pavulon) may be used at the dose of 0.06 mg per kg to 0.1 mg per kg, depending on the state of agitation and 0.06 mg per kg per hour used for maintenance. Patients must be monitored in an intensive care unit and the medication adjusted hourly if necessary. Sedation will also be necessary to prevent interference with passive ventilation. Diazepam (Valium), 0.2 to 0.3 mg per kg per hour, may be used or morphine sulfate, 0.1 mg per kg every 3 to 4 hours. Volume cycle respirators are preferred in order to provide adequate tidal volumes in the face of high pulmonary resistances. The inspired oxygen concentration should be sufficient to maintain a Pao_2 of 70 mm Hg. Arterial blood gases must be monitored frequently as well as the EKG, fluid intake and output, electrolytes, and vital signs. Tracheal cultures should be taken routinely if the patient is on the ventilator for a prolonged period, and suction and cleansing of the equipment should also be done frequently. A nasogastric tube is placed to prevent gastric distention. Extreme cases may require positive end expiratory pressure in order to maintain adequate oxygenation and bronchoscopy with pulmonary lavage in order to remove as much inspissated mucous plugs from the bronchi as possible. In some cases these modalities may be lifesaving.

General Principles

Immunotherapy. Hyposensitization with inhalant allergens may be appropriate under circumstances when a clear relationship exists between exposure and symptoms, such as with ragweed pollination in the early fall, a positive ragweed skin test, and symptoms exacerbating during the time of active pollination. Appropriate preconditions for treatment with allergen injection therapy include an unsatisfactory response to symptomatic therapy and unavoidability of the offending antigen.

Antibiotics. Most bronchitic infections associated with bronchospasm are viral. Ideally treatment should be predicated upon sputum culture, which may not always be possible. If the production of mucopurulent sputum is attendant to the illness, it may be appropriate to treat with broad-spectrum antibiotics for 1 to 2 weeks.

Hydration. Adequate hydration helps liquefy secretions and should be encouraged for all stages of the illness. Systemic antihistamines and anticholinergics may be drying and should be used with caution.

Emotional Support. Chronic asthma can be a disabling illness, requiring almost constant support and attention. Abilities, however, should be emphasized over disabilities, and the patient should be encouraged to take an active role in the surveillance and treatment of the illness. It is often helpful to point up the difference between emphysema and asthma and to stress the reversibility of the latter as well as how it may be managed. Active participation in daily activities and sports should be encouraged to the point that patients may be asked to take extra medication before an event such as a tennis game or a hike. For many patients asthma is a "condition" with which they live and to which they adjust, rather than a "disease" which presents a long-term insurmountable handicap.

ASTHMA IN CHILDREN

method of
HYMAN CHAI, M.D.
Denver, Colorado

Asthma is a common disease of childhood. It is characterized by the intermittence of its frequency in individuals and in different children, by the variability in its severity, and by a multiplicity of varying, unrelated precipitants which are known or, in a significant number of asthmatics, cannot be defined. Its onset rarely occurs at birth. The majority of children develop asthma between the ages of 6 months and 3 years. However, the first attack may occur at any age. The disease may remain mild and intermittent throughout life, it may steadily become worse, or it may become considerably alleviated as years go by. The onset of the so-called "growing out of asthma" appears to occur around puberty and to benefit girls less often than boys. However, despite the apparent disappearance of asthma in many children in time, the liability of recurrence is high and may remain so for life. Finally, the basic underlying cause that results in active disease remains unknown. There is little doubt about the genetic "liability" to develop asthma, but not all children in an asthmatic family get the disease, although the occurrence rate is higher than in nonasthmatic and nonallergic families. Furthermore, not all identical twins develop asthma; one of them might but the other might never develop the disease. My own experience corroborates the impression that the most common initiator of the first attack of asthma is a viral-like infection, commonly the "common cold." It thus appears that the genetic background to develop asthma requires a subsequent initial "switch," which may well be a virus infection more often than any other initiator.

Asthma, once the initial attack has occurred, can thereafter be precipitated by a variety of mechanisms, not necessarily related to each other. These include true allergy; exercise; the parasympathetic nervous system; possibly the nonsympathetic, nonparasympathetic nervous system; infections, which are almost always viral in the case of children and probably also in adults; emotional factors as an aggravating factor — rarely a primary cause in my view; exposure to cold; irritants such as perfume or paint; and some drugs such as aspirin or organic iodides, which may involve prostaglandins and release of other mast cell mediators by activating the alternative complement system. A small and usually very severe group are the so-called intrinsic asthmatics (better called idiopathic). Any asthmatic may have a single precipitant or may have them all. Most asthmatics have more than one, and 90 per cent of asthmatic children have exercise-induced asthma as a major component.

Available Drugs and Procedures for Therapy

All the following drugs and procedures will be discussed in relationship to the type of asthma the child may have, discussed later in this article, related to my personal views as to the indications for their use, the time period in which they should be used, and the expectations for such therapy.

Medication. CROMOLYN SODIUM. Cromolyn sodium is in worldwide use. It is an effective drug for many asthmatics, and for some the only medication necessary. Cromolyn requires a special apparatus for its administration, as the medication is inhaled as a powder consisting of 20 mg of active cromolyn in lactose. Usual therapy is an initial inhalation schedule of 1 capsule four times daily as preventive therapy. Education in the use of the Spinhaler is essential for success, and a simple indifferent explanation will not do. Its usefulness is also limited by the ability to teach the child to employ the Spinhaler correctly (the manufacturer's official directive states it is for children 5 years of age or older). In some children the inhaled powder produces bronchospasm. Some pediatricians and allergists utilize an inhaled beta-2 sympathomimetic (metaproterenol for example) prior to cromolyn inhalation to prevent the bronchospasm that occasionally occurs, and follow with cromolyn. I see little point in this. The sympathomimetic in its own right is a potent bronchodilator, and hence its use merely to prevent cromolyn-induced bronchospasm is an unnecessary maneuver. In such cases, the beta-2 sympathomimetic alone will be all that is necessary.

The Bronchodilators. THE SYMPATHOMIMETICS. These are available as tablets, liquids, liquids for inhalation, and Freon- (or other gas) propelled inhalants. Not all of them are available in all these formats. Two of them are injectable. Epinephrine is the only injectable available for use for children, although terbutaline is approved for use in adults and children over the age of 12 at this time. Isoproterenol is sometimes administered by intravenous drip for status asthmaticus and respiratory failure in children, but, as it is my view that its use requires experience, experienced personnel, and intensive care facilities, this procedure will be discussed only briefly for completeness.

Isoproterenol is an excellent bronchodilator but has just about equal cardiogenic (beta-1) and bronchodilator (beta-2) properties. It also is relatively short in duration (1½ to 2 hours). The

TABLE 1. **Sympathomimetics***

PRODUCT	AVAILABILITY	TYPE/DOSAGE	REMARKS
Metaproterenol	Tablets Liquid for oral use Freon inhaler	Beta-2 2 mg/kg per 24 hrs 1–2 inhalations/dose	A. Excellent bronchodilator in any of its formats; usual pediatric dose is 2 mg per kg per 24 hours given in divided doses
Terbutaline	Tablets Injectable	Beta-2	B. Not available for children under the age of 12; hence, dosage should be an initial 2.5 mg three times a day, or 5 mg for adolescents
Isoetharine	Tablets Liquid for use with Maximist Freon inhaler	Beta-2 0.5 ml + 0.5 ml water = 1 ml 1–2 inhalations/dose	C. Same as (A) above 6 years old +
Epinephrine	Injectable	Alpha, beta-1 and beta-2 0.01 mg/kg (1:1000) Maximum 0.3 ml	D. Only available injectable for children at this time (as in B); the only injectable to use if asthma and anaphylaxis are present at the same time

There are other sympathomimetics: Isoproterenol is a beta-1 and beta-2 agent and has been known to produce paradoxical responses in some patients (i.e., make things worse). There is a Freon-propelled format of racemic epinephrine available over the counter. The alpha and beta-1 effects are unnecessary. Metaproterenol given in any format lasts about 4 hours in my patients and is my personal choice.

*See also manufacturers' official directives for use in children.

cardiac stimulation, which will result in more blood being pumped through unventilated parts of the lung and hence increasing the "physiologic shunt," is of no advantage.

THE BETA-2 SYMPATHOMIMETICS. All of these have some degree of beta-1 effect on the heart but much less than isoproterenol or epinephrine. They also act for a longer period.

Metaproterenol, mostly beta-2, is an effective bronchodilator that will remain effective for 4 or more hours. Tremor in my experience is a very minor, relatively short-lived problem in children. Metaproterenol is available as a Freon-propelled inhaler, syrup for oral use, and tablets. (See also manufacturer's official directive for use in children.)

Terbutaline is very similar to metaproterenol in most aspects but tends to cause much more tremor than metaproterenol. This may reduce compliance, even though tolerance and decrease of the tremor develop in time for most children. It is also available as an injectable (SC), which is not approved at present for children under 12 years of age but may be in time.

Isoetharine is similar to metaproterenol and terbutaline. It is available in tablets, liquid for oral use, liquids for use in a delivery system such as a Maximist or IPPB apparatus, and Freon-driven inhaler.

Epinephrine, long in use for the treatment of asthma, has an alpha effect stimulating alpha receptors of the sympathetic system, thus causing vascular contraction and, in theory, bronchial muscle constriction, although this has never proved to be a disadvantage in practice. There is also some question as to whether there are many alpha receptors in the lung or any at all for that matter. In addition epinephrine has a beta-1 effect which is cardiogenic and a beta-2 effect which dilates the bronchi. It is the *only* sympathomimetic that should be used as the initial injection if hypotension and shock accompany the attack of asthma. It is the only injectable approved by the Food and Drug Administration (FDA) for use in children under the age of 12. Isoproterenol intravenously in status asthmaticus may be the only exception.

Epinephrine is available in its racemic form as a Freon-propelled inhalant as Primatene and as a subcutaneous injection. A retard format of epinephrine is available (Sus-Phrine). I personally have strong reservations about the use of an aqueous suspension (Sus-Phrine), as, once given, if another injection is needed for one reason or another before 4 hours, this adds epinephrine to epinephrine and may have dangerous consequences.

The Xanthines. These drugs are essentially theophylline and its salts. Most of the salts are converted to theophylline by liver enzymes before they become effective; hence they have no advantages over theophylline alone except for those children who do not tolerate theophylline's gastrointestinal irritation (nausea, vomiting, diarrhea, or all of these). It must be noted that salts of theophylline (aminophylline and oxtriphylline are examples) are dispensed as milligrams of the salt such as milligrams per tablet or per 5 ml liquid. The available theophylline will be less than the indicated milligrams of the salt. For example, aminophylline (theophylline ethylene diamine) as a 100 mg tablet will actually provide only 86 mg of

TABLE 2. **Theophylline Preparations**

PREPARATION	AVAILABLE FORMAT	DOSE	REMARKS
Aminophylline	Tablets Oral liquid Rectal enema Intravenous	86% Available theophylline	Under age 6, 10 mg per kg per 24 hours, over 6 years, 20 mg per kg per 24 hours, divided into 6, 8, or 12 hourly doses, depending on the clinical response and safe blood levels
Theophylline USP	Tablets, capsules	100% available theophylline	Same as above
Theophylline (anhydrous) timed release capsules (Slo-Phyllin)	Capsules	100%	Usually manage a dose every 8 hours; in some children with slow metabolism, might achieve 12 hr dosage
Theophylline (anhydrous) sustained action (Theo-Dur)	Tablets	100%	8 hour dosage usually achievable; 12 hour dosage more often than most preparations because of zero-order kinetics
Oxtriphylline (Choledyl)	Tablets	56% available theophylline	Medium-acting format because of type of manufacture but causes less gastric upset; often manage adequate blood levels with 6–8 hour schedule; has 56% of available theophylline, hence calculations must be based on this

There are many other theophylline preparations, some long-acting, some short. The important aspect here is to determine the amount of theophylline that will become available in the blood and calculate the amount given to arrive at an accurate theophylline dose per kilogram.

active theophylline and oxtriphylline only 56 mg per 100 mg. The xanthines act by prohibiting cAMP breakdown in the mast cell and thus preventing mediator release. This, in turn, prevents bronchospasm as well as relaxing respiratory smooth muscle by the same inhibition of cAMP in the smooth muscle cell.

Theophylline preparations are available as tablets, capsules, retard formats by varied manufacturing techniques, and liquid preparations of aminophylline (theophylline is relatively insoluble) for oral and intravenous use.

Glucocorticosteroids. Various forms of these glucocorticoids are available. It is important to

realize that their time half-lives in the bloodstream are not the same as their cellular half-lives. Prednisone, prednisolone, and hydrocortisone have relatively short cellular activity (24 to 36 hours) and hence can be used on an alternate day basis (i.e., 8 A.M. every 48 hours). Triamcinolone has much longer activity, while betamethasone and dexamethasone have still longer cellular activity and cannot be used on an alternate day basis. The advantage of alternate day therapy lies in its ability to achieve good control of severe asthma while at the same time minimizing adrenal suppression and other steroid side effects. Hydrocortisone is available for injection as a

TABLE 3. **The Glucocorticosteroids**

PRODUCT	ACTIVITY	FORMATS	REMARKS
Prednisone	Relatively short (24–36 hours)	Tablets 5 mg and 20 mg	A. Suitable for alternative day therapy 8 A.M. every 48 hours
Prednisolone	Relatively short (24–36 hours)	4 mg tablets	B. Same as (A) above
Hydrocortisone methylsuccinate (Solu-Cortef)	Short (24–36 hours)	100 mg injectable	C. Used every 6 hours IV in status asthmaticus
Methylprednisolone (Solu-Medrol)	Short	20 mg injectable	D. Same as (C) above
Betamethasone dipropionate (Vanceril)	Short	50 micrograms per inhalation	E. Normal use 400 micrograms per day in divided doses

There are other very potent steroids: betamethasone (Celestone) and dexamethasone (Decadron) in doses of 0.6 mg per tablet and 0.75 mg, respectively. Long-acting cellular activity (3 to 5 days) precludes their use in alternate day (QOD) therapeutic formats. Triamcinolone has the same long-acting cellular activity but lies in between prednisone and betamethasone. The steroids are lifesaving in asthma, given in the correct dose, at the correct frequency, and with an understanding of their side effects and the manner in which steroids can be used to minimize these sometimes unavoidable complications.

Experience over the years has shown that: (1) Short-term (4 to 5 days) of twice daily prednisone or prednisolone will rapidly control asthma with minimal side effects if these bursts are not used too frequently. (2) Short-term formats used on a QOD basis will achieve acceptable asthma control with acceptable side effects if the QOD dose is 30 mg or less. (3) In status asthmaticus intravenous high dose (200 mg of Solu-Cortef or 40 mg of Solu-Medrol) given every 6 hours is lifesaving. For very young children a dose of 2 mg per kg at the same frequency will achieve the same results. (4) Repeated efforts to reduce steroid intake over time should always continue, despite repeated failures.

TABLE 4. **Other Therapeutic Agents and Procedures**

Cromolyn sodium	20 mg in lactose; inhaled powder
Intravenous fluids	All that is necessary is replacement of fluid, based on daily requirements; pulmonary edema may occur if two or three times daily requirements are used in status asthmaticus
Antibiotics	Rarely indicated for asthma; virus infections invariably are the initiating agents of attacks precipitated by infections; bacterial infections rarely are
Humidification	Humidifiers are of questionable value in my experience; may cause mold overgrowth
Air filters	Electrostatic or HePA systems; only useful if one room is used and then only after the child goes to bed and keeps windows and doors closed; little value otherwise in my opinion.
Activity	Every asthmatic should be so treated as to allow unlimited physical activity
IPPB	Useful as a delivery system only; pressure is of little value
Maximist	Good delivery system for bronchodilators that are inhaled
Antihistamines	Not often very helpful; sometimes effective in purely seasonal asthmatics; its drying effect in my experience is more theory than fact
Postural drainage	May be lifesaving in severe status; little value for mild to moderate asthma; can exhaust child
Mucolytics	Of little value; adequate fluid intake is much more effective
Sedatives	There are no indications for sedatives at any time in the therapy of asthma
Psychosocial	Psychosocial consequences of the disease may be very severe; there is no evidence that psychologic factors are a primary factor in asthma

succinate salt, and prednisolone in similar fashion as methylprednisolone (Solu-Medrol). These can be given intravenously or intramuscularly, and their major application is in status asthmaticus. Retard formats such as injectable triamcinolone acetonide suspension have no place, in my view, in the treatment of asthma in children. The convenience of one injection once a month is totally negated by the accompanying total adrenal suppression for that period of time, as well as other side effects such as cushingoid features.

ACTH has found usefulness in Europe, particularly Great Britain, where it is said to reduce suppression of growth (compared to corticosteroids), but anaphylactic reactions have occurred, and by using adequate every other day prednisone therapy these side effects can be managed just as well and the discomfort and risks of injections can be avoided.

Other Drugs and Procedures. POTASSIUM IODIDE. Potassium iodide has had a long history in the therapy of asthma. A study done by colleagues and myself many years ago demonstrated that a dose of 50 mg per kg per day in divided doses controlled one asthmatic child in 20 remarkably well, when other medications at that time failed to do so. The risk to the thyroid by long-term use of iodides and the inescapable side effects (acne, metallic taste, salivation, rhinorrhea) occurred often enough to ensure lack of patient compliance. With more effective and easily administered medications available there should be little need for iodides.

COMBINATION DRUGS. Essentially these include theophylline and ephedrine with either phenobarbital or hydroxyzine to counter the stimulating effect of ephedrine. They were useful in their day, but with better drugs available and the freedom to adjust each component to suit the child, there is little need for continued use of these combinations.

BREATHING EXERCISES. I have found these of little help and inconvenient enough for the family and the children to almost ensure poor compliance. Except for the very severe asthmatics who never normalize their physiology with regard to airway function, asthmatics are normal or near normal between attacks, and these exercises, to my mind, serve little function. This cannot be compared to adults with obstructive lung disease in whom gross physiologic abnormalities are constantly present.

POSTURAL DRAINAGE. There are times when postural drainage is indicated. During severe attacks, unresponsive to therapy, the possibility of mucous plugs being a major source of airway obstruction is always present. In the absence of demonstrable radiologic evidence of atelectatic patches in the chest x-ray, their presence is difficult to prove. However, a trial of postural drainage carried out by experienced therapists may be worthwhile. Effectiveness must be demonstrable by an improvement in the clinical condition confirmed by objective lung function measurements when possible and the production of mucus. This is a tiring experience for children and leads to exhaustion in some of them; hence, the procedure must be accompanied by clear evidence of effectiveness; otherwise it should be discontinued.

MUCOLYTICS (SUCH AS N-ACETYL CYSTINE). In my experience these mucolytics have not been helpful, and their use has only aggravated bronchospasm.

REST AND A DRINK OF WARM WATER. When the attack is mild, many asthmatics do quite well if they rest awhile. The addition of drinking a glass of warm water, as used in some centers, seems to be effective. Whether this reduces the "cooling of the large airway" because of inhaling air through the mouth and bypassing the nose and, hence, acts by preventing bronchospasm caused by cool air reaching the carina and beyond (as has been shown in exercise-induced asthma) or is just the result of rest alone or a combination of both is difficult to ascertain, but the procedure appears to be effective for mild attacks.

SEDATIVES. I believe strongly that chronic asthma results in severe psychosocial problems for the child and the family. I find no hard evidence demonstrating that purely psychologic matters ever cause asthma, nor has my experience over the years ever convinced me that psychologic factors are even primary precipitants. Sedatives in my opinion are contraindicated for all asthma attacks and certainly for severe attacks, such as status asthmaticus and respiratory failure.

ACTIVE PHYSICAL LIFE. All asthmatics, regardless of severity, require to be so managed as to allow them to undertake a fully active life in childhood with no restrictions. Thus, their activity should not be confined to swimming, nor should they be restricted from undertaking any activities that might suit their personalities, from gymnastics to basketball. They may have to be pretreated before these activities, or they may be sufficiently controlled with effective routine therapy so that pretreatment is not necessary. In any event, they should be considered to be "normal" children leading normal lives with a peripheral problem of asthma with which they have to contend.

PSYCHOLOGIC CONSEQUENCES. The psychologic and social consequences of severe asthma in childhood may be serious and debilitating for the child and the family. Education of the family and the child as to the nature of the disease and, in my own view, behavioral therapy approaches to rectifying deficiencies resulting from the disease are extremely effective in returning the child to a normal psychosocial life.

EXERCISE. Exercise is a prominent precipitant in over 90 per cent of asthmatic children. The initial precipitant appears to be the arrival of cool air at the large airways, because exercise requires air to be inhaled through the mouth in large quantities in order to supply sufficient oxygen intake because of the physiologic demands of exercise beyond the anaerobic threshold and thus bypassing the warming ability of the nose. Prevention is essential for such patients. Prevention is obtained by one of the following procedures:

1. Those children who require around-the-clock medication may be sufficiently protected by this alone.

2. Those children who are not so protected, despite around-the-clock medication, will need preventive therapy utilized about 5 to 10 minutes prior to undertaking sustained physical activity. This can be achieved by the prior inhalation of 20 mg of cromolyn sodium or by the prior inhalation (2 inhalations) of metaproterenol. Metaproterenol is my preference because it provides longer bronchodilation, but any other beta-2 sympathomimetic would be adequate. Finally, if either cromolyn or the sympathomimetic is not totally effective, inhalation of both cromolyn and the sympathomimetic prior to exercise acts synergistically and may be better than either alone.

Should prior treatment fail to be successful, inhalation of a beta-2 (β-2) sympathomimetic (or its oral use for younger children) may be necessary to break the attack after the exercise.

EPINEPHRINE. Epinephrine is a sympathomimetic with alpha, beta-1, and beta-2 stimulating properties. It is an efficient bronchodilator and at this time is the only acceptable injectable bronchodilator for children under the age of 12 years. Children 12 years old and over can utilize terbutaline by injection. This has the advantage of avoiding the cardiogenic and alpha (vasoconstrictor) effects of epinephrine. It should be noted, however, that if shock accompanies an asthmatic attack, epinephrine is the only sympathomimetic that should be used. Asthma associated with anaphylaxis is an example of epinephrine being the only indicated sympathomimetic.

The Various "Faces" of Asthma and the Therapy Thereof

My personal approach to the therapy of asthma depends entirely on which of the following categories any single patient appears to be in at any particular time. All asthmatics may fall into any one of these categories at one time or another in their lives. A minority of them will stay in the severest group for the rest of their lives. My therapeutic approach is designed (1) for immediate relief, (2) for prevention in the future, and (3) to allow the asthmatic child to lead a fully normal active physical life.

Category I. The "Intermittent" Asthmatic. This is the child who has an attack of asthma once in a while, perhaps weeks apart. The attack may be of varying severity at the time but, once aborted, the child remains clinically free for long periods and is physiologically normal. It is obvious that providing such a child with "preventive" medication such as theophylline has little to commend it. These attacks are infrequent and intermittent and deserve the same format of therapy.

For children who cannot cope with an inhalation, an adequate dose of an oral beta-2 preparation is given when needed. This is repeated every 4 hours if necessary until the attack breaks and is then discontinued.

For children who can cope with an inhalation, two inhalations of Freon-propelled metaproterenol or isoetharine are given. I have found metaproterenol to last longer than isoetharine and hence tend to use this preparation. Two inhalations may be sufficient, or it may be necessary to repeat every 4 hours until symptoms do not return. Thereafter the preparation is used only whenever necessary.

For all children, if the attack is severe and requires rapid control and they are unresponsive to inhalation, epinephrine by subcutaneous injection is given, and repeated if need be. If the second response is still poor, the child falls into category III below, perhaps only temporarily.

Category II. The "Frequent" Asthmatic. The attacks occur three or four times a week. Each bout may vary in severity, but in general they occur frequently enough for medication to be more of a "stopgap" than therapy.

Preventive therapy is now indicated. A beta-2 sympathomimetic is my choice because theophylline blood levels are not required and control of symptoms will be more than adequate.

For the child who cannot manage an inhaler, oral isoetharine or metaproterenol in the correct dose, based on weight and given on a three or four times daily basis, may be all that is necessary. This should be provided daily regardless of clinical symptoms, as this is preventive therapy and is continued for some months. At any time this can be discontinued on a trial basis to determine whether the frequency has altered; but if symptoms return, this therapy should be reinstituted.

For the child or adolescent who can manage an inhaler, two inhalations of metaproterenol three or four times a day is my preference. Isoetharine could be used, if one wished, in the same manner. The same qualifications exist as those indicated in the paragraph above. Oral preparations of metaproterenol, terbutaline (above age 12), or isoetharine can be used if these are preferred. I personally prefer the inhalation when feasible, because relief occurs in 60 seconds, compared to 45 to 60 minutes for any oral preparation.

Over and above any medication, "breakthrough" attacks can always occur and cannot be anticipated. If they do occur, another oral dose of the beta-2 drug may be utilized or, in preference when feasible, two inhalations as necessary.

Category III. The "Continuous" Asthmatic. This child has asthma nearly all the time and, if pulmonary functions could be measured, is likely to have abnormal values in large and small airways regardless of clinical well-being. This child also has asthma at night or early morning and the symptoms can vary in severity.

THE MODERATE CONTINUOUS ASTHMATIC. This child requires around-the-clock therapy with an additional provision for "breakthrough" attacks. The basic ideal choice is a theophylline preparation, preferably one which will require the least number of doses per 24 hours and thus enhance compliance. Furthermore, adequate blood level control to normalize physiology (when this can be measured) or provide at least adequate clinical control (when physiology cannot be measured) is essential. There is some initial nuisance value in establishing the dose and the time interval between doses, because individuals utilize theophylline differently. Furthermore, the onset of complications (such as infection) change the manner in which theophylline is metabolized. In addition, the breakdown of theophylline can vary in any individual without any demonstrable cause. Thus the approach must be primarily to establish the correct dose and the correct time period between doses. (1) Very young babies (and adults) handle theophylline slowly. (2) Older babies and children generally handle theophylline with a fairly rapid theophylline metabolism and therefore require a higher dose than adults. (3) The preparation used may have to be limited to the dictates of the age of the child.

Young babies: Aminophylline (theophylline ethylenediamine) as a liquid preparation is used. The available theophylline is 86 per cent of every dose of aminophylline in the liquid preparation. Thus, if a preparation such as Somophyllin (90 mg of aminophylline per teaspoon) is used, the available theophylline per teaspoon (5 ml) will be 86 per cent of 90 mg or approximately 77.4 mg. Children below the age of 6 years tend to degrade and eliminate theophylline erratically. Hence, an initial dose of 10 mg per kg per 24 hours, provided in divided doses (no less than every 6 hours), is indicated in the interests of safety. The half-life of theophylline (about 4½ hours, depending on manufacturing format and hence absorption) means that at least 24 hours is necessary before blood levels are assessed. At this time dosage can be increased or decreased as indicated by clinical needs and safety. Children 6 years and older in my experience can safely be started on 20 mg per kg per 24 hours in divided doses with the same post–24 hour assessment for increase or decrease. This will inform you of the peak level and the trough level and will indicate whether (1) the drug has reached a therapeutic range and (2) how long in time this has been in the acceptable range. You may well decide that if the 2 hour level and 6 hour level are close, an 8 hour schedule will be adequate. It is unlikely that a 12 hour schedule will be possible with aminophylline in babies, although this does occur in some adults. Increments or reductions in dosage are then made in order to maintain the peak blood level below 20 micrograms per ml (it is much safer to go no higher than 15 micrograms per ml and a trough level not much under 10 micrograms per ml).

Children up to age 6 years: Much the same procedure is used as for young babies but, depending on age, a change could be made in a longer acting format of theophylline itself. The longer acting formats are pure theophylline in microlysed form and are manufactured so that availability in the gastrointestinal tract is retarded (either by coating portions of the theophylline granules with beeswax in various layers or by other procedures which delay absorption and thus spread the dosage over time). Slo-Phyllin and Theo-Dur are two examples of these retarded absorption formats. If your choice is the retarded formulas, then blood levels must be taken at 3 hours for a peak, at 8 hours, and at 12 hours for a trough. If the therapeutic criteria are met at any of these times, you will be able to prescribe theophylline at every 8 or 12 hours and hence provide a two or three times daily schedule, which is so much easier to manage and enhances compliance. The initial dosage that I use for children from 4 to 6 years is 10 mg per kg per 24 hours of long-acting preparation (Theo-Dur, Slo-Phyllin, Theolair) divided into three doses (every 8 hours). I then adjust it up or down after 24 hours for safe and therapeutic blood levels.

Adolescents: Adolescents should be handled the same way as children up to 6 years, except that the dosage schedule for older adolescents may be lower. Sixteen-year-old patients may require an initial test dose of 4 mg per kg rather than 5 mg as for the children.

Overall, these dose schedules are initial procedures and will have to be adjusted to suit individual needs. Repeated theophylline blood levels will be necessary if there is any evidence of toxicity (nausea, vomiting, headache, diarrhea, hyperventilation, sleeplessness, hyperactivity). These symptoms can be central or local or both. Any evidence of these problems requires an immediate blood level; otherwise toxicity may proceed to convulsive states. Regardless of the absence of any clinical evidence of toxicity, theophylline levels must be repeated routinely periodically, even if the control of the symptoms is going well, to exclude undetected toxic levels. A theophylline level must be obtained whenever a patient has lost stability of his or her asthma and when lack of compliance is suspected. A very low theophylline level will confirm the lack of compliance. For all these asthmatics at all ages, the addition of a beta-2 sympathomimetic for "breakthrough attacks," either oral or inhaled, depending on the age of the child, will be necessary.

Category IV. The Continuous, Moderately Severe Asthmatic. This asthmatic child or adolescent has all the therapeutic modalities included in his therapy as noted under Category III but still has inconsistent control. Theophylline levels are where they should be, but obviously theophylline is not enough. Lack of compliance is not the problem. The time has come for *additive* therapy.

Theophylline remains the basic therapy but now a beta-2 sympathomimetic (orally or by inhalation) is added to the therapy on a four times a day basis so that the last dose is given before bedtime. Therapy now consists of a theophylline long-acting preparation either every 8 or every 12 hours, plus an oral preparation (liquid for smaller children) such as isoetharine tablets for the child who is able to take tablets of metaproterenol, terbutaline, or isoetharine if that is your preference. My own preference for those children who can inhale a Freon-propelled beta-2 inhaler is to use this instead. The inhaled beta-2 is equally effective, provides a much lower dose, and is simple to take. In short, the therapy now is theophylline every 8 or 12 hours and a beta-2 sympathomimetic four times daily, plus additional beta-2 when unavoidable "breakthrough attacks" occur, as they will.

A variant in the additional drug is possible and could be tried before the addition of a beta-2 sympathomimetic. Cromolyn sodium could be added to the theophylline program, which would then consist of theophylline every 8 or 12 hours plus cromolyn four times daily instead of the beta-2 sympathomimetic. Alternatively, should the addition of the beta-2 to the basic theophylline be insufficient, cromolyn sodium could then be added, thus making a total of three preparations. Conversely, if theophylline and cromolyn were the initial two drugs, then the beta-2 could be added.

My own personal preference is for theophylline as the initial drug around the clock with the addition of metaproterenol by inhalation (if possible) or by tablet form if not. If this is still insufficient, cromolyn sodium is also used.

Category V. Severe Chronic Intractable Asthma. The patient in this category will have required the therapy delineated in Category IV. Failure of Category IV therapy now requires further additional therapy, namely, the addition of glucocorticosteroids. Two particular formats are available for therapy on a long-term basis: an inhaled form or tablets. At present, the available inhaled form is beclomethasone dipropionate, although triamcinolone acetonide may become available soon. The asthmatic patient at this point should have been on theophylline around the clock and taking a beta-2 sympathomimetic with or without cromolyn sodium. The next addition would be an inhaled steroid, beclomethasone dipropionate (Vanceril). In my view, this is applicable only to children who can adequately manage the inhaler. The initial inhaled dose added to therapy should be 100 micrograms (two inhalations) four times a day, making a total of 400 micrograms per day. It may take 2 or 3 days of such added therapy before it becomes apparent that this has been an effective addition. This dose should then be maintained for at least 1 week, thereafter being reduced by 100 micrograms a week until stability can be maintained by theophylline and a sympathomimetic plus cromolyn alone and the steroid stopped or held at whatever point in steroid reduction that stability has faltered. A dose just higher will be the maintenance dose thereafter and should be kept there for at least a month before trying reduction again. Two examples are cited for either of these eventualities:

1. The child is 12 years old, on theophylline every 8 hours plus 2 inhalations of metaproterenol and cromolyn sodium, both four times a day. Control is poor. Beclomethasone is now added, 2 inhalations (100 micrograms) four times a day. A week later all medications are maintained except the beclomethasone, which is reduced to 300 micrograms by eliminating the mid-afternoon dose. Stability continues, and a week later the mid-morning dose is eliminated, thus reducing the dose to 200 micrograms a day given twice daily. A week later the afternoon dose is dropped, stability remains, and a single morning dose of 100 micrograms is being given. Finally, a week later the morning dose is discontinued. The child remains well controlled and stable on the basic theophylline-sympathomimetic medication.

2. The same sequence is applied to this child as in example 1. However, on reduction of the second 100 micrograms (i.e., from 300 to 200 micrograms) the patient's asthma becomes unstable. Full four times daily dosage is then restarted and control gained. Beclomethasone is then reduced to 300 micrograms (100 micrograms three times daily) and maintained at this level but with repeated trials in reduction at 3 to 4 weekly intervals. Reduction could also be attempted with a 50 microgram reduction (1 inhalation), although it has not been my experience that single inhalation reductions are necessarily successful.

Should 400 micrograms of beclomethasone be of little help, then increments of 100 micrograms per day can be added; but as recent evidence has shown that daily inhalations of 500 micrograms and more may show indications of adrenal suppression equal to 30 mg of prednisone every other day, this may be self-defeating. In any event, any requirement of 1000 micrograms per day or more has no advantage over oral steroid therapy. Candida overgrowth may occur with any dose level and can be managed quite well by washing out the mouth with water after each inhalation (if the child can manage this) or by use of a nystatin mouthwash when evidence of Candida is apparent. There are asthmatics in this category who will not be controlled with the addition of inhaled beclomethasone. Oral steroids are now required, and certain goals have to be borne in mind:

1. The first objective is to obtain control of the asthmatic state.

2. The second objective is to convert the corticosteroid dosage to an alternate day schedule.

3. The next objective is to reduce the alternate day steroid dose to the lowest amount compatible with stability of asthma control.

4. The final objective is to manage attacks that "break through" therapy from whatever cause and to return to minimal alternate day dosage as soon as possible.

My procedure for achieving these four objectives is as follows: Oral steroids are now added to the therapy. A short-acting (in its effect on adrenal suppression) steroid must be used, and thus therapy is confined to prednisone or prednisolone. I use prednisone except for the extremely rare patient who cannot convert prednisone to prednisolone because of the absence of a converting liver enzyme. If this does ever occur, then prednisolone must be substituted. This is such an unlikely occurrence as to be of little concern.

Step 1: Immediate control of the asthma and an attempt to normalize pulmonary functions. Prednisone must be given in sufficient quantity twice a day until the objectives are achieved. For children under 6 years, 2 mg per kg is given twice daily. For children over 6 years, 20 mg is given twice daily. The prednisone is given morning and evening each day until the child is clinically better and free of asthma for at least 24 hours. It can then be stopped abruptly, and in my experience this covers about 4 to 5 days. If this short-term "burst" is successful in allowing return of the previous medication without oral steroids, that is all that is required. If such a "burst" procedure is needed on only a few occasions (months in between, for example), repetition is only necessary periodically.

Step 2: If, however, after stopping the steroids as outlined in Step 1, control breaks down again (usually within a week or 10 days), repeat Step 1. A third repetition of Step 1 can be tried, but if this also fails, then it is apparent that oral steroids will be needed on a continuous basis.

Step 3: I repeat Step 1 for the third time. However, once control has been obtained, then I proceed as follows: I reduce the steroid by half, i.e., 20 mg twice daily to 10 mg twice daily for 4 days. If the child remains stable, I convert this to a single 8 A.M. dose (20 mg) for a further 4 days. I then reduce this A.M. dose every third day by 5 mg until symptoms recur. The daily control dose is thus the dose just above the dose when symptoms occurred. This dose should then be tripled and provided on an alternate day 8 A.M. basis, reducing by 5 mg twice a week until the minimal amount of prednisone has been reached which still controls symptoms. This amount, in my own experience, has more often than not eventually been the same or less than the initial daily control dose.

A summary of the sequence of events indicated follows, using a 12-year-old child as an example:

1. Initial steroid, prednisone, 20 mg A.M. and P.M. (40 mg per day).

2. By the fourth day, the child has been well controlled for the last 24 hours. The dose is then reduced to prednisone, 10 mg twice daily.

3. Three days later, this is converted to 20 mg A.M. only, as control has been maintained. Thereafter this is reduced by 5 mg every 4 days, until a dose of 5 mg on alternate days results in the recurrence of minor symptoms. The daily dose is then increased to 20 mg twice daily to regain control and thereafter is switched to 30 mg given at 8 A.M. every 48 hours.

4. Thereafter every 3 to 4 days (essentially twice a week) this is reduced by 5 mg until symptoms begin to recur. Assume that this occurs at 15 mg on alternate day dosage. The dose is then increased to 20 mg on alternate day dosage and continued for the next 3 to 4 weeks and reduction again attempted. This process is continued thereafter either to establish the ability to remove steroids entirely from therapy (which happens often) or to significantly reduce the dosage in the passage of time.

5. Any severe breakdown in control at any time requires the utilization of the "short burst" therapy previously described, with an immediate return to the effective alternate day dosage schedule previously found to be effective. Infections, almost always viral and especially the common cold, are the main reasons for these "breakthrough" periods.

Category VI. This is the child, fortunately relatively uncommon, who cannot be maintained adequately on theophylline, a sympathomimetic, cromolyn sodium, inhaled steroids, and alternate day prednisone. Daily prednisone at the least dose possible is then inevitable, and side effects are unavoidable. The process of reaching this stage passes through all the categories (I to V) until it is obvious that no other procedure will be successful.

Other Therapies

Immunotherapy. Immunotherapy has been a controversial therapy for decades. There is little doubt that the principle of injecting an antigen to reduce the effects of the same antigen either being ingested or inhaled or otherwise injected into the body (such as insect stings) is effective. The usefulness of immunotherapy in the treatment of insect stings that have caused anaphylaxis attests to the effectiveness of the procedure. However, the difficulty in establishing the allergenicity of any particular extract of various antigens and the apparent variability of responsiveness in different patients who receive such injections make the outcome so variable as to suggest that the procedure lacks real value. This is not true in my experience. A positive skin test indicates the presence of the specific antibody to the specific antigen (usually IgE, perhaps very occasionally a homocytotropic IgG). The skin test does *not* define the target organ, and hence, unless the asthma history (seasonal ragweed asthma, for example) clearly correlates with the skin tests, failure is likely. Furthermore, there are so many factors involved in asthma other than the true allergic aspect that the addition of immunotherapy, even if demonstrated to be effective by pre- and postinhalation challenges, may show no clear clinical benefit, possibly because the other overriding factors are much more important or because, for the particular child, it did not prove to be effective. However, for those asthmatics with clear seasonal exacerbations supported by skin test evidence, and if the season is long or the symptoms severe enough to require massive medication therapy to control symptoms, a trial of immunotherapy is worthwhile. A year's initial therapy should provide evidence of improvement; if it does not, I tend to discontinue such treatment. Details of such therapy are not the purpose of this article. If immunotherapeutic procedures are required, these can be found in textbooks of allergy.

Maximist-Type Delivery System. This is essentially a pump that provides the force to nebulize medication in a nebulizer. It is useful for inhaled medication (other than cromolyn, which requires a special type of apparatus) and can be used for small children with a mask. The bronchodilator is placed in the nebulizer and administered by starting the pump. Off and on can be controlled by simple procedures such as maintaining or releasing positive finger pressure on the Y-tube in the system.

Intermittent Positive Pressure Apparatus (IPPB). This is actuated by inhalation and has mechanisms to control pressure of the air and the rate of flow. In my view, IPPB has little place in the treatment of asthma that the Maximist type does not provide. If real pressures are needed (such as in severe status asthmaticus), volume-cycled apparatus is essential.

Oxygen. Oxygen is always indicated if cyanosis is present. Flow rates can be reasonably high

(4 to 6 liters per minute), as asthmatic children in general have no abnormal hypoxic drives and hence will not develop apnea at high flow rates.

Sedatives. There is no role for sedatives in any form in the treatment of asthma. The asthmatic needs full control during severe attacks, and depression of these senses, including the respiratory center, can be dangerous.

Humidity. Humidification does help some asthmatics without a clear indication as to why. In my opinion the supportive role it achieves is very small unless mucus is a major problem, in which case it may be of some benefit coupled with postural drainage. But for general use the propensity for mold growth and the production of ozone (all electric motors produce ozone), which is an irritant to the lung with little overall benefit, precludes its usefulness.

Status Asthmaticus, Respiratory Failure

It is not the purpose of this article to detail the requirements for therapy for status asthmaticus. The child must be in an intensive care unit where facilities are available for intravenous fluids, theophylline blood levels, blood gases and blood chemistries, oxygen, intubation, volume-cycled apparatus for ventilation, and continuous electrocardiographic monitoring. Therapy may or may not easily reverse the status asthmaticus, and respiratory failure may then follow. However, in brief, the requirements are complete bed rest, continuous 100 per cent oxygen at 4 to 6 liters a minute, availability of effective postural drainage if this is needed, monitoring of blood gases, especially Pao_2 and $Paco_2$ as well as pH, maximized theophylline with or without additional beta-2 sympathomimetics by injection, intravenous corticosteroids such as Solu-Cortef, Solu-Medrol, or Celestone every 6 hours, and, in some cases, intravenous isoproterenol. The last-named agent has been generally abandoned in adults because of the occurrence of subendocardial hemorrhages, but it is still sometimes used for children. Recovery may take days.

Finally although this article is directed only to therapy and expresses my personal viewpoint, it goes without saying that the following axioms are necessary in any therapeutic program:

Avoid what one can avoid.

Investigate what can be investigated.

Measure what can be measured (pulmonary functions).

Cover what can be covered (if dust is important).

Remove what can be removed (pets, for example).

Filter what can be filtered (if this is indicated).

Above all, do not make demands on families that they cannot meet.

NASAL ALLERGY DUE TO INHALANT FACTORS

method of
LAWRENCE ZASLOW, M.D.
New Orleans, Louisiana

Allergic rhinitis is a very common illness. At least one person out of eight has symptoms and must seek medical assistance at some time during its course. Symptoms are caused by nasal membrane exposure to inhaled allergens and mediated by specific immunologic mechanisms.

Patients with allergic rhinitis have symptoms seasonally (hay fever) or nonseasonally (perennial allergic rhinitis). In over half, a positive history of allergy, including atopic eczema and bronchial asthma, may be obtained, as well as positive scratch and intradermal skin tests in almost all. The major inhalants causing seasonal allergic rhinitis are pollens and molds. The patient's symptoms are acute and correspond with the specific pollen count during the season. Symptoms recur yearly, with a tendency for worsening. Perennial allergic rhinitis refers to nasal allergy occurring chronically or year round and is caused by nonseasonal inhalants such as house dust, epidermoids, animal pets, and, in some instances, foods.

It must be kept in mind that symptoms of nasal allergy can be produced by mechanisms other than allergy. Patients with nonallergic vasomotor rhinitis become symptomatic after experiencing changes in temperature, humidity, emotion, anger, fatigue, fumes, or strong odors. Drugs such as rauwolfia, oral contraceptives, and the beta-adrenergic blockers such as propranolol hydrochloride (Inderal) can produce this state. Prolonged use of topical vasoconstrictors in the form of nasal drops or sprays can produce a chemical rhinitis (medicamentosa). Pregnancy, as well as myxedema, can cause a nonallergic vasomotor rhinitis, which will disappear following termination of pregnancy or upon approaching the euthyroid state. Patients with deviated septa or nasal polyps may experience chronic nasal obstruction. Treatment involves three modalities: (1) avoidance of the inhalant allergens, (2) symptomatic treatment, and (3) immunotherapy.

Avoidance of Inhalant Allergens

Once the specific inhalant allergens are determined, they should be avoided to bring about a lessening of the patient's symptoms. Avoidance cannot always be accomplished completely; however, some measures can be easily taken without much inconvenience.

Seasonal. In general, tree pollen predominates as a causative agent during the spring, grass pollen in late spring and early summer, and ragweed pollen in the late summer and early fall. The patient with hay fever caused by these pollens should decrease his outdoor exposure during the specific season. Most people take their vacations during the ragweed season, and those allergic to ragweed can benefit by going to areas free from this pollen. (These areas are described in standard allergy texts.) Since these patients have the inherent tendency to become easily sensitized, moving is not practical, as the chances are great that new sensitivities will develop in the new location.

Molds are found year round, with a tendency to peak in the spring, late summer, and fall. Patients with mold allergy should avoid damp and warm areas such as basements, closets, granaries, and areas of decaying vegetation. Old overstuffed furniture is an excellent reservoir for molds and should be removed. Dehumidifiers may decrease mold growth in areas of increased dampness and moisture. Certain chemicals can inhibit mold growth in the home. For cleaning walls and ceilings, as well as areas in the kitchen and bathroom, a mixture containing 1 ounce (30 ml) of benzalkonium chloride (Zephiran) added to 1 gallon (3800 ml) of water is effective in preventing mold regrowth for 2 to 3 months.

Nonseasonal. The most common offender is house dust. The home should be made as dust free as possible. Most people cannot avoid dust during the day, but the exposure to dust can be decreased in the bedroom of the home where the patient spends a great portion of his time.

The bedroom can be prepared by removing any overstuffed furniture, stuffed toys or animals, carpets, rugs, as well as other objects that tend to collect dust. A small rug made of synthetic material, such as nylon or Acrylon, may be used if it is washed weekly. The furniture should be wood, plastic, or metal so that cleaning can be thorough and easy.

Curtains or drapes may be used if they are washed frequently. Venetian blinds should not be used, since they trap dust. The closets, floors, and walls should be cleaned daily with a vacuum cleaner or damp cloth, preferably when the patient is not home. Feather pillows and mattresses should be replaced with foam rubber or Dacron material. Dust-proof encasings should be used to cover the pillows, as well as the box springs and mattresses. The bedding should be cotton or synthetic material and laundered frequently. Wool is to be avoided.

Patients allergic to epidermoids, i.e., the dust or dander from animals' fur or feathers, should not acquire any pet animals. If they have pets and are reluctant to give them up, the pets should be kept outside the home. Occasionally a patient may be extremely sensitive to epidermoids, and then it is mandatory that the animal be removed. Other sources of epidermoid allergens may be found in fur, as well as in fur linings for various garments. It is also found in some brushes, blankets, rugs, carpets, mattresses, upholstery, pillows, cushions, ropes, and stuffed toys. Avoidance measures for these patients will be similar to those listed for the dust-sensitive patient. These patients should avoid farms, barns, and zoos.

Air Filtration. Air conditioners reduce the pollen, molds, and dust simply by their filtering mechanism. The windows and doors can remain closed during the summer months, allowing a further reduction in the inhalant exposure. The humidity is also lowered, thereby inhibiting mold growth.

Electrostatic precipitators and HEPA (high energy particulate air) filters are more effective than air conditioners in removing particulate matter from the air. These units ionize particles that become attracted and are then disposed of by plates having opposite electric charges. These units can be installed into central heating and air conditioning systems.

Symptomatic Treatment

Antihistamines. Antihistamines act as competitive antagonists to histamine at the receptor sites on the effector cells. These drugs have local anesthetic as well as quinidine and atropine-like effects, producing side effects such as drowsiness, sedation, dizziness, nausea, vomiting, diarrhea, and dryness of the mouth, as well as difficulty in voiding and impotence. They exhibit variability in their clinical effectiveness, and therefore different preparations should be tried until one is found that gives the best clinical response with the least side effects. It is wise for the physician to familiarize himself with several preparations. These drugs should be used cautiously, if at all, in patients with asthma, because their atropine-like effects tend to dry out the bronchial secretions, producing inspissated plugs which cause airway obstruction. The type of antihistamine used should be changed from time to time to ensure continued effectiveness and to prevent tolerance. These drugs are quite effective for acute symptoms of nasal allergy, e.g., itching, sneezing, rhinorrhea. The following antihistamines are given three or four times a day: chlorpheniramine (Chlor-Trimeton), as a 4 mg tablet; chlorpheniramine-d form (Polaramine), as a 4 mg tablet; tripelennamine hydrochloride (Pyribenzamine), as a 25 mg tablet; brompheniramine maleate (Dimetane), as a 4 mg tablet; and diphenhydramine hydrochloride (Benadryl), as a 25 or 50 mg capsule. Benadryl, as well as promethazine hydrochloride (Phenergan), as a 12.5 or 25 mg tablet, may be used at bedtime; the side effect, sedation, will help ensure a restful sleep.

Sympathomimetics. Ephedrine sulfate, 25 mg tablet, as well as pseudoephedrine (Sudafed), 60 mg tablet, may be given three or four times a day. These drugs are used for symptoms of nasal obstruction and are useful in patients with associated asthma when antihistamines are undesirable. They should be used cautiously in patients with hypertension, heart disease, thyroid disease, or diabetes.

Most vasoconstrictors are combined with antihistamines for enhanced therapeutic effectiveness. Examples of these are phenylpropanolamine, pheniramine, and pyrilamine maleate (Triaminic) tablets, which should be given in the morning, midafternoon, and evening; brompheniramine, phenylephrine, and phenylpropanolamine (Dimetapp Extentabs), which should be given in the morning and evening; and triprolidine and pseudoephedrine (Actifed) tablets, which should be given three or four times a day. Cyclopentamine and pyrrobutamine phosphate (Co-Pyronil pulvules) should be given every 12 hours, and phenylpropanolamine, phenylephrine, phenyltoloxamine, and chlorpheniramine (Naldecon) sustained action tablets should be given on arising, in the midafternoon, and at bedtime.

If absolutely necessary, topical agents in the form of a spray or drops should be used for short periods of time so that rhinitis medicamentosa will not result. Oxymetazoline hydrochloride (Afrin) 0.05 per cent has been quite effective, because it has a prolonged action with minimal "rebound" effect.

Adrenocortical Steroids. Adrenocortical steroids act as anti-inflammatory agents. There are many relative contraindications, as well as important side reactions, which the physician must be aware of before using these drugs. Indications for use of the drugs in nasal allergy are limited to only the severest forms unresponsive to other conservative measures, i.e., during peak pollen season, or as therapy for chemical rhinitis. To avoid adrenal suppression, a 5 to 10 day short course is recommended.

ORAL ADRENOCORTICAL STEROIDS. The simplest and least expensive preparation is prednisone. It is given in the dose of 30 to 40 mg by mouth and then the dose is decreased by at least 5 to 10 mg a day every 2 days for a total of 5 to 10 days. Twenty-four to 48 hours are necessary for relief of symptoms to occur. When the patient's symptoms are relieved, conversion to topical adrenocortical steroids should be made. The long-acting preparations such as dexamethasone, as well as the deposteroids, should be avoided, since they cause prolonged adrenal suppression. It is not uncommon for allergic reactions to occur following the use of the peptide ACTH, and it is therefore not recommended.

TOPICAL ADRENOCORTICAL STEROIDS. Each metered spray of dexamethasone (Decadron Turbinaire) is equivalent to approximately 0.1 mg of dexamethasone phosphate. The recommended dose is 2 sprays in each nostril two or three times a day. When improvement occurs, the dose should be decreased to the minimum necessary for relief. This form of treatment is moderately effective in controlling allergic rhinitis complicated by polyps as well as severe nasal congestion. Side effects are rare; however, repeated use can cause adrenocortical suppression resulting from systemic absorption. More common side effects are nasal irritation and dryness. Reports demonstrate less adrenal suppression than with systemic use. The risk of long-term adrenal suppression from seasonal use appears to be small, since recent reports indicate that after this drug has been stopped, a prompt return of normal adrenal function occurs.

Beclomethasone (Vanceril) does not cause adrenocortical suppression at the usual dose and is favored over dexamethasone. (This use of beclomethasone is not listed in the manufacturer's official directive.) Vanceril should be used with a TR#40 DeVilbiss Nasal Adaptor. The dose is 1 spray in each nostril four times daily, and then the dose may be decreased for maintenance. Side effects over a long period of time are minimal and may consist of blood-tinged nasal secretion.

Intranasal Cromolyn Sodium. Cromolyn sodium (Intal) is available in capsules containing 20 mg as a powder. It appears to be more effective and less irritating to the nasal membranes when used as a 2 per cent solution for children and as a 4 per cent solution for adults. A 4 per cent solution is made by dissolving 30 capsules of the drug in 15 ml of distilled water. Several drops into each nostril may be used two to four times daily. (This use of cromolyn sodium is not listed in the manufacturer's official directive.) It is beneficial in a large majority of patients.

Immunotherapy

If avoidance and medication are not practical or effective in alleviating the patient's symptoms, then immunotherapy should be considered. The effectiveness of immunotherapy has been shown to be significant in lessening the progression and severity of the disease.

Immunotherapy involves injecting an aqueous mixture of specific proteins extracted from the inhalant allergens in gradually increasing amounts until a maintenance dose, or the patient's tolerance, is reached. Sensitivity, as well as the starting dose, is determined by the results of scratch and intradermal skin testing. The perennial method of treatment gives the best results. Injections are given twice a week until the maintenance dose is reached, and then the frequency of the injections is decreased to once a week and then to twice a month. Most patients should receive therapy for at least 3 years. However, the duration should be determined for each individual patient based on the type of sensitivity, the severity, and the clinical response. It is well known that the longer the patient receives therapy, the longer he remains symptom-free after immunotherapy is discontinued. Occasionally reactions may follow injections. A local reaction is a swelling at the site of injection of an area greater than the diameter of a 50 cent piece (3 cm), which does not subside in a 24 hour period. If this occurs, the next dose of extract must be reduced. A generalized reaction is manifest by an exacerbation of the symptoms of hay fever, asthma, or hives. This can be controlled by placing a tourniquet around the extremity above the site of injection and introducing 0.10 ml of epinephrine 1:1000 subcutaneously into the site of the injection, as well as another 0.10 to 0.20 ml of epinephrine injected subcutaneously into the opposite extremity. An antihistamine should be taken by mouth.

Atopic patients produce a skin-sensitizing antibody or IgE which causes generalized sensitization of skin and mucous membranes. In nasal allergy, IgE fixes to the nasal membrane and reacts with the specific inhalant mediators that produce the symptoms of nasal allergy.

Recent studies indicate that the first measurable immunologic change that occurs following immunotherapy is an increase in the IgG antibody. This antibody combines with the inhalant allergen so that it cannot react with IgE. IgG is responsible for early clinical improvement. These IgG antibodies increase and the peak titer is dependent on the total dose of antigen given to the patient. With continuous injection therapy there is a slow decrease in IgE occurring over months to years. Also, cell sensitivity of histamine-containing cells decreases, and this correlates well with clinical improvement and may be due to a decrease of IgE on the cell, displacement of IgE by IgG, or the interference with the cellular process needed for histamine release. Long-lasting relief of allergic symptoms is better correlated with the decrease in IgE and a decrease in cellular sensitivity than with the increase of IgG. Clinical improvement following immunotherapy must be the result of complex changes involving immunologic, as well as cellular, phenomena.

Pyridine-extracted, alum-precipitated extracts are available for immunotherapy. These extracts are absorbed more slowly and are associated with less local and systemic reactions. Recent studies have revealed that the active antigen in ragweed is denatured by pyridine extraction with resultant poor immunologic and clinical response. Therefore, it is recommended that aqueous pollen extracts be used for immunotherapy.

Complications

Nasal polyps are seen in patients with perennial allergic rhinitis commonly associated with chronic infection. These polyps should be treated conservatively with allergic management to inhibit growth as well as recurrence following surgery. Since the recurrence rate is quite high following polypectomy, surgery should be considered only in patients with severe obstruction. Surgery without allergic management and control may precipitate or worsen coexisting asthma.

Nasal and paranasal infection, especially sinusitis, is frequently associated with perennial allergic rhinitis and polyps. It is best treated with appropriate antibiotics based on culture and sensitivity studies along with vigorous allergic symptomatic therapy.

Intolerance to aspirin should be suspected in patients with perennial allergic rhinitis, nasal polyps, and bronchial asthma. Evidence of allergy to acetylsalicylic acid has not been demonstrated, and these patients have intolerance to other drugs, i.e., phenylbutazone (Butazolidin), indomethacin (Indocin), ibuprofen (Motrin), naproxen (Naprosyn), mefenamic acid (Ponstel), and tartrazine (F, D, and C yellow #5). Propoxyphene (Darvon) or acetaminophen (Tylenol) may be given to these patients without any untoward reaction. Acetylsalicylic acid must be avoided.

ADVERSE REACTIONS TO DRUGS: HYPERSENSITIVITY

method of
KENNETH P. MATHEWS, M.D.
Ann Arbor, Michigan

In addition to their common occurrence in ambulatory patients, several surveys have indicated that more than 15 per cent of patients on general medical services experience some type of adverse effect from drugs. As iatrogenic illnesses, these should be at least partly preventable. There are many types of drug reactions, including toxicity, intolerance, side effects, secondary effects, idiosyncratic reactions, psychogenic responses, and allergic or hypersensitivity reactions. The last group constitutes about 25 per cent of all significant adverse drug effects. To keep the term drug allergy or hypersensitivity meaningful, its use should be limited to those adverse drug reactions that are (or can reasonably be presumed to be) mediated by immunologic mechanisms. This discussion focuses on reactions of this type.

Prevention

Although there often is no way a physician can foresee that a patient will have an allergic reaction to a prescribed drug, the incidence of such difficulty can be minimized. By far the most important measure is to *routinely ask all patients whether they previously have taken the drugs one wishes to prescribe and whether there was any adverse effect therefrom.* One should be particularly concerned about reported ill effects of a type that suggests hypersensitivity. With the multiplicity of drugs available today, it usually is quite simple to substitute another preparation when the history is at all suggestive of drug allergy. Failure to heed such warnings is medically hazardous for the patient and legally hazardous for the physician. Another important preventive measure is to avoid the indiscriminate, intermittent, or topical use of potent sensitizers, particularly antibacterial agents.

Early Recognition

Most cases of drug hypersensitivity run a self-limited and fairly benign course if the offending drug is stopped promptly, but severe difficulty may ensue if the diagnosis is overlooked and the medication is continued. Unfortunately, however, the possible manifestations of drug hypersensitivity are numerous and protean, and none is pathognomonic for this condition. Thus, it is important to think of the possibility of drug allergy when one encounters one of its possible manifestations (Table 1), but all the conditions listed in this table can be also caused by other allergens or by nonimmunologic mechanisms.

Having considered drug hypersensitivity, a detailed history is the best means at present for assessing this possibility. The time interval between taking the drug and the onset of the suspected reaction is especially important, as is information about the frequency of reactions and the usual manifestations of hypersensitivity to the drug(s) in question. Also of relevance is whether the patient had taken the suspected preparation previously and whether the patient is known to have had reactions to any drugs previously. It is essential to ascertain *all* of the medicines being taken, remembering that patients are especially prone to forget drugs that are used habitually, purchased over the counter, or taken by routes other than by mouth or by injection. To be more certain that the patient is not overlooking some medicine, it is useful specifically to inquire about such drugs as aspirin, nose drops, cathartics, sedatives, tonics, ointments, contraceptives, penicillin, other antibacterial agents, and hormones. Particularly if the presenting reaction is often associated with a drug being taken and the time interval is suggestive, it is reasonable to assume that drug allergy is present until the diagnosis is supported or refuted by stopping the drugs and seeing if the symptoms disappear.

Unfortunately this procedure can lead to false diagnoses of drug allergy if a spontaneous remission coincides with withdrawal of drugs. It would be highly useful to have simple, objective tests for confirming drug hypersensitivity, but unfortunately such tests are not available for assessing most types of drug allergy. Skin tests

TABLE 1. **Some Manifestations of Drug Allergy**

Cutaneous	*Hematologic*
Urticaria and angioedema	Thrombocytopenia
Allergic contact dermatitis	Agranulocytosis
Erythema multiforme	Hemolytic anemia
Stevens-Johnson syndrome	*Hypersensitivity vasculitis*
Maculopapular eruptions	Serum sickness
Pruritus	Hypersensitivity angiitis
Fixed drug eruption	*Miscellaneous*
Purpura	Lupus erythematosus– like disease
Allergic photodermatitis	Drug fever
Respiratory	Anaphylactic shock
Asthma	Jaundice
Pulmonary infiltrative disease with eosinophilia	Others

generally are not reliable except for patch testing in patients with suspected allergic contact dermatitis to topical medications and prick or intracutaneous testing for IgE-mediated reactions to penicillin (see later discussion) or to high molecular weight biologicals such as adrenocorticotropic hormone (ACTH), equine antisera, or egg protein–containing vaccines. In patients with immunologically mediated hematologic drug reactions, various specialized tests are available involving the interaction of the drug, the patient's serum, and either platelets, red blood cells, or leukocytes. Other tests, such as radioallergosorbent test (RAST), antigen-binding measurements, skin windows, migration inhibiting factor (MIF) liberation, and lymphocyte cultures, have been employed on a research basis, but their results are not always relevant to the patient's clinical problem. Another basic difficulty is that the patient may well be reacting to a drug metabolite or degradation product. Of course, the diagnosis could be evaluated by readministering the drug, but this generally could not be justified on ethical grounds unless it is important for the patient to receive the drug in question; in such cases challenges should be initiated with only small amounts of drug under very careful surveillance.

Treatment

Needless to say, the primary treatment for most forms of drug hypersensitivity is to stop administration of the offending medication. Although there are some exceptions, most drugs are metabolized sufficiently rapidly that patients start to improve within 24 to 48 hours after discontinuing the offending medication. Of course, the patient should be informed about the diagnosis and advised about the increased risk of another reaction occurring if the same medication were used again in the future. Particularly in the case of drugs such as penicillin, which the patient might be given while unconscious after an accident, it may be advisable for the patient to obtain a Medic Alert emblem or other readily visible warning device. In cases of allergic contact dermatitis caused by topical preparations, the patient should be instructed about possibly occult sources of re-exposure to the offending agent; sometimes reference to specialized texts on contactants is helpful.

If the drug reaction is fairly mild, no further treatment other than stopping the drug is necessary or desirable. Appropriate symptomatic treatment for severe reactions is, of course, based on the type of symptoms. As discussed elsewhere in this book, urticaria, angioedema, and generalized pruritus frequently respond to therapy with antihistamines, particularly hydroxyzine. Supplementary injections of epinephrine or terbutaline may be helpful in severe cases. Aspirin or acetaminophen may be useful when fever, arthralgia, or malaise is prominent. Because of the self-limited nature of the disease, corticosteroids

TABLE 2. **Emergency Treatment of Anaphylaxis**

1. Immediately give subcutaneous aqueous epinephrine.
   Adult: 0.3 ml of 1:1000. May repeat 3 times every 10 to 15 minutes.
   Child: 0.005 ml per lb body weight of 1:1000. May repeat 3 times every 10 to 15 minutes.
2. Put patient in recumbent position, monitor pulse, blood pressure, and respirations, and start an intravenous infusion if not promptly responding.
3. When possible, limit further antigen absorption by a tourniquet.
4. Give parenteral antihistamine (e.g., 50 mg of diphenhydramine intravenously) especially if there is increasing urticaria or pruritus.
5. If patient is wheezing, give 5 mg per kg of aminophylline intravenously over 15 to 30 minutes. Omit if hypotension is developing.
6. For hypotension, give large amounts of intravenous fluids (saline or Ringer's solution). If this is insufficient, dopamine (Intropin) is suggested. Give intravenously in a dose of 200 to 500 mg in 500 ml isotonic saline solution (see package insert for details). An advantage of using dopamine is that it does not cause renal shutdown. Large doses can produce excess cardiac stimulation and a cardiac monitor should be used. Or consider use of levarterenol bitartrate (Levophed) and phentolamine (Regitine) for persisting hemodynamic shock. Mix 2 ampules levarterenol bitartrate (Levophed) (16 mg in 8 ml), and 1 ampule phentolamine (Regitine) (5 mg) in 1000 ml 5 per cent dextrose in water. Give intravenously at approximately 2 ml per minute. Titrate the blood pressure as it rises against the speed of flow of the intravenous infusion, repeatedly checking the blood pressure.
7. If the patient does not improve promptly, give intravenous corticosteroid (e.g., 200 mg hydrocortisone). For shock not responding to the aforementioned measures, some have recommended massive intravenous doses of corticosteroids (e.g., 30 mg per kg methylprednisolone sodium succinate (Solu-Medrol)), but an advantage of such massive doses is not well documented. Corticosteroids may prevent delayed anaphylactic deaths but are not rapidly efficacious. Hence, steps 1 through 6 should be considered first.
8. When other drugs are not available, intravenous epinephrine, 0.3 to 0.5 ml of 1:10,000 solution (a 1:10 dilution of the usual 1:1000 epinephrine preparation), should be given over 5 minutes. There is danger of cardiac arrhythmia.
9. Maintain airway, position to avoid aspiration, and be prepared to do endotracheal intubation or tracheostomy. Be prepared to treat cardiac arrest.
10. Release patient only after all parameters have largely returned to normal. Outpatients should not go home unattended. An oral antihistamine is often provided for the patient to take at home for the subsequent 24 to 48 hours.

seldom are required. The main exception is severe serum sickness–type reactions, in which a corticosteroid burst is especially to be considered if proteinuria or evidence of neurologic involvement is developing. Corticosteroids also are used for exfoliative dermatitis and for the Stevens-Johnson syndrome resulting from drugs. In allergic contact dermatitis they may be used topically or systemically, depending on the severity of the process. Anaphylaxis, most often caused by penicillin, requires immediate and energetic intervention. A suggested procedure is shown in Table 2.

Special Problems in Drug Hypersensitivity. An especially difficult situation arises when patients specifically require drugs to which they previously may have experienced an "allergic" reaction. Penicillin, insulin, and radiographic contrast media present common examples of drugs involved in this dilemma.

PENICILLIN. Another antibiotic can be substituted for penicillin in the vast majority of patients whose history is suggestive of penicillin allergy, but in rare instances, particularly in patients with subacute bacterial endocarditis, it may be desirable nevertheless to use penicillin. It is fortunate that skin testing is valuable in predicting immediate anaphylactic and other IgE-mediated reactions to this drug, since it not infrequently turns out that the patient is not at risk of developing a severe reaction after all;

previous hypersensitivity may have waned or the previous diagnosis may have been incorrect. A suggested procedure for skin testing is given in Table 3. Considerable prospective and retrospective data indicate that patients reacting negatively to these skin tests will not have an immediate, life-threatening reaction if given penicillin, though minor or delayed reactions could occur. Unfortunately the minor determinant mixture (MDM) still has not been released by the Food and Drug Administration for general use. Where this is not available, there is a slight chance of an immediate reaction in patients negative to penicillin G and penicilloyl polylysine. This has led to the suggestion that such persons initially be given low doses of penicillin, such as 100, 1000, and 10,000 units subcutaneously at 20 minute intervals before initiating full therapeutic doses. As a matter of prudence, some clinicians prefer to give an initial oral dose of 200,000 units of penicillin even when the skin tests are negative, but this should not be done on untested patients with a history of penicillin allergy since severe anaphylactic reactions can occur following oral administration of this drug. Patients allergic to penicillin G should be assumed to be allergic to the semisynthetic penicillins even though this actually is not always the case. There also is a lesser but nevertheless significantly increased risk of allergic reactions to cephalosporin antibiotics in such persons.

TABLE 3. **Penicillin Skin Testing***

PROCEDURE FOR SUSPECTED PENICILLIN ALLERGY		PROCEDURE FOR SUSPECTED SEVERE PENICILLIN ALLERGY	
Prick or Scratch Tests			*Prick or Scratch Tests*
1. Saline control	_____	1. Saline control	_____
2. PPL,† 6.0×10^{-5}M	_____	2. PPL, 6.0×10^{-5}M	_____
3. Penicillin G, 1×10^{-2}M (10,000 units/ml)	_____	3. Penicillin G, 1×10^{-5}M (10 units/ml)	_____
4. MDM,‡ 1×10^{-2}M	_____	Wait 15 minutes. Apply steps 4 and 5 only if step 3 is negative.	
		4. Penicillin G, 1×10^{-2}M (10,000 units/ml)	_____
		5. MDM, 1×10^{-2}M	_____

Wait 15 minutes. Apply intracutaneous (IC) tests only if the above are negative.

IC Tests (Use Volume of 0.02 ml)	IC
1. Saline control	_____
2. PPL, 6.0×10^{-5}	_____
3. Penicillin G, 1×10^{-2}M (10,000 units/ml)	_____
4. MDM, 1×10^{-2}M	_____

*Perform tests on an extremity so that a tourniquet could be applied if necessary.
†PPL-Benzylpenicilloyl polylysine (Pre-Pen) available from Kremers-Urban Company, Milwaukee, Wisconsin 53201.
‡Minor determinant mixture (MDM) contains penicillin G, sodium benzylpenicilloate, sodium benzylpenilloate, and sometimes sodium benzylpenicilloylamine.

In the very rare instances when penicillin therapy is mandatory in spite of positive skin tests, desensitization must be resorted to under extreme precautions, including placing an intravenous line, having appropriate drugs immediately at hand (Table 2), and constant attendance of the patient. A typical dosage schedule would call for starting with 0.1 unit (e.g., 0.1 ml of 1 unit per ml penicillin) subcutaneously in an extremity. If no reaction occurs, the dose is tripled every 20 minutes, if tolerated, until the therapeutic range is reached.

INSULIN. Localized itching, redness, and swelling occur not uncommonly at the commencement of insulin therapy but usually subside spontaneously after a few weeks; administering an oral antihistamine preparation 30 minutes before insulin may be helpful if the symptoms are more than trivial. In a few patients, however, the symptoms progress to generalized urticaria, angioedema, or other symptoms of anaphylaxis. With the preparations in use today, the insulin molecule itself usually is the allergen, although a few patients tolerate highly purified monocomponent preparations better than cruder materials. Prick testing followed (if negative) by intracutaneous tests with 0.02 ml insulin diluted to 8 to 10 units per ml with' saline solution are almost always positive in patients with IgE-mediated insulin allergy. They are not diagnostic, however, since positive results often are obtained in patients receiving insulin without manifesting allergic symptoms, but such testing may be useful in largely excluding the diagnosis or in attempting to select an insulin preparation that is most likely to be tolerated. Since the structure of pork insulin is more closely related to human insulin than the beef hormone, some patients will tolerate single-peak pork insulin in preference to beef or mixed insulins.

In the relatively rare situations in which no type of insulin is tolerated but therapy with this drug is necessary, desensitization often can be achieved quite readily employing procedures and precautions similar to those previously described for penicillin allergy. Employing diluted solutions, an average starting dose would be 0.001 unit (0.1 ml of 0.01 unit per ml insulin) subcutaneously followed by doubling or tripling of doses, if tolerated, given subcutaneously every 20 to 30 minutes until the therapeutic level is achieved. Once "desensitized," it is important for such patients to continue to take insulin regularly: a lapse of even 48 hours may lead to loss of tolerance. If desired, an insulin allergy desensitization kit can be obtained from Eli Lilly and Company.

RADIOGRAPHIC CONTRAST MEDIA (RCM). Another dilemma occurs when there are urgent indications for RCM injections in patients who previously had experienced anaphylactoid reactions from these materials. Although IgE antibodies have not been documented to cause these effects (complement activation with subsequent histamine release now is suspected), the fact is that there is about a 30 per cent probability that the patient will again react to another RCM injection. If further RCM injections seem mandatory, it has been empirically determined that the following procedure markedly reduces the incidence and severity of RCM reactions:

1. Give 50 mg prednisone orally every 6 hours for three doses beginning about 18 hours before the RCM injection, the last dose being 1 hour before the procedure.

2. Give 50 mg diphenhydramine intramuscularly 30 minutes before the procedure or intravenously 10 minutes before the RCM injection.

ASPIRIN. This drug may cause very severe or even fatal asthma. Most often this occurs in middle-aged patients, particularly those with nasal polyps. Aspirin also frequently causes urticaria, especially among patients suffering from chronic, idiopathic urticaria. As in the case of radiographic contrast media, it no longer is thought that these reactions are immunologically mediated even though the manifestations of the reactions are quite typical for allergy. Instead, inhibition of the cyclo-oxygenase enzymes involved in prostaglandin synthesis appears to be crucial. Consequently, these patients may have similar difficulties with other drugs that inhibit prostaglandin synthesis, such as indomethacin, phenylbutazone, mefenamic acid, and some other nonsteroidal anti-inflammatory drugs. Some also are intolerant of tartrazine yellow dye (FD&C Yellow No. 5), which is widely used for coloring medications and some foods. Patients with aspirin intolerance accordingly should be made aware of these possibilities as well as of the innumerable medications that contain aspirin itself. In short, they should be instructed that they should take no medicines unless they are certain that they do *not* contain acetylsalicylic acid (aspirin). Skin testing with aspirin is contraindicated, but the diagnosis usually (but not always) is obvious from the patient's history. When such patients require analgesics, acetaminophen usually is tolerated. In the very rare cases in which this drug also causes difficulty, sodium salicylate or propoxyphene hydrochloride can be used.

ALLERGIC REACTIONS TO INSECT STINGS

method of
WILLIAM W. BUSSE, M.D.
Madison, Wisconsin

Allergic reactions to insect stings occur in approximately 0.4 per cent of the population. While the severity of these allergic reactions is extremely variable, they are estimated to cause at least 40 deaths per year. Insects capable of producing these allergic reactions belong to the Hymenoptera order, which includes the honeybee, hornet, wasp, and yellow jacket. Venoms from these insects contain a number of allergenic proteins capable of generating an immediate allergic reaction. Allergic reactions are most frequently associated with stings of the yellow jacket and honeybee. Hypersensitivity reactions can also follow bites of the fire ants and harvest ants, although these are a lesser problem and regional in distribution.

Types of Reactions

Local Reactions. Pain, erythema, and swelling at the sting site are the usual response. These are self-limited reactions and do not usually require treatment. In some, local reactions may become more extensive and painful and may persist for days. A small portion of these reactions may be allergic or forewarn the development of anaphylaxis with subsequent stings.

Anaphylaxis. The systemic or anaphylactic reaction is potentially most serious. In the majority of patients, the generalized responses are cutaneous and involve erythema, pruritus, urticaria, or angioedema. These symptoms usually begin within 30 minutes after the sting. Systemic reactions are variable from patient to patient. In an extremely sensitive individual, fatal anaphylaxis can occur. These reactions tend to be sudden in onset and more explosive. Serious life-threatening or fatal reactions involve hypotension or respiratory obstruction from either laryngeal edema or lower airway bronchospasm. Circulatory collapse occurs with profound vasodilation. In other fatal reactions cardiac arrhythmias or cardiac arrest can develop. It is not known whether the allergic reaction escalates in intensity with each subsequent insect sting or if the allergic reaction pattern is likely to remain similar on each subsequent sting. Recognition of the variability of anaphylaxis is as important as awareness of its potential for a fatal outcome.

Delayed and Unusual Reactions. In rare situations following insect stings, neurologic or vascular symptoms may develop, including vasculitis, nephrosis, serum sickness, and encephalopathy. These reactions usually appear days after the sting and may be progressive. The allergic or hypersensitivity mechanism of these delayed reactions is not established.

Treatment

Local Reactions. These are usually self-limited and require no therapy. The local application of ice is helpful in reducing swelling, and oral antihistamines may relieve some of the pruritus. In extremely large and painful reactions, systemic corticosteroids may be beneficial (10 mg of prednisone three times a day for 3 days).

Generalized Systemic Anaphylactic Reactions (Table 1). TREATMENT OF ACUTE INSECT STING ANAPHYLAXIS. The initial treatment of choice in anaphylaxis, whatever the cause, is epinephrine. This is the same whether the clinical picture is generalized urticaria, angioedema, laryngeal edema, or hypotension. Aqueous epinephrine (1:1000), 0.3 to 0.5 ml (0.01 ml per kg), is given subcutaneously or intramuscularly. Local infiltration of the insect site with 0.1 to 0.3 ml of epinephrine will slow absorption of venom. If applicable, tourniquets are applied proximal to the sting site. After administering the initial epinephrine injection, subsequent therapy will depend upon the severity and progression of the reaction.

Isolated cutaneous symptoms will usually respond to epinephrine and an antihistamine. Following epinephrine, the administration of chlorpheniramine, 4 mg four times per day, over the next 24 hours is helpful. The presence of airway obstruction from laryngeal edema is more ominous and requires aggressive therapy. Epinephrine is administered every 15 to 20 minutes, as needed, along with intravenous antihistamines, diphenhydramine, 50 mg every 6 hours. Failure of this therapy to control the laryngeal edema requires a tracheostomy. The presence of laryngeal edema may make an endotracheal tube placement impossible. Although not effective in the acute situation, hydrocortisone (4 mg per kg per 4 hours) should be given in the treatment of protracted airway obstruction.

Severe bronchospasm is treated like status asthmaticus and requires a loading intravenous dose of aminophylline (6.0 mg per kg) and a constant infusion, approximately 0.5 mg per kg per hour, in addition to the aforementioned treatment.

Profound hypotension in severe anaphylaxis requires epinephrine to be given intravenously. One tenth ml of 1:1000 epinephrine is diluted in 10 ml of isotonic saline solution and given slowly intravenously, with repeat doses as needed. Intravenous volume expansion with isotonic saline solution is mandatory. With pro-

TABLE 1.   **Management of Systemic Insect Allergic Reactions**

I. Immediate therapy
  A. Administer 1:1000 epinephrine, 0.01 mg/kg (up to 0.5 ml) subcutaneously
  B. Infiltrate sting site with 1:1000 epinephrine, 0.1 to 0.3 ml, to retard venom absorption
II. Specific therapy for systemic reactions
  A. Isolated cutaneous reactions (urticaria, angioedema, or pruritus)
    1. Epinephrine in doses listed above; repeat if needed
    2. Chlorpheniramine, 4 mg PO every 4 hours for 24 hours
  B. Angioedema with airway obstruction
    1. Repeat epinephrine dose every 15 to 20 minutes as needed
    2. Intravenous antihistamine: diphenhydramine, 50 to 100 mg every 6 hours in adults; in children, diphenhydramine, 5 mg/kg/24 hours, is given in divided doses
    3. Hydrocortisone, 4 mg/kg/4 hours in the protracted situation
    4. Tracheostomy or placement of endotracheal tube
  C. Bronchospasm
    1. Repeat epinephrine as needed every 15 to 20 minutes
    2. Aminophylline, 6.0 mg/kg intravenously over 20 minutes; reduce dose if patient has been receiving oral aminophylline; after initial loading dose, continue intravenous aminophylline infusion as in treatment of status asthmaticus
    3. In persistent bronchospasm, hydrocortisone (4 mg/kg/4 hours) is given intravenously
  D. Hypotension
    1. Repetitive epinephrine subcutaneously or intramuscularly
    2. With profound or nonresponse hypotension, dilute 0.1 ml of 1:1000 epinephrine in 10 ml saline and give intravenously; repeat as necessary
    3. Intravenous fluid volume replacement with isotonic saline solution
    4. With protracted hypotension:
      a. Metaraminol, 100 mg in 1000 ml of 5% dextrose and water given by intravenous drip; *or*
      b. Levarterenol, 8 mg in 1000 ml of 5% dextrose and water given by intravenous drip
    5. Hydrocortisone, 4 mg/kg/4 hours intravenously
III. General measures
  A. With severe airway obstruction, be prepared to maintain an airway; tracheostomy may be necessary if endotracheal placement is not possible
  B. Oxygen administration
  C. Venous tourniquet distal to the sting site may reduce venom absorption

tracted and unresponsive hypotension, therapy will require administration of metaraminol or levarterenol. These patients should also receive hydrocortisone intravenously, 4 mg per kg per 4 hours. These patients shoud be monitored for arrhythmias and these treated as they arise. In most cases corrections of hypoxia and hypotension will reduce the likelihood of arrhythmias.

As a general rule, if the systemic allergic reaction is associated with laryngeal edema, hypotension, or airway obstruction, corticosteroids are also administered. This is not immediately beneficial in the acute episode. However, many of the severe anaphylactic reactions also have a late phase response occurring 4 to 6 hours after the initial symptoms. In addition to their other effects, corticosteroids may reduce the intensity of the late reaction.

IMMUNOTHERAPY. The commercial availability of Hymenoptera venom for treatment of the insect sting allergic patient represents an important advance. Venom immunotherapy has proved highly efficacious in preventing allergic reactions upon subsequent insect stings. In those patients appropriately selected for treatment, venom is administered weekly in progressively increasing doses until a venom equivalent of two venom sacs (100 micrograms) is received. The maintenance dose is administered every 3 to 4 weeks. Immunotherapy stimulates the production of IgG blocking antibodies toward venom. An increase in IgG venom antibodies is associated with protection against a subsequent systemic reaction when restung. However, there is no universal agreement as to which patients should receive venom immunotherapy (Table 2).

All patients with severe, life-threatening reactions to an insect sting should receive venom immunotherapy. Other situations are less clear. Considerable thought and concern are given to those persons with a mild, non-life-threatening reaction and positive venom skin tests. With time many of these patients may lose their allergic sensitivity, or, if restung, only experience a mild systemic reaction. Unfortunately there is no way to predict this situation. Within this group, children provide a unique situation. The child at risk during outdoor play, in many cases, may be unable to self-administer epinephrine if restung. Until the natural history of the non-life-threatening allergic reaction in

TABLE 2.   **Selection of Patients for Venom Immunotherapy**

REACTION	SKIN TEST REACTION	VENOM IMMUNOTHERAPY
1. None	Negative	No
2. Large local	Negative	No
3. Large local	Positive	No
4. Systemic	Negative	No
5. Non-life-threatening	Positive	Children: probably yes Adults: individual variability
6. Life-threatening	Positive	Yes

children is established, venom immunotherapy is recommended.

In adults with non-life-threatening allergic reactions and positive skin tests, it is important to review the advantages and disadvantages of venom immunotherapy. At present the duration of venom immunotherapy is unknown, but it is likely to involve years and entails a considerable expense. With the possibility that subsequent insect stings may not provoke a reaction or one that is mild, many patients may prefer to treat themselves with epinephrine if restung. This is a reasonable and probably safe alternative to venom immunotherapy.

All patients with insect sting allergy should carry an emergency kit containing injectable epinephrine. If these individuals are protected with immunotherapy, administration of the epinephrine may not be necessary when they are stung. However, with multiple stings the possibility of an anaphylactic reaction exists, even in the venom-treated individual. In patients not receiving immunotherapy at protective levels, epinephrine should be administered upon being stung. It is also practical to avoid these insects. In part, this can be accomplished by wearing shoes, not using scented perfumes and sprays, and eliminating floral pattern clothing.

Diseases of the Skin

ACNE VULGARIS

method of
PETER E. POCHI, M.D.
Boston, Massachusetts

Acne vulgaris is a common, inflammatory skin disease occurring chiefly in adolescence. Its cause is unknown, but several factors are known to be important in its pathogenesis. The basic defect is a retention hyperkeratosis in the epithelium of susceptible pilosebaceous follicles of the face, back, and chest. The cause of this hyperkeratosis and eventual occlusion of the follicular channel is unknown, but the ultimate result is follicular disruption and inflammation. The sebaceous glands of the skin, which develop in late childhood and early puberty, appear to be intimately related to the formation of the inflammatory papules and pustules. These lesions also appear to be dependent for their development upon the presence of intrafollicular anaerobic bacteria, *Propionibacterium acnes,* a source of a variety of enzymatic and chemotactic substances. Acne vulgaris is a self-limited disorder, and there is no evidence that early treatment will prevent its occurrence or shorten its duration. Nonetheless, therapy of the disease in its active phases will lessen its severity and help to prevent the formation of scars.

Local Treatment

Cleansing. While washing is stressed as being important in the management of acne, it is doubtful that meticulous hygiene is of any significant benefit. The pathologic changes in acne lie deeply within the follicles; surface cleansing can hardly be expected to be of much help. However, washing with soap or medicated cleansers does make the skin appear and feel less oily, and the use of lipid solvents (e.g., Seba-Nil) may enhance this effect. Excessive cleansing should be dis-couraged, since the physical trauma of doing so may actually aggravate the disease ("acne mechanica").

Medications. The use of topically applied preparations remains the cornerstone of acne therapy. Their action is directed toward either a reduction of the anaerobic bacterial flora or a reversal of the abnormal follicular hyperkeratosis. A frequent error made by patients using topical agents is limiting the application of medication to the erupted inflammatory lesions. This does little good, as the material must be applied to the entire acne-afflicted area in order to prevent new lesions from developing. Two of the most widely used topical preparations for acne are benzoyl peroxide and tretinoin (Retin-A). Benzoyl peroxide, available in numerous over the counter and prescription preparations and in various concentrations (2.5 to 10 per cent) and forms (lotions, creams, and gels), acts principally to reduce the number of intrafollicular bacteria and thereby to help prevent the formation of inflammatory lesions. These preparations may be applied once or twice daily, depending on skin tolerance. Benzoyl peroxide is somewhat irritating and on rare occasions may induce allergic sensitization. It may also bleach colored fabrics.

In addition to benzoyl peroxide, other topical antibacterial agents can be used in acne. Particularly popular in the past few years has been the use of broad-spectrum antibiotics. At present, only one agent, tetracycline (Topicycline), is marketed for topical use. This antibiotic has been found to be moderately effective in the treatment of mild to moderately severe cases of facial acne when applied twice daily. The medication may impart a slight yellowish but reversible discoloration to the skin; under ultraviolet (UV) light, it fluoresces a bright yellow. Experimental studies with topical erythromycin and clindamycin preparations have also been shown to lead to improvement in patients with acne. It is quite possible that these antibiotics, as well as others, will be marketed in the future. At present, extemporaneous formulations are employed, whereby erythromycin tablets or clindamycin capsule contents are dissolved in organic solvent vehicles, in concentrations of 1 to 3 per cent. A representative vehicle would contain 70 per cent isopropyl alcohol and 5 to 10 per cent propylene glycol. The solutions are generally applied twice daily.

Tretinoin (Retin-A), when applied topically, acts to reduce the follicular hyperkeratosis and indirectly to aid in reducing the formation of inflammatory lesions. It is most useful in comedonal and small papular and pustular acne. Because tretinoin is a strong primary irritant, its clinical effectiveness is mitigated by the low concentrations which must be used, i.e., from 0.01 to 0.1 per cent. Nonetheless, with careful instructions to the patient on reducing or avoiding other external irritants, such as solvent cleansers, medicated soaps, and overexposure to the cold and to sunlight, most patients can tolerate tretinoin reasonably well. I generally instruct patients to apply it at bedtime, initially only three times a week. After 2 to 3 weeks' observation, the frequency of application is increased to once or even twice daily. Occasionally, the acne may seem to worsen in the early weeks of treatment, but this flare-up usually subsides spontaneously. In some instances it does not, and if this is the case, the treatment should be discontinued. Tretinoin preparations, available only by prescription, are marketed as gels, creams, liquid, and saturated pads. In general, the creams are least irritating and the liquids and pads most irritating.

Other topical preparations for acne include more traditional remedies such as sulfur, resorcin (resorcinol), or salicylic acid, in various combinations and concentrations. Although the nature of their actions remains obscure, their beneficial effect has been established empirically from many years' experience. In studies in which they have been compared to benzoyl peroxide and tretinoin, they have proved to be somewhat less effective but have the virtue of being less irritating. I find them most useful in patients with sensitive skin, particularly atopic individuals. Examples of such preparations are Acnomel cream, Fostril cream, Sulforcin lotion, and Sulfacet-R lotion. They are applied to the affected areas once or twice daily.

Cosmetic use is common in women with acne and is often excessive. Prolonged daily use can in some cases aggravate the follicular hyperkeratosis. It is difficult to know, though, exactly which cosmetic is comedogenic and which is more so than another, since data are meager as to their effects on human skin. It is advisable to warn patients about the problem of aggravation by cosmetics and to suggest the use of water-based rather than oil-based formulations.

Acne Surgery. Blackheads, a common manifestation of acne, are not preinflammatory lesions, as had long been supposed. However, their extraction, particularly when they are numerous, will ordinarily improve the patient's appearance. The preferred instrument is the Unna comedo extractor, which has a wide, flat surface. The drainage of superficial pustules may also be carried out with the use of this instrument. Inflammatory nodules which undergo suppuration should be incised and gently drained with a needle or a No. 11 Bard-Parker blade. The patient should be warned against squeezing or picking lesions, since additional inflammation and possible scarring might ensue.

Intralesional Steroid Injection. The resolution of inflammatory lesions can be hastened by the intralesional injection of corticosteroid suspensions, e.g., triamcinolone acetonide suspension (Kenalog-10 Injection), diluted to 2 to 3 mg per ml. In large or persistent lesions, a higher concentration is often necessary (up to 10 mg per ml). The volume injected into a single lesion will vary from 0.05 to 0.25 ml, depending on the size of the lesion. Multiple lesions may be injected, without undue concern about any significant degree of steroid absorption into the general circulation. When patients show resistance to other forms of acne treatment, intralesional steroid injections remain as one of the few ways the patient's disease can be maintained with some degree of control.

Physical Treatment

Ultraviolet Light. Although it is generally accepted that sunlight is beneficial for acne, there are no scientific studies to support this view. Artificial ultraviolet light exposure, while seemingly helpful at times, is now deemed to exert little actual alteration in the number of inflammatory acne lesions. Its benefit seems to be related to the cosmetic camouflage of redness and pigmentation it produces. Ultraviolet light treatments are less commonly used than previously, primarily because of aggravation of the skin irritation, often a concomitant of topical benzoyl peroxide or tretinoin treatment.

X-Ray Treatment. Superficial x-ray treatment, which decreases sebaceous gland activity, is on rare occasions resorted to in cases resistant to other therapeutic measures. However, since the sebaceous glands eventually regenerate, improvement is often only temporary. There are several reasons why x-ray is little used today, the chief one being the advent of other methods for suppressing acne activity. In an older day, x-ray therapy stood alone in its comparative ability to reduce the severity of the disease.

Dermabrasion. Surgical planing may improve the appearance of facial, atrophic scars. For several reasons, however, enthusiasm for dermabrasion has waned considerably in the past decade. First, many patients seek a dermabrasion because of emotional conflicts and tend to lay the blame for their problems on their facial appearance. These patients constitute a poor-risk group and are almost invariably dissatisfied with the results despite objective evidence of improvement. Second, not all patients show improvement, and of many of those who do it is not always permanent, i.e., as the edema from the procedure slowly subsides over many months, the improvement is no longer as strikingly evident. Finally, in a patient with severe scarring, a second and third dermabrasion are often necessary. Nonetheless, it must be recognized that in selected patients, significant benefit could accrue from such treatment.

Systemic Treatment

Diet. Among foods which are traditionally prohibited in cases of acne are chocolate, nuts, fried foods, seafoods, and sweets. While patients may on occasion show some exacerbation from the ingestion of one or more of these foods, the great majority tolerate them without adverse effect. I proscribe only what appears by history or trial to have consistently or unequivocally worsened the condition.

Antibiotics. Acne is not an infection; bacterial culture of suppurative lesions yields no pathogens. However, antibiotic treatment does suppress the resident intrafollicular organisms, *P. acnes,* which elaborate numerous enzymes, e.g., lipases, proteases, hyaluronidase, neuraminidases, as well as yet unidentified chemotactic substances with cytotaxic and cytotaxigenic properties. Sebum, subjected in the follicle to the action of lipases, yields cytotoxic free fatty acids. Thus, suppression of *P. acnes* results in a lessening of inflammation. Tetracyclines, erythromycins, and the lincocins are all effective in reducing the numbers of these organisms, and frequently in less than conventional anti-infection dosages.

Tetracycline is the preferred antibiotic and the one most commonly used. I prefer to start with a dose of 250 mg two to four times daily, depending on the severity of the acne. Once a satisfactory response is achieved, usually within 2 to 5 weeks, the dose is reduced to the lowest effective level. Patients can often be maintained adequately on 250 mg daily. In severe, resistant cases, high-dose tetracycline therapy, i.e., 2 to 3 grams a day, may prove effective when lower, more conventional doses are wanting. The effect of antibiotic treatment in acne is suppressive, not curative; once stopped, activity will almost always return within a few weeks. Approximately 70 per cent of patients treated with tetracycline will show a favorable response. It is not always clear why some patients are resistant or gradually become worse again after long periods of good control. In such cases, resistance of *P. acnes* to the antibiotics cannot be demonstrated in vitro. With tetracycline, failures can sometimes be traced to the patient's taking the medication with food, antacids, or iron preparations, all of which interfere with the drug's absorption. Penicillin and sulfonamides are ineffectual in acne, although trimethoprim-sulfamethoxazole can reduce the intrafollicular bacteria and be helpful in treatment. (This use of trimethoprimsulfamethoxazole is not listed in the manufacturer's official directive.) However, since continuous therapy is required for controlling acne, the risk of allergic sensitization limits its usefulness.

Side effects from antibiotic treatment of acne are not too common, and when they occur are rarely serious. Most frequently encountered is a candidal vaginitis which often necessitates cessation of therapy. While desirable to do so, it is not absolutely necessary, as the vaginal infection can often be eradicated by treatment despite continuing tetracycline administration. Other side effects include gastrointestinal disturbances (nausea, stomach cramps, diarrhea, constipation) and, in high doses, increased sensitivity to sun exposure. A rare but troublesome problem from chronic antibiotic use is the development of a gram-negative folliculitis in which gram-negative organisms gain residence in the skin and result in a pustular folliculitis of the acne areas resembling the acne itself. Patients who develop "resistance" to antibiotic treatment could actually represent instances of this superimposed infection. Cultures should be done in such cases, and, if positive, appropriate antibiotic therapy utilized. The lincocin drugs, e.g., clindamycin, have proved to be effective antibiotics for acne, but the reports of pseudomembranous colitis occurring in patients treated with these drugs have sharply curtailed their systemic use in acne. (This use of clindamycin is not listed in the manufacturer's official directive.) It is best limited to those patients with severe, unremitting disease, not responsive to other treatments.

Hormones. In resistant cases, estrogen may be used in female patients to counteract the effect of the androgen-mediated sebaceous gland secretion. Such treatment is contraindicated in males because of undesirable feminizing effects which invariably ensue. A convenient method of estrogen administration is the use of oral contraceptive drugs. The higher the dose of estrogen, the greater the likelihood that some improvement will occur. However, with higher doses, there is a greater risk of side effects. Generally, I start patients on 75 micrograms of estrogen (Enovid,* 5 mg) and observe this response for three or four cycles. Sebaceous gland suppression from estrogen occurs slowly, and clinical improvement is not usually apparent until at least two or three cycles are completed. In addition, an initial but temporary flare-up of the acne may be observed in the early weeks of treatment. If after 4 months the acne has not improved, I increase the dosage to a 100 microgram preparation (e.g., Enovid-E,* Ovulen*) and continue to observe the patient. If there is no beneficial response after a further 4 months, treatment is discontinued. If a satisfactory response is observed in the initial months with Enovid,* 5 mg, the drug is changed to one containing 50 micrograms of estrogen (e.g., Demulen*). Treatment may be continued indefinitely. However, when drug therapy is stopped, sebaceous gland secretion returns to pretreatment levels, and as a result the acne may recur. Ovral,* a norgestrel-containing preparation, should best be avoided, since the progestational component is slightly more androgenic than that of other estrogen-progestin combination drugs.

Corticosteroids. When acne vulgaris is severe and has proved resistant to all treatments, the use of corticosteroids may be justified. The goal of such therapy is to reduce the severe inflammation with as low doses and as short courses as are possible. In addition to the well-known risks of systemic therapy, a corticosteroid folliculitis ("steroid acne") may result occasionally and complicate or confuse the clinical picture. I customarily begin with a dose of 20 to 30 mg of prednisone a day in a single A.M. dose, reducing it as soon as possible to lower levels. An attempt is made not to exceed 10 to 15 mg daily over any extended period of time; if more is required, treatment is almost invariably stopped. In most instances, I have not found alternate day steroid administration to be very satisfactory in controlling the inflammation in acne.

---

*This use of this agent is not listed in the manufacturer's official directive.

PSEUDOFOLLICULITIS BARBAE

method of
JOHN C. HALL, M.D.
Kansas City, Missouri

Pseudofolliculitis barbae is a disease primarily affecting the beard of black males. It does occur in white males also, but it is usually less severe. Women have also been affected in areas where they shave or pluck hairs such as the legs, pubic area, axillae, eyebrows, and face (in cases of hirsutism). Pseudofolliculitis pubis, pseudofolliculitis axillae, and pseudofolliculitis faciale (for females with facial involvement) have been proposed as additional designations for cases in women. Again, black females appear more often affected than white females.

Pathogenesis consist of curvature of the affected hairs that penetrate the skin near the follicle. The curved hairs may not exit the skin before turning inward, and therefore may not be visible above the skin. The resulting lesions are papules and pustules that are quite painful and unsightly. If looked for carefully, each one will show penetration by an ingrowing hair. The disease mimics acne, but comedones and cysts do not occur as in acne. Acne, of course, can occur concomitantly.

The ingrown hairs set up a foreign body inflammatory reaction that is relieved only when the distal end of the hair is removed. Sequelae include hyperpigmentation, scarring, keloids, and secondary infection.

The disease often flares after shaving and will improve if the patient does not shave, since, as the hairs become longer they lose the appropriate angle and bend rather than penetrating the skin. Some authors have suggested heredity as being important.

Short-Term Management

The purpose is to give the patient some immediate relief from the foreign body inflammatory reaction. Many modalities effective in treating acne are also appropriate in early management of pseudofolliculitis barbae.

1. Removal of ingrown hairs can be accomplished by removing the distal penetrating end of the hair by the physician with splinter forceps or by the patient with tweezers or a needle dipped in alcohol or gentle massaging with a Buff sponge. The skin may be too tender and inflamed for use of a Buff sponge.

2. Tetracycline or erythromycin, 500 mg by mouth twice a day or 250 mg by mouth four times a day, often reduces inflammation.

3. Modified Burow's solution (1 packet of Domeboro powder mixed with 1 pint of warm water) compresses for 10 to 15 minutes three times a day are soothing and help dry the lesions.

Long-Term Management

The purpose is to avoid repeated episodes of inflammatory lesions and the long-term effects of scarring. Most treatment modalities used for acne are ineffective.

1. Many suggestions have been made concerning appropriate shaving techniques. A razor is said to be worse than an electric shaver, and

chemical depilatories are often claimed to be helpful. Although in the acute phase of the disease it is often impossible to shave with a razor, I have not been impressed with long-term benefits of different methods of hair removal.

2. Growing a beard is curative but may not be socially acceptable. It is often difficult for the same patients that tend to have pseudofolliculitis barbae to be able to grow a full, attractive beard. I do not hesitate to recommend acceptance of beard growing to employers of patients if the patient chooses this form of therapy.

3. Permanent removal of hairs by electrolysis is also curative. This is particularly appropriate when associated with hirsutism.

4. Retinoic acid (Retin-A) is the single most effective agent. I begin with the 0.01 per cent gel and gradually work up to the 0.025 per cent, 0.05 per cent, and 0.1 per cent cream. The patient should apply the medication at night at least 30 minutes after washing the face to avoid excessive irritation. Morning application is usually avoided because of added irritation with sun exposure.

There are two important points for the patient to know: (1) There will be some redness, peeling, and irritation during the first few weeks of therapy, but this usually abates somewhat with time. (2) It takes prolonged treatment of about 6 weeks to determine the relative effectiveness. It is important to emphasize these two ideas to get appropriate patient compliance. It may be necessary to wait until the acute reaction has subsided before the patient can tolerate the topical retinoic acid. If the irritation is severe, I will apply 1 per cent hydrocortisone in a buffered aluminum acetate (Acid Mantle) cream to the treatment sites each morning in a thin coat.

5. Other therapeutic modalities that are advocated for treatment of acne, such as topical antibiotics, topical benzoyl peroxide, cryosurgery, ultraviolet light, and acne surgery not involving removal of the penetrating end of the hair, have not, in my experience, proved beneficial.

6. Treatment of resulting pigmentation, keloids, or secondary infection is no different than in other skin diseases, but these disorders must be recognized and treated accordingly.

Pseudofolliculitis barbae is a difficult disease to treat, and it is often helpful to warn the patient that his problem is at times recalcitrant to therapy of any kind except growing a beard. It is also important to make the correct diagnosis, since treating the patient for acne or folliculitis is ineffective in helping to avoid repeated episodes.

ALOPECIA

method of
NORMAN ORENTREICH, M.D.
New York, New York

The pathogenesis of alopecia can involve the living hair matrix and dermal papilla or the dead keratinized hair shaft. When only the shaft is involved, hair loss (breakage) is temporary and the follicle continues to produce hair without interruption. Involvement of the matrix and dermal papilla causes cessation of hair growth and shedding of the hair from the follicle. This may be followed by immediate regrowth of a new hair, temporary failure to regrow a hair, or persistent inability to regrow a hair from an existing follicle. If the total follicle or only the dermal papilla is destroyed, loss of hair is permanent.

Physiologic Shedding

Resting and growing hairs are randomly distributed throughout the scalp. Approximately 10 to 15 per cent of scalp hairs are in the telogen (resting) phase, while 85 to 90 per cent are in the anagen (growing) phase. This results in a shedding of 50 to 150 hairs a day with a seasonal cycle that reaches a maximum in November in the north temperate zone. Shampooing augments the number of hairs shed on that day, but shedding is reciprocally decreased on ensuing days.

There is a physiologic shedding in the early weeks of neonatal life that is spontaneous and temporary.

Congenital Alopecia

Congenital alopecia can be diffuse, complete, or patchy. It may occur with other congenital ectodermal anomalies such as defective teeth, nails, and other adnexae. Normal hair rarely develops after puberty.

Endocrinopathy-Associated Alopecias

The following endocrinopathies can produce alopecia: hyperpituitarism, hypopituitarism, hyperthyroidism, hypothyroidism, hypoparathyroidism, hypocorticoidism, diffuse adrenocortical hyperplasia, benign and malignant androgenic adrenocortical tumors, adrenogenital syndrome, benign and malignant androgenic ovarian tumors, polycystic ovaries, and diabetes. These conditions may be helped by appropriate endocrinologic medical or surgical therapy, but hair regrowth may not occur until many months later.

Puberty, menopause, and the postpartum period are frequently states of relative hyperandrogenism that can trigger androgen-dependent alopecia in genetically predisposed individuals.

Androgenetic Alopecia

Androgenetic alopecia (AGA) is the most common type of hair loss in both sexes. This alopecia occurs in those scalp hair follicles that have the genetic potential to be inhibited by androgens over a period of time. It is perhaps more appropriately called androchronogenetic alopecia. The converse of androchronogenetic alopecia is beard development or hirsutism.

AGA most frequently affects the hair follicles of the frontal and crown regions of the scalp; the anagen period becomes shorter with each hair cycle (with or without the telogen phase becoming longer). The end result for each genetically susceptible terminal hair is a reduction to the vellus state. In women AGA is milder, later in onset, and more diffuse because there is less of the inciting hormone.

Androgenetic alopecia is controlled by a single dominant sex-limited autosomal gene. Its genetic potential is expressed if the appropriate androgen enters the hair follicle cells, binds with the specific cytosol protein, and is translocated to the nucleus where it interacts with the cell's genetic material.

Genetic and endocrinologic evidence to date indicate that the inciting androgen is dihydrotestosterone (DHT), a 5-alpha-reduced metabolite of testosterone. Individuals with Type II pseudohermaphroditism (little or no DHT) do not develop AGA; neither do individuals with testicular feminization syndrome (absence of cytosol or nuclear androgen binding proteins).

Medical Treatment. Medical treatment is directed toward controlling the androgenic component of the alopecia, since treatment cannot be effectively directed against the chronogenetic components.

TREATMENT FOR MEN. Physical or chemical castration of transsexuals arrests but does not reverse the balding process. Any reduction of androgen levels in noncastrates sufficient to stop hair loss also produces a concomitant decrease in libido and sexual potency. Reduction of only plasma DHT levels, if it could be accomplished, would appear to be free of the undesired effects of lowering testosterone.

Scalp skin has the 5-alpha reductase enzyme that converts testosterone to DHT; reducing this local enzymatic production of DHT is possible by increasing the local tissue level of progesterone, a competitor for the 5-alpha-reductase enzyme.

In vitro evidence indicates that progesterone competes with testosterone for the 5-alpha-reductase; less DHT is made and more dihydroprogesterone (DHP) is made; DHP in turn competes with residual DHT for the cytosol/nuclear binding protein for a further reduction in the amount of DHT interacting with genetic material. Since progesterone can only partially inhibit DHT production and binding, it can only reduce the rate of AGA and not stop it.

TREATMENT FOR WOMEN. Plasma hyperandrogenism is not rare in women with multiple androgenetic dermatoses — acne, hirsutism, and alopecia. Estrogen therapy or surgery when indicated reduces ovarian hyperandrogenism. Excessive adrenal production of androgens and/or androgen precursors can be effectively and safely reduced by as little as 2.5 mg of prednisone at bedtime without significantly lowering cortisol levels. Eliminating exogenous androgens that precipitate AGA in genetically predisposed individuals is beneficial.

Testosterone and DHT circulate in the blood either free or bound to sex hormone binding globulin (SHBG), but only the free hormone can enter a cell. Deficient liver production of SHBG results in higher levels of free testosterone and DHT. Estrogens and thyroids stimulate liver production of SHBG and thereby reduce free androgen levels.

As noted above, topical progesterone can reduce skin DHT formation and cytosol–nuclear DHT binding. Menstrual irregularity from excess percutaneous absorption can occur if more than 2 ml of 2 per cent progesterone (40 mg) is applied daily.

Surgical Treatment. Sites of advanced AGA on properly selected men and women can be effectively and permanently corrected with 4 mm punch, free, full-thickness, hair-bearing autografts transplanted to it from the hairy occiput that is not susceptible to AGA. These grafts continue to produce hair at the same rate and of the same texture and color as the occipital (donor) site.

Neoplastic Alopecia

Benign and *malignant* neoplasms can produce hair loss by pressure, displacement, replacement, or systemic influences. Permanent alopecic areas that remain after the treatment of the neoplasm may be corrected with hair-bearing scalp transplants, as for AGA.

Acquired Traumatic Alopecia

Acute traction by plucking, combing, or brushing may break the hair shaft but does not disrupt continuity of growth; evulsing growing scalp hair from follicles induces telogen and produces a temporary (3 month) cessation of growth.

Chronic traction by tight "pony tails," "corn rowing" braids, curlers, hair pins, bobby pins, or styling combs and barrettes can cause alopecia at the sites of tension. Alopecia is temporary if the traction is brief, but permanent hair loss from follicle destruction can result from prolonged traction.

Avulsion is the forcible tearing away of scalp tissue and may, if untreated, cause not only loss of the hair-bearing skin but also injury to the underlying skull. If the avulsed area is small and the aponeurosis and subcutaneous fat are trimmed away carefully to avoid damage to the hair follicles, immediate replacement may "take" with partial or complete regrowth of hair. Advances in surgery now allow for microvascular anastomosis of an entire scalp, which, if performed promptly, prevents scalp avascular necrosis and permanent alopecia.

Friction from work or sporting gear can cause hair shaft breakage close to the scalp; frictional hair breakage is commonly seen on an infant's head at the point of maximal contact with the crib; it invariably improves after removal of the eliciting agent. Lichen chronicus circumscriptus (neurodermatitis) can produce a self-inflicted frictional alopecia.

Internal pressure, typically from a cyst, may cause a localized alopecia. Prolonged general anesthesia, especially in the Trendelenburg position, may cause a temporary alopecia in the area of dependent edema.

External pressure with or without laceration may cause an alopecia at the site of injury that can be permanent if there is scarring.

Electric burns which destroy the hair follicles produce permanent hair loss; superficial burns result only in temporary alopecia.

Thermal trauma from extreme heat or cold can cause permanent hair loss if there is deep necrosis with hair follicle destruction.

Chemical contactants of industrial or cosmetic origin usually produce only partial or complete disintegration of the hair shaft resulting in hair breakage and temporary alopecia. Severe primary irritant reactions or secondary bacterial infections that destroy hair follicles can produce permanent alopecia. Allergic eczematous contact dermatitis, which usually occurs in scalp-adjacent areas, does not produce permanent alopecia.

Ionizing radiation produces temporary alopecia when only the epithelial elements are affected; in 3 to 5 weeks hair loss is complete but regrowth may be seen as early as 10 weeks. When the radiation is sufficient to destroy the dermal papilla (more than 1500 r of a single dose of superficial x-rays with a half value of 0.9 mm Al or more), then alopecia is permanent and invariably associated with radiodermatitis. There is no safe permanent epilating dose.

Infections

Localized superficial infection seldom causes alopecia; deeper involvement can disrupt the follicular matrix and cause hair breakage or induce the telogen phase, causing temporary alopecia. Follicular destruction and permanent alopecia can be caused by viruses (herpes simplex, zoster, varicella, variola) and bacteria (tuberculosis, leprosy, pyogenic organisms). Most fungal infections involve the hair shaft and produce only breakage, although kerion and favus can cause total follicle destruction unless prompt and adequate treatment with griseofulvin is instituted.

Systemic infection associated with high fever frequently causes hair shedding 2 to 3 months later. This postfebrile hair loss is transient and requires only reassuring the patient. The shedding is frequently associated with a Beau line — a transverse depression in the nail plate growing out and representing matrix nail growth arrest at the time of peak illness. A corresponding narrowing in the hair shaft is called the Pohl-Pinkus mark.

Neurologic and Psychiatric Alopecia

There is insufficient evidence to establish direct neurogenic or psychiatric effects on follicular function.

Trichotillomania. This subconscious or conscious pulling out, twisting, or breaking off one's own hair from the scalp, eyebrow, or occasionally eyelashes is not uncommon and is frequently misdiagnosed as alopecia areata. The removed hair may be discarded, hidden, or ingested and occasionally results in trichobezoar formation. To confirm the diagnosis with the "trichotillo-test," apply a firmly attached occlusive substance or bandage to an affected area; hair outgrowth will be evident after removing the patch 4 to 8 weeks later. Psychiatric help should be recommended if the test is positive and the patient continues to deny this behavior or cannot stop this compulsion. Prolonged plucking may produce permanent alopecia.

Toxic Alopecia

Pharmacologic and occupational alopecias can be caused by non-follicle-specific toxins (e.g., lead, arsenicals, potassium sulfocyanate, quinacrine, quinine ethyl carbamate, general anesthetic agents) or by follicle-specific compounds (e.g., antineoplastics, folic acid antagonists, radiomimetics, unsaturated lipid-soluble agents (chlorbutadiene), substituted amino acids (leucenol), megadoses of vitamin A, and exogenous androgens (in the genetically predisposed). Entry may be by inhalation, injection, ingestion, or percutaneous absorption. Identifying and eliminating the cause usually is followed by regrowth. Antineoplastic alopecias can be ameliorated or prevented by tourniquet of the scalp or cooling during period of injection of the antineoplastic agent, but this carries the risk of preventing treatment of as yet undiagnosed scalp metastases.

Nutritional and Metabolic Alopecias

Caloric deprivation must be very severe (kwashiorkor, sprue, celiac disease) to produce hair loss. Increased shedding sometimes occurs after marked weight loss for obesity. Anemia, diabetes, hyper- and hypovitaminosis, and zinc deficiency may be associated with alopecia.

Dermatologic Alopecia

Alopecia areata is the name for a group of alopecias probably with an immunologic etiology. It may take many forms — areata, concentric, guttate, diffuse localized, diffuse generalized, ophiastic, totalis, or universalis. The hair loss is usually sudden and asymptomatic except for mild erythema and occasional premonitory paresthesia. Pathognomonic "exclamation point" hairs are present in the early active phase. Fine pitting of the nails occurs in about 20 per cent of the patients, and dermatoglyphics may show an increased number of arches. Although single patches frequently regrow spontaneously within a few months, the course is unpredictable (including the rare extension to totalis or universalis) and recurrences are common.

Hair growth in response to injection of anti-inflammatory corticosteroids into an alopecic site is both diagnostic and therapeutic. Usually only the most severe active phases of this disorder, or those in which there has already been inflammatory destruction of the hair papilla, do not respond to this treatment. Other causes for failure of regrowth are under- or overdosage of the injected corticoid. The corticoid of choice is short-acting triamcinolone acetonide (Kenalog) at 5 to 10 mg per ml; the long-acting triamcinolone hexacetonide (Aristospan) at 5 mg per ml may be substituted for some or all of the acetonide for a prolonged cutaneous depot effect. Between 0.05 and 0.1 ml at 1 to 2 cm intervals usually produces good regrowth within 4 to 6 weeks and little if any atrophy. Total dosage depends upon the severity of the condition, but even the most severe involvement can usually be treated with 50 mg or less per month. Ethyl chloride or Freon spray usually produces sufficient anesthesia; block an

esthesia of a scalp wedge can be achieved with lidocaine injections to the scalp perimeter through which the scalp's innervation passes. Hair regrown from treatment is usually of the same texture and color, but occasionally it is darker or curlier; spontaneously regrown hair may be hypopigmented. Pigmented hair is sometimes more susceptible to loss during recurrences; occasionally all pigmented hair is lost, creating apparent overnight graying, which is really partial and selective alopecia areata.

Oral anti-inflammatory corticosteriods have been given alone or in conjunction with intralesional injections for extensive alopecia areata or alopecia totalis and alopecia universalis, but are best avoided, since a safe and therapeutic regimen is rarely found.

Jet injector techniques are wasteful. Tattooing and iontophoresis usually fail to produce adequate regrowth. High potency topical steroids with occlusion sometimes produce good regrowth.

Immunotherapy with allergens such as dinitrochlorobenzene (DNCB) (investigational) is partially successful; since some of the allergens may be mutagenic and carcinogenic, and since none are curative, their use is rarely warranted.

Cicatricial alopecias, other than those already mentioned, include a number of cutaneous diseases with atrophy. There are pseudopelade, lupus erythematosus, lichen planus, and scleroderma. Intralesional steroids administered as for alopecia areata are usually effective in the active phase. Hair-bearing normal scalp may be transplanted into histologically confirmed "burned out" alopecic sites.

CANCER OF THE SKIN
method of
CHARLES S. LINCOLN, JR., M.D.
Berkeley, California

Cutaneous carcinomas are the most common of all malignancies. Of these, the basal cell carcinoma is the most common, followed in incidence by squamous cell carcinoma, Bowen's disease, melanoma, Paget's disease, and erythroplasia of Queyrat. The last three conditions should be referred to a physician well versed in their treatment or a medical center. Fortunately, metastatic carcinoma is primarily limited to the melanoma or badly neglected squamous cell carcinoma. There have been reports of metastatic basal cell carcinomas; however, they are very rare. At a recent medical convention the occurrence of metastatic basal cell carcinomas was presented with conclusive evidence that they do occur. Neglected, all the mentioned carcinomas are killers. Even the most benign basal cell carcinoma may become ulcerated and rapidly spread to invade the orbit or nostril with eventually a slow, lingering death. We seldom see such cases in private practice; however, if seen, such patients must be referred at once to a medical center or a physician skilled in chemosurgery (Mohs technique).

Many cutaneous malignancies are complicated because the initial treatment is inadequate or excessive. There are very few physicians still using radium (an unacceptable modality), which often results in chronic radiodermatitis. Radium cannot be calibrated. X-ray therapy in middle-aged and elderly patients is an excellent procedure if given properly by an expert after the diagnosis has been made by biopsy.

Prevention

Prevention is the name of the game, as in all disease, skin or otherwise. Dermatologists have an advantage, as they can see the disease, and often the skin will give a clue to internal disease such as diabetes, liver disease, mycosis fungoides, and metastatic carcinoma, to name a few.

Skin cancer may occur in all races, however, black or very dark-skinned persons are protected by their melanin pigmentation. Even eye color seems to play a part. For example, a black- or dark brown-eyed person with fair skin seems to be better protected than the fair-skinned, blue-eyed individual. It is almost hopeless to warn your patients (which all dermatologists I know attempt) that sunbathing only ages the skin. Sadly there are few things we can do because of poor patient cooperation. A hat is of some value, especially for a bald head; however, ultraviolet radiation is reflected off such things as snow, cement, water (unless very pure), and a fishing or pleasure boat, which is usually white.

There are many sun screens sold over the counter. Most contain para-aminobenzoic acid and its various esters (PABA). They really work, especially if applied 1 or 2 hours before sun exposure. I advise my sun-sensitive patients to use them as an after shave lotion or before applying makeup. PABA may cause an allergic contact dermatitis if the patient is allergic to such drugs as procaine and sulfanilamide, to name a couple. A true contact dermatitis to PABA is rare, but the alcohol preparations are drying. Let your patient pick out the sun screen most cosmetically acceptable according to the skin color. The average white-skinned person requires only 15 to 20 minutes to produce a sunburn or minimal erythemal dose (MED). Skin color has now been classified between 1 and 6. Briefly, number 1 always burns, and number 6 never burns. Sun screens recently have been labeled with a sun protective factor (SPF) which is rated 2 to 15. For your very sun-sensitive patients, advise an SPF range of 10 to 15 (Super Shade, Total Eclipse); for the person that tans well, an SPF of 2 to 4 may be advised (Coppertone, Sundare, RVP, and many others).

Precancerous Lesions

Next to prevention, the treatment of precancerous lesions is most important. The removal of deeply pigmented (black) nevoid (molelike) lesions, especially from the hands or feet, followed by a histopathologic examination will on a very rare occasion pick up an early melanoma. Usually the lesions are benign nevi (moles). Removal using a local anesthetic such as lidocaine (Xylocaine) or mepivacaine (Carbocaine) and "scalpel shaving" the lesion "off" for histopathologic examination is fast and simple. Hemostasis may be obtained by light electrodesiccation or the application of full strength trichloracetic acid (TCA). More radical surgery should follow the report of a malignancy such as wide excision or a more complete curettage and desiccation (C and D).

The majority of lesions seen are actinic keratoses (senile keratoses, solar keratoses) cutaneous horns, and seborrheic keratoses. Seborrheic keratoses in themselves are almost never malignant, but on occasion may turn out to be pigmented basal cell carcinoma. The so-called liver spots (a lay term), which are really actinic lesions, usually on the hands, arms, or face, are easily removed by the application of pure phenol (88 per cent) or the light application of liquid nitrogen on a cotton applicator. The thicker keratotic lesions may be frozen with Freon (Frigiderm) and curetted or "scalpel shaved" for biopsy. Again, the application of full strength TCA will give good hemostasis. On occasion I use a local anesthetic and "scalpel shave" off the lesion and curette the base followed by TCA for hemostasis or light electrodesiccation. Should the biopsy show squamous cell carcinoma, you may follow the patient closely or do an excision biopsy or perform a more complete curettement and desiccation. Squamous cell carcinomas arising from an actinic keratosis are said never to metastasize.

For the past 10 to 12 years, topical 5-fluorouracil (5-FU) has been in use with excellent results for the treatment of actinic keratoses! The use of 5-FU (Efudex, Fluoroplex) for precancerous lesions, especially when they are numerous, is in the scope of almost all physicians if they will follow a few simple rules.

Topical fluorouracil (Efudex) is available as a 2 or 5 per cent solution in propylene glycol and a 5 per cent cream in a vanishing cream base. After years of experimenting with the various preparations, I now use, with few exceptions, only the 5 per cent cream for the face, hands, and forearms. This simplifies the treatment routine, and the physician knows what to expect. Roche (Efudex) will supply directions; however, I prefer to give my own directions on the prescription: Apply the cream to the face morning and night. Avoid the eyes, angles of the nose, and mouth, and wash hands after each application. The old cream should be washed off before the application of new cream. Avoid the sun, and see the doctor at least weekly.

There can be hypersensitivity to 5-FU, which reduces the time of application. The physician should follow the patients closely to avoid a too severe reaction. Usually, in the first week there is little reaction. In 2 weeks erythema develops, and usually by the third week severe erythema with crusting and sometimes ulceration occurs. At this stage stop the 5-FU and use a topical steroid ointment (not cream). If the reaction is really severe, I resort to intramuscular steroids — betamethasone (Celestone Soluspan), dexamethasone acetate (Decadron LA) — and on occasion follow-up with oral steroids. This reduces the time period that the patients may be considered antisocial. For the hands and forearms a 1 week application of tretinoin (Retin-A) cream 0.1 per cent, followed by the application of 5-FU, will greatly enhance the effect of the fluorouracil. Some physicians mix the 5-FU with the tretinoin, with beautiful results, but as yet this is not commercially available.

Treatment

Treatment may be either surgical or by radiation. It is our feeling that the choice of therapy should not only be curative but also produce as little deformity as possible. Overdestruction of small lesions by chemosurgery, such as by the Mohs technique, is to be deplored. Choice of therapy must be geared to the capabilities and facilities available to the physician. For example, we would not expect a physician living far from a medical center to be able to give x-ray therapy even if this is indicated as the treatment of choice. He or she must use the method at hand except in rare cases.

Each malignancy is an individual problem, and such matters as age, distance of the patient from the office or medical center, and financial status must be considered, as well as the size and location of the lesion. An elderly person coming from a great distance at considerable expense may appreciate a three or four visit program even at some sacrifice in the cosmetic result. This should be discussed with the patient.

Surgical Excision. When possible, surgical excision is the preferred form of treatment. No other method is less painful, or is more certain of cure, and is within the ability of almost all physicians. Further, if the specimen is properly sectioned by the pathologist, the physician may be fairly certain of a cure if all margins of the tissue removed are free of tumor.

Surgical excision is especially valuable for treating the "botched" lesion that has recurred after improper x-ray therapy or electrosurgery.

Short of skin grafting, surgical excision depends upon the location of the lesion and the tissue available. In elderly persons with lax skin, large lesions may be excised with easy closure. The area of the lower eyelid is a danger area and should be excised with caution, because an ectropion is a very embarrassing surgical complication. Whenever possible, follow the wrinkle lines or the lines of elasticity of the skin when making an excision. Often the scar or excision line will fall in a wrinkle or skin fold and be imperceptible.

Electrodesiccation and Curettage. This is one of the best methods of treatment, but is often overlooked for the much more expensive and exotic procedures. In my office it is the most commonly used method. The tumor in question is infiltrated with a local anesthetic and is curetted or "scooped" out for the biopsy. An electrodesiccating device along with curettement is used to remove the remnants of the tumor (C and D). The curette is very selective, and the soft mushy substance of the malignancy may be easily differentiated from the firm texture of the normal skin. With experience, very large lesions may be removed with an excellent cure rate, statistically much better than cryotherapy.

Irradiation Therapy. Radiation is most frequently used on the more elderly patients, in particular those who are not good candidates for surgery. Also certain lesions, such as those on the rim of the eyelid or on the nose or near the inner canthus of the eye, are more easily treated by x-ray. From information obtained from many tumor conferences, it is my firm opinion that most skin malignancies are overtreated by radiologists. This is not so serious in the very old, but in patients of the younger to middle-age group, a chronic radiodermatitis may be anticipated years later. A total dose of 2000 r is considered by most therapists to be a lethal dose for most malignancies; yet doses of 5000 r to 6500 r or more are given. From long experience I have found that a dose of 3000 to 3200 r suffices, and with this dose a chronic radiodermatitis is unlikely. As a routine using a conventional superficial roentgen ray machine (80 to 100 KVP), half value layer (HVL) 0.7 to 1 mm aluminum, doses of 500 r each are given two to three times weekly for a total of six treatments, for a total dose of 3000 r. This routine reduces the number of office visits and the expense. There can be many variations in this routine, and only one trained in the use of x-ray therapy should consider using this type of therapy.

Cryotherapy. Cryotherapy, or the use of liquid nitrogen in a spray except for the cotton applicator, is at present, I feel, a fad. There are some specialists who insist that it is one of the best modalities but report only a 90 per cent cure rate. At best, this is only for experts in the use of liquid nitrogen. A given lesion is implanted with a thermocouple (a temperature measuring device) and frozen with liquid nitrogen. A deep freeze is produced with death of the malignant cells and some of the normal tissue. Cosmetic results are good, but in most cases are no better than excision, curettement and electrodesiccation, or x-ray therapy.

Chemosurgery. The Mohs technique of chemosurgery was developed by Dr. Frederick E. Mohs. This is not for the ordinary small skin malignancy seen by most of us in the office. The classic method utilizes zinc chloride paste and bichloracetic acid applied over the lesion in question, which upon fixation is removed level by level with a No. 15 Bard Parker blade. The removed fixed tissue is systematically examined under the microscope until no tumor cells are found in all the various levels or margins. This method has a reported incidence of cure of 98 per cent on basal cell carcinoma and is indispensable in the large invasive ulcerated carcinoma. Recently fresh tissue chemosurgery that utilizes no paste at all has been used. The true advantage of this technique is in the fact that a map of the lesion is made and the surgeon is also the pathologist, making a truly microscopically controlled excision possible.

Bowen's disease (intraepidermal carcinoma) is a slow growing, relatively benign skin lesion that may be treated surgically or by x-ray. At present 5-FU is the preferred treatment. Erythroplasia of Queyrat may be treated in the same manner as Bowen's disease.

Keratoacanthoma (KA) is a benign lesion that in the past was mistaken for squamous cell carcinoma, and can be a treatment problem, especially when multiple. Recently the injection of 50 mg of 5-FU directly into the KA has produced rapid regression with little or no scarring. (This use of 5-FU is not listed in the manufacturer's official directive.) Up to five injections may be required.

CREEPING ERUPTION

method of
MEYER YANOWITZ, M.D.
Miami, Florida

Creeping eruption or cutaneous larva migrans is caused most commonly by filariform larvae of the cat and dog hookworm, *Ancylostoma braziliense,* migrating through the skin. The larvae hatch from the droppings of these animals in warm, moist soil, and infestation occurs after exposure to contaminated areas, usually beaches, sandboxes, and under buildings.

Prophylaxis

Prevention is best accomplished by keeping animals off beaches, covering sandboxes, and wearing gloves while digging in the soil. Shoes should be worn outdoors, especially during the rainy summer season. Plastic dropcloths should be laid on the ground before working under buildings or under automobiles on damp soil.

Local Therapy

Thiabendazole (Mintezol) is the drug of choice, preferably topically, or orally if there is widespread infestation. (Topical use of thiabendazole is not listed in the manufacturer's official directive.) Mintezol suspension containing 100 mg thiabendazole per ml of vehicle is rubbed on with the fingers four times daily for 7 to 10 days. Cotton should not be used, as the suspension will be absorbed and will not be effective. This is the same product as used orally. A wide area around the advancing end of the track should be included, as the larvae are always ahead of any track which is visible. Relief of itching occurs within 1 or 2 days, but application should be continued for at least 1 week. The older methods of freezing, using ethyl chloride spray or liquid nitrogen, are painful and no longer necessary.

Systemic Therapy

When infestation is widespread, topical therapy may not be practical. Thiabendazole (Mintezol suspension or tablets) is given orally in doses of 22 mg per kg (10 mg per pound) of body weight every 12 hours for 2 days, not to exceed 3 grams per day. Side effects of headache, dizziness, nausea, and vomiting are common with systemic therapy but disappear within 24 hours. Any tracks remaining after systemic therapy may be treated with the suspension topically.

Supplementary Therapy

Itching is best treated with cold compresses of tap water or a 1:40 dilution of aluminum acetate solution USP. Antihistamines are not very helpful, although trimeprazine (Temaril) may be given for its sedative and antipruritic effect.

Secondary infection is managed by opening pustules, removing crusts with warm water and soap, and applying an antibiotic ointment. Systemic antibiotics, penicillin or erythromycin, may be necessary if there is extensive pyoderma. Curing the primary infestation hastens the resolution of the secondary infection.

DECUBITUS ULCER

method of
ROBERT JACKSON, M.D.
Ottawa, Ontario, Canada

Decubitus ulcers are ischemic ulcers resulting from pressure.

Local Care

1. Remove eschar if present.
2. Determine size, depth, and undermining.
3. Measure and record size of ulcer weekly. A palm-sized ulcer may take 8 months to heal.
4. Culture for bacteria. If there is redness, swelling, and tenderness, treat with appropriate antibiotic systemically. In my experience clinically significant secondary infections are rare.
5. X-ray for underlying osteomyelitis.
6. Dressing routine: (a) Terrycloth impregnated with isotonic saline solution, ¼ per cent silver nitrate solution, or 10 per cent benzyl peroxide lotion (Benoxyl). (If using Benoxyl, check for sensitivity reaction in surrounding skin. Also, put zinc oxide paste on 2 cm of surrounding normal skin.) Tuck terrycloth into all nooks and crannies of the ulcer. (b) Cover with plastic film. (c) Cover with large abdominal or amputation pad. (d) Attach with nonocclusive, hypoallergenic, adhesive tape (Dermicel) or binder. (e) Change

every 8 hours, cleaning the ulcer surface and undermined areas with 3 to 5 per cent hydrogen peroxide.

This routine requires knowledgeable and dedicated nursing care. My policy is to post these instructions clearly above the head of the patient's bed.

7. Granulation tissue can be destroyed by weekly application of 75 per cent silver nitrate stick.
8. If the ulcer does not show signs of healing in 1 month, consideration should be given to excision and full thickness grafting.

Removal of Pressure

Use your head. Use what is available. Ask for suggestions from the nursing staff.

1. Turn the patient every 2 hours night and day. This requires dedicated nursing.
2. Use pillows to keep pressure off the ulcer area.
3. Use plastic foam mattresses.
4. Use water bed flotation mattresses (Bard).
5. Get the patient out of bed.
6. Use support beneath legs for heel ulcers.

Many ulcers can be healed with the method outlined above, the patient's health notwithstanding. This does not imply that such findings such as cardiac edema, anemia, malnutrition, and control of diabetes should not be checked for and treated. It does imply that treatment of these general medical conditions alone will not cure decubitus ulcers.

CONTACT DERMATITIS

method of
MICHAEL J. KOWERTZ, M.D.
Sunnyvale, California

Contact dermatitis is an inflammatory response of the skin produced by external agents. Four types may occur: (1) primary irritant, (2) allergic, (3) phototoxic, and (4) photoallergic. The first two types are responsible for the majority of problems and will be discussed here.

1. *Primary irritant dermatitis* may be caused by short exposure to strong chemicals or by chronic exposure to weaker chemicals such as solvents and detergents. This condition is manifest by dry, scaling, often fissured skin, primarily of the backs

of the hands, interdigital spaces, and often the lower arms. The classic example of primary irritant dermatitis is "dishpan hands." On the thicker skin of the palms, the dermatitis is usually much less severe. When the palms are affected and the backs of the hands are spared, the condition is more likely to be another problem such as dyshidrosis.

Treatment consists of (a) removing or reducing exposure, (b) lubricating frequently with a heavy cream such as Eucerin or petroleum jelly, and (c) applying topical steroid ointments which do not contain propylene glycol, such as betamethasone dipropionate (Diprosone) or betamethasone valerate (Valisone), as needed for itching. Antihistamines and aspirin may be of limited value as adjunctive therapy to relieve itching.

2. *Allergic dermatitis* is an acquired, delayed allergic response which usually appears 12 to 72 hours after exposure and becomes more severe over the next 3 to 4 days, giving the patient the mistaken impression that it spreads. The primary reaction may vary from acute (erythema, edema, vesicles, weeping, and crusting) to subacute (erythema and edema). Frequently, because of chronic exposure or scratching, the lesions become lichenified and excoriated to resemble chronic eczema.

The most common sources of allergic dermatitis include Rhus oleoresins (poison oak, ivy, sumac, mango skin, ginkgo tree, and Japanese lacquer tree), nickel, neomycin, p-phenylenediamine (hair dye), ethylenediamine (a preservative found in Mycolog cream, for example, but not in the ointment), rubber, formalin, thimerosal (Merthiolate), and potassium dichromate (leather and many other products).

Treatment for acute allergic dermatitis consists of (a) applying cool, wet compresses of Burow's solution, saline, or water 15 to 30 minutes several times a day until the vesicles become dry, and (b) administering corticosteroid agents. If the dermatitis is generalized and depending on the severity, corticosteroid therapy must be given systemically for 1 to 3 weeks. Most patients with moderate to severe cases respond with 5 mg of prednisolone or prednisone in single or divided doses (7, 7, 6, 6, 5, 5, 4, 4, 3, 3, 2, 2, 1 tablets daily). I prescribe a single dose to be taken with food, preferably after breakfast. In my opinion, injectable steroids are not useful in the treatment of acute contact dermatitis. The long-acting preparations do not give a high enough initial blood level, and the short-acting agents do not maintain an adequate blood level long enough. In localized dermatitis, topical steroid therapy is preferred. In the vesicular stage, a preparation with a drying base such as betamethasone benzoate gel (Uticort), betamethasone dipropionate (Diprosone) spray or lotion, or fluocinonide gel (Topsyn) applied several times a day after the compresses should be used. In subacute dermatitis, any potent steroid in a cream base such as fluocinonide cream (Lidex) should be used. Corticosteroid therapy may be indicated in certain chronic dermatoses. For chronic dry dermatitis, a steroid cream in a water-in-oil base such as desoximetasone cream (Topicort) or in an ointment base such as betamethasone dipropionate ointment (Diprosone) should be used.

The treatment programs outined above assume that the etiology has been determined and that the contactant can be avoided except when it causes occasional sporadic outbreaks such as those seen in Rhus dermatitis. These recommendations are therefore based on the use of high-potency steroid treatment to clear the dermatitis in the shortest possible time, usually no longer than 2 to 3 weeks.

In those cases in which the offending agent has not been identified or cannot be avoided, long-term therapy may be required. For these patients, the adverse effects of using high-potency steroids such as atrophy (reversible) and striae (irreversible) must be considered, especially in intertriginous areas, face, eyelids, vulva, penis, and scrotum. Therefore, for long-term therapy, especially in these areas, hydrocortisone or the weakest preparation capable of providing reasonable control of the dermatitis should be used.

DERMATITIS HERPETIFORMIS
(Duhring's Disease)

method of
EDMUND D. LOWNEY , M.D.
Columbus, Ohio

The typical patient with dermatitis herpetiformis is an agitated middle-aged man who recurrently develops clusters of very itchy vesicles on the trunk. This is a polymorphous eruption, and inflamed papules, plaques, and wheals are also seen. All types of lesions are very pruritic. Quite often vesicles are absent or have been scratched away, making diagnosis difficult. Unfortunately, the atypical case is often confused with neurodermatitis, and response to specific therapy is often the only practical diagnostic measure. Dermatitis herpetiformis is occasionally associated with malabsorption, and atrophic changes suggestive of sprue are often seen on small bowel biopsy. If intact blisters are found, skin biopsy reveals subepidermal blisters associated with eosinophilia.

Although antibodies to skin components are almost never found in the serum, examination of skin by direct immunofluorescence techniques shows granular deposits of IgA in the dermal papillae of perilesional and uninvolved skin in many cases. Although linear IgA deposits may also be seen, granular deposits of IgA are more often associated with enteropathy and the HLA-B8 haplotype.

Sulfapyridine and Sulfones

Dermatitis herpetiformis is unique in that it often responds to systemic treatment with sulfapyridine or various sulfones. The mode of action of these drugs in this disease is unknown. The most common treatment is sulfapyridine. The drug should not be given to patients with sulfa allergy, and care must be taken to maintain hydration. Sulfapyridine can cause a number of adverse effects, including leukopenia, hemolysis, and renal damage, and a complete blood count, platelet count, urinalysis, and blood urea nitrogen (BUN) should be obtained at frequent intervals. Gastrointestinal symptoms are common, and it is best not to take the drug on an empty stomach. Therapy is usually begun with a small dose (e.g., 500 mg twice daily) and increased into the therapeutic range of 2 to 3 grams a day. If a therapeutic response is obtained, the dose should be lowered to the lowest amount that is effective. Sulfasalazine (Azulfidine), which is metabolized to sulfapyridine, is somewhat less effective than is sulfapyridine, but, when used in similar doses, is better tolerated by many patients. (This use of sulfasalazine is not listed in the manufacturer's official directive.)

Of the sulfones, diaminodiphenyl sulfone (Dapsone) is most commonly used. This is a toxic drug, which commonly causes, among other things, hemolysis and methemoglobinemia. Glucose-6-phosphate dehydrogenase deficiency should be ruled out before sulfones are given. It is a wise precaution to begin with a low dose such as 25 mg twice daily for the first week, and then to advance to the therapeutic range of 150 to 200 mg a day. (This use of diaminodiphenyl sulfone is not listed in the manufacturer's official directive.) Again, treatment must be monitored by repeated laboratory studies (complete blood count [CBC], platelet count, reticulocyte count, urinalysis, blood urea nitrogen [BUN], serum glutamic oxaloacetic transaminase [SGOT]). Methemoglobinemia may be clinically obvious. Further information about the toxicity of sulfapyridine and sulfones can be obtained by consulting package inserts and standard textbooks of pharmacology.

Other Agents

Many patients with dermatitis herpetiformis do better when on a gluten-free diet. The effect of this diet is often not seen for several months. Pyridoxine (50 mg twice daily) may decrease the amount of sulfapyridine needed and is harmless, at any rate.

When dermatitis herpetiformis does not respond to sulfapyridine or sulfones, the diagnosis is often in doubt. Many such patients respond to systemic corticosteroids, and these drugs are justified if the disorder is truly disabling and if other modalities have been exhausted. Thirty mg of prednisone a day is usually adequate, and some patients respond to much lower doses, or to alternate day therapy (e.g., 10 mg every other day).

Symptomatic Therapy

In all cases of dermatitis herpetiformis it is best to avoid systemic sulfonamides or steroids whenever topical therapy is adequate.

Mild and "burnt-out" cases of dermatitis herpetiformis can be treated as a mild neurodermatitis, with dilute topical steroid creams (e.g., triamcinolone cream 0.01 per cent), lubricants in the winter, and antipruritic psychoactive drugs such as hydroxyzine (Atarax, Vistaril), 25 mg three times daily, combined with adequate sedation at bedtime. Diazepam (Valium) may also be useful for short periods of time.

ATOPIC DERMATITIS
method of
MORRIS WAISMAN, M.D.
Tampa, Florida

Atopic dermatitis shows itself variously (and often consecutively) as oozing, crusted, excoriated infantile eczema, a less exudative papular eruption of childhood, and a dry, lichenified dermatitis of adolescence and adult life. The cardinal feature throughout is the genetically transmitted pruritic hyperreactivity of the skin to stress — physiologic, emotional, and environmental. Although asthma and hay fever are frequent accompaniments, an "allergic" or immunologic mechanism for atopic dermatitis is inconspicuous clinically, and indeed, as far as treatment is concerned, it may usually be ignored.

Infantile Eczema

Prevention requires bland bathing procedures, avoidance of diaper dermatitis, protection from contact with wool, elimination of soap and detergent residues from garments and bedclothes, and effective lubrication of dry skin.

Initiate treatment with cornstarch or powdered oatmeal (Aveeno) baths, 1 tablespoonful to the basin of tepid water, anointing afterward with a corticosteroid cream or ointment in quarter strength. If exudation is prominent, compresses of tap water or of Burow's solution diluted 1:30 are applied over the corticosteroid film and kept wet. (Corticosteroids extensively applied for prolonged periods may be absorbed and promote adrenal-pituitary suppression.) Subacute dermatitis often improves after a tar, such as coal tar solution USP (liquor carbonis detergens), is added to the corticosteroid ointment, starting with 3 per cent strength and increasing to 10 per cent if tolerated. Orally, an antihistamine, elixir of diphenhydramine (Benadryl), for example, may be antipruritic, and, if necessary, elixir of phenobarbital is additionally helpful for sedation.

Exclude from the household domestic pets, dust, and wool in the form of blankets, rugs, toys, and upholstery. Guard against diaper dermatitis, which may spread into an extensive eczema. Caution against exposure of the skin to potentially dangerous infection, pyogenic and herpetic. Even though in most cases dietary manipulation serves little practical use, it is prudent empirically to eliminate eggs from the diet. Infants with resistive dermatitis who are not being breast fed may benefit from changing the formula to goat's milk or a soybean substitute. Other possible offending foods singled out for suspicion include wheat, orange juice, chocolate, and fish.

Recommend hospitalization for patients unresponsive to these measures or when care is deficient at home. Lending psychologic support to the mother, who is often distraught, exhausted, and guilt ridden, is an essential component of the treatment of the infant. Withhold oral corticosteroids, if possible, unless everything else fails, and then administer only for short periods, say 2 or 3 weeks.

Adolescent and Adult Atopic Dermatitis

Acute and Subacute Dermatitis. The patient's comfort requires a room optimally air conditioned or heated, adequately humidified, and dust free. Prohibit the use of soap and hot water bathing. For exudative areas, thick gauze or soft cotton cloth compresses of cool tap water, or Burow's solution diluted 1:30, or magnesium sulfate or sodium chloride, 1 tablespoonful to 1 quart water, are applied for 1 hour or longer four or more times a day. The wet dressings may be left on almost continuously if the patient prefers, being removed every 4 hours to cleanse the skin of debris, and then reapplied anew. Tepid colloidal baths of cornstarch or powdered oatmeal, prepared by adding 1 cupful to the bath, are soothing and may be offered at frequent intervals for 30 minutes to several hours at a time. Mineral oil or an oily emulsion such as bismuth cream (4 per cent each of bismuth subnitrate and zinc oxide in equal parts of olive oil and freshly prepared solution of calcium hydroxide) should be applied immediately after the bath and every few hours thereafter for lubrication.

Corticosteroid creams, ointments, or lotions are the mainstay medications. Diluted with a suitable vehicle to half or one fourth strength or even less, they are still therapeutically active and afford increased safety and economy when extensive areas of the body are involved.

If the patient does not tolerate oils or greases, lipid-free skin cleaner (Cetaphil or Wibi) lotion is a serviceable emollient. Fluocinolone acetonide 0.01 per cent in propylene glycol (Synalar or Fluonid solution) is subsequently rubbed in twice a day or as often as required for pruritus.

Antihistamines are occasionally useful for relief of pruritus, especially if they tend to induce drowsiness. Such agents as diphenhydramine (Benadryl), 25 to 50 mg, or cyproheptadine (Periactin), 2 to 4 mg, or hydroxyzine (Atarax, Vistaril), 10 to 25 mg, or methdilazine (Tacaryl), 4 to 8 mg four times a day, are all appropriate. Barbiturates, chloral hydrate, glutethimide (Doriden, or flurazepam (Dalmane) are choices for inducing sleep at night.

When distress is severe and the eruption resists treatment with the foregoing measures, oral prednisone or intramuscular triamcinolone acetonide becomes necessary, unless contraindicated by other disease. It is essential to inform the patient that corticosteroids are suppressive and not curative, that side effects are frequent, that prednisone will be given only for a relatively short course (tapered off in less than 4 weeks) and not indefinitely, and that relapses commonly occur when medication is withdrawn. A single daily dose is administered in the morning. With improvement, a double dose on alternate days may be tried but is not often successful. In severe cases a change of environment, such as is offered by hospitalization, encourages a favorable response.

At all stages and ages, one must guard against bacterial and viral infection of the skin, miliaria, and allergic contact dermatitis from topical medication. Infrequent but noteworthy are hypersensitivity reactions to lanolin, neomycin, or ingredients of cream bases.

Chronic Dermatitis. Advise the patient to eliminate exposure to drying agents and external irritants, especially soap, detergents, alcohol rubs, and wool. He must also avoid the undesirable influences of environmental heat, humidity, and physical exertion. If he can change his residence, encourage a trial move to the warm, arid Southwest United States.

The skin, usually inherently dry, softens when hydration combines with a bath oil (Alpha Keri, Domol, Lubath, or Derma-Smoothe), ½ to 1 tablespoonful to the bath. (Warn about the danger of slipping in the bathtub!) Lowila Cake and Aveeno Bar are soap substitutes innocuous for most patients. Corticosteroid creams or ointments, diluted 1:2 or 1:4 or more as noted above and applied four times a day, lubricate and promote healing. Their effectiveness is enhanced by occlusion overnight with thin plastic film such as Saran Wrap.

If these measures fall short of achieving adequate control, tars should be introduced. The mildest form of tar medication is the tar bath. Balnetar or Polytar is mixed with barely tepid water, 1 tablespoonful to the tub, in which the patient soaks for 30 minutes to 1 hour or longer once or twice a day. One may add 5 per cent coal tar solution USP to bismuth cream or corticosteroid ointment, keeping alert for possible appearance of tar folliculitis. Additional relief of itching may be obtained by incorporating into the medication 0.25 per cent menthol, phenol, or camphor, or combinations of these.

Graduated, cautious exposure to sunlight and early morning or late afternoon sea bathing where available sometimes help, perhaps largely through psychic influences. Oral antihistamines may alleviate itching. For sedation, phenobarbital, 65 to 100 mg, or meprobamate, 200 to 400 mg, is often adequate. Useful also is the following:

> Chloral hydrate   15.
> Elixir Benadryl q.s. to make 120.
> Label: One or two teaspoonfuls at bedtime

Secondary infection demands an appropriate systemic antibiotic determined by bacteriologic culture and antibiotic sensitivity studies.

Office psychotherapy is an indispensable ingredient of treatment. Periodic brief discussions with the patient frequently spotlight emotional problems relating to home, school, job, or love life. The physician's interest, sympathy, support, encouragement, and advice can be consequential for initiating improvement. The aim is for the patient to identify and sublimate his inwardly directed aggressions. When problems are unsolvable, the understanding physican helps strengthen the patient's tolerance for his troubles and enables him to live more comfortably with the offending skin.

Diets, allergic skin testing, and hyposensitization, apart from the influence of suggestion, are generally useless in the management of atopic dermatitis.

NEURODERMATITIS

method of
MICHAEL J. SCOTT, M.D.
Seattle, Washington

Neurodermatitis is a psychosomatic disorder that may occur independently on normal skin or be superimposed on some prior-existing, nonrelated dermatitis. Pruritus is the main symptom; it may produce a seemingly endless cycle of pruritus causing scratching or rubbing, which in turn produces lichenification, which itself produces pruritus to complete the circle.

Neurodermatitis must be viewed as the patient's subconscious method of handling stress. If this stressful situation is just temporary, the acute neurodermatitis will usually clear even without therapy. If the stress is continuous over a long period of time, a chronic neurodermatitis may ensue. Patients in the latter category may have to develop a new perspective or direction in their lives to obtain a cure. Topical or parenteral therapy may otherwise afford only temporary relief in such patients. Occasionally the neurodermatitis may persist merely as a habit long after the initial stress has disappeared. These patients often respond dramatically to a variety of psychosomatic techniques, including hypnosis.

For successful therapy neurodermatitis should be viewed as a dynamic interplay of factors conducive to pruritus in a hereditarily predisposed surface. At present the immunologic aspects are not clearly defined.

The clinical manifestations vary considerably and result primarily from paroxysmal bouts of scratching. Since scratching is generally accomplished when the patient is idle, these paroxysms are most likely to occur in the evening or at night.

Therapy

The therapeutic approach must be comprehensive to be effective. Not only must the visible cutaneous irritation be treated but also the invisible psychic irritation. To treat one but not the other is to invite defeat. Cutaneous irritation may be relieved by topical applications, medicated compresses or baths, occlusive dressings, irradiation therapy, or oral or parenteral medication.

Depending upon the circumstances, I frequently employ the following:

Topical Therapy. A very soothing ointment is:

Rx 1:
Camphor	0.5 to 1%
Phenol	0.5 to 1%
Crude coal tar (Zetar)	2 to 5%
Hydrophilic ointment (USP)	
Lassar's paste	aa q.s.a.d.30.0

The percentage of Lassar's paste may be increased for oozing areas or decreased for dry areas. For oozing areas substitute liquor aluminum acetate in place of coal tar for its astringent effect. Hydrocortisone acetate 0.5 to 1.0 per cent may be added if desired.

Rx 2:
Menthol	0.5%
Phenol	0.5 to 1%
Iodochlorhydroxyquin	3%
Hydrophilic ointment (USP)	q.s.a.d.30.0

Various commercial "cortisone" ointments, applied either directly or beneath an occlusive plastic dressing (e.g., Saran Wrap), have been suggested. In my practice, I have found them expensive and no more effective than the above.

If a lotion is preferred, the following is beneficial:

Rx 3:
Menthol	0.5%
Phenol	1.0%
Aluminum acetate solution	15.0%
Zinc oxide	30.0%
Purified talc	30.0%
Glycerine	24.0%
Lime water	q.s.a.d. 120.0

An effective liniment is:

Rx 4:
Menthol	0.5%
Phenol	1.0%
Prepared calamine	8.0%
Zinc oxide	8.0%
Olive oil	50.0%
Lime water	q.s.a.d. 120.0

Occlusive Dressings. Lassar's paste covered by muslin and then wrapped with an adhesive elastic bandage (e.g., Elastoplast) is soothing and protects the affected areas from trauma of scratching. It is especially useful in localized neurodermatitis. This protective bandage may be changed every 3 to 5 days. A modified Unna boot (e.g., Gelocast, Dome Paste Boot) may also be employed to break the itch-scratch cycle.

Intralesional Injections. Intralesional injections of triamcinolone acetonide (10 mg per ml) mixed with equal volumes of 1 per cent lidocaine and injected intradermally through a 23 gauge needle have been recommended. A 2 inch square plaque could be injected at multiple sites with a total of 5 mg. I personally am not overly impressed with the overall effectiveness of this technique and seldom employ it.

Irradiation Therapy. In my opinion, the beneficial effects of ultraviolet, grenz ray, and x-ray therapy may be attributed as much to psychologic effect as to the activity of the irradiation per se. Certainly roentgen therapy should seldom, if ever, be employed. Natural sunlight has its advocates, but it must be remembered that if the patient is soaking up sunshine, he is generally on vacation or resting, and this factor is equally beneficial.

Oral and Parenteral Medication. Dosages must be individualized.

Mild Sedation. Mild sedation such as phenobarbital, 15 mg (¼ grain) at breakfast and supper and 30 mg (½ grain) at bedtime, is frequently as effective as more expensive medication. Rarely secobarbital (Seconal), 0.1 gram (1½) grains), or the combination of secobarbital and amobarbital (Tuinal), 0.1 gram (1½ grains), at bedtime is required temporarily.

Antihistamines. Promethazine hydrochloride, 12.5 mg twice or three times daily, is frequently very effective. No doubt the sedative effect is at least as important as the antihistamine aspect.

Tranquilizers. (1) Hydroxyzine (Atarax), 10 mg three or four times daily. (2) Meprobamate, 200 mg two or three times daily in divided dosage.

Hormones. Estrogens (Premarin, Gynetone, or equivalent) for women at or approaching the menopause may be advisable orally or parenterally.

Corticosteroids. Triamcinolone or prednisolone, 5 mg two or three times daily, is justifiable in severe generalized neurodermatitis, with gradual discontinuance as soon as possible. Corticosteroids may also be given intramuscularly.

Psychotherapy

Equally important as the foregoing conventional dermatologic therapy is the skillful application of psychotherapy. The combination of psychotherapy and conventional dermatologic therapy is the treatment of choice. Such combined or comprehensive therapy is best administered by one physician, whether he is a general practitioner, dermatologist, or psychiatrist. Psychotherapy is especially indicated to prevent recurrences, because emotional factors dominate as the trigger mechanism in exacerbations of neurodermatitis. Psychotherapy, to be effective, need be neither very time consuming nor highly complex. In some instances merely covering (or supportive) psychotherapy is all that is necessary. Reassurance, encouragement, persuasion, and suggestion belong in this category. Often merely patiently and attentively listening to the patients' reiteration of their personal troubles (catharsis) is unbelievably effective. I find that if you listen long enough, the majority will eventually tell you the actual source of their psychologic irritation that is frequently camouflaged by rationalizations on the initial visit. Employ empathy, not sympathy. In chronic or resistive cases uncovering forms of psychotherapy may be required to disclose the suppressed cause of emotional stress and tension. Hyperthyroidism and other systemic disorders should be ruled out.

Hypnotherapy. Since I, like most practicing physicians, do not have time for lengthy psychotherapy, I find hypnotherapy an ideal modality in judiciously selected patients for obtaining rapid and effective results. Orientation in psychodynamics is a basic prerequisite for successful hypnotherapy. Through the proper use of hypnosis one can circumvent the prejudices, rationalization, and argumentations that might normally impede other psychotherapeutic approaches. Hypnosis can be utilized in both covering and uncovering forms of psychotherapy. It is highly effective in relaxing the patient both physically and mentally. The principal methods by which symptoms may be relieved by hypnosis are the following:

DIRECT SUGGESTION. Direct suggestion is very effective for symptomatic relief of cutaneous itching, scratching, insomnia (precipitated by or aggravating the dermatitis), anxiety, and mental stress (associated with neurodermatitis as a causative, accompanying, or contributing factor). Direct suggestion is especially beneficial in cases of neurodermatitis that are perpetuated only as a habit.

SYMPTOM SUBSTITUTION. This implies replacing one habit pattern with another, more constructive pattern. Scratching, for example, may be replaced by a desire to pursue other physical activity. The effectiveness of this procedure is partially determined by how closely the substituted symptom equates symbolically and psychologically with the original symptom.

HYPNOANALYSIS. This is a recent improvement in hypnotherapy. In this procedure, hypnosis is combined with an analytic method of psychotherapy. Repressed emotionally traumatic incidents or thoughts may consciously be forgotten but forever remain in the subconscious, where they are capable of producing conflicts that may manifest themselves as neurodermatitis. The patient's conscious awareness of these causes can occasionally completely disintegrate a neurosis.

Haphazard use of hypnosis will render no better results than the haphazard use of any other modality of therapy. Biofeedback and autogenic training may also enhance the treatment of neurodermatitis.

Incongruous as it may seem, at times it is more discreet not to deprive the patient entirely of his dermatitis as a means of releasing nervous tension, because sometimes another more vital organ may become the target of his psychosomatic outlet.

In a relatively very small percentage of patients complete freedom from symptoms can be a bitter freedom indeed. Similarly, it must be remembered that however undesirable neurodermatitis may be, it originally fulfilled, and may yet fulfill, a psychologic need of the patient.

POISON IVY DERMATITIS

method of
ALBERT H. SLEPYAN, M.D.
Highland Park, Illinois

Poison ivy, poison oak, and poison sumac, members of the Anacardiaceae family of plants, produce by far the greatest number of plant dermatoses in North America. These are the public enemy number one of the plant world. The poisonous principles found in these plants are all closely related catechols producing identical symptoms. Very few patients are aware that the poison ivy plant is a great imitator. The leaves may on occasion take on the characteristics of their surrounding neighboring plants. Variations in shape and morphology of the individual leaflets account for the lack of recognition of the plant. Characteristically the leaves are three; however, sometimes the leaves are smooth, serrated, notched, or markedly indented. Occasionally an individual leaflet will suggest basswood, cottonwood, birch, or parsley; but on close examination there are always "leaves three, let them be."

Patients who repeatedly find themselves exposed and irritated by these plants are advised to make a trip or two to the library and thumb through a series of botanical atlases to become acquainted with the pictures of poison ivy growing in their respective areas.

Prophylaxis

The catechols can sensitize rapidly on contact and can be carried or remain a source of irritation for many months. The oily material extruded from the broken leaf or stem becomes tenacious and adherent to objects of contact such as shoes, boots, clothing, garden tools, auto tires, camping equipment, and a host of misplaced objects. Animals, especially dogs and cats, frequently carry the oleoresin to their unsuspecting hosts. Developing "the eye of a trapper" in recognizing the plant, is the best known preventive.

In highly sensitive individuals it is necessary to wash and clean the exposed areas with a degreasing agent, such as soap or detergent, within seconds or minutes to avoid an eruption.

Therapy

For the milder manifestations of the eruption, areas showing streaked erythema with beginning vesiculation, calamine lotion (USP XV) is soothing and drying. The lotion is applied every 4 hours. One must be sure that none of the vesicles are open or ruptured when the drying lotion is applied.

To areas showing erosive or ruptured vesicles, moist compresses of Domeboro packets, 1 packet to a pint of cold water, greatly reduce the itching and hasten the drying of the lesions. Prednisone is prescribed as outlined in Table 1. In the presence of oozing and pyodermic crusting, tetracycline (Achromycin) or erythromycin, 250 mg four times a day, is added to the steroid schedule. When the skin feels dry and scaling is evident, the calamine bentonite lotion is stopped and 0.1 per cent triamcinolone cream is substituted to reduce the remaining redness and act as a lubricant. Antihistamines such as chlorphenira-

TABLE 1. Prednisone Outline

DAY	NOON 12	P.M. 6	P.M. 10	A.M. 8
1	3	3	3	3
2	2 1/2	2 1/2	2 1/2	2 1/2
3	2	2	2	2
4	1 1/2	1 1/2	1 1/2	1 1/2
5	1	1	1	1
6	0	1	1	1
7	0	0	1	1
8	0	0	0	1
9	0	0	0	1

Five mg prednisone tablets are taken as outlined above. The patient is advised to cross out each dose as taken.

mine (Chlor-Trimeton), 4 mg every 4 hours, help relieve the pruritus and keep the patient comfortable. The patient is advised that tepid to warm water showering is permissible, without soaping, if care is taken in drying gently.

SEBORRHEIC DERMATITIS

method of
DONALD P. LOOKINGBILL, M.D.
Hershey, Pennsylvania

The clinical expression of seborrheic dermatitis ranges from dandruff (which some would view as a physiologic rather than a pathologic process) to a generalized exfoliative dermatitis. The classic expression of this common disorder, however, is one which is characterized by an erythematous scaling eruption in a characteristic distribution. The dermatitis is distributed in areas that are rich in sebaceous glands, specifically the scalp, retroauricular areas, eyebrows, eyelids, nasolabial folds, and presternal areas. The eruption can also appear as a confluent eruption over the malar areas; it is the most common cause of a "butterfly rash." Less commonly, seborrheic dermatitis can affect the larger flexural folds as in the axilla and inguinal areas. Rarely it can result in a generalized dermatitis.

The cause of this disorder is unknown. It can begin in infancy, in which case it usually clears before the first year of life. In adults, the disease often appears around the time of puberty. It is a chronic condition that waxes and wanes. Itching may be present. A specific cure is not available, but the condition is usually relatively easily controllable with the following measures:

Dandruff and Seborrheic Dermatitis of the Scalp

Dandruff flaking can usually be controlled simply with the use of a medicated shampoo. Tar shampoos may be helpful, but shampoos containing either selenium sulfide (Excel, Selsun) or zinc pyrithione (Danex, Head & Shoulders, Zincon) are preferred. In using these shampoos, it is critical that the patient understand two important concepts: (1) Shampooing is done as frequently as is necessary to control the scaling. Initially, every other day use may be needed. (2) It is the scalp, not the hair, that is being treated. The patient should be instructed to vigorously massage a thick lather of the shampoo into the scalp, rinse, repeat the application, let stand for 5 minutes, and finally rinse thoroughly.

Occasionally, additional measures are needed for resistant scaling or inflammation. Scales can be loosened by macerating them prior to the shampooing. For example, a traditional approach to seborrheic cradle cap is to apply mineral oil an hour before the shampooing. Tap water can be used equally successfully if the scalp is wetted and then covered with a shower cap to prevent evaporation 1 hour before shampooing. Daily use of lotions containing salicylic acid (Sebucare) can also be employed.

Inflammation is treated with cortisone lotions or solutions. Creams and ointments are impractical to use in the hairy scalp. A hydrocortisone lotion is usually sufficient. Preparations are available which combine hydrocortisone with salicylic acid (Barseb HC). These are simply applied to the scalp on a daily basis. Rarely, a stronger cortisone preparation is needed. For this, a number of the more potent fluorinated steroids are available in lotion or solution preparations.

Seborrheic Dermatitis of the Face

Currently, hydrocortisone cream in 0.5 to 1 per cent concentration represents the mainstay of therapy for seborrheic dermatitis affecting the nonscalp skin. A single daily application is usually sufficient. The patient is instructed to use the medication only when the disease is active. Once the condition is controlled, the medication can be, temporarily at least, discontinued. Usually, intermittent short courses of therapy are sufficient to control this spontaneously waxing and waning disorder. It is critical to emphasize that the more potent fluorinated steroid preparations are contraindicated in the treatment of seborrheic dermatitis of the face or flexural folds. These agents will rapidly control the inflammatory response on the face, but when they are discontinued there often is a rebound of the inflammation — resulting in an eruption that is frequently worse than the initial problem. Continuing cycles of use of medication ensue, and further side effects from the topical steroids may result. These include skin atrophy with thinning and telangiectases and the development of an acneiform dermatitis. In the flexural folds, prolonged use of the fluorinated steroids also results in skin thinning with development of striae. These side effects usually do not occur with the intermittent use of hydrocortisone cream.

Seborrheic Blepharitis

Treatment of seborrheic dermatitis of the eyelids presents a particularly difficult problem. Topical steroids, if accidentally rubbed into the eyes on a chronic basis, can result in cataracts and/or glaucoma. Erythromycin ophthalmic ointment may provide a helpful, and safer, therapeutic alternative for some patients. If topical steroid preparations are used, periodic ophthalmologic examinations should be considered.

Seborrheic Dermatitis of the Flexural Folds

The axilla and inguinal areas are much less frequently involved with seborrheic dermatitis. When it occurs, however, the judicious use of hydrocortisone cream is usually sufficient to control the problem. Sometimes, the addition of iodochlorhydroxyquin (Vioform) in combination with hydrocortisone (Vioform-HC) provides further benefit. In addition, if there is a complicating monilial or fungal infection in the flexural areas, particularly the groin area, the iodochlorhydroxyquin will provide coverage for these organisms. This medication may stain skin and clothing yellow.

In flexural folds, a cream (water-soluble base) rather than an ointment preparation is preferred. The cream should be applied sparingly and should be rubbed in until it "vanishes." Excessive amounts of cream, or use of ointments, may result in maceration in flexural areas and can be self-defeating.

Generalized Seborrheic Dermatitis

It is possible for seborrheic dermatitis to generalize, resulting in exfoliative erythroderma. This is exceedingly rare. The management includes those measures employed in treating exfoliative dermatitis from other causes. Systemic steroids may be needed.

In summary, seborrheic dermatitis in its usual form is a common, erythematous, scaling condition with a distinctive distribution. Control is usually easily achieved, but recurrences are common. Medicated shampoos are important for managing the scalp condition; hydrocortisone preparations provide the mainstay of therapy for the inflammatory component. Tars, salicylic acid–containing preparations, and iodochlorhydroxyquin can also be employed. The more potent topical fluorinated steroid preparations should be avoided.

STASIS DERMATITIS AND ULCERS

method of
IRWIN J. SCHATZ, M.D.
Honolulu, Hawaii

Chronic venous insufficiency of the leg is usually the result of thrombosis of the iliofemoral vein leading to stasis of venous blood flow. Inflammation of the venous wall reduces elasticity and damages previously competent venous valves; these changes lead to pooling and stagnation of blood. Occasionally, arteriovenous fistulas may produce a similar picture. Stasis results in a loss of fluid and red cells into the interstitial tissues, leading to induration, fibrosis, and hyperpigmentation. Minor injuries easily produce superficial ulcers (usually confined to the area around the malleoli) of irregular shape and size, shallow and often covered with an infected exudate. Such lesions are not excessively painful.

Treatment

Prevention. The sequelae of chronic venous insufficiency in great part may be obviated by a few simple measures taken immediately after an episode of acute deep vein thrombosis. These must include the prevention of postphlebitic edema by the use of a properly fitting elastic support, preferably of the pressure gradient type (Jobst), and the avoidance of long periods of standing in one position to prevent edema fluid from accumulating. These simple precautions are often sufficient to avoid the self-perpetuating cycle of stasis edema, poor nutrition of the subcutaneous tissues and the skin, ulceration, infection, and stasis dermatitis.

General Principles. DECREASE OR ELIMINATE EDEMA. Ulcers and dermatitis will not heal unless most or all of the tissue edema fluid is removed. In most cases, this may be accomplished with relative ease by simply placing the patient at bed rest, with elevation of the affected leg. Mobilization of fluid may occur within 48 to 72 hours; by the end of several days no detectable edema will be present. Unfortunately, those patients with considerable induration may require prolonged periods of bed rest with elevation of the extremity before any reduction in fluid occurs.

CLEAN THE ULCERS. Use intermittent moist dressings to soak the ulcers and the associated stasis dermatitis and permit natural mechanisms to begin the healing process.

STASIS ULCERS. Bed rest with intermittent soaking of the ulcers is essential. The solution may consist of saturated solution of boric acid (4 per cent), or isotonic saline, or ethanol-iodine complex (Wescodyne) solution (3 per cent). The choice of solution does not matter very much, as long as the compresses are applied intermittently in order to avoid maceration of the skin. Only rarely is antibiotic therapy necessary either locally or systemically; in most cases, simple cleansing by means of a sterile solution with intermittent drying and with the patient at bed rest will result in prompt healing.

For large ulcers, when secondary infection has cleared, the ulcer itself may be placed in an Unna paste boot, permitting ambulation. This is done by covering the ulcer with a piece of fine gauze, which is in turn padded with other gauze pads placed over the ulcer; the Unna paste boot (Dome-Paste), which consists of rolled bandages impregnated with zinc oxide, glycerine, gelatin, and calamine, is then applied. Such dressings may be changed one or twice weekly until the ulcer heals.

For very large ulcers, or those which do not heal promptly, split thickness skin grafting or pinch grafting may be necessary. Consultation with a plastic surgeon is then appropriate.

STASIS DERMATITIS. Again, the principle of bed rest to eliminate or diminish edema is mandatory.

1. Wet compresses applied four or five times daily for 1 or 2 hours will reduce the amount of inflammation and infection in the tissues. Between dressings, a drying spray or lotion should be applied (1 per cent hydrocortisone).

2. If secondary infection, as manifested by signs of cellulitis, lymphangitis, or bacteremia, is present, appropriate cultures should be taken and systemic antibiotics administered.

3. If chronic stasis dermatitis persists after the acute phase is treated, then an Unna paste boot (as described above) may be applied with some success. Occasionally, thickened indurated areas of dermatitis may require topical steroid medication such as triamcinolone acetate. When nodular areas develop and do not respond to topical steroids, then the occasional use of anti-inflammatory agents such as phenylbutazone (Butazolidin) may be necessary. When such agents are used, attention must be paid to periodic evaluation of hematocrit and red blood cell count, as well as stool guaiac examination.

It should be emphasized that the prevention of recurrence of either stasis ulcers or stasis dermatitis requires permanent and meticulous avoidance of accumulation of stasis edema. For this reason, pressure gradient type support stockings are necessary. These are individually made to measure for each patient and must be worn precisely according to instructions. Such garments require replacement every 2 to 3 months. If used properly, they will markedly diminish the likelihood of disability from chronic venous insufficiency.

DERMATOMYOSITIS/POLYMYOSITIS

method of
IVOR CARO, M.D.
Seattle, Washington

The following five major criteria have recently been recommended for a diagnosis of either polymyositis or dermatomyositis:

1. Symmetric weakness of the limb-girdle muscles with or without dysphagia and respiratory muscle weakness.

2. Elevation, in the serum, of the levels of skeletal muscle enzymes, particularly creatine phosphokinase, but also the transaminases, lactic dehydrogenase, and aldolase.

3. Electromyographic evidence of myositis.

4. Muscle biopsy changes of myositis; necrosis, regeneration, phagocytosis, and a mononuclear infiltrate.

5. Skin changes of dermatomyositis — including periorbital edema with a red/blue discoloration of the eyelids, erythematous scaling lesions over the knuckles of the hands, periungual telangiectasia with cuticular thickening, and a more generalized red and scaling rash over knees, elbows, upper trunk, and face.

For a "definite" diagnosis: three or four criteria (plus rash) for dermatomyositis; four criteria (without rash) for polymyositis.

For a "probable" diagnosis: two criteria (plus rash) for dermatomyositis; three criteria (without rash) for polymyositis.

For a "possible" diagnosis: one criterion (plus rash) for dermatomyositis; two criteria (without rash) for polymyositis.

Once the diagnosis has been made, it is useful to classify polymyositis/dermatomyositis as follows: (1) Polymyositis (PM). (2) Dermatomyositis (DM). (3) PM/DM with malignancy. (4) PM/DM in childhood. (5) PM/DM with overlap with other "connective tissue diseases."

The association of PM/DM with malignancy appears to be more common in patients over 40 years of age (particularly those over 60 years) and is more common in those with dermatomyositis than in those with polymyositis. It is slightly more common in females than in males.

Childhood PM/DM is rarely associated with malignant disease and may show a vasculitis as a prominent feature.

Treatment

Although there is no general agreement regarding the efficacy of corticosteroids and immunosuppressives, these agents are widely used in DM/PM.

Corticosteroids. Most patients with DM/PM are treated with corticosteroids, at least initially. It appears that better results are obtained if treatment is started within 2 months of onset of the disease. Children also appear to respond more favorably than adults. The usual precautions should be taken prior to instituting potentially long-term steroid therapy.

Prednisone is the corticosteroid of choice. It is inexpensive and less likely to cause a steroid-induced myopathy than are fluorinated steroids.

1. In adults, treatment should be begun at between 50 and 100 mg daily, depending on disease severity. Response to therapy should be measured by both improvement in muscle strength and fall in the serum levels of muscle enzymes. However, clinical improvement should be the most important index.

2. As improvement occurs, there should be a gradual reduction in the dosage of prednisone by 5 mg every 2 to 3 weeks.

3. If relapse occurs, the dose should be increased by 10 to 20 mg and a more gradual reduction attempted.

4. Maintenance therapy is usually required for months to years at doses between 5 and 25 mg daily. Alternate day therapy appears to have certain advantages and should be instituted at doses twice that of the daily dose, i.e., 10 to 50 mg on alternate days.

5. In children, high-dose (1.5 to 2.0 mg per kg per day) corticosteroid therapy is required to produce remission. As clinical improvement occurs, the dosage is gradually tapered (2.5 mg every fourth day). If evidence of relapse is noted (lessening of muscle strength or increasing serum levels of muscle enzymes), a return to the previous dose should be made. One should aim at maintaining patients in an independently functional state during the active phase of the disease, not at eradicating all manifestations of the condition. In most patients the duration of the active stage is 2 to 3 years, and maintenance therapy is recommended to prevent relapses. Corticosteroids have no role in the therapy of patients with "burnt-out" disease with muscle wasting and contractures unless active disease supervenes.

Immunosuppressive Agents. 1. In adults, after a 2 to 3 month trial of corticosteroids without significant response, immunosuppressive agents should be considered. Methotrexate is the agent most often used under these circumstances (this use of methotrexate is not specifically listed in the manufacturer's official directive). An initial intravenous dose of 10 or 15 mg is given. If this is well tolerated, it is gradually increased to 0.5 to 0.8 mg per kg per day at intervals of 5 to 7 days. After that, the patients are given weekly intravenous therapy.

After several weeks and with evidence of clinical and muscle enzyme improvement, the methotrexate is given once every 2 weeks, then once every 3 weeks, followed by once a month. Before and during therapy, the usual precautions for methotrexate treatment should be observed.

2. During this time, an attempt should be made to taper the steroid dose, as methotrexate has been shown to have a steroid-sparing effect.

3. Other immunosuppressive agents, particularly azathioprine, have also been used, although the most experience has been gained with methotrexate (this use of azathioprine is not listed in the manufacturer's official directive).

4. In children, methotrexate or azathioprine may have to be used if high-dose corticosteroids fail to control the disease after 3 to 6 months.

General Measures. During all phases of therapy, general measures play an important role.

1. Physical therapy to prevent contractures and respiratory and occupational therapy should be provided for all patients as indicated.

2. Treatment of the rash in dermatomyositis should include emollients and sun protection. Topical corticosteroids are often unnecessary, as the patients are taking systemic steroids.

The treatment of the calcinosis that may develop in childhood cases is difficult. Chelating agents such as the diphosphonates, aluminum hydroxide, and a low-calcium diet may be tried. Surgical excision of painful or infected calcium deposits may become necessary.

THE ERYTHEMAS

method of
E. WILLIAM ROSENBERG, M.D.
Memphis, Tennessee

It now appears likely that most of the group of skin eruptions classified morphologically as the erythemas represent the visible manifestation of a reaction to circulating immune complexes. These complexes ordinarily have two components: an antigen which may be microbial or chemical in origin, and associated antibody to the antigen. Because the presence of such complexes alters the rheologic properties of the plasma, and because the flow of blood tends normally to be somewhat slower in the naturally cooler skin than in the warmer internal organs, there is a tendency for such complexes to stick to the walls of venules in the skin with the resultant appearance of a rash. Considering the common mechanism of these various eruptions, it is not unusual that rashes of diverse causes look alike; it is remarkable that the clinical appearances are as distinctive as they are.

Looked at in this light, the management of these conditions becomes clear. First, look for the antigen: stop all possible offending drugs and look for signs of infection, especially ones that might be amenable to treatment. Second, and only then, consider the advisability or the necessity of inhibiting the antibody response. This can be accomplished to a degree with substantial amounts of systemic corticosteroid, provided that it is clearly understood that at the same time one is interfering with what might be a useful mechanism for removing foreign agents from the body.

Erythema Multiforme

Most cases of erythema multiforme are not serious and can be managed expectantly. All possible causative drugs must be stopped at once. Common triggering infections are antecedent herpes simplex attacks and coexistent mycoplasma pneumonia. There is nothing to be done about herpes, but mycoplasma pneumonia should be treated with a full course of erythromycin or tetracycline.

In some patients the mouth is so sore that eating becomes painful. In such patients lidocaine (Xylocaine) viscous syrup, used prior to eating, is helpful. Chilled formula-diet drinks (Metrecal, Sego) plus ice chips are usually well tolerated and may eliminate the need for hospitalization and intravenous alimentation. Lidocaine (Xylocaine) ointment applied prior to urination and cool water poured over the area during urination ease pain associated with vulvar erosions.

Occasionally patients suffer an explosive, very severe erosive form of erythema multiforme involving the eyes, oropharynx, and genitalia (Stevens-Johnson syndrome). Again, first be sure any offending drug has been halted. Frequently such patients require hospitalization and intravenous alimentation. Methylprednisolone (Solu-Medrol) is given by vein at a dose of 80 mg per day.

Erythema Nodosum

Erythema nodosum, another distinctive reaction pattern, is more likely to be infection related than is erythema multiforme. One is obliged to evaluate the patient for tuberculosis, deep fungus infection (especially coccidioidomycosis for those who have been in high prevalence areas), yersinia enteritis, lymphogranuloma venereum, streptococcal infection, sarcoidosis, and ulcerative colitis.

Drugs, including oral contraceptives, are a less likely cause of erythema nodosum than infection but should be asked about and when possible stopped.

Treatment is with bed rest and aspirin. Patients with subacute cases are helped by support hose. Because of the possibility of occult infection, the use of systemic corticosteroids should be resisted.

The Figurate Erythemas

The larger textbooks of dermatology list a variety of less severe and usually less distinctive patterns of erythema which merge into patterns resembling urticaria.

Again, one should inquire about a possible drug allergy and look for streptococcal infection, deep (and in these cases, superficial) fungus infections, viral infection, or granulomatous disease.

Erythema annulare centrifugum resembles a large spot of tinea corporis, frequently on the hip or flank. It may be benefited by a search for superficial fungus infection and the elimination from the diet of wine, beer, and cheese.

SUPERFICIAL FUNGUS INFECTIONS OF THE SKIN

method of
ANDREW H. RUDOLPH, M.D.
Houston, Texas

Superficial fungus infections of the skin can be divided into the superficial mycoses, dermatophytoses, and candidiasis.

Superficial Mycoses

Tinea Versicolor (Pityriasis Versicolor). Tinea versicolor is a very common superficial fungus infection caused by the organism *Malassezia furfur (Pityrosporon orbiculare)*. Lesions usually consist of asymptomatic, scaly patches characteristically located on the upper trunk and neck. The disease may involve large areas of the skin, and a Wood's light examination is often helpful in assessing the extent of involvement. In winter the lesions are usually fawn to brown in color; but in summer, because the presence of the fungus interferes with normal tanning, the lesions will often appear lighter than the surrounding skin. With increased ultraviolet exposure, this color difference becomes more prominent and is often the reason the patient seeks medical help. Although treatment may eradicate the fungus infection, the patient should be advised that it may take many months to resolve this color difference.

Griseofulvin is not effective in the treatment of tinea versicolor, but numerous topical agents have been used with varying success. A satisfactory treatment, especially in those patients with extensive involvement, is the use of selenium sulfide 2.5 per cent lotion (Exsel or Selsun). Following a bath or shower, the lotion is applied as a lather to all areas of the skin from the neck down to the waist. The lather is allowed to dry for 30 minutes and then is rinsed off thoroughly. The regimen is repeated at weekly intervals for 2 weeks, once every 2 weeks for 2 months, and then once a month for 3 months. Between treatments with the selenium sulfide lotion, a 25 per cent solution of sodium thiosulfate, used alone or in combination with 1 per cent salicylic acid in 10 per cent isopropyl alcohol and propylene glycol (Tinver lotion), should be applied twice daily to all visible scaly areas. Tolnaftate 1 per cent (Tinactin), haloprogin 1 per cent (Halotex), miconazole nitrate 2 per cent (MicaTin), or clotrimazole 1 per cent (Lotrimin) can also be used effectively, but these agents are expensive and for that reason are usually restricted to the treatment of limited infections.

The patient should be reassured that this is a benign disorder, but that recurrences, especially during the hot, humid months, are common in susceptible persons. These recurrences usually respond to re-treatment and can be minimized by having the patient use a soap containing salicylic acid and sulfur after the initial therapy.

Tinea Nigra. Tinea nigra is a superficial fungus infection caused by the organism *Cladosporium (Exophilia) werneckii*. The asymptomatic black or brownish-black macular lesions of tinea nigra generally occur on the palmar surface of the hand or, less commonly, on the plantar surface of the foot.

Treatment with a mild keralytic fungicide such as Whitfield's ointment is usually successful. Tincture of iodine, 2 per cent salicylic acid and 3 per cent sulfur ointment, topical 10 per cent thiabendazole, or one of the newer topical agents such as clotrimazole 1 per cent (Lotrimin) or miconazole nitrate 2 per cent (MicaTin) can also be used. Topical tolnaftate (Tinactin) is reportedly ineffective, as is oral griseofulvin.

Dermatophytoses

Tinea Capitis. Tinea capitis is a fungus infection of the scalp and hair which usually occurs in children. It is uncommon in adults. Depending upon the degree of inflammation present, tinea capitis may be classified into noninflammatory and inflammatory types. The epidemic, noninflammatory type is most commonly caused by an anthropophilic fungus such as *Microsporum audouini* or *Trichophyton tonsurans* and is characterized by patchy alopecia, broken hairs, mild scaling, and minimal inflammation. Sporadic, inflammatory tinea capitis is usually due to a geophilic (soil) or zoophilic (animal) organism such as *Microsporum gypseum, Microsporum canis,* or *Trichophyton mentagrophytes.* Inflammatory tinea capitis usually presents with hair loss, inflammation, and pustulation of the scalp. In certain patients a painful, elevated, boggy, erythematous mass (kerion) may develop. In severe inflammatory tinea capitis, permanent hair loss may result. The classification of tinea capitis into noninflammatory and inflammatory types is arbitrary, and exceptions are common; for example, *T. tonsurans* can induce either a noninflammatory or an inflammatory response. The presence of an inflammatory response seems to correlate well with the patient's development of delayed hypersensitivity (cell-mediated immunity) to the fungus.

Topical therapy alone is not effective in the management of tinea capitis, and griseofulvin is indicated in the treatment of all types. Griseofulvin in the microcrystalline form (Fulvicin-U/F, Grifulvin V, Grisactin) is most commonly used. A dose of 5 mg of the microcrystalline form of griseofulvin per pound (0.45 kg) of body weight per day is usually adequate for children. Thus, very small children can be treated with 125 mg of griseofulvin daily; children from 30 to 50 pounds (14 to 23 kg) with 125 to 250 mg daily, and children over 50 pounds (23 kg) with 250 to 500 mg daily. A dose of 1 gram daily of griseofulvin microsize is usually adequate in most adult patients. Better gastrointestinal absorption of griseofulvin may occur when it is ingested after high fat content meals and when the total daily dosage is divided into two equal doses with one dose given after the noon meal. Concomitant phenobarbital administration reduces the blood levels of griseofulvin. Griseofulvin should be avoided in patients with established porphyria or hepatic failure and should not be given to pregnant women. Ultramicrosize griseofulvin (Gris-Peg) can also be used in approximately half the total dosage recommended for microcrystalline griseofulvin. However, except for enhanced bioavailability, the ultramicrosize preparation does not seem to offer any significant advantage, increased effectiveness, or added safety over the microsize form.

The total dosage of griseofulvin must be individualized in both adults and children, and long periods of treatment may be required. Since incomplete treatment may be accompanied by relapse, it is best to continue the griseofulvin for 2 weeks after all clinical and laboratory examinations are negative. In most cases, the usual course of therapy is 6 to 8 weeks. Post-treatment follow-up should continue for an additional 6 to 8 weeks. Since griseofulvin is fungistatic rather than fungicidal, concomitant topical therapy is often helpful. The application of a mild topical antifungal agent may decrease dissemination of spores and infected particles and hasten resolution. Ointments can be used, but solutions are usually better accepted. Daily shampoos and other adjuvant measures, such as clipping the hair around the lesion to facilitate shampooing, removal or restriction of infected fomites, and a search for a source of the infection, are indicated. Siblings should be examined and treated if infected. With modern therapy there is no justification for extensive absences from school.

In inflammatory tinea capitis moist compresses and thorough but gentle daily shampooing are helpful to keep the scalp clean and to promote drainage. Although a kerion looks like a severe bacterial infection, it is not, and it should be regarded as an allergic inflammatory response of the scalp to the presence of fungi in the hair follicle. Kerions are treated with griseofulvin in the same dosage and duration as noninflammatory tinea capitis. In some patients, systemic steroids for 1 to 2 weeks may be necessary to calm the inflammation. Topical fungicides can be used as previously indicated but are ineffective by themselves.

Tinea Barbae. This is usually an inflammatory fungus infection of the bearded area of the face and neck caused by various species of Trichophyton and Microsporum, but most commonly by *Trichophyton mentagrophytes* or *Trichophyton verrucosum.*

Tinea barbae is managed similarly to tinea capitis of the inflammatory (kerion) type. Wet compresses should be used to remove any crusts or scales. A topical antifungal agent such as clotrimazole 1 per cent (Lotrimin) or miconazole nitrate 2 per cent (MicaTin) can be applied topically, and griseofulvin should be administered orally.

Tinea Corporis. Dermatophyte infections of the glabrous skin can be caused by many Microsporum and Trichophyton species or *Epidermophyton floccosum.*

These infections, if limited in area, can

usually be managed successfully by topical treatment alone. Miconazole nitrate 2 per cent (Mica-Tin), clotrimazole 1 per cent (Lotrimin), or halo-progin 1 per cent (Halotex) should be applied twice daily to all involved areas, taking into consideration that the advancing border of the fungal infection may extend up to 6 cm beyond the margin of the visible lesion. Following topical treatment, pruritus is usually relieved within 1 week and cures are usually obtained within 3 to 6 weeks. To reduce the possibility of relapse, treatment should be continued for 1 week after all the lesions have cleared. In exceptional cases, prolonged topical treatment may be required.

Extensive cutaneous involvement, lesions at hard-to-reach sites, involvement of the hair follicle, or chronic or recurrent infections may require the addition of oral griseofulvin. Griseofulvin microsize, 250 to 500 mg twice daily after meals for 1 month, is usually adequate. Incomplete treatment with griseofulvin may be followed by relapse.

Patients with extensive tinea corporis which is unresponsive to the use of topical antifungal agents and/or oral griseofulvin should undergo evaluation to determine a possible cause. This may include an immunologic work-up to determine if they have a deficiency of cell-mediated immunity to the organism. In addition, the dermatophyte should be cultured and subjected to griseofulvin sensitivities. Griseofulvin-resistant dermatophytes can be encountered, and these relatively resistant strains are affected only by large concentrations of griseofulvin which cannot be achieved therapeutically. Finally, in any failure of response to griseofulvin, poor patient compliance must be considered.

Tinea Cruris.   Tinea cruris is commonly caused by *Trichophyton rubrum, Trichophyton menta-grophytes,* or *Epidermophyton floccosum.* The crural area and inner thighs are usually involved; the scrotal skin is typically unaffected.

The treatment of tinea cruris is dependent upon the history and physical examination. In new, limited infections, a topical agent such as clotrimazole 1 per cent (Lotrimin) or miconazole nitrate 2 per cent (MicaTin) applied twice daily for 2 to 4 weeks is often sufficient. After clearing, maintenance therapy with one of these agents or dusting the involved area with tolnaftate (Tinactin) powder may help prevent recurrence.

Patients with chronic or recurrent tinea cruris unresponsive to topical therapy, those with extensive lesions, or those with follicular involvement should also be treated with oral griseofulvin, 0.5 to 1 gram daily for 30 days.

Severe inflammatory tinea cruris or tinea cruris which has become secondarily infected may require treatment with topical or systemic steroids and systemic antibiotics. Since tinea cruris may develop secondary to a dermatophyte infection of the feet, any concomitant tinea pedis should also be treated.

Tinea cruris is prone to recur, and instructing the patient on preventive local measures is important. Such factors as occlusion, wetness, and warmth contribute to recurrence or chronicity of the infection. Aeration of the involved area should be promoted. Tight underclothing or pantyhose should be avoided and the wearing of loose-fitting absorbent cotton clothing encouraged. Jogging and other physical activity should be avoided during acute flares. The use of powders (ZeaSORB, Tinactin) to decrease sweating and maceration may be helpful.

Tinea Pedis.   Tinea pedis is most commonly caused by *Trichophyton rubrum, Trichophyton menta-grophytes,* or *Epidermophyton floccosum.*

Tinea pedis may present clinically in the following ways: (1) as a chronic, dry, scaling eruption with or without hyperkeratosis involving the soles of the feet, often in a "moccasin" distribution; (2) as a vesicular or vesiculopustular eruption involving the arch of the foot (this type of tinea pedis is usually of an acute nature and often in the spring and summer months may complicate the chronic scaling type of tinea pedis); and (3) as an interdigital infection characterized by itching and scaling between the toes (the third-fourth and fourth-fifth toe webs are usually involved). The interdigital type of tinea pedis tends to be more chronic than the vesicular type and may be characterized by acute flares. The vesicular variety of tinea pedis and more often the interdigital variety of tinea pedis may be complicated by a superimposed bacterial infection. Finally, concomitant onychomycosis of the toenails may occur with any of the aforementioned varieties of tinea pedis.

The dry, scaly diffuse type of tinea pedis is particularly difficult to cure, and relapse is frequent. A good topical agent such as miconazole nitrate 2 per cent (MicaTin) or clotrimazole 1 per cent (Lotrimin) applied twice daily may be helpful in early mild infections. However, chronic infections usually require oral griseofulvin 0.5 to 1 gram for 30 days, along with a good topical agent. Antifungal therapy is continued until a clinical and laboratory cure is achieved. Treatment may have to be continued for up to 3 months, and it may be necessary to use a keratolytic agent such as 10 per cent salicylic acid in petrolatum along with the topical antifungal agent in treatment of the hyperkeratotic type of tinea pedis. In tinea pedis complicated by involvement of the toenails, especially the great toenail, the reservoir of infection in the toenail must also be eradicated if one wants to achieve a cure; however, often this is impractical or impossible.

In treatment of the vesicular variety of tinea pedis which is not secondarily infected, griseofulvin, 0.5 to 1 gram daily for 30 days, along with a topical antifungal agent such as miconazole nitrate 2 per cent (MicaTin) or clotrimazole 1 per cent (Lotrimin), may be applied twice daily. Uncomplicated interdigital tinea pedis may be treated in a similar manner but is somewhat more recalcitrant to treatment than the acute vesicular type.

The vesicular and more commonly the interdigital variety of tinea pedis are often complicated by a superimposed bacterial infection. This should be treated with bed rest, elevation of the foot, and wet compresses with Burow's solution (1:10 to 1:20) for 15 to 30 minutes three to four times a day. A systemic antibiotic, such as erythromycin, 250 mg orally four times a day for 10 days, is usually necessary, especially if the tissue reaction is severe or a lymphangitis is present. If autoeczematization is present, systemic corticosteroids may be required. After resolution of the bacterial infection, appropriate antifungal therapy should be initiated with the topical antifungal agents and dosages of griseofulvin described above.

Tinea pedis is difficult to cure and control because of the moist, warm environment of the feet. Efforts to reduce moisture and maceration and to keep the feet cool and dry are helpful; these include drying the feet thoroughly after bathing and frequently airing them; avoiding nylon hose or other synthetic fabrics which interfere with the dissipation of moisture and wearing instead cotton absorbent socks; and avoiding tennis shoes and wearing sandals, perforated shoes, or alternating pairs of shoes to permit their drying. Good foot hygiene is important, and a powder such as tolnaftate (Tinactin) may be used liberally twice daily. Despite these measures, recurrences are common, and some infections persist no matter what therapy is used or what precautions are taken.

Tinea Manuum. The management of the patient with tinea manuum is essentially the same as that recommended for tinea pedis of the chronic scaling type, although environmental factors do not play as critical a role. The infection may remain unilateral for many years, a phenomenon yet unexplained. Tinea manuum is usually accompanied by tinea pedis, and both sites of infection should be treated at the same time. If required, topical treatment may be supplemented by griseofulvin microsize, 0.5 to 1 gram per day

for approximately 4 to 8 weeks. The dry, scaly, diffuse type of palmar infection is difficult to cure, and relapse is frequent.

Candidiasis

Cutaneous Candidiasis. Superficial fungus infections of the skin can also be caused by *Candida albicans*. Candidiasis is usually made worse by a hot, humid environment, and therefore infection is often limited to areas of increased perspiration and maceration. Frequent sites of involvement are the intertriginous areas such as the groin, gluteal cleft, inframammary areas, and axilla. Since candidiasis does not respond to griseofulvin, it is very important to distinguish between lesions caused by *Candida albicans* and those caused by dermatophytes.

Initial therapy of acute intertriginous candidiasis should be similar to that of an acute contact dermatitis. Moist compresses with cool tap water for 15 minutes two or three times a day are both soothing and drying. After these compresses, the area should be allowed to dry thoroughly and then a topical steroid followed by or used in combination with nystatin (Mycostatin) or amphotericin B (Fungizone). A shake lotion containing these ingredients may also be used. Newer agents, such as miconazole nitrate 2 per cent (MicaTin) or clotrimazole 1 per cent (Lotrimin), are also effective. With acute infection of the intertriginous areas, the cream is usually better tolerated than the lotion. Paraben-free preparations should be used, as this preservative can sensitize an already aggravated site. In this regard, preparations containing ethylenediamine should also be avoided because of their potential sensitizing properties. In less acute cases it is probably best not to use a medication containing a topical steroid but to rely only on the anticandidal agent. Use of harsh soaps and vigorous scrubbing are contraindicated. In axillary candidiasis the patient should be instructed to avoid the use of deodorants and other irritating substances. The patient should be instructed on the role of environmental factors and the necessity of keeping the involved areas cool, dry, and well aerated both during treatment and after clearing to prevent recurrence. In women with candidiasis of the anogenital area, it may be necessary to treat for the presence of vaginal candidiasis with nystatin vaginal tablets, miconazole nitrate 2 per cent (Monistat 7) vaginal cream, or clotrimazole (Gyne-Lotrimin) vaginal tablets or cream. In both men and women, it may be worthwhile to suppress the reservoir of candidiasis in the gastrointestinal tract with oral nystatin tablets.

Candidiasis in patients receiving long-term

broad-spectrum antibiotics, systemic corticosteroids, cytotoxic agents, or immunosuppressive drugs is often severe and resistant to therapy.

A persistent candidal infection may be evidence of reinfection rather than treatment failure, and a search for a possible source of reinfection such as a marital partner should be made. Finally, patients with chronic, recurrent, or refractory candidiasis should be thoroughly evaluated to rule out any predisposing factors such as endocrine abnormalities, underlying malignancies, or immunologic defects.

HERPES SIMPLEX

method of
PATRICK CONDRY, M.D.,
and WILLIAM WELTON, M.D
Morgantown, West Virginia

Herpesvirus hominis infections are worldwide in distribution, with humans as the only natural host. Recent years have witnessed an upsurge in interest in these infections because of the seriousness of neonatal herpes and evidence of increasing incidence of genital herpes, which predisposes to the neonatal disease. The proliferation of treatment modalities, folklore, and over-the-counter remedies attests to the absence of any well-defined and successful management for these infections.

The virus itself is a double-stranded DNA virus with an icosahedral capsid possessing an envelope with antigenic potential. It is known to exist in two varieties. Type 1 virus, classically described as the agent of the "cold sore" and generally held responsible for herpetic infections above the waist, was contrasted with type 2, described as the agent of genital and other herpetic infections below the waist. These distinctions may well be losing their significance, as will be noted later.

Clinical Disease

Gingivostomatitis and herpes labialis are the most common expressions of this infection. The severity of the primary illness ranges from asymptomatic conversion of immune status recognizable only by the development of specific herpes antibodies to the profound febrile illness that may characterize this disease in children. Most common in children of ages 1 to 5 years, it evolves after an incubation period of 3 to 10 days and is characterized by fever and sore throat, followed by painful erosions on the tongue, palate, pharynx, gingiva, buccal mucosae, and lips. It may be accompanied by drooling, fetid odor, and regional adenopathy. It usually resolves in 2 to 6 weeks.

After healing, the child is subject to *recurrent episodes of herpes labialis* on the vermilion border of the lip. This more limited collection of grouped vesicles rapidly crusts and tends to heal in about a week. Although frequency and severity of individual episodes are not possible to predict, the overall pattern of the disease is one of gradual diminishing in frequency and severity over 2 to 3 years. Attacks may be precipitated by febrile illness, sun, trauma, and stresses in general. Occasionally recurrent bouts of erythema multiforme may follow clinical herpes in each recurrence.

Primary genital herpes may be a severe illness analogous to that described for primary gingivostomatitis, with genital swelling, pain, fever, and regional adenopathy. This may be accompanied by satellite lesions on the buttocks or other regional sites. Originally these infections were thought to be due to type 2 virus exclusively, but recent evidence implicates an increasing number of genital infections with type 1 herpesvirus, particularly among young college students. Again this infection may be asymptomatic, signaled only by rising antibody titers. Primary genital herpes may be accompanied by an aseptic meningitis with herpes antibodies demonstrable on the surface of white cells recovered from the cerebrospinal fluid.

Recurrent bouts of genital herpes may be painful and sexually disabling, or the virus may be asymptomatically shed. Particularly in women, it may be accompanied by lumbosacral herpes and an associated neuralgia. The major medical concern, however, is the danger of neonatal herpes in the infant of a mother shedding the virus in either an asymptomatic or a symptomatic episode of the disease.

Herpetic whitlow may occur in medical, nursing, or dental personnel whose hands come into contact with human saliva in which the virus has been shown to be shed asymptomatically in a small proportion of the adult population. After an incubation period of 5 to 7 days, a cluster of painful vesicles appears, usually on one finger. This can be accompanied by fever, regional adenopathy, and even lymphangitis with or without culture evidence of a secondary bacterial infection.

Kaposi's varicelliform eruption (or *eczema herpeticum*) may be caused by herpesvirus hominis as well as vaccinia virus. The crucial predisposing factor is an underlying skin disease, most commonly atopic dermatitis. It may also be seen in widespread burns, Darier's disease, epidermolytic hyperkeratosis, and pemphigus foliaceus. The virus, widely disseminated in the abnormal skin in these conditions, produces a generalized eruption composed of large erosions formed from rapidly coalescing vesicles, which then become secondarily infected. These patients may be quite ill, requiring intravenous antibiotics and other supportive measures.

Neonatal herpes may be increasing in incidence, paralleling the increases in genital herpes. The infant becomes ill, usually 6 days after birth, but infection may start at birth or up to 3 weeks later. Vesicles on the scalp, particularly the vertex, may be the first clue to this disease. The infection does not always disseminate and may be limited to the skin, eyes, mouth, or central nervous system. The disseminated infection has a high mortality rate and deserves aggressive therapeutics.

Herpes keratitis may arise with or without other herpetic lesions visible. It characteristically produces a dendritic lesion on the cornea, which must be stained with contrast agents in order to be seen. Eye examination by a trained ophthalmologist is preferable when this condition is suspected.

Persistent herpetic ulcer is being seen more commonly in the face of immunosuppression for organ transplantation or aggressive cancer management. Grouped vesicular lesions may be seen initially, but they tend to coalesce into a growing ulcer unresponsive to topical therapeutic agents.

Natural History

Recurrent lesions tend to decrease in size and severity over time. Most people cease suffering recurrences 1 to 3 years after the initial episode. Episodes tend to be sporadic, occasionally following some stress (e.g., sun, febrile illness), but often without recognizable precipitating events. Controlled studies of therapeutics often show placebo groups doing as well as test groups and occasionally better. Uncontrolled observations are thus of little value.

Treatment

There are four general approaches to therapy. Drying agents, such as ether and Campho-Phenique, are popular because they relieve some symptoms. Some specific antiviral agents are available, such as idoxuridine or adenine arabinoside. Physical agents have been tried, such as freezing (cryotherapy) and combinations of dyes and light. Finally, immunologic manipulation has had some popularity. Some investigational methods will also be discussed.

Drying agents are popular because they provide some local anesthetic-type relief. Ether applied hourly during the first 24 hours has had some proponents. Unfortunately ether is quite explosive and presents considerable storage difficulties. Both 4 per cent thymol in chloroform and 2 per cent glutaraldehyde (investigational) buffered to pH 7.5 are suggested, but both can be irritating and the latter stains the skin and is unstable, requiring same-day formulation for effectiveness.

Antiviral agents have proved quite useful in the management of herpes keratitis. Both idoxuridine and adenine arabinoside are available in commercial preparations. Unfortunately, they have not been shown to be beneficial in controlled studies in the skin. Five per cent idoxuridine in dimethyl sulfoxide (DMSO) may shorten individual episodes but apparently does not affect recurrences (this preparation is not available in the United States).

Physical agents are difficult to evaluate in controlled studies, owing to their nature. A light freeze (1 to 5 seconds of skin frost) with liquid nitrogen or topical refrigerant commercially available has been thought by some observers to decrease the frequency of recurrences. Proflavin or neutral red dyes followed by exposure to visible light enjoyed some popularity. Recent controlled studies have shown them to be ineffective, and multicentric Bowen's disease has been reported in the patients treated with this last modality.

Immunologic therapeutic agents have also been tried. Levamisole (anthelmintic), because of its ability to stimulate cell-mediated immunity, was tried, but controlled studies were unsuccessful in showing benefit. Bacille Calmette-Guérin (BCG) has been tried but failed to show success in controlled trials. Smallpox vaccination (since it is a related virus) has been tried, but in spite of its considerable risk, failed to show benefit in controlled study. Poliomyelitis vaccine is being used by some, but it has not yet undergone a controlled trial.

There are a number of newer agents and ideas being tried currently. Specific herpes vaccines are undergoing research trials. The German vaccine Lupidon has recently come under fire for possible carcinogenic properties of the modified virus. A second vaccine is also being studied, which uses a modification of the viral envelope rather than a live virus. It appears more promising. Two per cent phosphonoacetic acid in cold cream appears promising but is neither available commercially nor approved by the Food and Drug Administration. L-Lysine has been recommended in doses of 340 mg four times daily. It inhibits viral replication in vitro, but large amounts of arginine (e.g., peanuts, chocolate) must be avoided. Finally, acycloguanisine is being tested by Burroughs Wellcome. It acts by inhibiting viral thymidine guanase. It may become available commercially; preliminary data suggest it is safer and more effective than currently available remedies.

Treatment of Specific Syndromes

Severe primary gingivostomatitis may require hospitalization for supportive measures, such as intravenous fluids, antibiotics for bacterial secondary infections, topical anesthetics such as viscous lidocaine (Xylocaine), and soothing bicarbonate mouth rinses. Any of the topical drying agents may be used for relief locally (bearing in mind that "-caine" derivatives frequently cause contact dermatitis).

Herpes genitalis may be quite painful, and secondary urinary retention may require catheterization or hospitalization, or both. Sitz baths in tepid water or Burow's solution may be quite soothing, and micturition during the bath may obviate catheterization. It is crucial to warn female partners or patients of the risks of neonatal herpes so that they will discuss it with their obstetricians when appropriate.

Herpes keratitis should generally be managed by an ophthalmologist so that slit lamp examination and mechanical debridement are available to the patient when appropriate. The specific decision to use steroids in addition to the topical antiviral agents already mentioned should be made by the ophthalmologist.

Neonatal herpes should be treated aggressively because of its high morbidity and mortality rates. Exchange transfusion with type 1 or 2 specific donors and adenine arabinoside in a dose of 10 to 20 mg per kg per day (investigational) should be added to the usual supportive measures. This drug is also indicated in herpes encephalitis in a dose of 15 mg per kg per day and in chronic herpetic ulcers in the immunosuppressed patient at a dose of 20 mg per kg per day. The use of adenine arabinoside for chronic herpetic ulcers in the immunosuppressed patients is not listed in the manufacturer's official directive.

Epidemiology and Prevention

Positive herpes antibodies to herpesvirus hominis range from 30 to 40 per cent in the upper socioeconomic groups to 90 per cent in lower socioeconomic groups. This disease is highly transmissible, with one study showing seven of eight contacts developing an infection. Asymptomatic shedding of the virus has been demonstrated periodically in the saliva of some adults, from the cervix of asymptomatic women, and in the prostatic secretions of some men regardless of the history of clinical disease.

Males with genital herpes should avoid sexual contact from the earliest prodrome until crusts have fallen and the lesions have become re-epithelialized. They should be encouraged to use adequate lubrication and condoms in any questionable circumstances. Females should be advised to avoid intercourse for 1 week after a recurrent episode and for 2 weeks following a primary one. Contraceptive foam may have some antiviral properties. To prevent neonatal herpes, women with a history of genital herpes should probably undergo cesarean section if a clinical episode occurs close to the due date. Some would even advocate culturing the cervices of all such women and doing cesarean sections even in asymptomatic women with viral shedding.

Enhanced public and professional awareness of the significance of herpes simplex would undoubtedly improve the incidence of neonatal herpes until such a time as safe and effective systemic and topical antiviral medications are available or an effective vaccine obviates the problem entirely.

HIDRADENITIS SUPPURATIVA

method of
JAMES D. MABERRY, M.D.
Fort Worth, Texas

Hidradenitis suppurativa is a chronic, recurrent, suppurative, and scarring disease of the apocrine glands involving primarily the axillary, anogenital, and mammary areas. The initial lesions are tender, erythematous nodules later developing undermining and sinus tracts. The onset is usually at puberty or beyond. They are most often confused with furuncles or sebaceous cysts. The pathogenesis involves (1) keratinous obstruction of the apocrine duct; (2) dilatation of the duct; (3) intense inflammatory changes with neutrophil chemotaxis; and (4) secondary bacterial infection, usually of staphylococci, streptococci, *E. coli*, Proteus, Pseudomonas, or a combination thereof.

The cause is unknown, but hormonal factors and a predisposition to obesity and personal or family tendency toward acne are thought to be contributory.

Prognosis and course involve rupture of lesions and healing with scarring and sinus tracts.

Complications include anemia, interstitial keratitis, and squamous cell carcinoma in late, extensive cases.

Treatment

1. Explain to the patient the nature of the disease, and that simple antibiotic therapy and incision and drainage are not curative.

2. Obtain bacteriologic culture and sensitivity from the lesions.

3. Have the patient cleanse the areas twice daily with germicidal soap such as povidone-iodine (Betadine) or chlorohexidine gluconate (Hibiclens).

4. Institute appropriate systemic antibiotics, usually tetracycline, erythromycin, or minocycline. This therapy may have to be continued over a long period of time.

5. Apply topical antibiotic-astringent solutions twice daily, such as clindamycin (150 mg capsule) or erythromycin (250 mg tablet) in Vehicle/N (Neutrogena) or C-Solve lotion (Syossett) by adding four capsules of either antibiotic to 60 ml of either vehicle to make the appropriate concentration.

6. Wet compresses such as Burow's solution may be used if suppuration is present.

7. Intralesional corticosteroids (triamcinolone, 10 mg per ml), 6.5 ml per lesion, may resolve early small lesions quickly.

8. A short course of oral systemic corticosteroids (prednisone) or intramuscular triamcinolone (Kenalog), 40 mg, or betamethasone (Celestone), 6 mg, will be initially effective in controlling early lesions. Taper in 3 to 4 weeks.

9. Sulfones have been employed successfully in some cases. However, a glucose-6-phosphatate dehydrogenase (G-6-PD) must be obtained initially, and a complete blood count (CBC) initially and monthly during the course of treatment. (See manufacturer's official directive before using.)

10. Zinc sulfate, 220 mg twice daily, has shown encouraging results in early studies. This has also been proposed for acne therapy.

11. Superficial x-ray therapy of 1000 R total dose in divided weekly doses of 200 R each may be helpful in early cases.

12. Tight, restrictive clothing should be avoided.

13. Weight reduction should be vigorously instigated.

14. Hormonal therapy is of no benefit.

15. The surgical approach: (a) For early or localized lesions, simple incision and drainage with local 1 per cent lidocaine (Xylocaine) anesthesia will give immediate relief. (b) For late or extensive lesions, the exteriorization technique of Mullins is most satisfactory. A malleable palpebral probe is inserted into the lesions. There is often an exit site, as the lesions are extensively undermined. With a number 15 scalpel blade, the length of the tract is incised. Then, with use of a sharp dermal curette, the thick gelatinous material is completely removed. Cauterization with bipolar current seals the lesion. The wounds are left open to heal by granulation. Small areas may be done with local anesthesia, but in extensive areas general anesthesia must be used. (c) In some severely scarred patients, total en bloc surgical excision and skin grafting have been employed.

KELOIDS

method of
SAMUEL J. STEGMAN, M.D.
San Francisco, California

Successful treatment of keloids is related to selection of proper treatment and long-term follow-up, with re-treatment, as necessary. The success can be predicted somewhat by differentiating a true keloid from a hypertrophic scar. Keloids tend to overgrow the boundaries of the original injury, most frequently develop on the upper back and chest, shoulders, jaw, and earlobes, and are more common in young patients with darker skin. Occasionally, a keloid will form after injuries to the skin (acne, trauma, or surgery) during a rapid growth phase, i.e., the teenage years. Hypertrophic scars can occur anywhere, on patients of all ages, and are usually secondary to wounds poorly or not approximated, or wounds closed under tension from gravity or poor surgical design. They can even form from normal muscle pull across a wound which was properly approximated, such as in the deltoid area. Some individuals have a hereditary predilection to hypertrophic scars. Hypertrophic scars respond well to treatment (see below) or time, whereas keloids always have a questionably poor prognosis. Older keloids are less responsive than younger ones.

Surgery and Corticosteroids

The mainstay of keloid therapy is a combination of surgery and intralesional corticosteroids. Whenever possible, the keloid should be excised and the defect closed with the least possible tension across the wound. Appropriate surgical techniques include simple elliptical excisions with wide undermining and careful approximation of the wound edges, proximal flaps, Z-plasty scar revisions, or "shelling out" of the fibrous keloid, with use of the resulting redundant skin for closure. Unfortunately, there is always the risk of a second keloid forming, and it may be even larger than the first.

Wide keloids can be shaved off with a scalpel or razor blade without primary closure. Shave excisions must be treated immediately, and for a prolonged period of time, with intralesional corticosteroids. Linear keloids, or spheroidal keloidal masses (earlobes) can be excised and the scar revised simultaneously to reduce tension across the defect, thereby discouraging new keloid formation.

For intralesional injections, use triamcinolone acetonide (Kenalog) in concentrations of 5 to 40 mg per ml every 1 to 3 weeks, for as long as necessary to obtain flattening of the keloid. The width and length of the keloidal scar will not be altered by intralesional injections alone. A 30 gauge needle in a Luer-Lok syringe and a Dermajet are both effective for penetrating the keloid. The needle should be passed back and forth through the scar tissue to fill the entire keloid with medicine.

When injecting the area where a keloid was excised, infiltrate the triamcinolone acetonide around the suture line. The first injection can be given immediately after the wound is closed, or 1 week postoperatively, or even — as some physicians prefer — a few days before surgical excision. Continue the injections throughout the healing phase, until the wound shows no sign of keloid redevelopment.

Some keloids are extremely firm and difficult to inject. If a Dermajet is not available or will not penetrate the keloid, use hyaluronidase (Wydase) to help the solution permeate the thick collagen bundles. Mix the hyaluronidase on a one-to-one volume basis with the triamcinolone acetonide for injection. If prolonged pain occurs after injection, mix lidocaine (Xylocaine) with the triamcinolone acetonide. If needed, a mixture of triamcinolone acetonide, hyaluronidase, and lidocaine can be made into a single "cocktail." The final concentration of the triamcinolone is the only critical element.

Some patients experience severe pain during and after injection. For these patients, a field block using lidocaine 1 per cent with epinephrine will prevent or alleviate this type of pain. As the keloids soften with repeated injections, pain lessens and the block is not necessary.

Start the injections with triamcinolone acetonide at lower concentrations (5 mg per ml) and increase the concentration until softening or atrophy of the keloid occurs. Some patients are extremely sensitive and develop atrophy around the keloid. If the lower concentrations do not produce a therapeutic response, gradually increase the concentration up to 40 mg per ml.

Try to inject into the keloid itself. Repeated injections beneath the skin or into the nearby normal skin rapidly lead to atrophy of the surrounding tissues, and accentuate the appearance of the keloid itself.

Unintentional injection or the diffusion of the steroid into the surrounding skin and subcutaneous fat makes long-acting triamcinolone hexacetonide (Aristospan) unacceptable for this type of injection.

Liquid nitrogen cryotherapy 1 to 3 days prior to intralesional injections will help penetration of the steroid, probably because of the interstitial edema from the freezing injury.

Cryotherapy

Although some physicians use this for keloids, it appears to have its best results on hypertrophic acne scars on the chest, shoulders, and back. Several moderate to hard freezes, 4 to 6 weeks apart, on these acne scars will flatten them, although the outline of the scar will remain, as will its abnormal color and texture.

Radiation Therapy

Radiation therapy should be combined with excision of a keloid, to reduce the incidence of recurrence. Using 1.7 ml of aluminum half-value layer, a one-time only dose of 500 to 1500 R or 3 alternate day doses of 300 to 500 R are adequate. The radiation should be started on the day, or day following, excision surgery. Appropriate shielding is necessary, and radiation therapy should not be used on keloids on the neck. The radiation dose is dependent on the anatomic site, as well as on the size of the keloid. Radiation should not be used by someone not experienced in its use for this type of problem. For some resistant keloids, radiation therapy, intralesional injections, and excision surgery can be combined.

Constant Pressure

A successful treatment for certain keloids is to apply constant pressure over them. Use firm wrapping with a woven elastic bandage, or surgically designed straps and corsets, or even plastic buttons sutured in place. These will reduce keloid size, and help prevent recurrence; however, only a newly formed, soft keloid located in an appropriate anatomic site will respond to this type of treatment. To be effective, pressure must be in place 12 to 18 hours per day for several months — even up to a year.

Methotrexate

For some especially severe keloids located in areas which may hamper movement or function, oral or intramuscular methotrexate can be given, 12.5 to 15 mg every 3 days, for 3 weeks out of each month. The therapy is started approximately 1 to 2 weeks before surgical excision of the entire keloid, and continued for as long as necessary afterward — usually up to 6 months. The use of an antimetabolite, with all its ensuing risks, is justified only if the keloid is severe enough to hamper function and if the keloid has been refractory to other forms of therapy. (This use of methotrexate is not listed in the manufacturer's official directive).

LICHEN PLANUS

method of
PAUL R. GROSS
Philadelphia, Pennsylvania

Lichen planus is a papulosquamous eruption of unknown etiology. In typical cases there are symmetrically distributed 2 to 5 mm flat-topped polygonal erythematous papules. They tend to occur on the flexor aspects of the wrists and ankles, the genitalia, and oral mucosa, but may be generalized. The Koebner phenomenon of lesions occurring at sites of trauma may be observed. Severe itching is common. The histologic picture is distinct and biopsy confirmation is usually feasible if the clinical picture is not typical. Nail dystrophy may occur, as may scarring alopecia in severe cases.

The disease tends to be self-limited, with an average duration of about 8 months. Relapse is not infrequent, and chronic cases can persist indefinitely. In these cases, the lesions tend to coalesce into thickened plaques, especially on the lower legs. Hyperpigmentation, especially in black patients, can cause a severe cosmetic problem. This may persist long after the acute eruption fades. Of particular importance is chronic erosive oral lichen planus, which can lead to malignant degeneration after many years.

Allergic drug reactions can produce an almost identical picture, and the history must be taken in detail to exclude this possibility. Drugs most likely to cause lichen planus–like reactions include gold, thiazide diuretics, antimalarials, and barbiturates. There are usually histologic differences which allow one to discern true lichen planus from the drug eruptions which mimic it.

Treatment

Acute Lichen Planus. 1. Review drug history and discontinue possible causal agents.

2. For symptomatic relief of itching, sedate with antihistamines or hydroxyzine. Warn the patient about drowsiness as a side effect.

3. Cool baths and showers are less likely to provoke itching than hot ones.

4. Topical steroid creams such as triamcinolone 0.1 per cent should be applied to affected areas two or three times a day.

5. In severe cases unresponsive to topical steroids, consider a short course of prednisone to be used in decreasing doses over about 3 to 6 weeks, depending on severity and response. Based on the patient's size, a reasonable dose might be 40 mg a day as a single morning dose for 1 week, then 20 mg per day for 1 week, then 10 mg per day for 1 week. Avoid long-term systemic steroid therapy in chronic cases, because of the possibility of side effects such as hypertension, cataracts, diabetes, or osteoporosis.

6. Oral lesions may respond to triamcinolone acetonide in emollient dental paste (Kenalog in Orabase) applied topically or to intralesional injections of triamcinolone acetonide, 10 mg per ml.

Chronic Lichen Planus. 1. Topical steroids as above, with the possibility of occlusive polyethylene film dressings at night to increase the penetration of the steroid into the lesions.

2. Intralesional injections of triamcinolone acetonide, 5 or 10 mg per ml, into hypertrophic plaques.

3. Tranquilizers or antihistamines for symptomatic relief of itching.

4. Consideration might be given to the use of grenz ray therapy, a superficial type of ionizing radiation. However, this does have a tendency to increase the pigmentation, which may already be a problem in this disease.

5. A Goeckerman program, such as that used in psoriasis, is sometimes effective. Employ topical coal tar applications (e.g., 5 per cent crude coal tar cream) with graduated increasing doses of ultraviolet light.

6. Periodically review the drug history to be sure that a possible allergic drug reaction is not being overlooked.

SUNBURN AND PHOTOSENSITIVITY

method of
GUINTER KAHN, M.D.
North Miami Beach, Florida

From the beaches to the tanning salons, the public sun-craze goes on unabated. The result is sunburn and its sequelae, premature aging skin and premalignant keratoses. The sunlight that causes sunburn is found within the ultraviolet range of 290 to 320 nm (UV-B). Shorter wavelengths do not reach the earth.

Longer wavelengths (UV-A) augment sunburn erythema and are responsible for the erythema of photosensitivity from drugs, porphyrias, and instances of solar urticaria. The physician should determine whether a reaction is acute sunburn or the result of increased susceptibility to light, induced by an endogenous or exogenous photosensitizer.

Each sunlight-induced condition has its own UV range of activation. Sunburn (SB), lupus erythematoses (LE), and inherited polymorphous light eruption (PMLE) are incited by UV-B (290 to 320 nm). Many other sun-induced diseases are evoked by wavelengths longer than 320 nm (UV-A).

Basic to treating sunburn and photoeruption is *avoidance.* Know that:

1. Sunburn-producing UV is found only in daylight between 9 A.M. and 4 P.M. and far less at temperate, northern latitudes, especially in the winter. Window glass screens out UV-B, but allows passage of longer UV-A; therefore, sunburn is not produced through window glass, but drug photosensitivity is elicited.

2. Loosely woven clothing gives minimal protection. Tee shirts and other tightly knit clothing, even when wet, offer excellent cover and sun protection, as do a broad-brimmed hat, gloves, and long hair (to the neck and ears).

3. Sunscreens and protective cosmetics are now quantified by their protective capabilities, i.e., protective factor (PF). A product with a PF of 10 protects about twice as well as a sunscreen with a PF of 5.

Patients should be advised as follows: (1) Look for PF values on the label of sun protective materials. Values of 15 are excellent, but those below 5 are poor. (2) Seek out products that are water resistant, i.e., that do not come off during sweating, washing, or swimming. (3) Blow dry the area to which sunscreens are applied. (4) Drug or disease-induced photosensitization usually requires broad-spectrum light protection, i.e., a UV-B plus UV-A sunscreen aided by a clothing or cosmetic cover. (5) Stay indoors or behind window glass between 9 A.M. and 4 P.M. on sunny summer days. (6) Individuals vary in their resistance to sunlight. In general, light-complexioned persons with blue eyes burn easily and need to adhere most strictly to avoidance principles; a dark complexion helps, but does not guarantee immunity from sunburn, especially not from photosensitivity eruptions. (7) Avoid tanning, except for specific indications under the surveillance of a physician (PUVA therapy for psoriasis, mycosis fungoides, unrelenting atopic dermatitis, and polymorphous light eruption). Light protection from suntanning is minimal. Tanning without burning is almost impossible (contrary to sunscreen advertisements). Artificial tanning is produced rapidly but does not involve melanogenesis, and offers little UV light protection. (8) No sunblocker is adequate. Caution the patient against total reliance on light "blockers," because areas to which they are improperly applied or rubbed off soon become vulnerable to the sun's effects. (9) Begin sun protection in infancy. UV damage is cumulative, and childhood sun exposure adds to the solar insults of later years.

For patients needing total protection (endogenous or exogenous, i.e., chemical photosensitization) I recommend that they apply sunscreen, dry it, and cover it with make-up or clothing.

Systemic Agents Used Against UV Damage

Aspirin relieves both pain and redness of photodermatoses by its ability to block prostaglandin synthesis. UV-B erythema is mediated by prostaglandins, but UV-A is not.

Aminoquinolines (hydroxychloroquine sulfate, chloroquine, and quinacrine) suppress the inflammation of LE, PMLE, and solar urticaria. Because hydroxychloroquine sulfate and chloroquine can cause irreversible retinal damage, I recommend quinacrine, 100 mg twice daily, tapering the dose as improvement occurs. (This use of quinacrine is not listed in the manufacturer's official directive.)

TABLE 1.

1. Topical artificial quick tanning agents (all contain dihydroxyacetone): Man Tan, Q.T. Quick Tanning Foam/Lotion, Tanfastic, Tan-o-Rama
2. Sunscreens with high protective factor (PF)* and water resistance for UV-B protection:
   PreSun 15 }
   Total Eclipse } PF greater than 15
3. Sun blocks for full spectrum protection (PF):
   Solar Cream (16)
   A-Fil (8)
   RVPaque (8)
4. Cosmetics (PF):
   Fresh cover (7)
   Reflecta (7)
5. Lip sunscreens (PF):
   Pan Ultra (9)
   RVPaba (9)

General considerations:
1. Sunscreens work best if applied 1 hour before sun exposure.
2. Sunscreens that seem oily can be "dried in" with a fan or hair dryer.
3. An economical formulation when huge amounts of sunscreen are needed would be PABA 6 per cent, glycerine 6 per cent, q.s. in rubbing alcohol_____ml.
Sig.: Apply 1 hour before sun exposure. N.B.: Increase glycerine if more moisture is needed; increase PABA if more sun protection is needed.

*New products are appearing regularly; patients should check the sunscreen label (see text).

Cortisone benefits the patient with acute sunburn or photosensitization. The sooner after exposure it is given, the more rapid is the response. The dose varies with the severity, from 20 to 60 mg of prednisone per day. If prolonged administration is anticipated (more than 10 days), a single daily dose after breakfast is preferred. For long-term therapy (more than 30 days), I prefer the alternate morning regimen, to minimize side effects. The complete check list for physicians treating patients with systemic corticosteroids for prolonged periods is found in Lowney, E. D.: Arch. Dermatol. *99*:588, 1969.

Psoralens are used to melanize and thicken the epidermis. The method of choice is PUVA therapy, and this is discussed on page 742. It is useful for PMLE and for some cases of solar urticaria (safety in children under 12 years of age is not established).

Beta-carotene reduces the symptoms of erythropoietic protoporphyria. It is of questionable value in solar urticaria, PMLE, and porphyria cutanea tarda (PCT). Phlebotomy remains the therapy of choice for treating PCT. Beta carotene is available as Solatene in 30 mg capsules. Giving 30 to 300 mg per day in divided doses after meals causes no serious side effects. It takes about 6 to 8 weeks to deposit enough beta-carotene in the skin to achieve protection. Blood levels of 600 micrograms per 100 ml are needed. Beta-carotene imparts an orange color to the skin, especially to the palms and soles. The patient must be warned that stools might become orange and sometimes loose.

Management

Sunburn. Severe: prednisone, 20 to 60 mg orally per day; aspirin, 600 mg (10 grains) every 3 to 4 hours as tolerated.

Apply strong corticosteroid creams generously: desoximetazone (Topicort), amcinonide (Cyclocort), fluocinonide (Lidex) or betamethasone (Benisone). Apply cool tapwater compresses four times daily for about 30 minutes.

For mild or healing (desquamating) wounds, apply skin moisturizer (Keri) or colloidal oatmeal, petrolatum, and lanolin (Aveeno Oilated) to the skin while it is moist (after bathing). For pruritus or sensitivity add 0.5 per cent phenol to the oil or use ZeaSORB powder to the dry skin to avoid the frictional irritation of clothing. Note that the use of -caine medications is without value for post-sun itch or burn.

Topical and Systemic Chemical or Drug Photosensitization. 1. Know and discontinue all photosensitizers (see Table 2).

2. Utilize topical and systemic steroids as indicated above.

TABLE 2.

Systemic photosensitizers:
  Antibiotics
    Tetracyclines: demeclocycline is most common
    Nalidixic acid
  Tranquilizers and antihistamines
    Phenothiazines: chlorpromazine is most common
  Antifungal
    Griseofulvin
  Sulfonamides
    Chemotherapeutic agents
    Diuretics (thiazides)
    Hypoglycemic agents (sulfonylureas)
      Tolbutamide
      Chlorpropamide
  Quinidine
Topical photosensitizers:
  Salicylanilides and hexachlorophene were in soap,
    cleansing agents, and deodorants but are no longer
    used in the United States of America for this purpose
  Coal tar derivatives
    Pitch, tar, crude petroleum products, and topical and
    systemic medications for eczema and psoriasis
  Psoralens
    Perfumes, flavoring agents, and as topical and
    systemic medications to promote tanning and treat
    psoriasis and vitiligo (PUVA therapy)
  6-Methylcoumarin
    Synthetic psoralen flavoring and fragrance no longer
    used in the United States of America
  Sunscreens
    PABA, digalloyl trioleate (rare)
  Dyes
    Neutral red, proflavine, toluidine blue
  Heavy metals
    Cadmium (yellow tattoos)

3. Avoid light exposure as much as possible.

4. Apply high PF sunscreens to the exposed areas, and then cover with clothing or sun-blocking cosmetics.

A few photoreactions become chronic and persistent. The cause and mechanisms are not known. Therapy remains the same except that alternate morning prednisone is used (lowest oral dose that relieves symptoms).

Discoid Lupus Erythematosus. 1. Avoid 9 A.M. to 4 P.M. sunlight in the summer, and 10 A.M. to 3 P.M. sunlight in the winter.

2. Apply high PF sunscreens 1 hour before sun exposure, and cover the lesions with sunblock cosmetics or Covermark or Erase.

3. Use topical and alternate morning steroids if the lesions are progressing.

4. If progression continues in spite of steroids, give quinacrine, 200 mg per day on alternate mornings. Increase or decrease the doses as improvement occurs. (This use of quinacrine is not listed in the manufacturer's official directive.)

5. If all measures fail to stop the progress of discoid lupus erythematosus, I give gold thioglucose intramuscularly as recommended for rheumatoid arthritis (see p. 841). (This use of gold thioglucose for discoid lupus erythematosus is not listed in the manufacturer's official directive.)

Systemic Lupus Erythematosus. In the presence of sun-induced lesions stay indoors as recommended for discoid lupus erythematosus and apply a high PF sunscreen followed by sunscreening facial cosmetics and protective clothing to exposed areas. Apply full strength topical steroids to erythematous areas as for acute sunburn.

Systemic corticosteroid and immunosuppressive therapy is predicated upon physical and laboratory findings (see pp. 692 to 695).

Polymorphous Light Eruption. As above, avoid 9 A.M. to 4 P.M. sunlight, especially in the spring and summer, and use topical sunscreens and steroids. When the skin manifestations are not suppressed by this therapy, use alternate morning prednisone, 20 to 60 mg. If symptoms do not subside, give 200 mg of quinacrine every other morning, i.e., on the morning when prednisone is not taken. This use of quinacrine is not listed in the manufacturer's official directive.) If relief is not forthcoming, PUVA therapy is indicated (see p. 742).

Porphyria. ERYTHROPOIETIC PROTOPORPHYRIA. See above.

PORPHYRIA CUTANEA TARDA (PCT). Avoid alcohol, estrogen birth control pills, and low carbohydrate diets.

Utilize phlebotomy, removing 500 ml of blood every 2 weeks until symptoms and signs remit, or urinary total porphyrins are less than 500 mg for 24 hours, or hematocrit becomes less than 36 ml per 100 ml.

If phlebotomy is contraindicated, beta-carotene (Solatene) therapy can be tried. If it is not successful, cautious administration of 125 mg of chloroquine may be given one time per week. It is necessary to monitor temperature, complete blood count (CBC), and liver function tests until it is determined that the patient can tolerate chloroquine therapy, at which time the dose may be increased to 125 mg twice per week. (This use of chloroquine is not listed in the manufacturer's official directive.)

Solar Urticaria. Determine if light going through window glass prevents the eruption. If so, avoid only 9 A.M. to 4 P.M. sunlight. If impossible, apply a high PF sunscreen 1 hour before sun exposure, and consider PUVA therapy.

In cases of photosensitivity and solar urticaria to light going through window glass, all light must be avoided and the patient must apply a high PF sunscreen followed by opaque sunscreens, covering the exposed areas, as discussed above.

Occasionally antihistamines or quinacrine is effective against solar urticaria. (This use of quinacrine is not listed in the manufacturer's official directive.) Use them intermittently, because sometimes the disease is self-limited and may no longer have to be treated.

Herpes Simplex. Because cold sores can be brought on by exposure to six minimal erythema doses of ultraviolet light, the vulnerable areas (muzzle of face) should be covered by a high PF sunscreen prior to prolonged solar exposure.

Other Diseases. The relationship of light to many diverse and inherited and uncommonly rare diseases is beyond the scope of this text. Nevertheless, the general principles of therapy for photocutaneous diseases are applicable to all of them.

LUPUS ERYTHEMATOSUS

method of
EDMUND L. DUBOIS, M.D.
Beverly Hills, California

Lupus erythematosus (LE) is a disease of unknown cause which is usually classified as discoid or systemic. Studies during the past 20 years have shown a close interrelationship between the two types. No specific forms of therapy are available. The physician can merely manage the disorder and hope that prolonged remission will occur. Approximately 10 per cent of patients with discoid lupus erythematosus and at least 40 per cent of those with the systemic form will have spontaneous remissions. The incidence of transformation is high. Ten per cent of patients with discoid lupus will have overt dissemination, whereas 70 per cent with the systemic disorder will have cutaneous changes varying from slight erythema to classic discoid lesions. The skin manifestations in systemic LE may occur at a time when the internal manifestations are quiescent. Therapy for either form of the disease depends entirely upon the clinical manifestations. Therefore it is essential that patients with apparent localized skin changes have a complete general medical examination and routine laboratory studies. Details of all aspects of the diagnosis and management may be found in the author's monograph, *Lupus Erythematosus, A Review of the Current*

Status of Discoid and Systemic Lupus Erythematosus and Their Variants, 2nd ed. (revised). Los Angeles, University of Southern California Press, 1976.

DISCOID LUPUS ERYTHEMATOSUS

General Measures

1. A complete medical examination is performed with routine blood count and urinalysis at the time of diagnosis and at approximately 6 month intervals thereafter. A VDRL, antinuclear antibody or LE cell test, and chest x-ray should be done at the initial evaluation.

2. The patient is informed of the extent of the disease and importance of long-term follow-up.

3. If photosensitivity is a factor, excessive sun exposure should be avoided as well as other forms of ultraviolet light.

4. Lesions may appear at the site of trauma produced by burns or local irritation. Picking, scratching, and excoriating the skin in involved or noninvolved areas should be avoided, because these may produce exacerbations of the lesions.

5. If the skin lesions are extensive, cosmetic agents, such as Lydia O'Leary Covermark are psychologically useful, in addition to the local therapy outlined. If scalp lesions are extensive, a hairpiece or wig may be necessary.

Local Therapy

1. Since ultraviolet exposure may exacerbate the majority of lesions, it is advisable that sunscreens be employed when the patient has extensive sun exposure. I prefer either a menthyl anthranilate titanium dioxide preparation (A-Fil), which blocks both burning and tanning, or para-aminobenzoic acid (PABA) in alcoholic solution, which also blocks burning and allows slight tanning, as Pre-Sun or Pabanol. Brief periods of 5 or 10 minutes even in midday sun usually will not induce exacerbations of the lesions, and no sunscreen is necessary.

2. The mainstay of therapy for the small active lesion, characterized by erythema and scaling, is the use of local corticosteroid creams, ointments, and solutions. Betamethasone dipropionate 0.05 per cent ointment or cream (Diprosone) appears to be one of the most effective local agents. Medication will not affect atrophic depigmented scars. Fluocinolone acetonide 0.025 per cent (Synalar) cream, flurandrenolone 0.05 per cent (Cordran) cream or ointment, and betamethasone valerate (Valisone 0.1 per cent) cream or ointment are helpful. In resistant cases a higher concentration, such as triamcinolone acetonide topical cream 0.5 per cent (Aristocort), can

be used. Medication should be applied at least four times daily.

Occlusion with a plastic film such as Saran Wrap markedly increases absorption. (It is important to instruct the patient when using occlusive dressings to rub in as much of the material as possible, and then leave a depot layer about 1/16 inch thick over the lesion to be covered.) Slight continuous pressure over the dressing ensures better absorption. On the extremities this is easily done with elastic bandages. A translucent plastic steroid-impregnated tape with flurandrenolide, 4 micrograms per square cm (Cordran Tape), is useful for small lesions. Occlusive dressings should be kept in place 12 to 20 hours daily.

Areas which respond poorly to local creams and ointments may be benefited by the use of fluocinolone acetonide solution 0.01 per cent (Synalar Solution), or betamethasone dipropionate lotion 0.05 per cent (Diprosone). For mucous membrane or lip involvement, triamcinolone acetonide 0.1 per cent (Kenalog in Orabase) in a special vehicle is useful. It should be applied after each meal.

3. Intralesional corticoids are occasionally helpful in refractory lesions. Two useful preparations are triamcinolone diacetate, 25 mg per ml suspension (Aristocort), or triamcinolone acetonide, 10 mg per ml (Kenalog-10). About 0.1 ml is injected with a No. 27 needle into a 1 cm lesion. Transitory or possibly permanent subcutaneous atrophy may appear at the injection site.

4. Freezing the lesions with solid carbon dioxide or liquid nitrogen may temporarily control the skin changes, but permanent scarring frequently results.

5. Surgical procedures are ineffective. Recurrences may appear at the site of the skin grafts.

Systemic Therapy

Antimalarials. These drugs provide dramatic improvement in skin manifestations and low-grade systemic complaints, such as arthralgia and fatigue. They should be used when skin lesions are extensive or cannot be controlled by other measures. Antimalarials have recently fallen into disfavor because of retinopathy which occurs with excessive amounts. Newer studies suggest that if a dose of 400 mg per day of hydroxychloroquine (Plaquenil) or 250 mg per day of chloroquine (Aralen) (this use of chloroquine is not stated in the manufacturer's official directive) for patients weighing over 100 lbs is not exceeded, retinopathy is rare despite long-term treatment. Hydroxychloroquine (Plaquenil) is probably less retinotoxic than chloroquine (Aralen). Quinacrine (Atabrine) (this use of quinacrine is not stated in the manufacturer's official directive) has not been reported to produce retinal damage, but induces a yellow discoloration of the skin and, rarely, aplastic anemia. Treatment may be begun with one 200 mg hydroxychloroquine tablet twice daily for patients weighing over 100 lbs. In younger patients the dose should be adjusted by weight. If improvement is inadequate within 6 weeks, quinacrine, 100 mg per day, may be added. When improvement occurs the dose is gradually reduced to the minimum necessary for adequate control. No attempt is made to fully reverse all the lesions. If the patient cannot tolerate hydroxychloroquine (Plaquenil), one can try chloroquine (Aralen), 250 mg daily (currently, only 500 mg Aralen tablets are available and can be given every other day), or amodiaquine (Camoquin) (this use of Camoquin is not stated in the manufacturer's official directive), 200 mg daily. Quinacrine hydrochloride (Atabrine) may be used in combination with the other antimalarials to obtain a greater therapeutic effect. Do not combine chloroquine (Aralen), hydroxychloroquine (Plaquenil), or amodiaquine (Camoquin), because these are retinotoxic and the effects may be additive. Side effects include nausea, vomiting, diarrhea, dermatitis medicamentosa, and cycloplegia. Pigmentary changes of the skin, hair, and hard palate are occasionally noted during the long-term therapy.

A baseline ophthalmologic evaluation should be performed prior to therapy with all antimalarials and repeated at 4 month intervals during the course of therapy. If quinacrine hydrochloride (Atabrine) alone is used, annual examinations are adequate. A reversible corneal infiltrate caused by local deposition of the antimalarial may be noted. If symptoms occur from this, they will respond promptly to withdrawal or dosage reduction of the antimalarial drug. Hemoglobin, white blood cell count, and differential should be performed every 1 to 2 months.

Other Measures. Small doses of oral corticosteroids such as 5 mg per day of prednisone are frequently effective in controlling the skin lesions. There is no evidence that cytotoxic agents will affect discoid LE.

SYSTEMIC LUPUS ERYTHEMATOSUS

No specific therapeutic agent exists; therefore the major premise is that treatment depends upon the clinical severity of the illness. Systemic lupus may be a very chronic disorder, with multiple remissions and exacerbations. During periods of total remission or of very minimal activity no treatment is indicated. If the main complaint is mild rheumatoid arthritis or a rheu-

matic fever–like picture, this often can be adequately controlled by modified bed rest and salicylates. Frequent use of salicylates should be encouraged, since they reduce the requirements for antimalarials and steroids. Other nonsteroidal anti-inflammatory agents may also be useful and can be administered with salicylates. An increased amount of bed rest, in addition to other treatment, is usually helpful in controlling symptoms in the active stages of disease. If salicylates and rest fail, or if extensive cutaneous lesions are present, antimalarial therapy should be instituted. Minor skin lesions can be well controlled by the application of local steroids. If salicylates and antimalarials fail to control the disease, or if the patient is critically ill or has neurologic or significant renal involvement, steroid therapy should be started.

General Measures

1. A complete medical evaluation is made with routine blood count, urinalysis, and further studies as indicated by examination to determine the extent of the disorder. A careful medication history should be obtained. Systemic lupus erythematosus (SLE) may be induced by procainamide (Pronestyl), hydralazine (Apresoline), methyldopa (Aldomet), chlorpromazine (Thorazine), and other drugs. (For a complete list, see the author's monograph.)

2. The following points are discussed with the patient: the limitations on activities, the importance of long-term follow-up, and avoidance of sudden cessation of medications.

3. During active phases of the disease, it is best to avoid extreme sun exposure. (See Discoid Lupus Erythematosus.)

4. During active phases of the disease, particularly with fever and lethargy, the patient should be at modified bed rest. During minor exacerbations of the disease, activities should be restricted and work reduced, if possible, to half-time or less, so that the patient can rest for a couple of hours in the afternoon and obtain 10 or 11 hours' sleep at night.

5. For minor skin lesions, local therapy may be used. (See Discoid Lupus Erythematosus.)

6. Pregnancy should be avoided during the active phases of the disease. There is a 5 per cent incidence of the disease in parents and siblings. Abortion is indicated in the presence of severe renal and cardiac disease.

Systemic Therapy

Salicylates. For patients whose major disease manifestations include fever, polyarthritis, pleurisy with effusion, and pericarditis, a therapeutic trial with salicylates is indicated. Adults are usually given buffered aspirin, 0.9 gram (15 grains) three times daily immediately before meals and at bedtime with food. If improvement is inadequate within 48 hours, this dose is gradually increased to a maximum of 24 0.3 gram (5 grains) aspirin tablets a day or their equivalent. If there is insufficient clinical improvement or severe salicylism, the patient is maintained with the maximal dose tolerated which yields the best relief. If large doses of steroids are eventually required, salicylates and antimalarials are not used except in tapering the dose during steroid-induced remissions.

Indomethacin and Nonsteroidal Anti-Inflammatory Drugs (NSAID). If arthritis and arthralgia are the main clinical problems, these may often be alleviated by addition of indomethacin (Indocin), beginning with 25 mg once daily before meals and slowly increasing the dose to a maximum of 200 mg daily. (This use of indomethacin is not listed in the manufacturer's official directive.)

If indomethacin and salicylates are not helpful, then the patient may be given a trial of full dose salicylates plus one of the other NSAID such as ibuprofen (Motrin), 800 mg four times a day (occasional instances of aseptic meningitis have been reported with the drug), naproxen (Naprosyn), 250 mg three times a day, fenoprofen calcium (Nalfon), 600 mg four times a day, tolmetin sodium (Tolectin), 400 mg three times a day, or sulindac (Clinoril), 200 mg twice daily. None of these newer NSAID are approved for this use in the manufacturers' official directives.

There is evidence that NSAID may occasionally cause temporary renal impairment or hepatitis. Laboratory tests for this type of involvement should be monitored occasionally.

If salicylates cause changes in liver function tests, these may revert toward normal with continuation of therapy.

Antimalarials. Antimalarials are used if the disease is mild but inadequately controlled by salicylates, indomethacin, or other NSAID, or if extensive cutaneous lesions are present. They are also helpful in decreasing photosensitivity. In addition, they appear to act synergistically with steroids and permit reduction in the steroid dose. For adults, I prefer hydroxychloroquine (Plaquenil), one 200 mg tablet before breakfast and supper. Use of other antimalarials, precautions, and side effects are listed under Discoid Lupus Erythematosus. Antimalarials are helpful in reducing lethargy, arthralgia, pleuritis, and pericarditis but have no effect on severe systemic complaints such as renal lesions or hematologic or central nervous system (CNS) changes.

Corticosteroids. Steroids are used in the treatment of SLE in two types of patients. The first is the patient with a mild form of the disease whose arthritis or other symptoms are inadequately controlled by more conservative therapy. A small dose, such as 2.5 to 5 mg per day of prednisone is added to the therapeutic regimen of salicylates, NSAID, and antimalarials. The second type is the severely ill patient, who is immediately given large doses such as 40 to 80 mg per day of prednisone or its equivalent. Salicylates and antimalarial drugs are not initially employed in treating patients in this group. Indications for immediate institution of steroid therapy include thrombocytopenia, severe hemolytic anemia, significant nephropathy, central nervous system involvement, and marked toxicity from the disease. In critically ill patients, it may be necessary to increase the dose to as high as 800 mg daily of prednisone or its equivalent. I prefer to treat such patients who may be absorbing steroids poorly with parenteral hydrocortisone sodium succinate (Solu-Cortef), 250 mg twice daily. As much as 3000 mg per day may be required during critical situations, particularly in patients with central nervous system involvement. Methylprednisolone sodium succinate (Solu-Medrol), 50 mg intramuscularly or intravenously every 12 hours, is very useful in critical situations because it retains less sodium and causes less hypokalemia than hydrocortisone. There is no evidence that intravenous pulse dose Medrol (1 gram daily) is of significant benefit for the management of SLE compared with graduated dose treatment depending on the clinical urgency of the situation. As soon as clinical improvement appears, the dosages are reduced. It must be emphasized that the amount of corticosteroid varies with the severity of the disease. The endpoint usually employed in the critically ill patient is a sufficient dose to induce the typical "moon face." Remissions frequently appear in seriously ill patients when cushingoid side effects appear. Reduction of steroids should be done slowly by 10 to 20 per cent decrements every few days in those receiving extremely high doses, and by longer periods and smaller decrements in patients receiving lower doses. Mild rebound of fever and arthralgia may occur upon dose reduction. This usually disappears within a few days unless the dose reduction has been excessive. Peptic ulcer is the most common complication of long-term steroid therapy, and all patients receiving more than 10 mg daily of prednisone should at least have antacid therapy with a liquid aluminum hydroxide–magnesium trisilicate or aluminum hydroxide gel antacid such as Gelusil or Amphojel, 15 ml 1 hour after meals, between meals with food, and at bedtime. Alternate day steroid treatment reduces side effects but is primarily useful for management of lupus nephropathy and hematologic complications. The dosage of steroids should suppress major manifestations; no attempt should be made to give sufficient steroid to suppress all minor complaints. A good temperature response and low normal hemoglobin are the major guides to therapy. If nephropathy is present, there should be an adequate return of function and significant decrease in proteinuria. *This improvement may not be observed until steroid therapy is tapered following a 3 month course of 50 to 80 mg of prednisone per day for adults.* No attempt is made to reverse the elevated sedimentation rate, presence of LE cells, or antinuclear antibodies or to reduce anti-DNA binding levels. These may persist indefinitely in excellent remissions. Serum complement is depressed in active phases of SLE, and its return to normal may be a useful but not absolute guide for therapy.

Details of Management of Life-Threatening Complications of SLE Using Prednisone

Nonsteroidal anti-inflammatory agents are not used in critically ill patients because their effects are mild compared with those of steroids. Prednisone is given to febrile patients before meals in divided doses twice daily; it is given once daily to others except for those with hematologic and renal complications, for whom every other day treatment is satisfactory. The suggested doses are for adults. Children may require almost as much.

Hemolytic Anemia. Sixty to 80 mg of prednisone per day. If no improvement in clinical and laboratory features within several days to 1 week, increase the dose to 100 to 120 mg daily.

Thrombocytopenic Purpura. Eighty mg per day. Platelets may not rise for 6 or more weeks. The dose of prednisone can be increased to 125 mg daily.

Severe Polyserositis and Impending Cardiac Tamponade. Forty to 60 mg per day. Response begins within 1 or more days.

Acute Vasculitis. Forty to 100 mg per day. Response appears in a few days except for gangrene of the extremities when improvement occurs following several weeks. Once the process stabilizes, it is essential to reduce the dose of steroids in order to permit continued healing of the vascular lesion.

Acute Central Nervous System Damage. The possibility of steroid-induced psychosis must be ruled out in all such patients. If there is doubt about the etiology of the psychosis in patients receiving low dose corticoids, the simplest approach is to completely stop the steroids under hospital observation for 48 to 72 hours. In cases of steroid psychosis, dramatic subjective improvement will occur. If there is truly organic central nervous system involvement, small doses, such as 30 to 40 mg daily of prednisone, may be satisfactory for confusional states. If there is evidence of severe peripheral neuritis, transverse myelitis, mononeuritis multiplex, or other severe complications, 50 to 100 mg of prednisone should be given every 12 hours. If there is no response in 24 to 48 hours or if the patient is critically ill, change to a more physiologic glucocorticoid, such as hydrocortisone sodium succinate (Solu-Cortef), 250 to 500 mg intramuscularly or intravenously every 12 hours. Double the dose every 24 to 48 hours to 3000 mg daily, then maintain it at that level for several weeks until the patient is cushingoid. Another useful steroid with less mineralocorticoid alteration is methylprednisolone sodium succinate (Solu-Medrol), 50 mg intramuscularly or intravenously every 12 hours.

Renal Damage. Kidney biopsies are not routinely required for the management of lupus nephropathy. Routine biopsies in patients with normal renal function invariably show evidence of significant degrees of damage. The prognosis of steroid treatment does not necessarily correlate with biopsy appearance. The major indication for biopsy is to determine late in the course of the disease, with a creatinine level of 4 or more, whether additional therapy is warranted.

Treatment of nephropathy is begun with 50 to 60 mg daily of prednisone or 100 to 120 mg every other day. Improvement usually requires 8 to 12 weeks. During the initiation of steroid therapy, renal function may deteriorate temporarily and improvement may occur as the dose of steroids is tapered.

Steroid Withdrawal. A great deal of experience is needed to determine the amount and rapidity of reduction. In general, the more rapid the exacerbation and the faster the clinical improvement, the quicker the dose of steroid may be tapered. There is no evidence that the use of corticotropin aids decreasing steroid dosage. In those receiving large doses (50 mg or more of prednisone daily) for several weeks, 10 per cent of the dosage may be reduced at intervals as short as 4 days, whereas if the patient has been taking this dose for months (i.e., for renal disease), a 10 per cent reduction at intervals of a few weeks is recommended. This allows time for monitoring renal function as the medication is withdrawn. Patients whose illness is relatively stable and who are receiving small doses of steroids (10 to 20 mg daily of prednisone) should have reductions of about 10 per cent every 10 days. Some may note symptoms when reducing the dose of prednisone as little as 0.5 mg daily when they are receiving a total of 5 mg daily. The use of 1 mg tablets aids in the careful titration.

The majority of patients receiving 20 mg daily of prednisone or less will be benefited by the addition of antimalarial therapy, salicylate, and NSAID, which will help reduce their steroid requirement.

Attempts should be made to gradually and completely withdraw all steroid therapy if possible. The incidence of coronary atherosclerosis is greatly increased with maintenance doses of 10 mg per day.

Whenever possible, alternate day steroid therapy should be attempted. However, for patients who have active disease with arthralgia, vasculitis, or fever, small doses of steroids are required on the off day.

Immunosuppressives. If the renal lesion persists and progresses after tapering steroids following 3 months of 50 to 60 mg daily of prednisone, intravenous nitrogen mustard (Mustargen) should be used. (This use of nitrogen mustard is not stated in the manufacturer's official directive.) A baseline bone marrow test should be done. If this is normal, then adults can be given 15 to 20 mg intravenously at one time. The dose should not exceed the standard course of 0.4 mg per kg. This medication may be repeated in a minimum of 8 weeks if improvement is inadequate. Other immunosuppressives and cytotoxic agents are under investigation, but so far the benefits obtained from these agents are dubious. Azathioprine (Imuran) is of no proved value in management of SLE. Cyclophosphamide (Cytoxan) in doses of 50 to 100 mg per day for adults may be helpful in reducing steroid requirements for patients with acute vasculitic gangrene. A baseline bone marrow should be obtained. (This use of cyclophosphamide is not listed in the manufacturer's official directive.)

Use of Other Agents. Antibiotics, including sulfonamide derivatives, are used in the presence of any significant infection in patients with SLE. These should not be employed prophylactically or for treatment of minor viral infections, even in steroid-maintained patients. In the presence of an overwhelming progressive infection, gamma globulin in doses of 30 ml on one or more occasions may be helpful. Routine vaccination and immunizations such as smallpox, tetanus, typhoid, or poliomyelitis (Salk vaccine or Sabin live virus) can safely be performed, even when the patient is taking corticosteroids, provided that the disease appears stable.

DISORDERS OF THE MOUTH (BENIGN)

method of
C. THOMAS YARINGTON, JR.,
M.D.
Seattle, Washington

Benign disorders of the oral cavity include a variety of primary and secondary disease processes, the treatment of which will be described in some detail. Much of the material which follows has been adapted from previous articles on this subject by Manuel G. Bloom of Houston, Texas, as well as several current works by the present author.

Benign disorders of the oral mucosa include not only the oral manifestations of systemic and cutaneous diseases but also a host of processes related to the physiologic, histologic, anatomic, and mechanical conditions peculiar to the mouth. Consequently, correct diagnosis of oral problems, which must precede definitive therapy, also requires careful examination of the skin and, occasionally, a general medical evaluation.

In diagnosing oral disease it must be remembered that mucosal lesions are rapidly altered by chewing, nibbling, rubbing with the tongue, and irritation from malfitting dentures or carious teeth, as well as by the persistent use of tobacco, snuff, betel nut, and hard candies. Vesicles, bullae, and pustules rupture rapidly to leave erosions and ulcers. Poor dental hygiene permits rapid overgrowth of organisms and results in secondary infections.

Maximal therapy of oral disease frequently requires close cooperation between physician and dentist. The presence of plaque, calculus, periodontitis, caries, ill-fitting dental appliances, and malocclusion must be treated by a qualified dentist. Maintenance of good oral hygiene is the first step in treatment of oral disease. The patient should be instructed in the proper use of the toothbrush, unwaxed dental floss, interdental stimulation (rubber tip on a toothbrush or Stimudents), and perhaps use of an irrigation instrument such as the Water-Pic.

Lips

Fordyce's Disease. These very common (80 per cent of the population), asymptomatic, tiny, symmetrically grouped, yellowish tumors, lying flush with the surface, are due to hypertrophy of anomalous sebaceous glands of the mucous membrane. The lips as well as buccal mucosa and retromolar areas may be involved. No treatment is indicated except to assure the patient that the process is neither malignant nor premalignant.

Lip Pits. Congenital lip pits are bilateral, symmetrically located depressions occurring on the vermilion surface of the lower lip, one on each side of the midline. On occasion, the pits may be unilateral or present a nipple-like elevation. These blind sinuses represent persistence of developmental sulci. Occurrence is about 1 in 200,000 individuals.

The commissural lip pit, occurring at the angle of the mouth, is a relatively common developmental defect and is found in 12 per cent of whites and 20 per cent of blacks. Twenty-five per cent of the cases are bilateral. Lip pits are usually asymptomatic and require no treatment. Large or constantly draining lesions may be carefully excised for cosmetic reasons.

Cleft Lip and Cleft Palate. These occur with decreasing frequency owing to current parenthood planning measures. The cleft may be median, lateral, oblique, or bilateral and may vary from small depressions to extensive, deforming, and mutilating processes that involve the nostrils and the hard and soft palate. On rare occasions, the lower lip, tongue, and mandible may be involved. Associated anomalies of other organ systems are not uncommon. Surgical correction of cleft lip is started at 4 to 8 weeks of age. Palatal repair is usually deferred to avoid damage to growth centers and tooth buds. Specially designed nipples and palatal obturators are important for adequate nutrition, prevention of nasal or pulmonary infection, and overcoming speech problems. Extensive anomalies, especially with palatal or mandibular involvement, require long-term management by specialized teams of pediatricians, plastic surgeons, dentists, and speech therapists. If possible, infants with extensive clefts should be referred very early to a center specializing in long-term management of this defect.

Vascular Tumors. Capillary hemangiomas of infancy may involve the lips as well as other oral structures. Characteristically, most of the lesions involute spontaneously in several years and do not require treatment. However, the resolution may be slow and not completed until puberty. Cavernous hemangiomas are usually not apparent at birth but develop during childhood and may either reach a static size or show progressive enlargement. Mixed lesions occasionally occur. Management requires careful evaluation and frequent re-examination. Rapid growth, especially when vital functions are compromised, requires surgical intervention. Treatment is primarily surgical.

Mucoceles. Mucoceles arise from mucous extravasation into the adjacent tissue, usually with a pseudoenclosure of granulation tissue. Less commonly, they represent a true mucous retention cyst with surrounding epithelial sac, owing to obstruction of the excretory duct. They occur most often on the lower lip and occlusal line of the cheek. Some lesions drain spontaneously and involute. Persistent lesions are carefully deroofed under local anesthesia. The underlying granulation tissue or enlarged glandular tissue or both are carefully teased and squeezed out through the opening. The base is not desiccated. Postdesiccation granulation tissue may promote recurrence. Absorbable gelatin (Gelfoam) is used to control bleeding. Patients should be reassured that the lesions are not malignant or premalignant.

Trauma. Traumatic lesions of the lip are very common in contact sports and accidents. Lip lesions require careful debridement of devitalized tissue and accurate apposition of the vermilion border to preserve the lip line and prevent unnecessary scar formation. Nodules on the mucosal surface and even nodules deep in the lip tissues are a constant source of irritation. Radiographic examination is indicated when the wound is contaminated or associated with fractured teeth. Face bars on helmets and mouth guards reduce the incidence of injury to the lips and teeth in contact sports.

Mild thermal, electrical, and chemical burns of the lips respond to cool boric acid solution, compressing, and simple emollients such as 1 per cent hydrocortisone ointment (1 per cent Hytone; 1 per cent Cort-Dome, and others). Thermal burns of the lips, tongue, and especially the palate from hot foods are usually minor and heal uneventfully in about a week. One of the local anesthetic preparations, lidocaine (Xylocaine Viscous, and others), will relieve the pain and promote healing. Dry ice burns (seen in children who place dry ice in their mouths) can produce a severe slough. Deep and extensive burns require symptomatic and supportive therapy until definitive reconstructive surgery can be carried out. The dry and desquamating lips of severely ill patients should be kept greased with petrolatum or lanolin.

Acute sunburn of the lips is treated by frequent compressing with ice cold Burow's solution, containing one fourth teaspoonful of bath oil (Alpha Keri Bath Oil, Lubath) per pint, followed by application of 1 per cent hydrocortisone ointment. Further occurrences may be prevented by use of sunscreening lip pomades (Sun Stick

Lip Protectant; PreSun Sunscreen Lip Protection; RVPaba Lipstick). Windburn and cold chapping of the lips respond to the same routine.

Sucking-Licking Cheilitis. Some children and an occasional adult have the habit of constantly licking or sucking the lips and adjoining skin. Chapping (dryness and scaling) of the areas is soon followed by fissuring and secondary infection. Thumbsucking, with associated drooling, may produce a similar picture. After secondary infection is brought under control by an antibiotic ointment, the use of a silicone preparation (Silicote ointment) protects the skin from further maceration. Nighttime lipsucking may be partially alleviated by the wearing of mouth guards when sleeping. However, liplicking or sucking is a "tension" habit and is very difficult to cure. Psychotherapy for the parent is probably more important than treatment of the child.

Fissures. Lip fissures are chronic tears of the mucous membrane caused by dryness following sunburn, windburn, freezing, contact dermatitis, and so on. Secondary infection may modify the picture. The fissures are treated with a warm saline compress and an antibiotic ointment. If the lesion does not heal, press the margins of the fissure together and fix them in place with a wisp of cotton coated with flexible collodion. This is a tricky procedure and may require several attempts to carry out successfully. The fissure usually heals in several days. On rare occasions it is necessary to approximate the edges with 8-0 silk suture.

Biting and Chewing. Severe destruction of the lips and cheeks may result from involuntary biting and chewing in brain-damaged patients. If the brain damage is permanent, extraction of the teeth may be necessary to control the problem.

Loss of Vertical Dimension Dermatitis. Marked loss of vertical dimension and shortening of the face is found in all edentulous persons. Severe attrition of the teeth produces a similar but less severe condition. The lips overlap at the commissures to form intertriginous areas. Constant moisture leads to maceration, splitting, and secondary infection, producing the picture of perlèche. In edentulous patients, the wearing of properly constructed dentures will correct the loss of vertical dimension. Severe attrition is corrected by capping the teeth, or extraction and full dentures. Local treatment is the same as for angular cheilitis.

Actinic Cheilitis and Keratoses. These are potentially malignant. Sudden growth of a keratosis and prickly sensation when scratching the lesion or induration of the base, or both, suggest malignant transformation. Large lesions should be surgically removed for biopsy evaluation. Local application of 5-fluorouracil solution (Efudex, Fluoroplex) for 2 to 4 weeks is effective in many early lesions and does not leave scars but is exceedingly painful. The concomitant use of a corticosteroid ointment may decrease the discomfort without interfering with the action of fluorouracil. Note that after inadequate fluorouracil therapy, extensive squamous cell carcinoma may develop unnoticed beneath normal appearing skin. Cryosurgery and electrosurgical destruction are effective but likely to leave undesirable scars. Severe chronic lesions are best treated by a lip shave. All persons with active cheilitis should avoid unnecessary sun exposure and should carefully protect the lips with a sunscreen pomade.

Allergic Reactions. Allergic contact cheilitis and stomatitis are due to an exogenous allergen reaching the lips or mucosa by direct contact. Virtually any substance can produce the reaction in a susceptible person. Definitive treatment requires the identification and elimination of the allergen. This is not always possible. Whenever a contact allergy is suspected, eliminate lipstick, sunscreening pomades, local applications and medications, mouthwashes, toothpastes, chewing gums, hard candies, cough drops, spicy foods, acid foods, and sucking on citrus fruit, pencils, or vegetation. Contact dermatitis from reed mouthpieces of musical instruments has been described. Consider also substances used by the dentist before onset of the problem, such as antiseptics, antibiotics, phenolic derivatives, volatile oils, and cold sterilizing solutions used on instruments and denture materials. Allergic reactions develop occasionally to prosthetic materials and denture adhesives, as well as to nickel, cobalt, and chrome used in dental appliances. Local therapy is symptomatic. Inflammation is relieved by the frequent use of cool Burow's solution compresses for the lips and cool saline mouth rinses for the oral cavity, followed by a corticosteroid ointment (0.5 per cent) (Lidex, Kenalog, Aristocort) for the lips and Kenalog in a protective oral paste (Orabase) for mucosal surfaces. Note that Orabase is applied by gently pressing against the mucosa with a fingertip; it should not be rubbed in. Shreds of mucosal tissue are best removed by occasional rinsing with a sodium bicarbonate solution made by adding 1 teaspoonful of sodium bicarbonate to 250 ml (glass) of warm water. Systemic antihistamines and even systemic corticosteroids are indicated for severe cases. Compromise of the airway is very rare.

Allergic cheilitis and stomatitis are due to blood-borne allergens. The response may be cicatricial, eczematous, or combined. Urticaria of the lips and oral cavity is usually associated with a generalized reaction. Cold compressing and cold mouth rinses help in reducing the edema and inflammation. The general term urticaria includes idiopathic, hereditary, and allergic forms of angioedema. All these varieties may involve the oral tissues, esophagus, and trachea. If the airway is compromised or the patient presents other life-threatening symptoms, immediate injection of epinephrine (0.3 to 0.5 ml of 1:1000 solution) and, occasionally, a quick-acting corticosteroid, dexamethasone sodium phosphate (Decadron phosphate, 4 to 16 mg), are indicated. Severe laryngeal edema may require tracheostomy. Eczematous allergic cheilitis and stomatitis are rather rare allergic reactions caused by blood-borne allergens that present clinical manifestations almost identical with the contact variety. Every substance listed as a possible cause of acute urticaria may also produce an eczematous allergic reaction. Differentiation is made on the basis of history, negative patch test findings, exposure to the suspected allergen, or all three. Treatment requires search for and elimination of the causative factors if possible. Local treatment is identical with that used for the contact variety.

Macrocheilia. Many of the factors producing macroglossia may also cause enlargement of the lips. The most common causes of acute enlargement of the lips include trauma, angioedema, and infectious processes. Recurring lip swelling may be part of the Melkersson-Rosenthal syndrome (including a fissured tongue and recurrent facial palsy) or may be due to recurrent angioedema. Chronic macrocheilia is usually due to developmental defects, tumors, sarcoidosis, infectious processes, or interference with lymph drainage. In all these conditions, treatment is directed to the underlying cause.

Cheilitis Glandularis Apostematosa. This is a chronic idiopathic hypertrophy of groups of the vermilion border mucous glands and their ducts. Occasionally, mucous glands of the oral cavity, pharynx, and nose may be involved. Mild cases are relatively common. Everting and stretching the lower lip reveals erythematous duct openings, up to several millimeters in diameter, scattered irregularly over the vermilion and adjacent mucosal surfaces. In severe cases, the hypertrophied glands evert the enlarged lip. The patient must be assured that the condition is not malignant. Intralesional injections (0.2 to 0.3 ml) of a dilute triamcinolone solution (5 mg per ml) may be of some benefit. Surgical excision is reserved for very severe cases.

Angular Cheilitis (Perlèche). This is primarily an intertrigo and fissuring caused by maceration of the corners of the mouth, frequently complicated by chronic infection with *Candida albicans* or other organisms or both. Underlying factors include loss of vertical dimension, flaccid sagging cheeks, chronic riboflavin deficiency, Sjögren's syndrome, hypochromic anemia, and oral candidiasis. Primary treatment is directed to the underlying factors. Frequent applications of a nystatin, neomycin, gramicidin, triamcinolone (Mycolog) ointment are usually helpful.

Tongue

Glossodynia (painful tongue) or glossopyrosis (burning tongue) is usually a complaint of older adults, especially postmenopausal women. As with other subjective complaints, a variety of local and systemic factors must be evaluated. Obvious painful abnormalities such as allergic glossitis, vesiculobullous processes, and pyodermas are relatively easy to diagnose. Glossodynia may accompany macroglossia, xerostomia, and perversions of taste. Before making a diagnosis of idiopathic glossodynia, a thorough search must be made for underlying pathology. Dental problems to be considered include poor oral hygiene, periodontal disease, and referred pain from an occult dental abscess. Occasionally, an undiagnosed disease such as mild Candida glossitis (postantibiotic therapy), pernicious anemia, subclinical pellagra, diabetes mellitus, hypovitaminosis B, iron deficiency, or gastric reflux can be identified. Rare factors to be considered are trigeminal neuralgia, zinc deficiency, vascular disturbances in the central nervous system, and temporomandibular joint disease. It is reported that glossodynia has followed trigeminal nerve injury resulting from mandibular block injections. When there is definite evidence of nerve entrapment or neuroma formation, surgical intervention may be of value.

Unfortunately, no cause is discovered in most patients. The tongue appears normal except, perhaps, for the presence of mild asymptomatic conditions such as furring, migrating glossitis, or congenital fissures. Management is very difficult. Estrogens, vitamins (including vitamin B_{12}), and various other therapeutic agents are of little or no value. The patient's complaint must not be taken lightly. Assurance and reassurance that the problem is neither serious nor malignant, perhaps combined with judicious use of mild tranquilizers, are important. Good dental hygiene and adequate nutrition should be maintained. If the patient remains unduly disturbed or incapacitated or both, psychiatric consultation is indicated.

Coated tongue is due to more or less retention of normal desquamation of the filiform papillae. Mild coating is normal. The amount varies from day to day and from morning to night in the same person. Increased coating is associated with respiratory disease, fever, and smoking. It may be part of the "morning-after" syndrome. Gentle brushing with a soft-bristled toothbrush followed by thorough rinsing is usually effective therapy.

Smooth tongue is due to atrophy or absence of the filiform papillae. The finding is frequently associated with nutritional deficiencies such as iron deficiency anemia, Plummer-Vinson syndrome, malabsorption states (celiac disease, tropical sprue), pellagra, pernicious anemia, and nutritional macrocytic anemia. Treatment of the underlying process is indicated.

Fissured tongue (scrotal tongue) is a congenital anomaly that appears in 4 to 5 per cent of the population. Usually, the process occurs as an isolated defect. Fissured tongue is also part of the symptom complex of mongolism, Sjögren's syndrome, and Melkersson-Rosenthal syndrome. No treatment is necessary. However, the fissures should be pulled open and the bases carefully palpated. Small, asymptomatic carcinomas have been discovered in deep folds on rare occasions.

Geographic tongue is a benign, superficial, asymptomatic, migrating glossitis of unknown cause, occurring in about 2 per cent of the population. The tongue lesions of Reiter's syndrome are clinically and histologically identical. The patient is assured that the process is benign and self-limited. Gently cleansing the tongue with a soft toothbrush may be of value. Long-term corticosteroid therapy occasionally clears the process, but such potentially dangerous treatment is inadvisable for this minor condition.

Moeller's glossitis (glazed or slick tongue) is a very rare, chronic symptom complex, characterized by appearance of one or more discrete, glazed, beefy-red, painful lesions on the tongue. Causative factors include all the conditions listed under glossalgia plus nonulcerative galvanism if such a condition really exists. In most cases no cause can be identified, and no definitive treatment is available. Estrogens, androgens, corticosteroids, vitamins, trace elements, hydrochloric acid, and thyroid, individually and in combinations, have been tried with varying degrees of unsatisfactory response. Pain is controlled by the use of mild mouth rinses and anesthetic preparations.

Hairy tongue is usually black in color, but cases of yellow, dirty-gray, brown, blue, and even green have been reported. The cause for elongation of the filiform papillae is unknown. There is some evidence that activity of chromogenic bacteria or fungi produce the elongation and coloration. Suppression of competing organisms by long-term antibiotic therapy may be a predisposing factor. After local anesthesia with viscous lidocaine (Xylocaine Viscous), the elongated papillae can be carefully snipped away with sharp scissors. The area is then painted with 5 per cent trichloroacetic acid. Several such treatments usually clear the process. The patient is advised to brush the tongue gently when he brushes his teeth. The application of 40 per cent urea followed by vigorous brushing is also effective. A thin application of 25 per cent podophyllin in tincture of benzoin clears the process but is rather painful.

Median rhomboid glossitis is usually accepted as a developmental defect resulting from persistence of the tuberculum impar on the surface of the tongue. The process rarely appears before the age of 30. Median rhomboid glossitis is benign. Although squamous cell carcinoma has been reported to occur on the dorsal surface of the midtongue, this site is rarely affected by cancer. Recent work suggests that chronic infection such as chronic hyperplastic candidiasis may be a causative factor. On this basis, anticandidal preparations could be tried for a month or so. If the lesion shows change in size, shape, or consistency, a biopsy is indicated to exclude carcinoma.

In bifid tongue incomplete fusion of the lateral prominences of the embryonic tongue may leave a cleft at the tip of the tongue. A central tag consisting of muscle may be found in the cleft. The fissure requires no treatment. Occasionally, it is advisable to snip off the central tag under local anesthesia.

Oral Mucosa

The oral mucosa heals rapidly after acute trauma, usually without a scar. Chronic trauma frequently produces hyperplasia.

Denture stomatitis is a fairly common inflammatory process occurring beneath the dentures. Removal of the denture for a few days and then leaving the denture out only at night usually relieves the condition. If Candida is found on mucosal scrapings, nystatin ointment applied to the oral mucosa and the denture itself is of value.

Papillary hyperplasia is the hyperplastic response of palatal and gingival mucosa to chronic irritation from ill-fitting dentures. Mild cases regress spontaneously when the dentures are left out for 3 to 4 weeks. Severe cases require surgical removal of the lesions. When the mouth is healed, new properly fitting dentures are made. Reworking old dentures usually fails. Well-documented instances of carcinoma arising in papillary hyperplasia are exceptionally rare.

Nicotine stomatitis (smoker's palate) is a very common, reactive squamous metaplasia of the palatine ducts and a sialadenitis of the palatine glands caused by smoking. Previously considered a premalignant condition, the process is now classified as benign. The tissues revert to normal when the patient stops smoking.

Leukoplakia and Leukokeratosis. There has been much confusion in use of the word leukoplakia. Originally, it meant any white plaque. We feel that the term leukokeratosis should be reserved for white lesions that show no dyskeratosis on histologic examination. Leukoplakia is a histopathologic diagnosis implying premalignant potential. Unless the diagnosis is obvious (e.g., thrush, typical lichen planus), all keratotic lesions should be biopsied and treated on the basis of the histopathologic report.

Leukokeratoses are benign white plaques usually caused by chronic trauma, such as cheek-biting or nibbling, sucking mucosa between the teeth, sharp margins of carious teeth, malpositioned teeth, and ill-fitting dental appliances. Diagnosis should be confirmed by biopsy. Correction of dental abnormalities, good oral hygiene, and avoidance of tobacco are frequently followed by definite improvement. The inveterate cheek chewer is helped by a mouth-guard–like dental appliance that he wears at night to prevent cheek chewing while asleep. Most dentists are familiar with this appliance. As a rule of thumb, a biopsy must be taken if the process does not show marked clearing within 6 weeks after irritating factors are removed. The best site for the biopsy is a thin flaky margin or an erythematous area within the white lesion. Furthermore, any change in shape, consistency, or configuration, or the development of ulcers or erythroplasia-like areas, is an indication for additional biopsies.

Leukoplakia is a histopathologic diagnosis of premalignancy. It may be difficult for the pathologist to exclude carcinoma in situ, and multiple biopsies may be necessary to reach a definite diagnosis. Inasmuch as only a small percentage of these lesions develop into overt squamous cell carcinoma, they are treated as outlined for leukokeratoses. Resistant plaques are destroyed by cryosurgery. Frequent re-evaluation and additional biopsies are important. Histologic evidence of carcinoma in situ indicates the need of immediate complete surgical excision. Persistent lesions of the tongue and floor of the mouth have the greatest potential for malignant transformation. They should be excised early for histopathologic evaluation of the entire lesion.

Snuff dipper's keratosis (snuff-induced leukoplakia) develops in constant users of this tobacco combination. Development of snuff dipper's carcinoma must be kept in mind, and biopsies should be taken in all cases. The prognosis of this problem has not been definitely established. If the process does not resolve after termination of the habit, the lesion should be completely excised or destroyed by cryosurgery.

Pigmented Lesions of the Oral Cavity. Physiologic pigmentation is found routinely in blacks and other dark-skinned persons. No therapy is indicated.

Amalgam tattoos result from the submucosal inclusion of amalgam particles that spilled into periodontal tissues during filling of a gingival cavity or were thrown into the tissues by a slipped disc or bur. Soft tissue x-ray examination will reveal the metal within the dermis. No treatment is indicated. Occasionally, it may be necessary to take a biopsy to eliminate the possibility of melanoma. Similar areas of pigmentation follow accidentally introduced materials from lead pencils, ink, charcoal, dirt, asphalt, and so on. Pigmentary disfigurement of the vermilion borders of the lips may be improved by a lip shave and careful picking out of the foreign particles.

Cellular nevi are the most common human tumors. However, less than 0.1 per cent are intraoral. All varieties are found. Most lesions occur in dark-skinned persons, and many are not pigmented. Clinical differentiation between nevi and melanoma is frequently difficult. It is probably advisable to remove any suspected oral nevus for histopathologic examination. Excisional biopsy must be carried out on any lesion that becomes ulcerated or changes in color, size, shape, or consistency.

The presence of the mucocutaneous melanin pigmentation of Peutz-Jeghers syndrome necessitates search for concomitant intestinal polyps. Gastrointestinal roentgenograms should be taken every 2 years in order to detect developing polyps. Radical surgical procedures should be avoided in the absence of overt malignant change.

Oral lesions may be present in acanthosis nigricans, pityriasis rosea, psoriasis, amyloidosis, Rendu-Osler-Weber syndrome, Sturge-Weber syndrome, and Garner's syndrome. Therapy, when available, is directed toward the primary disease.

Vesicobullous Lesions

Pemphigus Vulgaris. This relatively uncommon and serious disease process manifests itself by the appearance of vesicles and bullae developing in a cyclic pattern in the oral cavity. Usually occurring in the fourth to sixth decade of life, most cases involve the mouth and pharynx, primarily with later cutaneous eruptions. The cutaneous lesions are thin-walled lesions which rupture easily, leaving a raw ulcer with progressive coalescence of the oral lesions, forming deep painful ulcerations with later cutaneous lesions.

Once the disease has been diagnosed, utilizing appropriate histologic techniques, treatment is undertaken with the use of systemic corticosteroids and immunosuppressive agents.

Benign Mucous Membrane Pemphigoid. This relatively uncommon lesion affecting the same age group as pemphigus involves the oral and ocular mucous membrane. The clinical and histologic pictures are identical to those of bullous pemphigoid, and the characteristic early diagnosis is made by observation of gingival involvement with severe desquamative changes and deep red and edematous membrane. Again, vesicular and bullous lesions involve all areas of the oral cavity and pharynx, and, in the majority of cases, the conjunctiva is involved as well. Topical and systemic corticosteroids are the treatment of choice.

Erythema Multiforme. Erythema multiforme is a symptom complex which occurs more commonly than the previously mentioned lesions and involves the development of cutaneous erythema with the eruption of vesicles and bullae on the skin and oral mucosa. The lips are usually involved, and in childhood, a variant, the Stevens-Johnson syndrome, is frequently seen in which genital lesions are prominent as well as the oral cutaneous problem. The gingiva is usually not involved.

This is a rather acute but self-limiting disease process accompanied by a high fever and general malaise. The exact cause is usually obscure, but is thought to be a hypersensitivity to a drug or an allergic response to some underlying disease process.

The treatment is the use of systemic corticosteroids and avoidance of any possible etiologic agent.

Erosive Lichen Planus. This process is a very common inflammatory disease process involving the skin and mucous membranes and classically manifests itself as white striations or plaques with reticulate formations, usually on the buccal mucosa, lateral tongue, or gingiva. In some cases, erosive or bullous lesions are seen, causing confusion with pemphigus or pemphigoid. Histologic evaluation easily differentiates the two, and no specific therapy is required, although topical steroids sometimes provide relief.

Aphthous Stomatitis. Recurrent aphthous stomatitis is the most common of the vesicobullous lesions of the oral cavity. Aphthous stomatitis is caused primarily by the pleomorphic transitional L-form of *Streptococcus sanguis*. There is no specific therapy for this lesion at present, but symptomatic relief can be achieved through a variety of local measures. The use of triamcinolone acetonide in emollient dental paste (Kenalog in Orabase) is very useful for symptomatic relief, merely coating the material over the ulcerated area with a fingertip, avoiding additional trauma, and thus protecting the area involved and decreasing the acute inflammatory reaction. Cautery of the lesions has been attempted, but the discomfort of the procedure rarely justifies the minimal relief which follows. The use of a tetracycline mouthwash, 250 mg per 5 ml used three to five times a day, has provided a good response in many patients and is to be considered, utilizing appropriate precautionary measures required for that particular medication.

Other general measures, such as ensuring adequate oral hygiene, eliminating dental irritants such as rough teeth or fillings, and avoiding unnecessary intraoral trauma or manipulation should be considered.

Recurrent Herpetic Gingival Stomatitis. Recurrent viral stomatitis is a well-known and common entity which plagues a great number of patients. The latent manifestations of the herpesvirus hominis may be triggered by exposure to ultraviolet light, intraoral manipulation, fatigue, dietary indiscretions, or a variety of other physical or emotional stresses. The small blisters appear, persist for several days, and begin to dry, forming a small ulcer or yellowish crust. All the therapeutic measures previously noted for the treatment of aphthous stomatitis have been attempted and include the use of ether, witch hazel, and alcohol on the cutaneous lesions (cold sores), and triamcinolone acetonide in emollient dental paste (Kenalog in Orabase) on the oral lesions. Recently, it has been recommended that the amino acid lysine, in doses of 300 to 1200 mg daily, may represent effective therapy for this disease process. In those patients who respond to this treatment, the response is rapid and, although the current lesions respond well, a cure is not produced, and the patient remains susceptible to the recurrent affects of the latent virus.

Gingivae and Periodontal Membrane

Normally, the eruption of deciduous and permanent teeth is associated with only local irritation and increased salivation. Primary dentition requires no treatment except reassurance of the parents, cold liquid food, and, occasionally, application of the topical anesthetic lidocaine (Xylocaine Viscous). Other symptoms associated with teething should be investigated for underlying respiratory or gastrointestinal causes.

Eruption cysts usually rupture spontaneously. When they do not, a wedge of gum tissue is removed to expose the crown of the tooth. A single incision may lead to scar formation and recurrence of the cyst.

Pericoronitis is the inflammatory reaction surrounding a partially erupted tooth, particularly a mandibular third molar. Warm saline mouth rinses suffice as treatment. Severe pericoronitis with facial or submaxillary swelling, cervical lymphadenopathy, elevated temperature, or trismus should be treated with systemic antibiotics. Extraction of the third molar and opposing third molar is indicated if x-ray examination reveals either tooth to be impacted.

Chronic marginal gingivitis and periodontal disease indicate the need for dental prophylaxis, correction of dental or occlusal abnormalities, and construction of proper fitting prosthetic appliances. Severe cases require gingivectomy for complete removal of calculus, debris, granulation tissue, and periodontal "pockets." When the process has resulted in loosening of the teeth, temporary or permanent (expensive) splinting by appropriate dental appliances may save the teeth. Full dentures are never as satisfactory as permanent prosthetics. Patients with rapidly progressing periodontal disease should be examined carefully for the presence of diabetes mellitus, hyperparathyroidism, hyperthyroidism, and collagen disease.

Chronic desquamative gingivitis is a diffuse inflammatory reaction limited to the attached gingiva. There is some question as to whether this condition is a specific disease or a variant of benign mucosal pemphigoid, bullous pemphigoid, or pemphigus. The histopathologic findings are not diagnostic and serve only to exclude other diseases. Management, as discussed under general therapeutic considerations, will give symptomatic relief. Application of a topical fluorinated corticosteroid may be of value. A gel preparation, fluocinonide (Topsyn Gel), is preferable to an adhesive oral paste (Orabase), which may strip the thin friable epithelium. Systemic corticosteroids and estrogens have been used with limited success.

Simple hyperplastic gingivitis has many causes. Some cases develop without apparent cause; others follow chronic irritation or inflammation (poor dental hygiene, ill-fitting dentures, extraction sites). Occasionally, the constant sucking of hard candies or sweet cough drops precedes severe hyperplastic gingivitis. The gingival hyperplasia associated with vitamin C deficiency is one variant of this condition. Pubertal hyperplastic gingivitis is related to a disturbed hormonal balance, probably associated with subclinical scurvy superimposed on poor dental hygiene.

Pregnancy gingivitis occurs in about 10 per cent of pregnancies. The relative ascorbic acid deficiency associated with pregnancy is possibly an underlying cause.

Treatment consists of the following measures:

1. Careful dental prophylaxis and maintenance of good oral hygiene.

2. Multivitamin preparations. Vitamin C, 500 to 1000 mg daily for 7 to 10 days, then slowly decreased to a maintenance dose of 100 mg daily. Smaller doses for children.

3. Elimination of use of hard candy and cough drops.

4. Gingivectomy for severe recalcitrant cases.

5. Removal of pregnancy tumors by electrocautery if severe ulceration or annoying hemorrhage occurs. But be conservative. Most of the pregnancy hyperplasia regresses spontaneously several months after parturition.

Phenytoin hyperplasia occurs in 6 per cent of patients who take phenytoin (Dilantin) to control their epilepsy. Poor dental hygiene underlies most cases. Treatment is as follows:

1. Careful dental prophylaxis should be carried out and good dental hygiene maintained as soon as phenytoin is started, because occurrence of hyperplasia does not justify stopping the drug.

2. Epileptic patients must be taught proper dental care, and a member of the family must oversee home treatment.

3. Early, local dental treatment may clear the process; later, gingivoplasty is indicated, especially if the hyperplastic tissue interferes with mastication or becomes an esthetic problem.

Leukemic gingivitis does not occur in edentulous patients. Local irritation, secondary to calculus, is probably necessary for development of clinical manifestations. Treatment is as follows:

1. Systemic therapy.

2. Local therapy: (a) Maintain best possible dental hygiene; (b) relieve pain with anesthetic preparations and soothing, warm, saline mouth rinses; (c) treat any associated bacterial or Vincent's infection; (d) be very careful when doing extractions, deep scaling, and biopsies, as serious hemorrhage may follow minor trauma; (e) treat pulpitis by adequate drainage.

Hereditary fibromatosis is a rare, congenital, gingival hyperplasia. Gingivoplasty is usually necessary. Severe cases may require extraction of several teeth to ensure complete removal of all hyperplastic tissue.

Teeth

Dental agenesis is diagnosed by x-ray evidence of absent tooth buds. The open space should be maintained by an orthodontic appliance until the jaw has reached adult size, at which time a permanent bridge can be constructed. Partial or complete anodontia of one or both dentitions is rare, but may occur as an isolated defect or may represent a facet of anhidrotic ectodermal dysplasia. Untreated anodontia leads to marked facial deformity. Removable and fixed dental appliances should be constructed as soon as the child will cooperate. Continuous modification of the appliance is necessary as the child grows. Every erupting tooth is saved to serve as a fixed abutment.

Early removal of supernumerary teeth, either erupted or impacted, is indicated. Impacted teeth should be removed because of the danger of pathologic fracture, infection, or development of a follicular cyst. Impacted third molars should be removed in order to prevent forward displacement of the teeth. The opposing third molar should be removed at the same time. Multiple unerupted and impacted permanent teeth and multiple supernumerary teeth are present in cleidocranial dysostosis.

Pigmentation of the teeth may result from neonatal jaundice, postinjury hemorrhage into the tooth pulp, or ingestion of excessive amounts of fluoride or tetracycline during the development of enamel. The pregnant mother should not be given tetracycline after the first trimester. Prolonged treatment with tetracycline should not be given to children before the age of 8 years. Children taking tetracycline for 1 year (such as for cystic fibrosis) present a 5 per cent incidence of staining. Attempts to bleach heavily pigmented teeth with oxidizing agents and ultraviolet light are only partially successful. Small areas can sometimes be corrected by carefully grinding out the stain and restoring the defect with a composite resin onlay. Only prosthetic replacement of the enamel with a ceramic or resin full crown gives good cosmetic results.

Developmental anomalies of the teeth in form, position, texture, and color are not uncommon. Orthodontics and prosthodontia afford excellent improvement for these patients. Malposition and malocclusion of the teeth can also be corrected by orthodontic treatment. However, severe overbite, underbite, or open bite requires orthognathic surgery. Orthodontic therapy is prolonged, time consuming, and expensive. Except in those patients in whom the deformity compromises the patient's appearance or oral function, advice on such treatment should be tempered by consideration of cultural, esthetic, and financial factors.

Posteruptive Dental Defects. Dental caries is the most common posteruptive dental defect. Treatment of caries belongs in a textbook on restorative dentistry, a field which is beyond the scope of this article. Maintenance of good dental hygiene and dietary restriction of refined carbohydrates are proved methods of reducing the incidence of caries. Gum chewers and hard candy devotees should be switched to sugarless products. Fluoridated drinking water (2 ppm) decreases caries by approximately 50 per cent. Fluorinated toothpaste is also beneficial in reducing decay. Rampant caries develops in patients with extensive dental hypoplasia, systemic lupus erythematosus, juvenile diabetes, chronic xerostomia, or very poor oral hygiene, and in children with high susceptibility to caries. Treatment requires maintenance of excellent dental hygiene, daily use of a fluoride gel (King's Gel-Tin), dietary control, and correction of underlying xerostomia if possible in addition to restorative dentistry.

Trauma. Loosened teeth are checked for vitality and stabilized by orthodontic bands. Occasionally, the root of a fractured tooth can be preserved by endodontic therapy and used as the base for an orthodontic appliance. Reimplantation of dislodged teeth may be attempted with a fair chance of success.

Tooth Substance Loss. Attrition is the wearing away of tooth substance by mastication. Toothbrush abrasion is the loss of tooth substances in V-shaped notches at cervical margins of teeth owing to horizontal brushing. Acid decalcification may follow long-term drinking of lemon juice in hot water, administration of hydrochloric acid in liquid form, and chronic vomiting. Loss of tooth substance caused by habits or occupation is seen in persons who open bobby pins with their teeth, the tailor who bites threads, and the carpenter who holds tacks or nails in his mouth. The patient with toothbrush abrasion is taught proper, vertical-stroke, brushing techniques. Other self-induced injuries are explained to the patient, and an attempt is made to break the habits. Restorative dentistry can correct the defects if expense is not a consideration.

Complications of Dental Extractions. Extraction of teeth is usually followed by uneventful healing. However, excessive bleeding, osteitis, perforation of the maxillary sinus, injury to the inferior alveolar nerve with resulting paresthesia, and even fracture of the mandible and osteomyelitis may occur. Bleeding and osteitis respond to accepted dental treatment and are seldom seen by the physician. Patients with severe bleeding should be examined for clotting defects. Paresthesia usually resolves spontaneously. A ruptured maxillary sinus will probably heal spontaneously if the opening is small (1 to 2 mm). Large openings are closed by surgical intervention. Tooth roots pushed into the sinus must be surgically extracted to prevent sinusitis. Broad-spectrum antibiotics are given during the healing stage.

Salivary Glands

Sialolithiasis. Salivary calculi are not uncommon. Prompt removal of the blockage is necessary to prevent sialadenitis and eventual obliteration of the gland. Small, superficial stones of the submandibular gland may be milked, probed, or surgically removed from the duct. Large or inaccessible stones may necessitate excision of the gland. Obstruction of the parotid gland is more frequently due to inspissated mucus secretion. A diagnostic retrograde sialogram occasionally dislodges the obstruction.

Acute sialadenitis usually is due to obstruction of a major duct by a mucous or bacterial plug. Most cases clear within several weeks on a routine of systemic antibiotics and oral rinses with dilute, hot lemon juice. If the symptoms persist, incision and drainage of a localized abscess or removal of the gland may be indicated.

Certain problems of the oral cavity occur with such frequency or cause such distress among patients that it is worthwhile to consider them from the standpoint of therapy even though they may present as general symptom complexes rather than a specific disease entity. Some of these various problems and general measures which might be considered in their management are discussed as follows.

Halitosis

Halitosis, or foul-smelling breath, is a minor but common complaint that has been magnified by advertising campaigns for mouthwashes, troches, and chewing gums. Usually, the problem is more noticeable to associates than to the patient. Most oral odors arise from the bacterial decomposition of food particles, desquamated mucosal cells, and salivary protein. Poor dental hygiene, carious or malpositioned teeth that collect food debris, xerostomia, mouth breathing, chronic periodontitis, and ulcerative oral processes contribute to such bacterial digestion. Bacterial decomposition of diseased oral tissues (e.g., severe bullous disease, necrotic tumors, noma) produces an extremely foul odor.

About 10 per cent of the causes are of extraoral origin, deriving from aromatic compounds circulating in the blood. Allyl disulfides (from garlic), aromas of alcoholic drinks, ketones (fruity odor of diabetic ketoacidosis), paralde-

hyde, and aromatic products from incompletely digested fats pass from the blood across the alveolar membrane and are exhaled. Rare cases of halitosis are due to inflammatory diseases of the nose, throat, lungs, and stomach.

Treatment. 1. Refer to a dentist for examination and correction of any dental problem.

2. Maintain good dental hygiene with frequent toothbrushing and use of dental floss.

3. Antiseptic mouthwashes are of some value. However, the effect lasts only a few hours, and prolonged use may damage oral mucosa.

4. Reduce or eliminate ingestion of aromatic, odor-releasing compounds.

5. Evaluate the cause of any associated xerostomia. Treat as indicated.

6. Correct any associated inflammatory or metabolic disease.

Xerostomia

Dryness of the mouth is not a disease but a sign of impaired salivary gland function, which may be temporary or permanent. Various drugs and infectious diseases of the salivary glands produce a transient xerostomia. When the drug is stopped or the primary disease resolves, the salivary flow returns to normal. Atrophic changes in salivary glands, such as those found in Sjögren's syndrome, senile atrophy, and postradiation atrophy, produce irreversible damage.

The principal conditions producing xerostomia are as follows:

1. Mouth breathing: excessive speaking, exercise, adenoids, deviated septum, nasal polyps, hypertrophic rhinitis, respiratory infections.

2. Agenesis of salivary glands.

3. Senile atrophy of the mucous glands.

4. Psychologic: tension (speaking or performing before an audience), menopause, depression, anxiety states.

5. Major salivary gland dysfunction: uncontrolled diabetes, diabetes insipidus, severe uremia, severe dehydration, radiation therapy atrophy, bilateral mumps, infection or fibrosis, chronic hypochromic anemia, systemic lupus erythematosus.

6. Drugs: sedatives, hypnotics, narcotics, tranquilizers, nicotine, atropine and related drugs, propantheline and related drugs, antiparkinsonian drugs, antihistamines, phenothiazines, tricyclic antidepressants, epinephrine or ephedrine and related drugs, amphetamines.

7. Syndromes with xerostomia as an important symptom: Sjögren's syndrome, Mikulicz's syndrome, Waldenström's syndrome.

Ptyalism

Excessive salivary flow is not a disease but a

symptom of many conditions, varying from simple local processes or drug reactions to serious organic lesions of the stomach, jaw, or brain. If the cause is not obvious, extensive diagnostic work-up is necessary before specific therapy can be given. The principal conditions producing ptyalism are as follows:

1. Any form of general stomatitis, including thermal and chemical burns.

2. Parkinsonism.

3. Drugs: mercury, iodides, bromides, pilocarpine, expectorants, phosphorus, arsenic, antimony, cantharides, digitalis intoxication, anticholinergic intoxication (roach poison), nicotine (excessive smoking).

4. Reflex stimulation of fifth nerve: sucking on small hard objects; impacted foreign body (e.g., fishbone) in gingiva; periodontal disease including parulis and epulis; new partial dentures, especially when ill-fitting; jagged caries and rough fillings; fungating oral lesions; expanding lesions of the jaws.

5. Esophageal-gastric and hepatic reflex: carcinoma of the distal esophagus, peptic esophagitis, acute gastritis, dilation of the stomach, gastric ulcer or carcinoma, duodenal ulcer or carcinoma, hepatitis, pancreatitis.

6. Organic lesions of the uncinate gyrus (one symptom of uncinate attacks).

7. Ptyalorrhea (functional?): tension; facet of a psychogenic aberration (e.g., manic-depressive neurosis); functional affection of the fifth nerve, analogous to tic douloureux; associated with pregnancy; associated with cerebral arteriosclerotic changes.

8. Pseudoptyalism (normal saliva production): Mechanical difficulties in swallowing — mumps, acute infections of oral cavity or pharynx; tumors of jaws, tongue, palate, or pharynx; actinomycosis of jaws or tongue; fracture or dislocation of jaw; osteoarthritis or other dysfunction of the temporomandibular joint; painful conditions of pharynx, larynx, or esophagus. Inability to swallow — botulism, myasthenia gravis, facial paralysis, bulbar and pseudobulbar paralysis, hypoglossal nerve paralysis. Lack of cerebral control (slobbering) — cerebral injury or inadequacy, epileptic convulsions, rabies.

Abnormalities of Taste

The sensation of taste is based on so many interacting factors that abnormalities are difficult to classify. Taste is related to (1) visual response to food, (2) psychogenic response to thoughts of food or drink, (3) taste bud stimulation, (4) olfactory component, (5) physical consistency of food, (6) passage of food over oral structures, (7) thermal stimuli, (8) integrity of nerves and central

receptor sites for taste, (9) ability to masticate properly, (10) sufficient saliva, and (11) general health. In addition, numerous local conditions, systemic diseases, metabolic dysfunctions, drugs, and trophic processes may affect taste. Therapy must be directed to the underlying factors.

1. Local conditions (loss of taste, foul taste): stomatitis, glossitis, coated tongue, gingivitis, severe caries, oral tumors, gummatous infiltration of tongue, xerostomia.

2. Gastrointestinal disease (foul taste: gastritis, pyloric stenosis, gastric ulcer or carcinoma, regurgital esophagitis.

3. Septic lung disease (foul taste): bronchiectasis, tuberculosis with cavitation, abscess.

4. Perverted taste: pregnancy (various complaints), menopause (altered salt or metallic taste), senility (decreased stimulation by sweets), hysteria.

5. Vitamin deficiencies (decreased taste associated with burning of the tongue): pernicious anemia, nutritional macrocytic anemia, pellagra, chronic vitamin B complex deficiency.

6. Drugs: gymnemic acid, present in leaves of *Gymnema sylvestre* (abolishes sweet and bitter but has no effect on salt or sour); stovaine (abolishes sweet and bitter); local anesthetics (abolish all taste); penicillamine effect (causes decrease to loss of all taste), possibly related to copper or zinc deficiency produced by chelation with penicillamine.

7. Trophic processes (decrease to loss of taste): peripheral lesions of lingual nerve (distal two thirds of tongue); chorda tympani lesions (distal two thirds of tongue); peripheral lesions of glossopharyngeal nerve (proximal one third of tongue); syringomyelia; migraine (temporary component); organic lesions involving the tractus solitarius or adjacent area of the medulla (e.g., tumors, local anemia, hemorrhage, syphilis, multiple sclerosis); organic lesions of the uncinate gyrus.

Macroglossia

Enlargement of the tongue results from hyperplasia of normal structures, neoplastic involvement, inflammatory and infectious processes, or infiltration of the tissues by fluids or abnormal cells. An unusually enlarged tongue associated with thick speech and a lowered pitch suggests cretinism or myxedema. Edentulous patients who do not wear dentures have a broad flat tongue that may be mistaken for macroglossia. The tongue returns to normal shape after dentures are constructed.

As with any symptom complex, therapy depends upon the underlying cause.

1. Trauma: bites, penetrating wounds, in-

sect stings, corrosive agents and burns, jaw fractures.

2. Allergic reactions: stomatitis venenata, allergic stomatitis, urticaria, angioneurotic edema, dermatitis medicamentosa.

3. Vitamin deficiencies: ariboflavinosis, pellagra, scurvy, beriberi.

4. Congenital syndromes: congenital macroglossia, mongolism (Down's syndrome), gargoylism.

5. Endocrine abnormalities: cretinism, myxedema, diabetes, amyloidosis, acromegaly, glycogen storage disease.

6. Tumors: epithelioma, fibroma, neurofibromatosis, lipoma, hemangioma, lymphangioma, myeloma, sarcoma, rhabdomyoma.

7. Cysts: mucocele, thyroglossal duct cyst, ranula, suprahyoid cyst.

8. Hemorrhage into tongue: scurvy, leukemia, rupture of lingual varicosity, rupture of blood vessel by trauma, purpura (many factors).

9. Infections: syphilis (gummata), actinomycosis, histoplasmosis, zoster, thrush, tuberculosis, smallpox, Ludwig's angina, leprosy.

10. Inflammations: erythema multiforme, pemphigus, bullous pemphigoid, severe glossitis.

11. Miscellaneous disorders: plumbism, mercurialism, cardiac decompensation, progressive muscular dystrophy, superior vena cava syndrome, sarcoidosis.

Hypomobility of the Tongue

Hypomobility of the tongue is so often a symptom of serious systemic disease that diagnostic procedures should be initiated at once if the cause is not immediately apparent. Consider the following differential diagnoses:

1. Physical disorders: ankyloglossia or traumatic glossitis.

2. Neoplastic diseases: infiltrative lingual malignancies or sublingual neoplasms.

3. Cysts: thyroglossal duct cyst, sublingual mucous gland cyst, ranula.

4. Oral infections: glossitis or sublingual infection.

5. Scleroderma.

6. Miscellaneous disorders (concomitant finding): pernicious anemia (loss of muscle tone), myasthenia gravis, amyotrophic lateral sclerosis, myotonia congenita, cerebrovascular accident, bulbar paralysis, syringomyelia, cardiac glycogen disease, severed hypoglossal nerve, bulbar poliomyelitis, hysteria, infiltrative processes listed under Macroglossia.

7. Senility (loss of muscle tone).

Dysphagia

Difficulty in swallowing is also a serious complaint. As with other oral dysfunctions with multiple causes, the underlying pathology must be determined before definite therapy can be started. Differential diagnosis is extensive.

1. Pharyngitis, tonsillitis and lingual tonsillitis, cancer.

2. Iron deficiency anemia: Plummer-Vinson syndrome and chronic gastrointestinal bleeding.

3. Pharyngeal muscle dysfunction.

4. Cricopharyngeal muscle hypertrophy.

5. Esophageal spasm (e.g., esophagitis, senility).

6. Conditions listed under Pseudoptyalism.

7. Macroglossia.

Infectious Diseases

Infectious diseases involved in the oral cavity include those processes which may be either primary or secondary as listed below.

Those diseases not primary to the oral cavity are only noted with a few pertinent clinical findings. The reader is referred to the appropriate articles for definitive therapy and general management. Local treatment has been discussed under general therapeutic considerations.

Bacterial Diseases. Impetigo may involve the vermilion surfaces and oral commissures.

Furuncles are common on the lip margins. Large furuncles of the upper lip may eventuate in cavernous sinus thrombosis.

Erysipelas can extend from the face into the oral cavity. Primary intraoral erysipelas is very rare.

Malignant pustule or malignant edema of anthrax occurs on the lips and occasionally on the tongue, palate, and pharynx. Involvement of the lips by the pustulous form has been reported a few times.

Cutaneous diphtheria of the upper lip is secondary to involvement of the nasal mucosa. Pharyngeal diphtheria may spread to the palate and rarely to the buccal mucosa.

Gingival abscess (parulis) results from the fistulous extension of a periapical or periodontal infection through the cortical plate to the gingival surface. Diagnosis is confirmed by x-ray examination. After several days of systemic therapy with penicillin or broad-spectrum antibiotics, adequate drainage is instituted by the dentist (e.g., apical curettage, apicoectomy, endodontic drainage, extraction of retained root). Today's dentist reserves tooth extraction as a last resort. The antibiotics are continued until the process has cleared. If the infection persists, culture and sensitivity tests are run to determine the more effective antibiotic. Frequent hot mouth rinses give relief of discomfort. The extraoral dental fistula (sinus) results from extension of the periapical or periodontal infection through the intervening tissue to the cutaneous surface of the maxillary-facial region. The resulting abscess and subsequent draining granulomatous lesion are frequently confused with a local infection. Local therapy and antibiotics are ineffective. After diagnosis is confirmed by x-ray examination of the teeth and culture to eliminate deep fungus or acid-fast bacillus infection, dental therapy is indicated as for the gingival abscess. Hot compressing of the cutaneous lesion promotes drainage and hastens healing. Occasionally, surgical debridement of the sinus tract is necessary.

Gonorrhea of the oral cavity has been reported very rarely. Increased incidence of oral sex and awareness of the problem should result in diagnosis of more cases. Clinically, the oral mucosa presents a fiery red appearance with scattered areas of epitheliitis partially covered by a yellow-white pseudomembrane. The patient complains of a burning sensation.

Granuloma inguinale occasionally develops on the lips and in the oral cavity. As with oral gonorrhea, the increasing incidence of oral sex should lead to more common occurrence.

Almost half of all patients with leprosy present with facial and oral lesions. Nodular infiltrations of the lips, tongue, and gingiva are fairly common. Perforation of the palate and severe faucial adhesions occur. Involvement of the trigeminal and facial nerves is common.

Lingual tonsillitis results from inflammation of the lymphoid, foliate papillae located on the sides of the base of the tongue. The process usually responds to hot saline gargles. Antibiotics are indicated for severe cases. A biopsy should be taken if there is a question of diagnosis.

Ludwig's angina is usually due to a hemolytic streptococcal infection of the floor of the mouth and submental areas. Most patients respond to adequate doses of appropriate antibiotics. If the airway is compromised, emergency treatment (e.g., tracheostomy) is necessary.

Melkersson-Rosenthal syndrome (cheilitis granulomatosa) is characterized by recurrent swelling of the lips, recurrent facial paralysis, and fissured tongue. This process is listed here because it may be an allergic reaction to various organisms. The course of the disease is recurrent and progressive. Intralesional corticosteroids (triamcinolone, 5 to 10 mg per ml, not over 0.2 ml per cubic cm of tissue) injected into the enlarged lip or tongue may be of value. Surgical revision of chronically enlarged lips has been successful in a few patients. Decompression of the facial nerve has been recommended for persistent paralysis of over 2 months.

Rhinoscleroma may slowly spread from the nostrils to the upper lip, and even lower lip, producing keloid-like hardness and adhesions to the alveolar process. Extension to the alveolar process, palate, and tongue is reported. After biopsy confirmation and identification of *Klebsiella rhinoscleromatis* by appropriate culture, sensitivity tests should be run to determine sensitivity of the particular species. Most strains are sensitive to chloramphenicol, tetracycline, and streptomycin. Antibiotic therapy is continued until bacteriologic cure is obtained. In severe cases, tracheostomy is necessary to maintain an adequate airway. Supportive therapy with adequate diet, multivitamin preparations, and attention to secondary systemic, pyogenic infections is utilized as indicated. When the active process is cleared, it may be necessary to reconstruct the respiratory tract or repair the cosmetic deformities.

An infectious cause for sarcoidosis has not been proved. Nonulcerating nodular infiltrates may extend from the lips to the oral mucosa. Repeated intralesional injections of dilute triamcinolone solution (5 to 10 mg per ml) at 3 to 4 week intervals frequently clear lip and mucosal infiltrates.

The chancre of syphilis occurs on the lips, tongue (especially the tip), gingiva, and less often on the oral mucosa and palate. Mucous patches appear on the lip, tongue, and cheeks. Split papules suggesting angular cheilitis may occur at angles of the mouth. Gummata develop on and around the lips and in the oral cavity. Gummatous infiltration of the tongue produces macroglossia. Diffuse interstitial glossitis first enlarges the tongue and then produces shrinkage. Painless perforation of the palate is almost pathognomonic. Congenital syphilis is stigmatized by Parrot's radial scars (rhagades) around the lips, an ill-defined vermilion-cutaneous line, Hutchinson's teeth, mulberry molars, and other dental abnormalities.

In tuberculosis, the primary tuberculosis chancre (Ghon lesion) occasionally develops on the lip and in the oral cavity. Lupus vulgaris may extend to the lips and oral mucosa. The tuberculous ulcer of the lips and oral cavity must be differentiated from squamous cell carcinoma. Scrofula has occurred on the tongue with drainage to the submandibular area.

In tularemia, oral involvement by the primary complex is fairly common in Europe. In Turkey and southern Russia, the mouth is the most common site for inoculation.

Vincent's disease (trench mouth, acute necrotizing ulcerative gingivostomatitis) is probably due to change in host resistance, permitting *Fusobacterium plautivincenti* and *Borrelia vincentii* to become pathogenic. Poor dental hygiene, stress, fatigue, and heavy smoking are predisposing factors. The disease presents as a necrotizing, ulcerative gingivitis that may become chronic and produce extensive alveolysis and bone necrosis. In severe cases the process extends to the buccal mucosa and pharynx, but in most instances the adjacent mucosa shows surprisingly little change. The acute, painful, bacterial stage is controlled by frequent mouth rinses with warm 1.5 per cent solution (50 per cent dilution with warm water) of hydrogen peroxide. The solution is forced between the teeth by action of the cheeks and tongue. Necrotic tissue on the interdental papillae is removed by very gentle rubbing with a hydrogen peroxide–moistened cotton swab. Local antibiotics such as polymyxin-bacitracin-neomycin mixtures (Neosporin) may be of some value. Do not use for more than 1 week because of potential hazard of nephrotoxicity and ototoxicity caused by the neomycin. Caustic preparations should not be used. Pain and discomfort are controlled by analgesics. In severe infections, especially when associated with ulcers on the fauces and tonsils, systemic antibiotic therapy with penicillin, tetracycline, or erythromycin is indicated. After the acute, painful stage has subsided, the dentist must instruct the patient in proper dental hygiene. The teeth are gently scaled, and periodontal pockets are opened. All dental defects, especially gingival caries and malocclusion points, must be corrected. If local predisposing causes are not corrected by the dentist, recurrences and unncessary loss of gingival tissue are to be expected.

The primary lesion of yaws is rare on the lips. The secondary stage frequently involves the perioral areas and lips. Tertiary stage lesions of the lips and oral cavity are similar to those found in tertiary syphilis but present much more destruction of the skin and adjacent bone.

Candida albicans and, to a lesser extent, other species of Candida are almost universal in distribution and can be found in most healthy mouths.

The organism is an opportunistic pathogen and may produce overt infection when stimulated by various factors such as debilitation, chronic infections, pregnancy, and hypovitaminosis B. Hypoparathyroidism, hypothyroidism, diabetes mellitus, thymoma, and low serum iron levels may be associated with chronic Candida infections. Long-term administration of antibiotics, corticosteroids, and estrogens increases the susceptibility to oral (and vaginal) infections. Immunosuppressed patients and children with immunodeficiencies may develop chronic, recalcitrant infections. Local factors such as severe caries, sharp tooth edges, ill-fitting dentures, and cheek nibbling promote and maintain the infection. Candida cheilitis of the vermilion border is almost never an isolated finding. Angular

cheilitis caused by Candida infection has been previously discussed. Thrush (moniliasis) is characterized by the presence of a somewhat adherent, coagulated milk-like pseudomembrane on the tongue, cheeks, or pharynx. Removal of the membrane by rubbing with a gauze pad leaves a raw, oozing surface. Oral candidiasis must be considered in every case of glossodynia, even when the tongue appears normal. Treatment consists of the following measures:

1. Identification and elimination, if possible, of all systemic factors. Correction of nutritional deficiencies.

2. Discontinuance of antibiotics and contraceptive pills.

3. Nystatin solution (Mycostatin Oral Suspension), 1 teaspoonful as a prolonged mouthwash, four times a day, before swallowing; or nystatin oral tablet or nystatin vaginal suppository as an oral troche, three times daily. Nystatin cream may be applied under the denture for resistant palatal infections in edentulous patients. Nystatin in Orabase may be released shortly and should prove to be an excellent therapeutic modality.

4. Dilute hydrogen peroxide mouth rinses for oral discomfort.

5. Gentian violet, 1 per cent solution, is messy but effective.

6. Dental prophylaxis. Dental restorative work, including attention to ill-fitting dentures and dental appliances.

7. A new product, clotrimazole tablet (Gyne-Lotrimin), may prove very effective as an oral troche but has not been approved by the Food and Drug Administration for this purpose.

Occasionally, the Candida organisms invade beneath the mucosa to produce a chronic, recalcitrant, submucosal infection. This appears as a pale, thickened, macerated, boiled-looking, firmly adherent pseudomembrane that is crinkled, rugose, and frayed. Characteristically, the areas remain soft and do not develop the firmness found in thickened leukoplakia. Recent investigative work indicates that some patients with recalcitrant and recurrent mucocutaneous candidiasis have a deficiency of an alpha$_2$ globulin anticandidal factor in their serum, and that others lack the enzyme myeloperoxidase in their leukocytes. Other recent work suggests a deficiency in the enzyme that cleaves β-carotene. At present, we have no specific therapy for such deficiencies. Many patients with submucous thrush respond satisfactorily but slowly to the routine for simple thrush. Failure to respond to therapy or rapid recurrence emphasizes the need to re-evaluate the case for underlying systemic disease and immunodeficiencies. Chronic, recalcitrant thrush and mucocutaneous candidiasis present a serious problem in therapy. Therapeutic procedures include the following:

1. Amphotericin B* and 5-fluorocytosine, intravenously, as individual drugs or at the same time for their synergistic action. (The intravenous use of 5-fluorocytosine is not listed in the manufacturer's official directive.)

2. Bone marrow transplants.

3. Leukocytes from HLA-compatible sibling.

4. Transfer factor in large doses.

Mycotic Diseases. Oral lesions of the deep fungus infections (e.g., actinomycosis, aspergillosis, blastomycosis, coccidioidomycosis, cryptococcosis, histoplasmosis, mucormycosis, nocardiosis, rhinosporidiosis, and sporotrichosis) are usually, although not always, part of the general infection. Cervicofacial localization is the most common manifestation of actinomycosis. South American blastomycosis almost always begins in the oral cavity.

Viral Diseases. Oral lesions may be present in chickenpox, cat-scratch disease, hand-foot-and-mouth disease, Kaposi's varicelliform eruption, infectious mononucleosis, lymphogranuloma venereum, measles, paravaccinia, variola, vaccinia, and zoster. Symptomatic local measures are instituted as indicated by the severity of the oral disease. Systemic therapy is directed to the primary disease.

---

*See manufacturer's official directive for this use.

DISORDERS OF THE MOUTH (MALIGNANT)

method of
J. WILLIAM FUTRELL, M.D.
Pittsburgh, Pennsylvania

Treatment of cancer of the mouth requires, first of all, consideration of the problems of the whole patient and likewise an understanding of the multidisciplinary approach to oral cavity malignancy. Curative treatment modalities usually involve surgery, irradiation, or a combination of the two. Adjuvant treatment methods include chemotherapy, cryotherapy, or various forms of immunotherapy. Approximately 90 per cent of intraoral cancers are histologically squamous cell lesions, and significant predisposing factors to development include excessive use of alcohol and tobacco, dental irritation and poor oral hygiene, and, in past years, syphilis.

Initial patient evaluation must include (1) a recognition of the psychologic impact of the process and its potential treatment, (2) a determination of the general health and nutritional status of the patient, and (3) an understanding of the need for pre- and post-treatment education of the patient and his family. Long-term follow-up is particularly important owing to the diffuse field changes and multiple primary cancer pattern of oral cavity malignancies. Specific means of patient evaluation include (1) thorough history and physical examination, including endoscopy, (2) biopsy of the primary lesion and frequently multiple biopsies to establish the extent of the disease, (3) facial roentgenograms for determining bone or sinus involvement, and (4) plain x-ray tomography and computed tomography (CT) scans to delineate involvement of areas such as the base of the skull, temporomandibular joints, or intracranial extension.

Intelligent discussion of extent of disease and treatment requires an accurate classification based upon the location, size, and histologic characteristics of the primary tumor, the extent of regional node disease, and the presence of distant metastases. The TNM system (Table 1) is valuable in determining both treatment and prognosis. Histologic determination of degree of anaplasia and vascular invasion is also important.

Treatment in the absence of systemic spread is essentially local-regional in that the primary tumor and its potential routes of spread, i.e., regional nodes, must be considered. The primary treatment choice of surgery, irradiation, or both is made according to whether or not the tumor can be adequately removed with a satisfactory margin, the radiosensitivity of the tumor, whether or not the tumor involves or is in close contact with bone or cartilage tissue, and the morbidity and mortality associated with each treatment method. Nutritional supplementation, often with preoperative hyperalimentation, is frequently an important treatment consideration. Improvement of dental hygiene by oral cleansing and tooth extractions as indicated together with optimization of pulmonary reserve is also important.

The anatomic boundaries of the oral cavity extend from the skin-vermilion junction of the lips to the junction of the hard and soft palate above, and to the circumvallate papillae below. Clinical behavior of the primary tumor and its route of metastasis differ, depending upon its anatomic location within the mouth. Treatment is

TABLE 1. **TNM Classification System for Squamous Cell Carcinoma of Head and Neck***

I. Primary tumor (T)
  TX No available information on primary tumor
  T0 No evidence of primary tumor
  TIS Carcinoma in situ
  T1 Greatest diameter of primary tumor less than 2 cm
  T2 Greatest diameter of primary tumor 2 to 4 cm
  T3 Greatest diameter of primary tumor more than 4 cm
  T4 Massive tumor more than 4 cm in diameter with deep invasion to involve antrum, pterygoid muscles, root of tongue, or skin of neck

II. Nodal involvement (N)
  NX Nodes cannot be assessed
  N0 No clinically positive nodes
  N1 Single clinically positive homolateral node less than 3 cm in diameter
  N2 Single clinically positive homolateral node 3 to 6 cm in diameter or multiple clinically positive homolateral nodes, none over 6 cm in diameter
    N2a Single clinically positive homolateral node 3 to 6 cm in diameter
    N2b Multiple clinically positive homolateral nodes, none over 6 cm in diameter
  N3 Massive homolateral node(s), bilateral nodes, or contralateral node(s)
    N3a Clinically positive homolateral node(s), none over 6 cm in diameter
    N3b Bilateral clinically positive nodes (in this situation, each side of the neck should be staged separately; that is, N3b: right, N2a; left, N1)
    N3c Contralateral clinically positive node(s) only

III. Distant metastasis (M)
  MX Not assessed
  M0 No (known) distant metastasis
  M1 Distant metastasis present (specify) _____

IV. Postsurgical treatment residual tumor (R)
  R0 No residual tumor
  R1 Microscopic residual tumor
  R2 Macroscopic residual tumor (specify) _____
  Stage grouping
    Stage I   T1 N0 M0
    Stage II   T2 N0 M0
    Stage III T3 N0 M0
              T1 or T2 or T3, N1, M0
    Stage IV T4, N0 or N1, M0
              Any T0, N2 or N3, M0
              Any T, Any N, M1

V. Histopathology
  A Cell type–squamous cell carcinoma
  B Tumor grade (G)
    G1 Well differentiated
    G2 Moderately well differentiated
    G3–G4 Poorly to very poorly differentiated

*Proposed by American Joint Committee for Cancer Staging and End Result Reporting (1979 Revision).

best discussed according to the following anatomic areas: (1) lips, (2) buccal mucosa, (3) lower and upper alveolar ridge and retromolar gingiva (retromolar trigone), (4) floor of the mouth, (5) hard palate, and (6) anterior two thirds of tongue (oral tongue). The posterior tongue tonsillar area and soft palate are classified with pharyngeal lesions.

Lips

Lower lip carcinomas outnumber those of the upper lip about 9 to 1 and occur in persons with prolonged exposure to actinic irradiation. Tumors can be exophytic, ulcerating, or verrucous with the ulcerating form the most aggressive. For small lower lip lesions, regional node metastasis is uncommon, but is more frequent with tumors of increasing size and less differentiation. Depending upon staging and biologic potential of the tumor, surgical treatment consists of wedge excision and primary reconstruction, at times combined with an upper neck dissection or occasionally with complete neck dissection. External radiotherapy is occasionally employed as primary treatment. Prognosis and functional rehabilitation are excellent, with a greater than 90 per cent 5 year survival. Upper lip lesions involve the same therapeutic considerations.

Buccal Mucosa

Primary carcinoma of the buccal mucosa has its highest incidence in males in their sixth decade and is frequently associated with tobacco chewing. Onset is often insidious, with pain, trismus, bleeding, and occasionally tumor extension throughout the cheek. Treatment often involves multimodality therapy, including irradiation and at times surgical excision of the entire cheek thickness. Not infrequently an en bloc resection of the cheek, including a portion of the mandible, combined with a radical neck dissection and cheek reconstruction is required. Prognosis is determined by clinical staging and there generally is a less than 50 per cent 5 year survival. Temporal artery methotrexate infusion has on occasion made unresectable tumors resectable.

Upper and Lower Alveolar Ridge and Retromolar Gingiva

The gingiva is mucosal tissue covering the bony alveolar ridge, with the retromolar trigone being the mucosa overlying the ascending ramus of the mandible from the last molar tooth to the apex superiorly at the maxillary tuberosity. The lower gingiva is most frequently involved, and tumors occur most often in persons 50 years of age or older. Exophytic lesions are generally less aggressive than ulcerated, invasive lesions. Retromolar trigone lesions tend to be invasive, with frequent node metastases such that surgical treatment often involves en bloc resection of the involved mucosa and mandible together with a neck dissection. With bone involvement, irradiation alone is rarely curative, although frequently it is useful as adjuvant therapy. Upper alveolar ridge lesions metastasize less frequently to cervical nodes, and appropriate therapy often involves combined surgery and irradiation.

Floor of Mouth

This anatomic area encompasses the semilunar space over the mylohyoid and hyoglossus muscles and extends from the inner surface of the lower alveolar ridge to the under surface of the tongue, and posteriorly to the anterior tonsillar pillar. Presenting tumor symptoms usually include a fissure or ulcer, and extension may occur to other anatomic areas, including the tongue, mandible, submaxillary gland, or cervical lymph nodes. Microscopic involvement of clinically negative neck nodes is frequent, and incontinuity resection of the primary lesion together with a radical neck dissection is frequently required. T1 tumors can be treated primarily by either surgery or irradiation, whereas T2 lesions most frequently involve combined therapy. Adjuvant chemotherapy may be useful in advanced lesions. Primary reconstruction is often possible with good rehabilitation. The 5 year survival rate is above 60 per cent.

Hard Palate

Squamous cell carcinomas of the hard palate are frequently slow growing and often of considerable size at initial presentation. Treatment is most often surgical and in the presence of cervical node metastases is frequently combined with irradiation therapy. Full tumor doses of irradiation to a primary palate lesion often leave uncovered bone, making the wearing of dentures after radiation therapy impractical. If preoperative irradiation is not carried to a full tumor dose, such complications are unusual. For advanced and unresectable lesions, cryotherapy is occasionally helpful. Rehabilitation after surgical resection usually requires wearing a palate obturator.

Anterior Two Thirds of Tongue

The oral or mobile portion of the tongue extends anteriorly from the circumvallate papillae to the junction of the floor of the mouth. More than 70 per cent of tongue cancers occur in the mobile portion, with a tendency toward less anaplastic histology for more anterior lesions. Involvement of the lateral tongue borders with infiltrative growth is most frequent, and with large lesions cervical metastatic disease is often present at initial evaluation. Bilateral metastases can also occur. T1 lesions can be treated by either surgical excision or radiotherapy, whereas larger lesions frequently require combined therapy. Surgical resection often involves removal of the affected portion of tongue, floor of mouth, and, on occasion, mandible. If mobile mucosa separates the primary tumor from the alveolus, direct bony involvement is rare and mandible resection is not indicated.

Posterior tongue and tonsillar lesions have a decidedly worse prognosis and are considered with pharyngeal cancers.

Rational Plan of Therapy

A multidisciplinary approach, including an understanding of surgical ablative and reconstructive techniques, the principles of irradiation therapy, and the potentials of chemotherapy, is important. Availability of additional support help from medicine, psychiatry, oral prosthodontics, and special nursing is essential. Little is new in the way of extension of surgical ablative procedures, although certain reconstructive techniques, particularly the use of myocutaneous flaps, have made rehabilitation considerably more attainable. Multimodality therapy has had the greatest impact on improved survival.

Specific points of optimal treatment include (1) accurate clinical staging, including multiple biopsies, fiberoptic endoscopy, and diagnostic x-rays as needed; (2) particular pretreatment attention to nutrition, oral hygiene, and cardiopulmonary status; (3) surgery, irradiation, or combined treatment designed to ablate the primary tumor and any existing regional metastatic disease; (4) primary reconstruction, which is immediately indicated following most extirpative procedures and which may require distant flaps, bone grafting, or skin grafting; (5) irradiation, given in various ways employing radium seed implants or external cobalt (^{60}Co) (tumor doses involving 5000 to 6000 rads for curative therapy are often fractionated to 200 rads in five treatments per week); (6) chemotherapy used as adjuvant therapy and in differing combinations, with bleomycin, methotrexate, vinblastine, doxorubicin (Adriamycin), and lomustine (CCNU) all having been shown to be effective against squamous cell carcinoma (most drug use now involves combinations of drug regimens according to tumor responsiveness and signs of toxicity; protocol therapy is most useful in determining efficacy of different treatment combinations); and (7) nursing and rehabilitation care, involving particular attention to the quality of life, including palliation efforts. Such considerations are an integral part of the therapeutic program and require communication and assistance from dietary service, speech therapy, social service agencies, chaplain service, and education of the patient and those in his own environment.

DISEASES OF THE NAILS

method of
MARGARET C. DOUGLASS, M.D.,
and EDWARD A. KRULL, M.D.
Detroit, Michigan

Acute Paronychia

Acute inflammation of the nail fold and surrounding tissue is most commonly due to staphylococci, streptococci, or *Pseudomonas aeruginosa*. Trauma or picking of a hangnail is frequently responsible for initiating the infection.

Treatment. 1. If possible, a bacterial culture and sensitivity should be obtained.

2. While results of the bacterial culture are pending or if a culture cannot be obtained, an antibiotic such as cloxacillin, 250 to 500 mg four times a day, or erythromycin, 250 to 500 mg four times a day, should be started, especially if the cellulitis is severe or lymphangitis is present.

3. Warm compresses with an agent such as Burow's solution (1:40 dilution) for 15 minutes four times a day give considerable relief, and for mild paronychia may be the only treatment necessary.

4. If fluctuation is present, the involved area may have to be incised and drained.

Chronic Paronychia

Chronic paronychia is often caused by a mixed infection of bacteria or *Candida albicans*. Trauma and frequent contact of the hands with water are often causative factors. These infections can be of long duration and are slow to respond to therapy.

Treatment. 1. Cultures obtained from between the nail fold and nail plate for both bacteria and fungi are important.

2. If bacteria are recovered on culture, treatment with an appropriate antibiotic should be initiated.

3. Warm compresses with Burow's solution (1:40 dilution), 15 minutes twice a day, may help decrease the inflammatory reaction and help dry the paronychial area.

4. Application of a drying agent such as Castellani's solution, colored or colorless, will decrease bacterial and fungal overgrowth. The antibacterial colored solution may be more effective, but many patients object to the bright fuchsia stain it will leave.

5. Four per cent thymol in alcohol, which has a drying and mild irritant effect, can be applied to the nail fold area twice a day.

6. If *Candida albicans* is present, use an antifungal agent such as 1 per cent clotrimazole solution (Lotrimin) twice a day to nail folds.

7. Surgical treatment may be needed on rare occasions in persistent paronychia. This would involve the excision of a strip of skin overlying the paronychia. Occasionally, if there is significant scarring, intralesional triamcinolone (Kenalog-10) may be beneficial.

Ingrown Toenail

The method selected for the treatment of ingrown toenails depends upon the degree of inflammation, the location of the injury in the lateral nail groove, and the number of recurrences.

Ingrown toenails occur more commonly in adolescents and young adults, especially those with sweaty feet. In older people, even with markedly curved nails, there is a decreased incidence of true ingrowing of the nails.. It is very uncommon in people who do not wear shoes. Therefore, it seems likely that a growing foot associated with sweating that allows the nails to lacerate the lateral nail groove more easily and the pressure of shoes on the nail are important factors in the etiology of ingrown toenails.

Treatment — Inflammatory Stage. In the inflammatory stage definitive scalpel surgery should not be undertaken because of the greater incidence of soft tissue infection and the possible occurrence of osteomyelitis if a matrix excision is undertaken. Soaking the foot in lukewarm water or in Burow's solution, 1:40 dilution (Domeboro 1 packet per pint lukewarm water), may be beneficial.

Antibiotics, erythromycin, 1 gram per day, or penicillinase-resistant penicillin such as cloxacillin, 1 gram per day for adults, may be indicated. Cultures and sensitivities from the inflamed site should be the basis for specific antibiotic selection.

However, ingrown toenails should be thought of in terms of a foreign body, i.e., the edge of the nail plate cutting through the lateral nail groove and permitting the entrance of bacteria. Therefore, the removal of the ingrowing wedge of nail or the protection of the lateral groove from the nail plate by some mechanical method is usually far more effective in the inflammatory stage than simply soaks and antibiotics.

1. If the ingrowth of nail is in the distal part of the lateral nail groove, then cotton pledgets separating the lateral nail edge from the groove may be helpful. Occasionally there is a small sharp point at the corner of the nail plate resulting from the failure of the patient to cut com-

712

pletely across the nail plate. This "fishhook" can be examined by completely visualizing the distal edge of the nail plate. If this "fishhook" is found, the point of the nail should be trimmed off.

2. If the more conservative methods of treating the inflammatory stage are ineffective, then a lateral wedge of nail plate should be removed. After administration of 1 per cent plain lidocaine (Xylocaine) or comparable local anesthetic, a small-nosed hemostat is inserted under the distal edge of the side of the nail and pushed proximally until there is a "give." This then separates the undersurface of the nail plate from the underlying nail bed and matrix. The small-nosed hemostat is then inserted between the proximal nailfold and the underlying nail plate. Then, using a nail splitter or similar nail-cutting instrument, a narrow wedge of nail is cut through the entire longitudinal length. By grasping the wedge of nail plate with a hemostat, the piece of nail is easily extracted. The wedge of nail is usually less than one quarter of the total width of the nail and does not have to extend any wider than a few millimeters beyond the edge of the lateral nail fold. Granulation tissue is gently curetted. A mild pressure dressing with Kling is applied. Systemic antibiotics are infrequently used and tend to be reserved for patients with a high susceptibility to significant bacterial infections, such as diabetics, or for those in whom surrounding inflammation is extensive. The patient begins soaks the evening of the surgery and continues soaking in Burow's solution 1:40 or Domeboro, 1 packet per pint of lukewarm water, twice a day for approximately 1 week.

Treatment — Definitive Stage. After about 4 weeks, a definitive procedure for an ingrown toenail can be undertaken. By this time the inflammatory response should have completely subsided. If it has not, then more time should elapse to allow the disappearance of the inflammation. If the toenail has ingrown on only one or two occasions, it may be better to allow the nail plate to regrow to ascertain whether ingrowing will recur. If, however, the ingrown toenail has recurred a number of times, or there seems to be some scarring which narrows the space through which the nail plate must grow, then a definitive procedure should be undertaken.

There are many methods of effecting permanent repair of an ingrown toenail. Almost all of them require the destruction or resection of the matrix corresponding to the wedge of nail plate that had previously been removed. Our method requires an incision through the proximal nailfold and then carried laterally to develop a flap of the proximal nail fold so as to visualize the entire extent of matrix. Then the nail bed and matrix are resected under direct visualization, with two anatomic landmarks looked for. One is the proximal invagination of the nail plate, and the other is the fibrofatty tissue in the lateral nail groove. If the excision is carried proximal to the apex of the nail groove, then it is very likely that the entire matrix in that wedge has been removed. The incision in the proximal nail fold is closed with nylon suture, and a nonadherent dressing (Telfa, petrolatum gauze) with modest pressure applied by Kling is used. The dressing is removed within 48 hours and a smaller dressing is applied. Sutures are removed in approximately 1 week.

Subungual Hematomas

Subungual hematomas usually occur shortly after trauma. Anticoagulants and bleeding tendencies may make the hemorrhage more significant. Pain usually results from the pressure produced by the bleeding underneath the nail. The treatment can be divided into two phases: treatment of the acute phase, and management of persistent subungual hematomas.

Acute. The most important aspect of treatment of subungual hematomas is to relieve pressure caused by the bleeding. The easiest method is to heat a copper paper clip to a red glow and apply the paper clip to the nail. The hot paper clip penetrates through the keratin easily, permitting the blood to egress from the underlying tissues. Because there is blood in a space beneath the nail, it would be difficult to push the paper clip through the hemorrhagic area into the toe, producing a burn in the underlying soft tissues. Occasionally if the hematoma is very extensive, it may be better to remove the entire nail plate. Other methods for relieving pressure include the use of nail drills or burrs on small hand-held drills.

Persistent Subungual Hematomas. Occasionally a subungual hematoma persists under a nail plate and does not migrate. This presents confusion in diagnosis, especially as to differentiation from other pigmented lesions. A reddish-blue color, an irregular shape, and an absence of color in the nail plate tend to differentiate nonmigrating subungual hematoma from nevi or other causes of nail pigmentation. However, to be certain, it is best to remove the part of nail overlying the subungual hematoma and identify and remove the old dried blood to establish that the cause is a nonmigrating subungual hematoma.

Verrucae (Periungual and Subungual)

Verrucae involving periungual and subungual tissues, in addition to being cosmetically unpleasant, can be very difficult to cure. A wide variety of treatment modalities have been used, all of which are effective in some patients, none being effective in all patients. Verrucae under the nail plate can be extremely painful, necessitating attempts at therapy.

Treatment. CHEMICAL METHODS (*All should be used with caution in the diabetic patient, especially on the feet*). 1. A commonly used technique consists of using a mixture of 16 per cent salicylic acid, 16 per cent lactic acid in flexible collodion (Duofilm) applied to the warts at night, with care taken not to apply it on normal tissue. The wart is then occluded with tape or a Band-Aid for 12 to 72 hours, depending on patient tolerance. When the tape is removed, the white macerated tissue can be scraped off. This must be repeated frequently for weeks or months.

2. Another method involves the use of 40 per cent salicylic acid plasters applied carefully to the warts and occluded with tape for 24 to 72 hours. After removal, the dead white tissue is pared and the plaster reapplied.

3. Another technique is the application of a mixture of 1 per cent cantharidin, 30 per cent salicylic acid, and 5 per cent podophyllin in penederm (Verrusol) by the physician. The mixture can be left on for up to 24 hours, but a lesser time (e.g., 1 to 2 hours) is recommended initially, since very large blisters can develop. It has the advantage of being painless when applied, although the resultant blister can be painful. Chemical lymphangitis can occur with severe reactions to the Verrusol. This mixture should not be used on mucous membranes or near the eyes. Several applications will probably be necessary. If used carefully, this is a particularly good technique for treating children, since the application is painless.

4. Glutaraldehyde 10 to 20 per cent, applied nightly to the verrucae, can also be used with some success, especially if combined with the application of liquid nitrogen in the physician's office. (This use of glutaraldehyde is not stated by the manufacturer.)

5. An alternative method involves the application of a mixture of 1 per cent salicylic acid, 5 per cent resorcinol, and 10 per cent formaldehyde in 70 per cent isopropyl alcohol applied twice a day for 5 days. This is followed by the application of a 40 per cent salicylic acid plaster for 48 hours under occlusion. The verruca is then pared, and the entire process is repeated for 6 to 10 weeks, or as long as necessary.

LIQUID NITROGEN. Liquid nitrogen, which has a temperature of about −200 C, applied to warts every 1 to 3 weeks is frequently effective. It can be applied by either a cotton swab or a spraying instrument such as a Cryac Unit. Since application is very painful, especially on hands and feet, it is difficult to use on children. It should be used only by physicians properly trained in its application. Blister formation is an expected result. Hypopigmentation can occur in darkly pigmented individuals, so great care should be used in cosmetically important areas. Patients with cold intolerance may have an increased risk of problems with cryotherapy. Caution should be used in applying liquid nitrogen over digital nerves, since permanent nerve damage can result from too much pressure or too deep a freeze.

SURGICAL MANAGEMENT. Some form of surgical management may be necessary for subungual and periungual warts. The technique employed by us is to use 1 per cent lidocaine (Xylocaine) or mepivacaine (Carbocaine) as a local anesthetic and remove enough of the nail plate to allow the accurate determination of the amount of soft tissue involved in the wart.

The wart is usually far more extensive underneath the nail plate than the clinical appearance suggests. Gentle and careful curettage of the wart should be carried out. Electrosurgery is usually avoided unless there are some very major bleeding points and then is gently done with low settings with electrofulguration type current. Usually a tourniquet is applied to the digit during the treatment of the wart so as to better visualize the surgical site.

With careful curettage and minimal electrosurgery, the likelihood of permanent damage and an adverse effect on either the attachment or the development of the nail plate is reduced. A nonadherent dressing such as Telfa and an external dressing of Kling can be used. The patient starts soaking the next day in lukewarm water. One of the antibacterial ointments such as povidone-iodine (Betadine) may be applied once or twice a day for approximately 1 week or until the crust comes off.

Fungal Infections of the Nail Plate (Tinea Unguium)

Dermatophyte infections of the nail plate are of at least two types: (1) leukonychia mycotica, in which white patches or pits are present on the surface of the nail, and (2) invasive subungual dermatophytosis, which begins at the edges of the nail and later can cause the nail to be thickened, friable, and discolored. The accumulation of subungual keratin and debris is characteristic. Almost all species of dermatophytes have been isolated from fungal infections of the nail, but the most common are *Trichophyton rubrum*, *T. mentagrophytes*, and *Epidermophyton floccosum*. Leukonychia mycotica is most often caused by *T. menta-*

grophytes. Since nail changes in psoriasis, Norwegian scabies, and certain other nail dystrophies can mimic tinea unguium, a KOH preparation and fungal culture obtained from the involved nail are important for diagnosis. The specimen can be obtained with a small curette at the juncture of normal and onycholytic nail or from shavings of the involved nail. It is important *not* to culture a specimen from the keratotic debris under the nail bed, since this does not contain fungal elements. Tinea unguium, especially of the toenails, is often resistant to treatment. Even if the lesions clear with therapy, recurrences are common.

Treatment. 1. Systemic griseofulvin therapy can result in complete resolution in some patients, more frequently with fingernail than toenail involvement. Griseofulvin dosage ranges from 250 to 500 mg twice a day of the microsize form or 125 to 250 mg twice a day of the ultramicrosize form. Although the point is controversial at this time, griseofulvin is still probably best taken with fatty foods such as bread and butter or peanut butter to increase absorption of the drug.

2. Topical preparations such as clotrimazole 2 per cent (Lotrimin) solution or 4 per cent thymol in alcohol may be helpful, especially with minimal involvement or with leukonychia mycotica.

3. Chemical debridement of the dystrophic nail can sometimes be accomplished with a preparation containing 40 per cent urea, 20 per cent anhydrous lanolin, 5 per cent white wax, and 35 per cent white petrolatum. This remains on the nail under occlusion for 7 to 10 days. The softened nail can then be removed by curettage. Application of an antifungal agent such as miconazole (MicaTin) or clotrimazole (Lotrimin) cream twice a day to the nail bed may eradicate the fungal infection.

4. Grinding down the thickened nail to relieve pressure from shoes gives dramatic relief to symptoms in many cases, and this may be the only treatment required.

5. In some instances, surgical removal of the nail plate prior to treatment may be beneficial.

6. Occasionally ablation of the matrix of the toenail by surgical methods may be indicated to remove the nail plate permanently because of the symptomatology and appearance of the nail.

Onycholysis

Onycholysis or separation of the nail plate from the nail bed has several causes, including psoriasis, fungal or bacterial infections, phototoxic reactions, contact allergy to nail hardeners and lacquers, and hyper- or hypothyroidism.

In psoriasis the onycholysis usually has a reddish-golden advancing line. In some industries requiring use of the nails to pick up heavy objects, such as bales of material, traumatic onycholysis may occur.

Treatment. 1. Fungal cultures should be performed. If positive, treatment is with topical or systemic antifungal preparations as described previously.

2. If there is a greenish material suggesting a chromogenic bacterium and perhaps candidiasis, the use of topical miconazole (MicaTin) or clotrimazole (Lotrimin), if candidiasis is suspected, and some antibacterial solution such as 15 per cent sulfacetamide in 70 per cent ethyl alcohol may also be tried.

3. If the process is related to psoriasis, one of the more potent topical steroids, such as fluocinonide gel (Topsyn) applied twice a day under the nails may also be beneficial.

4. The object of treatment of onycholysis not associated with specific underlying disease, is to develop reattachment of the nail plate to the underlying tissues; 4 per cent thymol in alcohol may contribute to this reattachment.

5. The nail plate should be trimmed back as far as possible to minimize the possibility of inadvertently catching the nail plate on extraneous objects and causing further onycholysis.

In addition, the patient should be warned against overvigorous cleaning with nail files under the onycholytic nail. If a patient with onycholysis is planning to undertake a greasy, dirty job, the application of a water-soluble ointment or soap under the nails may protect the underlying tissues and make the cleansing much easier.

6. If a phototoxic drug reaction is suspected, the causative agent should be discontinued (e.g., dimethylchlortetracycline, chlortetracycline, or chlorpromazine).

7. If a nail hardener or lacquer is suspected, the offending agent should be discontinued. In this case, corticosteroid lotions such as betamethasone valerate (Valisone) or betamethasone dipropionate (Diprosone) applied under the nail twice a day are helpful.

8. With idiopathic onycholysis a surgical procedure may be beneficial. The removal of the nail plate just proximal to the onycholytic area and removal of the subungual keratinous material allow the nail to reattach in about half the patients.

Onychogryphosis

Onychogryphosis, or thickened, claw-like nails, can be managed both surgically and conservatively. If the patient's medical status, especially the local circulatory status, is questionable, then conservative management of onychogryphosis is indicated.

Treatment. 1. Conservative management requires the use of a hand-held drill, such as a Dremel drill, and a carborundum pear-shaped grinder. Using a face mask and gloves to restrict the exposure to the nail grindings, the nail plate can be ground and clipped very quickly. The bulk of the nail can be reduced to relieve the symptoms from pressure on the nail plate. Occasionally on some of the older patients the pressure on the thickened onychogryphotic nail will initiate a subungual gangrene. The grinding down and clipping of the nail to prevent pressure at the site of the gangrene is important in its treatment.

2. A more permanent process when medical conditions allow would be to remove the nail plate permanently. This is achieved by a number of methods, some of which include the excision of the matrix and nail bed, which usually requires some surgery on the distal phalanx, or simply the removal of the matrix, which is essentially the sole nail-forming tissue. This then allows a pseudonail to form in the nail bed, but the onychogryphosis will not occur.

3. A medical treatment of nail destruction using urea may be successful. (See Fungal Infections of the Nailplate.)

Onychoschizia

Onychoschizia is the splitting of the nails in a transverse fashion. A successful treatment for this process is not known. Occasionally hydration, by soaking the nails for a number of minutes before bedtime, followed by the application of petrolatum or similar ointments to retain the moisture in the nail plate, may be successful.

The occupation of the patient — especially work requiring moisture followed by drying — and occasionally some nail cosmetics may contribute to the dryness and brittleness of onychoschizia.

Overcurvature of the Nail

Overcurvature of the nail along the longitudinal axis, also referred to as pincer nail or unguis constrictus, is not an uncommon problem. It is seen more often in adults than in children. Overcurvature of the nails of the smaller toes usually does not cause any symptoms. Overcurvature of the first toenail, by encircling tissue, may produce significant pain and discomfort and lead to an inflammatory ingrown toenail.

The degree of curvature and the extent of the nail plate that is involved in the curvature vary a great deal. In some patients the curvature is only on the lateral edge of the nail and may form an acute angle, curving back on itself as the edge is directed toward the mid-axis of the nail plate. In other instances the entire nail plate may be involved in the excess curvature.

The location of pain associated with overcurvature of the nail will vary to some extent but is usually situated in the lateral nail grooves. Patients whose nail plates are involved only at the lateral edge will feel pain in the lateral nail groove simulating an ingrown toenail. Patients with nails in which the entire plate is involved usually have pain along the lateral nail grooves as well, but on occasion they may develop pain just under the midpoint of the distal nail edge dorsal to the distal phalangeal tuft.

Partly because of the age of the patient and the lack of hyperhidrosis which seems to predispose to true ingrown toenail in the adolescent patient, a true ingrowing of nail with a laceration of the soft tissues by the edge of the nail plate, leading to an inflammatory response, is unusual in the overcurved nail plate.

The treatment of the overcurved nail to a great extent depends on the symptoms, the location of the pain, and the anatomic change in the nail. With the total nail involved, pressure over the plate should reproduce pain. It is important to identify whether the pain is in the tissue just beneath the midpoint of the nail or whether it underlies the nail edges in the nail grooves. If the pain is under the midportion of the nail plate, a much more complex procedure is required than with pain emanating from the edges.

Conservative management of the overcurved nail is the grinding down of the nail edges and clipping down the side as proximally as is comfortable. Sometimes the extent of the clipping can be increased by applying 3 per cent salicylic acid in petrolatum to the nail edge for 2 or 3 days before the procedure is undertaken. If the edges can be clipped significantly, the patient usually has relief of pain. In addition, if the nail plate is greatly thickened, a grinding down of the thickness of the nail plate will also reduce this discomfort by diminishing the nail mass upon which shoes exert a great pressure.

If conservative methods — grinding and clipping — are not successful and the pain seems to emanate from the edges, a trial of a wedge resection of the nail plate similar to that used for the inflammatory stage of ingrown toenail (see p. 713) can be tried. If this temporary procedure produces marked relief of pain, then a lateral wedge and corresponding matrix resection may be very successful. Those nails that have only the edges of the nail plate showing the marked incurvature respond to nail wedge resection and corresponding matrix.

If conservative methods and wedge resections of the nails are not successful, or the pain seems to be more central, then a far more complex procedure is necessary. Sometimes the curvature of the nail is so great that it actually captures within this curvature the tuft of the distal phalanx, and this can be verified by radiologic study. In these instances the ablation or resection of the matrix to prevent nail regrowth may be necessary. However, reconstructive procedures described for pincer nail in the literature may be attempted. Our method is to make incisions in the lateral nail folds and connect these with an incision 4 mm distal to the curvature of the nail plate but paralleling the curvature. Then the nail bed is dissected free of the underlying bone to approximately the level of the matrix. The distal tuft of bone is rongeured off and the nail bed then replaced and sutured in place. Usually there is an excess of tissue, which must be trimmed down on the sides. Appropriate dressings are applied. The procedure takes a number of weeks to heal because of the bone surgery. This flattening and reconstruction of the nail bed and matrix is successful in most but not all patients.

Psoriasis

Chronic nail changes are frequently associated with more generalized skin disorders such as psoriasis. Nail changes in psoriasis include thickening of the nail plate and buildup of subungual debris and onycholysis. The most typical change is the presence of multiple punctate pits in the nail surface. Psoriatic nail changes can be very similar in appearance to tinea unguium, causing confusion in diagnosis. Since therapy for the two conditions is completely different, it is important to consider both possibilities and perform appropriate cultures. Treatment of psoriatic nails can be difficult and unrewarding.

Treatment. 1. The application of one of the stronger fluorinated corticosteroid preparations around the nails twice a day, such as fluocinonide gel (Topsyn), fluocinonide (Lidex), or betamethasone (Diprosone), may give relief. Tar (e.g., 10 per cent liquor carbonis detergens or LCD) can be added to the topical corticosteroid preparation.

2. Injection of triamcinolone acetonide (Kenalog-10) directly into the nail matrix of involved digits can be successful. However, since injection into the nail matrix is extremely painful, this method is not popular with most patients and should be used only for severe cases.

3. PUVA therapy (psoralen plus long-wave ultraviolet light) can improve nails as the remainder of the psoriasis clears. However, it should be noted that PUVA should be reserved for the treatment of extensive psoriasis resistant to more traditional measures because of side effects such as the increased risk of skin cancer. Nail involvement alone is not an adequate indication for PUVA.

4. Cytotoxic drugs, such as systemic methotrexate, will often produce dramatic clearing of nails, but should never be used for nail disease alone.

Norwegian Scabies

Nail dystrophy is one of the manifestations of Norwegian scabies, a rare variety of scabies typified by the presence of a huge number of mites in keratotic and crusted skin lesions. Clinically, the nail changes are similar to those seen in psoriasis or tinea unguium. Diagnosis is easily made by finding the mite microscopically from a scraping of skin or nail lesions. Treatment is the same as for ordinary scabies.

Lichen Planus

Lichen planus may involve nails, resulting in longitudinal grooving, ridging, and splitting. More severe involvement may result in atrophy of the nail plate and the formation of a pterygium originating from the proximal nail fold. Usually lichen planus of the nail will be associated with involvement of skin or mucous membranes.

Treatment. 1. Mild nail changes of lichen planus are often reversible as the remainder of the disease resolves. There is no specific therapy for lichen planus, but topical corticosteroid preparations may hasten improvement. Spontaneous resolution after months or years is expected in the typical case.

2. Very severe cases with extensive cutaneous involvement and intractable pruritus may require systemic corticosteroids for relief of symptoms.

3. Injections of the nail matrix with triamcinolone (Kenalog-10), as in psoriasis, may be used for severe nail changes.

Hand Dermatitis (Atopic, Contact, Dyshidrotic)

Dermatitis involving the nail fold and surrounding area can lead to nail dystrophy regardless of the cause of the dermatitis. Often the nail will grow out normally if the dermatitis is controlled, but nail changes can be permanent if the dermatitis is severe enough to cause scarring of the matrix. Treatment is that of the primary dermatitis.

Alopecia Areata

Multiple small pits may be seen in the nails of patients with alopecia areata. This sign may at times be a diagnostic clue if the hair loss is not typical.

There is no specific treatment for the nail changes, but they may improve as the hair regrows.

Nevi and Pigmented Streaks

Subungual or periungual melanoma is not a common occurrence. Approximately 20 per cent of the malignant melanomas of the nail tissues are amelanotic and may be difficult to recognize.

Pigmentation extending into the soft tissues around the nail is strongly suggestive of melanoma. Multiple biopsies interpreted by an experienced pathologist may be needed to make the diagnosis.

A pigmented streak in the nail may be an early sign of acrolentiginous melanoma. These streaks are common in black patients. Unfortunately, although melanomas are uncommon in black patients, one of the more frequent sites and types is ungual acrolentiginous melanoma. Because pigmented streaks are common in black patients, the heavily pigmented and distinct streaks may be the only ones requiring biopsy. In white patients most pigmented nail streaks should be explored.

The technique involves removal of the nail plate and making incisions in the proximal nail fold so as to allow reflection of the nail fold and complete visualization of the nail tissues. Usually the lesion is not a distinct nevus but more of an irregularly colored, spotty pigmentation. It is therefore not always clear as to which site should be biopsied. Again, the most heavily pigmented or abnormal tissue should be sampled and usually at more than one site. A small ellipse, punch biopsy, or other technique may be used. As long as the proximal part of the matrix is not disturbed, there is usually no splitting of the nail plate. If the proximal matrix is divided, then repair, as for split nails, should be done. Multiple biopsies may be made or the entire area of pigmentation excised. Multiple sections should be made through the tissues. It is not uncommon to find only a few sites showing evidence of melanomas.

Tumors

Tumors of the nail can be divided into benign and malignant types. Fibromas which can be excised are not uncommon, especially in tuberous sclerosis. Myxomatous cysts, which may be related to the distal interphalangeal joint synovium (although this is contested), usually are best treated by intralesional corticosteroids (10 mg per ml of triamcinolone). Curettage of these cysts tends to leave a persistent draining area. Occasionally the myxomatous tissue may be excised, but this is not easily accomplished because there is no true capsule. Because myxomas can occur in the central part of the proximal nail fold, resulting in grooving of the nails, care must be taken in any surgical procedure to avoid the extensor tendon of the distal phalanx. Pyogenic granulomas are treated as they are in other sites, usually with scissor removal and light electrodesiccation. Glomus tumors are usually identified by the extreme tenderness of the tissues, especially with point pressure over the lesion or exposure of the digit to cold. It may not be easy to recognize the blue color until the nail plate has been removed and the proximal fold reflected. An incision over the tumor, which is usually encapsulated, a freeing up of the tumor, and a closure with sutures are all that is usually indicated.

Malignant lesions, such as Bowen's disease or squamous cell carcinoma, are not unusual around the nail tissue. Diagnosis may be difficult to make clinically, and any keratotic lesion or even a probable wart that persists in the subungual or periungual tissues should be biopsied to exclude Bowen's disease and squamous cell carcinoma. Surgery should be directed toward preserving the maximal function of the digit. Therefore, histopathologically controlled excision (Mohs' surgery) is desirable in order to minimize the amount of tissue removed while at the same time offering the greatest cure rate. These methods are preferable to amputation of part of the digit and offer a greater histopathologic reliability to the completeness of the excision. Basal cell carcinoma of the nail tissue is uncommon but may be treated also by the histopathologically controlled methods or by other methods such as excision, curettage and electrodesiccation, or x-ray.

The problem of melanomas is usually that of diagnosis and the histopathologic interpretation of the acrolentiginous lesion (see Nevi and Pigmented Streaks). About 20 per cent of melanomas of the nail-forming tissues are amelanotic, adding a further confusion to the diagnosis. Usually some level of amputation is necessary, but reference should be made to some of the more classic review articles on the selection of the level of surgery.

NEVI
(Moles)

method of
MURRAY C. ZIMMERMAN, M.D.
Whittier, California

Moles or nevi are multiple in type, and diagnosis is histologic rather than clinical. The major concern, since removal is usually incomplete, is that one is not unwittingly treating a malignant melanoma. If biopsy of every involved mole is not being taken, write on the chart, "Patient denies growth or change." The chance of a mole turning into a melanoma has been estimated at one per two million moles per year. If there is no history of growth or change, such transformation is most unlikely. Melanomas are discussed on page 662.

Classification

Junction Nevi. Junction nevi are those with increased clear cell numbers and activity at the dermoepidermal junction. In young children almost all nevi will show junctional activity. In a 90-year-old person such activity is extremely rare. Junctional activity is often present, extending down the epithelial cells lining hair follicles and sweat glands. It is the cause for "maculation" or a brown macule or freckle of pigment appearing in the center of a healed scar site after a mole is removed by shaving its top.

Compound Nevus. Here there is dermoepidermal junction activity plus intradermal nevus cells.

Dermal Nevus. This shows minimal or no dermoepidermal junction activity, only intradermal nevus cells.

Blue Nevus. This can be differentiated clinically because it actually looks blue. The blueness is due to the Tyndall effect of light dispersion on the brown granules in the cutis, which are very deep. A shallow removal of a blue nevus will dismay the unprepared doctor, because there will be sinister-looking brown pigment even at the base of a fairly deep scoop excision.

Juvenile Nevus. This is the spindle and epithelial cell nevus, usually a pink, raised nevus under 1 cm, diagnosed only microscopically. It may appear in adults.

Congenital Nevus. The patient is actually born with this type, frequently up to bathing trunk size or larger. These nevi have nevus cells extending down the full thickness of the skin and have an incidence of malignant change of up to 15 per cent. Their removal frequently is almost a career, rather than a job, for a team of plastic surgeons with multiple skin graft surgeries. Even this heroic therapy is unsatisfactory.

Halo Nevi. These are dark nevi, usually on the trunk, with a clear area of white depigmentation around them. The nevus is usually 5 to 10 mm in diameter and the clear area of depigmentation around it (halo) another centimeter or two. These are said to be the immune reaction to a malignant melanoma which the patient himself is destroying through his immune mechanism. On biopsy the cells look as if they have been through a blender and scrambled with inflammatory cells.

Epidermal Pigmentation Without Nevus Cells. A *freckle* or *ephelis* shows no increase in clear cells, only increased pigment. A *lentigo* shows more than the normal ratio of one clear cell to seven to nine dermoepidermal junction cells. *Melanosis* is a diffuse pigmentation such as that seen on the cheeks of pregnant women where, microscopically, no abnormality is seen. All of these are flat macules.

Epithelial Nevi. These include non–nevus cell nevi, such as linear epithelial nevus and seborrheic keratoses.

Malignant Melanoma. This may appear in all its various classifications.

Reasons for Removal of Nevi

1. If the patient gives a history of growth or change in a given mole, or a history of itching, or a history of bleeding without trauma, the mole should be removed.

2. Nevi on the palms, soles, or genitalia should be removed, according to some authors.

3. Any moles subject to chronic irritation by a shoulder strap, belt, bra strap, comb, or razor, may be removed.

4. Any mole which is unsightly, from a cosmetic point of view, may be removed for cosmetic purposes if this is desirable to the patient.

Since patients are said to have an average of around 30 moles per person, it would be impossible to remove all of the moles from all the population. The differential diagnosis of suspicious melanomas is given elsewhere.

Informed Consent

1. *Scar:* Before removal of the moles, tell the patient and have him sign a consent form, or write in the chart that (1) no matter how a mole is removed, it will leave a scar, and (2) the farther down on the body this is done, the more scarring it will leave. For example, on the face frequently the scars will be invisible and on the neck barely visible, whereas on the thorax there will always be

a permanent discolored scar, and progressively downward more and more scarring.

2. *Keloid:* Warn the patient, in multiple superficial mole removal from the trunk, that about 1 person in 20 will develop a hypertrophic scar or a keloid that may require x-ray or cryotherapy to flatten.

3. *Maculation:* Then warn the patient that in multiple mole removal "maculation" may develop in the scar. By "maculation" I mean a flat freckle of pigment, which should not rise but which will be present in the flat scar. In 2-year-old children, this will be present in 9 out of 10; in 20-year-olds, in about 1 out of 4; and in 90-year-olds, in about 1 out of 40. These pigmented macules cause a great deal of concern if not mentioned in advance.

My chart in a 20-year-old would express this as follows: "Pt. told: D 1:20M → scar ↑ scar c̄ ↓ locus. M̶ 1:4. Keloid 1:20." M̶ is my symbol for "maculation." It is said that juries believe everything that is in a chart and nothing that isn't. "D 1:20M" means "death, 1:20,000." If death is mentioned as a complication, lesser complications are covered (126 CAL. RPT. 976) even if not mentioned.

Biopsy. Biopsy is not recommended for all nevi, but for at least a random sampling if many are removed. If large numbers are being removed, several can be submitted in one specimen bottle, noted in the chart as "large," "medium," and "small." Another way to identify different nevi for biopsy is to dip the first one in Mrs. Stewart's Bluing, the second in India ink, and the third in merbromin (Mercurochrome). Enough of these will stick to the specimens to identify them as a specific mole, so that more can be put into the same specimen bottle of 10 per cent formaldehyde. As an alternative to this, old short end nonsterile pieces of suture material with armed needles can be saved, and as many as ten nevi can be strung on the suture like beads on a string. If the first one is identified with staining or because of its size, all the others will follow in sequence. This will not endear the doctor to the laboratory technician who has to align these in a block, but it is really not any more trouble than any other tissue specimen.

Techniques of Removal

Total. If there is a suspicion that a given mole might be a melanoma, excision biopsy with 0.5 cm margin around is the best technique, using the classic elliptical excision and suturing. The ellipse should have its long axis parallel to the tension lines of the skin. A wrinkle line or the direction of hair growth is usually a better indicator than a textbook picture. Buried sutures should be used to reduce the size of this wound,

since it will usually spread postsurgically to the same width as before skin sutures are put in. If the biopsy confirms the diagnosis of melanoma, a much wider, deeper excision with grafting is necessary.

Partial or Shaved Removal. This technique is recommended for at least 95 per cent of ordinary raised nevi. It is extremely fast, gives adequate tissue for biopsy, and heals with a minimum of surgical follow-up and a minimum of scarring. It is not suitable for a flat macule.

CLEANSING OF THE SKIN SITE. This can be undertaken with either 70 per cent alcohol or povidone (Betadine) solution.

ANESTHESIA. This is best administered with 1 or 2 per cent lidocaine with 1:100,000 epinephrine, in a lock syringe, through a ½-inch 30 gauge needle. The anesthesia should be injected back from the edge of the tumor. The epinephrine will produce physical blanching of the tumor. As an alternative to this, an extremely skillful operator can spray freeze with Freon 114 (Frigiderm) or Fluorethyl (a mixture of Freon 114 and ethyl chloride). This is sprayed on for about 10 seconds until the entire area turns white and is frozen solid. Total anesthesia and hemostasis are achieved, but these last only about 20 seconds. The operator who cannot complete the surgery in 20 seconds should use an injectable local anesthetic. As skill and speed are required, however, freezing will allow moles to be removed, even from apprehensive children, without a tear. A demonstration to an apprehensive child that the spray freezing on his hand will not hurt or harm him is usually enough.

SHAVING. After anesthesia, the skin around the mole is pinched up by the operator's left thumb and forefinger, and a scalpel with a *large* blade, either a No. 10 or a No. 21, is taken in the right hand. This is shaved across, parallel to the skin, from side to side, at the level of the normal surrounding skin. Since the area is raised in the operator's hand and is pinched, the mild pressure of the pinching prevents or minimizes capillary bleeding. When this is shaved off with the lesion pinched, there is automatically a slight concavity produced in the center of the mole site. This is desirable. The larger the mole, the more concave it should be. Otherwise the mole site, which is perfectly flat when the scab comes off, will be raised slightly in 3 months. A single masterful sweep is the best way, rather than nervously swinging back and forth and making a lot of tissue damage with multiple hesitant cuts.

HEMOSTASIS. The scalpel is then set down with the right hand, and the firm grip on the mole held with the left hand, so that bleeding is minimal. If this is bleeding, it should be touched once with a swab, to wipe away the blood; then a cotton-tipped applicator stick with either Monsel's solution (ferric subsulfate) or 80 per cent trichloroacetic acid is rolled onto the dry surface. Do not expect either of these agents to stop a gush of blood, because they will not do it. The lesion base *must* be dry. Then if these are rolled on, they will coagulate the cut ends of any blood vessels and prevent new bleeding. Gradually finger pressure can be released, in 10 seconds or so. If bleeding is seen, pinch again, with further rolling, until total control of bleeding is achieved. Trichloroacetic acid will stain the base of the wound white, and Monsel's solution, brown. An alternative to this is light electrodesiccation of the surface, again with the base first dried and then electrodesiccation to the *dry* base. This should be done not with the point of the needle, but with the flat. If the electric needle is being used, the skin should be dried of alcohol, since it is disconcerting to the patient and surgeon alike if alcohol fumes explode from the spark.

BANDAGING. Bandaging is required only where friction from clothing or something else is going to be a problem. The germ count stays lower on an unbandaged skin, and postoperative care should entail, in most cases, judicious neglect for at least 48 hours. The scab will fall off the face in about 7 days, on the trunk and arms in about 14 days, and on the legs in about 28 days.

HEALING. As healing proceeds, if the wound is not on this timetable or if there is erythema around the wound, a local antibiotic such as polymyxin B–bacitracin (Polysporin) ointment or polymyxin B–bacitracin–neomycin (NeoSporin) powder may be used, or an internal antibiotic such as tetracycline or erythromycin may be given. The presence of redness and scale in the scalp, indicating infectious dandruff, should be treated with selenium sulfide (Selsun, Exsel) shampoos twice daily; otherwise this low grade infection will slow healing of surgical sites near the scalp.

OCCUPATIONAL DERMATOSES

method of
FRANK C. KORANDA, M.D.
Iowa City, Iowa

Afflictions of the skin represent 40 to 65 per cent of reported occupational diseases. Occupational dermatoses are those skin problems which are aggravated or produced by the working environment.

In 90 to 95 per cent of cases, occupational dermatoses present as a dermatitis or an eczematous condition whose hallmarks are erythema, scaling, fissuring, edema, and often vesiculation and exudation. Most of these occupational contact dermatitis cases are due to contact irritation from chemical agents rather than to true contact allergy. The remaining 5 to 10 per cent of occupational dermatoses represent (1) infections, (2) occupational acne and chloracne, (3) mechanical trauma, (4) foreign body granulomas, (5) neoplasms, benign and malignant, and (6) pigmentary changes. The following skin diseases may predispose an individual to occupational dermatoses: atopic dermatitis, dyshidrosis of the hands and feet, nummular dermatitis, tinea infections, acne, psoriasis, and nonoccupational contact dermatitis. A careful history is essential for establishing whether a dermatosis is occupationally related.

Irritant Contact Dermatitis

Occupational contact dermatitis is usually an irritant reaction. Such a reaction is not an allergy. It is due to a physical change in the skin, which may occur in any person who is sufficiently and prolongedly exposed. Primarily the hands are affected. Dyshidrosis and other causes of hand eczema predispose. The most common occupational irritants are acids, alkalis, solvents, detergents, soaps, cutting oils, and heavy metals.

Treatment. 1. Personal hygiene and plant cleanliness are the major preventive measures.

2. Skin cleansing should be performed with a mild soap such as pHisoDerm.

3. Barrier creams provide little or no protection.

4. Gloves may be helpful as long as they are impenetrable and the irritant does not get inside them.

5. Daily or twice daily soaking of the hands in lukewarm water for 20 minutes, followed by the application of petrolatum jelly, Shepard's cream, or Bag Balm, helps prevent drying and fissuring.

Allergic Contact Dermatitis

Occupational contact dermatitis resulting from an allergic reaction, while much less common, is most frequently caused by rubber antioxidants and accelerators, epoxy resins, formaldehyde, nickel, chromates, and oleoresins. The only preventive measure is avoidance of contact with the allergen.

Treatment. 1. For chronic and subacute contact dermatitis, a topical steroid cream, triamcinolone acetonide 0.1 per cent (Aristocort A) cream or fluocinolone acetonide 0.025 per cent (Synemol) cream, is applied three to four times a day.

2. When the hands are affected, the more potent topical steroids, fluocinonide (Lidex E) or desoximetasone (Topicort), are required.

3. For extensive and severe dermatitis, a short course of systemic steroids is most expedient, efficacious, and cost effective. Prednisone, 40 to 50 mg every morning upon rising, may be taken for 10 to 15 days with no need for tapering the dose.

Infections

Skin affected by an occupational dermatitis is prone to secondary infections. Impetigo, folliculitis, or furunculosis may result.

Treatment. 1. Ten days of treatment with oral penicillin V potassium (Pen-Vee K) or erythromycin, 250 mg every 6 hours, is indicated.

2. Adjunctive therapy is with an antibacterial cleanser, chlorhexidine gluconate (Hibiclens), and with warm compresses.

Working in a warm, humid environment is conducive to superficial fungal infections and to candidiasis. Both conditions will respond to either haloprogin (Halotex) or miconazole (Mica-Tin) solution applied twice a day for 14 days.

Herpes simplex may occur in dental and medical workers from occupational exposure. Warm tea bag compresses may be used for 15 minutes every 4 to 6 hours, followed by povidone-iodine (Betadine) ointment until resolution.

Occupational Acne and Chloracne

Exposure to crude petroleum, cutting oils, greases, and coal tar may induce an occupational "oil acne." It starts as an inflammatory folliculitis from contact with contaminated clothing. Daily changes of work clothes, skin hygiene, 5 and 10 per cent benzoyl peroxide gels, and tetracycline, 500 to 1000 mg a day, make up the treatment.

Chloracne is a severe, recalcitrant disease produced by chlorinated aromatic hydrocarbons. These chemicals are used in some herbicides and pesticides and on some electrical devices. For any worker exposed to these chemicals, there should be the strictest skin hygiene, daily changes of work clothes, and separate lockers for street clothes and work clothes. If chloracne should ensue, the worker should be totally removed from the environment of exposure and conventional acne treatment begun.

Mechanical Trauma

Mechanical factors may induce alterations in skin. Acute exposure to pressure and friction can cause blister formation. Benzoin tincture may be applied. For prevention, mole skin and the wearing of gloves or two pairs of socks are helpful.

If the pressure and friction are of a gradually increasing or an intermittent intensity, thickening and hyperkeratosis of the skin surface occur. Treatment is with a 10 per cent urea cream (Aquacare HP or Nutraplus) or 20 per cent urea cream (Carmol), which should be applied to the skin every time after it is wet. Mechanical removal of the hyperkeratosis with a mildly abrasive sponge, Buf Puf, facilitates resolution.

If the pressure is more circumscribed, a callus can develop. It should be pared away with a scalpel or razor blade. A 40 per cent salicylic acid plaster, slightly larger than the callus, is applied and secured with cloth adhesive tape. It is left in place for 5 to 7 days. After removal, the callus is pared away again. This process is repeated as necessary.

Foreign Body Granulomas

Foreign body granulomas may be surgically excised. The specimen should be examined histologically. The causes are silica, zirconium, talc, beryllium, and magnesium.

Neoplasms

Benign and malignant growths may result from ultraviolet irradiation, x-irradiation, and topical carcinogens. After verification of the diagnosis by biopsy, these lesions are treated surgically. Sunscreens with the highest sun protection factor (SPF 15) should be recommended for those workers subject to solar exposure. These sunscreens (PreSun 15, Total Eclipse, Super Shade) should be applied every morning to the sun-exposed skin.

Pigmentary Changes

Alkyl phenols can cause permanent depigmentation of the skin. They are used as antioxidants in lubricating oils and plastics and as germicidal disinfectants. For limited areas of leukoderma, Vitadye solution and Covermark may be applied as camouflage. For more extensive depigmentation, therapy with oral psoralens and sunlight may be considered.

Hyperpigmentation may result as a postinflammatory response to dermatitis. Time and patience are the best prescriptions. Contact with tar and with certain plants and cosmetics may lead to hyperpigmentation. Much of this will resolve with sun avoidance and with the daily use of a sunscreen lotion with a sun protection factor of 15. If pigmentation still persists, Kligman's bleaching formula of 0.1 per cent tretinoin, 5.0 per cent hydroquinone, and 0.1 per cent dexamethasone in hydrophilic ointment may be applied daily for 6 to 8 weeks.

PEDICULOSIS

method of
HOWARD L. SALYER, M.D.
Nashville, Tennessee

There are three species of lice that naturally infest humans: (1) *Pediculus humanus var. capitis* (the head louse), (2) *Pediculus humanus var. corporis* (the body louse), and (3) *Phthirus pubis,* the pubic or crab louse. All three species feed on the skin, producing intense pruritus. They are worldwide in distribution and are on the increase clinically.

One per cent lindane (gamma benzene hexachloride) has been used in the United States for nearly 30 years to control lice. Until recent years this chemical was applied to the integument without regard to possible ill effects from percutaneous absorption. It is now known that 10 per cent of lindane can be absorbed from the skin into the blood after excessive or prolonged topical application and can have possible neurotoxic effects. Lindane is still in effect for treatment of lice, but the amount and duration of its use on the skin should be carefully monitored, and only the precise amount that is needed for treatment of the patient and contacts should be prescribed.

Pediculosis Capitis

Pediculosis capitis (head louse) is seen most frequently in children and women but can infest the scalp of any child or adult. There appear to be epidemics, especially in certain schools in the community, in which a large number of cases occur. Long hair encourages the condition, and communication may occur by shared hats, combs, or brushes.

There is usually an intense pruritus. The affected hairs become lusterless and dry. Secondary complications such as furunculosis and impetigo, especially at the nape of the neck and upper contiguous parts of the back, are common. In such instances the cervical nodes may become enlarged.

Diagnosis is made by identification of the oval nit (egg) cemented to a scalp hair, usually near the base. Microscopic examination allows ready differentiation from hair casts, seborrheic scales, and hair spray concretions.

Treatment. *Step 1:* Shampoo thoroughly with 30 ml (2 tablespoons) 1 per cent gamma benzene hexachloride shampoo for 4 minutes. Rinse well and dry.

Step 2: Don clean clothing.

Step 3: Secondary infection should be treated with appropriate systemic antibiotics.

Step 4: Contaminated clothing should be machine washed and dried with a 20 minute hot cycle. Nonwashable clothing should be dry cleaned, and combs, brushes, and so forth may be washed with 1 per cent gamma benzene hexachloride shampoo.

Step 5: Remaining nits may be removed with a fine-toothed comb or forceps. This is a tedious task, which may be facilitated by prior application of a solution of equal parts of white vinegar and water. This mixture softens the cement binding the nit to the hair.

Step 6: The shampooing should be repeated at the end of 1 week in order to kill any newly hatched lice (gamma benzene hexachloride is ovicidal, but may not be ovicidal to the entire nit population).

Step 7: Other persons in the family should be examined, but only those infested need be treated.

Pediculosis Corporis

Body louse infestation is usually associated with poor personal hygiene and wearing of clothing for prolonged periods without laundering. It is the least common form of lice seen in ordinary clinical practice.

The louse is found on the body itself only in cases of severe infestation; rather, it lives in the clothing, especially in seams, and leaves only briefly to feed on the skin. The resulting pruritus is responsible for the usual clinical picture, i.e., excoriations of the neck and trunk, and especially intrascapular areas.

Treatment. *Step 1:* Begin a program of good personal hygiene, with regular bathing and changes of clothing and bed linen. This is the most important step.

Step 2: Following the first bath, apply 1 per cent gamma benzene hexachloride lotion or cream over the entire body, and wash off after 4 hours. (This step should be omitted in children younger than 6 years.)

Step 3: Secondary bacterial infection should be treated with appropriate systemic antibiotics.

Step 4: Likely contacts should be examined, and treated when indicated.

Step 5: Lice and their eggs must be eradicated from clothing. Machine washing in hot water or drying at high heat for 20 minutes will destroy the parasites. Dry cleaning is adequate for nonwashable garments.

Pediculosis Pubis

The crab louse favors the hairy skin of the anogenital region, particularly the pubic area, but

723

may wander far afield, especially in hirsute persons, in whom infestation of body and axillary hair is not uncommon. Beards and mustaches are occasionally affected, and in children involvement of eyelashes and hairline zones of the scalp may be found. Pediculosis pubis is usually contracted by adults as a result of sexual intercourse, but it can also be acquired from bedding, toilets, and so on.

Pruritus is the usual complaint, and careful examination of the pubic hair will show the small, grayish nit cemented to the hair shaft near its base. The parasite itself, measuring 1 to 2 mm, can occasionally be observed, usually clinging to a hair and sucking blood, which gives it a rust color. It is an obligate parasite, living exclusively on human blood, and will die within 24 hours if separated from a host.

Treatment. *Step 1:* Following a thorough soapy shower or bath and drying, 1 per cent gamma benzene hexachloride lotion or cream is applied to the infested and adjacent hair areas, with particular attention to the mons pubis and perianal area. In a very hairy individual, application from the neck to the knees is advisable. No shaving is necessary.

Step 2: The medication should remain on the skin for 8 hours, following which a second shower or bath is taken.

Step 3: Fresh clothes should be donned, and the bed linen changed.

Step 4: Since this is almost always a venereal disease, a Venereal Disease Research Laboratory (VDRL) test for syphilis should be ordered.

Step 5: After 7 days, the treatment is repeated.

Step 6: Treatment of eyelash infestation is most safely accomplished by twice daily application of a thick coat of petrolatum for 8 days, followed by mechanical removal of remaining nits.

Step 7: Sexual contacts should be treated simultaneously in the same manner.

PIGMENTARY DISTURBANCES

method of
DAVID N. SILVERS, M.D.
New York, New York

Skin color is genetically determined. The number of pigment-producing cells (melanocytes) is the same in the skin of blacks and whites.

However, the number, size, and distribution of pigment granules (melanosomes) within the cells of the epidermis account for differences in skin color.

A form of pigmentary alteration considered desirable by many individuals is the suntan. Melanocytes respond to the ultraviolet rays of the sun, especially in the range of 2800 to 4000 angstroms (Å), by synthesizing an increased number of larger-sized pigment granules, resulting in a darker skin tone. Some fair-complexioned individuals do not tan but burn severely after even short exposures to sunlight.

Increased tolerance to sunlight and *enhanced pigmentation* can both be achieved by administration of trioxsalen (Trisoralen). Ten mg (2 tablets) are taken daily 2 hours before exposure to sun or ultraviolet irradiation. The initial exposure should be 15 to 20 minutes, and this is increased by 5 minutes per day. Although Trisoralen should be administered for no longer than 14 days (total dose, 28 tablets), increased sun tolerance and enhanced pigmentation can be maintained by periodic exposure to sunlight. This treatment is appropriate for therapeutic but not cosmetic purposes.

Hyperpigmentation

A variety of endocrinologic conditions can result in *diffuse hyperpigmentation* of the skin, presumably as a response to increased secretion of melanocyte stimulating hormone (MSH) and adrenocorticotropic hormone (ACTH) by the pituitary gland or through increased sensitivity of the melanocytes to normal amounts of these circulating hormones. The prototype of diffuse hyperpigmentation is Addison's disease (primary adrenal insufficiency). Hypermelanosis also occurs in patients with pituitary hyperplasia, adrenalectomy, and hypercorticism. Correction of the underlying condition does not necessarily result in a return to normal skin color. Generalized hypermelanosis may also be associated with diseases of the liver and biliary tract, including hemochromatosis, primary biliary cirrhosis, and porphyria cutanea tarda, and with a variety of nutritional deficiencies, including those of vitamin B_{12} and folic acid.

Melasma is a form of circumscribed hypermelanosis characterized by symmetrical, mottled hyperpigmented macules on the forehead, cheeks, temples, and upper lip. It occurs most commonly in pregnant women and women taking oral contraceptives. The condition is exacerbated by exposure to sunlight.

Postinflammatory hyperpigmentation is a common sequela of a wide variety of inflammatory dermatoses; it may fade spontaneously over a period of weeks or months. However, if it does not lighten satisfactorily, active treatment may be effective, provided that the hyperpigmentation is principally a manifestation of excess melanin within the epidermis and is not due, in large part, to deposition of melanin in the dermis, where it simulates a tattoo. While the aforementioned distinction can be made with certainty only by skin biopsy, it is more practical to assume that the pigmentation is primarily epidermal and to treat as such.

Treatment of Melasma and Postinflammatory Hyperpigmentation. 1. A cream containing equal parts of hydroquinone 4 per cent, tretinoin (Retin-A) 1 per cent, and hydrocortisone 2.5 per cent is applied to the hyperpigmented sites twice daily. If there is no significant irritation after 1 week, the frequency of application can be increased. A high potency fluorinated corticosteroid (i.e., triamcinolone acetonide 0.5 per cent) can be substituted for the hydrocortisone. However, its use over a period of several months can result in telangiectasias, thinning of the skin, and rosacea.

2. Use of the more potent depigmenting agent monobenzone 20 per cent (Benoquin) is not recommended, since the degree of lightening induced by this agent is difficult to control and irreversible depigmentation can occur, even at sites remote from the treated site.

3. Treatment should be continued until the desired skin tone is reached or until 6 weeks have passed without improvement.

4. Exposure of the hyperpigmented skin to sunlight must be avoided. Although opaque sunscreens (Reflecta, Covermark) which shield the skin from all wavelengths of light are most effective, their use is cosmetically unacceptable to most persons. The most practical and effective sunscreens are those containing para-aminobenzoic acid (PABA) (PreSun, Pabanol), PABA esters (Sea & Ski, Pabafilm, Block Out), or benzophenones (Solbar, Uval). Sunscreens are "rated" numerically according to their effectiveness in protecting the skin from exposure to ultraviolet light. Those rated 15 are virtually total blocking agents, reducing the amount of light in the burning wavelengths (2900 to 3200 Å) by nearly 95 per cent. If affected skin sites are not carefully protected from the sun, hyperpigmentation, especially in the case of melasma, is very likely to recur.

Hypopigmentation

Hypopigmentation may be secondary to a variety of inflammatory dermatoses. The same types of inflammatory processes which result in localized areas of hyperpigmentation may also cause hypopigmentation, which is usually temporary, requiring no treatment. While the melanocytes are not destroyed, they temporarily stop synthesizing melanin. A common example of postinflammatory hypopigmentation is *pityriasis alba,* a condition seen in children with atopic dermatitis and characterized by pale, oval patches of skin, especially on the cheeks. A common fungal infection, *tinea versicolor,* is characterized by hypopigmented macules on the skin of the chest, back, neck, and upper arms. This condition is controlled with the topical application of an antifungal agent such as miconazole nitrate (MicaTin) and clotrimazole (Lotrimin). The solution or cream is applied twice daily to the affected areas for 2 weeks, daily for 4 weeks, and then twice weekly for 3 months. Although treatment usually eradicates the organisms, the hypopigmented spots do not disappear until they are re-exposed to sunlight.

The most common condition resulting in a generalized loss of pigmentation is *vitiligo.* Although usually idiopathic, vitiligo may be associated with a variety of endocrinopathies and is characterized by progressive whitening of the skin, beginning most commonly on the extensor aspects of the extremities and around body orifices. Achieving repigmentation of vitiliginous sites is a difficult task often requiring many months of treatment.

Treatment of Vitiligo. 1. In the active stage of vitiligo, the condition is characterized by inflammation and erythema at the sites of pigment loss. Administration of systemic steroids (prednisone, 20 mg each morning for 1 week, then 15 mg every other morning for 2 weeks) may inhibit destruction of melanocytes. Application of topical corticosteroids is generally not effective in inhibiting the progression of the condition.

2. The most effective method for inducing repigmentation of vitiliginous sites is through the combined use of trioxsalen (Trisoralen) and measured exposure to ultraviolet light. Trioxsalen, 10 mg, is taken daily, approximately 2 hours before exposure to sunlight or fluorescent black light. Initial exposure should be approximately 15 minutes, and daily exposure can be increased by 5 minutes. Care should be taken not to get sunburned. Substitution for trioxsalen with 8-methoxsalen (Oxsoralen), a naturally occurring psoralen, is not recommended because it is more likely to produce severe phototoxicity (sunburn).

3. Repigmentation characteristically begins in a perifollicular fashion. Some repigmentation

should be noted within 3 months, or therapy should be stopped.

4. The patient should protect his eyes with sunglasses (plastic lenses with top and side panels to protect against reflected light).

5. The use of topically applied psoralen with subsequent exposure to ultraviolet light is discouraged. Although repigmentation may be induced, serious burns have resulted despite careful monitoring of the treatment.

6. Although various preparations have been specifically formulated to hide the vitiliginous sites, most patients do not find them satisfactory. Cosmetics available in department stores and pharmacies seem as well accepted.

7. Tattooing "flesh colored" pigment into the vitiliginous skin sites has produced poor results. Skin color changes with exposure to sunlight, thereby making it impossible to reproduce the appropriate skin shade for all seasons.

8. If the vitiliginous areas are truly extensive and repigmentation with psoralen is unsuccessful, total depigmentation of the skin may be acceptable. Total depigmentation can be achieved by the application of monobenzone 20 per cent (Benoquin).

Pigmented Lesions of the Skin

A wide variety of skin lesions typically are pigmented. Most are benign, including the following: freckle (localized site of hyperpigmentation), melanocytic nevus (focal proliferation of melanocytes), dermatofibroma (hyperpigmentation of the epidermis secondary to a fibrohistiocytic dermal proliferation), and seborrheic keratosis (focal proliferation of keratinocytes containing abundant melanin). Examples of malignant lesions that may be pigmented include basal cell carcinoma, Bowen's disease (squamous cell carcinoma), and malignant melanoma. Differentiation of the aforementioned lesions requires considerable clinical experience; histologic examination is recommended to confirm the diagnosis of any lesion in question.

Of the lesions mentioned above, the only one which is not a tumor is the freckle. It is histologically similar to postinflammatory hyperpigmentation, and lightening may be achieved by the application of a cream containing hydroquinone 4 per cent, tretinoin 1 per cent, and triamcinolone acetonide 0.5 per cent. The substitution of the fluorinated high potency corticosteroid for hydrocortisone will accelerate the lightening, and the potential adverse reactions should not be a problem when the preparation is being restricted to specific, small skin sites.

PEMPHIGUS AND PEMPHIGOID

method of
JOHN C. MAIZE, M.D.
Charleston, South Carolina

Pemphigus and pemphigoid are chronic vesiculobullous eruptions. The characteristic histologic feature of all forms of pemphigus is acantholysis of the squamous cells of the epidermis. The loss of cohesion between the epidermal cells results in vesicle formation. The acantholysis in pemphigus vulgaris and pemphigus vegetans occurs in the suprabasilar portion of the epidermis, and in pemphigus foliaceus and pemphigus erythematosus it occurs in the granular zone. Clinically, pemphigus vulgaris presents bullae that are flaccid and fragile, usually developing on uninflamed skin and mucous membranes. Downward pressure on a blister causes it to extend peripherally with ease; if friction is applied on normal-appearing skin, typical blisters can be induced (Nikolsky's sign). The blisters in pemphigus vulgaris rupture easily and reveal an oozing base. The resulting erosions show little tendency to heal spontaneously. The disease may begin with oral erosions or as a persistent scalp pyoderma. It may vary in severity from only a few relatively innocuous lesions to a generalized disease that can terminate in death. Pemphigus vegetans, which probably is a tumescent variant of longstanding lesions of pemphigus vulgaris, occurs predominantly in the intertriginous areas.

Direct immunofluorescence study of perilesional skin of patients with all forms of pemphigus generally demonstrates the presence of IgG antibodies in the epidermal intercellular spaces. The sera of 80 to 85 per cent of patients with active pemphigus have IgG pemphigus antibodies. There is a generally direct, although incomplete, correlation between the clinical extent of the disease and the antibody titer. Recent investigations demonstrating that pemphigus antibody is capable of inducing acantholysis in human epidermal cells grown in organ culture provide additional evidence for a pathogenic role of these antibodies.

Pemphigoid is a disease of older people. Its early lesions are urticarial papules and plaques, often with geographic shapes. Direct immunofluorescent examination of the perilesional area of pemphigoid blisters demonstrates the deposition of IgG and complement in linear fashion along the basement membrane zone.

TABLE 1. **Immunofluorescence Findings in Pemphigus and Pemphigoid**

DISEASE	DIRECT IMMUNO-FLUORESCENCE	SERUM ANTIBODIES
Pemphigus	+	+
Bullous pemphigoid	+	+
Cicatricial pemphigoid	+	Infrequent (10%)

Approximately 75 per cent of patients have circulating anti-basement membrane zone antibodies. The antibody titer, however, does not tend to show direct correlation with the severity of disease.

Cicatricial pemphigoid (benign mucous membrane pemphigoid) is an uncommon subepidermal bullous process that predominantly affects mucous membranes, but can also involve the skin. It usually begins in the mouth, but often extends to involve the eyes. Blindness is the most serious consequence of the conjunctival scarring, belying the title "benign mucous membrane pemphigoid." Direct immunofluorescence examination of perilesional areas of the mouth reveals basement membrane zone antibody in most cases, but serum basement membrane antibodies are detectable in only about 10 per cent of patients. The relationship to bullous pemphigoid is not currently known, although both conditions are characterized by subepidermal bullae and have associated anti-basement membrane zone antibodies.

Treatment

Pemphigus. Systemic corticosteroids are generally required to control pemphigus vulgaris; however, the morbidity induced by long-term, high-dose corticosteroid therapy has become a major clinical consideration in the management of pemphigus. The use of alternate day theapy has been proposed to minimize the incidence of corticosteroid-induced morbidity; however, alternate day therapy is usually not successful in achieving control in patients with extensive disease. Daily, single-dose therapy using a short-acting corticosteroid is usually as effective as daily divided doses in controlling the disease and reduces the risk of hypothalamic-pituitary-adrenal suppression. For patients with extensive disease, therapy is usually initiated in a dose of 2 mg of prednisone per kg of body weight every morning. Immunosuppressive agents (azathioprine, methotrexate, cyclophosphamide) usually require approximately 6 weeks to exert a beneficial effect. They are not as effective as prednisone for achieving control of pemphigus,

but they are useful for their steroid-sparing effect in long-term therapy. Immunosuppressive drugs should be used only by physicians who are thoroughly familiar with their complex effects. It should also be noted that these agents are not approved for treatment of bullous diseases by the Food and Drug Administration. Azathioprine may be started in a dosage of 1 to 2 mg per kg (or other immunosuppressive drug in appropriate dosage) at the same time prednisone therapy is begun, with careful monitoring of renal, hepatic, and hematologic functions. The patient must also be observed closely for intercurrent infection. Although the pemphigus antibody titer will generally correlate with disease activity in a given patient, careful clinical monitoring is the best indicator for adjusting the dosage of prednisone and the immunosuppressants. When the development of new blisters has ceased, tapering of the dose may be started. If both prednisone and an immunosuppressant are being used concurrently, the dosage of only one agent at a time should be adjusted, leaving at least a week in between to observe clinical activity. When the patient appears to be in complete clinical remission, repeated direct and indirect immunofluorescent studies should be done at approximately monthly intervals while the maintenance therapy is slowly tapered. When circulating and in vivo bound antibodies are no longer detectable, the corticosteroid and/or immunosuppressant therapy can be completely tapered and discontinued. Topical therapy is generally not helpful in controlling the disease, but daily baths are useful for removing crusts, and topical silver sulfadiazine (Silvadene Cream) is soothing and prevents bacterial overgrowth on denuded skin which can impede re-epithelialization.

Pemphigus erythematosus, pemphigus foliaceus, and pemphigus vegetans are usually more easily controllable than pemphigus vulgaris. Therapy for pemphigus erythematosus and pemphigus vegetans should be initiated with open wet dressings to remove accumulated scale-crusts, followed by the application of a fluorinated topical corticosteroid cream three or four times daily. Intralesional injection of triamcinolone hexacetonide (Aristospan), 5 mg per ml, is helpful for resistant lesions. It can be diluted 1:1 with sterile saline solution and administered in a dosage of 0.5 mg per square cm of lesional skin at monthly intervals. In pemphigus foliaceus and recalcitrant cases of pemphigus erythematosus and pemphigus vegetans, topical therapy combined with prednisone given in a single daily dose of 40 to 60 mg is usually adequate for control. The dose of prednisone can be tapered according to clinical response. As in the case of pemphigus vulgaris, the disappearance of pemphigus antibody from the serum and skin is a useful guide as to when maintenance therapy can be safely discontinued.

Intramuscular gold preparations, administered in the same dosage and with the same precautions as for rheumatoid arthritis, may be effective in the management of patients with pemphigus for whom corticosteroids are contraindicated, but it is not the drug of choice for pemphigus. (This use of intramuscular gold preparations is not listed in the manufacturers' official directives.)

Pemphigoid. Bullous pemphigoid is not generally as severe a condition as pemphigus vulgaris, and adequate treatment often culminates in prolonged remission. Treatment of generalized bullous pemphigoid is initiated with prednisone in a dose of 1 mg per kg given once daily. Immunosuppressants can also be used concurrently as in pemphigus vulgaris. Wet dressings or baths are useful for removing adherent crusts, and silver sulfadiazine (Silvadene Cream) can be applied after bathing to prevent bacterial overgrowth and thereby facilitate re-epithelialization. Hydroxyzine (Atarax, Vistaril), 25 mg three times daily, reduces pruritus. When new lesions have stopped forming, the dose of prednisone (and immunosuppressants) should be slowly tapered, adjusting the dose of only one drug at a time at weekly intervals. If new lesions develop, the dose should be raised to the level that was capable of controlling the disease before breakthrough occurred. When disease activity is completely controlled and the maintenance dose of corticosteroids has been reduced to low levels, repeat direct and indirect immunofluorescence should be done. If no anti–basement membrane zone antibody is detectable, maintenance therapy can be discontinued.

Localized pemphigoid usually does not require treatment with systemic corticosteroids. Open wet dressings for 15 or 20 minutes three times daily, followed by application of a potent topical corticosteroid cream, are often sufficient for control of the disease.

Cicatricial Pemphigoid. Oral corticosteroids and immunosuppressants are not reliably effective for control of this condition. If only oral lesions are present, triamcinolone in an emollient dental paste (Kenalog in Orabase) may be applied to the lesions after meals and at bedtime. Some patients prefer a corticosteroid cream or gel instead of the paste preparation because they are easier to apply. Pain is not usually a major problem, but discomfort may be relieved by viscous lidocaine (Xylocaine) solution or a 1:1 mixture of elixir of diphenhydramine (Benadryl) and kao-pectate used as a mouthwash or gargle before meals. Eye lesions should be managed in conjunction with an ophthalmologist. Contact lenses and intralesional corticosteroids may be helpful in preventing synechiae. In progressive cases that are unresponsive to local therapy, systemic corticosteroids and immunosuppressants may be used in the same way as for bullous pemphigoid.

PITYRIASIS ROSEA

method of
E. DORINDA SHELLEY, M.D.,
and SHARON G. McDONALD, M.D.
Peoria, Illinois

An oval pinkish-brown "herald patch," edged with fine scale, usually precedes by 1 to 2 weeks the development of similar smaller lesions. Lesions usually line up parallel to the ribs or along other dermatomes on the trunk and proximal extremities. Itching is variable during the 6 to 8 week course. Atypical vesicular, urticarial, and papular forms are difficult to diagnose, especially when confined to the arms or legs, but should be considered when three or more lesions appear in a row along a dermatome. Facial lesions are rare except in children. Alternative diagnoses include secondary syphilis, tinea corporis, viral exanthem, maculopapular drug eruption, guttate psoriasis, and pityriasis lichenoides chronica.

If lesions are present on the palms or soles, a serologic test for syphilis should be performed. A skin biopsy and/or KOH preparation may also help rule out other diagnoses in atypical forms.

Treatment

1. The patient should be reassured about the benign nature of the rash, which is nonscarring, disappears within 2 months, and is doubtfully contagious.

2. Ultraviolet light exposure on 3 consecutive days in natural sunlight or a tanning booth usually relieves itching and hastens resolution of the lesions. Sunbathing in a bikini until slightly pink (minimal erythema dose) is recommended.

3. Antihistamines such as hydroxyzine (Atarax, Vistaril), cyproheptadine (Periactin), or diphenhydramine (Benadryl) may help relieve itching, but are often not needed.

4. Lubrication with bland emollients such as water-in-oil emulsions (Eucerin, cold cream, USP) or buffered aluminum acetate (Acid Mantle Creme) may help relieve itching in patients with dry skin.

5. Topical steroid creams should be used only in extremely itchy and inflammatory cases.

For children: 1.0 per cent hydrocortisone cream (Hytone, Nutracort) two to four times daily.

For teenagers and adults: triamcinolone acetonide, 0.1 per cent cream (Kenalog, Aristocort) or fluocinolone acetonide (Synalar) four times daily.

6. If the rash persists longer than 3 months, perform a skin biopsy.

POLYARTERITIS NODOSA

method of
PEARON G. LANG, JR., M.D.
Atlanta, Georgia

Classic polyarteritis (periarteritis) nodosa is a leukocytoclastic vasculitis involving small and medium-sized muscular arteries. It tends to be segmental in distribution and has a particular propensity for the bifurcation of arteries. Adjacent veins also may be involved. Pathologically in its acute stages it is characterized by a panarteritis with necrosis of the vessel wall and infiltration by polymorphonuclear leukocytes with nuclear dust. Small numbers of eosinophils may also be present. Fibrinoid deposits may or may not be present in the vessel wall. With the passage of time these changes are replaced by a mononuclear infiltrate and fibrosis. Because of the recurrent nature of the disease, a biopsy may demonstrate coexisting healing areas and acutely inflamed areas in the same vessel.

There is also a cutaneous form of polyarteritis nodosa which is characterized by livedo reticularis, hemorrhagic nodules, and ulcerations (primarily on the lower legs). The typical pathologic changes of polyarteritis nodosa are seen in small arteries in the deep dermis and subcutaneous tissue. Although these patients may have a neuropathy and muscle involvement, severe internal organ involvement does not occur, e.g., renal, myocardial. This appears to be a limited and benign form of polyarteritis nodosa.

In reviewing the treatment of polyarteritis in the literature one finds much confusion. Despite attempts in the past to classify the vasculitides, there is still confusion and overlap. This is particularly true of polyarteritis nodosa, for there are no absolute diagnostic criteria. Even the aneurysms seen on angiography may not be diagnostic. A tissue diagnosis is the most reliable way of confirming the diagnosis; but once again, if there is small nonarterial vessel involvement, is this polyarteritis nodosa or simply a necrotizing vasculitis with polyarteritis nodosa–like features? Moreover, many of the cases reported as treatment successes appear to fall more in the catego-

ry of allergic granulomatosis than classic polyarteritis nodosa. This could be an important factor in drawing conclusions about the best therapeutic approach. Finally, because of its rarity, it is difficult to study large groups of patients with this disease in a prospective manner and to compare different modalities of therapy.

Treatment

Left untreated, polyarteritis nodosa is almost uniformly fatal, with only a 13 per cent 5 year survival. Renal and cardiac involvement are the major causes of death. It is felt by some, particularly in those patients in whom the cause can be linked to a drug or infection, that the disease may be self-limited and that if the patient can survive the acute phase, especially the first 3 months, the prognosis is good.

General measures include bed rest, nonsteroidal anti-inflammatory agents, suppressive therapy for hypertension, and compresses and debridement of cutaneous ulcers. For those with renal failure, dialysis may be required until the renal disease is brought under control. Physical therapy and rehabilitation may be required for certain patients. Diuretics and digitalis may be required in those with congestive heart failure and fluid retention.

The cutaneous form of the disease in general is much more responsive to treatment and usually can be controlled with lower doses of corticosteroids than can the more fulminant form of the disease.

Corticosteroids. The use of systemic corticosteroids in polyarteritis has improved the survival of these patients significantly, with a 5 year survival approaching 50 per cent.

The short-acting steroids should be used to avoid markedly suppressing the adrenal glands. Most clinicians employ prednisone. Once again, to decrease the amount of adrenal suppression, most clinicians prefer to give this as a single morning dose. There are some who feel, however, that with fulminant disease more efficacy is achieved by spreading the dosage over a 24 hour period.

The usual dosage of prednisone is 1 to 2 mg per kg. Most patients can be started on 60 mg per day and will respond; however, for the patient with fulminant disease a dosage approaching 2 mg per kg should be employed.

After the disease is under control, one can begin to taper the prednisone dosage by 5 mg per week. When a dosage of 40 mg per day is reached, administration should be changed to an alternate day steroid regimen, giving 80 mg every other morning. Depending on how long the patient has been on daily steroids, he may require 20 mg per day on his "off day" to avoid symptoms of adrenal insufficiency. At this point the "off day" dosage is decreased by 2.5 mg per week until the patient is solely on an every other day schedule. Then the steroids are tapered by 5 mg every 2 weeks until a dosage of 20 mg every other day is achieved. At this point one should taper the dose by 2.5 mg every 2 weeks either until the patient is completely off steroids or until the lowest possible maintenance dosage has been achieved.

The patient on steroids should be closely monitored for infection, gastrointestinal bleeding, osteoporosis, cataracts, glaucoma, glucose intolerance, hypertension, electrolyte imbalance, congestive heart failure, and fluid retention.

Immunosuppressive Agents. In one study the combined use of corticosteroid and immunosuppressives increased the survival of patients with polyarteritis nodosa to 80 per cent.

The two most commonly used agents have been cyclophosphamide and azathioprine.

Although in general these agents have been reserved for the patient not responding to steroids or for the patient with excessive side effects from steroids, this approach may have to be re-evaluated. It may well be that all patients with polyarteritis should be started on one of these agents along with their systemic corticosteroids.

It should be kept in mind that 2 or 3 weeks may be required before these agents have a significant effect, and therefore corticosteroids must be used in conjunction with them initially.

For induction of a remission the patient should be started on 1 mg per kg of prednisone per day in conjunction with 2 mg per kg per day of cyclophosphamide or azathioprine. (This use of these two agents is not listed in the manufacturers' official directives.) If there is no response, the dosage of the immunosuppressive agent may be increased, provided that this is tolerated. Although toxicity will determine the maximal dosage given, generally a dosage of 200 mg per day is not exceeded. Unless toxicity supervenes, the dosage of the immunosuppressive is not decreased until the patient is completely off steroids or until he or she has been tapered to as small a dosage of steroids as is possible. Tapering the immunosuppressive should be done gradually, e.g., 25 mg every 4 to 6 weeks.

After 2 to 3 weeks if a remission is achieved, the patient is switched to alternate day steroids and tapered in a manner outlined previously.

Cyclophosphamide and azathioprine share certain toxic features, but each of them also possesses distinctive features. Both may affect the hematopoietic system, but cyclophosphamide has a more depressing effect in general. The white cell count should be maintained at ≥3000 cells per cu mm, and the neutrophil count should be maintained between 1000 and 1500 cells per cu mm. Both agents are hepatotoxic but much less so than methotrexate. Gastrointestinal intolerance is not uncommon with these agents. Rashes and fever may occur in patients on azathioprine, and a reversible alopecia may be seen with cyclophosphamide. Cyclophosphamide also can cause irreversible damage to the gonads, resulting in anovulation and azoospermia. However, one of the greatest concerns with cyclophosphamide is its adverse effects on the bladder, which may result in a hemorrhagic cystitis. This may occur even after the drug has been discontinued. This cystitis may be followed by fibrosis and later carcinoma. If possible, the daily dose of cyclophosphamide should be given early in the day and fluids encouraged to prevent the drug and its metabolites from sitting in the bladder. Whether these drugs are oncogenic is still unclear, as many of the patients who develop malignancies while on these drugs may already be predisposed by their underlying disease. It should also be remembered that the toxic effects of these drugs may persist for several weeks after they are discontinued. Patients on immunosuppressives, especially in conjunction with systemic corticosteroids, also have an increased susceptibility to infections.

To monitor patients on cyclophosphamide and azathioprine, weekly complete blood and platelet counts, including a differential white count, should be obtained during the first month of therapy. The frequency of monitoring may then be decreased to once every 2 weeks for the next month. Subsequently these hematologic parameters need be checked only once every 3 to 4 weeks (unless the dosage is increased). Periodic urinalyses are also important, especially for patients on cyclophosphamide. A urinalysis and chemistry profile (including hepatic and renal parameters) should be obtained every two weeks for the first month, then monthly for several months, and then once every 2 to 3 months.

Drug interaction is important with both these agents. Allopurinol inhibits these drugs' degradation, especially of azathioprine, and can increase their toxicity. Phenobarbital stimulates those enzymes in the liver which activate cyclophosphamide and thereby may increase its toxicity. Finally, corticosteroids inhibit those enzymes in the liver which activate cyclophosphamide. Therefore, theoretically one may observe increased toxicity as the steroids are tapered.

Other Agents. Dapsone in doses of 100 to 200 mg per day has been reported to be helpful in a few patients with polyarteritis nodosa when used in conjunction with corticosteroids. (This use of dapsone is not listed in the manufacturer's official directive.) This agent, like the immunosuppressives, has a corticosteroid-sparing effect. Although having its own side effects, in general dapsone is much less toxic than the immunosuppressives and bears further evaluation, especially in those patients with the cutaneous form of the disease.

In those patients whose disease flares following streptococcal infections, prophylactic penicillin may be of value.

PRECANCEROUS LESIONS OF THE SKIN AND MUCOUS MEMBRANES

method of
HEIN J. TER POORTEN, M.D.
Richardson, Texas

A wide variety of dermatologic conditions may be precancerous. Included in this diverse group are conditions, such as actinic keratoses, Bowen's disease, erythroplasia of Queyrat, arsenical keratoses, and lentigo maligna, which are actually neoplasms in situ, confined to the epidermis. Leukoplakia is, strictly speaking, a descriptive term and is not always a neoplasia in situ or precancerous. Chronic radiation dermatitis may be characterized by neoplastic changes confined to the epidermis or by atypical cells in the dermis as well.

Another large group of dermatologic conditions includes several tumors, dermatoses, and genodermatoses, which have in common only the possible development of malignant tumors within them.

Among the tumors are giant condylomas of the genitalia, congenital sebaceous nevus of Jadassohn, usually confined to the head and neck region, and congenital giant hairy nevi, which are not always of the so-called bathing trunk variety. Giant genital condylomas may be associated with development of aggressive squamous cell carcinoma with regional adenopathy and are best treated by excision. Apparently successful use of autogenous vaccines has been reported. In case of sebaceous nevus, prophylactic excision is indicated, because various benign and malignant tumors may arise in an estimated 20 per cent of cases, usually after puberty. Although there is controversy as to the exact incidence of the development of malignant melanoma in giant hairy nevi, there is definite agreement that this occurs. Prophylactic excision is advisable whenever feasible. Smaller lesions may be excised primarily and larger ones in staged procedures.

Among the dermatoses are lichen sclerosus et atrophicus of the female genitalia, oral lichen planus, oral florid papillomatosis, and lupus vulgaris. Squamous cell carcinoma may arise in these cutaneous diseases. Careful follow-up is required of patients with these dermatoses, and this applies also to patients with chronic cutaneous ulcers, chronic draining sinus tracts as may be seen in osteomyelitis, old extensive scars, and even smallpox scars, in which various tumors rarely arise.

Among the genodermatoses with which cutaneous malignancies may be associated are albinism, the basal cell nevus syndrome, epidermodysplasia verruciformis, dyskeratosis congenita, xeroderma pigmentosum, and pachyonychia congenita. Regular follow-up and biopsy of new and suspicious lesions are required.

Actinic (Solar) Keratoses

These lesions are very common and are usually seen in normally sun-exposed areas, including the pretibial area in women. On occasion, they occur on normally covered areas of the body, because considerable light may be transmitted through clothing. A squamous cell carcinoma may arise in an actinic keratosis but is rarely deeply invasive and is not likely to metastasize.

Treatment. 1. Cryosurgery with liquid nitrogen is the treatment of choice for maculosquamous and papular lesions. The spray method is most practical and may require 5 to 15 seconds. Healing usually takes from 10 to 14 days, sometimes 21 days on the lower extremities, where great care must be taken, for excessive cryosurgery may eventuate in scarring in this area.

2. Light electrodesiccation followed by curettage or curettage followed by light electrodesiccation, under local anesthesia, may be used for papular, nodular, and hypertrophic lesions unresponsive to cryosurgery.

3. Topical chemotherapy with 5-fluorouracil is best reserved for multiple maculosquamous actinic keratoses or where extensive actinic damage is suspected but not readily detectable clinically. Usually the 5 per cent cream is used and applied twice daily. Since only the actinically

damaged skin will react to 5-fluorouracil, it is not important for the patient to apply it only to clinically obvious lesions.

To ameliorate the resultant intense inflammatory reaction, some patients may require concomitant use of 1 per cent or 2.5 per cent hydrocortisone cream, or even an intermediate strength fluorinated corticosteroid cream, for the remainder of the course of treatment, which may last a total of 3 to 6 weeks. Usually a corticosteroid cream is not added until after the maximal inflammatory response has been achieved and 5-fluorouracil has been discontinued. Sunlight should be avoided while 5-fluorouracil is being used, for it may accentuate the inflammatory reaction. Following the completion of treatment, regular use of an appropriate sunscreen having a sun protection factor rating in the 10 to 15 range should be encouraged.

4. Deep shave biopsy, to include the base of the lesion, or simple excision is at times indicated for nodular or hypertrophic lesions suspected of having progressed to squamous cell carcinoma.

For actinically damaged dry mucosa of the lower lip (actinic cheilitis) 5-fluorouracil may be used, but I prefer cryotherapy, which is usually quite effective. A lip shave is an alternative form of treatment.

Bowen's Disease

This is a squamous cell carcinoma in situ, more extensive in its epidermal involvement than an actinic keratosis, and it may give rise to an invasive squamous cell carcinoma with potential for metastasis. Typically, this lesion presents clinically as a banal-looking chronic eczematous plaque, on either sun-exposed or covered parts of the body, which does not disappear spontaneously or with topical corticosteroid treatment. The causation of Bowen's disease is unclear, although arsenic is suspected in at least some patients.

Treatment. 1. Topical chemotherapy with 5-fluorouracil, in a 2 per cent or 5 per cent concentration, is probably the preferred method of treatment, particularly for extensive lesions. Treatment must be continued twice daily for 4 to 6 weeks until the maximal inflammatory response is attained. Close follow-up with biopsy of remaining suspicious areas is required, since treatment may not be curative if the in situ neoplastic changes extend downward into hair follicles. Analgesics sometimes have to be given if there is extensive involvement of the glabrous skin of the penis, vulva, and perineum.

2. Surgical excision is frequently preferred for smaller, clinically well-circumscribed lesions.

3. Curettage and electrodesiccation, as well as cryosurgery with liquid nitrogen, may be effec-

tive but may not be curative if there is follicular involvement. Follow-up is required.

Erythroplasia of Queyrat

This carcinoma in situ is histologically essentially identical to Bowen's disease. Clinically, it presents as a chronic, shiny, red erosive patch on the mucous membranes of the penis and vulva and occasionally in the oral cavity, where it is most commonly seen in the floor of the mouth. Invasive squamous cell carcinoma may arise in these lesions and result in metastasis to regional lymph nodes.

Treatment. The introduction of topical 5-fluorouracil has largely replaced excisional surgery, because it usually results in preservation of structure and function. The weaker concentration of 5-fluorouracil, such as 1 per cent or 2 per cent lotion or cream, is preferred and may have to be used once or twice daily for 2 months or more, depending on individual reactivity to the medications and the severity of the induced inflammation. Analgesics are often required during the course of treatment, and hydrocortisone cream may have to be used concomitantly. Oral lesions are treated surgically. Regular follow-up is essential.

Arsenical Keratoses

These lesions have a characteristic clinical appearance and distribution, occurring most commonly on the palms and soles and palmar aspects of the fingers. When present on the trunk and extremities, arsenical keratoses may be indistinguishable from Bowen's disease. They are of low malignant potential but occasionally a squamous cell carcinoma arises which may grow rapidly. Basal cell carcinomas may also develop. Appearance of arsenical keratoses is usually preceded by many years by the ingestion of inorganic arsenic such as in the form of a tonic (Fowler's solution) or is due to industrial or occupational exposure. The possible development of visceral cancers warrants further evaluation of patients with arsenical keratoses.

Treatment. 1. Punch excision, using a 2 mm to 4 mm Keyes Punch, of miliary palmar and plantar arsenical keratoses provides definitive treatment. A punch slightly larger than the lesion should be utilized. A single suture can close the small defect in the skin.

2. Cryosurgery with liquid nitrogen for 15 to 30 seconds, using a double freeze-thaw cycle, can be effective, provided that there is good epidermal separation of the thick palmar skin.

3. Curettage and electrodesiccation, under local anesthesia, of palmar lesions.

4. Lesions on the trunk and extremities can

be approached as with Bowen's disease, using excision, topical 5-fluorouracil, cryosurgery, or curettage and electrodesiccation.

Leukoplakia

As a designation for a particular disease, leukoplakia is a poor term. To prevent unnecessarily aggressive treatment, biopsy is imperative to separate benign leukokeratoses from carcinoma in situ, since many dermatologic diseases may involve the oral and genital mucosa and be associated with leukoplakia. The changes of carcinoma in situ, which clinically may present as leukoplakia on a mucosal surface, are usually of uncertain and, no doubt, diverse etiology.

Treatment. 1. Avoidance of irritants such as tobacco in cigarette, cigar, and especially pipe smokers and by tobacco chewers should be stressed. Proper oral hygiene and correction of malocclusions and ill-fitting dental appliances are indicated. With involvement of the dry mucosa of the lower lip, a sunscreen should be used. Vitamin and iron supplementation may be required.

2. In cases of genital involvement, scrupulous hygiene is essential. Circumcision may be necessary. Hormonal insufficiency should be corrected in women.

3. Definitive treatment may require cryosurgery, which is effective on the lips and genital mucosa.

4. Excisional surgery and, less frequently, electrodesiccation may be used. Leukoplakia of the dry mucosa of the lower lip, not amenable to cryosurgery, may be treated with a lip shave.

Lentigo Maligna

This is an atypical melanocytic hyperplasia which remains confined to the epidermis for many years. It grows very slowly and may be seen anywhere on the skin, including the palms and soles, and even on mucosa. In more than 60 per cent of patients it occurs on the face. Definitive treatment is required to prevent possible development of malignant melanoma, seen in perhaps one third of patients.

Treatment. 1. Surgical excision, sometimes requiring grafting or even staged procedures, is the treatment of choice.

2. Radiation therapy, using soft x-rays, has been reported as successful.

3. Curettage and electrodesiccation, as well as cryosurgery, has been used but may not be curative if there is extension of atypical melanocytes down hair follicles. These modalities have been advocated for small early lesions, but such lesions can be managed well by excision.

Chronic Radiodermatitis

Atypical epidermal changes may give rise to actinic keratoses, basal cell carcinomas, and squamous cell carcinomas, whereas atypical cells in the dermis may give rise to radiation sarcomas. Actinic keratoses are usually clinically evident, but suspected tumors should be biopsied before deciding on treatment. Observation of patients with radiation dermatitis is normally sufficient, and prophylactic excision with grafting is not usually advocated.

Treatment. 1. Actinic keratoses respond to topical chemotherapy with 5-fluorouracil and cryosurgery.

2. Excision is definitive treatment for basal cell carcinomas and squamous cell carcinomas and is the treatment of choice for radiation sarcomas. Grafting may be required.

3. Curettage and electrodesiccation is effective for basal cell carcinomas and squamous cell carcinomas, but has the disadvantage that one is curetting within the confines of an altered dermis, and healing time may be greatly prolonged.

MILIARIA
(Prickly Heat)

method of
THOMAS L. PERRY, M.D.
Yakima, Washington

Miliaria is a cutaneous eruption resulting from occlusion of the sweat ducts. It usually occurs under environmental conditions of excessive heat and humidity. Miliaria is aggravated by occlusion of the skin with nonporous clothing or plastic material. It is most prone to arise in the intertriginous areas.

Maceration and hydration of the stratum corneum provide ideal conditions for the growth of bacteria. This proliferation of micrococci is thought to be a contributing factor in the production of miliaria, although actual secondary infection is rare.

Infants, bedridden patients, and those who have recently moved from a temperate to a tropical climate are most susceptible to miliaria. Pre-existing skin conditions, especially atopic dermatitis, may enhance the development of miliaria.

Extensive miliaria often impairs the thermoregulatory mechanism for at least 3 weeks. This may lead to hyperpyrexia and heat exhaustion.

There are four types of miliaria. Very superficial obstruction of the sweat duct results in miliaria crystallina. This is seen as crops of asymptomatic 1 to 2 mm vesicles. Often no treatment is required. Miliaria rubra, the most common type, appears as erythematous pruritic papules; often a very uncomfortable prickling sensation is felt by the patient. Miliaria pustulosa is usually associated with a pre-existing dermatitis. These tiny pustules are usually sterile if cultured. Miliaria profunda, caused by deep obstruction of the sweat ducts, is the least common variety. It is seen only in the tropics. Secondary infection, especially in malnourished children, may produce sweat gland abscesses.

Treatment

1. Removing the patient to a cool environment of moderate humidity is the single most effective treatment. Air conditioning is ideal.

2. Cool baths in fresh water are soothing. Soap should be avoided, but the addition of colloidal oatmeal (Aveeno) to the bath will help relieve symptoms.

3. Loose-fitting summer clothing is desirable.

4. Cholinergic drugs are contraindicated. Anticholinergic drugs, including antihistamines and phenothiazines, are not helpful.

5. Occlusive, greasy ointments should be avoided. Lipid-free skin cleanser (Cetaphil) lotion or calamine lotion with 0.25 per cent menthol is soothing. Cornstarch or talcum powder may be applied to intertriginous areas.

6. Topical steroids do not help. Topical antibiotics may be of some prophylactic value but are useless once the eruption starts.

7. When secondary infection occurs, *Staphylococcus aureus* is usually the predominant organism. Order culture and sensitivity reports, giving systemic antibiotics as indicated. Erythromycin, 250 mg orally four times daily, or cloxacillin, 250 mg orally four times daily, is usually the drug of choice.

8. Severe and prolonged postmiliarial anhidrosis may require the patient to move to a temperate climate.

PRURITUS

method of
DONALD J. MIECH, M.D.
Marshfield, Wisconsin

Pruritus is certainly the most common and often the most annoying symptom of skin disease. It is often associated with primary skin lesions in which there is usually an inflammatory process, but the pruritus can occur in clinically normal skin. The mechanism of pruritus is still poorly understood. No definite nerve receptors for the pruritic sensation have been demonstrated, although "penicillate" nerve endings have been seen at the dermal-epidermal junction and are thought to extend into the epidermis. These seem to conduct the sensation of pruritus superficially and to conduct pain within the deeper dermis; hence, the concept that itching is weak pain. A number of stimuli (e.g., mechanical, thermal, electrical) can cause itching if applied at the dermal-epidermal junction but can cause pain if applied more intensely or at deeper levels. Certain anatomic locations, such as the nape of the neck, periorbital area, and anogenital area, seem more responsive to the itch stimulus than others. This may account for some of the characteristic locations of certain itch-scratch reactions such as lichen simplex chronicus. Inflammatory skin diseases are often associated with pruritus. Whether this process is related to histamine release in the skin, prostaglandin E, proteolytic enzymes, kinins, or acetylcholine is not certain, although there is evidence that all these substances have pruritogenic activity.

A number of environmental factors can enhance the sensation of pruritus. Among these are temperature and humidity. Mechanical stimulation of the skin by the wool fibers in some clothing can increase itching, especially in the atopic person; and tiny spicules of fiberglass can be distractingly pruritic. Other factors such as stress and anxiety can also enhance pruritus. However, when external stimuli are reduced as they are prior to sleeping, the itch sensation may be increased.

Perhaps the most common cause of pruritus which can cause minimal associated skin changes is xerosis or dry skin. Elderly people and atopic persons often have dry skin, which plays a significant role in the subsequent development of their respective eczemas.

Among the other external factors are skin parasites such as lice and mites. Scabies can often be confused with other skin diseases, but its characteristic distribution and enhanced nocturnal itch should alert the physician to the diagnosis. Pediculosis can be identified by seeing the organism or its nit.

Essential Pruritus

The most challenging patients with pruritus are often those without primary skin lesions. This is sometimes referred to as essential pruritus and is frequently associated with underlying systemic disease. It is almost always a generalized pruritus. Localized pruritus is rarely a symptom of internal disease except for the pruritus vulvae associated with diabetes mellitus or pruritus of the nostrils associated with brain tumors. Essential pruritus occurs in a variable fashion and is not always related to the severity of the disease.

Essential pruritus can be a complaint of patients with endocrine, hepatic, renal, and hematopoietic diseases.

1. The endocrine diseases would include thyroid disease in which the frequency in both hypo- and hyperthyroid patients may be as great as 10 per cent. Diabetes and parathyroid abnormalities may also be corrected with generalized pruritus. Relief is usually derived from correction of the endocrine problem.

2. The hepatic diseases with cholestatic sequelae and retention of bile salts can sometimes be treated with cholestyramine (Questran), 9 to 12 grams three times daily. This can form an insoluble complex with the bile salts, leading to fecal elimination. Some drugs may also bind to the cholestyramine, thereby reducing their effect.

3. Patients with chronic renal disease can sometimes be very pruritic, especially those who have undergone dialysis. Often the most intense pruritus follows dialysis by several hours and is thought to be related to calcium metabolism and a secondary hyperparathyroidism, which occurs in many of these patients. Sunburn-spectrum ultraviolet (UVB) phototherapy administered two to three times weekly has recently been shown to be helpful in managing pruritus in these patients.

4. The hematopoietic diseases associated with pruritus include Hodgkin's disease, myelofibrosis, polycythemia vera, and occasionally myeloma. Some reports suggest that iron deficiency anemia can be associated with pruritus, the treatment for which would be correction of the anemia. Several reports have suggested a dramatic relief of the pruritus in patients with polycythemia and myelofibrosis with the use of cimetidine (Tagamet), 300 mg four times daily. (This use of cimetidine is not listed in the manufacturer's official directive.)

5. Psychogenic pruritus frequently suggests some psychiatric disturbance that would require evaluation and treatment by a psychotherapist.

General Treatment

Avoidance of factors which enhance pruritus, such as heat, irritating clothing fibers, and rapid changes in temperature and humidity, are necessary initial measures.

Sometimes avoidance of stressful situations will be helpful.

Topical Therapy

1. Hydration of the skin is very important for those patients with pruritus secondary to xerotic skin. This will include a substantial number of those patients living in northern climates who present with itching in the winter months. The stratum corneum easily absorbs water, but this is lost to evaporation if the surrounding air is dry. Therefore, a bath oil such as Lubath, Alpha Keri, or Robathol can be applied to the skin immediately after bath or shower before the skin can dry out. This retards the rapid evaporation of moisture. Some patients do very well with baby oil or heavier ointments such as Eucerin or Aquaphor. These latter two preparations are particularly helpful for dry hands or dry feet problems and, once again, are most effective when applied to damp skin.

2. Antipruritic lotions and creams can often be more effective than a topical steroid cream when there is no visible inflammation. Lotions containing menthol (0.25 to 1.0 per cent), phenol (0.5 to 1.0 per cent), or camphor (1.0 to 2.0 per cent) can produce a cooling, soothing sensation to the skin.

3. Topical steroids will help relieve the pruritus associated with inflamed skin, and many different types are available. It is important to avoid "overkill." Often 1 per cent hydrocortisone (Dermacort, Nutracort) may be helpful and should be considered initially when treating dermatoses on the face or on infants. Triamcinolone acetonide (Kenalog, Aristocort) 0.1 per cent and 0.025 per cent and flurandrenolide (Cordran) 0.025 per cent and 0.05 per cent are preparations with intermediate potency and are effective in most common inflammatory dermatoses. Sometimes camphor, menthol, or phenol can be added to the topical steroid for additional relief of itching.

Systemic Therapy

Antihistamines are the most frequently used and generally the most effective systemic treatment for pruritus. They are particularly effective in treating urticaria, which can be histamine mediated. Other patients with various types of pruritus may also respond to antihistamines, and many are available. The sedative side effect of most antihistamines may help relieve the pruritus almost as much as the antihistaminic action. Patients who must be alert during the day will often respond to a nighttime dose of antihistamine. Diphenhydramine (Benadryl), 25 to 50 mg, cyproheptadine (Periactin), 2 to 4 mg, or hydroxyzine hydrochloride (Atarax), 10 to 25 mg, may be given up to four times daily. Atarax has been used effectively as a mild tranquilizer, and part of its antipruritic effect may be so derived. Newer antihistamines such as clemastine fumarate (Tavist), 1.34 to 2.68 mg, and azatadine maleate (Optimine), 1 mg, may cause less drowsiness in some patients.

Systemic steroids should be used only in

those inflammatory conditions which are unresponsive to topical treatment. The patient should have no contraindications for use of these medications. Prednisone in doses of 40 to 60 mg with rapid tapering over 7 to 10 days may be given for acute inflammatory conditions such as widespread contact dermatitis. It must be emphasized that topical or systemic steroids will do little or nothing when an inflammatory process cannot be demonstrated.

Sedation can usually be achieved with adequate antihistamine dosage. However, some patients may need additional tranquilization or sedation.

Much still remains to be learned about itching. It is a symptom that deserves attention and understanding. The cause must be discerned if possible; then appropriate therapy can be instituted to relieve this symptom which causes so much human discomfort.

PRURITUS ANI AND VULVAE

method of
WESLEY KING GALEN, M.D.
New Orleans, Louisiana

Perianal, scrotal, and vulvar itching is a very distressing symptom complex frequently encountered in the practice of general family medicine, dermatology, proctology, and gynecology. Because this represents a symptom complex, the physician must separate and address multiple possible contributing factors and diseases in order to help the patient solve what most find a very embarrasing and stressful problem.

The predominant presenting complaint is usually itching, but on occasion burning or painful sensations will be mentioned. On examination signs may be extremely variable, including slight to intense erythema, bleeding or crusted papules and plaques, lichenification (mild to severe), nodules, or atrophy of the skin.

There are numerous factors that contribute to the itching in the genital and crural areas, including (1) abundant innervation with sensory nerve endings; (2) maceration caused by sweating and presence of urine and anal, vaginal, and apocrine gland secretions; (3) bacterial and candidal overgrowth of these secretions or urine affecting the pH and epidermal penetrability of the skin; (4) close apposition of skin surfaces and almost constant covering with multiple layers of clothes; and (5) environmental factors such as soaps involved in grooming and hygiene. Given all the above, it should be no surprise how common such problems are.

It is helpful to divide underlying causes into the following categories:

1. Primary causes, i.e., recognizable dermatoses of the skin or anatomic lesions.
2. Secondary causes such as diseases of the skin resulting from external factors: (a) Contact dermatitis — allergic, irritant. (b) Infestations and infections. (c) Systemic problems such as diabetes mellitus.
3. Pruritus with no evidence of the above.

Representative causes in those categories are included in Table 1.

All cases of vulvar or perianal pruritus require a thorough history and general examination of the skin. Additionally a 4 mm punch or small excisional biopsy may be needed to confirm the diagnosis. This can be easily performed with 1 per cent lidocaine (Xylocaine) for local anesthesia.

Primary or Endogenous Causes

Psoriasis rarely involves the genital or gluteal clefts without some other telltale lesions being present. A check of the scalp for scaling at the hair margins or occiput, or trauma points such as the knees and elbows for scaling plaques and the nails for pitting or onycholysis, may confirm the diagnosis of psoriasis. Similarly, seborrheic der-

TABLE 1. **Causes of Pruritus Ani and Vulvae**

1. Primary or endogenous causes:
   a. Psoriasis
   b. Seborrheic dermatitis
   c. Lichen planus
   d. Fox-Fordyce disease
   e. Hailey-Hailey disease (familial benign pemphigus)
   f. Atopic dermatitis
   g. Vulvar dystrophies
      (1) Lichen sclerosus et atrophicus
      (2) Postmenopausal atrophy
      (3) Hyperplastic plaques with or without atypia
   h. Carcinoma in situ and carcinoma of the vulva or anal canal or perianal skin
   i. Extramammary Paget's disease
   j. Anal fissures and/or hemorrhoids
2. Secondary or exogenous causes:
   a. Contact dermatitis
      (1) Allergic
      (2) Irritant
      (3) Intertrigo
   b. Infections or infestations
      (1) Viral: Herpes simplex, molluscum contagiosum, warts
      (2) Bacterial: *Hemophilus vaginalis*
      (3) Fungal: *C. albicans* or dermatophyte
      (4) Parasitic: Trichomonas, scabies, pinworms, pediculosis
   c. Associated underlying systemic problems, i.e., diabetes mellitus, Hodgkin's disease
3. Psychogenic causes:
   a. Lichen simplex chronicus without a precipitating cause or persisting well beyond the resolution of the underlying cause

matitis has usually been evident as erythematous, greasy scaling patches over the scalp, midface, chest, or axilla by the time it involves the perineum. Atopic dermatitis with lichenified skin at the posterior knees, posterior neck, and antecubital fossa will occasionally be associated with genital or perianal pruritus. All these conditions are well treated initially by topical steroids such as betamethasone valerate or triamcinolone acetonide 0.1 per cent. As they improve, lesser potency steroids such as 1 per cent hydrocortisone or desonide (Tridesilon Cream) 0.05 per cent should be utilized to reduce the chance of atrophy of the skin.

Lichen planus, while an uncommon cause of genital lesions, may occur as lilac papules with delicate net-like white surface ridging or frank erosions. These genital lesions may be associated with similar lesions of the oral mucosa, and a search for pruritic-like papules in other areas of the skin and nail dystrophy should be made. High potency topical steroids may be required here; fluocinonide (Lidex) 0.05 per cent, betamethasone (Diprosone) 0.005 per cent, or intralesional steroids (triamcinolone acetonide, 2.5 to 5 mg per ml) may be required to induce relief. This may be maintained by lesser potency topical steroids.

Fox-Fordyce disease, also known as apocrine miliaria, may be present as very subtle pink perifollicular papules of the perineum, axilla, or areola of the breast. This is intensely pruritic, and its treatment with topical steroids, estrogens, and antihistamines is moderately successful at least. Reports of intralesional steroids (triamcinolone acetonide, 2.5 to 5 mg per ml) and topical steroids under occlusion (Saran Wrap, Handy Wrap) for 12 hours have claimed greater success. The patients must be warned of possible local atrophy if these measures are required.

Hailey-Hailey disease or familial benign pemphigus is autosomal dominant in inheritance and appears as crusted and vesicular or vegetative plaques in the folds, especially the groin. The course of this disorder may be ameliorated by the judicious use of topical antibiotics (erythromycin [Ilotycin] ointment, bacitracin, gentamicin) and topical steroids. At times systemic antibiotics such as tetracycline hydrochloride, 250 mg orally four times daily, and even the use of systemic steroids will be required to induce remissions, but the physician must be cautious of rebound phenomenon and avoid the long-term use of steroids for a benign condition.

Postmenopausal vulvar atrophy may improve with the use of conjugated estrogen (Premarin) cream and the judicious use of topical steroids and lubricants. Vulvar lichen sclerosus et atrophicus, the male counterpart being balanitis xerotica obliterans, may require chronic use of topical steroid creams. Additionally 1 to 2 per cent testosterone cream has been reported to be helpful, as has the use of antihistamines (cyproheptadine [Periactin], 4 mg, hydroxyzine, 25 or 50 mg, or diphenhydramine, 25 to 50 mg, orally every 4 to 6 hours). Clear water compresses may lessen discomfort also.

Carcinoma in situ, Bowen's disease, and extramammary Paget's disease may present similarly clinically as white bands of epithelium on a red inflammatory base. These lesions as well as their red velvety equivalent, erythroplasia of Queyrat, require prompt diagnosis and treatment. Surgical ablation and topical 5 per cent fluorouracil (5–FU) cream have successfully treated erythroplasia of Queyrat and certain cases of carcinoma in situ. A diagnosis of bowenoid carcinoma in situ or extramammary Paget's disease requires a search for other occult malignancy — both visceral and adjacent to the lesions such as sweat gland cancer, cancer of cervix, or cancer of the colon or rectum. Both require thorough surgical removal when possible and will not respond to topical therapy.

Secondary or Exogenous Causes

Intertrigo occurs most freqently in obese patients, and particularly in diabetics. Maceration, produced in part by sweating in close body folds, allows the overgrowth of many microbes, especially *Candida albicans*. Therapy therefore must be directed at drying the area as well as treating *Candida albicans*. One very pleasant and frequently successful lotion consists of the following ingredients:

Nystatin cream (Mycostatin Cream, 100,000 units per gram)	30 grams
or	
Nystatin (Mycostatin) oral tablets	2 or 3 million units (4 or 6 tabs crushed)
Triamcinolone 0.1 per cent cream	15 grams
Milk of bismuth lotion	q.s. ad. 120 ml

When bacterial overgrowth is an additional problem, gentamicin cream, 15 grams, may be added to this mixture. Zinc oxide ointment may substitute for the milk of bismuth lotion when erosions are present.

Allergic contact dermatitis may be caused by numerous chemicals, including perfumes, hygiene sprays, contraceptive devices, nail polish, and medications applied to the area, particularly topical -caine anesthetics and neomycin. Treatment requires avoidance of the offending chemical and the use of compresses and topical steroids. Irritant dermatitis may be caused by soaps and detergents, perfumes, and hygiene sprays and their propellants, as well as by perfumed and dyed toilet paper. This, too, requires avoidance of the irritant, compresses, and the topical use of steroid emollients.

Herpes simplex may initially present with pruritus, but this rapidly evolves into tender or painful ulcers. The diagnosis may be confirmed with Tzanck smear or viral culture or immunofluorescent stains of smears from the lesions. Compresses with povidone-iodine (Betadine) solution and warm water, followed by milk of bismuth lotion for drying, may minimize the discomfort. Some physicians apply topical idoxuridine 1 per cent solution or adenine arabinoside 1 per cent ointment (investigational) to specific lesions, but evidence is lacking that this abbreviates the duration of herpes simplex or is adequately absorbed through the epidermis to help. Condylomata acuminata have a fairly typical verrucoid appearance and are treated by many means, including surgical excision, cautery, and cryosurgery. Additionally, the application of 20 per cent podophyllin in tincture of benzoin for 2 to 4 hours, followed by careful washing of the area, has been quite successful. Molluscum contagiosum is distinguished by smooth dome-shaped papules with central puncta. A keratotic plug known as a molluscum body can be expressed from the lesion by pressure of curettage. Treatment with curettage is frequently successful.

Vulvar pruritus of fungal causes requires a potassium hydroxide preparation and appropriate cultures to establish the etiology. Numerous anticandidal regimens can be used, including the mixture mentioned for intertrigo, as well as vaginal preparations of miconazole and clotrimazole (Lotrimin). Tinea cruris may be adequately treated with the latter two creams, but it is rarely a cause of true vulvar pruritus.

Pinworms (*Enterobius vermicularis*) may be proved by the "Scotch Tape test," in which tape applied to the perineum upon waking before washing is examined under oil for characteristic ova. This disorder is well treated with oral piperazine, but it may require treating family members as well. Trichomonas may be evident in the urine or on a saline preparation of vulvar skin or vaginal discharge. Treatment with oral metronidazole is usually successful, but for complete success the patient's sexual partner must also be treated.

Scabies and pediculosis pubis may also cause perineal and perianal discomfort and pruritus. Diagnosis of scabies with microscopic examination of scrapings reveals the causative mite, whereas the diagnosis of pediculosis may require indirect signs such as ova attached to a hair (nits) and excoriated papules. Scabies is well treated with 1 per cent gamma benzene hexachloride (lindane) lotion applied as a lotion for 12 hours and then rinsed off, or as a shampoo used 4 to 8 minutes in pediculosis and thoroughly rinsed out. Also crotamiton (Eurax) cream may be very soothing and helpful in treating scabies. Eurax is applied for 24 to 48 hours and then washed off.

Psychogenic Causes

Psychogenic overlay is present in many patients suffering from genital or perianal pruritus. As long as all possible endogenous and exogenous problems have been ruled out or addressed adequately, the physician may feel some confidence in the causal role this plays in the patient's problem.

Hydroxyzine, 50 mg orally every 4 to 6 hours, used for both its antihistamine and ataractic benefits, may be very helpful. The patient must be informed of the role chronic rubbing has in prolonging the problem. Topical steroids to help with the lichenification and excoriations should be used, and the patient should wear cool loose clothing when possible. On occasion, however, the patient will require psychiatric consultation to resolve this disorder.

PSORIASIS

method of
WILLIAM WATSON, M.D.
Stanford, California

Psoriasis tends to be a lifelong disease. The physician should emphasize to the patient that although there is no known cure for psoriasis, it is treatable and in most cases can be well controlled. The patient should be encouraged and given an optimistic outlook. This is necessary, since compliance with topical regimens that are often messy and time consuming is essential for good control of the disease.

As a general principle, therapy should be conservative and topical whenever possible. Systemic therapy with potentially toxic drugs, such as cytotoxic agents, should be reserved for crisis situations such as exfoliative erythroderma or generalized disease that has failed to respond to topical therapy. One should always be aware of the fact that the course of psoriasis is unpredictable. Spontaneous remissions are common, and exacerbations may be triggered by infection or by physical and emotional stress.

Therapy of psoriasis can be divided into nonspecific soothing measures and specific therapy aimed at slowing down the rapid proliferation rate of psoriatic epidermis.

Nonspecific Measures

Daily baths containing oil emulsions are very soothing and useful for gentle mechanical removal of thick scales. This is often necessary before applying active antipsoriatic medicines, since they will not penetrate adequately if placed on a lesion covered with scale. There are many commercial, cosmetically elegant bath oils available for this purpose (Alpha Keri, Domol, Nutraspa, Lubath). Tar preparations for the bath (Zetar, Polytar, Balnetar) are also useful if the patient is going to be receiving ultraviolet or natural sunlight therapy, since the thin coating of tar will sensitize the psoriatic plaques to ultraviolet light and enhance the antipsoriatic effect.

Bland emollients are an extremely important part of psoriasis therapy. They hydrate the skin, aid in removal of scale, and alleviate pruritus secondary to dryness. In general, ointments such as petrolatum or Aquafor are most effective in hydrating the skin, but many patients prefer the less effective, more esthetic oil in water emulsion creams or lotions such as Nivea cream, Albolene, and Lubriderm. Since acutely inflamed psoriatic skin tolerates active antipsoriatic agents poorly, in acute inflammatory psoriasis or generalized pustular psoriasis bland emolliation and bed rest constitute the treatment of choice.

Nonspecific systemic therapy includes tranquilizers, if the psoriasis seems to be stress aggravated, and salicylates or antihistimines (hydroxyzine, 10 to 25 mg, cyproheptadine, 4 mg, or diphenhydramine, 25 to 50 mg, three to four times daily) for relief of pruritus.

Specific Topical Therapy

Keratolytic Drugs. Salicylic acid ointments in concentrations varying from 3 to 10 per cent are useful in psoriasis when there is an extremely thick scale, particularly on the palms and soles. This preparation is more effective if the affected area is first soaked in warm water for 10 to 20 minutes. Six per cent salicylic acid in a propylene glycol gel (Keralyt) is extremely effective in hyperkeratotic psoriasis when applied overnight under an occlusive dressing (Saran Wrap). Creams containing 10 to 20 per cent urea (Carmol, Aquacare H.P.) are keratolytic, hydrate dry skin, and enhance penetration of active compounds such as topically applied corticosteroids and tar. A 40 per cent aqueous urea soak for 15 to 20 minutes daily aids in severe adherent hyperkeratosis. Lactic acid creams and lotions, 5 to 10 per cent (LactiCare), have a similar action and may be combined with urea in extremely resistant hyperkeratotic palmar-plantar psoriasis.

Topically Applied Corticosteroids. Topically applied corticosteroids are the most widely prescribed drugs for psoriasis. They act in a number of ways. They are epidermal mitotic inhibitors, anti-inflammatory, and vasoconstrictors. They are available in cream, ointment, gel, and lotion bases and gain good patient acceptance and compliance because they are cosmetically elegant and nonmessy and do not have an unpleasant odor. Topical corticosteroid therapy is particularly effective if applied under occlusive plastic wraps, which increase their penetration through the skin up to 100-fold. When this method is used, there is prompt resolution of psoriatic plaques, often in as short a period as 1 week. Unfortunately there is usually prompt rebound if treatment is discontinued, and tachyphylaxis is common if treatment is continued beyond 2 to 3 weeks. Adverse side effects of prolonged local use of corticosteroids, particularly the more potent fluorinated compounds, include atrophy, atrophic striae, telangiectasia, and vascular fragility with resulting ecchymoses. Such undesirable effects are usually seen on the face and in intertriginous regions, or when the drugs are used with occlusion. There is evidence of systemic absorption with resultant adrenal suppression when fluorinated corticosteroids are used topically with occlusion for prolonged periods of time. The risk is remote, however, if they are used without occlusion.

The selection of a topically applied corticosteroid and vehicle depends largely on the location and type of psoriasis. The face, axillae, and anogenital region permit increased penetration, and the use of potent compounds in these areas should be limited to short periods of time, usually 4 weeks or less. Nonfluorinated compounds (hydrocortisone 0.5 to 1 per cent; desonide 0.05 per cent) can be used in these areas for prolonged periods of time with no adverse local effects. Unfortunately the weaker compounds are often not effective antipsoriatic drugs. Potent flourinated corticosteroids with plastic occlusion are particularly useful in patients with extremely thick psoriatic plaques and in palmar-plantar psoriasis.

Corticosteroid lotions (fluocinolone solution 0.01 per cent; betamethasone valerate 0.1 per cent [Valisone]), gels (Topsyn, Flurobate), and sprays (triamcinolone [Kenalog]) are particularly useful in the treatment of psoriasis of the scalp, since they do not leave the hair greasy. Psoriasis of the nails occasionally responds to the daily application of an occlusive plastic tape impregnated with flurandrenolide (Cordran tape). Atrophy of the periungual skin and fingertips is a potential complication with prolonged use. Other indications for the topical use of corticosteroids include highly inflammatory psoriasis and pustular psoriasis in which other topically applied antipsoriatic compounds such as tar or anthralin cannot be tolerated.

Since topically applied steroids do not induce remissions of psoriasis, become less effective with prolonged use, promote local rebound, or have potentially adverse local effects, I seldom use them alone, and restrict their use to the following situations: in highly inflammatory psoriasis in which other antipsoriatic compounds cannot be tolerated until the inflammation subsides; in facial, intertriginous, and scalp psoriasis in which tar or anthralin is not used (in these areas nonfluorinated compounds are preferable); as adjunctive therapy in resistant lesions, on a short-term basis, in combination with tar or anthralin compounds; and in palmar-plantar psoriasis, with occlusion.

Intralesional Corticosteroids. Intralesional injection of corticosteroids beneath localized thick psoriatic plaques usually induces prompt, but usually temporary, resolution of the lesions. Triamcinolone acetonide or triamcinolone diacetate 2.5 mg per ml) or betamethasone is usually used. This type of treatment should be used only in small isolated areas, since systemic absorption does occur.

Severe psoriasis of the nails can be treated by intralesional injection of the proximal nail folds (area of the nail matrix) with corticosteroids; the success rate is about 50 per cent. This has to be done at biweekly intervals for 2 to 6 months. It is not a practical treatment, because it is an extremely painful procedure and has poor patient acceptance. Local atrophy is a common complication, particularly if the same area is injected repeatedly.

Coal Tar Products. Tar has been used for centuries for the treatment of many skin disorders. Over the past century, coal tar preparations have been the most popular and most effective treatment for psoriasis. Coal tar is a byproduct of the destructive carbonization and distillation of coal and the redistillation of its intermediary products. Even after all the complicated processes of chemical extraction, crude coal tar is still a heterogeneous mixture of some 10,000 different compounds. Only about 55 per cent of the tars, representing approximately 400 compounds, have been identified. Crude coal tar (USP) is defined in the eighteenth U.S. Pharmacopeia only as a "nearly black, viscous liquid, heavier than water, having a characteristic naphthalene-like odor, and producing a sharp, burning sensation on the tongue." Different batches of tar contain varying proportions of constituent compounds, which may explain the variation in therapeutic results in psoriasis. The actual mechanism of action of coal tar in psoriasis has not been determined, nor have the components that are the most active been identified. Tar is photosensitizing and seems to have its greatest therapeutic effect when combined with ultraviolet light, either in the form of natural sunlight or from artificial ultraviolet sources.

The classic method of treating severe and extensive psoriasis is the modified Goeckerman regimen. This consists of daily tar baths, exposure to increasing increments of ultraviolet light in suberythema doses, and the application of 1 to 5 per cent crude coal tar (USP) in an ointment or zinc oxide base several times daily. This is an extremely messy treatment, since the crude coal tar ointment is black and stains clothing permanently. Because of this, use of the Goeckerman regimen is usually limited to a hospital or day care center setting and is reserved for patients with extensive psoriasis. Total remission of psoriasis lasting for months can be obtained after 3 to 4 weeks of a Goeckerman regimen.

Cosmetically acceptable tar preparations can be made by using liquor carbonis detergens, a 20 per cent tincture (alcoholic solution) of crude coal tar. It can be mixed in a cream or ointment base in concentrations varying from 3 to 15 per cent and has one fifth the potency of equivalent concentrations of crude coal tar. The color of such a cream or ointment is a deep beige rather than black, but the smell of tar is still present. Liquor carbonis detergens cream applied two to three times daily in conjunction with ultraviolet light often gives excellent results. After the psoriasis has cleared, the patient can often maintain remission with a daily tar bath plus ultraviolet light. Scalp psoriasis responds well to the overnight application of 5 to 10 per cent liquor carbonis detergens in Nivea oil, worn under a shower cap.

Currently, even more cosmetically elegant gels (Estar gel, psoriGel) containing coal tar are available on a nonprescription basis. They seem to have a therapeutic effect equivalent to that of 5 per cent crude tar and have the advantage of being nongreasy and nonstaining since they do not rub off on clothing. They tend to have a drying effect, however, and adjunctive emollient therapy is usually necessary.

It is well known that crude coal tar is highly carcinogenic when applied to the skin of laboratory animals. There have been no reports of an increased frequency of skin cancer in psoriatic patients treated for many years with coal tar and ultraviolet light (also carcinogenic): in fact, Jacobs reported a lower frequency of skin cancer in tar-treated psoriatic patients than in age-matched control subjects.

Despite being unpleasant treatment, coal tar therapy of psoriasis has proved effective and has the advantage of inducing remission, which corticosteroids and various systemic therapies, to be discussed later, do not.

Anthralin (Dithranol). Anthralin is a synthetic drug, trihydroxyanthracene, that has proved to be very effective in psoriasis since its introduction in a stiff paste formulation in 1953. Anthralin causes a more rapid resolution of psoriatic plaques than crude coal tar and induces remissions lasting from weeks to as long as 2 years. The mode of action is believed to be a reduction of DNA synthesis caused by intercalation of the anthraline molecule between DNA pairs.

Anthralin is most effective when incorporated into a stiff paste. It is carefully applied to the individual psoriatic lesions where it remains for a period of 6 to 10 hours, usually overnight. The formulations used at Stanford are as follows:

Anthralin hard paste: Anthralin 0.1 to 0.8 per cent, salicylic acid 0.4 per cent, hard paraffin (candle wax) 10 to 15 per cent, and Lassar's paste USP.

Test areas for the 0.1 per cent formulations are used initially to ensure that the patient does not develop a primary irritant reaction, which happens with moderate frequency. The concentration is then increased to tolerance. Complete resolution of psoriatic plaques is usually attained in 10 to 14 days as opposed to 3 to 4 weeks for the Goeckerman regimen.

The main disadvantage of the anthralin hard paste regimen is that the paste is not water soluble and must be removed with copious amounts of mineral oil. Anthralin stains clothing a purplish brown and also temporarily stains the skin. For these reasons, as with the Goeckerman regimen, it is used mainly in a hospital or day care center setting.

A pomade with the following formulation is available commercially as *Lasan pomade:* anthralin 0.4 per cent, salicylic acid 0.4 per cent, mineral oil 76.0 per cent, cetyl alcohol 21.9 per cent, and sodium lauryl sulfate 2.1 per cent. This is the most effective treatment for severe scalp psoriasis. It is massaged carefully into the scalp and left on for 6 to 8 hours under a shower cap, and then shampooed out. Great care must be taken to avoid contact with the eyes, since severe conjunctival irritation can occur.

Anthralin is also available in an ointment base (Anthra-Derm), which is more suitable for outpatient use. It is a useful alternative in psoriasis that is resistant to topical corticosteroid therapy or tar preparations. The main disadvantages are staining and primary irritant reactions. Because of potential irritant reactions, anthralin should not be used on intertriginous regions or the face, or in psoriatic erythroderma and acute pustular psoriasis. Primary irritant reactions from anthralin are treated topically with corticosteroids.

Systemic Therapy

Systemic Administration of Corticosteroids. Systemically administered steroids are initially effective in controlling psoriasis, but increasing daily doses are usually required to maintain control, and since psoriasis is a chronic disease, severe systemic side effects are common. Severe rebounds of psoriasis generally occur on cessation of systemic steroid therapy. Approximately half the patients with inflammatory exfoliative erythroderma and acute generalized pustular psoriasis seen at Stanford are admitted because of rebound following systemic corticosteroid therapy. For this reason, systemic steroid therapy in psoriasis is almost always contraindicated. The few exceptions include life-threatening acute generalized pustular psoriasis, acute erythroderma, and rapidly progressive and destructive psoriatic arthritis. In these instances systemic corticosteroid therapy should be used only when all other measures, including hospitalization and methotrexate therapy, have failed.

Methotrexate. Methotrexate given by the oral, intramuscular, or intravenous route is effective in 90 per cent of psoriatic patients in totally controlling the skin lesion and is considered the most useful drug in life-ruining psoriasis that has resisted all other modes of therapy. Needless to say, the associated risks of such therapy must be carefully weighed against the potential benefits. The indications should be strict and should follow the guidelines for the use of methotrexate in psoriasis published by the National Program for Dermatology Psoriasis Task Force. In these guidelines, the indications include severe disabling psoriasis that has not responded to conventional treatment, recalcitrant psoriatic erythroderma, localized debilitating pustular lesions of the palms and soles, acute generalized pustular psoriasis, and severe psoriatic arthritis.

Methotrexate acts in psoriasis by inhibiting epidermal DNA synthesis during the S phase of the cell cycle. It does this by blocking dihydrofolate reductase and preventing the conversion of deoxyuridylate to thymidylate in the de novo pathway of DNA synthesis. Because the proliferative compartment is so much greater in the psoriatic epidermis than in normal tissues, a selective therapeutic action with little systemic toxicity can be attained with relatively small doses of methotrexate. Many dosage schedules for methotrexate have been used in psoriasis. Currently preferred schedules include a single weekly oral dose of 7.5 to 25 mg or three 2.5 to 7.5 mg doses at 12 hour intervals over a 24 hour period once weekly. Small daily doses seem to be associated with increased adverse side reactions. Higher dosage may be indicated in the treatment of severe psoriatic arthritis. If oral administration causes gastrointestinal side effects, weekly intramuscular or intravenous doses of 25 to 50 mg can be used. Bone marrow suppression may be more common with parenteral administration.

Methotrexate is the most effective systemically administered drug for severe psoriasis. It should be reserved for crisis situations and preferably should be used on an intermittent basis, with a return to more conservative therapy when the psoriasis or arthritis or both are controlled. The need for pretreatment and follow-up liver biopsies in order to detect early fibrosis (often not detectable by routine liver function tests) is a negative factor in the prolonged use of methotrexate in psoriasis. It should be noted that patients taking methotrexate should abstain from drinking alcoholic beverages, since there is evidence that this combination increases the risk of hepatic damage.

Hydroxyurea. Hydroxyurea is a fair second line candidate for systemic therapy in psoriasis if there are contraindications to the use of methotrexate, such as hepatic fibrosis or cirrhosis. It acts as a DNA inhibitor. (This use of hydroxyurea is not listed in the manufacturer's official directive.) Hydroxyurea is about 60 per cent effective, as opposed to 90 per cent of methotrexate. Psoriasis also tends to become refractory with prolonged hydroxyurea therapy, and there is a narrow margin between therapeutic effectiveness and toxicity, particularly bone marrow suppression. Psoriatic patients respond slowly to hydroxyurea. If clearing of psoriasis is going to occur, it usually takes about 2 months. The recommended dosage of 0.5 gram three times daily for 4 weeks. It then may be reduced to 0.5 gram once or twice daily. The white blood cell count should be monitored weekly, and if the count drops below 4000 per cu mm, the dosage should be decreased or the drug discontinued. Adverse side effects include leukopenia, anemia, and thrombocytopenia. Macrocytosis of red blood cells has been found

in over 80 per cent of the patients treated with hydroxyurea. A "flulike" syndrome consisting of fever, malaise, joint pain, and headache has been reported. This reaction is not dose dependent.

Photochemotherapy

Photochemotherapy is a term used to indicate that the therapeutic effect is a result of the interaction of a systemically administered drug and ultraviolet light. It is systemic treatment with an effect localized to the skin. PUVA is the acronym for psoralen (P) and long wave ultraviolet light (UVA). This new approach uses 8-methoxypsoralen, a photosensitizing furocoumarin, given orally in a dosage of 0.65 mg per kg, followed in 2 hours by exposure to an artificial long wave ultraviolet light source. Two large multicenter clinical trials have established the efficacy of this treatment in over 2000 patients; in over 80 per cent of the patients complete clearing of the psoriasis occurred. Clearing occurred after an average of 25 treatments given two to three times weekly. Maintenance treatments are given as needed, varying from once weekly to once monthly. Immediate side effects from PUVA therapy are rare and are manifested as a phototoxic reaction of redness and occasional blistering of the skin. Some patients experience severe pruritus and nausea. There have been no detectable effects on other organ systems. PUVA has the advantage of being a systemic treatment and is easy to administer, without producing systemic side effects. It has great patient acceptance, since the need for applying messy topical preparations is eliminated.

The effect of PUVA in psoriasis is believed to result from the ultraviolet light–mediated interaction of psoralen with epidermal DNA, thereby halting DNA synthesis in the hyperproliferative psoriatic lesions. The binding of a drug to DNA after ultraviolet irradiation poses a theoretical risk of cytogenetic changes with resultant carcinogenesis. For this reason approval of this therapy for psoriasis by the Food and Drug Administration has been delayed pending long-term follow-up studies on PUVA-treated patients. Increased sister chromatoid exchanges have been reported in human lymphocytes exposed to 8-methoxypsoralen and ultraviolet light in vitro. The significance of this is not understood. Because of the potential for long-term adverse side effects, PUVA treatment should be limited to patients with severe and extensive psoriasis that has not responded to conventional topical therapy. Many believe that PUVA is the treatment of choice over all other systemic therapies for refractory and disabling psoriasis.

INFLAMMATORY ERUPTIONS OF THE HANDS AND FEET

method of
W. DAVID JACOBY, Jr., M.D.
Tucson, Arizona

Many dermatologic diseases may have prominent and distinct manifestations involving the hands and feet. In these diseases, e.g., secondary syphilis, erythema multiforme, scleroderma and other collagen diseases, psoriasis, photosensitivities, and porphyria cutanea tarda, usually other systemic and cutaneous findings are present. In this article we will deal only with those inflammatory skin conditions that have their primary cutaneous manifestations limited to the hands or the feet. These include the following:

Specific Diseases

Primary Irritant Contact Dermatitis (Housewife's Eczema). This is probably the most commonly seen inflammatory dermatitis, involving usually only the hands. It presents as erythema, occasionally with vesiculation but more often with dryness, scaling, and cracking and may involve only a few fingers on one or both hands. If web spaces are involved, suspect liquids or soapy cleaning solutions as the cause.

Allergic Eczematous Contact Dermatitis. Twenty-five per cent of all hand dermatitis may be allergic (cell-mediated type IV) in nature. It presents with bright erythema, vesiculation, and bullae if acute, or as cracking, scaling, and fissuring if chronic. If on hands suspect occupational exposure to an allergen and if limited to the feet suspect a shoe component (particularly rubber) as the allergen.

Dyshidrosis. Dyshidrosis presents as intensely pruritic crops of discrete clear vesicles, which appear on the palms and soles; characteristically the sides of the digits are involved. It is frequently precipitated by worry, stress, and anxiety.

Tinea Pedis and Palmaris. This may occur as (1) a dry, scaling dermatitis involving the "moccasin" area of the feet, (2) a vesicular or bullous eruption involving the arch of the foot or plantar surfaces of the toes (this more inflammatory type may cause an id reaction on the hands that mimics dyshidrosis), or (3) a white, macerated, intertriginous dermatitis in the web spaces. Occasionally one hand may be involved simultaneously with a dry, scaling tinea palmaris, the so-called "two feet–one hand" syndrome.

Recalcitrant, Recurrent Pustular Eruption of the Palms or Soles. This presents with recurrent crops of clear vesicles appearing on the palms or soles. These vesicles rapidly become pustular and then dry out, forming the characteristic and diagnostic red-brown crusts.

Localized Atopic Dermatitis. This dermatitis may occur on the hands but is especially common on the dorsum of the toes, especially the large toe in young atopic children. It presents as an erythematous dry, scaling dermatitis and must be differentiated from an allergic contact dermatitis to shoe components.

General Principles of Therapy

1. *Eliminate exposure to the cause* if it is an irritant or allergic contact dermatitis. Hand protection with gloves is a must.

2. *Wet compresses:* Their purpose is to dry and soothe, if dermatitis is vesicular, bullous, oozing, and weeping. Use aluminum sulfate and calcium acetate (Domeboro). Dissolve 1 packet or tablet in 1 or 2 pints of water. Soak a clean cotton cloth in solution and then compress affected area for 10 to 15 minutes. Repeat every 4 to 6 hours until lesion becomes dry.

3. *Oil and water soaks:* The purpose of these is to soften, hydrate, and lubricate if the dermatitis is dry, cracking, and fissuring. Use water-dispersible antipruritic oil (Alpha Keri Oil), 4 capfuls in one pint of lukewarm water. Soak hands or feet for 15 minutes in solution three or four times daily.

4. *Antibiotics:* Antibiotics clear secondary bacterial skin infection that is due almost always to either coagulase-positive staphylococci or streptococci, or both, as evidenced by the presence of honey-yellow shellac-like crusts. Use systemic, not topical, antibiotics. Choices are (1) erythromycin, 250 mg, (2) dicloxacillin, 250 mg, or (3) cephalexin (Keflex), 250 mg, four times daily for 10 days.

5. *Antihistamines:* Their purpose is to relieve pruritus. Choices are (1) hydroxyzine (Atarax), 10 to 25 mg, (2) diphenhydramine (Benadryl), 25 to 50 mg, or (3) cyproheptadine (Periactin), 4 mg, four times daily as necessary.

6. *Topical corticosteroids:* The purpose of these is to reduce inflammation and clear the dermatitis. The choice of vehicle, i.e., cream or ointment, is dictated by the type of dermatitis: if it is moist, use a cream, if it is dry and cracked, use an ointment. On the hands and feet a strong fluorinated preparation is needed. Plastic occlusion will increase effectiveness approximately tenfold. Choices are (1) fluocinonide (Lidex) cream or ointment, (2) halcinonide (Halog)

cream or ointment, or (3) diflorasone diacetate (Florone) cream or ointment. Apply two times a day sparingly.

7. *Systemic corticosteroids:* These provide dramatic anti-inflammatory action in *severe* dermatitis, provided that there are no contraindications to their use. Systemic steroids are used only for short periods of time (7 to 21 days) to gain control, never for maintenance therapy. Choices are (1) prednisone, 60 mg orally initially, and then decrease the daily dose by 5 mg each day over the next 11 days until discontinued, (2) dexamethasone (Decadron-LA), 8 mg intramuscularly, or (3) triamcinolone acetonide (Kenalog), 40 mg intramuscularly.

Specific Therapy

Primary Irritant Contact Dermatitis (Housewife's Eczema). 1. Hand protection is essential. The patient must avoid irritants, particularly soap, cleaning solutions, and vegetable and meat juices. Use rubber gloves with separate cotton liners for all housework.

2. Treat secondary bacterial infection, if present.

3. Compress with aluminum sulfate–calcium acetate (Domeboro) solution if the dermatitis is weeping or, if dry and cracked, use oil and water compresses.

4. Usually topical corticosteroid therapy with occasional overnight plastic glove occlusion will suffice.

5. Isolated painful fissures may be "glued" together with flexible collodion.

Allergic Eczematous Contact Dermatitis.
1. Avoid suspected allergen.

2. Do patch testing with the screening series and for suspected allergen when acute dermatitis has resolved.

3. Use wet aluminum sulfate–calcium acetate (Domeboro) compresses for lesions in the vesicular or bullous phase, or oil and water soaks for dry and chronic lesions.

4. Use topical corticosteroid preparation after compresses.

5. For severe eruption as evidenced by pronounced edema, vesiculation and bullae, marked pruritus, and discomfort, or beginning autoeczematization, use a short course of a systemic corticosteroid initially.

Dyshidrosis. Since this condition is frequently triggered by stress and anxiety, it is for many patients a chronic, intermittently recurrent one.

1. A stress reduction program may be helpful, e.g., yoga, transcendental meditation, counseling, and so forth, in the long-term overall management.

2. For mild cases, a topical corticosteroid cream will control most flares.

3. Antihistamines may be used for pruritus, especially hydroxyzine hydrochloride (Atarax).

4. For severe flare-ups, systemic corticosteroids are the means of gaining control.

Tinea Pedis and Palmaris. The diagnosis must always be substantiated by either a positive KOH preparation or a fungal culture before initiating therapy.

1. For the dry, scaling variety or the macerated, intertriginous type use miconazole nitrate (MicaTin), 2 per cent cream twice daily for 1 month. Topical therapy may be ineffective in some patients, and systemic griseofulvin (Grisactin), 500 mg a day or griseofulvin ultramicrosize (Gris-PEG), 250 mg twice a day for 30 days, should be tried. In some patients, even with systemic griseofulvin it is impossible to clear this fungal infection.

2. For the vesicular, bullous variety use (a) Domeboro compresses, (b) systemic griseofulvin for 1 month, (c) systemic corticosteroids if a severe id reaction or autoeczematization has occurred, and (d) systemic antibiotics for secondary bacterial infection.

3. For the "two feet–one hand" syndrome use systemic griseofulvin.

Recalcitrant, Recurrent Pustular Eruption of the Palms or Soles. This is probably a localized variety of pustular psoriasis. One bacterial culture probably should be done to rule out pyoderma. It will be negative in this condition.

1. A tar gel (psoriGel or Estar Gel) twice daily.

2. Corticosteroid ointment twice daily. Apply directly over the aforementioned tar gel.

3. Occasionally, overnight plastic occlusion with corticosteroid ointment only (not the tar) will be helpful. For failures, and there will be many, for this is a difficult condition to treat, try (a) grenz ray therapy, (b) PUVA (psoralen–ultraviolet light) therapy (investigational), or (3) anthralin* ointment 0.1 to 0.5 per cent at bedtime.

Localized Atopic Dermatitis. 1. Have child go barefoot around the house.

2. Wear thick cotton socks and leather shoes.

3. Avoid rubber tennis shoes.

4. Use oil and water soaks if dermatitis is cracked and dry.

5. This, plus a topical corticosteroid cream or ointment, will clear most.

6. If the eruption fails to clear or persists, a patch test to rule out an allergic contact dermatitis to a shoe component should be performed.

---

*This use of this agent is not listed in the manufacturer's official directive.

BACTERIAL DISEASES OF THE SKIN

method of
BAYLOR KURTIS, M.D.
Houston, Texas

Nonbullous Impetigo

Depending on environmental and anatomic factors, nonbullous impetigo may be caused by Group A beta-hemolytic streptococci, *Staphylococcus aureus,* or a combination of both.

Treatment. TOPICAL THERAPY. Topical antibiotic therapy is now rightfully regaining popularity after a period of disfavor. It is particularly useful for lesions covering a limited area.

1. The lesion is compressed three to four times daily with tepid water, after which loosened crusts are gently removed.

2. After compressing, a topical antibiotic such as neomycin, bacitracin, or a neomycin-bacitracin-polymyxin combination is applied. (The sensitizing potential of neomycin is reduced when used for short periods of time in limited areas.)

3. I do not recommend gentamicin, as it has been associated with the emergence of resistant strains.

SYSTEMIC THERAPY. 1. Penicillin V, 250 mg orally four times daily. This should be continued for 7 to 10 days.

2. Benzathine penicillin G, 600,000 to 1,200,000 units intramuscularly.

3. Erythromycin succinate, 250 mg orally four times daily.

4. In those cases of nonbullous impetigo not responding to penicillin, a culture should be taken to determine whether the cause is a penicillinase-producing Staphylococcus. In that case, a semisynthetic penicillinase-resistant penicillin such as cloxacillin, 250 mg orally four times daily, is recommended.

5. In endemic areas in which nephritogenic strains are known to be present, multiple urinalyses should be performed at weekly intervals.

Bullous Impetigo

Bullous impetigo is caused by *Staphylococcus aureus* Group II, which is usually penicillin resistant. Culture and sensitivities should be taken; however, because of the potential seriousness of this condition, therapy with a semisynthetic penicillin should be started immediately.

Treatment. 1. Cloxacillin, 500 mg orally four times daily.

2. Erythromycin succinate, 250 to 500 mg orally four times daily, may be used in a patient allergic to penicillin.

3. Clindamycin, 150 to 300 mg orally three times daily, may be used as an antistaphylococcal agent only when both of the aforementioned drugs are contraindicated. Patients must be warned to stop the drug at the first sign of diarrhea.

4. Compresses may be used as outlined above.

5. Topical antibiotics do not have any significant effect in bullous impetigo.

Ecthyma

Ecthyma begins as a superficial pyoderma similar to impetigo; however, the process extends beyond the epidermis, producing a shallow ulcer, often with a thick crust. The legs are most often involved. Group A beta-hemolytic Streptococcus is almost always the offending organism.

Treatment. 1. Warm compresses 15 to 20 minutes three to four times daily with subsequent removal of loose crusts are a helpful adjunct to systemic therapy. Topical antibiotics are ineffective in ecthyma.

2. Penicillin V, 250 mg orally four times daily.

3. Benzathine penicillin G, 600,000 to 1,200,000 units intramuscularly.

Erysipelas and Cellulitis

Erysipelas is a superficial cellulitis which demonstrates a marked erythema with well-defined borders. It usually involves either the face or the legs. It is occasionally accompanied by fever and toxicity and may be recurrent.

Erysipelas is a potentially serious infection, with sporadic instances of mortality still being reported.

I, therefore, treat all such cases with procaine penicillin, 600,000 units intramuscularly twice daily. I would consider 600,000 units of procaine penicillin daily the absolute minimal dosage.

The patient should be under close supervision.

In those patients with recurrent disease preventive therapy with penicillin or erythromycin, 250 to 500 mg orally daily, may be beneficial.

Cellulitis is similar to erysipelas in that it is a diffusely spreading, often streptococcal infection. However, the involvement in subcutaneous tissues is deeper than in erysipelas, and the diffuse brawny inflammation demonstrates less sharply defined borders. Regional lymphadenopathy is commonly present. Occasionally red streaks extending proximally from the area of inflammation are seen and represent ascending lymphangitis.

1. A patient with constitutional symptoms or extensive disease should be hospitalized.

2. The involved area should be immobilized and elevated with intermittent warm packs applied four times daily.

3. Depending on the severity of the infection, either oral penicillin, 250 to 500 mg four times daily, or intramuscular procaine penicillin, 600,000 to 1,200,000 units daily, may be used. Mild disease may be treated with one intramuscular injection of benzathine penicillin G, 1,200,000 units.

4. In those occasional cases caused by Staphylococcus, appropriate antibiotics must be used.

Folliculitis

Folliculitis is a superficial, virtually always bacterial infection of the hair follicle. *Staphylococcus aureus* is almost always the offending organism in both folliculitis and furunculosis. For mild cases, daily washes with an antibacterial soap such as hexachlorophene (pHisoHex) is sufficient. Not infrequently keratin plugging of the follicle is the precipitating event. This can be removed by daily scrubbing with an abrasive sponge (Buff-Puff) or by applications with topical retinoic acid solution 0.1 per cent (Retin A) or other peeling and drying compounds such as those used in acne, e.g., benzoyl peroxide preparations (Persa-Gel). Occasionally, systemic antibiotics are also needed. I use erythromycin succinate, 250 mg orally four times daily, or tetracycline, 250 mg orally four times daily.

Furuncles and Carbuncles

A furuncle is a deep form of folliculitis with involvement of subcutaneous tissue. When multiple continuous hair follicles are involved, in particular on the neck and the upper back, the lesion is known as a carbuncle. Persistent and recurrent disease is known as recurrent furunculosis.

Treatment. TOPICAL. For recurrent disease, preventive measures such as twice daily showering with an antibacterial soap (pHisoHex) and twice daily applications of a topical antibiotic (bacitracin) to the anterior nares are beneficial.

SYSTEMIC. 1. The antibiotic of choice is cloxacillin, 250 mg orally four times daily. Since the percentage of penicillin-resistant "community strains" of Staphylococcus continues to rise, penicillin V is not advised.

2. Erythromycin succinate, 250 mg orally four times daily.

3. Tetracycline, 250 mg orally four times daily, is sometimes helpful.

4. Large lesions may need incision and drainage.

5. Some patients with recurrent disease require daily administration of low dose antibiotics such as erythromycin succinate or tetracycline, 250 mg orally once to twice daily, as a preventive measure in addition to those topical measures mentioned above.

Cysts and Abscesses

For small infected abscesses which are pointing, drainage is sufficient. Care must be taken to break all fibrous bands within the cavity, allowing the entire lesion to drain. I usually insert an iodoform wick to maintain drainage. Occasionally, I will withdraw the wick slowly, e.g., one quarter to one half inch, to assure obliteration of cyst cavity. For deeper nonpointing abscesses, hot compresses and antibiotics are used until the lesion either resolves or presents itself for drainage.

Ruptured epidermoid (sebaceous) cysts result in inflammation secondary to a foreign body (keratin) rather than bacteria; therefore antibiotics are not necessary for these lesions. I use drainage procedures only. In cases of recurrent cyst rupture, I excise the cyst in toto after the inflammation has subsided.

Bacterial Infections of Toe Webs

When interdigital spaces of the feet are macerated or boggy, there is usually a bacterial cause which must be treated prior to evaluation for fungal involvement. These are often gram-negative organisms. Wood's light will produce a green fluorescence if Pseudomonas is present.

Treatment. 1. Toes must be separated with cotton pads or cigarette filters, allowing air to enter the web spaces.

2. Whenever possible, the patient should walk barefoot or wear open-toed sandals.

3. Aluminum chloride solutions may be applied to the web spaces without occlusion to ensure drying. I use aluminum chloride in anhydrous ethyl alcohol (Drysol), which may be applied daily for 5 days and then weekly or biweekly as needed. It should not be applied if open wounds are present. Antiperspirant aerosols (Right Guard, silver can) also contain aluminum chloride and are often effective when sprayed locally.

4. Gentian violet 0.1 per cent and Castellani's paint (full strength, half-strength, or colorless) are good drying agents with antibacterial properties.

5. Acetic acid soaks 0.25 to 1.0 per cent when the offending organism is known to be Pseudomonas.

Erythrasma

Erythrasma is a chronic superficial bacterial infection presenting as reddish-brown sharply marginated macules in intertriginous areas or as boggy macerated toe webs. These lesions will fluoresce coral-red under Wood's light.

Treatment. 1. Topical antibiotics, in particular topical erythromycin, applied two to four times a day.

2. Kerolytic agents such as salicylic acid, sulfur ointments, or a salicylic acid gel (Keralyt gel).

3. Erythromycin succinate, 250 mg orally four times daily for 10 to 14 days.

External Otitis

Etiology of external otitis is multifold. Bacteria, especially gram-negative bacilli and occasionally *Staphylococcus aureus,* play a significant role secondary to a primary inflammation.

Treatment. 1. I will frequently use a corticosteroid spray alone (Kenalog spray) applied from 3 inches three times daily for 3 seconds to reduce the inflammation. Often this is sufficient to suppress the primary inflammation and antibacterial measures are unnecessary.

2. Cotton tip applicators or other instruments inserted by the patient should be strictly forbidden.

3. Gentian violet 2 per cent in alcohol 2 to 3 drops in each ear nightly.

4. A colistin–neomycin–hydrocortisone–acetic acid compound (Coly-Mycin S otic), 2 to 3 drops three to four times daily, or colistin B suspension, *or*

5. Two percent hydrocortisone–0.1 per cent polymyxin B (Aerosporin) may be inserted with a dropper three to four times daily, *or*

6. Desonide 0.05 per cent–acetic acid 2 per cent (Otic Tridesilon) 2 to 3 drops in each ear three times daily.

When drops are used, care must be taken that the head remains tilted to one side after insertion to prevent immediate spillage of the medicine. A gauze wick may be inserted by the physician and kept saturated by the patient to prevent loss of medication.

Atypical Mycobacteria

Cutaneous granulomatous infections may be acquired in swimming pools or while cleaning tropical fish tanks. The most frequent offending organism is *Mycobacterium marinum (Mycobacterium balnei).*

Treatment. 1. Untreated lesions may spontaneously resolve, although this may take months or even years.

2. Surgical excision.

3. Electrosurgical or cryosurgical destruction.

4. Tetracycline, 250 to 500 mg orally four times daily for 4 to 12 weeks.

5. Minocycline, 100 mg twice daily for 8 weeks or longer.

6. These organisms do not respond well to first line antituberculous therapy. The so-called second line antituberculous drugs may be effective; however, they are expensive and therapy is prolonged.

Staphylococcal Scalded Skin Syndrome (SSS)

SSS is a widespread erythematous eruption accompanied by large flaccid bullae and skin which easily separates, giving a burned or scalded appearance. It occurs in infants and children up to 6 or 7 years of age. All patients but those with the mildest cases should be admitted to a hospital. It is caused by Group II Staphylococcus, which is usually resistant to penicillin treatment.

Treatment. 1. Skin, nasal, and nasopharyngeal cultures should be performed.

2. Oral antibiotics usually suffice. (a) Cloxacillin, 12.5 mg per kg per day in four equally divided doses. (b) Erythromycin, 50 mg per kg per day in four equally divided doses.

3. If the child appears toxic, the antibiotics should be given intravenously with intravenous fluids as a supportive measure.

4. Corticosteroids are contraindicated.

ACNE ROSACEA

method of
JAMES F. GREGORY, M.D.
Belleville, Illinois

Acne rosacea is a chronic idiopathic disorder which involves primarily the central vertical third of the face and consists of three components: (1) papulopustular lesions, (2) telangiectases and flushing, and (3) hypertrophy of the sebaceous and fibrous components of the nose ("rhinophyma"). A keratitis and/or seborrhea are less frequent accompaniments of the other manifestations. Any of these components may occur alone or in any combination with the others.

Rosacea differs from acne vulgaris in several respects: it occurs almost exclusively in the 30 to

50 year age group, is more common in women (although rhinophyma occurs almost exclusively in men), and is associated with no demonstrable infectious component, no increase in sebum production, and no significant hormonal influence.

Treatment is designed to control the disorder, since no definitive therapy is available.

Systemic Therapy

1. Tetracycline remains the mainstay of therapy. Initial dosage should be 1 gram per day given for 10 to 14 days, after which 500 mg per day is frequently adequate to maintain control. Tetracycline improves not only the papulopustular component but also the telangiectatic and ocular components. Occasionally a return to 1 gram per day may be necessary to control acute flares. In giving the higher dosage, compliance may be improved by encouraging twice a day administration, since it is a rare patient who finds his stomach appropriately empty four times a day. Higher dosages, up to 2 grams per day, may be necessary in severe cases.

2. When the patient is unable to take tetracycline, erythromycin may be tried in dosages equal to those of tetracycline. Another alternative is minocycline, 50 mg orally twice daily. These medications offer the advantage of flexibility in time of administration (minocycline and the enteric coated forms of erythromycin may be taken at meals), but usually are not as efficacious as tetracycline.

Topical Therapy

1. Topical therapy is of limited value. If a significant erythematous, scaly component is present, as with associated seborrhea, 1 per cent hydrocortisone or 1 per cent hydrocortisone with iodochlorhydroxyquin (Vioform HC) may be used. Potent steroids, whether fluorinated or not, should not be used on the face for conditions as chronic as acne rosacea. Initial improvement may result from their use, but subsequent worsening and significant atrophy will eventually result.

2. Although other topical treatments, e.g., drying agents, topical antibiotics, and retinoic acid, have been anecdotally touted, they have been of little or no benefit in my experience.

3. Telangiectases may benefit from low-voltage electrocautery administered with a fine-tipped needle.

Preventive Measures

Preventive measures are largely based upon the theory that vasodilatation worsens the condition; therefore, extremes of heat and cold, spicy foods, alcohol, caffeine, and excessive anxiety should be discouraged. Great individual variation exists among patients in their response to these factors; most identify no external provoking factors.

SCABIES

method of
STEPHEN A. ESTES, M.D.
Cincinnati, Ohio

Despite effective therapies for scabies, epidemics continue without clear explanations. Scabies can be a difficult diagnosis to make. It is a great imitator of numerous other skin conditions and at times eludes even the best dermatologist. A high index of suspicion is critical in recognizing scabies. The diagnosis should be based on one or more of the following: epidemiologic pattern, prominent nocturnal pruritus, consistent cutaneous eruption, and a positive skin scraping.

Treatment

Treatment of scabietic patients must include asymptomatic family members and sexual contacts, who may not develop symptoms for 6 weeks.

Gamma Benzene Hexachloride (Lindane), 1 per cent. Lotion or cream is applied over the entire skin surface from neck to soles of feet, left on overnight, and washed off in the morning. This exposure should be in the 6 to 12 hour range. It is important to stress that the medicine be applied to the eruption *and* normal skin as well. The same procedure is repeated the next night. Two ounces of either the cream or lotion is adequate to treat an adult twice. One correct application of lindane will give a 96 to 98 per cent cure rate. The second application is used to provide for patient error in application.

Between applications the patient's sheets, towels, and clothing should be put through a hot cycle in the washing machine. Although fomites are thought to have minimal significance in the spread of scabies, this laundering is considered a reasonable precaution.

Bathing prior to application of lindane is no longer recommended, since it may potentiate percutaneous absorption of the drug.

Central nervous system (CNS) toxicity can result from percutaneous absorption of lindane. However, most reported cases of possible CNS toxicity represent drastic overuse or misuse of the drug. Severe cutaneous disruption caused by scabies, excoriations, and secondary pyoderma may potentiate the possibility of neurotoxicity occurring, especially in children who have a large surface area–to–mass ratio. Such considerations cause some physicians to use alternative therapies in infants, small children, and pregnant women.

Crotamiton, 10 per cent. While this medication has the advantage of being an antipruritic agent, its efficacy is less than that of lindane. Cream or lotion is applied after a bath in a similar manner to lindane. Twenty-four hours later a repeat application is made, and a cleansing bath is taken at 72 hours. Since infants and children may have scabies on the scalp and face, this preparation or sulfur can be used on these areas.

Sulfur, 5 or 10 per cent in Petrolatum. Five per cent sulfur is used in infants and children and 10 per cent in adults. It is applied two or three times at 24 hour intervals, and a cleansing bath is taken 24 hours after the last application. The efficacy of sulfur has not been critically evaluated. Irritant dermatitis and adverse CNS effects have been reported on occasion. This preparation is not esthetically pleasing and may cause patient noncompliance.

Complications

Postscabietic Pruritus. The aforementioned therapies kill mites and eggs, which, along with mite feces, remain in the stratum corneum and presumably are antigens which cause continued pruritus and dermatitis. Treatment with oral antihistamines, topical corticosteroids, and, rarely in severe cases, a short course of oral prednisone will control symptoms. Postscabietic pruritus may last days to weeks. Patient education with regard to this entity is indicated in order to prevent the patients' overuse of potentially toxic scabicides.

Pyoderma. Mild to severe pyoderma is frequently seen in conjunction with scabies and should be treated with systemic antibiotics.

Nodular Scabies. A few patients may develop persistently pruritic nodules that remain for months after adequate therapy for scabies. Such nodules represent a continued hypersensitivity reaction and may respond to topical corticosteroids. Recalcitrant nodules will respond to intralesional corticosteroid injections.

Keratotic Scabies. Crusted or keratotic scabies represent a tremendous overgrowth of the mite population on patients who are compromised on an immunologic or neurologic basis. The keratotic debris scraped or desquamating from these patients is loaded with live mites. Such cases, although rare, are frequently the cause for local epidemics in hospitals, nursing homes, and mental institutions. The recommended treatment schedules with scabicides should be doubled, application of medication should include the face and scalp, and fomite precautions should be instituted. Symptomatic or asymptomatic primary contacts should be treated to contain the spread of this more contagious form of scabies.

Psychologic Consequences. Infestations of any sort are psychologically uncomfortable for many people. Emotional reactions may range from shame and anxiety to persistent delusions of parasitosis. A straightforward educational approach coupled with sensitivity minimizes most problems and assures patient compliance with therapy.

SCLERODERMA
(Systemic Sclerosis)

method of
THOMAS A. MEDSGER, JR., M.D.
Pittsburgh, Pennsylvania

Scleroderma (systemic sclerosis, progressive systemic sclerosis [PSS], or systemic scleroderma) is one of the diffuse connective tissue disorders and is characterized by fibrotic, degenerative, and occasionally inflammatory lesions involving the skin, joints, muscles, gastrointestinal tract, and other internal organs such as the lungs, heart, and kidneys. Understanding current concepts of the pathophysiology of scleroderma is crucial to an appreciation of the rationale for the various therapeutic regimens presently employed. The following steps are considered to be involved:

1. Microvascular injury occurs for unknown reasons, leading to ischemia and necrosis of tissue.
2. This event evokes a response of the immune system with both cell-mediated and humoral components: (a) Peripheral blood (and possibly skin) lymphocytes produce lymphokines capable of stimulating fibroblasts to produce collagen. (b) Plasma cells produce a variety of antinuclear and other antibodies.
3. Fibroblast stimulation is uncontrolled, resulting in poorly regulated production of collagen in skin and other connective tissues, such as blood vessels.
4. Organ system dysfunction occurs as a result of accumulation of collagen in the parenchyma of organs and replacement of normal and ischemic cells.

General Therapy

Management of the patient with PSS first requires the establishment of a strong relationship between patient and physician. It is essential to discuss the variable nature of the disease and to differentiate between the diffuse form (with widespread cutaneous involvement, including both extremities and trunk) and the CREST syndrome (limited skin changes [sclerodactyly] in association with calcinosis, Raynaud's phenomenon, esophageal dysfunction, and telangiectasia) and their respective prognostic implications. Detailed instruction, using diagrams of the skin, blood vessels, and esophagus, for example, and a rational approach to each problem posed by the patient help achieve such rapport.

A number of factors make the evaluation of potential therapeutic agents extremely difficult. These include the variable and slowly progressive course, lack of easily quantitated indices of improvement or deterioration (especially of viscera), difficulty in objectively judging changes in skin thickening, and the influence of psychologic factors.

Unfortunately, the pathogenetic steps considered above are by and large speculative. Thus, therapeutic programs are most often concerned with complications of the illness rather than its underlying cause. Nevertheless, in considering the events cited above, at least three theoretical mechanisms of drug action are possible: (1) suppression of the appearance and/or function of lymphocytes, (2) blockade of the overactive fibroblast, and (3) increased solubilization and/or metabolism of the excessive extracellular collagen deposited.

The influence of corticosteroids on both cutaneous and visceral scleroderma has been disappointing, although they are effective for certain problems most often encountered when PSS is found in overlap with other related disorders (e.g., mixed connective tissue disease). Manifestations such as active proliferative synovitis, acute pericarditis, and inflammatory myopathy respond impressively to corticosteroids, and many patients may even show some regression of cutaneous changes. A few investigators have expressed concern that the indiscriminate use of corticosteroids (e.g., prednisone, 20 mg per day or more) in patients with diffuse skin involvement may precipitate renal scleroderma. Potassium para-aminobenzoate (Potaba) and dimethyl sulfoxide (DMSO) have been prescribed, but evidence for their effectiveness is unconvincing.

Several centers have been impressed with the beneficial effects of D-penicillamine, a compound known to interfere with the intermolecular cross-linking of collagen. This drug appears indicated only in instances of rapidly progressive diffuse skin involvement, and close monitoring for toxicity is required. Initial dosage of 250 mg daily is suggested with gradual increase every 2 to 4

months to a maximum of 1000 mg per day. (This use of D-penicillamine is not listed in the manufacturer's official directive.)

The use of colchicine (0.6 to 1.8 mg daily) has been advocated on the basis of its ability to prevent extracellular accumulation of collagen by inhibiting the release of procollagen from fibroblasts. Although its safety is acknowledged, no confirmatory studies have yet supported the initial enthusiasm regarding the efficacy of this agent.

For reasons cited above, the participation of immune mechanisms in PSS pathogenesis has kindled interest in the use of immunosuppressive drugs. The literature in this regard is still meager and largely anecdotal, but some physicians use such agents in patients with rapidly progressive disease who appear destined to develop disabling contractures or life-threatening internal organ involvement.

Supporting Measures

Raynaud's Phenomenon. A common sense approach to Raynaud's phenomenon should be suggested, including dressing warmly and avoiding, if possible, unnecessary or prolonged cold exposure and cigarettes. Vasodilating drugs have proved disappointing, although some patients appear to improve on oral reserpine, 0.25 to 0.50 mg daily, or methyldopa, 500 to 1500 mg daily. (This use of these agents is not listed in the manufacturers' official directives.) Intra-arterial reserpine (1.0 mg injected directly into the brachial artery) has had variable results, but some patients report sustained improvement lasting several months or more. A number of new agents with peripheral vasodilating properties are being used without dramatic success. Intermittent cervical sympathetic blockade may help diminish pain and increase circulation to digital infarctive lesions. Surgical thoracic sympathectomy usually results in only transient relief of vasospasm, and has no significant influence on the course of cutaneous or visceral sclerosis. Some voluntary control over vasospasm can be achieved using biofeedback training.

Uninfected painful digital tip infarcts or gangrenous areas are best left alone and dry to demarcate by autoamputation. Pain induced by minor trauma may be minimized by the use of protective and immobilizing finger casts, which our patients are taught to make themselves. Adequate oral analgesics should be used; codeine up to 360 mg daily or the equivalent may be needed. Surgical intervention is rarely required, and then only for drainage or debridement of nonviable, secondarily infected tissue. Open finger ulcers should be kept clean and fibrinous exudate removed several times daily after soaking in half-strength hydrogen peroxide. Although local pain may be relieved by topical antibiotic and corticosteroid ointments, these compounds do not appear to aid healing.

Skin. Excessive skin dryness and pruritus may be partially relieved by the use of special lotions, soaps, and bath oils rubbed thoroughly into thickened areas. Occasionally, oral preparations such as antihistamines or phenothiazine derivatives may be helpful. Household detergents should be avoided. Patients with diffuse scleroderma are unable to disperse heat adequately and are thus predisposed to heat stroke after excessive sun exposure.

Joints and Muscles. Arthralgias, arthritis, and tenosynovitis often respond adequately to the use of salicylates or other nonsteroidal anti-inflammatory agents. Corticosteroids are seldom required, but some clinicians prefer to utilize them during the acute "puffy hand" stage. An occasional patient with proliferative synovitis must be treated as if he had rheumatoid arthritis. A vigorous exercise program is helpful in maintaining an adequate range of motion and improving the muscle tone required for personal and occupational activities. We teach our patients such stretching exercises to improve motion in the upper extremity joints, especially hands. Subcutaneous calcinosis cannot be dissolved by chelating agents, and surgical removal of these deposits is occasionally complicated by persistent draining fistulous tracts which uniformly become secondarily infected.

The typical "fibrotic" myopathy of PSS is mild and only slowly, if at all, progressive and is unaffected by corticosteroid therapy. In contrast, steroids are definitely indicated in the few cases in which there is marked weakness, high serum muscle enzymes, and severe degenerative and inflammatory change on biopsy.

Gastrointestinal Tract. Oral problems may prove exasperating in PSS because of decreased oral aperture, loosening of teeth related to resorption of the lamina dura with thickening of the periodontal membrane, or the xerostomia of associated Sjögren's syndrome. Regular prophylactic dental care and good oral hygiene are essential. Patients with dysphagia for solid food must learn to avoid tough meat and dry bread and to masticate completely. Reflux esophagitis usually can be minimized by the routine use of antacids and elevation of the head of the bed. In resistant cases, cimetidine has proved efficacious. The development of esophageal stricture may require periodic dilatation. Successful excision of strictures and correction of gastroesophageal reflux by gastroplasty have been reported. When malabsorption syndrome results from small intestinal involvement, the use of broad-spectrum antibiotics reduces bacterial overgrowth and often dramatically improves (although never eliminates) symptoms. Ideally, the proper antibiotic choice is made after duodenal intubation for quantitative aerobic and anaerobic cultures. We have often used intermittent (2 to 3 week) courses of tetracycline or ampicillin, followed by rest periods of 1 to 2 weeks. Mycostatin may also be prescribed to reduce Candida or other fungal overgrowth. Replacement therapy is recommended for inadequately absorbed substances such as iron, vitamin B_{12}, and calcium. A direct gastrointestinal smooth muscle stimulant, metaclopramide, has been shown to increase esophageal motility, but in our experience it has proved ineffective in small bowel scleroderma. Colonic involvement is generally asymptomatic or causes only constipation.

Lung and Heart. No established primary therapy is available for pulmonary fibrosis or for pulmonary arterial hypertension. An occasional patient may show a diffuse interstitial pulmonary infiltrate with chronic inflammatory cells, although usually the biopsy suggests fibrosis as the dominant feature. Thus, theoretically, both corticosteroids and D-penicillamine could have a role, but only anecdotal information on their efficacy is available in the literature. Prompt antibiotic administration is necessary in the event of superimposed bacterial pneumonia.

The treatment of congestive heart failure resulting from PSS is difficult because of a poor response to digitalis, digitalis toxicity, and arrhythmias related to fibrosis of the conducting system and/or working myocardium. A greater reliance is placed on diuretics in this situation. Several cases have been reported in which D-penicillamine seems to have been helpful. As noted above, acute pericarditis is a clear-cut indication for the use of corticosteroids in standard doses.

Kidney. Several advances have been made in the treatment of patients with malignant arterial hypertension and renal failure caused by "scleroderma kidney." This complication, appearing almost exclusively in patients with "diffuse" scleroderma, is heralded by headache, blurred vision, microscopic hematuria and proteinuria, and, often, congestive heart failure. Very aggressive antihypertensive therapy appears to decelerate the progression of azotemia, and in some instances may abort the process completely. Agents directed against the hyper-reninemia, such as propranolol, appear to be useful, and a recently used group of inhibitors of angiotensin converting enzyme seems promising.

Prompt bilateral nephrectomy should be performed if hypertension cannot be controlled medically. Many patients have now been successfully carried on hemodialysis, although vascular access has been a limiting feature because of scleroderma involvement of vessels and poor flow through fistulas. Several successful renal transplants have been performed, but in one case scleroderma changes were subsequently detected in the donor kidney on biopsy.

Related Disorders

Scleroderma in Overlap. Scleroderma is frequently found in patients who also have manifestations of other connective tissue diseases; such difficult-to-classify situations are termed "overlap syndromes." The recently described "mixed connective tissue disease" is a disorder with shared features of systemic lupus erythematosus, polymyositis, and scleroderma. It is characterized by the presence of large amounts of serum antibody to ribonucleoprotein (anti-RNP). Although not a benign condition, many of the signs and symptoms respond promptly to low or moderate dose corticosteroid therapy.

Eosinophilic Fasciitis. This variant of scleroderma results in sclerosis and chronic inflammatory cell infiltration of the deep fascia and subcutis, with lesser involvement of overlying skin and muscle. Unusually vigorous physical exercise has been implicated in precipitating the disease in a number of patients. The extremities (and trunk) are most commonly affected, although often the digits are spared. Raynaud's phenomenon is absent, as are visceral stigmata of PSS. Important clues are the presence of moderate to marked peripheral (and tissue) eosinophilia and hypergammaglobulinemia. Although the disorder is most often self-limited, with gradual resolution of the indurative changes over several years, low dose corticosteroid therapy (prednisone, 5 to 15 mg daily) often leads to prompt symptomatic improvement and abolishes the eosinophilia.

Localized Scleroderma. Morphea (patches) and linear scleroderma are forms of skin thickening noted for their distribution pattern and absence of visceral changes. These conditions are predominantly found in children. An arthropathy may be associated, and some patients have eosinophilia and serum anti-DNA antibodies. Treatment is considered when there is rapid enlargement or progression of an individual lesion, or the development of multiple patches. Intralesional injection of one or another corticosteroid preparation is generally recommended.

URTICARIA AND ANGIOEDEMA

method of
LENNART JUHLIN, M.D.
Uppsala, Sweden

Urticaria is a localized edema of the skin as a result of histamine release. In the order of frequency it can be separated into acute, physical, and recurrent urticaria. Swelling of subcutaneous tissues is called angioedema and is common in the lips and around the eyes, but is also seen in the hands, feet, and genitals and around the knees. Angioedema can occur alone or together with any type of urticaria. A special type of angioedema is hereditary angioedema (HAE).

Acute Urticaria

Causes. Acute urticaria is often caused by an antigen-antibody reaction occurring within some hours after taking a drug or a special type of food such as eggs, seafood, nuts, berries, or fruits. After penicillin the urticaria can appear as late as 1 to 2 weeks after stopping treatment. Inhalants such as pollen, dust, molds, and sprays occasionally cause hives. Urticaria produced by histamine releasers or antigens penetrating through the skin is most common in children and atopic patients. The wheals appear where the skin is thin and has been exposed to various contactants such as plants, cosmetics, or the licking of a dog. Injections of drugs or stings from insects should not be forgotten.

Treatment. ELIMINATION OF CAUSE. Take a careful history of the patient's intake of drugs, foods, and drinks. Ask about special habits. Does the patient eat a lot of candies, licorice, or menthol tablets? Ask again about such drugs as cough medicine or salicylates. Name trade names. Has the patient had urticaria before? What was the cause then? Eliminate all possible offenders.

ANTIHISTAMINES. For daytime use a type with low central nervous system depressant action such as dimethindene (Forhistal, Fenestil*), especially if the patient must drive a car. Patients should nevertheless be warned that they might react with tiredness. Dexchlorpheniramine maleate (Polaramine Repetabs) or brompheniramine maleate (Dimetane, Dimotone*) has a prolonged and good antihistaminic effect, but sedation can occur initially. Clemastine furamate (Tavigil*, Tavist) has similar effects and is preferred by some patients. A few pa-

---

*May not be available in the United States of America.

tients have noticed that, especially when taking clemastine, they do not care what happens around them or do not follow orders properly. We therefore do not prescribe it, for example, for hospital or military personnel. A noncolored antihistamine should be used. The use of azo-dyes with antihistamines is forbidden in many countries, as they might worsen the urticarial reactions. The treatment usually must be continued for 1 to 2 weeks.

EPINEPHRINE. If the patient also has signs of asthma or has a very extensive and severe urticaria, 0.3 to 0.5 ml (0.3 to 0.5 mg) of epinephrine 1:1000 subcutaneously is recommended except in elderly patients with heart problems. The effect is prompt and lasts for some hours, but the treatment should be followed by antihistamines as mentioned above.

CORTICOSTEROIDS. If the antihistamine has no or insignificant effect after 2 to 3 days and if I am almost sure of what has provoked the attack of urticaria and that further exposure can be avoided, I often prescribe a short course of corticosteroids such as prednisone, 40 mg the first morning and then decreased by 5 mg per day.

Physical Urticaria

This is the group of urticarial disorders which is common in persons between 17 and 40 years of age and in which the cause and diagnosis are often missed by both the patient and the doctor. It should therefore always be excluded first when examining a patient with urticaria. We will consider each of the four most common types separately.

Dermographism. Strike the skin firmly with a blunt object both on the inside of the forearm and on the back. The localized whealing called dermographism is usually evident within 20 minutes. In rare cases there is initially a normal response but the wheals appear 6 to 24 hours later as delayed dermographism. The patient is often not aware of the fact that the urticaria is caused by scratching or by pressure from clothes or from leaning against a chair. Why such patients suddenly react with whealing is often not known, but it has been found after infections, after treatment with penicillin, and in patients with scabies. When the scabies has been treated, the dermographism can disappear within a month.

TREATMENT. 1. *Itching* may start the scratching and is often felt in the evening when undressing. If the skin is dry, an emollient such as an oil in water emulsion (Lubriderm) should be used after hydration.

2. *Antihistamines, including hydroxyzine* (Atarax, Vistaril), reduce the immediate dermographism considerably. In delayed dermographism the response is poor.

3. *Ultraviolet-B (UV-B) irradiation:* In some patients the condition remains for years. Many are better in summertime, and irradiation with a lamp emitting UV-B can be of value.

4. *Rubbing the skin with a brush* has been advocated to deplete the skin of histamine. The patient then decides himself when to produce urticaria with the hope of reacting less for some days to further scratching. This treatment is of value only in very special cases.

Pressure Urticaria. This deep-seated urticaria appears some hours after pressure. It is common on the hands, which feel stiff, or on the shoulder after carrying something heavy.

TREATMENT. Avoid pressure. Antihistamines are of limited value, as are epsilon-aminocaproic acid (EACA)* and tranexamic acid.† Check and avoid worsening factors mentioned under Recurrent Urticaria, below. A diet free of salicylates or azo-dyes can be helpful.

Heat Urticaria or Cholinergic Urticaria. The wheals are small, often of pinhead size, and itching. Sometimes there is only itching. The best method to provoke the symptoms is for the patient to get warm by heavy physical exercise such as running up stairs. The symptoms can also follow a hot bath but are rarely seen after a sauna.

TREATMENT. Avoid overheating and emotional stress. Prescribe hydroxyzine (Atarax, Vistaril), 10 mg two to three times daily.

Cold Urticaria. The hives appear on cold exposed areas, usually during the warm-up period. They disappear within an hour or less. Tests with ice cubes for some seconds to 10 minutes are of value for diagnosis and prognosis. Delayed cold urticaria is rare. Always warn the patients of the risk of shock when swimming even in a warm pool (18 to 26 C [64 to 79 F]).

TREATMENT. 1. Arctic clothing and a warm garage for the car.

2. *Antihistamines:* If urticaria is seen after contact with an ice cube for 2 minutes or less, antihistamines are of no practical value. If the hives first appear after a positive ice cube test of 3 to 12 minutes, antihistamines should be tried. They should also be tried in patients not reacting to ice cubes but reacting to cold wind or

*This use of this agent is not listed in the manufacturer's official directive.

†May not be available in the United States of America.

water. There are individual preferences. We have let the patients try one type of antihistamine per week and have tried to evaluate the effects, including possible negative effects. Three drugs were preferred more than others: dexchlorpheniramine maleate (Polaramine Repetabs), clemastine fumarate (Tavigil, Tavist), and cyproheptadine (Periactin). The patients mainly used them on the days when they had to be outdoors.

3. *Desensitization* with cold water on exposed areas has been tried, but the treatment is unpleasant, the effect is often poor, and there is a risk of producing vasculitis from the repeated cold challenge.

Hereditary Angioedema (HAE)

Hereditary angioedema is transmitted as an autosomal dominant trait and characterized by nonitching swellings of the subcutaneous tissue of the skin and mucosae. The edema can affect any area such as an arm, lips, tongue, larynx, or urinary or gastrointestinal tract. In the last-mentioned case there are symptoms of ileus. HAE can start in childhood or later and can continue with periods of attacks. The patients are deficient in a glycoprotein, which is an inhibitor of the activated first component of complement (C1 esterase inhibitor). The episodes of edema appear when it falls under a certain level, and they are often initiated by trauma. Death in laryngeal edema is a threat to the patient.

Treatment. 1. *Hospitalize* the patient when there is a severe acute episode. It is difficult to interrupt spontaneous attacks, but when swelling of the larynx occurs tracheostomy might be necessary. Injection of C1 esterase inhibitor concentrate or plasma infusion is helpful to prevent further edema.

2. *Danazol,** 400 to 600 mg daily initially to an adult, is the treatment of choice. It is an antigonadotropic hormone with only weak androgenic effects. It increases the level of C1 esterase inhibitor within a week. Most patients experience an effect on the first day. The minimal maintenance dose needed to stop future attacks varies from patient to patient. In some patients 200 mg three times a week or less can be enough. When they feel that an attack might come, they may increase the dose for a day by 200 to 400 mg. The side effects seen are a certain increase in weight, amenorrhea, and, in a few patients, slight virilization with a change of voice. Blood pressure should also be controlled.

Recurrent Urticaria

Here the hives have continued to appear several times a week for more than 6 to 8 weeks without known cause. The term chronic urticaria is used when periods with hives dominate, and recidivating urticaria is used when there are more free periods. In these patients one should control thyroid function, erythrocyte sedimentation rate (ESR), and any evident or hidden infection such as of the sinus, gallbladder, or teeth. If the patient has been to tropical areas, check for parasites.

Treatment. ANTIHISTAMINES. The patients have as a rule tried some of the antihistamines discussed under Acute Urticaria, but the effect has been of limited value or the hives have reappeared when they decrease treatment.

DIET. It is very common for attacks to be precipitated by anti-inflammatory drugs such as salicylates and also food additives such as preservatives and azo-dyes. Give the patient a list of foods in which these items occur and do not occur. Think of additives in drugs. Tartrazine is the most well known azo-dye, but others are also important. Ask for special habits. Heavy milk drinking or drinking of wines and other alcoholic beverages should be stopped as a test. Also, yeast-containing products such as beer, soft bread, cheese, vinegar, ketchup, grapes, and yeast itself should be avoided. Antioxidants such as BHT/BHA are found in milk and cream powder, mayonnaise, dressings, animal fats, and oils. The positive effect of a change in diet is usually seen within a few weeks. If the patients are taking antihistamines, they should try to reduce the dose. After improvement test items are avoided one by one.

HOSPITALIZATION. If patients continue to have hives despite a controlled diet for over a month, hospitalization is recommended for better control of environmental factors and a restricted diet that avoids certain food additives and yeast. Check for C1 esterase inhibitor in blood. If it is low and there is no family history of this deficiency, investigate for malignancy. If it is normal, try a 1 week course of nystatin.* On suspicion of a hidden infection, we give tetracycline for 2 weeks.

DAPSONE. Mark the individual wheals. If they do not disappear within 12 hours, take a biopsy, ask for evidence of vasculitis, and think of systemic lupus erythematosus. Do the same if the erythrocyte sedimentation rate remains elevated. If methods are available, control complement, C1 subcomponents, and complexes. In patients with

---

*This use of danazol is not listed in the manufacturer's official directive.

*This use of this agent is not listed in the manufacturer's official directive.

signs of vasculitis and complement disorders, a trial with dapsone* and antihistamines might be considered.

B₂-AGONISTS. If there is no or poor help from antihistamines, try a B_2 adrenergic stimulator such as terbutaline (Bricanyl,* Brethine*), 2.5 mg three times daily, and after some days double the dose to get optimal effect. We have seen complete disappearance of longstanding urticaria in a few cases after some days' treatment. In most patients no beneficial effect is found.

BE CURIOUS. Try not to give up, and try to do better than the natural healing tendency of urticaria. Have the patient back within half a year for a new check-up if the hives continue.

---

*This use of this agent is not listed in the manufacturer's official directive.

WARTS

method of
H. V. ALLINGTON, M.D.
Oakland, California

In choosing treatment for warts, one should bear in mind that they are harmless and will in all probability ultimately disappear spontaneously. Thus one should choose a method that will leave as litle scar as possible. Scars are unsightly and may be sensitive for long periods, even permanently, if they occur at sites of pressure or weight bearing. Factors such as discomfort, temporary inconvenience and disability, and efficiency should also be considered. At times a decision to withhold treatment entirely is best. However, one cannot predict how large existing warts may become or how many more may develop if left untreated.

It is well to explain to the patient that warts are the result of infection by a virus, that we have no medication effective against the virus, and that no vaccine is available. Treating warts can be exceedingly frustrating. They have been compared to weeds. One can thoroughly destroy all those visible at one time, but he cannot assure the patient that others have not already been "reseeded" and will develop weeks or months later.

I treat most warts with liquid nitrogen. We have a storage container that is filled for us once a week. Each morning we siphon the liquid from it into a pint thermos bottle further insulated in a box, which is easily carried from room to room. If one wishes to use it only occasionally and if a source is close by, it may be got a pint or a quart at a time. Usually, in an insulated bottle, it will last 24 hours or more. I apply it with cotton-tipped applicators of various sizes and shapes. (For details, see Allington, H. V.: Cryosurgery. *In* Epstein, E. [ed.]: Skin Surgery. 4th ed. Springfield, Ill., Charles C Thomas, 1977, p. 635.) The applicator saturated with liquid nitrogen is applied continuously until the wart is frozen to its full extent and depth, and then intermittently as needed to maintain freezing for the time decided upon. The ideal reaction is one that produces enough damage to the wart that it will die and do as little harm as possible to the underlying normal skin. Usually it is necessary to produce a blister that forms at the dermoepidermal junction and separates the wart from the underlying dermis.

Little or no pressure is used for juvenile plane warts or small common warts on areas where the skin is thin, and a freezing time of 20 to 45 seconds may be adequate. Some pressure is required, and treatment time is increased to as much as 3 minutes for warts embedded in palmar or plantar skin or for those of considerable thickness or capped by a hyperkeratotic crust. If hyperkeratosis is pronounced, preliminary paring is helpful.

One of the major advantages of liquid nitrogen is that it has a somewhat selective destructive action, tending to spare the dermis. Even with intense or repeated freezing one rarely produces true scarring, although some degree of hypopigmentation and atrophy may result. A keloid rarely develops.

Following treatment the site may be left alone to heal and the resultant blister top or crust allowed to shed spontaneously. In some cases I ask patients to return in approximately 2 weeks. If a crust or blister top is present, it is removed. If some viable wart remains, it may be touched with bichloracetic acid. If an adequate reaction to freezing has not occurred, liquid nitrogen may be reapplied.

Occasionally, excessively large hemorrhagic blisters may result. This may be expected if several warts in close proximity are treated at the same time, one confluent reaction resulting. Such blisters may be drained early, and a sterile dressing or one using a mild antibiotic ointment may be applied. If blisters are not large enough to be annoying or do not rupture spontaneously, no dressing is needed and normal bathing is allowed.

Liquid nitrogen causes pain, roughly proportional to the duration and depth of freezing. Treatment to the tips of the fingers and toes, palmar and plantar surfaces, lips, and other normally hypersensitive areas hurts most. Burning or stinging occurs as freezing is begun. Once thoroughly frozen, the lesion becomes relatively numb. Pain is most severe when freezing is stopped and thawing occurs. For most lesions it is mild to moderate and lasts for only a few seconds or a minute or two. In some instances it may be sufficiently intense to require analgesics more potent than aspirin for the first 24 to 36 hours. A local anesthetic may be injected before treating periungual or plantar warts, for example, but the injection is also painful.

A rare but significant complication is one of nerve damage, resulting in paresthesia or numbness. This is usually temporary, and occurs where the skin is thin and there is little subcutaneous tissue. One way to ensure against this is to avoid freezing to a depth that will cause the skin to adhere to the underlying tissue, being sure that the skin is mobile throughout treatment.

The failure rate is greatest for deeply embedded warts such as those beneath the nails and on palmar and plantar surfaces. In many cases when the initial treatment fails, prompt retreatment with liquid nitrogen will succeed.

When liquid nitrogen has failed, or for primary treatment in some patients, I use a method similar to that described by Dr. George Lewis. The area is injected with lidocaine (Xylocaine) and the wart "shelled out" with a curet. If the wart resists curettage, it can be softened by the momentary use of an electrodesiccating spark, care being taken not to damage surrounding normal skin. Curettage must be thorough. Ragged or overlying marginal skin is removed with scissors. When all wart tissue is removed, a smooth, almost glistening surface or pocket will result. Hemorrhage is stopped with pressure or the application of 50 per cent aluminum chloride solution, and the area dressed with a mild antibiotic ointment. If this has been done carefully, healing will occur with minimal scarring. The failure rate may be less than that with liquid nitrogen, especially in deeply embedded lesions.

When scarring is not important, I occasionally follow curettage with light electrodesiccation.

When warts are large or confluent into mosaic patches, the area may be divided into two or more sections and these treated with liquid nitrogen at intervals of 2 or 3 weeks to avoid excessively large reactions. In these, however, I often use 40 per cent salicylic acid plaster. This is cut to the size of the lesion, applied, and held in place with adhesive tape. It is usually left in place for 5 to 7 days. The patient removes it, soaks the foot in hot water, and gently pares or scrapes away softened keratotic material before reapplying the plaster. I usually ask to see the wart at intervals of 2 or 3 weeks. The area is carefully debrided and progress assessed. At times bichloracetic acid is applied to thicker areas of remaining

wart before the plaster is reapplied. Progress is often slow, but most warts eventually will yield and disappear.

Juvenile plane warts may be moistened with 3 to 5 per cent salicylic acid in isopropyl alcohol once or twice daily, interrupting the treatment if too much dryness or irritation develops.

In patients who have many warts or large embedded or periungual lesions or in persons fearful of treatment, I have for many years occasionally advised that the involved area be soaked in water as hot as can be comfortably tolerated (La Crecchio and Haserick advised 45 to 48 C [113 to 118.4 F]) for up to a half hour once or twice daily as time permits. A plastic foam or other insulated container will help maintain heat. Salicylic acid (5 to 10 per cent) in isopropyl alcohol is usually applied to the warts twice daily after soaking and drying. This appears to hurry involution and disappearance in a significant number of patients.

It has been observed that in patients with many warts, treating one or a few will be followed shortly by the disappearance of the others. For this reason, when patients are being treated by a conservative method such as salicylic acid plasters or hot water soaks, I may treat isolated lesions with liquid nitrogen. It may be that releasing antigen from the treated lesion acts as a vaccination.

Verruca acuminata occurring on moist areas such as body folds and genitalia will often respond to the application of podophyllin. I apply 25 per cent podophyllin in acetone to the lesions and ask that it be left in place for 6 hours and then washed off with mild soap and water. For the inflammatory reaction and sloughing that follow, warm sitz baths are helpful. Analgesics are frequently needed during the period of peak reaction when there is extensive involvement. This is most effective for warts on frank mucosal surfaces. Re-treatment is often required. When the lesion is significantly keratinized, as on marginal skin, success is less likely. In such lesions liquid nitrogen is often effective. Occasionally curettage and electrodesiccation may be preferable.

I usually use liquid nitrogen for warts on the lips and eyelids.

In patients with many small warts, such as those on bearded areas or legs where they are spread by shaving, I frequently use a fine electrodesiccating spark. In most instances this can be applied momentarily without the use of an anesthetic. I also use this occasionally on small warts in other areas, such as the "satellites" that sometimes appear about a larger lesion. It is easier to confine the effect of electrodesiccation used in this way to a small lesion than that of liquid nitrogen.

In recent years, sparked by newer developments in immunology, a number of attempts have been made to treat warts by stimulating the body's defense mechanisms. Some success has been achieved. However, no routine, simple, uncomplicated, and reliable method has yet been developed. Until an effective and safe antiviral agent is found or a specific vaccine is available, warts will continue to be, at times, a frustrating problem for both patient and physician.

HERPES ZOSTER

method of
GORDON MacDONALD, M.D.
Riverside, California

In its typical form, herpes zoster presents a well known classic picture. There are groups of vesicles on erythematous bases, situated in a dermatomal pattern. The eruption is usually preceded for several days by burning or aching pains in the affected zone. The eruption is unilateral, and is associated with regional lymphadenopathy. Diagnostic problems do arise during the prodrome when the pain may simulate an acute surgical abdomen, a cardiovascular disease, or an intracranial lesion. It also appears that there may be viral neuralgia and neuritis without any eruption.

The pain and the eruption of herpes zoster are produced by ganglionitis that in turn results from the activation of a hitherto dormant varicella-zoster virus, which has remained without replication in a dorsal ganglion since the patient suffered from chickenpox, possibly as many as 6 or 8 decades previously. It has been postulated that the zoster-varicella virus travels from the skin to the involved ganglion along the course of a sensory nerve during the attack of varicella. Frequently the trigger factor is not apparent, but it appears that activation may be precipitated by trauma, by intercurrent infection, by malignant disease, or by immunosuppressant drugs. With the diminution of immunologic restraint the virions replicate in vast numbers, setting up an acute inflammation in the ganglion, and streaming down the axon to the skin.

Underlying malignant disease may precipitate a disseminated form of the disease, with lowered immunity and viral replication in the central nervous system as well as in internal organs. Disseminated zoster has been defined as 25 or more lesions in at least two noncontiguous dermatomes. This complication should be treated with vidarabine (ara-A) or interferon (investigational) if available. (This use of vidarabine is not listed in the manufacturer's official directive.)

Herpes zoster is age dependent, being rare in children, and prevalent in older people. The severity is also age dependent, with very few symptoms in young patients and effects that can be quite devastating in the older age group.

In younger patients with relatively mild manifestations the treatment may be largely symptomatic. A high school student, for instance, may require only a diagnosis and reassurance. Below the age of 60 years patients do not ordinarily suffer from postzoster neuralgia, and in this age group simple symptomatic treatment will suffice. A shake lotion or wet dressings in the acute phase followed by a steroid cream during the dry scaling period should be useful. Analgesic agents may be prescribed as required.

Older patients (usually past 60 years of age) are candidates for postzoster neuralgia. The physician has an opportunity to prevent or minimize this complication in the majority of patients by the institution of early and adequate systemic corticosteroid therapy. Prednisone appears to be the most suitable drug, and it should be given in dosage of 60 mg each morning for 1 week, followed by 40 mg each morning during the following week. The 20 mg tablets are the most convenient.

Postzoster neuralgia always poses a formidable problem. Numerous successes (and a few failures) have been reported with a series of intracutaneous injections of a suspension of triamcinolone acetonide, giving 40 mg per injection. If there is persistent suffering, consultation with a neurosurgeon should be sought. Surgical excision of the affected dermatome may give dramatic relief, and this procedure should be considered in patients with life-ruining postzoster neuralgia for which other treatment has failed. Patients of any age with ophthalmic zoster should also receive prompt systemic corticosteroid therapy to prevent corneal scar formation as well as postzoster neuralgia.

HERPES GESTATIONIS

method of
THOMAS J. LAWLEY, M.D.
Bethesda, Maryland

Herpes gestationis is an uncommon blistering disease of pregnancy and the puerperium. The onset is most often in the second and third trimesters of pregnancy. The term herpes gestationis is a misnomer, since the disease is not associated with any known viral infection. The eruption usually begins on the abdomen, but it may become widespread; it consists of grouped erythematous plaques and vesicles which are usually intensely itchy. It tends to remit within a few weeks to a few months post partum, although exacerbations frequently occur within 24 to 48 hours after delivery. Herpes gestationis tends to recur in subsequent pregnancies, and in some patients it may recur with the use of oral contraceptives. This disease is associated with an increased risk of fetal morbidity and mortality. Rarely infants may be born with skin lesions similar to those of the mothers, but they tend to resolve within a few days. Herpes gestationis appears to be immunologically mediated, since direct immunofluorescence of perilesional skin will reveal the presence of the third component of complement and occasionally IgG in a linear band along the basement membrane zone. The presence of these deposited immunoreactants will clearly distinguish herpes gestationis from the other pruritic eruptions of pregnancy.

Treatment

1. The aim of therapy is to prevent the eruption of new lesions and to relieve the severe pruritus. Treatment with prednisone, 20 to 40 mg per day, is usually adequate to achieve these ends within 2 to 3 days. Prednisone should then be tapered 5 mg per week until a level is reached at which only an occasional lesion occurs.

2. Severe exacerbations of itching and the appearance of new blisters frequently occur at the time of delivery, even in patients with well controlled disease. Therefore it may be necessary to administer hydrocortisone sodium succinate, 100 mg intravenously, to patients who have been receiving systemic corticosteroids.

3. Some patients with mild herpes gestationis can be adequately controlled by treating with topical corticosteroid creams and oral antihistamines.

4. Open wet dressings with a saline solution or tap water applied for 15 or 20 minutes three to four times per day are effective in drying oozing and weeping lesions.

PRURITIC URTICARIAL PAPULES AND PLAQUES OF PREGNANCY

method of
THOMAS J. LAWLEY, M.D.
Bethesda, Maryland

Pruritic urticarial papules and plaques of pregnancy (PUPPP) is an extremely itchy eruption that occurs in the last trimester of pregnancy. Although it has been described only recently, it is probably the most common pruritic dermatosis of pregnancy. The clinical manifestations include erythematous urticarial papules and plaques that begin on the abdomen and spread to involve the thighs and buttocks and occasionally the arms. The primary lesions are small (1 to 2 mm) papules that are often surrounded by a narrow pale halo. The numerous papules tend to merge into plaques over the course of a few days, especially on the abdomen. Although the eruption is pruritic enough to keep most patients awake at night, excoriated lesions are extremely rare. The condition usually resolves within a few days to a week following delivery. No specific diagnostic test exists for PUPPP. The eruption does not appear to recur in subsequent pregnancies. The small number of cases reported to date precludes evaluation of the risk of fetal and maternal morbidity or mortality in PUPPP.

Treatment

1. Lesions and symptoms usually respond within 2 to 4 days to frequent (five to six times daily) topical applications of fluorinated corticosteroid creams.

2. In some cases, the intensity of symptoms and the lack of response to topically applied corticosteroids may necessitate the use of prednisone, 20 to 40 mg per day, which should be given in divided doses. The dosage can be tapered by 5 mg every 2 to 3 days.

3. Oral antihistamines have been ineffective.

The Nervous System

BRAIN ABSCESS

method of
ROBIN P. HUMPHREYS, M.D.
Toronto, Ontario, Canada

Microorganisms capable of inciting brain abscess may arise from an adjacent sinus, soft tissue, or bony source of infection, or from a remote site of infection and spread to brain by the bloodstream. Alternatively, they may be implanted in the brain as a consequence of compound trauma. By whatever means these bacteria arrive in brain, their reception is characterized by a focus of ischemia in which the organisms, especially the anaerobes, flourish.

The signs and symptoms of brain abscess may be any combination of infection (primary site perhaps included), meningismus, intracranial hypertension, convulsions, and deteriorating neurologic function. The diagnosis can be strongly suspected by a high voltage delta slow focus obtained from the suppurative region on electroencephalogram (EEG), or by focal accumulation of radiopharmaceutical (with or without the peripheral "doughnut" sign) on radiotracer brain scan. But nothing is more definitive than computed tomography (CT) of the head, which certifies the diagnosis of brain abscess or its antecedent cerebritis.

Nevertheless, the evolution of the subsequent inflammatory process is often accompanied by changing clinical signs. It can be effectively interrupted at any stage by the appropriate therapeutic program.

Prophylaxis of Brain Abscess

That prophylaxis of brain abscess is of some importance has been substantiated by the declining numbers of abscesses related to dental and otogenic sources of infection, now subject to vigorous antibiotic and/or surgical treatment. The clinician is advised therefore to anticipate brain abscess as a potential complicating factor in patients with sinus-otitic infection, chronic pulmonary suppuration, previous compound brain wounds, or skull osteomyelitis, and in children with congenital cyanosing heart disease, especially when a cerebrovascular ischemic event has been suffered. Obviously, the diagnosis and control of the primary infection will limit the possibility of secondary cerebral spread.

Principles of Treatment

Notwithstanding the potency of contemporary antibiotic programs, the mortality statistics for brain abscess treatment have not declined as expected during the past 2 decades. Thus the *early diagnosis* of suspect cerebral suppuration is still the linchpin to successful treatment. This diagnosis is now greatly facilitated by the remarkable exactness of computed tomography.

An *aggressive* and *appropriate antimicrobial drug regimen* is then instituted, preferably based on the analysis of pus from the primary source of infection and/or aspirate of the cerebral lesion. Simultaneously, the clinician must institute measures to *combat the brain's response to the focus of infection*, namely the bulk of the abscess, its peripheral edema, and seizures.

Treatment of the Primary Source of Infection

The discovery of a cerebral abscess should not totally divert attention from the primary source of infection. It may be much easier to identify the microorganism in the infected sinus, ear, or bloodstream than in the brain, with this information then used to guide the appropriate chemotherapy. Moreover, the cerebral thrombophlebitis and/or suppuration will not easily resolve as long as they are being fed by the primarily infected site. If operation on the brain becomes necessary, then the neurosurgeon will proceed with greater security, knowing that an appropriate antibiotic screen has been instituted and that the original site of infection has also been identified and perhaps drained.

This is not to imply that neurosurgical treat-

759

ment must await complete eradication of the initiating focus of infection. In these situations, life is threatened not usually by bacteria but by the brain's reaction to infection with edema and resultant mass effect. The patient desperately ill with increasing intracranial pressure will thus require early drainage of the brain abscess perhaps at a stage before the primary source of infection has been isolated. Hence, treatment scheduling is determined by the patient's response to the focus of the infection in the brain.

Antibiotic Management of Brain Abscess

CT head scans performed in patients with brain abscess provide a rapid, accurate diagnosis of this lesion and its anatomy, numbers, size, loculation, and capsule properties. During the phase of inflammatory cerebritis, the CT study will demonstrate the area of edema, shift of ventricular structures, and focal accumulation of the injected contrast agent. While these features are not necessarily specific for cerebral inflammation, this diagnosis is established given the preceding history and physical signs. The infectious process can be halted at this stage by providing broad antibiotic coverage, as the bacteriologic analysis often is not known.

As chloramphenicol remains the drug with the most potent antibacterial range and also best transgresses the blood–cerebrospinal fluid (CSF)–abscess barriers, it is recommended as the first choice for treatment of organism-type-unspecified brain abscess. Chloramphenicol is prescribed, 6.0 to 8.0 grams per day given intravenously every 6 hours in adults, or 100 mg per kg per day administered intravenously every 8 hours in children. Perhaps because of the gravity of an infection in the nervous system, it is tempting to add a second drug, notably penicillin G, which should be effective against streptococci if present. This is administered to adults as 10 million units per day every 6 hours intravenously and to children as 250,000 to 500,000 units (depending on organism sensitivity) per kg per day every 4 hours intravenously. However, penicillin's penetrance of infected nervous tissue, like that of many other antibiotics, does not match the record of chloramphenicol.

If this antibiotic plan has been effective, then the patient's condition will improve and subsequent CT scans outline disappearance of contrast enhancement and features of mass effect. It will be necessary to continue therapy for 2 to 4 weeks. But the infection may not resolve, and instead the region of cerebritis undergoes central liquefaction and becomes surrounded by a dense, collagenous wall. This produces the "ring" or "doughnut" sign on an enhanced CT scan. Surrounding brain edema can be massive and even more threatening than the infection. At this stage, pus must be obtained from the abscess for analysis (see below). However, the ultimate, specific antibiotic choice does not often differ from those drugs already mentioned, with the exception of cloxacillin, which is used against penicillinase-resistant staphylococci. Cloxacillin is given to adults as 2.0 grams every 4 hours intravenously and to children as 200 mg per kg per day every 4 hours intravenously. (Cloxacillin for intravenous use may not be available in the United States of America.) Antibiotic treatment is continued until the lesion has resolved on CT scan (usually within 4 weeks), or for a period of 2 to 3 weeks following abscess excision.

Pharmacologic Management of Abscess Epiphenomena

With the exception of the abscess rupturing into the ventricular system or the development of septic thrombophlebitis, patients with brain abscess usually do not die of the infection. Rather, their deteriorating clinical condition is a measure of worsening brain edema and rising intracranial pressure (ICP). These epiphenomena must be treated early and aggressively. When minutes count, and when the patient is to be transferred to a neurodiagnostic and/or operative facility, then ICP can be managed with the intravenous administration of 20 per cent mannitol, 2.0 grams per kg given over 15 to 30 minutes. This *single* dose of the hyperosmotic agent will *temporarily* relieve the situation and facilitate penetrance of antibiotic into brain. Simultaneously, dexamethasone, given as a 10 mg intravenous push and then 4 to 6 mg every 6 hours, will also relieve brain edema. Arguments which pertain to their anti-inflammatory properties should not militate against the use of glucocorticoids in this established infectious process. There seems little doubt that dexamethasone is quite effective in reducing edema about a brain abscess, and, as already stressed, it is usually edema, not pus, which kills. But one is obligated to the correct choice of antibiotic for simultaneous chemotherapy and to continue this program much longer (as previously noted) than the steroid administration, which is seldom given for more than 10 to 14 days.

Epilepsy is a frequent concurrent problem requiring immediate and long-term attention. Seizures occurring during the acute illness usually imply a combination of inadequate infection control, spreading edema, and/or the development of cortical thrombophlebitis. Thus, the treatment plan for the preceding is reviewed, in addition to prescribing anticonvulsants. The risk of chronic epilepsy following abscess treatment is 35 to 70 per cent and bears no relationship to the patient's age, abscess site, mode of surgical treatment, or presence of residual neurologic deficit. Nevertheless, the seizures, although often infrequent, can linger for years, and will require delicate manipulation of anticonvulsant drugs. Phenytoin (diphenylhydantoin sodium), 5 to 7 mg per kg per day, is used to begin therapy.

Operative Treatment of Brain Abscess

There is no single surgical stratagem best for all brain abscess patients. Some, namely those with early cerebritis, will not require operation if their antimicrobial program is effective. The formation of a classic abscess will have been aborted. However, a patient harboring a well-formed deep basal ganglia abscess will likely require its aspiration, but certainly not its excision, whereas another patient with a cerebellar abscess will be subject to early surgery for its total removal.

The CT scan is the prelude to abscess surgery. It will outline its site, depth, and relationship to nearby vital structures in addition to demonstrating the characteristic stage of evolution of a formed abscess. When operation is decided upon for pus identification and internal decompression, then the first maneuver is burr hole aspiration performed via the most direct but innocuous route to the capsule. It is a moot point whether the instillation at this time of a barium-antibiotic mixture is of any advantage. The abscess size can be followed just as readily with enhanced CT scans, although the placement of a radiopaque substance may outline abscess contents streaking away from the capsule into brain and perhaps to the ventricle. The need for local instillation of antibiotics directly into abscess cavities has been questioned, as the penetration of the abscess by systemically administered chloramphenicol and penicillin has been shown to be quite adequate when blood levels are high.

After the early, diagnostic burr hole assay of a brain abscess, its contents can be liberated further by repeat aspiration or continuous catheter drainage. Seldom will one aspiration serve to completely eradicate the abscess and its purulent debris. However, its shrinkage becomes apparent by the diminishing volumes of aspirate obtained from repeat samplings and by the collapse of the capsule noted on successive CT studies. The information obtained on CT examinations, however, should be matched with the patient's overall response to treatment, as it is not unknown for CT to suggest complete resolution of the abscess when, in fact, such was not the case.

Craniotomy and operative removal of the abscess capsule and contents is recommended for all patients with cerebellar abscesses as well as accessible supratentorial lesions. This recommendation applies especially for abscesses which are chronic and thick walled or multiloculated (some of which loculi may be promoting continuing infection), for abscesses which are of post-traumatic origin and contain fragments of bone or foreign bodies, or finally, for those in the acute stage which are not responding to aspiration.

The craniotomy is sited to permit approach to the abscess via the shortest route through noneloquent cortex. The abscess is obliterated with its excision, a guarantee which does not obtain when it is aspirated. In the latter circumstance the mixed glial and fibroblastic capsule may collapse, yet remain as a possible source for recrudescence of infection or as a potent epileptogenic focus. While the risk of epilepsy is not abolished after abscess excision, it is certainly no greater and may be less than that which results after abscess aspiration.

The excision of a brain abscess will certainly hasten the resolution of the infectious process and its antibiotic management. However, one must remember, when reviewing the various mortality and morbidity statistics, that the more favorable results obtained in patients who have had abscess excision reflect in part the more chronic nature of their infection and the location of the abscess.

Failure to Control the Infection

In spite of a thorough treatment program, the brain infection may be unyielding. If the microorganism has been identified, and its sensitivities matched to the antibiotic(s) administered in the correct dosage, then the patient's continuing symptoms reflect persisting prima facie infection or spread of infection to adjacent CSF spaces or venous channels. In the former instance, a persisting loculus of infection remains despite the obliteration of its neighbors. This is cause for operative excision of the entire abscess.

The ventricular spinal fluid may become contaminated when the abscess tracks to the adjacent ventricle or the latter is unwittingly entered at the time of aspiration. When CSF infection is proved, the effectiveness of antibiotic delivery to the CSF should be examined. It may be necessary to institute a direct means of drug introduction to the ventricle.

Septic cortical thrombophlebitis is a most serious consequence of the spread of infection from a brain abscess. The patient's condition worsens dramatically, usually in association with a marked seizure disorder. The entire drug program — antibiotic, anticonvulsant, antiedema agents — must be reviewed and renewed, with intensification of dosages and routes of administration.

Conclusion

It is anticipated that CT and not antimicrobials will be responsible for improving the statistics for brain abscess care. Patients will survive because the abscess is so identified and localized, thus permitting an early, aggressive, planned management program.

PARENCHYMATOUS HEMORRHAGE OF THE BRAIN

method of
J. P. MOHR, M.D.
Mobile, Alabama

The diagnosis of parenchymatous hypertensive hemorrhage is best accomplished by computed tomography (CT scan), which is uniformly positive in cases scanned within the first week. Beyond that time, changes in the CT scan appearance render some hemorrhages isodense or low dense, causing diagnostic confusion with ischemic infarction. Lumbar puncture, the former mainstay of laboratory diagnosis, is now no longer relied upon, since it is frequently normal in cases of small hematoma and can be expected to reveal blood only in the larger hemorrhages in which the patient is in a stuporous or comatose state. Cerebral angiography has also proved an unreliable diagnostic method, since the mass of the hematoma is frequently too modest to cause displacement of vessels; further, the hemorrhage is almost always completed before angiography can be performed, which eliminates the chance of seeing the actively bleeding vessels.

The general medical approach to parenchymatous hemorrhages is similar regardless of the site and size of the hematoma. It is uncertain whether any of the measures employed actually change the course of the condition, but it all too often proves irresistible to try to stop the hemorrhage, reduce the cerebral edema and risk of seizures, and lower the blood pressure usually found elevated on admission.

1. Most hemorrhages have ceased before the patient has arrived at the hospital and do not require either acute surgical decompression or coagulant therapy such as epsilon-aminocaproic acid. The rare hemorrhages which are indolent and continue after arrival in the hospital should give rise to the suspicion that the patient has a significant coagulopathy. If the bleeding time is excessively prolonged, fresh platelet infusions up to 4 to 8 units in an effort to restore the bleeding time to normal appear worthwhile. A prolonged prothrombin time on patients taking oral anticoagulants would prompt therapy with several units of fresh frozen plasma or 15 mg of vitamin K.

2. Cerebral edema is rarely sufficiently severe to require steroid therapy, and when it is, the hematoma is often life threatening. Steroids are frequently employed, however, and when used are given in the order of 10 mg of dexamethosone intravenously, followed by 4 mg intramuscularly every 6 hours for the first week to 10 days.

3. The hypertension present on admission is sometimes higher than was present before the hemorrhage and will often restore itself toward normal levels after several days of bed rest. Since the presence of the hypertension does not contribute to continuation of the bleeding and serves only to place the patient at risk for other hemorrhages later, an approach to lowering the blood pressure should be undertaken with the long range future in mind. The conventional program of diuretics, propranonol, and/or hydralazine (Apresoline) is a prudent long-term program. Short-term use of nitroprusside and other acute measures to lower the blood pressure do not appear to have an impact on the clinical course and may actually complicate matters if the blood pressure is reduced below normal levels.

The outlook for the hematoma and its potential surgical management are greatly influenced by the location and size of the hematoma.

1. Very small hematomas in the putamen, thalamus, or individual cerebral lobes may easily be misdiagnosed for ischemic disease in the absence of CT scanning performed early in the course of the disease. Anticoagulant therapy should be withheld in such patients unless CT scan settles the diagnosis. Clinical recovery for such patients within weeks or months is usually excellent if the initial neurologic examination shows only incomplete abnormalities: preservation of even a slight degree of motor movement on the affected side provides a good outlook for eventual functional recovery of the affected limbs; somatosensory, visual, and language and memory disturbances are frequently only short-lived in such cases. Active rehabilitative programs

are deferred for the first week to enable the hematoma to stabilize, following which the patient should be able to participate in such programs without fear of hemorrhage recurrence.

2. Hematomas that produce a complete deficit in one or more major neurologic parameters can be expected to be of moderate to large size and to have a poor prognosis for eventual functional neurologic recovery. Surgical intervention to remove the hematoma does not appear to shorten the clinical course or improve the eventual outcome, but in instances of threatened cerebral hemisphere herniation in the first few days after the hemorrhage has occurred, such surgery can be lifesaving. For the patient with paralyzed limbs, passive range of motion exercises must be undertaken for protracted periods of time in hopes of preventing pulmonary embolism from clinically unrecognizable thrombophlebitis. Because of the recent hemorrhage, low-dose heparin therapy would be ill advised.

3. Huge hematomas causing coma within the first 24 hours ordinarily take life despite every therapeutic effort. They can be treated expectantly in all instances except when the hemorrhage has been encountered in the first hour or so, when attempted surgical evacuation of the clot is worthwhile.

The single exception to these management plans is in a setting of cerebellar hemorrhage. Here, the hemorrhage disrupts cerebellar function at its outset to such a great extent that clinical recognition of continuing hemorrhage is all but impossible. A clinical syndrome of sudden onset of nausea, vomiting, inability to stand and walk, and the less frequently encountered conjugate eye deviation, facial paresis, and sixth nerve pseudopalsy are features suggesting this diagnosis. When CT scanning is available, hemorrhages below 3 cm in size may be safely treated medically in most instances. Evacuation of the larger hematomas is advised to prevent clinically unrecognized brainstem compression from developing to the point at which the patient undergoes sudden cardiorespiratory arrest. The clinical outlook is usually excellent following surgical evacuation when undertaken before the patient reaches the state of coma. This state is frequently reached within the first few hours, so that patients admitted acutely must be prepared for surgery within the first 24 to 48 hours. If the patient's state of consciousness remains satisfactory beyond the period of 48 hours, surgery is usually not required. If coma is allowed to develop before surgery is undertaken, the chance for reversal of the clinical deficit is extremely low.

ACUTE ISCHEMIC CEREBROVASCULAR DISEASE

method of
LOUIS R. CAPLAN, M.D.,
and DANIEL B. HIER, M.D.
Chicago, Illinois

Ischemic cerebrovascular disease is a general term that includes heterogeneous pathophysiologies. Diverse vascular pathologies may produce ischemic infarction, including (1) atheromatous stenosis or occlusion of a large intracranial or extracranial vessel; (2) lipohyalinotic change in penetrating cerebral vessels related to hypertension; (3) atheromatous plaque formation; (4) hemorrhage into an atheromatous plaque; (5) dissection of a large vessel; (6) fibromuscular dysplasia; (7) thrombosis of a cerebral vessel secondary to abnormalities of hemostasis; and (8) cardiac lesions (myocardial infarction, valve disease, aneurysm, endocarditis) with embolization.

Mechanisms of brain ischemia also differ and include (1) the reduction of blood flow distal to a severe stenotic lesion, (2) the propagation of a thrombus into distal vessels, (3) the embolization of a plaque fragment, platelet aggregates, or an organized clot, and (4) vascular spasm. Important as well are a variety of defense mechanisms which tend to diminish the ischemia and its consequences. These protective mechanisms include (1) the development of effective collateral circulation, (2) the passage of cerebral emboli, (3) clot lysis, and (4) the ability of brain tissue to recover from an ischemic insult. The responsibility of the physician is to aid the patient's natural healing tendencies, to prevent progression of existent ischemia, and to minimize the probability of stroke recurrence.

General measures that pertain to all ischemic strokes include the following:

1. Bladder care. Initially, indwelling catheters are useful in preventing bladder overdistention. Subsequently intermittent catheterization with a straight catheter is useful in assisting the patient in re-establishing normal bladder function.

2. Skin care. Pressure ulcers may be avoided by frequent position changes, reduction of skin irritation, and use of air or water flotation mattresses.

3. Passive range of motion. Even before formal physical therapy is initiated, the nursing staff

may begin ranging exercises on the paralyzed limbs in order to prevent contractures.

4. Early physical therapy.

5. Frequent movement of legs and the use of elastic stockings, which may help prevent venous thrombosis. However, careful surveillance for pulmonary embolism and thrombophlebitis is essential. In cases of severe hemiplegia, a short-term course of low-dose heparin therapy (5000 units subcutaneously every 12 hours) is useful in preventing phlebothrombosis.

6. Careful attention to the shoulder on the paralyzed side. This may help prevent painful dislocation at this joint.

7. Emotional support. Attention must be paid to those psychologic reactions to the stroke (especially depression) that may interfere with the rehabilitation process. Supportive psychotherapy and short-term tricyclic antidepressant therapy are sometimes of benefit.

More specific treatment will depend on (1) the location and nature of the vascular lesion, (2) the extent of the clinical deficit, (3) the presence of other serious medical or neurologic disease that might contraindicate a given therapy, (4) the availability of technology and qualified personnel to carry out a particular treatment, and (5) the reliability and cooperativeness of the patient in following a specific therapy. One might follow a particular course of therapy depending on the answers to a series of questions posed for each patient diagnosed as having ischemic stroke.

Has the Patient Had a Small Cerebral or Subdural Hemorrhage Rather Than an Ischemic Infarct?

Recent studies of patients with cerebral hemorrhage have dispelled many of the old axioms. Patients with cerebral hemorrhage may (1) have no headache, (2) develop their deficit gradually, (3) have a minor degree of neurologic deficit, (4) be older than 60 years, (5) not be suffering from a severe degree of hypertension, and (6) have only minimal or no blood in the cerebrospinal fluid on lumbar puncture. Since most treatments used for the patient with ischemic stroke (for example, warfarin, carotid surgery, aspirin) are either harmful or not of benefit to patients with cerebral hemorrhage, it is important to exclude this diagnosis before treatment is initiated. Careful attention to the clinical course may reveal features incompatible with a diagnosis of hemorrhage (hemorrhage does not usually produce transient attacks or a deficit of sudden onset with rapid clearing). Computed tomography (CT) demonstrates intracerebral hemorrhages as well as an occasional subdural hematoma that may mimic an ischemic stroke. Lumbar puncture is helpful in excluding significant subarachnoid hemorrhage, especially in the patient with a prominent headache but little clinical deficit.

Is the Patient a Candidate for Any Specific Treatment?

Having excluded the diagnosis of hemorrhage, the physician must proceed to select treatment for the patient with ischemic stroke. If the patient has a severe neurologic deficit, the chances of preventing further ischemia in the same vascular territory are generally less than the chances of doing the patient harm by surgical or anticoagulant therapy. The risk:benefit ratio rises with severity of the deficit. Severe coexistent medical or neurologic disease may contraindicate certain therapies. Since effective specific therapy depends on precise diagnosis, the absence of appropriate technology (CT scan, arteriography, carotid noninvasive flow tests) should lead to either the use of general supportive measures only or the transfer of such a patient to a tertiary center equipped for the diagnosis and treatment of stroke patients.

Is the Ischemic Lesion Secondary to an Embolus Arising from the Heart?

Surveillance of patients with ischemic stroke has taught us that emboli do not always produce a sudden deficit that is maximal at onset (the deficit may develop more gradually or stepwise, although the time of progression does not generally exceed 48 hours) and that cardiac disorders of diverse types (not just rheumatic heart disease with mitral stenosis or recent myocardial infarction) may be associated with cerebral embolism. These cardiac disorders include prolapsed mitral valve, calcified mitral annulus, "benign" atrial fibrillation, atrial myxoma, cardiomyopathy, and ventricular aneurysm.

It has been our practice to routinely obtain a cardiac echocardiogram and electrocardiographic monitoring in patients with ischemic stroke. In patients with an ischemic stroke secondary to an embolus of cardiac origin, we generally suggest immediate anticoagulation for patients with high risk for subsequent emboli. For example, early anticoagulation is usually indicated for patients with rheumatic heart disease and mitral stenosis or an acute myocardial infarction when no medical contraindication is present (Table 1). Anticoagulation is begun with an initial intravenous bolus of 5000 units of heparin, followed by

TABLE 1. Drugs Which Effect Hemostasis

DRUGS	INITIAL DOSE	MAINTENANCE DOSE	CONTROL PARAMETERS
Heparin	5000 units IV	1000 units IV	Partial thromboplastin time 2 × normal control
Warfarin	15 mg orally	5–15 mg qd (depending on body size and prothrombin time)	Prothrombin time 1½–2 × normal control
Aspirin		5 grains (330 mg) tid–qid	
Dipyridamole*		75 mg qid	
Sulfinpyrazone*		200 mg qid	

*This use of this agent is not listed in the manufacturer's official directive.

continuous infusion of 1000 units of heparin per hour. The dose is then titrated to keep the partial thromboplastin time at approximately twice the control. Clotting time is also followed. After a few days, warfarin is begun. When the prothrombin time is one and a half to two times the control, we discontinue the heparin and maintain the prothrombin time at this level in order to minimize the bleeding risk. In patients with a relative or absolute contraindication to anticoagulation (severe hypertension or active duodenal ulcer) or in those patients with a lesser but perhaps longer term risk of embolism (for example, chronic atrial fibrillation without known ischemic or rheumatic heart disease), we have used aspirin, 5 grains (330 mg) three times daily, and dipyridamole, 200 to 400 mg each day. (This use of dipyridamole is not listed in the manufacturer's official directive.) In the latter group, further embolization has provided the impetus to switch to warfarin therapy.

Is the Ischemic Lesion Secondary to a Lacunar Infarction?

Among patients with ischemic strokes who do not have a cardiac source of emboli, some will have lacunar infarcts produced by disease of small penetrating blood vessels. The arteropathy underlying lacunae is a medial hypertrophy associated with lipohyalinosis of the walls of penetrating blood vessels supplying the deeper regions of the brain. This lesion is seen almost exclusively in hypertensive patients. Lacunar syndromes are characterized by (1) development of the deficit over 1 to 7 days (rarely longer), (2) past or present hypertension, (3) absence of prominent headache, (4) retained alertness, (5) a normal or nonfocal electroencephalogram (EEG), (6) a clinical deficit compatible with a small deep lesion (for example, isolated motor hemiparesis, pure sensory stroke, dysarthria–clumsy hand syndrome, or ataxic hemiparesis), (7) absence of a higher cortical function deficit, and (8) a CT scan showing either a small deep infarct or no lesion at all.

Lacunae are the most common ischemic lesion found in the brain at postmortem examination. If lacunar infarction can be diagnosed with confidence, it is our practice to omit angiography and to treat the patient conservatively with a brief period of bed rest. After clinical stabilization (2 to 3 weeks) we urge careful reduction of blood pressure and long-term monitoring of blood pressure. Neither anticoagulants nor antiplatelet aggregation drugs seem warranted.

The Patient Without Hemorrhage, Embolism, or Lacunar Infarction

Among the remaining patients the diagnosis of hemorrhage, cardiac embolus, and lacunar infarction has been excluded. In patients with mild to moderate neurologic deficits, optimal treatment will depend upon the location and severity of the vascular lesion. At present this can be determined only by cerebral angiography. It is our practice to pursue angiography as soon as the patient stabilizes. If the patient has no deficit or stabilizes with a slight degree of dysfunction, angiography is performed immediately. If the patient's deficit is fluctuating, heparin is administered (using guidelines set out in Table 1) until the deficit stabilizes or it is clear that the patient is worsening despite the treatment. Angiography is recommended at this point. Further treatment then depends upon the angiographic findings:

1. Occlusion of the internal carotid artery at its origin. Treatment includes a period of bed rest for 1 to 3 weeks, depending upon stability of the deficit and maintenance of systemic blood pressure. If the patient's deficit is worsening, short-term heparin treatment is recommended (2 to 3 weeks).

2. Severe stenosis of the carotid artery at its origin (residual lumen less than 1 mm). This is a surgical lesion. If a patient has no deficit, endarterectomy is performed urgently. If the patient has a deficit (or a lesion on CT or radionuclide scan), surgery is delayed for 6 weeks while the patient is given heparin or warfarin (see Table 1). During this 6 week period, if transient ischemic attacks (TIAs) or an additional slight deficit develops, surgery is urged without further delay.

3. Nonstenosing plaque (either at the carotid origin or intracranially). It has been our practice to treat patients with plaque disease with antiplatelet aggregating agents (aspirin, 5 grains [330 mg] three times daily, with or without dipyridamole, 75 mg four times daily). If TIAs or a new deficit develops, warfarin or endarterectomy is considered.

4. Stenosis of the carotid artery intracranially at the carotid siphon or stenosis of the middle cerebral artery. Warfarin is administered for a period of 6 months to 1 year, maintaining the prothrombin time at one and a half to two times the control. If the symptoms persist despite this treatment and facilities are available, creation of a surgical shunt (usually from the superficial temporal to middle cerebral artery) is advised.

5. Occlusion of the carotid artery, one of its major branches, the vertebral artery, or the basilar artery intracranially. Bed rest, maintenance of systemic blood pressure, and short-term anticoagulation using heparin or warfarin for 3 weeks to 3 months are suggested.

6. Severe stenosis of the vertebral arteries or basilar artery. Warfarin is prescribed for at least 6 months. If repeated transient attacks occur or if the clinical deficit is mounting, the patient is considered for a surgical shunt (usually from the occipital artery to the posterior-inferior cerebellar artery or to another long circumferential cerebellar artery).

In patients not having angiography for one reason or another, it is our practice to use aspirin, 5 grains (330 mg) three times daily, often with dipyridamole, 200 to 400 mg each day. It has not been our practice to use long-term warfarin treatment without angiographic confirmation of the lesion except in some patients with clinically severe disease of the vertebrobasilar system. In some patients who are suboptimal candidates for surgery or anticoagulation (older patients or those with coexistent severe medical or neurologic disease), noninvasive tests of the carotid circulation may help the physician decide on whether to pursue angiography.

REHABILITATION OF THE HEMIPLEGIC PATIENT

method of

DAVID B. KING, M.D.

Halifax, Nova Scotia, Canada

Introduction

For this discussion I am going to emphasize hemiplegia secondary to cerebrovascular disease, although hemiplegia from other causes will utilize many of the same principles if the hemiplegia is fixed and not progressive.

Most hemiplegic patients in medical practice have had a stroke. About 200,000 deaths per year are directly attributed to stroke, but ten times this number survive stroke, often with significant disability. Spontaneous recovery may take place up to 2 years, but the maximal recovery is usually within 6 months. Most start to recover within 4 weeks, and those destined to recover good strength will show some recovery within that time.

In addition to the hemiplegic deficit, other neurologic disabilities occur, which significantly interfere with rehabilitation. These include (1) dementia, (2) aphasia, (3) apraxia, (4) homonymous hemianopia, (5) sensory distortion, and (6) sensory loss.

Statistics as to the outcome of stroke vary quite considerably. One study implied that 40 per cent of patients became independent without a cane, 20 per cent required a cane, 13.5 per cent were not independent, 11 per cent were bedridden, and 12.5 per cent died. These figures relate mainly to occlusive stroke.

Management of the Acute Stroke

Respiratory Status. Attention is first directed to the preservation of life. Cerebral edema associated with stroke may secondarily affect the respiratory center, or indeed the primary vascular lesion may involve it. The patient may have to be intubated and placed on a respirator. Steroids and hyperosmolar agents are used for the control of cerebral edema with varying success.

Hypostatic pneumonia and pulmonary emboli may complicate stroke. Physiotherapy directed toward postural drainage and the encouragement of coughing are indicated. Low dose heparin should be employed in an attempt to prevent pulmonary emboli. Besides the morbidity and mortality associated with these conditions, they may worsen the neurologic deficit by complicating hypoxia.

Cardiovascular Status. If an underlying rhythm disturbance is detected on physical examination, the patient should be monitored and the arrhythmias treated appropriately. Cardiac failure should be treated promptly. Ischemic heart disease is a frequent accompaniment of cerebrovascular disease, and the obtunded patient cannot complain of chest pain. An electrocardiogram should be done on all stroke patients with a view to excluding an underlying myocardial infarction.

Hypertension may produce stroke secondary to hemorrhage. Hypertension may also be present in ischemic stroke. Its management in the acute situation is subject to some controversy. As a rule of thumb a diastolic pressure over 120 should be lowered gradually to 100.

Atrial fibrillation, recent myocardial infarction, and murmurs detected on physical examination suggest embolic stroke. A controversial issue here is when to introduce anticoagulant therapy. Computed tomography scanning now allows rapid exclusion of the hemorrhagic stroke. Anticoagulation should be commenced within 24 hours to prevent further emboli after ruling out cerebral hemorrhage by computed tomography or lumbar puncture.

Specific Cerebrovascular Disease. The most common underlying vascular disease is atherosclerosis. However, not all strokes are secondary to this entity, and in elderly patients over 55 years of age temporal arteritis should be considered. If the clinical picture is suggestive of temporal arteritis, a sedimentation rate should be obtained immediately. Steroids should be employed as soon as the diagnosis is made. Hemorrhage secondary to arteriovenous malformation, berry aneurysm, or hypertension may require surgical intervention. Computed tomography scanning has been of significant value in this regard.

The Central Nervous System. Cerebral edema secondary to cerebrovascular disease does not respond well to steroids and hyperosmolar agents, but they should be employed. Hyperventilating the patient by use of a respirator will remove carbon dioxide and lessen intracranial pressure. One should consider withholding therapy if the dominant hemisphere is involved with significant brain swelling, since the prognosis for recovery of neurologic function is so poor. Seizures will occasionally complicate acute stroke,

embolic in particular. Anticonvulsant therapy should be employed, but only under circumstances in which a clinical seizure has occurred. The patient should be rapidly treated using intravenous phenytoin (Dilantin) therapy. Attention should be paid to the cardiac status while this is done. Approximately 1 gram of phenytoin (Dilantin) is given over 10 to 15 minutes (not to exceed 50 mg per minute) intravenously. The drug should not be used intramuscularly.

Metabolic Problems. Diabetes is associated with cerebrovascular disease, and a stroke superimposed on diabetes often results in poor control. Consideration should be given to using a sliding scale under these circumstances until the clinical situation is stabilized. Careful attention must be paid to fluid and electrolyte balance, since inappropriate antidiuretic hormone (ADH) secretion may complicate a stroke. Renal and hepatic status should be assessed. If the clinical situation dictates, endocrine disturbances should be excluded.

Genitourinary Tract. Urinary retention is the usual acute problem. This is not likely to be a permanent event with unilateral cerebral lesions. Intermittent catheterization should be employed, although staff limitations may sometimes require that an indwelling catheter be used. In this circumstance bladder irrigation should be carried out.

Gastrointestinal Tract. Constipation should be managed with enemas every second day, switching subsequently to stimulatory suppositories such as bisacodyl (Dulcolax). Acute gastric dilatation may present as a cardiovascular crisis. A nasogastric tube will rapidly relieve this situation. Stress ulcers may be a complication of an acute cerebral event, particularly with the use of high dose steroids, and may require management with cimetidine (Tagamet), antacids, and nasogastric tube. Recent work has suggested the superiority of hourly antacids over intravenous cimetidine.

Hematologic Status. A number of hematologic disorders may be associated with stroke syndromes, such as polycythemia and sickle cell disease. These require specific management.

Surgical Considerations. Surgery has a limited role in the acute situation. The evacuation of a superficial hematoma from the nondominant hemisphere in an obtunded patient would be an exception. Extracranial progressive carotid ligation for berry aneurysm would be another such instance. The major role of surgery in cerebrovascular disease would be prevention of fur-

0# 768

ther insults to the brain. Cardiac surgery directed to valvular problems, left ventricular aneurysms, and left atrial myxomas will prevent further embolic events. Lesions of the carotid artery, in which there is greater than 50 per cent stenosis or ulceration or thrombus formation, may be grounds for carotid endarterectomy. The subclavian steal syndrome is a surgically correctable cause of vertebrobasilar insufficiency. The surgeon's role in subarachnoid hemorrhage secondary to berry aneurysms is well known. After a delay of 7 days to prevent the consequences of cerebral vasospasm, a direct attack on the aneurysm is usually carried out. Surgery for arteriovenous malformations with en bloc resection has been performed.

General Principles of Stroke Rehabilitation

Stroke rehabilitation involves an evaluation of the patient, planning of the therapy, and careful ongoing multidisciplinary assessment.

The first decision is whether or not the patient should be rehabilitated. There are clinical situations familiar to all physicians in which a maximal effort on the part of a multiplicity of personnel is likely to be unrewarding.. A clear-cut example would be an elderly, demented patient with significant underlying medical disease. Once the decision has been made to rehabilitate the patient, a functional classification of his neurologic deficit should be worked out. His mental status must be assessed in some detail. The presence or absence of aphasia is important. Some effort must be made to obtain an idea of his premorbid personality. This may often best be done by interviewing the family. One of the most important aspects of stroke rehabilitation is that of motivation, and pre-existing psychologic problems in the patient may be detrimental. The degree of his motor and sensory deficits should be quantitated. As soon as possible his gait should be assessed.

Rehabilitation for some years has employed a team concept because of the number of medical and allied personnel involved in the program. Under the direction of a physician, a physiotherapist, an occupational therapist, a speech therapist, and a social worker all have parts to play in the eventual rehabilitation of the hemiplegic patient.

Ongoing evaluation should include bed activities, ability to rise and sit, ability to transfer, ability to bathe, locomotion, ability to dress, personal hygiene, bowel and bladder function, and feeding. Later on, an assessment of homemaking activities and vocational abilities is required. It is important that any program be modified to deal with specific problems of an individual patient. The program should be flexible.

It is likely that prognosis for rehabilitation will be poor in the presence of dementia, dense hemiplegia with no early improvement, severe spasticity, emotional instability, significant impairment of sensation, and severe cardiovascular disease. Most patients will have reached their maximal achievement within 6 months, and a decision to discontinue therapy must be made realistically.

Specific Principles of Stroke Rehabilitation

Current physical therapy programs depend on the following principles: (1) Therapy should be introduced early. (2) Younger patients have a better prognosis. (3) A muscle that is not used atrophies. (4) Tendons tend to shorten unless stretched. (5) Paralyzed muscle must be protected against overstretching. (6) Joints not moved are subject to contracture. (7) Habit patterns are difficult to break, so good habits should be established early. (8) Repetition is important in the learning process, and therefore the more often the patient is shown how to do something, the better is the eventual response. (9) Patients who are not rehabilitated are worse off than those who are. (10) Patients require ongoing evaluation and a restructuring of the program to deal with specific problems.

The Rehabilitation Program

It is perhaps easiest to discuss the program in terms of some arbitrarily defined phases relating to the motor activity of the patient. These may be conveniently listed and discussed independently: (1) the bed phase, (2) the wheelchair-dependent phase, (3) the wheelchair-independent phase, (4) the ambulatory-dependent phase and (5) the ambulatory-independent phase.

Bed Phase. The objects of the bed phase are the following: (1) to maintain range of motion, (2) to prevent contractures, (3) to maintain and improve strength in the nonparalytic limbs, and (4) to prevent the hazards of prolonged bed rest. The following actions should be carried out in order to achieve these objectives:

1. Generally in ischemic stroke the bed rest should be for 2 days. In the case of hemorrhage, perhaps the period of time should be longer —up to 3 weeks. Mobilization should be arranged in keeping with the level of consciousness of the patient and his underlying cardiac status.

2. An adequate fluid intake should be ensured, initially by intravenous therapy and subsequently by oral or nasogastric feeding. Intake and output should be followed carefully.

3. Low dose heparin should be employed in the early management of stroke in order to prevent deep vein thrombosis.

4. Patients on bed care should be turned every 2 hours. Hemiplegic limbs should be put through passive movement on a regular basis.

5. Some attempt should be made to prevent pressure sores by the introduction of sheepskins or air mattresses. Constant nursing vigilance is the most important factor preventing such sores.

6. A monkey bar should be in place, which is primarily designed to strengthen the nonparetic limbs.

7. All beds should be equipped with side rails.

8. A cradle should be employed to keep sheets off the patient's feet.

9. The patient's arms should be placed in the so-called Statue of Liberty position, slightly elevated on pillows, to encourage drainage. The arms should be elevated, abducted, and externally rotated. A wrist splint may be used.

10. Efforts should be made to keep a good postural alignment of the body.

11. An attempt should be made to prevent eversion of the leg and to prevent as much as possible plantar flexion at the ankle. A trochanter role and the drop foot brace or bed board are useful. These are attempts to prevent the overstretching of muscle and the complication of pressure palsies.

12. When the patient is being positioned on one side, a pillow between the thighs is useful.

13. A systematic program of passive exercise of the paretic limb should be instituted. As early as possible, the patient should be encouraged to move his paretic limbs with his nonparetic side.

14. Intermittent catheterization is preferable to an indwelling catheter, but staff and other practical conditions may necessitate the use of an indwelling catheter, at which time bladder irrigations are employed.

15. An enema should be employed every 48 hours if necessary. Bisacodyl (Dulcolax) suppositories may be gradually introduced and subsequently glycerine suppositories used.

16. It is important to emphasize that exercises should be carried out with the nonparetic side as well.

17. Psychologic support is critical. Many patients have gone from a role of major activity to one of complete dependence. There is a great deal of fear and anxiety. This is best dealt with on a person-to-person basis rather than by medication.

18. Early involvement of the family is important. They can be a source of psychologic support to the patient. If willing and able, they should be part of the rehabilitation program.

Wheelchair-Dependent Phase. The wheelchair-dependent phase may sometimes be ignored. The standard metal chair with detachable arms and foot rests with heel and toe loops to prevent foot slippage is important. The patient must be taught wheelchair transfer from bed to chair and from chair to bed. A cushion in the chair may add comfort and prevent pressure sores. The early mobilization to a wheelchair may allow spontaneous voiding. The patient may also be able to carry out self-care activities in a more productive fashion in the sitting position. The early use of a wheelchair with the mobility that it provides may give the patient a psychologic boost.

Wheelchair-Independent Phase. The patient enters the wheelchair-independent phase when he can transfer unassisted and use the vehicle alone. This furnishes him with his first major independence.

Ambulatory-Dependent Phase. In the ambulatory-dependent phase there are a number of principles to be emphasized:

1. Spasticity is helpful in the leg for walking, except for the spastic plantar flexors at the ankle. Because of this, consideration might be given to a lift for the opposite shoe or a drop foot brace.

2. Exercises to the nonparetic side are important, because that is the side that is going to do most of the weight bearing.

3. Passive exercises should be employed to the paretic side.

4. Introduction of the standing phase should be performed slowly, because after prolonged bed rest postural hypotension may be a complication. This could lead to further cerebral ischemia and increasing neurologic deficit. The blood pressure therefore must be carefully followed by the nursing staff.

5. Mechanical assistance to walking is employed—first parallel bars and subsequently a walker.

6. Gradually increasing weight should be taken on the paretic leg and instruction given in walking synergies and posture. Besides the guidance of the physiotherapy staff, a mirror may be helpful.

7. In the future electric aids may prove of value; these include rhythmic stimulation of the peroneal nerve to improve walking synergies or electric stimulation to overcome a drop wrist.

Ambulatory-Independent Phase. The ambulatory-independent phase involves the following measures:

1. The concept of using the cane and the paretic leg together.

2. Transfers from bed to cane.

3. How to utilize the cane in walking up steps. Close attention must be paid to the patient's use of the bannister; he may find it more helpful to drag his paretic side up to the nonparetic side. The patient may find it easier to go down stairs backward utilizing the same technique.

4. While still under supervision, the patient should be taken out for walks.

5. Under certain circumstances it would be impractical and dangerous to introduce the ambulatory-independent phase. This obviously includes situations in which the patient is demented or has very severe spasticity and major clonus or has significant incoordination.

Special Problems in the Rehabilitation Program

Certain special problems are met with throughout the rehabilitation program. These include (1) ataxia, (2) spasticity, (3) anesthesia, (4) aphasia, (5) incontinence, (6) impairment of the activities of daily living, (7) visual complications, (8) occupational retraining, and (9) psychosocial problems.

Ataxia. The problem of ataxia is an extremely difficult one, and in many instances little can be done to correct it. A program of lying, sitting, and subsequently walking exercises has been devised, and in some patients it is of benefit and should be tried. Pharmacotherapy for ataxia has not been particularly useful. It may be that certain types of ataxia related to cerebellar cortical disease may respond better to cholingergic analogues than the cerebellar ataxia arising secondary to the cerebrovascular disease which involves cerebellar nuclei.

Spasticity. Various techniques in physiotherapy have been applied to the problem of spasticity, including heat, cold, and ultrasound, which are effective only for short periods of time. They may allow the mobilization of a spastic limb and range of motion while the therapy is being applied, and this in itself is of value. The medications that are commonly employed in this circumstance are diazepam (Valium), although the doses often reach sedative levels before reducing any spasticity, and dantroline sodium (Dantrium), which is a useful antispasticity drug but does have limiting side effects. It also results in the universal problem with antispasticity agents, which is the removal of useful spasticity that provides support to walk. Baclofen (Lioresal) has also been a useful compound. (This use of baclofen is not listed in the manufacturer's official directive.) These agents would seem to have their major role in treating painful spasms and in removing spasticity in the bedridden patient to make nursing care easier. A number of surgical

procedures have been designed to relieve spasticity, such as the anterior and posterior rhizotomies, neurectomies, cordotomies, and lengthening tenotomies.

Anesthesia. Anesthesia and dysesthesia following stroke are major problems. The patient should use his vision as much as possible when there is significant impairment of position sense. Thalamic pain, a severe burning pain, often associated with hyperpathia and dysesthesias in a hemidistribution may respond to pharmacotherapy. Carbamazepine, phenytoin (diphenylhydantoin), chlorprothixene, and, most recently, baclofen have been used with some success. (This use of these agents is not specifically listed in the manufacturer's official directives.) The use of chlorprothixene is based on the successful treatment of postherpetic neuralgia with this agent. In my hands, this has been a moderately effective therapy, but careful attention should be paid to blood pressure and level of consciousness in elderly patients. I have also had considerable success with baclofen. It is employed in conventional doses not greater than 60 mg a day, but it must be taken on a long-term basis.

Attention must also be paid to the shoulder and arm because of the development of the so-called "shoulder-hand syndrome." This may be primarily a postural syndrome secondary to relative anesthesia of the limb. The shoulder should be kept in a sling, movement of the part should be encouraged, and an arm rest should be employed in any wheelchair. Treatment of the problem, once it begins, consists of heat, ultrasound, either local or systemic steroids for short courses, or mild analgesics.

Aphasia. Aphasia is a controversial issue. Some sources suggest that the early introduction of speech therapy is beneficial in aphasics. In my experience it is certainly of benefit to concentrate on this aspect, which is really the most devastating complication of stroke. The patient's past educational and cultural background is obviously important. The utilization of visual stimulation and a slow, intense, and clear repetitive diction may benefit the patient. All staff looking after these patients must be aware of this, and this approach should be taken by the attending staff as well as the speech therapist. A great deal of encouragement should be given the patient, even for small gains. All forms of communication must be utilized. Any conversation that takes place at the bedside should use simple language. It is important to note that language improvement may occur after a year of deficit, although most often the maximal recovery is made within the first month. Patients under age 55 have a better prognosis.

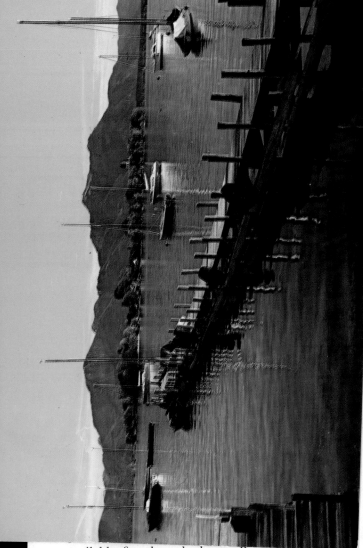

available for the telephone. Prior to discharge, the patient should be thoroughly assessed by occupational therapy and appropriate plans made for his living conditions at home.

Visual Complications. Patients with hemianopia should never be addressed or nursed from their blind side. Tasks should be arranged in the good visual field. The patient should not be placed with his intact field to the wall.

Refractive errors, while not complications of stroke, unless recognized may jeopardize an otherwise carefully thought out program.

Brainstem lesions produce diplopia. This is very distressing for the patient. Use occlusion of one eye and switch it periodically.

Occupational Retraining. Occupational retraining may be a major hurdle for the patient. Auxiliary services and even his place of employment may be mobilized for the patient's benefit. Social service should be requested to assess the community resources and the family's situation well prior to discharge.

Psychologic Problems. Psychiatric problems may complicate the rehabilitative program. Depression is managed in the conventional ways with psychotherapy and antidepressants. The family should be involved and the patient offered constant encouragement. It is important to build up his self-esteem and self-confidence. Even the smallest successes should be praised. Anxiety in reference to what the future holds for him may be managed with anxiolytics, but they should be used with caution, particularly in the elderly patient, because they may have additive effects with antispasticity drugs. The disorders of higher cerebral function, such as dementia, significant personality changes, marked denial, and anosognosia are only too familiar as problems complicating stroke. It is too early to comment on the current status of cholinergic analogues in the management of dementia.

On occasion it is necessary for a social worker to work with the family prior to discharge. Consideration should be given to the emotional responses of the family and their responsibilities. Education is an important aspect of this, and the family should understand the patient's disease, the prognosis, and how to assist the patient in the home environment. Alternatives to home care also should be discussed.

The Potential of Rehabilitation

In a disease such as stroke, in which there is a large component of spontaneous recovery, it becomes extremely difficult to assess the benefits of a rehabilitation program. One may very legitimately ask the question of whether the expenditure of time and money is justified by the results.

Space does not permit us to review the data in detail, but certain important facts emerge from the literature. Younger patients tend to do better than older ones. The sooner the rehabilitation program starts, the better the results. There is no one physical sign that is an absolute indicator of a poor prognosis. Persistent hypotonus and hyporeflexia on the hemiplegic side, however, suggest a poor outcome. A delay of more than 4 weeks in the initiation of voluntary activity is also a poor prognostic sign. Severe sensory dysfunction does not result in as good an outcome as pure motor problems. Also to be considered are the accompanying illnesses, such as hypertension, cardiac decompensation, obesity, and obstructive lung disease.

On the other side of the coin, good prognostic indicators are personal motivation and a productive premorbid personality. Support of a spouse is valuable. Good bladder control, good visual-motor coordination, minimal sensory loss, and an early return of tone, of deep tendon reflexes, and of voluntary activity are signs of a probable successful outcome.

EPILEPSY IN ADOLESCENTS AND ADULTS

method of
ROBERT G. FELDMAN, M.D.
Boston, Massachusetts

Therapy for epilepsy includes certain medications, in appropriate dosages, intended to reduce the frequency and severity of recurrent attacks. To be a successful participant in his own therapy program, the epileptic patient must be helped to accept the diagnosis and the various psychologic and social ramifications that accompany it. For an epileptic patient to be willing to take medicine every day, tolerate occasional side effects, and still run the risk of having another seizure, he must be provided with information that will enable him to believe he has some degree of control over what happens to him. Control of seizures is affected by the behavior and attitude of the person with epilepsy as well as the physician directing the therapy.

The willingness of physicians and nurses to be available to answer questions about why a seizure has occurred eventually provides the patient and his family with an understanding of the circumstances which can lower seizure threshold — an understanding which can contribute to better control. To simply "add another pill" when a seizure occurs leads to overmedication and contributes little to preventive therapy. Managing epilepsy on an expedient or crisis basis is never satisfactory. A continuing patient-doctor relationship must exist in which the physician commits himself to help the patient learn ways to reduce, if not eliminate, the frequency and severity of the epileptic attacks. In addition he must provide guidance for psychosocial and vocational achievement. By being indifferent to these matters, medical personnel omit an important aspect of the management of epilepsy.

The event of a seizure is a symptom of instability of the neuronal membrane. The initial seizure in a person, occurring at any age, must be explained. An etiology must be sought and necessary measures must be taken to prevent the recurrence of such seizures. Anyone who has a brain is potentially an epileptic. It is simply a matter of lowering the threshold enough. Symptomatic convulsions will occur in most people when (1) their blood sugar is lowered quickly to below 40 mg per 100 ml, (2) blood pressure falls abruptly below a critical level, (3) there is not sufficient oxygen, and (4) the body temperature

rises to over 105 F (40.5 C). Normally, there are mechanisms which prevent spontaneous neuronal discharging, and seizures are not easily produced. In individuals prone to epileptic attacks, the threshold may be lowered by a variety of circumstances. Seizures are controlled by maintaining a balance between those factors which precipitate them and those which prevent them. Avoidance of seizure threshold-lowering events and the addition of medication to raise the threshold make seizures less likely to recur (Fig. 1).

Clinical Manifestations

In epilepsy spontaneous electrical discharging of a group of neurons, localized or propagated to other groups of neurons, produces changes in the patterns of the electroencephalogram (EEG). The anatomic location of the abnormally firing cortical neurons will determine the clinical manifestation of a seizure. Such a topographic relationship is most obvious when a group of spontaneously firing epileptogenic neurons produces a seizure characterized by a specific behavior or sensation attributable to the function of cells in a specific area of the brain. If this focus is in the motor area, a motor seizure occurs. If it is in the sensory area, a focal sensory seizure results. A seizure arising from a temporal lobe focus may cause certain subjective experiences, specific cognitive phenomena, or automatic behaviors.

When using the International Classification of the Epileptic Seizures, those seizures during which consciousness is lost are referred to as *generalized seizures*. In this category are grand mal seizures with tonic-clonic movements and petit mal or absence seizures. *Partial seizures*, on the other hand, include seizures in which consciousness is not lost. Such partial seizures include elementary partial (focal, jacksonian) and complex partial (psychomotor, temporal lobe) seizures. Consciousness may occasionally be clouded but is not lost. The diagnostic differenti-

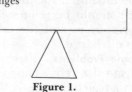

Inadequate antiepileptic
  medication
Threshold lowering events:
  Emotion, trauma, fever   Natural seizure threshold
  illness, lack of sleep,   Correct antiepileptic
  hydration/electrolytes,   medication
  hyperventilation, photo-   Adequate amount of
  sensitivity, alcohol/drugs,   medication
  hormonal changes

Figure 1.

ation of epilepsy as partial or generalized is important because of the differences in therapeutic response to specific medications in each type of epilepsy. In some patients there may be both partial and generalized attacks, and they should be treated accordingly.

The First Seizure. The occurrence of a generalized convulsion is a frightening experience for the patient's family and for anyone witnessing it. For the patient, loss of consciousness and amnesia for the episode can be devastating to his self-image and esteem. For this reason, the manner in which the initial attack is handled is important to the future well-being of the patient. Anxiety about the cause of the seizure and the possibility of its recurring can be relieved somewhat by following through with a thorough workup, including an EEG and a computerized axial tomogram (CAT).

The age at which a person has his first seizure may give a clue as to the etiology of the condition. A genetic predisposition will reveal itself at any time. During growing years the underlying tendency for a seizure may be precipitated by threshold-lowering effects of endocrine imbalances and changes associated with pubescence. Likewise, the effects of an early birth trauma, hypoxic event, or infantile febrile illness may not make its appearance as a seizure until adolescence. Vascular malformations are often recognized by the associated epileptic seizure. Most patients have no clearly identifiable structural abnormality to explain their epileptic tendency, and yet there may be those in whom a brain tumor must be suspected and may be detected with complete investigation. Primary and metastatic brain tumors must always be ruled out as a cause of seizures in all age groups. Between 20 and 40 years of age, epilepsy develops most frequently as a result of trauma to the head in which cerebral contusion has occurred. Inflammatory conditions such as vasculitis, meningitis, and neurosyphilis are common causes for seizures which develop in middle age. After cerebrovascular accidents, infarctions may develop a margin of neurons and gliosis which become epileptogenic. Whenever possible, treatment of seizures must begin with diagnosis and treatment of specific underlying conditions such as tumors, infections, or systemic illness. However, regardless of the cause, it is the recurrent seizure disorder which requires ongoing monitoring and therapy.

Prevention of recurrence of seizures is desirable, not only because of its effect on the life style and safety of the patient, but also because there is reason to believe that the longer a person is seizure-free the better will be the prognosis for future control of seizures. Conversely, the development of "mirror foci" or spread of epileptic activity experience by the recent concept of "kindling" makes the likelihood of seizure recurrence even greater. Therefore, early diagnosis and institution of appropriate therapy are extremely important.

Drug Management

Drug management of the epilepsies involves (1) selection of an effective drug for the particular seizure type; (2) determination of proper dosage for the patient's size and requirement to achieve a therapeutic blood level of specific drug; (3) observation for side effects; (4) adjustment of medication to optimal levels for achievement of seizure control with minimal side effects; and (5) choice of alternative drugs if initial selection fails to stop the seizure or produces untoward effects.

Generalized Epilepsy. EMERGENCY TREATMENT (STATUS EPILEPTICUS). For generalized tonic-clonic (grand mal) convulsions, and for partial seizures which become secondarily generalized, phenytoin (Dilantin) is the most reliable primary drug. Phenytoin is extremely effective in stopping status epilepticus involving tonic-clonic convulsions. An intravenous loading dose can be safely given (14 mg per kg), followed by maintenance doses of 100 mg orally or intravenously every 6 to 8 hours to achieve a therapeutic phenytoin serum concentration throughout the first 24 hours after the loading dose. Phenytoin does not depress respiration as much as intravenous doses of diazepam or phenobarbital, nor does it deeply depress the level of consciousness, allowing better evaluation of mental status after the seizures have been brought under control. Most cases of status epilepticus caused by poor patient compliance in taking medicine will usually respond to a loading dose. When tonic-clonic status epilepticus appears to be refractory, attention must be directed to other possible threshold-lowering factors: (1) a new acute central nervous system process such as meningitis, encephalitis, trauma, or subarachnoid bleeding; (2) metabolic disturbances such as hyponatremia, hypocalcemia, hypoglycemia, or hepatic or renal failure; (3) withdrawal from sedative drugs, including alcohol; (4) drug intoxication; (5) sleep deprivation; or (6) fever.

To control status epilepticus and to prevent its recurrence, a therapeutic serum concentration must be achieved quickly and maintained effectively. When the patient has a series of seizures or prolonged status even though he has been faithfully taking medication, and an emergency laboratory determination of the serum level is in the low or middle part of the therapeutic range, then a loading dose sufficient to produce a higher level should be given. In those rare instances in which the serum level of phenytoin is found to be in the high therapeutic range, a loading dose of another drug should be given.

Precaution must be taken, when giving phenytoin in emergency situations, to avoid side effects. It should never be given intramuscularly, because it is so slowly absorbed. Furthermore, phenytoin crystals may precipitate in the muscle. Serious complications of intravenous phenytoin sodium include hypotension, atrial and ventricular conduction disturbances, ventricular fibrillation, and cardiorespiratory collapse. These complications occur more frequently in the elderly. If phenytoin is given at the recommended rate of 50 mg per minute, it will take approximately 20 minutes to administer a full loading dose to an adult. Brain and cerebrospinal fluid levels of phenytoin reach a peak 1 hour after completion of the infusion. It is therefore helpful to use an adjunctive drug, such as diazepam, which has a brief duration of action but which can temporarily control seizures while the loading dose of phenytoin is being administered and absorbed. Intravenous diazepam, phenobarbital, or paraldehyde may be needed to stop an ongoing seizure or to control status epilepticus when a full loading dose of phenytoin fails.

Phenobarbital is given to patients who have had allergic reaction to phenytoin, who cannot take phenytoin because of abnormal cardiac conduction or autorhythmicity, or who continue to seize despite a full loading dose of phenytoin. The therapeutic range of phenobarbital serum concentration is 15 to 40 micrograms per ml. A proper intravenous loading dose is 8 to 20 mg per kg, and this should be followed by a maintenance dose of 5 mg per kg per day. Peak serum levels occur up to 12 hours after an intramuscular injection and therefore should not be administered intramuscularly for treatment of status epilepticus for several reasons: (1) there is a slow time to peak serum concentration; (2) toxic quantities will accumulate if patient is given repeated injections; (3) the patient will continue to seize until the peak serum concentration and therapeutic level are reached; and (4) if the seizures do not stop, adjunctive use of diazepam, which may be necessary, can cause serious cardiorespiratory depression, as the depressant effects of diazepam and phenobarbital are additive.

Diazepam (Valium) reaches maximal brain concentration 1 minute after the end of an intravenous infusion. The usual initial adult dosage of intravenous diazepam for status epilepticus is 5 to 10 mg, given over 1 to 2 minutes. Serum concen-

tration reaches a peak quickly, and then disappearance occurs in two phases, the distribution phase and the elimination phase. The distribution phase half-life is 16 to 90 minutes; the elimination phase half-life is much slower. The serum concentration of diazepam has fallen by 50 per cent 20 minutes following intravenous injection, accounting for the failure of diazepam to control serial seizures of status epilepticus when given as the only drug. Intravenous diazepam is most helpful if used when generalized tonic-clonic activity has continued without interruption for 3 to 5 minutes and a patient is receiving a loading dose of phenytoin which has not yet reached peak effect. The decision to use intravenous diazepam to treat refractory tonic-clonic status epilepticus after a full loading dose of phenytoin or phenobarbital must be given serious consideration because of possible cardiorespiratory depression and hypotension. For this reason other agents, including paraldehyde, may be tried.

Paraldehyde in a dosage of 0.1 to 0.15 ml per kg by intravenous or intramuscular route may be helpful in controlling status epilepticus. Peak blood levels are reached 20 to 60 minutes after an intramuscular injection, which must be given deep into the buttocks, 5 ml at a time in an injection site. The elimination half-life is 3 to 10 hours.

General anesthesia may eliminate seizures for the duration of administration, only to have the seizures return after the anesthesia wears off. General anesthesia does have value, however, when time to reach peak effect is needed after giving a loading dose of phenytoin. Similarly, curarization can be used to reduce the muscle activity of seizures and reduce the stress of status epilepticus upon the heart and the effects of apnea, while awaiting the effects of a loading dose to take hold.

MAINTENANCE THERAPY FOR GENERALIZED TONIC-CLONIC SEIZURES. Phenytoin is the most effective drug for preventing recurrent generalized seizures of the tonic-clonic type. Success of the prescribed dosage depends upon the pharmacokinetic principles which characterize the drug, including (1) absorption, (2) distribution, (3) biotransformation, and (4) excretion. In recommending an oral dose for an adult, one should take into consideration that, depending upon the manufacturer, different oral preparations of the same generic drug (e.g., phenytoin) may have different times to peak concentration. Absorption from the gastrointestinal system will be affected by the formulation of the capsule, changes in pH of the gastric contents, or competition of the drug with other substances for metabolic enzymes. The rise and fall of serum concentration of the drug will be reflected in the quantity distributed to the brain, presumably the site of action of its antiepileptic effects. Because different antiepileptic drugs follow common metabolic pathways, there may be an interference with the eventual serum concentration of the individual drugs when administered together (Table 1). Enzyme induction and/or decreases in protein binding are suspected as the mechanisms for decreasing serum concentration of the first administered drug, and inhibition of hepatic metabolism is presumed to be responsible for increases in serum concentration. Excretion of drugs is decreased when there is renal failure and, in patients with hepatic disease, when the rate of inactivation is slowed.

Initiation of therapy should be done with one drug, preferably phenytoin. If one begins therapy with a maintenance dose of 300 mg per day, steady state serum concentration is not reached for 7 days. If an oral loading dose of 400 mg, 300 mg, and 300 mg given at 4 hour intervals (i.e., 1000 mg over 8 hours) is administered, therapeutic blood levels are reached within 24 hours. It is possible to prescribe phenytoin once a day, since its half-life is 22 hours. Some patients prefer it twice a day because of gastric irritation when taking 300 mg or more all at once. A daily intake of 300 to 400 mg usually provides a therapeutic serum concentration of 15 to 20 micrograms per ml. Some patients obtain therapeutic levels with less oral intake than others, and a daily dose of 200 mg may be sufficient to produce a level of 10 to 20 micrograms per ml in some. There are many epileptic patients who remain completely seizure free with serum concentrations well below the so-called therapeutic range despite an intake of 300 to 400 mg per day. In several of these patients, to push the drug dosage higher in order to increase the serum concentration results in toxic side effects. It is absolutely necessary to regulate each patient's medications according to his own needs for seizure control and not depend upon the serum concentration alone, i.e., to treat the patient, not the blood level.

Increases in doses of phenytoin can be made until seizure control and adequate serum concen-

TABLE 1. **Antiepileptic Drug Interactions***

ORIGINAL DRUG	ADDED DRUG	EFFECT OF ADDED DRUG TO SERUM CONCENTRATION OF ORIGINAL DRUG
Phenytoin	Phenobarbital	Decrease, increase, or no change
	Primidone	No change
	Carbamazepine	No change
	Ethosuximde	No change
	Methsuximide	Increase
	Clonazepam	Data conflicting
	Valproic acid	Decrease
Phenobarbital	Phenytoin	Increase
	Carbamazepine	No change
	Clonazepam	Data conflicting
	Methsuximide	Increase
	Valproic acid	Increase
Primidone	Phenytoin	Increase in concentration of derived phenobarbital
	Ethosuximide	No change
	Clonazepam	No change
	Valproic acid	Increase in concentration of derived phenobarbital
Carbamazepine	Phenytoin	Decrease
	Phenobarbital	Decrease
	Primidone	Decrease
	Valproic acid	No change
Clonazepam	Phenytoin	Decrease
	Phenobarbital	Decrease
	Valproic acid*	No change
Valproic acid	Phenytoin	Decrease
	Phenobarbital	Decrease
	Primidone	Decrease
	Carbamazepine	Decrease
	Ethosuximide	No change
	Clonazepam*	No change

*Modified from Browne, T. R.: Am. J. Hosp. Pharm. 35:1048, 1978.
†Absence status epilepticus has been reported with concomitant use of valproic acid and clonazepam.

tration are achieved. Toxicity may be evidenced by nystagmus, ataxia, lethargy, and slurred speech (usually at a level over 20 micrograms per ml). If the seizures are not controlled while a therapeutic serum level is maintained, reconsideration must be given to the selection of the drug for treating the seizure. Two drugs may be necessary to control seizures in some patients. In such instances, plasma concentrations of each agent should be within its therapeutic range. A second drug should be added one dose at a time, recognizing that additional side effects may develop. Simultaneous reduction of the first drug should not be done. When a second drug is added and control is achieved, the original ineffective medication can be removed cautiously.

Since it is most desirable that therapy be maintained with adequate doses of a single agent, or a single primary drug and an adjunctive second one, care must be taken to avoid polypharmacy. Accumulation of previously tried and unsuccessful prescriptions results in confusion for the patient and the unnecessary additive side effects of several drugs. Reduction can begin when the second drug has reached a therapeutic level. Phenobarbital, usually the second drug introduced, can be given as a single dose (90 to 180 mg) because of its long half-life (96 hours). Once a day dosing is convenient, and it reduces noncompliance by avoiding the patient's tendency to forget to take the middle of the day dose. Furthermore, it eliminates the problem of daytime sedation when a single dose is taken before going to sleep. Another advantage of long half-life and once a day dosage of phenytoin and/or phenobarbital is the ability to maintain serum levels despite times when oral administration may be impeded, such as for medical tests (gastrointestinal [GI] series) or operations. One can "catch up" before the protective level falls too far.

MAINTENANCE THERAPY FOR ABSENCE (PETIT MAL) SEIZURES. The absence variety of generalized epilepsy responds poorly to phenytoin. Although absence seizures are usually found in children, this type of seizure is often mixed with tonic-clonic seizures when absences occur in adults or late adolescents.

Clonazepam (Clonopin), a benzodiazepine structurally related to diazepam, has been shown to be effective against absence seizures, as well as infantile spasms and myoclonic or atonic attacks. Peak serum concentrations of clonazepam occur 1 to 3 hours after oral administration, and the elimination half-life is 20 to 40 hours. Most patients whose seizures are controlled with clonazepam have serum blood levels of 5 to 70 nanograms per ml. Unfortunately, the levels of patients who do not respond or who have side effects (drowsiness, ataxia, behavior changes) with clonazepam also usually fall into the same range. The starting dose for adults is 1.5 mg per day or less, given preferably in three divided doses. The dosage may be increased by 0.5 mg every 3 days until a maximum of 20 mg per day or seizure control is achieved.

Clonazepam, although effective in the treatment of absence seizures, should be used after unsuccessful trials of ethosuximide or valproic acid (see below), because of side effects and the development of tolerance to its antiepileptic effects.

Ethosuximide (Zarontin) is one of the several succinimide derivatives which have antiepileptic activity. The others include methsuximide (Celontin) and phensuximide (Milontin). Ethosuximide, the most effective drug for absence seizures, has side effects (drowsiness and gastrointestinal disturbances) which are less severe or frequent than those of methsuximide or phensuximide. Furthermore, it has fewer interactions with other antiepileptic medications. Ethosuximide is specifically useful in absence seizures and has little beneficial effect on tonic-clonic seizures (in fact, it may increase tonic-clonic sei-

TABLE 2. **Characteristics of Commonly Used Drugs**

DRUG	SEIZURE TYPE	TIME TO STEADY STATE	SERUM HALF-LIFE	THERAPEUTIC SERUM LEVEL
Phenytoin	Generalized (tonic-clonic), partial (focal, complex)	7–8 days	24 ± 12 hours	10–20 micrograms/ml
Phenobarbital	Generalized (tonic-clonic), partial (focal, complex)	14–21 days	96 ± 12 hours	15–40 micrograms/ml
Ethosuximide	Generalized (absence)	7–10 days	30 ± 6 hours	40–100 micrograms/ml
Valproic acid	Generalized (absence)	1–4 days	10 ± 2 hours	40–150 micrograms/ml
Primidone	Generalized (tonic-clonic), partial (focal, complex)	4–7 days	12 ± 6 hours	5–12 micrograms/ml
Carbamazepine	Generalized (tonic-clonic), partial (complex)	3–4 days	12 ± 3 hours	4–12 micrograms/ml

zure frequency), and therefore must be used along with phenytoin in those patients who have mixed types of generalized epilepsy.

Dosage of ethosuximide is introduced slowly because of possible gastric irritation. In adolescents or adults introduction of therapy while avoiding the initial sedative effect can be accomplished by giving 250 mg at bedtime for 3 days and then adding a second dose about 8 hours later. Patients usually develop tolerance to the sedative and gastric side effects as the dosage is gradually increased. Although the half-life would permit once a day administration, the gastrointestinal irritation and drowsiness are bothersome. There is seldom need to give the drug in three or more doses. The usual daily maximal dosage is 1500 mg per day. After increases are made gradually over several weeks to reach a serum level of 40 to 100 micrograms per ml, maintenance dosage with ethosuximide usually produces good control of absence seizures for many years without significant decrease in effectiveness in a given patient, while methsuximide seems to lose its ability to control absence seizures at the same dose level after 18 to 24 months of therapy. Ethosuximide and the other succinimides can cause bone marrow depression, and complete blood counts should be done monthly for the duration of succinimide therapy.

Methsuximide (Celontin) reaches peak serum levels in man 1 to 4 hours after one oral dose, but it has a very short half-life (1 to 2.6 hours). However, a metabolite, N-desmethyl-methsuximide (NDM), has a longer half-life of 34 to 48 hours and is probably the active antiepileptic substance resulting from administration of methsuximide. Higher blood levels of phenytoin and phenobarbital result when given in conjunction with methsuximide. After the initial dosage of 300 mg per day, increments of 150 mg per week should be made until seizures are controlled or toxicity is observed. The side effects include drowsiness, irritability, and ataxia. Acute psychotic-like reactions have occurred. A therapeutic serum concentration range of 10 to 40 micrograms per ml of NDM reflects the steady state of methsuximide.

Phensuximide (Milontin) has a half-life of 4 to 8 hours with a prompt time to peak serum level of 1 to 4 hours after an oral dose. Like methsuximide, phensuximide has an active metabolite, N-desmethyl-phensuximide (NDP). However, the metabolite has a very brief half-life, and it does not accumulate during chronic administration. Even on daily doses of 1000 to 3000 mg per day in divided doses, phensuximide is a weak antiepileptic agent for absence type seizures. Its side effects are similar to those of the other succinimides. Phensuximide has little value in treating absence seizures when compared to ethosuximide and methsuximide or the new agent, valproic acid.

A simple eight-carbon branched-chain fatty acid, *valproic acid* (Depakene) is effective in suppressing generalized seizures, mainly absence attacks. Unlike any other antiepileptic agent in structure, it has been useful as the sole drug and as adjunctive therapy along with phenytoin and phenobarbital.

Valproic acid has been considered equally effective to ethosuximide. There is some evidence that a combination of valproic acid and ethosuximide together may be more effective than either drug alone. And yet valproic acid may be more effective than ethosuximide for treating patients who have mixed absence and tonic-clonic seizures. Valproic acid is the most effective agent against atonic seizures for which other drugs have had little effect.

Valproic acid reaches a steady state in plasma after 1 to 4 days of oral administration. Its short half-life (6 to 15 hours) makes compliance difficult because of the need for frequent dosing. A plasma concentration of more than 50 micrograms per ml is usually necessary to achieve control of absence seizures. Therapeutic levels should be approached slowly, as side effects develop easily and interactions with other drugs being taken can produce additive untoward effects, including drowsiness, irritability, and gastrointestinal disturbances. Acute coma has been observed in patients receiving phenobarbital when valproic acid is added, since the blood level of phenobarbital rises 20 to 50 per cent. The serum level of phenytoin drops as valproic acid dosage is increased because of competition for protein-binding sites. Tonic-clonic seizures have increased in some patients as a result of this interaction, a result caused by the decrease in phenytoin level. Although there is conflicting evidence as to its frequency, it should be noted that absence status epilepticus has been reported with concomitant use of valproic acid and clonazepam.

There are at least 14 recorded deaths from valproic acid hepatotoxicity. This, plus the possibility of persistent nausea, alopecia, and interference with clotting mechanisms, necessitates careful supervision in using valproic acid. It should be used mainly in those patients whose seizures have been refractory to ethosuximide, and monthly liver function studies should be performed.

Partial Epilepsy. Treatment of partial epilepsy of a focal nature depends upon the location of the epileptogenic area. Focal motor and focal sensory seizures arising from lesions in cortex of the pre- or postcentral gyrus are best controlled by adequate doses of phenytoin and/or phenobarbital, as in the treatment for generalized epilepsy. If the focus is in the cortex of the temporal lobe, it may produce auditory or olfactory hallucinations. More complex symptoms occur when the seizure arises in the deeper limbic structures of the temporal lobe. These may result in automatisms, memory disturbances, and changes in affect. Such attacks fall into the category of complex partial (psychomotor) epilepsy, which is the most difficult type of epilepsy to control. Many patients do not respond to phenytoin, and others are made worse with phenobarbital. Primidone (Mysoline), however, which has phenobarbital as one of its metabolites, may be more effective. Carbamazepine (Tegretol) has become a major therapeutic agent in the treatment of complex partial epilepsy.

Primidone (Mysoline), a desoxybarbiturate derivative, is rapidly absorbed from the gastrointestinal tract and is converted by the liver to phenobarbital and phenylethyl malonamide (PEMA). The half-life of primidone is from 6 to 18 hours, while that of its metabolite (PEMA) is longer (24 to 48 hours). The latter has an antiepileptic action of its own. A daily dose of primidone of 300 to 750 mg is needed to achieve a therapeutic plasma level of 5 to 15 micrograms per ml. Primidone has been effective by itself, but when given with phenytoin it may be even more beneficial. The sedative effect of primidone which results may be so unpleasant upon initiation of therapy that patients are unable to tolerate more than 1 tablet of 250 mg. Severe lethargy and gastrointestinal upset occur in sensitive individuals. It is best to introduce the medication gradually by giving a bedtime dose of 100 mg or half of a 250 mg tablet for 3 or 4 nights, gradually increasing the dosage to a full tablet. Increments of 125 mg should be made when dosage is increased.

Carbamazepine (Tegretol), an iminostilbene derivative, is an effective agent for complex partial epilepsy in doses of 800 to 1600 mg per day (plasma level of 4 to 10 micrograms per ml). Carbamazepine can be used alone or in conjunction with phenytoin, when indicated for secondarily developing generalized seizures. Since, as with primidone, initial dosage may produce such unpleasant side effects that the patient will not want to continue the therapy, gradual introduction and dosage adjustment are required. Dizziness, drowsiness, somnolence, headache, and visual disturbances may occur after only one dose of 200 mg in some individuals. The half-life of carbamazepine is 14 to 17 hours, and therefore it can be given in two administrations within 24 hours, to facilitate compliance.

In some patients carbamazepine cannot be tolerated because of serious hematologic effects such as leukopenia or marked decrease in platelet count resulting in poor blood clotting. The clotting problems seem to occur more frequently in older age groups.

Nonpharmacologic Treatments for Epilepsy

Therapy for epilepsy which does not involve the use of drugs has been necessary in some patients. The main nonpharmacologic treatments are surgical intervention and behavioral therapies. If a patient has seizures which are refractory to all available medical therapy, neurosurgical procedures may be helpful if properly selected for the individual patient. Surgical treatment should never be used unless the patient has been thoroughly studied for response to all conventional medications, at maximal tolerable levels. The paucity of experienced epilepsy surgical centers makes this type of therapy accessible to relatively few patients at present. In some patients behavioral therapies may be of great value as adjunctive therapy along with pharmacologic agents.

Neurosurgical Intervention. Surgical therapy is useful only when it can be proved that the epileptic disorder arises from a specific lesion of the brain and it is assumed that removal of the lesion (malformation, cyst, residual scar from inflammation on scar, or neoplasm) will reduce or eliminate the likelihood of recurring attacks.

Several techniques have been found useful in altering the nature of the seizure disorder and thus rendering the patient more responsive to pharmacologic treatments. These approaches have included (1) temporal lobectomy for localized focal epileptogenic lesion in the temporal lobe; (2) subtotal hemispherectomy, removing at least three lobes of the brain; (3) subtotal resection of cortex; and (4) sectioning of the corpus callosum.

Most neurosurgeons will not consider a patient a suitable candidate unless it is shown that the epileptic seizures are of such severity and frequency that they interfere with the patient's existence so much that he is willing to undergo risk of possible permanent deficit as a result of the surgery. Furthermore, it is often difficult to ascertain that the seizure arises from a single operable site. Detailed electroencephalographic techniques, using depth electrodes, may be necessary to establish the source of epileptogenicity. Cortical and subcortical recording is then done during the procedure to delineate the areas. It has been estimated that with careful selection no more than 5 per cent of epileptic patients might benefit from surgical therapies.

Behavioral Therapies. Behavioral methods

of seizure control, whether drawn from learning theory, conditioning, psychodynamic process, or various biofeedback techniques, have usually been used as adjuncts to pharmacologic treatments. The success of behavioral methods can be measured accurately only when variables, such as the drugs prescribed, their absorption and excretion, and intercurrent illness affecting seizure threshold, are considered. Evidence worthy of consideration by clinicians is accumulating that suggests some behavioral methods may be useful in treating selected patients who have seizure disorders.

Behavioral therapies have three theoretical targets: (1) the seizure as a response to specific environmental triggers (internal and external), (2) the seizure as a reinforced behavior, and (3) the seizure as a symptom of the emotional state of the patient. Treatment programs can be directed toward antecedent events, stimulus, or postictal behavior response. When seizures occur as a symptom of underlying emotional conflict or psychosocial maladaptation, the personality structure of the organism (O) requires attention as a probable cause of poor seizure control. The paradigm of stimulus-organism-response (S-O-R) provides a structure for systematically reviewing the various techniques used in treating patients with epilepsy.

THE SEIZURE AS A RESPONSE TO A SPECIFIC ENVIRONMENTAL STIMULUS (S-o-r). These behavioral therapies focus on precipitants to seizures, emphasizing identification of antecedents. The stimulus-organism-response chain may be either learned or unlearned, and it is usually distinguished by the close timing of antecedent event and seizure occurrence. Often, the triggering stimulus is highly specific, although not necessarily simple. The aim of treatment in these approaches is to alter the seizure threshold by manipulating the presentation of stimuli. The sensory-induced or reflex epilepsies are the most exquisite examples of seizures induced by specific environmental stimuli. Various techniques have been tried and described in the literature, including (1) systematic desensitization, (2) habituation, (3) conditioning, (4) adversive conditioning, (5) relaxation, and (6) biofeedback-sensorimotor rhythm training. Some patients who are able to identify antecedent events that serve as a stimulus to onset of seizure activity experience better control using these techniques in conjunction with medication.

THE SEIZURE AS REINFORCED BEHAVIOR (s-o-R). In this aspect, seizures are viewed as behavioral responses that either increase or decrease in frequency as a consequence of their occurrence. Neither antecedents nor the organism itself is of great concern. Emphasized are the consequences of seizures, i.e., whether they are followed by reinforcement. Behavior that is not reinforced tends to become extinguished. New behavior repertoires are built by shaping, a method by which successive approximations of a desired behavior are reinforced. These approaches are often drawn from the technique known as operant conditioning.

The frequency of some seizures depends on the responses elicited from others that tend to reinforce the behavior. This reinforcement often takes the form of oversolicitous attention from parents, teachers, and peers after a seizure. When such attention or favor becomes an end in itself, it can increase the number of seizures a patient has. Some behavioral methods have been used in attempts to reduce the frequency of seizures by changing their consequences. The methods often used are planned ignoring or extinction of behavior by providing no reinforcement of it and/or positive reinforcement for not having seizures.

THE SEIZURE AS A SYMPTOM OF EMOTIONAL STATE (s-O-r). These methods focus on behavior that is generally thought to be learned, though not necessarily consciously, within the individual (the organism). They emphasize analysis of defenses and restructuring of personality in an effort to promote tension reduction and altered ways of coping with life events. The methods may also attempt to identify seizure antecedents such as emotional triggers, but they differ from the first category in that triggers are viewed as representing information input that reflects unresolved conflicts within the seizure patient. Therefore, the triggers are related thematically rather than by specific physical stimulus properties. Moreover, these approaches can be distinguished by the commonly held view that modification of a specific behavior without addressing the underlying problem will be of little benefit to the patient. Dynamic psychotherapy and family and group therapies are examples of these. The nature of the relationship between the occurrence of seizures and emotional stress is neither completely understood nor generally agreed on.

Prognosis

Does a person "outgrow" his epilepsy, or does the occurrence of an epileptic attack mean that the individual is committed to a lifelong prescription of antiepileptic medications? Should a person be placed on prophylactic therapy following a single seizure? If the patient has had no seizures while taking medicine for over 5 years, can the dose requirement be reduced or the medication discontinued? Do persons with epilepsy have unique personalities? These are common questions that are encountered in the management of persons with epilepsy. Each patient must be evaluated separately, but there are generalizations which might be useful.

Epilepsy and Personality. Evidence suggests that the frequency of emotional disturbance is higher in patients with epilepsy and that increases in stress relate to frequency in seizures. However, the association between a specific personality pattern of disturbance and a specific seizure disorder has yet to be clearly established. A more reasonable view in light of current evidence is that patients with partial complex seizures are more vulnerable to effects of emotional activation because limbic system structures are involved. This involvement has consequences in two ways: (1) control of behavior is more problematic, and (2) memory is affected, which in turn influences the way persons cope with the disorder. Because of the retrograde amnesia in these patients, the identification of emotional precipitants is more difficult for them. Personality patterns in these patients may reflect the role that seizures have played in their lives and the way in which they have been viewed by others, particularly family members. Moreover, patterns within the family served to reinforce their status as "sick" persons, and such a status perpetuates dependency. The recurrence of seizures reduces self-confidence in a patient whose epilepsy is poorly controlled. He is dependent on others during an attack when consciousness is affected. Embarrassment and fear of being rejected by those who witnessed the seizure may follow recovery. Behavior patterns may develop as a result of longstanding, poorly controlled epilepsy. What have been considered unique characteristics of the epileptic personality in cases of temporal lobe epilepsy may simply reflect the person's prolonged accumulation of learned responses to the feeling of having no control over his environment. Parents, teachers, and medical personnel contribute to the patient's view of himself by their behavior and reactions to him and his seizures. Parents must be supportive but not overly protective to the point of being suppressive. Teachers and family members must accentuate the abilities of a person with epilepsy, rather than his limitations and handicaps. Those who witness seizures often must know how to be helpful both during and after the attack. Through counseling and medical advice, they must be prepared for the possible occurrence of a seizure and to accept the sense of helplessness when it happens. Frustration of failed therapies

and interrupted family plans must be met with understanding rather than anger and rejection toward the seizure patient. A thoroughly open program of information and expression of feelings by all members of the family, as well as the patient, may alleviate behaviors that complicate seizure control and lead to future problems of social and personal adjustment.

A Single Seizure. A symptomatic epileptic attack in association with high fever, toxic encephalopathy, alcohol withdrawal, meningitis, or syncope will probably not recur. In these instances acute circumstances can explain the single seizure. There are otherwise healthy individuals who have a seizure after an all-night party or cramming for examinations because of sleep deprivation. The decision to treat or not to treat the initial single seizure is based on (1) detailed information about the circumstances surrounding the event; (2) adequate laboratory data at the time to identify low blood levels of sugar or electrolytes or other toxins; and (3) presence of electroencephalographic (EEG) evidence of epilepsy at least 2 weeks after the seizure. In the absence of confirmatory evidence of a seizure disorder, one would be reluctant to commit a patient to long-term medication, with its inconveniences and potential side effects, for prevention of another attack which might not occur anyway. However, if there is sufficient information to make a diagnosis of epilepsy, adequate therapy must be instituted and continued. Periodic observation and repeat electroencephalograms should be done. Often, a single seizure remains as such on medication. In some individuals medication can be discontinued after a seizure-free period of 5 years or more. At that time, on no medication and with a normal EEG (best with sleep deprivation stress), the patient can be allowed to go without medication. Yearly normal electroencephalograms for 3 to 5 more years should be done to help the physician decide that the "single seizure" was just that and that lifelong medication will not be necessary.

"Outgrowing" Epilepsy. The presence of a specific brain lesion such as congenital cysts, post-traumatic changes, vascular malformations, or tuberous sclerosis in a child with epilepsy is a definite basis upon which to commit treatment for a lifetime; when no structural condition is identified, then the prognosis is better. Focal seizures occurring in early life have a more favorable prognosis, but no remissions can be expected when the first seizure occurs after the age of 7 to 9 years. When petit mal type seizures are considered, children may follow the course of one third having more seizures after puberty, one third continuing to have absence seizures of various types, and one third developing tonic-clonic seizures as well. There are many adults who have what they think is their "first" seizure, but who find when checking with their parents or previous medical records that they had been told that they had "outgrown" their childhood epilepsy. The prolonged period of being seizure free may simply be a matter of increasing threshold with increasing age. A person with a history of epilepsy may go through life on no medication whatsoever, as long as he is not faced with sufficient threshold-lowering factors (Fig. 1) to precipitate an attack at a particular time.

Stopping Medication. Many patients begin to feel confident when their seizures have been controlled for a year or more. Forgetting that it is because of the medication that the seizures are under control, a patient might miss one dose now and then. If nothing happens, the patient begins to question the need for as much medicine as he was taking, and begins to take one less pill a day or so. When the plasma level falls below the protective level for the patient's personal seizure threshold, an attack will occur. Eighteen months is a frequent period of time for this to happen, unless the patient is seen at least every 6 to 10 months and reminded of the need for medication. When seizures are well controlled for 5 years or more on medication, the patient must be reminded about the protective nature of the proper dose of the correct medication. The data from a Scandinavian study showed that 30 per cent of such "controlled" patients will have occurrence of seizures within 2 years of stopping medication. If no untoward effects develop, prophylactic medication can be relatively "inexpensive insurance" for maintaining a desired life style.

The expectations of the physician and the patient (and the family) will determine the outcome of the therapy. An optimistic yet realistic attitude has better results than one which accepts recurrent seizures as inevitable. Realistic optimism with a good understanding of seizure threshold and how to keep it elevated is the way to approach treatment of persons with epilepsy.

Acknowledgment

Appreciation is expressed to Dr. Thomas R. Browne for providing much of the pharmacologic data concerning antiepileptic drugs and to Miss Anne Fidler for assisting in preparing the manuscript.

EPILEPSY IN CHILDHOOD

method of
W. EDWIN DODSON, M.D.
St. Louis, Missouri

Introduction

Convulsions result from the abnormally synchronous discharge of neurons, which cause sudden interruptions of normal motor, cognitive, or sensory brain activities. Convulsions or seizures are symptoms of many brain disorders. Although the cause of a seizure should always be investigated, in more than half of patients the cause cannot be identified. Epilepsy is recurrent seizures, excluding convulsions caused by transient metabolic disturbances.

The principles of treating children with epilepsy are straightforward. First the seizure is documented. Documentation involves a careful description of the behavior or experiences during the seizure and a careful attention to the sequence of events. Documentation also involves recording where, when, and how many seizures occurred. Determining the baseline seizure frequency is valuable for evaluating future therapy. The description of the seizure is used to classify the seizure type. Classification is important because it is the basis for selecting drug therapy. After specifically treatable causes are excluded, an antiepileptic drug is started. Children taking anticonvulsant drugs must be followed closely, because the doses of anticonvulsants which control seizures are often close to the doses which produce neurologic side effects. Periodic reevaluations are required to adjust drug dosage.

The importance of identifying and treating the specific cause of seizures cannot be overemphasized. Failure to identify and treat promptly a metabolic or infectious cause of seizures may lead to permanent brain damage. For this reason the initial management of children with seizures should be directed at identifying treatable causes. Is there sufficient glucose, oxygen, and blood pressure? Are fluids and electrolytes in balance? Does the patient have meningitis? When a treatable disorder is causing seizures, specific therapy is essential; giving antiepileptic drugs to control seizures is of secondary importance. Even when seizures are severe and life threatening, one must remember that anticonvulsant drugs are only symptomatic therapy which does not treat the cause of seizures.

Classification of Seizure Types in Older Children and Adolescents

The classification of seizure types helps one select the appropriate antiepileptic drug. Among older children and adults the International Classification is the most widely used scheme (Table 1). Unfortunately this system has deficiencies for categorizing certain types of pediatric seizures such as neonatal seizures, febrile seizures, and the Lennox-Gastaut syndrome. These groups of seizures are thus considered separately.

The International Classification divides seizures into two main types, *partial* and *generalized*. Partial or focal seizures have a focal origin in the brain and involve a relatively restricted amount of nervous tissue. Partial seizures can spread to involve the entire cortex, secondarily producing a generalized seizure. A partial seizure may cause simple motor or sensory symptoms, so-called partial seizures with *elementary* symptoms. When the convulsion originates in the temporal lobe or limbic structures, the seizures may include psychic symptoms, patterned, complex behavior, and sensory symptoms, so-called partial seizures with *complex* symptoms (previously called psychomotor seizures). Any normal motor, sensory, affective, or cognitive experience may be reiterated by the convulsion. Epileptic seizures are usually stereotyped. The epileptic movement, sensation, perception, or behavior pattern recurs suddenly from a background of normal behavior. In par-

TABLE 1. **Classification of Seizures in Childhood**

  I. Neonatal seizures
 II. Infantile spasms
III. Multiple types of seizures with encephalopathy (Lennox-Gastaut syndrome)
 IV. Febrile convulsions
  V. Status epilepticus
 VI. The International Classification of epileptic seizures*
    A. Partial seizures (focal)
       1. Seizures with elementary symptoms
       2. Seizures with complex symptoms
       3. Seizures secondarily generalized
    B. Generalized seizures
       1. Major seizures†
         a. Tonic-clonic (grand mal)
         b. Tonic
         c. Clonic
       2. Absence seizures
       3. Minor Motor†
         a. Atonic-Akinetic
         b. Bilateral massive myoclonic
    C. Unilateral seizures
    D. Unclassified

---

*From Gastaut, H.: Epilepsia 11:102, 1970.
†These "traditional" headings are not part of the International Classification.

tial complex seizures, an aura, a sensory or psychic experience, sometimes occurs first, warning of the impending convulsion. Typical auras include emotional apprehensiveness, epigastric discomfort, or visual, olfactory, or auditory hallucinations. The most common movements in partial complex seizures are repetitive swallowing, licking, or chewing movements. Other movements in complex partial seizures include repetitive picking at clothing and staring. Because partial seizures may be secondarily generalized, it is important to inquire repeatedly about features of partial seizures, even among patients felt to have generalized tonic-clonic seizures. Partial seizures often respond to the same drugs used to treat generalized tonic-clonic seizures.

Generalized convulsions begin bilaterally without sensory, motor, or psychic evidence of a focal onset. The *generalized tonic-clonic* grand mal seizure and partial seizures respond to the same drugs, including phenobarbital, phenytoin, and carbamazepine. *Absence* seizures are a second type of generalized seizure. Absence seizures interrupt consciousness with variable but minimal amounts of associated movement. Typical movements in absence seizures include head nodding and blinking. Medications effective in absence include ethosuximide, acetazolamide, valproic acid, and clonazepam. The last two medications also have activity against major seizure types, especially partial seizures with complex symptoms. Absence behavior may be associated with different types of electroencephalographic (EEG) abnormalities. *Petit mal* epilepsy is absence seizures associated with an EEG pattern of 3 per second spike and wave. Absence behavior also occurs as a manifestation of partial seizures with complex symptoms (psychomotor seizures). Absence seizures can occur in association with other types of seizures in the Lennox-Gastaut syndrome.

Akinetic, atonic seizures, infantile spasms, and bilateral massive epileptic myoclonus form another group of generalized seizures, which differ in their responsiveness to antiepileptic medications. These seizure types have been called *minor motor* seizures although they are by no means minor problems. These seizures sometimes respond to a benzodiazepine, acetazolamide, valproic acid, or the ketogenic diet.

Neonatal Seizures

Neonatal seizures are often caused by identifiable disorders, many of which are associated with traumatic or premature birth. Asphyxia, electrolyte disorders, intracranial hemorrhage, and infection are common causes of neonatal seizures. Less frequently brain malformations, inborn errors of metabolism, drug abstinence syndromes, and drug intoxication cause neonatal seizures. Because treatable causes are prevalent, the initial management of convulsing newborns is directed at metabolic causes. The infant is quickly assessed for hypoglycemia, hypocalcemia, and hypomagnesemia. If hypoglycemia is suspected from a blood glucose test tape (Dextrostix), the infant should be treated promptly without awaiting results of laboratory glucose determination. The initial therapy of neonatal hypoglycemia is 25 per cent dextrose given intravenously at a dose of 2 to 4 ml, providing 0.5 to 1 gram per kg. The initial dose is followed by the continuous infusion of 10 per cent dextrose. Follow-up measurements of blood sugar are essential to assure that treatment elevates the blood glucose to or slightly above normal levels. Hypocalcemia is treated by the intravenous infusion of 5 per cent calcium gluconate, 4 ml per kg (200 mg per kg), while monitoring cardiac rhythm. Hypomagnesemia is treated by giving 50 per cent magnesium sulfate intramuscularly, 0.2 ml per kg. Pyridoxine dependency or deficiency very rarely causes continuous seizures in infants. In infants having continuous convulsions, 50 mg of pyridoxine can be given intravenously while observing the electroencephalogram for a response.

Ongoing, continuous neonatal seizures which are not reversed by specific metabolic remedies should be treated with anticonvulsant drugs. Phenobarbital is the first drug of choice and is given in two divided doses of 10 mg per kg each, slowly intravenously. If seizures are not controlled by these doses of phenobarbital, the next drug of choice is phenytoin. Phenytoin is given intravenously in two doses of 10 mg per kg. Phenytoin is given slowly, with monitoring of the electrocardiograph because of the risk of cardiac arrhythmias. After 20 mg per kg of both phenobarbital and phenytoin has been given, most newborns have drug concentrations above 15 micrograms per ml. If seizures continue, the next therapy is somewhat debatable. The best options include paraldehyde given per rectum in dose of 0.15 ml per kg or additional doses of phenobarbital.

Phenobarbital and phenytoin are the principal medications used for maintenance therapy or prevention of chronic convulsions in newborn infants. Maintenance therapy is started at 3 mg per kg per day of phenobarbital and 6 mg per kg per day of phenytoin. Because newborns vary greatly in their ability to eliminate anticonvulsants and because their drug-eliminating capacity increases during the first months of life, it is necessary to re-evaluate these infants frequently. Drug levels in blood are an important aid in adjusting dosage.

Infantile Spasms

Infantile spasms are a form of epilepsy unique to early childhood. These convulsions appear between 4 months and 4 years of age, usually before 12 months of age. Infantile spasms can be caused by many different brain disorders and are often associated with widespread brain pathology. The principal treatment is adrenocorticotropin (ACTH). The dose is 40 units of ACTH gel intramuscularly daily. Retrospective studies suggest that ACTH should be started promptly. When ACTH was initiated within a month of onset of spasms, patients were more likely to have lasting seizure control than if ACTH was begun later. The optimal duration of ACTH therapy has not been well defined, although most authorities recommend at least 6 weeks. If there is no response to ACTH, prednisone or dexamethasone may be tried. Conventional anticonvulsant therapy is usually needed, too. Among more conventional anticonvulsant drugs, benzodiazepines particularly may be helpful. Clonazepam is available in the United States, whereas in Europe nitrazepam is used. The doses of clonazepam should be low initially, and increased as rapidly as possible, avoiding sedative side effects. The initial dose is 0.25 mg at bedtime. Although serum concentration does not correlate well with therapeutic response, it is reasonable to aim for concentrations of 50 nanograms per ml.

The prognosis of infantile spasms is best for those children who develop normally before the spasms begin, patients in whom no etiology can be discerned. Unfortunately, controlling infantile spasms does not assure normal neurologic development. After 6 weeks of therapy with ACTH many of the patients who were controlled will relapse, in which cases another course of ACTH is indicated. Unfortunately these patients are less likely to respond to a second course of ACTH than to the first.

Lennox-Gastaut Syndrome

The Lennox-Gastaut syndrome is a severe form of epilepsy in which children have multiple types of seizures, especially akinetic seizures. Some patients develop this syndrome after infantile spasms. The Lennox-Gastaut syndrome consists of multiple seizure types, diffuse encephalopathy, usually with mental retardation, and often an EEG pattern of slow spike and wave. The different seizure types include akinetic drop attacks, partial seizures, absence seizures, and generalized tonic-clonic seizures. Mild akinetic seizures may cause only brief head nodding, whereas more severe ones cause a complete drop to the ground.

Seizures associated with the Lennox-Gastaut syndrome are often difficult to control. Often children with this disorder require several antiepileptic drugs, including a benzodiazepine and a major anticonvulsant. The ketogenic diet or valproic acid has been used with variable success. Because of the complexity of handling these severe seizure disorders, neurologic consultation is indicated.

Febrile Seizures

Seizures associated with fever occur in approximately 4 per cent of children. Less than 10 per cent of the children who convulse with fever have epilepsy which is activated by the fever. Febrile seizures are rare after 4 years of age. Thus brief generalized seizures with fever are usually a benign, self-limited condition.

The initial evaluation is directed at distinguishing between epilepsy and simple febrile seizures, being certain to rule out treatable causes, especially meningitis. Guidelines about therapy in febrile seizures have been controversial. In prospective studies simple febrile seizures are rarely associated with serious neurologic problems. However, when certain risk factors are associated with febrile seizures, the chance of a child's later developing epilepsy is increased. The so-called risk factors are (1) a family history of epilepsy, (2) an abnormal developmental history or neurologic examination, and (3) the occurrence of a complicated seizure, *complicated* meaning prolonged for more than 20 minutes, recurrent within 24 hours, or focal. With two or more risk factors, the incidence of epilepsy at age 7 years is 10 per cent. Fifteen per cent of the children who have complicated seizures with focal features and abnormalities on neurologic examination will have epilepsy at age 7 years. The risk of recurrent febrile seizures is greatest among young children. When all ages are considered, the risk of a recurrent febrile seizure is about one in three, but if the first febrile seizure occurs before the age of 13 months, the risk of recurrence is 50 per cent. Thus many authorities recommend treating patients younger than 18 months and treating patients with two or more risk factors.

Phenobarbital given daily, producing blood levels of 15 micrograms per ml or more, reduces the chance of recurrent febrile seizures. Continuous administration of valproic acid also reduces the risk of recurrent febrile seizures, but valproic acid has serious hepatotoxicity. Intermittent therapy with phenobarbital has variable success; probably it does not work in most cases. A major drawback to phenobarbital is the high incidence of behavioral toxicity. Depending on the child's prior behavioral status, between 20 and 80 per cent of children develop behavioral problems. When therapy is given, it is usually continued for 1 year or until age 4 years when the chance of a recurrent seizure becomes very low.

Status Epilepticus

Status epilepticus is repeated or continuous clonic convulsions lasting more than 1 hour. Because the chances of serious metabolic disturbances and death increase after 20 minutes of convulsions, aggressive but careful therapy is indicated to stop seizures lasting more than 20 minutes. Status epilepticus is an emergency best treated with intensive supportive care and the intravenous administration of antiepileptic medications. In treating status epilepticus it is important to have a plan such as the one in Table 2. If the patient was not treated previously with antiepileptic medicines, diazepam is a good first choice. When diazepam is used, it is necessary to follow up with a longer acting anticonvulsant such as phenytoin, because diazepam is short acting. If the patient was previously treated with barbiturates, phenytoin is a better first drug because the combination of diazepam with a barbiturate has a heightened potential for causing respiratory and cardiovascular depression. Whenever diazepam is given intravenously there is a risk of apnea and hypotension and one must be prepared to support the patient.

Both diazepam and phenytoin must be given intravenously because they are poorly absorbed

TABLE 2. **Treatment of Status Epilepticus**

	Route	Dose
1. Maintain vital functions and substrates		
Airway and oxygen		
Blood pressure		
Blood glucose		
2. Search for a treatable cause		
Medications		
Diazepam (Valium)	IV	0.25 mg/kg or 1 mg/yr age, maximum of 10 mg/dose
Phenytoin (Dilantin)	IV	10 mg/kg slowly, twice
Phenobarbital (Luminal)	IV	10 mg/kg slowly, twice
Paraldehyde	PR	0.3 ml/kg in oil per rectum

after intramuscular administration. Phenytoin should be given intravenously at rates slower than 50 mg per minute with monitoring of the cardiac rhythm. Phenobarbital can also cause apnea and hypotension, especially when combined with high doses of diazepam. If treatment with phenytoin and phenobarbital does not control seizures, paraldehyde can be given rectally in a dose of 0.3 ml per kg. Paraldehyde is an organic solvent which should be diluted in vegetable oil. It should not be given in mineral oil, which prevents its absorption.

In most patients status epilepticus stops after the first or second medication. As emphasized previously, if diazepam stops the seizures, a longer-acting antiepileptic drug, usually phenytoin, should be given to maintain seizure control. If seizures are not controlled by the medications listed in Table 2, it may be necessary to consider general anesthesia. A variety of agents may be effective, but my preference is phenobarbital. Continuing seizures despite vigorous therapy often indicates progressive brain disease. Repeated assessment until the cause is found is an essential part of management.

Absence status, including petit mal, is not an emergency comparable to major status epilepticus. Absence status can be treated more deliberately. If desired, a benzodiazepine, diazepam, can be given intravenously while one observes the EEG. Alternatively, oral medication can be used. The patient is given loading doses of ethosuximide or valproic acid or a benzodiazepine, all of which are rapidly absorbed from the gastrointestinal tract. Intravenous acetazolamide is also available for treating absence status. Because absence status is almost never life threatening, medication should be administered prudently.

The Initial Management and Evaluation of the Child with Seizures

Patients having convulsions should be evaluated carefully with history, physical examination, and selected laboratory tests. Laboratory tests are directed at rapidly identifying specific, treatable causes of convulsions. The evaluation includes measurement of serum electrolytes, blood sugar, calcium, magnesium, and blood urea nitrogen to rule out metabolic causes of seizures. Because meningitis can cause seizures, one should always consider lumbar puncture for the infant or young child with a convulsion and fever. If the history suggests recurrent hypoglycemia, it may be necessary to carry out a carefully supervised fast to evaluate this possibility. Inborn errors of metabolism are a rare cause of seizures in newborns and young infants which can be detected by screening tests for disorders of amino acid and carbohydrate metabolism. Not all children who have a seizure need skull x-rays, computed tomography (CT) brain scans, or radionuclide scans. Children who have febrile seizures should be evaluated first with an electroencephalogram and receive roentgenographic evaluation only if there is evidence of a focal abnormality. However, if the seizures are partial or focal, if there is trauma, or if there is focal neurologic abnormality, progressive neurologic disease, or no response to usual anticonvulsant therapy, radiographic investigation is indicated. Radionuclide scanning is especially sensitive to brain inflammation and vascular malformations.

Principles of Long-Term Management of Epilepsy with Drugs

Selection of an antiepileptic drug is made after the seizure type is classified. In the case of major seizures therapy is initiated with barbiturate, phenytoin, or carbamazepine. For absence seizures ethosuximide, valproic acid, clonazepam, or acetazolamide is used. In so-called minor motor seizures, often difficult to control, therapy is initiated with a benzodiazepine or with a major drug if the child is having a significant number of generalized major seizures.

After the antiepileptic therapy is chosen, it is important to instruct the child's parents about the seizure process and its therapy. Anticonvulsant medication must be taken consistently. Parents should be told when the medication will begin to work. They should be warned about common early side effects which abate after a few days with the development of tolerance. These expected, transient side effects, such as mild sedation, are not an indication to stop therapy. The family should also be warned about certain idiosyncratic side effects and notify the physician promptly if these occur.

Family members should be instructed how to care for and position the convulsing child. The child should be placed on his side with the head in a dependent position so that secretions drain from the mouth and throat. A soft cushion under the head prevents bruises and bumps. There should be no attempt to forcefully restrain the convulsing child, and the parents should not try to force open the mouth to place an airway, a procedure which is likely to break teeth and injure the child.

If seizures are infrequent, therapy can be initiated on a deliberate, nonurgent basis with low doses to minimize early side effects. Most antiepileptic drugs are eliminated slowly. As long as 1 to 3 weeks is required for medications to become fully active, because five half-lives must elapse before drug concentrations stabilize. If it is necessary to begin therapy more rapidly, loading doses rapidly produce high drug concentrations but have a greater chance of early side effects.

Because children vary in their ability to eliminate drugs, there is great variability in dosage requirements. Follow-up examinations assessing both potential effectiveness and toxicity are essential components of good care. Drug level measurements can indicate how to adjust drug dosages and help optimize therapy for individual children. The best practice is to begin therapy with low or average dosage such as the doses indicated in Table 3 and then re-evaluate the child when sufficient time has permitted drug levels to stabilize.

Certain treatments require extra time before they become fully effective. The ketogenic diet and valproic acid may not become fully active for 6 weeks, despite the fact that chemical or pharmacologic equilibrium occurs more rapidly.

Principal Medications Useful for Treating Seizures

Phenobarbital, Primidone, Mephobarbital. These medications are effective in major seizures. Phenobarbital in adequate concentrations reduces the risk of recurrent febrile seizures. Primidone is metabolized to phenylethylmalonimide and phenobarbital and is used to treat complex partial seizures. Because primidone is metabolized to phenobarbital they usually should not be given simultaneously. Because of its long half-life phenobarbital can be given in a single daily dose. Primidone should be given in two or more doses.

The most frequent and troublesome side effects of the barbiturates are adverse behavior. In young children, barbiturates can cause hyperactivity, irritability, and irascibility. Sedation is usually transient, abating with tolerance. Behavioral side effects are major problems in older patients with complex partial seizures. Allergic, idiosyncratic side effects are relatively rare.

Phenytoin. Phenytoin is the most widely used hydantoin to treat seizures. It is active against major seizures, including partial seizures with either elementary or complex symptoms. Phenytoin may prevent absence behavior when it is a manifestation of partial complex seizures. Phenytoin dosage is sometimes tricky to regulate in children, because phenytoin is eliminated by enzymatic biotransformation, which is partially saturated at usual concentrations. As the concentration increases, it is important to make small dosage changes to avoid unpredictably large changes in concentration.

The neurotoxicity of phenytoin correlates with the concentration. When levels are above 20 mg per liter, most patients have a nystagmus; above 30 mg per liter, there is ataxia; above 40 mg per liter, mental changes and lethargy occur. At very high concentrations phenytoin may cause seizures or choreoathetosis.

Phenytoin usually should not be given intramuscularly because the absorption is erratic and slow, although eventually complete. When phenytoin is given by mouth it usually can be given twice daily, and in many cases a single dose works. Different brands of phenytoin are not equivalent, and levels should be checked before and after the patient switches brands.

Carbamazepine. Carbamazepine is effective in treating major types of seizures, partial elementary and partial complex seizures, and generalized tonic-clonic seizures. Carbamazepine has low behavioral toxicity but may cause troublesome sedation when therapy is initiated at fairly high doses. It is preferable to begin at low doses, 5 to 10 mg per kg, and increase the dose gradually. A few patients cannot tolerate carbamazepine even at low dosage because of idiosyncratic vertigo and diplopia.

The most frequent side effect of carbamaze-

TABLE 3.

DRUG	$T_{1/2}$ RANGE (HOURS)	AVERAGE TIME TO REACH STABLE CONCENTRATION (WEEKS)	DOSAGE RANGE (MG/KG/DAY)	THERAPEUTIC CONCENTRATION RANGE (MICROGRAMS/ML)
Phenobarbital	31–150	2–3	1–5	10–20
Primidone	6–8	2–3	10–25	8–12
Carbamazepine	10–30	1	15–25	4–12
Phenytoin	3–60*	1	4–12	10–20
Ethosuximide	24–42	1	20–40	45–100
Valproic acid	4–15	1/2	10–70	50–100
Clonazepam	16–60	1	0.03–0.10	0.02–0.10

*Effective half-life varies with level.

pine is a concentration-related depression of the polymorphonuclear leukocyte count. It is important to obtain baseline and follow-up white blood counts and differentials when carbamazepine is used. Hepatotoxicity is rare. Idiosyncratic fatal aplastic anemia is exceedingly rare in childhood. If the absolute poly count is less than 2000 or the white cell count is less than 4000, they should be repeated and additional investigations made. Carbamazepine can usually be given in two daily doses, although some patients may develop side effects. If high doses are required, giving three or four daily doses minimizes the fluctuation in blood levels.

Ethosuximide. Ethosuximide is effective for absence convulsions, including petit mal, but has no activity against major types of seizures. Because ethosuximide causes a transient reduction in white blood count, it is important to obtain a baseline complete blood count (CBC) and follow-up blood counts periodically during the first months of therapy. Unusual side effects related to ethosuximide are hiccups and hallucinations. Severe idiosyncratic side effects are rare.

Valproic Acid. Valproic acid is effective in both absence seizures and major types of seizures. It is also effective for myoclonic seizures. Although valproic acid has a relatively low behavioral toxicity, it may interact with other medications such as phenobarbital to cause adverse behavior. Gastrointestinal upset, partial alopecia, and skin rash are rare and not usually significant side effects. The most serious side effect is hepatotoxicity, which may be fatal. Most of the hepatotoxicity has occurred in the first 6 months of therapy, usually in patients with severe epilepsy treated with multiple antiepileptic drugs. Before starting valproic acid, baseline liver function tests should be normal, and liver tests should be re-evaluated periodically. Unfortunately, it is not clear which liver test is best for the early detection of this dangerous toxicity. The serum glutamic oxaloacetic transaminase (SGOT) was only mildly increased in some of the fatal cases and did not always provide sensitive or early warning. Because valproic acid has a short half-life, it may be necessary to give it three or four times a day.

Benzodiazepines. Clonazepam and diazepam are the most frequently used benzodiazepines for treating seizures. Clonazepam is useful in absence and akinetic seizures. Diazepam is used principally in treating status epilepticus. When clonazepam is started, transient sedation is a frequent problem. Thus it is best to start with low doses and gradually increase the dose to allow tolerance to develop. Serious side effects are rare with the benzodiazepines. Rarely they may cause alterations in mood and behavior. Withdrawal of clonazepam in some patients may cause increased seizure frequency.

Acetazolamide. Acetazolamide (Diamox) is a carbonic anhydrase inhibitor effective in absence seizures and some akinetic seizures. Because this compound is a sulfonamide, it should be avoided by patients allergic to other sulfonamide compounds. The usual dosage is 10 to 20 mg per kg per day. Levels of acetazolamide are not routinely monitored, but the serum bicarbonate can be followed. Chronic therapy with this drug can cause a form of renal tubular acidosis.

Drug Concentration Measurements

Drug levels should be measured whenever the patient develops unexpected toxicity or fails to respond at average doses. If seizures are not frequent, drug therapy should be initiated at low or average doses. The patient should be re-evaluated after drug concentrations stabilize. If seizures are prevented without side effects, it is not necessary to measure levels. If seizures continue or if there is toxicity, drug levels help one decide whether to increase or reduce dosage or go to another medication. The therapeutic ranges indicate drug levels below which most patients do not respond and the levels above which many patients have side effects. Therapeutic ranges are based on relatively few patients. They are general guidelines which must be supplemented by repeated observations of the patient. Drug levels are not an absolute indication for changing drug dosage but are only a part of the total picture. For example, certain patients with difficult to control seizures require concentrations above the therapeutic range to prevent serious seizures. But if these patients are free of side effects, then dosages should not be reduced even though the concentrations are above the so-called therapeutic range.

It is best to give as few drugs as possible when treating epilepsy because of the problems of cumulative and subtle drug side effects. When an initial medication is ineffective, it should be discontinued. If it reduces seizure frequency without complete control, it should be retained while a second medication is tried. Prevention of all seizures without side effects is the goal of treating epilepsy, but for some patients this is not realistic. When the process causing the seizure is severe, doses of medications high enough to control seizures often cause toxicity. In certain patients a reduction of seizure frequency without side effects is better than complete seizure prevention with chronic drug intoxication.

HEADACHE

method of
W. PRYSE-PHILLIPS, M.D.
St. John's, Newfoundland, Canada

Pain felt in the head may be referred from other structures, may be due to distortions of intracranial pain-sensitive structures (traction headache), or may be due to excessive or prolonged tension in the head musculature or to vascular disturbances. Since the treatment of the first two classes is that of the underlying cause, symptomatic therapy not being appropriate, this discussion will center entirely upon tension and vascular headaches.

VASCULAR HEADACHES

Headaches determined as being of a vascular nature but not due to the usual subclasses of migraine occur in association with fever, hypoxia, hangover, or hypoglycemia, and during severe hypertension, following the administration of vasodilating drugs, and after concussion or seizures. Here again, treatment is of the cause, so these will not be discussed further. There remains a large group of headaches subsumed under the category of migraine which may be categorized as follows:

1. *Classic* migraine, in which a throbbing unilateral headache follows some kind of aura.

2. *Complicated* migraine, in which transient neurologic signs accompany the classic variety.

3. *Cluster* migraine, in which severe unilateral retro- and periorbital pain occur in association with evidence of major parasympathetic discharge in the eyes, nose, and face.

4. *Common* migraine, in which the headache is usually ill localized, has both steady and throbbing components on both sides of the head, and is unaccompanied by neurologic signs. With this are frequently combined the symptoms of a tension headache.

In an attack of classic migraine, the aura is associated with diminution of cerebral blood flow, while the subsequent throbbing head pain is associated with its increase. However, the temporal and spatial patterns of blood flow do not always correlate with the clinical features of an attack. It may be that impaired autoregulation of the cerebral vessels forms a final common pathway whereby the features of the attack are produced. The roles of serotonin in plasma and platelets, and of numerous tissue amines, including bradykinin and various prostaglandin fractions, are likely to be highly relevant.

Treatment of Classic and of Complicated Migraine

General Principles. When a patient with migraine is first seen, a complete history and physical examination (the latter including an extended examination of the nervous system) are mandatory. This may be enough to allow the patient to accept reassurance that he does not have a brain tumor or other serious disease, but in some cases both the physician and the patient require further reassurance, which can be gained by noninvasive investigations — e.g., some combination of skull x-ray, radionuclide brain scan, or computed tomography (CT) scan. Most patients who give a typical history do not need such investigations at all. No reassurance should ever be given without explanation, and no explanation is adequate unless backed by confident diagnosis based upon the clinical interview and, if necessary, the aforementioned investigations. Reassurance, while unlikely to reduce the number or severity of headaches the patient suffers in the future, may nevertheless allow him to accept them without added anxiety. The explanation given him will also help assure his cooperation in the treatment regimens proposed below.

A second principle is that one should try to treat the patients without drugs whenever possible. Every headache is the product of a combination of the patient's constitution (which presumably cannot be changed) and some set of internal or external trigger factors, which are often subject to influence by the physician. Through the history one must find the trigger factors which singly or in combination precipitate each particular headache. The patient is seldom aware of them until he is told what they are and then observes the occurrence of his own headaches for a period, noting which factors operate in his case.

To prescribe drug therapy on a continuing basis without attempting to alter the external triggers listed in Table 1 is unwise. A patient with vascular headaches should at some time be put through a period of dietary self-surveillance. While a number of people recognize that such foods as cheese, chocolate, beer, or red wine cause some of their headaches and therefore avoid them, they are seldom aware of the other foods which allow build-up of tissue levels of vasoactive amines, sufficient to reach a predetermined point at which the ingestion of any one of them triggers a headache.

The patient therefore should be asked at the initial interview if he is aware of any dietary triggers and, if not (since there is usually no great

TABLE 1. **Factors Capable of Triggering Vascular Headaches**

1. Chronic loss of sleep
2. "Sleeping-in"
3. Menstrual periods
4. Bright lights, loud noise, and other physical stresses
5. Fall in barometric pressure
6. Hypoglycemia (missing a single meal will sometimes be sufficient)
7. Dietary factors (See Table 2)
8. The birth control pill, chloroquine, indomethacin, ethosuximide (these drugs should not be taken by people with vascular headaches)

urgency in treatment), is instructed to go away without treatment and to note in a diary the foods eaten in every 24 hour period prior to all headaches experienced during the subsequent 2 months. On his return, the diary is inspected, the foods and headaches are noted, and the patient henceforth avoids the foods which seem to have regularly triggered headaches, as listed in Table 2. If that is insufficient, all the foods so listed may be excluded for a 2 month period. With the avoidance of trigger factors whenever possible, the frequency and/or severity of vascular headaches is likely to be markedly reduced in about half of all patients seen. In the remainder, whose attacks are frequent enough, some form of drug prophylaxis is required.

Drug Prophylaxis. If, after the elimination of as many trigger factors as possible, the patient is still having headaches at an unacceptable level of frequency or severity, then long-term prophylaxis will be necessary. I prefer the following drugs for this purpose, in the order given below:

AMITRIPTYLINE. This tricyclic drug has sedative, antidepressive, and anticholinergic properties and also raises pain thresholds. It is presented in tablets of 10, 25, and 50 mg, and the usual single nightly dose of between 10 and 75 mg continued for up to 9 months is my usual first choice of therapy.

It is contraindicated in patients with cardiac failure, those who have had a recent myocardial infarction, or those who have taken monoamine oxidase inhibitor (MAOI) drugs in the last 2 weeks. Its usual adverse effects are sedation, anticholinergic effects, and a tendency to potentiate alcohol and sedative drugs if taken concomitantly. It also lowers seizure thresholds. The patient should be warned about postural hypotension, dry mouth, and mild sedation for the first few days of therapy or after increasing the nighttime dose.

PIZOTYLINE (SANDOMIGRAN). This drug (investigational in the United States of America) is a strong serotonin antagonist and also has antihistaminic, anticholinergic, antidepressant, and sedative properties. It is presented as a 0.5 mg tablet, and the starting dose should be 0.5 mg daily for 2 days, increasing to 0.5 mg twice daily for 2 days, after which a three times daily dose is prescribed. A maximum of 1 mg three times daily may be taken.

Contraindications include the presence of prostatism, glaucoma, or other conditions in which the anticholinergic effect would be damaging, and the ingestion of MAOI drugs in the previous 2 weeks. Adverse effects include drowsiness and stimulation of appetite leading to a gain in weight. If the drug is effective for 4 or 5 months, it may be tapered off to see if the migraine cycle has been broken; if it has not, the drug can be reinstituted. It has not been in use

TABLE 2. **Dietary Precipitants of Vascular Headaches**

Monosodium glutamate	Soy sauce, some Chinese foods, packet soups, canned foods
Nitrites	Hot dogs, ground beef, glyceryl trinitrate
Tyramine, B-phenylethylamine, and other vasoactive amines	Cheese—all forms except cottage cheese
	Pizza
	Chocolate
	Chicken livers
	Nuts
	Onions, mushrooms
	Broad, navy or lima beans
	Citrus fruits
	Smoked and pickled meat and fish
	Beef concentrates, stock cubes
Individual idiosyncrasies	Beer, red wine
	All forms of alcohol
	Fried foods
	Yogurt
	Eggs

long enough for one to be certain that there are no long-term dangers.

PROPRANOLOL (INDERAL). This agent blocks catecholamines at beta-adrenergic receptor sites. It is presented as 10 and 40 mg tablets, and a reasonable starting dose would be 40 mg twice daily, increasing to 80 mg twice daily if necessary. (This use of propranolol is not listed in the manufacturer's official directive.)

Contraindications include the presence of bronchial asthma, allergic rhinitis, any degree of heart block worse than first degree, sinus bradycardia, right ventricular failure with pulmonary hypertension, and a tendency to hypoglycemic attacks. Adverse effects include dizziness and epigastric distress, but the drug is usually well tolerated. If it is effective, long-term use appears to have no contraindications.

CYPROHEPTADINE (PERIACTIN, VIMICON). This drug has antiserotonin, antihistamine, and anticholinergic properties. It is presented as 4 mg tablets. The starting dose would be 4 mg three times daily, increasing to a maximum of 20 mg daily.

Contraindications include the presence of prostatism, glaucoma, or stenosing pyloric ulcer. Adverse effects include appetite stimulation with gain in weight, and drowsiness. The drug is of only moderate effect, and in my experience it works best in patients who have an allergic history as well as vascular headaches.

CLONIDINE (CATAPRES). This drug is generally marketed as an antihypertensive having a central effect in diminishing sympathetic activity at the vasomotor center. It is presented as 0.1 and 0.2 mg tablets. Daily doses of up to 150 micrograms have a moderate effect in reducing vascular headaches. (This use of clonidine is not listed in the manufacturer's official directive.) The drug is contraindicated in patients with renal failure or Raynaud's phenomenon and in those who are taking antidepressant treatment. Adverse effects include drowsiness, thirst, and a dry mouth.

METHYSERGIDE (SANSERT). There is no doubt that this strong serotonin antagonist is an excellent prophylactic against vascular headaches of all types. Many physicians regard it as a drug of early if not of first choice, and others have suggested its use as a diagnostic test. It is presented in tablets of 2 mg, and a recommended regimen might be to start with 2 mg a day, increasing to 4 mg and then 6 mg per day over a 4 week period and continuing for up to 4 months. After that the drug should be tapered slowly to nothing and a 1 month drug holiday given. The reason for this is the rare but frightening occurrence of retroperitoneal, myocardial, or pleuro-pulmonary fibrosis, arterial insufficiency, or symptoms of phlebitis or deep vein thrombosis, all of which require careful supervision of the patient. Although the retroperitoneal fibrosis may be reversible with time, it is by no means certain that the fibrosis induced elsewhere is only transient. The drug is absolutely contraindicated in pregnancy and in patients with any form of pulmonary or cardiovascular disease or hypertension.

Although methysergide works, one has to decide in every case whether it is right to treat a disease which is not life threatening and for which there are many other therapies with a drug which, even in rare instances, is capable of producing life-threatening complications. The decision must be left up to the individual physician faced with his patient in the clinical setting. I hardly ever use methysergide.

OTHER MEASURES. Some other prophylactic measures have been suggested. In patients who have electroencephalographic evidence of a "low convulsive threshold," the use of carbamazepine or phenytoin (Dilantin) in normal antiepileptic dosage (even though the patients do not have seizures) may bring relief of headaches. Sodium chloride restriction has been suggested as a useful measure in prophylaxis, and headaches have also been reduced in patients who have attended biofeedback sessions whereby they have learned to control the blood flow in, for example, their hands.

Treatment of the Acute Attack. Although it may be possible to diminish the symptoms of the aura, thought to be due to reduced cerebral blood flow, by the inhalation of small amounts of amyl nitrite or the ingestion of glyceryl trinitrite, the value of this is uncertain. The subsequent headache will certainly not be relieved by such measures.

The patient having an acute attack of migraine is in severe pain and should be allowed to lie on a bed in a quiet, dark room for as long as necessary. As early as possible in the attack, a combination of either acetylsalicylic acid or acetaminophen, 325 to 650 mg, should be taken by mouth with metoclopramide, 10 mg, to aid absorption.

Acetaminophen is a nonsalicylate analgesic and antipyretic without anti-inflammatory action. It is contraindicated in patients with anemia and renal or hepatic disease.

Metoclopramide has its main effects on gastrointestinal motility, acting through local acetylcholine enhancement, and it is also a dopamine antagonist. Its effect on gastrointestinal motility is to increase absorption of those drugs absorbed in the small intestine, such as acetaminophen. It has also antiemetic properties. Tablets contain 10 mg. Metoclopramide is contraindicated in patients taking MAO inhibitors, tricyclics, or sympathomimetic drugs, and it is unwise to give it to patients with epilepsy. Adverse effects include drowsiness, lassitude, and extrapyramidal signs such as parkinsonism and dystonias. In single doses, however, these adverse effects are less important.

If the aforementioned measures are not effective, or if nausea, prolonged headache, or the patient's agitated mental state demands alternative therapies, a combination of a single dose of dexamethasone, 10 to 20 mg orally or by intramuscular injection, and promazine, 50 to 100 mg, or prochlorperazine, 5 mg orally or 25 mg by rectal suppository, is recommended.

Dexamethasone is a synthetic glucocorticoid with 25 times the glucocorticoid effect of hydrocortisone but with diminished sodium-retaining properties. It is presented in tablets of varied strength and as an injection (4 mg per ml). It is contraindicated in patients with peptic ulcer disease.

Prochlorperazine (Compazine, Stemetil) is a phenothiazine with antiemetic, anticholinergic, and sedative properties. It is presented as tablets of 5 mg, rectal suppositories of 25 mg, and a preparation for deep intramuscular injection.

Contraindications include the presence of glaucoma or prostatism, and epilepsy. The drug potentiates central nervous system (CNS) depressants and produces sedation and other side effects.

As an alternative to the combination of dexamethasone and promazine or prochlorperazine, chlorpromazine, 50 to 100 mg orally or by intramuscular injection, has been recommended for use by itself in the circumstances of the acute attack. However, I prefer the combination mentioned above.

A glaring omission in the discussion so far has been that of ergotamine tartrate and its various preparations. Although numerous patients and their physicians have over the years sworn by its use, five points must be made: (1) No controlled clinical trial known to me has shown ergot to be better than a placebo. (2) It is seldom taken at the right time in the attack, and it is usually prescribed in combination with other agents which are independently valuable in the treatment of migraine. (3) It frequently produces intolerable side effects, including malaise, cramps, nausea, and vomiting. (4) It is frequently subject to extreme abuse, particularly when ill-advisedly taken as prophylaxis; when the drug is stopped, rebound headaches occur, necessitating further administration of the drug, (5) It is absolutely contraindicated in pregnancy and in patients with hepatic, renal, coronary, or peripheral vascular disease or with hypertension.

While it is a kind of medical folklore that ergotamine is a specific treatment for migraine, this can be no longer accepted as true; whatever beneficial action the drug has in patients with migraine, it is not due to its vasoconstrictor capacity, since it has been shown that the drug does not significantly constrict the extracranial vessels, the dilatation of which is thought to be the cause of pain in migraine. Possibly some antiprostaglandin effect may be held responsible. I have not used ergot preparations for my patients for the last 10 years, but for those who do wish to use it the following notes are added.

A number of preparations of ergotamine tartrate are available, in most of which it is combined with caffeine, an antihistamine antiemetic, and/or sedative agents.

In patients who have been tried on the aforementioned treatments without success, a trial of ergotamine is warranted. To find his effective dose, the patient should take 1 mg of ergotamine orally (either alone or in a combined preparation) at the first intimation that an attack is developing. If there is an unacceptable adverse effect such as peripheral, coronary, or arterial constriction, ergotamine should never be used again. If no adverse effects occur and there is prompt adequate relief of the pain, then subsequent attacks may be treated with the same dose taken in the same manner. If there are no serious adverse effects but relief is not adequate, then the dose should be doubled to 2 mg at the onset of the next attack; and if that fails, one might either give up on the drug or on a subsequent occasion administer it by deep intramuscular injection of 0.25 or 0.5 mg ergotamine tartrate. Additional agents such as antiemetics, analgesics, and metoclopramide may still be needed.

Ergotamine will work at the first dose or not at all. Repeated doses are not advised in any one attack, and in my opinion ergotamine has no place in the prophylaxis of migraine headaches of any variety.

The use of narcotic analgesics in migraine is debatable. Certainly, it is difficult to withhold them from the patient in extreme distress. My practice is to allow an injection of meperidine (Demerol), 50 to 100 mg intramuscularly, to a patient once, on the first occasion of his presentation during an acute headache, but after that to give no more, and to rely on prophylaxis and other forms of therapy to dispense with it. Patients who repeatedly come to a hospital complaining of migraine headaches and requesting meperidine should be identified and treated in a standard manner by all the physicians likely to come in contact with them according to a prearranged plan such as that outlined above and not employing the use of narcotic analgesics at all. Addiction both to narcotics and to non-narcotic analgesics is a very real problem in some migraine patients, and tolerance, habituation, and both physical and psychologic dependence are frequently seen among subjects used to taking ergotamine, barbiturates, caffeine, and minor analgesics or tranquilizers on a regular basis. The frequency of such analgesic and other drug abuse must be remembered by every physician called upon to treat patients in acute migraine attacks.

Treatment of Common Migraine ("Tension-Vascular" or "Combined" Headaches)

Most migraine headaches lead to a phase of muscle tension headache when the acute attack remits, but in the combined headache both tension and rather ill-defined vascular components are present from the outset.

Prophylaxis. Preventive measures of value are much the same as those which apply to classic migraine and should be adopted in the same way. Probably more emphasis should be placed upon the psychologic triggers and the patients' response to various types of life stress. Depending on the quality of the pain, the physician may choose to use more of the antimigraine or more of the antitension therapies described, respectively, above and below. When alterations in life style and avoidance of trigger factors are impossible to achieve or are ineffective, I rely first and most upon amitriptyline whether or not there is any element of depression of mood, combined in many cases with some of the measures to be outlined below in the treatment of tension headaches.

Treatment of the Acute Attack. With combined headaches, severe pains comparable in severity to those occurring in classic migraine seldom occur. Should they do so, then they may be handled in the same way with the proviso that narcotic analgesics not be used. In my experience, the possibility of drug abuse is greater in the group of patients with combined headaches than in those with classic or complicated migraines.

A variant of common migraine is the syndrome of severe, localized, unilateral temporal pain with marked tenderness along the superficial temporal artery. The relative youth of the patient and normal erythrocyte sedimentation rate (ESR) differentiate this from cranial arteritis. Local anesthetic infiltration around the artery provides temporary relief and may be repeated

three or four times until the other measures described have time to work.

"Carotidynia" is a term used to describe a syndrome of tenderness over the carotid artery in the neck, with an added aching pain spreading up into the neck and lower jaw. The cause is unknown. It may be relieved by steroids or by antimigraine agents as outlined above, although it usually clears in a short time if left alone.

Treatment of Cluster Migraine

Since by their nature these headaches tend to occur in temporal proximity to each other for a period of a few weeks in a year only, therapy should not be continuous throughout the year but should start only when the first headache of a series begins.

Prophylactic Therapy. INDOMETHACIN (INDOCIN). This nonsteroidal anti-inflammatory, antipyretic, and analgesic drug is presented in tablets of 25 and 50 mg. A suitable dose would be 25 mg twice daily taken with a meal or an antacid and increasing if necessary to a maximum of 100 mg per day. (This use of indomethacin is not listed in the manufacturer's official directive.) Contraindications include the presence of peptic ulceration, gastrointestinal inflammatory disease, and aspirin sensitivity, but it is usually well tolerated and adverse effects are uncommon.

LITHIUM CARBAMATE. The mode of action of this drug is uncertain. While effective in prophylaxis, it has a narrow therapeutic range, so facilities for careful monitoring of blood levels are essential. Between two and four 300 mg tablets may be taken each day in divided doses to achieve a blood level of between 0.6 and 1.2 mEq per liter. (This use of lithium carbamate is not listed in the manufacturer's official directive.) Contraindications include renal or cardiovascular impairment. The more common adverse effects are muscle irritability and weakness, incoordination, tremor, fatigue, diarrhea, nausea and vomiting, and involuntary movements.

METHYSERGIDE. See above.

ERGOT PREPARATIONS. See above.

Treatment of the Acute Attack. 1. Chlorpromazine, 100 to 700 mg per day orally in divided doses.

2. Prednisolone, 30 mg ordered as a stat dose, followed by 20 mg on alternate days for 10 doses. (For details of administration see above.)

3. If the patient is in agony with retro-orbital pain resulting from cluster migraine, he may be given a single dose of meperidine by intravenous or intramuscular injection if the other drugs have not had time to take effect. Morphia, which further constricts the pupil and may increase the pain, should not be used in this circumstance.

Treatment of Cranial Arteritis. The diagnosis of migraine applied to a patient's headache with onset after the age of 50 years is almost always a mistake. In all elderly patients with headaches, cranial arteritis must be considered and diagnosis achieved almost upon an emergency basis, because of the risk of visual loss. After blood has been taken for ESR and temporal artery biopsy planned, high dose dexamethasone (100 mg daily in divided doses with meals or antacids, and with potassium supplements) should be continued for a few days until the ESR falls to normal. The use of low dose steroids before the ESR has fallen is, in my opinion, inadequate and potentially dangerous.

Temporal artery biopsy may also relieve pain but is not adequate treatment alone; high but later tapering doses of steroids *must* be prescribed and continued for a year or until the ESR has been normal for at least 3 months — whichever is longer.

MUSCLE TENSION HEADACHE

Although the majority of tension headaches occur because of psychologic problems or following mechanical disturbances in the region of the cervical spine, many patients who later develop traction headaches caused by intracranial tumors start off with a tension headache, and this also occurs in association with vascular headaches. By the time a patient comes to a doctor complaining of symptoms of tension headaches, he has usually tried most of the common remedies himself without success, and therefore, as in other headache problems, a full history and both general and neurologic examination are mandatory before the diagnosis is confirmed and treatment attempted. Again, this practice allows reassurance and explanation of the nature of the pain in uncomplicated cases. Sometimes this will break the pain-spasm-pain cycle and is all the patient needs. If not, one must go farther.

Prophylaxis

Anxiety-tension and depressive states which are commonly associated with tension headaches must be treated. Depressive symptoms are frequently somatic and not psychologic, and therefore such features as early waking, weight loss and anorexia, and loss of energy must be inquired for carefully. Depression with major somatic and minor psychologic symptoms is very responsive to treatment with tricyclic drugs.

The treatment of anxiety states is outlined elsewhere in this volume. Sometimes simple psychotherapy and social manipulation are sufficient to relieve the tension which produces headaches, but such is not often the case and formal psychotherapy is often required, commonly combined with the temporary use of minor tranquilizers.

Behavioral therapy has proved very helpful in those centers where it is available. Either deconditioning to a hierarchy of more and more anxiety-provoking stimuli or direct inhibition of muscle tension may be learned. In the latter case, relaxation or electromyogram (EMG) biofeedback techniques are commonly employed; when anxiety symptoms cannot be found and there is no structural cause evident for the tension headache, it is worthwhile to refer the patient to a department of psychology in which such techniques are available.

The use of continuous prophylactic tranquilizers for tension headaches is not recommended; they represent no more than suppressive therapy and do nothing to treat the underlying cause of the problem, which should be handled as outlined above.

Treatment of Pain

At times when patients are more than usually disabled by their tension head pain, a combination of simple analgesics such as acetaminophen, usually supplemented by metoclopramide as outlined above and (so long as steps are being taken to treat the underlying cause) a single dose of a minor tranquilizer, is of value.

If tension headaches do not respond to these measures, then one should check again that the diagnosis is really correct and that there is no underlying intracranial or cervical disease present. If none is found, then one might suspect that the patient's tension headache is being perpetuated by recurrent attacks of migraine that are wholly or partly concealed in the continuing background headache. A trial of therapy for vascular headaches as outlined above may then be given.

EPISODIC VERTIGO

method of
ROBERT W. BALOH, M.D.
Los Angeles, California

Vertigo — A Symptom of Vestibular System Disease

Dizziness is a nonspecific term used by patients to describe a sensation of altered orientation in space. It can result from damage to any of the body orienting systems, although it most commonly occurs with lesions of the visual, proprioceptive, or vestibular systems. Vertigo, an illusion of rotation, is a special type of dizziness associated with disease of the vestibular system (including visual-vestibular and cervical-vestibular pathways). Although some physicians use a broader definition for vertigo, this more specific use of the term has both historical precedence and practical benefit. The word vertigo is derived from the Latin word *vertere,* meaning "to spin," and most classic neurologists used the term to describe a sensation of spinning. When its use is thus restricted, vertigo represents a subclass under the more general class of dizziness. Because of this specificity the presence of vertigo has important diagnostic and therapeutic implications.

Therapy

Treatment of vertigo can be divided into two general categories: specific and symptomatic. Specific therapies include, for example, antibiotics for bacterial or syphilitic labyrinthitis, anticoagulants for vertebrobasilar insufficiency, and surgery for an eighth nerve tumor. Many of the specific therapies for lesions of the vestibular system are discussed in other articles in this volume. Obviously, whenever possible, treatment should be directed at the underlying disorder. In the majority of cases, however, specific therapy is not available and the clinician must rely on symptomatic treatment.

Drugs Used for Symptomatic Therapy. The commonly used antivertiginous medications and their dosages are listed in Table 1. It is apparent that many different classes of drugs are used. As a general rule, the usefulness of each of these drugs has been determined by empiric observation, and in any given individual it is difficult to predict which drug or combination of drugs will be most effective. A patient may respond to one drug but not to others in the same class.

Mechanism of Action. Numerous animal studies have documented that drugs with anticholinergic activity diminish the excitability of vestibular nucleus neurons. These drugs suppress both the spontaneous firing rate and the response to vestibular nerve stimulation, suggesting a cholinergic transmission from primary to secondary vestibular neurons. The antivertiginous properties of the antihistamines may be due at least in part to their weak anticholinergic activity. Both the anticholinergic and antihistaminic drugs also have parasympatholytic activity, which may account for their effectiveness in relieving the autonomic symptoms associated with vertigo.

Several tranquilizers are effective in suppressing vertigo. Diazepam decreases the resting activity of vestibular nuclei neurons, possibly by decreasing the reticular facilitatory system. It also affects crossed vestibular and cerebellar-vestibular inhibitory transmission. The phenothiazine chlorpromazine, in addition to its well-known dopaminergic blocking effects, also displays weak antihistaminic and anticholinergic actions. It was initially developed from the antihistamine promethazine. Chlorpromazine and its derivative prochlorperazine are effective in suppressing nausea and vomiting, presumably through direct action on the chemoreceptive trigger zone in the brainstem. Trimethobenzamide, an ethanolamine-substituted antihistamine, appears to have a similar mode of action without having as bothersome extrapyramidal and sedative effects as the phenothiazines. The butyrophenone tranquilizers droperidol and haloperidol have dopaminergic blocking and antiemetic properties similar to those of the phenothiazines and also have the same undesirable extrapyramidal side effects.

Strategy of Symptomatic Treatment of Several Common Types of Vertigo

The strategy concerning which drug or combination of drugs to use is based on the known effects of each drug (see Table 1) and on the severity and time course of symptoms.

An episode of *prolonged severe vertigo* is one of the most distressing symptoms that one can experience. The patient prefers to lie still with eyes closed in a quiet, dark room. In this setting, sedation is desirable and the tranquilizing medications listed toward the bottom of the table are most useful. Of these, I prefer diazepam because it has less troublesome side effects than the phenothiazines or butyrophenones. The initial dose of 10 mg is given intravenously, followed by 5 to 10 mg orally every 4 to 6 hours. If nausea and vomiting are prominent, an antiemetic can be combined with diazepam (prochlorperazine or trimethobenzamide). Parenteral use of diazepam can cause respiratory depression and hypotension, and therefore the patient must be closely observed with emergency resuscitory equipment available.

Chronic recurrent vertigo is a different therapeutic problem, since the patient is usually trying to carry on normal activity and sedation is undesirable. The antihistamines, sympathomimetics, and anticholinergic medications are useful in this setting. Of the antihistamines, promethazine has the most sedating effect and is therefore useful only in situations in which moderate sedation is desirable. The administration of promethazine

Table 1. **Dosage and Important Effects of Several Commonly Used Antivertiginous Medications**

CLASS	DRUG	DOSAGE	SEDATION	ANTIEMETIC	DRYNESS OF MUCOUS MEMBRANES	EXTRA-PYRAMIDAL SYMPTOMS
Antihistamine	Meclizine	25 mg orally q4–6h	±	+	+	−
	Cyclizine	50 mg orally or intramuscularly q4–6h *or* 100 mg suppository q8h	+	+	++	−
	Dimenhydrinate	50 mg orally or intramuscularly q4–6h *or* 100 mg suppository q8h	+	+	+	−
	Promethazine	25 or 50 mg orally or intramuscularly or suppository q4–6h	++	+	++	−
	Trimethobenzamide	250 mg orally or intramuscularly, q6–8h	±	+++	±	±
Anticholinergic	Scopolamine	0.6 mg orally q4–6h	±	+	+++	
	Atropine	0.4 mg orally or intramuscularly q4–6h	−	+	+++	
Sympathomimetic	Amphetamine	5 mg orally q4–6h	−	−	+	±
	Ephedrine	25 mg orally q4–6h	−	−	+	−
Phenothiazine	Prochlorperazine	5 or 10 mg orally or intramuscularly q6h *or* 25 mg suppository q12h	+	+++	±	++
	Chlorpromazine	25 mg orally or intramuscularly q6h	+++	++	±	+++
Benzodiazepine	Diazepam	5 or 10 mg orally, intramuscularly, or intravenously q4–6h	+++	+	−	−
Butyrophenone	Haloperidol	1.0 or 2.0 mg orally or intramuscularly q8–12h	+++	++	±	++
	Droperidol	2.5 or 5 mg intramuscularly q12h	+++	++	±	++

and the sympathomimetic ephedrine (25 mg of each) produces less sedation than promethazine alone and is more effective in relieving associated autonomic symptoms. This combination has been shown to be particularly effective in preventing *motion sickness*. Meclizine, cyclizine, and dimenhydrinate are effective in treating mild episodes of vertigo and also for prophylaxis of motion sickness.

Treatment of *positional vertigo* is a difficult therapeutic problem because, although the vertigo is very severe, it usually lasts only a few seconds. In order to completely suppress these brief episodes the patient would have to be heavily sedated throughout the day, usually an unacceptable circumstance. The most common variety, benign paroxysmal positional vertigo, has the characteristic features of short duration (usually 15 seconds or less) and decreasing severity with repeated positional changes. As the term implies, it is usually a benign disorder of the labyrinth most often unassociated with other symptoms. More than 90 per cent of patients have a spontaneous remission within 6 months, although the vertigo recurs in a small percentage of patients. Once the diagnosis is clear, a simple explanation of the nature of the disorder and its good prognosis provides a great deal of relief for the patient. Because the fear and anxiety that accompany the distressing symptom of vertigo are decreased, all forms of treatment become more effective.

MENIERE'S DISEASE

method of
MICHAEL E. GLASSCOCK, III, M.D.
Nashville, Tennessee

Meniere's disease is a disorder of the endolymphatic system of the inner ear characterized by a triad of symptoms consisting of episodic attacks of vertigo, tinnitus, and fluctuating hearing loss. A fourth symptom, fullness or pressure in the involved ear, is seen in the majority of patients. The pathophysiology of Meniere's disease is thought to be a hydrops of the endolymphatic system giving rise to dilatations of Reissner's membrane in the cochlea and the saccule of the vestibule. The cause of this hydrops is not known, but there is convincing new evidence that the endolymphatic sac may play some role.

The diagnosis can be made by history alone, but because of the unilateral nature of the sensorineural hearing loss, it is important to perform a thorough neuro-otologic evaluation to rule out the possibility of a cerebellopontine angle tumor. This should consist of a careful history and physical examination, including a neurologic examination. Air and bone conduction audiograms with speech discrimination scores are vital to establish the nature of the hearing loss. In most cases, the low tones are involved in Meniere's disease, whereas the high tones are affected by angle tumors. X-rays of the internal auditory canal should be obtained and the vestibular response documented by means of a caloric test. Should any of these tests suggest a cerebellopontine angle lesion, a computed tomography (CT) scan and possibly a posterior fossa myelogram should be performed.

The natural course of Meniere's disease is as follows:

1. The patient develops fullness and tinnitus in one ear, the hearing drops, and very shortly thereafter the patient begins to experience vertigo with nausea and often vomiting. Untreated, the acute attack may last from 10 minutes to 1 hour. The patient then becomes very sleepy, and, if he lies down and rests, will often feel better after 3 to 4 hours of sleep. Upon awakening, the hearing may have returned to normal.

2. As the next stage evolves, the patient continues to have fluctuations of hearing with each attack, but the hearing does not return to normal between episodes. The tinnitus and fullness become constant and the vertigo more frequent. In some patients the hearing loss stabilizes at a given level and does not fluctuate.

3. The final stage (burned-out) is characterized by a profound deafness, constant tinnitus, and fullness in the involved ear. The patient may have no vertigo or frequent vertigo at this time. When the attacks do come, they are without warning, often throwing the patient to the ground violently. Many patients experience a chronic unsteadiness in this stage.

In the first two stages of Meniere's disease, there is a natural tendency toward spontaneous remission and exacerbations. Involvement of the opposite ear occurs in 15 to 20 per cent of the cases. Most bilateral disease occurs simultaneously; however, the opposite ear may be affected as long as 10 to 15 years after the first.

While stress is not thought to be the underlying cause of Meniere's disease, it has long been known to be a factor in precipitating attacks. In this sense any type of stress is important whether it be emotional or physical (e.g., overwork, loss of sleep, influenza, upper respiratory infection).

Treatment

The treatment of Meniere's disease is either medical or surgical. All patients should have a medical trial prior to surgical intervention.

Medical.   Assuming that the histopathology of Meniere's disease is a hydrops of the endolymphatic system, the logical medical regimen should be based upon salt restriction and diuretics. Each patient is requested to refrain from eating ham, bacon, sausage, peanuts, corn chips, potato chips, saltines, and other such foods, and to use a salt substitute for cooking and serving at the table. Triamterene and hydrochlorothiazide (Dyazide) is given on a daily basis. These two measures will, in many instances, reduce the fullness and tinnitus and stabilize the hearing. Patients with Meniere's disease will have to remain on a low-salt diet for the rest of their lives. Once the pressure and tinnitus have lessened, the diuretics may be discontinued until the symptoms recur. For this reason, the individual may expect to take diuretics off and on for years.

A combination of diazepam (Valium) and glycopyrrolate (Robinul) is effective in controlling the vertigo. At first it might be necessary to use these drugs daily for 2 to 3 months; however, once the cycle of attacks has been broken, they can be employed only when an episode occurs.

On occasion, patients with an acute attack of Meniere's disease will present to a hospital emergency room. In such a case, the vertiginous attack is usually severe and requires immediate attention. Diazepam (Valium) should be administered intravenously. The exact dose depends upon the individual; therefore, it should be titrated slowly until the vertigo lessens. In addition, atropine sulfate (0.4 to 0.8 mg) should be given subcutaneously. These two drugs will stop most acute attacks of Meniere's disease.

Surgical. Patients are considered for surgical intervention only after they have had an adequate medical trial and yet continue to have disabling attacks. There are two types of surgical procedures available: those that preserve residual hearing (conservative), and those that destroy residual hearing (destructive).

Those patients who have serviceable hearing (30 dB pure tone level with 70 per cent discrimination score) should be considered for a conservative procedure only. When the hearing is not serviceable (60 dB — 40 per cent) a destructive operation is acceptable.

In choosing a procedure, the hearing in the opposite ear must be considered as well. For instance, if one is dealing with a dead ear on the opposite side, a destructive operation would never be considered in the only hearing ear even if the ear is affected by Meniere's disease.

The two most commonly used conservative surgical operations are the endolymphatic sac drainage procedure and the middle fossa section of the vestibular nerve. The sac operation attempts to mechanically drain the endolymphatic system of the excessive fluid. The middle fossa operation allows the surgeon to denervate the inner ear balance system (semicircular canals and utricle) while at the same time preserving the hearing nerve.

When a destructive procedure is indicated, the labyrinth is destroyed by drilling away the three semicircular canals and removing the neuroepithelium.

Shunt (drainage) operations give 50 to 65 per cent relief of vertigo, while vestibular nerve section patients can expect to be symptom free 95 per cent of the time. The latter procedure carries more risk and is a bigger operation. For these reasons, most surgeons will perform a shunt first and, if it does not work, then will go on to a nerve section.

Labyrinthectomy (destructive) patients can expect relief of vertigo approximately 93 to 96 per cent of the time.

One of the most important things the physician can do for patients with Meniere's disease is to show compassion and to make them understand that their disease can be treated and that they do not have to go through the rest of their lives disabled by episodic attacks of vertigo.

VIRAL MENINGOENCEPHALITIS

method of
HILLEL PANITCH, M.D.
San Francisco, California

Acute viral infections of the central nervous system vary greatly in severity from relatively mild "aseptic" meningitis to fulminant and often fatal encephalitis. Additional forms of virus-induced disease include post- or parainfectious encephalomyelitis (an immune-mediated process usually occurring 1 to 2 weeks after infection), chronic persistent viral infections, such as subacute sclerosing panencephalitis, and progressive multifocal leukoencephalopathy. The diagnosis of viral meningoencephalitis is frequently one of exclusion. Since in most cases no specific antiviral therapy is available, other causes of meningoencephalitis for which specific modes of treatment exist must be excluded before the diagnosis of viral disease is made. Such conditions include partially treated bacterial meningitis, granulomatous meningitis (including tuberculosis, fungal infections, sarcoidosis, and toxoplasmosis), cerebral vasculitis, and brain abscess. Until bacterial or tuberculous infection can be ruled out, it is often advisable to treat the patient with antibiotics or antituberculous drugs, depending upon the clinical status and results of examination of the cerebrospinal fluid, particularly the number and type of cells present. Brain abscess may be excluded by computed tomography (CT). In vasculitis, fungal meningitis, and toxoplasmosis, initiation of specific treatment is less urgent and should not be undertaken without a definite diagnosis obtained by culture or biopsy.

In uncomplicated viral meningitis, cerebrospinal fluid pressure is usually normal, whereas in encephalitis it is almost always increased. Cell counts range from 10 to 2000 per cu mm, although very high counts are unusual. Polymorphonuclear leukocytes appear in the first 24 to 48 hours, followed by a mononuclear pleocytosis. In some viral infections, particularly herpes simplex encephalitis, a small number of red blood cells are frequently present. Protein concentration is slightly elevated, but is usually less than 100 mg per 100 ml. Cerebrospinal fluid glucose level is most often normal, but may be low in mumps meningitis, lymphocytic choriomeningitis, and herpes encephalitis. Routine cultures are of course negative for bacteria or fungi.

Supportive Care

Treatment of viral meningoencephalitis is determined to a great extent by the state of consciousness of the patient. In uncomplicated viral meningitis, the patient is fully conscious or only slightly obtunded and usually complains of severe headache, stiff neck, and photophobia. Hospitalization and bed rest are indicated. Patients should be isolated until the nonbacterial nature of the infection can be ascertained. Isolation may also be necessary for patients returning from abroad who may have been exposed to exotic viral agents. Headache should be relieved with aspirin, acetaminophen, or codeine, and fever above 39 C (102 F) should be treated with aspirin.

In viral encephalitis, the state of consciousness is almost invariably altered and may range from agitation to delirium to increasingly severe obtundation to deep coma. Seizures often occur, as do metabolic derangements and increased intracranial pressure. An adequate airway must be established and the patient should be placed in a semiprone position or on his side. Endotracheal or nasotracheal intubation should be performed if the patient is unable to clear secretions or if respiration is impaired. Vital signs, including blood pressure, pulse, pupillary light reaction, and state of consciousness, should be recorded every 1 or 2 hours. Oral feedings and fluids should not be given until the level of consciousness is normal, and the patient must therefore be maintained on intravenous fluids. Five per cent dextrose in isotonic saline solution or half-isotonic saline solution should be used in order to avoid further increasing the intracranial pressure. For longer-term management, tube feed-

ings may be required. Male patients should be fitted with a condom catheter, and if urinary retention develops, an indwelling Foley catheter should be inserted. Female patients with impairment of consciousness also require catheterization. Intake and output must be carefully monitored to prevent fluid overload. Serum electrolytes should also be obtained frequently, as inappropriate secretion of antidiuretic hormone often occurs, and fluid restriction or use of hypertonic saline solution may be necessary. Bowel function may be regulated by stool softeners or bisacodyl suppositories. Alternating-pressure air mattresses, foam pads, or sheepskin pads should be used to prevent decubitus ulcers, and patients should be turned every 2 hours. Physical therapy, including passive movement of the extremities and footboards or boots to maintain the feet in dorsiflexion, should be used to prevent contractures. A moderate degree of hyperthermia may be tolerated, but patients with temperatures above 40 C (104 F) should be treated with aspirin and cooling blankets or alcohol sponge baths.

Specific Therapy

Seizures. Status epilepticus may occur and should be treated with either phenytoin or phenobarbital. A loading dose of 1 gram of phenytoin should be given intravenously at the rate of 50 mg per minute, and treatment should then be continued at a dosage of 300 to 400 mg per day in adult patients. Phenytoin should never be administered intramuscularly. In patients with known cardiac problems, phenobarbital may be preferable, although it tends to produce greater depression of the sensorium. One hundred milligrams should be given initially over a 4 to 5 minute period, and loading should be continued until seizure activity stops or until 500 to 700 mg has been given. Respiration must be well controlled, and artificial ventilation must be immediately available if needed. Diazepam given intravenously in 10 mg increments may also be used if initial drug therapy fails. The patient must subsequently be maintained on phenytoin or phenobarbital, and serum drug levels should be monitored frequently. After recovery, and establishment of normal electroencephalographic (EEG) activity, treatment should continue for 6 months to 1 year.

Cerebral Edema. Increased intracranial pressure with brain herniation is the most frequent immediate cause of death in severe viral encephalitis, especially that caused by herpes simplex type 1. Acute impending herniation should be managed with osmotic diuretics and corticosteroids. Five hundred milliliters of 20 per cent mannitol given over a 30 minute period lowers intracranial pressure for 3 to 8 hours; however, repeated administration is decreasingly effective, and a rebound phenomenon of increased pressure may occur. Corticosteroids should therefore be started simultaneously. When intracranial pressure is elevated but herniation is not imminent, the patient may be treated with steroids alone. The risk of potentiating infection has proved to be small compared to the benefit derived from steroid therapy. When steroids are used, 10 to 20 mg of dexamethasone should be given intravenously, followed by 4 to 8 mg intravenously or intramuscularly every 4 to 6 hours. This schedule should be maintained for 48 to 72 hours or until signs of elevated intracranial pressure abate. Steroids should then be gradually tapered over a 7 to 10 day period. Cranial decompression has been used in the past in the presence of severe cerebral edema. It may sometimes be accomplished in conjunction with brain biopsy, but is an approach of last resort in severely ill patients, and has rarely been associated with a favorable outcome.

Antiviral Agents. Specific agents for treatment of viral infection comparable in potency to antibiotics for bacterial infection are not available. The only type of viral encephalitis in which antiviral chemotherapy has been moderately successful is that associated with herpes simplex type 1. Initial anecdotal reports describing improvement with idoxuridine (IUDR) or cytosine arabinoside (ara-C) have not been confirmed, and ara-C, which acts as an immunosuppressant, may in fact cause a more severe or prolonged course of disease. A clinical trial in disseminated herpes zoster showed ara-C to be ineffective. Recently, vidarabine (adenine arabinoside, ara-A, Vira-A) has been shown to exert a beneficial effect in herpes simplex encephalitis and to be relatively nontoxic. In a well controlled study, mortality was reduced from 70 to 28 per cent, although many of the surviving patients had severe incapacitating residua of their disease. The drug is given in a dose of 15 mg per kg per day intravenously over a 12 to 24 hour period for a total of 10 days. Side effects are usually restricted to nausea, vomiting, and diarrhea, although at doses over 20 mg per kg bone marrow depression may occur. Treatment must be started early, before the onset of coma, in order to be effective. Initial reports of success have now been confirmed in a much larger number of patients with biopsy-proved disease. Although severe neurologic deficits often remain, up to 40 per cent of patients are said to have returned to normal activities. Vidarabine, administered in the same dosage, has also been effective in neonatal herpes with involvement of the central nervous system (CNS).

The availability of vidarabine should not be allowed to lead to a reduction in the thoroughness with which patients are evaluated and specific viral diagnoses sought. Acute and convalescent sera must be obtained for antibody testing. In addition, brain biopsy should be performed in patients with suspected herpes simplex encephalitis, and special diagnostic studies (histologic staining, immunofluorescence, and viral culture) must be done to confirm the diagnosis. Treatment may be initiated at the time of biopsy, but should be stopped after 5 days if studies prove negative in order to avoid unnecessary toxicity and to prevent fluid overload, which may contribute to brain edema.

Other antiviral agents such as vidarabine monophosphate and acyclovir (acycloguanosine) may turn out to have even greater therapeutic value. Acyclovir is more active than vidarabine against herpes simplex type 1 in vitro and in experimental animals, and toxicity appears to be minimal. Preliminary clinical reports of efficacy against herpes simplex and herpes zoster have been encouraging, but results of controlled studies in viral encephalitis are still pending. The drug is not yet commercially available. Another experimental agent that may prove to be useful in CNS viral infections is human leukocyte interferon, which has recently been shown to be effective in localized herpes zoster and in preventing reactivation of herpes labialis in patients undergoing surgical procedures on the trigeminal root for treatment of trigeminal neuralgia. Its usefulness in other viral infections is currently under investigation.

MULTIPLE SCLEROSIS
method of
LABE SCHEINBERG, M.D.,
and AARON MILLER, M.D.
Bronx, New York

Multiple sclerosis (MS) is a common cause of disability coming on in the productive period of adult life between the ages of 15 and 50 years, ranking in frequency after trauma and the rheumatologic disorders. Other disabling disorders such as cardiovascular and cerebrovascular disease are more common but usually have onset after age 50 years. Neurologic disorders such as headache and epilepsy are more prevalent but do not have the unpredictable disabling features of MS.

The cause and cure of MS are unknown at present, and therefore the long-term management of MS is often a dynamic process depending on a continuing interaction between the patient and the physician.

Ideally the management of most disorders requires both specific and symptomatic therapy. Since the cause and pathogenesis are unknown, there is no accepted specific treatment of MS. Many treatments have been proposed, based primarily on an immunologic hypothesis of the pathogenesis, but well controlled studies have reported equivocal results. While short-term administration of ACTH or steroids may bring about earlier relief of acute symptoms and signs, the ultimate results are the same as in untreated or placebo-treated patients. There seems to be no role for the long-term use of ACTH or steroids to prevent recurrences. Other immunosuppressive agents such as azathioprine or cyclophosphamide have been advocated, but at present the risks seem to outweigh the possible benefits.

Other therapies directed to alter the natural history have been advocated from time to time, as is to be expected with any chronic disorder with an unpredictable course in desperate patients. These are based on tenuous hypotheses and have not been proved to have any benefits in well controlled trials. Some that are currently fashionable are mentioned only as caveats to practitioners.

Unproved Therapies

The most common of these are diets. These include various supplementary or elimination diets such as linoleate supplementation, gluten-free diets, low animal fat diet, natural food diets, and megavitamin therapy. Since diet therapy gives the patient a feeling of participation in regular active treatment, one may recommend any low fat, well balanced diet which will keep the patient's weight optimal for the present or anticipated disability.

Other unproved therapies include cobra venom injections, acupuncture, dorsal column stimulators, transcutaneous neural stimulators, hyperbaric oxygen therapy, and decompression of arterial supply to the brain. These are usually costly; some have inherent surgical risks, e.g., dorsal column stimulation; and the occasional remissions noted are no more frequent than those seen in untreated patients. The argument that patients need to have hope and should be encouraged to try new therapies must be weighed against the costs, the risks, and the resultant despondency which may result from therapeutic failure. Most of those who administer these treatments seek early cases, since it is well established that remissions occur in 75 per cent of patients during the first 5 years irrespective of the treatment.

Experimental Therapies

Experimental protocols involving treatment with myelin basic protein, copolymer I, or interferon are based on the viral-immunologic hypotheses, and they are currently under investigation. The effectiveness of these agents will not be known for several years.

General Therapeutic Guidelines

We recommend some general guidelines in the management of the patient with MS:

1. The patient and significant others should be informed of the diagnosis when it is established. It should be specifically named "multiple sclerosis" and not given a euphemistic label. The physician should also discuss the categories of "suspect" and "probable" when appropriate. This is important for establishing trust for a long-term relationship and immediate benefits such as disability insurance.

2. The patient should be given a definite return appointment and followed at regular intervals. The frequency of visits depends on such factors as severity, progression, and complications. This is important to provide counseling, to prevent, detect, and treat complications, and to determine the course and rate of progression for long-term planning. This is important also in advising patients seeking fad treatments or "cures" from charlatans.

3. The patient should be counseled not to expect a cure but to understand that with effort the painful, disabling complications can often be prevented.

4. The patient should receive instruction in the rationale of any treatment, possible side effects, and especially the limitations. The patient is usually anxious and intelligent, but often desperate.

5. The patient should participate in the therapy, e.g., adjusting dosage of such drugs as baclofen or carbamazepine to the optimal levels. Schedules, which are often empiric, should be flexible.

6. The patient should not be reproached for deviating from the neurologist's recommendations or advice, since it probably did not affect the course of the disease.

7. The patient with MS has complex problems and usually requires management at various times by a multidisciplinary team consisting of physicians, nurses, social workers, rehabilitation

counselors, physical therapists, and other health professionals.

8. The patient with MS often has problems with disability benefits, architectural barriers, and job discrimination, and legal counsel may be required. This concept should be introduced early to the patient and significant others.

Specific Therapy

The specific therapy of MS can be divided into prophylactic, curative, and restorative. Since the cause is unknown, there is no prophylaxis. Once the disease occurs, there is no effective means of preventing recurrences or exacerbations. Stress (both physical and psychologic), trauma, infections, exposure, climate, and other factors have been incriminated as precipitants but without sufficient proof to warrant that one advise patients other than to continue their normal life pattern. Certainly some occupations or professions are incompatible with the disability present or anticipated, and counseling is important.

There is similarly no cure or means to eliminate the causative agent and arrest the progress at present, although many have been advocated.

Finally, there is no restorative agent or means to repair destroyed myelin sheaths, although some remissions appear to be greater than that expected from resolution of inflammation and edema in acute lesions.

It is difficult for the average physician to avoid treating the acute exacerbation even though the ultimate results are the same as in untreated patients. We employ the following arbitrary regimens, since they can be employed easily on the outpatient basis with minimal side effects:

ACTH gel (40 units per ml), 2 ml intramuscularly each day for 5 days, then 1 ml intramuscularly each day for 5 days.

Prednisone, 40 mg per day in divided dosage on alternate days for 1 month with appropriate safeguards.

Symptomatic Therapy

The most common problem in MS is disturbance of gait. It may be secondary to weakness, incoordination, spasticity, or any combination of these. If the spasticity is excessive and the major cause of difficulty, baclofen may be administered up to 80 mg per day in divided doses, with care taken not to remove the rigid column of support provided by the spasticity. Should this occur, the dosage should be lowered and adjusted by the patient to a satisfactory level.

Flexor spasms may be very disturbing to the patient and are similarly relieved by baclofen. Physical therapy, e.g., passive range of motion

activity, is often helpful but only when applied in a baclofen-treated patient.

Weakness or incoordination of the legs may be so severe as to make independent walking impossible. Patients should have gait training and assistance of canes, crutches, braces, walkerettes, or even wheelchairs as needed. The need for these assistive devices varies from time to time, and if the patient is severely paraparetic, training in transfer techniques should be provided. Electric wheelchairs (Amigo or Porto-scooter) help many patients and may preserve energy for other activities.

Weakness or incoordination of the upper extremities is extremely disabling, and the response to any drugs or other therapy is discouraging. Some have employed propranolol, but it is generally useless.

Complications of these motor deficits are contractures and decubiti, and the management is preventive with baclofen, passive range of motion exercises, and frequent changes of position using water mattresses and egg crate foam pads. Should these develop, nerve blocks, neurectomies, tenotomies, and skin grafting may be necessary to treat the infection and general debilitation and prevent recurrences.

In the management of motor symptoms of MS, physical and occupational therapy play an important role. The important principles to guide one in this area are as follows:

1. Physical therapy will not in itself strengthen or coordinate denervated parts but will assist other parts in replacing the lost or impaired functions.

2. Patients should avoid overexertion with concomitant fatigue and elevation of body temperature, which lead to aggravation of symptoms.

3. Physical therapy coupled with antispasticity agents, i.e., baclofen, is important in maintenance of function and prevention of contractures and decubiti.

4. Occupational therapy is important in assisting patients with the activities of daily living and vocational rehabilitation.

5. Premature anticipation of disability is an important consideration in planning total rehabilitation programs.

6. The disability of MS may fluctuate, and the total program should be flexible depending on frequent re-evaluation. Wheelchairs and transfer training may be needed at one stage and gait training or active exercise at other times.

Valuable modalities in physical therapy are gait training in walkerette or parallel bars as indicated, active strengthening exercises to the arms and transfer training, swimming, and use of an exercise bicycle to increase endurance. Massage, hot packs, electrical stimulation, whirlpool baths, and similar modalities are of little value. Local application of ice packs may be transiently beneficial in relief of spasticity. Immersion in tanks with turbine-agitated water and detergent is useful in the cleansing of decubiti and leads to more rapid healing or preparation for plastic surgery.

An important aid for patients and others is *The Source Book for the Disabled;* New York, Paddington Press, 1979.

Other motor symptoms such as dysarthria, scanning speech, or dysphagia respond poorly to any form of therapy. If the last is severe and protracted, a feeding gastrostomy may be a life-saving measure.

Lassitude and easy fatigability are nonspecific motor symptoms often seen even in the absence of other symptoms or signs. These may be managed by appropriate periodic rest periods, general toning exercises, e.g., swimming or exercise bicycle, and brief (2 to 4 weeks) courses of prednisone, pemoline, or even dextroamphetamine.

Sensory symptoms are usually transient and not disabling. However, if the paresthesias are painful or radicular pain, e.g., trigeminal neuralgia, is severe, carbamazepine, up to 1600 mg per day in divided dosage, is usually effective. Other sensory complaints such as vertigo, diplopia, or blurred vision are usually self-limiting and not disabling. Diplopia may be alleviated by patching.

Bladder, bowel, and sexual problems are extremely common among patients with MS, and fortunately the first two are amenable to management. Among males, impotence and decreased libido may occur in the presence of few other disabilities, may be persistent, and generally defy all efforts at correction. Counseling of the married couple is important. Among females frigidity is common, may be related to loss of sensation in the perineum, and is often transient.

Bladder symptoms with associated tract infections are among the most important problems of the patient with MS because of the disability, the social stigma, and the tendency of these complications to shorten life expectancy. Fortunately there is a great deal that can be offered in the management. It must first be recognized that based on the nature of the symptoms (frequency, urgency, incontinence, or retention) alone, one cannot correctly diagnose these as a result of either failure "to store urine" or "to empty urine." In many instances there is detrusor-sphincter dyssynergia. In every case one should perform urodynamics (combined cystometry and

sphincter electromyography), which can be done on an outpatient basis using only simple catheterization of the urinary bladder and surface electrodes inserted into the anus. Cystoscopy is often not necessary unless urinary obstruction is suspected, and intravenous urograms should be performed every 2 years or so. As a minimal screening diagnostic work-up, the residual urine should be measured following as complete voluntary voiding as is possible, along with culture and sensitivity testing of the urine.

If the urodynamic study reveals a large capacity bladder with an excessive residual and significant detrusor-sphincter dyssynergia, one should begin treatment with small doses of baclofen (5 mg three times daily) and gradually increase this to a level that will not produce undesirable hypotonicity of the legs. This should be accompanied by bladder training with regular voiding on a toilet if possible, employing Credé maneuvers, and percussion of the suprapubic region with the side of the hand. If measurement of residual urine at an interval of weeks reveals an excessive amount (more than 100 ml), then the patient should be instructed in the practice of clean intermittent self-catheterization. The frequency will depend on the amount of residual, symptomatology, and fluid intake.

If the study reveals a small capacity bladder with residual, then one should initiate treatment with propantheline bromide, 15 mg three times a day, or imipramine, 50 to 150 mg a day. (This use of these agents is not listed in the manufacturers' official directives.) When this is accompanied by significant detrusor-sphincter dyssynergia, then baclofen should be administered before initiation of anticholinergic therapy. The latter could be added when there is adequate evidence of decreased dyssynergia.

Periodic follow-up with checking residual urine, urinalysis, culture, and sensitivity should be performed routinely, guided by the symptomatology. The fluid intake should be adequate to maintain a daily urine output of at least 1000 ml. Acidification of the urine should be attempted with ascorbic acid, 1.0 gram four times a day, and urinary antiseptics such as methenamine mandelate or hippurate, 1.0 gram four times a day, may be used to counteract infection and stone formation.

Many patients have constipation as a result of decreased fluid intake, limitation of activity, and diet. Loss of bowel control also occurs, although less frequently. These are best managed by a diet high in roughage, increased fluid intake, bulk formers such as psyllium hydrophillic mucilloid (Metamucil), softeners such as dioctyl sodium sulfosuccinate (Colace), suppositories, and small enemas as needed. Bowel training with regular evacuation is indicated for loss of control.

As indicated, sexual problems are common in men and women. In the female without major spasticity, frigidity is usually transient and responds to simple counseling. In the male sexual problems are often more persistent and require more intensive counseling of both partners. The psychologic impact is apparent when it is considered that the majority of patients are between 20 and 40 years of age. Recently the use of various implants in the male to achieve erection has been advocated, but this is questionable in unstable disorders, and the results are often unsatisfactory.

Psychologic problems are common in patients with MS, while euphoria is frequently described as typical. However, it is often seen in later stages associated with dementia, and depression is more common. The patient is often intelligent and well educated, and is frequently desperate. Upon learning the diagnosis, anxiety and depression are common, and often transient. With the passage of time and perhaps onset of disability, with the associated social and vocational problems in a productive period of life, the patient is subjected to a variety of stresses. Professional counseling, either individually or in groups, is frequently supportive during periods of strain. This is preferable to the use of "rap sessions," wherein MS patients meet without professional supervision or guidance, although these may be of some value when no trained therapists are available.

Certain problems and situations are common enough to warrant special attention. First among these is pregnancy, since MS is most prevalent in women in the child-bearing years. There is still controversy about the effects of gestation and delivery upon the course of MS, but other factors, such as desire for children, progression of the disorder, psychosocial supports for the patient, and degree of disability, must be taken into account in helping the patient and spouse reach their own decisions about family planning.

Vocational problems are similarly of major importance and within the purview of the physician. One can predict that, because of motor problems in a significant proportion of cases, jobs requiring skill, strength, and stamina may be impossible for many. Fortunately, the majority of patients are of high intelligence and young enough to alter career goals. Early discussion between the physician, family, and vocational counselor are of great value.

In conclusion, MS is a common disease of unknown cause which produces disability in some patients by motor symptoms. Although there is no cure and nothing alters its natural history, with persistence and understanding the physician can help the patient achieve a productive life span of average duration with minimal complications.

MYASTHENIA GRAVIS

method of
J. E. TETHER, M.D.
Indianapolis, Indiana

A rapidly rising diagnosis rate, especially in centers where awareness of the symptomatology of myasthenia gravis exists, has taken this condition out of the "rare disease" category.

General Considerations

Myasthenia gravis is a condition of unusual fluctuating fatigability and weakness of voluntary muscles, aggravated by exertion, emotion, menstruation, infection, or any kind of stress, and relieved in part by rest.

Although extraocular muscles are frequently but not always involved, causing ptosis of one or both eyelids and difficult focusing or diplopia, any voluntary muscle group may exhibit weakness or fatigability of varying degree.

Therapy is aimed at improvement in strength and endurance to a level as near normal as possible by means of specific drugs and manipulation of environment. The mortality rate of almost 90 per cent before the use of effective therapy has fallen to nearly zero in some clinics.

Anticholinesterase Drugs

Successful treatment of myasthenia gravis can be achieved only if both physician and patient have some knowledge of (1) the disturbance of neuromuscular transmission present, (2) the action and side effects of drugs used in overcoming this disturbance, and (3) its variability.

There is mounting evidence that myasthenia is an autoimmune disease — i.e., that abnormal serum antibodies interfere with acetylcholine (ACh) muscle receptors. Anticholinesterase (anti-ChE) drugs decrease the destruction of ACh by cholinesterase (ChE), allowing ACh to rise to a level sufficient to stimulate the receptors. This may result in a return of strength and endurance up to 90 per cent of normal in myasthenic patients.

If, however, ACh rises too high, muscle fasciculation, or even muscle paralysis (cholinergic weakness), may occur, which is sometimes difficult to distinguish from myasthenic weakness. This is usually, but not always, accompanied by signs and symptoms of parasympathetic overstimulation. These include flushing, sweating, salivation, lacrimation, miosis, nausea, abdominal cramping, diarrhea, and bradycardia.

The patient should be warned of these symptoms and should always be supplied with and instructed to take 1 to 2 tablets of atropine sulfate, 0.4 mg each, at the onset and to repeat this dose every 15 minutes until relief, or a dry mouth, occurs. If these side effects do not occur but an increasing dosage of anti-ChE drug fails to improve strength or even seems to diminish it, the patient is instructed to reduce the dose below its previous level. No patient is given atropine or belladonna regularly with anti-ChE drugs to reduce their side effects unless he understands this rule. It is rarely necessary to block these side effects; indeed, it is inadvisable because they serve as valuable warning signs of overdosage.

Since myasthenia is variable and remissions or relapses may occur at any time, each patient must be instructed to vary anti-ChE drugs according to side effects.

Most myasthenics have a higher than normal tolerance to anti-ChE drugs and a broad range between good results and side effects. However, a few, the "brittle" myasthenics, have a very narrow range between effective dose and side effects, with poor response even within this range.

Fortunately, no organic toxicity or habituation has ever occurred with any of the anti-ChE drugs in current use. When remissions occur, side effects appear, and dosage must be lowered or the drug discontinued. A myasthenic in remission may be more sensitive to anti-ChE drugs than a normal person. In an occasional case, drug resistance occurs, and, unfortunately, a patient resistant to one drug is usually resistant to others.

Dosage may vary, depending on the drug used, from ½ tablet two or three times daily in mild myasthenics to 100 tablets daily in extreme cases of myasthenia gravis. In most cases, medication is better tolerated and has a longer duration of action when given with protein meals, or with protein food between meals. Patients with severe dysphagia or jaw weakness may benefit by a small dose 1 hour before meals. Such patients should avoid talking for an hour before eating to rest the pharyngeal muscles.

Anticholinesterase Drugs in Current Use

Neostigmine (Prostigmin). Neostigmine is available in 15 mg tablets of the bromide salt and the methylsulfate solution for parenteral use in strengths of 1:1000 (1 mg per ml), 1:2000 (0.5 mg per ml), and 1:4000 (0.25 mg per ml). The oral:parenteral dosage ratio is about 30:1. Onset of action of intravenous injection is immediate, of intramuscular injection 5 to 15 minutes, and of oral ingestion about 30 minutes. Duration of action, depending on amount given, route of administration, and degree of myasthenia, is 2 to 5 hours.

For recently diagnosed patients and as an oral therapeutic test, it is best to begin with ½ tablet (7.5 mg) after meals, and to increase the dose every day or two by ½ tablet after meals until side effects, usually abdominal cramps, occur. These are counteracted with atropine, and the dose is reduced by ½ tablet. If this dose fails to hold until the next one, ½ tablet is given between meals and at bedtime with a glass of milk, and this dose is increased by ½ tablet increments until side effects again appear.

In severe cases, hourly doses are occasionally necessary for good control, but larger doses at less frequent intervals are usually more desirable. Such patients may require medication during the night, or they may be unable to swallow their morning dose. When dysphagia is severe, an oral or even a parenteral dose a half hour before meals may be necessary.

Pyridostigmine Bromide (Mestinon). This is available in 60 mg tablets. In our experience this drug has the following advantages over neostigmine: (1) it has a slightly longer duration of action, 3 to 6 hours during the day, and a bedtime dose will often last all night; (2) gastrointestinal side effects are much less severe; and (3) it seems to be slightly more effective on the smaller bulbar muscles.

Since 60 mg of pyridostigmine bromide is roughly equivalent to 15 mg of neostigmine, patients may be transferred from one drug to the other on a tablet-for-tablet basis. For new patients, or as an oral therapeutic test, ¼ tablet (15 mg) is given after meals, and this dose is increased every day or two by ¼ tablet after meals until a slight reaction occurs, which is also counteracted with atropine. Then, if necessary, smaller doses are added between meals and at bedtime with milk.

Prolonged action pyridostigmine (Timespan Mestinon) is available in scored tablets of 180 mg. It increases the duration of action to one third longer than that of 60 mg tablets. We give the same, or slightly higher, milligram dosage after meals and at bedtime. Because of the slower release of medication, fewer peaks are encountered, and therefore some patients on prolonged action pyridostigmine seem to have steadier strength and fewer side effects. However, a few patients seem to absorb the drug poorly.

Pyridostigmine syrup contains 60 mg per 5 ml. This preparation is useful in treatment of myasthenic infants or children, in dysphagic patients, or in patients requiring fine dosage adjustment.

Ambenonium Chloride (Mytelase). This drug is available in half-scored 10 mg tablets. Ten mg of ambenonium chloride is roughly equivalent to 60 mg of pyridostigmine or 15 mg of neostigmine orally. In transferring patients from these drugs to ambenonium chloride, however, it is advisable to use half this proportionate amount and to increase by no more than 5 mg increments.

In our experience, ambenonium has a more rapid onset of action than neostigmine or pyridostigmine. It has fewer gastrointestinal side effects. Muscle fasciculation, with a peculiar "stiff" weakness of tongue and pharyngeal muscles to the point of total inability to speak or swallow, may be the first sign of overdosage. Our patients are given 0.4 mg soluble hypodermic tablets of atropine sulfate and are told to take 4 tablets at the onset of this reaction, or to place them under the tongue if unable to swallow, and to repeat this dose every 15 minutes until either relief or dry mouth occurs.

Ambenonium chloride is often the drug of choice for patients requiring large dosage of neostigmine or pyridostigmine or those with a duodenal ulcer or an irritable bowel. We feel, however, that patients should have experience with the milder drugs before they try ambenonium chloride.

Edrophonium Chloride (Tensilon). This is available in 10 ml vials, 10 mg per ml, and in ampules of 1 ml (10 mg). Because of its brief action, it is unsuitable for treatment, but this very factor makes it ideal as a diagnostic agent, or as a means of regulating treatment with other anti-ChE drugs. In either case, we first check the degree of weakness and myasthenic signs. (For diagnosis, these are also measured after a placebo.) Then edrophonium chloride, in a tuberculin syringe, is injected at the rate of 0.1 ml or 1 mg every 30 seconds intravenously, leaving the needle in place. In the intervals, we watch closely for muscle fasciculation, especially about the eyelids, or for nausea, "tightness" in tongue or throat, or abdominal cramping. Injection is stopped immediately if these occur. After they cease, which usually takes only a minute or two, the degree of improvement is measured.

With this procedure, improvement in an untreated patient, exceeding that of a placebo, is indicative of myasthenia, whereas in a treated patient it usually indicates underdosage. Lack of improvement at 0.1 to 0.3 ml usually indicates adequate dosage or overdosage in a treated patient. However, should improvement occur in skeletal muscles but not in bulbar muscles, it is best to decrease the dose of anti-ChE drug.

Steroid Therapy

Patients who respond poorly to anticholinesterase therapy, especially those with residual bulbar symptoms such as persistent ptosis, diplopia, dysarthria, and dysphagia, should be given a trial of alternate day prednisone. In our experience, 90 per cent of over 300 such patients have improved on prednisone compared with their previous therapy.

Patients with difficulty in swallowing or breathing, or requiring high dosage of anti-ChE drugs, should be hospitalized for high-dose prednisone. We start with 100 mg daily at 8 A.M. for 5 days, after which the dose is reduced by 25 mg every other day to reach 100 mg on alternate days. Prednisone usually reduces the need for anti-ChE drugs and cholinergic weakness, and reactions may occur unless they are reduced. We have not seen weakness resulting from prednisone alone, although others have reported it.

In some cases, the need and tolerance for anti-ChE drugs are reduced to zero, while in others they are still necessary. Usually the dosage is higher on the "off day" of prednisone.

We use a high protein, 3 gram sodium, potassium-rich diet. We have had little difficulty with electrolyte imbalance, and have seen elevated blood sugars only in potential diabetics. Several known diabetics with dysphagia on anti-ChE drugs could swallow well on prednisone. Their blood sugars were controlled by raising insulin dosage on the prednisone day.

Only a few patients have developed peptic ulcer, osteoporosis, glaucoma, cataracts, or cushingoid syndrome on even high-dose alternate day therapy.

As soon as patients do well, or even better, on the "off day," the dose is gradually reduced until symptoms reappear, at which time it is slightly increased.

Ocular myasthenics with resistant diplopia or eyelid ptosis may be treated as outpatients with low dose (20 to 30 mg) alternate day prednisone. We have had excellent results in such patients.

Preoperatively, patients on prednisone should be given 100 to 150 mg of methylprednisolone sodium succinate (Solu-Medrol) intramuscularly. Postoperatively, they should be given the same dose daily at 8 A.M. until swallowing well, when they may go back on their previous prednisone dose.

Myasthenic vs. Cholinergic Crisis

When patients with myasthenia gravis are unable to swallow, to clear secretions from pharynx or trachea, or to breathe adequately without artificial aid, they are said to be in myasthenic crisis.

Another type of crisis, caused by excess of anti-ChE drugs, is called cholinergic crisis, and may be difficult to distinguish from true myasthenic crisis. Patients most likely to develop this type of crisis are the "brittle" myasthenics, who have a narrow therapeutic range between underdosage and overdosage, and whose response within that range is only partial. In such patients, dysphagia is often a serious problem, sometimes leading a desperate patient or his physician to administer a further overdose of anti-ChE drug with disastrous results.

We have seen several instances of cardiac arrest after the too-rapid administration of intravenous edrophonium chloride or an injection of neostigmine in such patients.

In any patient with impending or existing crisis, the first considerations are adequate airway and assistance to breathing. After aspiration, intubation may be necessary.

If excess secretions, miosis, or other signs of parasympathetic overstimulation are present, atropine, 1.2 mg, should be given parenterally. Atropine will at least relieve oversecretion and will not cause additional weakness, even if the crisis is myasthenic and not cholinergic. However, it should not be pushed to excessive dryness, or a bronchial plug may result.

Should no improvement occur after atropine, edrophonium should be given intravenously at the rate of 0.1 ml (1 mg) every 30 seconds. If improvement occurs before side effects, the crisis is myasthenic, and neostigmine, 0.25 mg, is given intramuscularly. At 2 hour intervals, edrophonium chloride is again given as described, and more or less neostigmine is given according to the patient's response.

Should side effects occur with edrophonium, should there be no improvement, or both, the crisis is presumed to be cholinergic, and anti-ChE therapy is stopped until the patient first improves and then relapses, when edrophonium is again tried.

In patients who have developed an apparent anti-ChE drug resistance, we have found that the best course is to stop all anti-ChE therapy and let the respirator do the work. Usually, after several days the patient will again show a response to edrophonium, and anti-ChE therapy may then be resumed. Should the patient then respond poorly, steroid therapy should be started.

Patients should be encouraged to breathe on their own for longer and longer periods until they no longer need the respirator. Anti-ChE drugs should be regulated according to needs or reactions. Dosage is often much lower after a crisis, and total remission may occur, especially after a cholinergic crisis.

We have seen a sharp drop in crises since the advent of steroid therapy.

Surgical and Obstetric Management

We give severe myasthenics, about to undergo surgery or labor, an intramuscular steroid as described previously, regardless of whether or not they have been on steroid therapy. We withhold anti-ChE drugs until they have a positive edrophonium response postoperatively or post partum.

Mild myasthenics are given no anti-ChE drugs preoperatively as they generally do as well without them. They may continue oral anti-ChE drugs during labor. If an enema is required, the preceding anti-ChE dose is omitted to avoid a cholinergic reaction.

The anesthetic for either surgery or delivery should be either spinal or saddle block when possible. We feel that intubation should be done with all general anesthesia in myasthenics so that the airway may be kept clear and respiration assisted when necessary. Succinylcholine may be used cautiously, especially in patients on anti-ChE medication, because both are depolarizing. Curare may be given in a much smaller than usual dosage if relaxation is necessary. Edrophonium or neostigmine will reverse a curare block. If the patient is slightly underdosed, however, he will seldom require any muscle relaxant.

Should respiration fail or blood pressure drop during surgery or delivery, edrophonium should be given intravenously, 0.1 ml every 30 seconds, until the patient breathes normally. Then neostigmine, 0.5 mg, is given intramuscularly.

Postoperatively or post partum, a respirator, an aspirator, and emergency tracheostomy and bronchoscopy sets should be immediately available. Edrophonium, parenteral neostigmine, and atropine should be kept at the patient's bedside. Intramuscular or oral medication should be regulated according to the patient's needs. Underdosage is often indicated by abdominal distention, at times to the point of paralytic ileus, and by inability to empty the bladder. After surgery or delivery, either a severe relapse or a remission may occur, resulting in considerable change in the patient's dosage requirements. It is best to begin with about half the previous dosage.

Pregnancy

There may be improvement, aggravation, or no change in myasthenic symptoms during pregnancy. Often, those patients who improve during pregnancy have a severe relapse post partum, and vice versa. Cesarean section need be done only if there is an obstetric indication.

Neonatal Myasthenia

Neonatal myasthenia may occur occasionally in infants born of severely myasthenic mothers. The child may seem normal at delivery, but symptoms may occur within 24 to 36 hours after delivery. Therefore the infant should be placed in the premature nursery, where it can be watched. Symptoms include weak cry, shallow respiration with cyanosis, inability to suck, dysphagia with regurgitation of water through the nose, and flaccidity of all muscles. Such an infant should immediately be given 0.125 mg of neostigmine methylsulfate intramuscularly. If improvement occurs, neostigmine methylsulfate, 0.125 mg or more, should be given a half hour before each feeding, six times daily. The dose should be lowered if diarrhea occurs. Neonatal myasthenia lasts only a few days to a few weeks, which would seem to indicate that the autoimmune factor from the mother had entered via the placenta. The prognosis is good for complete and permanent recovery, but the infant would almost surely die unless the condition were recognized and treated.

Thymectomy

Our patients are given a thorough trial on steroid therapy before thymectomy is considered, even those with thymomas. Preoperatively they are given 100 to 150 mg of methylprednisolone sodium succinate (Solu-Medrol) intramuscularly. Many of them actually show improvement in the recovery room.

Rather than a transsternal or transcervical approach, we use a lateral thoracotomy approach, which may be another reason for the rapid recovery of our patients.

In most cases anti-ChE drugs are withheld postoperatively until patients show a positive response to edrophonium. Intramuscular steroid is continued at 8 A.M. daily until patients are eating, when they return to oral prednisone.

Contraindications and Cautions

No myasthenic should ever be given curare, quinine, or quinidine without full knowledge of their provocative effects and adequate facilities to combat them. Morphine, ether, and chloroform are also contraindicated. We have had no difficulty with meperidine or codeine in the usual dosage range.

Aspirin, in some myasthenics, seems to bring about cholinergic reactions when given in conjunction with anti-ChE drugs. Others tolerate it well. Each patient should be cautioned concerning its use.

Most antibiotics are well tolerated, but increased weakness has been observed with streptomycin, neomycin, and gentamicin.

Sedatives, when used at all, should be given only in small amounts. Because of the frequent association of anxiety with myasthenia, we have found tranquilizers to be a good adjuvant in treatment. They are not given on a regular schedule, but only when anxiety is experienced.

We usually advise against use of alcohol by myasthenics, because it may cause increased weakness or side effects. High enemas should be avoided in treated myasthenics, because they frequently precipitate cholinergic reactions. Strong laxatives may have a similar effect. Should a barium enema be required, oral medication should be stopped, and 0.5 mg of neostigmine should be given intramuscularly every 3 hours before and during the procedure if necessary.

Limitation of Activity

Myasthenics are likely to overdo when they first experience an increase in strength and endurance from anti-ChE drugs. This may bring about a relapse lasting several days and requiring heavier dosage.

They are therefore advised to increase activity only gradually and to take intermittent rest periods, especially in midafternoon. They are, however, cautioned regarding too much inactivity, because disuse weakness is the inevitable penalty.

Myasthenics should avoid jobs requiring excessive standing or use of the arms, especially above shoulder level. Positions subjecting them to excessive tension or quota demands are also undesirable. Sufficient time should be allotted for rest periods.

Emotional Considerations

Myasthenia is aggravated more by emotion than by any other type of stress. Also, before the diagnosis is made, the patient may be criticized as "lazy," which leads to guilt, anxiety, or depression, thus further worsening his or her condition.

During treatment, optimistic encouragement

and even psychotherapy often speed the patient's response.

TRIGEMINAL NEURALGIA

method of
JOHN D. LOESER, M.D.
Seattle, Washington

The management of trigeminal neuralgia (tic douloureux) has become standardized in the past decade; pain relief can be obtained by medical or surgical therapy in over 98 per cent of the patients. The first step is, of course, accurate diagnosis. Classic trigeminal neuralgia is characterized by (1) electric shock-like pains, (2) intervals without pain, (3) unilateral pain during any one attack, (4) pain restricted to the distribution of the trigeminal nerve (rarely, glossopharyngeal or nervus intermedius), (5) pains of sudden onset and abrupt termination, (6) non-nociceptive triggering of pain, usually from ipsilateral anterior face, and (7) minimal, if any, sensory loss in the trigeminal distribution. A longlasting burning component of pain is frequently seen after neurodestructive procedures. Patients with atypical features do not respond as well to therapy as those with classic trigeminal neuralgia.

Management

The initial therapy is always medical. Two drugs have proved value: carbamazepine (Tegretol) and phenytoin (Dilantin). Carbamazepine is the drug of choice, as it will provide relief of pain in 70 per cent of patients. The initial dose is 100 mg orally daily, with 100 mg increments daily until a level of 200 mg three times daily is reached. Carbamazepine should always be taken with meals, never on an empty stomach. After a week at this dosage level, it may be increased gradually until either pain relief or toxicity occurs. Sixteen hundred to 1800 mg daily is an adequate dosage level to consider this drug a failure. Side effects include gastric irritation, lethargy, ataxia, confusion, and, very rarely, liver or blood dyscrasia. For this reason, I obtain a complete blood count (CBC) monthly for the first year and quarterly thereafter. Of the 70 per cent who obtain good pain relief, approximately 15 per cent will discontinue the drug because of side effects.

If carbamazepine is not successful, the next step is phenytoin (Dilantin),* initially at a dosage of 100 mg orally three times daily. After 1 week the dosage may be increased to four times daily, and thereafter gradually increased until pain relief or side effects occur. Phenytoin toxicity is usually manifested by lethargy, ataxia, and nystagmus. If carbamazepine or phenytoin individually does not provide relief, a combination of the two is occasionally successful; I recommend an initial dosage of phenytoin, 100 mg orally three times daily, and carbamazepine, 200 mg three times daily, gradually increasing one or the other as needed.

Short-term palliation can usually be obtained by blocking the region of either the trigger area or the pain with local anesthetics. Repeated blocks usually do not provide long-term relief. While the effects of pharmacotherapy are being awaited, nerve blocks may allow the severely afflicted patient to eat, drink, perform oral hygiene, and relax. Narcotics may be used for short-term amelioration, but should never be utilized on a chronic, recurrent basis. Non-narcotic analgesics are rarely of value. No other medications are known to stop the pain of tic douloureux.

Surgical Therapy

Two approaches can be utilized to manage trigeminal neuralgia after medical therapy has failed: exploration of the trigeminal nerve via suboccipital craniectomy with the goal of mobilizing an aberrant artery (occasionally vein) from the nerve, or percutaneous radiofrequency trigeminal gangliolysis. The former is a major operation, but age alone is not a contraindication. It has the unique advantage of pain relief for 90 per cent of the patients without sensory loss. Hence, there is no risk of corneal anesthesia or anesthesia dolorosa. When an offending vessel is not identified, the trigeminal nerve is partially sectioned; this has an 80 per cent success rate but does produce partial facial numbness.

Gangliolysis is a minor operation performed under local anesthesia and requiring patient cooperation. An insulated needle is placed through the cheek into the foramen ovale and trigeminal semilunar ganglion; after physiologic and fluoroscopic localization, a radiofrequency lesion is used to partially destroy the trigeminal nerve. This produces partial numbness in a restricted region of the face. The 1 year success rate is 80 per cent, with some drop off in subsequent years.

---

*This use of phenytoin is not listed in the manufacturer's official directive.

The complication rate is very low (less than 0.5 per cent). Other surgical procedures may be necessary on a very infrequent basis.

OPTIC NEURITIS OR NEUROPATHY

method of
JOHN B. SELHORST, M.D.
Richmond, Virginia

Optic neuritis is a term applied to a relatively rapid loss of vision caused primarily by an arrest or disruption of conduction along the optic nerve. Its inflammatory nature either is inferred from the history of a similar process elsewhere in the body or is assumed as a matter of exclusion from other optic neuropathies. Thus the condition must be distinguished from other acute or subacute optic neuropathies as well as chronic but recently discovered ones. This differential diagnosis is of utmost importance, for if the diagnosis of optic neuritis is incorrect, a genuine opportunity to treat the patient is passed over or perhaps lost altogether.

The function of the optic nerve is to transmit impulses along its more than 1 million axons from the retinal ganglion cells to the lateral geniculate body. A primary optic neuropathy is one that initially involves the nerve proper, i.e., the segment extending from the optic disc to the chiasm. Conditions which also interfere with transmission in ganglion cell axons but are excluded from the discussion of primary optic neuropathies are intraocular diseases affecting the retina and disorders at or posterior to the chiasm. Consequently attention to ophthalmoscopy of the symptomatic eye and visual field examination of the fellow eye is needed to define the disorder to the optic nerve proper. Compromise of the optic nerve from contiguous processes, i.e., dysthyroidism, orbital hematoma, papilledema from increased intracranial pressure, is not primary but secondary optic neuropathy.

Recognition of An Optic Neuropathy

Improper transmission of impulses along the optic nerve is perceived by the patient as loss of contrast (foggy, cloudy, or blurry vision), reduction in light intensity (dimness), or inappropriate perception of color (dyschromatopsia, color desaturation). Complaints pertaining to suppression in the extrafoveal or peripheral visual field are much less common. Positive visual phenomena are also common and include glare, mistiness, and bright or multicolored sparks of light (phosphenes). The latter occur spontaneously, with eye movement or in conjunction with other sensory stimuli, i.e., sound or pain.

Each eye is tested separately. Pertinent tests of optic nerve function are (1) best corrected visual acuity, (2) color plate discrimination, (3) visual field examination, and (4) swinging flashlight test. An abnormality in any of these tests is consistent with an optic neuropathy, but quite often they are all abnormal. The first three are subjective tests, and several guidelines apply to their use. The better of near or distance vision reflects optimal optic nerve function. In testing for acquired loss of color plate discrimination, one must recall that about 5 per cent of males have a hereditary color deficiency involving cone function in each eye. Careful confrontation visual fields are very helpful as a preliminary assessment but do not replace conventional perimetry. The swinging flashlight test is the only objective measure of optic nerve function, and as such its performance is invaluable. As a flashlight is swung from the normal or less affected eye to the fellow eye, dysfunction is indicated by the first response of the pupil: dilation rather than constriction or no response. This paradoxical response is known as an afferent pupillary defect because it uncovers a relative imbalance in the afferent arc of the pupillary light reflex. It is frequently referred to as the Marcus Gunn pupil. In the presence of normal optic media and retina the Marcus Gunn pupil is to the optic nerve what the Babinski sign is to the pyramidal tract, an unequivocal pathologic sign. Ophthalmoscopy of the optic disc and retinal nerve fibers does not estimate function but is helpful. Gutter-like defects, thinning and atrophy of the retinal nerve fiber layer and pallor of the optic disc, imply a chronic process. Swelling of the optic papilla accompanied by loss of vision (papillitis) suggests possible intraocular inflammation and prompts a search of the overlying vitreous for a cellular reaction.

Visual evoked responses, a recent development in electrophysiology, measure the conduction of retinal stimuli through the optic nerve and along visual pathways to the occipital cortex. This is a sensitive method in demonstrating normal optic nerve conduction, delayed transmission in demyelinating disorders, and impairment or failure of conduction in various optic neuropathies. Visual evoked responses, particularly to small pattern stimuli, are useful in three types of patients: (1) malingerers or hysterics, (2) multiple sclerosis suspects, and (3) those with indefinite optic neuropathies.

Once a deficit in optic nerve function is established, the physician must determine the nature of the process. Lessell (N. Engl. J. Med. 299:533, 1978) has aptly pointed out that the most important factor in this determination is the temporal profile of the visual loss. Traumatic and vascular insults are abrupt. The inflammatory or demyelinative process of optic neuritis results in deterioration of vision over several days before reaching maximal deficit and then improving in the weeks ahead. Toxic and metabolic disorders have a subacute presentation. Compressive or infiltrative processes are insidious and progressive. Thus a major point in the history is the time of onset, duration, and changing quality of the deficit. The physician must decide if visual loss occurred recently or was simply recently discovered. This is not always determinable, since monocular deficits are sometimes appreciated only when the better eye is closed or covered.

Treatment

After identification of an optic neuropathy and recognition of its probable nature by its temporal profile, appropriate treatment is undertaken. This is best discussed by dividing the processes into unilateral and bilateral optic neuropathies.

Unilateral Optic Neuropathies. VASCULAR OPTIC NEUROPATHIES. The syndrome of sudden visual loss accompanied by optic disc edema is known as ischemic optic neuropathy. Infarction with swelling in the optic disc occurs because of occlusive disease or impaired flow in the small retrolaminar arteries which supply the disc head. The upper or lower half of the optic disc is often selectively involved and results in an altitudinal visual field defect, but arcuate nerve fiber and central visual field defects are not uncommon. As elsewhere in the body, there is no direct treatment for infarction, but rather efforts are made against its recurrence. Recently attention was brought to an association between ischemic optic neuropathy and systemic hypertension (Ellenberger: Am. J. Ophthal. 88:1045, 1979). Perhaps more deliberate management of hypertension will reduce the incidence of ischemic optic neuropathy occurring in the opposite eye of a small number of patients (approximately 1 in 5).

Another association of ischemic optic neuritis that cannot be overemphasized is with systemic giant-cell arteritis (temporal arteritis). Whenever ischemic optic neuropathy appears, particularly after age 50, a history for malaise, arthralgias, weight loss, jaw pain with chewing, or headache is sought, and the patient is sent immediately for a sedimentation rate. It is good to recall that salicylates are frequently used without consultation for assorted pains and may suppress the sedimentation rate of a patient with temporal arteritis. If either the history is suggestive or the sedimentation rate is elevated, there remains a serious threat to further arterial occlusions, especially in the heart or opposite eye. Therefore, corticosteroids are started promptly. Prednisone, 20 mg orally four times a day for 1 month, is recommendable. Relief of pain often occurs within a day and tends to confirm the diagnosis. Dosage may be gradually decreased by 20 mg per day per month once the sedimentation rate is reduced to and maintained at near normal levels and constitutional symptoms are completely ar-

rested. Monthly visits are recommendable, along with pre-visit sedimentation rates. Therapy generally extends over 6 to 12 months. Alternate day steroids are not used. Rarely ischemic optic neuropathy of the fellow eye develops despite corticosteroids. Because skip lesions along the superficial temporal artery (STA) have been documented, the prospect of a negative biopsy has caused some observers to suggest that STA biopsy is unnecessary if the clinical diagnosis is sufficient to warrant treatment. Yet to justify the prolonged, careful management that this disorder and its corticosteroid program require, many practitioners prefer to document the diagnosis by histologic proof of arteritis. The benignity of the procedure says much for its general recommendation.

Occasionally collagen vascular diseases, particularly systemic lupus erythematosus, involve the optic nerve in their early stages. Since these are treatable disorders, a search for their symptoms is included in an appropriate history. A sedimentation rate and antinuclear antibody (ANA) titer are reasonable in patients with a sudden, idiopathic optic neuropathy, and particularly so if there is an undiagnosed systemic disorder.

INFLAMMATORY-DEMYELINATIVE OPTIC NEUROPATHIES. These neuropathies are caused by known infectious agents, by postinfectious immunologic sequelae, or by unknown processes. They are grouped together because they are often indistinguishable. The best opportunity to identify one or the other is by involvement elsewhere in the body. Meningitis, syphilis, sarcoidosis, a preceding viremia (especially the childhood exanthems), and multiple sclerosis are good examples. If a precipitous loss of vision occurs over 1 to 2 days, a history to exclude these illnesses is necessary. Most often, however, no systemic basis for the optic neuritis is apparent.

Optic neuritis occurs chiefly between ages 20 and 50. Women are more often affected than men (2:1). Pain about the eye, especially with eye movement, occurs in a majority of patients with optic neuritis. Pain is most common with far abduction, apparently because the S-shaped intraorbital optic nerve is pulled taut. Fortunately this pain is infrequently severe. Pain with eye movement and positive visual phenomena in the affected eye assist in the diagnosis and occasionally precede the visual loss by several days. The globe is sometimes tender, and previously mentioned signs of optic nerve dysfunction are necessarily present. Patients are occasionally completely blind, albeit temporarily. Mild optic disc edema not uncommonly occurs in the days following maximal visual loss. To fully evaluate an idiopathic optic neuritis, skull roentgenograms to exclude clinically silent processes in the paranasal sinuses (ethmoidal or sphenoidal mucocele) are desirable, along with sedimentation rate, antinuclear antibody (ANA) titer, and fluorescent treponemal antibody (FTA). After a review of the history and performance of a general physical examination and careful neurologic examination to exclude systemic disorders, idiopathic optic neuritis is diagnosed.

The natural history of idiopathic optic neuritis includes recovery of good vision in the affected eye in 70 per cent of patients within 2 months and 85 per cent in 6 months. The subsequent development of multiple sclerosis occurs in 20 to 50 per cent of patients (Perkins and Rose; Oxford University Press, 1979). The variable reports of patients developing multiple sclerosis are apparently dependent upon the nature of the referral base, its geographic location, and duration of each study. From this information several points are nonetheless made. First, a majority of patients with optic neuritis have an uncomplicated, monophasic illness. Second, a large number recover near normal and very useful vision, although the quality of contrast, brightness, and color are altered. Third, since there is no current treatment for multiple sclerosis, little is achieved by raising this possible eventuality with the patient. Should the patient raise the question of demyelinative disease or the physician perceive a true need from the history or presentation to pursue an investigation, evoked potential and cerebrospinal fluid studies are perhaps useful. However, the diagnostic yield of such studies in early presentations of multiple sclerosis is lower than in those patients with a well-established clinical diagnosis. Additionally, several investigators have suggested that the course of multiple sclerosis in patients presenting with optic neuritis is more benign.

A major difficulty encountered by the practitioner is determining whether or not to use corticosteroids. Studies have yet to show any difference in ultimate visual function among those receiving and those not receiving corticosteroids for optic neuritis. In all likelihood the axonal disruption that accounts for the ultimate visual function months ahead has occurred by the time maximal visual deficit is attained in the first several days. Very often the patient does not see a doctor until this period is reached. Correspondingly, little information is available regarding very early treatment of optic neuritis with corticosteroids. There are indications, however, that pain is relieved promptly and visual recovery occurs sooner in those receiving corticosteroid treatment.

Given this information a number of clinicians forthrightly dismiss the use of corticosteroids altogether. Other physicians believe that there remain several limited indications: (1) progressive visual loss within 36 hours, (2) distressing ocular pain, (3) poor vision in the fellow eye, and (4) bilateral, simultaneous visual impairment. A suggested oral regimen of prednisone is (1) 20 mg three times a day for 7 days, (2) 20 mg twice a day for 3 days, (3) 20 mg daily for 3 days, (4) 10 mg daily for 3 days, (5) 5 mg for 3 days, and (6) discontinue. Since there is little evidence that the basic pathologic process is altered by this treatment, efforts to do no harm remain paramount. A history of tuberculosis exposure, brittle diabetes mellitus, or recent gastrointestinal ulceration precludes judicious corticosteroid use. Furthermore, to avoid side effects, corticosteroids are employed for a short period, extending no more than 3 weeks or just beyond the period of presumed active inflammation. A seemingly beneficial response permits longer use but should raise the possibility of a tumor or infiltrative causes of optic neuropathy. Intraorbital injections are used by some authors. The results offer no improvement over oral administration. Furthermore, to be certain that the drug reaches the optic nerve, it should be injected near the retrobulbar muscle cone. This technique hazards occasional penetration of the globe or impalement of the optic nerve itself and is, therefore, not recommended for such marginal benefits. Some clinicians advocate adrenocorticotropin (ACTH) instead of oral corticosteroids. The pharmacologic basis for any difference in the response is uncertain.

Regular follow-up examinations of optic neuritis are essential until improvement is recorded, because the expected recovery confirms the diagnosis. Occasionally improvement does not follow; this should suggest the possibility of an alternative diagnosis. If visual function declines, investigation for a compressive or infiltrative optic neuropathy is strongly recommended.

COMPRESSIVE-INFILTRATIVE OPTIC NEUROPATHIES. The hallmark of these processes is their progressive nature. They include giant aneurysms, suprasellar masses, meningiomas or gliomas of the optic nerve, and eccentric intrasellar tumors among a host of less frequent causes. Once a progressive optic neuropathy is suspected, investigation proceeds along the anatomic divisions of the optic nerve: intraorbital, canalicular, and intracranial. Cranial-orbital computed tomography (CT) scan, plain roent-genograms of the skull and optic foramen, po-lytomography of the optic canal, carotid angiog-raphy, and cerebrospinal fluid (CSF) for cytology and chemical analysis are carried out, in this order, until a pathologic process is un-covered. Neurosurgical intervention is often needed.

TRAUMATIC OPTIC NEUROPATHY. A history or self-evident signs of trauma about the head are usually present. Fractures are often found in one of the bones composing the anterior fossa. The optic nerve is usually avulsed or con-tused. Visual loss is immediate. Either the whole nerve or its superior portion (causing a lower altitudinal visual field defect) is involved. For-ward momentum causes contusion of the supe-rior optic nerve from displacement against the upper proximal lip of the optic canal.

One concern in traumatic optic neuropathy is that small contusions or penetrating bone fragments of the nerve within the optic canal promote its swelling. Loss of optic nerve func-tion with progressive visual loss follows. In such instances some surgeons advocate immediate decompression of the optic canal via a cranial or transethmoidal approach. To warrant such intervention, progressive visual loss should be clearly documented and surgery promptly under-taken. A short high dosage of corticosteroids is recommended by others. Dexamethasone, 4.0 mg every 6 hours orally for 3 days is used.

HEREDITARY OPTIC NEUROPATHIES. Most of these involve central vision, are insidious from early life, and manifest in both eyes. One, however, is notorious for its mimicry of optic neuritis and unilateral presentation up to 1 year before involvement of the second eye. This is Leber's hereditary optic neuropathy. It general-ly occurs in males in their teens or twenties and is distinguished by the family history and by the appearance of a full, congested, hyperemic optic disc. By inference it is linked to an unu-sual sensitivity to minute amounts of cyanide. Some advocates claim occasional good results with hydroxycobalamin injections. Since visual recovery is variable, this regimen has little cause to recommend it.

Bilateral Optic Neuropathies. Any of the unilateral optic neuropathies may occur bilater-ally and sometimes simultaneously. Asymmetric involvement is the rule. If the eyes are equally involved, a Marcus Gunn pupil is not found by the swinging flashlight test. Signs and symptoms with bilateral occurrence are otherwise similar to those occurring in one eye.

TOXIC-METABOLIC OPTIC NEUROPATHIES. Toxic or metabolic derangements affect both optic nerves equally, although asymmetry of involvement is not uncommon. Occasionally detection in one eye precedes that in the other. Strictly unilateral toxic-metabolic neuropathies are suspect, for these may be examples of optic neuritis. Central visual function is commonly impaired, particularly within the papillomacular bundle. Scotomas, therefore, involve the central visual field and the blind spot (centrocecal sco-toma).

Known metabolic deficiencies causing an optic neuropathy include those of thiamine and vitamin B_{12}. Thiamine deficiency is usually asso-ciated with a severe, generalized nutritional deprivation, most commonly that of chronic al-coholism. Thiamine in conjunction with a good diet is recommendable, preferably before visual loss has developed in the chronic alcoholic. A vitamin B_{12} level, with appropriate replacement if low, is suggested in any idiopathic bilateral optic neuropathy. Many toxic agents and drugs have been incriminated in the causation of optic neuropathy. Too often the implication is based on only one or several isolated examples. None-theless, if a bilateral optic neuropathy of acute or subacute onset presents, a drug or toxic ex-posure history is mandatory. Any possibly of-fending agent should be withdrawn.

ACUTE PERIPHERAL FACIAL PARALYSIS
(Bell's Palsy)

method of
JOSEPH MOLDAVER, M.D.
New York, New York

Bell's palsy, also called idiopathic cryptogenic palsy or palsy "a frigore," is an acute neuropathy of the seventh cranial nerve. Its cause has been debated. Two main theories are postulated. Some believe that it is due to vascular damage resulting in either ischemia or anoxia. Another group of workers claim that it is the result of a viral in-fection. Regardless of the cause, it was formerly generally thought that there was a swelling of the nerve in the fallopian canal, which is relatively narrow. The trend was for most otolaryngologists to open the canal and explore the nerve; in many instances the nerve was slit, with the assumption that it would remove the intraneural pressure. For many years this was the usual approach, and

Bell's palsy was considered an emergency problem. Those who believed very strongly that the problem was basically vascular even had the patients hospitalized for better observation. They were subjected to all kinds of vasodilating medications: intravenous injections of procaine hydrochloride (Novocain), sympathetic block, or large doses of nicotinic acid. Often the patient was treated with histamine. Others preferred to use antihistaminic drugs. There was great confusion in the therapeutic approach to the disease. Everybody was claiming good results with different techniques. Statistics shown were favorable, which is understandable, as 90 per cent of the patients recovered completely with or without treatment.

Nevertheless, it was decided that the patient should be observed, since there were still about 10 per cent who could develop severe sequelae such as synkinesia, misdirection of impulses, and mass movements. If, after one week or so, or sometimes longer, there was no significant change, the patient underwent surgery as described above.

Surgeons indicate that the electrodiagnostic tests were of no value to them, as they could not be guided by such tests and could not select patients with severe cases from those who might recover spontaneously. This is correct, as the tests consisted of only electromyography (EMG) and conduction time; this technique is insufficient, and unfortunately other methods were not used as a rule, such as the strength-duration curve or chronaxy measurement. In all facial palsy, and especially in Bell's, with the combined techniques of electrodiagnosis one can differentiate at an early stage the patients with complete wallerian degeneration from those who are less affected. This can be detected 4 days after onset. On the other hand, with EMG, fibrillation of denervation can only be seen after 2 to 3 weeks, and at that time the damage to the nerve is complete and it could be too late. With direct stimulation of the nerve and the muscles and using square wave current, such tests can be performed every day without any damage. This is very well tolerated. Patients can be followed regularly and safely, and the proper selection of the patients who require eventual surgery can be done. From my experience, regardless of the severity of Bell's palsy, there has been no significant difference in the patients who were operated upon and those who were not. At any rate, the nerve should never be slit.

The viral theory of Bell's palsy is the one most accepted at present. It has become clear that the nerve is affected not only in the fallopian canal but all along its course. Bell's palsy frequently occurs in epidemics, but it is possible that we are not dealing with a single virus for all patients. We might recollect that in the past poliomyelitis was also considered as being due to one virus until it was discovered that several could be responsible for the disease. It is useful to mention that a facial paralysis can also occur with herpes zoster, as well as in acute infectious mononucleosis or Guillain-Barré syndrome; in the latter condition it is often bilateral and sometimes may be the major manifestation of the disease.

Treatment

The diagnosis of Bell's palsy does not usually give any difficulty, but it is advisable to have a complete neurologic examination. With any facial paralysis there is always a psychologic trauma. It should be explained to the patient that the majority of patients recover completely, but that if after 3 months there is no significant improvement, there is the possibility of sequelae of variable degree. The usual treatment advocated is with steroids, provided that there is no contraindication. Prednisone is prescribed, 60 mg daily for 4 days; this is progressively reduced to 30 mg for another 4 days, and then 10 mg for 1 or 2 weeks. My own feeling is that this type of treatment has not proved to be better than a antihistaminic medication such as diphenhydramine (Benadryl), 25 mg two or three times a day, mostly at night, with the assumption that the swelling of the nerve could be reduced.

Exposure keratitis or conjunctivitis can occur because of the eye's blinking action being markedly affected. Protection is afforded by the use of an eye shield, and drops of 0.5 per cent methylcellulose can be instilled in the eye several times daily. As for electrotherapy, there is no benefit to be gained by it; it is both costly and a waste of time. Gentle massage can be performed by the patient for a short time twice a day. Decompression of the nerve is very seldom indicated, and its value is questionable. If after 2 years there has been no significant return of motion, which can happen in 1 or 2 per cent of the patients, the crossing of the twelfth to the seventh nerve could give favorable results. The crossing of the spinal accessory to the facial nerve should never be done. When reconstruction is contemplated, it is good to know that 25 per cent of the patients, according to my statistics, can have a supply of the facial nerve from the nonaffected side in the lower part of the face.

During the past decade great developments have taken place in the reanimation, reconstruction, and rehabilitation of the facial musculature, not only from an esthetic point of view but also from the point of view of improvement of the general function of the muscles. For instance, nerve grafting and tendon-muscle unit graft, with the utilization of the extensor digitorum brevis, the palmaris longus, or a segment of the gracilis muscle, have been developed. At times part of the masticator muscles can be used. With these techniques, properly selected, even regaining a trace of contraction can make a great difference in the expression of the face. If all those techniques fail to give a satisfactory result, muscles from the nonaffected side can be transferred, but these are the muscles of the midline. Face-lifting or suspension could be a last resort. Each case is a specific problem to be studied properly. The experience, skill, and wisdom of the surgeon enters into play, and the patient even in the most severe cases can be given some hope for improvement.

PARKINSON'S DISEASE

method of
MELVIN D. YAHR, M.D.
New York, New York

It is now well established that the major biochemical abnormality in patients with parkinsonism is a loss or inhibition of activity of dopamine in the striatum (caudate nucleus and putamen). The physiologic consequence of this deficiency is a disturbance of neurotransmitter relationship in this structure, particularly that which exists between dopamine and acetylcholine. These two neurotransmitters, which have opposing actions, are functionally interdependent and normally in exquisite balance. The decrease in dopaminergic activity allows for functional overactivity of acetylcholine, which is presently felt to be the underlying basis for the symptoms of parkinsonism. Hence, the current approach to its treatment is directed to reestablishing normal relationships between these two neurotransmitters. This can be accomplished by pharmacologic agents whose action is to decrease striatal cholinergic or increase dopaminergic activity.

The major symptoms of parkinsonism — tremor, rigidity, and akinesias — may occur in a variety of disorders and conditions which affect the nervous system. Toxic agents such as manganese, neuroleptic drugs such as reserpine and haloperidol, and viral infections such as those encountered in von Economo's disease and degenerative disorders have all been known to produce the parkinsonism syndrome. These forms of parkinsonism with a definable causative factor are separable from idiopathic parkinsonism or Parkinson's disease, the cause of which is unknown. The latter is the type most frequently encountered and is distinguishable by its onset in adult life, usually above 50 years of age; a course which is slowly but relentlessly progressive, leading over a variable period of time to total disability; and a combination of symptoms that include varying degrees of tremor, rigidity, and akinesia. Parkinson's disease has been encountered in all races in every region of the world, and shows no preference for either sex. It is one of the leading causes of neurologic disability in persons over 60 years of age. Although its exact frequency is unknown, it has been estimated to have a prevalence rate of 100 to 150 per 100,000 with an incidence of 20 cases per 100,000 annually. With the world population showing an increase in numbers of people in the older age groups, Parkinson's disease can be expected to be encountered with increasing frequency in the years to come. To date, attempts to discover its cause and pathogenesis have been unsuccessful.

In view of the present state of our knowledge, the treatment of parkinsonism must be considered as symptomatic, supportive, and palliative. It is only in the exceptional case of secondary parkinsonism resulting from the use of drugs or occurring in association with specific disease processes that treatment of the causative factor may result in eradication of symptoms. The more frequently encountered patient will require lifelong treatment, consisting of the administration of specific medications, supportive psychotherapeutic measures, and physical therapy.

As is often the case in a chronic disease of unknown cause with protean manifestations and no curative therapy, hard and fast rules regarding treatment, when applied indiscriminately to all patients, give less than optimal results. Indeed, we have found it wise in Parkinson's disease to use highly personalized treatment programs, using as a guide not only the patient's symptomatology but also the degree of functional impairment and the expected benefits and risks obtainable from presently available therapeutic agents.

Judiciously employed treatment may control the symptoms of parkinsonism in a large proportion of patients for extended periods of time. In most it allows relatively normal activities of living during most phases of this disorder. The introduction of new pharmacologic approaches to its treatment has markedly reduced mortality and forestalled the progressive disabling nature of this disorder.

In general, Parkinson's disease is a slowly evolving process in which early symptoms are subtle and minimal in nature, with progression occurring over a variable period of time. The rate of progression may be roughly correlated with the degree of dopamine deficiency in the brain and has a bearing as to the types of pharmacologic agents to be used. During the initial phase of Parkinson's disease dopamine deficiency is minimal despite damage to the nigral cells responsible for its production, since those surviving are in a state of overactivity, synthesizing and releasing more dopamine per unit time than normally. This phase of parkinsonism may be considered as a partially compensated one and is best treated with agents capable of enhancing the existing state of striatal dopaminergic activity. As the disease progresses owing to continued degeneration of dopaminergic cells in the nigra, with resultant increased degree of dopamine deficiency, a decompensated phase of parkinsonism ensues. Treatment here relies on the production of dopamine in the striatum itself by administration of its immediate precursor levodopa or direct stimulation of dopamine receptor mechanisms by ergoline derivatives.

Compensated Phase Treatment

The decision to utilize drug therapy is determined by the patient's symptoms and functional impairment. In those in which these are mild and little if any functional impairment exists, reassurance and periodic examination may suffice. For example, such an approach is applicable when mild tremor at rest involving a limb is present. When some degree of akinesia and rigidity develops with minimal impaired coordinated movements, the use of one of the following, either alone or in combination, is indicated.

Anticholinergic Agents. A number of drugs, closely allied in chemical structure, whose primary action is to counteract the muscarinic effects of acetylcholine in the central nervous system, are presently available. There is little reason aside from personal preference for choosing one over the other. When used in appropriate dosage, they can produce a moderate degree of improvement in all symptoms of parkinsonism. However, their usefulness is restricted by a number of side effects which prevent administration in full dosage. Among those most often encountered are dryness of the mouth, blurred vision, urinary retention, obstipation, and psychic phenomena ranging from mild behavioral abnormalities to overt psychotic episodes.

The order of presentation of these compounds is not necessarily the sequence in which they are used. A rule of thumb is that for mild cases and those patients in older age groups the less potent agents may be preferred. For example, diphenhydramine (Benadryl) is often used in preference to one of the piperidyls or benztropine, since it is less likely to produce disturbing side effects. In such instances less than optimal improvement results, but on balance this is more acceptable than annoying side effects. In general, initiating therapy with one of the piperidyl compounds, preferably trihexyphenidyl (Artane), and adding an agent from one of the other groups is the desirable form of therapy.

PIPERIDYL COMPOUNDS. Trihexyphenidyl (Artane) is the oldest but still the drug of choice in this group of compounds. It should be started in dosage of 2 mg three times a day and slowly increased to tolerance. Most patients will tolerate up to 10 mg a day with only minor annoying side effects. Occasional patients may take 20 mg a day. A modest decrease in all symptoms of parkinsonism can be expected from its use.

Similar effects may be obtained from cycrimine (Pagitane), which is begun in doses of 1.25 mg three times a day and increased to a total daily dose of 20 mg; procyclidine (Kemadrin), begun in doses of 5 mg twice a day and increased to 30 mg; and biperiden (Akineton), beginning with 2 mg three times a day and increasing to a total daily dosage of 20 mg.

TROPANE. Benztropine mesylate (Cogentin) is a potent anticholinergic compound whose pharmacologic action closely mimics atropine. Because of this it cannot be used in full dosage without producing undesirable side effects. It is extremely useful in patients receiving full dosage of one of the piperidyl compounds or L-dopa. When given in 1 or 2 mg doses at bedtime, its long duration of action eases symptoms during the night and when arising in the morning. It is also available as a parenteral preparation and can be used in 1 mg doses to reverse the symptoms of parkinsonism arising from the use of neuroleptics.

Antihistamines. These agents have a mild degree of antiparkinson action as a result of their anticholinergic properties. They are useful in patients unable to tolerate the more potent drugs or when given in combination with them. They are frequently started simultaneously with L-dopa or one of the piperidyls or soon after starting them.

Diphenhydramine (Benadryl) is preferred because it is well tolerated. Administered in starting dosage of 25 mg three times a day, it can be increased to 50 mg four times a day. A major limiting side effect is its soporific action.

Orphenadrine (Disipal), 50 mg, or chlorphenoxamine (Phenoxene), 50 mg, each given three times a day, can be used in its stead.

Amantadine. Introduced as an antiviral

agent, amantadine hydrochloride (Symmetrel) was accidentally found to have beneficial effects on the symptoms of parkinsonism. Its mechanism of action is controversial, some feeling that it acts directly on striatal dopaminergic mechanisms and others, that it blocks cholinergic action. When used alone in doses of 100 mg twice or three times a day, its therapeutic effects are evident within 48 to 72 hours, consisting of a mild reversal of symptoms of parkinsonism. More effective action can be achieved when it is combined with an anticholinergic agent such as trihexyphenidyl. The effects of amantadine are short lived, tending to diminish after a few months. Many of its side effects are similar to those of the anticholinergic agents, particularly the induction of confusional and delusional states. In some patients after long-term use, edema and a form of livedo reticularis develop over the limbs.

Tricyclic Compounds. The antidepressants imipramine (Tofranil) and amitriptyline (Elavil) are useful agents in early phases of parkinsonism. Not only do they block the reuptake and storage of dopamine, hence making it more available at the synaptic cleft in the striatum, but they have anticholinergic action. Used alone or in combination with one of the above, they may improve akinesias, rigidity, and the not infrequent associated depressive symptoms of early parkinsonism. Imipramine, 10 mg, or amitriptyline, 25 mg, given three or four times a day, may be safely administered for extended periods without encountering the untoward side effects of their use.

Decompensated Phase

Patients with well established signs and symptoms of parkinsonism, experiencing difficulties in their routine activities of daily living and their business or social obligations, fall into this category. They are best treated initially with agents capable of replenishing striatal dopamine and, as the disease progresses, the addition of those which modify its catabolism or those which mimic its pharmacologic effects.

Levodopa plus Carbidopa (Sinemet). The best available means for making levodopa available to the brain for conversion to dopamine is its administration with a peripheral decarboxylase inhibitor (carbidopa). Available as a combination tablet, it contains fixed ratios of carbidopa, 10 or 25 mg, to levodopa, 100 or 250 mg. Treatment is best started with low doses, utilizing Sinemet 10:100 given three times a day and increased by 1 tablet every 3 days. The dosage at which therapeutic responses occur is variable. In general, patients will begin to show improvement when a total daily dose of Sinemet 50:500 mg is reached. Further increases are then made at monthly

intervals with the goal of finding the minimal dosage which gives an acceptable degree of functional improvement. In most instances this will be between 70:700 mg and 100:1000 mg, with exceptional patients requiring 150:1500 mg daily. Sinemet is best administered in four equally divided doses during the waking hours, although on occasion more frequent scheduling is found to be desirable.

At onset of treatment with Sinemet side effects are infrequent. Some patients experience nausea and vomiting, which may be obviated by using the combination tablet containing 25 mg of carbidopa and 100 mg of levodopa. Alternatively, reducing the dosage by half may be effective. Those in the older age groups may experience confusional states, primarily nocturnal, necessitating lower doses or discontinuation of the drug. Indeed, toxic psychosis may occur at any time in patients taking this drug, and it is of some importance that it be recognized and appropriate readjustment of dosage be carried out. The most frequent and therapeutically limiting side effects produced by levodopa are abnormal involuntary movements. These may be mild, choreiform movements limited to a bodily segment or severe, generalized, and dystonic in nature. They are dose as well as time related in that they occur more frequently in patients on high doses of levodopa and in those to whom it has been administered for extended periods of time. Indeed, abnormal movements may be induced in patients on long-term therapy at daily dosage levels that were previously tolerated without such effect. The only effective measure for their control is reduction of dosage of Sinemet. In general, one gradually reduces the daily dosage, seeking a level at which the movements are tolerable and a degree of control of parkinsonism symptoms possible. Equally difficult to manage is the development of erratic and variable responses to therapy, the so-called "on-off" phenomena. These consist of episodes in which patients alternate between having full-blown parkinsonism symptoms and being asymptomatic. They may occur precipitously and in random fashion or be gradual and predictable in onset, related to a shortened duration of action of a given dose of Sinemet. This latter variety, often termed an end-dose "off" response, may be controllable by rearrangement of the dosing schedule so that time intervals of 2 to 3 hours are used rather than 4 to 5. More often than not this will prove to be less than completely satisfactory and one has to resort to the use of ancillary agents. Those that have proved most effective are still considered as investigational in this country but are generally available abroad.

Bromocriptine   (Parlodel). This   semisynthetic ergoline compound, which is capable of activating dopamine receptors, has been shown to have antiparkinsonism properties. In comparative studies with Sinemet it is less potent with a lower therapeutic index, since it has additional side effects. These consist of a greater tendency to nausea and vomiting and an increased incidence of toxic psychosis and limb edema as well as phlebitic phenomena. Although it is not recommended for use as the primary drug in treating parkinsonism, it can be useful as an adjunctive agent. In limited daily dosage of 20 to 50 mg it has been found helpful in decreasing the severity and frequency of "on-off" phenomena. It is our practice to add Parlodel to an existing regimen of Sinemet, beginning with doses of 2.5 mg four times a day and gradually increasing by doubling the dose at weekly intervals. Parlodel is available in 2.5 mg tablets but has only been recommended by the manufacturer for use in galactorrhea. It should be noted that a number of newer analogues of this compound, which may be more effective, are now undergoing trial.

L-Deprenil. This compound is an inhibitor of monoamine oxidase B (MAO-B), the form in which this enzyme is present in the striatum. Dopamine is a major substrate for MAO-B and the pathway by which it is primarily metabolized. Inhibiting MAO-B allows dopamine to accumulate, enhancing and prolonging its action. In contrast to other MAO inhibitors, such as tranylcypromine (Parnate), which inhibit MAO-A and B, it can be administered in conjunction with Sinemet without fear of producing hypertensive crises. Its usefulness at present is as an adjunct to Sinemet in the control of "on-off" phenomena, especially those of the end-of-dose variety, as well as in patients experiencing a loss of benefit from their existing therapeutic program. When it is added in 5 mg doses twice a day, patients may experience considerable benefit from its use, but unfortunately it tends to accentuate the side effects owing to the action of dopamine as well. L-Deprenil is presently available only on an experimental basis.

In summary, the patient with established parkinsonian symptoms is best treated with levodopa combined with carbidopa. Its dosage should be individualized for each patient, limited to the lowest level which gives functional improvement rather than that which attempts to erase every vestige of the disease. When it is appropriately used, as many as 80 per cent of those with Parkinson's disease can expect to experience benefit. This will be optimal during the first 3 years of use, following which many will enjoy less but still substantial benefit and side effects will occur in a significant number. At present, no completely satisfactory means of treatment exists for this phase of the disease, although a number of ancillary agents show promise of being helpful.

Ancillary Therapeutic Measures

Physical Therapy and Exercise. The general tendency of patients with Parkinson's disease to become inactive and dependent can in part be overcome by the judicious use of physiotherapeutic methods. These need not be extensive, nor is elaborate gadgetry required. The regimen should be individualized, with thoughtful attention given to the patient's abilities and disabilities and specific programs established for each. By and large physiotherapy is directed toward the maintenance of joint mobility, correction and prevention of postural abnormalities of trunk and limbs, and maintenance of normal gait. Passive stretching of the limbs, muscle massage, resistive exercises, and gait training are all utilized to accomplish this objective. As a rule, treatment is given anywhere from one to five times a week, depending on the individual needs. In addition, all patients are advised to establish a daily program of exercises. Patients are encouraged to take long walks, utilize a stationary bicycle, and practice the exercises outlined by the physiatrist. Constant reminders of the concept that disability can be prevented or at least delayed by physical activity should be given to the patient, with emphasis that much of this must be done by himself.

Supportive Psychotherapy. Few patients accept the diagnosis of parkinsonism with equanimity. More often than not the realization that one is suffering from this disorder evokes visions of total disability with confinement to wheelchair or bed. The attendant anxiety and depression in the early stages of the disease contribute as much to the disability as do the symptoms of parkinsonism. It is, therefore, of utmost importance that at the time of initial contact with the patient he be properly indoctrinated as to the nature of the disease with regard to its variability, its slowly progressive course, and what can and cannot be done to control the symptoms. It must be emphasized that the disease is slowly progressive and interwoven with periods when it is stationary. Much can be accomplished by dispelling fears, usually acquired from hearsay rather than reliable sources, concerning sanity, inheritance, and the like. Realistic goals concerning business and family life must be discussed with each patient. Every attempt must be made to maintain the patient as a social being, since there is often a tendency in many patients to withdraw from interpersonal relationships as a consequence of their altered outward appearance. It cannot be overemphasized that the successful treatment of parkinsonism is dependent on the physician's ability and willingness to offer a total care program to the patient. When this is done, there are only rare instances when the need arises for referral of patients for specific psychiatric treatment.

PERIPHERAL NEUROPATHY

method of
W. C. WIEDERHOLT, M.D.
La Jolla, California

Many physicians are frustrated in their therapeutic approach to peripheral neuropathies because in many etiologic factors are unknown, and in others no specific treatment is available. It should be remembered, though, that a substantial proportion of all neuropathies occur secondary to compression of a peripheral nerve or secondary to endogenous and/or exogenous toxic-metabolic disorders. Consequently, many neuropathies will improve significantly when trauma is avoided, deficiencies are corrected, exogenous toxins removed, and systemic illnesses treated. When dealing with peripheral neuropathies, it is helpful in diagnosis and also in planning appropriate treatment to think in broad categories, such as entrapment or compressive neuropathies, mononeuritis and mononeuritis multiplex, and subacute and chronic polyneuropathies. Using such broad categories very often will immediately suggest specific entities and hence lead to appropriate management. While no classification of the overwhelmingly large number of subacute chronic polyneuropathies is entirely satisfactory, one based on the pattern of functional involvement is helpful. Such a classification reflects the mode of clinical presentation; it allows the physician, in many instances, to narrow the possibilities to just a few, to be further studied; and it very often suggests appropriate therapy. Such a classification is given in Table 1. It must be remembered that both entrapment neuropathies and mononeuropathies may be seen as part of, or as an early manifestation of, a more generalized neuropathy. Since the management of many neuropathies —regardless of the etiology — is similar, a discussion of general principles of management and management of complications of neuropathies will follow the classification. Finally, some common specific entities will be dealt with.

General Considerations

It is essential to try to establish a proper etiologic diagnosis, because specific treatment of underlying conditions will, in most instances, alleviate a neuropathy. When axonal degeneration has occurred, the time-frame for treatment should be in months to years rather than in a few weeks. In many neuropathies, regardless of the cause, certain complications occur, and pain or discomfort is a frequent accompaniment.

Treatment of Systemic Illness or Malignancy. The treatment of the primary illness or removal of a malignancy will very often be followed by alleviation or resolution of symptoms and signs referable to the neuropathy.

Removal of Exogenous Toxins. Often no specific therapy is available. Removal and meticulous future avoidance of toxins are beneficial.

Replacement Therapy in Deficiency Disorders. In specific deficiency disorders, appropriate therapy is obvious. In some instances such as vitamin B_{12} deficiency, therapy has to be lifelong. Except in situations in which the neuropathy is directly related to malnutrition, malabsorption, or both, diet is not a major factor, but patients should be instructed in a well-balanced diet. While there is no good evidence to suggest that additional vitamin therapy has any additional benefit, it appears prudent that the patient with a neuropathy receive at least an ample complement of vitamins through a well-balanced diet, or, if that cannot be assured, by adding a multivitamin preparation to the diet.

Removal or Reduction of Certain Medications. If a therapeutic agent is responsible for a neuropathy, optimally the drug should be discontinued. In some instances such as with vincristine, reduction of the total daily dosage may alleviate the neuropathy. In other instances, the ill effect of the drug may be counteracted by adding another medication. Examples are folate in phenytoin (diphenylhydantoin) neuropathy and pyridoxine in isoniazid neuropathy.

Management of Pain. Patients with neuropathies may have two types of pain, singly or in combination. One is usually diffuse and may have a burning quality and often is present continuously. The other is an intermittent, severe, lancinating type of pain which may be sharply localized. Factors which will either bring on or aggravate a given pain, such as pressure of clothing or bedsheets or drafts, can be identified and should be removed. Frequently, just wearing socks or gloves may reduce burning paresthesias. In patients in whom the pressure of the bedsheet worsens the symptoms in their feet, a cradle over the feet is indicated.

TABLE 1. **Classification of Peripheral Neuropathies**

I. Entrapment and compressive neuropathies
II. Mononeuropathies and mononeuritis multiplex
III. Subacute and chronic polyneuropathies by pattern of functional involvement
    A. Predominantly motor: inflammatory (Guillain-Barré), lead, porphyria, Charcot-Marie-Tooth disease
    B. Predominantly sensory
        1. Proprioception and vibration most affected: remote effects of malignancy, tabes dorsalis, hereditary sensory neuropathies type 2
        2. Pain and temperature most affected: amyloidosis, diabetes, leprosy, Fabry's disease, hereditary sensory neuropathy type 1
    C. Predominantly autonomic: diabetes, amyloidosis, Riley-Day syndrome
    D. Mixed sensory motor and autonomic
        1. Systemic diseases
            a. Endocrine: diabetes, thyroid dysfunction, acromegaly
            b. Collagen-vascular: rheumatoid arthritis, periarteritis nodosa, systemic lupus erythematosus
            c. Dysproteinemias: myeloma, macroglobulinemia
            d. Remote effect of malignancy
            e. Renal failure
            f. Liver failure
        2. Medications
            a. Antibiotics: isoniazid, nitrofurantoin, ethambutol, chloramphenicol, chloroquine
            b. Anti-cancer agents: vincristine, vinblastine, nitrogen mustard
            c. Immunizations: rabies, typhoid, smallpox, rubella, pertussis
            d. Others: Dapsone, phenytoin (diphenylhydantoin), disulfiram, glutethimide, gold, hydralazine
        3. Environmental toxins
            a. Solvents: carbon disulfide, N-hexane, methyl N-butyl ketone
            b. Heavy metals: lead, mercury, arsenic, thallium
            c. Others: carbon monoxide, hexachlorophene, tri-ortho-cresyl phosphate, glue, acrylamide
        4. Deficiency disorders: alcoholism, thiamine, pyridoxine, pantothenic acid, riboflavin, vitamin B_{12}, folic acid, malabsorption
        5. Hereditary disorders: Refsum's disease, metachromatic leukodystrophy

While no absolutely satisfactory approach exists to management of discomfort from diffuse, burning-type pain, some patients respond quite well to management with standard pain medications. Pain relief may frequently be achieved with acetylsalicylic acid (0.6 gram every 4 hours while awake) and with additional propoxyphene (32 to 64 mg every 4 hours as needed) or codeine (32 mg every 4 hours). In some patients, a combination of fluphenazine (2 to 5 mg per day) and amitriptyline (50 to 100 mg per day) may significantly reduce discomfort. In other patients, intermittent use of minor tranquilizers such as diazepam (5 mg three or four times daily) may be beneficial. Since patients are very often much more uncomfortable during the night hours, the short-term use of a nighttime sedative is indicated. If pain is severe and persistent, the use of meperidine or morphine must be considered. In chronic situations, other measures such as percutaneous nerve stimulation or acupuncture should be explored.

The diffuse burning-type discomfort in peripheral neuropathies occasionally responds to therapy with phenytoin or carbamazepine. The therapeutic benefit of these two drugs is usually much better in those patients who suffer from intermittent, lancinating-type or neuritic-type pain. Carbamazepine, in doses of 200 mg three to four times a day, appears to be the drug of choice. (This specific use of carbamazepine is not listed in the manufacturer's official directive.)

In patients with no hope of recovery or in patients with a fatal illness, after all medication attempts at controlling pain have been unsuccessful, destructive surgical procedures such as rhizotomies and cordotomies can be considered.

Management of Respiratory Failure. Unfortunately, a few neuropathies are accompanied by respiratory failure, which may develop within a few hours. It is, therefore, essential that the patient be alerted to the early warning signs, which include increasing anxiety, restlessness, and a weak cough. In situations in which respiratory failure may occur, frequent determinations of vital capacity and blood gases are indicated. Patients whose vital capacity is less than 25 per cent of the expected normal require ventilatory assistance. Such patients must be transferred to intensive care units, and the type of ventilatory assistance will depend on the specific situation. If ventilatory assistance is required for many days to weeks, tracheostomy is indicated. Oxygen without ventilatory assistance should not be used, because it may depress the respiratory center.

Avoidance and Management of Complica-

tions. Patients with entrapment neuropathies, either as a primary entity or as a manifestation of a more generalized neuropathy, should be meticulously instructed in the avoidance of additional trauma to nerves most vulnerable at the elbow and at the knee. It is frequently helpful, particularly in patients who are confined to bed, to apply appropriate padding at the elbows and knees. This is aided by frequent turning in those bedridden and paralyzed. This latter measure and meticulous skin care will also avoid development of decubitus ulcers. If no improvement occurs with just avoiding additional trauma, surgical lysis must be considered.

Patients with neuropathies which produce loss of pain sensation are extremely vulnerable to injuries to skin and joints and superimposed infections and should be appropriately warned about these complications.

Fortunately, bladder involvement is rare. If it occurs, condom catheter drainage, urethral catheter drainage, and prompt treatment of superimposed infections are all very important. Similarly, involvement of the gastrointestinal system with constipation, diarrhea, ileus, or gastric distention is rare. Nevertheless, these complications do occur and should be treated appropriately.

In some neuropathies, orthostatic hypotension may be a minor, or even a serious, complication. Minor degrees are easily handled with elastic stockings, while in the more severe cases mineralocorticoids must be administered.

Bed Rest. Patients with severe paralytic neuropathies may be confined to bed because of weakness. As mentioned above, padding of elbows and knees, frequent turning, meticulous skin care, and a cradle over the feet are all important measures to reduce the patient's discomfort and to avoid unnecessary complications.

Physiotherapy. Patients may not move their limbs appropriately because of paralysis or because movement will aggravate discomfort. In both situations, in order to avoid contractures, passive range of motion early in the course of a neuropathy — twice a day for 10 to 20 minutes — is important. In patients with severe weakness, overstretching of limbs should be avoided, because it may lead to inadvertent injury of muscle, tendons, ligaments, and joints. In the patient with a severe disabling neuropathy, passive range of motion is essentially all that has to be done early in the course of the illness. In some patients, hot moist or dry packs to their legs and/or back may reduce discomfort. As soon as there is evidence of improvement, a graded exercise program is instituted, of course taking into account the patient's

individual progress. The aims of this graded exercise program are several-fold. One is to teach the patient better utilization of remaining functions, strengthening of muscles which are still functioning, and avoidance of contractures. The rate of recovery is not affected by any of these measures per se. Patients with footdrop are greatly helped by a short leg brace. This should also be worn at night or while bedridden if contractures occur. Patients with wristdrop may benefit by a splint which keeps the hand in slight extension, because grasp becomes much more effective in this position.

Specific Neuropathies

No attempt has been made to be all inclusive. Only those conditions which are relatively common or for which a specific form of therapy is available will be dealt with.

Entrapment Neuropathies. It cannot be overemphasized that an entrapment neuropathy may be the only manifestation of a more generalized neuropathy, may be part of an obvious generalized neuropathy, or may be a complication of a systemic illness. It is obviously important for the institution of appropriate therapy to sort out these various possibilities. As an example, some women during pregnancy develop symptoms and signs of a carpal tunnel syndrome, which requires no specific therapy because almost all resolve following delivery of the baby.

The most common entrapment neuropathies are compression of the ulnar nerve at the elbow, compression of the median nerve in the carpal tunnel, compression of the lateral cutaneous femoral nerve at the ilioinguinal ligament, and compression of the peroneal nerve at the head of the fibula. Very often, avoidance of trauma is all that is needed to relieve the patient's symptoms and restore normal neurologic function. Padding of the elbow in ulnar nerve compression, a wrist splint at night in the carpal tunnel syndrome, and avoidance of crossing legs and use of knee padding at night in peroneal nerve compression may all suffice. If, after a reasonable period of time (usually measured in terms of 1 to 2 months), no improvement has occurred, surgical lysis and/or transposition of the nerve must be considered. Local perineural injection of corticosteroids, while sometimes giving dramatic temporary relief, is to be discouraged because of the high rate of complications. In patients with compression of the lateral cutaneous femoral nerve (meralgia paresthetica), simple pain medication, as outlined above, usually suffices. In chronic situations in which the patient may be very much disturbed by the persistent paresthesias, surgical decompression may be indicated.

Mononeuritis and Mononeuritis Multiplex. In almost all instances, this condition is due to occlusion of the vasa nervorum, secondary to systemic vasculitis or atherosclerosis. No specific therapy is available except for measures as can be directed against the underlying disease process. Mononeuritis multiplex, which commonly develops in patients with periarteritis nodosa, may respond to therapy with corticosteroids.

In those patients who develop mononeuritis or mononeuritis multiplex caused by direct invasion of nerves by primary or secondary malignancies, localized x-ray therapy frequently is of great benefit in temporary relief of symptoms and improvement of neurologic function. Diffuse involvement of peripheral nerves resulting from malignancies may respond to appropriate chemotherapy.

Subacute and Chronic Polyneuropathies. DIABETIC NEUROPATHIES. The most common neuropathy in diabetes is symmetric, usually involves the feet more than the hands, and has a slowly insidious progression with its onset several years after diabetes has been diagnosed. Simple supportive measures, as outlined above, usually suffice. Whether or not rigid control of the diabetic condition is helpful in the treatment of the neuropathy is unknown. The consensus is that control may have some beneficial effect. Less commonly, diabetic neuropathy may predominantly involve the autonomic nervous system with an atonic bladder, impotence, anhidrosis, constipation alternating with diarrhea, and even ileus. This condition is rather serious, and management is limited to proper drainage of the bladder, treatment of superimposed bladder infection, relief of constipation and control of diarrhea, relief of ileus, and nasogastric drainage in situations of gastric distention. A small group of diabetics, usually elderly patients with late onset diabetes, is afflicted by mononeuropathies, presumably secondary to occlusion of the vasa nervorum. Commonly, a sixth nerve paresis, a third nerve paresis, or an L4-type radiculoneuropathy is seen. The prognosis is usually excellent over a span of 3 to 6 months, with complete recovery the rule rather than the exception. In the L4 radiculoneuropathy, pain is usually an early and disabling feature and should be treated as outlined above. Reassurance as to the relatively good prognosis is important.

UREMIC NEUROPATHY. Because of the longer survival time, uremic neuropathy is now much more common than in days past. In addition to the primary uremic neuropathy, patients should be watched for the development of a deficiency neuropathy as a complication of renal dialysis. Frequent renal dialysis appears to control the neuropathy to some degree, while renal transplantation very often produces a rather dramatic and longlasting beneficial effect.

ARSENIC AND THALLIUM INTOXICATION. Arsenic and thallium intoxication still occur with sufficient frequency, often as an expression of a rather complex family feud, to warrant brief mention. The diagnosis of both conditions, as long as one considers the possibility, is relatively easy, with typical white transverse banding of the nails (Mee's lines) and brownish cutaneous pigmentation and demonstration of abnormal amounts of arsenic in hair and fingernails in arsenic intoxication, and the typical loss of hair in thallium intoxication. Elimination of the offending agent and supportive therapy usually are all that is needed. The treatment of either condition with dimercaprol is controversial.

ALCOHOLIC AND NUTRITIONAL DEFICIENCY POLYNEUROPATHY. Nutritional polyneuropathies are almost always due to multiple dietary deficiencies. It is therefore imperative that adequate dietary therapy and vitamin supplementation be instituted. In countries where malnutrition is no problem, alcoholic polyneuropathy is probably the most common form of neuropathy, and it is generally acknowledged that it is due to an insufficient diet, specifically a thiamine deficiency. It is uncertain to what degree alcohol contributes to the neuropathy as a direct toxin. Ideally, anyone with alcoholic polyneuropathy should abstain from alcohol consumption, should receive a well balanced diet, and should take supplemental multivitamins. In addition, patients with alcoholic neuropathy, or for that matter with any complication of alcoholism when seen acutely, should receive thiamine (100 mg daily), preferably via the intravenous route initially, and later by the oral route.

REFSUM'S DISEASE (HEREDOPATHIA ATACTICA POLYNEURITIFORMIS). This is a relatively rare, recessively inherited disorder caused by a single autosomal recessive gene. The disease is characterized by accumulation of phytanic acid in various tissues of the body, including the peripheral nervous system. The precise relationship between phytanic acid accumulation and symptoms remains obscure. It has been demonstrated in a small number of patients that a diet free of phytanic acid, over a prolonged period of time, produces definite clinical improvement and avoids relapses of symptoms and signs.

INFLAMMATORY POLYNEUROPATHY (GUILLAIN-BARRÉ SYNDROME). Mortality in this syndrome is rather low, principally because of aggressive management during the acute phase of the illness of respiratory insufficiency, superimposed infections, and cardiac arrhythmias. The long-term prognosis is relatively good, with few if any residual neurologic deficits, most of which are of a minor nature, such as footdrop. From this it follows that diligent management of respiratory insufficiency, if such occurs during the acute phase of the illness, is of paramount importance. The fact that no consensus exists about the efficacy of steroid therapy indicates that its benefits in this condition are at best slight. Since an occasional patient on steroid therapy may make a remarkable, rapid recovery and, furthermore, since short-term steroid therapy entails little risk, it appears that those patients who develop progressive paralysis and/or respiratory failure could be treated with prednisone. The suggested regimen is prednisone, 100 mg per day in divided doses for 3 to 4 days, and then gradual reduction over 6 to 7 days to a total daily dose of 40 mg. If, during this course of therapy, further progression is noted, the dosage may again be increased. Whether or not continuation of steroid therapy after approximately 2 weeks of treatment, on either a daily basis or an alternate day basis, is justified is unknown. It is also not established that patients with the chronic progressive or chronic stable form are benefited by long-term steroid therapy.

CHRONIC RELAPSING POLYNEUROPATHY. In its clinical manifestations, this neuropathy is very similar to the inflammatory polyneuropathy, except that there are recurrent bouts of a polyneuropathy which, in most instances, responds quite well to steroid therapy. As a matter of fact, many patients with this syndrome will have a relapse when steroid therapy is discontinued, and sometimes when steroid therapy is reduced. The optimal level of alternate day prednisone treatment must be determined individually. Some patients can be maintained and do well on 20 mg every other day, while others may need as much as 60 to 100 mg every other day.

PORPHYRIA POLYNEUROPATHY. This polyneuropathy of acute intermittent porphyria very often runs a self-limited course but may occur repeatedly. Although there is no specific therapy for this condition, it is important to recognize that barbiturates, sulfonamides, and griseofulvin may precipitate acute attacks and, therefore, have to be avoided. Chlorpromazine, from 25 to 50 mg four times per day, is extremely effective in the management of the severe pain often seen in patients with porphyria. In addition, this phenothiazine frequently will control mental symptoms such as delirium often seen in porphyria. If sedation is needed, chloral hydrate or paraldehyde may be used, because no ill effects from these two drugs have been reported in porphyria. If the severe neuritic pains are not controlled

with chlorpromazine, meperidine may have to be used.

LEPROSY.   See pages 34 to 38.

ACUTE HEAD INJURIES IN ADULTS

method of
GEORGE T. TINDALL, M.D.,
and SUZIE C. TINDALL, M.D.
Atlanta, Georgia

Introduction

Accident prevention is the obvious solution to the problem of head trauma. However, despite aggressive preventive measures, the morbidity and mortality from head injury will always be a significant problem. It is estimated that in 1976, 3.6 per cent of the total population, or 7,560,000 persons, suffered head trauma of some sort. Of this number 1,255,000 injuries could be classified as major. Approximately 50 per cent of the injuries occur at home; 16 per cent are secondary to motor vehicle accidents; 33 per cent occur at play, in school, or in the public domain; and only 2 per cent occur at work, the area which has received the most constructive thought regarding protection against accidental head injury. The estimated cost of head injuries in 1976 was $2.24 billion in wages lost and medical expenses. In addition to the high mortality rate following serious head injury, unknown numbers of patients suffer socially and financially devastating sequelae of head trauma that range from the total dependency of vegetative survival to minor psychomotor deficits.

Significant advances have been achieved in the diagnostic and therapeutic aspects of head injury in recent years. The development of sophisticated emergency medical services in many communities and public awareness of cardiopulmonary resuscitation techniques have contributed to prevention of prolonged apnea at the scene of the accident and permitted rapid transportation of head injury patients to an appropriate medical facility for definitive care. The development of the multifaceted approach to critical care medicine with intensive nursing care, monitoring techniques, respiratory support systems, and availability of a wide array of potent pharmaceuticals has positively affected the outcome in many patients with severe head injury. Perhaps the most significant advance has been the discovery and widespread use of computed cranial tomography (CT scanning). This technique has revolutionized diagnosis in patients with head injury, permitting rapid identification of intracranial mass lesions. It has become the diagnostic procedure of choice in head-injured victims.

In this article the current diagnostic and therapeutic management of closed head injury is discussed in the light of these recent diagnostic and therapeutic advances. Particular stress will be placed on the use of the CT scan not only in establishing a specific anatomic diagnosis in head injury but also in making therapeutic decisions in these patients. Additionally, the indications and the expected therapeutic benefits of medical treatments developed in recent years, including corticosteroids, hyperventilation, intracranial pressure monitoring, dehydrating agents (e.g., mannitol), and pentobarbital, will be discussed in an attempt to place these modalities in a practical perspective.

Mechanisms of Closed Head Injury

The majority of severely head-injured patients die from one of the following causes:

1. Irreversible parenchymal damage in vital cerebral areas such as the brain stem.

2. Uncontrolled intracranial hypertension with cerebral shifts and herniation secondary to either sizable intracranial hematoma or diffuse cerebral swelling.

3. An intercurrent undesirable systemic medical complication such as hypoxia, hypotension, or acidosis.

An understanding of the mechanism of *coup* and *contracoup* injury is important in understanding the pathology of head injury. At the site of a blow to the head, some degree of skull deformation occurs, causing the coup injury. Since the intracranial contents have a different consistency from the skull, following impact there is a tendency for the skull to accelerate more rapidly than the intracranial contents, thus generating a negative pressure in areas removed from the actual site of impact. If this negative pressure is great enough, there may be cavitation and hemorrhage in the cerebral tissue, thus creating the contracoup injury. This mechanism of cerebral injury explains the occurrence of polar contusions in the frontal, temporal, and occipital lobes in head injury. Differential rates of movement of the skull and cerebral contents are also responsible for the shearing of bridging veins over the

convexities, the etiology for most traumatic subdural hematomas.

Brain shifts and herniations are common in traumatic intracranial lesions and are frequently accompanied by characteristic clinical manifestations. One of the more important of these syndromes is that of supratentorial brain herniation through the tentorial incisura. This condition results from a unilateral supratentorial mass lesion that causes increased intracranial pressure, which in turn forces the medial edge of the ipsilateral temporal lobe (i.e., uncus) into the incisura. This results in compression of the upper brain stem and presents a dangerous situation. The earliest clinical signs of such an event include a change in the level of consciousness, change in respiratory rhythms (e.g., Cheyne-Stokes variety), and evidence of pupillary dilatation and third cranial nerve dysfunction. As herniation progresses, coma deepens and the patient may exhibit decerebrate or decorticate responses to noxious stimuli. Both pupils become fixed at midposition, and respiratory efforts progress through central neurogenic hyperventilation to irregular patterns frequently with prolonged periods of apnea. If untreated, the course of transtentorial herniation is usually fatal. Thus therapeutic efforts should be aimed at preventing this situation.

A hemiparesis in a patient after trauma is most often due to destruction or compression of the contralateral cerebral cortex, but in at least 30 per cent of patients the hemiparesis is a "false" lateralizing sign and will be *ipsilateral* to the side of the traumatic lesion, causing mass effects. This situation is caused by compression of the contralateral cerebral peduncle against the free edge of the tentorium, the displacement resulting from unilateral herniation of the uncus through the incisura.

Classification of Head Injury

A useful, practical classification of craniocerebral trauma is given in Table 1.

TABLE 1. **Classification of Craniocerebral Trauma**

A. Scalp injuries—lacerations, abrasions, avulsions, and hematomas
B. Skull fractures—several classifications are employed
  1. Simple—closed with skin intact
  2. Linear or stellate
  3. Nondepressed or depressed
C. Intracranial injury
  1. Concussion—a clinical syndrome implying loss of consciousness in the absence of identifiable gross traumatic pathology
  2. Contusion—a noncoalescent hemorrhagic area of cerebral substance; these lesions vary in severity and may or may not be associated with loss of consciousness or neurologic deficit
  3. Epidural hematoma—usually secondary to laceration of the middle meningeal artery with bleeding confined to the epidural space
  4. Subdural hematoma—may be acute, subacute, or chronic, and is often secondary to tearing of cortical bridging veins; the acute lesion is usually associated with extensive underlying brain damage (e.g., contusion, lacerations, edema), and it is this damage that accounts for the high mortality of acute subdural hematoma
  5. Intracerebral hematoma—may be acute or delayed
  6. Diffuse cerebral swelling — frequently associated with high velocity motor vehicular trauma
D. Gunshot wound to the head
E. Penetrating wounds of the head (e.g., knife, icepick)
F. Miscellaneous
  1. Arterial injuries—both intra- and extracranial
  2. Traumatic cerebral aneurysms
  3. Carotid cavernous traumatic fistulas
  4. Traumatic cerebrospinal fluid fistulas

Clinical Evaluation

The initial evaluation and treatment of the patient with an acute head injury should not be delayed until a history is obtained, although historical information can be obtained concomitantly. Historical information of importance would include a detailed description of the accident, knowledge of whether or not the patient lost consciousness, the degree of amnesia both preceding and following the injury, and knowledge of ethanol or drug abuse. The usual aspects of a general history, including past and present medical and surgical illnesses, allergies, medications, and the like, should not be overlooked.

Complete physical and neurologic evaluation of the patient should be done rapidly on head-injured patients and should include appraisal of the airway, vital signs, and associated injuries. (See Acute Evaluation and Treatment in the Emergency Room, below.)

Alteration in the level of consciousness (LOC) is the single most important indication of the severity of head injury. Immediate and frequent serial evaluations of the level of consciousness are mandatory for following the head-injured patient, and to this end a simple, practical classification of coma is useful for recording findings and communicating findings to other members of the health care team. In use for the past 8 years at our institution, the Grady Coma Scale is useful for this purpose. References to levels of consciousness in the remainder of this article will be according to this scale (Table 2).

Another coma scale used widely in many centers handling head-injured patients is the Glasgow scale developed by Jennett and associates as an aid for prediction of outcome in head-injured patients. This scale ranks best patient responses in terms of eye opening, motor response, and verbal response. Maximum score is 15. This grading system is shown in Table 3.

In addition to establishing the level of coma, there are other important aspects of the neurologic and general physical examination. The scalp and skull should be inspected for contusion, laceration, and com-

TABLE 3.   **Glasgow Scale**

Eye opening	Spontaneous	4
	To speech	3
	To pain	2
	Nil	1
Best motor response	Obeys	6
	Localizes	5
	Withdraws (flexion)	4
	Abnormal flexion	3
	Extensor response	2
	Nil	1
Verbal response	Oriented	5
	Confused conversation	4
	Inappropriate words	3
	Incomprehensible sounds	2
	Nil	1

pound or depressed fractures. Basilar skull fracture is suggested by the presence of otorrhea, rhinorrhea, hemotympanum, Battle's sign (bluish discoloration over the mastoid), and/or periorbital ecchymoses.

Pupillary signs should be noted. A unilateral dilated pupil usually indicates brain stem or oculomotor nerve compression (see above). On the other hand, bilateral dilated pupils reflect intrinsic damage to the upper brain stem and are usually regarded as an ominous sign. The optic fundi should be examined; however, the examiner should avoid the use of mydriatic drugs to facilitate this examination. The position of the eyes with attention to forced gaze deviation or gaze palsies should be noted. Corneal and vestibulo-ocular (doll's eyes) reflexes should be tested, as these reflexes reflect the integrity of the required brain stem structures in the comatose patient. The rapid rotation of the head necessary to induce the vestibulo-ocular reflex should not be performed until cervical spine x-rays have eliminated the possibility of an associated cervical fracture.

Examination of the motor system includes a search for appropriate and inappropriate responses to superficial and deep painful stimuli. Unilateral or bilateral decorticate or decerebrate posturing is an important observation. Evidence of a hemiparesis may be subtle or obvious. Sensory examination is usually less informative. The lack of response to pinprick or pinching in a patient in less than Grade IV coma should raise the suspicion of an accompanying spinal cord injury.

Methods of Diagnostic Evaluation in Head Injury

Important neurodiagnostic aids in evaluating head injury include plain skull and cervical spine x-rays, CT scanning, and cerebral angiography. A brief description of each of these diagnostic procedures follows:

Plain X-Rays. It is our practice to obtain portable anteroposterior and lateral skull films and a single lateral cervical spine film in addition to an anteroposterior chest x-ray on all patients with head injury in a Grade III status or worse immediately upon arrival in the emergency room. Such x-rays may or may not be obtained at the discretion of the physician in patients less severely injured. The value of the practice of obtaining routine skull x-rays in head-injured patients

TABLE 2.   **Grady Coma Scale**

GRADE	STATE OF AWARENESS
I	Drowsy, lethargic, indifferent and uninterested, and/or belligerent and uncooperative; does not lapse into sleep when left undisturbed
II	Stuporous; will lapse into sleep when not disturbed; may be disoriented to time, place, and person
III	Deep stupor—requires strong pain to evoke movement; may have focal neurologic signs but will respond appropriately to noxious stimuli
IV	Does not respond appropriately to any stimuli; may exhibit decerebrate or decorticate posturing; retains deep tendon reflexes; may have dilated pupil or absent corneal or oculocephalic reflexes
V	Does not respond appropriately to any stimuli; flaccid—no deep tendon reflexes; usually apneic

has recently been questioned, primarily from the standpoint of cost effectiveness. Nevertheless they should be a routine part of the evaluation of any patient suspected of having a depressed or compound skull fracture.

Plain radiographs demonstrate skull fractures and visualize foreign bodies (bone or missile fragments) within the cranial cavity. Fractures extending across the meningeal arterial channels are often associated with acute epidural hematomas. A shift in the midline structures, such as a calcified pineal body, may be indicative of an intracranial mass lesion. Cervical spine films may show an associated cervical spine fracture, a finding in 3 to 10 per cent of all severely head-injured patients.

Computed Tomographic Scanning (CT Scan). Head injury patients admitted in Grade II coma or worse should undergo emergency CT scanning of the head as soon as the airway is assured and vital signs are stabilized. Intubated ventilated patients are paralyzed as necessary with pancuronium bromide (Pavulon), 2 to 4 mg intravenously, to prevent motion artifact. A noncontrasted scan is obtained; if there is no major lesion, then contrast enhancement is performed. The CT scan has virtually revolutionized neurologic diagnosis in head injury. The degree of depression of a skull fracture is easily ascertained. Subarachnoid blood may be visualized within cerebral cisterns. Acute epidural hematoma is seen as a biconvex high density lesion along the inner table of the skull (Fig. 1). Acute subdural hematoma appears as a high density lesion concave to the cerebral convexity adjacent to the inner table of the skull. Subacute subdural hematomas may be isodense to brain and their presence inferred only by associated shifts of midline cerebral structures or membrane enhancement following iodinated contrast injection. Chronic subdural hematomas show as low density lesions over the convexity. Intracerebral hema-

tomas and contusions "light up" owing to the fact that blood density is greater than the surrounding cerebral density. Cerebral swelling is seen as low density regions with ill-defined margins. Cerebral shifts are ascertained by visualizing shifts of midline structures, including the pineal gland and third and fourth ventricles. Distortion of lateral ventricles may be seen secondary to nearby mass lesions or swelling. Signs of tentorial herniation include torsion of the brain stem structures in association with marked dilatations and shifts of the contralateral lateral ventricle.

The importance of serial CT scanning in the head-injured patient has recently been emphasized in the literature as a means for detecting two entities: (1) a delayed intracerebral hematoma as a result of head injury, now a well-recognized entity; and (2) post-traumatic hydrocephalus. Failure of a patient to improve and/or neurologic deterioration are definitive indications for repeat CT scanning.

Cerebral Angiography. Formerly the mainstay of the diagnostic evaluation of the severely head-injured patient, cerebral angiography is now used only as a supplement to CT scanning and usually under limited circumstances. Indications for its use include absence or malfunction of a CT scan, suspected extracranial or intracranial large vessel injury, and equivocally abnormal CT scan findings.

Other Diagnostic Studies. Echoencephalography and radioisotope brain scan have essentially no role in the modern diagnostic evaluation of the head-injured patient. If immediate access to a CT scan is not available, some neurosurgery centers perform a ventriculogram with measurement of intracranial pressure in the emergency room in patients with Grade III coma or worse. We have had limited experience with this method of diagnosis. It should be emphasized that *lumbar puncture is contraindicated* in the diagnostic evaluation of head-injured patients, as it may exacerbate intracranial shifts, can precipitate transtentorial herniation, and, importantly, yields little useful information.

Therapeutic Management of Head Injury

The Alert or Grade I or II Patient. The physician's clinical judgment is often taxed more fully in dealing with this category of patient than with the severely injured patient. The decision regarding hospitalization as opposed to outpatient care depends upon an estimate of the intracranial damage and the possibility of the patient's developing an intracranial mass lesion. The neurologic evaluation outlined above should be expanded to include detailed evaluation of the gait, cranial nerves, coordination, and sensory systems. Patients with alterations in consciousness or neurologic deficit, no matter how minor, should be hospitalized for observation. The patient who is stuporous or in a Grade II state should undergo immediate CT scan evaluation; this examination in the more alert patient may be performed at a later time or not done at all at the discretion of the physician. Likewise, skull x-rays are not man-

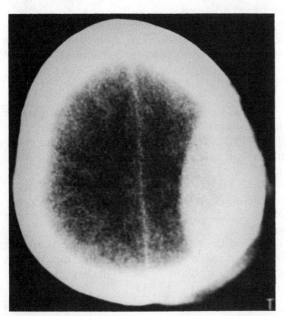

Figure 1. CT scan showing an acute epidural hematoma.

datory in all patients, but should be performed if a skull fracture is suspected.

In evaluating the patient who is neurologically normal and well oriented, note should be taken of the mechanism of injury and the course of the patient immediately after injury. A period of unconsciousness lasting for more than 5 minutes and associated with amnesia for the event of injury and/or retrograde amnesia should prompt careful controlled observation of that patient for the next 12 to 24 hours. A decrease in consciousness level, however minor, that develops after the period of initial trauma should be a warning sign to the physician to institute careful observation for impending brain decompensation.

The Grade III or Worse Patient. EMERGENCY MANAGEMENT. At the scene of the accident the patient suffering severe head trauma should be placed in the horizontal supine position. Movement of the patient should be carried out with careful attention to maintaining stability of the cervical spine. This can be accomplished with the use of sandbags.

The primary concern is for the *airway*. Prolonged apnea in the early stages after injury is a significant cause of early mortality and morbidity in the head-injured patient. After clearing the mouth, assisted ventilation is indicated immediately in the form of mouth-to-mouth ventilation or positive pressure ventilation, using an oral airway and Ambu bag. Oxygen should be supplied in transport. In our opinion, endotracheal intubation should be performed only under controlled circumstances in an emergency room after a lateral cervical spine film has documented the absence of a fracture.

A rapid assessment of the patient's neurologic status, including a determination of vital signs, should be made and periodically checked thereafter. Scalp bleeding can be controlled with a pressure dressing. An intravenous infusion is started (isotonic saline solution), but care should be taken to restrict fluids, as excessive administration may augment existing cerebral edema as well as create difficulties in coping with the syndrome of inappropriate secretion of antidiuretic hormone, which is not uncommon in the head-injured patient.

As soon as the patient is stable, transfer to the nearest hospital facility equipped to handle victims of serious head trauma (i.e., a facility with availability of a neurosurgeon, CT scanner, and intensive care unit equipped with appropriate monitoring equipment) should be effected.

ACUTE EVALUATION AND TREATMENT IN THE EMERGENCY ROOM. Upon arrival in the emergency room the patient should be placed in a large, well-equipped room. Adequate trained personnel should be available to institute the following medical measures.

1. A satisfactory airway should be a concern of first priority. Ventilation is continued initially with aid of an oral airway, Ambu bag, and supplemental oxygenation. Following a lateral portable cervical spine x-ray to exclude cervical spine fracture, endotracheal intubation should be performed and assisted ventilation instituted in all patients in Grade III or worse coma. The assistance of an anesthesiologist is invaluable. The patient is initially hyperventilated to a Pco_2 of 25 to 30 mm Hg and Po_2 is kept at about 90 torr until the severity of injury is further defined.

2. Vital signs and associated injuries: Blood pressure, heart rate, and respiratory rate should be recorded and frequently rechecked thereafter. A careful search is made for possible multiple injuries (e.g., chest or abdominal injuries, long-bone fractures). Hypotension and tachycardia are rarely associated with primary brain injury; consequently, the presence of these signs raises the possibility of concomitant injuries or long-bone fractures. An accompanying spine fracture with spinal cord injury may also account for a hypotensive state. Occasionally excessive blood loss may result from large scalp lacerations. If hypovolemic shock is present, a central venous pressure (CVP) line is inserted and treatment is carried out in the conventional manner while searching for the source of the shock.

3. A careful neurologic evaluation and general physical examination are made and the patient's condition recorded so as to direct immediate investigation and to serve as a reference for later examinations.

4. Portable anteroposterior and lateral skull films, lateral cervical spine film, and anteroposterior chest films are obtained. Also, an electrocardiogram is recorded, as cardiac arrhythmias frequently accompany severe head trauma.

5. Complete blood count (CBC), platelet count, SMA-6, SMA-12, serum osmolality, and blood alcohol levels are drawn. A type and cross-match for several units of whole blood is secured.

6. A Foley catheter is inserted in the urinary bladder in order to exclude urinary injury and to provide an accurate monitor of urinary output.

7. If the patient does not require treatment for hypovolemic shock, 5 per cent dextrose in 0.45 per cent saline solution is begun intravenously at 80 ml per hour.

8. If the patient is decerebrate or showing

signs of rapid neurologic deterioration, 500 ml of 20 per cent mannitol may be given over the first hour or so.

9. The following medications are administered: (a) Tetanus prophylaxis. (b) Dexamethasone, 10 mg intravenously at once and 6 mg intravenously every 6 hours. (c) Phenytoin (Dilantin), 200 mg intravenously hourly for five doses, followed by 200 mg every 12 hours maintenance. (d) Cimetidine, 300 mg intravenously every 6 hours.

10. With this emergency therapy accomplished, the patient is transported immediately to the CT scan, and triage to the operating room or intensive care unit is determined on the basis of CT scanning results.

Surgical Management

Surgical procedures for craniocerebral trauma range from repair of scalp lacerations to extensive craniotomies. Conventional neurosurgical indications include the following types of injury:

Scalp Injuries. Abrasions and contusions require routine wound care. Subgaleal and subperiosteal hematomas usually absorb spontaneously and practically *never* require needle aspiration. The underlying bone should be palpated through lacerations to detect skull fractures. In closing lacerations, interrupted monofilament sutures should be placed through all layers of the scalp after thorough cleansing and debridement.

Skull Fractures. Nondepressed skull fractures require no surgical treatment. Depressed fractures are managed according to the degree of compression and location. Compound depressed fractures require elevation of the indriven bone fragments, debridement of necrotic brain, and repair of dural lacerations.

Acute Traumatic Hematomas. As a general rule, all acute epidural and subdural hematomas should be surgically evacuated as soon as possible. The decision for surgical intervention in the case of a traumatic intercerebral hematoma is dependent upon the size and location of the hematoma, the amount of mass effect and shift of adjacent cerebral structures, and the clinical condition of the patient.

Acute traumatic intracranial hematomas are generally evacuated through large craniotomies. Details of these surgical procedures and the accompanying anesthetic techniques are beyond the scope of this article. The interested reader should consult standard neurosurgical reference material for further details.

Intracranial Pressure Monitoring

Intracranial pressure monitoring (ICP) is an adjunctive measure frequently employed in the care of the head-injured patient. Although it has never been shown conclusively to have a positive effect on patient outcome, it does serve to alert the physician to early intracranial decompensation secondary to increased ICP and aids in planning rational medical and surgical therapeutic intervention. Three basic systems are employed for such monitoring: (1) ventricular cannulation, (2) subarachnoid hollow metal cannulas, and (3) epidural transducers. All can be set up using transducers and monitoring equipment available in most intensive care units. Monitoring is associated with minimal morbidity when used by neurosurgeons familiar with the techniques. We prefer to place a ventricular catheter connected to a subcutaneous Rickham reservoir. This reservoir can then be punctured by a 25 gauge needle and connected to a monitoring transducer. This system allows for intermittent monitoring over a prolonged period of time and also permits quick access to the ventricular system for drainage should this become necessary. To date ICP monitoring seems to be helpful in two clinical situations: (1) in the patient harboring a traumatic intracerebral hematoma of questionable surgical significance, and (2) in the patient with intractable increased ICP from cerebral swelling.

Medical Management and Supportive Care

As in most critical care situations, intensive, intelligent, and well planned nursing care is imperative for optimal care of the patient. A simple but comprehensive daily care sheet should be kept on each patient. It should include a continuous record of vital signs; ICP values; neurologic status; intake and output; blood gas, hematologic, and electrolyte values; ventilator settings; and medication administered. The nursing staff must be cognizant of neurologic assessment and critical care principles.

Many of the principles of the treatment of head injury are directed at normalizing ICP, maintaining of satisfactory cerebral perfusion pressure, and sustaining of an appropriate intra- and extracellular metabolic state for recovery to take place. The severely head-injured patient should be kept in a physiologic and metabolic state as near normal as possible. To this end the early recognition and correction of intracranial and systemic difficulties are of utmost importance. The following discussion emphasizes the areas of greatest importance in intensive care of the head-injured patient.

Pulmonary Care. Controlled ventilation is maintained as long as there is any threat of increased ICP, aspiration secondary to obtundation, or pulmonary complications such as contusion or pneumonia. The endotracheal tube is left in place for the first 5 to 7 days. At this point the patient is evaluated; if it seems controlled ventilation will be needed for a longer time, an elective tracheostomy is performed in the operating room. Prolonged use of an endotracheal tube is associated with long-term complications from tracheal stenosis. A volume ventilator is used with settings at a slow rate (10 to 12 per minute) and high tidal volume (15 ml per kg of body weight). The P_{CO_2} should be kept in a range of 25 to 30 mm Hg, and supplemental oxygen is given to maintain a P_{O_2} above 80 mm Hg. Positive end-expiratory pressure (PEEP) up to 10 cm is employed if adequate oxygenation cannot be maintained in other ways. Pancuronium bromide (Pavulon), 2 to 4 mg intravenously as needed, is used to produce patient compliance to continuous ventilation. An arterial line is used not only to monitor systemic blood pressure but also to serve as a port for obtaining blood samples for analysis. Blood gas determinations are obtained at least daily, and more often as required. The systemic arterial pH should be maintained at approximately 7.4.

Cardiovascular Care. Daily hematocrit determinations are made and transfusions of packed red cells given to maintain the hematocrit above 30. A central venous pressure (CVP) line is employed routinely, and CVP should be kept at 2 to 5 cm of water. Blood pressure is kept within normal ranges, using antihypertensive medication as necessary. We prefer to use methyldopa (Aldomet) or hydralazine (Apresoline) in appropriate dosages, but will employ a sodium nitroprusside intravenous drip if blood pressure becomes dangerously elevated. Cardiac arrhythmias are best handled in consultation with a cardiologist. Most arrhythmias seen in association with severe head injury occur in the acute stages of trauma and do not pose long-term problems.

Fluid and Electrolyte Balance. A Foley catheter is placed in the urinary bladder, and careful monitoring of intake and output is accomplished. Dextrose 5 per cent in 0.45 per cent saline solution with 20 mEq KCl to each liter is given at 80 ml per hour. There is a tendency for personnel involved in the initial emergency treatment of the patient to be overzealous in fluid administration, and this should be guarded against. The goal should be to keep the patient "on the dry side" but not hypovolemic. Urinary output should exceed 30 ml per hour. Daily electrolyte and serum and urine osmolality values are monitored. Serum sodium should be maintained at 140 ± 5 mEq per liter. Hyponatremia should be avoided, as it serves to increase brain edema. Although hyponatremia may be secondary to iatrogenic fluid overload, its most frequent cause in the severely head-injured patient is the syndrome of inappropriate antidiuretic hormone secretion (SIADH). Criteria for diagnosis of this syndrome include hyponatremia with hypo-osmolarity of serum, urine that is less than maximally dilute (usually 50 to 80 mOsm per kg) when compared with plasma osmolality, inappropriately large amounts of urinary sodium even during water loading, normal renal and adrenal functions, no evidence of volume depletion, and disappearance of all abnormalities following adequate restriction of water. SIADH is best corrected by restriction of free water administration, but under circumstances of severe hyponatremia the use of potent intravenous diuretics (e.g., furosemide) with hourly replacement of sodium and potassium loss in the urine, using 3 per cent saline solution to which potassium is added, is acceptable therapy. Serum osmolality should be monitored frequently for detection of early trends toward a hyperosmolar nonketotic state. We delay institution of nasogastric tube feedings until the patient's condition is quite stable, usually 8 to 10 days after the injury.

Medications. We routinely administer phenytoin sodium (Dilantin) as a prophylactic anticonvulsant. A total of 1 gram in divided doses is given intravenously over the first 24 hours, and a maintenance dosage of 400 mg each day is given thereafter. Serum phenytoin blood levels are checked 5 days after starting therapy and the maintenance dosage altered accordingly.

Although there is no conclusive evidence that corticosteroids are helpful in the head-injured patient, we routinely administer dexamethasone (Decadron), 10 mg intravenously upon arrival in the emergency room and 6 mg intravenously every 6 hours thereafter. Cimetidine, 300 mg intravenously every 6 hours, is also administered to inhibit gastric acid secretion.

Control of Increased ICP. Control of increased ICP is a primary goal in treatment of the head-injured patient. The previously discussed surgical removal of traumatic intracranial mass lesions is mandatory in this regard. If a patient with initially normal ICP shows elevations at a later time, a repeat CT scan should be obtained to ascertain the reason. Frequently a delayed intracerebral hematoma or cerebral edema will be found. The following methods for control of ICP are useful in the order presented:

1. Use of controlled ventilation as previously

described to lower the P_{CO_2} to 20 to 25 mm Hg.

2. Infusion of mannitol in a dose of 25 grams intravenously every 6 hours. Serum osmolality should be kept under 320 mOsm per liter and should be monitored closely.

3. Ventricular drainage may be employed if there has been ventricular cannulation for measurement of ICP.

4. In patients with severe increased ICP refractory to other modes of therapy the induction of barbiturate coma may be tried. A loading dose of 200 to 400 mg of pentobarbital (Nembutal) is given intravenously, and further dosage is titrated to keep the blood barbiturate level at 2.0 to 3.5 mg per 100 ml. Blood pressure is monitored closely to assure prevention of hypotension.

Therapeutic intervention for ICP may be slowly withdrawn after ICP has been normalized for a period of at least 48 hours.

Serial CT scans are an important part of management. We perform follow-up scans on day 3 or 4, at 2 weeks, and at 3 months. Delayed intracerebral hematomas and post-traumatic hydrocephalus can be detected in this manner. Early and vigorous use of rehabilitation services such as physical and occupational therapy is employed for those patients exhibiting satisfactory recovery.

Outcome

There are no absolutely reliable criteria for prediction of outcome in the individual head-injured patient. The older the patient, the less likely the outcome will be satisfactory. The presence of a surgically significant mass lesion makes prognosis poorer than in a similar group of patients without mass lesions, although this may only reflect the fact that surgical mass lesions are more common in the older patient. As it is to date impossible to predict the outcome in the individual patient, we employ vigorous and sustained supportive treatment in all patients as outlined above.

Sequelae of Head Injury

Sequelae of head injury include (1) postconcussive syndrome; (2) cerebrospinal fluid leak; (3) carotid cavernous traumatic fistulas; (4) post-traumatic epilepsy; (5) anosmia, blindness, deafness, and facial palsy; and (6) post-traumatic hydrocephalus.

Of these, the postconcussive syndrome is the most common sequela. It is characterized by headaches, difficulties with concentration, dizziness, memory disturbances, irritability, and various other psychomotor difficulties. Resolution of the syndrome is gradual and there is no specific treatment, although an understanding, sympathetic, and supportive approach on the part of the physician is usually beneficial.

HEAD INJURIES IN CHILDREN

method of
DAVID G. McLONE, M.D., PH.D.
Chicago, Illinois

Impact to the skull is an inevitable part of childhood play. The automobile, high-rise buildings, increased participation in contact sports, and the apparent increase in battered children have added to the frequency and severity of head injuries in children. In the vast majority of cases, the injury to the nervous system is insignificant. Occasionally the brain is primarily injured or processes are set in motion which will secondarily injure the nervous system. Little can be done about the primary injury, but a great deal can now be done about the secondary injuries. The secondary event will compound the primary injury or initiate a process leading to irreversibility or death if intervention is not prompt. Because intracranial pathology is so often a part of general trauma, physicians must have an understanding of the various consequences of head injury, typical clinical presentations, diagnostic tools available, and emergency therapy. Fortunately, expanding intracranial hematomas are rare, but children still die from them.

Trauma may account for one third of all pediatric surgical admissions, and half these children have incurred a head injury. One child in ten will suffer a significant head injury during school years, and one third of these children will be hospitalized.

There are some obvious physiologic differences in the response to trauma of adults and children. The very young child has an open fontanelle and sutures, in combination with a subarachnoid space and cisterns which are large. Brain extracellular space is also greater in young children. All these structural features enable the child to tolerate a rapidly expanding intracranial mass better than an adult. These structural differences also delay the onset of signs and symptoms which would reveal the impending disaster and lull the medical personnel to a false state of security.

Extensive classification of head injuries serves little clinical purpose. The child who is alert may be the child in critical condition in a short period of time. Comatose children with spontaneous respirations should be vigorously treated and are likely to survive in good condition. The children, rather, will be grouped based on need for observation, diagnostic study, and surgical intervention.

Management

The fact that half the children who will die from a head injury are awake when admitted to the hospital supports more liberal criteria for admission. Seventy per cent of the deaths will occur in the first 48 hours. No perfect criteria exist for those who should be hospitalized for observation. Most criteria result in the admission for observation of a large number of children who will recover completely without any treatment. This is done in the hope that those children who deteriorate later will be included in this larger group. This should place the child with an impending intracranial disaster in the situation in which the diagnosis will be made early and appropriate therapy administered.

The admission to a hospital of a child with a head injury requires that the hospital have a facility for constant observation, personnel conversant with the care of cranial trauma, emergency equipment available for pediatric patients, and readily available neurologic surgery. Pediatric endotracheal tubes and volume respirators are essential for the admission of these children. The absence of any of these capabilities precludes admission and demands transfer to another hospital.

Effective criteria for admission of a child with a head injury include the following points: (1) any loss of consciousness, (2) skull fracture, (3) persistent vomiting, (4) convulsion, or (5) bleeding or cerebrospinal fluid leak. The presence of irritability or lethargy or the lack of an adequate history should influence the decision in favor of admitting the child. Children not admitted should be watched closely at home and their parents instructed to return them to the hospital if the level of consciousness deteriorates or one of the other criteria for admission is now met.

Assuming a child meets one of the criteria for admission, what are the various steps taken to ensure prompt diagnosis and treatment? First, all children seen with a head injury should be suspects for a concomitant spinal injury. The child with a depressed level of consciousness is assumed to have a spinal injury until proved otherwise. The child should be maintained flat with the head in a neutral position on a firm surface, and a search for evidence of spinal trauma, a neurologic examination, and spine films are indicated prior to transfer to a regular hospital bed.

The children can be divided into two groups following admission: Group 1 would include the child who is alert to lethargic and who has stable vital signs and no focal neurologic deficit. Group 2 would include the child who has any of the following: stupor or coma, unstable vital signs, focal signs, an open or penetrating wound, a depressed skull fracture, or a cerebrospinal fluid leak.

All children admitted with the diagnosis of head injury should have skull films, because depressed fractures need repair and linear fractures which cross major dural venous sinuses and/or the middle meningeal artery or cranial pneumatized sinuses require close observation or further diagnostic procedures. An occasional linear fracture will expand over weeks because of the herniation of intracranial contents through the fracture, and skull films should be obtained at 6 weeks after injury. It is also prudent, when possible, to obtain computed tomography scans on all significant head injuries.

Frequent neurologic examinations are of paramount importance in children admitted for observation.

Group 1 patients will comprise the largest number. Observation by an informed observer is essential in the management of these children. They should be admitted to areas of the hospital where frequent vital signs can be obtained and the nurse-to-patient ratio is such that close observation is possible.

Observations should include: (1) level of consciousness, (2) blood pressure and pulse, (3) pupils (size, equality, reaction) and, (4) movement of the extremities. The significance of changes in these observations should be understood by the nurse. Deterioration of any one of these moves the child into Group 2.

Obviously, progression toward coma should alert one to the possibility of an expanding intracranial mass. Inequality of the pupils and/or developing weakness of one side of the body herald the onset of a rapid sequence of events caused by brain shift. The brain shift may result from the focal edema, an expanding hematoma, or post-traumatic hydrocephalus.

A very useful but often neglected or misinterpreted method of monitoring the child is a frequent determination of blood pressure and pulse. A shock-like state in children, hypotension and tachycardia, except in the infant, is almost never the result of intracranial events. The very young child can occasionally lose enough blood intracranially to produce shock. Other sources of blood volume loss should be sought when this occurs in older children. The cardiovascular system of children is quite resistant to shock, and decompensation occurs late and is rapid. The antithesis of shock, hypertension and bradycardia, together or separately, is an early indicator of an expanding intracranial mass. This may occur with only minimal change in the child's level of consciousness. The changes in blood pressure and pulse are usually progressive, and a decrease in pulse or an elevation in blood pressure should increase the frequency of taking vital signs or move the patient to Group 2.

Children with persistent vomiting should have intravenous fluids started. The recording of accurate intake and output with urine specific gravities is important in children with head injuries. Inappropriate ADH (antidiuretic hormone) syndrome is common following head injuries in children. Confusion, alterations in level of consciousness, and seizures can be precipitated by an ensuing hyponatremia. Profound hyponatremia and seizures can cause irreversible damage to the central nervous system. Monitoring serum electrolytes, serum and urine osmolality, and fluid restrictions are the most effective means of preventing this syndrome. If profound hyponatremia exists and the child is symptomatic, 3 per cent saline solution may be used to restore normal serum osmolarity.

Occasionally diabetes insipidus (DI) occurs following a head injury. Rarely the child will progress from inappropriate ADH syndrome to true DI and not just diuresis following water retention. It is usually transient and only rarely requires the use of antidiuretic hormone.

Group 2 patients include those children who have obviously surgical lesions or need immediate further diagnostic studies to determine if a surgical lesion exists.

Little can be done to correct tissue destruction and cell death occurring as part of the primary event. The secondary events are amenable to treatment. Continued bleeding, advancing edema, ischemia, hypoxia, and hypercarbia, as well as open wounds and depressed fracture, can be controlled and corrected.

If the airway is even questionably inadequate, steps must be taken to ensure the patency of the airway. Clearing the airway and the insertion of an oral or endotracheal tube should be done immediately. (Remember that there is the possibility of a cervical spine fracture.) Tracheostomy is usually not needed acutely, but is often preferable for long-term care of the airway. Serial blood gases should be determined to show that not only is the airway open but ventilation and exchange are adequate.

Tissue hypoxia and hypercarbia compound any intracranial insult. Cerebral vasculature dilates in response to the fall in pH resulting from hypercarbia. As the Pco_2 increases, so does intracranial pressure, and a previously delicate balance may shift toward rapid deterioration.

This cerebral vascular response can be used for the child's benefit. Hyperventilation leads to a decline in the Pco_2, an increase in the pH, and cerebral vascular constriction. Hyperventilation is an effective way to rapidly reduce intracranial pressure. Unlike that of adults, the cerebral vasculature of children remains sensitive to hyperventilation for several days, and controlled ventilation may be used to reduce intracranial pressure for long periods.

After the airway is secure, ventilation demonstrated to be adequate, and any obvious hemorrhage controlled, it must be determined if there is a nonintracranial impending catastrophe, and priorities set.

Routine laboratory studies, including complete blood count (CBC), electrolytes, blood urea nitrogen (BUN), creatinine, sickle cell preparation (black children), prothrombin time, partial thromboplastin time, urinalysis, and blood type and cross-match, should now be obtained.

The care of a child with a severe head injury requires a sophisticated intensive care team approach. Modern transducer technology has made it possible to monitor intracranial pressure continuously with great benefit and little risk to the child. The signs and symptoms of deterioration from intracranial pressure often occur late, and the effectiveness of therapy may be impossible to evaluate without an intracranial monitor.

A logical sequence in an approach to the management of increased intracranial pressure would first involve a recognition of the signs and symptoms that might indicate the presence of intracranial hypertension. Second, an understanding of the anatomy and physiology of the intracranial contents is essential, so that, third, a rational therapy can be instituted to restore and maintain intracranial pressure within limits compatible with normal brain function.

Monitoring intracranial pressure is very important in the evaluation of response to therapy. The dose of mannitol needed, usually 0.5 gram per kg every 4 to 6 hours, or the effect of hyperventilation, Pco_2 25 to 30 torr, can be determined only by monitoring intracranial pressure. Intracranial pressure can be monitored either by a bolt in the skull or by a catheter in the lateral ventricle.

An arterial line is also an integral part of managing these children. Not only does the arterial line make serial arterial blood gases easier, it also allows the monitoring of mean systemic arterial pressure so that cerebral perfusion pressure (the difference between mean intracranial pressure and mean systemic arterial pressure) can be maintained at a level to ensure brain perfusion, usually greater than 50 torr.

The number of patients needing intracranial pressure monitoring is about the same as the number requiring surgery, which is a small minority of the patients with head injuries admitted to the hospital.

If a seizure has occurred or the child is in status epilepticus, anticonvulsants — phenobarbital, 5 mg per kg, and/or diazepam (Valium), 1 to 10 mg intravenously slowly — are indicated to prevent further seizures or stop them. Patients with open or depressed fractures and comatose patients should also be started on anticonvulsants. The physician should be prepared to deal with the depressed respirations that frequently follow as a result of the postictal state and the direct action of the medication. Phenytoin (Dilantin) has a delayed effect if given orally and is absorbed poorly from intramuscular depots, and therefore larger doses must be used acutely for seizures.

Analgesics or narcotics that alter the child's state of consciousness should be used only when absolutely necessary. Obviously seizure medication is needed, but it would be a mistake to sedate a child to "make him more comfortable" and, by altering the level of consciousness, to lose this vital sign of assessing neurologic deterioration.

The use of large doses of barbiturate, "barbiturate coma," is of benefit in the most severely injured children. Phenobarbital, 5 mg per kg, is given every hour to attain a serum level of 3 mg per 100 ml. This can be done only by a team of physicians and nurses in an intensive care situation. The efficacy of steroids in small or large doses is yet to be established.

If we now again divide the Group 2 children into two groups, Group 2A includes children without surgical lesions and Group 2B includes children with surgical lesions.

The use of hyperosmolar agents, mannitol and urea, has precise indications and contraindications in both Group 2A and 2B patients. Prior to determining if a patient has a surgical lesion, mannitol is indicated only if the patient is deteriorating rapidly and not responding to hyperventilation or if the child will not survive the time needed for diagnosis. A neurosurgeon must be on hand and an operating room available within a reasonable period of time. The administration of mannitol to all patients with severe head injuries is definitely contraindicated. Hyperosmolar agents dehydrate the normal brain. They usually decrease intracranial pressure and increase cerebral blood flow. They also allow intracranial hematomas to expand and compound pre-existing cerebral vascular congestion. Within hours, if prompt surgical decompression is not carried out, the rebound associated with these agents makes the second state of the child with a mass lesion even worse. In those children without surgical lesions and intracranial pressure within normal limits, mannitol is not indicated.

Children with evidence of dangerously increased intracranial pressure without a surgical lesion benefit from controlled ventilation and the prolonged use of hyperosmotic agents. Mannitol is usually effective for only about 72 hours because it slowly leaks across the blood-brain barrier and decreases the effective osmotic gradient. Serial blood gases and intracranial pressure monitoring in an intensive care facility are essential parts of this management.

Diagnostic Procedures

From Group 2 will come those patients who require further diagnostic studies.

The single most significant technical innovation in diagnostic neuroradiology in recent years is computed tomography (CT scanning). This tool enables the neurosurgeon to make rapid accurate diagnosis of intracranial hematomas, brain edema, and brain shift. The dose of x-ray to the child is about that received during a regular skull series. CT scanning has also shown us that the vast majority of even the most severely injured children do not have surgical lesions. Because of the noninvasive nature of the study, repeated studies to follow the child's progress can be done with little risk.

Cerebral blood flow studies, when available, have diagnostic and prognostic value in the management of children with head injuries.

Specific Management

Scalp Lacerations. Lacerations of the scalp without evidence of underlying injury to the skull should be treated by shaving the area around the laceration; the wound should be scrubbed and any foreign material removed. The skin edges may be bleeding profusely from multiple points, in which case rapid hemostasis is needed. Rather than attempting to close off individual bleeding points, hemostats should be applied to the galea aponeurotica and this layer everted over the skin edge. This maneuver is almost always successful in preventing further hemorrhage. No attempt should be made to probe the wound to determine if there is a depressed skull fracture or defect. A linear fracture needs no treatment, and a depressed fragment should be managed in the operating room. Both fractures should show on appropriate skull films or CT scanning. Probing through a skull defect could result in unnecessary injury to or contamination of the brain and its coverings.

After the wound is debrided and cleansed, the skin edges are closed in one or two layers. We prefer a single layer closure with a monofilament suture.

Skull Fractures. LINEAR FRACTURE. Linear skull fractures are important because they indicate that there has been significant trauma and alert one to the possibility of intracranial bleeding. Fractures that cross major dural sinuses or the middle meningeal artery or that pass into the foramen magnum are the most dangerous fractures for delayed intracranial hematomas. Forty-eight to 72 hour observation is needed for this group of children.

Fractures extending into the cranial sutures will frequently continue in the line of the suture, producing diastasis, especially if the squamous suture is involved.

If the linear fracture is associated with a laceration of the underlying dura mater and the pia-arachnoid enters this defect, the fracture may not heal and may grow wider with time. This "growing fracture" is produced by the pulsation of cerebrospinal fluid between the bone edges. A follow-up skull film 4 to 6 weeks after the injury is indicated if a palpable mass is developing along the fracture line.

PING-PONG FRACTURE. Trauma to the skull at delivery or during the neonatal period may result in a dent in one of the cranial bones rather than a fracture. The depression may be small or may involve an entire cranial plate. We elevate all these depressions by making a small skin incision, introducing a periosteal elevator extradurally, and applying pressure on the depressed segment until it is level with the surrounding bone.

DEPRESSED FRACTURE. Depressed skull fractures that are displaced greater than the thickness of the skull should be surgically elevated. Tomograms of the area may be necessary to determine the extent of the depression. If there is a rent in the dura mater, it should also be repaired. The onset of early or late epilepsy is correlated with the severity of injury as determined by the duration of amnesia and the presence of the dural tear.

We have not elevated minimally depressed fractures over major dural sinuses unless they are occluding the sinus as determined by angiography. All depressed fractures should have CT scan or angiography prior to surgery to rule out other lesions.

COMPOUND-DEPRESSED FRACTURES. All these fractures should be repaired in the operating room. The hair should be removed from the surrounding scalp and the wound scrubbed in the usual manner for an intracranial procedure. Debridement of the skin edges and removal of loose, contaminated bone fragments are important. Depressed pieces of bone which are not grossly contaminated can simply be elevated. Any dural laceration or injury to the underlying brain is then dealt with. The field is irrigated with large volumes of saline solution, and the wound is closed with monofilament suture.

BASAL SKULL FRACTURES. Fractures which pass into the basicranial area are certainly more common than are detected by x-ray or clinical signs. As with linear fractures over the convexity of the skull, the vast majority are benign.

Some of these fractures will traverse foramina of cranial nerves and transiently or permanently interrupt the function of these nerves. Surgical decompression of these nerves in most cases is not indicated.

Fractures of the petrous bone or frontal, ethmoidal, and sphenoid can result in a direct communication between basal cerebrospinal cisterns and the ear or cranial air sinuses. The presence of glucose in clear fluid draining from the nose or ear is evidence that it is cerebrospinal fluid (CSF). Almost all traumatic CSF leaks will close spontaneously, usually within 14 days. Persistent or recurrent leaks, as with spontaneous leaks, require a craniotomy and closure of the fistula and dural repair. Occasionally air will enter the cranial cavity through the defect. The pneumoencephalos can be seen on plain skull films.

CSF draining from an orifice should not be occluded by a dressing. We prefer treating the patient flat in the bed for 2 weeks with an antibiotic such as nafcillin, 100 mg per kg per day. This favors the flow of CSF from inside to out and decreases the possibility of contamination of CSF pathways. Some advocate repeated lumbar puncture and maintaining the patient in the sitting position. This creates a negative intracranial pressure and prevents flow across the defect, allowing it to seal. Both are effective, but the former method seems less hazardous.

The presence of periorbital ecchymosis, raccoon eyes (bilateral black eyes), or a contusion over the mastoid process, Battle's sign, should alert one to the possibility of a basilar skull fracture or a CSF leak.

Hematomas of the Scalp and Cephalohematomas. The subgaleal hematoma results from bleeding into the space above the periosteum. The distinguishing clinical feature between subgaleal and cephalohematoma is that the confinements of cephalohematomas feel like depressed skull fractures, because the outer rim of clotted blood feels firm and elevated while the center is liquid and soft. Skull films show that the bone is usually not depressed. Scalp hematomas are usually associated with a linear skull fracture. Only rarely will either of the lesions in themselves require treatment. One should resist the urge to needle these fluid cavities. Infection in this space leads to an open draining wound, a scalp defect, and prolonged hospitalization for the child.

All children with a significant scalp hematoma should have a CT scan. Some of these children are bleeding on both sides of the skull from open diploë in the fracture line, and significant epidural hematoma can develop.

Rarely the hematoma will calcify and require cosmetic surgery.

Intracranial Hematomas. SUBDURAL HEMATOMA. The diagnosis of a subdural hematoma is made by CT scanning or angiography. If a subdural hematoma is a possibility, a contrast enhanced scan should be done to reveal the occasional isodense hematoma. Diagnostic subdural taps into the subdural space often give erroneous results and are dangerous. Acute subdural hematomas cannot be aspirated, and the extent of chronic subdural hematomas cannot be determined by this method. We have seen CSF aspirated and interpreted as hygroma fluid, clear fluid converted to grossly hemorrhagic fluid by lacerating a cortical vein, and several cases of subdural hematomas converted to subdural empyemas.

EPIDURAL HEMATOMAS. The epidural hematoma is the prime example of an occult intracranial lesion which, if unsuspected, will cost the child's life. This more than any other lesion requires that the surgeons taking care of these children have an understanding of intracranial pathophysiology and its management.

The diagnosis is made quickly by CT scanning, and rapid surgical decompression by removing the blood clot through either a craniotomy or craniectomy is lifesaving. Angiography in the absence of CT scanning is also an excellent means of diagnosis. If angiography is used and the child has a dilated pupil, the side of the dilated pupil should be studied first. If diagnostic studies are not available or the child has deteriorated and is not responding to hyperventilation, an attempt at diagnosis and decompression should be made, again first on the side of the dilated pupil. Diagnostic burr holes are the least acceptable means for management and should be used only in extreme cases.

Intracerebral Hematomas. Extravasation of blood into brain parenchyma following a head injury is not uncommon. CT scanning has identified these previously unsuspected lesions. Most of these are small and do not require surgery. Some of these intracerebral hematomas present with a picture very similar to that of an epidural hematoma and require emergent surgery. Surgery is indicated for those lesions which act as mass lesions with evidence of increased intracranial pressure or brain shift. The frontal, occipital, and temporal tips are the most common sites. Lesions under the motor cortex or left parietal lobe should be managed conservatively if possible.

Penetrating Wounds. Objects that penetrate the skulls of children come from a wide variety of sources.

If the object is still projecting from the child's head, no attempt should be made to remove it until the child is prepared in the operating room. The projectile may be temporarily obstructing bleeding from a major source such as a dural sinus.

CT scanning or angiography should be performed to rule out sinus injuries or intracerebral hematomas.

We debride the entrance wound and site of exit if it is a through wound. No attempt should be made to debride the tract through cerebral substance. This only extends the injury. Readily accessible bone, hair, and clothing should be removed, the wound irrigated, the dura closed watertight, and the skin sutured. If a dural graft is needed for closure of the dura mater, pericranium should be used. Postoperative antibiotics and anticonvulsants should be given.

Post-traumatic Hydrocephalus. Bleeding into cerebrospinal fluid pathways can produce obstruction to circulation of CSF. It may be acute and transient and is relieved when the blood is absorbed. Occasionally it results in permanent scarring in the arachnoid villi, leading to malabsorption of CSF and transient or permanent hydrocephalus.

Children who are making progress and then deteriorate should be investigated for the possibility of acute hydrocephalus.

The diagnosis can be established by CT scan or angiography. Diversion of CSF to a body cavity or to an external drainage system will control the progression, and, if done early, it will prevent brain damage.

BRAIN TUMORS

method of
DONALD R. OLSON, M.D.
Reno, Nevada

Traditionally, the subject of brain tumors has been approached through the application of standard neurosurgery. With the advent of computed axial tomography, the diagnosis can now be made with definitude early in a patient's work-up and, in many cases, long before the neurosurgeon is called. In the separate categories usually recognized, malignant and nonmalignant tumors must be discussed individually. By utilizing modern microsurgical techniques, nonmalignant brain tumors can be removed with great accuracy from most areas of the brain with minimal sequelae. Over the past few years our approach to the malignant tumor has changed, with programs presently going on in areas of chemotherapy and tumor immunology in addition to surgical reduction in tumor volume.

Nonmalignant Tumors

We must categorize nonmalignant tumors of the brain not only as to their cell type but as to their location and, thereby, their symptom complexes related directly to secondary effects on other structures or tissues. Of the nonmalignant tumors, the most frequently seen is the meningioma, which may be of various cellular types and degrees of aggressiveness. In the usual situation, the meningioma is found in standard locations — parasagittal, sphenoid wing, olfactory groove, foramen magnum — and less commonly in other areas. The diagnosis of a meningioma may be readily made with contrast-enhanced computed axial tomography. Meningiomas readily take up contrast and show with computed axial tomography as a dense mass lesion. As well, small calcium deposits might be seen within the tumor substance itself. By utilizing microsurgical techniques, meningiomas in most areas may be completely removed. In the area of the base of the brain, meningiomas are a more difficult problem, invading the bone and causing potential recurrence if this invaded bony material is not totally removed. Derome et al., in France, have written extensively as to the radical removal of meningiomas of the base. Their technique, in addition to removing the soft tissue aspects of the tumor, is designed to reflect backward the anterior aspects of the brain, reinforcing the dura, and removing, in effect, the more central aspects of the skull base until all tumor is completely removed and then replaced, with bone grafts rebuilding the base of the skull. This type of surgery surprisingly does not carry major risk, but is very lengthy and tedious. Another area of importance because of location is the area of the cerebellopontine angle, where the acoustic neuroma is most commonly seen. Acoustic neuromas may also be of different cell types, but surgically, after appropriate diagnosis, are approached through microsurgical techniques. House et al. have had excellent results utilizing a neuro-otologic approach.

Other benign tumors of the base frequently encountered are tumors of the sellar-parasellar area. The great majority of these tumors are adenomas, either functional or nonfunctional in type. Here we list Guiot's conclusions:

Pituitary Tumors. Hyposecretory tumors are considered surgically on the basis of their size, their shape, and whether they are invasive. For the nonfunctional pituitary (chromophobe adenoma), systematic postoperative cobalt therapy is indicated. The functional adenomas (acromegaly, prolactin, and Cushing's disease) are managed on the basis of endocrinology. Growth hormone in acromegaly less than 5 ng per ml and prolactin levels less than 30 ng per ml in amenorrhea-galactorrhea syndrome should be strived for. ACTH levels may now be measured, as well, by immunoassay analysis to accurately appraise the

results in Cushing's disease. Cerebrospinal fluid rhinorrhea and postoperative diabetes insipidus are the most frequent surgical complications. With microsurgical technique and utilization of the transsphenoidal route, a complication rate below 4 per cent should be expected. The mortality rate in a series reviewed comprising over 1400 cases remains below 1 per cent.

Malignant Tumors

Of the malignant tumors of the brain, glioblastoma multiforme or high grade astrocytoma is the most frequently occurring primary brain tumor, and metastatic tumor is most common. Metastatic tumors account for approximately 50 per cent of all tumors of the brain. The traditional tumors that metastasize to the brain are lung, breast, thyroid, kidney, and gastrointestinal. The management of the metastatic tumor is based upon the degree of primary symptomatology. A single metastatic tumor clinically symptomatic with a high Karnofsky scale (Table 1) should be surgically removed.

Of the primary malignant tumors of the brain, namely, astrocytoma, medulloblastoma, ependymoma, and glioblastoma multiforme, there is some variance in that some centers recommend biopsy followed by chemotherapy and x-ray therapy, but more commonly surgical debulking of the tumor is considered to increase the

TABLE 1. **Criteria of Performance Status (Karnofsky)**

Able to carry on normal activity; no special care is needed	100%	Normal; no complaints; no evidence of disease
	90%	Able to carry on normal activity; minor signs or symptoms of disease
	80%	Normal activity with effort; some signs or symptoms of disease
Unable to work; able to live at home; cares for most personal needs; a varying amount of assistance is needed	70%	Cares for self; unable to carry on normal activity or to do active work
	60%	Requires occasional assistance but is able to care for most needs
	50%	Requires considerable assistance and frequent medical care
Unable to care for self; requires equivalent of institutional or hospital care; disease may be progressing rapidly	40%	Disabled; requires special medical care and assistance
	30%	Severely disabled; hospitalization indicated, although death not imminent
	20%	Very sick; hospitalization necessary; active supportive treatment necessary
	10%	Moribund; fatal processes progressing rapidly
	0%	Dead

effectiveness of chemotherapy and/or x-ray therapy at appropriate dose levels. Nitrosourea (BCNU, CCNU) is the most effective and most often used chemotherapeutic agent for primary brain tumors.

Management of Primary Malignant Brain Tumors. Cancer of the brain is a frequent entity and is the second most common cancer in children. As reported in 1977, there were 10,900 new cases of primary cancer of the brain, with 8800 deaths. Of the 690,000 new cases of cancer in the United States, 385,000 patients died; 50 per cent of these deaths were directly associated with cancer metastatic to the nervous system, mostly from lung cancer, breast cancer, malignant melanoma, lymphomas, and leukemia.

Brain Tumor as Cancer. Shapiro (Memorial Sloan-Kettering Cancer Center) states that when a patient develops cancer systemically, his body must deal with a cancer burden. When a cancer mass becomes equal to 1000 grams of systemic tumor burden, the situation is considered lethal. This amount of tumor is equivalent to 1×10^{12} cells. In contrast, brain tumors share a space within the skull with the total mass of the brain already occupying 1200 to 1300 ml. Therefore, a 100 gram tumor is equivalent to 1×10^{11} cells, thereby becoming almost 100 per cent lethal. Most tumors when they become symptomatic are generally in the range of between 30 and 60 grams. In order to cure cancer, it is necessary to reduce the bulk of the tumor to a size at which the natural body mechanisms can effectively handle the tumor burden. In general, the reduction in tumor bulk to approximately 10 grams or 1×10^{10} cells, assuming an initial malignant burden of 100 grams or 1×10^{11} cells, represents a subtotal surgical resection of 90 per cent. A so-called "total resection" might actually reduce the tumor to 1 gram of tissue, which still leaves 1×10^9 cells, which, thereafter, must be killed by radiation therapy. Radiation therapy, by definition, is effective but only to a limited degree in brain tumors. The best radiation therapy to brain tumors can account for only two logs of killed cells; therefore, a postoperative tumor burden of 1 gram would be reduced to only 0.01 gram or 1×10^7 cells by radiation therapy. It is then left for chemotherapy to reduce the population of cells two more logs to 0.0001 gram or 1×10^5 cells. Such a scenario obviously is seldom fulfilled, since most subtotal resections limit the reduction to only 30 or 40 per cent bulk reduction of the tumor. The best chemotherapeutic agents currently available produce only one log net cell kill, thus permitting the tumor to grow at a rate faster than can be killed by the drugs.

Surgical Considerations. Although for many years classic resection of the primary brain tumor had been taught, for the past 20 years the utilization of corticosteroids has greatly influenced and reduced the surgical mortality, which is presently now listed as 1 to 2 per cent. By utilizing computed axial tomography, early diagnosis can now be established. Among some oncologists and radiotherapists, there is a trend to suggest that biopsy plus radiation therapy and/or chemotherapy is sufficient and adequate therapy. Jelsma and Bucy have shown without question that patients undergoing extensive surgical resection or reduction of the tumor bulk survive more than 1 year, whereas patients undergoing minimal resection or needle biopsy all die within the first year. The same holds even with the advent of symptomatic therapy, including chemotherapy.

At this time, five surgical indications can be identified that on the whole favor an active role for the neurosurgeon: (1) To establish a diagnosis. (2) To provide symptomatic therapy, especially by reducing intracranial pressure. (3) To permit time for anticancer therapy, specifically radiation therapy and early chemotherapy, which require a minimum of 8 to 10 weeks. (4) To remove tumor bulk as a form of anticancer treatment. (5) To convert tumor cells not actively growing into those in an active growth phase, making these tumor cells more susceptible to treatment.

Radiation therapy, utilizing whole head treatment delivering 5500 to 6000 rads, has been shown more effective than the previous traditional 5000 rad treatment. However, there is good evidence that in experimental animals dose levels in the range of 6000 rads do produce damage to the normal brain.

Discussion of chemotherapy is based upon the 1962 article by Rall and Zubrod, which describes the pharmacologic characteristics of drugs required for central nervous system neoplasms. The basis of their observation was patients having meningoleukemia, with which, for the most part, the blood-brain barrier is preserved. Since that time, there has been much evidence, including uptake seen with radioactive isotope brain scan, that in the primary brain tumor the functional blood-brain barrier does not exist. It is estimated that 90 to 95 per cent of primary brain tumors do not have a functional barrier to the entry of molecular sizes consistent with the most common chemotherapeutic agents. The remaining 5 to 10 per cent of tumor exists as a single infiltrating cell or cluster of cells that occupy an area of the brain adjacent to the bulk of the tumor and are supplied by normal blood vessels. That is to say, tumor cells receive their nutrients from the normal brain blood vessels, and the chemotherapeutic agents that normally do not cross the blood-brain barrier presumably must then find their way to the clusters by diffusion from the main bulk of the tumor. Nitrosourea, the main chemotherapeutic agent used for the brain, readily crosses the blood-brain barrier. The most commonly used agents for malignant brain tumors are 1,3-bis(2-chloroethyl)-1-nitrosourea (BCNU) and 1-(2-chloroethyl)-3-cyclohexyl-1-nitrosourea (CCNU). These drugs, all of which cross the blood-brain barrier, are rapidly metabolized in vivo and produce a delayed form of bone marrow toxicity, namely, thrombocytopenia and leukopenia. This may not become evident for 3 or 4 weeks. Another commonly used agent is procarbazine, a monoamine oxidase inhibitor, which also crosses the blood-brain barrier and produces bone marrow depression as a major toxicity. Vincristine sulfate has been used against brain tumors for over 15 years, but its efficacy is still not well established. It is known to have difficulty crossing the blood-brain barrier. Its major adverse effects are peripheral neuropathy, ileus, and jaw pain (Table 2).

Summary

Patients receiving chemotherapy, radiation therapy, or any other modality for brain tumor should be evaluated on the Karnofsky grading scale at least once a month. When combining these data with computed tomographic scans done at 2 to 3 month intervals and utilizing steroid therapy as recommended by the Brain Tumor Study Group, 17 weeks appears to be the expected median survival of patients following resection for primary malignant brain tumors. Adding radiation therapy increases median survival at least two-fold. There is also evidence that adding chemotherapy further prolongs the survival of such patients to exceed 18 months. For patients in a normal community, full radiation therapy and placement on a chemotherapeutic program are recommended following surgical debulking of the tumor.

TABLE 2.   **Chemotherapeutic Agents in Malignant Brain Tumors***

DRUG	USUAL DOSE†	ROUTE	TOXICITY
BCNU	80 mg/M² per day for 3 consecutive days; repeat every 6–8 weeks	Intravenous	Delayed (3 weeks) Thrombocytopenia Leukopenia Abnormal liver function tests
CCNU	130 mg/M² every 6–8 weeks	Oral	Same as BCNU
MeCCNU	220 mg/M² every 6–8 weeks	Oral	Same as BCNU
Procarbazine	150 mg/M² daily for 28 days; repeat after 28 day rest	Oral	Leukopenia beginning 3–4 weeks Rarely may induce severe rash, probably associated with phenytoin
Vincristine	1 mg/M² every 1–2 weeks	Intravenous	Peripheral neuropathy
Streptozotocin (experimental use only)	1.25 grams/M² every week	Intravenous	Renal acidosis picture (serum uric acid decreased,· serum phosphates decreased) Creatinine clearance should be 50 ml/min and should be determined every 6 weeks

*These agents have undergone controlled clinical trials or are now under active investigation in brain tumor patients.
†Combination chemotherapy has been valuable. If contemplated, drug dosage must be reduced by about half.

SECTION 13

The Locomotor System

RHEUMATOID ARTHRITIS

method of
DANIEL E. HATHAWAY, M.D.,
St. Paul, Minnesota

and RONALD P. MESSNER, M.D.
Minneapolis, Minnesota

Rheumatoid arthritis remains a disease of unknown cause for which there is no cure. Despite this, there are numerous therapies that can be used, which in most cases will allow the patient to sustain a normal life style. Less than 15 per cent of the patients become bed or wheelchair bound. Between 30 and 50 per cent of patients with rheumatoid arthritis never require any medical therapy more aggressive than aspirin. These facts make patient education an extremely important foundation on which to build therapy when dealing with a newly diagnosed patient with rheumatoid arthritis.

Once the diagnosis is established, one must make a determination as to the level of activity of the inflammatory process. Patients may vary from the young woman with normal x-rays but who on examination has red, warm joints with palpable thickening and effusions, to the elderly patient who has had arthritis for many years, with deformity, contractures, and dramatic radiologic changes but no active synovitis. The goal in the first patient is to reduce her pain through reduction of the inflammatory response. The goal in the second patient would be to provide analgesia and develop a program which best allows her to meet the demands of daily life in an independent fashion.

In the patient with active inflammatory synovitis, one must stress the importance of adequate rest. Patients should be encouraged to get 8 to 10 hours of sleep per night and to get off their feet for a minimum of 1 hour during the middle of the day. Bed rest during hospitalization without other therapy will result in a dramatic reduction in active disease. In this era of stringent cost controls and bed utilization review, this form of therapy is rarely used, but it does emphasize that rest plays a role in routine management of these patients.

With active disease it is important that patients be encouraged to put their joints through daily passive range of motion to maintain joint flexibility and prevent the development of contractures. As the activity of the disease subsides, more exercises can be encouraged to maintain muscle strength, which will improve joint stability.

Aspirin remains the initial drug of choice for most patients with rheumatoid arthritis. Except for the rare patient with true aspirin hypersensitivity in association with nasal polyps and asthma, there is almost no such thing as an aspirin-intolerant patient. This, however, requires the physician to educate patients on the rationale behind the therapy so that they will be compliant in trying the various forms of aspirin that will almost always allow the achievement of anti-inflammatory levels (20 to 30 mg per 100 ml). Patients with no history of gastrointestinal intolerance to aspirin are instructed to start with 3 regular 5 grain (325 mg) aspirin tablets to be taken immediately after meals and before bed with a snack and a full glass of liquid. Should gastrointestinal intolerance be noted, they are instructed to switch to a buffered product. If this still results in symptomatic gastrointestinal distress, 1 tablespoon of liquid antacid is added to their regimen, taken 90 minutes after meals, before bedtime, and at any other time that they are symptomatic. Enteric-coated aspirin is expensive and is reserved for those patients who continue to have difficulty. The patient should receive an adequate trial (6 to 8 weeks) of high dose aspirin before consideration of alternative drugs. In children and the elderly with some impairment of hearing, it is necessary to follow salicylate levels in the blood in order to avoid aspirin intoxication. For most patients, however, one can simply have them increase their dosage by 1 tablet every 3 to 5 days until they note tinnitus or reach 20 tablets per day. Most patients will develop tinnitus with an acetylsalicylic acid (ASA) level in the range of 28 to 30 mg per 100 ml. If they then reduce their total daily dosage to 2 tablets less than that which causes tinnitus, they will be in an anti-inflammatory range. An ASA level drawn at this time will confirm the adequacy of the dose or alert the physician to the occasional patient in whom tinnitus is an unreliable sign. The usual range is between 12 and 20 aspirin tablets per 24 hours.

If after an initial 2 month trial of rest, physical therapy, and aspirin, the patient continues to have marked morning stiffness and active synovitis, one can turn to the nonaspirin, nonsteroidal anti-inflammatory drugs (NSAIDs). In direct comparative studies these drugs have an anti-inflammatory potential equal to aspirin. In the individual patient, however, it is impossible to predict who will respond to what drug. These drugs must therefore be tried in a sequential fashion in anti-inflammatory dosages. A 2 to 4 week trial is sufficient to judge effectiveness.

The NSAIDs generally fall into two chemical families. The first is the propionic acid derivatives, including naproxen (Naprosyn), ibuprofen (Motrin), and fenoprofen (Nalfon). The other family is the indole derivatives, including indomethacin (Indocin), tolmetin sodium (Tolectin, and sulindac (Clinoril). These drugs can be tried either in place of aspirin or in addition to full anti-inflammatory dosage of aspirin. The commonly used dosages of these drugs in rheumatoid arthritis are naproxen, 500 mg in the morning, 250 mg in the evening; ibuprofen, 600 mg four times daily; fenoprofen, 600 mg four times daily; tolmetin sodium, 400 mg four times daily; and sulindac, 200 mg twice daily. The maximal dosage of indomethacin is 50 mg four times daily. It is frequently necessary, however, to begin at a reduced level (either 75 or 100 mg per day) and increase gradually to the maximal tolerated dosage. Many patients will have central nervous system (CNS) toxicity, including headache and dizziness, if the drug is introduced at too great a dosage or dosage increase is advanced too rapidly. Of the aforementioned drugs, in-

domethacin also has the greatest potential of gastrointestinal intolerance. The pyrazolone derivative phenylbutazone (Butazolidin) is rarely used in the routine management of patients with a lifelong problem such as rheumatoid arthritis because of potential bone marrow toxicity. However, it can be effective in a dosage of 100 mg three or four times per day for 10 days to control a flare of the disease. Although the NSAIDs will cause some gastrointestinal intolerance, headaches, or rash in some patients, they are in general well tolerated and cause few side effects. In rare instances, propionic acid derivatives, especially fenoprofen, have been associated with the development of interstitial nephritis. All these drugs are prostaglandin synthetase inhibitors and through an effect on the kidney can induce salt and water retention.

Intra-articular steroids have become a widely accepted and commonly used therapy for specific joints, which have not responded to aspirin, the nonsteroidal anti-inflammatory drugs, physical therapy, and rest. They are also used while one is waiting for the remittive drugs (which will be discussed below) to take effect. The crystalline preparations such as triamcinolone hexacetonide (Aristospan) have been shown to be more efficacious than the more soluble preparations. One occasionally sees a crystalline response following this injection, which can last up to 24 hours and mimic an attack of gout. Therapy includes use of ice packs on the involved joint and a nonsteroidal anti-inflammmatory agent.

Remittive agents are those which can induce a true remission in the disease and which have been shown to influence the natural history of the disease with decreased evidence of bony destruction on x-ray. The indication for the use of a remittive agent is progressive rheumatoid arthritis, uncontrolled by more conservative measures, including aspirin, the nonsteroidal anti-inflammatory drugs, intra-articular steroids, physical therapy, and adequate rest. This group would include the gold salts, penicillamine, hydroxychloroquine, and the cytotoxic agents azathioprine* and cyclophosphamide.* With these drugs it takes between 2 and 6 months before the patient begins to notice any benefit. Gold, penicillamine, and the cytotoxic agents all have a high chance (75 to 80 per cent) of being beneficial for the patient. The response can vary from pain relief without any objective improvement in synovitis to a complete remission. Hydroxychloroquine can also be this efficacious, but the frequency of good response is somewhat lower.

---

*This use of this agent is not listed in the manufacturer's official directive.

In 1981 the gold salts remain the first of the remittive drugs that would be utilized by most rheumatologists. The two preparations currently available are gold thiomalate (Myochrysine) and gold thioglucose (Solganal). There is some evidence that gold thioglucose is somewhat more effective and less toxic. It does not produce nitritoid (nitrate-like) reactions, including flushing, tachycardia, and occasionally vasomotor collapse. Both are given by intramuscular injection. The initial 10 mg test dosage is to make sure that the patient does not have an anaphylactic response. This is followed 1 week later by 25 mg and thereafter 50 mg per week until the patient has received 1 gram of gold, or has developed toxicity or an excellent response. If the patient has shown improvement after receiving the initial loading course of 1 gram, the injections are decreased in frequency while maintaining the same dosage. One can go initially to every 2 weeks for 3 to 6 months, then every 3 weeks, and finally once per month. If the patient's disease flares, one again must increase the frequency of the injections. Attempts have been made to correlate the gold levels in blood, urine, and synovial fluid with the clinical response, but these have been unrewarding.

Approximately 30 per cent of the patients who are started on gold will develop an unacceptable toxicity. The most common toxic reaction is a nonspecific pruritic dermatitis. One occasionally sees lichenoid eruptions or a rash which mimics pityriasis rosea. In the past when larger doses of gold were used and the patients were less closely followed, an occasional patient would develop an exfoliative dermatitis. Mucous membrane lesions with stomatitis are also seen. As a rule of thumb, an unexplained rash on a patient who is receiving gold is a gold rash until proved otherwise. With evidence of mucocutaneous toxicity, the gold should be withheld and not restarted until the reaction has totally resolved. Therapy is then reinitiated with a 5 mg injection, and the dosage is increased by 5 mg per week until the patient is receiving 25 mg per injection. Many patients will be able to tolerate this dosage with improvement in their arthritis, but without recurrence of the toxicity.

Transient proteinuria is seen in between 3 and 10 per cent of the patients. An occasional patient will develop the nephrotic syndrome. The proteinuria almost always clears spontaneously in less than 1 year once the gold has been discontinued. Renal biopsies have revealed membranous nephropathy with evidence of immune complex deposition. In general, the proteinuria is more transient than mentioned above, and one simply holds the gold until it has cleared and then restarts gold as mentioned above following a mucocutaneous reaction.

The most serious potential complication of gold therapy is hematologic. The development of mild leukopenia is quite common. The injections should be withheld if the white count drops below 4000. Eosinophilia is also common; although it frequently correlates with toxicity, it can also be seen without other problems, and therefore one need not change the therapy on the basis of this parameter. Thrombocytopenia (less than 100,000), either alone or in association with leukopenia, may herald the onset of an aplastic anemia and necessitates permanent discontinuation of gold therapy. Serious but unusual complications include colitis, hepatitis, peripheral neuropathy, and hypersensitivity pneumonitis. Because of toxicities the patient must be carefully monitored for proteinuria or hematologic problems. Patients should get a complete blood count (CBC), platelet count, and urinalysis once a month. During the other weeks of the month prior to the injections, they should have a white blood cell count and a dip stick urine test to check for protein. Gold should be withheld if there is a 1+ or greater proteinuria. With sustained benefit and without evidence for toxicity, gold injections can be continued indefinitely.

The patient who is refractory to gold or who has developed an unacceptable toxicity should be switched to one of the alternative agents. There is no uniform agreement at present as to the next drug of choice. Possibilities would include low dose prednisone (less than 7 mg per day), D-penicillamine, or hydroxychloroquine.

D-Penicillamine has been approved for the therapy of rheumatoid arthritis by the Food and Drug Administration. It is widely used in Europe and has become very popular in this country. Some rheumatologists are now using penicillamine prior to gold because as an oral agent it is easier on the patient than weekly injections. However, it has a somewhat higher incidence of toxicities, with several studies showing up to 50 per cent of the patients tried on this agent will have to discontinue it because of an unacceptable reaction. The incidence of toxicity has been decreased by the "go slow, go low" dosage schedule as popularized by Dr. Israeli Jaffe. The patient is started on either 125 or 250 mg initially. At 1 to 3 month intervals the dosage is raised by similar increments. One should maintain the patient on the lowest dosage that produces an appropriate clinical response. Although dosages in excess of 1000 mg per day are occasionally used in rheumatoid arthritis, most patients who are going to respond to this agent will do so on 750 mg per day or less. A history of penicillin allergy is not a contraindication to use of this drug.

The toxicities of D-penicillamine are similar to those of gold, including rashes, stomatitis, proteinuria, and hematologic complications. Rash and stomatitis can be managed by dosage reduction and sometimes are benefited by cyproheptadine (Periactin). If this does not relieve the problem, penicillamine should be temporarily discontinued and restarted at a lower dosage once the reaction has cleared. Stomatitis, unfortunately, tends to recur and may require discontinuation of therapy. Ten to 15 per cent of the patients will develop proteinuria, and some become nephrotic. Moderate proteinuria, up to 2 grams per 24 hours, is acceptable. Greater protein loss than this should result in discontinuation of the drug. The earliest hematologic problem tends to be thrombocytopenia. This may be transient and self-limited if the drug is discontinued. We do not restart penicillamine after observing significant thrombocytopenia (less than 100,000), but others will reinitiate the drug at a lower dosage once the platelet count has returned to normal. Leukopenia less than 3000 may herald the development of aplastic anemia and requires permanent discontinuation of the drug. With the initiation of therapy, many patients will complain of loss of taste. This will resolve spontaneously despite continuation of the therapy. Reactions requiring permanent discontinuation are drug fever, usually seen early in the course of therapy, breast enlargement, and a number of autoimmune syndromes, including Goodpasture's syndrome, myasthenia gravis, polymyositis, pemphigus, drug-induced systemic lupus erythematosus, and obliterative bronchiolitis. Because of the renal and hematologic complications, the patient should have a complete blood count (CBC), platelet count, and urinalysis every 2 weeks while the dosage is being altered and monthly once a good clinical response has been obtained and the dosage is stabilized.

An alternative to penicillamine would be the antimalarial hydroxychloroquine (Plaquenil). This drug may also be useful in the patient who has had to stop gold because of persistent proteinuria and in whom the physician does not want to use penicillamine because of proteinuria. The dosage of hydroxychloroquine is 200 mg per day. The primary toxicity is ocular and is dose and age related. Most toxicity occurs with an accumulative dose greater than 600 grams and in patients older than 60. Hydroxychloroquine may be deposited in the cornea and can be seen on slit lamp examination. This is not an indication to stop the drug. The primary serious toxicity is deposition in the pigmented layer of the retina. This can result in macular degeneration and ultimately blindness. The patient should be evaluated by an ophthalmologist initially and then at 4 to 6 month intervals. Besides funduscopic examination, visual field determination with both red and white objects is indicated. Loss of peripheral red vision is an early sign of retinal toxicity, and the drug should be discontinued. Other than the ocular problem, hydroxychloroquine tends to be well tolerated by the patient.

Since rheumatoid arthritis is a chronic illness, corticosteroids in doses which cause adrenal suppression or other toxicity, such as osteoporosis, cataracts, hypertension, diabetes, and decreased resistance to infection, should be avoided. The one indication for high dose prednisone is rheumatoid vasculitis. Many patients, however, will note significant improvement in their joint discomfort and morning stiffness on low dose prednisone (2 to 7 mg orally every morning). Unfortunately, corticosteroids do not alter the progression of the joint destruction, and not all patients will have an objective reduction in their synovitis. It is also common in patients who had an initial good response to low dose prednisone to subsequently have a flare of their disease while remaining on the same dose. Resuppression of symptoms and active synovitis will frequently require a dosage that is unacceptable on a long-term basis. Because of the effectiveness of low dose steroids in symptomatic control, many physicians will utilize them early in the course of the illness while waiting for the remittive agents such as gold or penicillamine to take effect. They then will attempt to wean the patient from steroid therapy.

The other remittive agents are the cytotoxic drugs azathioprine (Imuran)* and cyclophosphamide (Cytoxan).* Their indication would be severe, ongoing, destructive rheumatoid arthritis, refractory to conventional therapy, including gold, penicillamine, hydroxychloroquine, and corticosteroids. Azathioprine is converted in the body to 6-mercaptopurine, an antimetabolite which is both immunosuppressive and anti-inflammatory. Cyclophosphamide is an alkylating agent which is perhaps our most potent immunosuppressive agent. The primary toxicity of these drugs is bone marrow suppression. Cyclophosphamide can cause sterility, alopecia, and hemorrhagic cystitis. Cyclophosphamide has been implicated in the induction of malignancies. This is less clear with azathioprine but remains a very real consideration when one is anticipating the use of

---

*This use of this agent is not listed in the manufacturer's official directive.

these drugs for nonmalignant diseases. These drugs should be used only by physicians who are familiar with their toxicities, and the patient must be carefully informed as to the potential risks of the therapy.

Multiple experimental therapies for rheumatoid arthritis are currently being evaluated, including plasma- and leukapheresis, radiation, several immunostimulant drugs (e.g., levamisole), and an oral gold preparation. There are also newer nonsteroidal anti-inflammatory drugs on the horizon whose mechanisms of action differ from the prostaglandin synthetase inhibitors. Only time and further testing will show their proper place in the therapy of rheumatoid arthritis.

Patients with rheumatoid arthritis need a consistent sympathetic physician who will offer psychologic as well as medical support in the therapy of their chronic disease. There are numerous allied fields that can be very helpful in the management of these patients, including the physiatrist, the orthopedic surgeon, the physical and occupational therapist, and the social worker. The physiatrist and physical therapist will work to maintain and increase joint mobility and muscular strength. The occupational therapist can frequently and ingeniously devise new ways for even very crippled patients to remain independent as far as their activities of daily living are concerned. The social worker can provide psychologic support as well as being helpful in the management of the significant economic problems which can be caused by chronic illness. The orthopedic surgeon plays a role throughout the course of the disease. This ranges from synovectomies, primarily of knees, wrists, and metacarpophalangeal joints that are refractory to medical therapy, to later joint replacement in those patients with persistent pain secondary to joint destruction. The best artificial joints currently are those of the hip and the knee. The patient should achieve pain relief following these operations, and most have improved mobility. Other arthroplasties are being utilized more frequently but remain experimental as to design.

There are a number of pamphlets and books, written in easily understandable terms, which may be helpful to patients with rheumatoid arthritis. These can be obtained from either a local or the National Arthritis Foundation. Other books for patients include *Coping with Arthritis*, by Dr. Timothy G. Johnson, and *Arthritis: A Comprehensive Guide*, by Dr. James F. Fries.

JUVENILE RHEUMATOID ARTHRITIS

method of
BERNARD F. GERMAIN, M.D.,
TOMAS S. BOCANEGRA, M.D.,
FRANK B. VASEY, M.D.,
and LUIS R. ESPINOZA, M.D.
Tampa, Florida

The treatment of juvenile rheumatoid arthritis, as in any disease, begins with an accurate diagnosis. The diagnosis of juvenile rheumatoid arthritis may be difficult. The disease may begin as either of three distinct forms: (1) systemic onset, (2) pauciarticular, and (3) polyarticular.

The treatment of juvenile rheumatoid arthritis may be divided into (1) medical management (drugs), (2) physical therapy, (3) surgery, and (4) education and counseling.

Drug Therapy

Nonsteroidal Anti-inflammatory Drugs. Many children with juvenile rheumatoid arthritis respond to a nonsteroidal anti-inflammatory drug, and aspirin remains the nonsteroidal anti-inflammatory drug of choice. Most children require 65 to 100 mg per kg per day divided into four or five doses. A child weighing more than 25 kg should be started on the lower dose. Each dose should be taken after a meal or snack. Thus a 25 pound child (11.3 kg) would require 10 to 15 baby aspirin tablets (75 mg) per day in divided doses. An older child can use adult aspirin (325 mg). Two parameters should be used in determining proper aspirin dosage: the clinical response and the serum salicylate level. A serum salicylate level of 20 to 25 mg per dl (100 ml) 2 hours after the last dose is about right; serum levels of 30 mg per dl and above are dangerous. Small children may tolerate choline salicylate (Arthropan) better. Choline salicylate is a liquid; each teaspoon contains salicylate equal to 650 mg of aspirin (10 grains). Buffered aspirin such as Ascriptin or Bufferin can be used in older children who experience gastrointestinal irritation with plain aspirin. Tolmetin (Tolectin) is the only other nonsteroidal anti-inflammatory drug approved by the Food and Drug Administration for use in children (20 to 30 mg per kg per day), although others are being tested for safety and efficacy, e.g., sulindac (Clinoril) and ibuprofen (Motrin).

Aspirin side effects include gastric irritation (heartburn, nausea, gastric ulceration), tinnitus, dizziness, and, at high serum salicylate levels, behavior and learning problems. Respiratory alkalosis followed by metabolic acidosis may occur at high serum salicylate levels. Aspirin frequently causes a rise in serum liver transaminase levels, particularly at serum salicylate levels of 35 mg per dl or greater. This is reversible with discontinuance of the aspirin. Residual liver damage has not been reported, but cases of severe acute hepatitis with encephalopathy have been reported.

Acetaminophen may be used for additional analgesic and antipyretic effect, but it has no anti-inflammatory action.

The use of indomethacin (Indocin) in children has been discouraged in the United States because of reports of hepatic toxicity and peptic ulceration. It is used in Great Britain. Phenylbutazone (Butazolidin) and oxyphenbutazone (Tandearil) should not be used in children because of the frequency and severity of side effects (peptic ulceration, hepatitis, and bone marrow suppression).

Gold Therapy. Gold therapy should be used in children who continue to have active synovitis despite adequate treatment with aspirin; gold may induce a remission in these children. Aurothioglucose (Solganal) or gold sodium thiomalate (Myochrysine) is used at a dose of 1 mg per kg per week given intramuscularly. A test dose is given initially. Thus a 20 kg child would receive a test dose of 5 mg, followed by 10 mg the subsequent week, and 20 mg per week thereafter. (See also manufacturer's official directives for use of these agents in children.) The major side effects of gold therapy include bone marrow suppression (leukopenia, anemia, thrombocytopenia, bone marrow aplasia), glomerulonephritis, and mucocutaneous lesions (oral ulcers, pruritus, rashes). Rarely hepatitis, colitis, and pulmonary fibrosis have been reported as gold side effects. Consequently complete blood counts, urinalysis, and careful questioning should precede each injection. Gold should be withheld if any evidence of a side effect is present. Gold may be restarted at a lower dose if minor problems occur but clear with cessation of the drug (such as mild leukopenia, pruritus, oral ulcers, or mild proteinuria). Weekly injections should be continued until a remission or significant improvement occurs; the injections can then be given at intervals of up to 1 month. If a total dose of 500 to 750 mg has been given without improvement, gold therapy is probably unsuccessful and should be stopped.

Adrenocorticosteroids. Systemic corticoste-

TABLE 1. **Major Side Effects of Corticosteroid Treatment**

Posterior subcapsular cataracts
Growth arrest
Glucose intolerance
Hyperosmolar coma
Obesity
Increased risk of infection
Hypothalamic-pituitary-adrenal suppression
Acne
Purpura
Myopathy
Osteoporosis
Aseptic bone necrosis
Peptic ulceration
Hypertension
Sodium and water retention
Hypokalemic alkalosis
Psychosis

roids may be necessary if aspirin and gold therapy are unsuccessful, or if the child is too sick to wait for a response to gold therapy. Indications for corticosteroid therapy include (1) unremitting severe synovitis causing the child to be bedridden; (2) severe unresponsive fever; (3) pleuritis, pericarditis, and myocarditis; and (4) uveitis if topical corticosteroid therapy is unsuccessful. In general the lowest possible dose that will allow the child to function should be used (e.g., 5 to 15 mg of prednisone or prednisolone each morning). High dose corticosteroids may be necessary in the extremely sick child. Later alternate day corticosteroids may be feasible. The large number of corticosteroid side effects should be kept in mind when prescribing these drugs (Table 1).

D-Penicillamine. D-Penicillamine (Cuprimine, Depen) is used successfully in the treatment of adult rheumatoid arthritis, but its use remains experimental in children. Ten mg per kg per day is given on an empty stomach. Side effects include bone marrow suppression, glomerulonephritis, mucocutaneous lesions, lupus-like syndromes, myasthenia gravis, myositis, and others. This drug should be administered only by those experienced in its use and side effects.

Hydroxychloroquine. Hydroxychloroquine (Plaquenil) may be used at a dose of 5 to 7 mg per kg. Retinal toxicity is the most serious potential side effect (ophthalmologic examinations, including visual field examinations, are required at 6 month intervals). This would limit the use of hydroxychloroquine to older children able to cooperate during an eye examination (see also manufacturer's official directive). Accidental ingestion of as little as 1 gram of chloroquine has been reported to be fatal in children. As with

D-penicillamine, the administration of this drug should be limited to those familiar with its use.

Cytotoxic Drugs. Cytotoxic drugs are agents of last resort. Their potential side effects are so serious as to make their use questionable in all but the most severe and recalcitrant cases.

Physical Therapy

Physical therapy is as important as medical management. A physical therapist should be involved in the child's care from the onset of joint symptoms. The application of heat to involved joints helps relieve pain and improve range of motion.

Splints are used to rest involved joints and to maintain positions of maximal function. The physical therapist should recognize and ideally prevent early joint contractures. If limitation of joint motion has occurred, the physical therapist institutes exercises to improve ranges of motion. The prevention and alleviation of contractures at the hip, knee, and ankle are of vital importance to the future unimpeded mobility of the child. Early recognition, prevention, and alleviation of flexion contractures at the wrist and metacarpophalangeal and proximal interphalangeal joints of the hands are vital for the child's future functional ability.

Positions of most useful function vary with each joint. Maximal dexterity and strength of the fingers require the wrist to be at least in the neutral position, i.e., 0 degree, but 15 to 20 degrees dorsiflexion is the position of optimal function. Forty-five degrees of flexion is required at the metacarpophalangeal joints. A mild flexion contracture at the elbow presents no functional problem. The shoulder should have at least 90 degrees of abduction, flexion, and external rotation. Full extension and 90 degrees of flexion should be maintained at the hip. The same range of motion is necessary at the knee. The ankle should be maintained in a neutral position.

Surgery

Surgery plays a secondary role in the management of a child with juvenile rheumatoid arthritis. Synovectomy is rarely indicated. On the other hand, joint reconstruction has become important for those children who are left with residual function loss. Total hip replacement and even total knee replacement may be required when the child is no longer growing. Jaw reconstruction markedly improves the appearance of those patients with micrognathia. At the ankle an osteotomy may be necessary to restore the foot to a neutral position. Excision of the metatarsal heads relieves metatarsophalangeal subluxation. Wrist fusion in a position of function may be required if a flexion deformity is present. Flexible implants are available for severe deformities of the metacarpophalangeal and proximal interphalangeal joints.

Education and Counseling

Education and counseling of both the parents and the child are very important. A chronically ill child is challenging (1) because of the uncertainty of the diagnosis and (2) because of the uncertainty of the prognosis. Often the normal pattern of family life is greatly disrupted. Parents need time to ask questions, and they need sources of information. The local chapter of the Arthritis Foundation can provide pamphlets and often has a children's arthritis club. These clubs allow parents to meet other parents with similar problems and to learn more about the disease. Books written for patients and relatives of patients can be very helpful. (Calabro and Wykert: *The Truth About Arthritis Care;* New York, David McKay Company, Inc., 1971. James F. Fries: *Arthritis; A Comprehensive Guide;* Reading, Mass., Addison-Wesley Publishing Company, 1979.) The child may have difficulty relating to his or her peers and to school. Often help from someone trained in the difficulties experienced by children with chronic disease is necessary.

Eye Care

Asymptomatic uveitis may occur in children with juvenile rheumatoid arthritis, especially children with pauciarticular arthritis. Young girls with a positive fluorescent antinuclear antibody test are at particular risk. This chronic smoldering inflammation leads to synechiae (adhesions) between the iris and the lens and between the iris and the cornea. The lens and cornea become coated with inflammatory debris. Ultimately cataracts, glaucoma, and band keratopathy result. Only a slit lamp examination will reveal the early signs of inflammation. A slit lamp examination should be performed at least every 6 months, and more often for the pauciarticular group. The treatment of chronic anterior uveitis is difficult and should be done by an ophthalmologist. Topical, intraconjunctival, and oral corticosteroids are used with an appropriate topical mydriatic.

Prognosis

The prognosis of juvenile rheumatoid arthritis should be kept in mind. In 75 per cent of children with juvenile rheumatoid arthritis the disease will remit and the child will be normal or have only minimal functional disabilities. Since the prognosis is in general good, treatment should be careful and conservative. On the other hand, physical therapy should be utilized at its fullest to avoid preventable joint deformities.

ANKYLOSING SPONDYLITIS

method of
ROBERT M. BENNETT, M.D.
Portland, Oregon

Ankylosing spondylitis is a chronic inflammatory disease which principally affects the axial skeleton but can also involve peripheral joints, usually the hips, knees, and shoulders. In its classic form it is a disease of young men (M:F ratio about 9:1), with a prevalence of 0.1 per cent in Caucasians; it is relatively uncommon in blacks. More recent epidemiologic studies, using the HLA-B27 genetic marker, have indicated that about 20 per cent of B27 positive individuals will have evidence of low grade sacroiliitis, with an equal distribution between men and women. For Caucasians this translates into a prevalence of 1.6 per cent. Sacroiliitis is therefore a rather common affliction, with most patients having a mild course, but only 10 per cent, mainly males, will develop significant spondylitis. An understanding of this considerable variation in disease severity is essential in a balanced approach to treatment. A majority of patients, with minimal disease, present with a history of inflammatory low back pain and will benefit from appropriate drug treatment. A minority of patients, mainly young males, will have a potentially crippling form of spondylitis. Early diagnosis is particularly important in such patients, as much can be accomplished in ameliorating symptoms and preventing progressive spinal deformity.

General Considerations

There is no curative therapy available for ankylosing spondylitis. The aims of effective management are five-fold: (1) amelioration of pain and stiffness, (2) maintenance of spinal mobility, (3) prevention of progressive spinal deformity, (4) recognition and treatment of disease complications, and (5) maintenance of a minimally restricted life style. These objectives can be accomplished only by patient cooperation and a lifelong self-discipline in medication and remedial exercises. The necessary motivation will be achieved only by the patient's full understanding of the nature and potential disability of his illness.

General advice as to occupation and recreational activities is often required. Except for those patients with the mildest disease, occupations involving heavy manual labor should be avoided. On the other hand, unduly sedentary jobs with minimal opportunity for moving around and stretching the spine are also to be discouraged. Certain recreational pursuits such as long distance running, competitive weight lifting, high diving, and road cycling may be deleterious to many, but not all, patients. Walking and swimming are excellent forms of exercise. In those patients with more severe disease, a close collaboration is required between a rheumatologist and experts in the fields of ophthalmology and orthopedic surgery.

Physical Therapy

A lifelong exercise program is the cornerstone of the successful management of ankylosing spondylitis. Drug therapy, by reducing pain and stiffness, is a complementary prerequisite that facilitates the successful completion of daily physical therapy.

1. Careful attention to correct posture is mandatory. (a) Patients should always hold themselves erect when standing, being mentally atuned to adopting a "military presence." (b) They should not slouch in chairs, but seek out chairs with a straight back and a headrest. (c) Sleeping posture should be "stretched-out" on a firm mattress with only a small pillow (or none at all), to minimize cervical and thoracic flexion.

2. A self-disciplined exercising regimen should become as routine an activity as shaving or brushing the teeth: (a) Range of motion exercises to maintain flexibility of the spine and peripheral joints. (b) Isometric muscle contraction exercises to strengthen the abdominal muscles, the rhomboids, the quadriceps, and the gluteus. (c) Breathing exercises to promote diaphragmatic breathing and maintain costovertebral joint mobility.

This posture and exercise program should initially be taught by a physical therapist and continued at home. It is important for the physician to routinely re-evaluate the patient's perseverance and the effectiveness of the program at periodic examinations.

Drug Therapy

Appropriate medication aims at giving symptomatic relief by reducing inflammation and minimizing pain, stiffness, and muscle spasm. There is no evidence that drug therapy influences the natural history of the disease, but by facilitating a regular physical therapy program it helps in maintaining spinal mobility and normal function.

1. Phenylbutazone is the most effective drug in providing symptomatic relief. However, the potential complication of bone marrow dyscrasia limits its justifiable use to those patients with particularly active disease or those unresponsive to other medications. Serious toxicity is unusual in the normal dosages used in ankylosing spondylitis: agranulocytosis in 3:10,000 patients (often an idiosyncratic reaction unrelated to total dosage); aplastic anemia in 1:10,000 patients (related to duration of treatment and seen more in the

elderly). These problems necessitate a full blood count every 6 or 8 weeks, and patient education to report fever, rash, sore throat, or bleeding. Other toxic effects include dyspnea, peptic ulceration, stomatitis, edema, hepatitis, and cardiorenal dysfunction. Phenylbutazone is strongly bound to plasma proteins and can interfere with concomitantly administered drugs such as warfarin sodium and oral hypoglycemic agents. Its usual dosage is 100 mg given three or four times daily. Total daily doses of more than 400 mg should not be given on a long-term basis.

2. Indomethacin is the drug of choice for the long-term management of most patients with ankylosing spondylitis. It is usually given in a dosage of 25 mg three times a day. Unacceptable headache, dizziness, or obtunded mentation can occur at any dosage. In such patients the restriction of indomethacin to a dose of 50 to 100 mg, just before retiring to bed, often results in pain-free sleep and a gratifying reduction in morning stiffness without concomitant cerebral side effects. During the daytime the use of some other medication may be required. Other side effects of indomethacin include dyspepsia, peptic ulceration, psychosis, corneal deposits, edema, hepatitis, asthma, antiplatelet antibodies, peripheral neuropathy, and rashes. In the doses recommended for ankylosing spondylitis indomethacin is a remarkably safe drug with a wide therapeutic-toxic ratio.

3. Aspirin is seldom effective in providing good symptomatic relief in ankylosing spondylitis; this is in marked contradistinction to its use in rheumatoid arthritis. Some patients with mild disease may gain some benefit from aspirin, and in these patients it is often preferred on account of its inexpensiveness and relative safety. Other nonsteroidal anti-inflammatory agents, used in higher dosages than usually recommended in the package inserts, may be tried in patients intolerant of indocin: ibuprofen (Motrin),* 2400 mg to 4800 mg per day; naproxen (Naprosyn),* 500 mg to 1000 mg per day; tolmctin (Tolectin),* 1200 mg to 1800 mg per day; and sulindac (Clinoril), 300 to 600 mg per day.

4. Corticosteroids have only a minor role in most cases. Those with persistent peripheral joint involvement may be helped by prednisone, 7.5 mg to 10 mg per day; dosage of 10 mg per day of prednisone should not be exceeded for more than a few days. However, patients with severe ocular inflammation may require high dose corticosteroids on a rapidly tapering dosage regimen.

Intra-articular corticosteroid injections are sometimes indicated in a hip, knee, or shoulder; the steroid of choice is an insoluble preparation such as triamcinolone hexacetonide (Aristospan).

5. Gold, pencillamine, antimalarial agents, and cytoxic drugs are not of proved value in ankylosing spondylitis.

Radiotherapy

This form of treatment provides excellent symptomatic relief and may slow disease progression. However it has now fallen into disrepute on account of the increased incidence of leukemia, aplastic anemia, and other malignancies in patients so treated. Another complication is transverse myelitis. Radiotherapy should not now be used except in exceptional circumstances. A case in point is progressive neck involvement with severe limitation of motion. If used judiciously, in selected cases, before bony fusion has occurred, it may enable the patient to regain enough movement to follow through with a carefully tailored physical therapy program. In such cases the radiotherapist will take care to shield the thyroid gland, and the total dose should not exceed 600 rads.

Surgery

Sometimes surgery is required on the spine and peripheral joints. In those patients with a severe fixed flexion deformity of the spine, so that their field of vision encompasses only a small area in front of the feet, a vertebral wedge osteotomy should be considered. Patients who have developed significant degenerative changes in the hips or knees, secondary to previous inflammation, will usually be helped by appropriate arthroplasties. Destructive arthritis of the temporomandibular joint, causing severe pain on mastication or inadequate jaw opening, can be helped by arthroplasty. Surgical synovectomy of a persistently inflamed peripheral joint is virtually never required; the period of postoperative immobilization invariably leads to a significant deterioration in function. Such patients are best managed with a "medical synovectomy," using a long-acting corticosteroid preparation such as triamcinolone hexacetonide (Aristospan) injected into the joint.

Complications of surgery are common:

1. There is a tendency for bony ankylosis to occur after joint replacement.

2. Intubation is made difficult by jaw involvement or a rigid cervical spine.

3. Atlantoaxial joint involvement can lead to high cervical cord compression during anethesia.

4. Costochondral joint involvement, with a

---

*This use of this agent is not listed in the manufacturer's official directive. See also manufacturer's dosage recommendations.

reduced chest expansion, results in an increased incidence of postoperative pulmonary problems.

5. Wedge osteotomy may be complicated by gastric dilation (caused by stretching of the superior mesenteric artery over the third part of the duodenum), and general immobility poses a real risk from aspiration of vomitus. One experienced surgeon in this area has a 13 per cent mortality.

Special Problems

1. Iritis is treated with atropine and topical corticosteroids. In severe cases systemic steroids are required. Chronic or relapsing iritis is best treated with continuous low dose corticosteroids.

2. Motor vehicle accidents and other trauma may result in fracture of the fused spine. Sudden death and tetraplegia have been reported. Persistent localized pain after an accident should alert one to the possibility of a fracture; radiographs are often difficult to interpret if there is extensive ligamentous calcification. Treatment of a spinal fracture is along conventional lines.

3. Neck fusion poses significant functional problems from the aspect of reading, negotiating street crossings, and driving a car. Reading can be helped by using prismatic spectacles; driving may be made safer by the installation of a right-angled convex mirror on the car hood (bonnet) about 3 feet in front of the driver.

4. A cauda equina syndrome with incontinence of urine, muscle wasting of the lower limbs, and pain in a sciatic distribution may occur in patients with severe longstanding disease. There is no effective definitive treatment to date, and the symptoms must be managed on a purely symptomatic basis.

5. Pulmonary problems should be minimized by refraining from smoking, keeping out of dusty atmospheres, and using appropriate vaccines, e.g., pneumococcal vaccine (Pneumovac), when appropriate. The prompt diagnosis and treatment of chest infections is mandatory. A chronic fibrotic reaction sometimes occurs in the upper lobes; it is often mistaken for tuberculosis. There is no specific treatment.

6. Cardiac problems in the form of conduction disturbances and aortic regurgitation may occur. If significant aortic insufficiency develops, the placement of a prosthetic valve must be considered.

Genetic Counseling

With the new-found knowledge of the association of ankylosing spondylitis with HLA-B27, a gene product of the sixth chromosome, many patients now request genetic counseling. Assuming normal mendelian segregation of a single B27

locus, 1 in 2 children would be B27 positive. About 8 per cent of B27 positive males and 1 per cent of B27 positive female children will later develop significant ankylosing spondylitis. Therefore, the risk of a B27 heterozygote parent having a child who will later develop significant ankylosing spondylitis is 4 per cent for a male child and 0.5 per cent for a female child.

BURSITIS AND CALCIFIC TENDINITIS

method of
RONALD A. RESTIFO, M.D.
San Jose, California

Bursae are small, serous sacs interposed between moving parts to lessen friction effects; tendons are specially arranged cords of fibrous tissue which unite muscle with some other part, most often transmitting force through their attachment with the periosteum of bone. Inflammatory changes in these sites are usually caused by mechanical and degenerative factors, but may be associated with arthritic (rheumatoid arthritis, rheumatoid variants, gout, pseudogout) or septic processes. Common sites of bursitis are the subacromial (lateral aspect of the shoulder), olecranal (circular swelling at the tip of the elbow), and trochanteric (lateral aspect of the hip); the descriptive terms "weaver's bottom" and "housemaid's knee" describe ischiogluteal and prepatellar bursitis, respectively. The anserine bursa is located along the medial aspect of the knee, and, when inflamed, produces localized erythema and swelling. Achilles bursitis occurs at the heel, often from shoe pressure, but requires the exclusion of a rheumatoid variant, particularly in a young male. Tendinitis, with or without calcific deposits, may accompany subacromial bursitis or trochanteric bursitis, but is also seen in the bicipital tendon (anterior aspect of the shoulder), as an epicondylitis (lateral aspect of the elbow), as de Quervain's syndrome (thumb side of the wrist), or involving the inferior aspect of the heel.

Treatment

The objectives of treatment are the relief of pain and inflammation, the restoration of function, and the prevention of degeneration.

1. *Rest:* The patient may simply require general rest or limited weight bearing, but in the

acute and subacute phases a sling, splint, or padding may be indicated.

2. *Cold vs. heat:* Cold helps reduce swelling during the first 24 to 48 hours of the acute phase. Heat with moist hot packs, or by more formal ultrasound or diathermy, is usually more helpful thereafter and in the chronic phase.

3. *Anti-inflammatory medications:* Phenylbutazone, 100 mg four times daily, is often effective. Side effects include gastric irritation, peptic ulcer, decrease in blood count, and fluid retention. Sulindac (Clinoril), in doses of 150 to 200 mg twice a day, has shown similar effectiveness. Although not listed in the indications, anti-inflammatory effects have been noted with indomethacin (Indocin), 25 mg four times a day or 50 mg three times a day, and would be expected with other nonsteroidal anti-inflammatory agents such as fenoprofen (Nalfon), ibuprofen (Motrin), naproxen (Naprosyn), and tolmetin (Tolectin) in therapeutic doses. On occasion, the attack may be so acute as to require oral steroid therapy; start with prednisone, 40 mg, and taper by 5 mg each day.

4. *Analgesics:* The acute and subacute phases usually require moderate analgesia such as propoxyphene napsylate with acetaminophen (Darvocet N), 100 mg every 4 hours, aspirin or acetaminophen (Tylenol) with 30 to 60 mg of codeine every 4 hours, or pentazocine (Talwin), 50 mg every 4 hours as needed. The episode may be sufficiently severe to require meperidine, 50 mg, or oxycodone, aspirin, phenacetin, and caffeine (Percodan), 1 tablet every 6 hours.

5. *Local steroid therapy:* The injection of 40 to 80 mg of methylprednisolone acetate (Depo-Medrol), using a 23 gauge, 1 inch or 25 gauge, 5/8 inch needle at the point of maximal tenderness, can be extremely helpful. The procedure is better tolerated if the area is first sprayed with ethyl chloride. Prior to injecting an acutely inflamed bursa, an attempt should be made to aspirate fluid, which, if obtained, is sent for appropriate analysis. The patient should be informed that a small number of injections result in increased pain and swelling, but that these symptoms are limited to 24 to 48 hours and are tolerated with the use of analgesics and cold packs.

6. Surgery, with bursal resection or removal of calcific deposits, or multiple punctures in an attempt to aspirate calcium or needle the bursa, is necessary in only a small percentage of patients.

7. Treatment with dimethyl sulfoxide (DMSO) or acupuncture, despite popular interest, has not been proved to be effective. Potential future complications have essentially curtailed the use of radiotherapy.

8. Exercises should be avoided in the acute phase, but once healing begins, passive exercises followed by active exercises for muscle strengthening are usually helpful.

9. Long-term goals should include protection of the affected part by muscle-strengthening exercises and elimination of those activities which produce undue stress on the involved area.

OSTEOARTHRITIS

method of
GERSON C. BERNHARD, M.D.
Milwaukee, Wisconsin

Osteoarthritis, whether primary or secondary, develops as a result of biochemical abnormalities and physical stresses in articular cartilage. Alteration of matrix components or impact loading of subchondral bone may initiate the process. Erosion of cartilage follows. A proliferative bone response at joint margins produces osteophytes. A similar subchondral bone response in areas of extra physical stress produces increased thickness (eburnation). The bony changes are easily identified radiographically, but may not correlate with the patient's symptoms. Pain — the cardinal clinical feature of osteoarthritis — can result from early inflammation at joint margins where osteophytes are beginning to form, capsular or tendon sheath irritation, muscle spasm, or, less frequently, intermittent synovitis. Pain arises from periosteum, joint capsule, synovial membrane, and muscle where pain receptors are found — not cartilage. Loss of motion occurs as a result of pain, muscle contracture, and scarring of joint capsule, but rarely from osteophytes. Limited motion alters joint biomechanics, aiding the development of further cartilage degeneration. Other causes of pain in osteoarthritis are neurologic, such as peripheral nerve entrapment or radiculopathy, secondary to osteophyte formation.

General Principles

Patients should be informed of the nature of this disease, distinguishing it from inflammatory destructive arthritis. They can be reassured that terrible deformity and crippling or fatal complications are not likely to ensue. Only selected severely involved joints become destroyed. At the same time, the responsibility for the most effective treatment is shared between the patient and physician. Periods of daily joint rest and avoidance of abuse should be viewed not as a restriction or deprivation but as a rational positive approach to continued function and a safe way to modify pain. Many patients need to be disabused of the notion that more work or physical activity will keep them limber or "work the arthritis out." Excess weight is mechanically hindering to large joint function and back care. Hence, weight reduction for the obese patient is desirable and should be both a goal and responsibility of the patient, with a dietitian's guidance. Sport activities in moderation should not be interdicted, but altered or modified for the specific patient. Many with osteoarthritis of the hip or knee can continue to play golf, but use a motorized cart. Similarly, the jogger should change to swimming. Other activities, such as crocheting or knitting, should be done in moderation, allowing periods for joint rest.

Physical and Occupational Therapy

A range of motion regimen should be taught to most patients by a therapist and performed daily at home. This tends to keep normal joint motion, or regain some lost motion, and prevents progressive contractures, but it does little to relieve pain. Similarly, the occupational therapist can instruct patients in small hand joint motion. Both physical and occupational therapists can introduce principles of joint protection, work simplification, and rest, while instructing in the home range of motion program. A cane, used properly in the contralateral hand of a patient with an afflicted knee or hip, can reduce needless weight bearing, relieve pain, provide stability, and thus enhance independence. Isometric muscle exercises of large groups (such as quadriceps), done regularly, tend to maintain function and joint stability. If the exercised joints hurt for more than an hour after exercising, the therapy program should be modified. Heat — especially moist — offers some analgesia, aids mobility, and reduces muscle spasm. Again, a therapist can instruct patients in home heat techniques, including bathtub whirlpool, that are safe and simple. Since the lumbar spine is frequently afflicted with osteoarthritis and degenerative disc disease, principles of back care and positions of rest should be explained to most patients.

Drugs

There are three reasons for employment of drugs in treating osteoarthritis: analgesia, suppression of inflammation, and relief of muscle spasm. It may be possible to avoid drugs, or to use them intermittently.

Analgesics. Aspirin, plain or with antacids (Ascriptin, Bufferin, Cama) or enteric-coated (Ecotrin, Enseals) are the mainstay of nonnarcotic analgesia. Other salicylate combinations such as salicylsalicylic acid (Persistin), magnesium salicylate (Magan, Mobidin), calcium salicylate (Calurin), choline salicylate (Arthropan), disalicylate (Disalcid), trisalicylate (Trilisate) may be equally effective analgesics, and sometimes have better gastrointestinal tolerance. Doses of 650 to 975 mg of aspirin or its equivalent every 4 to 6 hours as needed for pain are usually effective. Acetaminophen in similar doses can be substituted in patients who cannot tolerate or should avoid salicylates. For more severe pain, narcotics may be necessary temporarily, such as propoxyphene (Darvon, Dolobid), codeine, or oxycodone (Percodan). The group of nonsteroidal anti-inflammatory drugs (NSAID) have some analgesic effect, but are generally less potent than salicylates or acetaminophen.

Anti-inflammatory Agents. During the inflammatory phases of osteoarthritis, or in those patients with a chronic inflammatory component, an anti-inflammatory drug regimen, coupled with other measures, will relieve stiffness, pain, and swelling, and may slow the degenerative process. Aspirin or the other salicylates are again the cornerstone of this drug treatment, but in larger and more constant doses. A maintained salicylate blood level of 15 to 25 mg per dl (100 ml) is considered anti-inflammatory. This usually requires 975 to 1300 mg (15 to 20 grains) of aspirin four times per day, or its equivalent in other salicylate preparations. Changing from one salicylate preparation to another every 2 to 4 weeks to ascertain the most effective and tolerated drug for a specific patient is occasionally justified. The nonsteroidal anti-inflammatory drugs (NSAID) may produce the same or better results in a given individual. Their chief advantages are generally fewer pills required per day and good gastrointestinal tolerance. Each, however, has the potential of rash, headache, modest sodium retention, and gastrointestinal irritation. To obtain the equivalent anti-inflammatory effect of salicylates, one requires 400 to 600 mg four times per day of ibuprofen (Motrin); 600 mg four times per day of fenoprofen (Nalfon); 250 mg two or three times per day of naproxen (Naprosyn); 150 to 200 mg two times per day of sulindac (Clinoril); 75 to 100 mg per day divided doses of indomethacin (Indocin); 100 mg three or four times per day of either phenylbutazone (Butazolidin, Azolid) or oxyphenbutazone (Tandearil, Oxalid); or 400 mg three to four times day of tolmetin (Tolectin).

Adrenal Corticosteroids. Systemic use (oral or parenteral) of these agents is rarely of any value in treatment of osteoarthritis. The serious side effects of their prolonged use make them contraindicated.

Intra-articular injection of anti-inflammatory corticosteroids can suppress severe superimposed inflammation in a specific joint. Aspiration of the excess fluid, as well as putting the joint at rest, may be equally effective. Furthermore, the inhibitory effect of corticosteroids on cartilage polysaccharide synthesis tends to promote the fundamental lesion of osteoarthritis. Repeated intra-articular steroid injections may augment cartilage damage, causing the development of a severe, disorganized form of osteoarthritis or pseudo–Charcot joint. Hence, intra-articular steroids should rarely be used in the treatment of osteoarthritis, and, if used, followed by a period of 2 to 4 weeks of joint rest until cartilage has recovered.

Muscle Relaxants. Relief of muscle spasm is important to pain control and maintenance of joint motion. Rest, heat, splints, gentle massage, and passive motion exercises may accomplish this goal. Muscle relaxing agents may augment this effort. Several drugs can be tried, including diazepam (Valium), 2 to 5 mg three or four times per day, meprobamate (Equanil, Miltown), 400 mg three to four times per day, or methocarbamol (Robaxin), 0.5 to 1 gram four times per day. These drugs should be prescribed for only a short time, and not very frequently, for fear the patient may become habituated.

Surgery

A wide variety of surgical procedures may relieve pain, realign joints, or remove irritative worn cartilage. Removal of torn menisci or loose cartilage bodies may slow the degenerative process by removing the mechanically irritating factors. Redistribution of weight bearing onto less worn cartilage can be accomplished by osteotomy of a hip or knee, but may be only temporarily effective. Total joint replacement or resurfacing has become popular with the advent of new adhesive materials. However, this reconstructive surgery does not reconstitute the degenerated joint to normal, and is not without complications of failure and infection. It should be reserved for the patient with advanced disease who has severe pain on only mild activity and/or disabling deformity with loss of motion. It should not be offered to patients as a means of returning to previously vigorous physical activity. Techniques and hardware are still developing, but are now available for ankles, knees, hips, shoulders, elbows, and wrists.

Measures in Osteoarthritis of the Spine

Rest in the supine position is best for painful osteoarthritis of the lumbar spine, as well as back sprain. The cervical spine is best rested with a small pillow rolled under the neck and/or a semi-soft cervical collar. Traction of either cervical or lumbar spine may have its major effect by putting the affected part at complete rest. This conservative therapy, coupled with analgesics and muscle relaxants, may require many days to a few weeks for maximal benefit. It should be followed by rehabilitation of motion and muscles, with careful attention to principles of back or cervical spine care. Surgical procedures are very infrequently indicated. One such indication, however, is cord compression, with slowly advancing quadriparesis, or lumbar spinal stenosis.

Obstetrics and Gynecology

ANTEPARTUM CARE

method of
RICHARD P. BENDEL, M.D.
Minneapolis, Minnesota

Introduction

The objective of antepartum care is to ensure the delivery of a healthy baby to a healthy mother. This objective is not always obtained, but good care, utilizing current knowledge and techniques, is working to reduce perinatal mortality and morbidity rates, and maternal mortality is nearing an irreducible minimum.

In the past, prenatal visits consisted mostly of checking maternal weight, blood pressure, and fetal heart rate, and answering a few questions the patient had about minor concerns, such as "stretch marks," swollen feet, and backache. These remain important functions of a prenatal visit, but in addition, today we are concentrating on identification of the high-risk patient — if possible even before pregnancy — careful education, sophisticated methods of fetal surveillance, appropriate interference when indicated, and noninterference in the majority of patients.

Pregnancy as a Planned Event

Today, the majority of young married women are using contraception. Unmarried women and teenagers are also increasingly utilizing contraception and visiting private physicians and family planning clinics. The wide acceptance of contraception plus yearly visits for a Papanicolaou smear has given physicians an opportunity to discuss future pregnancy with patients. High-risk patients can be identified, and the importance of planning the pregnancy can be discussed. For example, a patient with diabetes can be told of some of the problems she will face if she decides to become pregnant. A patient with oligo-ovulation can be appraised of the importance of basal body temperatures in documenting ovulation and contraception. Patients with a family history of genetic disorders can be counseled or sent to a genetic counselor, depending on the knowledge and expertise of the physician. The importance of avoiding all drugs, cigarettes, and excessive alcohol in pregnancy should be discussed with all women.

The evidence against cigarette smoking is growing, implicating this habit as an important cause of poor reproductive outcome. Cigarette smoking increases the chances of early abortion, stillbirth, and premature labor. The newborns of smokers weigh an average of 8 ounces less than the infants of nonsmokers, and are at an increased risk of sudden infant death syndrome (SIDS). Recent data released by the United States Collaborative Perinatal Project implicate smoking in placental abruption and heart defects. Surprisingly, women who were smokers but stopped smoking before pregnancy also had an increased risk. Therefore, it is important to continue the efforts to discourage smoking at any time.

Since the report of Jones and Smith in 1973, numerous reports of the "fetal alcohol syndrome" have been published. It appears clear that severe dysmorphic and mental defects can result from chronic alcohol ingestion during pregnancy. As little as 3 ounces of absolute alcohol per day (six drinks or the equivalent in beer or wine) may cause the syndrome. Smaller amounts of alcohol may also be harmful. Currently, the Department of Health, Education, and

Welfare has recommended that pregnant women have no more than two drinks per day. "Binge" drinking should be completely avoided, as high levels of blood alcohol even for a short time may be harmful to the fetus.

All drugs should be avoided during pregnancy, especially during embryogenesis. Women who may possibly become pregnant in the near future should be cautioned to communicate with their physician before taking any medication if there is a chance they may be in early pregnancy.

Women discontinuing the use of oral contraceptives should be advised to wait at least one cycle before trying to conceive. There is at least a suggestion in the literature that conception in the month following discontinuance of oral contraceptives results in a slightly higher rate of congenital anomalies. Also, since there may be a delay in resuming regular cyclic ovulation, dating of the pregnancy will be easier.

Confirmation of Pregnancy

Women should be told to have an early examination in suspected pregnancy. The first appointment should be 2 to 4 weeks after missing a menses. Early examination is extremely helpful in calculating an accurate estimated date of delivery. Rapid tests of urine for HCG (human chorionic gonadotropin) can be done in the office, and are reasonably reliable at 40 to 42 days after the last menstrual period (LMP). Radio Receptor Assays (RRA) for HCG can now be obtained in most larger laboratories for about $15. These tests become positive as early as 8 days following conception. The RRA for HCG has been helpful in cases of suspected early ectopic pregnancy, whereas urinary HCG tests are falsely negative in 50 per cent of ectopic pregnancies.

Many physicians and clinics now have smaller Doppler units for early detection of the fetal heart. With careful scanning, the fetal heart beat can be positively identified at 10 to 12 weeks. Some offices even have ultrasound. Positive identification of a beating fetal heart can be made at 8 weeks. These modalities are very helpful when the patient is spotting or bleeding in the first trimester and the diagnosis is threatened abortion. If a living embryo is demonstrated by either of these techniques, there is a much higher chance of the pregnancy continuing.

When the pregnancy is confirmed, the patient can be cautioned against medication and drugs (as noted previously), questions answered, and the "due date" calculated. Pregnancy lasts an average of 280 days (40 weeks) from first day of LMP until delivery, or 266 days (38 weeks) from conception. Clinicians always talk of pregnancy in menstrual weeks, whereas embryologists and others often speak of weeks from conception. For example, when a clinician states that a genetic amniocentesis is best done at 15 to 16 weeks, he or she means 13 to 14 conception weeks. The estimated date of confinement (EDC) can be calculated by Naegele's rule. From the date of the LMP, subtract 3 months, then add 7 days and a year to get EDC. An LMP of August 10, 1980 would be given an EDC of May 17, 1981.

First Prenatal Visit

A careful and complete history, physical examination, pelvic evaluation, initial laboratory work, diagnosis of high-risk factors, and discussion of findings and recommendations should be done.

History. In addition to the usual historical data, a concentrated search for high-risk factors should be made. This is facilitated by using one of the new high-risk scoring prenatal forms, such as the American College of Obstetricians and Gynecologists (ACOF) approved form from the Hollister Company.

Menstrual History. Age at menarche and frequency, duration, and regularity of menses are determined. Patients with a history of oligoovulation will need careful assessment of uterine size and possibly sonography to accurately set EDC. Note the recent history of contraceptive use. Is the pregnancy a failure of a vaginal barrier method? Is it the result of an IUD failure? If the IUD is still in the uterus, it should be removed if the suture is available to grasp with a forceps. Pregnancy with an IUD in the uterus is subject to approximately 50 per cent loss if the IUD is removed and 50 per cent loss if the IUD is left in place. However, if the IUD is left in place, there is increased danger to the mother, as these patients have increased risk of late second trimester losses along with severe pelvic infection and maternal death. A woman who becomes pregnant immediately after stopping oral contraceptives may have had delayed ovulation, and the LMP cannot be used uncritically to set the EDC. Some patients may have been taking oral contraceptives haphazardly and will have taken them during early pregnancy. According to the reports of Janerich and coworkers and of Nora and Nora, these women have a two-fold risk above that of the general population of having a child with a congenital heart defect. Patients should be made aware of these increased risks on their initial visit.

Past Obstetric History. Careful recording of all previous pregnancies, including any losses, complications of labor and delivery, and fetal outcome should be done. Past records of pelvimetry and cesarean section should be obtained.

A history of any pregnancy loss (other than one early spontaneous abortion) places the patient at increased risk for a poor outcome in the current pregnancy.

Past Medical History. This must include at least the following: (1) General health. (2) Hypertension. (3) Heart disease. (4) Diabetes. (5) Kidney disease (infection, calculi, glomerulonephritis). (6) Anemia. (7) Venereal disease. (8) Surgery. (9) Blood transfusions. (10) Allergies. (11) Drug abuse. (12) Alcohol and cigarette use. (13) Psychiatric illness. (14) Other serious illnesses.

Present Pregnancy. (1) Bleeding. (2) Cramping. (3) Pelvic pain. (4) Fetal movement — "quickening." (5) Breast soreness, fullness. (6) Urinary symptoms. (7) Weight change. (8) Medication (both prescribed and "over the counter"). (9) Nausea or vomiting.

Family History. Special attention should be paid to any history of chromosomal defects, neural tube defects, and other birth defects. A family history of diabetes is also important. Hypertension, heart disease, cancer, and so forth, are included for completeness of the record. The occurrence of twins in the family, as a rule, is simply due to normal chance. Occasionally, a family will have a strongly positive history of several generations of frequent multiple gestations.

Physical Examination

A thorough physical examination must be done and includes the following:

1. Blood pressure and pulse.
2. Weight and height.
3. Eyes, ears, nose, and throat (EENT) — includes careful funduscopic evaluation of blood vessels.
4. Teeth — good teeth are important for good nutrition. There is still a common misconception that teeth deteriorate during pregnancy. Teeth will not be harmed if the patient has proper dental care. Bleeding and swollen gums are secondary to the accumulation of scale (tartar) at the gum line. The patient should see a dentist for complete cleaning and removal of scale; she should be taught proper brushing and massaging of gums and do these each day, which will prevent these problems.
5. Thyroid.
6. Heart — flow murmurs are heard in 50 per cent of pregnant women. Other murmurs, arrhythmias, and cardiac enlargement must be evaluated as in the nonpregnant person.
7. Breasts — self-examination should be taught to all women.
8. Abdomen.

9. Extremities — varicose veins, edema.
10. Neurologic — deep tendon reflexes (DTR), toe signs.
11. Pelvis. *External genitalia and Bartholin's, Skene's, and urethral glands (BSU):* look for evidence of inflammation, discharge, excoriation.

Vagina: look for discharge, erythema, lesions; Candida vaginitis is more frequent in pregnancy — diagnosis is by KOH preparation and treatment is with miconazole nitrate (Monistat Cream).

Cervix: description of length, external os, internal os, defects from past obstetric trauma, conization, etc.

Corpus: size, consistency, mobility. Estimating size in the first trimester is very important, and the accurate setting of EDC can play an extremely helpful role in management of late pregnancy complications. From 6 to 12 weeks' menstrual age, the experienced examiner should be able to set the size of the uterus within ± 1 week. (This excludes patients with gross obesity, uterine myomas, and uterine anomalies.)

Adnexa: ovarian size and mobility. Frequently a corpus luteum of pregnancy can be palpated; usually it is not any larger than 5 to 6 cm.

Rectum: hemorrhoids and masses.

Mensuration: clinical mensuration should be done on all patients on the first visit. Occasionally a patient will not tolerate complete evaluation until later in pregnancy. (a) Ischial spines: note whether sharp, blunt, prominent, or widely spaced. (b) Sacrosciatic notch: >2½ fingerbreadths (fb) is normal. (c) Sidewalls: parallel or convergent. (d) Sacrum: deep, average, flattened. (e) Diagonal conjugate: >12.0 cm. Obstetric conjugate is 1½ cm less than measured conjugate diameter (CD). (f) Arch: two fingers should fit under arch; inferior rami of pubic bones should make an angle >90 degrees. (g) Intertuberous (TI): should measure >9.0 cm. (h) Coccyx: movable, fixed, angulated from past injury.

If any measurements are questionable, make a notation to recheck at 36 weeks. Clinical pelvimetry ought not to be discarded, even though in recent years it appears to be not as important as in the past. The true test of pelvic adequacy obviously comes during labor and delivery. Most clinicians prefer to follow the course of labor, with careful continuous electronic fetal monitoring as well, and if labor progresses normally with continuous cervical dilatation, descent of the presenting part, and normal fetal heart rate recordings, the pelvis is considered adequate for this fetus.

X-ray pelvimetry has been greatly overused in the past. Unnecessary x-ray exposure to the fetus and mother should be avoided whenever possible. Antepartum x-ray pelvimetry should be done only in the following clinical situations:

1. History of fractured pelvis.

2. Breech presentation.

3. Past history of difficult forceps delivery and clinical suspicion of contracted pelvis.

4. Previous cesarean section for nonrecurring indications when subsequent vaginal delivery is being considered.

Joyce and others have shown that antepartum x-ray pelvimetry for a high head almost never influences the management of labor. When a patient is admitted in labor with a questionable abnormal presentation, a fetogram and pelvimetry are indicated. Some clinicians will perform x-ray pelvimetry during labor before using oxytocin stimulation, whereas others, in recent years, have been relying more on continuous fetal monitoring (as noted previously).

Laboratory Studies

1. Hematocrit or hemoglobin level. Obtained initially and (if within normal range) repeated every 2 months. If hematocrit level is 30 mg per 100 ml or less, or hemoglobin level less than 10.5 grams per 100 ml, red cell indices and serum ferritin determinations are done for evaluation of type of anemia and iron stores.

2. Blood type, Rh type, and screen for irregular antibodies. If patient is Rh negative and unsensitized, repeat at 26, 34, and 38 weeks. If irregular antibodies are found, consultation is needed — see below.

3. Urinalysis and urine culture. Tests for bacteriuria, such as Culturia, are simple and inexpensive and can be done in the office. Urine "dip stick" test for protein and glucose is performed at each subsequent visit.

4. VDRL test.

5. Gonococcus (GC) culture from cervix.

6. Papanicolaou smear.

7. Rubella titer. If less than 1:10, patient is not immune and should be vaccinated after delivery.

8. Sickle cell screen on black patients.

9. Fasting blood sugar (FBS) and 2 hour postprandial blood sugar determinations for selected patients with these factors: (a) Glucosuria. (b) Previous infant weighing more than 4000 grams (9 pounds). (c) Family history of diabetes. (d) Unexplained pregnancy losses. (e) Previous infant with congenital anomalies. These studies should be done initially, at 28 weeks, and when glucosuria is found.

Counseling

Weight and Nutrition. More and more attention is rightly being paid to proper nutrition. Hand in hand with good nutrition is appropriate weight gain during pregnancy. In the past, physicians gave ill-advised recommendations to restrict weight gain, to the detriment of some patients. The average and desirable weight gain during pregnancy is 11 kg (24 lb). Women underweight at the beginning of pregnancy should gain more. Women significantly overweight may restrict weight gain to 7 kg (15 lb). No pregnant woman should lose weight. Weight gain is usually 2 kg (4 to 5 lb) in the first 12 weeks, then 0.34 kg (0.75 lb) per week until term.

Poor nutrition may result in poor reproductive performance and low birth weight infants. Risk factors for poor nutrition are the following:

1. Adolescence, especially less than 15 years of age.

2. Three or more pregnancies within 2 years.

3. Economic deprivation.

4. Food faddism.

5. History of poor reproductive outcome.

6. Heavy smoking, alcoholism, or drug addiction.

7. Prepregnancy weight less than 85 per cent of normal, or less than 100 pounds. Also, persons who are obese with weight more than 120 per cent of normal for height.

These patients should have consultation with a dietitian or nutritionist. For economically deprived women, "WIC" (Supplemental Food Program for Women, Infants and Children) and United States Department of Agriculture (USDA) food stamps are available. Information on eligibility can be obtained from local health departments or the regional office of the USDA.

Smoking. As noted previously, patients should be encouraged to stop smoking if at all possible or to cut it down to the minimum.

Alcohol. Abstain from alcohol completely if possible. The pregnant woman should have no more than two drinks per day (or equivalent in wine or beer), and no binge drinking should be done.

Exercise. Exercise is good for the normal healthy patient. Studies have shown that the pregnant patient in good physical condition has a shorter, easier labor with fewer complications. The patient should not exercise to complete exhaustion, nor should she engage in dangerous exercise. As the uterus enlarges in the second half of pregnancy, agility and balance are impaired, and exercise or sports requiring fine coordination and delicate balance may not be possible.

Work. Pregnancy disability for most patients does not begin until the onset of labor.

Obviously, complications may arise, e.g., twins, hypertension, and placenta previa, that will require restriction of activities.

Sex. The usual coital practices of most patients may continue throughout pregnancy until labor begins, membranes rupture, or an obstetric complication intervenes. In the last few months, the couple may find coitus more comfortable lying on their sides.

Travel. Travel is not restricted during pregnancy. The most serious problem is that premature labor and other complications may occur in the course of travel, and the patient is then caught away from familiar physicians and hospital and without her medical record being available. When traveling, the patient should be cautioned to stand up and walk about every 2 hours to minimize venous stasis.

Drugs. The only medication that needs to be prescribed for most patients is oral iron supplements. Pregnancy requirements for iron are approximately 800 mg, which amounts to 3 mg per day. Most women do not absorb that much from a normal diet, so 30 to 60 mg daily of ferrous sulfate or gluconate should be prescribed. Three tablets a day is excessive. Also, the patient does not have to start taking iron tablets until the second trimester, when nausea has disappeared and embryogenesis has been accomplished.

Occasionally folic acid may be needed for a patient with anemia and evidence of folate deficiency on work-up.

Prenatal vitamins are not needed for most patients. If the patient has one or more of the high-risk factors noted earlier under Weight and Nutrition, a multiple vitamin capsule may be prescribed prenatally.

The nausea of early pregnancy is often so severe that patients need treatment. Doxylamine succinate and pyridoxine hydrochloride (Bendectin) may be prescribed for this. It has been used for several decades and appears to be safe. If it has any teratogenic effect, it is minuscule. All other drugs are given only for very serious medical conditions.

Genetic Counseling

Midtrimester transabdominal amniocentesis is now the accepted standard of practice for prenatal detection of a variety of genetic diseases. United States courts have held physicians responsible for not informing high-risk patients of the availability of these studies. The amniocentesis is done as an outpatient procedure at 15 to 16 weeks' menstrual age (13 to 14 weeks' conception age). It is preceded by ultrasound to confirm the stage of gestation, localize the placenta, diagnose

multiple gestation, and select the puncture site. There is essentially no risk to the mother from the procedure. There is an increased abortion risk, in the range of 0.5 to 1.0 per cent. The following groups of patients should be made aware of the availability of genetic amniocentesis:

1. Women aged 35 years and older.
2. Parents who have a previous child with Down's syndrome or other chromosomal defect.
3. Known translocation carriers.
4. Carriers for metabolic errors.
5. Previous child with neural tube defect, or when either parent has survived despite a neural tube defect.

Subsequent Prenatal Visits

Traditionally, after the initial work-up, the timetable has been to see patients every 4 weeks until 30 weeks, every 2 weeks until 36 weeks, and then once each week. Do not hesitate to see patients more often if there is any complication; e.g., if there are suspicious signs of early preeclampsia at 32 weeks, have the patient return in 1 week or sooner.

All patients should be seen at 18 to 20 weeks to document fetal heart tones with the fetoscope. This helps date the pregnancy, as experienced examiners should be able to detect fetal heart tones (FHT) by 20 weeks' menstrual age. If FHT are not heard, sonography should be done.

On each visit, the following items are assessed:

1. Weight and blood pressure.
2. Urine for glucose and protein.
3. History of untoward symptoms since previous visit.
4. Abdominal examination with FHT and measurement of uterine fundus. The most accurate and reproducible way to measure uterine growth is to use a tape measure in the midline and record the distance in centimeters from symphysis pubis, over the prominence of the uterus, to the fundus in the plane of the sternum. From 22 weeks until 36 weeks, growth averages 1 cm each week; i.e., at 28 weeks the uterus measures 28 cm. A discrepancy of more than 2 cm should make one suspicious of uterine size inappropriate for dates.
5. Palpation of fetal presentation and fetal parts.
6. Pelvic examination should be done on several visits in the last month. This is to confirm diagnosis of presentation and assess status of the cervix. Pelvic examination should be done at any time when indicated by history of contractions, discharge, etc.
7. Edema.

8. Answer questions the patient may have.

On one or more of the prenatal visits, the following must be discussed.

Breast Feeding

Fortunately for the baby, breast-feeding has come back into vogue. For years, most practitioners believed that breast-feeding was best but that there really was not *that much* difference between mother's milk and commercial formula. In addition, physicians did not want the new mother to feel guilty if she chose not to nurse.

In actuality, human breast milk and cow's milk are very much different except for water and lactose content. Protein composition and aminogram are very different. Lactoferrin and lysozyme are missing from cow's milk, and the casein systems are different. Cow's milk is hypernatremic and hyperosmolar.

Breast-fed babies have fewer infections, particularly diarrhea, than bottle-fed babies. This is due to both lack of chances for contamination of the milk (compared to prepared formula) and a variety of host resistance factors contained in breast milk. These include IgA, lysozyme, and bifidus factor, as well as many macrophages and lymphocytes. These white cells are protected in the stomach by the whey clot and pass into the small intestine. There they migrate into the gut mucosa and take up positions along the lamina propria and confer passive immunity on the baby.

Another benefit of breast milk is the antiallergic effects. Cow's milk protein, namely betalactoglobulin (not present in human milk), is the single most common food allergen in infancy. Breast-feeding and avoiding semisolid foods until 6 months of age are the best prophylaxis against infant food allergies.

Successful breast-feeding appears to depend heavily on the attitude of patient and her close friends and relatives. Anatomic reasons for failure are few. Maternal anxiety is probably the most common reason for failure. All pregnant women should be actively encouraged to breast-feed. Local LaLeche League groups are most helpful in providing woman-to-woman instructions in techniques.

Childbirth Preparation

Classes conducted by Lamaze groups and Childbirth Education Association are now available throughout the country. All patients and prospective fathers (significant other) are encouraged to participate in these classes. "Preparation for Parenting" classes are also becoming available in many communities. Experience has shown that the woman who enters labor well informed and emotionally prepared tolerates labor much better and requires less analgesia and anesthesia than the ill-prepared patient.

Labor and Delivery Expectations

More and more patients are expecting their delivery experience to differ significantly from the traditional sterile labor and delivery as practiced in most United States hospitals over the past 40 to 50 years. Women want their husbands with them throughout labor and delivery. They are asking for delivery in a birthing room. They want to handle their infants immediately and to nurse them immediately. They are asking for a delay (for 1 to 2 hours) of instillation of $AgNO_3$ drops so that they can make "en face" contact with the infant. They are decrying the traditional enema and perineal shave. In the usual situation, when there are no medical complications, the physician should cooperate with and be the leader in encouraging these changes to make childbirth as humane and family centered as possible. Obviously, if the patient expects some of these changes, and the physician or hospital is tradition bound, there will be conflicts. These must be discussed and settled ahead of time if the time of delivery is to be a joyful experience for all concerned.

Intrauterine Fetal Assessment

Ultrasound. Sonographic studies of the uterine contents have become increasingly more helpful at all stages of gestation. The time is approaching when nearly every gravid woman will have one or more ultrasound studies during pregnancy. Some of the current indications are the following:

1. First trimester bleeding — fetal movement or fetal heart activity confirm living pregnancy.

2. Diagnosis of hydatidiform mole.

3. After 14 weeks, fetal biparietal for calculation of gestational age.

4. Diagnosis of twins.

5. Placental localization. (a) Preceding amniocentesis. (b) Placenta previa. (c) Abruptio placentae.

6. Intrauterine growth rate retardation (IUGR) — serial biparietal studies to assess growth.

7. Diagnosis of fetal anomalies.

8. Diagnosis of fetal death in utero.

Amniocentesis. Transabdominal puncture of the amniotic sac with aspiration of fluid for analysis has also become a common procedure in the practice of obstetrics. Amniocentesis is used in the following situations: (1) prenatal detection of genetic disorders, (2) evaluation of isoimmunized pregnancies, (3) determination of fetal lung maturity, or (4) amniography (rare cases).

Oxytocin Challenge Test (OCT) or Contraction Stress Test (CST). Following the report by Ray and colleagues in 1972, the Oxytocin Challenge Test (or Contraction Stress Test) has become one of the most useful of all tests to evaluate fetal well-being. It is used for any patient suspected to be at high risk for uteroplacental insufficiency, e.g., maternal diabetes, hypertension. In general, it is not used before 28 weeks' gestation.

CONTRAINDICATIONS. Certain clinical conditions may contraindicate the OCT, and these include previous classic cesarean section, placenta previa, and those conditions under which possible premature labor from the OCT would outweigh its advantages, such as multiple gestation, incompetent cervix, and premature rupture of membranes.

PROCEDURE. The test is performed in the labor suite. The bed is elevated 30 degrees, and the patient tilted slightly to the left to reduce the possibility of supine hypotension. An intravenous infusion of dextrose solution is started and blood pressure and pulse rate are obtained every 20 minutes. The external tocodynamometer and fetal monitor are attached, and uterine contractions and FHR are recorded. The fetal signal can be obtained by ultrasound, phonocardiogram, or external fetal electrocardiogram (ECG).

After a baseline observation period of at least 30 minutes, dilute oxytocin is begun at 1.0 milliunit per minute and increased progressively until uterine contractions are occurring every 3 to 4 minutes. Arbitrarily, three contractions in a 10 minute period has been selected as sufficient for an adequate OCT.

INTERPRETATION. The results can fall into one of five categories:

1. Negative. No late decelerations are noted.

2. Positive. Repetitive late decelerations.

3. Suspicious. At least one definite late deceleration.

4. Unsatisfactory. Either the technical quality of the recording is such that late decelerations cannot be ruled out or there is a failure to stimulate sufficient uterine activity. An unsatisfactory test is of no help and usually should be repeated the next day.

5. Hyperstimulation. There is excessive uterine activity present along with heart rate deceleration. When the contractions occur more often than every 2 minutes or last longer than 90 seconds or there is increased baseline tonus, this is called hyperstimulation and is not suitable for clinical purposes.

EVALUATION. Accumulated experience has shown that a normal OCT is very reassuring. There will be no more than two or three fetal deaths per thousand during the week following a negative OCT. A positive OCT is more difficult to interpret. If no action is taken, 20 per cent or more fetuses will die in utero during the next week. However, if labor is induced, approximately 60 per cent of the fetuses will tolerate labor and can be delivered vaginally.

Nonstress Test (NST). The NST has been evaluated over the past 3 or 4 years and is now the single most useful antepartum test of fetal well-being. Compared to the OCT, it is easier, faster, and more economical, and it is noninvasive. There are no contraindications to its use.

PROCEDURE. The patient lies on her side in the semi-Fowler position and the monitor belts are applied. The fetal heart rate (FHR) is recorded for 15 to 30 minutes, and fetal movement is also noted on the tracing. If the fetus is healthy, there will be a FHR acceleration of 15 beats per minute lasting for at least 15 seconds associated with fetal movement. Two accelerations in a 30 minute period constitute evidence of fetal well-being. A reactive fetus is just as reassuring as a negative OCT. Depending on the high-risk population being evaluated, 80 to 90 per cent will have reactive tests, and an OCT will not have to be done. If the fetus is nonreactive, then proceed to OCT (see previous discussion).

Hormone Assays. Tests for determining urinary or serum estriol levels are available and are especially useful for following patients with chronic hypertension, preeclampsia, intrauterine growth retardation, and diabetes. Both have wide day-to-day fluctuations as high as 40 per cent. Therefore, serial determinations are mandatory to follow the trends. Determinations of estriol levels are most often used in conjunction with NST and OCT.

Determinations of human placental lactogen (HPL) have not proved to be useful and have generally been discarded.

Lecithin to Sphingomyelin (L/S) Ratio. Determination of amniotic fluid surface-active phospholipids has come to be the premier test of fetal lung maturity. It has replaced creatinine determinations and Nile blue sulfate staining. If the lecithin to sphingomyelin ratio on the acetone precipitable fraction (this is primarily dipalmitoyl lecithin) is 2 or more, the respiratory distress syndrome (RDS) will be extremely rare in the neonate — <2 per cent — if the fetus does not become acidotic during labor and delivery. Most reports of falsely mature L/S leading to a higher percentage of RDS were the result of determining the L/S ratio on amniotic fluid without going through the cold acetone precipitation step. Presence of phosphatidyl glycerol (PG) can also be determined as an additional help. Although PG makes up less than 10 per cent of the surface-active phospholipids, it does not appear in amniotic fluid until 37 to 38 weeks and, therefore, is a sure sign of fetal lung maturity.

Prevention and Treatment of Complications

Here, a variety of complications will be discussed. The problems selected are primarily those that develop during the antepartum course, not maternal medical complications that antedated the pregnancy, e.g., maternal diabetes, which would require a complete monograph of its own.

Multiple Pregnancy. Twins occur in slightly more than 1 per cent of pregnancies, yet account for about 10 per cent of perinatal mortality. Multiple gestation must be diagnosed prenatally in order to be treated. Approximately one half of twin gestations are not diagnosed until labor and delivery. The more suspicious the practitioner is, the higher the percentage of antepartum diagnosis. In some clinics, an ultrasound study is done on all patients at 20 weeks to diagnose multiple gestation. If twins are found, the following program is recommended:

1. Begin frequent rest periods as soon as diagnosis is confirmed.

2. The patient should stop working at 26 to 28 weeks.

3. Modified bed rest at home from 26 to 36 weeks.

4. Frequent cervical checks.

5. Instruct patient to report any unusual uterine activity.

6. If any sign of cervical effacement or premature labor occurs, start isoxsuprine, 20 mg four times daily, and begin strict bed rest.

7. If labor begins before 35 weeks, deliver in a Level III perinatal center.

8. If triplets or more than three fetuses are present, hospitalize in a Level III perinatal center starting at 28 weeks or sooner if indicated.

9. Neonatologist or pediatrician should be present at delivery.

Intrauterine Growth Retardation (IUGR). This occurs in approximately 5 per cent of births and is very frequently (50 per cent) not diagnosed antenatally. Be suspicious — if the uterus is small for dates, it should not automatically be attributed to poor dating. Obtain an ultrasound measurement of fetal biparietal diameter. Results are most accurate if the initial study is done before 26 weeks. Serial studies to follow growth will usually be needed. If diagnosis seems likely, then the fetus is followed with weekly nonstress test (NST) and estriol determinations, and is delivered when the lungs are mature. (See previous discussion of current testing of intrauterine fetal status).

IUGR is the most common cause of neonatal hypoglycemia. Anytime this diagnosis is suspected, or whenever the physician delivering a baby is surprised by its small size or scrawny appearance, a pediatrician should be notified immediately and the neonate tested serially for blood glucose levels. The initial glucose level should be obtained within 1 hour on IUGR babies.

Infections. Approximately 5 to 6 per cent of women have asymptomatic bacteriuria. During pregnancy, acute pyelonephritis occurs in 1 per cent of patients. Most of these acute episodes occur in women with bacteriuria. When asymptomatic bacteria are found, the patient should be treated with a 10 day course of antibiotics and follow-up monthly urine cultures should be obtained. If repeated cultures are positive, retreatment and continuous prophylaxis are instituted. If an acute urinary tract infection occurs, treatment consists of the following:

1. Hospitalization.

2. Parenteral antibiotics (appropriately selected by sensitivity testing).

3. Intravenous fluids.

4. Uterine and FHR monitoring to detect fetal distress or onset of premature labor.

5. Measures to stop premature labor (if there is no evidence of fetal distress).

6. Continuous treatment with oral antibiotics until labor. Sulfisoxazole (Gantrisin),* 500 mg four times daily, and nitrofurantoin (Furadantin),* 100 mg four times daily, have proved to be safe and effective. Gantrisin must be used carefully near term if hyperbilirubinemia of the newborn is expected, e.g., blood group isoimmunization. Furadantin should not be used in persons with G6PD deficiency (2 per cent of black women).

Isoimmunization. Thirteen per cent of whites, 8 per cent of blacks, and 1 per cent of Asian peoples are Rh negative. Therefore Rh incompatibility is by far the most serious potential cause of isoimmunization. However, since 1968, the availability of Rho(D) immune globulin (human) (RhoGAM) has greatly reduced the perinatal loss secondary to erythroblastosis from anti-D antibody. There are many other red cell surface antigens, and virtually all can cause se-

---

*See manufacturer's official directive before using for this purpose.

vere hemolytic disease. Some of these are the Kell, Duffy (Fy), M, and others. Lewis antigens (Le^a and Le^b) are notable exceptions. Since the fetal red cells do not have this antigen, anti-Le antibodies will not destroy the fetal red cell. Rh positive women can also become sensitized, usually to c of the Rh system.

When antibody screening is negative, repeat screening at 26, 34, and 38 weeks.

If antibody titers develop, screening must be repeated every 2 to 4 weeks during the second half of pregnancy. As long as titers remain 1:8 or less, there is virtually no chance of fetal hydrops and death, and the patient may be allowed to progress to term.

When the titer reaches 1:16, amniocentesis must be done and the excess optical density at 450 millimicrometers plotted on the Liley graph. The first amniocentesis should be done at 22 weeks if titers are significant. Intrauterine fetal transfusion can begin at 24 to 25 weeks if the fetus is severely affected. Because of availability of RhoGAM, Rh disease is much less common, but it still remains responsible for significant perinatal mortality. Because of the decreased incidence, fewer physicians are knowledgeable in this field, so when it occurs consultation with an expert is necessary for the average practitioner.

Approximately 1.5 per cent of Rh negative women will become sensitized during their first term pregnancy, usually in the last trimester. Bowman of Winnipeg has shown that this can be prevented by giving an injection of RhoGAM at 28 weeks' gestation (and again following delivery if the newborn is Rh positive). Prophylaxis at 28 weeks will soon become standard antepartum care.

Varicose Veins. About 20 per cent of pregnant women suffer from varices. There is a familial tendency for these to occur. They tend to appear in late first trimester, gradually become worse, and resolve fairly quickly after delivery, leaving some residual problem. The severity of varicose veins increases with each pregnancy.

TREATMENT. 1. Rest with legs elevated several times each day.

2. Use elastic support.

3. During periods of standing or inactivity, perform exercises such as repetitive flexing of ankles or rising up on tiptoes.

Pregnancy leotards that are measured for each individual patient have proved extremely effective in eliminating the discomfort and aching of varices of both lower extremities and vulva. These can be obtained from Jobst Institute, Inc. (653 Miami Street, Toledo, Ohio 43695).

ABORTION

method of
PAUL OGBURN, M.D.,
and WILLIAM E. BRENNER, M.D.
Chapel Hill, North Carolina

Abortion is defined as removal of the products of conception from the uterus prior to the time that the fetus is sufficiently developed for extrauterine survival. Abortions may be divided into those that are spontaneous and those that are induced. Spontaneous abortions may be divided into the following groups: (1) complete abortion, (2) incomplete abortion, (3) inevitable abortion, (4) threatened abortion, (5) missed abortion, and (6) habitual abortion.

Induced abortions may be divided according to the gestational age of the pregnancy and the techniques available for pregnancy termination.

Spontaneous Abortion

Pregnancy that terminates prior to the time of fetal viability without instrumentation or medical induction is termed spontaneous abortion.

Complete Abortion. Complete abortion is when all the products of conception are evacuated from the uterus. This may be either diagnosed by identifying the complete products of conception or presumed, if the products of conception are not available for examination, by finding the uterus contracted, firm, and with minimal bleeding from the cervical os.

THERAPEUTIC CONSIDERATIONS. 1. Pelvic examination should be performed to identify abnormal pelvic masses and signs of products of conception, such as uterine atony, significant bleeding per the cervical os, and tissue in the cervical os.

2. Vital signs and hematocrit should be determined to evaluate sepsis, excessive blood loss, and impending shock.

3. Blood type and Rh sensitization should be determined. If the patient is Rh negative and unsensitized, 75 micrograms of Rh immune globulin (MicRhoGAM) should be given intramuscularly.

4. Passed tissue should be examined grossly and microscopically to assure completeness of abortion and presence of fetal tissue to rule out ectopic pregnancy and trophoblastic disease.

5. Contraception and counseling should be offered.

6. Methylergonovine (Methergine), 0.2 mg

orally every 6 to 8 hours for a total of six to eight doses, may be given if the patient is not hypertensive or allergic and has no history of peripheral vascular disease. This helps involution of the uterus and decreases postabortal bleeding.

Incomplete Abortion. In incomplete abortion the products of conception are only partially expelled. There is uterine bleeding and an open cervical os. Frequently the uterus is enlarged and boggy.

THERAPEUTIC CONSIDERATIONS. 1. The abortion frequently can be completed by removing the remaining products of conception (usually the placenta) from the lower uterine segment with ring forceps under sterile conditions. If the abortion is easily completed, the same procedures listed for complete abortion can be performed and the patient can usually be discharged from the clinic or emergency room.

2. If the remaining products of conception are not easily extracted or the patient continues to have a boggy uterus, bleed, or show signs of infection, shock, or hypovolemia, she should be admitted to the hospital. Intravenous infusion of lactated Ringer's or isotonic saline solution should be started with 20 to 30 units of oxytocin in every 1000 ml.

3. If the uterus is less than 12 weeks' size, the remaining products of conception usually can be evacuated by suction curettage under sterile conditions. This should be followed by sharp curettage to check for completeness.

4. After 12 weeks' gestation, special forceps (Biere forceps) are useful for removing the fetus and the placenta.

5. Once fetal tissue has been expelled from the uterus, the cervix has usually dilated enough for the suction curettage to be done without mechanical dilatation.

6. In patients who have not expelled the fetus and are over 16 weeks pregnant, induction with intravenous oxytocin may be preferred (see manufacturer's official directive concerning induction with oxytocin). If infection occurs, the fetus may have to be extracted with special abortion forceps followed by suction curettage. After 16 weeks' gestation, the placenta is usually more easily removed with forceps than by suction or sharp curettage.

7. Paracervical block or a 25 to 50 mg dose of intravenous meperidine (Demerol) given slowly may give adequate pain relief. Rarely it is necessary to perform the curettage under general anesthesia.

8. Methylergonovine (Methergine) may be used in the aforementioned manner.

9. Seventy-five micrograms of Rh immune globulin (MicRhoGAM) should be given to un-

sensitized Rh negative women by intramuscular injection.

10. Blood should be transfused when indicated by vital signs or hematocrit level.

11. Patients may usually be discharged safely 4 to 12 hours after the procedure if their conditions are stable.

12. The incidence of endometritis requiring subsequent hospitalization may be decreased by treating the patient with tetracycline, 250 mg four times daily for 5 days.

Inevitable Abortion and Threatened Abortion. Inevitable abortion is characterized by uterine bleeding, cramping, and progressive cervical dilatation. The inevitable abortion should be completed in the same manner as that noted for the incomplete abortion.

Threatened abortion is characterized by uterine bleeding and cramping *without* cervical dilatation or passage of any products of conception. Ectropion, erosions, cervicitis, and vaginal trauma can cause these signs and symptoms and should be diagnosed by speculum examination of the cervix and vagina with appropriate Papanicolaou smears and therapy.

THERAPEUTIC CONSIDERATIONS. 1. The uterine size should be documented. No intercourse or vaginal instrumentation should occur for 2 weeks.

2. Bed rest, until 24 hours after the bleeding has ceased, is frequently utilized. Progestins should not be used because they are probably teratogenic. Neither bed rest nor use of progestins has been proved to be of benefit.

3. Patients should be informed of the potential risks and the need for close medical followup. They should also be reassured, since approximately 20 per cent of normal pregnancies have first trimester bleeding without known deleterious effects.

Missed Abortion. In missed abortion there is fetal death in utero prior to 20 weeks' gestation and there is no bleeding or apparent spontaneous uterine contractions or expulsion of the products of conception.

DIAGNOSIS. 1. Failure of the uterus to grow over the course of 4 weeks.

2. Loss of fetal heart tones using the Doppler apparatus.

3. Ultrasound examination that documents loss of fetal definition.

4. Absent fetal cardiac movement.

5. Conversion of the pregnancy test to negative.

THERAPEUTIC CONSIDERATIONS. 1. Abortion should be induced with the appropriate methods previously discussed for completing other types of abortion.

2. In patients from 16 to 20 weeks gestation, the vaginal administration of 20 mg of prostaglandin E_2 every 4 to 6 hours is usually more satisfactory than intravenous oxytocin or primary vaginal surgical removal (dilatation and evacuation [D&E]), even with Biere forceps.

3. Failure to promptly and adequately treat death in utero usually results in patient anxiety and depression and may occasionally result in diffuse intravascular coagulation.

Habitual Abortion. Habitual abortion has been defined as three consecutive abortions.

ETIOLOGIC AND THERAPEUTIC CONSIDERATIONS. 1. Any defect that alters the size and shape of the endometrial cavity may cause repeated abortions and should be looked for at the time of uterine evacuation. If this is not done, hysterosalpingogram or hysteroscopy may be used after involution.

2. Fetal tissue should be closely observed grossly for signs of genetic abnormalities. Genetic counseling may be beneficial to the patient with habitual abortion. Karyotyping of the fetus or of both marital partners may uncover balance translocations or other genetic abnormalities that may cause repeated abortions. Chronic diseases such as hypothyroidism or diabetes mellitus should be diagnosed and treated.

3. Inadequate luteal phase is suspected if the endometrial dating in the secretory phase of the cycle is 2 days or more behind the ovulation date. Some success has been reported by using progesterone, 25 mg rectally twice a day, or 12.5 mg daily intramuscularly continuously for 8 weeks after ovulation. Another method includes induction of ovulation with clomiphene citrate, 50 to 200 mg per day orally for 5 days (this dose may be higher than that listed in the manufacturer's official directive) started on menstrual day 5, followed by 10,000 units of human chorionic gonadotropin (HCG) every 2 to 4 days following ovulation for one to three doses, followed by 5000 international units twice a week for 1 to 2 weeks. Because of the difficulty in making the diagnosis, the need for special tests, and the hazards of using clomiphene citrate and HCG, the syndrome of inadequate corpus luteum should probably be treated only by physicians who are very familiar with the syndrome.

4. Cervical incompetence is characterized by second trimester abortion of more than one pregnancy after painless cervical dilatation. Painful uterine contractions may occur only as a terminal event or after rupture of membranes. Treatment consists of the placement of a cerclage suture (Shirodkar or McDonald types) in the subsequent pregnancy, preferably between 14 and 17 weeks' gestation. The Shirodkar method includes the placement of Mersilene tape in the submucosal tissue around the cervix at the level of the internal os. Both procedures should be done under sterile conditions with adequate anesthesia in the Trendelenburg position by physicians skilled in their performance. The Shirodkar suture can be left in place for future pregnancies and the fetus delivered by cesarean section. Alternatively, the suture may be removed in early labor to permit vaginal delivery and then be replaced with the next pregnancy. The McDonald suture should be removed at the time of labor.

Induced Abortion

Induced abortion is the removal of the products of conception from the uterus before viability by either surgical or medical means. It may be termed *therapeutic abortion* if it is performed to aid or maintain the health of the patient or *elective abortion* if it is performed only at the wishes of the patient. The general considerations outlined under Spontaneous Abortion (regarding use of Rh immune globulin [human] [RhoGAM] in the Rh negative unsensitized woman and maternal status and treatment) should serve as guidelines for patients undergoing induced abortion. The gestation age is usually the determinant for the best method (see Fig. 1).

Therapeutic Considerations. 1. See list under Spontaneous Abortion.

2. A positive pregnancy test is mandatory.

3. Accurate assessment of uterine and fetal size is mandatory to determine the safest method and to prepare for possible complications.

4. Extensive counseling to ensure that the patient is (a) appraised of the alternatives to abortion, (b) aware of the risks and benefits of abortion, (c) aware of her feelings about abortion, (d) not being coerced into having an abortion, and (e) informed of appropriate contraceptive methods.

5. Prior to 8 weeks' gestation, vacuum aspiration can be performed with a no-touch technique, using a 4 to 6 mm pliable cannula and a specially adapted Karman type syringe. Although cervical dilatation is rarely necessary, paracervical block anesthesia usually makes the procedure more comfortable. Microdoses of RhoGAM may be used when indicated. Intravenous oxytocin or oral methylergonovine (Methergine) is rarely indicated.

6. Prior to 14 weeks' gestation, vacuum aspiration (suction curettage) with a 12 mm or less flexible or rigid cannula and a high volume suction pump is ordinarily used. It is usually preferable to use a no-touch technique on an outpatient basis rather than in an operating room or an inpatient basis. Mechanical cervical dilata-

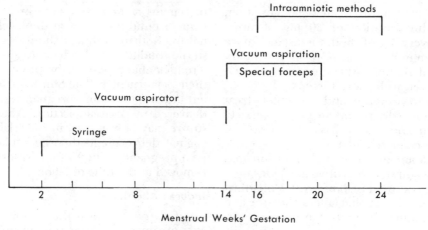

Figure 1.

tion with either rigid dilators or laminaria tents is usually necessary. Intravenous oxytocin (30 units in 1000 ml of electrolyte solution) may assist hemostasis. The products of conception should be identified for completeness before considering the curettage complete. Some physicians also check the uterine cavity with a sharp curettage.

7. Between 14 and 20 weeks' gestation, evacuation can be performed after more complete dilatation with laminaria tents or larger Pratt dilators with the aid of special forceps (such as Biere forceps). Specialized training is usually necessary to perform safe uterine evacuation at this gestational age. Completion of the abortion is mandatory. All portions of the fetus should be identified before considering the abortion complete. If vital signs are stable for 4 hours of close observation after evacuation, the patient may be discharged on treatment with methylergonovine and tetracycline, as described in the treatment of incomplete abortion.

8. Between 16 and 24 weeks' gestation, abortion may be medically induced on an inpatient basis. Because surgical intervention with general anesthesia may be necessary, preoperative precautions (including nothing by mouth and determinations of hematocrit, blood type, and Rh factor) should be taken.

a. The following agents in the doses given are commonly used intra-amniotically: (1) 40 mg of dinoprost tromethamine ($PGF_{2\alpha}$) (5 mg test dose followed by 35 mg after five minutes); 20 mg repeated dose in 24 hours; (2) 250 ml of 20 per cent hypertonic saline solution; (3) 250 ml of 20 per cent hypertonic saline solution with 5 to 20 mg of dinoprost tromethamine ($PGF_{2\alpha}$); (4) 80 grams of hypertonic urea with 5 to 10 mg of dinoprost tromethamine ($PGF_{2\alpha}$) after removal of as much amniotic fluid as possible.

b. Pretreatment or concomitant placement of intracervical laminaria tents is probably useful to shorten the induction to abortion time and probably decrease the incidence of cervical trauma, including lacerations and cervical fistulas.

c. Augmentation with constant infusion of intravenous oxytocin may be hazardous because of overstimulation and should be avoided unless there is inadequate uterine contractility.

d. After a transabdominal amniocentesis using a no-touch technique is performed under local anesthesia, the agents are either introduced directly through the needle or, if repeated administration is anticipated, introduced through a catheter that is threaded through the needle. In the latter instance, when the needle is removed, the catheter can be left in place and additional doses administered without repeated amniocentesis.

e. Prostaglandin E_2 in 20 mg vaginal suppositories and 15S, 15 methyl-$PGF_2\alpha$ tromethamine salt for intramuscular use are also approved by the Food and Drug Administration for inducing midtrimester abortion. However, because these agents often cause nausea and vomiting, they are usually used only when amniocentesis is not feasible.

f. If abortion is incomplete after 2 hours or hemorrhage occurs, surgical removal of the placenta is indicated unless there are extenuating circumstances.

9. Hysterotomy for abortion should be reserved for patients in whom other methods have failed and alternative methods are contraindicated. Morbidity and mortality rates are much higher with hysterotomy than with the aforementioned techniques in patients without complications. Even when concomitant sterilization is planned, the other methods of abortion followed

by minilaparotomy or laparoscopy sterilization are usually safer than hysterotomy and bilateral partial salpingectomy.

10. Because of the high rates of complication, hysterectomy as a means of abortion should be performed only when there is pathology indicating the need for hysterectomy. For example, severe, acute infection, which cannot be controlled by evacuation and antibiotics, or uterine tumors are possible indications for hysterectomy.

Criminal abortions are those performed under conditions that are not allowed by law. The law may regulate who performs the abortion and where it is performed.

Complications

About 90 per cent of the serious complications of abortions are due to hemorrhage, infection, or uterine injury.

Hemorrhage. Hemorrhage is defined as more than 500 ml blood loss. Hypotension, tachycardia, dizziness, anemia, and estimates of the amount of blood lost are signs and symptoms that guide the physician in determining the need for intravenous fluids or blood replacement. Early hemorrhage may result from incomplete abortion, uterine damage, uterine abnormalities, and functional causes. Oxytocics may attenuate functional atony.

Prolonged or heavy bleeding after abortion may be functional or result from uterine pathology or incomplete abortion. A repeated dilatation and curettage (D&C) to complete the abortion and determine uterine pathology or hormonal treatment may be useful.

Infection. Fever, leukocytosis, neutrophilia, positive blood cultures, and other cultures are diagnostic. Endometritis, pelvic inflammatory disease, cystitis, and pyelonephritis are the most frequent infections. Aerobic and anaerobic organisms are common. Therapeutic considerations include the following:

1. Minor infections can often be treated on an outpatient basis (ampicillin, 500 mg four times daily, or tetracycline, 250 mg four times daily for 10 days).

2. More severe infections can be treated with hospitalization, bed rest, semi-Fowler position, and intravenous antibiotics such as penicillin, 2.4 million units every 4 hours, gentamicin, 80 mg three times daily intravenously or intramuscularly, and clindamycin (Cleocin), 300 mg intravenously every 6 hours. An intravenous regimen is continued for 4 days, or until the patient is afebrile. This is followed by a regimen using oral antibiotics, such as tetracycline or ampicillin for another 10 to 14 days.

3. Rarely, hysterectomy may be lifesaving in the patient who does not respond to antibiotics or who has clostridia infection. Clostridia should be suspected if free gas is noted in the myometrium by x-ray or if there is hemolysis.

4. Repeat curettage may be necessary because those with infection often have retained tissue.

Uterine Trauma. Gross cervical and uterine traumas may occur with all methods. Uterine perforation may occur with mechanical dilators and uterine sounds and curettes. Cervical lacerations, false passages, and fistulas can occur with mechanical dilators, laminaria tents, and abortion induced with medications. After perforation, possible trauma to the abdominal and pelvic structures, including bladder, bowel and ovaries, must be evaluated. This may require laparoscopy, laparotomy, or prolonged observation.

Other Rare Complications. These include anesthesia complications, disseminated intravascular coagulation (DIC), and other traumas.

1. Local anesthesia is used under most circumstances because it is usually adequate and safer than general anesthesia. Allergic and hypersensitivity reactions can occur with local anesthetics. With local anesthetics, tinnitus, headache, excitability, and convulsions may occur with toxic systemic doses that can occur from rapid absorption.

2. Inappropriate bleeding from disseminated intravascular coagulation can occur from hypertonic saline solutions, necrosis, and sepsis. Elevated levels of fibrin split products, decreased platelet count, and decreased prothrombin levels with prolonged thrombin clotting time and prolonged partial thromboplastic time are often the initial changes in the peripheral blood. Replacement of blood coagulation factors with fresh frozen plasma and of platelets with platelet transfusions, and treatment of inciting factors, such as sepsis, are mandatory.

RESUSCITATION OF THE NEWBORN

method of
ROBERT G. MENY, M.D.
New Brunswick, New Jersey

Birth asphyxia complicates approximately 10 per cent of all births and requires rapid reversal so that brain damage can be avoided. Resuscitation of the newborn is mainly respiratory in nature, in contrast to that of the adult, which is usually cardiac. It therefore follows that the most vital aspects of the treatment of birth asphyxia are those directed at ventilating the lungs.

The occurrence of birth asphyxia can often be predicted from the maternal history both before and during labor and from signs of fetal distress (see Table 1). However, not all cases of birth asphyxia can be anticipated, a fact which weighs heavily against the practice of home delivery.

Personnel and Equipment

A person skilled in all aspects of resuscitation should always be available in the delivery suite. Skills, particularly endotracheal intubation, should be perfected in workshops on resuscitation. The use of anesthetized kittens for the teaching of endotracheal intubation is especially important.

The basic equipment needed is listed in Table 2; its availability and function should be checked on every shift.

When severe birth asphyxia is encountered, adequate help should be summoned immediately. Three people may be needed (one each for ventilation, cardiac compression, and drug administration).

Whom To Resuscitate

All babies should be resuscitated, with these possible exceptions: (1) Infants with birth weights of 500 grams or less who do not respond to bagging. (2) Infants who have an Apgar score of 0 at 1 minute, who have had an absent heart rate for over 10 minutes prior to delivery, and who do not respond to bagging. (3) Infants with multiple severe congenital anomalies.

As a general rule, when there is a question as to whether to begin or continue resuscitation, the patient should be given the benefit of the doubt. In this regard, a recent study shows that of 31 patients with an Apgar score of 0 at 1 minute or 4 or less at 5 minutes, 29 were without serious neurologic or mental handicap after a follow-up period of at least 5 years.

Procedure

Evaluation of the status of the newborn infant is best objectified by immediately assigning an Apgar score. If this is 7 or more, simply perform the following measures:

1. Suction the anterior mouth and then the nose, using a No. 5 French suction catheter for preterm babies and a No. 8 French for term babies. Do this gently and bear in mind that overly vigorous suctioning produces bradycardia.

TABLE 1. **Factors Associated with Birth Asphyxia**

Maternal conditions:
  Chronic hypertension
  Toxemia
  Diabetes
  Placenta previa
  Abruption
  Rh sensitization
  Heart disease
Intrapartum conditions:
  Cesarean section (especially with general anesthesia)
  Cord prolapse
  Opiates given within 2 hours of delivery
  Prolonged rupture of membranes when associated with amnionitis
Fetal conditions:
  Pre- or postmaturity
  Intrauterine growth retardation
  Passage of meconium (other than breech)
  Fetal tachycardia
  Fetal bradycardia (especially Type II dips)
  Multiple births
  Hypoxia (as demonstrated by transcutaneous oxygen monitor)

The stomach does not have to be suctioned except in infants delivered by cesarean section and in those deliveries complicated by the passage of meconium.

2. Keep the baby warm by drying off and placing under a radiant warmer servocontrolled to 36.5 C (97.7 F).

3. Stimulate the baby, if need be, with a few slaps on the sole. If the Apgar score is less than 7, go through the aforementioned steps quickly, using no more than 30 seconds. If there is no response, begin:

4. Ventilation with bag and mask. Give the

TABLE 2. **Resuscitation Equipment**

Radiant heated bed
Aspiration equipment: Nos. 5, 8, and 10 French catheters
O_2 source
Ventilation bag: nonrebreathing valve, capable of delivering >80% O_2
Face masks: newborn and premature sizes
Laryngoscope: blade sizes 0 and I
Orotracheal tubes, straight: 2.5, 3.0, 3.5, and 4.0 mm
Oral airways: sizes 000, 00, and 0
Stethoscope
Umbilical catheter tray: Nos. 3.5 and 5.0 French catheters
Drugs:
  Glucose 10%
  $NaHCO_3$, 1.0 mEq/ml
  Epinephrine, 1/10,000
  Naloxone (Narcan), 0.02 mg/ml
  Calcium gluconate, 10%
  Plasma protein fraction (human) (Plasmanate)
  Dextrostix
Portable x-ray available 24 hours
Blood gas equipment available 24 hours

maximal percentage of oxygen possible, using a self-inflating bag with tail or reservoir to increase the percentage of oxygen delivered.

Pressures of up to 40 cm H_2O may be necessary for the first few breaths, so a tight-fitting mask is essential. After the lungs have been expanded, pressures of more than 20 cm H_2O are not usually needed.

The baby should be ventilated at a rate of 30 to 40 breaths per minute, allowing time for expiration between each inspiration. Too often, one sees forced overaeration because the patient is not allowed to breathe out.

Efficacy of bagging is indicated (in this order) by (a) increase in pulse rate, (b) increase in blood pressure (pulse becomes palpable), and (c) improvement in color.

If there is no response after 30 seconds, intubate.

5. Orotracheal intubation (see Table 3 for tube size): (a) Suction the trachea with a No. 8 French catheter, if necessary. (b) After visualizing the cords, pass the orotracheal tube 2 cm beyond the vocal cords. Because this is sometimes forgotten while intubating, the "tip to lip" rule is a valuable aid in avoiding intubation of the right main bronchus. For an infant with a birth weight of 1.0 kg, the distance from the distal tip of the tube to the lip is 7 cm; for a 2.0 kg infant, 8 cm; and for a 3.0 kg infant, 9 cm. Use of this rule usually assures that the tip of the tube is near the midtrachea. (c) After intubating, auscultation over the lungs and the stomach will reveal if the esophagus has been entered by mistake. This occurs only when visualization of the tip of tube is not maintained during intubation. (d) Ventilate at a rate of 40 per minute and with pressures identical to those for bag and mask ventilation. Observe for response in heart rate and improvement in color.

6. If heart rate has not increased to >70 beats per minute after 10 lung inflations, start external cardiac massage at a rate of 120 per minute. For every three compressions, ventilate once. Do not ventilate and compress at the same time. There are two methods of cardiac compression: (a) The hands are placed around the thorax with the fingertips at the spine, and both thumbs compress the midsternum to a depth of 1 to 2 cm. (b) If the surface on which the infant lies is firm, the tips of the index and middle fingers of one hand may be used for compression. This should result in palpable femoral pulses if properly performed and if the infant is not hypovolemic.

7. If the measures listed above have not produced the desired response: (a) Give a 1:1 mixture of sodium bicarbonate (1 mEq per ml) and 10 per cent dextrose in a dose of 6 ml per kg via an umbilical catheter, preferably arterial. This mixture is hypertonic, and its rapid injection may lead to cerebral intraventricular hemorrhage, so that its use should be confined to the newborn in dire need: the infant with an Apgar score of 5 or less at this point who has not shown a response to the earlier stages of resuscitation. (b) If bradycardia still persists, give 0.5 ml of a 1:10,000 solution of epinephrine via an umbilical catheter. If asystole is present, this same dose is given as an intracardiac injection. Should there be poor response, give 1 ml per kg of 10 per cent calcium gluconate. (c) Obtain arterial blood gases, pH, central hematocrit, blood glucose, and calcium if the infant has received any of the aforementioned medications, and keep the patient under close observation for at least several hours. During this time frequent vital signs, including blood pressure determinations, are advisable. (d) For all infants who fail to respond to resuscitation or who, although successfully resuscitated, continue to show signs of respiratory distress, a chest x-ray is useful to detect tension pneumothorax, diaphragmatic hernia, or other congenital anomalies. Pneumothorax can also be detected by the use of high intensity transillumination.

8. Occasionally an infant will have suffered acute blood loss sufficient to induce hemorrhagic shock. This is often associated with vaginal bleeding prior to delivery. These infants may respond only to specific therapy with volume expanders, which, in order of preference, are as follows: (a) Whole blood — low titer, type O, Rh negative. If possible, cross-matched against mother prior to delivery. However, uncross-matched blood may be used. Give 10 to 20 ml per kg. (b) Plasma or plasma protein factor (human) (Plasmanate), 10 to 20 ml per kg. (c) Albumin (5 per cent), 10 to 20 ml per kg.

When possible, monitor blood pressure while giving any of the agents cited above.

9. For depressed infants whose mothers received opiates during labor, especially in the 2 hours prior to delivery, give naloxone (Narcan), 0.01 mg per kg by the intravenous or intramuscular route. This may be repeated twice.

10. Meconium-stained amniotic fluid: 60 per cent of these infants have meconium below their

TABLE 3. **Endotracheal Tube Size**

BIRTH WEIGHT (KG)	INSIDE DIAMETER OF TUBE
Under 1.0	2.5 mm
1.0–2.0	3.0 mm
2.0–3.0	3.5 mm
3.0 and over	4.0 mm

vocal cords. In those cases in which the meconium is particulate or pea-soup in nature, meconium aspiration syndrome can occur unless a combined obstetric-pediatric approach is taken. (a) Prior to the delivery of the chest, clear the mouth and nose of meconium. (b) Immediately after birth, intubate the trachea and, while withdrawing the endotracheal tube, apply suction with the mouth. A paper face mask can be placed between your mouth and the endotracheal tube adapter. (c) If meconium is recovered, repeat (b) until the trachea is free of meconium. Ventilation prior to complete removal of meconium will result in its being forced down into smaller airways, with subsequent atelectasis and emphysema.

ECTOPIC PREGNANCY

method of
JOHN J. STANGEL, M.D.
Valhalla, New York

General Comments

An ectopic pregnancy is any gestation occurring outside the uterine cavity. It usually occurs in the fallopian tube, but may be found implanted on the ovary, on any of the abdominal viscera, or on the uterine cervix. Delay or inaccurate diagnosis of an ectopic pregnancy can result in acute life-threatening intra-abdominal hemorrhage. Three to 5 per cent of maternal deaths per year are due to ruptured ectopic pregnancy.

Primary Tools

History and Physical Examination. The key to the management of this condition is to maintain a high index of suspicion. Any woman of reproductive age with a history of a missed period (with or without atypical vaginal bleeding), lower abdominal pain, and a unilateral adnexal mass must be considered to have an ectopic pregnancy until proved otherwise.

Tests. Biocept-G. This is a radioreceptor assay for human chorionic gonadotropin (HCG) done on blood. The test is extremely sensitive, giving a positive test down to 40 MIU per ml of HCG. The results are available in 2 hours. At the time of the missed period a positive test is consistent with pregnancy; a negative test is consistent with a nonpregnant state. An ectopic pregnancy is usually positive or borderline positive Biocept-G.

Ultrasound Scan. Ultrasound can be used to locate the gestational sac of an early pregnancy and check the adnexal areas for cystic structures suggestive of an ectopic gestation. Before the sixth week of pregnancy it may be difficult to actually locate a pregnancy outside the uterus. But if sonar studies fail to show a gestational sac within the uterine cavity in a patient with a positive Biocept-G, one should be very suspicious of an ectopic pregnancy. This is especially true if a separate extrauterine mass is found. Grey scale is the most appropriate technique for ectopic evaluation.

Laparoscopy. In the hands of an experienced endoscopist this procedure will definitively rule in or out an ectopic pregnancy. If a patient is in hypovolemic shock with an acute abdomen, there is no need to perform laparoscopy since it is apparent that the patient probably has an acute hemoperitoneum and requires immediate surgery. The accompanying flow sheet (Table 1) indicates the utilization of these tests and the recommended management based on the data generated.

Management

Tubal Gestations. Patients with ectopic gestations may be divided into three categories, depending upon the severity and acuteness of their presentation.

Category I: Acute Ruptured Ectopic Pregnancy. This patient usually presents with a history of amenorrhea and acute abdominal pain followed by signs of acute hypovolemic shock. She must be admitted to the hospital for immediate emergency surgery.

1. Start one or more intravenous lines with a large bore needle or catheter (16 or 18 gauge).

2. Type and cross-match for 2 to 4 units of whole blood. Begin transfusion as soon as possible. In a severe emergency, type O negative blood may be given until the patient's typed blood is available.

3. Intravenous plasma expanders such as albumin and Ringer's lactate should be started through a separate intravenous line.

4. Obtain hemoglobin and hematocrit immediately.

5. Insert a Foley catheter and measure intake and output. If the output drops despite apparently adequate intravenous input, a central venous pressure (CVP) line should be started.

6. Obtain appropriate surgical consent from patient and/or family.

7. Notify the anesthesiologist about the patient, emphasizing the acute hypovolemic state. Inhalation and not conduction anesthesia must be used.

TABLE 1.

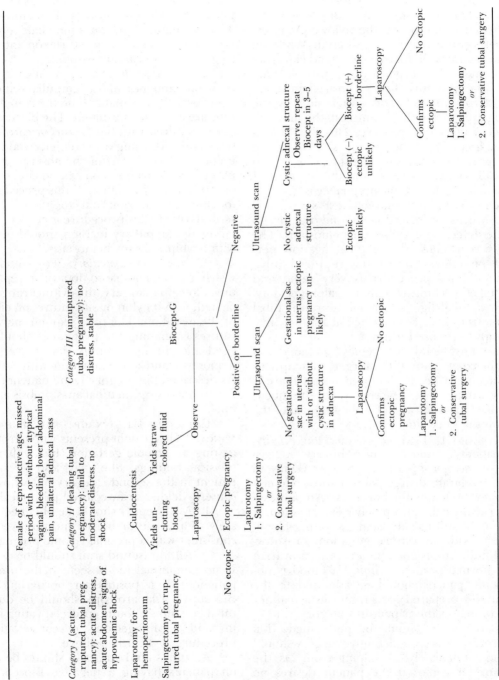

8. Surgery: The abdomen must be entered rapidly, usually through a midline or paramedian incision. The surgical procedure selected must be the most rapid to stabilize the patient. The usual procedure is the removal of the affected tube, a salpingectomy with a cornual resection. If the contralateral tube is absent and the patient desires further childbearing, the following conservative procedure may be considered. While an assistant aspirates all the free blood and clot from the abdomen, the surgeon raises the bleeding tube in the operative field. Tonsil clamps are placed across the tube on either side of the bleeding area so that the tips meet in the mesosalpinx below the site of rupture. This should stop the bleeding. The tube on the side of clamp facing away from the site of rupture is ligated with 0 silk or nylon suture, and the segment of tube containing the ectopic pregnancy is resected and the tonsil clamps removed. Next, several 3–0 Dexon sutures are placed in the mesosalpinx to close the defect created and for hemostasis. The result is very much like a tubal ligation performed on either side of the ruptured tubal pregnancy. This procedure is very rapid and indeed takes less time to do than a salpingectomy. As with a tubal ligation, a microsurgical tubal anastomosis can be accomplished at another time to attempt to restore fertility.

Care must be taken to remove all blood and clot at the completion of the surgery. The ipsilateral ovary must not be removed unless there is intrinsic damage to it. The removal of the tube is not, by itself, an indication for the removal of the ovary on the same side.

CATEGORY II. LEAKING ECTOPIC PREGNANCY. This patient presents with a history suggestive of an ectopic pregnancy. She is usually in mild to moderate distress with a soft abdomen and lower abdominal tenderness. An adnexal mass is usually palpable on pelvic examination. A culdocentesis will usually yield unclotting blood, consistent with an ectopic gestation, or straw-colored fluid, consistent with a ruptured ovarian cyst or normal peritoneal fluid. If blood is obtained, the patient should be admitted to the hospital and prepared for surgery in a manner similar to that of the patient in Category 1.

A laparoscopy should be performed. If a tubal pregnancy is seen, definitive surgery should be done immediately. A salpingectomy is the procedure of choice if the patient desires no further childbearing. Conservative surgery can be performed if the patient desires the preservation of her fertility. Conservative surgery should be considered regardless of whether or not the woman has a normal contralateral tube, since both tubes are necessary for optimal chances for future pregnancy.

A choice of one of three conservative procedures may be made, depending upon the location of the tubal gestation and the experience of the surgeon.

1. *Isthmic pregnancy:* A segmental resection of the tube can be carried out, using a needle point electrode and low unipolar cutting current. This is followed by an immediate end-to-end tubal anastomosis, using 8-0 Dexon and magnification (loupes or a microscope).

2. *Ampullary pregnancy:* A linear salpingotomy (an antemesenteric ampullary incision) is made over the pregnancy, and the contents of the tube are carefully evacuated. The bleeding points can be sutured with 6-0 Dexon or carefully electrocoagulated, using a needle electrode and low unipolar current. After hemostasis is accomplished, the tubal incision can be closed with 6-0 or 8-0 Dexon. A variation of this procedure is not to close the incision but to allow it to close secondarily. If this procedure is chosen, the margin of the ampullary incision should be sutured with a whipstitch for hemostasis.

3. *Isthmic or ampullary:* For situations in which it is not feasible to do a tubal repair at the time of ectopic surgery, the oviduct can simply be ligated, with 0 nylon or silk suture, on either side of the gestation. The tube segment between the sutures containing the pregnancy should be excised and the mesosalpinx defect oversewn for hemostasis and approximation with 3-0 Dexon. As described in Category I, the patient then may have a microsurgical tubal anastomosis at another time.

CATEGORY III: UNRUPTURED TUBAL PREGNANCY. This patient presents with a history suggesting an ectopic gestation, but with very few physical findings. She may also present as a patient in the second category but whose culdocentesis yielded straw-colored peritoneal fluid.

1. A Biocept-G should be obtained immediately. A positive or borderline positive result is consistent with a possible ectopic pregnancy.

2. An ultrasound scan should be done next. If no gestational sac is seen in the uterus in a patient with a positive or borderline positive Biocept-G, a laparoscopy should be done. If a tubal gestation is found, proceed with a laparotomy and a salpingectomy or conservative tubal procedure as described above.

An ultrasound scan also should be obtained on patients having a negative Biocept-G. If a cystic adnexal structure is seen, the Biocept should be repeated in 3 to 5 days. If the test becomes positive or borderline positive, laparoscopy should be done.

Ovarian Pregnancy. A wedge resection of the affected area of the ovary should be attempted. The defect created should be closed with 3-0

Dexon and the capsule repaired with 4-0 Dexon. If it is clear that a wedge resection and repair will not yield sufficient hemostasis, a unilateral oophorectomy should be performed. The ipsilateral tube should be preserved if it appears to be normal.

Cervical Pregnancy. Cervical pregnancies can be evacuated by suction curettage. If significant bleeding occurs, ligation of the cervical branches of both the uterine arteries should be performed. If hemorrhage continues, a hysterectomy may be necessary.

Abdominal Pregnancy. The gestation should be removed, but the placenta must be left untouched. Removing the tissue of the site of implantation can produce abdominal hemorrhage that is extremely difficult to control.

Postoperative Care. 1. Rh immune globulin (human): Women who are Rh negative should receive RhoGAM within 72 hours of surgery.

2. Adjunctive therapy: No special use of steroids, antibiotics or hydrotubation is necessary.

General Principles. 1. At the time of surgery, always evacuate all blood and clot from the abdomen, using suction and continual irrigation.

2. Handle the tissues gently. Do not abrade tissue surfaces or allow them to dry. Particular attention must be directed to keeping the tubal serosa moist through constant irrigations.

3. When in doubt of the diagnosis of persistent lower abdominal discomfort in a female of reproductive age, consider laparoscopy to rule out an ectopic pregnancy.

4. Uterine suspension is not appropriate, helpful, or necessary as part of ectopic pregnancy surgery.

5. For conservative tubal surgery for ectopic pregnancy, no indwelling tubal stents or other prosthetic devices should be used.

Summary

1. A patient with a ruptured ectopic pregnancy presents with an acute abdomen and hypovolemic shock. Laparotomy with salpingectomy or a ligation and excision of the ruptured tube segment is the appropriate therapy.

2. A patient with a leaking ectopic pregnancy presents with milder discomfort. A culdocentesis yields nonclotting blood. A laparoscopy makes the diagnosis of ectopic pregnancy. The treatment is laparotomy with a salpingectomy or a conservative procedure.

3. A patient with an unruptured ectopic pregnancy is frequently discovered by her physician's high index of suspicion. Women with a high risk history (previous ectopic pregnancy, tubal surgery, tubal ligation and/or pelvic inflammatory disease [PID]), and a history of a missed period should have a Biocept-G and an ultrasound scan. A positive Biocept-G with no gestational sac is an indication for laparoscopy, and further surgery is appropriate.

For details of conservative techniques for the treatment of tubal gestations, see Stangel and Gomel: Clin. Obstet. Gynecol., *23*:251, 1980.

HEMORRHAGE IN LATE PREGNANCY

method of
ISADORE DYER, M.D.
New Orleans, Louisiana

Patients will vary in reporting vaginal bleeding both as to promptness and as to appraisal of the amount. All vaginal bleeding in late pregnancy should be considered abnormal and the source thereof determined as quickly as possible.

Sources of Mild Bleeding

1. Often accompanies the onset of labor.
2. Contact bleeding (cervical) following coitus, attempts at douching, or examination.
3. Endocervical polyps, condylomata acuminata, cervical malignancy, or vaginitis.
4. Rarely, ruptured varices or lacerations.

Sources of Profuse Bleeding

1. Low-lying (implanted) placenta (placenta previa).
2. Placental separation (abruptio placentae).

Examination for Cause

Patients who have experienced mild bleeding may safely be examined in the office. It is essential that vital signs be determined, including blood values, blood pressure, and pulse. Uterine tone, or its absence, is valuable to ascertain, as well as the attitude of the fetus and fetal heart rate. The size of the uterus measured in centimeters from the brim of the symphysis pubis to the uterine fundus will be of diagnostic worth in assessing intrauterine hemorrhage should the measurement increase.

A speculum examination will reveal the cause of vaginal or cervical bleeding, and proper measures can be instituted.

Finally, if the bleeding source is intrauterine, the amount of a mild nature, and the bleeding not active, steps should be taken to confirm the diagnosis of placenta previa or low-lying placental implantation, the most likely diagnosis.

With the advent of ultrasound, studies have shown that almost half of pregnant women have some degree of placenta previa present up to the third trimester. As the uterus enlarges, the attached placenta is lifted away from the cervical os and causes no problem with regard to separation, bleeding, or delivery. Ultrasound remains a most valuable clinical tool to aid in the diagnosis of placenta previa.

Placenta Previa

Expectant Treatment. A placenta previa which blocks the lower uterine segment can be resolved safely only by cesarean section. Once the diagnosis has been made, efforts should be directed to secure a mature fetus. Since the first episode of bleeding will rarely be severe enough to demand intervention, blood values should be maintained (we have transfused several patients on occasion), and the patient should remain quiescent with restriction of activity in order to reduce uterine irritability. This includes restriction of coitus.

This plan will be successful if the patient can be immediately transported to a hospital at any hour of the day or night, and if the hospital is equipped with an obstetrical operating room available at any hour and a blood bank. Should these not be available in a given community, either hospitalization for observation will be mandatory or the patient can be transferred to a community where ideal care is available.

Active Treatment. 1. With low placental implantations, in which the fetus presents as a vertex, a simple rupture of the membranes can be performed through a thin, partially dilated cervix. This will often resolve the condition. Oxytocic stimulation is permissible.

2. Complete placenta previa can be resolved with safety only by cesarean section.

Pitfalls to Avoid. 1. The amount of hemorrhage is unpredictable. Blood must be available and ready to replace the estimated loss.

2. An operating room must be available 24 hours a day.

3. Placenta previa may occur more commonly in multiple births.

4. Placenta previa accreta is recognized as a common entity. To control postpartum hemorrhage, be prepared to perform a hysterectomy.

5. The fetus often loses blood through the placenta; anticipate fetal anemia.

6. One of the most dangerous conditions is a placenta previa with anterior implantation in a patient who has undergone one or more previous low cesarean sections. The placenta has been found to erode through the transverse scar, implant partially extrauterine, or, on occasion, rupture into the bladder. Only heroic measures, multiple units of blood, and adequate assistance can resolve these emergencies.

Abruptio Placentae

There are variations in the degree of placental separation, in the underlying acute or chronic disease in the mother, and in the amount of visible bleeding observed by the clinician. Although the exact cause remains unknown, the following factors are significant in statistical analysis of abruptio placentae:

1. There is an increased incidence noted in women who have inadequate nutrition. Studies have pointed out the possible relationship of poor folate metabolism.

2. Although the mechanism is not clear, repeated studies tend to show a correlation between alcohol consumption and smoking, both of which are considered "risk" factors for abruptio placentae, and certain other fetal and placental problems. The incidence of abruptio placentae has been reported to increase in proportion to the number of cigarettes smoked, although the mechanism of action is unclear.

3. The severe types occur in women with chronic cardiovascular renal disease, in severe toxemias of pregnancy, and with eclampsia.

4. Abruptio placentae has been observed in women of high social status, in the absence of any acute or chronic disease, whose diets were considered adequate.

5. Although we have observed and reported placental separation as a result of trauma, it is not a common factor in a large experience with severe trauma in pregnancy.

Course of the Condition. Ernest Page in 1954 outlined the effects of placental separation on the mother as follows: (1) a degree of shock which is frequently out of proportion to the hypotension, (2) a disseminated "fibrin embolism," (3) an in vivo defibrination resulting sometimes in incoagulable blood, (4) an ischemia of the renal cortex which leads to varying degrees of necrosis, and (5) the activation of the fibrinolytic system in the plasma.

Since any or all of these events may occur rapidly, it has been our aim to empty the uterus as soon as possible after the diagnosis is made. The mild and limited partial separations of the placenta that occur in labor are usually of no great clinical concern.

Treatment. 1. Obtain blood and attempt to replace loss.

2. Collect 5 ml whole blood in a test tube.

Note whether the clot will lyse or is well formed.

3. If a bleeding diathesis has occurred (no clot is observed), one must keep in mind the seriousness of disseminated intravascular coagulation. If it is profound enough within a relatively short period of time, uncontrolled bleeding will occur. While the prime interest is concerned with correction of the underlying cause of the events, attempts should be made to keep the fibrinogen level as close as possible to 150 mg per 100 ml. Whole fresh blood should be administered freely, always keeping in mind that fresh frozen plasma per unit can improve the fibrinogen level 25 mg per 100 ml. Although there have been many reports concerning the use of heparin, this has not been a treatment of choice in my experience.

4. Attempt to empty the uterus. If feasible, simple membrane rupture plus stimulation with a dilute intravenous drip of 10 units of oxytocin injection (Pitocin) in 1000 ml of 5 per cent glucose in distilled water will resolve the condition by early delivery. This is possible only in an "inducible" multigravida or the occasional primigravida in labor.

5. There is evidence from some studies that massive transfusion has yielded excellent results; in others, predominant vaginal delivery is the vogue. In spite of these conservative approaches, it remains our policy to deliver promptly the patient with abruptio placentae as soon as the diagnosis is confirmed. In this respect, cesarean section is commonly performed on the patient who, in the estimation of the clinician, cannot be delivered shortly by induction. In this manner we have eliminated the use of fibrinogen and avoided disseminated intravascular coagulation but have lowered maternal losses and complications from the sequelae common in this condition.

Rupture of a Marginal Sinus

For completeness, this entity must be considered. Although bleeding may occur as a result of a ruptured marginal sinus several weeks before term, more commonly it occurs just prior to or at the onset of labor. The initial amount of bleeding may be brisk and then cease as labor progresses, or some recognizable bleeding may persist throughout labor. In any event, placenta previa can be ruled out, the fetus is rarely in jeopardy, and the diagnosis can be made only after the third stage when the affected area can be seen at the junction of membranes and placenta.

Vasa Previa

This condition is rare. It represents a fetal vessel traveling along the membranes, usually in a velamentous cord insertion, and the vessel is ruptured as the membranes break. The maternal status remains stable; the fetus immediately dies unless delivery is instant. Determination of the blood as fetal will prove the predelivery diagnosis.

PREGNANCY-INDUCED HYPERTENSION*

method of
DONALD A. G. BARFORD, M.D.,
and ROBERT J. SOKOL, M.D.
Cleveland, Ohio

Introduction and Definitions

Hypertension, regardless of etiology, is a major pregnancy complication and risk factor for the fetus. Pregnancy-associated hypertensive disorders may be categorized as follows:

Chronic Hypertension. (1) Evidence of hypertension during previous pregnancy or between pregnancies. (2) Underlying disease, e.g., chronic pyelonephritis or glomerulonephritis, predisposing the patient to hypertension, which is manifest during pregnancy.

Preeclampsia — Hypertension Specifically Related to Pregnancy. Preeclampsia is characterized by the development of hypertension, proteinuria, and extracellular fluid retention, although the development or worsening of hypertension alone during pregnancy should be considered adequate to make the diagnosis. Preeclampsia may be categorized in two ways:

BY CHRONICITY. (1) Pure — no previous evidence of chronic hypertension. These patients are typically nulliparous and develop hypertension late in the third trimester. Occasionally, pure preeclampsia occurs earlier in pregnancy in association with hydatidiform mole or multiple gestation. (2) Superimposed on chronic hypertension. Preeclampsia develops in a patient who meets criteria for chronic hypertension. These patients are more often multiparous, develop more severe hypertension, and do so earlier in gestation.

BY SEVERITY. (1) Mild preeclampsia — pregnancy-induced hypertension to levels less than those necessary to diagnose severe preeclampsia. Proteinuria of <3+ on dipstick determination may be present, as may edema, al-

*Supported in part by USPHS Grant No. 5M01-RR00210.

though neither proteinuria nor edema is necessary to make this diagnosis. (2) Severe preeclampsia — criteria for mild preeclampsia plus (a) blood pressure of ≥160 mm Hg systolic or ≥110 mm Hg diastolic on at least two occasions, 6 hours apart, with the gravida at bed rest, using cuff of appropriate width for the determination; or (b) proteinuria of ≥5 grams per day (≥3+ on dipstick determination); or (c) cerebral or visual disturbances, e.g., scotomas; or (d) epigastric pain, suggestive of intrahepatic edema or subcapsular hemorrhage; or (e) oliguria of <500 ml per day. (3) Eclampsia — grand mal seizure(s), complicating preeclampsia.

In managing patients with pregnancy-induced hypertension, keep the following points in mind:

1. Because blood pressure tends to fall during the second trimester, measurements taken for the first time during this period may be misleading. Failure to observe this decrease is an important predictor of later severe hypertension.

2. Preeclampsia is a multisystem disease which probably does not have a single cause. Nonetheless, it is clear that it is associated with generalized small artery spasm and markedly diminished uteroplacental flow. These two features, respectively, can be thought of as accounting for (a) maternal complications — severe hypertension, hepatic damage, renal damage (acute tubular necrosis, cortical necrosis), coagulopathy (thrombocytopenia, microangiopathic hemolysis), and/or cerebrovascular accident; and (b) fetal complications — intrauterine growth retardation, decreased fetal reserve ("fetal distress"), abruptio placentae, or intrauterine fetal demise.

3. The earlier in pregnancy preeclampsia develops, the more severe it should be considered, regardless of the precise criteria listed above.

4. Clinically, it is often difficult, if not impossible, to be certain whether a given patient has pure or superimposed preeclampsia, the latter indicating chronic hypertension. This is not, however, a major problem, because the treatment of preeclampsia is based on its severity.

Principles of Treatment

The treatment of preeclampsia may be *conservative* if the disease is mild. Pregnancy is carried either until the patient enters labor spontaneously or until pregnancy reaches term (at least 38 weeks). Delivery is then effected. If, on the other hand, the disease process is severe or mild disease worsens while being treated conservatively, *active* treatment is undertaken. The patient is stabilized and delivery is effected. Regardless of

how mild the disease may seem initially, three categories of information must be considered to determine appropriate therapy. These are (1) maternal condition, (2) pregnancy duration and fetal maturity, and (3) fetal condition.

Conservative Therapy for Mild Preeclampsia

Assess and Treat Maternal Condition. 1. *Admit the patient to the hospital.* Mild chronic hypertension can often be treated on an outpatient basis. If blood pressure increases, if there are signs of end-organ compromise, e.g., renal, or if there are signs of intrauterine growth retardation or fetal compromise, immediate hospitalization is warranted. In our experience, treatment at home under these circumstances is inadequate; early hospitalization is the single most important factor in reducing the incidence of severe disease.

2. *Place the patient at bed rest with bathroom privileges* in order to improve renal blood flow and uteroplacental perfusion.

3. *Place the patient on a "no-salt-added diet"* (4 grams salt). Severe salt restriction may worsen depletion of intravascular volume. Excess sodium may worsen hypertension in preeclampsia.

4. To be assured that the disease process is remaining "mild" and is under control *follow* (a) blood pressure every 6 hours; (b) deep tendon reflexes twice each day; (c) patient weight and the appearance of finger and facial edema daily; and (d) serial laboratory determinations, the frequency determined by patient condition: (1) initial urine culture; (2) initial complete blood count with platelet count; followed by (3) hematocrits for hemoconcentration; (4) platelet counts for intravascular coagulation; (5) blood urea nitrogen (BUN), uric acid, creatinine clearance, and 24 hour urinary protein for renal function; and (6) serum electrolytes and enzymes for hepatic damage.

5. *Avoid sedatives.* Although many clinicians use phenobarbital to make it easier for the patient to remain at bed rest, delivery may become necessary on short notice. Sedatives could affect fetal and neonatal monitoring findings and produce neonatal depression.

6. *Do not use antihypertensive medications,* specifically for mild preeclampsia. However, in situations in which chronic hypertension is the issue, the following guidelines are of use: (a) The patient may have discontinued medication herself when she found she was pregnant. Also, it is occasionally possible to discontinue medication early in pregnancy if the patient is very reliable, limits salt intake, and is able to rest at home. This avoids fetal exposure to drugs, but is only possible in mildly hypertensive patients. (b) More often, therapy for chronic hypertension is war-

ranted or should be continued. We recommend alpha-methyldopa (Aldomet), generally in the range of 750 to 1500 mg per day, often with chlorthalidone (Hygroton), 50 mg per day, or hydrochlorothiazide, 50 mg per day. Higher doses of alpha-methyldopa are frequently associated with considerable patient malaise. Potassium supplementation is usually unnecessary with chlorthalidone. (c) We avoid propranolol because of effects on the uterus. It may increase uterine tone. Fetal complications, including intrauterine growth retardation, neonatal hypoglycemia, and pre- and postnatal bradycardia, have been reported.

Assess Pregnancy Duration and Fetal Maturity. Arriving at as accurate an estimate as possible of pregnancy duration–fetal maturity is a central component of the conservative treatment of preeclampsia. A careful review of the patient's records for the date of the last menstrual period, early assessments of uterine size, the date of the first appearance of the unamplified fetal heart tones, and identification from the record of the date of quickening can be helpful. If the patient has been referred for care, the referring physician's records should be obtained. A history of ultrasound examinations performed during the second trimester can be most helpful. Ultrasound examination for biparietal diameter, abdominal circumference, total intrauterine volume, and placental grade may also be useful and must be interpreted carefully in view of the risk of intrauterine growth retardation.

If the patient remains stable and does not commence labor spontaneously, amniocentesis for evaluation of fetal maturity is often indicated prior to the induction of labor. Amniocentesis is best performed at or after 38 weeks' gestation, since there is a greater likelihood of being able to act upon the results of a "mature" test. In addition to determining the L/S ratio and/or foam ("shake") test, fetal fat cells, and amniotic fluid creatinine, determination of phosphatidylglycerol may add precision in estimating gestational duration and predicting pulmonary maturity.

Assess Fetal Condition. 1. *Perform serial non-stress tests* two to three times per week. In our experience, if it is normal, the test reassures one of fetal well-being. If it is suspicious, the test should be repeated, as a quiet period of fetal inactivity may have been sampled. Near term, a test should not be considered abnormal unless the fetus remains quiet for a minimum of 1 hour. We have taken a minimum of two fetal heart rate accelerations of at least 15 beats per minute, in association with fetal movements, as constituting a normal nonstress test. Some clinicians follow the nonstress test, particularly if it is equivocal,

with an oxytocin challenge test. We have not found the oxytocin challenge test useful in making management decisions above and beyond those provided by the nonstress test.

2. *Determine urinary estriols daily.* In conjunction with the creatinine clearance, serial estriols are a helpful adjunct to the nonstress test. Persistently low estriols (less than a value on a straight line from 8 mg at 32 weeks to 12 mg per 24 hours at 40 weeks) or a fall of greater than 35 per cent below the mean of the last 3 days is of concern. This test has a higher false positive rate than the nonstress test. Interpret these tests as follows: (a) If both the nonstress test and estriols remain normal, conservative therapy may continue. (b) If the nonstress test is normal but the estriols are abnormal, it is usually safe to defer definitive action for a day to obtain another nonstress test and estriol determination. (c) If the nonstress test is abnormal, even on repeat testing, but the estriols are normal, fine clinical judgment is needed and intervention may be warranted. (d) If both the nonstress test and estriols are abnormal, active therapy is indicated.

3. *Perform serial amnioscopies* every other day, if cervical dilatation permits. This is a particularly helpful technique near term. The finding of meconium is an indication for delivery.

Comment. Conservative therapy is appropriate for mild hypertensive disease. It is most important to recognize that the condition is never ablated in pregnancy, except by delivery of the infant and placenta. Although the clinical signs tend to resolve with conservative therapy, it is, in our opinion, inappropriate to decrease the level of surveillance and treatment by discharging the patient from the hospital. The majority of patients with mild preeclampsia are near term, and the length of maternal hospitalization is generally not excessive. Patients with preexisting hypertension may require considerably longer stays. Discharge of these patients from the hospital may be associated with the unwarranted development of severe preeclampsia and stillbirths.

Active Therapy for Severe Disease

Stabilize the Patient. This is the first task in treating severe pregnancy-induced hypertension. Based on the older literature, immediate delivery by cesarean section is not warranted, since it is associated with an increased risk of maternal and fetal mortality. The goal is to obtain baseline studies (see above) and to begin the process which will lead to prompt delivery. The patient's condition can usually be stabilized within 6 to 12 hours.

IMPROVEMENT OF MATERNAL CONDITION. Prevent the development of eclampsia, severe hypertension (i.e., diastolic blood pressures of greater than or equal to 110 and systolic greater than 180 mm Hg), the serious sequelae of coagulopathy), renal and hepatic failure, and cerebrovascular accidents.

1. *Transfer the patient to the labor and delivery suite.* If there is evidence of hyperexcitability of the central nervous system, magnesium sulfate (as indicated below) should be given prior to any other therapeutic manipulations.

2. *Obtain vital signs every 15 minutes.*

3. In addition to a peripheral venous line, *place a central venous pressure (CVP) line.* Keep open with 5 per cent dextrose and half isotonic saline. Avoid lactated Ringer's solution.

4. *Place a Foley catheter.*

5. *Record intake and output hourly.*

6. *Determine hematocrit every 4 hours* to assess hemoconcentration.

7. *Bring the CVP to 5 to 10 cm water* by intravenous hydration. The initial CVP is often ≤0 cm water. The initial hematocrit is often in the 40 to 45 per cent range, but will fall to the 30 to 35 per cent range with treatment. Overhydration can lead to congestive heart failure.

8. *Assess clotting.* Often the simple clinical test of observing a tube containing a few ml of blood for adequate clotting, retraction, and the absence of lysis is adequate.

9. *Type and cross for 2 units of blood.*

10. *Infuse magnesium sulfate* ($MgSO_4$). For the loading dose, we prefer the intravenous route; 2 to 4 grams of magnesium sulfate (50 per cent solution — 4 to 8 ml) should be given *by slow intravenous injection over a 5 minute period.* It is critical that this medication be given slowly, as respiratory and cardiac arrest may occur. One ampule of calcium chloride (10 ml of 10 per cent solution) should be available in case of overdosage. Following the administration of a bolus dose of magnesium sulfate, *begin a constant infusion.* (a) Add 4 grams $MgSO_4$ (8 ml of a 50 per cent solution) to 230 ml of D_5W. This solution contains 1 gram $MgSO_4$ per 60 ml. (b) Use a standard infusion set with a large dropper (10 drops per ml). (c) Use a constant infusion pump. The rate should be from 1 gram per hour = 60 ml per hour = 10 drops per minute, to 2 grams per hour = 120 ml per hour = 20 drops per minute. The rate of infusion is titrated by frequent evaluation of the patient's deep tendon reflexes. The only indication for discontinuing the infusion is the disappearance of the patient's deep tendon reflexes. In our experience, oliguria will often respond to the magnesium sulfate infusion and increases in the fluid load, monitored by the central venous pressure.

11. *Treat hypertension* specifically only if the diastolic ≥110 and the systolic ≥180 mm Hg. *Hydralazine* is effective in lowering the blood pressure in the majority of these patients. Some patients exhibit marked sensitivity to the drug. The usual loading dose is 10 to 20 mg by intravenous injection. We recommend giving 2.5 to 5 mg intravenously initially and measuring the blood pressure every 5 minutes for 15 minutes. Provided that the blood pressure does not fall rapidly to very low levels, the remainder of the dose can be administered. Intermittent intravenous bolus doses may be given, or a constant infusion according to the following protocol: (a) Add 40 mg hydralazine to 100 ml D_5W or 20 mg hydralazine to 50 ml D_5W. (b) Use a "mini dropper" infusion set (60 drops per ml). (c) Use a constant infusion pump to deliver 10 mg hydralazine per hour = 25 ml per hour = 25 drops per minute. The rate of infusion should be determined by frequent monitoring of the patient's blood pressure.

12. In general, diuretics are not indicated for severe preeclampsia, and more potent antihypertensive agents are seldom necessary.

PREGNANCY DATING–FETAL MATURITY. If a patient requires prompt delivery, assessment of fetal maturity is not warranted. However, if delivery of a preterm infant is anticipated, transfer of the patient to a tertiary level center is warranted prior to delivery to assure intensive care of the neonate. The use of maternal steroids to attempt to induce fetal pulmonary maturity is not indicated under these circumstances.

ELECTRONIC MONITORING. Begin electronic monitoring, using fetal abdominal electrocardiography or Doppler ultrasound, as well as a tocodynamometer for uterine activity, prior to beginning maternal medication. This provides baseline data concerning fetal heart rate, fetal heart rate variability, and the presence of any decelerations with uterine activity. Fetal monitoring should be continued until delivery. Internal fetal monitoring should be instituted when practical to provide the most reliable data for fetal assessment.

Start Medical Induction of Labor. This is accomplished with intravenous oxytocin after the maternal condition has been stabilized and if, on the basis of fetal monitoring, it appears that the fetus will tolerate labor. The finding of a cervix that is favorable for induction is helpful; an unfavorable cervix does not change the necessity for delivery. It is often possible to induce labor successfully in severe cases even with unripe cervices. Induction of labor if the fetal presentation is not cephalic is not warranted, and cesarean section constitutes a better choice. This problem is more frequently encountered in preterm pregnancies.

If eclampsia has occurred, it is generally believed that the induction of labor tends to be relatively easy. This has been the case in our experience. With meticulous attention to detail during these inductions, many cesarean sections can be avoided. This is clearly an advantage to the mother and very possibly to the fetus.

Should seizures occur despite adequate therapy with magnesium sulfate, the use of intravenous diazepam (Valium) is appropriate. Intravenous bolus doses of 10 to 20 mg can be given and repeated as necessary with assessment of the degree of central nervous system depression.

Effect Delivery. Gentle spontaneous or low forceps delivery under pudendal or local anesthesia is ideal. Generally, we prefer not to utilize epidural anesthesia for these patients for either vaginal delivery or cesarean section. In our experience, the risk of maternal hypotension and worsened fetal condition caused by decreased uteroplacental perfusion constitutes an unnecessary and unwarranted risk. Other clinicians believe that epidural anesthesia with sympathetic blockade represents an ideal form of delivery anesthesia for these patients. This may well be appropriate in mild to moderate degrees of the disease. For cesarean section, we prefer balanced general anesthesia (thiopental sodium, nitrous oxide, and succinylcholine) with endotracheal intubation; however, the choice must be made in conjunction with the available anesthetic services. A pediatrician should be present in the delivery room.

In vaginally delivered patients, the patient should receive 120 mg of phenobarbital (Sodium Luminal) intramuscularly immediately after cord clamping.

Continue to Treat Post Partum. The same regimen may be used after the patient has recovered from general anesthesia. The patient should remain in the labor and delivery suite for a minimum of 24 hours. Often a 48 hour stay is warranted, unless there is a specific obstetric intensive care unit available. Magnesium sulfate should be maintained, together with a long-acting barbiturate, for a minimum of 12 to 24 hours. Phenobarbital, 30 to 60 mg intramuscularly every 4 to 5 hours, is often necessary to assure appropriate sedation. Diazepam (Valium), 10 mg intramuscularly, is an alternative. Diuresis and signs of decreased central nervous system irritability will often be observed within 24 to 72 hours post partum.

While it is crucial for signs of central nervous system irritability to have disappeared prior to discharge, it is not necessary for the patient to be entirely normotensive. Generally, these patients will be ready for discharge by the end of the first postpartum week. It should not be inferred, however, that the clinician's task is completed upon hospital discharge. If there is any reason to suspect that the patient did not have "pure" preeclampsia, i.e., disease related only to pregnancy, then further investigations may be warranted at the 4 to 6 week postpartum examination. These investigations might include repeat urine culture and intravenous pyelography, together with renal function tests. This is particularly important if the patient is elderly or multiparous, situations in which an increased incidence of renal abnormalities has been identified.

ANESTHETIC CARE OF THE OBSTETRIC PATIENT
method of
PAUL J. POPPERS, M.D.,
and MICHAEL N. SKAREDOFF, M.D.
Stony Brook, New York

In recent years there has been considerable progress in obstetric anesthesia and analgesia, which in no small part is attributable to the clinical and research efforts of obstetric anesthesiologists. They have become integral and indispensable members of the perinatal team. The team members must be conversant with the dangers and difficulties associated with anesthetic procedures during labor and delivery. They care for two patients, one of whom, the parturient, has an altered physiologic status and is usually not adequately prepared for anesthesia. The second patient, the fetus, may be affected, directly or indirectly, by both the anesthetic procedure and the drugs administered. A thorough comprehension of the physiologic and pharmacologic effects of anesthesia and analgesia is therefore an absolute prerequisite for anesthesiologist and obstetrician. Armed with this knowledge, they must cooperate closely. Only then are the hazards of obstetric anesthesia and analgesia minimized and the advantages fully realized, and only then is obstetric management facilitated and perinatal mortality and morbidity significantly decreased. The ultimate benefit lasts a lifetime.

Maternal Considerations

Aspiration. Anesthesia accidents today are the fourth major cause of obstetric death. Approximately one half of anesthetic fatalities are caused by inhalation of vomitus. Gastric emptying time is significantly increased in pregnant women in the third trimester. Vomiting occurs frequently during labor and delivery, and because general anesthesia or heavy sedation obtunds the laryngeal reflexes, any regurgitated food or gastric juice may be aspirated into the tracheobronchial tree. The laryngeal or bronchial spasm that results may lead to acute anoxia. Moreover, undigested food particles cause airway obstruction. The acidic aspirate destroys the bronchial epithelium. Pulmonary edema and intra-alveolar hemorrhage follow this disruption of the alveolar capillary membrane. Bacterial pneumonitis is a normal sequela.

Labor pain, anxiety, dehydration, or starvation ketosis produces sympathetic excitation that slows gastric emptying. Administration of analgesics and sedatives potentiates this effect. Therefore, one must consider every parturient to have a full stomach.

Patients in labor must be fasting, the fluid requirements being met by parenteral fluids. Antacids and cimetidine raise the pH of gastric contents and are, by sole exception, allowed to be taken orally. Anesthetic techniques that greatly reduce the danger of gastric aspiration are preferred. They are conduction or nerve block (spinal, epidural, paracervical, or pudendal block) or, if general anesthesia is required, rapid induction and tracheal intubation with a cuffed tube. Chances of regurgitation are minimized if the endotracheal tube is inserted with the patient in a slightly head-up position, with simultaneous application of digital pressure on the cricoid cartilage (Sellick's maneuver) to occlude the esophagus.

Should aspiration occur, vigorous therapy is called for. Food particles must be removed by means of a bronchoscope. A good airway should be immediately established by intubation of the trachea, and 100 per cent oxygen administered by intermittent positive pressure breathing. Large doses of corticosteroids may reduce inflammatory reaction. Bacterial pneumonitis is to be prevented or treated with massive doses of antibiotics. Saline irrigation of the tracheobronchial tree is ineffective and pushes the aspirate toward the distal bronchioles. In addition, it washes out surfactant, thus contributing to the occurrence of atelectasis. Any patient suspected of having aspirated gastric material, particularly if symptoms of aspiration are present, should be placed in an intensive care environment for close monitoring and ventilatory care until resolution of the process. The respiratory status should be monitored by chest x-rays and arterial blood gas determinations. The circulation must be carefully watched and supported. Vigorous chest physiotherapy must be instituted as early as possible.

Hypoxia. The second major cause of anesthetic mortality in parturients is hypoxia with associated hypercarbia. It results from poor airway management, accidental esophageal or endobronchial intubation, improper ventilation, or an unsuspectedly low inspired oxygen concentration. Other mechanical factors, such as disconnection of the endotracheal tube from the anesthesia circuit, may be involved.

Hypotension. Sudden, severe hypotension following regional anesthesia is the third most frequent cause of anesthetic maternal mortality. Two factors are responsible for this catastrophe. One is aortocaval compression (or the supine hypotensive syndrome). In a pregnant patient at term who lies supine, the weight of the uterus may compress the major blood vessels, diminishing venous return to the heart. Hypotension and tachycardia result. The other factor is sympathetic blockade, which is a physiologic consequence of regional anesthesia. In addition to magnifying the effects of the supine hypotensive syndrome, it produces pooling of blood in the pelvis and lower extremities.

Maternal mortality caused by hypotension is preventable. A wedge of folded towels, sheets, blankets, or foam plastic placed underneath the right buttock of the patient shifts the uterus and relieves the aortocaval compression. It is an absolute indication for every parturient who lies supine. Expansion of circulating volume with lactated Ringer's solution, 500 to 1000 ml given 30 minutes before the block, is required. When cesarean section under spinal block is planned, a prophylactic intramuscular injection of ephedrine, 50 to 100 mg, is mandatory. For vaginal delivery with low spinal anesthesia, such injection is advisable.

Despite these precautions, sudden hypotension may still occur. Therefore, the blood pressure must be taken every minute for 15 minutes following the administration of a regional anesthetic. Thereafter it suffices to determine the blood pressure once every 5 minutes for the duration of the block. Immediate correction of hypotension is indicated whenever the systolic pressure falls to or below 100 mm Hg. As a first step one should displace the uterus to the left, either manually or by turning the patient on her left side. In addition, intravenous injection of ephedrine, 15 to 25 mg, may be necessary to restore the blood pressure. Oxygen by mask should be administered and lactated Ringer's solution infused.

In the exceptional patient in whom cardiac arrest resulting from "shock" occurs after administration of the spinal anesthetic, the baby must be delivered by immediate cesarean section. The aortocaval compression thus having been relieved, normal cardiorespiratory resuscitation can be successfully instituted.

Toxic Reactions to Local Anesthetics. Inadvertent intravenous injection of local anesthetic is a potential hazard in regional anesthesia. Rapid intravascular injection may result in convulsion and cardiovascular collapse. It is therefore important to perform tests to ensure that bolus doses of local anesthetic are not accidentally administered into the vascular system.

For subarachnoid block anesthesia, the endpoint is easily defined: the flow of clear cerebrospinal fluid through the spinal needle. If the fluid exiting from the hub of the needle is bloody, that blood may have originated from the puncture of an epidural vein during needle passage through the dura. The strategy of choice is: if in doubt, allow the fluid to clear. If it fails to do so, the likelihood of the needle being in an epidural vessel is high and it is necessary to attempt another lumbar puncture. If the fluid clears, it is most likely cerebrospinal fluid. It then is safe to administer the local anesthetic.

Cannulation of a vein during administration of epidural anesthesia during labor occurs at a rate of 1 per cent. It is more likely to occur if the puncture is made in the lateral part of the epidural space where the veins are more densely clustered than in the midline.

In order to diminish the risk of intravascular injection of local anesthetic, one should (1) insert the catheter in the midline rather than in the lateral portions of the epidural space; (2) aspirate carefully through the catheter before taping it in place; (3) use a test dose through the catheter; and (4) before every reinforcement dose, aspirate through the catheter.

The anesthesiologist should be on the alert for the following symptoms of local anesthetic toxicity: (1) paresthesias or "tingling" in the lips or hands; (2) a metallic taste in the mouth; (3) ringing in the ears; (4) feeling of faintness, dizziness, nausea, or anxiety; (5) prodromal twitching of the hands or feet; or (6) diplopia and nystagmus.

When convulsions do occur, the treatment strategy has as its ultimate goal adequate oxygenation of the maternal-fetal unit. Therefore immediate therapy should consist of the following steps:

1. Ventilation with oxygen by bag and mask, or, if unconsciousness seems imminent, rapid tracheal intubation facilitated with succinylcholine, 60 to 80 mg intravenously. (An assistant applies cricoid pressure to prevent aspiration.)

2. Turning the parturient into the left lateral position.

3. Use of intravenous thiopental, 50 to 75 mg, or diazepam, 5 mg.

4. Vasopressor therapy with ephedrine sulfate if arterial hypotension supervenes or persists despite having the patient in the left lateral decubitus position.

5. Generous administration of intravenous fluids.

6. Maternal vital signs to be taken at least once a minute until blood pressure stabilizes.

7. The fetal monitor to be immediately connected and the fetal heart rate and uterine contractions to be monitored for signs of uteroplacental perfusion insufficiency (late or Type II decelerations).

8. Preparation for immediate cesarean section to be made.

9. Finally, in the case of cardiovascular collapse, standard protocols of cardiopulmonary resuscitation to be immediately instituted.

Fetal and Neonatal Depression

Several factors may cause or contribute to depression of the fetus and newborn. One of the most important is asphyxia consequent to inadequate placental function caused by toxemia, renal disease, or diabetes. Acute asphyxia of the fetus may result from maternal hypotension, placental abruption, a hypertonic or tetanic state of the uterus, or umbilical cord compression. Prolonged or precipitate labor and operative obstetrics are traumatic causes of infant depression.

Obstetric anesthesia and analgesia are the third cause, in order of frequency, of neonatal depression. They may also aggravate the effects of the aforementioned conditions. On the other hand, judiciously selected pain relief diminishes patient anxiety and lowers circulatory catecholamine levels. As a result, uterine blood flow increases and the fetal oxygenation improves. By themselves, these drugs may produce depression, either directly or indirectly. The direct effects result from placental transfer of drugs. Maternal hypotension (as a result of regional vasodilatation) or uterine vasoconstriction (caused by peripherally acting vasopressors) may be indirectly responsible for depression of the neonate, because either decreases placental perfusion.

Placental drug transfer occurs mainly by simple diffusion. The rate of diffusion is determined by the degree of ionization, lipid solubility, plasma protein binding, molecular weight, and concentration gradient of the compound. All sedative, analgesic, and anesthetic drugs administered during labor cross the placental barrier. Clinical doses of muscle relaxants, with the exception of gallamine, cross in such small quantity that they do not measurably affect the fetus. Inhalation anesthetics in analgesic concentrations do not cause fetal depression. Anesthetic concentrations of potent inhalation agents may cause fetal depression after 5 to 6 minutes of administration to the mother. This time lag is due to the presence of a three-compartment type of circulation, which slows drug uptake in fetal brain tissue: maternal alveolar-arterial equilibration precedes maternal-fetal circulatory equilibration. The latter lags because only 55 per cent of the fetal cardiac output goes to the placenta via the umbilical artery, with the remaining 45 per cent perfusing the fetus. Nitrous oxide, since it is a weak anesthetic, is usually well tolerated for up to 15 minutes by the mature fetus. However, it can depress the fetus of less than 36 weeks' gestational age.

Thiobarbiturates are the preferred induction agents for general anesthesia. A single intravenous injection, not exceeding 250 mg, does not significantly depress the fetus, and is by far the safest induction method for the mother. In asthmatic patients injection of thiopental may induce an asthmatic attack. For these patients, ketamine, 1.0 mg per kg intravenously, should be given as an induction dose (see manufacturer's official directive before using).

Long-acting barbiturates, given by mouth or by intramuscular injection for sedation, may cause significant respiratory depression in the neonate. These sedative hypnotic drugs possess no analgesic action and indeed may produce an antianalgesic effect. Furthermore, they cannot be specifically antagonized, and should be avoided.

Promethazine (Phenergan) in 25 mg doses is a useful sedative that does not appear to cause fetal depression. Diazepam (Valium) should not be used. It causes prolonged depression of the neonate, with hypotonia and hypothermia.

Narcotics administered during labor are known to cause respiratory depression in the neonate. In general, very little preference can be expressed for one particular drug, because in equianalgesic doses they all cause the same degree of respiratory depression. Only the duration of the depressant effect is different for each, and this is related to the length of its narcotic action. Narcotic drugs can be specifically antagonized by naloxone (Narcan). However, the total amount of narcotic administered during the course of labor should be kept to a minimum, and narcotic antagonists should be given only when indicated.

Administration of large quantities of local anesthetics is associated with a gradually increasing circulatory drug concentration that may ultimately lead to respiratory or circulatory depression of the fetus, or both. Therefore, whenever these are used, the smallest possible quantity of the least toxic anesthetic in its lowest effective concentration should be employed.

Safety Measures and Equipment

All patients in labor must have an infusion via a large bore intravenous plastic cannula. For each, a blood pressure cuff with manometer and a stethoscope must be available. No oral food or fluid intake is allowed, with the exception of 3 hourly ingestion of liquid antacid.

Each individual labor room must be provided with suction apparatus, oxygen supply, and positive pressure breathing apparatus. Oral and endotracheal airways, a laryngoscope, thiopental, succinylcholine, and vasopressors, with syringes and needles for their administration, should be close at hand. In addition, the delivery room must be equipped with a modern, well-working anesthesia machine which delivers oxygen and nitrous oxide, and allows vaporization of volatile anesthetics.

Appropriate neonatal resuscitation equipment, such as apparatus for positive pressure breathing, infant-size laryngoscope, endotracheal tubes with stylettes, oral airways, and suction catheters, must be present. The availability of umbilical catheterization sets for administration of sodium bicarbonate is also indicated.

Anesthesia for Labor and Vaginal Delivery

The cooperation of the patient is essential to achieve satisfactory pain relief during labor and delivery. It can be obtained only if the normal process of childbirth is explained and the discomfort that it involves is discussed, so that the mother's fear of the obstetric events is allayed. This preparation, a task for both obstetrician and anesthesiologist, may be just as important as the administration of drugs.

Psychoprophylaxis is helpful because it puts emphasis upon the physiologic character of childbirth. The breathing techniques that are taught occupy the mind of the patient during labor, and reduce the amount of pain that is being experienced.

The patient should be told that natural childbirth techniques may frequently not be entirely adequate and that a conventional anesthesia technique may become necessary during the course of her labor. Without this instruction, the patient might otherwise experience frustration and a sense of guilt for having failed to have her baby without receiving anesthesia.

Nerve Block and Conduction Anesthesia

Paracervical block relieves pain of the first stage of labor. The block is performed during active labor, preferably in the phase of maximal slope, when the cervix is at least 4 cm dilated and the presenting part engaged. Bilateral injections of 5 to 10 ml of 1 per cent lidocaine are made in the lateral fornices at an approximate depth of 1.5 cm. Because of its limited duration the block may have to be repeated in 1 to 1½ hours.

Careful aspiration is necessary to prevent injection into a paracervical vein with subsequent systemic toxicity in the mother. In order to avoid direct injection into the fetus, a needle guard must be used; the needle must be directed laterally, and the block should not be performed when cervical dilatation exceeds 8 cm.

Fetal complications occur frequently. The incidence of bradycardia may be as high as 50 per cent, and of acidosis, 100 per cent. The fetal distress occurs on the basis of uterine arterial vasoconstriction that is provoked by the local anesthetic. A fetus that is already distressed may suffer fatal consequences. For these reasons, paracervical nerve block is not recommended.

Pudendal nerve block eliminates pain of the second stage of labor and provides anesthesia for performing an episiotomy and its repair, and for operative delivery by forceps or vacuum extraction. Pudendal blocks can provide a patient with a comfortable delivery that includes forceps maneuvers.

The ischial spine is palpated and the needle introduced through the sacrospinous ligament immediately below and medial to the spine. After careful aspiration to prevent injection into a pudendal vessel, 5 to 10 ml of 1 per cent lidocaine is injected. The transvaginal approach is preferable to the transperineal approach because it allows direct guidance of the needle point to the ischial spine by the index and middle fingers. Injection into the presenting part of the fetus is thus avoided. For the same reason, use of a needle guide ("Iowa trumpet") is obligatory. If descent of the fetal head makes vaginal insertion of fingers and needle guide impossible, one should not administer a pudendal block but resort to local infiltration of the perineum.

Saddle block is a low spinal block technique. The extent of the anesthesia is limited to the sacral and lower lumbar nerves. This type of block abolishes the pain of an episiotomy and outlet or midforceps delivery.

Saddle block anesthesia should be administered within one half hour of estimated delivery. The lumbar puncture is performed with a small-bore spinal needle, with the patient in the sitting position. A hyperbaric solution containing either a mixture of tetracaine, 3 to 5 mg in 10 per cent dextrose, or lidocaine (Xylocaine), 30 to 50 mg in 7.5 per cent dextrose, is injected. The sitting position is maintained for 30 to 45 seconds to allow the spread of local anesthetic to the sacral and lower lumbar segments.

Despite the low level of sensory anesthesia, hypotension occurs in a significant number of patients. Frequent blood pressure determinations are therefore indicated. Hypotension is to be treated as outlined previously. A prophylactic intramuscular injection of ephedrine, 50 mg, is useful.

Epidural block anesthesia, using a catheter for intermittent injection of a local anesthetic agent, provides continuous, flexible, and complete pain relief during labor and delivery with minimal adverse effects upon the mother and fetus. Two types of epidural anesthesia are commonly used: the lumbar epidural block and, less frequently, the sacral or caudal epidural block. Lumbar epidural anesthesia is probably the safest and certainly the most effective regional block that can be offered to the patient in normal labor. Danger of hypotension requires careful monitoring of blood pressure at 5 minute intervals.

Anesthesia can be started when the cervical dilatation is 4 to 5 cm in a multiparous patient, and 5 to 6 cm in a primiparous patient. Labor should be well established, with strong and regular contractions (and the presenting part in a normal presentation engaged in the pelvis without cephalopelvic disproportion). The epidural catheter should preferably be placed early in active labor, when the patient is still comfortable and able to cooperate. The complete block can thereafter be quickly established at any given time when required.

For lumbar epidural anesthesia, the epidural space is entered with a 16 or 17 gauge needle in the interspace of L2-L3 or L3-L4. A plastic catheter is gently threaded rostrally or caudally.

The preferred agent is bupivacaine (Marcaine), 0.25 or 0.5 per cent. The use of epinephrine-containing solutions of local anesthetics is not advisable. Even in low concentrations, epinephrine diminishes uterine blood flow, slows labor, and may cause profound hypotension. A test dose of local anesthetic is injected to rule out subarachnoid injection and to prevent massive spinal block that would result if the full dose were injected. If, after waiting for 5 minutes, there are no signs suggestive of spinal anesthesia, an additional 5 to 10 ml can be injected to obtain a satisfactory level of analgesia. Before each injection of local anesthetic, aspiration should be attempted to avoid intravascular or subarachnoid injection.

For continuous caudal anesthesia the sacral

epidural space is entered via the caudal hiatus with a 16 or 17 gauge needle, through which a catheter is advanced. A rectal examination is mandatory prior to withdrawing the needle to rule out its placement anterior to the sacrum and possibly in the fetus, thus preventing anesthetic intoxication of the fetus.

A test dose of anesthetic is required. Its effect should be evaluated in 5 to 10 minutes for the absence of subarachnoid anesthesia. However, rectal sphincter muscle relaxation on digital examination and loss of the rectal sphincter reflex indicate that the perineum is anesthetized. (If these objective signs cannot be found, no additional anesthetic drug should be given but another block should be attempted.) In the presence of perineal analgesia, injection of an additional 12 to 15 ml of anesthetic establishes the complete caudal block.

A single caudal injection must be administered through a large-bore needle (16 or 18 gauge) to allow easy aspiration of blood or cerebrospinal fluid. Aspiration must be attempted in two planes. Again, a rectal examination must be done before the anesthetic is injected. The usual dose is 25 ml of 0.5 per cent bupivacaine.

Sacral and lumbar epidural blocks require that they be performed by experienced physicians for their success and safety, and additional personnel must be available for constant supervision of the patient. The techniques involved are relatively difficult to perform.

Total spinal anesthesia as a complication of epidural anesthesia is rare, provided that a test dose is administered and its effect carefully evaluated. Massive inadvertent subarachnoid local anesthetic administration may occur when an epidural needle or epidural catheter has penetrated the dura. It is followed by immediate total spinal anesthesia, which is characterized by loss of consciousness, apnea, and vascular hypotension.

The best treatment is, of course, prevention. Avoidance of subarachnoid needle puncture can be effected by care and good needle control. However, if clear fluid does appear in the hub of the needle (a glucose reagent strip can be used to determine if the fluid is indeed cerebrospinal fluid), the epidural needle should be removed and reinserted in an adjoining interspace.

Treatment of a massive subarachnoid injection should be directed toward supporting the patient until the effects wear off:

1. The patient, if unconscious and apneic, should be immediately intubated to avoid aspiration, and ventilated with air or oxygen until spontaneous respiration recommences.

2. Generous amounts of fluids should be given to counteract hypotension.

3. The uterus should be immediately displaced by turning the patient on her side, to avoid aortocaval compression.

4. If fluid load and uterine displacement are inadequate to prevent hypotension, 10 to 25 mg of ephedrine sulfate should be injected intravenously.

5. In the event that the patient does not become unconscious or apneic, management would be that of a spinal anesthetic.

The lumbar epidural anesthetic technique is more physiologic than the caudal approach. Faster onset of pain relief in the first stage of labor is obtained from lumbar epidural anesthesia, and with less anesthetic. Also, the total dose of anesthetic required throughout the course of labor and delivery is much smaller than that for the caudal block. This may be an important consideration in terms of drug toxicity in mother and fetus when a prolonged labor is anticipated. Lumbar epidural block is preferred if cesarean section is a distinct possibility.

Caudal epidural anesthesia is rarely associated with accidental dural puncture, whereas this complication is not exceptional in the performance of lumbar epidural anesthesia. Immobility of the patient is less a requirement in the initiation of a caudal epidural block. Relaxation of the perineum is more profound with caudal anesthesia, which is of special importance in prematurity. A test dose given through the catheter in the caudal canal produces objective signs indicating proper placement of that catheter.

Inhalation Analgesia and Anesthesia

Analgesic concentrations of inhalation anesthetics provide a fair measure of pain relief during delivery. A cooperative patient experiences little or no discomfort at childbirth when inhalation analgesia is supplemented with pudendal block or local infiltration of the perineum, and preceded by a small dose of narcotic, e.g., meperidine, 50 mg. It does not cause cardiovascular or respiratory depression in either mother or fetus. The pushing reflex is not abolished, and the patient can consciously bear down with contractions during the expulsion phase.

Perhaps the greatest pitfall of inhalation techniques is their apparent simplicity. This is particularly dangerous because anesthesia is induced more easily in the parturient for several reasons. Physiologic changes in pregnancy include a reduction in functional residual capacity and an increase in alveolar ventilation, which result in more rapid induction of anesthesia. Pregnancy is also associated with reduced anesthetic requirements. Narcotics given during labor may further reduce the minimal alveolar concentration (MAC) required and so contribute to the risk of inhalation analgesia with inadvertent anesthetic overdose and loss of protective reflexes. Vomiting and/or silent regurgitation may occur, resulting in immediate respiratory obstruction or aspiration syndrome. In addition to the physiologic alterations of pregnancy noted above, the pregnant patient has a higher metabolic rate and increased oxygen consumption, predisposing her to the rapid development of hypoxia in the event of respiratory depression or airway obstruction. Hypercapnia and acidosis can then develop very quickly, and these changes are exaggerated in the obese parturient who has additional derangements of pulmonary function.

Administration of nitrous oxide and potent inhalation agents is deceptively simple and should be left to those practitioners who are skilled in this technique — it is not for the inexperienced!

General anesthesia must be administered when regional anesthesia is contraindicated or has failed, and when inhalation analgesia is inadequate. After the patient has breathed oxygen for several minutes, induction is accomplished with thiopental, 250 mg intravenously. The trachea is intubated after intravenous injection of succinylcholine, 100 mg. Anesthesia is maintained with nitrous oxide, 50 per cent in oxygen.

Deep halothane anesthesia is indicated whenever uterine relaxation is required. Internal podalic version and extraction, delivery of the aftercoming head, which is trapped by the cervix in a breech delivery, and manual removal of a retained placenta are indications for uterine relaxation with halothane (2 to 4 per cent in oxygen). Because deep halothane anesthesia may lead to severe depression of the maternal circulation, the blood pressure must be taken at 1 minute intervals. Under no circumstances should the administration of halothane be continued when the systolic pressure falls to 80 mm Hg. Since halothane relaxes the uterus, it may cause postpartum atony and hemorrhage.

Anesthesia for Cesarean Section

Spinal anesthesia is very effective and technically simple for cesarean section. The incidence of neonatal depression is low. The mother is not exposed to an increased risk of aspiration of vomitus. However, hypotension occurs frequently, which could be life threatening if severe and precipitate. Prophylactic intramuscular injection of ephedrine, 50 to 100 mg, 10 to 15 minutes prior to the subarachnoid puncture is mandatory. It is helpful to infuse rapidly at least 1000 ml of an electrolyte solution shortly before performing the spinal block. Further, it is absolutely indicated to tilt the patient's uterus to the left immediately following the administration of subarachnoid block. These precautions prevent a disaster, but some degree of hypotension may still occur. Immediate correction with intravenous administration of ephedrine, 15 to 25 mg, is then indicated, followed by rapid infusion of electrolyte solution. Spinal anesthesia is contraindicated in the presence of hypotension, moderate to severe hypertension, placenta previa, abruptio placentae, borderline placental perfusion or suspected umbilical cord compression, certain neurologic diseases, or skin infection. Acute fetal distress indicates immediate abdominal delivery under general anesthesia.

Tetracaine in hyperbaric solution is the agent most commonly used for cesarean section. Dosage depends upon the patient's height (Table 1). For cesarean hysterectomy, 1 mg should be added to each dose listed in the table. As soon as the anesthetic has been injected, the patient should be placed on her back in a 10 to 15 degree left lateral tilt.

Continuous lumbar epidural anesthesia is an excellent choice for cesarean section. The incidence of hypotension is lower, the onset slower, and the degree less severe compared with spinal anesthesia. Thus, epidural block is actually safer for cesarean section. It also yields better control of level and duration of anesthesia than the single subarachnoid injection. Epidural anesthesia pro-

TABLE 1. **Dosage in Milligrams of Tetracaine in 5 per cent Dextrose for Spinal Anesthesia in Obstetrics**

	HEIGHT OF PARTURIENT			
	5'–5'2" (150–155 cm)	5'2"–5'6" (155–165 cm)	5'6"–6' (165–180 cm)	>6' (>180 cm)
Vaginal delivery, saddle block	3–4	4–5	5	5
Cesarean section, patient in lateral decubitus position	6	7	8	9
Cesarean section, patient in sitting position	7	8	9	10

vides the surgeon with excellent operating conditions, and is very well tolerated by mother and fetus. The volume of local anesthetic required for epidural block is variable, but is in general 5 to 15 ml greater than that for vaginal delivery.

General anesthesia is well established for cesarean section. Studies on placental transfer of anesthetics and their distribution in fetal tissues have led to a technique of general anesthesia which has excellent results for mother and neonate, rivaling those of regional anesthesia. Surgical dispatch is desirable. Within 10 minutes after induction of anesthesia, the fetus should be delivered. Therefore the patient is anesthetized only after the operative site is prepared and draped, and the surgeon stands ready to make the incision. After 3 to 5 minutes of preoxygenation, induction is accomplished with thiopental, 3 to 4 mg per kg of body weight, in a single dose intravenously, to be followed by succinylcholine, 100 mg. Surgery is started immediately after the trachea has been intubated. Anesthesia is maintained with nitrous oxide, 50 per cent in oxygen. It may have to be supplemented with a succinylcholine infusion before the infant is delivered. Thereafter, narcotics may be used to supplement the inhalation anesthesia. With all techniques, a prolonged UD (uterine incision–delivery) interval greater than 180 seconds has been found to be directly related to fetal hypoxia and acidosis.

Anesthetic Management of Obstetric Complications

Prematurity. Conduction anesthesia is preferred for vaginal delivery and for cesarean section. It obviates the need for sedatives, narcotics, hypnotics, and inhalation anesthetics. It also allows the mother to breathe oxygen; raising the maternal arterial oxygen tension to 300 mm Hg provides optimal fetal oxygenation. Perineal relaxation obtained with regional block is an added benefit in vaginal delivery of a premature infant.

Breech Presentation. Only minimal doses of narcotic or sedative drugs should be given in order not to jeopardize the fetus. It is important that one not interfere with the progress of labor and the maternal expulsive effort. Thus, it is often better to give small doses of local anesthetic in low concentrations. One must be prepared for rapid induction of deep halothane anesthesia to relax the uterus in case the aftercoming head becomes trapped. The parturient is especially susceptible to overdosage with inhalation anesthetics, and utmost caution must be exercised during controlled ventilation with potent agents.

Multiple Pregnancy. Prematurity and abnormal presentation frequently occur in multiple pregnancy. Interference with labor by medication or anesthesia should be avoided. Uterine relaxation may be required to allow a podalic version and extraction of the second infant in twin births or to deliver the aftercoming head of a fetus in breech presentation. The mother may experience respiratory embarrassment and also hypotension if the uterus is very large. Many anesthesiologists believe that if analgesia is required, continuous epidural is ideal. In some circumstances there may exist a maternal indication for general anesthesia that outweighs the fetal considerations.

Fetal Distress. Obstetric causes of fetal distress generally dictate *immediate* delivery of the fetus. If a conduction block has been established, oxygen should be administered. An increase in fetal arterial oxygen tension, however slight, may significantly increase hemoglobin saturation. Because of the time factor, it is not feasible to initiate regional anesthesia. General anesthesia is rapidly induced with thiopental and succinylcholine, and maintained with nitrous oxide in oxygen as described above.

Anesthetic causes of fetal distress do not necessarily require that the fetus be delivered immediately. Maternal hypotension as a cause of distress can be corrected. Fetal bradycardia caused by high blood levels of a local anesthetic following inadvertent intravascular injection of the agent is often temporary. Drug distribution in maternal tissues enables the fetus to transfer the local anesthetic to the mother, after which the fetal heart rate recovers.

Toxemia and Preeclampsia. In nonsevere cases lumbar epidural anesthesia is the anesthetic of choice for labor and vaginal delivery. It causes less depression of a fetus that is compromised by a borderline placental circulation. Regional anesthesia is not to be used to lower the blood pressure to "normal" levels, and hypotension must be avoided. Spinal anesthesia for cesarean section is thus a poor choice in patients with high blood pressure. In addition, should spinal anesthesia produce severe hypotension, vasopressor therapy is poorly tolerated. For cesarean section, general anesthesia is preferred in severe cases of preeclampsia, and epidural block in mild cases. It should be borne in mind that magnesium sulfate, although it is a very valuable component of toxemia therapy, potentiates the muscle relaxants. A suggested technique for general anesthesia for cesarean section in the toxemic parturient who has had magnesium sulfate therapy is the following:

1. Placement of patient in supine position with left lateral tilt.

2. Preoxygenation for 3 minutes.

3. The use of hydralazine, 80 mg per 125 ml of 5 per cent dextrose in water, to be administered in an intravenous infusion until the diastolic pressure is approximately 85 to 90 mm Hg.

4. Induction with thiopental, 4 mg per kg intravenously, followed by succinylcholine, 50 to 75 mg intravenously, during which time Sellick's maneuver is employed.

5. Rapid sequence intubation of trachea.

6. Nitrous oxide, 50 per cent in oxygen inhalation anesthesia.

7. Monitoring of neuromuscular blockade with a nerve stimulator.

Continuous lumbar epidural anesthesia may be successfully used in preeclamptic patients to prevent the blood pressure from rising to dangerous levels. It should not be considered a treatment of hypertension. Postpartum preeclampsia can be treated and serious complications avoided by gradually lowering the blood pressure with intravenous infusion of hydralazine. Once the blood pressure has fallen significantly, magnesium sulfate, long-acting barbiturates, and diazepam can be substituted.

Tetanic Uterine Contractions. This condition interrupts placental perfusion for a prolonged period of time and causes fetal asphyxia. It is usually produced by oxytocin, used to induce or augment labor, but it may occur spontaneously. A tetanic contraction calls for immediate therapy. Intravenous injection of magnesium sulfate, 2 to 6 grams, relaxes the uterus. Deep general anesthesia with halothane is an alternative, but only if immediate delivery is desired.

Cardiovascular and Pulmonary Disease. The great stress of the second stage of labor is to be avoided in patients with significant disease of heart and lungs, or with vascular anomalies. Continuous regional anesthesia abolishes the pain and associated maternal tachycardia. It can be administered as soon as a labor pattern has been established. It is preferable in the majority of vaginal deliveries. However, hypotension is dangerous in a patient with a fixed cardiac output, and therefore regional anesthesia is not a preferred technique in this instance.

For cesarean section, regional block is the anesthesia of choice in patients with asthma and other forms of obstructive pulmonary disease. For emergency cesarean section, better control of respiration and circulation can be achieved with general anesthesia.

Effect of Anesthesia and Analgesia upon Labor

Uterine muscle relaxants, such as halothane and magnesium sulfate, decrease the strength of contractions. Increased blood levels of catecholamines, whether endogenously produced by pain and anxiety or exogenously administered, retard the progress of labor.

Regional anesthesia in the form of epidural block inhibits labor in the presence of maternal hypotension, fetopelvic disproportion, or dysfunctional labor, or when it is superimposed on excessive systemic medication. On the other hand, it enhances labor by relieving maternal anxiety. The second stage of labor may be prolonged because of paresis of the abdominal musculature and elimination of the expulsion reflex. The intelligent and informed patient, however, is able to push better when pain is abolished by epidural anesthesia. Nonetheless, regional anesthesia does cause an increase in the rate of low forceps deliveries. On occasion internal rotation of the fetal head does not occur because the regional anesthesia has relaxed the pelvic floor. Epidural anesthesia may be of great benefit in preventing tumultuous labor and precipitous delivery, both important causes of birth trauma and subsequent neurologic deficit.

Vasopressors

Considerable controversy still exists as to the use of vasopressors during labor and delivery relative to their effect upon the fetus. Animal experiments and clinical studies support the view that ephedrine is a safe and useful agent in the prophylaxis and treatment of hypotension. In contrast, peripheral vasoconstrictors have been found to further decrease the uterine blood flow in hypotensive animals. They may also be the cause of a uterine tetanic state.

Ephedrine can be safely used in conjunction with synthetic oxytocics. However, together with ergot preparations, it causes dangerous hypertension.

Post–Spinal Anesthesia Headache

Although it is without pathologic importance, a post–spinal anesthesia headache is most distressing. Obstetric patients are particularly prone to develop this following dural puncture because they are young, healthy, active women who have gone through a period of increased cerebrospinal fluid pressure during the second stage of labor. The incidence of post–spinal anesthesia headache can be lowered to about 2 per cent by use of a small bore (25 or 26 gauge) spinal needle. Intravenous hydration and bed rest (with bathroom privileges) in the first 24 or 48 hours after delivery are also helpful. Treatment may consist of further bed rest, preferably in the lateral decubitus or even prone position to lower the hydrostatic pressure of cerebrospinal fluid on the puncture site, epidural injections of 30 ml of isotonic saline solution every 3 hours for 24 hours, a tight abdominal binder, and, especially, explanatory reassurance. Common analgesics can be prescribed. Dramatic and longer-lasting improvements have been observed after epidural injection of 5 to 10 ml of autologous venous blood under strictest asepsis. An expectant attitude is very often best. An epidural blood patch should be done only if the patient is still prostrate after 2 or 3 days. The technique requires that it be performed by an experienced physician.

POSTPARTUM CARE

method of
CHARLES D. KIMBALL, M.D.
Seattle, Washington

Currently postpartum care is undergoing rapid and drastic change as a result of new concepts relating peptide neurotransmitter hormones and emotional experience to development of neuronal functions and initiation of the biologic affectional bond between mothers and infants early in the neonatal period. This trend is reflected by structured alterations and revisions of obstetric routine in many maternity units in order to comply with patient demands. Alternative childbirth programs and increasing numbers of hospital and do-it-yourself home deliveries (many of which are inadequately supervised) have caused Public Health officials deep concern and apprehension that the perennial 15 per cent of high risk mothers and infants who need skilled and experienced obstetric or pediatric care will suffer preventable disaster.

Physical Problems. Postpartum hemorrhage and puerperal sepsis, which have always been life-threatening complications of maternity, require expedient anticipatory management. Prevention and prompt recognition and treatment of these major maternal hazards must still be the main consideration as soon as the third stage of labor is completed.

Postpartum Hemorrhage. Routine examination of the cervix, vagina, and placenta by direct visual inspection and (if indicated) by gentle bimanual palpation of the intrauterine cavity will ascertain existence of any retained placenta or significant anatomic trauma that should be repaired promptly. There is no good excuse for failure to take time to determine the presence of tissue damage so that remedial and preventive measures can avoid further trouble.

After the placenta is delivered, intravenous oxytocic drugs should be given as indicated: oxytocic injection (Pitocin or Syntocin), 0.5 ml by intravenous push or 2 ml in 500 ml of 5 per cent glucose by intravenous drip, or ergonovine (Ergotrate), 0.2 mg by slow intravenous push. An intravenous drip of 5 per cent glucose via a polyethylene catheter is especially indicated when any vasodilating block anesthesia is used. It should be started prior to delivery to secure intravenous access as a precautionary measure against a sudden, worrisome fall in blood pressure. This occurs in some patients, probably because of intense anxiety reaction, producing a surge of endogenous epinephrine with the resultant uterine and transient vasomotor atony. Transabdominal aortic compression by pressure of the closed fist at the level of the umbilicus or bimanual compression of the uterus against the symphysis will stem blood loss, and can be lifesaving until vasomotor tonus can be stabilized and blood loss replaced by balanced intravenous fluids or whole blood as indicated. The aortic compression maneuver is also helpful to achieve clear visualization of the birth canal when brisk bleeding obscures vision following expulsion of the placenta.

Puerperal Sepsis. As with fire in the wastepaper basket, the sooner the infection is discovered and extinguished, the less damage occurs. Temperature elevation of 38 C (100.4 F) for two or more consecutive 8 hour readings signals impending morbidity and alerts need for diagnostic tests. Before any antibiotic therapy is given, blood count, blood culture, cultures of lochia and catheterized urine, and sometimes chest x-ray are mandatory. As soon as these are done, one of the cephalosporins or ampicillin should be given in doses of 1 gram every 4 hours by piggyback in intravenous balanced dextrose solution. Too much too soon is better than too little too late. In most instances laboratory reports and patient response will confirm this choice of medication. If fever, elevated pulse rate, and other signs of toxicity persist, Bacteroides anaerobes should be suspected and no time lost in giving chloramphenicol, 1 gram every 6 hours intravenously, or clindamycin in carefully adjusted recommended doses. Gentamicin in place of a cephalosporin can then be considered with precautions taken regarding neurotoxicity.

When early treatment of sepsis has not been given and pelvic thrombophlebitis, parametrial abscess, or other localized tissue infection is suspected, consultation and appropriate surgical intervention should be considered.

Postpartum Breast Function. Stimulation and inhibition of lactation is a genetically built-in biocybernetic mechanism of mammalian evolution. It actually needs little if any therapeutic management despite the voluminous market that has been created for breast pumps, nipple shields and creams, and lactation-suppressing hormones. Milk production depends on prolactin (lactogenic) hormone from the anterior pituitary, and letdown flow of milk is stimulated by oxytocic hormone from the posterior pituitary. Prolactin hormone output is triggered by the sudden decrease in placental estrogen and progesterone when polypeptide endorphin release is generated by the nerve cells in the hypothalamic centers. Milk production is sustained physiologically until dopamine, a suppressor of prolactin, is activated by feedback of reabsorbed excess milk in the lacteal glands. If there is no reabsorption feedback, the milk supply will increase to meet the demands of the growing infant appetite. Administration of estrogen hormones simply delays output of the endorphin release for prolactin until the blood estrogen level drops. Lactation then usually occurs with less acute breast engorgement.

Caked breasts and painful engorgement in nursing mothers can be relieved by local application of heat for 15 to 20 minutes, followed by ice cold compresses for 5 minutes and immediately putting the baby on the breast or otherwise emptying the swollen lacteals. Painful engorgement in non-nursing mothers nearly always subsides within 18 to 24 hours when the reabsorbed milk has suppressed prolactin.

Emotional Behavior Problems. Most emotional and behavioral problems of postpartum patients are manifested by distorted perceptual attitudes based on neuroendocrine dysfunctions. Impressive evidence now indicates that the postpartum period may be a critical time in the mother-infant relationship when ongoing neuroendocrine functions responsible for lactation, maternal feelings, and behavior are initiated. Based on reliable reports that both umbilical cord and maternal blood levels of endogenous opium-like peptides (endorphins) and prolactin hormone rise significantly during labor and breast feeding, it has been suggested that nurturing behavior and formation of the so-called affectional bond between mother and infant are motivated by these hormones. This pleasurable mood of contentment, well-being, and affection evidenced by most mothers at their infants' births is ostensibly due to the elevated endorphin peptides and the well-known influence that opiates exert on affect and intimate behavior. The added facts that both exogenous and endogenous opiates evoke prolactin secretion and that both of these hormones are reported to be suppressed by the opium antagonist naloxone tend to support this contention. It is also known that prolactin is suppressed by reabsorption of milk from engorged breasts and by dopamine agonists such as bromocriptine mesylate (Parlodel).

Postpartum blues and maternal depression, which usually occurs in conjunction with prolactin suppression are often responsive to dopamine receptor blockers such as prochlorperazine (Compazine), trifluoperazine (Stelazine), and triflupromazine (Vesprin), as well as to tricyclic antidepressants such as nortriptyline (Aventyl), desipramines (Norpramine), and amitriptyline (Elavil), which increase norepinephrine activity. Postpartum mental and emotional disturbances are nearly always self-limited and respond well to medication and to time. Traditional psychotherapy has not been found to be of much help.

The ultimate therapeutic importance of including behavioral science concepts and methodology in the management of obstetric patients is to prevent serious damage to the newborn brain circuits at the critical period when initial neuronal programming for affectional basic trust and autonomic visceral physiology is being set. Sufficient evidence from the primate laboratories and other sources is at hand to indicate that the neurobiologic quality of the infant's early contact is vital to the development of character structure and prevention of remote emotional illness and sociopathic behavior. Childhood autism and depression and adolescent drug addiction and self-destruction appear to be closely correlated with separation of mothers and newborns and perinatal pair bond hormonal deficiency.

CARE OF THE LOW BIRTH WEIGHT INFANT

method of
MARTIN H. GREENBERG, M.D.
Savannah, Georgia

Organization and regionalization of perinatal care have significantly contributed to the amelioration of outcome for the low birth weight (LBW) baby during the past decade.

Whenever possible, antepartum identification of high risk situations, with delivery in a facility offering mother and baby the best potential outcome, should be sought. Red flags such as toxemia, diabetes, thyroid disease, fetal growth retardation, previous prematurity, or other poor obstetric history may assist in alerting the physician to the case in need of consultation. Diagnostic measures are available to assist in detection of fetal maturity and malformations. Each delivery facility must be equipped for emergency and support efforts to minimize problems for mother and baby.

All LBW babies are *not* created equal. Some are very low birth weight (VLBW) and are under 1500 grams. Even in this latter group, the prognosis for survival and outcome appears brighter as advances are made in diagnosis, treatment, and technology.

Confusion in terminology from the early days of neonatology and relics of designation from health department statistics still equate LBW solely with prematurity. Figure 1 focuses on maturity or ripeness with appropriate prefixes to designate the spectrum of its deviations.

All four states may coincide with LBW. Immaturity can be total or restricted to a vital organ (such as the lung) and may not be compatible with life. The VLBW baby frequently falls into this group. The premature baby is just born too soon, for whatever reason. Prematurity is strictly a *temporal* definition and must not be equated with a fixed weight definition, however convenient. The postmature baby is one who stays in utero too long (beyond 42 weeks from the estimated date of confinement). Some lose weight and become LBW secondary to malnutrition caused by placental failure. Postmaturity, however, may be compatible with normal fetal growth (and even result in large-for-gestational age infants) if placental function and other parameters remain stable. Dysmaturity may occur at any stage of pregnancy and relates to *dysfunction*. This may be anatomic, metabolic, endocrine, or functional, and leads to intrauterine growth failure and therefore LBW.

It is important to properly define the type and seek a cause for LBW in order to anticipate

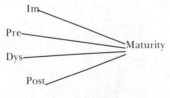

Figure 1.

problems. LBW babies who are small for gestational age (SGA) (using standard charts of intrauterine growth by Lubchenco et al.) can be divided into two groups: the environmental and the genetic. The former are babies who were destined to be normal in size, but somewhere in pregnancy (any trimester) dysmaturity occurs. Placental dysfunction may be chemical (fetal alcohol syndrome), metabolic (toxemia, diabetes), or infectious. Here the nuclear material is normal in quantity but cytoplasm is reduced. Catch-up growth may occur. Intrauterine growth is frequently disproportionate in this group. In the second, genetic, variety, the nuclear matter is impaired but cytoplasm remains normal in quantity. These babies frequently have familial syndromes, chromosomal abnormalities, and birth defects.

Antenatal Care

A high risk pregnancy may be identified by previous obstetric or family history, or by danger signals during the current gestation. Consultation with an obstetrician who is knowledgeable in current methods of diagnosis and treatment of the high risk patient should be sought.

Labor presents many potential problems. When delivery of a low birth weight baby is imminent, analgesia should be nil or held to a minimum. It must be understood that even small amounts of meperidine, scopolamine, hydroxyzine, or similar products significantly depress the baby at birth and that residual effects may last up to 24 hours. Magnesium sulfate must also be used with caution, since accumulation in the fetus produces depression and lethargy lasting as long as 72 hours. When it is completely metabolized, seizures caused by rebound hypomagnesemia can occur.

It is imperative for the sake of the fetus that an intravenous solution with dextrose and *minimal daily requirement of electrolytes* be provided to the laboring mother. Maternal ketosis resulting from starvation produces acidemia in the baby. Infusion of excessive water (without electrolytes) depresses fetal serum sodium levels, leading to seizures soon after birth.

Electronic monitoring is of great value, especially when fetal compromise caused by placental insufficiency occurs. Amnioscopy can alert the delivery team to meconium staining prior to rupture of membranes, and may help prevent meconium aspiration syndrome by early intervention in the delivery room.

Blood from the vagina should be analyzed by the Apt test to determine if it is fetal or maternal in origin. The labor and delivery suite should be equipped to do the test as follows: Mix the blood with water to obtain a pink-red supernatant hemoglobin solution, centrifuge, and decant the supernatant fluid. To five parts of this fluid, add one part of 1 per cent sodium hydroxide. If a yellow-brown color develops, the blood is maternal in origin; a red color shows that the blood is from the infant.

Moderate bleeding from a cervical erosion or tear is of little hemodynamic consequence to the mother, but similar amounts of blood from the fetal circulation secondary to vasa previa or premature placental separation may deplete the baby's blood volume and lead to stillbirth or fetal shock.

Delivery Room

At delivery, the low birth weight baby needs the greatest obstetric expertise available. The fetal head must be protected from rapid expulsion, which may lead to intracranial vascular tears. Low outlet forceps placement to protect and guide the head is most helpful. The obstetrician must be prepared to suction meconium from the nasopharynx of the emerging fetus to prevent meconium aspiration syndrome.

An individual who can properly resuscitate the baby must be present at the delivery. In fact, *all* persons on the delivery team should be currently versed in the basic needs of neonatal resuscitation. The mnemonic *"save him"* (Table 1) is a good way to remember the step-by-step sequence in an orderly resuscitation.

In case of specific narcotic depression, naloxone hydrochloride (Narcan) is used, 0.005 mg per kg per dose intravenously. This dose may be

TABLE 1.

S *Suction* and clearance of the airway; extend the head, using a neck roll

A *Airway:* Use properly fitting airway compatible with the baby's size

V *Ventilation:* Bag and mask; a number 2.5 to 3.0 Portex tube should be available if endotracheal (ET) tube is needed (or bag and adapter to ET tube)

E *Evaluation* by a second person or electronic devices

H *Heat and heart:* Keep the baby warm and dry in a radiant warmer; cardiac massage with thumb pressure over the sternum 80 to 100 beats per minute if needed

I *Intravenous solution:* Use umbilical vein; isotonic saline solution or 5 per cent dextrose in water (D_5W) may be infused and serves as an open line for medications

M *Medications:*
  a. Epinephrine 1:10,000, 0.5 ml per kg per dose
  b. Bicarbonate (7.5 per cent $NaHCO_3$), 2 mEq per kg plus 1 ml sterile water
  c. Calcium gluconate (10 per cent solution), 100 mg per kg per dose slowly (over 10 minutes) intravenously

---

repeated with little risk of secondary respiratory depression.

The Apgar score should be accurately recorded at 1 and 5 minutes by an individual trained in neonatal physical diagnosis and not relegated to an inexperienced trainee.

Admission Nursery Care

All newborn nurseries should be designed to provide a specialized area for initial observation of the baby during the period of stabilization. This may be a designated area in a single nursery, or a specific room created for that purpose. Trained personnel and adequate equipment must be available. The following steps will assist in caring for the baby:

1. Place the dried baby in a warm environment (neutral thermal environment), preferably in a radiant warmer with servo-control skin thermistor.

2. Monitor the vital signs, including temperature, pulse, respirations (including respiratory patterns), and blood pressure at frequent intervals.

3. In the absence of an adequate history, detailed physical and neurologic examination of the baby aids in determining the degree of maturity and anticipating problems (i.e., preterm, small for gestational age [SGA]).

4. "Routine" care includes instillation of silver nitrate drops into the eyes and administration of 0.5 mg of vitamin K (aqueous) intramuscularly, plus weight, length, and head circumference measurements.

5. Delay bathing until the infant's condition is stable.

6. Obtain blood for baseline studies. (Many tests may be derived from a sample of cord blood.) These should include type and Rh (and Coombs' test when the mother is Rh negative or has type O blood), hematocrit, total protein, white blood count, and bilirubin.

7. A transfusion may be necessary for the pale baby with a hematocrit below 40 per cent, or shock demonstrated by blood pressure less than 35 to 40 mm Hg. Fresh frozen plasma or human plasma protein fraction (Plasmanate), 10 ml per kg, will improve perfusion by blood volume expansion. Such expansion is frequently followed by a drop in hematocrit. Transfusion with packed red blood cells restores hemoglobin to acceptable levels for tissue oxygenation.

8. High hematocrit levels are common in SGA babies, leading to apnea, respiratory distress, or seizures. If the peripheral hematocrit is above 65 per cent, a central hematocrit determination is necessary. If this, too, is 65 per cent or above, and the infant is symptomatic, partial

transfusion (rather than simple phlebotomy) reduces red blood cell mass and reverses adverse signs.

9. Blood sugar levels are determined by reagent strips (Dextrostix) hourly for the first 6 hours, at 3 hour intervals for the next 24 hours, and every 6 to 8 hours thereafter. A range of 45 to 120 mg per 100 ml is acceptable. It must be remembered that babies may remain asymptomatic with blood sugar levels of 0; therefore, clinical criteria alone are unreliable. Dextrostix must be fresh to be accurate and offer reliable results.

10. An intravenous line should be established, since the LBW baby rapidly loses fluid, is prone to hypoglycemia, or may need rapid blood product replacement. In the event alterations in acid-base or electrolyte balance are detected, correction will be required. During the first hours, 10 per cent dextrose in water ($D_{10}W$) will be sufficient. By 24 hours of age, sodium (2 to 5 mEq per kg) and potassium (2 to 3 mEq per kg) will be added unless otherwise indicated.

11. Respiratory distress can occur at birth or shortly thereafter. In preterm infants, this will most often be due to lack of anatomic and/or biochemical maturity. The following steps are taken when respiratory distress is present: (a) Thorough physical examination, including auscultation (best done in the axillae) and careful observation of respiratory patterns. Asymmetry caused by underlying pneumothorax or thoracic anomaly may be demonstrated. Transillumination of the chest is helpful prior to radiographic confirmation. A 25 gauge scalp vein needle attached to a three-way stopcock and syringe, placed in the third interspace at the anterior axillary line, will temporarily relieve pressure from a pneumothorax, pending definitive treatment. (b) Chest x-ray assists in differential diagnosis. Classic appearance of "ground glass lung" is not pathognomonic of hyaline membrane disease, but could also represent pneumonia (especially caused by group B Streptococcus), congenital heart disease (hypoplastic left heart syndrome), or hemorrhage. (c) Since "sepsis" can masquerade as respiratory distress, cultures of blood, tracheal aspirate, and spinal fluid should be obtained. Treatment with aqueous penicillin G, 100,000 to 200,000 units per kg per day, or ampicillin, 100 to 200 mg per kg per day, intravenously, plus gentamicin, 5 mg per kg per day intramuscularly, may be started until culture results are confirmed. (d) Administer just enough humidified, warmed oxygen in order to abolish cyanosis. The percentage and duration of oxygen used must be carefully recorded. Document daily calibration of oxygen monitoring equipment. Determine the initial arterial blood gas status and at frequent intervals when oxygen therapy is sustained. The arterial oxygen tension (Po_2) should be maintained at 50 to 70 mm Hg and pH above 7.2.

Blood gases may be obtained by arterial puncture (radial or temporal) or umbilical artery catheter. The catheter tip at T8 (1 cm above the diaphragm) is the preferred site; however, L3 to L4 may be used, but dislodging of the catheter occurs more frequently. Continuous oxygen monitoring via skin transducers is excellent, but the current cost is prohibitive for the majority of hospitals. Blood from a warmed heel may be used, but is the least reliable because of variation in blood-drawing technique. Multiple sticks may also permanently inflict damage to the foot, especially on weight-bearing surfaces. Blood gas levels are obtained whenever a change in environmental oxygen is made or respiratory status of the patient is altered.

12. Progression of respiratory difficulty may require addition of continuous positive airway pressure by means of a tight-fitting mask, nasal prongs, or placement of an endotracheal tube. Ventilatory assistance is considered when arterial Pco_2 approaches 60 mm Hg or the pH falls below 7.2. Long-term ventilatory support is best done in well equipped and staffed centers. Ventilation during transport may be achieved by a portable respirator, mask, or endotracheal tube and bag. Penlon or Hope bags designed for neonatal use are preferable, since they do not create excessive pressures and reduce the risk of airway (lung) rupture.

Continuing Nursery Care

After the initial period of stabilization and in the absence of obvious sepsis, respiratory distress, major anomalies, or other contraindications, the baby may be fed by the oral route.

1. Nipple feeding should be relegated to the stable infant of 32 weeks' gestation or more, and performed by the most expert member of the nursing staff. When feasible, these babies may breast feed.

2. The vast majority of LBW babies will best be fed via an indwelling nasogastric tube. This may be by continuous drip (using an infusion pump) or by intermittent feedings at regular intervals. Transpyloric feedings or jejunostomy techniques are performed in centers where close monitoring is available.

3. Sterile water (15 to 30 ml) is used for the first feeding. Breast milk from the infant's mother should be used when possible. Recent studies demonstrate specific differences in breast milk of the mothers of prematures that may be advantageous to the baby. Banked breast milk is

of value, but strict criteria for use and handling are necessary. Commercial "premature" formulas are available. When utilized, a protocol for gradual increase in both concentration and volume of feedings is recommended.

4. Fluid and caloric requirements may not be easily met by either the oral (gastrointestinal) or intravenous route. Usually, the infant requires 100 to 120 ml per kg per day of water. This may be decreased to 80 ml per kg per day in a baby with fluid retention, or increased for the baby requiring long-term radiant warmth or phototherapy (120 to 180 ml per kg per day or more). An average intake of calories of 110 to 130 cal per kg per day will promote growth and a weight gain of 20 to 30 grams per day, but achievement of this level may take many days. Weight, length, and head circumferences are recorded and graphed daily, along with urine specific gravity.

5. In those infants in whom long-term intravenous feedings will be required, parenteral alimentation with amino acids, high dextrose levels, and fats (plus essential trace minerals and vitamins) will permit growth and provide adequate nutrition. This may be achieved using peripheral or central venous routes. It is critical to have expert nursing, pharmacy, and surgical back-up, in order to minimize the potential risks and complications of this mode of nutrition.

6. Electrolytes (especially sodium, potassium, and calcium) must be monitored on a regular basis. Hypocalcemia is a frequent complication in the LBW baby. One hundred mg per kg per day of calcium gluconate slowly intravenously may be given, but one must be certain that the infusion is well established in the vein because of the deleterious effects of extravasated calcium. When possible, oral calcium gluconate, 200 to 400 mg per kg per day, is administered.

7. Apnea is frequently seen in the LBW baby. The preterm baby has an immature central nervous system, and apnea may occur at the low end of a Cheyne-Stokes respiratory cycle. Apnea is often associated with bradycardia. It may also herald sepsis or represent seizure activity. Appropriate investigation is necessary to determine the cause.

In most instances, the baby will respond to stimulation. Oxygen should not be used as a routine measure to relieve apnea, since it is easy to give a baby too much oxygen and lead to toxicity.

A variety of apnea alarms, continuous rocking devices, water beds, and agitators are available to treat or prevent apnea, but there is no substitute for a well-trained nurse at the bedside.

Theophylline treatment of apnea has received much interest, but caution in its use is urged. First, the underlying cause of apnea must be determined. Laboratory determination of serum theophylline levels maintains a margin of safety.

8. Jaundice is a universal problem in newborns, but is potentially more dangerous for the LBW baby. In the face of liver enzyme immaturity, acidosis, hypoxia, and hypoproteinemia, the LBW baby is prone to bilirubin toxicity (kernicterus) at very low levels of bilirubin.

Early use of phototherapy, especially when bruising is extensive, is warranted. Blood type, Rh, Coombs, complete blood count, and total and indirect bilirubin levels are determined before phototherapy is begun. Modest rises in bilirubin may also be due to sepsis. Infection may produce increases in both direct and indirect bilirubin fractions. Phototherapy must be discontinued if the *direct* bilirubin is above 2 mg per 100 ml, or the bilirubin is far below the level of an anticipated exchange transfusion. Serial determinations of bilirubin by standard or newer albumin binding techniques will assist the clinician in management. Early exchange transfusion at relatively low bilirubin levels (less than 10 mg per 100 ml) may be necessary. A rise of 0.75 mg per hour or more is a good indication for imminent exchange transfusion. Babies undergoing phototherapy require careful scrutiny of their fluid requirements because of increased insensible water loss. The hematocrit is followed frequently during and after phototherapy. Small booster transfusions of packed red blood cells may be necessary when the hematocrit falls below 30 to 35 per cent and there is no apparent reticulocyte response.

8. Necrotizing enterocolitis (NEC) is a common problem in LBW babies, especially those who have had shock, respiratory distress, or sepsis. Monitoring of the stool for occult blood, abdominal distention, and intolerance of feedings are early indications of NEC. Serial x-rays of the abdomen to detect immobile segments of bowel, pneumatosis intestinalis, or free air in the portal system or abdominal cavity will assist in therapeutic considerations. Medical management includes discontinuing feedings and administration of parenteral antibiotics. Close cooperation with a pediatric surgeon is important, since surgical intervention may be required on an emergency basis.

9. The LBW infant is at high risk for seizures because of intrauterine and extrauterine difficulties such as anoxia, hypoxia, birth trauma, sepsis, or shock. These seizures seldom have the "tonic-clonic" appearance seen in older children. Yawning, apnea, staring, unilateral shaking, peculiar mouth or excessive sucking movements,

and/or limb or eye twitching may all represent seizure activity. The electroencephalogram (EEG) is of limited value. The computed axial tomography (CAT) scan is most helpful in diagnosis of hydrocephalus, areas of atrophy, anomalies, hemorrhage, or intracranial calcifications as underlying causes for seizures.

The treatment of choice for seizures is phenobarbital at 10 mg per kg per day. Higher doses, up to 25 mg per kg per day, may be necessary to initially control seizure activity. Monitoring of phenobarbital levels assists the clinician in treatment. Thirty to 45 mg per liter is an effective therapeutic range, but must be correlated with clinical findings. Drowsiness in the first week after use is expected and is not a reason to discontinue its use. It abates after the infant remains on the medication.

10. During some course of hospitalization, many LBW babies will have a heart murmur resulting from a patent ductus arteriosus. In most cases the patent ductus will close spontaneously as the infant matures. Some will cause symptoms of heart failure or be associated with prolonged pulmonary problems such as bronchopulmonary dysplasia. Consideration must be given to closure by surgical or pharmacologic means (i.e., indomethacin) after consultation with a cardiologist and adequate diagnosis. (This use of indomethacin is not listed in the manufacturer's official directive.) Only the surgical approach is consistently effective in closure. Although there are reports of considerable success with pharmacologic closure, long-term follow-up studies are not yet available, and this mode of therapy is not recommended without strict adherence to a study protocol in well trained hands.

11. The importance of good skin care of the small baby is often overlooked. The LBW baby seldom is endowed with vernix caseosa at birth and has little subcutaneous tissue protection. Electrodes from monitoring devices easily damage the fragile skin. Material applied to the skin is easily absorbed. Injured integument is frequently the portal of entry for sepsis.

Lanolin or other material that protects the skin but does not provide an occlusive layer may be used. Petroleum jelly or baby oil should be avoided, since bacteria trapped beneath them easily multiply and underlying moisture promotes breakdown of the vulnerable skin.

12. Access to the nursery for parental contact with the baby is recognized as essential. It enables free communication between the nursery staff and parents. The family is better equipped to cope with their infant's difficulties. Parents should not, however, be forced to accept too much information too soon from overzealous staff members. Gradual contact with the baby and his environment permits the parents to understand circumstances at their own rate of assimilation. Intensive staff training to deal with parents and their problems prevents misunderstanding and enables the nursery team to offer compassionate assistance.

Preparation for Discharge

1. Predischarge planning sessions are attended by physicians, nurses, social worker, and public health follow-up members. The attending physician responsible for the continuing day-to-day care of the baby must receive detailed information and instructions before the baby leaves the hospital.

2. Use of a predischarge room for parent education by the nursing staff and routine care of the baby aids in the transition from hospital to home care.

3. Provision for medicines, formulas, follow-up schedules, and any equipment used for the baby is clearly outlined to the family.

4. Eye examination for *all* LBW babies is essential. Retinopathy of prematurity may compromise a baby's vision without exposure to oxygen therapy. All babies who required oxygen need regular examinations during the first year, since retrolental fibroplasia may not be seen until several months after discharge.

5. Check hematocrit and hemoglobin at discharge and at follow-up visits.

6. Vitamins, especially C and D are given (1 ml per day of Tri-Vi-Sol drops), in addition to formula, since the LBW baby does not ingest enough vitamin-fortified formula per day to prevent rickets and/or scurvy.

Follow-up

The LBW baby is at high risk of developmental disability. Expert follow-up is important. An individual with specific training in the subtleties of child development, and independent of the neonatologist's bias, will assist in early detection of problems and act by instituting therapy when indicated. When cerebral palsy, language, vision, or hearing defects occur, they can be minimized by prompt intervention. Support of the family on a continuing basis is important.

The Gesell Developmental Screening Inventory, as modified by Knobloch, Stevens, and Pasamanick (1980) offers the clinician an effective and conveniently administered instrument to test the adaptive behavior and development of the infant from as early as 4 weeks after the expected date of confinement (EDC). It is most important to calculate a correction for prematurity early in the baby's life, since prejudice against the infant's performance and milestone achievement may preclude meaningful acceptance by the baby's caretaker.

Family follow-up is just as important when a baby dies during the perinatal period. Indication of cause of death by autopsy examination and laboratory tests, such as chromosome determination or biochemical studies, helps the family overcome grief by understanding. This information is necessary in genetic counseling and future family planning for the immediate and peripheral relatives. Parent support groups exist in many cities and are most helpful.

Babies who have been in neonatal intensive care units are frequently victims of sudden infant death syndrome (SIDS) and child abuse. Nursery personnel should assist in early identification of the child and family at greatest risk. Medical and nursing specialists, social agencies, and support groups offer guidance and education to those engaged in care of babies at all levels. We must all be receptive to a continuum of knowledge, innovations, and options available by open communications from perinatal centers to their regional constituents and partners. The well informed primary physician must remain the focal point for continuity of medical care.

NORMAL INFANT FEEDING

method of
WILLIAM J. CASHORE, M.D.,
and WILLIAM OH, M.D.
Providence, Rhode Island

Besides fulfilling the infant's nutritional requirements, feeding time is an opportunity for interaction and bonding between the mother and her infant. Breast feeding, in particular, may increase the mother's satisfaction and the infant's sense of being loved and secure. In this regard, however, the time spent together and the sense of communication developed may be more important than the specific technique of feeding in fostering a smooth emotional relationship. The busy mother should try to relax mentally and physically, if only for a few minutes, before starting to feed her baby. Attitudes of haste, muscular tension, or resentment at interruption of chores may interfere with lactation and are also transmitted to the infant, with possible adverse effects on feeding behavior.

The physician should discuss feeding thoroughly with the new mother. The primiparous mother may have many questions and some anxieties; the experienced mother may also welcome helpful suggestions based on the physician's own observations and practices. Specific questions about breast feeding and about additives and preservatives in artificial infant foods are now more common than they once were, so the physician is obliged to keep well informed on these matters. Time spent shortly after birth in the discussion of feeding will often lead to fewer feeding problems during the first year.

Whether an infant is breast fed or bottle fed, a modified demand schedule, with feedings approximately every 3 to 4 hours, is most adaptable to the normal gastric emptying time (2 to 3 hours) of most infants and to the individual needs of most newborns and their families. A flexible schedule will avoid the extremes of too-rigid scheduling and too-frequent small feedings. Most mothers quickly learn to recognize a hunger cry as distinct from other reasons why their babies cry, and should be encouraged not to use milk as a pacifier if the baby is crying for other reasons.

Method of Breast Feeding

The appropriate source of nourishment for human infants is human milk. Breast feeding for most or all of the first year has been strongly supported in recent statements by several national pediatric societies, expert committees on infant nutrition, and individual authorities on infant feeding. The marked decline in breast feeding which began before World War II and continued for some years after has been reversed; the resurgence of interest in breast feeding is obvious from the increased percentage of nursing mothers found in all maternity services, in the more supportive attitude of physicians and nurses, and in the existence of medical and nonmedical support groups for breast-feeding mothers both inside and outside hospitals.

Although breast feeding should be encouraged, a mother should nurse her baby because she is convinced that it is best for her baby to do so, and not because she has been pressured by friends, relatives, or physicians to act against her own inclinations. The physician should be encouraging and supportive toward breast feeding, but should be careful to avoid imparting guilt feelings (possibly counterproductive) to the mother who strongly prefers artificial feeding.

Adequate preparation for breast feeding should begin prenatally. Matters such as (1) the advantages of breast feeding, (2) conditioning of breasts and care of the nipples, (3) characteristics of colostrum and breast milk, (4) type of diet, and (5) effects of medications, alcohol, and daily routines on breast milk and the baby should be explained to the mother. Time spent on detailed instruction and answering the mother's questions may help make the difference between success and failure of breast feeding. Instructional booklets, trained nurses, and other breast-feeding mothers may all serve as useful sources of information. The mother should be sure that she herself is well nourished, follows a well balanced diet, and consumes enough extra nutrients for her infant. The period of breast feeding is not an appropriate time for "starvation" diets to lose weight during her postpartum period.

Feeding schedules vary in different hospitals. In our hospital, babies are usually given a first feeding of sterile water after 8 hours of observation, and then nursed at the next feeding time if the first feeding of water is tolerated. However, there is no compelling reason why nursing could not be started earlier, as soon as the mother and infant have recovered from the immediate effects of labor and parturition. Infants are usually nursed at 4 hour intervals during the first weeks and are usually nursed at both breasts for each feeding. As a general guideline, the infant should be nursed approximately 3 to 5 minutes at each breast on the first day, 5 to 10 minutes on the second, 10 to 15 minutes on the third and fourth days, and 15 to 20 minutes thereafter. Prolonged sucking may contribute to cracked nipples and mastitis. If the milk is abundant, the newborn will usually stop nursing when satisfaction occurs.

There is no sound scientific basis for the practice, common in many hospitals, of offering supplemental feedings of water after each nursing period. If there is objective evidence of undernutrition or underhydration such as excessive weight loss, slow weight gain, a persistent hunger cry, or scanty stool, then supplementary feeding with water or an appropriate commercial formula is indicated until the mother's milk supply increases. If necessary, most infants will readily accept a combination of formula and breast milk — a common situation when working mothers cannot nurse their babies throughout the day.

Rarely, it becomes necessary to restrict nursing to shorter periods or a more structured schedule if feedings become too frequent or if intake becomes too large, as evidenced by excessive weight gain. At these times and at the time of weaning from the breast, the physician's support, encouragement, and reinforcement of previous instructions may be needed.

Premature infants may be breast fed as soon as they are well enough and strong enough to suck adequately. In our premature nursery, we make extensive use of donated milk for gavage feedings of our smaller prematures, and we encourage mothers who wish to breast feed their premature infants to express or pump their milk and donate it to be fed to their own or other infants until their infants become strong enough to nurse. However, we do not hesitate to supplement breast milk with prepared formula if the weight gain of a premature infant on breast milk alone appears unsatisfactory.

Breast feeding is probably overrated as a cause of neonatal jaundice. In several reported series of cases, the documented incidence of "breast milk" jaundice in white infants is between 0.5 and 2.5 per cent. However, average bilirubin levels may be considerably higher in infants of Oriental, Mediterranean, or American Indian parents. In some mothers, pregnane-3 (α) 20(β)-diol in the breast milk may inhibit glucuronyl transferase in the liver, producing hyperbilirubinemia, which is usually of late onset and of several weeks' duration. These infants should be followed with periodic bilirubin determinations. In most cases, the serum bilirubin is only moderately elevated and no treatment appears necessary. If the indirect (unconjugated) bilirubin fraction exceeds 15 mg per dl (100 ml), it is advisable to discontinue breast feeding for approximately 48 hours. If breast feeding itself is the cause of the jaundice, there will usually be a prompt fall in the serum bilirubin level, after which nursing can safely be resumed in nearly all cases.

Entry of maternal medications into breast milk is variable and somewhat unpredictable because of individual differences in drug absorption, metabolism, and pharmacokinetics. Usually, drug concentrations in breast milk are not high enough to pose a serious risk to nursing infants. Breast feeding should be discontinued if the mother is required to take anticoagulants, antithyroid drugs, iodides, bromides, antimetabolites, radioactive preparations, diethylstilbestrol, or tetracycline.

Artificial Feeding

Although the frequency of breast feeding has increased in recent years, many mothers still prefer formula feeding, while some others use formula for part of the day or after cessation of breast feeding. Whatever formula basis is used, it is prepared to provide enough water, calories, protein, carbohydrates, fat, and minerals to sustain normal metabolism and growth. During the first 6 months, the 24 hour requirements for normal infants are as follows: (1) Water: 130 to 190 ml per kg (2 to 3 oz per pound). (2) Calories: 100 to 120 kcal per kg (45 to 55 kcal per pound). (3) Protein: 3 to 4 grams per kg (1.4 to 1.8 grams per pound). (4) Carbohydrate and fat should constitute 50 per cent and 35 per cent of the caloric intake, respectively.

Calculation and Preparation of Milk Formula. To prescribe a formula it is necessary to know the infant's nutritional requirements and the approximate caloric, protein, carbohydrate, fat, and mineral content of the milk preparation used. For example, either of the following would be adequate for a 1-week-old infant weighing 7 pounds (3.18 kg):

1. *Evaporated milk* (See Table 1).

2. *Commercially prepared milks* (e.g., Enfamil, Similac, SMA) are available in different forms such as powder, liquid concentrate, and "ready to feed"; the instruction for each type of formula must be observed. The liquid concentrates of the commercial formulas are quite popular, and are prepared by mixing one part concentrated formula with one part water to achieve an isocaloric formula of 20 kcal per oz (30 ml). The total amount prepared and placed in each bottle and the feeding schedule should be the same as in the example given above.

Sterilization. Formula should be sterilized until the infant is at least 4 months old. There are two methods of sterilization:

1. Aseptic sterilization, in which the formula, utensils, bottles, and nipples are sterilized separately. This method may be somewhat cumbersome.

2. Terminal sterilization avoids excessive handling of already-sterilized equipment. In this method, the bottles and nipples are first washed and the formula prepared in a clean container. A 24 hour supply of formula is divided into six to eight individual feeding bottles, which are then capped with the nipples turned upside down. The bottles are placed in a closed container of boiling water for 25 to 30 minutes. Formula can be stored in the refrigerator and warmed just before feeding. Leftover formula should not be used after 24 hours.

Infants readily tolerate formula at room temperature. Ready-to-use commercial formulas, prepackaged in sterile nursing bottles, can safely be stored and fed at room temperature. The expiration date of the formula should be noted, and hospital stocks should be rotated to avoid waste.

Schedules. A modified demand schedule, with feedings approximately every 4 hours, is appropriate for breast or formula feeding. In our hospital we observe and teach the following routine for artificially fed infants: (1) Nothing by mouth for 8 to 10 hours. (2) Twelve to 24 hours: after a first feeding of sterile water, 1 to 2 oz (30 to 60 ml) of formula every 4 hours. (3) Second and third days: 2 to 3 oz (60 to 90 ml) of formula (20 kcal per 30 ml) at each feeding. (4) Fourth to seventh days: increase to 3 to 4 oz (90 to 120 ml) at each feeding. (5) Second to sixth weeks: slowly advance the amount of formula as needed, up to 7 or 8 oz (210 to 240 ml) per feeding.

Most infants will feed approximately six times daily for 2 to 4 weeks, with a decrease in frequency to five per day by the end of the sixth week. A change from formula to whole milk can be made at 5 to 6 months of age.

Feeding time usually should not exceed 30 minutes, although many mothers and infants like to use feeding time as a "play period" in addition to feeding. The baby should be held, the bottle should not be propped, and the baby should be "burped" at the middle and end of each feeding.

Water may be given to supplement milk at any time, and unsweetened juices after 3 to 4 months of age. Early feeding of juices may be associated with contact rashes of the face and buttocks. Sugar water should not be used as a supplementary fluid or as a pacifier.

Solid Foods

Here, again, there has been a change in attitudes during the past few years. Accompanying the strong recommendations in favor of breast feeding noted above are observations by many of the same authorities on infant nutrition that, if the mother is well nourished, breast milk alone appears nutritionally adequate for at least the first 4 to 6 months of life. While the necessity

TABLE 1. **Evaporated Milk Formula**

	FLUID	CALORIES	PROTEIN (GRAMS)
Evaporated milk	7 oz (210 ml)	308 kcal	14.7
Water	11 oz (330 ml)	—	—
Karo Syrup	1 tbsp (15 ml)	60	—
Total	18.5 oz (555 ml)	368	14.7

Four oz (120 ml) of formula should be placed in each of six bottles and 3 to 4 oz (90 to 120 ml) fed every 4 hours.

for early introduction of solid foods has been called into question, the fact remains that in many families the introduction of solid foods to infants is often a matter of individual preference or cultural background. For babies receiving formula, a reasonable procedure is to start precooked rice cereal twice a day when the child is no longer satisfied with 30 oz (900 ml) of milk in 24 hours. Strained fruits and vegetables may follow a month or so after the introduction of cereal. Strained meats and eggs are not indicated before age 6 months. Many pediatricians prefer to start one new type of animal protein at a time, so that possible sources of protein allergy may be more readily recognized.

When the child at 7 or 8 months of age shows interest in chewing coarser foods, zwieback, toast, crackers, or cookies may be given. Peanuts, hard candy, and all other foods with small hard particles should be avoided until after the toddler years.

For the introduction of solid foods, commercially prepared strained baby foods are convenient, but can be replaced by puréed or finely strained table foods without added salt or sugar, once solid feedings are well established. "Junior foods" and "mixed meals" (mainly cereal) offer no advantage over carefully prepared table food, especially for infants with teeth. The ready preference· of many infants for highly sweetened desserts and fruits must be counteracted by careful attention to a balanced diet.

Vitamin and Mineral Supplements

Growing breast-fed infants should receive supplements of vitamins A, C, and D; these are usually prescribed at the time of discharge from the hospital. The need for vitamin supplements in artificially fed infants depends mainly on the vitamin content present in, or added to, the formula during preparation. Many physicians prefer vitamin supplementation for the formula-fed as well as the breast-fed infants. After the infant has begun to take a variety of solid foods (usually between 6 and 12 months), vitamin supplements are not usually necessary.

Infants who are totally breast fed absorb iron extremely well and probably do not need iron supplements in the first 6 to 8 months. Infants who are totally or even partially fed on formula do require iron supplements, whether added to the formula or given separately. Formula-fed infants receive adequate fluoride if the local water supply is fluoridated, but should receive a fluoride supplement if the fluoride content of the water is very low. Since fluoride does not cross readily into breast milk, breast-fed infants should also receive a fluoride supplement, especially in nonfluoridated areas, where the mother's fluoride intake will also be low.

DISEASES OF THE BREAST
method of
DOUGLAS J. MARCHANT, M.D.
Boston, Massachusetts

Careful breast examination should be part of every routine office visit. It is at least as important as the pelvic examination and perhaps more so, because those factors that result in the early diagnosis of pelvic malignancy, i.e., the Papanicolaou smear and abnormal vaginal bleeding, are independent of the examining technique. It is especially important in the evaluation ·of the pregnant patient.

Breast conditions requiring medical consultation can be grouped under the following four categories: (1) Abnormalities of physiology, including galactorrhea, with or without amenorrhea, mastodynia, and fibrocystic changes. (2) Benign neoplasms, i.e., a dominant mass, fibroadenoma, cysts, intraductal papilloma. (3) Inflammations or infections — fat necrosis, plasma cell mastitis, postpartum mastitis. (4) Cancer.

The breasts are a subspecialization of the skin and are of ectodermal origin. At birth, the breast consists almost entirely of ducts, but with the rise of estrogen levels at puberty, enlargement occurs with pigmentation of the areolae. The duct system enlarges, and following ovulation and the production of progesterone, the alveoli make their appearance. Breast growth and development, however, are not totally dependent upon levels of estrogen and progesterone; insulin, cortisol, thyroxine, growth hormone, and prolactin are required for complete functional development. Minor deficiencies of these hormones can be compensated for by an increase in prolactin.

Abnormalities of Breast Development

Anomalies include accessory breast tissue and supernumerary nipples. The milk ridge, which develops in the embryo, extends from the axilla to the groin. Accessory breast tissue, including ducts, alveolar tissue, and nipples, may develop along this ridge. Interestingly, supernumerary breasts occur more often in the male. Micromastia, i.e., small breasts, and macromastia, large breasts, as well as the absence of the mammary gland, have been reported.

Physiologic Alterations

Physiologic changes, such as inappropriate lactation, with or without amenorrhea, may be due to a decrease in the luteinizing hormone–releasing hormone (LHRH). This results in, first, a decrease in pituitary production of gonadatropin and amenorrhea, and second, a decrease in the hypothalamic pituitary inhibiting factor (PIF). This produces an excess of prolactin and lactation. In addition to a careful history, the physical examination should include a careful search for signs of abnormal thyroid function and the evaluation of visual fields and the optic fundi. Gonadotropins (LH and FSH) and serum prolactin levels should be obtained. The higher the prolactin level, the more likely there is a pituitary tumor. In this situation, an x-ray of the sella turcica and polytomography are recommended to rule out pituitary neoplasia.

Nipple discharge may be associated with tranquilizers, particularly the phenothiazines, with oral contraceptives, and with manual stimulation. It is important to note if the discharge is bilateral or unilateral. The character of the discharge is important in the differential diagnosis. Clear or milky discharge usually is associated with physiologic alterations, including manual stimulation. Serosanguineous or bloody discharge most often indicates an intraductal papilloma and rarely a malignancy. Bilateral clear or milky discharge, with or without amenorrhea, should be investigated to rule out pituitary neoplasia. Patients with unilateral serosanguineous or bloody discharge, in addition to careful palpation of the breast, should have the fluid examined by a Papanicolaou smear. For those patients with grossly bloody discharge, a mammogram or xeromammogram is indicated. Patients with bloody discharge seldom have a palpable mass, although the quadrant involved may be identified by careful palpation. Exploration of the duct system is recommended. The majority of patients will have a benign intraductal papilloma. Approximately 10 per cent will have carcinoma.

Mastodynia, or significant pain in the breast, particularly when it occurs in the premenstrual phase, is a frequent complaint among women of childbearing age. It is a common symptom in the perimenopausal patient as well. In the absence of a palpable lesion, this condition is best treated with reassurance, analgesics, and the wearing of a properly fitted bra. Salt restriction, diuretics, and hormones, including androgens, are seldom effective. More recently, danazol, in doses of 100 to 400 mg per day or less, has been suggested as

treatment. The long-term effects of this drug have not been evaluated, and it has not been approved by the Food and Drug Administration for this purpose.

The term fibrocystic disease probably is a misnomer. Alterations which are described under this heading include a spectrum of anatomic and physiologic changes. The lesions usually are bilateral and multiple. They are characterized by pain and tenderness and an increase in symptomatology premenstrually. Clinically, fibrocystic changes occur in three different stages; however, there is overlapping of the symptomatology at any stage. Early changes occur in the late teens and early twenties and include painful, tender breasts, particularly in the axillary tail and occurring premenstrually. Examination discloses tenderness and a sensation of fullness or a pseudo-lump in the axilla. This is followed by a multinodular breast. Examination discloses multinodular changes, and occasionally a dominant mass is palpated. This is difficult to differentiate from carcinoma, although only 1.5 per cent of breast cancers occur in persons less than 30 years of age. The final change may be described as cystic alterations. Occasionally, the patient may complain of pain or a burning sensation, along with the appearance of a mass in the breast. The cyst may rapidly increase in size. It is well circumscribed, generally tender and mobile, and clear on transillumination. The fluid aspirated is usually clear or yellow. With cysts of longer duration, the fluid may be green to dark brown or black. Cystic changes are important because they are common, are symptomatic, and require judgment when recommending treatment. The peak incidence occurs in women between the ages of 30 and 50 and may be the result of excess estrogen stimulation and the absence of cyclical corpus luteum formation and the production of progesterone.

Reports vary, but most authors agree that the risk of breast cancer is increased two to four times in the patients with cystic changes. The risk increases with the degree of dysplasia. In advanced lesions, there may be discrete, tender cystic masses. If there is increased duct proliferation, the term adenosis is employed. One variant associated with dense fibrosis is commonly called "sclerosing adenosis."

When lactation has been suppressed, the inspissated milk may produce a galactocele. This essentially is a cyst containing thick, creamy milk. Palpation reveals a well delineated, round, movable mass, usually located near the center of the breast tissue. A galactocele should be suspected whenever a mass develops in a woman who has lactated within the past year. Aspiration usually reveals milky fluid, and no additional treatment is required.

Miscellaneous abnormalities of physiologic or developmental origin include failure of development of the breasts, commonly associated with ovarian agenesis, precocious development of the female breasts, adolescent hypertrophy, and, rarely, massive breast hypertrophy in pregnancy.

Inflammations and Infections

Mondor's disease probably is superficial thrombophlebitis. Physical examination reveals a dimpling and string-like band. This is not a common lesion and the cause is not clear, although most authorities believe that trauma may be responsible. The patient complains of pain, and examination reveals the tender cord-like area. The pseudoretraction associated with the process may be confused with retraction caused by carcinoma, and, of course, if there is any question, appropriate diagnostic studies, including mammography, should be performed. The disease is self-limited and requires no treatment. The tenderness usually diminishes over a period of 3 to 4 weeks.

Duct ectasia or plasma cell mastitis may be manifested by nipple discharge. It is usually multicolored, sticky, bilateral, and from multiple ducts. Frequently, it is associated with burning, itching, or pain around the areolae. Palpable swellings are noted under the areolae. With chronic inflammation there is fibrosis, which results in thickening of the walls of the ducts and occasionally in retraction of the nipple. At this stage, there may be a hard retroareolar mass. It may be necessary to excise the entire duct system, not only as a therapeutic maneuver but also to rule out carcinoma.

Postpartum mastitis results in a localized area of inflammation which is tender and indurated to palpation. There may be a slight elevation in temperature. The treatment is to stop nursing and, rarely, to give antibiotics. Occasionally, the process continues to breast abscess formation. Fluctuation may be observed, and there is considerable elevation of temperature. The abscess should be drained and the patient treated with antibiotics. Most of the abscesses are caused by coagulase-positive *Staphylococcus aureus*. The antibiotics to which the organism is sensitive should be given in full dose for a week to 10 days after adequate drainage. A curved incision should be used, following the skin lines, and a Penrose drain should be left in the cavity for 2 to 3 days.

The breasts occasionally are the site of fat necrosis. The lesion is important because it may obscure the diagnosis of carcinoma. Most of the patients give a history of trauma and complain of pain or tenderness. In about a quarter of the patients there is some ecchymosis and redness of the skin, and in almost all cases a mass can be palpated. One half of the cases are associated with retraction, and in some series axillary adenopathy has been reported. The treatment is local excision.

Sebaceous cysts are common in the skin over the breast. They are superficial, are quite circumscribed, and contain a dilated sebaceous duct in the overlying skin. These cysts, when they become infected, may be associated with induration, inflammation, and abscess formation. They may be confused with carcinoma. Treatment is local excision.

Benign Neoplasms

The common benign neoplasm is the fibroadenoma. This appears predominantly in young women and presents as a firm, painless mobile mass. It may attain a very large size, especially in adolescence. Lesions tend to be multiple but bilateral in only 10 to 20 per cent of the cases. The lesions are discovered accidentally by the young patient and, unlike fibrocystic alterations, do not change in the menstrual phase. They may grow rapidly during adolescence, pregnancy, or the menopause and with exogenous estrogen stimulation. If the mass increases dramatically in size, one must consider cystosarcoma phylloides.

The predominant symptom of a solitary intraductal papilloma is nipple discharge. Patients with a solitary intraductal papilloma tend to be older than patients with other benign breast lesions. Most patients present with a spontaneous nipple discharge, which may be bloody. Surgical exploration is required. These are benign lesions, and simple excision is all that is required.

Because it may be confused with a benign fibroadenoma, or a giant adenofibroma, cystosarcoma phylloides is discussed here. This is a neoplasm containing both mesenchymal and epithelial elements arranged in a very characteristic pattern. The initial symptoms include a mobile, rounded mass. In most cases, there is a history of rapid increase in size. Pain and tenderness are rare. The majority occur in the central or upper part of the breast. The skin usually is mobile over the mass, and the nipple is not retracted. Dilatation of subcutaneous veins is common, even with relatively small masses. The mammographic appearance is very similar to that of a fibroadenoma. Both are spherical or lobulated and form a dense mass sharply demarcated from the surrounding breast tissue. Treatment is wide, local excision.

Breast Aspiration and Biopsy

A dominant mass may be cystic or solid, benign or malignant. If the lesion is solid and the patient is under 25 years of age, observation or excision biopsy, depending on the size of the mass, is recommended. If the patient is over 25 years of age, mammography and excision biopsy are recommended. If the mass appears to be cystic, an attempt should be made to aspirate the lesion with a 20 to 21 gauge needle. If the fluid is clear or cloudy and no residual mass is palpated immediately following the aspiration, follow-up examination in 1 month with reassurance and monthly breast self-examination is recommended. If the mass remains immediately following aspiration, or if the fluid is bloody, the patient should have a mammogram and a biopsy. If there is a residual mass on the first follow-up examination, mammography and biopsy are recommended.

Outpatient breast biopsy is becoming increasingly popular. With properly selected patients it is uncomplicated and cost effective. The lesion should be small (not subclinical, as noted on a mammogram), relatively superficial, and clinically benign. Surgery is best performed in a regular operating room setting with assistance, but it may be performed in a properly equipped office. Local anesthesia is employed and, if possible, a circumareolar incision which follows the lines of Langer is employed. An inframammary incision is rarely justified and a radial incision, never. Meticulous hemostasis is employed. A minimal number of sutures should be utilized to reconstruct the breast tissue, and these should be of fine, plain catgut. Many surgeons allow the breast tissue to be approximated without sutures once hemostasis is achieved. The incision is closed with fine nylon, a fine subcuticular suture of polyglycolic suture material, or Steristrips. As a general rule, a minimal amount of suture material should be left in the breast.

Biopsy and definitive diagnosis are becoming more popular for lesions which appear clinically malignant. Available data suggest that delay of definitive treatment for 1 or 2 weeks does not adversely influence survival. However, it is absolutely essential that this type of surgery be carefully performed with minimal manipulation of breast tissue, sharp dissection, meticulous hemostasis, and absolute asepsis. Infection or marked ecchymosis will greatly interfere with definitive surgical treatment for breast cancer. Biopsy and delay of treatment can be justified only under ideal conditions, which means careful biopsy

technique and immediate consultation with the surgeon responsible for the definitive treatment.

For lesions of suspicious origin, at least 500 mg of tissue should be sent to the pathologist with a note that estrogen-binding studies should be performed. This will require a frozen section to determine whether the lesion is benign or malignant. Therefore, for all but the most obvious lesions, it is advisable to request the frozen section diagnosis to determine whether or not estrogen-binding studies should be performed.

Breast Cancer

Breast cancer is the most common cancer in women, representing 28 per cent of all malignancies. Every year more than 100,000 women in the United States develop breast cancer, and 34,000 will die of metastatic disease. One out of every 13 newborn girls will develop breast cancer. It is the leading cause of death of women at any age and the most common cause of death in women aged 39 to 44. Eighty per cent of the lesions are clinically detected in patients over 40 years of age and less than 1.5 per cent in those under 30. A significant number of early breast lesions are found in patients 40 to 50 years of age. This has been dramatically demonstrated in breast cancer detection programs in which one third of the clinically occult lesions have been found in patients in this age group.

The proper evaluation of the breast begins with an accurate and thorough history, including the age of the patient, menstrual history (particularly the date of the last menstrual period), family history of breast disease, the use of medication, pregnancy history (including date of birth of the first child), and surgery (including history of previous breast disease). For specific symptoms such as nipple discharge, it is important to note the date of onset, the character of the discharge, whether it is spontaneous or produced by manipulation, the association with menstrual irregularities, and the use of medications, including tranquilizers, especially the phenothiazines. Breast self-examination should be taught and continued by the patient at monthly intervals 1 week after the menses or on a regular schedule noted on the calendar for the postmenopausal patient. This examination by the patient is done in a systematic manner and consists of palpation and inspection, noting any change in breast size, contour, and consistency.

Adjuncts to the physical examination include thermography and mammography. The scientific basis of thermography rests on the fact that infrared radiation emitted by a surface is proportional to its temperature. Thus, the thermogram is a pictorial display of multiple, simultaneous pressure measurements. While thermograms are not a specific test for cancer, they are useful markers and may direct the examiner's attention to a particular area of the breast. They should always be used as an extension of the physical examination and confirmed by mammography.

It is important to distinguish between screening and the diagnostic evaluation of the symptomatic patient. Women with clinical signs of cancer should always have a mammogram regardless of age. Every woman with *obvious* cancer should have a mammogram, since the rate of synchronous bilateral cancer approximates 4 per cent. In patients under 30 years of age, there is controversy concerning the efficacy and safety of mammography. The young breast is dense, and unless the cancer is associated with microcalcifications it is difficult to detect by mammography. In screening, mammography has a sensitivity rate of about 90 per cent. Forty-five per cent of all cancers are detected by mammography alone, that is, they are clinically occult. Physical examination discovers 55 per cent of the breast cancers, but physical examination is positive alone in 10 per cent of the cases (false negative mammography in 10 per cent). It is important to use both physical examination and mammography in screening for breast cancer.

A negative mammogram in the presence of a real three-dimensional mass which does not yield fluid on aspiration should not deter the surgeon from biopsy. From 10 to 15 per cent of the palpable carcinomas may be missed by mammography. Conversely, a suspicious mammogram in the absence of clinical findings deserves biopsy.

An evaluation of the patient with breast cancer includes, of course, a complete physical examination, chest x-ray, liver function tests, and, as mentioned previously, mammography. Radionuclide scanning and films for metastatic disease are obtained on the basis of symptoms and for lesions greater than 2 cm in diameter. In the assessment of a malignant tumor, the TNM system provides for the pre- and postoperative categorization of primary lesions and the extent of involvement. Three capital letters are used: T = primary tumor; N = regional nodes; M = distant metastasis. T0 indicates no evidence of primary tumor, TIS, carcinoma in situ, and T1, T2, T3, T4, progressive increase in tumor size. TNM assignments may be grouped into a smaller number of clinical stages, as follows: Stage 0: the lesions are too small to palpate but found by mammography. Stage I: the lesions are palpable but less than 2 cm in diameter. Stage II: the

lesions are 2 to 5 cm in diameter. The axillary nodes may be thought to be involved but are movable. There is no chest wall fixation, edema, infiltration, or ulceration of the skin. Stage III: the lesions are greater than 5 cm in diameter. The lesion is fixed to the chest wall and is associated with edema, infiltration, or ulceration of the skin of the breast. Stage IV: the lesion shows evidence of distant metastasis.

Selective Treatment. Cancer of the breast is often a systemic disease, with perhaps 50 per cent or more of the patients presenting with metastatic disease, and it is entirely proper that previously held concepts for therapeutic approaches based on this be reassessed and placed in proper perspective.

Total mastectomy with axillary dissection (modified radical mastectomy) has largely supplanted the radical operation and is the operation of choice for most surgeons for Stage I and II curable breast cancer. A total removal of the breast and axillary dissection is common to both procedures, although it is recognized that a complete axillary dissection is technically more difficult when the chest wall muscles are not removed. Cosmetically, the preservation of the bulk of the pectoralis major muscles leads to a less deformed chest wall. Functionally, arm strength and mobility may be preserved more fully and with less swelling and arm edema. Psychologically, preservation of the chest wall musculature permits better plastic reconstructive procedures later, if desired by the patient.

Radiation therapy as an alternative to surgery has the chief advantage of better functional and cosmetic results with equal or less morbidity. Complete tumor excision, although not necessarily a wide surgical resection, is important for good local control with radiation therapy. Following gross removal of the tumor, modest doses of radiation of 5000 rads can control microscopic disease with adequate function and cosmesis. Boost therapy to the area of excision can be done with electron beam or with interstitial implantation of radionuclides. If primary radiotherapy is recommended, it should be restricted to patients with lesions that are relatively small in comparison to the size of the breast. In premenopausal patients who are clinically Stage I, it is important to have axillary sampling to determine those women with positive nodes who may benefit from adjuvant chemotherapy.

Adjuvant Therapy. With optimal combinations of surgery and radiotherapy, less than 5 per cent of patients with breast cancer will have local recurrence. However, more than 70 per cent of all breast cancer patients will die of or with active breast cancer in a 30 year period following initial diagnosis. It is clear that a significant increase in the survival of breast cancer patients will depend upon earlier diagnosis prior to the occurrence of metastasis or treatment of such micrometastases immediately following local therapy.

Adjuvant radiotherapy, particularly for lesions in the upper outer quadrant of the breast, has not resulted in any increase in survival, and therefore it is not recommended following routine modified radical mastectomy. However, for patients with medial or areolar lesions, in which case there is a possibility of internal mammary gland involvement, adjuvant postoperative radiotherapy is recommended to the internal mammary chain area.

Recent studies have indicated that adjuvant chemotherapy is most effective in premenopausal patients with significant axillary involvement. No single form of adjuvant therapy may be considered an established form of therapy. Patients with clinical Stage I and Stage II lesions with no histologic evidence of nodal involvement should not be treated with antineoplastic agents at present. Adjuvant regimens, designed for individual patients, that significantly differ from published regimens should be discouraged.

Use of Estrogen Receptors in the Management of Breast Cancer. It is now well established that estrogen-positive tumors are associated with clinical response to therapeutic hormone manipulation and to a prolonged interval between diagnosis of breast cancer and recurrence. If the estrogen receptor (ER) is positive (greater than 10 femtomoles per mg of protein), the likelihood of response is greater than 50 per cent. If the ER is negative (less than 10 femtomoles per mg of protein), the response is less than 8 per cent. Furthermore, a high content (greater than 100 femtomoles per mg of protein) is associated with an increased response, that is, greater than 80 per cent. The estrogen receptor assay should be utilized, along with other clinical factors that predict response, to select patients for hormone treatment. These clinical factors include a tumor-free interval of greater than 2 years, postmenopausal status, prior response to hormone treatment, and metastatic or recurrent disease predominantly in skin or lymph nodes.

The relationship of the estrogen receptor assay of breast cancer to clinical response to cytotoxic chemotherapy remains controversial. However, current opinion appears to be that no such predictive relationship exists for chemotherapy response.

Tumor specimens collected for estrogen receptor should include at least 500 mg of tissue and should be placed on dry ice or liquid nitrogen within 20 minutes of surgical removal, since the estrogen receptor protein is very heat labile. A representative specimen must always be submitted for histologic verification.

Results of Selective Treatment. Seventy-two per cent of patients with Stage I disease survive 10 years and 40 per cent of patients with Stage II have a similar 10 year absolute survival. It should be noted, however, that after a 20 year period, only 20 per cent of patients in Stage I still survive. Thus, more than half of the patients presenting with so-called "early" breast cancer actually have systemic disease. Cure must depend upon the diagnosis of subclinical disease and appropriate systemic therapy.

Metastatic Disease or Recurrent Carcinoma. Treatment of recurrent or metastatic cancer consists of hormone manipulation based upon endocrine receptor values, the menopausal status of the patient, and the location of the metastatic disease. Oophorectomy is indicated, possibly followed by adrenalectomy or hypophysectomy if there is a response in the premenopausal patient who is estrogen positive. If the estrogen receptor is negative, or if there is *rapidly* advancing visceral disease, chemotherapy should be started immediately. If there is no response to oophorectomy or other hormonal manipulation, chemotherapy should also be used.

For the postmenopausal patient who is estrogen positive, estrogens or tamoxifen may be employed, followed by adrenalectomy. If there is failure, the patient is treated with chemotherapy. Combination chemotherapy, e.g., CMF—cyclophosphamide, 50 mg daily by mouth; methotrexate, 25 mg intravenously weekly; and 5-fluorouracil, 500 mg intravenously weekly—seems to achieve the highest response rate, the greatest complete response, the longest remission duration, and the greatest increase in survival. Single drugs, either as part of a sequence or randomly used, appear to be less effective than combination chemotherapy.

Recently it has been shown that tamoxifen offers the best choice of therapy for the patient with metastatic breast cancer after conventional endocrine therapy and combination chemotherapy have failed. The recommended dosage of tamoxifen is 10 mg orally twice a day. Most patients have no serious side effects; however, the majority experience hot flashes. Some patients report increased appetite and weight gain.

Localized bone metastasis may be treated

with radiation therapy, or, if weight-bearing bones are involved, orthopedic intervention with internal fixation is recommended.

ENDOMETRIOSIS

method of
CHARLES C. TSAI, M.D.,
and H. O. WILLIAMSON, M.D.
Charleston, South Carolina

Endometriosis is the presence of endometrial tissue outside the uterine cavity. It is divided into endometriosis interna (adenomyosis) and endometriosis externa. The incidence of endometriosis externa appears to be on the increase. The factors responsible for the apparent increase are related to improved endoscopic techniques resulting in more frequent diagnosis and to longer reproductive years in women owing to early menarche, late menopause, and fewer pregnancies in modern times. Endometriosis is found in 20 to 35 per cent of infertile patients and 5 to 50 per cent of pelvic laparotomies. In a recent report, endometriosis was found in 46 per cent of adolescents with chronic pelvic pain. It is usually stated that there are racial differences in the incidence of endometriosis in that it is prevalent in whites but not in blacks. This concept, however, has been refuted by two recent reports. A Hawaiian study revealed that women of Japanese origin had the highest incidence, followed by non-Japanese-Orientals, whites, and blacks. Another study revealed that over 22 per cent of black women who underwent laparoscopy for a variety of pelvic symptoms had endometriosis.

Presenting symptoms include infertility, dysmenorrhea, dyspareunia, pelvic pain, irregular menses, rectal pain, and hematuria. These symptoms occur in varying frequency. The diagnosis of endometriosis is usually established by laparoscopy with or without biopsy. Endometriosis is found most frequently in the cul-de-sac, followed by the uterus, ovary, rectosigmoid, urinary bladder, and fallopian tube.

Methods of Therapy

Surgery. Endometriosis can be surgically managed by either definitive or conservative surgery. Definitive surgery is indicated when the symptomatic patient does not wish to have any more childbearing. If the patient is 40 years of age or older, or if her endometriosis is severe, a total abdominal hysterectomy and bilateral salpingo-oophorectomy may be performed. If the patient is young and the endometriosis is of limited extent, the ovaries can be preserved after any ovarian implants are carefully removed.

A recurrence rate of about 7 per cent in patients with ovarian conservation has been reported. This seems to justify preserving the ovarian tissue for the benefits of endocrine function in young patients.

Conservative surgery, consisting of excision and occasionally fulguration of all visible implants and other procedures as outlined, is intended to preserve and improve fertility potential. Anterior uterine suspension and plication of the utero-ovarian ligaments are useful preventive procedures when retrofixation of the uterus or prolapse of adnexa to the cul-de-sac are likely to occur. Division of the uterosacral ligaments and presacral neurectomy may be effective in relieving dyspareunia or midline pelvic pain but do not improve pregnancy rates. Dilatation of the uterine cervix is not beneficial except in cases of cervical stenosis. Appendectomy is not indicated for a normal-appearing appendix, as it is rarely involved by endometriosis and fecal contamination of the operative field is a potential hazard. Inhibition of adhesion formation should be sought by careful hemostasis and meticulous reperitonization of raw surfaces. Medications such as glucocorticoids and promethazine have shown inconsistent effects and are not currently recommended. Intraperitoneal instillation of 32 per cent dextran 70 in 10 per cent dextrose (Hyskon) at 2.5 ml per kg of body weight at the time of abdominal closure in animal experiments seems to diminish adhesion formation. However, the use of dextran 70 for this purpose is not approved by the Food and Drug Administration, and there is as yet lack of clinical confirmation. Recent interest in microsurgery, using refined instruments, has greatly improved the outcome of infertility surgery on tubal diseases, including endometriosis.

Hormones. These include medroxyprogesterone acetate, estrogen with a progestogen, and danazol. Oral medroxyprogesterone acetate is given as 10 mg three times daily for 3 to 6 months (this use is not officially recommended by the manufacturer). It is less effective, but may remain a useful alternative if the patient is not an appropriate candidate for other hormonal therapy. Breakthrough bleeding during the treatment is the major disadvantage, but this is usually scant and may be controlled by addition of small doses of estrogen.

Estrogen with a progestogen ("pseudopregnancy") can be given conveniently in the form of a progestogen-dominant oral contraceptive with 50 micrograms or less of estrogen. It is started with 1 tablet daily and continued without interruption for 6 to 12 months. (This use of these agents is not specifically listed in the manufacturers' official directives.) It may be escalated to a maximum of 4 tablets daily if breakthrough bleeding occurs. Side effects are those associated with the use of oral contraceptives and include nausea, vomiting, headache, weight gain, mood changes, thromboembolic phenomena, and breakthrough bleeding during the first few months. The symptoms from endometriosis may become worse, as estrogen with progestogen can stimulate the growth of the implants during the first few months before atrophic changes occur.

Danazol, a derivative of testosterone, has antigonadotropic action which results in a hypoestrogenic state referred to as pseudomenopause. It is given as 200 to 800 mg daily in two divided doses starting on the first day of a menstrual cycle and continued for 3 to 9 months. Although the dosage approved by the Food and Drug Administration is 800 mg per day, lower dosages have been found effective in several clinical trials. If the disease is mild, 200 to 400 mg may be started and the dose escalated if breakthrough bleeding occurs. If severe, a higher dosage is preferred. The duration of therapy depends upon the extent of the lesions as well as the rapidity of the disappearance of signs and symptoms. Danazol does not possess estrogen or progestogen effects; therefore, it exerts an immediate suppressive action on endometriosis implants. Its side effects include edema, weight gain, acne, hirsutism, and deepening of the voice. Thromboembolic phenomenon, however, has not been reported. The androgenic side effects can be lessened by decreasing the dosage. Breakthrough bleeding may occur during the first few months and can usually be alleviated by increasing the dosage or by office curettage. Addition of an estrogen preparation to control the breakthrough bleeding is not indicated. While the cost of danazol therapy is substantial, a recent prospective report revealed a corrected pregnancy rate of 83 per cent in mild endometriosis and an overall rate of 72 per cent. Although danazol appears a promising compound, its definitive role in the treatment of endometriosis cannot be settled until more long-term studies are completed.

Methyltestosterone, 5 to 10 mg per day orally, is effective in the relief of symptoms of endometriosis such as dysmenorrhea and dyspareunia, but its use is now limited because of significant androgenic side effects and the recent availability of danazol. Although serial injections of depo-medroxyprogesterone acetate (150 mg intramuscularly every 2 weeks for two doses, then 150 mg monthly for a total of 4 to 6 months) have been utilized in the management of endometriosis, this is not currently approved by the Food and Drug Administration, and the usefulness of this agent in infertile patients is severely curtailed because of the often prolonged anovulation following discontinuance.

Combinations. Preoperative treatment with danazol for 3 to 6 months may cause disappearance of small implants and also make conservative surgery easier. Postoperative therapy with hormones may be indicated if a significant amount of implants were not removed surgically, but one should bear in mind that the immediate postoperative period offers the highest chances of pregnancy.

Factors Affecting the Selection of Initial Therapy

Presence or Absence of Symptoms. Initial treatment depends upon the presence or absence of symptoms such as infertility, dysmenorrhea, dyspareunia, and pelvic pain. If the patient is asymptomatic, she may be observed or treated with hormones. If she is symptomatic, her desire to preserve fertility potential is the determinant for therapy. If childbearing is no longer an issue, she may be managed by hormonal therapy or, preferably, by definitive surgery of resection of implants and total abdominal hysterectomy with or without bilateral salpingo-oophorectomy. If she desires preservation of fertility, her choices include conservative surgery, hormonal treatment, or combination therapy.

Severity and Extent of Endometriosis. Because of multiple sites of involvement, a classification system based on the severity and extent of endometriosis is not only helpful in selecting the initial mode of treatment but also valuable in predicting and comparing the outcome of different therapies. Among several systems devised, the most widely used has been that of Acosta et al. (1973), which divides endometriosis into mild, moderate, and severe degrees. The American Fertility Society in 1979 published a classification system which quantitates the severity by assigning numerical values to lesions found in the pelvic cavity. If endometriosis in an infertile patient is of severe degree with involvement of the internal genital, urinary, or gastrointestinal systems, conservative surgery with appropriate procedures is indicated. On the other hand, if endometriosis is of mild degree, hormonal therapy is preferred. However, factors such as the patient's age, duration of infertility, financial means, attitude, and understanding of the disease should also be taken into consideration in selecting the initial therapy. For example, a 20-year-old with 1 year of infertility and moderate to severe endometriosis may be treated initially with hormones and then conservative surgery if hormonal therapy fails.

Pregnancy Rate. In several series with long-term follow-up, estrogen with progestogen therapy seems to offer the least overall success among different modes of treatment. Although the overall pregnancy rates between danazol and conservative surgery are comparable, danazol fares better in mild endometriosis and conservative surgery better in more severe forms. About half the pregnancies occur within 6 months following completion of either danazol therapy or conservative surgery. This suggests that postoperative hormonal therapy should not be routinely given to the patient who desires immediate pregnancy. The pregnancy rate of 50 to 60 per cent following initial surgery falls to only 12 per cent after a second conservative surgical procedure. This suggests that the best chances of achieving pregnancy are with the first conservative surgery.

Recurrence Rate. If patients are followed for an average of 3 years, the recurrence rates of endometriosis following different forms of initial therapy increase to as high as 25 to 45 per cent. Recurrence following estrogen with progestogen therapy seems to be the highest, whereas that after danazol or conservative surgery is lower and comparable. The more severe the degree of endometriosis, the higher the chances of recurrence. The patient should be advised to fulfill her fertility desires as soon as is feasible, since a significant number of patients are not curable short of definitive surgery.

Recommendation of Initial Therapy

Asymptomatic. *Mild:* Observation. *Moderate and severe:* Cyclic or continuous progestogen-dominant oral contraceptives.

Symptomatic. NOT INTERESTED IN CHILDBEARING. Age is another important factor in selecting the mode and nature of therapy. *Mild:* Hormonal therapy. *Moderate and severe:* Definitive surgery. Ovarian ablation by ovariectomy without extensive resection of implants may be indicated for patients who are poor surgical risks.

DESIROUS OF FUTURE CHILDBEARING. The therapy of choice is principally hormonal, as the recurrence rates following hormonal therapy and conservative surgery are comparable. *Mild and moderate:* Either danazol, estrogen with progestogen, or medroxyprogesterone acetate. *Severe:* Danazol is the drug of choice, as estrogen with progestogen therapy has been reported to cause the rupture of endometriomas. *Urinary or gastro-*

intestinal (GI) involvement: Reconstructive surgery may be preferred over hormonal therapy.

DESIROUS OF CHILDBEARING NOW. *Mild:* Danazol. *Moderate:* Conservative surgery or danazol. The choice depends on the severity and extent and the individual factors as discussed above. *Severe:* Conservative surgery alone or danazol for 3 to 6 months, followed by conservative surgery.

DYSFUNCTIONAL UTERINE BLEEDING

method of
LORRAINE C. KING, M.D.
Philadelphia, Pennsylvania

Dysfunctional uterine bleeding (DUB) is defined as abnormal bleeding or out-of-phase uterine bleeding for which no organic cause can be found by routine history and physical examination, including screening coagulation profiles, blood chemistries, Papanicolaou smear, endometrial biopsy or uterine curettage. It is, therefore, a diagnosis made by the exclusion of local and systemic disease. Dysfunctional uterine bleeding is bleeding that occurs because of a disturbance in normal cyclic hormonal secretions.

The term DUB is still frequently used to connote abnormal bleeding as the result of anovulatory menstrual cycles. This refers to abnormal bleeding from an endometrium stimulated by estrogen alone. However, in recent years, Yen and others have shown that DUB may indeed occur in ovulatory as well as anovulatory cycles. Indeed, anovulatory bleeding is approximately 10 times more common than ovulatory dysfunctional bleeding. However, consideration must be given to the possibility that DUB may result from disturbed corpus luteum function, as commonly uncovered in infertility evaluations. In such instances, corpus luteum insufficiency and, less commonly, prolonged corpus luteum activity may be found in an otherwise ovulatory patient. It should be remembered that the diagnosis may be readily made between irregular ovulatory and anovulatory dysfunctional uterine bleeding with a well timed endometrial biopsy, aspiration, or dilatation and curettage (D&C). Certainly, D&C will also rule out the presence of intrauterine pathology (endometritis, polyps, submucous myomas, undiagnosed derangements associated with early pregnancy losses, and cancer). Although it should be emphasized, D&C may not always be necessary in the management of this problem.

Classification of Dysfunctional Uterine Bleeding

Ovulatory. This type accounts for approximately 10 per cent of all cases of DUB and usually presents as persistent mid-cycle spotting or polymenorrhea with unusually short cycles of only 18 to 21 days, owing to either a *short proliferative* or *short luteal* phase.

DUB may also result from abnormal corpus luteum function, ranging from insufficiency to prolonged activity.

Anovulatory — "Classic Type." Progesterone is absent. There are two predominant patterns:

1. *Menometrorrhagia*, resulting from fluctuating levels of estrogen with subsequent breakdown of proliferative endometrium with estrogen falls, resulting in heavy irregular bleeding until renewed follicular activity raises the estrogen level again.

2. *Oligomenorrhea and hypermenorrhea*, associated with prolonged cycles, usually greater than 45 days. In this state there are gradual prolonged rising estrogen levels, followed by a rapid fall in estrogen levels with prolonged heavy bleeding from an endometrium that is proliferative and generally hyperplastic.

Treatment Goals

1. Prompt arrest of bleeding.
2. Assured maintenance or control of bleeding for several weeks.
3. Relatively diminished bleeding upon withdrawal of hormonal treatment.
4. Prevention of recurrent hemorrhage after the initial treatment cycle.

Hormonal Treatment of DUB

Following the diagnosis of DUB, by whatever means necessary, the hormonal management of this problem centers on (1) progestin therapy, (2) estrogen and progestin therapy, or (3) estrogen therapy only. In considering therapy with these agents, the comparative effectiveness of the sex steroids should be fully understood.

A purely progestational hormone will *not* arrest active bleeding. If the dosage is sufficient, it will initiate shedding of the proliferative endometrium. When the endometrial shedding is complete, the bleeding will stop, at least temporarily, but the process requires several days, and blood loss may be profuse.

Estrogen alone will arrest DUB by causing active proliferation of the endometrium. However, since the endometrium is still proliferative, breakthrough bleeding will begin to occur after several days of therapy, and, when discontinued, severe hemorrhage will occur.

Progesterone and estrogen will promptly arrest DUB, because it converts the anovulatory endometrium to a stable secretory endometrium; therefore, breakthrough bleeding is unlikely to occur, and when hormone therapy is discontinued, the withdrawal bleeding should be similar to a normal menstrual flow. This may be achieved by the proper use of one of the combined oral contraceptives.

However, the combination of progesterone, estrogen, and androgen gives the promptest arrest of DUB, and the secretory endometrium produced is *exceptionally* stable. The ultimate endometrial shedding is also significantly diminished. A 19-nor steroid, norethindrome (Norlutin), contains these three properties (estrogenic, progestational, and androgenic). It is very efficacious, if used properly, in the management of DUB.

Many hormonal treatment regimens incorporating estrogenic, progestational, and/or androgenic substances are present in the literature and are undoubtedly equally effective, if properly administered.

Progestational Therapy

A treatment regimen utilizing norethindrone (Norlutin) is proposed here, based upon the severity of the uterine bleeding. This therapy is extremely reliable and effective and is based on sound therapeutic principles.

Severe Hemorrhage. Ten mg every 4 hours until bleeding stops, then 10 mg three times daily for 3 days, then 10 mg twice daily for 3 weeks. After withdrawal bleeding, cycle with 5 mg twice daily from day 5 to 25 for 3 months.

Moderate Bleeding. Ten mg twice daily for 3 weeks, then, after withdrawal bleeding, cycle with 5 mg twice daily from day 5 to 25 for 3 months.

Mild DUB. Five mg twice daily for 3 weeks, then, after withdrawal bleeding, cycle with 5 mg twice daily from day 5 to 25 for 2 to 3 months.

Combined Estrogen plus Progestin Therapy (Oral Contraceptive Treatment)

The use of almost any estrogen and progestin combination oral contraceptive (e.g. Ovral, Ovulen, Norlestrin 2.5, Enovid) may be administered as 1 tablet four times a day for a total of 20 days. Obviously, if the bleeding does not abate within 24 to 36 hours, an organic cause for the dysfunctional bleeding (e.g., polyps, submucous myomas, neoplasia, pregnancy complications) must be considered, and an examination under anesthesia with a uterine dilatation and curettage should be performed.

If the bleeding diminishes with the aforementioned treatment, investigation of possible hemorrhagic tendencies and the evaluation of the underlying cause should be initiated while restoring hematologic stability, if so indicated, with blood replacement or the initiation of iron therapy.

With such oral contraceptive therapy, for the moment, endometrial stability is established by the production of a compact pseudodecidual reaction. The patient must be warned, however, to anticipate heavy bleeding and severe cramping 2 to 5 days after therapy is discontinued.

If the treatment is successful, the same combined oral contraceptive may be restarted on the fifth day of the flow in a normal cyclic fashion and continued for several months. In the patient who does not require contraception, cyclic oral contraceptive therapy may be discontinued after 3 months. In such patients, if spontaneous menses do not resume on a regular basis, it is recommended that medroxyprogesterone (Provera) in a dosage of 10 mg orally be administered daily for 7 to 10 days every 8 to 12 weeks to avoid excessive endometrial buildup.

Estrogen Therapy

Dysfunctional uterine bleeding may be found associated with *low* estrogen stimulation, with resultant minimal endometrial stimulation. In this situation progestin treatment is of no benefit, since the tissue base is insufficient for progesterone to exert its action. The same endometrial status may exist following prolonged hemorrhagic desquamative bleeding, resulting in little residual tissue.

The arrest of acute bleeding may be achieved with the administration of conjugated equine estrogen injection (Premarin intravenous) in a dosage of 20 mg intravenously every 4 hours until bleeding abates (up to three doses). Progestin treatment must be initiated with the estrogen therapy and continued to ensure the arrest of uterine bleeding for the desired treatment period in an effort to prevent recurrence of hemorrhage.

Clomiphene Citrate (Clomid) Therapy

The use of clomiphene citrate (Clomid) may be useful in the anovulatory patient desirous of pregnancy, or in the infertility patient with DUB who has a corpus luteum defect. In addition, one occasionally encounters a patient with anovulatory bleeding with DUB who is either nonresponsive or poorly responsive to hormonal therapy. In such patients, many of whom have coexistent endometrial hyperplasia, clomiphene citrate (Clomid) may be used to induce three to six consecutive ovulatory cycles. This treatment will help "entrain" the hypothalamic-pituitary-ovarian mechanism and convert the endometrium to a normal state, both effects helping to reduce the incidence of recurrent abnormal bleeding.

AMENORRHEA

method of
WILLIAM C. PATTON, M.D.
Loma Linda, California

Definition

Amenorrhea which requires proper diagnosis and treatment exists under the following conditions: (1) No menses by age 14, with absent pubertal growth spurt and absence of secondary sexual development. (2) No menses by age 16 despite normal pubertal growth spurt and normal secondary sexual development. (3) In a previously menstruating woman, no menses for an interval equivalent to three usual cycle lengths or a total period of 6 months. (4) Exclusion of the physiologic amenorrhea of pregnancy, lactation, or the postpartum period.

Therapy: General Considerations

Since amenorrhea is not a diagnosis, but is a symptom of an underlying disorder, precise diagnosis is required before instituting therapy. The diagnostic scheme shown in Figure 1, when applied to amenorrhea as defined above, will allow the physician to precisely place each patient into one of the six major categories listed in Table 1.

It is also useful to review the general organization of the reproductive endocrine system as shown in Figure 2, and to note that the disorders relate to a failure of function at one of the four general levels of this system.

Five specific regimens of endocrine therapy for amenorrhea will now be described. Under the heading Therapy: Specific Entities, these will be referred to by number. They are as follows:

1. Estrogen Replacement. This is indicated for the treatment of the symptoms of estrogen deficiency — hot flashes and vaginal dryness — and to prevent osteoporosis. A progestin is also given to protect the endometrium from the hyperplastic or possible neoplastic effect of unopposed estrogens, and there is increasing evidence that progestins so given substantially reduce or

AMENORRHEA
TSH

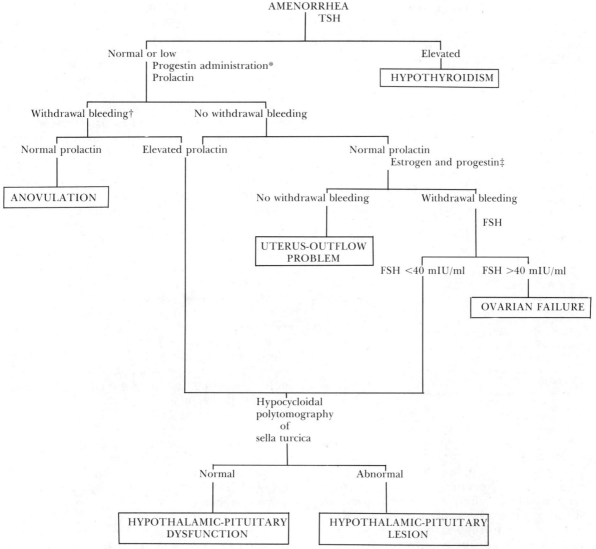

Normal or low
Progestin administration*
Prolactin

Elevated
HYPOTHYROIDISM

Withdrawal bleeding†   No withdrawal bleeding

Normal prolactin   Elevated prolactin

ANOVULATION

Normal prolactin
Estrogen and progestin‡

No withdrawal bleeding   Withdrawal bleeding
                                           FSH
UTERUS-OUTFLOW
PROBLEM

FSH <40 mIU/ml   FSH >40 mIU/ml

OVARIAN FAILURE

Hypocycloidal
polytomography
of
sella turcica

Normal   Abnormal

HYPOTHALAMIC-PITUITARY   HYPOTHALAMIC-PITUITARY
DYSFUNCTION   LESION

*Progesterone in oil, 100 mg IM, or medroxyprogesterone acetate (Provera), 10 mg daily × 5 days.
†Any bleeding or spotting detected by the patient is adequate.
‡Conjugated estrogens (Premarin), 5 mg daily × 21 days, plus medroxyprogesterone acetate (Provera), 10 mg daily during the final 7 days of Premarin.

Figure 1.

eliminate the risk of endometrial cancer associated with unopposed estrogen therapy. Conjugated estrogens (Premarin), 0.625 mg, are given each day for the first 25 days of each calendar month. Some patients may require 1.25 or 2.5 mg for relief of symptoms. It is likely that 0.3 mg will relieve symptoms in most patients, but may not be enough to prevent osteoporosis. Medroxyprogesterone acetate (Provera), 10 mg, norethindrone (Norlutin), 5 mg, or norethindrone acetate (Norlutate), 5 mg, is also given on days 16 through 25 of each calendar month. Most patients will experience withdrawal bleeding on about the twenty-seventh of the month. The administration of the hormones on a calendar month basis allows the physician to know what his patient is taking on any given day if a problem develops, and also avoids more complex regimens in which the days of administration change from month to month.

2. Progestin Replacement. This is indicated when chronic anovulation with adequate or increased endogenous estrogen production is present. It will substitute for the corpus luteum function which is lacking in these patients, and will prevent the untoward effects of prolonged unop-

TABLE 1.   **Causes of Amenorrhea**

Hypothyroidism—1–3%
Anovulation—75–80%
   Polycystic ovary syndrome—common
   Hypothalamic-pituitary dysfunction—common
   Cushing's syndrome—very rare
   Functioning ovarian tumor—very rare
   Hyperthyroidism—rare
Hypothalamic pituitary dysfunction—5–10%
   Weight loss
   Emotional stress
   Hyperprolactinemia
   Sheehan's syndrome
   Drugs
Hypothalamic pituitary lesion—5–10%
   Neoplasms
   Granulomas
   Empty sella syndrome
Ovarian failure—5%
   Premature ovarian failure
   Gonadal dysgenesis
   Resistant ovary syndrome—very rare
Uterus-outflow problem—2–5%
   Obstruction
     Imperforate hymen
     Cervical stenosis
   Absent uterus and vagina
     Congenital agenesis
     Testicular feminization
   Asherman's syndrome
   Tuberculosis

posed estrogen stimulation of the endometrium — endometrial hyperplasia or neoplasia and anovulatory dysfunctional uterine bleeding. Medroxyprogesterone acetate (Provera), 10 mg, norethindrone (Norlutin), 5 mg, or norethindrone acetate (Norlutate), 5 mg, is given once daily for the first 10 days of each calendar month. Withdrawal menstruation can be expected on about the twelfth of the month.

3. Gonadotropin Suppression. Administration of pharmacologic amounts of estrogen and progestin to produce gonadotropin suppression is indicated only for the treatment of chronic anovulation when there is also a need to control hirsutism or a need for contraception. Any of the combined oral contraceptives currently on the market will accomplish this purpose. Contrary to popular opinion, it is not necessary to consider the "estrogenicity" or "androgenicity" of any of the particular contraceptives in the treatment of hirsutism, since the therapeutic effect is provided by suppression of LH-dependent androgen excess, and not by any intrinsic steroid effect of the preparation. The lower dose preparations are recommended because most of the serious side effects of oral contraceptives are dose related. The usual 21 days "on," 7 days "off" method of administration is recommended.

4. Bromocriptine (Parlodel). This new drug is indicated for the treatment of amenorrhea that is accompanied by hyperprolactinemia with galactorrhea of sufficient magnitude to be troublesome to the patient. This drug has not yet been approved by the Food and Drug Administration for use in the presence of a known pituitary or hypothalamic tumor, or for induction of ovulation when infertility is a problem. It will usually result in the return of cyclic ovulatory cycles, and the patient should be advised to use a mechanical or intrauterine form of contraception. The dosage is 2.5 mg once daily for a week and then 2.5 mg twice daily. The initial dose is lower so that the patient can develop tolerance to the most common side effect of the medication, nausea. Unfortunately, most patients will have a recurrence of amenorrhea and galactorrhea when the drug is discontinued, and the manufacturer recommends that the drug be used only for a period of 6 months at a time.

5. Induction of Ovulation. With the exception of bromocriptine, none of the other endocrine therapies mentioned above will result in normal cyclic ovulation. Induction of ovulation is indicated in amenorrhea only when the patient desires to become pregnant, and can be accomplished by using various regimens or combinations of clomiphene citrate (Clomid), human chorionic gonadotropin (A.P.L.), bromocriptine (Parlodel), or human menopausal gonadotropins (Pergonal). These potent medications have potentially serious side effects, and patients who are candidates for ovulation induction should be referred to physicians who are familiar with the use of these regimens.

It should be re-emphasized that therapy is directed toward the specific cause of amenorrhea, the induction of ovulation when pregnancy is desired, or control of the problems of estrogen deficiency, unopposed estrogen, hirsutism, or galactorrhea. Very few patients will request induction of cyclic menses for psychologic reasons when they are told the reason for amenorrhea

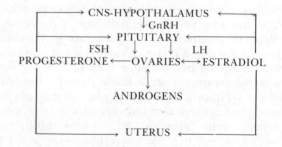

Figure 2. The reproductive endocrine system. GnRH = Gonadotropin-releasing hormone (LRF, LH-RH). FSH = Follicle-stimulating hormone. LH = Luteinizing hormone.

and a few facts about the basic nature of the menstrual shedding of endometrium, and are reassured that menses are not necessary for the elimination of any "poisons." Amenorrhea resulting from *anovulation* or *hypothalamic-pituitary dysfunction* should be re-evaluated annually, because the true cause may be an occult *hypothalamic-pituitary lesion* that becomes apparent with the passage of time. This re-evaluation should not be neglected just because one of the five endocrine therapies is used with resulting cyclic menses, because they do not treat the underlying cause of amenorrhea.

Therapy: Specific Entities

Hypothyroidism. Primary hypothyroidism is characterized by elevated thyroid-stimulating hormone (TSH), and return of TSH levels to normal with thyroid hormone therapy indicates adequate replacement of thyroid hormone. L-Thyroxine (Synthroid, Letter), 0.05 mg, is given daily for 2 weeks and then increased to 0.10 mg daily. TSH is measured after 6 weeks of therapy. If the TSH is elevated, the dose is increased in 0.05 mg increments every four weeks until the TSH becomes normal. Secondary hypothyroidism is usually due to Sheehan's syndrome or to a hypothalamic-pituitary lesion. These problems are discussed below.

Anovulation. The polycystic ovary syndrome probably affects 2 or 3 per cent of all women in the reproductive age group, but does not always result in amenorrhea. The basic disturbance is chronic anovulation with excessive extraovarian estrogen production. The estrogen leads to elevated luteinizing hormone (LH) levels and reduced follicle-stimulating hormone (FSH) levels. This gonadotropin imbalance perpetuates anovulation and stimulates ovarian androgen overproduction. The patient thus has progesterone deficiency and excessive production of estrogens and androgens. The clinical manifestations include various combinations of infertility, hirsutism, amenorrhea, intermittent abnormal bleeding, and endometrial hyperplasia or neoplasia. If amenorrhea or abnormal bleeding is the only problem, endocrine therapy No. 2, progestin replacement, is used to protect the endometrium from the excessive estrogen. Progestins reduce the number of estrogen receptors in the endometrium and thus reduce the proliferating effect of estrogen. If the patient desires pregnancy and infertility is the major problem, endocrine therapy No. 5, ovulation induction, is indicated. It is possible to induce ovulation by medical means in the overwhelming majority of the patients, and ovarian wedge resection should never be done in this condition except as a therapy of

last resort. The chief disadvantages of ovarian wedge resection are that therapy is not permanent and that there may be signficiant peritubal adhesions following surgery, which may further impair fertility. If hirsutism is a problem, or contraception is needed, endocrine therapy No. 3, suppression of gonadotropins with an oral contraceptive, is indicated, since the androgen overproduction depends on stimulation by LH, and oral contraceptives will normalize LH levels. This is one of the few indications for use of oral contraceptives in the treatment of amenorrhea.

The patient with hypothalamic pituitary dysfunction has amenorrhea because the overall production of gonadotropin-releasing hormone (GnRH) is reduced, or because the pituitary does not provide an adequate LH surge to trigger ovulation. In the former case overall estrogen production is relatively low, and in the latter case overall production is reasonably normal. In both cases, the patient is usually asymptomatic, and no therapy is indicated unless pregnancy is desired, in which case endocrine therapy No. 5, ovulation induction, is indicated. These patients should not receive oral contraceptives, because the oral contraceptives may further reduce the level of hypothalamic-pituitary function and perpetuate the problem. The patient with hypothalamic-pituitary dysfunction anovulation can be differentiated from the patient with polycystic ovary syndrome anovulation by measurement of the LH level. LH is elevated in the latter, and normal or low in the former. These two conditions will account for the overwhelming majority of patients with amenorrhea who are encountered by the practicing physician, and their management, except for ovulation induction, is straightforward and simple.

If the patient has any of the signs or symptoms of Cushing's syndrome, this very rare condition can easily be excluded by performing the overnight dexamethasone suppression test. The patient is instructed to take two 0.5 mg tablets of dexamethasone (Decadron) at 11:00 P.M., and then to report to the laboratory for a plasma cortisol level at 8:00 A.M. the following morning. If the plasma cortisol level is less than 5 micrograms per 100 ml, Cushing's syndrome is excluded. If the cortisol is greater than 5 micrograms per 100 ml, consultation with an endocrinologist for further diagnosis and management is indicated.

Functioning ovarian tumors that produce androgens are usually accompanied by obvious virilism. Functioning ovarian tumors that produce estrogen are usually palpable as ovarian masses. If the hirsute patient has a total serum testosterone less than 200 nanograms per 100 ml and if the amenorrheic patient has no palpable ovarian mass, functioning ovarian tumors can be positively excluded. Further comments about diagnosis and treatment of these rare lesions is beyond the scope of this discussion.

Hyperthyroidism is relatively common, but usually presents with abnormal bleeding rather than amenorrhea. Other signs and symptoms are usually obvious in the woman of reproductive age. Therapy is directed at the cause of the hyperthyroidism, and menses usually return.

Hypothalamic-Pituitary Dysfunction. This category of hypothalamic-pituitary dysfunction differs from that described above under Anovulation in that estrogen levels are lower and/or there is hyperprolactinemia.

Amenorrhea associated with weight loss is becoming increasingly common. Anorexia nervosa represents the extreme of this condition and is a medical emergency requiring intensive medical and psychiatric therapy. More commonly, a teenager, even though her weight is normal, decides she must lose weight. The usual pattern is sudden cessation of menses, weight loss of 5 to 15 pounds, and then failure of menses to return even when the weight is regained. No treatment other than explanation and reassurance is needed. While menses often eventually return, amenorrhea may persist for a prolonged time. A similar situation is seen in the nonobese woman who loses weight by engaging in strenuous athletics or running considerable distances each day. Patients with weight loss amenorrhea seldom have estrogen deficiency symptoms, but some of the younger ones may note distressing loss of breast size. Endocrine therapy No. 1, cyclic replacement of low doses of estrogen and progesterone, may be of benefit in this instance. Oral contraceptives should not be used, because their pharmacologic amounts of estrogen and progestin will further reduce gonadotropin-releasing hormone (GnRH) production and low GnRH is the underlying problem in the dietary amenorrheas. Endocrine therapy No. 5, ovulation induction, is possible if infertility is present.

The amenorrhea that is tied to obvious social, occupational, and life situations is usually also due to GnRH deficiency. If there are symptoms of estrogen deficiency, endocrine therapy No. 1 will be helpful, but most patients are asymptomatic and require only explanation and reassurance. Again, oral contraceptives should not be used, because they suppress GnRH. Ovulation induction is indicated if pregnancy is desired.

Amenorrhea in patients with hyperprolactinemia and a normal sella turcica may be treated with endocrine therapy No. 4, bromocriptine (Parlodel), if there is troublesome galactorrhea. Ovulation induction, No. 5, is indicated for infertility. These patients may be harboring a small, as yet undetectable prolactin-producing pituitary adenoma and require annual coned-down views of the sella turcica after the initial hypocycloidal sellar polytomography.

The diagnosis of Sheehan's syndrome should be suspected when there is a history of shock in association with abortion, ectopic pregnancy, or delivery. Failure of lactation is usually the first sign. Consultation with an endocrinologist is indicated for evaluation of pituitary reserve, since secondary hypothyroidism and secondary hypoadrenalism may be present. Estrogen deficiency symptoms are troublesome and may be treated with endocrine therapy No. 1. Induction of ovulation and normal pregnancy are usually possible if desired.

A number of drugs may cause disturbances of hypothalamic-pituitary function, resulting in amenorrhea, but only the most common of these will be discussed. About 1 per cent of women who discontinue oral contraceptives will have amenorrhea that persists more than 6 to 12 months. Such patients must be evaluated for amenorrhea in the usual way, but no therapy is necessary unless they desire pregnancy or have symptoms of estrogen deficiency. In these situations therapies No. 5 and No. 1, respectively, are useful.

Patients who take phenothiazine tranquilizers for psychoses will frequently have amenorrhea associated with galactorrhea and hyperprolactinemia. If no associated hypothalamic-pituitary lesion is found on evaluation, no treatment is necessary unless the patient desires pregnancy. In that case, the drug should be discontinued, and cyclic ovulation and fertility may be expected to return. The use of bromocriptine in such a patient who must continue the phenothiazines would not be indicated.

We still see patients who have received an injection of depo-medroxyprogesterone acetate (Depo-Provera) who have prolonged amenorrhea because of the suppression of GnRH that this drug produces. However, evaluation of amenorrhea is indicated even though the drug seems to be etiologic. It should be emphasized that Depo-Provera and Provera have considerable pharmacologic differences. The effect of Depo-Provera lasts for a number of months, and the drug should not be used as a progestational agent in any of the situations described in this article.

Hypothalamic-Pituitary Lesions. If the hypocycloidal polytomography of the sella turcica is abnormal in the patient being evaluated for amenorrhea, appropriate endocrine and neuro-surgical consultation should be obtained, as the management of various lesions of the hypo-thalamus-pituitary is beyond the scope of most physicians and of this discussion. The important point to emphasize here is that none of these lesions will be missed if the amenorrhea diagnosis flow chart (see Fig. 1) is followed.

Ovarian Failure. Some patients will have normal menarche with normal menses for a vari-able number of years, and then will develop amenorrhea because of exhaustion of ovarian follicles and premature ovarian failure. Elevated FSH is the key to the diagnosis. These women are permanently infertile, and treatment is directed toward relieving the symptoms of estrogen defi-ciency and prevention of osteoporosis. Estrogen deficiency symptoms are almost always present in this group of patients, and are almost always absent in all the other amenorrhea patients. En-docrine therapy No. 1, estrogen replacement, will provide safe and satisfactory relief.

Patients who have gonadal dysgenesis will have no secondary sexual development or puber-tal growth spurt. After the diagnosis is made, endocrine therapy No. 1 will provide estrogen for growth and secondary sexual development. It may be necessary to use doses of conjugated estrogens (Premarin) in the 2.5 to 5 mg range to accomplish adequate growth and secondary sex-ual development. A karyotype should be per-formed if there is premature ovarian failure or gonadal dysgenesis. Removal of the gonad is indicated if there is a Y chromosome present in the karyotype because of the increased risk of malignant neoplasms of the gonad in patients with a Y chromosome.

The resistant ovary syndrome is very rare and will present in exactly the same fashion as premature ovarian failure. Treatment is exactly the same, and the only difference is that the resistant ovary may occasionally lose its resistance to FSH and LH with spontaneous resumption of cyclic menses, ovulation, and unexpected preg-nancies. The resistant ovary can be differentiated from premature ovarian failure only by ovarian biopsy, but it is so uncommon that it probably does not justify routine ovarian biopsy in cases of ovarian failure.

Uterus-Outflow Problem. The imperforate hymen will be obvious on physical examination of the young woman with normal secondary sexual development but no menses. A palpable mass may be found representing a vagina filled with menstrual blood. A cruciate incision of the hymen will relieve the obstruction. This can sometimes be done in the office under local anesthetic, but frequently will require a brief anesthetic in the operating room.

Cervical stenosis may follow conization of the cervix or the use of abortifacients, and if it is complete with resulting obstruction of menstrual outflow, it can be treated by repeated dilation of the cervix.

When the vagina is absent, the uterus is usually absent also, since both depend on the müllerian ducts for their normal formation in the embryo. The young woman with absent vagina and uterus will usually have normal secondary sexual development, and the diagnosis will be made by physical examination. Such a patient is either an otherwise normal young woman with congenital agenesis of the müllerian duct, or is a genetic male with the testicular feminization syn-drome. In the testicular feminization syndrome, there is lack of receptors for androgens through-out the body. This leads to failure of masculiniza-tion of the embryo and consequent development of a normal female phenotype. At puberty, the testes produce increasing amounts of androgen, which has no effect since the body is resistant to it, and also normal amounts of testicular es-trogen, sufficient to feminize the patient when there is no androgen to antagonize it. Congenital müllerian agenesis and testicular feminization syndrome can be differentiated by a karyotype (XX in the former, and XY in the latter) or by measuring the serum testosterone concentration (normal female level in the former, normal male level in the latter). Removal of the gonad should be accomplished in the testicular feminization patient after puberty because of the risk of neo-plasia when a Y chromosome is present in an undescended gonad. Estrogen replacement ther-apy (hormone therapy No. 1) would then be necessary. The patient with congenital agenesis of the vagina does not require any endocrine therapy, because she has normal ovaries that function in a normal way. Both patients require the formation of a vagina if coitus is desired. This can be done by applying pressure to the rudimen-tary vaginal pouch that is usually present, using thick-walled test tubes available from chemical supply houses as dilators. One starts with a tube about 1 cm in diameter and gradually increases it as the neo-vagina deepens and develops. The patient is instructed to apply pressure in a slightly dorsal, cephalic direction for 15 to 20 minutes each day. A functioning vagina can usually be created in 3 or 4 months by a motivated patient. The advantage of creating a vagina this way rather than with a surgical procedure involving a skin graft and mold is that the vagina created by dilators will be lined with epithelium that has its origin from estrogen-sensitive tissue. Secretions will be more physiologic, with less problem of desquamation and odor than with the vagina created surgically. There is also less scarring and contracture.

Asherman's syndrome results from destruction of the endometrium with adhesion formation between the front and back walls of the uterus. The endometrium of pregnancy (the decidua) is uniquely susceptible to the trauma of curettage and infection, and the diagnosis may be suspected when a patient develops amenorrhea following therapeutic or spontaneous abortion or delivery, particularly when there is an associated history of infection or curettage. The diagnosis can be confirmed by hysteroscopy or hysterosalpingography. No treatment is necessary unless the patient wishes to become pregnant. In this case the adhesions are lysed under direct hysteroscopic visualization, or by performing a dilatation and curettage. A Lippes loop IUD is placed in the uterine cavity at the conclusion of the procedure, the patient is given tetracycline, 250 mg four times daily for 7 days, and conjugated estrogens, 5 to 7.5 mg per day for 60 days, to promote endometrial proliferation. The Lippes loop, used to prevent adhesions during healing, is removed after 30 days.

Tuberculosis that destroys the endometrium is distinctly rare in the United States, but should be suspected if there is obliteration of the endometrium and no good history to suggest Asherman's syndrome. The tuberculosis should be treated, but the prognosis for subsequent pregnancy is very poor.

DYSMENORRHEA

method of
JAY S. NEMIRO, M.D.,
and ROBERT J. STILLMAN, M.D.
Washington, D.C.

The term dysmenorrhea is derived from the Greek word meaning difficult monthly flow, and is one of the most common complaints seen by the gynecologist. Approximately 52 per cent of postpubescent females are in some degree affected by this condition, with about 10 per cent incapacitated for 1 to 3 days each month. It is the greatest single cause of lost working hours and school days among young women.

Almost all ovulatory women experience some abdominal discomfort around the time of menstruation as part of the moliminal complex, which may also include breast tenderness, bloating, irritability, and fatigue. However, the mild cramp-like pains subside soon after the menstrual flow begins, and most women have no further problems. When abdominal symptoms become more severe and persistent, often coupled with systemic complaints, we label this dysmenorrhea.

Dysmenorrhea is termed primary in the absence of gross pathologic conditions of the pelvic organs.

Secondary dysmenorrhea is pelvic pain associated with established genital tract pathology such as endometriosis, endometrial polyps, adenomyosis, submucous and intramural fibroids, cervical stenosis, pelvic inflammatory disease, blind uterine horns, and intrauterine devices.

Primary dysmenorrhea has also been attributed to a variety of causes, including uterine hypoplasia, uteroflexion, cervical stenosis, and even errors in posture, allergic states, and psychologic factors. Specific therapies utilized for each were rarely efficacious. More recently, evidence has accumulated to implicate prostaglandins (PGs) as the cause of primary dysmenorrhea. Support of this theory is based on the following evidence: (1) Exogenous PGs cause the same symptoms as seen in primary dysmenorrhea. (2) Serum metabolites of PGs, 15-keto-13,14-dihydro-$PGF_2\alpha$, are higher in patients with dysmenorrhea. (3) PG levels are increased in the luteal phases near onset of menses. (4) No cyclic rise in PGs and no dysmenorrhea occur in anovulatory cycles. (5) Elevated PG levels have been demonstrated in the endometrium and menstrual extracts of patients with primary dysmenorrhea. (6) Myometrial hyperactivity associated with dysmenorrhea can be markedly reduced with PG inhibition. (7) PG synthetase inhibitors are efficacious in treatment of painful menses.

PGs are produced from triglycerides in a rapid process initiated by the activity of the lysosomal enzyme phospholipase A_2. At the time of menstruation, lysosomal breakdown from decidual tissues releases the phospholipase A_2, resulting in the production of arachidonic acid. This PG intermediate combines with eicosanoic acid in the presence of a second enzyme, prostaglandin synthetase, to form $PGF_2\alpha$ and PGE_2, among others. The former two are the most common PGs associated with dysmenorrhea. Local PGs markedly increase uterine tone by increasing myometrial cell excitation and contraction through their influences on calcium membrane transport and binding. This local hypertonicity results in ischemia and the painful contractions characteristic of dysmenorrhea. Systemic absorption produces the gastrointestinal and cardiovascular effects often associated with the syndrome.

It is speculative as to what factors predispose some patients to the development of primary dysmenorrhea. It is likely due to a combination of factors ranging from increased synthesis to increased sensitivity and altered metabolism. Whatever the predisposing factors, the current understanding of PG's role in the etiology of primary dysmenorrhea has led to more direct and efficacious therapeutic intervention.

Treatment

The treatment of dysmenorrhea should include the following points:

1. A thorough history and physical examination to rule out causes of secondary dysmenorrhea. Once the diagnosis of primary dysmenorrhea is established:

2. Physician support, reassurance, and elucidation of the causes and treatment possibilities to the patient assume importance. The use of placebos and the assumption of psychogenic cause are not warranted.

3. If contraception is desired and no contraindications to contraceptive use exist, any combined (low dose) oral contraceptive usually offers effective relief.

4. If contraception is not desired or is contraindicated, then mild symptoms may be relieved by local application of heat, bed rest, and aspirin (a PG inhibitor). For more severe or unrelieved symptoms, we recommend the use of a more potent prostaglandin inhibitor, such as naproxen sodium. Since little PG is stored, and is released only around the time of menstruation, prolonged prophylactic use before the predicted onset of distress is usually not necessary. Naproxen sodium, 500 mg orally at the first sign of menstrual distress, then 250 mg four times daily for 2 to 3 days, is effective. (This use of naproxen is not listed in the manufacturer's official directive.) Ibuprofen, 400 mg three to four times daily for 2 days, can be used alternatively. (This use of ibuprofen is not listed in the manufacturer's official directive.) No loading dose has been recommended. Our personal experience with mefenamic acid is limited. We do not recommend the use of indomethacin because of a higher incidence of serious side effects.

5. Because of the effectiveness of the PG synthetase inhibitors, the likelihood of other organic cause must be seriously considered if relief is not obtained with their use. Rarely are narcotics or β-mimetic agents warranted to control pain or uterine contractions.

Side effects of naproxen and ibuprofen include occasional nausea, indigestion, heartburn, headaches, and decrease in menstrual flow. Rarely bronchospasm, angioedema, skin rashes, and fluid retention occur. However, in the dosages and treatment schedules outlined, they are generally both safe and effective in the treatment of dysmenorrhea.

MENOPAUSE
method of
HAROLD L. KAYE, M.D.
Dallas, Texas

The physiologic and psychologic changes associated with the sudden cessation or progressive reduction of estrogen production require medical understanding and care. Menopausal symptoms may occur after surgery, after radiotherapy, or physiologically. These symptoms result directly from estrogen deficiency.

Surgical menopausal symptoms may be sudden and dramatic. Some of the effects of long-term estrogen deprivation are still unknown. Whether or not all people undergoing surgical castration will need estrogen replacement is debatable. It is my policy that all women under age 40, some between age 40 and 45, and all symptomatic women who have bilateral oophorectomy receive cyclic estrogen replacement.

The physiologic menopause may be defined as the normal physiologic processes leading to the failure of the ovaries to manufacture and secrete estrogens. This deficiency accounts for the well known menopausal symptoms. Patients may have psychologic as well as physiologic changes. These psychologic symptoms may be most disturbing to the patient and must also be evaluated and treated.

Objects of Therapy

1. Evaluation of abnormal bleeding by endometrial biopsy or dilatation and curettage (D&C).

2. Elimination of hot flushes and flashes (vasomotor symptoms).

3. Improvement of psychologic symptoms: anxiety, apprehension, insomnia, depression, crying, emotional outbursts.

4. Improvement of headaches.

5. Avoidance of senile vaginitis with its concomitant decrease in vaginal lubrication and dyspareunia.

Estrogens and Carcinoma

Estrogen is the drug of choice in treating the menopausal symptoms. In view of recent publications concerning the carcinogenic properties of estrogen, a word on that subject is warranted. Unfortunately, more on this subject has been written in newspapers and magazines than in scientific journals. Estrogens, when used cyclically in the lowest effective dose, are highly effective toward improving the quality of life. Abnormal bleeding, such as markedly irregular cycles, profuse short cycles, or bleeding between menses, should be studied histologically in order to diagnose the cause prior to the initiation of therapy. *All postmenopausal bleeding* must be evaluated by office biopsy or curettage. If the patient has had a hysterectomy, she cannot get endometrial carcinoma. Posthysterectomy patients can thus be reassured. Occasional Papanicolaou smears from the vaginal vault should be taken.

Estrogens have stimulating effects on breast tissue, but there has never been clear evidence reported of estrogens causing cancer of the breast. It is ill advised to prescribe estrogens for patients with proved carcinoma of the breast. Although estrogens are safe and effective drugs when used properly, they should never be forced upon a reluctant patient who has predetermined that they are dangerous.

Drugs, Dosage, Administration

Basically, since menopausal symptoms are the result of a hormone-deficient state, they should be treated by proper estrogen replacement. This may be done by oral administration, injection, or pellet implantation.

Oral administration is the preferred route because it is the most easily implemented, least expensive, and least troublesome, and dosages can be easily altered. For most patients 0.625 mg of conjugated estrogen or 1 mg of estradiol daily will be sufficient. When it is not, or in patients under age 40 with surgical menopause, 1.25 mg of conjugated estrogen or 2 mg of estradiol daily should be used. My standard regimen is for patients to take their daily dose from calendar day 6 until the end of each month. She does not take medication for the first 5 days. This eliminates the need to count weeks and the confusion that arises because months are unequal in length.

Injection may be used when rapidity of effect is important. In the immediate postoperative period 20 to 40 mg of 17-valerate estradiol (Delestrogen) intramuscularly may be used. The patient can then begin oral replacement at home. Other than this, there is little use for this route of administration. There may be an occasional patient who cannot tolerate oral estrogen or in whom injections offer a psychologic advantage.

*Pellet implantation** is a satisfactory route for the rare patient who cannot take this oral medication. Since it is difficult to nullify the effects,

---

*Pellets of estrogen have temporarily been withdrawn from the market by the Food and Drug Administration, which feels that proof of activity and safety has not been presented, even after many years of use. Present research may result in permission to market the pellets again. They are now available only to physicians with investigation numbers.

bleeding may be a disturbing complication even after it has been clearly explained to the patient. I limit this procedure to posthysterectomy patients. Estrogen pellets as 25 mg. pure estradiol are available. Implantation of 2 or 3 of these pellets along with 1 pellet of 75 mg of pure testosterone will last 4 to 6 months. (This use of estrogen pellets is not listed in the manufacturer's official directive.) They are placed into the fatty tissue of the anterior abdominal wall.

Estrogen cream may be used for topical effect in atrophic vaginitis. There is absorption of estrogen from the vaginal mucosa, and this mode should not be used if there is a contraindication to estrogen.

Tranquilizers or psychoenergizers are rarely needed. These may be used occasionally in small doses for a short period of time. Phenobarbital, belladonna, and ergotamine tartrate (Bellergal-S) provides occasional relief and may be used in patients in whom estrogens are contraindicated. Often a few minutes of the physician's time and his careful listening are more therapeutic than a whole bucket of pills.

How Long Can Estrogen Replacement Be Continued?

In the postsurgical patient, I reduce the dosage at about age 45 and eliminate it at age 50 to 55. If symptoms persist, the drug is continued and the symptoms are re-evaluated every year or two. In other patients the drug is stopped at age 50 to 55 and, again, if symptoms persist, the estrogen is continued. Often in women over age 50, just 0.3 mg of conjugated estrogen or its equivalent can be used. There are some who recommend the use of estrogen to age 60 and others forever.

In summary, most of the menopausal symptoms are caused by decreasing estrogen secretion. As with any deficiency disease, the hormone should be replaced. The lowest therapeutic dose should be used cyclically. Any bleeding in the postmenopausal female must be investigated.

VULVOVAGINITIS

method of
FREDERICK J. FLEURY, M.D.,
and RANDOLPH WM. ROLLER, M.D.
Springfield, Illinois

The common diseases of the vulva and vagina can be easily diagnosed using simple office methods and effectively treated in most cases with little difficulty. The most frequent causes of vulvar inflammation are (1) candidiasis, (2) herpetic infections, (3) dermatophyte infections, (4) poor perineal hygiene, (5) chemical or allergic reactions, and (6) the vulvar dystrophies, lichen sclerosus and hypertrophic dystrophy. The most common causes of vaginal discharge are (1) *Hemophilus vaginalis* (recently renamed *Gardnerella vaginalae*), (2) Candida, (3) *Trichomonas vaginalis*, (4) cervicitis, (5) atrophic vaginitis, and (6) excessive quantities of normal secretions. "Nonspecific vaginitis" is not a separate entity. Use of the term indicates either no appreciation of the common vulvovaginal diseases or a poor diagnostic effort.

The most common symptoms of Candida infection are vulvar pruritus and vaginal discharge. When a patient complains of vulvar itching, Candida infection is suspect until proved otherwise. This infection also presents with vulvar burning and soreness, dyspareunia, and occasionally splitting of the vulvar skin. Patients often demonstrate erythema and edema with small reddish punctate areas on the periphery — the so-called "satellite lesions." In severe or chronic cases, self-inflicted excoriations, which can be confused with herpetic ulcerations, may be present.

The diagnosis of Candida vulvitis is virtually certain when patients present with a typical clinical picture and the organism is identified in wet smear of vulvar secretions. Clinicians must be careful not to assume that Candida vulvitis is accompanied by Candida vaginitis. Not infrequently patients have no vaginal symptoms and microscopic examination of *vaginal* secretions may fail to demonstrate the organism. In these cases it is helpful to do a Nickerson culture of the vulvar skin, demonstrating the organism as small dark brown colonies.

The treatment of choice for Candida vulvitis is miconazole cream (Monistat) or clotrimazole cream (Gyne-Lotrimin or Mycelex-G). With a single prescription, the patient has a topical treatment for the vulva and a cream for the vagina. Patients with a history of chronic, recurrent infections can be given multiple refills to use as needed. They should be instructed to apply the cream to the vulva two or three times a day at the first sign of itching. One applicator of the same cream can be placed vaginally at bedtime for 5 to 7 nights as well. Twice daily vaginal application for three days, approved recently, is equally effective.

In the last decade, genital herpes virus infections have become commonplace. The diagnosis can usually be made on clinical history and the finding of shallow, exquisitely tender ulcers. It is usually impossible and *unnecessary* to determine if there is vaginal or cervical involvement.

Severe primary infections are usually accompanied by genital ulceration with exquisitely tender inguinal adenopathy, tenderness, labial edema, malaise, and low grade fever. If the diagnosis must be confirmed, a Papanicolaou smear of one of the ulcers may demonstrate multinucleated giant cells or intranuclear inclusion bodies. If available, tissue culture can provide virus isolation. Antibody studies are of little value in clinical practice.

Despite innumerable treatment regimens for herpes, none are truly effective. The patient can be greatly helped by providing strong oral analgesics and recommending frequent warm soapy sitz baths. A suprapubic catheter to avoid irritation of urethral ulcers can be used when urination is very difficult or impossible. When suprapubic catheterization is required, hospitalization and a brief anesthetic are usually necessary. At this time, the patient can be examined painlessly, wet smears and appropriate cultures can be taken, and the vulva can be scrubbed with a povidone-iodine solution. Povidone-iodine has been shown to be a virucidal and is one of the most commonly recommended topical antiseptics in the palliation of this disease.

At least 35 per cent of patients infected with the herpes virus will have recurrent lesions. These are reactivations of dormant virus and not reinfections. Typically, these reactivations are far less severe than the initial infection. Patients with recurrent genital herpes should be told they are infectious for up to 7 days after the onset of their recurrence. Additionally, they may rarely shed virus when there are no apparent lesions and they should not deliver vaginally when recurrent lesions are present. Contrary to the popular understanding that patients with herpes should have frequent examinations, annual Papanicolaou smears are sufficient.

Tinea cruris can cause pruritus and soreness of the vulvar skin, although it spares the labia minora and vagina. Most cases are relatively mild and may be overlooked by the patient. Occasionally, severe infection results when the disease involves the crural folds. After a prolonged itch-scratch cycle, there is a secondary bacterial infection. The organism can be easily identified by scraping loose skin onto a glass slide, mixing it with 10 to 20 per cent KOH, and examining it under a microscope. The small short curved hyphae confirm the presence of this infection. Miconazole or clotrimazole cream massaged into the affected areas at least three times a day until complete resolution is the best treatment. In severe cases, 2 to 3 weeks of treatment may be required, even though symptomatic relief occurs very quickly.

Poor perineal hygiene may be directly related to showering in preference to tub bathing. Careful interlabial cleansing with soapy water during a tub bath is not only important for healthy vulvar skin but is extremely beneficial to virtually all vulvar maladies except neoplasia. Folklore notwithstanding, it is extremely rare for a woman to react to soaps, bubble bath, or other substances in tub water.

The direction of perineal wiping is not as important as myth would suggest. Fecal organisms, other than Candida, are harmless to healthy vulvar skin. When the itch-scratch cycle causes breaks in the vulvar skin, lengthy exposure to vulvar smegma and rectovaginal secretions may initiate infection followed by more scratching and inflammation. The inevitable, temporary urinary and fecal contact with the vulva is totally harmless when women cleanse the vulva carefully during regular bathing. Chronic vulvitis secondary to poor hygiene is best treated by a short course of topical corticosteroids as an adjunct to soapy sitz baths.

An occasional patient will react adversely to chemicals or medications applied to the vulva. In most cases, a history of contact to a new substance is all that is necessary to make the diagnosis. Occasionally, however, it takes great effort to determine the causative agent.

A great many substances have been described as causing vulvitis, including soap, fabric softener, scented or colored toilet tissue, and nylon undergarments. Such diagnoses are usually invoked when the clinician has been unable to make a specific diagnosis. One truly common cause of vulvar contact dermatitis is "feminine hygiene spray." This complication has been helpful in preventing the widespread acceptance of these unnecessary sprays.

The mainstay of treatment of a true vulvar contact dermatitis is withdrawal of the offending agent, careful cleansing of the vulvar skin with soapy sitz baths, and careful rinsing, followed by the application of topical corticosteroids.

The vulvar dystrophies should be considered during the evaluation of all patients with chronic vulvitis. There are two broad categories of vulvar dystrophy. The first includes those atrophic diseases that are variations of lichen sclerosus. These patients present with pruritus and splitting of the vulvar skin. Although this disease can be suspected clinically, the diagnosis rests with histologic confirmation. The second category includes hypertrophic or hyperplastic conditions. These are often called leukoplakia, leukoplakic vulvitis, or neurodermatitis. Hypertrophic dystrophy may be clinically suspected, but, again, the diagnosis must be made on histologic examination. In vir-

tually all cases, vulvar biopsy should be performed in the office under local anesthesia. The biopsies serve not only to confirm the diagnosis but also to rule out more ominous dysplastic or frankly malignant lesions.

The treatment for lichen sclerosus is topical testosterone propionate in petrolatum. This medication should be massaged into the involved skin three times a day. Although symptomatic relief may come in a few weeks, histologic improvement takes many months. Even after patients are feeling better, they should continue the medication three times a day until dramatic improvement has resulted. Later, the frequency of application can be gradually reduced, based on the patient's needs. Patients with lichen sclerosus, however, must continue to use the medication at some interval for the rest of their lives to prevent recurrence. Patients with hypertrophic dystrophy respond promptly to topical fluorinated corticosteroids. As an adjunct, patients with either vulvar dystrophy should be carefully evaluated for other causes of their chronic vulvitis, including urinary incontinence, poor hygiene, and chronic vaginal discharge.

Hemophilus vaginalis has been renamed *Gardnerella vaginalae* because careful study of this organism has shown it is not of the Hemophilus genus. The hallmark of this infection is malodorous discharge. Signs of irritation are characteristically absent, as this organism is not a tissue pathogen. Gardnerella infection is a sexually transmitted disease. Because untreated women may harbor this organism in the vagina indefinitely, a recent acquisition of this infection should not be assumed.

The diagnosis can be made with ease by identifying the characteristic "clue cells" on microscopic examination of the vaginal secretions mixed with saline. These cells represent numerous small bacilli as they cling to the surface of vaginal epithelial cells. Another reliable method of detecting this infection is the sudden burst of a fishy odor released when the discharge of *Gardnerella vaginalae* is mixed with potassium hydroxide. Confirmation of this infection, however, relies on the identification of the clue cells in the secretions.

The treatment of *Gardnerella vaginalae* infection is in a state of chaos. The only medication approved at present is triple sulfa vaginal cream, but studies currently in progress do not seem to support this approval. Ampicillin and cephalosporins given orally to the patient and her consort (500 mg four times daily for 5 to 7 days) have been recommended for many years, but the effectiveness of these two medications is far inferior to that of metronidazole. Metronidazole in a dosage of 250 mg three times daily for 7 days or 500 mg twice daily for 5 days for the patient and her consort is effective in 95 to 98 per cent of patients. Unfortunately, metronidazole has not yet been approved for this indication.

Trichomonas vaginalis is another sexually transmitted disease. It commonly presents with vaginal discharge and soreness but is also associated with intermenstrual spotting, postcoital spotting, and other forms of abnormal vaginal bleeding. This organism causes great tissue inflammation and friability, and it is not unusual for these patients to bleed freely after a simple Papanicolaou smear.

The diagnosis of this infection rests with microscopic examination of the vaginal secretions and demonstration of the motile trichomonad. The diagnosis should not be made by simple visualization of a frothy green discharge, because in the majority of patients there are no bubbles and the discharge is gray-white.

The only drug approved for this infection in the United States at present is metronidazole. There are currently two approved dosage schedules: metronidazole, 250 mg three times daily for 7 days, and metronidazole, 1000 mg for two dosages in 1 day. The patient and her consort should be treated. Metronidazole should be avoided in the first trimester of pregnancy, and perhaps in the second and third trimesters if symptoms can be relieved with local measures such as povidone-iodine gel. Since Trichomonas causes severe tissue injury accompanied by secondary bacterial infection, this disease should be eradicated when discovered. With the dosages of metronidazole listed above, 95 to 98 per cent of patients respond after a single course of therapy. A similar number of treatment failures respond after a second course of medication. In the rare patient requiring repeated dosages of metronidazole, it has been recommended that the patient's hematologic profile be monitored.

Cervicitis is a frequent cause of vaginal discharge and is often confused with vaginal infection. At examination, however, patients with cervicitis can be readily differentiated from women with vaginitis by noting the purulent cervical mucus emanating from the endocervical mucosa. On microscopic examination, patients with cervicitis show many leukocytes but lack inflammation of the vaginal mucosa as evidenced by the absence of immature vaginal squamous cells. Conversely, clear cervical mucus and immature vaginal cells connote vaginitis and not cervicitis. Many of the causes of cervicitis have not been identified. Those most frequently mentioned are gonorrhea, *Chlamydia trachomatis,* herpes simplex, and *Trichomonas vaginalis.* Accordingly, any patient with a purulent endocervical mucosa should

have a culture for gonorrhea. If there is no evidence of herpes or *Trichomonas vaginalis* and the culture for gonorrhea is negative, the patient should be treated empirically for presumed *Chlamydia trachomatis* infection, especially if the patient is symptomatic. The treatment of Chlamydia infection is tetracycline or erythromycin, 250 mg four times daily for 7 to 14 days. Both the patient and her consort should be treated. Unfortunately, in most communities the diagnosis of this infection is still one of exclusion. In time, culture capability of this organism or other diagnostic methods will be widely available.

Atrophic vaginitis is not as common as is generally believed. Most patients actually have uncomplicated, asymptomatic vaginal atrophy. This is especially true in premenarchal children and breast-feeding patients who have atrophic changes virtually identical to those of the postmenopausal woman.

Significant inflammation of the atrophic vagina, true atrophic vaginitis, causes vaginal soreness and spotting. The spotting is a worrisome symptom, and prior to treatment with topical estrogens, neoplasia of the genital tract must be excluded. The diagnosis of atrophic vaginitis is made not only by the exclusion of other infections but also by the demonstration of an absence of mature vaginal squamous cells and the preponderance of parabasal and intermediate cells in the secretions. The number of white and red cells is proportional to the degree of inflammation.

The treatment of *symptomatic* atrophic vaginitis is topical estrogen cream applied daily or every other day for up to 2 weeks. Prolonged use may cause breast tenderness, nausea, and occasionally uterine bleeding when the medication is withdrawn.

Two groups of patients complain of vaginal discharge but actually have no infection. They are women with excessive mucoid secretions from an otherwise healthy endocervical mucosa and those with an excessive epithelial discharge of the squamous cells of the vagina. Both discharges are harmless, and in most patients reassurance is all that is necessary. In the rare patient with excessive mucorrhea, it may be necessary to ablate some of the endocervical mucosa by use of silver nitrate sticks or cryotherapy in the office. Surgical conization in the absence of dysplasia is not indicated in the management of this problem.

An occasional patient will have excessive quantities of mature squamous cells and present with a profuse, nonirritating paste-like discharge. Cultures and biopsies of these patients are normal, and yet such patients produce truly great quantities of this epithelial paste. Presently there is no cure for this problem. Palliation is available in the form of intermittent douching, tampons, or mini-pads. Douching is preferred, and patients can determine the frequency of douching, depending on their symptoms.

URINARY TRACT INFECTIONS DURING PREGNANCY

method of
ROBERT E. HARRIS, M.D.
San Antonio, Texas

Introduction

Urinary tract infections during pregnancy are commonly seen and require special attention. They produce considerable morbidity and are important complications of pregnancy. Such infections are not isolated events but present as a variety of clinical situations and manifestations. Urinary tract infections are diagnosable and treatable such that prevention of more serious renal disease is possible following adequate therapy of early onset infections, e.g., asymptomatic bacteriuria.

Urinary tract infections are usually manifest in one of three ways during pregnancy. Asymptomatic bacteriuria is defined as a recovery of $\geq 100,000$ bacteria per ml of urine (on two consecutive samples) from a patient with no complaints. Acute cystitis is manifest by urinary urgency, frequency, dysuria, and bacteriuria, with absence of fever and costovertebral angle tenderness. The diagnosis of acute pyelonephritis, an inflammation of the renal parenchyma, is based upon history, symptoms and signs, physical findings, and laboratory reports.

Etiology

The most frequent causative agents for urinary tract infections during pregnancy are the aerobic gram-negative bacilli normally residing in the gastrointestinal tract. *Escherichia coli* (the most common microorganism isolated, accounting for approximately 85 per cent of initial urinary tract infections), *Proteus mirabilis, Klebsiella pneumoniae,* and the enterococci are usually isolated from pregnant patients with uncomplicated urinary tract infections. By contrast, complicated urinary tract infections, seen in those patients with previous urologic surgical procedures and/or those who have been treated with a multiple course of antimicrobial agents, tend to be caused less often by *E. coli* and more often by other microorganisms such as *Pseudomonas aeruginosa*.

Diagnostic Evaluation

Screening of all pregnant patients by means of quantitative urine cultures at the initial visit and at least once during the remainder of the pregnancy has been strongly recommended for detection of bacteriuria. However, the detection of asymptomatic urinary tract infections in the general population by means of screening programs has not become an established preventive measure primarily because of the cost to the individual. Therefore, simple, economic, and feasible tests have been developed for detection of bacteriuria. Whenever a screening test is positive, a clean-catch, midstream urine sample is obtained for culture.

Asymptomatic Bacteriuria

Asymptomatic bacteriuria is one of the most commonly diagnosed urinary tract infections during pregnancy. The prevalence is associated with the presence of sickle cell trait, lower socioeconomic status, reduced availability of medical care, and increased parity. Depending upon the population studied, bacteriuria occurs in 2 to 10 per cent of all pregnant women. Eradicating these infections is important, as 25 to 40 per cent of asymptomatic bacteriuric patients will develop symptomatic infection (i.e., pyelonephritis) during the gestational period. Almost 50 per cent of pregnant bacteriuric patients have asymptomatic upper tract infection as demonstrated by fluorescent antibody-coated bacteria and bladder washout techniques.

The antimicrobial therapy for asymptomatic bacteriuria should be based upon the sensitivity of the microorganism isolated from the urine sample. Those drugs considered to be safe during pregnancy include sulfisoxazole* (Gantrisin) — during the first and second trimesters — ampicillin,* cephalexin* (Keflex, Ancef, Duricef), and nitrofurantoin macrocrystals* (Macrodantin). Generally we have employed one of the following regimens:

1. Nitrofurantoin macrocrystals,* 100 mg orally three times daily for 10 days. The nitrofurantoin macrocrystals are highly concentrated by the kidneys and do not change the natural sensitivity for 90 per cent of the fecal *E. coli,* thus rarely causing resistant bacteria to arise in the fecal flora.

2. Ampicillin,* 250 mg orally four times a day for 10 days.

3. Cephalexin,* (Keflex), 250 mg orally four times a day.

4. Sulfisoxazole* (Gantrisin), 500 mg orally four times a day for 10 days.

A repeat urine culture should be obtained upon completion of therapy to ensure eradication of the bacteriuria. If this repeat urine culture is positive for bacterial growth, therapeutic fail-

---

*See also manufacturer's official directive regarding use in pregnancy.

ure has occurred (persistence or relapse) and re-evaluation of microorganism sensitivities and antimicrobial therapy should be accomplished. Recurrent infection, following asymptomatic bacteriuria, occurs for approximately 25 per cent of patients during the same gestation. Therefore, asymptomatic bacteriuric patients should be closely monitored throughout the remainder of the gestation by some type of urine screening method to detect such a recurrence. Should reinfection occur, the patient should be re-treated according to the microorganism sensitivities. At our facility those patients with recurrent asymptomatic bacteriuria during the same gestation have been maintained on suppressive antimicrobial therapy throughout the remainder of the gestation and for 2 weeks post partum. Our choice for suppressive therapy has been nitrofurantoin macrocrystals (Macrodantin), either 50 mg orally three times a day or 100 mg every evening. Both have been used satisfactorily to eradicate bacterial growth. An effective alternative antimicrobial is methenamine mandelate, 500 mg orally three times a day, which, unfortunately, interferes with urinary estriol evaluations. These values of urinary estriol are used at many medical centers for assisting in the determination of fetal well-being.

It has been previously recommended that each patient with asymptomatic bacteriuria during pregnancy should have a postpartum intravenous pyelogram (IVP) evaluation to rule out urinary tract abnormalities, e.g., renal or ureteral calculi or chronic pyelonephritis. By this method, 28 per cent of patients are found to have urinary tract abnormalities. However, it has been demonstrated that those patients with the more significant abnormalities are those who had recurrent infection. If a patient has asymptomatic bacteriuria on more than two occasions during the same gestation, the chance of her having an abnormal IVP rises to 66 per cent. Thus, all patients with recurrent infections during the same gestation definitely should be evaluated by an IVP in the postpartum period. The IVP should be done approximately 6 weeks after delivery to allow the normal physiologic changes of the urinary tract to nonpregnant status.

Women who previously have been bacteriuric during pregnancy have been found to have recurrent urinary tract infections and IVP abnormalities several years after the initial episode of asymptomatic bacteriuria. For this reason, we screen our patients at the 8 week post partum check-up for bacteriuria. Each of these patients who have had asymptomatic bacteriuria is instructed to have an annual screening test for bacteriuria.

Acute Cystitis

The incidence of acute cystitis during pregnancy is 1.3 per cent. The pregnant patient with acute cystitis should be begun on immediate therapy with nitrofurantoin macrocrystals, sulfisoxazole, or ampicillin. The most commonly isolated microorganisms in patients with acute cystitis in our population have been equally sensitive to these antimicrobial agents. Frequently a contaminated urine culture is obtained from the pregnant patient. Therefore, the initial urine culture should be obtained by catheterization prior to the onset of therapy to ensure an acceptable urine sample for identifying microorganisms and drug sensitivities. Our therapy is one of the following:

1. Ampicillin, 250 mg orally four times a day for 10 days.
2. Nitrofurantoin macrocrystals, 100 mg three times a day for 10 days.
3. Sulfisoxazole, 500 mg four times a day for 10 days.

A urine culture should be obtained 2 days after onset of therapy and also 1 week after completion of therapy to ensure eradication of the microorganism, or that no resistant microorganisms or persistent infection is present. The patient should be followed for the remainder of the gestation for recurrence of urinary tract infections. Should there be recurrence, the patient is treated with suppressive therapy, as noted for those with recurrent asymptomatic bacteriuria. Intravenous pyelograms are not indicated for patients who had acute cystitis during pregnancy. However, whenever there has been recurrent urinary tract infection during pregnancy, postpartum urologic evaluation is necessary to rule out the presence of urinary calculi, urethral stricture, or other abnormalities. In our population 20 per cent of those selected patients with recurrent infection have had ureteral or renal calculi.

Acute Pyelonephritis

The diagnosis of acute pyelonephritis during pregnancy is reported to occur in 1 to 2.5 per cent of patients. As screening for and treatment of asymptomatic bacteriuria have increased, the incidence of pyelonephritis, in those particular medical centers with screening programs, has decreased. It has been reported that early detection and elimination of bacteriuria during gestation should prevent antepartum pyelonephritis in at least two thirds of all patients who would otherwise have been admitted to the hospital. Our medical center experience has confirmed these earlier data, and this is the main reason for the treatment of asymptomatic bacteriuria during pregnancy. Another predisposing factor for pyelonephritis is the presence of urinary calculi during pregnancy, which often cause acute infection episodes. Thus, any patient with acute pyelonephritis during pregnancy may have a coexisting calculus (ureteral or renal).

For the pregnant patient who is seen with acute pyelonephritis, hospitalization is strongly advised. Immediate antimicrobial therapy is necessary prior to the return of the urine culture report, as this disease may lead to maternal sepsis and shock with resultant maternal death and/or fetal wastage. The urine specimen for culture should be obtained by catheterization upon admission and prior to the initiation of intravenous antimicrobial therapy. Intravenous antimicrobials are continued until the patient is afebrile and can tolerate oral medications. The antimicrobial agent is continued orally for a total therapy course of 3 weeks. The usual microorganisms isolated are *E. coli*, which in our medical center are predominantly sensitive to ampicillin, our first drug of choice. Each physician must be aware of the hospital laboratory sensitivities and the particular microorganisms usually present for that patient population with pyelonephritis. A repeat urine sample for culture is obtained on the second day of treatment. Following intravenous antimicrobial therapy, 85 per cent of patients should become afebrile within 48 hours and 97 per cent within 96 hours. If the patient does not respond to the initial therapy, two factors should be considered: (1) an underlying obstructive uropathy (as by stone formation); (2) the presence of resistant microorganisms. The initial urine culture report should be available, with sensitivities, within 48 hours. If the patient is not responding, owing to resistant microorganisms, switching to another antimicrobial agent can be accomplished. If the patient is responding (in vivo) to the antimicrobial agent being used, but the in vitro laboratory testing reveals resistant microorganisms, we do not automatically change antimicrobial agents. The urine should be examined for the presence or absence of pyuria and bacteria. However, if the patient is not responding and the microorganisms are resistant, it is necessary to change the antimicrobial agent. Most often a cephalosporin is selected. Many physicians will begin initial therapy with cephalexin (Keflex) because of the microorganisms sensitivities usually seen for their particular population.

The outline for a patient with pyelonephritis includes the following:

1. Hospitalization.
2. Hydration.
3. Lowering the elevated temperature.
4. Monitoring renal functions and measuring intake and output. There is a transient renal dysfunction with acute pyelonephritis during pregnancy. Thus, renal function is lower as measured by a marked lowering of the creatinine clearance. Hence it is important to realize that certain antimicrobial agents, such as the aminoglycosides, must always be used with caution.

5. Intravenous antimicrobial agents. Antimicrobial agents utilized include (a) ampicillin, 1 to 2 grams every 6 hours, (b) cephalothin sodium (Keflin), 500 mg to 1 gram every 6 hours, or (c) gentamicin (Garamycin), 50 mg every 8 hours if renal function is adequate.

Erythromycin and nitrofurantoin macrocrystals (Macrodantin) have both been used in the treatment of acute pyelonephritis but are not our choices for the acutely ill patient.

6. Continued suppressive antimicrobial therapy (nitrofurantoin macrocrystals, 50 mg three times a day or 100 mg at night, or methenamine mandelate, 1 gram three times a day) to prevent recurrence of pyelonephritis during the remainder of the pregnancy is important. The pregnant patient who has an episode of pyelonephritis is very likely to experience a recurrence during her pregnancy if she is not maintained on suppressive antimicrobials. As the normal physiologic changes of the urinary tract persist for 2 weeks postpartum, therapy is continued not only for the entire pregnancy but for the first 2 weeks following delivery. Furthermore, of those patients who were hospitalized for pyelonephritis during the eighth week of post partum period, the majority were hospitalized during the first 2 weeks. Of these patients who had antenatal pyelonephritis, 30 per cent will develop recurrent bacteriuria, 18 per cent will develop recurrent pyelonephritis (75 per cent of those who were not given suppressive therapy), and 40 per cent will have abnormal postpartum intravenous pyelograms. Therefore, we feel it is preferable to follow the initial therapy with suppressive antimicrobial therapy. Suppressive therapy is begun following the initial 3 week course of antimicrobial therapy. An acceptable, but not optimal, alternative to suppressive therapy is diligent examination every 2 weeks of the results of urine cultures to detect recurrent urinary infection. Should bacteriuria or recurrent pyelonephritis occur, the patient is re-treated and refollowed.

Postpartum Bacteriuria and Urinary Retention

Postpartum bacteriuria occurs in 3 per cent of noncatheterized patients and in 6 per cent of catheterized patients. The most valid day to obtain urine cultures for true bacteriuria is the third postpartum day. The incidence of positive urine cultures is significantly higher in those patients who were catheterized for urinary retention. Approximately 40 per cent of patients who have postpartum urinary retention for longer than 24 hours will develop asymptomatic bacteriuria with the possibility of ensuing symptomatic infection. Thus, these patients are treated prophylactically during the catheterization and for 2 days following catheter removal. During the postpartum period different antimicrobial agents may be utilized that would not have been used during the gestation. Thus, either trimethoprim-sulfamethoxazole (Septra), or nitrofurantoin macrocrystals are drugs of choice, but ampicillin or cehalosporins are not recommended. Ampicillin and cephalosporins should be reserved for first-line therapy of active infections and not for prophylaxis for urinary retention.

PELVIC INFECTIONS

method of
G. ERIC KNOX, M.D.
Minneapolis, Minnesota

Female pelvic infections involve — singly or in combination — the uterus, fallopian tubes, ovaries, and surrounding peritoneal surfaces. Rarely, the upper abdomen and its contents can be involved via extension of a primary pelvic infection. For classification purposes, pelvic infections may be divided into either lower tract infections which involve only the cervix (uncomplicated gonococcal disease) or acute pelvic inflammatory disease involving the intraabdominal portions of the reproductive tract and peritoneal surfaces. In addition, infections occurring post partum or after gynecologic surgery microbiologically resemble acute pelvic inflammatory disease (PID), but, because of the different clinical setting in which they occur, are usually addressed as separate entities.

Uncomplicated Cervical Gonococcal Infections

Although most of these infections are discovered by culturing an asymptomatic carrier or sexual partner of a person with known gonorrhea, clinically they may present as cervical discharge, dysuria, low grade temperature, or generalized cervical discomfort. Treatment should begin with a well documented diagnosis.

1. Endocervical and rectal cultures for gonorrhea must be obtained.

2. Treatment of choice consists of aqueous procaine penicillin G (APG), 4.8 million units injected intramuscularly at two sites, with 1.0 gram of probenecid by mouth. Should the patient be allergic to penicillin, tetracycline hydrochloride, 0.5 gram by mouth four times a day for 5 days (total dosage 10.0 grams), should be given. Patients allergic to penicillin and who cannot tolerate tetracycline may be treated with spectinomycin hydrochloride, 2.0 grams in one intramuscular injection.

3. Sexual partners should be examined, cultured, and treated at once in a manner as outlined above.

4. Patients with incubating syphilis (seronegative, without clinical signs of syphilis) are likely to be cured by all of the aforementioned regimens except spectinomycin. All patients should have a serologic test for syphilis at the time of diagnosis. Patients with gonorrhea who also have syphilis or are established contacts to patients with syphilis should be given additional treatment appropriate to the stage of syphilis present.

5. Follow-up cultures should be obtained from both cervix and rectum 3 to 7 days after completion of treatment to rule out the presence of penicillinase-producing *Neisseria gonorrhoeae*. These patients should be treated with 2 grams of spectinomycin intramuscularly. All organisms isolated on post-treatment cultures should be tested for penicillinase production. Should penicillinase-producing gonorrhea be found, sexual contacts with gonorrhea should likewise receive spectinomycin, 2 grams intramuscularly in a single injection. It should be remembered, however, that most infections present after treatment with the initial recommended antibiotic schedules are due to reinfection rather than to penicillinase-producing organisms. This type of infection, therefore, indicates a need for improved contact tracing and patient education.

Acute Pelvic Inflammatory Disease (PID)

Acute PID occurs when cervical pathogens such as *Neisseria gonorrhoeae, Chlamydia trachomatis,* or other nongonococcal bacteria gain access to the fallopian tubes or other intra-abdominal portions of the reproductive tract. Nongonococcal flora include aerobic gram-positive cocci and gram-negative enteric bacteria, anaerobic gram-positive cocci, and Bacteroides, including *Bacteroides fragilis*. Bacterial access to the upper reproductive tract occurs as a consequence of surgical manipulations such as dilatation and curettage, cervical conization, hysterosalpingogram, or intrauterine device (IUD) insertion. Alternatively, cervical vaginal bacterial organisms may gain access to the fallopian tubes because of a breakdown in local barriers to infection, presumably a consequence of prior gonococcal infection. The following management sequence can be used when acute PID is suspected:

1. A careful history, together with general, abdominal, and pelvic examinations, should be performed to rule out other pathology which may be mistaken for PID. Because therapy for conditions such as urinary tract infections, nonbacterial pelvic pain, appendicitis, ectopic pregnancy, ovarian cysts, early pregnancy, or endometriosis is vastly different from that for PID, a correct diagnosis is mandatory.

2. An endocervical culture for *Neisseria gonorrhoeae* must be obtained.

3. Patients without complications dictating hospitalization (see below) should be treated with a loading dose of 1.5 grams of tetracycline hydrochloride, followed by 500 mg of tetracycline every 6 hours for 10 days. Alternatively, a loading dose of either 4.8 million units of intramuscular aqueous procaine penicillin G or 3.5 grams of oral ampicillin together with 1 gram of oral probenecid, followed by 500 mg. of ampicillin every 6 hours for 10 days, may be used.

4. If an IUD is present, it should be removed at the onset of treatment.

5. All recent sexual contacts of women with acute PID should be examined and have cultures taken for *Neisseria gonorrhoeae*. Treatment for asymptomatic contacts is the same as outlined above for uncomplicated gonorrhea.

6. All patients should be compulsively followed up with re-examination at 48 hours, 7 days, and 21 days after beginning therapy to document a satisfactory clinical response and to repeat cervical gonorrhea cultures. If a patient is not responding satisfactorily to outpatient therapy, hospitalization and further diagnostic consideration are strongly recommended.

7. Hospitalization is strongly recommended under the following conditions: (a) An unclear diagnosis. Laparoscopic confirmation of the diagnosis should be considered for patients with an unclear diagnosis or in patients who fail to respond to antibiotic therapy. (b) Presence of an adnexal mass or suspicion of a pelvic abscess. (c) Any suggestion that the patient will not be able to complete the prescribed antimicrobial regimen on an outpatient basis. (d) Peritoneal signs. (e) Severe illness suggested by vomiting, temperature greater than 100.4 F (40 C), or pain requiring analgesics. (f) Pregnancy. (g) Failure to respond to outpatient therapy.

8. In addition to cervical cultures, hospitalized patients should have blood cultures obtained. Serial and frequent recording of temperature, white counts, and vital signs is mandatory. In a severely ill patient, consideration to baseline blood gases should be given as well.

9. Treatment of hospitalized patients with severe peritonitis but without adnexal masses consists of either crystalline penicillin G, 20 million units daily, or 2 grams of ampicillin every 4 hours. Once the patient is afebrile, oral ampicillin, 500 mg orally four times a day to complete a 10 day course of antibiotics, is required. Should a positive blood culture be found, then parenteral antibiotics should be given for at least 5 days following defervescence. Alternatively, tetracycline, 250 mg given intravenously four times a day until improvement occurs, followed by 0.5 gram orally four times a day to complete 10 days of therapy may be used. This latter regimen is not suggested for patients with positive blood cultures. Patients with either severe peritonitis or adnexal masses should be treated with a combination of drugs designed to cover the presumed polymicrobial infection, and this combination should always include an antibiotic that inhibits *Bacteroides fragilis*. Either penicillin or ampicillin in the doses given above, together with gentamicin, 3 to 5 mg per kg in three divided doses daily, and clindamycin, 600 mg every 6 hours, is recommended. Alternatively, chloramphenicol, 1 gram every 8 hours, can be substituted for clindamycin. These complex antibiotic regimens should be monitored with drug levels when available, measurement of renal function, and serial determinations of serum iron to detect bone marrow inhibition should chloramphenicol be used. Parenteral antibiotics should be continued for a minimum of 5 days following defervescence.

10. If rupture of an abscess is suspected, immediate antibiotic therapy and exploratory laparotomy are mandatory. Patients who respond to antibiotic therapy will usually have a gradual reduction in peritoneal tenderness, reduction of white blood cell count and pulse, and return of gastrointestinal function, and an increased sense of clinical well-being. Clinical follow-up on at least a daily basis is necessary to ensure that appropriate cure is being effected. A temperature elevation that continues in the face of otherwise good clinical improvement does not by itself indicate that treatment is ineffective.

11. Patients should be re-examined every 48 to 72 hours for the emerging presence of an abscess that can be drained. Drainage should be undertaken when the abscess is fluctuant, well adherent to the vagina, present in the midline, and well down in the rectal vaginal septum.

12. Worsening peritoneal signs, vital sign instability, or documentation of a pulmonary embolus at any time following initiation of antibi-

otic therapy requires surgical exploration. Likewise, patients who continue to be severely ill beyond 72 hours of intensive medical therapy may also require surgery. At the time of exploration, no firm recommendation as to the extent of the surgery can be made; instead, the procedure selected should be tailored to the particular clinical situation at hand.

Postpartum Infection

Chorioamnionitis and endomyometritis may occur following either vaginal delivery or cesarean section. The bacteria involved are the same as those that cause pelvic inflammatory disease, with the important addition of the group B Streptococcus. In general these organisms are normal inhabitants of the cervical vaginal flora and are found in patients who do not acquire postpartum infection as well. Manifestations of postpartum endometritis may range from an isolated fever to prolonged ileus, marked abdominal tenderness, and localized cervical uterine tenderness on pelvic examination. Because an elevated white blood count may accompany labor, its diagnostic validity is limited in this situation. Blood cultures will be positive in approximately 10 to 15 per cent of all patients and should be obtained. Endometrial cultures are usually contaminated by the normal cervical vaginal flora and, as noted above, do not distinguish infected from noninfected postpartum patients; therefore, they are indicated only when a prompt response to antibiotics is not obtained.

1. Before initiation of antibiotic therapy, elimination of other causes of fever, such as urinary, breast, pulmonary, or wound infection, is necessary.

2. Prophylactic antibiotics at the time of either premature rupture of membranes or prior to cesarean section without amnionitis do not reduce the incidence of serious postpartum infection and therefore are not indicated.

3. Infants of mothers with an endomyometritis do not need to be isolated from the mother or from other infants in the nursery.

4. Intravenous antibiotic therapy should consist of ampicillin or penicillin, together with either kanamycin or gentamicin. If a prompt clinical response is not obtained, either clindamycin or chloramphenicol should be added to the antibiotics already employed. Alternatively, gentamicin with clindamycin is an effective initial regimen.

5. Guidelines for therapy should mirror those of the treatment of pelvic inflammatory disease, with serial examinations performed to rule out the presence of an abscess, to monitor the clinical response, and to detect the presence of an emerging wound infection. Surgical exploration should be considered in any patient who fails to respond to medical therapy.

Postgynecological Surgery Infection

Preoperative prophylactic antibiotics are indicated in premenopausal women undergoing vaginal hysterectomy. A short course of almost any broad-spectrum antibiotic (e.g., ampicillin, cephalothin) administered as one dose prior to surgery and two doses in the next 12 hours provides sufficient prophylaxis at minimal cost and with minimal complications. The efficacy of prophylactic antibiotics for abdominal hysterectomy and other gynecologic procedures that do not involve a vaginal transection or the cervical vaginal cuff is not well established, and therefore such use of these agents is not recommended. Infections following all gynecologic surgery involve the same organisms as those involving pelvic inflammatory disease, and therefore the antibiotic clinical approach is, in general, the same. Cultures should be taken, patients monitored closely, abscesses drained when possible, and the same antibiotic regimens used. It should be stressed that the lack of a prompt response to adequate antibiotic therapy should indicate the need for additional diagnostic steps, including ultrasound and/or laparotomy.

MYOMA OF THE UTERUS

method of
ALBERT B. GERBIE, M.D.
Chicago, Illinois

Myomas, the most frequent uterine tumors, are usually asymptomatic and almost always benign. Bleeding is the predominant symptom and, when present, usually occurs between the ages of 40 and 50. Menstrual periods which have increased in amount, duration, and frequency are characteristic. Continuous flow or intermenstrual spotting, if caused by myomas, is usually submucosal or polypoid. Other symptoms such as pressure or discomfort are unusual, because myomas may become very large before these are noted. If pain is present, additional investigation is necessary, as pain is not a symptom of an uncomplicated myoma. Usually it results from an accident to one of the myomas such as torsion or degeneration. Electrophoretic types of the X-linked enzyme glucose-6-phosphate dehydrogenase used as cell markers have demonstrated that each human myoma is most likely unicellular in origin.

Active treatment of myomas is usually not indicated, because symptoms are not usually present or, if so, are very mild and surgical therapy can be delayed. The need for active treatment is dependent upon (1) the presence and severity of symptoms, (2) the potential danger or risk to the patient because of myomas, or (3) the presence of coexisting lesions that require treatment.

Slight increase in the amount or duration of menstrual flow does not necessitate active treatment. Profuse bleeding or hemorrhage usually indicates that active therapy should be instituted. One must individualize therapy for each patient, as there are many factors which modify treatment. These are the size and position of the myomas, the age of the patient, history of complications during previous pregnancy, desire for future pregnancies, the presence of other pelvic pathologic lesions, and symptoms.

Symptoms of pressure, discomfort, or abdominal fullness are seldom, if ever, severe enough to indicate surgical treatment. On the other hand, pain associated with myomas may indicate an acute accident, which makes treatment urgent.

Tumors that are large in size (more than 12 weeks of gestation) may degenerate and thus jeopardize the patient's health and life. Pedunculated tumors, because of their high incidence of torsion, should be removed, as torsion may result in peritonitis. A rapidly growing tumor indicates either degeneration or malignant change; treatment definitely is indicated. Interligamentous myomas may cause urinary tract disabilities and should be removed. Submucous tumors are apt to cause bleeding, and are prone to interfere with implantation. Polypoid tumors may cause the uterus to attempt to expel them, thus opening the cervical canal to infection and causing pain of uterine contractions. A cervical myoma, even if only moderate in size, should be removed, as it may obstruct the birth canal.

If a patient is being operated on for some coexisting lesion, such as uterine prolapse, cystocele and rectocele, endometriosis, or pelvic inflammatory disease, it may be desirable to treat the lesion and the myomas simultaneously.

Although the presence of myomas may indicate therapy, there are times when they also present a contraindication to the most desirable treatment of one of these coexisting lesions. Carcinoma of the cervix is usually treated with radiation. One might choose to perform a radical hysterectomy and node dissection rather than radiation because of the danger of degeneration to the myomas. This would also be true if one ordinarily uses preoperative radium for adeno-carcinoma of the endometrium. If large myomas are present in such a patient, the preoperative radiation would be contraindicated. If the patient has a complication of pregnancy, particularly incomplete abortion, this should be treated prior to the management of the myomas.

Myomas may occasionally interfere with implantation, particularly submucous myomas, or may degenerate during pregnancy as they apparently increase in size. Occasionally they do cause malposition or obstruct the birth canal, or interfere with the forces of labor itself. Usually they remain asymptomatic and do not interfere with pregnancy.

Two other indications for operation must be listed: (1) Uncertainty of diagnosis; this is true particularly with a pedunculated myoma, which may be confused with a solid ovarian tumor. Because of the danger of overlooking an ovarian malignancy, operation is indicated. (2) Excessive fear of tumors. Occasionally a woman may have a real cancerophobia, and the knowledge that myomas are tumors and are present in her may be so disturbing to her that surgical removal is indicated.

There are two acceptable methods of management of these patients: nonoperative procedures and operative procedures.

Nonoperative methods are used in all patients who do not require definitive surgical treatment. They should be examined every 3 to 6 months; cytosmears for cervical malignancy are performed once a year. Slight anemia can be treated with iron. Most patients with uterine myomas are so treated, continue to be followed, and never come to operation. Profuse bleeding, which may be associated with myomas, can be controlled by continuous or cyclic progestational agents. This is a temporary procedure that may be done to build the blood count while waiting for definitive surgical therapy. One must recognize, though, that growth of the uterus and myomas may be stimulated by these agents.

Operative procedures are the most satisfactory treatment if definitive therapy is indicated. Curettage may relieve bleeding and allow examination of tissue for possible uterine malignancy. Myomectomies are performed in young patients and in those who wish to retain childbearing function. These patients must be told that there is a 25 per cent risk of a second operation at some time in the future for recurrence of myomas. Myomectomy is also indicated for the rare fibroid polyp that may project through the cervical os. The offending myoma is removed; hysterectomy at this time is contraindicated because of the hazard of infection. If indicated, hysterectomy may be performed 6 to 8 weeks later. If a surgical procedure is being performed for endometriosis and myomas are also present, myomectomy may be indicated. In the rare circumstances in which myomas may cause disturbances in childbearing function (particularly in a uterus of more than 6 months' size in a patient who has had repeated spontaneous late abortions), or when a large cervical myoma or a pedunculated myoma obstructs the birth canal, myomectomy should be performed. If during pregnancy an accident or degeneration occurs within a myoma, a myomectomy may be indicated. Management is very conservative; operative procedures are avoided if possible, and are done only for progressive symptoms of degeneration and impending peritonitis. At the time of operation only the offending myoma is removed.

Women in the climacteric are usually treated surgically, because abnormal bleeding is more disturbing, tumors are usually large, coexisting lesions are more frequent, and childbearing has usually been completed. Postmenopausal patients seldom require treatment for myomas unless abnormal bleeding occurs or the tumor continues to increase in size.

For definitive treatment of myomas, either vaginal or abdominal hysterectomy is the procedure of choice if there are no contraindications to operation and if the patient's family is complete. This will permanently rid the patient of her myomas, will obviate further surgical procedures, and will remove the hazard of future uterine tumors. The ovaries are usually conserved in premenopausal women unless they are abnormal. These will continue to function normally after hysterectomy and therefore should be retained.

CANCER OF THE UTERUS

method of
PAUL B. HELLER, M.D.,
and ROBERT C. PARK, M.D.
Washington, D.C.

Carcinoma of the uterus is used as a general term for carcinoma of the endometrium and carcinoma of the cervix uteri. The histologic type of cervical carcinoma is mainly squamous; however, a small percentage may be adenocarcinoma, adenosquamous, and adenoid cystic (cylindroma). The main histologic category of endometrial disease is adenocarcinoma. Again, a small percentage may be adenoacanthoma, adenosquamous carcinoma, and clear cell carcinoma.

Until recently, the greater percentage of genital cancer consisted of carcinoma of the cervix, and at Walter Reed Army Medical Center the incidence of cervical carcinoma is still greater than that of endometrial carcinoma. However, some institutions now report that endometrial carcinoma has equaled or exceeded cervical carcinoma in incidence. The American Cancer Society has completed anticipated incidence and death figures for these diseases. Estimated new cancer cases for the past year include 37,000 of the corpus and endometrium and 16,000 of the cervix. An additional 16,000 new cervical cancer cases will be in situ lesions, making the total figure for both in situ and invasive cervical carcinoma 32,000. Estimated cancer deaths for endometrial cancer are 3300 and for cervical cancer, 7400. According to a survey from 1930 to 1976, the death rate for cancer of the uterus has progressively decreased.

CARCINOMA OF THE ENDOMETRIUM

Adenocarcinoma of the endometrium is now the most frequent invasive carcinoma of the female genital tract. Its precursor states are thought to include cystic and adenomatous hyperplasia. These diseases may arise from unopposed estrogen stimulating the uterus. The postmenopausal female who has the correct constitutional characteristics may be at risk. Classically, these include diabetes, hypertension, and obesity. Other factors may be nulliparity, anovulation, and liver disease. Ovarian stromal tumors may be associated in up to 15 per cent of cases. The common denominator here seems to be an excess of estrogenic hormone, not modified by progesterone effect. A paradoxical situation exists in that a postmenopausal female is envisioned as having symptoms related to estrogen lack; therefore, where does the estrogen arise if not exogenously given? In the early to mid-1970s, a theory was formulated by MacDonald and Siiteri, based upon the premise that the estrogen involved was estrone derived as a conversion product from androstenedione. Androstenedione is produced in the adrenals; when the proper circumstances exist (i.e., obesity), there is an excessive conversion to estrone, and the target organ receptor sites affected by this have a neoplastic reaction. The precursor states, cystic and adenomatous hyperplasia, develop in conditions of unopposed estrogen and may take from 5 to 20 years to envolve into invasive adenocarcinoma.

Staging

The staging of endometrial carcinoma is based upon clinical and, in some cases, radiographic findings. If a pathology report from an endometrial sampling reveals carcinoma, the other examinations to be performed would include (1) physical examination, including nodal evaluation; (2) chest x-ray; (3) intravenous pyelogram; (4) cystoscopy; (5) proctoscopy; (6) barium enema; and (7) liver/spleen scan (if conditions dictate).

Operative staging, as done in ovarian cancer, is not acceptable for statistical purposes in this disease. Therapy for endometrial carcinoma is dependent upon staging (Table 1). This schema is the one described by the FIGO (International Federation of Gynecologists and Obstetricians) in 1971. It takes into consideration the uterine size (sounding is used) as a parameter of tumor growth. The endocervical canal must be separately and carefully sampled. Various radiographic studies, as mentioned, are necessary as part of the diagnostic work-up. One must consider the differentiation of the carcinoma, as this enters into the staging. Spread of the endometrial carcinoma is by lymphatics. It may go through the lower uterine segment into the parametrium. From the fundus, the lesion may spread along the lymphatics associated with the ovarian vessels. Rarely, spread may occur along the round ligaments to the inguinal nodes. Lymphatics are present deep in the myometrium (greater than one third to one half) and the subserosal tissue. Deep myometrial invasion appears to be associated with a greater incidence of positive nodes. In 1973, a study by Morrow, DiSaia, and Townsend revealed 3.4 per cent pelvic node metastasis without deep myometrial penetration, whereas 14.1 per cent of the same group of nodes were involved if there was deep myometrial invasion in Stage I. The incidence of pelvic node metastasis also was seen with increasing stage (10.6 per cent was noted in Stage I, and 36.5 per cent was noted in Stage II). Nodal metastasis was noted to increase with loss of differentiation in a study in 1976 by Creasman, Boronow, and Morrow. Spread to the cervix is evaluated because it will indicate the more extensive therapy. In cases of deep myometrial penetration and dedifferentiation upwards of 10 per cent incidence of post-treatment vaginal cuff metastasis is noted if pre- or postoperative radiation is not given. Spread to the ovaries and tubes is not uncommon, which is an important reason for the modality of total abdominal hysterectomy and bilateral salpingo-oophorectomy. Additionally, the ovaries may be a source of estrogen. Metastatic spread may include pelvic peritoneum, serosal implants, cul-de-sac nodules, para-aortic nodes, and lung lesions.

Therapy

Stage IA, G1. A small uterus with a well differentiated tumor can probably be effectively treated with a total abdominal hysterectomy and bilateral salpingo-oophorectomy. At Walter Reed, if pathologic examination of the surgical specimen reveals superficial residual disease, a radium/cesium application is given to the vaginal cuff.

Stage IA, G2, G3, and Stage IB, All Grades. These lesions are treated with preoperative pelvic irradiation to 5000 rads, followed in 1 to 4 weeks by extrafascial total abdominal hysterectomy and bilateral salpingo-oophorectomy. Certain centers are presently investigating the benefits of surgical staging by performing an extrafascial total abdominal hysterectomy, bilateral salpingo-oophorectomy, and pelvic and para-aortic node sampling in both Stage I and Stage II lesions. If there is greater than 50 per cent myometrial penetration or pelvic or para-aortic node involvement, external and possibly internal radiation may then be tailored to the spread of the disease, dependent upon these pathologic findings. Approximately 75 per cent of endometrial carcinoma is discovered as a Stage I lesion.

Stage II. This involves 5 to 15 per cent of all cases of endometrial carcinoma. Stage II disease may be treated by external radiotherapy to 5000 rads whole pelvis dose and approximately 3500 rads given by intracavitary application. This is followed by a simple extrafascial total abdomi-

---

TABLE 1.   **Classification and Staging of Carcinoma of the Corpus Uteri**

Stage 0:   Carcinoma in situ; histologic findings suspicious of malignancy; cases of Stage 0 should not be included in any therapeutic statistics

Stage I: The carcinoma is confined to the corpus

Stage IA: The length of the uterine cavity is 8 cm or less

Stage IB: The length of the uterine cavity is more than 8 cm

The Stage I cases should be subgrouped with regard to the histologic type of the adenocarcinoma as follows:

G1 Highly differentiated adenomatous carcinoma

G2 Differentiated adenomatous carcinoma with partly solid areas

G3 Predominantly solid or entirely undifferentiated carcinoma

Stage II: The carcinoma has involved the corpus and the cervix, but has not extended outside the uterus

Stage III: The carcinoma has extended outside the uterus but not outside the true pelvis

Stage IV: The carcinoma has extended outside the true pelvis or has obviously involved the mucosa of the bladder or rectum; a bullous edema as such does not permit allotment of a case to Stage IV

Stage IVA: Spread of the growth to adjacent organs

Stage IVB: Spread of the growth to distant organs

---

nal hysterectomy and bilateral salpingo-oophorectomy as in Stage I. Primary radical abdominal hysterectomy, bilateral salpingo-oophorectomy, and pelvic lymphadenectomy may be performed as an alternative method. Again, as mentioned in the Stage I disease category, there are ongoing studies involving simple extrafascial abdominal hysterectomy and oophorectomy and pelvic and para-aortic node sampling, followed by tailored irradiation.

Stage III. Various combinations of surgery and chemotherapy or radiotherapy may be used here. The disease has spread beyond the uterus but is not outside the pelvis. If the extension is to the parametrium and/or to the pelvic wall, the modality of pelvic radiotherapy is useful. Tubal and ovarian involvement may be treated by combinations of radiotherapy and surgery (total abdominal hysterectomy, bilateral salpingo-oophorectomy). Vaginal involvement allows consideration of internal and external radiotherapy in combination. Various regimens of progestational agents are also used. About 10 per cent of endometrial lesions are confined to Stage III.

Stage IV. In this instance, the cancer has histologically involved the bladder and/or rectum (Stage IVA) or is outside the pelvis (Stage IVB). Pelvic radiation therapy may be used to control local disease, whereas progestational agents (megestrol acetate [Megace], medroxyprogesterone [Depo-Provera]) are given for distant lesions. Occasionally, multidrug chemotherapy regimens are used: doxorubicin (Adriamycin), cyclophosphamide (Cytoxan), fluorouracil (5-FU), and megestrol acetate (Megace).

Recurrent Carcinoma. Recurrent carcinoma of endometrial origin, if not responsive to usual therapy, may be treated with medroxyprogesterone acetate (Depo-Provera) or megestrol acetate (Megace). This is helpful, especially in disease found in the chest. If single agents do not effect a response, three and four drug regimens, as mentioned in Stage IV disease, may be administered.

Progesterone receptors, as suggested by Ehrlich, may indicate degree of response to progestational agents in metastatic and recurrent endometrial carcinoma. Evidence of a greater amount of receptor sites for progesterone would indicate a better response. It has been noted that the well differentiated lesions appear to have a larger number of receptor sites.

Survival

Most females with endometrial carcinoma, when found, are in an early stage of the disease. As noted, 75 per cent of this disease is confined to Stage I. Unfortunately, survival in Stage I is quite variable, depending upon the size of the lesion and the differentiation. For instance, Stage IA, G1 lesions will be associated with a 90 per cent or better 5 year survival rate, whereas Stage IB, G3 has about 50 per cent 5 year survival. Overall, Stage I has a survival rate of about 75 per cent. Stage II endometrial carcinoma has a survival rate of approximately 50 per cent, the range being from 35 to 55 per cent, and Stage III about 20 per cent. Stage IV disease has a 5 year survival in the range of 10 per cent. In general, 20 per cent of women with all stages of endometrial carcinoma will die of the disease. Adenoacanthoma appears to be associated with a better prognosis, and the glandular portion of the lesion is well differentiated. Adenosquamous carcinoma of the endometrium, unfortunately, has poorer survival, in the range of 35 per cent.

Medically Inoperable Patients

Patients who are inoperable for medical reasons in Stage I and Stage II are initially treated with radiation alone. If the uterus is small with a well differentiated tumor, two 72 hour applications with tandem to a dose of 6000 mg/hours are given, and the vagina will receive 8000 rads surface dose in two applications with colpostats. With an enlarged uterus and a well differentiated tumor, three applications of internal irradiation with tandem at 2500 mg/hours for a total of 7500 mg/hours, plus 8000 rads to the vaginal surface with two applications of a colpostat, are used. For an enlarged uterus with an anaplastic tumor, 4000 to 6000 rads external irradiation is given, plus one or two radium applications as necessary. Four thousand rads surface dose to the vagina may be given with colpostats if the external irradiation has not exceeded 5000 rads. For carcinoma involving the corpus and cervix (Stage II), 4000 rads whole pelvic irradiation, plus tandem and colpostats in two applications for 48 hours, is given.

CERVICAL CARCINOMA

Cervical carcinoma is now second in frequency to endometrial carcinoma in the United States. At Walter Reed, the percentage of cervical carcinoma found as Stage I disease has been on the increase. It now accounts for approximately 65 per cent of the cervical cancers examined at this institution. The finding of disease at this early stage is in large part due to early detection methods. These include both Papanicolaou smear and colposcopy. If a Papanicolaou smear is suggestive of dysplasia or malignancy, a colposcopic examination with biopsy is performed. Under colposcopic visualization, abnormal lesions are sought. If the lesion is visualized and biopsied but is less than an invasive cancer, it may be treated in one of several ways. Dysplasias of mild and moderate types are usually excised or treated with cryotherapy. Severe dysplasia and carcinoma in situ can be treated by cone biopsy or cryotherapy. If, on colposcopic visualization, the extent of the lesion cannot be seen or endocervical curettings are positive, a cone biopsy is performed. Most important is to rule out invasive carcinoma.

Staging

Staging in cervical carcinoma, as in endometrial cancer, is based upon pretreatment clinical and radiographic findings. The pelvic examination may be performed with or without anesthesia but should be uniform within an institution. At Walter Reed, the method of determination is an examination by the senior radiotherapist and gynecologic oncologist at a pretreatment conference. Staging does not change if the disease advances or if surgery gives additional information. Table 2 indicates the most recent International Federation of Gynecology and Obstetrics (FIGO) staging for cervical carcinoma. Stage 0 or carcinoma in situ is an intraepithelial disease that

TABLE 2.   **Clinical Staging for Cancer of the Cervix (FIGO)**

Stage 0:   Carcinoma in situ, intraepithelial carcinoma
Stage I: Carcinoma confined to the cervix (extension to the corpus should be disregarded)
Stage IA: Microinvasive carcinoma (early stromal invasion)
Stage IB: All other cases of Stage I; occult cancer should be marked "occ"
Stage II: The carcinoma extends beyond the cervix but has not extended to the pelvic wall; the carcinoma involves the vagina, but not the lower third
Stage IIA: No obvious parametrial involvement
Stage IIB: Obvious parametrial involvement
Stage III: The carcinoma has extended to the pelvic wall; on rectal examination there is no cancer-free space between the tumor and the pelvic wall; the tumor involves the lower third of the vagina; all cases with hydronephrosis or nonfunctioning kidney (tumor related)
Stage IIIA: No extension to the pelvic wall
Stage IIIB: Extension to the pelvic wall and/or hydronephrosis or non-functioning kidney
Stage IV: The carcinoma has extended beyond the true pelvis or has clinically involved the mucosa of the bladder or rectum; a bullous edema is not classified as Stage IV
Stage IVA: Spread of the growth to adjacent organs
Stage IVB: Spread to distant organs

does not require work-up beyond determination that no invasion is present. If invasive carcinoma is discovered histologically, several additional diagnostic procedures will be initiated in order that the staging may be more accurately defined: (1) careful pelvic examination and nodal evaluation; (2) chest x-ray; (3) intravenous pyelogram; (4) cystoscopy; (5) barium enema; (6) liver scan and bone scan and survey (if determined necessary); and (7) lymphangiogram—although not part of staging, this is done on any patient thought to be in greater than Stage IB.

If patients are medically suitable for surgery, a staging laparotomy will be performed on those who have a positive lymphangiogram. A study by Leman, in 1975, indicated that negative lymphangiograms at Walter Reed correlated very well with clinical findings; however, positive lymphangiograms were correct in only about 57 per cent of the patients. If positive para-aortic nodes are found on staging laparotomy, then the left scalene node is biopsied. Tailored radiation may be used if the para-aortic nodes are positive, whereas scalene node positivity would indicate a need for systemic therapy. Nodal involvement in general has been noted to be about 15 per cent for Stage I, 25 to 30 per cent for Stage II, and 50 to 60 per cent for Stage III.

Treatment

Stage 0 or Carcinoma in Situ or Intraepithelial Carcinoma. Hysterectomy by the abdominal or vaginal route has been the standard therapy in the United States. The upper vagina should be evaluated and removed if abnormal. If the patient desires further childbearing, therapeutic cervical conization with careful follow-up is a valid management. Recently a large number of clinics have begun to use cryosurgery. This technique is still to be evaluated. Local excision with colposcopic guidance has been recommended but may not be an adequate treatment. Radiation therapy, utilizing tandem and ovoids for 6000 to 7000 mg/hours, may be used in patients not medically suitable for surgery. Most important is that invasive disease be ruled out before treatment is initiated.

Stage IA. There has been a controversy about the definition and treatment in this category. Many feel that if there is a single lesion of less than 3 mm penetration from the basement membrane, no lymphatic involvement is seen in capillary-like spaces, and cone margins are clear, a total abdominal hysterectomy with wide vaginal cuff is adequate treatment. At Walter Reed, a radical hysterectomy is still the treatment of choice. In this circumstance, nodal dissection and ureteral unroofing may be less aggressive than in more advanced lesions. If a patient is not a surgical candidate, radiation therapy may be employed. Usually two radium or cesium insertions of 72 hours each for about 10,000 mg/hours is the treatment of choice.

Stage IB. The main modality of therapy in the United States for this stage is radiotherapy. Both external and internal therapy are used. Four thousand rads whole pelvic irradiation, followed by two 48 hour radium insertions or cesium insertions, totaling approximately 6000 mg/hours, is used. Complications of radiotherapy include bowel injury (e.g., sigmoiditis) and bladder complications (e.g., cystitis). There is also hematopoietic suppression because of marrow irradiation. Fistula formation occurs occasionally. Another method of treatment is radical surgery. Radical hysterectomy and pelvic lymphadenectomy with or without salpingo-oophorectomy is a reasonable alternative. If positive nodes are found on the final specimen, 5000 rads of pelvic irradiation may be added. The advantages of radical surgery include removal of cervix and uterus, which are sites of the disease. If tissue is radioresistant, recurrence is not possible in these removed tissues. In radical surgery, ovaries may be left, thereby eliminating the need for exogenous hormones. Patients with previous pelvic inflammatory disease do not tolerate radiotherapy well. With radical hysterectomy, radiation of other tissues in the pelvis is avoided. The disadvantages of radical surgery are several. This surgery must be reserved for those who can tolerate the procedure. All acute complications of surgery are possible. Fistula formation is noted more commonly than with radiation. The survival in either type of treatment is equal.

A special consideration for preplanned radiation and surgery is given to Stage IB barrel or large endophytic lesions. In this instance, 4000 rads of whole pelvic irradiation with a slightly reduced internal dosage of about 5500 mg/hours, followed by simple total extrafascial hysterectomy in 4 weeks, is the treatment of choice. This special case of combined therapy is necessary, because eradication of the disease by radiation alone is difficult. Radical radiation and radical surgery are never used in a planned combination.

Stage II. Stage IIA is a rare entity. If extension into the upper lateral fornices of the vagina is the only involvement, radical surgery, as in Stage IB, may be used. Anterior or posterior extension in the vagina would suggest radiation therapy such as in Stage IB. Patients with Stage IIB, in general, would receive 4000 to 5000 rads of whole pelvic irradiation, followed by two radium or cesium insertions for 48 hours, using tandem and ovoids. The internal dosage would equal 5000 mg/hours.

Stage III. Stage III cervical carcinoma is treated by radiation. The treatment may be individualized. The geometry of the lesion is important in designing the treatment plan. The treatment will consist of a greater emphasis on external portions of the radiation dosage. Six thousand rads may be given as the external dose, with the addition of 3000 to 4000 mg/hours as the internal application. Consideration may be given to parametrial boosts if there is need on one or both sides. The doses may be 500 to 1000 rads. Whole pelvic irradiation may occasionally be given to 7000 rads without intracavitary application.

Stage IV. In Stage IV the disease confined to the pelvis may be treated in a similar manner to Stage III. If the disease is widespread, radiation can be used only for palliation. Treatment may vary in this situation. Combinations of chemotherapy and irradiation may be used. Cisplatin has recently begun to be used in advanced squamous carcinoma of the cervix, with some moderate response. Methotrexate and bleomycin have also been used in the past with some success.

Survival

Survival in early disase is excellent. Stage I survival has been noted to be 80 to 90 per cent at 5 years. Stage IIA has a good survival rate in the 75 to 80 per cent range. Stage IIB survival is about 66 per cent at 5 years. Stage III ranges about 35 to 45 per cent 5 year survival. Stage IV is noted to be from 10 to 14 per cent, depending upon the study cited.

Recurrent Cervical Carcinoma

Although carcinoma of the cervix is curable if found early, treatment may not be successful in about half of the patients. Most failures, as expected, occur in patients in the more advanced stages. About 95 per cent of deaths resulting from treatment failure occur by 5 years. Exenterative surgery may be used for central pelvic failures. Anterior exenteration, removing the uterus if present, anterior vagina, and bladder, may be used for central recurrence involving the bladder. If the rectum is the site of recurrence, a posterior exenteration, removing uterus, vagina, and rectum, is performed. Recurrence involving both bladder and rectum is treated with total exenteration. Ultraradical surgery is usually reserved for recurrence after radiation. If radical hysterectomy was the first modality of therapy, radiation is used initially to treat a recurrence.

SPECIAL CONSIDERATIONS

Special consideration is usually made for carcinoma in pregnancy. If severe dysplasia or carcinoma in situ is discovered while a patient is pregnant, careful follow-up is the rule. However, one must not overlook invasion. With the aid of colposcopy, the patient is seen during each trimester of pregnancy. At 6 weeks after delivery, a re-evaluation is performed, at which time therapy is planned. Occasionally, if the limit of the lesion cannot be seen on colposcopic examination, a shallow cone biopsy will be performed after the first trimester.

If invasive disease is found late in pregnancy, delivery by cesarean section occurs as soon as fetal viability is determined. After this, treatment for the carcinoma is initiated. Early in pregnancy, either radical hysterectomy or radiation therapy is used without regard to fetal salvage.

CARCINOMA OF THE VULVA

method of
ERNEST W. FRANKLIN, III, M.D.
Atlanta, Georgia

Carcinoma of the vulva remains primarily a disease of the geriatric population, although it is increasingly diagnosed at an earlier stage. Approximately 95 per cent of the lesions will be epidermoid carcinoma, whereas the remaining 5 per cent represent a diverse group extending from melanoma and sarcoma to adenocarcinoma or transitional cell carcinoma of the Bartholin's glands or skin appendages, basal cell carcinoma, or Paget's disease. In addition to the invasive carcinoma of the vulva, an increasing number of patients are seeking medical attention because of chronic or acute inflammatory lesions or irritations of the vulva, which are of concern because of their premalignant potential.

Potentially Malignant Lesions

Included under the potentially malignant conditions are (1) granulomatous disease, (2) vulvar dystrophy, (3) intraepithelial neoplasia, and (4) nevi. Delay on the part of both patient and physician signficantly affects prognosis in carcinoma of the vulva. For this reason, any vulvar lesion that does not heal promptly with appropriate therapy or that is ulcerated, indurated, or nodular should be biopsied immediately. Selection of the site for biopsy, given a diffuse process, can be improved by the combined use of acetic acid and toluidine blue stain. This technique involves the following measures:

1. Cleanse the suspicious area with 1 to 3 per cent acetic acid. Colposcopy may be of some assistance at this point, although it is of less value on the vulva than in the vagina or cervix owing to the keratinization of the epithelium of the vulva.
2. Dry.
3. Paint with 1 per cent toluidine blue.
4. Dry.
5. Decolorize with 1 per cent acetic acid.

Toluidine blue is a nuclear stain. Those areas that remain blue have nuclear hyperactivity and are suspect. Biopsy of the vulva is an office procedure, easily performed under local anesthesia with or without suturing with absorbable material (preferably polyglycolic acid synthetics for less tissue reaction).

Precise histologic diagnosis is essential both to exclude malignancy and to prescribe appropriate treatment. Chronic granulomatous disease, especially granuloma inguinale, is not as frequent a precursor of vulvar malignancy as in past decades, when it was more prevalent. Among populations in which chronic granulomatous disease is present, however, vulvar malignancy is a frequent sequela. Any area that is ulcerated or nodular and occurs in the presence of such chronic irritation and scarring should be biopsied. Another lesion that predisposes to malignant degeneration, seemingly on the basis of longstanding chronic irritation, is the occasional malignancy occurring within a condyloma acuminatum. Although this is predominantly a benign papillomatous lesion, when the lesions are of exceptionally long duration and large in size they should be treated by excision to rule out the possibility of malignant degeneration. A distinct entity that has a similar appearance is the rare verrucous carcinoma, which may occur anywhere in the lower genital tract.

The vulvar dystrophies include lesions previously described as leukoplakia, kraurosis, and lichen sclerosus et atrophicus. There has been some confusion regarding terminology utilized for gross and histologic description. Recent recommendations regarding classification of these lesions defines them as epithelial dystrophies, either atrophic or hypertrophic or mixed, and with or without atypia. Such lesions have been thought to be premalignant, but more concise studies show that only a small percentage, approximately 5 per cent, undergo malignant degeneration, and these are primarily the hypertrophic lesions. After initial biopsy of the lesion to rule out malignancy and appropriately classify the entity, therapy will be directed toward relief of symptoms that are chronic and cannot be permanently relieved. These symptoms, including itching and dyspareunia with easy laceration of the skin, can be alleviated by the following measures:

1. Keep the area clean and dry.

2. For the atrophic, easily fissured lesion, apply a combination of 1 per cent hydrocortisone and 2 to 3 per cent testosterone proprionate in white petroleum jelly two to three times daily. When symptoms are controlled, application may be reduced to daily.

3. If only itching and irritation are present, use of 1 per cent hydrocortisone daily may be sufficient; observe every 4 months for ulcerations or nodularity.

4. Surgery plays only a limited role in relief of this condition. The introitus may be contracted due to the dystrophy. A perineorrhaphy may be of benefit, but this usually leads to further tissue breakdown and scarring as a hazard of the procedure. Vulvectomy or excision of the infected skin is usually of only limited benefit because the lesions will occur at the skin margins, particularly with the atrophic dystrophies, including lichen sclerosus et atrophicus.

The preinvasive lesions include Bowen's disease, intraepithelial carcinoma, and Paget's disease. Bowen's disease denotes a specific histologic variant of intraepithelial neoplasia whose true malignant potential is limited. It is rarely observed to progress into invasive carcinoma but seems to be becoming increasingly frequent, particularly among the younger population in the third and fourth decades. Any form of intraepithelial neoplasia may well be multifocal over the entire anogenital tract, including the vagina, vulva, anus, and intergluteal crease. This area represents a unique skin organ subject to increased risk of developing both epidermoid carcinomas and melanomas.

Planning of therapy following biopsy depends upon the extent of the disease, be it unifocal or multifocal. When possible, wide local incision of single or multiple lesions with careful examination at margins and primary closure is preferable. Complete simple vulvectomy for a limited unifocal lesions is not necessary. Some authors have advocated removal of the entire vulva as a "high-risk site" when a single or several discrete lesions are present. Such a procedure does not really remove the entire area at risk, however, as the vagina and anus are at equal risk. Conversely, when the entire vulva is involved by a diffuse multifocal process, including possible extension to the anus, removal of the full thickness of involved epithelium with a superficial vulvectomy while retaining underlying structures, including labial fat pad and clitoris, is appropriate. Both functional and cosmetic results following this procedure can be excellent, with decrease in vulvar irritation and improved coital function.

The use of topical 2 or 5 per cent 5-fluorouracil applied twice daily has been effective in some patients, although recurrence has been frequent. Erythematous reaction to this treatment causes significant morbidity with the treatment during its use. As the results are somewhat limited and the disease may recur, this program cannot be recommended as enthusiastically as previously.

Treatment of Paget's disease must involve a deeper resection. An invasive carcinoma lying below the epithelium has been reported in approximately 10 per cent of patients, and the disease may represent an intraepithelial spread of invasive adenocarcinoma. It also has a tendency to penetrate hair follicle shafts. After simple vulvectomy, bilateral groin dissection should be performed if invasive carcinoma is discovered. As with all intraepithelial neoplasia, the neoplastic cells may involve the epithelium far beyond the gross lesion. In any surgical removal of such lesions, frozen sections should be obtained from the margins to confirm adequacy of excision.

The perineum, which makes up 1 per cent of the body surface, is also a preferential site for the occurrence of melanoma; 5 to 8 per cent of melanomas occur there.

All nevi should perhaps be excised from this area if such an opportunity is available. Treatment of melanoma in this site follows the general guidelines laid down for treatment of melanomas elsewhere in the body regarding resection of the primary lesion and regional lymphatics. Prognosis seems related primarily to depth and pattern of invasion.

Invasive Carcinoma

The prognosis in invasive epidermoid carcinoma of the vulva is determined mainly by the character of the primary lesion, its grade of differentiation, and its location. These will be determinants in success or failure of removal of the primary lesion and in prevention of local recurrence, and they will also affect the probability of lymph node metastasis. Control of the primary lesion as well as regional lymphatic metastasis should be achievable in a high percentage of patients with epidermoid carcinoma of the vulva, the majority of which carcinomas are well differentiated with a less aggressive spread pattern. The more anaplastic lesions do behave in a more aggressive fashion, with a higher frequency of regional metastasis. With early superficial invasion of the stroma, particularly in a focal area of no more than 3 mm depth, the well-differentiated lesions may be managed by a wide local incision or vulvectomy alone. When the lesion is anaplastic or has demonstrable lymphatic involvement, however, it is necessary to undertake regional lymphadenectomy. The size and histology of the lesion will determine the probability of regional metastasis more than the extent of anatomic involvement. It is my opinion that lesions involving the clitoris are no more likely to metastasize directly to the pelvis than lesions in other locations of similar histology and size. Involvement of anatomy adjacent to the vulva will predispose the patient to an increased frequency of local recurrence if the surgeon does not excise adequate margins, which should be evaluated at the time of surgery by frozen section.

The majority of epidermoid carcinomas of the vulva should be eminently curable. The first challenge is adequate excision of the primary lesion. The majority of the patients can be salvaged with adequate surgery because the disease follows a rather predictable pattern of dissemination with spread to the regional lymphatics, which are amenable to en bloc resection. The first pathway of spread is to the inguinal and femoral nodes. The lesions in the anterior vulva will cross to the medial nodes within the groin area; lymphatics draining the posterior vulva will proceed along the labiocrural fold to the more lateral nodes within the groin. The subsequent pattern of spread is through the femoral canal via Cloquet's nodes, the lymph node(s) lying medial to the femoral vein and beneath the inguinal ligament but representing the lowest of the external iliac lymph node chain, and thence to the deep pelvic nodes. Epidermoid carcinoma of the vulva metastasizes directly to the pelvic nodes only rarely, if ever, but the same may not be true for sarcomas and melanomas. Carcinomas will usually proceed to the ipsilateral groin and rarely will involve the contralateral lymph nodes unless the ipsilateral nodes are involved, although a lesion involving the midline may, of course, involve either of both lymphatic chains.

The probability of lymph node metastasis will depend on the size and histologic grade of the primary lesion as well as the clinical status of the inguinal nodes. The frequency of clinically occult metastasis is significant and varies from one series to another, with an overall frequency of approximately 11 per cent. It is therefore not advisable to plan therapy simply on the basis of presence or absence of palpable metastases within the groin. The fundamental procedure for the patient with invasive epidermoid carcinoma of the vulva is en bloc radical vulvectomy and bilateral groin dissection. Cloquet's nodes should be removed and submitted independently for frozen section. If results are positive, a deep pelvic lymphadenectomy should be undertaken. It will be rare to find pelvic lymph node metastasis in the absence of a positive Cloquet node and also in

the absence of a clinically suspicious or positive inguinal node discernible at surgery. This operative procedure will cure the great majority — better than 90 per cent — of patients with N_0 N_1 node status (nonpalpable or unsuspicious nodes) so long as adequate local excision of the primary lesion is undertaken.

Conversely, problems arise with the patient who has enlarged nodes, with or without fixation, owing to the presence of metastases (N_2, N_3). As the peripheral sinuses of these lymphatics become obstructed with tumor, the malignancy enters surrounding collaterals and there is an increased risk of cutaneous recurrence. Following resection of N_0 N_1 nodes, such recurrence should be nil; with clinically suspicious and positive nodes, the recurrence rate may be as high as 40 per cent, however. This can be partially countered by wide excision of skin overlying the lymphatics with use of skin grafts to cover the groin defect. My preference is to evaluate whether metastases are present in these enlarged lymph nodes by needle biopsy. If tumor is confirmed, there is a significant risk of pelvic lymph node metastases and possibly of more distant spread of disease. Under this circumstance, an extraperitoneal exploration of the periaortic lymph nodes is undertaken, with occasional findings of such distant metastasis, thus making local treatment of disease of the vulva and groin alone futile. If no disease spread is found beyond the pelvis, preoperative radiation to the pelvis and groin is carried out, delivering 5000 rads to the midplane of the pelvis and to a depth of 2 cm below the skin within the groin bilaterally. This radiation therapy does increase problems of wound healing. After the groin dissection, if the incision does not close easily without tension, a myocutaneous flap utilizing either tensor fasciae latae or gracilis muscle is used to cover the groin defect. Surprisingly, in many of these patients the incision can still be closed primarily with successful healing.

Surgical Technique

The technique involves an en bloc dissection of inguinal lymphatics and vulva specimens with overlying skin. The width of the excision of the skin in the groin area is determined by the degree of suspicion regarding underlying disease, as noted previously. Points are defined 3 cm inferior and 3 cm medial to the anterior superior iliac spine bilaterally. A gentle crescentic incision is made passing just above the mons pubis. For anterior lesions, this incision will be more cephalad. The risk of metastasis to this area is not great with a posterior lesion, and in this case the incision is extended well down onto the mons, approaching the base of the labia in such fashion that subsequent mobilization of the flap will permit primary closure of the incision. The inferior line of excision will encompass the lymphatics of the groin, with excision of overlying skin, and will extend to the labiocrural fold, then posteriorly across the perineal body or to a point even more posterior if this does not allow sufficient margin about the invasive malignancy. Occasionally, of course, when extensive lesions are present, it will also be necessary to remove the rectum with a concurrent diverting colostomy.

Superior and inferior skin flaps are developed by undermining of the skin and subcutaneous tissue in the plane of the superficial fascia. From the beginning of the operation, one must pay strict attention to avoidance of trauma to the margins of the skin flaps to assure the best probability of healing. Thus, traction is placed on these only by the use of skin hooks, not by using digital pressure or other retractors. The undermining extends to approximately 7.5 cm above the inguinal ligament and beneath the skin of the thigh to the apex of the femoral triangle. Fatty and lymphatic tissue overlying the external oblique fascia is mobilized by extension of the incision to the fascia, allowing mobilization of the specimen to the inguinal ligaments. The lateral margins of the dissection are defined along the fascia lata, which is identified. Remaining intact are the lymphatics and fatty tissues at the upper outer angle of the groin dissection. It is in this area that the superficial circumflex iliac vessels will pass. A hemostat is used to dissect along the fascial plane, and the bundle is clamped, divided, and sutured. The medial clamp is utilized for traction, as the lymphatic and fatty specimen is reflected medially. This proceeds across the plane of the external oblique fascia. The fascia on the medial aspect of the sartorius muscle is incised from the inguinal ligament to the apex of the femoral triangle and placed on medial traction. Dissection proceeds medially, with reflection of the fatty specimen. Along the inferior aspect of the specimen medial to the apex of the femoral triangle will be found the saphenous vein, which is identified and clamped in such a fashion as to include surrounding lymphatics from the lower extremity. Inclusion of these lymphatics in the ligature is important in order to avoid lymphocyst formation by continued drainage from these channels.

With medical traction on the upper outer aspect of the groin specimen, sharp dissection of the specimen across the femoral nerve is carried out. The femoral artery is identified by palpation, and dissection is extended to the vessel. Depending on point of origin, the superficial circumflex iliac vessels may be preserved or sacrificed. The anterior aspect of the femoral artery is dissected free of surrounding lymphatics and fatty tissue, and the origin of the superficial external pudendal artery is identified and secured. This identifies the approximate location of the adjacent saphenous vein arising from the femoral vein, both of which are defined by sharp dissection. The saphenous vein is clamped, divided, and secured deep to the fossa ovalis, with reflection of the specimen further medially over the adductor muscle and preservation of the small artery and vein entering that muscle on its lateral aspect. The specimen is then boldly reflected off the fascia of the adductor muscle and across the mons

pubis, utilizing dissection on the fascia overlying the symphysis. Care must be taken to identify the lymphatic bundle as it enters the femoral canal. This is clamped and remains isolated during the course of reflection of the specimen across the anterior aspect of the vulva. After hemostasis is assured, the femoral canal is explored, with identification and removal of lymph nodes present, which are submitted as Cloquet's nodes.

During the course of frozen section evaluation of these lymphatics, the femoral canal is closed securely to avoid subsequent femoral hernia but in such fashion as not to impinge on the femoral vein. In order to protect the femoral vessels, which may become exposed if the groin incision does separate during the postoperative period, the sartorius muscle is transplanted to overlie them. This is accomplished by placing the lateral skin flaps on anterior traction. A finger is passed posterior to the belly of the sartorius muscle, and the fascia lata lateral to the sartorius muscle is incised superiorly to the anterior superior iliac spine. The muscle is dissected from this point and its tendon is sharply excised. The muscle is then dissected from its lateral and posterior attachments, taking care to preserve the blood supply, which enters on the deep aspect of the muscle somewhat laterally. This muscle is sutured to the inguinal ligament overlying the femoral vessels.

The vulvectomy is carried out by inserting a finger along the adductor muscle fascia deep to the labiocrural fascia and carrying out blunt dissection along this plane. This specimen is reflected posteriorly across the mons to the base of the clitoris, which can be the site of profuse bleeding. It is therefore clamped and secured in a closed fashion. In similar way, the origins of the bulbocavernosus muscle are identified, clamped, divided, and secured. The specimen is then reflected posteriorly, with only incidental bleeding occurring, which is controlled by the Bovie until the pudendal artery and its vaginal and vulvar branches are approached posteriorly. This vessel is carefully secured and the incision extended posteriorly over the perineal body. All vulvar tissues external to the urogenital diaphragm are removed. The exact extent of this dissection will vary, depending on the localization of the lesion, the incision usually being terminated just external to the hymenal ring. If the lesion is on the inner aspect of the vulva, with extension perhaps to the vagina, the vaginal incision is made on the contralateral aspect to improve exposure of the lesion prior to its incision in order that an adequate margin may be obtained. Similarly, a deeper dissection along the posterior vaginal wall and rectum may be necessary for removal of the entire lesion.

A decision regarding whether it is necessary to carry out pelvic lymphadenectomy will then be made based on the findings of the frozen section of Cloquet's node. Approximately 20 to 25 per cent of patients with pelvic lymph node metastasis can be cured, but it is necessary to select the patients who will be at risk for such metastasis, as defined by the presence of metastases to inguinal or Cloquet's nodes, or both. If pelvic lymphadenectomy is elected, it is begun by opening the external oblique fascia along the course of the round ligament in the inguinal canal. The round ligament is placed on traction in order to pull the peritoneum medially. The inferior epigastric artery and vein are identified at their origin, transected, and secured. The peritoneum is reflected medially, allowing access to the peritoneal space. Dissection is begun along the anterior face of the external oblique vessels and proceeds deep into the obturator fossa in continuity with the lymphatics entering the femoral canal, which were previously transected. The obturator nerve and vessels are identified and preserved as the specimen is reflected superiorly. The ureters are evident on the peritoneal reflection medially along with the hypogastric vessels. The lymphatics are usually removed along the external iliac vessels and in the obturatory fossa to the level of the iliac bifurcation, at which point the upper margin of the lymphatics is secured to avoid lymphocyst formation, and the specimen is removed. After hemostasis is assured, it is my preference to insert a sump drain into the extraperitoneal space through a stab incision higher in the lateral abdominal wall prior to closure of the fascia in order to decrease postoperative morbidity.

Closure of the incision can be quite a challenge. It will be of no benefit to close the incision in a traumatic fashion with tension on the suture lines; similarly, it is important to avoid simply closing it by suturing skin to skin with tension, thus causing the closure to be elevated above the underlying structures and creating "dead space." The skin over the anterior abdominal wall, thighs, and perineum and the vaginal mucosa are mobilized to a maximal degree. Some patients have a remarkable degree of mobility of the skin in this area. Closure is begun on the lateral aspect of the groin incisions, tacking the deeper aspect of the subcutaneous tissue to the underlying muscle. Only when the skin is thus brought into close apposition are skin sutures placed in such fasion as to avoid undue tension. Although the vagina may be drawn outside with some tension and sutured to the fascia external to the introitus, care must be taken to avoid undue tension on the urethra, as elongation of this structure may produce not only stress incontinence but also an unusual pattern of voiding, with spraying and deviation of the stream.

Sump suction catheters are placed beneath the groin flaps through skin incision superiorly. It is then appropriate to consider the use of skin flaps or split thickness grafts after the skin has been closed to the maximal degree possible. Z-plasties as well as mobilization of flaps from the posterior aspect of the thigh have been used successfully; the flaps are relocated from the lateral position to overlie the symphysis pubis anterior to the urethra, on frequent occasions resulting in primary healing. Pressure dressings are avoided, as these further traumatize suture lines. Immediately prior to the final placement of skin sutures, the edges are sharply debrided to remove any devitalized tissue at the margins. It is also well to inject fluorescein to check on the blood supply of these skin flaps prior to their closure.

Meticulous care of the vulva and groin incisions is carried out during the postoperative period. Emphasis is placed on cleansing of all suture lines every 8 hours with hydrogen peroxide. Use of a warm air blower (hair dryer) afterward decreases moisture and maceration of the incisions. Prior to surgery, the patient received prophylactic antibiotics (penicillin or cephalosporin) as well as heparin, both of which should be continued postoperatively. The suction drains to the groin and the catheter remain in place for a period of approximately 5 days. Prophylactic cultures are obtained from the groin suction catheters at 48 hours.

If necrosis develops in the skin flaps, an attempt is made to keep these dry and to avoid secondary infection in order that the underlying flaps may have a chance to adhere. Debridement may subsequently be carried out. Wet to dry dressings with 50 per cent peroxide are then utilized, as well as sharp debridement, to allow for establishment of granulation tissue and secondary healing of the groin. Rarely, skin grafts may also be utilized.

Utilizing these techniques, the majority of patients have had healing of their groin and vulvar incisions with an average hospitalization of 2 to 3 weeks. The patients are discharged with elastic stockings to be worn during waking hours for at least 3 months. Lymphangitis contributes to long-term lymphedema in the leg. It is primarily due to streptococcal infection. Prophylactic penicillin or erythromycin therapy is therefore continued for 1 year following surgery. Recurrent lymphangitis and/or leg edema are both infrequent with this regimen.

PREOPERATIVE AND POSTOPERATIVE CARE FOR ELECTIVE GYNECOLOGIC SURGERY

method of
ROBERT L. DEATON, M.D.
New Castle, Indiana

Successful surgery requires a qualified surgeon and a well informed patient. Gynecologic surgery is, the majority of the time, elective in nature. The surgeon must make every effort to anticipate and prevent the potential complications of surgery. Only by performing a thorough preoperative evaluation and by adequately counseling the patient can optimal care be provided.

Preoperative Evaluation

Each patient must be fully counseled as to the indications for the surgery, the proposed surgical procedure to be performed, and the potential risks of the proposed surgical procedure. The risks should be outlined in detail, with emphasis on the more frequent complications. Alternative procedures or therapy should be discussed, along with the results that can be expected from surgery. Length of hospitalization and expected convalescence should be detailed to the patient. The diagnosis of the condition requiring surgery and its prognosis should be explained in layman's terms. The patient should be given every opportunity to ask questions regarding the proposed surgery.

Adequate patient evaluation is required prior to surgery. A thorough history and physical examination is completed prior to hospital admission. Factors which might increase the patient's surgical risk, such as smoking, obesity, previous history of thromboembolism, or poor nutrition, should be noted and dealt with prior to surgery. A comprehensive gynecologic history, along with breast, pelvic, and rectal examination, is a mandatory prerequisite. Cervical cytology (Papanicolaou smear) should be performed within 3 months of surgery. Any abnormality should be investigated with colposcopy and cervical biopsy. In patients with abnormal menstrual bleeding, an endometrial biopsy or curettage is required to rule out carcinoma before a hysterectomy or exploratory laparotomy is performed. Patients undergoing surgical treatment for stress urinary incontinence should have additional work-up to rule out other forms of incontinence that may not benefit from surgery. An intravenous pyelogram, cystoscopy, urethroscopy, cystometrography, urinalysis, urine culture, and, when indicated, glucose tolerance test should be performed prior to surgery. Any patient undergoing surgery for a known or a suspected malignancy should be evaluated for metastatic disease. The possibility of pregnancy in a female patient in the reproductive age range must always be considered.

If possible, gynecologic surgery should be scheduled during the proliferative phase of the cycle, avoiding surgery during the menses. Hysterectomy is performed either within the first 48 hours or 6 weeks after a diagnostic procedure (cone biopsy or dilatation and currettage [D&C] of the uterus) in order to avoid the effects of inflammation or healing.

Preoperative Orders

"Routine" orders are to be avoided. All orders should include the following:
1. Diagnosis.
2. Doctor or service to which the patient is being admitted.
3. Proposed surgery.
4. Diet, including nothing by mouth for at least 8 hours before surgery.

5. Activity.
6. Vital signs each shift.
7. Abdominalperineal shave for major abdominal or vaginal surgery (no shave required for minor vaginal surgery, such as D&C).
8. Providone-iodine (Betadine) douche the night prior to major procedures.
9. Antibacterial shower the evening prior to major surgery (providone-iodine or hexachlorophene).
10. Cleansing enema (soapsuds or Fleet's).
11. Type and cross-match for 2 units of whole blood if indicated.
12. Medications: Pain and sleep medications as well as patient's usual medications. Prophylactic antibiotic treatment with cephalothin sodium (Keflin) for patients undergoing vaginal hysterectomy in the reproductive age groups. Use preoperatively and for 24 hours postoperatively — e.g., cephalothin sodium, 1 gram intravenously or intramuscularly on call to the operating room, followed by 1 gram intravenously every 6 hours for 24 hours. Mini-dose heparin in patients with high risk for thrombosis (sodium heparin, 5000 units subcutaneously every 12 hours until ambulatory). Preoperative medications as ordered by the anesthesiologist. Systemic bacterial endocarditis (SBE) prophylaxis if indicated by history.
13. Appropriate operative permit signed by the patient, indicating the proposed procedure, the operating surgeon, and indication that the patient was counseled.
14. Special orders such as bowel preparation and catheterization are individualized.

Operative Evaluation

Every patient after being given her anesthetic and prior to being prepared for surgery should have a thorough bimanual examination. Naturally, the bowel and bladder should be empty in order to obtain an adequate examination. The importance of this examination cannot be overemphasized. It allows for a change in the surgical approach to the patient if findings differ from those of the preoperative examination.

The surgeon should be in the room while the patient is being positioned on the operating room table. This will prevent injuries that would otherwise go unrecognized until the postoperative period (mainly nerve injuries).

Postoperative Care

Just as there are no "routine" preoperative orders, there can be no "routine" postoperative orders. There are, however, many things that must be considered in the postoperative period. Postoperative orders void all prior orders. Areas which must be considered postoperatively and noted on the orders are the following:

1. A statement of the operative procedure performed and the condition of the patient.

2. Diet. This depends on the type of the surgery and anesthesia. Normally, patients are usually kept on no oral intake (NPO) until bowel activity is present.

3. Intravenous fluids are ordered to maintain good fluid and electrolyte balance until the patient is tolerating oral feeding.

4. Vital signs. Vital signs should be recorded every 15 minutes until stable, then hourly for 2 hours, and then every 4 hours.

5. Intake and output record, if indicated.

6. Medications: medications for sleep, pain, sedation, and nausea are needed. Antibiotics are ordered if indicated or if used prophylactically. If low-dose heparin is used, it should be continued until the patient is ambulatory (5000 units subcutaneously every 12 hours). Blood transfusions should be given when indicated. Normally, packed cells are used in the postoperative period in order to prevent pulmonary edema. With large blood volume loses, whole blood rather than packed cells is preferred.

7. Laboratory tests. Primarily, hemoglobin-hematocrit level is monitored postoperatively. Other tests are obtained as indicated by the patient's condition.

8. Special instructions. Usually, the Foley catheter can be removed the day following surgery except in patients in whom urethropexy has been performed. Inspiratory respirometry and pulmonary toilet are used routinely on all major procedures. If drains or packs are used, special instructions should be included on the order sheet to make the staff aware of their proper care. If infection is present, appropriate infection control measures are needed.

In addition to the postoperative orders, all patients undergoing surgery should have a brief operative note written in the chart. This operative note should include the diagnosis, the procedure performed, type of anesthesia, surgeon and assistants, operative findings, blood loss, fluid replacement, presence of drains, complications, packs, and condition of the patient. This allows the staff taking care of the patient postoperatively to know the general nature of care that is going to be required. A formal dictated operative note is required for all surgeries.

General Remarks About Postoperative Care

1. In the immediate postoperative period, blood loss and fluid balance are best evaluated by changes in urinary output, pulse, and blood pressure. Hemoglobin-hematocrit determinations may not reflect acute blood loss during this period of time.

2. With extensive gynecologic surgery, central venous pressure monitoring may be needed for fluid management.

3. Early ambulation is preferred postoperatively. Preferably, ambulation should be resumed the evening of surgery.

4. Incentive respirometry should be used routinely on all major surgical cases, beginning the evening of surgery.

5. Diet should be withheld until spontaneous passage of flatus occurs. Ice chips and sips of water may be given if bowel sounds are present but no spontaneous flatus has yet occurred.

6. Drains should be left in place until output is negligible.

7. In patients at high risk for thrombosis, in addition to low-dose heparin, full-length support hose are indicated.

8. Urinalysis and culture should be obtained whenever a Foley catheter is discontinued.

9. A postoperative fever requires investigation for a source of infection. Mild elevations of temperature within the first 24 hours postoperatively are usually caused by atelectasis and respond to improved pulmonary toilet. Elevated temperatures beyond the first 24 hours postoperatively require a thorough search for the cause. The usual sequence for infection is pulmonary, urinary, and wound infection. Other but less common causes of fever are abscess formation, thrombophlebitis, sepsis, or drug reaction. Antibiotics should be used only to treat infection, not fever.

Meticulous wound care is important. Serosanguineous drainage from an abdominal wound subsequent to the first 24 postoperative hours is virtually pathognomonic of wound dehiscence. Most wound dehiscences do not manifest themselves clinically until the fifth postoperative day. If evisceration occurs, the patient should be returned to the operating room for a second operative closure.

Discharge Instructions

On release from the hospital, the patient should be fully counseled as to the diagnosis, pathologic findings, procedure performed, and complications. It is imperative that time be taken to explain fully the patient instructions regarding her activity postoperatively, her medications, and when she should return for her follow-up postoperative appointment. In addition to discussing the postoperative instructions, it is helpful to give the patient a written copy of the important postoperative instructions on discharge. This greatly reduces postoperative misunderstanding once the patient is home. The patient is advised, upon discharge, to contact the physician if any problems arise in the postoperative period prior to her scheduled appointment.

THROMBOPHLEBITIS IN OBSTETRICS AND GYNECOLOGY

method of
JAY D. COFFMAN, M.D.
Boston, Massachusetts

Thrombophlebitis is a frequent complication of gynecologic surgery, and occurs during pregnancy but is more common post partum. Usually thrombi form in the deep veins of the calves, thighs, or pelvis, but superficial veins may also be involved. Septic phlebitis may accompany pelvic organ infections. Deep vein phlebitis presents the immediate danger of a pulmonary embolus and the future possibility of disability from development of a postphlebitic limb. Deep venous thrombosis of the upper extremity (axillary or subclavian veins) also has a significant incidence of pulmonary emboli. The goal of intensive treatment is to prevent these complications that result from the thrombi embolizing to the lungs and/or the thrombus extending to destroy valves in the veins or block collateral veins. The importance of treating superficial phlebitis, in which emboli to the lungs rarely occur, is to prevent extension to the deep venous system.

Thrombophlebitis of the Deep Veins

1. Anticoagulation with aqueous heparin (sodium or calcium preparations) is the most important part of therapy and requires hospitalization for adequate control.

a. Continuous infusion of intravenous heparin is the method of choice. There is probably a decreased incidence of bleeding with the continuous infusion method compared to intermittent intravenous therapy. The aim is to prolong the activated partial thromboplastin time (APTT) to 2 to 2.5 times the normal control. The patient should be given an initial loading dose of 5000 units and then an infusion of 750 to 1000 units per hour. The APTT should be checked in approximately 4 hours. If the APTT is low, another bolus of heparin may be necessary. Adjustments in heparin should not be made more often than every 8 hours thereafter (five half-

lives). After the correct dose is determined, the APTT should be determined once daily to be sure of adequate anticoagulation and to avoid excessive prolongation of the APTT. Occasionally a large dose of heparin is needed during the first 2 or 3 days, when active thrombosis is occurring, and a decrease in dose later becomes necessary. If continuous infusion pumps are not available, intermittent intravenous heparin may be given, starting with 10,000 units for the average weight adult. With this method, the APTT should be prolonged to 2 to 2.5 times normal one half hour before the next dose. This requires a dose usually every 4 to 6 hours. Clotting times may also be used to follow heparin anticoagulation or to check on the APTT; the clotting time should be prolonged to 20 to 30 minutes. When the continuous infusion method is used and/or if small indwelling catheters are used, needles or catheters should be changed every 48 hours to prevent infection.

b. If veins cannot be used, heparin may be given subcutaneously (15,000 to 20,000 units of concentrated aqueous heparin every 12 hours). It must be injected with great care; stretching of the skin or rubbing the site of injection induces hematomas.

c. On approximately the fifth day of heparin treatment, warfarin therapy should be started at 10 mg per day (and increased if necessary) until the one stage prothrombin time is 1.5 to 2 times normal. Then a daily maintenance dose (usually 2.5 to 7.5 mg daily) is determined. Warfarin or other oral agents must be given at least 5 to 7 days before heparin is discontinued to depress blood factors important in clotting which are not measured by the prothrombin time. If a large loading dose is given, factor VII is depressed within 36 hours but the other factors are not yet depressed. The patient therefore is in danger of bleeding but is not protected against clotting. After stabilization of the prothrombin time, the test should be performed at least every 3 weeks. Anticoagulation for calf phlebitis is usually continued for 6 weeks and for iliofemoral phlebitis, 3 months. In patients resistant to warfarin or who develop rare sensitivity reactions (skin rashes, loss of hair), phenylindandione (phenindione) preparations may be used. During pregnancy, warfarin is not used. Warfarin may cause congenital defects during the first 3 months of pregnancy; also, it passes the placenta barrier and may be associated with hemorrhage in the fetus or in the placenta. Long-term anticoagulation after phlebitis during pregnancy can be treated with subcutaneous heparin every 12 hours. The dosage range is between 5000 and 15,000 units every 12 hours, but sometimes the dose must be increased around the twenty-eighth week. The patient can be taught to administer the heparin in the same manner that diabetics learn to take insulin.

d. Daily hematocrits, urinalysis for red cells, and stool guaiac tests should be performed for evidence of bleeding complications while the patient is on heparin in the hospital.

e. Intramuscular and subcutaneous injections of other medications should be avoided in anticoagulated patients, for hematomas often occur at the injection site. Aspirin and other anti-inflammatory agents or drugs that decrease platelet effectiveness are also contraindicated.

f. Since elderly females show a greater tendency than others to bleed during heparin therapy, the APTT must be more closely monitored and kept as close as possible to two times the control level.

g. If there is a history of a gastrointestinal ulcer, a bland diet and antacids should be administered throughout the anticoagulation period. For the same reason, drugs that irritate the gastric mucosa should not be used during anticoagulation.

h. Anticoagulants should be used cautiously in patients with liver disease, uremia, or thrombocytopenia. In hypertensive patients, the diastolic pressure should be lowered below 105 mm Hg before anticoagulants are given.

i. If anticoagulation is contraindicated because of active bleeding, recent prostatic, brain, or spinal cord surgery, or blood dyscrasias, phlebitis of the calf may be treated only with heat and elevation. However, since the incidence of fatal pulmonary emboli is much greater in iliofemoral disease than in calf phlebitis, inferior vena cava plication and ovarian vein ligation are indicated if anticoagulation cannot be used. If the patient is too ill for this procedure, an umbrella may be inserted in the inferior vena cava.

2. The involved extremity is elevated above heart level to promote edema absorption and increase venous flow velocity. The Trendelenburg position or elevation of the limb on pillows is best; jack-knifing of the body must be avoided. Elevation of the extremity is contraindicated if arterial insufficiency is also present.

3. Constant warm, wet packs or "Aquamatic K-pak"* (100 to 105 F [37.5 to 40.5 C]) is applied to the affected area to increase venous flow velocity. The skin beneath the warm pack should be protected by a suitable ointment (petrolatum or lanolin) against maceration. Even so, the skin of the limb usually peels following treat-

*Gorman-Rupp Industries, Bellville, Ohio.

ment. Local heat should not be applied to the limbs with arterial insufficiency.

4. Complete bed rest is ordered, but the use of a bedside commode is allowed for bowel movements. Range of motion exercise is encouraged to prevent Achilles tendinitis.

5. Bed rest is usually continued until deep tenderness has disappeared and swelling of the extremity has been stablized (average of 10 days). By this time, the thrombus is adherent to the vein wall. In iliofemoral disease, some swelling of the limb may persist for months.

6. The patient is then allowed to walk with elastic support (bandages or stockings) and instructed not to sit for more than 30 minutes without some exercise. If pain and swelling do not recur within 1 to 2 days, hospitalization can be ended. If the patient's arterial circulation is normal, heavy elastic stockings (not support hose) should be worn for a 3 month period or until swelling no longer occurs during ambulation. Panty girdles which impede the venous circulation should never be worn. Resumption of full activity is usually allowed 1 to 2 weeks after hospital discharge. During that time, the patient is instructed to elevate the affected limb above heart level for 30 minutes four times a day, and whenever the limb feels tired or heavy.

7. Oral contraceptives are contraindicated for patients who have had thrombophlebitis.

8. If the patient develops thrombophlebitis after warfarin is stopped or within the following year, long-term anticoagulation with warfarin should be considered.

9. If acute bleeding occurs during anticoagulation (gastrointestinal bleeding, retroperitoneal hemorrhage, gross hematuria), heparin may be neutralized by intravenous protamine sulfate given as 1 mg per 100 units of heparin considered still to be present. With continuous infusion heparin, half the calculated protamine dose, should be given slowly; the APTT can be checked within a short time. With warfarin, 5 mg of vitamin K_1 is given intravenously but will not normalize the prothrombin time for 6 to 24 hours; fresh whole blood, plasma, or fresh frozen plasma can be given for an immediate effect. For patients whose hemodynamic status may not tolerate volume expansion, clotting factor concentrates can be administered in doses of 500 to 1000 units, but there is a greater risk of serum hepatitis than with whole blood or plasma. Minor bleeding (microscopic hematuria, spontaneous ecchymoses, bleeding gums, nosebleeds) usually stops with reduction in the dose of the anticoagulant. In an occasional patient taking warfarin, spontaneous ecchymosis may appear over the body,

despite a prothrombin time in the therapeutic range. This is usually due to a depletion of factor IX, which is not measured by the prothrombin time, and also warrants a reduction of the anticoagulant dose.

10. If a pulmonary embolus occurs after adequate treatment with heparin for 48 hours, inferior vena cava interruption should be performed. Since a high incidence of thrombi is found in the more proximal veins, even when the phlebitis appears limited to the calf, interruption of the inferior vena cava is indicated. A pulmonary embolus occurring within 48 hours of the start of therapy is not considered an anticoagulation failure, for heparin has no effect on pre-existing thrombi.

11. The use of fibrinolytic agents, streptokinase or urokinase, given intravenously for an acute venous thrombosis for 2 to 3 days (followed by heparin therapy) is a recent advance in therapy. However, the danger of bleeding from these drugs is so great that they should be reserved for the unusual cases of iliofemoral phlebitis with ischemia of the foot (phlegmasia cerulea dolens). When there is ischemia of the foot with iliofemoral phlebitis, venous thrombectomy may be considered. Although thrombosis of the vein usually recurs following surgical removal of clots, the circulation of the limb improves. Anti-inflammatory drugs (phenylbutazone, indomethacin) or dextran is not used in the treatment of deep thrombophlebitis.

Prophylaxis of Deep Venous Thombosis

Mini-dose heparin, 5000 units subcutaneously every 12 hours, has been shown to reduce the incidence of postoperative venous thrombosis, especially in patients over 40 years of age undergoing major surgery. It should be used in all patients undergoing cesarean section because of the increased incidence of phlebitis with this surgery. Although excess bleeding during surgery has been reported in some patients on this dose, it is a safe and effective prophylactic measure if the APTT is checked 4 hours after a 5000 unit subcutaneous dose and is not prolonged. However, it must be started at least 2 hours before surgery, for it has been shown that most venous thromboses begin during the operation. Mini-dose heparin is not effective in patients with fractures or joint replacements. Anticoagulation with therapeutic doses of heparin or warfarin is also effective, but bleeding becomes a problem. Dextran has been shown to be effective in some studies. Antiplatelet agents have not been thoroughly investigated for this use. Boots that intermittently compress the feet and calves during and after surgery may also protect against venous thrombosis.

Superficial Thrombophlebitis

1. Phlebitis of the superficial veins is usually not treated with anticoagulation, because the incidence of pulmonary emboli is negligible.

2. If phlebitis of the greater saphenous vein in the thigh ascends to the junction with the superficial femoral vein, the tail of the clot may extend into the femoral vein, and pulmonary emboli may occur. Therefore, phlebitis in the upper half of the thigh is usually treated with anticoagulation and/or by ligation of the saphenous vein flush at the junction with the superficial femoral vein.

3. Moist heat is applied to the affected veins for 30 minutes four times a day, with the limb elevated above heart level.

4. The patient remains ambulatory, but elastic support is worn if the lower extremities are involved.

5. The phlebitis will usually heal (disappearance of tenderness, redness, and heat) in 5 to 21 days. In resistant cases, a course of phenylbutazone (200 mg every 6 hours for 3 days and then 100 mg every 6 hours for 4 days) may be given to attenuate the inflammation and relieve the symptoms; however, phenylbutazone treatment may conceal the signs of deep vein thrombus development with the danger of a pulmonary embolus. Phenylbutazone has not been shown to have any effect on the thrombus. If the superficial phlebitis continues to extend proximally in the leg despite conservative treatment, then anticoagulation should be instituted.

6. If recurrent episodes of superficial phlebitis occur (idiopathic, associated with malignancy or thromboangiitis obliterans), long-term anticoagulation is used. It may be unsuccessful in preventing future episodes, especially in patients with malignancies.

7. Phlebitis resulting from intravenous therapy usually disappears after removal of a needle or catheter; applications of local heat may be necessary. If the deep veins are involved, as evidenced by swelling of the limb and the development of collateral veins, anticoagulation should be instituted. If infection is present as indicated by fever, leukocytosis, and excess inflammation, by culture of the needle or catheter after removal, or by culture of fluid or pus from the local tissues, appropriate systemic antibiotics (according to sensitivity studies if possible) are administered. Occasionally, septic phlebitis must be treated by the removal of the involved segment of vein surgically. Septic pelvic phlebitis is

treated with heparin and antibiotics; ligation of the inferior vena cava is necessary if pulmonary emboli occur. All patients suspected of this disease should have a lung scan because of the danger of pulmonary abscesses.

8. Patients with thromboangiitis obliterans will often cease having episodes of superficial phlebitis if they stop smoking.

CONTRACEPTION

method of
GARY S. BERGER, M.D.,
Chapel Hill, North Carolina
and LOUIS G. KEITH, M.D.
Chicago, Illinois

Much has been written in recent years about the proper prescription of the medical means of contraception. Nonetheless, patients and physicians often have questions regarding problems which occasionally arise. The following is a list of frequently asked questions; their answers represent our approach to the therapy of these situations.

What To Do About Breakthrough Bleeding?

When a patient reports breakthrough bleeding while taking oral contraceptives, the first question which comes to mind is whether she is taking her pills every day as scheduled. When pill taking is intermittent, the likelihood of breakthrough bleeding is extremely high. This situation can be corrected easily be adhering to a rigid time schedule for administration of the contraceptive. It might be recommended that the woman use some technique such as keeping her pills next to her toothbrush so that each morning she takes the tablet at the same time. On the other hand, for women who are regular and consistent pill takers, the likelihood of breakthrough bleeding or spotting is highest among those who take the very low dose oral contraceptives, that is, pills containing less than 50 micrograms of estrogen. The mechanism for the breakthrough bleeding or spotting probably reflects a relatively hypoestrogenic state in which the integrity of the endometrium cannot be maintained throughout the cycle. In this situation, the physician and patient can make one of a number of choices. First of all, the patient can be assured that the breakthrough bleeding does not indicate any sign of uterine pathology or an increased likelihood of pregnan-

cy, and, therefore, no adjustment in the contraceptive dose need be made. If, however, the patient is uncomfortable with the notion of continued breakthrough bleeding or spotting, then the estrogen dose can be increased. Some physicians advise simply continuing with the same contraceptive preparation and adding a second exogenous estrogen such as conjugated estrogen (Premarin), 1.25 mg, for the first 21 days of one or two consecutive cycles.

Finally, it should be recognized that if these complaints occur during the first few cycles of pill taking, the probability of continued breakthrough bleeding or spotting in subsequent cycles is reduced by approximately 50 per cent during each of the first 3 months of pill taking.

What To Do About Pill Amenorrhea?

When a woman develops amenorrhea while taking oral contraceptives, the basic mechanism is the same as that when she develops breakthrough bleeding or spotting. First of all, the most important question to ask is: " Is she taking her pills regularly?" If not, pregnancy must be considered as the first possibility in the differential diagnosis. If she is a regular pill taker, and presents with the history of gradually decreasing amounts of withdrawal flow and eventual cessation of flow, this indicates a situation in which the endometrium is being inadequately stimulated by estrogen and, in relationship to the dose and potency of the estrogen, has excessive progestational effect. Therefore, a switch to an oral contraceptive with a higher dose of estrogen relative to the progestin component is indicated. Some studies have shown that certain oral contraceptive preparations are more likely than others to lead to predictable endometrial control, in that patients are more likely to experience withdrawal flow as scheduled in the absence of breakthrough bleeding or spotting.

Is There a Time Limit to Using Oral Contraceptives?

When the high dose combination birth control pills were in common use in the past, there was widespread concern among prescribing physicians that uninterrupted long-term oral contraceptive therapy might permanently suppress the normal function of the hypothalamic-pituitary-ovarian axis. Because of this, it was a common practice a decade ago for physicians to enforce a "rest period" among oral contraceptive takers after 1 or more years of continuous contraceptive use. This practice led in many instances to unwanted pregnancies.

With the use of current formulations, there is no good evidence that the length of contraceptive administration itself is associated with the likelihood of post-pill amenorrhea and/or anovulation. The most common reason for malfunction of the ovulatory mechanism after discontinuation of pills is the woman's own endogenous hormonal cycle, which existed *prior* to pill administration. While there are many types of side effects and certainly a variety of major complications associated with the pill, the risks of occurrence of these complications do not appear to increase with increased duration of use of the pill. An exception to this statement may be made in the case of the hepatic adenoma, in which dose and duration of oral contraceptive use may be associated with the likelihood of this rare condition. However, this is such a rare entity that it does not seem to make sense to restrict the duration of use of contraceptive pills for several million women in the hopes of avoiding one or two cases of hepatic adenoma.

An important concept regarding the maximal duration of pill taking is that of the "reproductive life plan" of the individual patient. Since the risk of serious vascular complications, such as myocardial infarction, is associated with increased age, the woman who has been taking oral contraceptive pills for many years and who does not plan any future pregnancies should discuss with her physician the best method for continued birth control until the time of menopause. In most cases, for the older woman in this situation, sterilization or the use of barrier contraceptives would be preferable to continued use of orals.

Who Are the Patients Most Likely To Have Problems with the Pill?

The major complications associated with pill use are those of the vascular system, i.e., thrombophlebitis, stroke, and myocardial infarction. Any woman with a pre-existing abnormality such as a past history of thrombophlebitis or coronary artery disease should avoid pill use. Other risk factors for myocardial infarction are older age, obesity, hypercholesterolemia, a history of smoking, and diabetes. While these factors are associated with increased risk of death from myocardial infarction at all ages, the risk increases rapidly after age 35.

Is Sterilization Reversible?

Any woman contemplating sterilization should view this as a permanent procedure. However, since recent publications reporting a high degree of success (up to 70 per cent) in reversing prior tubal sterilization by using microsurgical techniques, the concept of "reversible" sterilization has been discussed by many, particularly in the lay press. In selected instances, it is technically possible to re-establish tubal patency and for pregnancy to occur after a previous sterilization operation. However, no currently available method of sterilization is designed to be reversible, and there is no guarantee for any particular patient that such an operation can be successfully reversed at a later time.

After less destructive operations such as Pomeroy ligation or clip or ring sterilization, the likelihood of re-establishing tubal patency probably exceeds 90 per cent. Tubal patency, however, is not the end result desired by the patient, and normal tubal function cannot be guaranteed even when patency exists. In most studies, the pregnancy rates among women undergoing reversal operations are in the range of 50 per cent at best. This is in the hands of those most expert in microsurgical techniques; it cannot be assumed that these success rates would apply to any physician who attempts to reconstruct the fallopian tubes after sterilization. Furthermore, the cost to the public is high (roughly in the range of $5000 per case) for an attempt to re-establish fertility after sterilization, and the concept of reversible sterilization cannot be supported as a viable approach to contraceptive prescription at present.

What Is the "Post-Sterilization Syndrome"?

Over the past 20 years, a number of investigators have reported that after sterilization some women may experience increased pelvic pain and/or irregular uterine bleeding. These studies have been reviewed by Rioux (J. Reprod. Med. *19*:329, 1977). While such symptoms indeed may occur among some women after sterilization, the evidence has not been provided that the sterilization is associated with such problems. The difficulties in performing an adequate study to resolve this question are enormous. It is obvious to any physician who provides care to women that most women who develop menometrorrhagia or who have pelvic pain have not undergone previous sterilization. It is necessary to take into account all other causes of these symptoms before one can attribute the occurrence of symptoms to an operation which may have occurred weeks, months, or years prior to their onset. There is suggestive evidence that ovarian function may change to a degree after sterilization. Investigators found lower mean plasma progesterone levels in the midluteal phase of the menstrual cycle among 40 women after sterilization as compared to a similar number of women seen in an infertility clinic with only the diagnosis of male factor (Obstet. Gynecol. *54*:189, 1979). At present, the existence of a "post-sterilization syndrome" remains questionable.

The term "post-sterilization syndrome"

should not be used as a diagnostic term. Any woman who demonstrates pelvic pain or menometrorrhagia requires appropriate diagnosis and treatment regardless of whether she has previously undergone a sterilization. Further research is required in order to determine whether any true association, much less a causal relationship, exists between these symptoms and a sterilization operation.

What To Do About the Intrauterine Device (IUD) User Who Develops Amenorrhea?

The most common reason for amenorrhea among IUD users, as among nonusers, is pregnancy. Since, like all contraceptive methods, the IUD is not infallible (it carries a 2 to 4 per cent failure rate per year), any woman who misses a period with an IUD in situ must be immediately investigated for the possibility of pregnancy. If pregnancy is diagnosed, then the IUD should be removed as promptly as possible regardless of the patient's desire for continuation of the pregnancy. If she desires to terminate the pregnancy, this should be done at the time of IUD removal. Even if she wishes to continue the pregnancy, the risks of spontaneous abortion (septic or nonseptic) will be lower if the IUD is removed than if the IUD is allowed to remain in utero.

Since the IUD provides its maximal contraceptive effect at the endometrial site, there is a 2 to 5 per cent probability that a pregnancy may be extrauterine for the woman who becomes pregnant while using an IUD. This fact must always be kept in mind by the physician who sees an amenorrheic patient who has an IUD. It is important to remember that even though the ectopic pregnancy rate is high, this does not mean that IUDs *cause* ectopic pregnancy. It simply reflects the fact that IUDs do not prevent extrauterine pregnancy with the same high degree of success that they prevent intrauterine pregnancy.

Which Patients Are at Highest Risk of Infection Associated with IUD Use?

Many epidemiologic studies now have consistently demonstrated an increased risk of pelvic inflammatory disease associated with IUD use. A number of risk factors have been identified. These include most importantly a previous history of pelvic inflammatory disease (PID) and the number of sexual partners. While some studies show higher rates of PID among young nulliparous women, other studies have not confirmed these findings.

When advising a new IUD accepter about the risk of pelvic inflammatory disease, it should be stated that the IUD is a risk factor, but that exposure to sexually transmitted diseases is an even greater risk factor. The patient should be instructed to contact her physician immediately if she develops any symptoms of pelvic infection, which include abdominal pain, fever, or a foul-smelling vaginal discharge.

What Is the Safest IUD?

There is no currently available intrauterine device that is free of medical risks or side effects. Every IUD has a range of reported side effects and efficacy. The variation depends upon such factors as the number of persons in the study, the duration of follow-up, the method of data analysis, and the inherent skills of those inserting the IUD. Careful review of the literature reveals that problems are not associated with any one particular IUD but are common to all IUDs.

ALCOHOLISM

method of
CHARLES L. WHITFIELD, M.D.
Baltimore, Maryland

Alcoholism is a highly treatable illness, contrary to what we learned in medical school and residency training. Successful treatment depends on a positively motivated health professional who is armed with specific diagnostic and treatment skills, many of which are outlined below. Treatment success can be defined as the *achievement of abstinence from alcohol and other psychoactive drugs, or longer and longer periods of abstinence, and helping the patient and his family improve in life functioning.* Using this definition, when treatment is initiated and maintained for about 3 years, 70 per cent of alcoholic patients will recover successfully from alcoholism.

The spontaneous recovery rate from alcoholism is about 8 per cent. If a patient is motivated into accepting treatment, about 40 to 50 per cent will recover. If in addition a treatment plan is initiated and regular follow-up is maintained, about 70 per cent will recover. The appropriate terms for an alcoholic in recovery are *recovered* (public or polite) alcoholic or *recovering* (personal or clinical term) alcoholic; the terms "ex-," "reformed," "former," or "cured" are misnomers and are inappropriate.

General Treatment Principles

It is no surprise that many of us are pessimistic about the treatment outcome and prognosis for recovery in alcoholism, given the stereotype of the "skid row" alcoholic. Indeed, the "skid row" alcoholic with no family, social support, or motivation to stop drinking has a poor prognosis. However, he accounts for only about 3 per cent of the total population of alcoholics.

However, 97 per cent of alcoholics have some sort of support system *available,* although it must often be discovered and activated. Potentially they have a good prognosis. If *all* major supports are present, there is probably an 80 to 90 per cent success rate.

Avoid a "Psychoanalytic" Approach. It has repeatedly been shown that treating alcoholics as though their abnormal drinking behavior were secondary to underlying psychopathology is not only usually doomed to failure but often countertherapeutic. Thus, insight-oriented or in-depth psychotherapy early in the treatment of alcoholism is contraindicated. By contrast, general office supportive and directive counseling or psychotherapy, using the treatment methods outlined below, and focused on the alcoholism as a *primary* illness, is usually effective in helping the alcoholic patient reach a successful recovery.

Specific Treatment Methods

Treatment consists of (1) motivating the patient into treatment, (2) initiating a treatment plan, and (3) providing regular follow-up.

Motivating into Treatment. Breaking down *denial,* which is a cardinal feature of the disease, is the most difficult part of treatment. Doing so is an ongoing process. By using the following motivational techniques in a *persistent* and *patient* manner, breaking down denial can be accomplished, and surprisingly it can be enjoyable for the physician.

What at first appears to be simple "denial" is actually a complex of ten possible mechanisms. These are (1) conscious lying (one of the least common mechanisms), (2) classic denial, (3) a blackout (alcoholic amnestic response), (4) euphoric recall (the patient remembers only the good times when drinking), (5) the fact that no one points it out, (6) wishful thinking, (7) denial on the part of family and other close people, including helping professionals, (8) ignorance of what an alcoholic is (Bissell, 1980), (9) toxic effects on information processing and memory, and (10) a complex thinking quandary. This last mechanism consists of a genuine confusion by the patient. He knows that something is wrong in his life, but somehow cannot connect it with drinking alcohol (Wallace, 1977). I have never met an alcoholic who wanted to be one. Indeed, the person usually struggles painfully *not* to be alcoholic, all the while falling more and more prey to the illness. One alcoholic patient said, "The chains of alcoholism are so light that you cannot feel them, until they are so strong you cannot break them." Also, those people around and close to the alcoholic deny, cover up, and make excuses for the drinking behavior, thus perpetuating the vicious cycle of denial and alcoholic drinking. This is why it is so important for family members as well to be referred to the fellowship of Al-Anon, explained below.

There are three common techniques to break down denial in patients and in their family members if necessary. These are by (1) confronting, (2) empathizing, and (3) offering hope. *Confronting* is telling the person what you observe, including that you have diagnosed the disease alcoholism. This may be the most difficult of the three actions, but for the motivation to be effective it must be accomplished. The patient will usually deny the diagnosis, and may even get angry. However, with persistent and patient use of motivation and treatment techniques, the patient will eventually admit that he has a problem with alcohol. Empathizing and offering hope help allay the person's denial, anxiety, and anger.

Empathizing means the ability to experience with another person, to perceive accurately what the person is experiencing, and then to communicate that experience. Examples of empathic statements are: "I might guess that you don't want to be alcoholic," and: "It must be frustrating not to be able to drink normally."

Offering hope is crucial. The physician must deliver a clear message that there is a way out, and that there is relief from the misery and bewilderment of the patient's condition. The way out is through treatment, which consists of abstinence from alcohol and other sedative drugs, and the liberal and regular use of treatment aids, described below.

Motivation is an ongoing process. In follow-up, denial will recur, and it can be dealt with by using the same three techniques. It can be useful to refer to your original notes or to the patient's Michigan Alcoholism Screening Test results in the medical record to help break down the recurring denial.

Another effective motivational technique is to "fight the disease and support the patient" (V. Fox, 1978). Since they are not taught this in their training, most professionals fight both the disease and the patient, which tends to destroy the rapport and trust so needed for acceptance of treatment. Some examples of this technique are shown in Table 1. There are several other effective motivational techniques available (see below).

Initiating a Treatment Plan. The steps which have proved most effective in initiating alcoholics into treatment can be described as "eight minimal actions." These are as follows: (1) Tell the patient his *diagnosis:* alcoholism. (2) Tell him it is a *disease.* (3) Tell him it is *not his fault* for having it. (4) Tell him (a) it is *treatable,* (b) *with treatment recovery is likely,* and (c) you or someone else will tell him how to treat it. (5) Tell him it is his *responsibility* to accept treatment for his disease. (6) Offer him a specific *treatment* "*menu*" or treatment alternatives, and *initiate a treatment plan.* (7) Interview the *spouse* or closest family member. (8) Provide *regular follow-up.*

Whether the patient admits to having a drinking problem or not, it is most effective if the term *alcoholism* is used. The term "drinking problem" may be used early in the discussion, before the patient's feelings regarding alcoholism are known. Some patients will be relieved to have the subject dealt with openly. Most alcoholics have at

TABLE 1.　**Examples of Supporting the Patient and Fighting the Disease**

SUPPORTING THE PATIENT	FIGHTING THE DISEASE ALCOHOLISM
Denial	
I guess you don't want to be alcoholic	Tell diagnosis, a disease
(Patient says, "I can quit anytime" or "don't need it," etc.)	
I know you can, and	if you can't, there is a way out
Trust	
(Patient says, "Don't you trust me?")	
I trust you completely	I don't trust that disease alcoholism you've got
Drunk on telephone	
I want to talk to you	when you're not drinking

some level suspected their problem, but do not know exactly what it is. Many believe their problem to be hidden from others. However, even in the most denying and uncooperative patient, telling the diagnosis is useful, because it "plants a seed" that is likely to grow, given time and motivation.

Concerning whether the patient admits to being alcoholic, there is a difference between the terms admit and accept. The term *admit* implies a more intellectual process, i.e., weighing the facts regarding one's drinking experiences and coming to the conclusion that it is a problem. At first the alcoholic may admit that he is "an alcoholic." Eventually he may admit he is powerless over alcohol and that his life has become unmanageable, the first of AA's 12 suggested steps. The term *accept* implies the emotional realization that it is all right to be an alcoholic. To the alcoholic, acceptance of his illness is like saying good-bye to an old friend — alcohol. Thus it is not surprising that early recovery alcoholics go through a difficult process, like a grief reaction, of denial, anger, depression, bargaining, and finally acceptance. Part of acceptance is the discovery that being a recovering alcoholic has decided rewards and is a positive experience. While admission usually comes relatively early in the course of recovery, acceptance may not occur for from months to years.

Telling the patient that he has a disease and that it is not his fault for having it is a powerful motivator for patient cooperation. I and others have seen countless denying patients become receptive to treatment after hearing these words. The statements act to relieve guilt, a powerful and painful emotion in most alcoholics. If the patient tries to avoid responsibility for further drinking because he "has a disease," one should use step 5 and tell him it is his responsibility to seek treatment.

Telling the patient his disease is treatable and that with treatment recovery is likely offers hope to the depressed alcoholic, who tends to think that there is no way out of his frustration and misery. The therapist tells him, "There is a way out." It is often worthwhile to say, "You can get better, others have done so." Next, tell the patient specifically how to get better by explaining the treatment options or "menu."

These treatment options consist of Alcoholics Anonymous (AA), group therapy, individual supportive psychotherapy and follow-up, disulfiram (Antabuse), family treatment (Al-Anon and/or family therapy), and inpatient treatment.

It is helpful to take some time to explain each of the possible treatments. If the patient is in a crisis and no time is available during the first visit, I suggest scheduling a return appointment as soon as possible within a few days, or referring the person immediately to a competent alcoholism therapist.

AA AND GROUP THERAPY. Alcoholics and other chemically dependent people seem to recover best in group therapy settings. Groups effectively break down the denial process through a combination of confrontation and support. Every alcoholic should be strongly encouraged to attend Alcoholics Anonymous. Many physicians who are specialists in alcoholism consider it the single most important aspect of treatment. Formal alcoholism group therapy is also successful. I give my patients a "choice" of going to either group therapy or AA — or both — but not to neither one.

COUNSELING AND PSYCHOTHERAPY. Individual supportive psychotherapy, which all physicians can provide, is useful to (1) continue the patient's education about the disease of alcoholism and the recovery process; (2) monitor the patient's functioning in important life areas, such as family, job, and interpersonal relations; (3) provide support for anticipated stresses during recovery; (4) evaluate the patient's ego strength and psychopathology; and (5) assist the patient in change and growth.

Psychotherapy should be supportive, directive, or crisis oriented, especially during detoxification and the first weeks and months of treatment. In-depth, insight-oriented, or dynamic psychotherapy will usually add to the patient's stress during this early period of abstinence, when major life changes are occurring, and thus it is contraindicated. The physician can also use these supportive psychotherapy sessions to monitor the anticipated improvement in the medical consequences of alcoholism and thus provide objective feedback to the patient of the recovery process.

The method of referral and the selection of a group are crucial. The referral should be made with enthusiasm and clarity. Many patients will be reluctant to attend AA or a group. Therefore, the physician should be familiar enough with these treatments to be persuasive. Perhaps the best way to learn about them is for the physician to attend one or more AA meetings and an open group therapy meeting. To locate such a meeting, call the local AA office listed in the phone book. Also, call the local Council on Alcoholism to find an open group therapy meeting.

INTERVIEW WITH THE SPOUSE OR CLOSEST FAMILY MEMBER. An interview with the spouse or closest person is helpful for the following reasons: (1) to gather additional information to establish the diagnosis; (2) to ensure that the family agrees with the goal of abstinence; (3) to explore the drinking pattern of the spouse; (4) to discern any special problems occurring in any of the close family members, including the children; (5) to educate the spouse about the enabling process; (6) to refer the spouse to Al-Anon, and teenage children to Alateen, or some other available family resource; and (7) to schedule a follow-up visit or telephone call (Williams, 1980).

It is best to interview the spouse directly. However, in some cases, the interview can be conducted over the telephone. If this is impossible, educational reading material is available. It is important to provide a follow-up visit in a month or two in the office after the spouse has attended several Al-Anon meetings.

In most difficult cases, the spouse should be seen in the office early, preferably a few days after the physician sees the patient. One should also explore the drinking pattern of the spouse, since about 20 per cent are heavy drinkers or alcoholics themselves. If this is the case, they may require treatment for their own alcoholism before going to Al-Anon. This is one reason why it is important to interview the spouse in person if possible. Treating the family in these ways helps both the alcoholic and the family member.

DISULFIRAM (ANTABUSE). Consideration should be given for every alcoholic patient to take disulfiram (Antabuse). Experience with this drug now covers over 32 years and includes hundreds of thousands of patients. Athough physicians with the most experience in prescribing disulfiram consider it to be safe, many who have never prescribed it are fearful of using it. The dangers have probably been overemphasized. Very few deaths attributed to it have been recorded in medical literature. Most of these occurred early in the drug's history and usually at daily doses exceeding 1000 mg (approximately four times the present recommended daily dose of 250 mg). The dose range is 125 to 500 mg per day.

Disulfiram should be prescribed with the patient's full knowledge and consent. To assist the physician in this educational process, Ayerst Laboratories has published a helpful patient education booklet entitled "Now that you're on Antabuse." I have also compiled a separate patient education handout about it and about the disease alcoholism (Whitfield, C. L.: *The Patient with Alcoholism;* Chicago, Year Book, 1981).

There are several advantages for the patient's recovery by using disulfiram: (1) since the drug is taken daily, it is a daily reminder that the person cannot safely drink; (2) it provides evidence of compliance in an alcoholism treatment program; (3) it saves the alcoholic the energy of worrying about whether to drink; (4) it is compat-

ible with other forms of treatment; and (5) it can also provide family and employer with reassurance that the alcoholic cannot get drunk. With disulfiram use the patient must plan his drinking many days in advance. Persons have been known to experience alcohol-disulfiram reactions as long as 2 weeks after stopping the drug. Most alcoholics do not drink this way. The decision to drink is commonly a spur-of-the-moment, impulsive decision (Williams, 1978). Thus, disulfiram acts as a sort of "insurance policy," protecting the person against drinking on impulse. There is some evidence that patients without cirrhosis of the liver can stop taking disulfiram and safely drink by as few as 3 days later. Likewise, there is evidence that those with liver cirrhosis can safely drink 5 to 6 days later. However, a "safe period" is probably somewhere between 1 and 2 weeks or, to make it simple, 10 days. Many patients say that a benefit of disulfiram therapy is that it saves them previously lost energy from frequent, compulsive thoughts and ruminations as to whether or not they might drink. They simply make a daily decision to take disulfiram, and thereafter they cannot safely drink.

Monitoring whether a patient is taking disulfiram as prescribed is done mostly by patient self-report and by observing the patient and his recovery. With this method, about 20 per cent of patients who tell you they are taking it will not actually be doing so. However, many of these patients will not be drinking. Urine and breath tests to measure disulfiram metabolites have been developed, although they are not presently commercially available. A decision to stop the drug is best made jointly by the physician, other therapist, spouse or close person, the AA sponsor, and the patient. It should be based on the strength of the person's recovery. Important guidelines in this decision are as follows: (1) active AA participation, (2) coping with crises without recourse to drinking, (3) improved family relationships, (4) dissolution of denial, (5) social ease (diminution in social anxiety), (6) growth in self-esteem, and (7) in excess of 1 to 2 years of abstinence (Zuska and Pursch, 1980).

DETOXIFICATION. It has been shown that most alcoholics can be detoxified from alcohol by outpatient or social setting procedures. Probably 95 per cent can be detoxified in this way, leaving only about 5 per cent requiring hospitalization for detoxification. While most alcoholics can be detoxified at home, some will benefit from a community social setting detoxification center. A detailed discussion of alcohol withdrawal and detoxification is provided in the reference book cited above.

OUTPATIENT TREATMENT. I believe that

outpatient treatment is most appropriate for most alcoholics. It is more economical, it allows the patient to keep working and carrying on daily activities, and it promotes recovery in the more realistic environment of the patient's unique day-to-day life. However, if outpatient treatment is to be relied upon and successful, it must be *intensive, thorough, and monitored by consistent and regular follow-up.*

INPATIENT TREATMENT. Inpatient treatment does not appear to be associated with better treatment results than does outpatient treatment. Indications for hospitalization are the same as those for any general medical patient being evaluated for admission. Also, if the patient particularly wants to be admitted to the hospital, or if the patient has a severe alcohol-disulfiram reaction, hospitalization is indicated. During the long course of outpatient alcoholism treatment, perhaps 25 per cent of patients will require inpatient treatment.

I caution against using a general hospital for treatment of alcoholism per se unless the hospital unit to which the patient is admitted has demonstrated expertise in helping alcoholics recover. I also caution against admitting a patient to general psychiatric units, or, in the case of adolescent alcoholics, to a general adolescent treatment unit. On such units alcoholics tend to be given purely medical or psychiatric labels, and the alcoholism itself tends not to be addressed. The major reason for this deficiency appears to be the lack of training of most physicians and hospital staff. Fortunately, this deficiency is slowly changing, as now about one third of the United States' 120 medical schools are beginning to teach about this area of medicine. A few nursing and other schools are also starting to require learning in these areas as a requirement for graduation.

FORMAL TREATMENT PROGRAM. Inpatient treatment may also be delivered outside a hospital but in a formal, live-in treatment center, or for outpatients at a "day hospital." Caution should be used in selecting such a treatment facility or program. One can obtain useful information about such facilities by using any of the following: (1) word of mouth from a trusted colleague who has expertise in the field of alcoholism; (2) telephoning the chairman of the local medical society's committee on alcoholism; (3) telephoning the local Council on Alcoholism; (4) using similar criteria, listed below, for selecting a referring consultant; or (5) consulting the *Alcoholism Treatment Facilities Directory* (usually available from the local Council on Alcoholism).

During the 1970s, many alcoholism treatment units were established. Some of these were part of health care "chains," and their efficacy remains to be established. While some may have a record of successful alcoholism rehabilitation, others do not. It is up to the referring helping professional to investigate thoroughly any referral facility before sending a patient to it (see suggestions above and below).

The duration of inpatient treatment is variable, depending on the patient's needs. While 1 week may be adequate for some, 2 months may be needed for others. There is no evidence that prolonged inpatient treatment contributes to higher rates of success than a short inpatient stay. Criteria for selecting patients tending to require shorter inpatient stays are (1) first time in treatment, (2) short duration of relapse, and (3) a relative absence of complications. An "ideal" duration of inpatient treatment has been suggested as varying from 9 to 28 days.

REFERRAL. The helper may elect not to treat the alcoholic but to refer him elsewhere. This decision, arrived at after careful self-scrutiny, is commendable. It is better to refer than to become involved with alcoholics in a negative and antitherapeutic manner. If such a decision is made, responsibilities may be limited to recognizing the disease of alcoholism, referral to other sources of help, and avoiding placing problems in the path of the recovering patient by avoiding prescriptions of sedative medication or advising him to cut down his drinking (Williams, 1980).

For this important referral, one should select a physician or other caregiver who has demonstrated skills and expertise in helping alcoholics recover. One way to find such an expert is to call the local Council on Alcoholism (listed in the Yellow Pages of the phone book under Alcoholism) or to ask a trusted colleague who has had some *success in treating alcoholics.* In selecting a skilled consultant, look for the following characteristics: The competent and effective caregiver tends to (1) be abstinence oriented; (2) use AA and /or group therapy as one mainstay of treatment; (3) offer disulfiram to most patients; (4) avoid the use of psychoactive drugs in long-term treatment, especially the sedative-hypnotics; (5) refer the spouse to Al-Anon or family therapy; (6) provide regular follow-up; and (7) avoid insight-oriented psychotherapy, unless indicated later in the course of recovery. The helper who makes the referral should *follow the patient periodically and enforce an abstinence-oriented program, as well as full use of any agreed-upon treatment aid.*

The physician who assists his patients by providing long-term treatment gains the *satisfaction of seeing the patient recover.* Indeed, most physicians who have participated in the long-term treatment of an alcoholic find it to be a most rewarding experience. Indications for referring a patient to a psychiatrist are suicidal ideation and psychosis.

SEDATIVE DRUG PRESCRIBING. Although many alcoholics present to the physician with symptoms that will probably be helped by sedatives, such as anxiety, insomnia, and tremors, in actuality these drugs probably interfere with successful recovery. Sedative drugs have a role in acute detoxification, and major tranquilizers and lithium have usefulness in helping treat the schizophrenic and manic-depressive alcoholic. However, other psychoactive drugs are usually contraindicated, especially sedatives, hypnotics, and "minor tranquilizers." There are at least nine reasons for avoiding psychoactive drugs in treating alcoholics: (1) all the sedatives are cross-tolerant with alcohol, and thus have a "built-in" escalation factor; (2) combining sedatives with alcohol is often dangerously synergestic; (3) loss of control, a cardinal feature of alcoholism, occurs with prescribed sedative drugs; (4) blackouts, or amnestic reactions, also may occur with other sedatives and minor tranquilizers; (5) patients may alter the prescription you write to receive more drugs; (6) prescribing these drugs reinforces sedative ingestion as a coping mechanism; alcoholics already have difficulty in using another sedative, alcohol, in this way; (7) they prevent the patient's developing his own individual coping mechanisms; (8) they interfere with learning to relate to others in a healthy manner; and (9) using the drugs may alienate the patient from perhaps the best treatment he could receive, i.e., Alcoholics Anonymous. Bissell (1975) has said, "I do think we need to give our patients a substitute for alcohol, but I don't think that substitute can be another sedative. I think it has to be our concern, our time, our caring, and ourselves."

Follow-up. Next to dealing with denial and motivating the patient, follow-up is the most difficult part of treatment. One reason is that when an alcoholic recovers there may be an early "honeymoon period," during which the patient feels and looks so good that the physician is lulled into believing that regular follow-up is not necessary. However, because it takes about 3 years before solid recovery can be secure, regular follow-up is indicated.

During the first 6 weeks after stopping drinking, the patient is most likely to relapse. Therefore, at least weekly visits are indicated for this time, with a gradually decreasing frequency thereafter. During this early period many patients are fragile and need much support and some direction. Therefore, it is useful to spend 30 minutes with them at each of these early visits.

High risk times for potential relapse may include special days and occasions, such as vacations, holidays, business trips, birthdays, anniversaries, separation, divorce, death of a close person, and illness in the family. Other relapse danger times are when a patient stops taking disulfiram (Antabuse) or stops going to AA or group therapy meetings. Finally, symptoms or situations that may lead to a relapse, and thus that are to be avoided without using other drugs, are exhaustion, dishonesty, impatience, argumentativeness, righteousness, depression, self-pity, complacency, expecting or wanting too much, loosening disciplines, using psychoactive drugs, and feelings of omnipotence.

The "dry drunk" is also a danger time. A dry drunk is a flare-up of negative emotions and behavior reminiscent of that when the patient was drinking. It may be an anxiety or panic attack, or the patient may be depressed, be having a flare-up of held-in hostility, be feeling a wish to drink and not accepting the disease, be a schizophrenic hearing voices, or be having a plain bad day. Dry drunks may last from a few hours to several weeks or even months, and they are frequently part of the natural history of recovery. Treatment is by recognition, education, and alteration of the diet and other current life habits. Dry drunks are often associated with the patient's eating much "junk food." A nutritious diet should be prescribed. Caffeine intake, including coffee, tea, colas, and chocolate, should be markedly decreased or discontinued. Sweets and sugar should be avoided, and a substantial breakfast is often helpful. Moderation in the patient's work, recreational activities, and rest should be advised.

Although it should not be telegraphed to the patient, *relapse is part of the natural history of successful recovery,* and the physician should not become discouraged. Instead, he should *immediately recruit the patient back into treatment.* Relapse is a time for both the patient and the physician to learn about their mistakes.

Paradox in Alcoholism and Recovery

Many paradoxes exist about alcoholism and recovery. Recognizing and accepting them can make work with alcoholics easier and more pleasant. One paradox has to do with self-recognition of having a problem. The paradox is that while the alcoholic may have some degree of knowledge that he has a problem related to drinking, he does not know that he has a problem. A second paradox is that while the alcoholic cannot recover on his own but needs help from others to get better, the only way he can recover is by his own internal resources. A third paradox is that while alcoholics cannot drink normally or safely without losing control, they sometimes can. A fourth paradox is that the disease alcoholism, its treatment, and its follow-up are at the same time simple and complex. A paradoxical statement heard at AA meetings is that "Alcohol was my best friend and my worst enemy." Another is that you can only help an alcoholic when he wants help, while if you help early, treatment is more effective and can save a lot of misery. Still another paradox is that understanding or insight about one's problems is helpful, and it is worthless (e.g., "Utilize, don't analyze," from AA). Then there is the idea that during recovery it is "bad" to be an alcoholic, while it is also wonderful to be in the growing process of recovery. Finally, there is the issue of whether alcohol is a "good" or "bad" substance. The paradox is that it is neither and it is both. For some people under some circumstances alcohol use can bring about positive results, while for others, or under certain circumstances, using alcohol brings about negative results.

An ancient Chinese saying suggests that to get inside the temple of truth one must pass by two pillars or guardians of the entrance. These guardians are confusion and paradox. Recognizing and accepting that alcoholism, its recovery, and its treatment may be confusing and paradoxical for both the helper and the victim can make understanding and the helping process go more efficiently and enjoyably. These paradoxes are part of those that exist throughout anyone's life and throughout the universe.

NARCOTIC POISONING

method of
JOYCE H. LOWINSON, M.D.
Bronx, New York

The possibility of encountering a patient with a narcotic overdose should be anticipated by all physicians, especially those working in emergency rooms. However, with the spread of heroin availability to the suburbs and even rural areas, every physician should be well prepared to treat such a problem when the need arises. A narcotic overdose constitutes an acute emergency and calls for prompt evaluation and action to avert death, which can occur within a matter of minutes. A knowledge of how to handle this life-threatening situation will determine whether or not a patient will survive.

Most narcotic overdoses are accidental, and the single narcotic drug most frequently responsible is heroin. However, pharmaceutical drugs (especially hydromorphone [Dilaudid], meperidine [Demerol], and pentazocine [Talwin], among others) are also widely used by street addicts. An overdose may also be seen in a clinical setting and occasionally may be the result of a suicide attempt. In addition to the aforementioned drugs, methadone may be the cause of an overdose in a relative or friend of a patient on methadone maintenance. In very rare cases, *l*-alpha-acetylmethadol (LAMM or levomethadyl) may be the responsible agent.

It behooves all physicians to have a basic knowledge of how to diagnose and treat a narcotic overdose. Diagnosis must be swift, and there must be no delay in implementing treatment.

Although morphine is the prototypic drug, we shall in general be speaking of heroin, since this is the drug most frequently encountered in emergency room overdoses. The symptoms and treatment are fairly representative of those of other opiates and opioids, except that symptoms differ slightly for meperidine and propoxyphene and the course is considerably longer for methadone.

The typical victim has traditionally been described as young, male, black or Hispanic, and poor. However, this stereotype does not always hold true. With the increasing availability and purity of heroin, more white, more female, more middle class, and even more older persons are turning to heroin. Moreover, given the changing geographic distribution of these drugs, more overdoses will turn up in the emergency rooms of suburban hospitals as well as in the urban medical centers.

Diagnosis

A depressed respiratory rate, miosis, and a reduced level of consciousness or coma constitute a clinical triad which is the hallmark of an opiate overdose. The patient may also be cyanotic. Of paramount importance is a history of narcotic intake, but time is too short to postpone treatment until laboratory tests confirm the diagnosis.

The pulse rate, blood pressure, and temperature may be normal even in the presence of apnea. In a study of 149 patients at the Montefiore Hospital and Medical Center, 88 per cent of the patients had normal or low blood pressure, and 90 per cent had normal or low temperature; of the 10 per cent who had elevated temperature, all but four developed relatively severe medical complications.

Respiration was depressed or absent in almost all patients. A few had shallow, rapid breathing. Pulse rate and rhythm were regular in most cases, although six patients had irregular rhythms.

Miosis was present in 85 per cent. Dilated pupils are associated with use of meperidine and pentazocine, or with development of cerebral anoxia.

Shock or pulmonary edema — or a combination of both — may be present. With a history of ingestion of meperidine or propoxyphene, convulsions may also occur.

Most heroin addicts present with the stigmata of intravenous use or "mainlining" (i.e., old and fresh tracks) and fresh puncture marks. Since some addicts use the intranasal route (snorting), the nasal mucosa may show evidence of edema, inflammation, or ulceration; in extreme cases, the septum may be perforated.

Auscultation of the chest may reveal rhonchi, wheezing, or rales, alone or in combination. These findings indicate the possible presence of pulmonary edema or pneumonia.

Although the liver may be enlarged, the abdominal findings are generally unremarkable.

Laboratory Tests

Routine blood tests usually show a normal hematocrit (except in the presence of pulmonary edema, which may be associated with an elevated hematocrit). White cell counts are usually elevated, with a marked lymphocytosis. Liver function tests are frequently abnormal, reflecting the high incidence of hepatitis among heroin addicts. Sodium, potassium, blood urea nitrogen (BUN), and calcium are usually normal. Blood glucose levels are slightly elevated, although occasionally they may be markedly reduced to 50 mg per 100 ml or less. The bicarbonate level is low relative to the degree of acidosis. Arterial blood gases usually show mild hypoxia, hypercapnia, and acidosis. These abnormalities are increased in the presence of pulmonary edema. X-rays of the lungs may reveal infiltration which cannot be definitively diagnosed as edema or pneumonia. In such cases, a patient should be treated for both. Hypoxia may produce atrial fibrillation, which generally responds to proper oxygenation.

Treatment

As indicated above, a narcotic overdose is an acute emergency requiring rapid diagnosis and immediate implementation of treatment. There is no time to delay, as the course of events can progess rapidly and can be irreversible. While laboratory tests can be used to confirm the diagnosis, treatment cannot be delayed pending the outcome of these tests. The primary rule in treating narcotic overdose is to support vital functions and establish an adequate airway. If the patient is apneic, he should be intubated and attached to a respirator. An intravenous line should be started; a bolus of 50 ml of 50 per cent glucose should be given in the event that hypoglycemia is responsible for the coma. Gastric lavage should be attempted only after an endotracheal cuff has been inflated; this precaution will eliminate the possibility of aspiration.

The first task is to re-establish and maintain vital functions and support the patient. If breathing has stopped or has slowed to a rate at which ventilation is inadequate, an airway tube should be inserted and a respirator mask applied. If the patient is comatose, it is advisable to use an endotracheal tube with an inflatable cuff to avoid aspiration. Artificial respiration should be started immediately whenever respiration is severely depressed.

One of the most dramatic effects produced in medicine is the reversal of a narcotic overdose with the use of naloxone (Narcan), one of the few — if not the only — specific antidotes known.

Naloxone is a pure antagonist competing with and displacing heroin from the opiate receptor sites. The administration of intravenous naloxone in the treatment of coma and apnea can produce an almost immediate reversal of all narcotic effects with prompt stimulation of respiration. Prior to the development of naloxone, nalorphine (Nalline) and levallorphan (Lorfan) were used to treat narcotic overdose. Because naloxone has no agonist properties, it is safe to use when the overdose is due to a mixture of drugs, or when the possibility exists that a narcotic is not the responsible agent; in such situations naloxone cannot exacerbate the respiratory depression caused by the non-narcotic drug. Also, it will narrow the diagnostic possibilities. However, levallorphan has agonist as well as antagonist properties and tends to increase respiratory depression. If the diagnosis is in error (i.e, if the depression is due to the intake of a sedative-hypnotic or alcohol), levallorphan will intensify the respiratory depression. Because naloxone lacks these agonist properties, it can be used without concern for complications. Naloxone is the drug of choice, and whenever possible it should be used.

Morphologically, the two antagonists are based on the morphine molecule and are quite similar. Both have greater affinity for the opiate receptor sites and therefore displace heroin, leading to the reversal of respiratory depression as well as of other narcotic effects. Naloxone has the additional advantage of being twice as potent as levallorphan. Both agents act within 3 minutes; naloxone is said to act within 2 minutes when administered intravenously. The onset of action is only slightly less rapid when administered subcutaneously or intramuscularly.

Despite the presence of coma, a narcotic antagonist should be used only if the patient is apneic. However, a prepared syringe containing naloxone should be kept available near the patient's bed in the event that respiration should cease. Mofenson considers the semiconscious state to be protective, because it reduces oxygen consumption. In addition he points out that it is needless and cruel to precipitate severe withdrawal symptoms in a narcotic-dependent patient as long as his breathing is satisfactory.

The essential issue is to implement measures that will prove to be lifesaving. If withdrawal symptoms are produced in a narcotic-dependent patient, one might consider using clonidine hydrochloride, which has proved effective in attenuating withdrawal symptoms in methadone-maintained patients. Clonidine should be considered only after vital signs have been stabilized, and the patient should be carefully monitored for a drop in blood pressure. (This use of clonidine is not listed in the manufacturer's official directive.)

Naloxone (Narcan) is available in a solution of 0.4 mg per ml. A dose of 0.4 mg should be administered intravenously. A second dose of 0.4 mg can be administered within 3 minutes. If respiration fails to improve, it is unlikely that the cause of respiratory depression is a narcotic overdose, and other causes must be sought without delay. To reverse postoperative narcotic depression, lower doses of naloxone are usually effective.

Since naloxone is considerably shorter acting than heroin, it is necessary to watch the patient closely for the next 24 hours and to be ready to administer repeated doses in the event of a relapse. If the drug responsible is methadone, the patient must be watched for 48 to 72 hours. Because the recovery is so dramatic, both the patient and the physician may be deceived into believing that it is safe for the patient to be discharged from the hospital. However, it cannot be overstressed that because of the very real possibility of a relapse, it is essential that the patient remain in the hospital where he can continue to be observed and his vital signs monitored. In addition, abstinence syndromes resulting from discontinuance of sedative-hypnotics and/or alcohol must be considered. Toxicologic studies of urine or blood will indicate the presence of the former. If such a syndrome develops, treatment should begin immediately.

Narcotic Overdose in Children

When the possibility of a narcotic overdose exists in a child, there is need for even more careful attention. The course of events in children can be even more rapid than in adults.

According to Dole, if a child — aged 2 to 6 years — has ingested an adult's dose of methadone, he may become progressively comatose in a period of a half hour to 3 hours and, in the absence of treatment, may die of respiratory failure within this time. There should be no delay in initiating artificial respiration. If an airway tube is available, it should be inserted and a respiratory mask applied. Whenever possible, an anesthesiologist should be called to insert an endotracheal tube with an inflatable cuff to protect against aspiration. Only then should lavage be considered. If more than an hour has passed since ingestion of the drug, it is not likely that lavage can be beneficial, and it may interfere with adequate ventilation.

As with adults, naloxone is the antidote of choice and should be administered intravenously in a dose of 0.01 mg per kg. If the child is comatose but respirations are adequate, the narcotic antagonist should be withheld, although it should be prepared and ready at the bedside. If respiration improves, but not adequately, the same dose should be injected in 5 minutes and again in another 5 minutes. In the absence of a response, other causes of coma must be sought without delay. If subsequent doses of naloxone are given intramuscularly, the initial intravenous dose should be increased by 50 per cent.

Since methadone is much longer acting than naloxone, naloxone must be repeatedly administered for at least 24 hours. It is imperative that the child remain in the hospital where he can be observed for 72 hours and treated if necessary.

As with all emergencies, the patient should be kept close to the nurse's station for continuous observation, and a syringe should be prepared with the antidote near the bed in the event of a recurring need.

Naloxone has also been found to be of life-saving value following the accidental ingestion of diphenoxylate hydrochloride with atropine sulfate (Lomotil) by children. It is also the ideal agent to treat opioid overdose in the newborn, and the Food and Drug Administration (FDA) has approved its use for this purpose.

PSYCHONEUROSIS
method of
LOUIS A. CANCELLARO, Ph.D., M.D.
Johnson City, Tennessee

The psychoneuroses, unlike physical illnesses, are not well defined disease states, traceable usually to identifiable pathologic lesions in specific organs or organ systems. A more fitting description would be to consider them as aggregates of symptoms, grouping in clusters much like a syndrome, having boundaries which at times are not clearly delineated, resulting in a degree of overlapping. In choosing a particular diagnosis, the physician is guided by the predominant symptomatology, as manifested by the patient seeking help. Anxiety, being ubiquitous, is present in varying degrees in most all of the psychoneurotic syndromes, namely, anxiety, phobic, obsessive, and depressive neuroses. Since no specific neuropathologic lesions account for the syndrome, psychologic factors are proposed as an etiologic basis. We then take into consideration numerous constitutional and environmental factors that impact upon an individual, such as varied stresses found in one's environment, the emotional responses to these stresses, and the ego defenses that are mobilized to deal with the stresses. The process is a dynamic one. Vulnerability to a psychoneurosis is generally related to one's premorbid personality structure. We cannot dismiss the input from infancy to maturity. However, in treatment, focus can be placed on changes that are needed to be made for conflict resolution and symptom relief and not on total understanding of past experiences.

Anxiety is ever present in our lives, the symptom being widely shared by all persons. Nevertheless, it can be handled successfully and be used as an alerting mechanism for the individual. The predominant feeling associated with anxiety is apprehension, generally a concern about some unexpected future threat. This feeling may vary considerably, ranging from minimal apprehension on the one hand to panic at the other end of the continuum. Fear, in contrast to anxiety, is a response to real precipitating factors which can be readily identified and often may be associated with dramatic physiologic responses. Anxiety may serve as a signal alerting a person to an impending threat to his or her well-being — for example, the jitters one experiences before taking an examination. If failure is the apprehension and study was less than adequate, corrective action might be taken — more study.

There is no single approach to the treatment of the psychoneuroses. At one time, psychoanalysis was considered the preferred method of treatment. At times, the final outcome fell short of the desired expectation. Although insight was gained, the patient seemed unable to function other than maladaptively. Since this book is geared to the nonpsychiatric physician, I would like to address three approaches the physician might find helpful and to comment briefly on other modes of treatment that are useful, as well as when referral to a psychiatrist would be indicated.

The first approach I would like to discuss is that of supportive psychotherapy. Since patients presenting with anxiety in its variety of manifestations are usually seen first by the primary care physician, treatment can be accomplished in an office practice utilizing this modality. Treatment is effective only if there is established a good rapport and a positive attitude of listening. This entails providing an explanation of what is happening commensurate with the patient's level of understanding. When this occurs the patient can be enlisted to participate in the treatment process. Patients should be encouraged to verbalize their apprehensions, fears, and concerns, and be permitted to ask questions, regardless of how ridiculous these might appear. In so doing, this fosters a good doctor-patient relationship and often diminishes many of the unnecessary phone calls and unscheduled office visits the physician will received if the patient is left in a state of ambiguity. Clarification serves also to dispel many of the misconceptions patients have concerning illness, as well as providing an excellent opportunity to reveal other misbeliefs or distortions that otherwise might not be discovered and discussed. Since anxiety in itself is stress, it is swift to respond to the assurances of a supportive physician — one who shows empathy and communicates this by positive actions.

Sometimes patients have anxiety so intense that it renders them unable to profit by any insightful approach until the anxiety state is reduced. With this in mind, I would like to proceed with a discussion of a second modality of treatment, that of pharmacotherapy.

In electing pharmacotherapy, the physician must have an awareness and full understanding of the harmful stresses impacting on the patient and the degree to which they incapacitate daily functioning, if the choice of treatment is to be successful. The choice of an agent is most important. Often, physicians become somewhat timid in the prescribing of tranquilizing drugs because of the bad publicity given them in the lay press and because of misunderstanding as to how best to utilize these drugs. The drugs that have proved more efficacious in the treatment of the neuroses, given the conditions described above, are the benzodiazepines. These drugs produce less unwanted drowsiness, and are capable of reducing anxiety at nontoxic dosages. Drugs such as barbiturates and meprobamate should not be used. Besides oversedation, these drugs more readily lead to physiologic dependence, and varied drug interactions are common. Barbiturates in the geriatric group tend to have a paradoxical stimulating effect instead of sedation that might be desired at bedtime. Chlordiazepoxide (Librium), diazepam (Valium), and oxazepam (Serax) are examples of benzodiazepines commonly used. I will comment briefly on the use of these three compounds. It must be remembered that drug therapy in itself should not be expected to produce a cure. Drug treatment should be a time-limited, highly controlled modality, used only to return the patient to a level of functioning wherein he or she might then learn to cope with stressful situations in some form of psychotherapy. If anxiety is eliminated to the point at which the patient becomes complacent and dependent on the medication, very little productive change would occur. A major criticism of pharmacotherapy is that it may be construed to be a lifelong sentence, with the patient trading the anxiety state for one of a drug state. When benzodiazepines are chosen, the physician's awareness of class differences enables him to individualize his treatment in an effective manner. A thorough knowledge of drug half-life and active metabolites permits the physician to have total control over the medication and tailors the therapy to fit the patient's needs.

Drugs with a longer half-life require a longer time to reach a steady blood level and, when reached, have a long period of drug accumulation. This provides the physician with an indication of how frequently a drug ought to be administered. These drugs can be administered once a day following attainment of a steady state. This is in contrast to drugs with a shorter half-life, which achieve a prompt steady state, have shorter periods of accumulation, and require administration at much more frequent intervals. Another characteristic of significance for effective therapy is the awareness of pharmacoactive metabolites. This information can be utilized in reducing the amount of drug prescribed. Chlordiazepoxide and diazepam are examples of drugs with long half-lives, the former being from 6 to 30 hours and the latter, 20 to 50 hours. They possess active metabolites, and frequent administration of the drugs produces increased cumulative effects resulting from both the drug and its active metabolites. To illustrate diazepam's long half-life, an active metabolite has a half-life in excess of 45 hours. Examples of drugs with shorter half-lives are lorazepam (Ativan) and oxazepam, half-life being approximately 10 to 15 hours in the former and 7 hours in the latter. Both these drugs do not have active metabolites. Thus, the physician is able to prescribe lorazepam at least three times daily and oxazepam a maximum of four times daily. Patients in the geriatric age range, as well as those with severe hepatic disease, metabolize these drugs more slowly; therefore, in such cases less drug is required. I suggest starting with the smallest possible dosage — for example, diazepam, 2 mg three times daily until a steady state is achieved, approximately 5 to 10 days of therapy, graduating to a single daily dosage, being guided by objective therapeutic response. It is noteworthy that there have been no deaths reported with the use of benzodiazepines in isolation. When deaths are reported, these drugs are found to have been used in combination with a variety of others, particularly the tricyclic antidepressants.

Despite the fact the benzodiazepines are superior to the barbiturates and meprobamate, significant therapeutic risks are evident. They potentiate the action of other central nervous system depressants, such as ethanol or barbiturates; they can cause physiologic dependence at significant high doses over long periods of time, resulting in withdrawal following abrupt discontinuation; and their sedation can impair skills that require manual dexterity and concentration. The risk to the elderly has already been pointed out. It is prudent to see patients on benzodiazepine therapy initially 1 week following the start of medication and subsequently at 2 week intervals. The patient should be advised from the onset that drug therapy is time limited. Four to 6 weeks is generally sufficient for the majority of patients treated in the nonpsychiatric physician's office. It should be pointed out that prolonged use of diazepam over a period of several months may lead to the development of depressive symptoms; therefore, an in-depth drug-taking history is essential for every patient seen initially. As the patient begins to feel better, tapering of the medication can be accomplished with relative ease, provided that the patient was prepared for this eventuality. When poor or no response is encountered, increasing the medication does not prove effective, and referral to a psychiatrist is advisable.

The aim of medication is not to obliterate all anxiety but to enable the patient to function more effectively in his environment. Medication should be instituted only after a careful diagnostic evaluation of the patient, in which it is determined whether the symptom complex seen is a primary syndrome or secondary to another disorder. If indeed the symptom complex is secondary to a disorder, the underlying disorder should be treated, not the presenting symptoms; for example, the anxiety associated with schizophrenia is not relieved by the benzodiazepines.

Major phenothiazines or other psychotropic drugs such as butyrophenones or thioxanthene derivatives should not be routinely utilized in the treatment of the psychoneuroses. In situations in which the state of anxiety is of such intensity that it is not alleviated by the benzodiazepine chosen, the utilization of small doses of a phenothiazine could be considered. In this situation, I find helpful trifluoperazine (Stelazine), 2 mg two to three times daily. A major consideration for not using these drugs is the side effects of the extrapyramidal type that might be encountered with high doses and the possibility of the occurrence of tardive dyskinesia. In the treatment of phobic neurosis associated with spontaneous panic attacks and anxiety neuroses with panic attacks, small doses of antidepressants (particularly imipramine) have proved effective in alleviating the panic state.

The third modality to be considered is that of group psychotherapy. The primary care physician might well wish to consider a twice monthly or monthly group composed of long-term patients wherein the opportunity is provided for them to see each other's problems and see that they are not alone or unique. A significant degree of anxiety can be diminished if one is exposed to a variety of coping mechanisms, the number of which is determined by the people in the group. This approach provides an unusual opportunity for reinforcement of positive aspects of the patient's personality, and has a direct effect upon the physician in that his frustration tolerance does not become overwhelming. In the group setting, the physician can address the medication needs of his patients, and the need for additional individual appointments can be reduced or eliminated. Another utilization of group psychotherapy is along the lines of insight direction. This is more effectively conducted by those skilled in group dynamics. The need for these skills cannot be overemphasized. It can be quite dangerous for patients to be stripped of their defenses without replacement. These defenses serve to protect the individual from overwhelming anxiety and possible decompensation. Referral can be made by the primary care physician. Often the physician, being unfamiliar with group psychotherapy for whatever reason, might not support the patient's interest in group psychotherapy as a modality of treatment. The concern here is with what group psychotherapy can do when everything appears to have been tried.

Other approaches that have demonstrated usefulness require specialized skills and are generally not provided by the primary care physician.

Psychoanalytically oriented psychotherapy is aimed at assisting the patient to develop insight by directing attention to an understanding of the underlying conflict thought to give rise to the problem. This is particularly effective when the personality structure is reasonably intact.

In addition to psychoanalysis, varied modifications are employed today which utilize basic psychodynamic principles, placing the emphasis on the here and now, or — stated another way — on how the neurotic symptoms affect the individual in his or her daily routine. The patient in this process is encouraged and aided in learning new methods of adjusting to stressful life structures.

Behavioral therapies have been effectively applied in the treatment of phobias and a variety of anxiety states, compulsions, and obsessions. Most of the techniques utilize a graduated exposure to the phobic object. This involves, for the most part, experiencing sequences in imagination followed by real life experience.

Systematic desensitization after the method of Wolpe is predictably effective and generally used. Simply put, the technique involves a graduated exposure to the phobic stimulus along a hierarchy constructed after the patient has learned to experience muscle relaxation. Most behavioral therapies do not attempt to uncover dynamic mechanisms. Focus is on what can be done about the problem, not on how it came to be.

Biofeedback, still somewhat in its infancy, has demonstrated effectiveness in reducing chronic muscle tension. It uses technology to assist the patient in self-education regarding bodily function. It is believed that by altering physiologic behavior a decrease in anxiety will result. The reverse is also considered to be true.

A variety of relaxation techniques have proved beneficial in some patients. According to Jacobsen's method, patients are trained to relax their muscles in a progressive fashion, thereby diminishing anxiety.

Transcendental meditation enables a person to have a positive mental experience. The act of meditation 20 minutes twice a day is in itself an anxiety-reducing response.

These approaches are not incompatible with such standard modalities as group, individual, and supportive psychotherapy and pharmacotherapy. These techniques serve to enhance self-esteem, for they tend to emphasize and reinforce the patient's assets and positive attributes.

The primary physician must be mindful that these patients who prove refractory to treatment methods provided, including pharmacotherapy, who present with complex symptomatology that challenges the treating physician beyond reason, and who are in need of more specialized treatment intervention should be referred to the psychiatrist. In some instances, appropriate consultation may be utilized in lieu of direct referral. When referral is made, preparation of the patient for this is essential. Informed patients, who understand the reasons why a psychiatrist is to be seen, are relieved of a tremendous amount of unnecessary concern and are better able to channel their energies constructively.

DELIRIUM

method of
ROBERT O. PASNAU, M.D.
Los Angeles, California

The most commonly occurring psychosis in medical practice is delirium. In fact, one of every five psychiatric consultations in the general hospital is requested for the evaluation and management of a patient with delirium. Yet, many physicians claim that they rarely see psychiatric patients, and many consultations requested for patients who are suffering from delirium include the request to "rule out schizophrenia." It must be kept in mind that there are many mildly to moderately delirious patients who are treated successfully without the involvement of a psychiatric consultant.

Often, the request for consultation is for help with the management of disturbed behavior. Many delirious patients are noisy and troublesome and occasionally become assaultive and/or suicidal. However, there is evidence that there are at least an equal number of delirious patients who lie in bed quietly and, although perplexed, make polite and normal responses to superficial social remarks. Thus they may not be recognized as delirious and may even be considered "good patients."

It appears that the number of delirious patients is increasing. It seems that our ability to produce delirium is increasing far more rapidly than our ability to diagnose or treat it. With an increase in the potency of the drugs that are frequently toxic to cerebral tissue, with more prolonged surgical procedures, and with an aging population, we can expect delirium to increase in severity as well as frequency.

The causes of delirium usually come from outside the central nervous system. They include metabolic disorders such as hypoxia, hypercarbia, hypoglycemia, ionic imbalances, renal or hepatic disease, or thiamine deficiency; systemic infections; alcohol or drug intoxication and/or withdrawal; and postoperative states. Delirium may also occur following seizures, on regaining consciousness after head injury, and in cases of encephalopathy caused by hypertension. Certain parietal lobe epilepsies may present as cases of delirium.

Several categories of patients seem to be at risk for the development of delirium. Although it can occur at any age, it is especially frequent in childhood and after the age of 60. The group at greatest risk is those who have already had some degree of brain damage. This includes aging people with arteriosclerotic or senile brain changes. One has only to give such a patient a low dose of a barbiturate as a sleeping medication to produce an extremely convincing delirium. Also at risk are patients who come to the hospital frightened and lonely. Often they have no supportive relationships with the staff or the physician, and they may be cut off from their own families. Others at risk are those suffering from sensory deprivation. Ophthalmologists are particularly aware of the effect of "black patch" on the production of delirium. Experience with patients in intensive care units indicates that delirium may develop more frequently in a "sensory-deprived" unit than in one with much staff contact, many windows, and a high degree of personal interaction. The patient who has lost a great deal of sleep is also at increased risk.

The new classification of organic mental disorders in the Diagnostic and Statistical Manual of Mental Disorders (3rd ed.), DSM-III, lists delirium as one of seven organic brain syndromes. It describes the acute failure of integrated cerebral functioning resulting from a wide range of possible factors, which is manifested at the behavioral level by the syndrome of delirium. Five diagnostic criteria are listed for this disorder:

1. Clouding of consciousness. This term implies a demonstrable disorder of "grasp," i.e., an inability to comprehend a relationship among the elements of one's environment and relate them meaningfully to one's self and one's past experience and knowledge. This clouding also is manifested by a reduced capacity to shift, focus, and sustain attention to environmental stimuli.

2. At least two of the following behavioral disturbances: (a) perceptual disturbances, including illusions, hallucinations, or misinterpretations; (b) incoherent speech; (c) disturbance of the sleep cycle with insomnia and/or daytime drowsiness; or (d) change in psychomotor activity, either increased or decreased.

3. Memory impairment and disorientation.

4. Fluctuating course of clinical features over a short period of time, usually hours to days. Included in this are "lucid intervals" and "sundowner" phenomena.

5. Evidence of a specific organic factor or factors judged to be etiologically related to the disturbance. This evidence may be obtained from the history, from physical examination, or from laboratory tests.

The duration of an episode of delirium is usually brief. It is rare for it to persist for more than 1 month, and if the underlying disorder is promptly corrected, recovery may be complete. On the other hand, if the underlying disorder persists, delirium gradually shifts to one of the other organic brain syndromes, occasionally to dementia, sometimes to coma and death. With a definite history of preexisting dementia, it may be necessary to decide whether a patient with delirium also has dementia. When there is any question, it is wise to assume that the patient has a delirium. This should lead to a more active therapeutic approach. The wise clinician will assume that the condition is reversible and, if at all possible, will attempt to correct the organic brain syndrome.

Treatment

1. Protect the patient. This is the first and most necessary step. Occasionally, delirious patients are suicidal, but even if not, they may get into serious trouble. They may become fearful, mistake a window for a door, and step through it.

We have found that "sitters," usually staff who are comfortable with the patient, will take responsibility for his care and provide the best protection. In the absence of continued observation, soft restraints are sometimes needed.

2. Provide continuous good nursing care. We have found that one person spending a significant amount of time with the patient may quiet his fears, help keep him oriented, and attend to his physical and psychologic needs. It is also important to reassure the patient, informing him of the situation and that the way he perceives things may be altered by drugs, toxins, and diseases. The patient should also be told that his state of consciousness will improve, that it is not a serious or permanent situation, and that it can be treated. The patient should have an equal opportunity to communicate his fears and concerns to the staff member. Family visitation and regular medical visits are extremely important. Frequent statements of a general orienting nature by whoever is present are helpful. The patient should be told the hospital, the ward number, the date, and the time. Repeated, careful explanations of all diagnostic and surgical procedures may help. This is particularly important at sundown when especially elderly patients tend to become disoriented — the so-called "sundowner syndrome." During the "lucid intervals," it should be possible to reassure and inform the patient.

3. Take care of the general medical condition. During the period of delirium it is extremely important to pay attention to the patient's general medical condition. Nutritional needs, vitamin supplements, adequate hydration, and electrolyte balance are all important. It is possible to correct one underlying cause, only to have another factor complicate or continue the delirium after the original etiologic agent has been identified and eliminated.

4. Identify the causative factor or factors and treat them. Unfortunately, causative factors are often not found. One of the most frequent offenders is the patient's drug regimen. Almost any drug in a susceptible person may precipitate a delirium.

5. Sedate the restless and fearful patient. Sedation should be used in as small doses as possible, but in most patients some sedation will be necessary. Because most patients are worse at night, sedation should be saved for that period if possible. Haloperidol (Haldol), with a few notable exceptions, has emerged as the drug of choice in delirium. It is remarkably effective in calming restless, agitated, fearful, and hallucinating patients. It is apparently safe in the presence of a wide range of physical illnesses and is not likely to increase delirium. (We have recently seen a case in which 60 mg was used in an elderly patient, which potentiated an anticholinergic delirium. However, if the principle of small dosages in elderly patients is adhered to, it is unlikely that such side effects will occur using this drug.) With the exception of the anticholinergic delirium, for which physostigmine is the drug choice, it should also be noted that for alcohol and drug withdrawal delirium, as well as hepatic encephalopathy, the benzodiazepines are the most preferred agents.

Haloperidol may be used in doses of 2 to 5 mg orally or parenterally. Parenteral physostigmine may be used in doses of 1 to 4 mg given intramuscularly every 30 minutes until the patient's condition has stabilized. Increased acetylcholine side effects must be carefully monitored. These include bradycardia, hypertension, and gastrointestinal disturbances. For delirium associated with alcoholism, chlordiazepoxide (Librium) may be used, up to 100 mg intravenously every 4 hours for 24 to 40 hours.

6. Prescribe an adequate convalescent period. It is important to remember that the patient with delirium needs adequate convalescent time. Relapse is common when treatment is discontinued and responsibility returned to the patient too soon.

Delirium is an extremely common illness that every physician must recognize and treat. Awareness of its frequency and skill in its treatment are necessary tools in the armamentarium of the practitioner of medicine in every field.

AFFECTIVE DISORDERS
method of
DAVID L. DUNNER, M.D.
Seattle, Washington

Affective disorders is a term denoting disorders of mood with particular reference to depression. Although the incidence of the depressive disorders is unknown, several estimates suggest that depression is perhaps the most frequent psychiatric condition and that 15 to 20 per cent of the population will experience a significant depression at some time. Most depressions are extremely responsive to treatment. However, inaccurate clinical diagnosis results in many depressed patients being inadequately treated. In this article we will review classifications of depression which are useful in delineating specific treatments for depressed patients, with emphasis on the new nomenclature (DSM III).

Definition

Depression is a word which has both psychiatric and commonplace meanings. Thus, people will use the word "depression" to mean that they are upset about a particular life event. Depressed mood in the absence of specific symptoms of depression is essentially not of sufficient significance to be clinically treatable. Depression as a psychiatric disorder consists of depressed mood plus depressive symptoms. Other terms for depressed mood include feeling sad, blue, hopeless, low, down in the dumps, and irritable. Typical depressive symptoms include change in appetite and weight, with either poor appetite and weight loss or increase in appetite and weight gain; change in sleeping habits, with either insomnia or hypersomnia; change in motor activity, with either agitation or motor retardation; loss of interest in usual activities, and in sexual relations; loss of energy; feelings of worthlessness, of self-reproach, or of guilt; decreased ability to think or concentrate; and recurrent thoughts of death or suicide or suicide attempts. In this article we will use depressed mood plus symptoms to define psychiatric depression in contrast to depression without symptoms.

Subclassification

It is generally recognized that there is an affective response to the death of a close friend or relative. This depression, which is termed "uncomplicated bereavement," is associated with depressed mood and depressive symptoms. Bereavement tends to be prompt in onset and relatively short lived. Feelings of worthlessness and psychomotor retardation are uncommon with this disorder. In general, bereavement is not treated by psychiatrists but is usually treated by internists or family physicians. Bereavement is often not treated except with supportive care. Brief courses of small doses of antianxiety agents may be of benefit. It is unusual for psychiatrists to treat bereaved persons. However, when the syndrome fails to respond to brief therapy, one should consider a major affective disorder as a diagnostic possibility.

Although "reactive depression" has been a commonly used diagnosis for depressions which appeared to be the result of environmental stress, the approach in DSM III is to define the affective state independently of presumed etiology, either as a "major depression" or as an "atypical depression." A useful alternative is to classify depressions as "secondary" if the depression occurs in the course of another psychiatric illness or as "primary" if there is no prior psychiatric condition. Although the primary-secondary distinction has been superseded by DSM III, in this article we will discuss treatment using the primary-secondary classification and will indicate how the DSM III interfaces.

Primary affective disorder can be separated into those patients who have a history of mania (bipolar) and those patients who have depression only (unipolar). Mania is defined as a change in mood state (euphoria or irritability) and presents symptoms such as increase in activity, increase in talkativeness, flight of ideas or racing thoughts, grandiosity, decreased need for sleep, distractability, and impulsive behavior. The severe form of this disorder, which is often accompanied by delusions of grandeur or frank psychosis, usually results in the patient being hospitalized specifically for the manic condition. Such patients are termed bipolar I. In DSM III these patients would be termed bipolar disorder. Patients who have manic symptoms but not to the degree resulting in hospitalization (i.e., hypomanic symptoms) are termed bipolar II. Bipolar II patients typically have recurrent depressions and hypomania. Their hypomanic symptoms are rarely incapacitating and may be productive or beneficial to their life status. In DSM III, some bipolar II patients (approximately half) would be termed bipolar disorder and the other half would be termed atypical bipolar disorder. Less severe forms of bipolar and unipolar depression, cyclothymic personality and depressive personality, respectively, were defined as patients who had mood disorder but not of sufficient severity to require treatment. The DSM III terms "cyclothymic disorder" and "dysthymic disorder" would probably correspond well to the older terms cyclothymic and depressive personality, respectively. It should be noted that "secondary" depressions will probably be considered "major depressions" in DSM III.

One other point of diagnostic clarification regards the presence of schneiderian first rank symptoms in the primary affective disorders. These symptoms, such as bizarre delusions, somatic delusions, auditory hallucinations such as a voice commenting upon the patient's behavior or two or more voices conversing with one another, and delusions such as audible thoughts and thought broadcasting, represent psychotic symptoms which in the past have been used synonymously with schizophrenia. However, there has been a tendency in diagnosis in the past few years to define schizophrenia as a chronic illness with insidious onset and a poor prognosis. Other data suggest that schneiderian first rank symptoms can be present in primary affective disorder, particularly during mania. This point is in some contention, and in DSM III the presence of schneiderian symptoms creates a distinct problem. In DSM III, "mood incongruent" delusions would ordinarily result in the patient being classified as a schizoaffective disorder. However, because of the realization that the term schizoaffective disorder is poorly defined and probably overlaps considerably with bipolar disorder, schizoaffective disorder is not defined by criteria in DSM III. It is our preference not to use the term schizoaffective disorder because of the lack of consensus about the meaning of this term. Instead we prefer the term atypical psychosis for patients who have an admixture of schneiderian first rank symptoms, affective symptoms, and a chronic course. Indeed, most patients who have schneiderian symptoms, affective symptoms, and an episodic course seem to meet criteria for major affective disorder and are often not generally distinguishable from patients with bipolar affective disorder.

In contrast to the rather clearly defined bipolar and unipolar disorders, there are other disorders in which the illness is presumably affective, although the data to support this may be scant. An example is "masked depression," in which a patient will present clinically with somatic complaints rather than depressive symptoms. Masked depressions may be more frequently seen among older patients. The recognition of this problem is important, since it is felt that masked depression represents a significant portion of patients with depression and that most frequently such patients do not have their psychiatric problems adequately recognized or treated. Another less well defined illness is depression occurring in a patient whose psychiatric disorder becomes complicated by a second psychiatric illness, for example, alcoholism or polydrug abuse. An underlying depression is often suspected in such patients, particularly if they have positive family histories of depression and if there are atypical features to the course of their secondary illness. The disorders, i.e., alcoholism and depression, would have to be treated.

Bipolar-Unipolar Differentiation

Recent data support the separation of bipolar from unipolar primary affective disorder. In general, bipolar I illness is a well characterized clinical condition in comparison to other primary affective disorder subtypes. Patients with bipolar I illness tend to have extreme psychomotor retardation and often have hypersomnia when depressed, whereas patients with unipolar depression may either be agitated or have psychomotor retardation. Furthermore, the age of onset of illness tends to be earlier in life in bipolar disorders than in unipolar disorders, with the former occurring at a mean age of approximately 30 years and the latter occurring at a mean age of 40 years. Of some interest is the fact that bipolar disorders may have a more frequent postpartum onset than unipolar disorders. Although there is considerable evidence relating genetic and biologic factors to the etiology of bipolar depression, these factors have not been elucidated to the point at which a clear biologic-genetic etiology has been determined. However, in general, bipolar depression tends to be familial, and approximately 40 per cent of first degree relatives of a patient with bipolar disorder will experience either bipolar or unipolar depression. In contrast, unipolar depression probably represents a very heterogeneous group of patients, with various causes for their disorders. For example, the genetic and biologic factors associated with bipolar disorder are not nearly as well delineated among families of patients with unipolar disorders, and the relationship of unipolar disorders to other psychiatric illnesses such as alcoholism is often striking.

Clinical Course

The course of affective disorders can be recurrent attacks or single episodes. The bipolar disorders tend to be marked by recurrent episodes, sometimes on a regular cyclic basis in such a way that the timing of subsequent attacks is quite predictable. Unipolar disorders tend not to be as recurrent, and the frequency of attacks tends to be much reduced in unipolar depression as compared to bipolar depres-sion. Rapid cycling (four or more episodes per year) occurs in about 10 per cent of bipolars, and such patients present particular treatment problems. Mania usually begins early in bipolar illness, with about 80 per cent of patients having experienced a manic attack at the onset of their disorder. About a third of patients have a significant premanic depression, and almost 100 per cent of patients have a significant postmanic depressive episode. Indeed, the concept of "unipolar mania" (defined as patients who have only recurrent manic episodes) was studied and found not to be useful in that most patients who have recurrent manic episodes also have some depressive features. Between episodes of illness, patients with bipolar and unipolar illness tend to be free of affective symptoms.

Treatment

Treatment considerations should relate to diagnosis, current mood state, and the clinical history. For example, one could be treating a patient with bipolar disorder who is manic or who is depressed or who is euthymic but prone to recurrent cycles. Similarly, one could be treating a patient with unipolar disorder who is depressed or who is prone to recurrent attacks.

Finally, it should be noted that the suicide risk in depressive illness is considerable. About 15 to 20 per cent of patients with depression die from suicide, and approximately 30 to 50 per cent of primary affective disorder patients have a history of suicide attempts. Suicide generally occurs during the depressed phase of illness. Although it has been stated that suicide is unusual early in the course of depression and more common later in the course of depression, we suggest that the clinician should be carefully aware of suicidal behavior during any phase of the depressive illness. Suicide during mania and during the interim euthymic phases between depressions is unusual. Suicidal behavior tends to occur more frequently among men, among older patients, and among patients who are single, widowed, or divorced. It should be noted that there has been a considerable increase in the reported suicides among adolescents in the past few years.

Most patients who have committed suicide have indicated their intent to suicide to other people, and such communication of suicidal intent should be taken quite seriously in the depressed patient. In terms of assessing suicidal risk in an individual patient it is important to have an underlying assumption that all patients with depression are suicidal but that their tendency to suicide at any given point in time may be contingent upon a number of factors. For example, very few patients with depression will have active suicidal plans. A higher percentage of patients will have thoughts of death or suicide, and a majority of patients with depression will wish they wouldn't wake up in the morning or wish they were dead. The recognition of this hierarchy of suicidal behavior is important in order to establish rapport with the patient, have the patient feel he is understood by the therapist, and apply appropriate treatment. It should be stressed that hospitalization should be advocated for any patient in whom the suicidal risk is felt to be high at that period of time. Depression is a highly treatable disorder, and the suicide of a patient during the course of a severe depression should be looked upon as a mistake in treatment.

Under the following heading we will discuss modes of treatment for various types of depression. In general these modes include electroconvulsive therapy, pharmacotherapy, and various forms of psychotherapy. The decision about which mode or combination of modes to use is often based upon the severity of the depressive symptoms as well as the state that the patient is in. It should be emphasized that the best guide to treatment is the past response or lack of response of a given patient to treatments he has received for prior episodes.

Modes of Treatment

Electroconvulsive Therapy. Electroconvulsive therapy (ECT) was widely used in the 1940s, but the beneficial effects of other forms of treatment, as well as some attempts to legally regulate its use, have resulted in decreased use of ECT. However, it should be noted that ECT is the most effective of all the forms of antidepressant treatment.

ECT is usually administered to hospitalized patients, although patients who have family members to take care of them can receive this treatment on an outpatient basis. A course of therapy usually consists of a series of 8 to 12 treatments, with a frequency of approximately one every other day. Before the treatment is administered the physician should have good knowledge of the patient's medical condition, including cardiovascular and pulmonary status. The only absolute contraindication to ECT is a space-occupying brain lesion. During ECT there is a temporary increase of intracranial pressure, which could result in brainstem herniation if a space-occupying lesion is present.

The patient is prepared for ECT by maintaining an empty stomach at least 8 hours prior to ECT. Approximately half an hour before ECT a small dose of atropine is administered in order to reduce bronchial secretions. Prior to ECT, the patient should void and dentures should be removed. Furthermore, hairpins should be removed, and any constricting garments around the chest should be removed or loosened. Imme-

diately before administering ECT the patient should receive an anesthetic intravenously, usually a short-acting barbiturate. The patient is then given succinylcholine in a dose sufficient to cause relaxation of all muscles but not so excessive as to reduce spontaneous respiration for too prolonged a period after ECT. The usual dose of succinylcholine is about 20 to 40 mg intravenously. It is important to maintain the airway and respirate the patient during the succinylcholine-induced paralysis. With bilateral ECT the electrodes are placed on both temples. With unilateral ECT both electrodes are placed over the nondominant hemisphere. In either case a short period of electrical current is applied to the electrodes, usually at the point of maximal muscle depolarization from the succinylcholine. This current application induces a grand mal convulsion characterized by a tonic phase, followed by a clonic phase which usually is over in about 20 seconds. It is important to respirate the patient with oxygen until the effects of succinylcholine wear off and the patient begins to breathe spontaneously. At this point the patient will be drowsy and somewhat confused. The patient's airway should be protected and the patient should be observed for approximately half an hour after ECT or until such time as the patient's confusion has cleared sufficiently to enable the patient to resume usual functioning. There is a considerable amount of confusion, which occurs just after each treatment; as the number of treatments increases, the patient may become confused for longer periods of time between treatments. Usually a course of eight treatments suffices to treat a severe depression, at which time a few days are necessary to enable the confusion to clear up sufficiently that the patient can return home. Although much has been made recently of permanent brain damage resulting from ECT, ECT remains the safest and most effective treatment for severe depression. ECT is useful in the treatment of acute depression. There is no reliable evidence that chronic ECT prevents occurrence of future attacks of depression.

Antidepressant Medication. Antidepressant medication can be divided into two types: the tricyclic antidepressants and derivatives, and the monoamine oxidase inhibitors (Tables 1 and 2). The tricyclic antidepressants have become the most widely used treatment of depression and are efficacious in approximately 80 per cent of depressed patients. Recently, measurement of these compounds in the blood has become available, and for most compounds there seems to be some relationship with either a threshold or range of blood levels and therapeutic response. Thus, if a patient is not responding to a tricyclic antidepres-

TABLE 1. **Tricyclic Antidepressant Medication**

GENERIC NAME	TRADE NAME(S)	DOSE RANGE*
Amitriptyline	Amitid, Amitril, Elavil, Endep	150–300 mg/day
Imipramine	Imavate, Janimine, Presamine, SK-Pramine, Tofranil	150–300 mg/day
Nortriptyline	Aventyl, Pamelor	50–150 mg/day
Desipramine	Norpramin, Pertofrane	150–200 mg/day
Protriptyline	Vivactil	10–60 mg/day
Doxepin	Adapin, Sinequan	150–300 mg/day

*Some doses may be higher than those listed in the manufacturer's official directive.

sant and is felt to have an adequate dose, it would seem advisable to obtain a plasma tricyclic level approximately 12 hours after the last dose of tricyclic medication to determine if the blood level is in the adequate range.

The tricyclic antidepressants can be generally divided into two types: those which are sedating (such as amitriptyline, nortriptyline, and doxepin), and those which are more alerting (such as imipramine, desipramine, and protriptyline).

As a general principle of psychopharmacology it is inadvisable to use fixed dose regimens. Thus patients who are outpatients should be encouraged to alter the dose frequently, within certain guidelines, depending on symptoms or side effects, and for hospitalized patients the physician should carefully assess the dose on a daily basis, balancing therapeutic effect with side effects.

In treating unipolar depression one should be cognizant of two general types of depression: those with agitation and insomnia, and those with psychomotor retardation and hypersomnia. For the former inpatients, who also may experience anxiety as a prominent feature of the depression, a sedating antidepressant often given at bedtime seems to be most effective. For the latter patients, a more alerting antidepressant, often given toward morning hours in divided doses, seems to be the most logical choice of medication. The target dose for hospitalized patients should be approximately 3.5 mg per kg (imipramine or amitriptyline). It should be noted that protrip-

tyline is given in approximately one fifth the dose of the other tricyclic antidepressants.

In considering the starting dose one should take into account previous responses to antidepressants, the general medical state of the patient, and the patient's age. Patients who are older should be started on lower doses of antidepressants than younger patients, and older patients have a lower target dose. The initial dose should be increased progressively toward the target dose with an attempt to achieve the target dose within the first week of treatment. During the first week of treatment there is usually no apparent improvement in depression. Toward the end of this period the patient, when questioned carefully, may experience very brief periods of feeling well, followed by a feeling of sinking back into the depressive condition. The patient should be encouraged to see this as a beneficial sign that the antidepressant will be working and the dose should be increased appropriately. For outpatients the general starting dose of amitriptyline or imipramine is approximately 25 to 100 mg per day, and the dose should be increased by the patient over the course of 3 to 4 days.

It is advisable, considering the suicidal potential of such patients, to have the patient seen or phone in during the first week of treatment so that the dose can be adjusted upward or downward, depending on therapeutic response or side effects. In general outpatient depressives have less severe depression than hospitalized patients and often require less antidepressant total dos-

TABLE 2. **Monoamine Oxidase Inhibitors**

GENERIC NAME	TRADE NAME	DOSE RANGE
Hydrazine		
Isocarboxazid	Marplan	10–30 mg
Phenelzine	Nardil	15–75 mg
Nonhydrazine		
Tranylcypromine	Parnate	10–60 mg

age, although many depressed outpatients will require doses in the range of 3.5 mg per kilogram.

At times inpatients or outpatients will not respond to antidepressants at the target dose, and the dose will have to be increased, perhaps even above the therapeutic levels recommended in the Physician's Desk Reference. For example, it is not uncommon to have patients respond to 350 mg of amitriptyline, whereas they had not responded to a daily dose of 300 mg. Special attention should be paid to the patient's cardiovascular status when doses are increased, and in general outpatients should be told that they should reduce the dose and increase their salt and food intake if they feel dizzy. The typical side effects of tricyclic antidepressants are dry mouth, constipation, blurring of vision, and orthostatic hypotension (experienced as dizziness when one changes position). Later in the course of treatment patients may experience a craving for sweets and weight gain.

Patients tend to respond within 2 to 4 weeks of instituting treatment, although on close questioning they may not feel 100 per cent back to normal. At this point the patient should be maintained on the antidepressant for 2 to 6 months. Frequently toward the end of this interval the dose can be gradually reduced with approximately 10 per cent reduction in dose every week or every other week. Having the patient reduce the dose by 10 to 25 per cent and then waiting a week or two to see if symptoms recur is a satisfactory way of determining whether the patient still requires that dose of medication. The patient should be advised not to stop the dose suddenly, as a brief confusional episode may ensue. Perhaps the most serious side effect is orthostatic hypotension. The patient should be advised about the occurrence of this symptom and told to decrease the dose slightly and to increase fluid and salt intake should dizziness occur.

The acute depressions of bipolar patients are often somewhat refractory to treatment with tricyclic antidepressants. In general, such patients have retarded depression, and imipramine-like drugs seem to be more indicated than amitriptyline type drugs. The patient often will improve somewhat but not completely, and the depression in general will take several months to improve in spite of using maximal doses. For this reason it may be preferable to treat the acute postmanic depressive phase of a bipolar patient with a monamine oxidase inhibitor rather than with a tricyclic antidepressant. The premanic depressive phase of bipolar patients often spontaneously ends in manic or hypomanic episodes. Thus, the patient should be alerted to the possibility of a manic occurrence during the course of tricyclic treatment, and it may be advisable to treat the patient simultaneously with lithium carbonate. In general, tricyclic antidepressants seem to accentuate mania and are contraindicated during manic or hypomanic episodes. Lithium carbonate has an antidepressant effect, but treatment of the acute depressed phase of bipolar or unipolar depression with lithium carbonate alone is not recommended.

It has been claimed that low doses of antipsychotic agents may be useful in treating some depressive episodes. Furthermore it has been suggested that patients with psychotic depression often are nonresponders to antidepressant therapy and that antipsychotic drugs should be added to the tricyclic antidepressant. In general, antipsychotic drugs are not the treatment of choice for depression. The addition of an antipsychotic drug to antidepressant therapy in psychotic depressives is of clinical benefit at times. However, ECT should also be considered in these patients.

Monoamine oxidase inhibitors (MAOI) were introduced into psychiatry before the tricyclic depressants and were noted to be quite effective in the early years of their use. A potentially serious side effect of these drugs results from inhibition of MAO in liver. Tyramine, which is present in many food substances, is ordinarily metabolized by liver MAO. If tyramine-containing foods are ingested while the patient is treated with an MAOI, tyramine enters the bloodstream and sudden increases in blood pressure may occur. Because of their serious side effect (headache, strokes), MAOI were little used for many years. They have been reintroduced recently and are gaining considerable popularity for the treatment of postmanic depressive episodes of the bipolar type.

There are two general types of MAOI. Tranylcypramine has a structure very similar to that of amphetamine and is stimulating, whereas phenelzine is somewhat less stimulating. MAOI drugs have the usual side effects of tricyclic antidepressants, and orthostatic hypotension is the most frequent serious side effect. Hypertensive crisis can be avoided completely if patients watch their diet and associative use of medication. The appropriate dose of the medication can be determined by the dose required to inhibit MAO in platelets. In general, a dose of 45 mg a day of phenelzine inhibits this enzyme in about 50 per cent of patients, and thus a somewhat higher dose is required of this medication.

PROPHYLAXIS OF DEPRESSION. Recently tricyclic antidepressants such as amitriptyline and imipramine have been administered on a long-term basis to patients with recurrent unipolar depression to effect a reduction in the frequency of future attacks of this disorder. Such reduction in frequency and/or severity of future episodes with long-term treatment is termed prophylaxis or maintenance therapy, and several studies support the efficacy of chronic tricyclic antidepressants in unipolar recurrent depression. However, it should be noted that some of these studies report a high incidence of manic or hypomanic failures while supposedly unipolar patients are being treated with tricyclic antidepressants. The bipolar II category includes patients who have brief hypomanic episodes before or after their depression, and such patients probably were included as unipolar in those studies mentioned above, resulting in the reported hypomanic failures with chronic tricyclic treatment. Lithium carbonate has also been shown to have a prophylactic effect for recurrent unipolar and bipolar depression, and lithium carbonate is preferred over tricyclic antidepressants for such treatment.

The appropriate dose of tricyclic antidepressants in prophylactic treatment has not been established, although most physicians seem to prefer a maintenance dose of approximately 100 to 150 mg daily of amitriptyline or imipramine. Other antidepressants have not been systematically studied for their long-term prophylactic effect. Lithium carbonate maintenance will be discussed later in this article. Maintenance efficacy for recurrent depression may not become clinically apparent until the patient has been in treatment for about 2 years.

Patients with the rapid cycling form of bipolar illness will experience recurrent depressions and hypomanic episodes. Their depressions are seen as illness, whereas the hypomanic episodes are not viewed by the patient as being clinically significant. However, treating such patients with tricyclic antidepressants alone or in combination with lithium carbonate seems to result in a perpetuation of the cyclic process, whereas treating rapid cyclers with lithium carbonate alone or perhaps with a small dose of antipsychotic agent (such as thioridazine) may be of benefit.

SPECIAL USES IN DEPRESSION. The use of tricyclic antidepressants in the secondary depressions and in bereavement has not been systematically studied. In our experience if such patients require an antidepressant based on the presence of depressive symptoms, they usually respond at relatively low doses of the antidepressant such as 50 mg daily of amitriptyline. One should be cautious in treating depression associated with alcoholism, since the antidepressants are sedating as is alcohol, and the sedative effects of alcohol may be potentiated. Also, particular attention

should be paid to treating depression in the elderly, as such patients are particularly prone to the hypotensive and cardiovascular effects of tricyclic antidepressants. The beginning dose for elderly patients is low, on the order of 10 to 25 mg of amitriptyline daily, and very slow increments of the dose are advised, along with careful assessment of blood pressure and cardiovascular status.

An important drug-drug interaction of the tricyclic antidepressants is with guanethidine, an antihypertensive agent. The antihypertensive effects of guanethidine can be blocked with the administration of tricyclic antidepressants. Thus, if patients are hypertensive and prone to depression, it is advised that they be treated with an antihypertensive agent other than guanethidine. In addition, tricyclic antidepressants are not advocated during the first trimester of pregnancy.

Acute Mania. Acute manic disturbances may present particular problems because the patient may not be willing to be hospitalized for treatment. Treating manic patients on an outpatient basis is difficult because of the lack of control regarding medication that can be exercised in such circumstances. Thus, the optimal plan is to hospitalize the patient for treatment of an acute manic disorder. ECT is effective in the treatment of acute manic disturbances, although the usual method of treating acute mania is with lithium carbonate, antipsychotics, or a combination of lithium carbonate and antipsychotics. In general, treatment of acute mania consists of beginning an antipsychotic drug and instituting lithium carbonate as soon as the patient is willing to take medication orally. The severity of the acute manic disorder and cooperation of the patient are the critical factors in the choice of the antipsychotic drug. For example, patients who are uncooperative in taking oral medication will require intramuscular medication, such as haloperidol or chlorpromazine. Chlorpromazine can be given in 25 to 50 mg doses intramuscularly every 1 to 3 hours, with careful attention being paid to blood pressure, since orthostatic hypotension often accompanies this route of administration. Haloperidol has been used more recently as an acute antimanic drug and is often given as 5 to 10 mg intramuscularly every 1 to 2 hours. Haloperidol has a great propensity for causing parkinsonian symptoms, which should be treated with antiparkinson drugs. Haloperidol has very little effect on blood pressure, and although haloperidol is not as sedating as chlorpromazine, manic patients can be successfully sedated with haloperidol. For patients who are more cooperative or whose manic episode is less severe, thioridazine is an excellent drug in that it has very few blood pressure effects or parkinsonian side effects. The thioridazine dose should not exceed 800 mg per day. Starting doses on the order of 200 to 400 mg a day can be used in combination with lithium carbonate to treat the acute manic episode. It should be stressed that the patient's general medical and in particular cardiovascular status should be known prior to treatment with these drugs.

Lithium carbonate is perhaps more effective in treating acute manic episodes than are the antipsychotic agents. However, lithium carbonate cannot be given in an intramuscular form, and thus the patient must be cooperative to be treated with lithium carbonate. Prior to treatment with lithium carbonate it is advisable to have a medical work-up, which would include physical examination, electrocardiogram, thyroid studies, white blood count, urinalysis, blood urea nitrogen, and creatinine. There have been several regimens described for determining the dose of lithium carbonate. These involve giving a "test dose" of 600 to 900 mg of lithium carbonate and determining a blood lithium level at a fixed time thereafter. This blood level is used to select a "therapeutic" dose. In our experience these projected doses often result in a high daily dose being administered to the patient with resulting lithium toxicity. We prefer to start lithium carbonate at 300 to 600 mg the first day and increase the dose daily until therapeutic blood lithium concentrations result. This method requires frequent blood levels but is safe for the patient and produces fewer acute side effects, such as nausea and vomiting. The therapeutic blood lithium concentration for acute mania is about 1.0 to 1.5 mEq per liter. Blood levels should be taken frequently on hospitalized patients who are undergoing increasing doses of lithium treatment, particularly older patients or patients with borderline renal function. Patients should be examined daily for the presence of lithium side effects, such as nausea, vomiting, diarrhea, or tremor. Signs of neurotoxicity for lithium should also be observed; these would include confusion, gross tremor, ataxia, slurring of speech, and sedation. These neurotoxic symptoms may occur in some patients at doses within the therapeutic range, particularly if the patient is receiving high doses of antipsychotic drugs concomitantly. It is vital that the patient have an adequate fluid and salt intake during lithium treatment, because lithium urinary excretion is dependent on sodium metabolism. In many but not all cases, manic symptoms will improve at about 10 to 14 days, at which time the dose of the antipsychotic drug can be tapered. The dose of lithium may also have to be reduced somewhat, as the patient while manic may be drinking copious amounts of fluid and this phenomenon will decrease as the mania abates. The physician should be cautioned about premature discharge of the manic patient from the hospital, as insight and judgment seem to be the last manic symptoms to improve in contrast to sleep and activity. Patients who are discharged from the hospital prematurely may stop their medication and have a relapse of manic symptoms. As a general guide, the manic episode has not been completed until the patient enters into a postmanic depressive phase.

LITHIUM CARBONATE MAINTENANCE. Prophylaxis of manic episodes is the most striking reason why lithium carbonate has become the accepted drug of the 1970s. It was found that the administration of this simple salt on a long-term basis reduced the frequency and intensity of subsequent manic episodes in patients who are prone to bipolar cyclic manic depressive illness. The maintenance dose is that dose sufficient to produce a blood level of 0.7 to 1.0 mEq per liter. The drug should be given in divided doses in order to minimize the acute effect on the kidneys. During proper administration of chronic lithium treatment there are minimal side effects, mainly occasional diarrhea or occasional tremor. A slight polyuria is frequently found, but this is usually not of clinical significance.

There are several medical concerns about long-term administration of lithium. An antithyroid effect is often noted early in the course of administration and can be corrected by giving thyroid supplements if clinical manifestations of hypothyroidism persist. Cardiac effects, especially in older patients, have been noted during lithium treatment. Sinus node dysfunction may be accentuated during lithium therapy. A third effect has been related to severe polyuria and the possibility of renal disease in patients undergoing chronic lithium treatment or who have experienced lithium toxicity. For this reason patients should have monitoring of medical status, including thyroid tests, blood urea nitrogen, creatinine, and electrocardiogram at least yearly while undergoing lithium treatment. If symptoms develop referable to a primary medical illness, appropriate consultations should be obtained. It should not be too lightly stressed that patients must be carefully monitored during long-term lithium treatment and that it is important to obtain blood lithium levels at least every other month in patients who are being chronically maintained. Blood for lithium concentrations should be obtained 8 to 12 hours after a lithium dose. It is best to have the interval between the patient's taking the medication and the blood level remain constant from visit to visit. During steady state lithium treatment the blood level generally does not vary more than 0.1 mEq per liter, and variations greater than this are probably due to irregularities in the patient's taking the medication. The most likely time for a relapse during lithium treatment is in the initial 6 months of treatment, based on actuarial life table statistics. Patients have a risk of developing an affective episode when starting lithium treatment of about 5 per cent per month through the initial 6 months of treatment, and subsequent to that the risk is about 1 per cent per month. Maintenance lithium treatment for outpatients (who are generally euthymic) is usually initiated with low doses, i.e., one capsule per day. The dose is increased on a weekly basis until the therapeutic blood level is achieved. Patients are generally seen every 1 to 2 weeks initially, and when they are stable the interval between visits can be lengthened to once per month.

While it is clear that lithium has an effect on reducing manic and hypomanic episodes very dramatically in the first year of treatment, its effect against depression in both bipolar and unipolar recurrent depression is less clear. Recent data suggest that it takes approximately a year and a half to 2 years of treatment before the prophylactic effect of lithium against recurrent depression can be statistically demonstrated. However, the data also suggest that there may be subclinical beneficial effects on mild mood states during this initial period. Thus, in starting patients on lithium one should carefully explain that it is likely that they will have recurrent depressions at least for 1 to 2 years in spite of treatment and that these depressions initially may seem as severe as their prior depressions before they went on lithium. Secondly, the patients should notice a decrease in the frequency and severity of manic and hypomanic attacks, although manic episodes may not be completely obliterated during lithium treatment. Those patients who have had a recurrence of severe manic episodes at least once every 7 years or at least two recurrent depressive episodes in 5 years are candidates for lithium prophylactic treatment. It should also be noted that the prophylactic efficacy of lithium carbonate in unipolar recurrent depression is controversial, although supported by several research studies. The comparative efficacy of lithium versus tricyclic antidepressants in this patient population in particular is worthy of further study.

Patients frequently feel well for long intervals during lithium treatment, and some may wish to stop their medication. This should not be advised, since on stopping medication patients tend to return to their previous rate of episodes, and the failure rate on stopping lithium treatment seems to be the same as if the patient never was on lithium treatment.

Although there are few drug-drug interactions with lithium, diuretics should be avoided. Lithium excretion requires sodium, and concomitant diuretic administration often results in lithium retention and can provoke episodes of lithium toxicity. Thus, patients should be cautioned not to change their sodium intake or their sodium metabolism in any way while taking lithium carbonate. Lithium toxicity, in contrast to lithium side effects, tends to be a fairly acute onset illness. Usually the symptoms occur over a week or so, and these symptoms are characterized by polyuria, confusion, agitation, and tremor, and may eventually progress to coma and death. As the patients continue to take lithium they become progressively dehydrated because of polyuria resulting from lithium toxicity. The treatment of lithium toxicity is to stop lithium and to rehydrate the patient, particularly with water, sodium, and potassium. The potassium is probably the most important, since lithium toxicity seems to result in an intracellular hypokalemia, which, if not corrected, can lead to cardiac arrhythmia.

Psychotherapy. Although psychotherapy is generally felt to be of importance in the treatment of depression, there has been a considerable change in the emphasis on psychotherapy for depressed patients over the past several years. In the late 1960s in some centers, analytically oriented psychotherapy was considered the treatment of choice for both bipolar and unipolar affective disorders. The efficacy of psychopharmacologic agents resulted in the need for greater specificity and efficacy in the psychotherapies employed for affective disorders. We favor an approach toward psychotherapy that is relatively low keyed and basically educational. It is very important to have the patient understand his illness as thoroughly as possible and to understand the need for and the role of medication. The patient should be taught to recognize early symptoms and to adjust medication according to agreed-upon guidelines. Decisions which could alter life situations, such as job changes, marital changes, moves, and the like, should be avoided if at all possible until the depression is over.

It is important to have the patient try to get out of the house as much as possible, even if only for an hour a day. Physical exercise, such as jogging, may be of benefit to some patients. However, patients should be cautioned that physical exercise is usually of only brief benefit in depression.

In addition to educational psychotherapy, supportive psychotherapy may be of benefit in depression. More specific psychotherapies, such as cognitive-behavioral psychotherapy, have been used successfully with some depressives.

Psychotherapy of a manic patient during such episodes is extremely difficult, as the patient usually attempts to maintain control of the therapy situation. Family and/or marital therapy may be indicated in some manic patients after remission of the manic episode.

A flexible approach to psychotherapy is probably best. Some patients may benefit from certain types of therapy but not other types, and some patients may need little psychotherapy.

Barbiturates and Stimulants. Barbiturates should be avoided as sleeping medications for patients with depression. Barbiturates are totally unneeded for treatment of depressed patients with insomnia because such patients can be treated with a sedating antidepressant such as amitriptyline. In addition barbiturates tend to activate liver enzymes which metabolize tricyclic antidepressants. Thus, the effect of a barbiturate in combination with a tricyclic antidepressant would be to lower the dose of the antidepressant. Stimulants such as methylphenidate or amphetamine are of only temporary benefit in depression and should be avoided.

SCHIZOPHRENIA

method of
BRUCE M. COHEN, M.D., Ph.D.,
and JOSEPH F. LIPINSKI, M.D.
Boston, Massachusetts

Schizophrenia is a chronic disease that profoundly affects the thinking, emotions, and behavior of the afflicted individual. Although the cause of schizophrenia is unknown, there is considerable evidence supporting a genetic predisposition, at least in some patients. Some environmental factor or factors also may be important, as with most inherited diseases, but whether such factors are physical or emotional in nature is undetermined. Criteria for the diagnosis of schizophrenia are at present much in dispute. The following suggestions regarding treatment assume that the diagnosis has been made by the criteria of Feighner and associates (Arch. Gen. Psychiatry 26:57, 1972) or the new and similar criteria of the Diagnostic and Statistical Manual, Edition III (DSM III) of the American Psychiatric Association.

Treatment: General Principles

There is no cure for schizophrenia, but there are treatments that can ameliorate symptoms and minimize disability. These treatments can be divided into two classes:

1. Specific treatment for the symptoms of schizophrenia, which involves the proper use of antipsychotic medication (APM).

2. Adjunctive treatment to protect the patient and society and to help the patient cope with his or her illness. Such treatment includes hospitalization when necessary and various forms of counseling and support.

As stated, APM is the specific treatment of choice in schizophrenia. Unlike mania or depression, in which recovery with time and rest alone may be seen, profound improvement in schizophrenia rarely occurs without such treatment. With such treatment considerable restitution can be seen in many patients, in distinction to the generally chronic deteriorating course of untreated schizophrenia. Sedatives and antianxiety drugs (so-called minor tranquilizers) have no specific effect on the symptoms of schizophrenia and ordinarily have no place in treatment of this syndrome. "Orthomolecular" and "megavitamin" therapies have no demonstrated efficacy. Electroconvulsive therapy (ECT), so useful in treatment of the acute psychoses, is of no proved benefit in schizophrenia.

Use of Antipsychotic Medications

There are a great many APM agents, and these fall into a variety of chemical classes. At present there is no evidence that they differ in efficacy when used at equivalent doses, and all *may* work by the same mechanism (central dopamine blockade). The only proved differences between agents are in side effects. Thus, the physician should familiarize himself with a handful of APM drugs with different side effects and from a range of chemical classes. A rough estimate of comparative antipsychotic potency (with chlorpromazine arbitrarily given a value of 100) is given in Table 1. How the various APM agents differ in side effects is presented in more detail later in this article, but it is generally true that medications with high antipsychotic potency per milligram (high-potency APM) have more motor side effects, whereas medications with low antipsychotic potency per milligram (low-potency APM) have more anticholingeric, sedative, and autonomic side effects.

There are no absolute criteria for selecting a specific APM for any given patient. Past history is often helpful, as medications that have worked in the past are likely to work again. Medications that

TABLE 1.   **Equivalent Doses of Commonly Used Antipsychotic Agents, by Chemical Type***

GENERIC NAME	TRADE NAME	APPROXIMATE EQUIVALENT DAILY DOSE (MG)
Phenothiazines		
Aliphatic		
Chlorpromazine	Thorazine, etc. (generic)	100
Triflupromazine	Vesprin	30
Piperidines		
Mesoridazine	Serentil	50
Piperacetazine	Quide	12
Thioridazine	Mellaril	95
Piperazines		
Acetophenazine	Tindal	20
Butaperazine	Repoise	12
Carphenazine	Proketazine	25
Fluphenazine	Prolixin, Permitil	2
Perphenazine	Trilafon	10
Trifluoperazine	Stelazine	5
Thioxanthenes		
Aliphatic		
Chlorprothixene	Taractan	65
Piperazine		
Thiothixene	Navane	5
Dibenzazepines		
Loxapine	Loxitane, Daxolin	15
Clozapine	(Leponex, experimental)	60
Butyrophenones		
Haloperidol	Haldol	2
Diphenylbutylpiperidines		
Pimozide	(Orap, experimental)	0.3–0.5
Penfluridol	(experimental)	2 (1 week dose)
Fluspirilene	(experimental)	—
Indolones		
Molindone	Moban	10
Rauwolfia alkaloids		
Reserpine	Serpasil, etc. (generic)	1–2

*From Baldessarini, R. J.: Chemotherapy in Psychiatry. Cambridge, Massachusetts, Harvard University Press, 1977.

have not been beneficial despite adequate doses or that have caused distressing side effects in the past are best avoided. In addition, expected side effects should always be considered in choosing a medication. In patients requiring sedation, a low-potency APM is often helpful. In older patients or patients with concomitant medical illness, a high-potency APM is usually safer, avoiding the marked autonomic side effects of the low-potency agents.

An effective dose of APM is frequently the equivalent of 400 to 800 mg of chlorpromazine per day. There is, however, marked variability in tissue levels from patient to patient for the same dose of medication. There may also be marked differences in individual sensitivity to the APM. Unfortunately, at this time, determining blood levels of the APM is not helpful because there is no adequate body of information establishing a therapeutic range of blood levels for any APM. Instead, it is best to monitor dosage by gauging clinical effect and side effects. Few patients will improve without experiencing some side effects, but severe side effects usually indicate that dosage is too high.

Generally, therapy can be started with the equivalent of 100 to 200 mg of chlorpromazine per day and medication can be increased as tolerated to the equivalent of 400 to 800 mg of chlorpromazine per day over the next few days. High-potency APM often are tolerated especially well in this early period. Initially, medication should be given in divided doses for patient comfort, but when the daily dose is stable, the entire day's medication may be taken at bedtime.

APM drugs are slow acting. Improvement *may* take weeks to begin and may continue over months. Therefore, changes in medication regimen should not be made too hastily. If a patient seems to be getting no benefit from APM, dosage may be increased if side effects are mild or moderate. Often patients become physiologically tolerant of side effects over the course of weeks or months and can tolerate higher doses. There is, however, no evidence that *very* high doses of medication (e.g., 4 to 5 grams of chlorpromazine per day) are of benefit for most patients with schizophrenia. Occasionally a patient may require very high doses owing to individual peculiarities of absorption, distribution, metabolism, or sensitivity. In such patients it is probably wise to try two or three APM drugs that are chemically very different before trying extremely high doses of any one medication. In any case, as with most other medications, the lowest effective dose is the best dose.

Intramuscular medications may be useful and may even be necessary if the patient is dangerous to himself or to others and is uncooperative. Comparatively, intramuscular APM may be two to three times as potent as oral APM. In particular, autonomic side effects (see discussion later in this article) may be especially troubling after intramuscular medication. In patients with a poor history of medication use and multiple relapses, intramuscular depot APM may be useful. Only two such medications are presently available in the United States; both are esters of fluphenazine that are slowly hydrolyzed and released after injection. Equivalent doses are poorly established but fluphenazine decanoate is generally given as 0.5 to 2.0 ml (12.5 to 50 mg) every 2 to 4 weeks; fluphenazine enanthate is generally given in similar dosage every 1 to 2 weeks. The use of depot medication should be carefully discussed with the patient, and the patient should agree to this course of treatment as a means of preventing relapse. In patients whose medication intake is supervised (in the hospital) but whose compliance is suspect, APM may be given as an elixir, since such medication is difficult to sequester in the mouth.

Long-Term Use of Antipsychotic Drugs

Schizophrenia is one of the few psychotic syndromes for which controlled studies indicate the efficacy of maintenance antipsychotic medication. As always when using a medication with serious side effects, the potential benefits must be weighed against the potential risks. Also, the lowest dose that is effective should be used, and periodic "holidays" off drugs should be tried yearly to determine the need for continued drug treatment (see discussion of tardive dyskinesia later in this article).

Side Effects of Antipsychotic Medications

A considerable amount of discussion will be given to the description and management of the various side effects of antipsychotic drugs. The reasons are several. Although most of the side effects mentioned are not dangerous in themselves, they can cause marked discomfort. Since APM agents are likely to be taken for many years, if not for a lifetime, early recognition and treatment of these conditions will do much to improve the quality of the patient's life. Compliance is another issue. Convincing patients with schizophrenia of the benefit of medications is often a difficult task. The presence of side effects, especially if minimized or ignored by the physician, is frequently enough to cause patients to surreptitiously discontinue their medication and risk all the attendant miseries and dangers of a reemergent psychosis.

Motor Side Effects

Motor side effects (also called extrapyramidal side effects, or EPS) of the antipsychotic drugs are common, occurring in approximately 5 to 60 per cent of patients, depending upon the medication used. They can be separated into five general categories: dystonias, parkinsonism, akathisia, withdrawal dyskinesias, and tardive dyskinesia. These will be discussed according to the temporal order in which they occur.

Dystonias. Dystonias commonly present as acute, persistent, and sometimes painful contractions of the muscles of the tongue, eyes, face, neck, or back. They usually appear within the first few days of treatment and are more common with the high-potency drugs, such as the piperazine class of phenothiazines and haloperidol. They are most common in young male patients. A typical picture is that of a person who has been receiving the drug for several days, who suddenly begins to find his tongue protruding uncontrollably, interfering with speech, or his eyes deviating upward conjugately (oculogyric crisis), or who begins to experience acute torticollis or retrocollis (which, when severe, can approach opisthotonus), or any combination of these. These very distressing symptoms can be treated effectively with any of the available anticholinergic drugs such as benztropine mesylate, trihexyphenidyl, or diphenhydramine, usually given parenterally. For example, 25 to 50 mg of diphenhydramine given intravenously or intramuscularly usually provides complete relief within minutes. As the dystonia may well reappear after the anticholinergic drug's effect has worn off, institution of treatment with oral anticholinergic agents at that time is advisable. This should be continued for at least several days.

Parkinsonism. Antipsychotic drugs produce a syndrome essentially indistinguishable from idiopathic parkinsonism: slowed movements, rigidity, mask-like facies, stooped posture, small-stepped, shuffling gait, resting tremor of the hands ("pill-rolling") and feet, and sometimes the head, and drooling. Uncommonly, the rigidity can be severe enough to produce muteness and the inability to move. The symptoms usually begin sometime between the first and fourth week but may appear at any time during treatment. At times, because of the slowed movements and impassive facies, this drug-induced syndrome is incorrectly diagnosed as depression or catatonia. Treatment consists of administration of one of the anticholinergic (antiparkinsonism) drugs. As the latter can themselves produce a toxic psychosis, the physician should use the lowest dose that is effective.

Tolerance to the EPS of antipsychotic drugs develops in several months in some, but not all, patients. A common practice is to discontinue antiparkinsonism medications after 3 to 4 months and observe the patient closely for re-emergence of symptoms, reinstituting treatment if necessary. Some patients will require antiparkinsonism drugs even after years of therapy with antipsychotic medications.

Akathisia. Akathisia is a syndrome marked by motor restlessness, a sense of vague but severe discomfort, particularly in the lower extremities, which is partially relieved by movement, and anxiety. Affected patients commonly complain of being inexplicably anxious, of being unable to sit still or concentrate, and of feeling comfortable only when moving. They will often continually pace or fidget by tapping their feet or crossing and uncrossing their legs, and usually appear quite distressed. Akathisia first occurs at about the first to the fourth week, as with parkinsonism. This is a very common syndrome, and one that is frequently missed by physicians. It is sometimes diagnosed as simple anxiety or as a worsening of the psychosis. If the latter diagnosis is made, the dose of antipsychotic drug is usually increased, with resultant worsening of the akathisia.

Treatment is often less successful than in either the dystonias or drug-induced parkinsonism. Akathisia may subside if the dose of the APM used is lowered. Antiparkinsonism drugs are sometimes effective, as is switching from a high-potency to a low-potency APM, such as thioridazine (Mellaril). Antianxiety drugs such as the benzodiazepines are of unproved benefit in this syndrome but may be tried if other measures fail. At times, nothing is effective, and the akathisia persists. In these patients, the effect of the drug on the psychosis must be weighed against the distress caused by the drug. One strategy is to ask the patient to tolerate the symptoms for 1 or 2 months or until the psychosis remits. At this time the antipsychotic drug is discontinued in the hope that the psychosis will not soon recur.

Prompt recognition and treatment of dystonias, parkinsonism, and atkathisia are critical if one is to obtain patient cooperation. Lack of treatment of EPS often leads to the patient's discontinuing medication, followed by re-emergence of florid psychotic symptoms.

Withdrawal Dyskinesia. Withdrawal dyskinesia usually occurs after discontinuation of antipsychotic drug treatment when treatment has continued for one or more years. It consists of a choreoathetoid movement disorder developing 1 to 3 days after medication is stopped and lasting only several days or a week. This condition *may* represent the early form of tardive dyskinesia (see below). No treatment is necessary in most patients.

Tardive Dyskinesia. Tardive (late-appearing) dyskinesia is a syndrome consisting of involuntary choreoathetoid movements involving the tongue, orofacial and neck muscles, extremities, and trunk muscles, in order of frequency. It is called *tardive* dyskinesia because of its tendency to occur after years of antipsychotic drug treatment. The first sign of the illness may be a twitching of the tongue (seen best with the tongue at rest and while observing with a transverse light), which has been likened to "a bag of worms." Chewing movements, pursing or smacking of lips, and protrusion of the tongue into the cheek also are found early in the illness as are "piano-playing" adventitious movements of the fingers and toes. In some patients there may be pelvic thrusting, grunting abnormalities in gait, and other evidence of major muscle group involvement. It is reported that the prevalence of this syndrome approaches 20 per cent in patients treated with antipsychotic drugs over long periods. Although it is reported to occur more frequently in older age groups, it can occur in adolescents, at times after only a few months' treatment with APM. It may make its appearance while the patient is still receiving the drug, but frequently it is seen after the dose of the drug is decreased or discontinued.

There is no treatment for this disorder. Perhaps 60 per cent of people with this syndrome have irreversible cases, although symptoms may diminish in severity with time. Young persons with relatively short exposure to antipsychotic medication appear to have better chances of remission. Treatment with drugs used for parkinsonism usually produces either no effect or a worsening of the syndrome. Reinstituting antipsychotic drugs or increasing the dose of these drugs may decrease (mask) the symptoms, but in such patients one runs the risk of worsening the underlying dyskinesia. "Breakthrough" dyskinesia with re-emergence of dyskinetic symptoms 6 to 8 weeks after an increase in dose is not uncommon; thus, increasing the dosage is not recommended.

Again, although a large number of drugs have been tried to treat tardive dyskinesia and varying levels of efficacy have been claimed, there is no medication that has been found to be clearly effective in this syndrome. Prevention, early diagnosis, and trials off medication form the basis of management. Schizophrenic patients receiving antipsychotic drugs chronically should have yearly evaluations off medications. A reduction in dose of 10 per cent every week until the drug is discontinued or the psychosis worsens significantly is recommended. This will allow the physician to determine if tardive dyskinesia has developed and if there is a continuing need for the drug. When dealing with a patient with tardive dyskinesia whose schizophrenia worsens off drugs, a clinical judgment must be made as to which course — drug versus no drug — is the safest and best for the patient.

Other Side Effects of Antipsychotic Medication

Anticholinergic Side Effects. Although motoric effects may be the most striking common side effects of APM, there are a host of other side effects to be monitored, as with many medicines. All APM drugs are to a greater or lesser degree anticholinergic agents. Low-potency APM drugs are relatively strong anticholinergic agents. Further, anticholinergic (antiparkinsonism) agents are often given with high-potency APM to counteract extrapyramidal side effects (EPS). Thus, most patients on APM experience anticholinergic side effects. The side effects are both peripherally and centrally mediated.

Peripherally mediated anticholinergic side effects include dry mouth, blurred vision (from partial paralysis of the ciliary muscles), constipation, urinary hesitancy, and increased pulse rate. These side effects are usually mild, and some tolerance develops to them. Anticholinergic agents, however, must be used with caution in patients with a variety of medical conditions, including narrow angle glaucoma, cardiac disease, bladder outflow obstruction, or impaired gut motility. Also, patients with dry mouth from medication should be advised not to chew or suck on sugared gum or candy, as they are at increased risk of developing infections of the soft tissues of the mouth, especially candidiasis. If peripheral anticholinergic side effects are severe but medication is otherwise well tolerated and a change to an APM with less anticholinergic effect or a reduction in antiparkinsonism medication is not indicated, bethanechol chloride (Urecholine), 25 mg

three times daily, may be given. This treatment may be effective for urinary hesitancy, constipation, dry mouth, and blurring of vision.

Central anticholinergic side effects include disorientation, confusion, poor memory, agitation, or frank delirium. These side effects, mild to severe, are usually seen along with peripheral anticholinergic side effects and should not be mistaken for a worsening of the patient's underlying illness. If there is confusion on this point, anticholinergic medication should be reduced or stopped or, in severe cases, a challenge dose of physostigmine, an anticholinesterase that crosses the blood-brain barrier, may be given (this procedure is described in Baldessarini, R. J.: Chemotherapy in Psychiatry; Cambridge, Mass., Harvard University Press, 1977).

Autonomic and Sedative Side Effects. APM, especially low-potency APM (see Table 1), cause sedation and have diverse effects on the autonomic nervous system mediated by cholinergic, adrenergic, dopaminergic, and perhaps other central and peripheral mechanisms. The most common such effect is hypotension, which can be severe. Frequently but not invariably, this hypotension is postural and the patient may complain of lightheadedness only on standing. This is often most severe in the morning on rising, and patients should be so warned. Treatment usually consists of reassuring the patient and waiting for tolerance to develop. In severe cases it may be necessary to switch to an agent less likely to produce this side effect, with bed rest and use of support stockings as necessary until symptoms subside. Blood pressure monitoring, of course, can be of benefit. Patients with cardiac disease are best treated with high-potency APM, which have less effect on pulse, blood pressure, and cardiac conduction and repolarization. If a cardiovascular pressor agent is needed (a very rare event) by a patient taking APM, an alpha-pressor (e.g., metaraminol) should be used. Beta-pressors (e.g., isoproterenol) or mixed pressors (e.g., epinephrine) should be avoided, as they may further lower blood pressure.

Allergic Reactions. As with all medication, patients can develop a variety of allergic reactions to APM. Rashes secondary to APM are ordinarily mild and time-limited reactions, but it is wise to change medication to an APM from a different chemical class. Should rash or specific evidence of hepatic dysfunction develop, liver function tests must be monitored, as cholestatic jaundice may develop in patients taking APM. This reaction is rare and is most often seen with low-potency APM. APM drugs may depress white blood cell (WBC) count (leukopenia) and may cause agranulocytosis. The latter is extremely rare and, again, is more likely to occur with low-potency APM. Routine monitoring of white blood cells (WBC) is not of any proved benefit in early detection of agranulocytosis, and it is better to monitor potential symptoms. Patients are at greatest risk in the first months after starting a new medication. They should be advised to report any evidence of infection (especially sore throat, fever, or malaise) and a WBC must be obtained should such symptoms arise.

Miscellaneous Side Effects. APM drugs may cause photosensitivity, and patients should be instructed to avoid extensive exposure to ultraviolet radiation, to use a tanning agent with a sunscreen if they are outdoors for any extended period in the summer, and to wear protective clothing. Pigment deposits in skin, lens, and cornea have been reported, although rarely, in patients taking low-potency APM agents, and regular eye examinations are important in patients receiving large doses over many years. Thioridazine is apparently unique in being able to cause a degenerative pigmentary retinopathy when used in doses exceeding 1200 mg daily. Treatment is preventive, with this medication never being used in doses exceeding 800 mg daily. Thioridazine and occasionally other low-potency APM drugs may cause ejaculatory failure or impotence.

All APM drugs may lower the seizure threshold, but this effect again is most marked for low-potency APM. Patients taking anticonvulsants may need to increase their dosage of these medications. Rarely, individuals experience a first seizure while taking APM. Neurologic consultation is required, but usually treatment can be continued with a change to a higher potency APM and, often, the addition of anticonvulsants.

APM drugs often cause weight gain, which should be treated by diet alone, as appetite suppressants are contraindicated in schizophrenia. APM agents also impair temperature regulation, an effect that is of particular importance in elderly persons, who should be advised against undue exposure to excessive heat or cold. Although there is no clear evidence that APM drugs cause dysmorphogenesis, use of these agents should be avoided during pregnancy and especially during the first trimester, if at all possible.

Withdrawal Syndromes. In addition to motor symptoms, which occasionally occur with abrupt withdrawal of high doses of antipsychotic drugs (see Withdrawal Dyskinesia, above), nausea and vomiting, gastritis, dizziness, and tremors may occur. The latter can usually be avoided by a gradual reduction of the dosage over several weeks.

Drug Interactions and the Use of Other Drugs in Schizophrenia

APM drugs show mild antagonism of guanethidine action but potentiate the effects of most other antihypertensives, including diuretics, hydralazine, alpha-methyldopa, and propranolol. They have a variable but often profound influence on the effects of insulin or oral hypoglycemics. In turn, many agents, including antacids, may affect the absorption and thus the efficacy of APM. Finally, the sedative and anticholinergic effects of APM drugs and various other medications are additive, requiring caution in simultaneous use.

Because of drug interactions, increased exposure to potentially toxic agents, and increased difficulty in drug management, the simultaneous use of other pharmacologic agents should be avoided. Common exceptions to this rule include the addition of antiparkinsonism medications to APM drugs producing EPS and drugs added for the treatment of other medical conditions. Thioridazine, with its own remarkably potent anticholinergic effects, probably should never be used together with antiparkinsonism drugs such as benztropine, trihexyphenidyl, and so forth, because of the possibility of anticholinergic toxicity. The use of two or more APM drugs at the same time has no support in the literature and is not recommended. The use of anxiolytic agents is rarely indicated and if apparent cause arises, one must look for situational problems, requiring counseling and practical help, mild worsening of symptoms of the underlying illness that require an increase in APM, or akathisia.

Patients with schizophrenia, like any persons with chronic debilitating illness, may become depressed. Again, counseling and practical help may be of benefit. An akinetic syndrome, often a late-occurring EPS of APM, must be considered. Treatment by reduction of medications or an increase in antiparkinsonism medication may be strikingly effective. Should the patient develop a full syndrome of endogenous depression, the diagnosis of schizophrenia should be questioned and a diagnosis of affective illness considered. In chronic schizophrenia, treatment with an antidepressant drug is only infrequently necessary or helpful, but such medication can be added to the treatment regimen for persistent or severe symptoms of depression. There is conflicting evidence regarding the effect of antidepressants in schizophrenia, but the patient should be warned about and monitored for the reappearance of symptoms of psychosis. In addition, the sedative, anticholinergic, and other autonomic and cardiac side effects of the tricyclic antidepressants, APM, and antiparkinsonism medication are additive.

Thioridazine, chlorpromazine, or an antiparkinsonism agent should virtually never be used in conjunction with a tricyclic antidepressant, and patients taking such medications should have their therapy switched, if possible, to a high-potency APM and a tricyclic antidepressant alone.

Adjunctive Treatment

Patients with schizophrenia can benefit from a variety of adjunctive treatments designed to maximize their role in society, their enjoyment in life, and their self-esteem on one hand, and to reduce stress, help them cope with their illness, and protect them from the consequences of that illness on the other hand.

Hospitalization should be used as needed. Commonly this happens when the patient is unable to care for himself and there is no one who can adequately help, or when the patient explicitly represents a risk to himself or others. Hospitalization should always be kept as short as possible to prevent the syndrome of complete dependence on the hospital ("institutionalization"). As with many illnesses, but especially those involving thinking and perception, the patient's social and intellectual abilities are compromised during exacerbations of schizophrenia. Thus, during hospitalization (or during relapses in general) the patient's activities and responsibilities should be kept simple. Activities and responsibilities should be increased as improvement allows, with the goal of an early return to as full a social functioning as is feasible.

Most patients with schizophrenia require supportive efforts. As with other patients with chronic, debilitating illness, they require an understanding, active physician ready to serve as a counselor and an expeditor. Often a schizophrenic patient will want and need regular counseling on family, social, and job-related matters. This can be provided by the treating physician or other medical or allied health personnel. There remains no clear evidence, despite multiple studies, that "insight-oriented psychotherapy" is of benefit in schizophrenia.

An evaluation of occupational ability, including a determination of the patient's skills and highest former level of functioning, is important. Job counseling on a continuing basis is often of help, especially as recovery may be slow, incomplete, and marked by occasional relapses.

Just as the patient needs supportive therapy, so the patient's family may need counseling and support. Schizophrenia is an illness that engenders fear, misunderstanding, impatience, and mistrust in the patient, his family, and the community. However, if family members understand the nature and course of the illness, the family can be a major resource in caring for the schizophrenic patient. Family members often feel guilty and embarrassed about the illness, and it is important to address this issue directly. There is no adequate evidence that family members or their behavior is responsible for the production of schizophrenia. The assignment of blame is unwarranted and harmful and, occasionally, malicious. Maladaptive behavior in family members should be approached as maladaptive per se, not as causal of schizophrenia.

Physical and Chemical Injuries

BURNS

method of
WILLIAM W. MONAFO, M.D.
St. Louis, Missouri

Annually in the United States, more than 2,000,000 patients sustain burn injuries severe enough to require medical care. There are about 300 hospital emergency department visits per 100,000 United States population resulting from burns; about 20 of these patients, or about 70,000 per year, are burned so severely that they require hospital admittance.

Etiology

Scalds from hot liquids or steam account for about one third of burn injuries; flames, contact with hot surfaces, and caustic chemicals together cause another third. American dwellings are dangerous places, judging from the fact that 20 to 30 per cent of all burn injuries are sustained there. Including those injuries to housewives, about a third of all burns are job related.

Estimation of Severity

An estimate of the severity of a given burn is important in determining how and where the patient can best be treated and — in extensive injuries — for determination of the prognosis. Age and concomitant significant injury or illness are important co-determinants of outcome.

Depth of Burn

First Degree Burns. Erythema, pain, and tenderness exist. There are no blisters or blebs. These injuries, of which sunburn is the common example, are of no physiologic consequence and require only symptomatic treatment with oral analgesics or with topical ones such as 0.5 per cent dibucaine cream (Nupercainal).

Second Degree Burns. These injuries are subdivided on the basis of the depth of tissue necrosis into superficial and deep ("deep dermal") varieties. *Superficial second degree burns* are characterized by the presence of fluid-filled blebs or blisters and by their exquisite hypersensitivity. These burns heal spontaneously by proliferation of viable epithelial rests, which remain within the dermal appendages. Re-epithelialization is complete within 10 to 20 days. Severe hypertrophic scarring is rare. Minor, patchy depigmentation is often the only permanent residual.

Deep Dermal Burns (Deep Second Degree Burns). Necrosis extends deep into the lower, reticular layer of the dermis, which contains relatively few epithelial rests. Blebs and blisters may be present. These burns are insensate to pain and are usually ivory or off-white in color without demonstrable capillary blood flow. Distinguishing such burns initially from ones that are truly full thickness may be impossible. Spontaneous healing requires 21 to 60 days or even longer. Wound contraction, which may result in limitation of joint motion, and hypertrophic scarring are regular sequelae.

Third Degree (Subdermal, Full Thickness) Burns. The vasculature of the dermis is destroyed. The exposed dermis ("eschar") appears leathery and is inelastic, tending to wrinkle over bony prominences. The burns are insensate. Interstitial hemorrhage is usually present and may impart a red, blue, or green color to the eschar. Thrombosed subcutaneous veins may be visible. Hemoglobinuria may be present when there are extensive full thickness burns. Skin grafting is necessary for permanent wound closure unless the wound is small, in which case it can be allowed to close spontaneously by *contraction,* a process now known to be due to the presence of myofibroblasts, cells containing contractile protein, which proliferate in the granulation tissue in the base of the wound.

Estimating the Extent of Injury

The "rule of nines" is a satisfactory method. In adults, ascribe 9 per cent of the total body surface area (BSA) to the head and neck and to each upper limb; 18 per cent to each lower limb; 18 per cent each to the anterior and posterior aspects of the torso; and 1 per cent to the perineum and genitalia. In infants, the head and neck constitute proportionately more (close to 20 per cent) of the body surface area. To approximate the extent of patchy burns, the area encompassed by the flat of the patient's hand accounts for about 1 per cent of his skin surface.

First Aid at the Scene

Extricate the victim from the heat source, taking care that the rescuers themselves do not incur injury. Record the vital signs and state of consciousness. Ensure the airway. Check for associated injury. In moderate or major burn injuries (see below) start a peripheral, large bore intravenous line through unburned skin if possible and administer lactated Ringer's solution at the rate of 500 to 1000 ml per hour (adults), depending on injury severity, estimated 24 hour fluid needs, and the time that will be required for transportation to a facility where a physician is present. Wrap the patient in a sterile or clean dry sheet. If associated problems, such as fracture or central nervous system trauma, are suspected, appropriate splinting and other precautions designed to minimize additional trauma during transport should be taken (Table 1).

Emergency Department Assessment

Three burn injury severity groups are generally readily discernible:

1. *Minor burns:* Second degree burns of less than 15 per cent of BSA in adults, or less than 10 per cent BSA in children, which do not involve the face, hands, or perineum.

2. *Moderate burns:* Fifteen to 30 per cent BSA in adults, 10 to 20 per cent BSA in children. The third degree component is less than 5 per cent BSA. The hands, face, or perineum are not included.

3. *Severe burns:* Total second and third degree burn area greater than 30 per cent BSA; or third degree burns cover greater than 10 per cent

TABLE 1. Immediate Care of the Severely Burned

1. Complete history and physical examination with special emphasis on the circumstances of injury and any subsequent treatment.
2. Insert a secure, large-bore intravenous catheter, preferably through unburned skin. Begin crystalloid infusion.
3. Insert urinary catheter. Hemoglobinuria suggests the presence of much full-thickness burn.
4. Insert Levin tube; secure in place; empty the stomach.
5. Remove dirt and loose debris from wounds; culture them.
6. Estimate extent and depth of wounds; assess need for escharotomy.
7. Weigh the patient now and daily.
8. Dress the wounds
9. Obtain baseline blood gas and chemical determination; repeat at 12 or 24 hour intervals.
10. Tetanus prophylaxis; penicillin for streptococcal prophylaxis.
11. Analgesia—only if necessary and then intravenously.

BSA; or somewhat smaller burns involving the vital areas; or many electrical or chemical burns of smaller extent (because they tend to be deep).

Those with minor burns can usually be treated as outpatients. Patients with moderate burns in general require hospital admittance. Patients with severe burns are best treated in a specialized center with beds reserved for the care of burn injuries. An organized team of professional and paraprofessional personnel is necessary to provide the necessary spectrum of care to such individuals.

Treatment of Minor Burns

Most such injuries are second degree and therefore tender and painful, because the exposed cutaneous nerve endings are viable. Before manipulating the wounds, allay pain with ice water compresses. An injection of codeine or meperidine may also be necessary.

Cleanse the wounds gently of loose skin, dirt, or debris, using sterile instruments and sterile isotonic saline solution. If there is gross contamination, a surgical soap should be used and thoroughly rinsed away. Puncture intact blisters and trim them away unless, as is sometimes the case on the palms or soles, the blisters are very thick, Apply a sterile occlusive dressing. Properly done, this provides comfort, avoids subsequent bacterial contamination, and maintains involved joints in a functional position. Topical antibiotics or antiseptics are unnecessary in superficial second degree burns and may cause annoying allergic reactions. A layer of petrolatum-impregnated gauze should be placed over the burn. Next, apply absorbent gauze pads, preferably those without a cotton lining, in generous numbers, followed by a thick absorbent pad such as a standard abdominal dressing pad. Complete the dressing with a cotton roll of appropriate width such as Kling or Kerlix or bias cut stockinette. The wrappings should commence distally to avoid undesirable constriction. The most common errors in dressing minor burns are (1) too thin a dressing that becomes saturated with the wound exudate and is thus subject to contamination from without, and (2) improper binding or constricting of the part, which causes pain and/or distal edema.

For previously immunized patients who require a booster, 0.5 ml of tetanus toxoid should be given subcutaneously; in the nonimmune, hyperimmune human antitetanus globulin (TIG), 250 to 500 units, should be given. A course of active immunization should be started simultaneously.

For superficial second degree burns, dressing changes at 4 to 5 day intervals are adequate. The inner components of the old dressing are best soaked away with sterile isotonic saline solution. Bacterial cultures of the wound should be taken if the appearance of the wound warrants it. If infection is judged to have supervened, a topical antibiotic cream such as silver sulfadiazine (Silvadene) or an ointment containing polymyxin B sulfate, neomycin, and bacitracin (Polysporin) can be applied to the wound surface. Infected burns should be dressed at least once daily. Admittance to the hospital for more intensive local treatment may be necessary and should be done promptly if the infection is severe or the patient uncooperative. Topical or systemic oral antibiotics with activity against beta-hemolytic Streptococcus and *Staphylococcus aureus* can be instituted while awaiting the results of the culture, particularly if the unburned skin surrounding the wound displays evidence of cellulitis or lymphangitis.

Patchy second degree burns of the face may be treated without dressings, which are difficult to maintain in satisfactory position, particularly in children. In this instance, one of the aforementioned topical antibiotics is applied once or twice daily after the wound has been cleansed.

Debridement of the eschars of small, deep second degree burns and of full thickness burns may be carried out in stages at the time of the dressing change. Split thickness skin grafts can be applied to small wounds in outpatients as necessary.

Careful follow-up is important in patients with minor burns, which, although they do not endanger life, may cause significant loss of time from work and lead to serious disability if improperly treated. Burns in normally dependent portions must be continuously elevated initially, which means that patients with burns of the feet or lower limbs should not attempt to resume their usual activities. Care must be taken to ensure that normal joint motion is preserved, particularly in the elderly, who may require more frequent observation for this purpose.

Treatment of Moderate and Major Burns

Initial Evaluation and Procedure. Unless there is stridor, cyanosis, inspiratory retraction of thoracic muscle, delirium, coma, or other evidence of acute hypoxia, there is time for a careful and complete history and physical examination. Particular attention should be paid to the circumstances of the accident, because this information may provide the best clue as to depth of injury (clinical criteria for differentiating deep dermal from full thickness burns are gross) and the presence of otherwise unsuspected inhalation injury or of significant associated trauma. Record the extent, location, and estimated depth of the burns on a schematic diagram of the body. In larger injuries it may be more convenient to estimate unburned parts.

Secure intravenous access is essential. If an intravenous line has already been placed, it should be checked for size (18 gauge at least), patency, and the absence of leaks. If no intravenous line exists, one should be inserted either percutaneously or by "cutdown," through unburned skin if possible. The intravenous line need not be placed centrally in the vena cava initially. An indwelling urinary catheter should be inserted. Urine flow, the best single indicator of adequacy of resuscitation, should be measured at hourly intervals after the bladder has been emptied of its initial contents. If the urine is red in color, it should be centrifuged immediately and the sediment examined for the presence of red blood cells, which in large amounts may herald the presence of an associated, hitherto unsuspected injury to the genitourinary tract. Alternatively, the color may be due to hemoglobin or myoglobin pigment, which should be measured quantitatively and which, if present, indicates that there is a large component of full thickness injury.

A large nasogastric tube with a sump attachment should be inserted into the stomach and secured in place and its patency maintained by frequent irrigation, because adynamic ileus and gastric dilatation are common. The risk of aspiration and asphyxia is real, especially in patients who are to be transported. Adynamic ileus is generally over after 48 hours. After baseline determination of arterial blood Po_2, Pco_2, and pH have been drawn with the patient breathing room air, nasal oxygen is routinely administered at 4 liters per minute pending completion of the initial assessment or if the patient is to be transported.

Analgesia. One of the most frequent errors in the initial management of the severely burned is the inappropriate and unnecessary administration of large doses of narcotics or hypnotics by the intramuscular or subcutaneous route to unresuscitated patients. Deeply burned patients have little pain, as the cutaneous nerve endings are destroyed. The second degree components of the burn may cause extreme complaints of pain, however. Patients with extensive painful injuries should be given intravenous morphine or meperidine slowly in small amounts (10 to 15 mg of meperidine, 2 to 3 mg of morphine) until the desired effect is achieved in order to avoid respiratory depression caused by cumulative absorption of previously administered narcotics from erratically perfused peripheral injection sites.

Resuscitation. Extensive burns result in hypovolemic shock that is caused by the spontaneous accumulation of edema in the injured tissue. The rate of edema formation is rapid — the majority of the fluid shift occurring during the first 8 to 12 hours following the injury; during the subsequent 12 to 24 hours, edema continues to form, although at a lesser rate. Subsequently, there is variable resolution of the edema, which may require several weeks, especially in patients over the age of 40.

In general, adults with second and third degree burns with 20 per cent BSA or more and children with somewhat less extensive injuries will require intravenous resuscitation. In many instances, fluid therapy is precautionary, in that, although hemoconcentration, oliguria, and tachycardia exist, the blood pressure remains normal and the sensorium grossly intact. Overt shock may be present at the outset in patients with massive injury or may develop more slowly during the first 4 to 10 hours in patients with smaller injuries who are not provided the necesssary precautionary fluid replacement.

The common denominator in successful resuscitation from actual or impending burn shock is the prompt administration of "crystalloid" (i.e., sodium salt) solution in adequate amounts. Several "formulas" have been proposed which are intended to provide a rough estimate of the volume of crystalloid which will be required, but it must be remembered that considerable variability exists and that the individual response to resuscitation, monitored at hourly intervals or even more frequently, provides the only sure guide to the progress of therapy.

During the first 24 hours after injury, from 2 to 4 ml of crystalloid (lactated Ringer's solution is the most widely used) per kg of body weight per per cent body surface area burned is necessary; about half of this volume is given during the first 8 hours following injury, when the rate of fluid sequestration in the wounds is maximal. Children of less than 20 kg, who have a larger surface area–body weight ratio, may require somewhat more fluid as reckoned on this basis. The monitoring of central venous pressure provides little useful information. In about 10 per cent of cases, usually in the elderly or in patients with a combination of massive burns and severe inhalation injury, we insert a Swan-Ganz catheter into the pulmonary artery for the recording of pulmonary artery and wedged capillary pressures and for the serial determination of cardiac output.

Burn shock is characterized by decreased cardiac output, increased peripheral resistance, increased (and sometimes persistent) pulmonary vascular resistance, decreased renal plasma flow and glomerular filtration rate with accompanying oliguria, and metabolic acidosis that is roughly proportional to the severity of the injury. Blood volume is decreased, but even in the most severe injuries red cell mass is 90 per cent or more of normal. Striking elevations of the hematocrit and the hemoglobin reflect the acute loss of plasma and interstitial water. Measured plasma volume may be as much as 40 to 50 per cent subnormal.

In most patients, resuscitation can be satisfactorily monitored by adjusting the rate of crystalloid infusion as necessary to maintain an hourly rate of urine flow of 30 ml in adults. In children of 20 kg or less, 1 ml per kg per hour is adequate. The systolic blood pressure should be monitored, even if the limbs are burned, using a Doppler ultrasonic probe. A pulse of 110 or less in adults and a stable level of consciousness are also important signs. Restlessness or agitation may denote cerebral hypoxia caused by inadequate resuscitation, associated inhalation injury, or previously unrecognized head injury.

Careful titration of the rate of fluid administration, using the aforementioned criteria, provides adequate volume and so avoids acute renal failure, which is the most common result of inadequate or undue delayed resuscitation, yet minimizes the risks of interstitial pulmonary edema, of cardiac failure, and of unnecessarily augmenting edema in the injured tissues.

The administration of plasma or albumin during the acute phase of resuscitation has largely been abandoned because of the demonstration that these "colloids," which have undesirable side effects and which are costly, do not promote the intravascular retention of water. The leak-rate of colloid-containing solutions from the circulation is identical to that of colloid-free ones during the first 24 hours following injury.

Baseline determinations of arterial Po_2, Pco_2, pH, and lactate and of blood electrolytes, urea, and creatinine, as well as a complete blood count, should be obtained and repeated at 8 to 12 hour intervals as resuscitation progresses. Acidosis may require supplementary administration of sodium bicarbonate. Severe hyperglycemia is not infrequent and may require intravenous insulin. Paradoxically, profound hypoglycemia occasionally occurs in burned infants. Hyperkalemia is not a frequent problem acutely unless renal failure has supervened.

The hematocrit and hemoglobin should *not* be used to gauge the adequacy of resuscitation, as these values typically continue to rise or remain elevated despite a satisfactory clinical course. Similarly, attempts to raise the central venous pressure of the pulmonary capillary wedge pressure from their expected low values into the normal range can result in unnecessary fluid loading.

Escharotomy. Circumferential burns of the limbs may result in a constricting eschar that impedes tissue blood flow, both distally and in the subcutaneous and muscular compartments subjacent to the burn. Normal interstitial pressure is actually slightly negative. It has repeatedly been demonstrated that, following circumferential burns, the tissue pressure may exceed 40 mm of mercury, a point at which capillary blood flow is absent. If the distal part is unburned, peripheral cyanosis, edema, coldness, and paresthesias appear as comparatively late clinical signs. The Doppler ultrasonic probe should routinely be used to monitor the presence of peripheral (including digital) pulses in both burned and unburned areas distal to circumferential burns. We and others now continuously monitor subcutaneous and intramuscular pressures during the first 24 to 48 hours, using a soft wick catheter attached to a pressure transducer. Our present criterion is to perform escharotomy if tissue pressure reaches 40 mm of mercury. Palpable or audible distal pulses are often still present with pressures in the dangerous zone above 20 mm of mercury. The linear escharotomy should be done with aseptic technique along the medial and lateral aspects of the limb, using a scalpel or cutting cautery. Care should be taken not to cross the flexion creases of joints. The incisions should extend proximally for at least 1 inch. The success of escharotomy is signaled by prompt separation of the wound edges, fall in interstitial pressure, and return of previously absent pulses. Careful hemostasis should be secured, as considerable oozing can result. Circumferential or near circumferential burns of the chest and/or abdomen may impair respiratory excursions and also require escharotomy; these should be done in the anterior axillary lines and connected anteriorly across the costal margin and in the infraclavicular area as necessary. Escharotomy is sometimes necessary in very deep thermal burns and is frequently required in high voltage electrical injuries, which induce massive muscle edema.

Carbon Monoxide Poisoning, Inhalation Injury. Acute carbon monoxide poisoning should be suspected in all patients found unconscious at the scene of a fire in a closed space, whether or not they have associated cutaneous burns. If apnea exists, artificial respiration should be carried out until endotracheal intubation can be instituted. The treatment is controlled ventilation, using 100 per cent inspired oxygen and high minute ventilation. Under these circumstances, the half-life of carboxyhemoglobin is 30 minutes to 2 hours. Permanent central nervous system injury can result from protracted hypoxia in severe cases of carbon monoxide poisoning.

The term inhalation injury implies that toxic, gaseous incomplete products of combustion have been inhaled. Formaldehyde, acrolein, and a variety of other toxic aldehydes and acids may be generated, depending on what is being combusted. True thermal injury to the respiratory tract mucosa is rare because of the insulating effect of the humid gas normally present. Carbon monoxide poisoning may coexist. Inhalation injury is a severe complication of burns and raises the mortality probability appreciably. The diagnosis of the presence of inhalation injury should be suspected when the injury has occurred in a closed space, when the burns involve the face and neck and have singed the vibrissae, when there is carbon visible in the pharynx and sputum, and when there is pharyngeal edema and stridor. If the diagnosis of inhalation injury is suspect and particularly if stridor or increasing hoarseness and dyspnea suggest impending occlusion of the upper airway, it is wise to carry out fiberoptic laryngobronchoscopy immediately. This procedure serves to document the degree of edema in the upper airway as well as to visualize the trachea and bronchi, which are inflamed, injected, and/or ulcerated; usually these are visible carbon particles as well. If the endoscopist sees significant edema, it is proper to insert an endotracheal tube at that time, because, especially when there are also extensive burns, airway edema may be expected to increase during the ensuing hours.

It is important to realize that arterial blood gas determinations and chest x-rays may be completely normal on admittance in patients with inhalation injury. Hypoxemia and tachypnea are present from the outset in only the most severe inhalation injuries; rather, these signs typically appear insidiously during the first 12 to 24 hours. When occlusion of the upper airway is the principal problem, endotracheal intubation alone for several days may be all that is necessary. If, however, progressive hypoxemia supervenes, as monitored by serial determination of arterial blood gases, mechanical ventilatory support with increased concentrations of oxygen in the inspired gas mixture may be necessary. A volume controlled ventilator is mandatory. We frequently employ 4 to 8 cm of positive end-expiratory pressure from the outset in patients who require ventilatory support, in an effort to minimize small airways closure. After several days, bacterial infection of the respiratory tree occurs nearly universally, usually by a mixed flora of organisms. Frequent cultures of the tracheal aspirate are taken, and, if the aspirated secretions disclose the presence of pus on Gram stain, systemic antibiotics are given in full dose according to in vitro susceptibility testing. Because the clearance from the blood of antibiotics, particularly aminoglycosides, is often rapid in burned patients, measurements of peak and trough blood antibiotic levels are helpful in adjusting dosage. Recent prospective studies have shown that the administration of corticosteroids, which have been recommended in the past as a means of decreasing the inflammatory response in the respiratory mucosa, is in fact associated with an increased incidence of severe septic complications in patients with coexisting cutaneous burns and inhalation injury.

Weaning from mechanical ventilatory assistance may not be possible for several weeks. Extensive slough of the tracheobronchial mucosa may cause serious problems in the maintenance of airway toilet. Frequent endoscopy may be necessary to adequately clear the airway.

Tracheostomy should not be done routinely or as a precaution, because it carries with it severe complications such as sepsis, tracheal erosion with hemorrhage, tracheoesophageal fistula, or tracheal stenosis. However, tracheostomy may be necessary in patients with inhalation injury, despite its disadvantages because of inability to maintain airway patency owing to voluminous secretions, or because relentlessly worsening hypoxemia dictates the necessity for prolonged mechanical ventilatory assistance. Endotracheal intubation should generally precede formal tracheostomy; depending on the severity and duration of the respiratory complication, it often suffices.

Wound Management. The ischemic nature of burn wounds provides the rationale for treating them topically with agents intended to prevent or suppress bacterial growth, as systemically administered antibiotics would not be expected to reach poorly vascularized wounds in adequate concentration. Normal human skin contains comparatively few bacteria, ones that are ordinarily considered saprophytes, such as *Staphylococcus epidermidis, Bacillus subtilis,* and diphtheroids. But extensive burns frequently become densely colonized with a variety of aerobic gram-negative bacteria and with *Staphylococcus aureus* within 5 to 10 days. Bacterial infection originating in the wound is responsible for more than one half of the deaths from extensive burns.

BACTERIOLOGIC SURVEILLANCE. Systematic bacteriologic surveillance of burn wounds should be performed at least twice weekly, preferably using a technique that permits quantitation as well as speciation of the resident flora. A quantitative culture performed on a homogenized wound biopsy is probably the best method, but is relatively expensive and may be painful. We reserve this for instances in which invasion of infection is thought likely. A bacterial density of 10^5 or greater per gram of tissue is consistent with invasion infection, but clinical correlation is necessary. Lesser densities are frequently observed in patients who are progressing satisfactorily. We routinely use a quantitative gauze-capillarity surface culture technique: a sterile gauze pad of known surface area is placed on the wound for 5 minutes; the bacteria are eluted from it into a broth culture medium of known volume; serial dilutions in pour plates are then made. Consistent bacterial surface densities greater than 10^5 per sq cm may mean that treatment failure is impending, but, as with the biopsy cultures, clinical correlation is necessary.

TOPICAL BACTERIOSTASIS. The current topical antibacterial agent of choice is silver sulfadiazine cream (Silvadene). This drug is reasonably efficacious in patients with moderate injuries, but fails to adequately suppress bacterial growth in many deep burns that exceed 50 per cent BSA. Probably because it is highly insoluble, and therefore poorly absorbed, the drug is relatively nontoxic, although it does exaggerate the leukopenia that occurs during the first 3 to 7 days after injury. Allergic reactions to the sulfadiazine moiety are infrequent and usually can be ignored.

The white cream is applied to the wound surface at the time of the dressing change with a sterile-gloved hand. Meticulous removal of spontaneously separating eschar and the unroofing of subescharotic spaces and of excess cream and other detritus, a process which may require several hours in a patient with extensive burns, are completed before the cream is applied.

We then wrap the wounds in loose-weave, thick cotton dressings that provide comfort, minimize evaporative water loss from the wound, and protect it from further environmental bacterial contamination. The malar areas of the face and the perineum are ordinarily treated without dressings, which are awkward to maintain in those areas. The cotton dressings are conveniently held in place with bias-cut stockinette which serves as an inexpensive elastic bandage and can be laundered and reused if desired.

We avoid immersion hydrotherapy in patients with large open wounds because of the risk of inoculating bacteria from the perineum or from densely colonized local areas of the wound to ones that are sterile or only sparsely colonized.

If the clinical and bacteriologic evidence indicates that invasive wound infection is present, we will substitute topical mafenide cream (Sulfamylon) for the silver sulfadiazine. This sulfonamide, which is readily absorbed and has significant toxicity, owing primarily to its inhibitory effect on the enzyme carbonic anhydrase, is nevertheless useful for short periods, particularly in infections caused by *Pseudomonas aeruginosa*. Acid base imbalance and hyperventilation, its principal toxic effects, can be avoided by applying the drug only to the involved areas and limiting the duration of its use.

During the past several years we have collected clinical evidence suggesting that the modification of silver sulfadiazine by the addition to it of the rare earth metal cerium in the form of its nitrate salt, $Ce(NO3)_3.6 H_2O$, so that the final concentration of cerium is 0.05 molar (2.2 per cent), appreciably increases its efficacy, particularly with respect to the suppression of gramnegative bacteria on the wounds of patients with extensive, ordinarily lethal burns. We have observed a statistically significant improvement in mortality of about 50 per cent compared to that obtained by most observers using silver sulfadiazine alone. The only toxicity attributable to this modification that has been recognized has been methemoglobinemia, which is presumably due to bacterial reduction of the topically applied nitrate. The absorbed nitrite causes conversion of native hemoglobin to methemoglobin. This complication, which has occurred only in patients with burns greater than 65 per cent BSA, is ordinarily rapidly corrected by discontinuing the offending agent. Methemoglobinemia (which can also supervene following the use of topical 0.5 per cent silver nitrate solution) is recognized clinically by the presence of cyanosis or a slate gray hue of the skin in patients with a normal arterial Po_2.

WOUND CLOSURE. Prompt wound closure is the ultimate goal of acute burn care. But the necessary skin grafting procedures, which are traumatic and commonly involve severe blood loss, must be appropriately timed and of such magnitude that they can be tolerated without a significant incidence of perioperative complications. A tentative therapeutic program should be formulated for each hospitalized patient. The following examples outline our approach to the most common categories of injury:

1. *Third degree burns of less than 10 per cent BSA.* These are excised and closed with full thickness skin grafts as soon as is practicable, but generally within the first week following injury, before significant bacterial infection of the wounds has occurred. Except for the extremes of age, the mortality probability in these injuries is low. Most of the morbidity relates to bacterial infection and/or the prolonged convalescence required if the eschar is permitted to separate spontaneously.

2. *Second degree burns, irrespective of extent.* The mortality probability is comparatively low. Treatment is essentially supportive, as spontaneous healing will occur provided that serious infection does not supervene. But, since deep dermal (deep second degree) burns result in considerable hypertrophic scarring and in compromised joint function, such burns, when they involve the hands or face, are not allowed to epithelialize spontaneously, but are instead treated surgically between the fifth and fifteenth days after injury, using the technique of laminar or tangential excision; this procedure involves the sequential shaving away of the superficial layers of devitalized dermis. Using a knife with a calibrated guard (Goulian, Humby), the excision is continued progressively deeper into the dermis until brisk capillary bleeding occurs from the exposed reticular dermis. Hemostasis is secured, sometimes with topical thrombin solution, elevation, and local pressure. The wounds are immediately covered with autologous skin grafts, which, except on the face, are usually first modified by passing them through a "meshing" instrument (Zimmer Company), which delivers a geometric pattern of intercalated incisions onto the sheet of split thickness skin. The skin can then be expanded laterally to a given ratio. On the dorsum of the hands, a 1.5 to 1 expansion ratio is used, which leaves small interstices for the escape of clot, thus

aiding graft take, and gives a satisfactory cosmetic result, or the small interstices of the minimally expanded graft heal rapidly in a few days by epithelial outgrowth.

3. *Extensive (greater than 50 per cent BSA) burns; third degree component greater than 10 per cent BSA; mortality probability 50 per cent or greater.* Injuries such as these require a coordinated approach that permits progressive wound closure with grafting priority being given to functionally and cosmetically important areas. After shock has been treated, a period of 7 to 10 days is allotted during which intensive efforts are made to provide the necessary caloric intake, using tube feedings if necessary. Clinical differentiation of deep dermal from full thickness burns is more accurate after such a delay. Areas of superficial second degree burns are healed or nearly so by now, and if inhalation injury is present, pulmonary function is often improving, or at least stable. Full thickness burns of the back and buttocks, which are functionally of low import, are given last priority.

Full thickness burns of other areas are then sequentially excised and covered immediately with autologous skin, the grafts being meshed and expanded, usually to a 3 to 1 expansion ratio in order to conserve donor sites, which may include the scalp and posterior neck. Each operative procedure is limited to 2 hours in adults and 1 to 1½ hours in small children. The procedures are spaced at 7 to 10 day intervals to allow for the orderly recropping of donor sites when three or more procedures are necessary. Intensive physical therapy and progressive splinting are employed concomitantly. In our hands, the topical use of cerium nitrate–silver sulfadiazine cream has appreciably decreased the incidence of invasive infection originating in the eschars of such full thickness burns. Instead, these eschars remain firm, dry, and conveniently in place until they are electively excised.

Systemic Antibiotics. Fresh burns are prone to infections with beta-hemolytic streptococci. We administer aqueous penicillin for streptococcal prophylaxis during the first 5 days following injury in inpatients and in outpatients with injuries of appreciable size or depth. Bacteremia is known to be frequent in hospitalized burn patients. Blood cultures are obtained frequently, their procurement coinciding with abrupt elevations in body temperature. Persisting or recurrent bacteremia is treated by the administration of an appropriate antibiotic in full dosage based on in vitro susceptibility tests. Perioperatively, we administer systemic antibiotics selected on the basis of the resident wound flora, because surgical manipulation of these contaminated wounds is known to result in transient bacteremia. Some pulmonary infections, particularly in patients with inhalation injury, also require systemic antibiotics. *Prophylactic* systemic antibiotics are not used except as described. Specifically, the mere recovery of microorganisms from the wound surface is not an indication for the administration of systemic antibiotics unless there is unequivocal evidence that invasive wound infection is occurring.

Nutrition. Major burns are characterized by hypermetabolism. Resting metabolic expenditure in patients with burns of greater than 50 per cent BSA may be twice normal. The hypermetabolism is due in part to the increased evaporative water loss that is known to occur through even superficially burned skin. Lipids in the epidermis provide the normal cutaneous barrier to water vapor, so that even superficial injuries result in increasing rates of evaporative water that may approach 10 times normal. At body temperature, 0.58 kcal is required for the evaporation of each ml of water. In addition, catecholamine secretion rates are often markedly elevated. Finally, sepsis itself, a common complication in the burn patient, is known to provoke hypermetabolism.

Nutritional support is essential for the management of the burn patient. Lacking this, wound healing will slow, host defense mechanisms, particularly those involving neutrophil and lymphocyte function will be suppressed, and the probability of lethal infection will increase.

In addition to basal caloric needs, burned patients require approximately 40 kcal per day per per cent burn.

We have found that the negative nitrogen balance that characterizes the catabolic state of the burn patient can be satisfactorily met by using hen's eggs as a protein source. We give up to 36 eggs per day in adults with extensive burns, administering them by nasogastric feeding tube if necesssary (6 grams of high quality protein per egg). Powdered rice, a caloric source of low osmolality, is a convenient way to provide additional carbohydrate through feeding tubes. We attempt to meet the estimated caloric requirement within 96 hours following injury. It is essential that the importance of the nutritional state be carefully explained to the patients, many of whom will spontaneously ingest 50 or 60 calories per kg per day without the necessity for tube supplements. Intravenous hyperalimentation carries increased septic risks in burn patients because catheter access sites are often burned. If intravenous hyperalimentation is used, the central catheters should be rotated at 72 hour intervals.

DISTURBANCES DUE TO COLD

method of
CAMERON C. BANGS, M.D.
Oregon City, Oregon

HYPOTHERMIA

Importance and Incidence

In the past few years there has been a definite increase in the severity of winter weather in the United States. This fact, coupled with the increased use of the wilderness for winter recreation, has skyrocketed the number of cold weather injuries being treated medically. In the United States there are no statistics as to the incidence, but in England, where hypothermia is probably more common and definitely more appreciated, it is estimated that there are 20,000 to 100,000 cases annually. In one study, 11.4 per cent of elderly British people living alone at home were found to have body temperatures of 35 C (95.0 F) or below. Prior to the development of our modern techniques for managing hypothermia, the mortality rate for severe hypothermia ranged as high as 85 per cent. With the development of improved therapy, the mortality rate should be nearly negligible.

Pathophysiology

Human beings are warm weather animals, having evolved in the tropics and neither tolerating the cold well nor, with rare exceptions, adapting to it well. Until they developed a microclimate (clothing, shelter) to keep skin temperatures close to 32.8 (91.0 F), they could not survive at temperatures much below 21 C (70 F).

Our body temperature is controlled by a "thermostat" located in the hypothalamus. The thermostat is responsive to as little as 0.5 C change in blood temperature and is responsive to the nerve impulses it receives from the temperature-sensitive nerve endings in the skin. When the body is influenced by either a heat or a cold stress, the hypothalamus responds in either of two general ways, by increasing or decreasing heat production or by increasing or decreasing heat losses.

As we sit comfortably at basal metabolic rate we are producing approximately 50 kcal per square meter of body surface, or roughly 100 kcal per hour for the average-sized person. Under maximal cold stimulation, we have the ability to increase heat production approximately five-fold by shivering, or roughly 500 kcal per hour. This maximal heat production can last but a few hours and then, owing to glycogen depletion and fatigue, it tapers off to a lower level. There is a significant individual variation in ability to shiver, with one study showing that one third of persons were deficient in ability to shiver intensely. Because of increased shunting of warm blood to the extremities during shivering, the body's natural insulation is decreased about 25 per cent. Shivering is suppressed by many factors, including hypoglycemia, hypoxia, fatigue, voluntary muscle activity, and intense mental concentration. Shivering is also suppressed by drugs, particularly phenothiazines, barbiturates, and, under some circumstances, alcohol. The major physiologic defense against cold stress is to prevent heat loss by doubling the peripheral insulation through peripheral vasoconstriction.

In animals adapted to the cold, the major defense against cold stress is to greatly increase the natural insulation. The arctic fox, for example, can tolerate temperatures to −34 C (−30 F) without having to increase heat production to stay warm. Nude persons can tolerate temperatures only to 21 C (70 F) before having to increase heat production to stay warm. The human's major defense against the cold is an intelligent ability to increase the temperature of the microclimate through the use of shelters or clothing.

The major (60 to 65 per cent) route for heat loss is via radiation. About 85 per cent of our body surface is available for heat loss via this mechanism, but this surface area can be reduced somewhat by assuming a compact position. Evaporation accounts for 20 per cent of heat loss, with two thirds coming from the skin and one third from respiration. Convective air currents aid in the loss of heat to an extremely variable degree. Normally we lose very little heat via direct contact or conduction, but in most survival situations conductive heat loss is increased through direct contact with ground, snow, ice, or water.

Subdivision of Cases

For practical purposes hypothermic victims can be divided into those with core temperatures above 32 C (90 F) and those with core temperatures below. This arbitrary division is convenient for treatment purposes because those with temperatures above 32 C (90 F) have favorable mortality rates and require less intense therapy. Those with temperatures below 32 C (90 F) require very careful medical management or an appreciable mortality rate will occur.

The arbitrary division at this level is of value for clinical evaluation also. Patients with temperatures above 32 C (90 F) may be lethargic and slow mentally, but for the most part they should be generally oriented and have no marked mental derangement. Their movements may be stiff and somewhat uncoordinated, but they should still be able to function with some meaningful ability. Those with temperatures below 32 C (90 F) will be disoriented, confused, and very lethargic, and as the temperature falls toward 29.4 C (85 F), stupor or coma may develop. In several patients we have observed a peculiar affect in which the patient appeared puzzled and confused, but acted as if this were almost voluntary. Severe hypothermic patients will be extremely uncoordinated and unable to perform any meaningful physical task; they may be quite stiff, with muscle rigidity simulating rigor mortis. In extreme hypothermia — core temperatures below 26.6 C (80 F) — death may be mimicked. These patients will be totally unresponsive, with no obvious vital signs, and will appear as if rigor mortis had set in. It is extremely important that these people not be pronounced dead prematurely, as warming and resuscitation may still be effective. Follow the adage that no person is dead until he is warmed and dead.

In taking the core temperature it is, of course, extremely important to use low recording clinical thermometers (available from ZEHL, 8 Lombard Street, London) or battery-operated thermocouples, e.g., "Yellow Springs." Taking deep rectal or esophageal temperatures is preferred to oral temperatures.

Clinical Presentation

It is important to appreciate that it is not necessary to be lost in the snow for several days to acquire accidental hypothermia. In fact, the majority of instances occur in cities among elderly persons and frequently when the temperature is above freezing, as in poorly heated or unheated dwellings. Alcoholism is probably the most common associated factor, more because of the resulting altered sensorium and judgment than because of its pharmacologic effects. Associated medical disorders, include diabetic ketoacidosis, myxedema, old age, and general debilitation secondary to chronic diseases such as malignancy. Erythematous skin diseases that increase heat loss may result in hypothermia. Trauma, particularly head trauma or that associated with blood loss and shock syndrome, enhances the onset of hypothermia.

Laboratory Assessment

1. *Arterial blood gases.* These should be determined immediately and followed carefully as the patient rewarms. Po_2 is usually depressed and Pco_2 elevated, and pH is invariably decreased. The pH should be corrected to temperature by adding 0.0147 pH unit for each degree Celsius below 37 C.

2. *Complete blood count (CBC).* Hematocrit and hemoglobin levels are usually elevated secondary to hemoconcentration. Platelet counts may be depressed secondary to sequestration and will return to normal on rewarming. White blood cell counts are variable, frequently elevated. Bicarbonate, O_2 saturation, and total CO_2 should then be recalculated, using the corrected pH. Blood viscosity is elevated.

3. *Blood sugar levels.* These may be elevated in the 200 to 400 mg per 100 ml range, presumably owing to inactivation of insulin by low temperatures. Occasionally hypoglycemia results from decreased glucogenesis and glycogen depletion secondary to shivering.

4. *Serum potassium concentration.* This is generally normal at the onset of therapy but may rise to dangerous levels because of influx from peripherally damaged tissues. Potassium level should be followed closely during the rewarming.

5. *Serum enzymes.* Concentrations of serum glutamic oxaloacetic transaminase (SGOT) and creatine phosphokinase (CPK) are frequently elevated to a marked degree secondary to tissue destruction, particularly if frostbite is present.

6. *Electrocardiogram.* The patient should be on continuous cardiac monitoring and a baseline 12-lead cardiogram obtained. The initial electrocardiogram (ECG) may be of poor quality because of muscle tremor. It should be repeated during the rewarming.

7. *Chest x-ray.* This is important early in the treatment owing to the frequent pulmonary complications, particularly pneumonia.

Treatment

Mild Hypothermia (Core Temperatures Above 32 C [90 F])

General Principles. This group should have a favorable prognosis. It is important to look for associated metabolic illness and trauma, particularly frostbite. Further hypothermia should be guarded against by getting the patient into dry clothing, out of the wind, and well insulated against cold.

Specific Therapy. The aforementioned baseline blood studies should be obtained, an intravenous line established, and cardiac monitoring started. If there are no cardiac contraindications, intravenous volume expansion is started with crystalloid solution, such as 5 per cent dextrose in lactated Ringer's or saline solution. Most cardiac arrhythmias do not require specific treatment, as they will subside with rewarming.

Techniques of Rewarming. These mildly hypothermic patients may be rewarmed externally. The most effective application of heat is to the three areas of the body least insulated from the core, which includes the inguinal area, the lateral chest, and the head and neck. The use of heated humidified oxygen (see discussion later in this article) is a good adjunct to rewarming.

Severe Hypothermia (Core Temperatures Below 32 C [90 F])

General Principles. This should be considered to be a medical emergency and patients treated properly and carefully or rewarming fatalities may occur. Because of the lack of well-controlled clinical studies, there remains some controversy as to the rate and technique of rewarming. The method discussed below is certainly not the only technique available. It has been used extensively with good results and can be done in any hospital by most physicians. The rewarming is best carried out by a team, including a respiratory therapist, acute care nurses, several orderlies, and several physicians, with one physician acting as overall supervisor. A prearranged protocol is of great value.

A thorough initial evaluation is done to rule out associated medical problems, keeping in mind the frequently associated metabolic disorders of trauma and frostbite. The baseline blood studies are done, an intravenous line is established, and cardiac monitoring is started.

Volume Expansion. Rapid intravenous volume expansion using crystalloid solution is perhaps the single most important modality of management. This should be started in the field by paramedical personnel prior to transportation. Five per cent dextrose in lactated Ringer's or saline solution is the preferred solution. Three hundred milliliters should be given as rapidly as possible, and the remaining part of the liter given during the first hour. This should be followed by another liter, with the rate adjusted to the patient's condition. The solution should be at least at room temperature but may be warmed to 37.7 C (100 F). The amount of heat supplied by 1 liter of warmed solution is not great enough to warrant such inconvenience or delay in volume expansion.

The intravenous volume expansion is felt to prevent "rewarming shock," occurring because of core temperature afterdrop and hypovolemic hypotension secondary to fluid shifts during rewarming.

Cardiac Arrhythmias. The patient should be on continual cardiac monitoring, and a baseline 12-lead electrocardiogram obtained. In general, most cardiac arrhythmias subside with the rewarming and do not require therapy. Atrial fibrillation will convert spontaneously to sinus rhythm as core temperature approaches normal, or shortly thereafter. It is rare that antiarrhythmic agents or electrocardioversion is necessary. The bradycardia of hypothermia is physiologic, and it may be dangerous to increase the rate artificially. If the rate is increased with drugs or electrical pacing, the oxygen demands of the myocardium may be increased to a greater extent that the hypothermic patient's circulation can supply. Isoproterenol is contraindicated because of its fibrillogenicity. Frequent premature ventricular contractions, particularly those occurring near the T wave, have been treated safely with lidocaine.

The ventricular fibrillation threshold is lowered with hypothermia, and trauma to the heart should be avoided. Cardiac catheterization and temporary pacemaker wires do carry increased risk and in general should be avoided. Swan-Ganz catheters are of less danger and may be indicated, but usually the patient can be managed without them. Central venous pressure monitoring may be useful. If ventricular fibrillation does occur, it should be managed in the usual manner, but the patient will usually not convert to sinus rhythm until core temperature is well above 32 C (90 F). Cardiopulmonary resuscitation (CPR) should be continued while the patient is being rewarmed. With fibrillation, rewarming is slowed because of decreased circulation, and extreme measures, such as total body immersion in water to 43.3 C (110 F), may be necessary. Monitoring and CPR are obviously difficult to carry out with a patient submerged in water.

Acidosis. There is some evidence that rapid correction of the acidosis may result in ventricular fibrillation. In most circumstances acidosis will correct itself during rewarming and it is unnecessary to give intravenous sodium bicarbonate. Our general principle is to obtain a baseline pH and repeat pH measurements as the temperature starts to rise; only if there is no improvement in the pH is bicarbonate administered.

Management of the Airway. Endotracheal intubation has been shown to cause ventricular fibrillation and should be avoided or undertaken very cautiously. With pure hypothermia the airway can generally be managed without intubation. If intubation is necessary it should be done carefully by a skilled anesthesiologist, and even in the comatose patient the airway should be anesthetized to avoid reflexes that could lead to ventricular fibrillation. Hyperventilating the victim is believed also to lead to ventricular fibrillation and should be avoided. These patients are hypoxic, and 100 per cent oxygen is indicated.

Techniques of Rewarming. GENERAL PRINCIPLES. If the victim is warmed externally, peripheral vasodilatation will occur, shunting cold blood back to the core. This may result in a core afterdrop of up to 3 C. Because of this rapid influx of cold blood to the heart, the conducting system of the endocardium may be cooled more than the myocardium, causing conduction disturbances, particularly ventricular fibrillation. The shunting of core blood to the periphery in an already volume-depleted circulatory system may result in hypovolemic rewarming shock. For these reasons, external rewarming is generally to be avoided. (It should be noted, however, that some centers are successfully utilizing this meth-

od.) By rewarming the core initially the aforementioned problems are avoided.

PERITONEAL DIALYSIS. A rapid and readily available technique of core rewarming is use of heated peritoneal dialysis (Fig. 1). One trocar may be inserted in the usual manner and heated dialysate infused and then drained through the same trocar. A more effective method is to insert two trocars, one into each lateral gutter. Heated fluid is infused through one trocar and removed via the other. Commercially available dialysate fluid (5 per cent dextrose) is used starting with potassium-free solution and adding potassium as indicated. In addition to supplying heat to the core, the alkaline solution will assist in correcting the acidosis.

The temperature of the solution entering the peritoneal cavity should be 37.7 C (100 F) and never exceeding 45 C (112 F). The solution may be warmed in a water bath or circulated through a 44 foot blood rewarming core submerged in water between 48.8 and 54.4 C (120 to 130 F). Temperature of the solution may be measured simply by detaching the plastic adapter near the

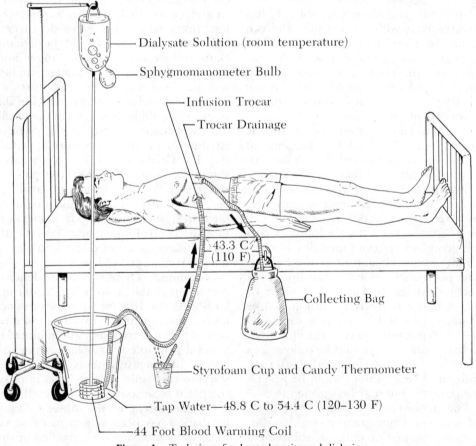

— Dialysate Solution (room temperature)

— Sphygmomanometer Bulb

— Infusion Trocar

— Trocar Drainage

43.3 C (110 F)

—Collecting Bag

—Styrofoam Cup and Candy Thermometer

— Tap Water—48.8 C to 54.4 C (120–130 F)

—44 Foot Blood Warming Coil

Figure 1. Technique for heated peritoneal dialysis.

trocar and running the solution into a Styrofoam coffee cup and checking it with a candy thermometer. Owing to the resistance of the blood warming core, the flow will be very slow unless pressure is increased in the hanging dialysate fluid by pumping air into the bottle using a bulb from a sphygmomanometer. Using this technique 2 liters of dialysate fluid may be infused in 10 to 15 minutes, and if two trocars are used a continuous flow can be provided.

The core temperature will rise 8.5 C (15 F) within 1 or 2 hours, requiring 10 to 20 liters of dialysate. The core temperature will usually rise rapidly during the early rewarming and then more slowly as the core temperature approaches 34 to 36 C (93 to 97 F). We generally stop rewarming when core temperature reaches 96 F (35.5 C) to avoid overshooting.

HEATED HUMIDIFIED OXYGEN. A good adjunct to core rewarming is provided by heated humidifed oxygen. Although the amount of calories delivered is relatively small, the heat is delivered directly to the core through the lungs. This technique is extremely safe and is being increasingly utilized as an early prehospital treatment for immersion hypothermia by the United States Coast Guard. One thoretical hazard may exist because the drive to respiration in hypothermic patients is hypoxia rather than hypercapnia, and this theoretically could be abolished with 100 per cent oxygen.

Heated humidified oxygen is produced by utilizing any Cascade humidifier, readily available in most respiratory therapy departments. Both heat and oxygen can be conserved by recycling through soda lime (see Fig. 2). The tubing between the humidifier and the patient's mask should be as short as possible to avoid heat loss and water condensation. Water condensation is a definite problem, and the mask should be higher than the humidifier to avoid water aspiration. A thermometer at the mask is necessary to avoid exceeding 46.1 C (115 F). Oxygen is most effective if delivered at 46.1 C (115 F). At this temperature, no evidence of tracheal irritation has been observed.

Patients tolerate the heated humidified oxygen readily until the core temperature reaches 35 C (95 F). If necessary, ventilation is easily assisted through manual compression of the bag. Using the soda lime recycler, 100 per cent oxygen will be delivered by an oxygen flow rate of about 2 liters per minute.

EXTRACORPOREAL CIRCULATION. A most rapid and successful technique of rewarming is through the use of extracorporeal circulation, in which blood is removed, rewarmed through a heart-lung machine, and then recycled. This technique is unfortunately available only at centers routinely doing open heart surgery.

AFTERCARE. After the patient has been rewarmed, he or she should regain normal mentation. If this does not ocur, other causes should be sought. Temperatures should be monitored for 24 hours, but rarely does the patient fail to maintain normal temperature. Fevers following hypothermia are usually associated with other illnesses, particularly pneumonia. Pneumonia has been reported as the most common cause of death following hypothermia and should be carefully watched for through periodic examinations and chest x-rays. Prophylatic antibiotics may be indicated. Other diseases frequently associated with hypothermia, as mentioned previously, should be ruled out.

The rewarmed patient generally requires at least 48 hours of hospitalization for nutritional and volume stability.

FROSTBITE

Frostbite is simply defined as ice crystal formation within tissue. It occurs primarily in humans (rather than animals) secondary to cold-induced intense vasoconstriction in the extremities, which decreases peripheral heat flow. It is generally confined to the hands and feet, rarely occurring in the ears and other tissues. Subfreezing temperatures are required for its occurrence, and the exact incidence is unknown. It can cause small loss of tissue or loss of entire appendages. Even minor frostbite leaves a lifelong decreased tolerance to cold. Experience in military populations shows that more frostbite occurs in the upper extremities than in the lower, but in civilian practice it is much more common in the feet and toes.

Clinical Presentation

The most common description of frostbite by patients is that their extremities become cold, and then painful, with the pain gradually changing to numbness, causing the extremities to feel club-like. There is individual variation, with some victims never suffering much pain and others never having their pain subside. When pain loss or numbness is present, it frequently is replaced by extreme pain during the thawing process. Again there is individual variation, with some finding the thawing process relatively painless.

The appearance of the frostbitten area varies with the severity and duration of exposure. While still frozen, the extremity may be pale or violaceous and feel hard as wood and frozen. It is important to realize that even severely frostbitten

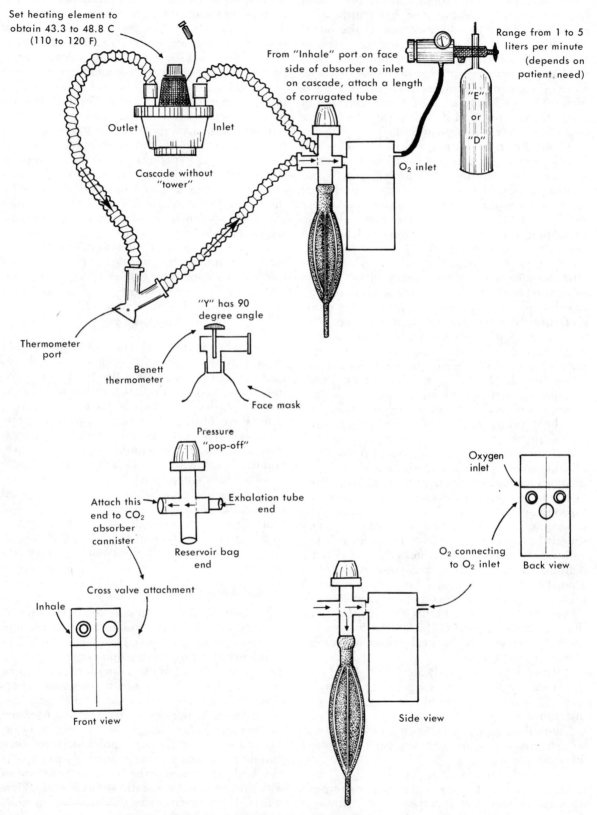

Set heating element to
obtain 43.3 to 48.8 C
(110 to 120 F)

From "Inhale" port on face
side of absorber to inlet
on cascade, attach a length
of corrugated tube

Range from 1 to 5
liters per minute
(depends on
patient need)

Outlet   Inlet

Cascade without
"tower"

O_2 inlet

"E"
or
"D"

Thermometer
port

"Y" has 90
degree angle

Benett
thermometer

Face mask

Pressure
"pop-off"

Attach this
end to CO_2
absorber
cannister

Exhalation tube
end

Reservoir bag
end

Cross valve attachment

Inhale

Front view

Oxygen
inlet

O_2 connecting
to O_2 inlet

Back view

Side view

Figure 2.   Technique for heated humidified oxygen.

tissue may initially appear relatively normal and undramatic.

Within 12 hours of thawing, the extremity will be red or violaceous, and if the skin blanches at all, color will return very slowly. Swelling may be mild or may be severe enough to impair circulation. With more severe frostbite, blistering will occur, which usually is more severe distally. Blisters may be clear or red and dark owing to hemorrhage. Hemorrhagic blisters carry a poorer prognosis.

As the weeks go by, black eschar forms, usually distal to the initial superficial skin changes, and a definite line of demarcation will become apparent. Without infection, the injury remains dry, but with infection moisture and exudate will appear.

Evaluation

Determining the severity of frostbite when it is seen initially remains an inexact science. Appearance may be misleading, because the skin changes do not reflect the underlying vascular damage. If freezing is severe, the occluded vessels may not provide enough flow to allow blister formation, resulting in a less dramatic initial appearance.

Trying to evaluate the duration and degree of cold exposure is unreliable because of many variables, including ambient temperature, wind chill factor, moisture, and insulation, as well as the multiple factors that influence heat flow to the injured part, such as constricting boots or garments, cigarette smoking, and individual vasospasticity. Some help in determining severity may be obtained through angiography, nuclear scanning and uptake, x-rays, and thermography. Recently plethysmography has been used effectively to evaluate circulatory status. Muscle enzyme levels will be elevated, with creatine phosphokinase (CPK) level above 1000 mg per 100 ml. There is a crude correlation between level of CPK and tissue damage.

Therapy

Rapid Thaw. The definitive treatment for frostbite remains somewhat controversial and unsettled because of the inability to compare cases. There is little controversy over the advantage of rapid thaw. It is believed that less tissue morbidity results when the extremity goes through the thawing process rapidly.*

Rapid thawing is carried out by immersion in hot water with temperatures ranging from 37.8 to 43.3 C (100 to 110 F), not to exceed 44.4 C (112 F). This should be done in large vessels of water

---

*Note: If the frostbite has thawed before being examined, do not immerse the extremity in hot water.

with the temperature monitored by a thermometer. The temperature of the water will fall rapidly, and hotter water will have to be added from time to time. The water should be circulated either manually or mechanically, and the extremities should not be traumatized by the vessel wall. The involved extremity should remain submerged until it is clinically thawed, being pliable and having good skin circulation, which generally requires 30 to 60 minutes.

Nonsterile water is adequate but once the extremity is thawed, treatment should be as aseptic as possible.

Early Medications. Although no well-controlled human clinical studies are available comparing the advantages of early medication, there are animal studies and clinical observations to support the use of some medications immediately after thawing. The general principle of early medication is to prevent or diminish the previously described complications of arterial spasm and vascular coagulation.

Intra-Arterial Reserpine. Administration of intra-arterial reserpine depletes the myoneural end plates of norepinephrine, resulting in a "medical sympathectomy" and arterial dilatation. Intra-arterial injection of 0.5 mg proximal to the lesion is done using the femoral arteries for the lower extremity and the brachial or radial artery for the upper extremity (this use of reserpine is not listed in the manufacturer's official directive). This should be administered as close to thawing as possible and repeated every several days for 2 to 3 weeks

This modality is particularly effective in relieving the symptoms of minor frostbite when seen several days after the injury. It should be repeated once or twice at weekly intervals. Immediately after injection, a local warm flush must be experienced to verify actual arterial injection.

Phenoxybenzamine. This drug is a long-acting adrenergic blocking agent that also causes a "medical sympathectomy." It is given orally in doses of 10 to 60 mg daily, and its effects can be monitored by partial thromboplastin time (PTT). There are clinical impressions that it reduces morbidity in cases of acute frostbite and may be useful chronically to reduce vasospastic symptoms.

Antiplatelet Drugs. Heparin and dextran have been shown in animal experiments to decrease tissue loss from frostbite and these also should be started with the thawing process. Heparin can be administered as an initial dose of 5000 units and continued as an intravenous infusion of 1000 units per hour with the results being followed by PTT determinations. Low molecular weight dextran is given as an intravenous infusion of 500 ml, repeated daily for the first week or two (this use of these agents is not listed in the manufacturers' official directives).

After Thawing

Sterile Technique. Because of the danger of infection it is believed that a sterile environment is indicated for several weeks until the infectious period is past. This is particularly important when large areas of frostbite are present. Sterile technique is carried out, using sterile bed sheets with a blanket cradle to protect the extremity. The person is placed in protective isolation. When the frostbitten area is handled the personnel should wear sterile cap, gown, and gloves. After several weeks, when the extremities are well demarcated and dry, sterile technique may be abandoned.

Whirlpool Bath. Whirlpool baths twice daily with tap water in antiseptic solution such as hexacholorophene in a stable emulsion (pHisoHex) or povidone and iodine (Betadine) greatly decrease the chance of infection, aid in the debridement, and decrease discomfort. These should use tepid water of 37.8 C (100 F). During the whirlpooling, the extremities should undergo active physical therapy of moving the toes, fingers, and feet.

Antibiotics. Antibiotics are not indicated prophylactially, but if infection occurs, they should be used according to culture results.

Amputation. It is becoming more and more clear that early amputation is contraindicated, and no amputation should be carried out until it is obvious that nonviable tissue is present. Frequently the overlying eschar may be superficial, with viable tissue beneath. Under most circumstances 8 weeks is the absolute minimum before amputation is considered. Sometimes 6 to 8 months should elapse before amputation is undertaken.

Fasciotomies. There is some evidence that subcutaneous fasciotomies will increase tissue blood flow, therefore decreasing tissue loss. They should be carried out only in extremely swollen extremities and done as soon as marked swelling occurs.

Coexisting Hypothermia. When severe hypothermia and frostbite coexist, both entities probably are best treated by leaving the extremities frozen until the core temperature approaches normal; then rapid thawing of frostbite and use of medications are instituted.

General Principles. Cigarette smoking should not be allowed owing to its vasoconstrictive effect. Alcohol and marijuana have not been shown to be harmful in the postfrostbite period. All efforts should be made to provide the patient with a pleasant environment, and visitors should be allowed, but during the early phase they should be dressed for protective sterility. With severe frostbite, the extremities should not be used. If the damage is to the feet, walking should be avoided; if the hands are involved, the patient may have to be fed and assisted with general care.

After Hospital Care. Patients should be reminded that they will always be more susceptible to cold owing to continued vasoconstriction, and if at all possible they should avoid further cold stress. It is not necessary for them to remain hospitalized during the entire demarcating process, but after discharge, the extremity should be protected from the clothing and excessive use avoided.

Minor Frostbite

The most common cold injury seen by a physician will be minor frostbite. Frequently the physician will be contacted several days after the injury with the complaint that the digits are numb or painful.

On examination there may be minor skin changes or discoloration, small blisters, or even some minor eschar formation. Generally the major pulses are palpable, but capillary filling may be delayed. These people can be treated as outpatients by soaking their digits in tepid water at 37.8 C (100 F) with added antiseptic solution for 20 to 30 minutes three times a day. While soaking the digits the patient should wiggle them actively. Patients should avoid cigarette smoking and prolonged use of the extremity. These victims have been found to benefit greatly from intra-arterial reserpine injections (this use of reserpine is not listed in the manufacturer's official directive). Their symptoms may subside immediately after the injection, and frequently one injection is adequate. The majority of changes will subside in about 8 weeks, but decreased tolerance to cold may last several years or longer. Wintertime use of phenoxybenzamine has been shown to decrease cold intolerance.

DISTURBANCES DUE TO HEAT

method of
JOHN F. RYAN, M.D.
Boston, Massachusetts

Patients who present with excessive heat storage abnormalities can be classified into three categories: (1) heat cramps, (2) heat exhaustion, and (3) heat stroke. A differential diagnosis is made by symptoms. Heat cramps are the mildest form of the hyperthermic syndrome. Increased disturbances lead to a diagnosis of heat exhaustion, whereas the most severe situation is heat stroke. All are stages of the same heat storage dysfunction.

Heat cramps are characterized by localized muscle cramping. The treatment consists of rest in a cool environment and electrolyte determination and replacement either orally or parenterally, depending on whether the patient is vomiting.

Heat exhaustion is accompanied by water depletion and hypovolemia. The symptoms are severe headache, lassitude, vomiting, tachycardia, and hypotension. Treatment is similar to that of heat cramps, i.e., rehydration and rest.

Heat stroke is a medical emergency. The mortality of heat stroke has been reported as ranging from 17 to 70 per cent. It is recognizable by three signs: (1) neurologic abnormalities, (2) hyperthermia, and (3) hot dry skin, either pink or ashen in hue.

Rectal temperature has been reported usually in excess of 41 C (105 F). Core temperature is higher. Sweating is frequently, but not always, absent. Consumption coagulopathy associated with petechiae and gross hemorrhage has been reported.

Central nervous system symptoms are initially those of headache, dizziness, and confusion. These are followed by coma associated on occasion with such findings as convulsions, hemiplegia, decorticate posturing, or fecal incontinence. In fatal cases, cerebral edema has been present at autopsy.

High fever appears related to increased heat storage in the body caused by decreased radiation and convection related to a high ambient temperature. Evaporation by sweating is usually reduced also owing to a high relative humidity.

The hot dry skin owes its variation in color to peripheral perfusion. Pink color is present when perfusion through skin and skeletal muscle is increased. Ashen color usually represents low cardiac output and hypotension.

Treatment of heat stroke is aimed at reducing body temperature, maintaining or restoring a high cardiac output, and correcting any electrolyte derangement present.

Clothing should be removed, and an intravenous line, a central venous catheter, and a Foley catheter inserted. An electrocardiogram and suitable pulse detector (precordial stethoscope) should be monitored continuously. If the patient is unconscious, an arterial blood sample should be drawn. Oxygen administration, endotracheal intubation, and ventilation may be indicated by the clinical situation or by the hypoxemia and/or hypoventilation noted in the arterial blood.

Cooling can be accomplished by administration of previously refrigerated Ringer's lactate and by ice bath immersion. Once the temperature is lowered to 38 C (100 F), cooling measures should be terminated to prevent inadvertent hypothermia. Rehydration will be accompanied by increased urinary output. If anuria occurs and persists despite hydration, electrolyte correction, and diuretic administration, then early dialysis should be considered.

A recently noted complication of anesthesia, malignant hyperthermia, is characterized by tachycardia, tachypnea, and dark blood in the surgical field; arrhythmias are common. Rigidity may follow succinylcholine administration during intubation, or it may or may not occur later in the syndrome. Fever is usually a later sign and commonly rises rapidly to 43 to 45 C (110 to 113 F). It is most important to stress the need for noting and diagnosing any unexplained sharp rise in pulse rate during anesthesia, especially when the more common causes of tachycardia are not present or have been eliminated from the differential diagnosis. The mortality rate is 58 per cent. Malignant hyperthermia occurs suddenly and unexpectedly, usually during an otherwise uneventful anesthesia and surgery. The cause appears to be related to an inability of calcium transfer from the sarcoplasm of muscle to its primary storage area, the sarcoplasmic reticulum. The increasing calcium concentration in muscle leads to a marked increase in aerobic and later anaerobic metabolism, causing a severe respiratory and metabolic acidosis. Later cellular membrane integrity is impaired, leading to hyperkalemia and high plasma levels of intracellular muscle constituents.

Treatment consists of stopping the anesthetic, administering 100 per cent oxygen, hyperventilation, administering dantrolene sodium (1 to 10 mg per kg by rapid intravenous infusion over 5 to 10 minute intervals) (this use of dantrolene sodium is not listed in the manufacturer's official directive), correcting the acidosis, treating the hyperkalemia, cooling, procainamide therapy (an intravenous infusion of 15 mg per kg administered over 10 to 15 minutes is suggested), and maintaining urine output. Dantrolene sodium has been uniformly successful in treating this syndrome. Side effects of rapid intravenous infusion are a 5 to 10 per cent increase in pulse rate and cardiac output. Procainamide is still recommended for its antiarrhythmic properties. Indices to be monitored include electrocardiogram, temperature, and the use of a Foley catheter, arterial line, and central venous pressure line. Complications have been reported as consumption coagulopathy, renal failure, inadvertent hypothermia, pulmonary edema, hyperkalemia, muscle necrosis, and neurologic sequelae.

SPIDER BITES AND SCORPION STINGS

method of
JAMES A. ROLLER, M.D.
Hannibal, Missouri

Of the many spider species found in the United States, only a few cause harm to humans. The bites of orb weavers, jumping spiders, wandering spiders, running spiders, and wolf spiders may result in local edema, erythema, vesiculation, and pain. Ecchymosis, lymphadenopathy, and ulceration may occur infrequently. These bites should be treated with analgesics as required, cool soaks, soothing lotions, and reassurance. Secondary infection following a spider bite is uncommon, and routine antibiotics are unwarranted. Precautionary warning to the patient, however, is wise; tetanus prophylaxis should be administered following any bite.

The two spiders of greatest medical importance in the United States are *Loxosceles reclusa* (the brown recluse spider) and *Latrodectus mactans* (the black widow spider). Envenomation by either species may result in disability and rarely death.

Brown Recluse Spider

Loxosceles reclusa bites are most common in the south-central United States, but elsewhere bites of several other Loxosceles species can result in typical clinical findings of the brown recluse bite.

Investigation of brown recluse venom is being carried out, but the causes of severe systemic complications are as yet unclear. Evidence suggests that autopharmacologic reactions may be involved.

Brown recluse bites are usually unremarkable, resulting in mild clinical findings which cannot be distinguished from those of other spider bites. Uncommonly, however, Loxosceles envenomation may cause the recognizable, well-demarcated, cyanotic macule, followed by eschar formation and ulceration. Hemolysis resulting in hemoglobinuria, myoglobinuria, and acute renal failure, as well as disseminated intravascular coagulation, are the most serious systemic complications of loxoscelism. Children are at particular risk of developing these complications, but death is rare.

Most brown recluse spider bites can be treated as any trivial bite and managed conservatively. Clinical experience indicates that systemic corticosteroids given within the first 24 hours following a brown recluse bite may lessen the severity of systemic complications. Envenomation resulting in a necrotic area 2 cm in diameter or larger should be treated with prednisone, 50 mg orally every 12 hours for 5 days. As in other bites, tetanus prophylaxis is advisable. The patient should be observed closely for signs of hemolysis, and initial laboratory data should include complete blood count and urinalysis. Platelet count, fibrinogen level, and fibrin split products may be indicated. Disseminated intravascular coagulation complicating loxoscelism has been successfully treated with heparin, and hemolytic anemia has been treated with packed red cells and exchange transfusion. Bites resulting in renal failure have been successfully managed with peritoneal dialysis or hemodialysis.

Although surgical excision and grafting have been recommended by several authors, one must remember that brown recluse bites are quite benign, and heal with little if any scarring. Early grafts are often rejected, and repeated procedures may be necessary. Healing of large, ulcerated lesions may take many weeks, but when spontaneous healing is allowed, the results are often surprisingly good and far less disfiguring than grafts.

Cool soaks and light superficial debridement of the eschar may be helpful. The wound may heal quite slowly, and patients should be reassured.

Black Widow Spider

The black widow spider is found throughout most of the Unites States, but bites occur most frequently in the South. The usual bite creates only minor discomfort; however, the young, the elderly, and the hypertensive may have complicated reactions. Within an hour after the Latrodectus bite, the neurotoxic effects of the venom may produce severe cramps, fasciculations, muscle spasm, and marked abdominal rigidity without tenderness. Headache, chest tightness, sweating, paresthesia, nausea, fever, and hyperative reflexes may also occur. Most patients' symptoms are relieved by intravenous diazepam (Valium). If patients are asymptomatic after observation for a few hours, they may be sent home, and diazepam (Valium) may be continued by mouth for a few days. Other muscle relaxants such as methocarbamol (Robaxin) may be used. A specific antivenin is available for high risk patients suffering severe envenomation, and the response is often dramatic. The antivenin is administered intravenously after appropriate skin testing for allergy to horse serum is found to be negative.

Scorpions

Scorpions are found in many areas of the United States. The stings of most species are of little significance, causing only local pain and edema lasting up to several hours. Reassurance is usually indicated and cool soaks or soothing lotions may be helpful.

The only scorpion of medical importance in United States is *Centruroides exilicauda (C. sculputuratus),* which is found throughout Arizona and occasionally adjoining parts of California and New Mexico. Deaths caused by this scorpion's sting are rare, and most serious envenomations occur in young children. Local application of an ice cube to the bite site may relieve pain; however, ice packs carry the risk of tissue damage through freezing, and prolonged exposure to cold should be avoided. Morphine and meperidene (Demerol) are contraindicated, since they may potentiate Centruroides venom. Although barbiturates have been recommended, there is little good evidence that they are helpful. Small doses of diazepam (Valium) are helpful in controlling excitability and convulsions. Administration of the specific antivenin manufactured in Mexico is the most effective treatment for severe Centruroides stings. Physicians should consult with local public health officers.

PORTUGUESE MAN-OF-WAR (JELLYFISH) STINGS

method of
BRUCE W. HALSTEAD, M.D.
Colton, California

There are several hundred species of coelenterate jellyfishes capable of inflicting stings. The symptoms vary in nature from a mild skin irritation to death. One of the more severe coelenterate stingers is the Portuguese man-of-war, which in the strict sense of the term is not a jellyfish, but is a colonial hydroid. True jellyfishes are members of the class *Scyphozoa,* whereas the Portuguese man-of-war (*Physalia*) is a member of the class *Hydrozoa.* There are two species of *Physalia, P. physalis* of the tropical Atlantic Ocean and *P. utriculus* of the Indo-Pacific region. Both species are capable of inflicting extremely painful stings with their nematocyst apparatus.

The venom of *Physalia* is a highly labile protein complex having neurotoxic properties. The venom is readily destroyed by heating to 60 C, by drying, or by alcohol, ether, acetone, or most other organic solvents.

The clinical effects most commonly reported from the stings of *Physalia* are intense local pain extending along a pattern corresponding to the lymphatic drainage (i.e., axillary lymph nodes) and joint and muscle pain. The pain varies from moderate to severe, sharp, shooting, or throbbing, depending upon the description given by the patient. The pain has sometimes been described as similar to that of an electric shock. The usual lesion is a discontinuous line of small papules, each surrounded by a small zone of erythema. There may be well-defined linear welts or scattered areas of punctate whealing and redness. Whealing is prompt and rarely massive, and usually disappears within a few hours. The erythema may remain for about 24 hours. However, slow-healing skin ulcers may continue for a period of time. The intensity of the sting appears to vary, depending upon the length of time that the tentacle remains in contact with the skin. Lesions caused by the multiple-tentacled Atlantic species *P. physalis* are usually more extensive than those produced by the single-tentacled *P. utriculus.* The local effects may be accompanied by headache, malaise, primary shock, collapse, faintness, pallor, weakness, cyanosis, nervousness, hysteria, chills and fever, muscular cramps, abdominal rigidity; nausea, vomiting, respiratory distress, backache, throat constriction, collapse, coma, and so on. No authenticated deaths from *Physalia* stings have been reported.

Therapy

Prompt first-aid measures are of particular importance in *Physalia* stings, as well as in all other types of jellyfish stings, because as long as the tentacles adhere to the victim's skin they continue to discharge their venom. The following procedures are therefore recommended: (1) Remove adhering tentacles with the use of gloves, bathing towel, seaweed, gunny sack, dry sand, salt, sugar, or any dry powder. This should be done immediately. (2) Pour alcohol over the wounded areas as soon as possible. Rinse the skin off with salt water after at least 2 minutes have elapsed. Do not rub the wounded area with sand. (3) Apply a corticosteroid-analgesic balm, preferably by aerosol.

Priority of treatment must be governed by such problems as shock, respiratory arrest, cardiac complications, and skin reactions. For the most part treatment is symptomatic. There are no known specific antidotes. The application of compresses moistened with aromatic spirits of ammonia has been found to be effective. In the absence of all other medicinals, native islanders apply urine, with surprisingly good results.

The Commonwealth Serum Laboratories, Melbourne, Australia, have recently developed a jellyfish antivenin for the deadly sea wasp *(Chironex fleckeri)*. The stings of this jellyfish are extremely painful, and may cause death. Although *Chironex* is an Australian jellyfish, there are closely related species inhabiting West Indian waters. Any victim who has received the first aid measures mentioned above and continues to have difficulty in breathing, swallowing, or speaking, or continues to be in severe pain may require sea wasp antivenin. The antivenin is supplied in containers of 20,000 units. Complete instructions as to its use are supplied by the manufacturer.

ACUTE MISCELLANEOUS POISONING

method of
JAY M. ARENA, M.D.
Durham, North Carolina

The basic treatment for acute poisoning, whether drug or chemical, is mainly symptomatic and supportive. Overtreatment of the poisoned patient with large doses of nonspecific and questionably effective antidotes, stimulants, sedatives, and other therapeutic agents often does far more harm and damage than the poison itself. A calm attitude, with the judicious use of drugs, parenteral fluids, and electrolytes for homeostasis, and the maintenance of an adequate airway are far more effective than heroic measures, which usually are unnecessary. As a matter of fact, it is often difficult to tell whether recovery from an acute poisoning occurred because of or in spite of the treatment used. Remember: "Treat the patient, not the poison."

Severe Poisoning

1. Establish adequate airway by inserting an oropharyngeal or endotracheal tube. Often, however, extension of the head and forward displacement of the mandible are sufficient. The situation may require mouth-to-mouth breathing or mechanical respiratory equipment. Physiologic improvement of the patient's condition is often notable when tissues receive adequate oxygen.

2. Empty the stomach with a large nasogastric tube and analyze a sample of the contents. Assess the patient's general condition and obtain pertinent information.

3. Generally, legs and head are elevated to the level of the right atrium to allow venous drainage of the lower extremities and promote circulatory pooling in the head and thorax. Cardiac failure may necessitate alterations in position.

4. Elastic bandaging of the legs prevents venous stasis. Passive leg exercises are advisable if depression is extreme. The patient is turned from side to side every 2 hours to promote pulmonary drainage and reduce atelectasis.

5. Homeostasis is maintained by parenteral fluid according to blood electrolyte concentrations and urine output. An indwelling catheter is placed in the bladder to permit accurate hourly measurement of output. When the kidney is not damaged, fluid therapy is aided by hourly measurement of urine specific gravity.

6. If oliguria is associated, electrocardiographic examination and frequent measurement of serum potassium levels are required.

7. Vital signs are recorded every 15 minutes or more frequently if values are labile or vasopressors are administered.

8. Drugs should be given only when specifically required. Rarely is therapy with an antidote significantly urgent; an example would be cyanide poisoning. Intensive supportive therapy reduces the need for medication.

9. Central nervous system stimulants should not be used to improve respiration. These drugs impart a false sense of security, and harmful reactions, such as rebound depressions or convulsions, may occur. If the myocardium is hypoxic, epinephrine may induce fatal ventricular fibrillation.

10. Intravenous vasopressors such as phenylephrine, methoxamine, or other adrenergic drugs may be required if the patient has tachycardia above 110 pulse beats per minute, prolonged capillary filling time, pallor, or diaphoresis. Moderate hypotension as low as 80 mm Hg does not necessitate vigorous therapy with vasopressors unless urinary output is depressed. Extremely potent agents, such as levarterenol bitartrate, are used for severe shock, but vasoconstrictors may significantly depress urinary output.

Oral Poisons

Attempt to recover the unabsorbed poison when the poison has been taken by mouth. Many poisons are in themselves emetics, but if vomiting does not occur spontaneously, it should be induced. However, emesis should not be attempted in caustic, corrosive, and petroleum-distillate poisoning, or if the patient is semiconscious or comatose.

In children emesis can best be induced by

having them drink a glass of water or milk (never carbonated fluids), after which they should be gagged with the finger or the posterior pharynx stroked with a blunt object. Use of warm saline solution or mustard water as an emetic is impractical. An overdose of salt in a child could be dangerous (hypernatremia) and even fatal.

Syrup of ipecac (not the fluid extract) can be given in doses of 10 to 15 ml and repeated in 15 to 30 minutes if emesis does not occur. For best results, 1 or 2 glasses of water (milk should not be used, as it will delay emesis) should be given after the administration of the syrup of ipecac, because emesis may not occur on an empty stomach. Activated charcoal should never be given simultaneously with ipecac, because it will absorb the ipecac and prevent its emetic effects. Recent studies indicating that induced vomiting empties the stomach of ingested poisons more effectively than does gastric lavage have produced increased enthusiasm for its use. Nevertheless, the ipecac that fails to effect vomiting either remains in the gastrointestinal tract as an irritant or is absorbed and exerts actions concomitantly with any toxins already present, and its cardiotoxic effects must be kept in mind. Syrup of ipecac or apomorphine should not be used when antiemetic drugs have been ingested, if more than an hour or two has elapsed. Gastric lavage would be safer and more effective.

If syrup of ipecac is not available, the mechanical method, gagging with fingers or spoon, is the safest and the most logical form of treatment in the home and should be tried first.

The use of table salt as a home emetic, particularly in children, should be discouraged. Fatal salt poisoning has occurred in children and adults from this obsolete method.

Apomorphine, 0.066 mg per kg (0.03 mg per lb), given subcutaneously, usually causes prompt vomiting. Since it is a respiratory depressant, it should not be given if the patient is comatose, if the respirations are slow or labored, or if the poisoning is by a respiratory depressant. Naloxone hydrochloride (Narcan) preferably, or other narcotic antagonists (see Table 4, pp. 998 to 1001), will rapidly terminate the emetic effects of apomorphine and help diminish the subsequent depression (their use, however, is not mandatory, and is often unnecessary). The combined proper use of these drugs for emptying the stomach in acute poisoning has already been shown to be effective and safe, both experimentally and clinically. The advantages are (1) rapid emesis with removal of all gastric contents, (2) no obstruction of lavage tubes, producing delays and incomplete emptying, and (3) reflux of contents (such as enteric-coated tablets) from the upper intestinal tract into the stomach.

Gastric Lavage. Gastric lavage is indicated within 3 hours after ingestion of a poison and even several hours later if large amounts of milk or food were taken beforehand or if enteric-coated or stomach-emptying delaying drugs (especially the anticholinergics) have been ingested. Gastric lavage is contraindicated after the ingestion of strong corrosive agents such as alkali (concentrated ammonia water, lye) or mineral acids (considered safe here if done within 30 to 60 minutes). Strychnine poisoning, because of the danger of producing a convulsion, and the ingestion of petroleum distillates (danger of aspiration pneumonia) are also contraindications, unless containing toxic insecticides or chemicals. In semicomatose or comatose patients gastric lavage should be attempted only after an endotracheal tube with inflatable cuff (unnecessary in infants) has been inserted. Consult toxicology texts for specific instructions and techniques in performing a gastric lavage, especially in children.

General Rules. 1. Identify the poison.

2. Administer a specific antidote and a local antidote for residual poison not removed by evacuation of stomach contents.

3. Give an antagonist when available.

4. Administer symptomatic treatment as indicated.

5. When the nature of the poison is unknown, give activated charcoal. Two to 4 tablespoonfuls to a 240 ml (8 oz) glass of water is suitable for oral use or lavage. The "universal antidote" is not effective and is not recommended.

6. In massive ingestions (suicide attempts), when therapeutic results fail to reach expectations, rule out concretions in the stomach (x-ray, gastroscopy, or surgery if necessary). Give castor oil as a solvent and to hurry the material through the intestinal tract. Follow with activated charcoal.

Antidotes. Antidotes may be given to render the poison inert or to prevent its absorption by changing its physical nature (see Table 1).

Inhaled Poisons

Remove the victim from the gas atmosphere and apply artificial respiration if necessary.

Injected Poisons

Apply tourniquets central to the point of injection. If feasible, remove as much of the poison as possible by surgery and suction.

TABLE 1. **Therapeutic Agents**

TO NEUTRALIZE ACIDS*

1. Magnesia magma (milk of magnesia), 100 to 300 ml (3 to 10 ounces)
2. Sodium bicarbonate (dilute solution)
3. Calcium hydroxide solution (lime water), 200 ml (6⅔ ounces)
4. Aluminum hydroxide gel, 60 ml (2 ounces)
5. Precipitated calcium carbonate (chalk), 100 grams (3⅓ ounces)
6. Wall plaster—crushed in water
7. Soap solution

TO NEUTRALIZE ALKALIS*

1. Vinegar (2% acetic acid), 100 to 200 ml
2. Lemon juice, 100 to 200 ml
3. Orange juice, 100 to 300 ml
4. Dilute (0.5%) hydrochloric acid, 100 to 200 ml

DEMULCENTS

1. Olive oil, 200 ml (6⅔ ounces)
2. White of egg, 60 to 100 ml (2 to 4 ounces)
3. Any vegetable oil, 200 ml (6⅔ ounces)
4. Milk
5. Starch water
6. Liquid petrolatum (mineral oil)
7. Butter

EMETICS

1. Syrup of ipecac, 10 to 15 ml repeated in 15 to 30 minutes if necessary (do not allow to remain in stomach)
2. Apomorphine, 6 mg for adults, 1 or 2 mg for children 1 to 2 years old, subcutaneously (0.066 mg per kg). Respiratory depressant effect may be counteracted by Narcan, 0.01 mg/kg.
3. Household mustard or table salt used for emetic purposes should be discouraged. Fatal salt poisoning in children and adults has been documented.

STIMULANTS

1. Caffeine and sodium benzoate, 0.5 gram (7½ grains) subcutaneously
2. Nikethamide (Coramine), 5 ml intravenously or subcutaneously
3. Pentylenetetrazol (Metrazol), 0.1 gram (1½ grains)
4. Black coffee by rectum

SEDATIVES

1. Phenobarbital, 0.03 to 0.1 gram (½ to 1½ grains)
2. Pentobarbital sodium, 0.1 gram (1½ grains)
3. Barbital sodium, 0.3 to 0.6 gram (5 to 10 grains) orally or subcutaneously
4. Chloral hydrate, 0.5 to 1 gram (7½ to 15 grains) orally
5. Sodium bromide, 0.3 to 1 gram (5 to 15 grains) orally
6. Paraldehyde, 3 to 15 ml by mouth (double dose by rectum)

*It is unlikely that serious exothermic effects will occur from the use of well diluted, mild neutralizing agents.

Absorbed Dermal Poisons

Flush skin with large quantities of water after all clothing has been removed.

Chemical Burns

Flush skin with water thoroughly and repeatedly. Consult ophthalmologist for eye care as soon as possible after thorough flushing. Do not use chemical antidotes in the eye.

Supportive Measures

Adequate amounts of fluids by mouth or parenterally are important, especially if poison is excreted by the kidney (See articles on Parenteral Fluid Therapy, pp. 488 to 508). Use of blood transfusions, exchange blood transfusions (small children), and hemodialysis if an artificial kidney is available may be helpful. Lipid dialysis is a useful technique in the treatment of poisonings by glutethimide, pentobarbital, secobarbital, phenothiazines, camphor, and other lipid-soluble substances that cannot effectively be removed by hemodialysis using an aqueous dialysate. Peritoneal dialysis with its inexpensive disposal equipment and easy technique may also be indicated and is particularly valuable for use in children. In nondialyzable poisons, plasmapheresis is an effective measure.

Shock

Therapy of shock requires careful consideration of the action of the poison ingested, the administration of vasopressor agents and steroids, the replacement of fluids, and transfusion of blood when needed.

COMMON POISONS AND THERAPY*

1. Acetaldehyde

See Methaldehyde.

2. Acetaminophen

This compound with a half-life of 1 to 2 hours does not produce the gastrointestinal hemorrhagic or acid-base disturbance of acetylsalicylic acid, but it has a more subtle form of hepatic toxicity which can be serious. Treatment is symptomatic and supportive.

Oral methionine (Pedameth), 2.5 grams every 4 hours up to 10 grams, has recently been found effective in reducing the frequency and severity of acetaminophen-induced liver damage (this use of methionine is not listed in the manufacturer's official directive). Although this compound has few side effects and is of low toxicity, it does have the potential to aggravate a preexisting hepatic disease, and therefore should only be given early (before 12 hours) after inges-

*Modified from Arena, Jay M.: *Poisoning: Toxicology, Symptoms, Treatment,* 4th ed. Springfield, Ill. Charles C Thomas, 1979; and *Davison's Compleat Pediatrician,* 9th ed., Philadelphia, Lea and Febiger, 1969.

tion, before the likely acetaminophen hepatic effects take place.

N-acetylcysteine (Mucomyst), based on preliminary evaluation, appears to act as a glutathionine substitute and to combine directly with the toxic acetaminophen metabolite. It is presently being recommended as the oral drug of choice (loading dose of 140 mg per kg, followed by 70 mg per kg every 4 hours, for a total of 18 doses), if given within 12 hours after ingestion (this use of N-acetylcysteine is not listed in the manufacturer's official directive).

3. Acetanilid

Gastric lavage or emesis. Saline cathartic. Methylene blue for methemoglobinemia. Discontinue drugs in chronic poisoning or idiosyncrasies.

4. Acetic Acid (Glacial)

Magnesium oxide. Demulcents. For inhalation, treat pulmonary edema. Shock therapy.

5. Acetone

Gastric lavage or emesis. Analeptics and respiratory stimulants if necessary. Artificial respiration and oxygen.

6. Acetylsalicylic Acid (Aspirin)

See Salicylates.

7. Alkalis

Give milk and force water, followed by diluted vinegar or fruit juices by mouth. *Do not use strong acids.* Demulcents. Corticosteroids to prevent stricture. Esophageal dilatation after fourth day. Broad-spectrum antibiotics.

8. Aminophylline

See Xanthines.

9. Ammonia (Ammonium Hydroxide)

See Alkalis. Force water.
Do not dilute with strong acids, because heat may be generated.

10. Amphetamine

Gastric lavage or emesis. Activated charcoal. Sedation or short-acting barbiturates with caution. Chlorpromazine (Thorazine), 1 to 2 mg per kg intramuscularly and repeat if necessary. Haloperidol (Haldol), 0.5 to 2.0 mg three times daily, has been used effectively recently.

11. Amyl Acetate (Banana, Oil, Pear Oil)

See Acetone.

12. Aniline and Derivatives (Dimethylaniline, Nitroaniline, Toluidine)

Gastric lavage or emesis. Artificial respiration and oxygen. For skin contact, thorough cleansing. Methylene blue for methemoglobinemia.

13. Antihistaminics

Gastric lavage or emesis. Activated charcoal. Saline cathartic. Do not use stimulants. Levarterenol for hypotension. Short-acting barbiturates with caution.

14. Antimony

Gastric lavage with 1 per cent sodium bicarbonate solution. Demulcents. Dimercaprol (BAL). Maintain fluid and electrolyte balance.

15. Antipyrine (Phenazone)

See Acetanilid.

16. ANTU (Alphanaphthylthiourea)

Gastric lavage or emesis. Saline cathartic. Oxygen. Avoid oils (more readily soluble).

17. Arsenic Trioxide (White Arsenic)

Gastric lavage or emesis. Thirty milliliters of tincture of ferric chloride and 30 grams of sodium carbonate in 120 ml of water as antidote in lavage (remove precipitant). Dimercaprol (BAL). Shock therapy.

18. Arsine Gas

Move from environment. Exchange transfusion. Dimercaprol (BAL) is ineffective. Industrial prevention with education, ventilation, etc.

19. Aspidium (Male Fern) Oleoresin

Gastric lavage or emesis. Activated charcoal. Saline cathartic. Demulcents. Short-acting barbiturates. Artificial respiration and oxygen. Avoid fats and oils.

20. Atropine

Gastric lavage with 4 per cent tannic acid solution or emesis. Pilocarpine or physostigmine (preferable) for parasympathomimetic effects. Miotic for eyes. Oxygen. Small doses of barbiturates, chloral hydrate, or paraldehyde for delirium or convulsions. Cold packs or alcohol sponging for hyperpyrexia. Indwelling catheter.

21. Barbiturates (Table 2)

There is no specific antidote for the barbiturates. In acute poisoning, current practices in most centers with much experience consider the imme-

TABLE 2. **Treatment of Barbiturate Intoxication**

CONDITION	TREATMENT	GUIDES
Respiratory insufficiency	Airway, suction; endotracheal intubation, cuffed tube, lavage; humidified oxygen; mechanical ventilation, pressure- or volume-controlled ventilator	Arterial Po_2, O_2 saturation, Pco_2, pH, minute ventilation; x-ray film of chest; airway pressure
Hypovolemia	Albumin, 5% solution, 1 liter, then dextrose, 10% in sodium chloride 0.9 per cent solution; potassium chloride supplement, 40–120 mEq	Central venous pressure, arterial pressure, urine output, and osmolality
Low urinary output	Fluid infusion; furosemide, 40 mg IV, or ethacrynic acid, 25 mg IV	Urinary output and osmolality
Heart failure	Digoxin, 0.5 mg IV, followed by 1–4 doses of 0.25 mg digoxin at 1–2 hour intervals	Central venous pressure, ECG
Pneumonia	Ampicillin sodium, 1 gram every 4 hours IV; methicillin sodium, 1 gram every 6 hours IV; chloramphenicol sodium succinate, 500 mg every 6 hours IV; gentamicin sulfate, 0.75 mg/kg every 6 hours IM	Sputum and blood culture, with antibiotic sensitivity; chloramphenicol after aspiration of gastric contents; gentamicin for gram-negative bacteria resistant to other antibiotics
Dialysis	Peritoneal; lipid; hemodialysis (preferred)	Barbiturate levels of 3.5 mg/100 ml for short-acting drugs and 8–10 mg/100 ml for long-acting agents; impaired hepatic and renal function

diate establishment of adequate pulmonary ventilation as well as control of shock of prime importance, whereas analeptics are considered subsidiary, if not actually contraindicated. The evidence indicates that the most favorable results are obtained by careful attention to respiratory and circulatory functions.

Forced diuresis by giving large amounts of fluids intravenously and also giving diuretics (acetazolamide [Diamox] or mercurials) reduces the need for vasopressor drugs, prevents renal complications and hyperthermia, and lessens crust formation in the respiratory tract. Contraindications are cardiac and renal disease. Pulmonary edema does not seem to be a serious hazard. Hemodialysis should be resorted to when indicated.

In addition to supportive measures, treatment for intoxication with this group of drugs should include forced diuresis with alkalinization of the urine. Dialysis need be considered only in the presence of renal function compromise. Alkalinization of the urine should be considered if intermediate or long-acting barbiturates have been ingested. The nonionized form of these drugs is highly lipid soluble and easily crosses the tubular membranes in the kidney; the ionized form is not lipid soluble and does not cross the tubular membrane. Since alkalinization of the urine increases the ionized form of the intermediate and long-acting barbiturates, tubular reabsorption is decreased, resulting in more rapid clearance of the drug. Administration of intravenous sodium bicarbonate raises the urine pH to about 8.0, a point at which the action of the

ionized form of the intermediate and long-acting barbiturates is significantly increased.

The nonbarbiturate hypnotics include glutethimide and methyprylon. The history is of paramount importance in the diagnosis of overdoses with these agents. Physical signs are not specific and may be confused with signs of overdosage of other types of central nervous system (CNS) depressants. If lethargy, mydriasis, hypotension, flaccid paralysis, and respiratory depression are present, intoxication with these drugs should be considered. Determination of serum and urine levels may also be helpful in confirming the diagnosis. Glutethimide also produces alternting periods of coma and relative alertness; this effect is due to the periodic increases in blood levels of glutethimide resulting from its excretion via the biliary tract with reabsorption into the circulation from the gastrointestinal tract. Lethal plasma levels of glutethimide and methyprylon are not known. The approximate fatal dose of glutethimide is 10 to 12 grams and that of methyprylon is more than 6 grams. Supportive measures, forced diuresis, and dialysis are the most effective measures for treating overdoses of these drugs. Large doses of activated charcoal have also been shown to be beneficial.

Immediate gastric lavage with a solution of saline and activated charcoal. Continue lavage with isotonic saline until the return is clear. Use castor oil for instillation and withdrawal to increase solubility of sedatives and dissolve concretions. Ensure clear airway. Respiratory stimulants such as picrotoxin or pentylenetetrazol (Metrazol), administered in subconvulsive doses, are not often used in present-day therapy. Artificial respiration. Administration of 100 per cent oxygen. For circulatory depression and shock caused by depression of vasomotor center, as well as direct action on smooth muscle in blood vessel wall: pressor amines such as levarterenol (which acts directly on vascular smooth muscle). Intravenous hydrocortisone. Blood transfusions. Trendelenburg position. For water loss from skin and lungs, decrease in urine, electrolytes variable: adequate hydration with 5 to 10 per cent glucose in water to facilitate renal elimination of barbiturates. Use of electrolytes based on analysis of plasma. After the vital signs have been stabilized and adequate renal function has been ascertained, urea or acetazolamide (Diamox)-induced (forced) osmotic diuresis with alkalization of urine has proved to be effective and successful therapy in reducing mortality, severity of intoxication, and duration of treatment and hospital stay, and is now the treatment of choice in most centers. For hypostatic pneumonia resulting from hypotension and hypoventilation: prophylactic antibiotics. For depression of kidney function resulting from hypotension and central antidiuretic action of barbiturates: exchange transfusion (children). Intermittent peritoneal dialysis. Artificial kidney (lipid dialysis). For cerebral edema: mannitol or urea. (See also Narcotic Poisoning, pp. 949 to 951.)

22. Barium (Soluble Salts)

Gastric lavage with 2 to 5 per cent solution of either magnesium or sodium sulfate. Ten ml of 10 per cent sodium sulfate intravenously, repeat-

TABLE 3. **Treatment of Convulsions Due to Poisoning**

DRUG	METHOD OF ADMINISTRATION AND DOSAGE	ADVANTAGES	DISADVANTAGES
Ether	Open drop	Dosage easily determined. Good minute-to-minute control. No sterile precautions	Difficult to give in presence of convulsion. Requires constant supervision by physician
Thiopental sodium (Pentothal sodium)	Give 2.5% sterile solution IV until convulsions are controlled. Maximum dose: 0.5 ml/kg	Good minute-to-minute control. Can be given easily during convulsion	Doses larger than recommended may cause persistent respiratory depression. Requires sterile equipment and administration
Pentobarbital sodium (Nembutal sodium)	Give 5 mg/kg by gastric tube, rectally, or IV as sterile 2.5% solution at a rate not to exceed 1 ml/minute until convulsions are controlled	Good control of initial dose	No control of effects after drug has been given. Requires sterile precautions. May produce severe respiratory depression
Phenobarbital sodium	Give 1–2 mg/kg IM or by gastric tube and repeat as necessary at a 30 minute interval up to a maximum of 5 mg/kg	Effects last 12–14 hours	Causes severe persistent respiratory depression in overdoses
Succinylcholine chloride	Give 10–50 mg IV slowly and give artificial respiration during period of apnea. Repeat as necessary	Will control convulsions of any type. Effect lasts only 1–5 minutes. Circulation not ordinarily affected	Artificial respiration must be maintained during use. No antidote is available. Apnea may persist for several hours in some cases
Trimethadione (Tridione)	Give 1 gram IV slowly. Maximum dose: 5 grams	Little depression of respiration	Not effective in all types of convulsions
Tribromoethanol (Avertin)	Only by rectal instillation. 50–60 mg/kg causes drowsiness, amnesia; 70–80 mg/kg produces light unconsciousness and analgesia	Ease of administration and pleasant induction without mental distress and respiratory irritation	A nonvolatile anesthetic given by a route which prevents adequate control once it is administered. Contraindicated when renal or hepatic injury exists
Amobarbital sodium (Amytal)	Give 2% sterile solution. Dose range 0.4–0.8 gram	Immediate action and lasts 3–6 hours	Inhibits the cardiac action of the vagus. May produce severe respiratory depression
Phenytoin (Dilantin)	Give slowly IV 150–250 mg from Steri-Vial and repeat in 30 minutes with 100–150 mg if necessary	Lack of marked hypnotic and narcotic activity	Solution is highly alkaline and perivenous infiltration may cause sloughing. Not always effective, and other anticonvulsants frequently must be used. Cardiac arrest has been reported after IV therapy
Paraldehyde	Give 5–15 ml by gastric tube, rectally or IM	Little depression of respiration. Effects last 12 hours	Harmful in presence of hepatic disease. Old and loosely stoppered solutions can break down to acetic acid and produce serious intoxication
Diazepam (Valium)	Give 2–5 mg IM or IV. Repeat in 2 hours if necessary	More effective for relieving muscle spasm associated with seizures	Hypotension and respiratory depression or muscular weakness may occur if used with barbiturates

TABLE 4. **Antidote Chart***

ANTIDOTE	DOSE	POISON	REACTION (ANTIDOTE) AND COMMENTS
Acids, weak Acetic acid, 1% Vinegar, 5% acetic acid (diluted 1:4 with water) Hydrochloric acid, 0.5%	100–200 ml	Alkali, caustic	
Activated charcoal Darco G (Atlas Chem.) Nuchar C (W. Va. Pulp & Paper; Merck) Norit A (Amer. Norit Co.)	2–4 tbsp to glass of water or a mixture of soupy consistency	Effective for virtually all poisons, organic and inorganic compounds of large and small molecules*	Broad spectrum of activity No reaction except staining
Alcohol, ethyl	IV as 5% solution in bicarbonate or saline solution PO as 3–4 oz of whiskey (45%) every 4 hours for 1–3 days	Methyl alcohol Ethylene glycol	Metabolizes methyl alcohol and prevents formation of toxic formic acid; glycols into oxalates
Alkali, weak Magnesium oxide (preferred) Sodium bicarbonate	2.5% solution (25 grams/liter) 5% solution (50 grams/liter)	Acid, corrosive	Gastric distention from liberated carbon dioxide
Ammonium acetate	5 ml in 500 ml water	Formaldehyde (formalin)	Forms relatively harmless methenamine
Ammonium hydroxide	0.2% solution Both are for gastric lavage		
Antivenins *Specific*	See package insert for dosage instructions		
Antivenin *(Crotalidae)* Polyvalent (Wyeth)		N. and S. American snakebite venoms	
Antivenin *(Latrodectus mactans,* and *L. curacaviensis)* (Merck)		Black widow spider venom	
Antivenin *(Micrurus)* (Wyeth and C. Amaral and Cia L.T.D.A. Cloria 34, PO Box 2123, São Paulo, Brazil)		Coral snake venom	
Nonspecific		Black widow spider venom	
Adult (may be used without antivenin, *for adult only*)			
Methocarbamol (Robaxin)	On diagnosis, 1 ampule (1 gram, 10 ml) IV in 15 ml isotonic saline solution over 5 minute period or in IV drip. Follow in 12 hours with 2 tablets (1500 mg) 3 times a day for 2 days		Muscle relaxant
Orphenadrine citrate (Norflex)	On diagnosis, 1 ampule (2 ml, 60 mg) IV in 5 ml isotonic saline solution followed in 12 hours by 1 tablet (100 mg) 2 times a day for 2 days		Muscle relaxant
Child Antivenin	Antivenin IV followed in 1 hour by methocarbamol, 1 tablet (500 mg) and 1 tablet every 12 hours for 2 days		In children the antivenin should be used; this may be supplemented with the muscle relaxant when necessary
Atropine sulfate	1–2 mg IM and repeat in 30 minutes	Organic phosphate esters: Guthion, malathion, parathion, mushroom, TEPP, trithion, etc., other cholinesterase inhibitors	Atropinization
Bromobenzene	Adult: 1 gram Child: 0.25 gram (in lavage solution)	Selenium	
Calcium EDTA or Versene (ethylenediamine tetraacetate) (DPTA [diethylenetriamine pentaacetic acid], more promising analogue)	25–50 mg/kg 2% solution 2 times a day for 5 days 50 mg/kg, 20% solution (0.5% procaine) IM daily for 5–7 days Repeat these courses after 2 day rest period	Cadmium Cobalt Copper Digitalis Iron Lead (combined therapy with dimercaprol [BAL] for encephalitis) Nickel, and other metals	Nephrotoxic Increases urinary potassium excretion Use sodium salt (Na EDTA) for digitalis in place of Ca EDTA, which chelates Ca ion, producing hypocalcemia, and reduces synergistic action of the Ca and digitalis, converting dangerous arrhythmias to sinus arrhythmias (other specific therapy preferred) Oral EDTA should not be used until all lead has been removed or absorbed from the GI tract

*Exceptions are cyanide, alcohols, boric acid, corrosives, and ferrous sulfate.

TABLE 4. **Antidote Chart** (*Continued*)

ANTIDOTE	DOSE	POISON	REACTION (ANTIDOTE) AND COMMENTS
Calcium gluconate	10% solution 5–10 ml IM or IV, may be repeated in 8–12 hours	Black widow spider and insect venom	Muscle relaxant Bradycardia Flushing Local necrosis from perivenous infiltration (methocarbamol, etc., also effective)
Calcium lactate	10% solution (in lavage solution)	Chlorinated hydrocarbons Fluoride Oxalates	
Chlorpromazine (Thorazine)	1–2 mg/kg IM	Amphetamine*	Drowsiness Hypotension Neuromuscular (parkinsonian)
Copper sulfate	0.25–3.0 grams in glass of water	Phosphorus	Forms insoluble copper phosphide
Cyanide poison kit (Eli Lilly stock #M76)			
Amyl nitrite pearls Sodium nitrite	0.2 ml (inhalation); follow with 3.0% solution (10 ml) in 2–4 minutes *and*	Cyanide	Hypotension
Sodium thiosulfate	25% solution (50 ml) in 10 minutes through same needle and vein (repeat with ½ doses if necessary)	Iodine	Sodium thiosulfate used alone for iodine; forms harmless sodium iodide
Deferoxamine B (Desferal, Ciba) Deferoxamine isolated from *Streptomyces pilosus*	1–2 grams IM or IV (adults, repeat if necessary every 4–12 hours); also 5–10 grams via nasogastric tube following gastric lavage†	Iron Hemochromatosis	Diarrhea Hypotension
Dimercaprol (BAL)	*Severe intoxication* Day 1: 3.0 mg/kg every 4 hours (6 injections) Day 2: Same Day 3: 3.0 mg/kg every 6 hours (4 injections) Days 4–13 (or until recovery): 3.0 mg/kg every 12 hours (2 injections) *Mild intoxication* Day 1: 2.5 mg/kg every 4 hours (6 injections) Day 2: Same Day 3: 2.5 mg/kg every 12 hours Days 4–13 (or until recovery): 2.5 mg/kg daily (1 injection)	Antimony Arsenic Bismuth Gold Mercury (acrodynia) Nickel Lead (combined therapy with EDTA for encephalitis) Contraindicated for iron	Flushing Myalgia Nausea and vomiting Nephrotoxic Hypotension Pulmonary edema Salivation and lacrimation Temperature elevation (especially in children)
Diphenhydramine hydrochloride (Benadryl)	10–50 mg IV or IM	Phenothiazine tranquilizers (for extrapyramidal neuromuscular manifestations)	Atropine-like effect Drowsiness
Dithizon	10 mg/kg twice a day PO with 100 ml 10% glucose solution for 5 days	Thallium	Diabetogenic Not available for therapeutic use. May be obtained through a chemical company
Household antidotes Milk Raw eggs Flour Starches		Arsenic Mercury and other heavy metals Same as above Iodine	These are useful and readily available antidotes that can be used in an emergency. All have demulcent properties
Hydrogen peroxide	3% solution (10 ml in 100 ml water as lavage solution)	Potassium permanganate Oxidizing agent for many other compounds	Irritation of mucous membranes Distention of abdomen from release of gas
Iodine, tincture	15 drops in 120 ml water	Precipitant for: Lead Mercury Quinine Silver Strychnine	Precipitants must be thoroughly removed by gastric lavage
Magnesium sulfate Sodium sulfate	2.5% solution for lavage 10% solution IM and repeat in 30 minutes Also as catharsis for rapid elimination of toxic agent from GI tract	Precipitant for: Barium Lead Hypervitaminosis D Hypercalcemia (glucocorticoid therapy preferable)	

*Recent reports have indicated that haloperidol (Haldol) is more effective in smaller doses than chlorpromazine for amphetamine intoxication.
†Some reports suggest that large oral doses of deferoxamine can be absorbed and result in systemic toxicity, and its oral use is being questioned.

999

TABLE 4. **Antidote Chart** (*Continued*)

ANTIDOTE	DOSE	POISON	REACTION (ANTIDOTE) AND COMMENTS
Methylene blue	IV: 1% solution given slowly (2 mg/kg) and repeat in 1 hour if necessary PO: 3–5 mg/kg (action much slower)	Methemoglobinemia produced by over 100 drugs and chemicals: Acetanilid Aniline derivatives Chlorates Dinitrophenol Nitrites Pyridium, etc.	Perivenous infiltration can produce severe necrosis
Monoacetin (glyceryl monoacetate)	0.5 ml/kg IM or in saline solution IV. Repeat as necessary	Sodium fluoroacetate "1080"	Not available commercially. If parenteral therapy not feasible, can give 100 ml of monoacetin in water
Nalorphine (Nalline) or Levallorphan (Lorfan) or Naloxone (Narcan)	Adult: 5–10 mg IM or IV and repeat in ½ hour Child: 0.1–0.2 mg/kg IM or IV and repeat in ½ hour Adult: 0.5–1.0 mg IM or IV Child: 0.02 mg/kg IM or IV 0.01 mg/kg IV, IM, or SC	Codeine Demerol Dionin Heroin Methadone Morphine Pantopon (For respiratory and cardiovascular depression)	Withdrawal symptoms Depression effects in other than narcotic compounds Produces no respiratory depression, psychotomimetic effects, circulatory changes, or miosis
Penicillamine and its derivatives (Cuprimine)	1–5 grams PO	Mercury and other heavy metals	Fever Stupor Nausea and vomiting Myalgia Leukopenia, thrombocytopenia Nephrosis, reversible Optic axial neuritis, reversible Ineffective when severe vomiting is prominent
Petrolatum, liquid (mineral oil)			Solvent Demulcent
Physostigmine salicylate (Antilirium)	1–2 mg IM or IV*	Atropine and related alkaloids; anticholinergic compounds; particularly effective for the cardiac arrhythmias and CNS toxic effects of the tricyclic antidepressant drugs Atropine and related alkaloids	Excess can produce diarrhea, bradycardia, hypersalivation, rhinorrhea, and cholinergic crisis; Rx with propantheline bromide (Pro-Banthine) preferable to atropine
Pilocarpine (not being marketed in tablet form in U.S.)	PO: 2–4 mg IM: 0.25–0.5 mg		Antagonizes the parasympathetic (mydriasis and dry mouth), not central nervous system, effects of atropine
Potassium permanganate	1:5000 and 1:10,000 solution for gastric lavage	Nicotine Physostigmine Quinine Strychnine Oxidizing agent for many alkaloids and organic poisons	Strong irritant and should not be used in strong dilutions or with any residual particles
Pralidoxime iodine (2-PAM iodine) Pralidoxime chloride (2-PAM chloride)	Adult: 1–2 grams Child: 25–50 mg/kg IM or IV as 5% solution	Organic phosphate esters Cholinesterase inhibition by any agent: chemical, drug, etc.	Diplopia Dizziness Headache
Protamine sulfate	1% solution IV slowly (mg/mg) to that of heparin	Heparin	Sensitivity effects
Sodium chloride	1 tsp salt to 1 pint water (approximately isotonic saline solution) 6–12 grams PO in divided doses or in isotonic saline IV	Silver nitrate Bromides	Forms noncorrosive silver chloride Hypernatremia
Sodium formaldehyde sulfoxalate	5% in lavage solution (preferably combined with 5% sodium bicarbonate)	Mercury salts	Dimercaprol (BAL) therapy should follow gastric lavage
Sodium thiosulfate	PO: 2–3 grams or IM: 10 or 25% solution Repeat in 3–4 hours	Iodine Cyanide	
Starch	80 grams/liter water	Iodine	

*Not approved by Food and Drug Administration for intravenous use in children.

TABLE 4. **Antidote Chart** (*Continued*)

ANTIDOTE	DOSE	POISON	REACTION (ANTIDOTE) AND COMMENTS
Tannic acid	4% in lavage solution Never use in greater concentrations	Precipitates alkaloids, certain glucosides, and many metals	Hepatotoxic Tannates formed should not be allowed to remain in the stomach Because of its hepatotoxicity, should be used cautiously and in no greater than 4% solution
Universal antidote (activated charcoal alone preferable)	Two parts pulverized charcoal (burned toast); One part magnesium oxide (milk of magnesia); One part tannic acid (strong tea)	Obsolete for any use	Overrated and ineffective. Can actually be harmful in that it may give false sense of security to those who use it
Vitamin K₁	5–150 mg IV Rate not to exceed 10 mg/min	Coumarin derivatives: Coumarin Marcumar Warfarin, etc.	Bleeding Focal hemorrhages

ed in 30 minutes for serious symptoms. Artificial respiration and oxygen. Procainamide for ventricular arrhythmias. Potassium.

23. *Benadryl* (Diphenhydramine HCl)
See Antihistaminics.

24. *Benzene* (Benzol)
Gastric lavage or emesis. Artificial respiration and oxygen. Shock therapy. Blood transfusion if necessary. Avoid fats, oils, alcohol, and epinephrine or related drugs (these induce ventricular fibrillation).

25. *Benzene Hexachloride* (BHC)
Gastric lavage or emesis. Wash skin thoroughly. Short-acting barbiturates. Avoid fats, oils, and epinephrine.

26. *Benzine* (Petroleum Ether, Naphtha)
See Kerosene.

27. *Beryllium*
Calcium disodium edetate (edathamil). Corticosteroids for chemical pneumonitis. Excision of skin granulomas and ulcers. Prevention with education of beryllium-using workers or operators.

28. *Bismuth* (Soluble Compounds)
Gastric lavage or emesis. Activated charcoal. Saline cathartic. Dimercaprol (BAL). Discontinue medication at first sign of toxicity. Methylene blue for methemoglobinemia.

29. *Boric Acid* (Boracic Acid)
Gastric lavage or emesis. Saline cathartic. Shock and convulsive therapy. Peritoneal dialysis or exchange transfusion.

30. *Botulism*
See pages 23 to 32 and 1005.

31. *Bromides*
Discontinue all sources of bromides. Six to 12 grams of sodium chloride in divided doses with 4 liters of water daily for 1 to 4 weeks (adult dose). Isotonic salt solution or ammonium chloride intravenously in more serious cases. Hemodialysis with artificial kidney.

32. *Cadmium*
Gastric lavage or emesis. Remove patient from exposure. Saline cathartic. Calcium disodium edetate (edathamil). Dimercaprol (BAL) contraindicated (BAL and cadmium combination is nephrotoxic). Artificial respiration and oxygen. Antibiotics and corticosteroids for chemical pneumonitis and pulmonary edema.

33. *Caffeine*
See Xanthines.

34. *Camphor*
Gastric lavage or emesis. Demulcents. Short-acting barbiturates. Artificial respiration and oxygen. Shock therapy. Avoid fats, oils, alcohol, and opiates. Lipid dialysis.

35. *Cantharidin* (Spanish Fly, Russian Fly)
Gastric lavage (cautiously because of corrosive effects) or emesis. Demulcents. Therapy for shock. Short-acting barbiturates. Adequate fluids for diuresis. Avoid morphine because of respiratory depression.

36. *Carbon Dioxide*
Terminate exposure; move patient to fresh air. Artificial respiration and oxygen. Respiratory and blood pressure stimulants.

37. Carbon Disulfide

Gastric lavage or emesis, if ingested. Move from exposure. Artificial respiration and oxygen. Pulmonary edema and therapy for shock. Short-acting barbiturates. Prevention: maximum allowable concentration (MAC) must be observed at all times. For skin contact, wash thoroughly.

38. Carbon Monoxide

Move patient from exposure immediately. Artificial respiration and oxygen. Administration of 100 per cent oxygen in a pressure chamber, if available. Hypothermia. Blood transfusion or washed red blood cells given early. Chronic carbon monoxide poisoning and therapy are questionable.

39. Carbon Tetrachloride

Gastric lavage or emesis, if ingested. Move from source of exposure. Remove contaminated clothes. Artificial respiration and oxygen. Shock therapy with special emphasis on fluid and electrolytes in face of oliguria or anuria. Avoid fats, oils, alcohol, epinephrine, and related compounds. Prevention: use of less toxic chemicals, such as methyl chloroform.

40. Chloral Hydrate

See Barbiturates.

41. Chlorates

Gastric lavage with care, or emesis. Demulcents. Shock therapy. Methylene blue for methemoglobinemia.

42. Chlordane

Gastric lavage or emesis. Short-acting barbiturates. For skin contamination, thorough washing of skin and removal of contaminated clothing. Avoid fats, oils, demulcents, and epinephrine, which should not be used in any halogenated insecticide poisoning.

43. Chlorinated Alkalis (Hypochlorites, Chlorine)

Careful gastric lavage or emesis for large amounts only. Diluted vinegar and fruit juices. Demulcents. Move from exposure and wash skin thoroughly. Antibiotics and corticosteroids for pulmonary edema and pneumonitis from chlorine inhalation. Oral magnesium oxide (paradoxic as it may sound) to prevent formation of irritating hypochlorous acid in the stomach.

44. Chloroform

Gastric lavage or emesis. Demulcents. Artificial respiration and oxygen. Respiratory and cardiac stimulants. Ten per cent calcium gluconate intravenously (slowly).

45. Chlorothiazide (Diuril)

Discontinue use of drug. Correct fluid and electrolyte imbalance.

46. Chromium (Potassium Salt, Chromic Oxide)

Gastric lavage or emesis. Demulcents. One per cent aluminum acetate wet dressings for skin contamination. Ten per cent edetate (edathamil) ointment for skin ulcers. Remove from source of exposure, whether it be from inhalation or skin contact.

47. Cocaine

Gastric lavage or emesis. Remove drug from skin or mucous membranes. Short-acting barbiturates. Artificial respiration and oxygen.

48. Codeine

Gastric lavage or emesis. Saline cathartic. Nalorphine (Nalline), levallorphan (Lorfan), or preferably naloxone (Narcan). Artificial respiration and oxygen. Maintain body heat and fluid balance.

49. Colchicine

Gastric lavage or emesis. Saline cathartic. Artificial respiration and oxygen. Shock therapy. Discontinue or reduce dosages of drugs at first sign of toxicity.

50. Copper

Gastric lavage or emesis if vomiting has not occurred. Demulcents. Shock therapy. Calcium disodium edetate (edathamil). Penicillamine derivatives.

51. Cosmetics

Deodorants (aluminum salts, titanium dioxide, antibacterial agents); depilatories (soluble sulfides or calcium thioglycolate): gastric lavage or emesis, if large amount ingested.

Hair tints and dyes: discontinue use if allergy develops.

52. Curare

Discontinue drug immediately. Endotracheal catheter and use a positive pressure artificial respirator with oxygen until muscle function returns. Neostigmine or edrophonium chloride.

Cold packs or alcohol sponging for temperature elevation.

53. Cyanides (Hydrogen, Potassium, Sodium)

Gastric lavage or emesis, if ingested. See Table 4 for cyanide poison kit. Kelocyanor (dicobalt tetracemate) is being used effectively in Europe but is not approved for United States use at present. Artificial respiration and oxygen. Remove contaminated clothing and wash skin thoroughly.

54. DDT (Chlorobenzene Insecticide, TDE, DFDT, DMC, Methoxychlor, Neotrane, Ovotran, Dilan, Dimite)

Gastric lavage or emesis. Saline cathartic. Short-acting barbiturates. Artificial respiration and oxygen. Remove contaminated clothing and wash skin thoroughly. Avoid fats, oils, demulcents, epinephrine, and related compounds.

55. Demerol HCl (Meperidine HCl)

See Morphine.

56. Detergents (Anionic and Nonionic Surfactants, Phosphate Salts, Sodium Sulfate and Carbonate, Fatty Acid Amides)

Unless taken in large quantities, no serious toxic symptoms other than gastrointestinal symptoms; at present causing havoc with public water supplies. Milk, egg whites, mild soap solution by mouth.

57. Diamthazole (Asterol)*

Use as directed only or discontinue use. Should not be used in children under 6 years of age. Short-acting barbiturates.

58. Dichlorohydrin

See Carbon Tetrachloride.

59. Dichlorophenoxyacetic Acid (2,4-D; 2,4,5-T Esters or Salts)

Gastric lavage or emesis. Quinidine sulfate to relieve myotonia and suppress ventricular arrhythmias. Antipyretic for hyperpyrexia.

60. Dieldrin

See Chlordane (Indane Derivatives).

61. Diethyltoluamide (Dimethylphthalate, Indalone)

---

*This product was discontinued in the United States (1966), but is still available in Europe.

Gastric lavage or emesis. Demulcents. Short-acting barbiturates.

62. Digitalis (Purple Foxglove) (Digitoxin)

Discontinue use. Gastric lavage or emesis for accidental or suicidal ingestion. Artificial pacemaker. Potassium chloride, orally or intravenously, under electrocardiographic observation. Procainamide, quinidine, phenytoin (Dilantin), propranolol hydrochloride, lidocaine, or atropine.

63. Dilantin Sodium

See Phenytoin.

64. Dimethyl Sulfate

Moves to fresh air; eyes, skin, and mucous membranes should be washed thoroughly with water. Weak alkali wet dressings for skin burns. Antibiotics and corticosteroids for pneumonitis. In contaminated areas deactivate by spraying with water or 5 per cent sodium hydroxide solution.

65. Dinitro-ortho-cresol (Dinitrophenol Derivatives)

Gastric lavage with sodium bicarbonate solution or emesis. For skin contamination, wash thoroughly with weak alkaline solution. Oxygen and circulatory stimulants. Reduce temperature with cold packs or alcohol sponging. Maintain fluid and electrolyte balance.

66. Dioxane

See Acetone.

67. Diphenhydramine HCl (Benadryl HCl)

See Antihistaminics.

68. Diphenylhydantoin Sodium (Dilantin Sodium)

See Phenytoin.

69. Dithiocarbamate (Ferbam)

Discontinue use of spray. Avoid alcohol.

70. Doriden

See Barbiturates.

71. Emetine (Alkaloid of Ipecac)

Gastric lavage if emesis has not taken place. Maintain fluid and electrolyte balance. Cautious digitalization. Cardiac pacemaker until ECG is normal and pulse regular.

72. Ephedrine

Gastric lavage or emesis. Activated charcoal. Short-acting barbiturates. Phentolamine (Regitine) early, to block hypertensive effects.

73. Epinephrine (Adrenalin)

See Ephedrine.

74. Ergot Derivatives

Gastric lavage or emesis. Activated charcoal, 1 to 2 tbsp in water. Saline cathartic. Atropine sulfate for abdominal pain and spasm, 10 per cent solution of calcium gluconate for myalgia, and papaverine HCl or methacholine (Mecholyl) as vascular antispasmodic. Short-acting barbiturates and artificial respiration and oxygen, if necessary.

75. Essential (Volatile) Oils

One hundred milliliters of castor oil, then remove by gastric lavage. Saline cathartic. Demulcents. Short-acting barbiturates. Artificial respiration and oxygen. Maintain fluid and electrolyte balance.

76. Ether

Artificial respiration and oxygen. Maintain adequate airway, blood pressure, and body temperature.

77. Ethyl Alcohol (Pure) (Whiskey = 40 to 50 Per Cent Alcohol; Wines = 10 to 20 Per Cent Alcohol; Beers = 2 to 6 Per Cent Alcohol)

Gastric lavage or emesis. Sodium bicarbonate, 1 tsp to 1 pint water, every 1 to 2 hours to prevent acidosis. Intravenous bicarbonate for acidosis. Caffeine and sodium benzoate or strong coffee. Hypertonic glucose or urea for cerebral edema. Intravenous glucose for hypoglycemia. Avoid depressant drugs (barbiturates interfere with enzymatic action of alcohol dehydrogenase) and potent respiratory stimulants.

78. Ethylene Chlorohydrin (Ethylene Dichloride)

Gastric lavage or emesis. Move from exposure. Artificial respiration and oxygen. Thorough washing for skin contact. Epinephrine or levarterenol for maintaining blood pressure.

79. Ethylene Glycol (Diethylene Glycol, Propylene Glycol)

Gastric lavage or emesis. Artificial respiration and oxygen. Ten per cent calcium gluconate intravenously to precipitate metabolic product, oxalic acid, and oxalates. Maintain body temperature, fluids, and electrolytes. Short-acting barbiturates. Dialysis. Oral and intravenous ethyl alcohol (see Methyl Alcohol).

80. Ferrous Sulfate (Copperas, Green Vitriol; Approximately 20 Per Cent Elemental Iron)

Clearance with suction and maintenance of open airways. Control of shock with available intravenous fluids, blood, plasma, and oxygen. Gastric lavage with concentrated solution of sodium bicarbonate, 5 per cent disodium phosphate, or milk until returning fluid is clear. Critically ill patients should receive calcium disodium edetate (edathamil) intravenously; if none is given orally, intravenous dose should be 70 to 80 mg per kg per 24 hours in dextrose or isotonic saline solution in an 0.5 to 2 per cent concentration; if used orally (and rate of its absorption through a gut wall damaged by iron is not known), only half the aforementioned dose should be used intravenously, 35 to 40 mg per kg per 24 hours. Guided by the clinical picture and daily iron levels in serum, and, if measurements are available, by the urinary output of edetate (edathamil) and iron, intravenous and/or oral calcium disodium edetate (edathamil) is continued in a total daily dose of no more than 70 to 80 mg per kg; duration of treatment with this drug should not be, and need not be, longer than 5 days. Deferoxamine (Desferal), a chelating agent, has been demonstrated to be effective in the treatment of acute iron poisoning. Dosage recommended is 5 to 10 grams by mouth or nasogastric tube* and 1 to 2 grams intravenously (slowly to avoid hypotensive effects) or intramuscularly. Parenteral therapy can be repeated if serum iron levels remain high. Follow-up liver function tests and study of gastrointestinal tract with a radiopaque medium for strictures.

81. Fluorides (Fluorine, Hydrogen Fluoride, Fluorosilicates [Insoluble])

Gastric lavage or emesis with lime water (0.15 per cent calcium hydroxide), calcium chloride solution (1 tsp per liter water), or milk. Ten per cent calcium gluconate intravenously or intramuscularly. Demulcents. For inhalation move to fresh air. Artificial respiration and oxygen. Prophylactic antibiotics and corticosteroids for pulmonary irritation and edema. Wash skin immediately and thoroughly with water and apply magnesium oxide paste with 20 per cent glycerin.

---

*There are some studies suggesting that large doses of deferoxamine can be absorbed and result in systemic toxicity, and its oral use is now being questioned.

82. Fluoroacetate Sodium

Gastric lavage or emesis. Saline cathartic. Ten per cent calcium gluconate or sodium glycerol monoacetate (Monacetin). Short-acting barbiturates. Procainamide for arrhythmia. For skin contact, wash thoroughly.

83. Food Poisoning (Botulism)

See also pages 23 to 32.

Types A and B polyvalent antitoxin (inadequately processed vegetables and meats) or Type E antitoxin (fish and marine products). Trivalent (A, B, E) antitoxin now available.* Maintain an airway. Parenteral fluids.

84. Formaldehyde (Formalin)

Gastric lavage with 0.1 per cent ammonia or 1 per cent ammonium carbonate solution. Saline cathartic. Combat shock or collapse; levarterenol if necessary.

85. Glutethimide (Doriden)

See Barbiturates.

86. Gold

Discontinue use of parenteral therapy. Dimercaprol (BAL). Antihistaminic therapy. Supportive therapy for renal and hematologic effects.

87. Hydralazine (Apresoline, Phthalazine Derivates)

Gastric lavage or emesis. Discontinue use or reduce dosage. Maintain blood pressure.

88. Hydrochloric Acid (Muriatic Acid)

Do not use gastric lavage after 1 hour past ingestion. Neutralize acid with magnesium oxide, milk of magnesia, or lime water. Give demulcents. Maintain blood prsessure, fluids, and electrolytes. Antibiotics and corticosteroids to prevent infection and strictures. Thorough washing of skin and application of magnesium oxide paste. Gastroscopy for determining corrosive injury to the stomach.

89. Hydroquinone

Gastric lavage or emesis. Saline cathartic. Methylene blue for methemoglobinemia.

90. Hypochlorites (Clorox, etc.)

See Chlorinated Alkalis.

---

*U.S. Center for Disease Control, Atlanta, Georgia. Telephone number for day coverage is (404) 329–3753; for night and weekends, (404) 329–3644.

91. Iodine (Iodoform, Iodides)

Give suspension of starch or flour or 1 to 5 per cent solution of sodium thiosulfate. If not available, use milk or egg whites. Follow by gastric lavage. Regulate fluids and electrolytes, depending on degree of renal involvement. Epinephrine, diphenhydramine (Benadryl), or hydrocortisone for anaphylactoid reaction.

92. Isoniazid

Prompt gastric lavage or emesis (symptoms appear within 30 minutes). Discontinue drug or reduce dosage. Pyridoxine, 200 to 400 mg intravenously. Short-acting barbiturates intravenously for convulsions. Parenteral sodium bicarbonate for acidosis. Hemodialysis. Osmotic diuresis (mannitol, urea, furosemide, or ethacrynic acid) hastens excretion.

93. Isopropyl Alcohol (Rubbing Alcohol)

See Ethyl Alcohol.

94. Kerosene (Petroleum Distillates: Benzine, Gasoline, Naphtha, Mineral Seal Oil, etc.)

Prevent aspiration. Gastric lavage or emesis to be avoided. Oxygen and antibiotics. Corticosteroids for pulmonary edema and chemical or lipoid pneumonitis (particularly for mineral seal oil aspiration). Results are equivocal, yet since therapy is short range, it may benefit those with severe pulmonary distress and "shock" lung.

95. Lead

Gastric lavage with 1 per cent sodium sulfate solution, followed by saline cathartic for immediate ingestion. Calcium disodium edetate (edathamil) intravenously or intramuscularly for 5 days and repeat if necessary. Four per cent urea (30 per cent in severe cases) intravenously for encephalopathy with increased intracranial pressure: craniectomy may be necessary. Mannitol or adrenal corticosteroids are also used for this purpose and often preferred. Ten per cent solution of calcium gluconate or morphine for severe abdominal pain (colic). Early diagnosis and treatment are paramount in preventing death or serious sequelae in children. Dimercaprol (BAL) combined with calcium disodium edetate (edathamil) therapy is more effective in lead encephalitis than use of edetate (edathamil) alone. Penicillamine (Cuprimine) as an oral chelating agent has recently been reported to be effective and may be used in adjunctive therapy as an investigational drug.

96. Mace (Anti-Riot Gas)

See Tear Gases.

97. Manganese

Remove from further exposure. Antibiotics and corticosteroids for pneumonitis. Calcium disodium edetate (edathamil) may be beneficial if given early. Antiparkinsonian drugs. Diphenhydramine (Benadryl), biperiden hydrochloride (Akineton), or methylphenidate hydrochloride (Ritalin).

98. Marihuana

Removal of drug exposure (characteristic "burnt rope" acrid odor on clothes and body). There are no withdrawal symptoms except with extreme cases of habituation.

99. Meperidine HCl (Demerol HCl)

See Morphine.

100. Meprobamate (Equanil, Miltown, etc.)

Gastric lavage or emesis. Saline cathartic. Artificial respiration and oxygen. Maintain blood pressure with methoxamine hydrochloride. In massive ingestion, use castor oil (for possible concretion) as solvent and purge.

101. Menthol

See Phenol.

102. Mercury Compounds

Gastric lavage immediately with egg white solution or with 5 per cent sodium formaldehyde sulfoxylate; if unavailable, a 2 to 5 per cent solution of sodium bicarbonate may be used. Magnesium sulfate as cathartic (early only). Dimercaprol (BAL). Penicillamine derivatives (oral antidote). Maintain fluid and electrolyte balance and nutrition. Spironolactone (Aldactone) has prevented renal tubular necrosis in experimental animals (rats).

103. Metaldehyde (Converts to Acetaldehyde)

Gastric lavage or emesis. Demulcents. Short-acting barbiturates. Artificial respiration, oxygen, and antibiotics. Parenteral chlorpromazine and calcium gluconate.

104. Methadone (Dolophine)

See Morphine.

105. Methyl Alcohol

To prevent the formation of formic acid and formates, 10 ml ethyl alcohol per hour can suppress the metabolism of methyl alcohol. In severe poisoning, ethyl alcohol can be given intravenously in 5 per cent concentration in bicarbonate or saline solution and 90 to 120 ml (3 to 4 oz) of whiskey (45 per cent alcohol) orally every 4 to 6 hours for 1 to 3 days. Combat acidosis. Hemodialysis is paramount in serious poisoning.

106. Methyl Bromide (Chloride, Iodide)

Move from exposure. Artificial respiration and oxygen. Epinephrine for bronchospasm; antibiotics and corticosteriods for pneumonitis. Prevention: safety dispensers for fumigant use.

107. Methyl Salicylate (Oil of Wintergreen)

See Salicylates. Gastric lavage, however, may be worthwhile, even several hours after ingestion, because methyl salicylate is poorly absorbed.

108. Metrazol

See Pentylenetetrazol.

109. Morphine (Codeine, Heroin, Propoxyphene [Darvon], Meperidine [Demerol], Dihydromorphinone [Dilaudid], Opium Alkaloids [Pantopon])

Gastric lavage (before loss of consciousness). Do not use syrup of ipecac or apomorphine. Activated charcoal. Saline cathartic. Delay absorption of intramuscular drug with tourniquet and cryotherapy. Maintain adequate airway, body temperature, fluids, and electrolytes. Give narcotic antagonists, nalorphine (Nalline) or levallorphan (Lorfan). Naloxone hydrochloride (Narcan) is preferable (see Table 4). Ephedrine for hypotension and bradycardia — methoxamine or phenylephrine if pulse is rapid. Doxapram hydrochloride (Dopram), 3 to 5 ml intravenously, is the respiratory stimulant of choice, but it has short-lasting effects (3 to 5 minutes).

110. Muscarine (Some Mushrooms)

Artificial respiration with oxygen. Atropine, 1 to 2 mg every hour until free of respiratory effects. Melphalan (PAM) or pralidoxime chloride (Protopam) chloride may be useful adjunct therapy. Gastric lavage or emesis if vomiting has not occurred. Thiotic acid, an investigational compound, has been reported to be effective in European trials.

111. Naphthalene (Mothballs, Repellents, etc., Paradichlorobenzene, Camphor)

Gastric lavage or emesis for ingestion. Give sodium bicarbonate every 4 hours to maintain alkaline urine and prevent renal blockage with acid hematin crystals. Blood transfusions as necessary. Short-acting barbiturates. Avoid use of milk, oils, or fatty meals. In prevention, these products should be kept out of hands and away from clothes of children (symptoms produced not only by ingestion but also by inhalation and transcutaneous absorption).

112. Naphthol

See Phenol.

113. Nickel (Nickel Carbonyl)

Remove from skin by thorough washing. Artificial respiration and oxygen. Dimercaprol (BAL). Antibiotics and corticosteroids for pneumonitis.

114. Nicotine

Gastric lavage or emesis. Activated charcoal. Short-acting barbiturates. Artificial respiration and oxygen; use of positive pressure resuscitator through period of respiratory failure may prevent death. Thorough washing of skin and removal of clothing will be necessary for skin contamination.

115. Nitrates, Nitrites

Gastric lavage or emesis. Saline cathartic. Methylene blue for methemoglobinemia. Maintain blood pressure with levarterenol. Short-acting barbiturates for convulsions.

116. Nitric Acid

Give large amounts of water. Neutralize with lime water, magnesia, etc. Gastric lavage cautiously if seen within the first hour after ingestion. Gastroscopy to detect caustic burns of the stomach. Demulcents. Morphine for pain, but avoid large doses and possible depression. Shock therapy. Corticosteroids to prevent stricture formation. For eye and skin contact wash thoroughly with water: *do not use chemical antidotes in the eye.*

117. Nitrobenzene

Gastric lavage or emesis. Artificial respiration and oxygen. Methylene blue, 1 per cent solution for methemoglobinemia. Avoid fats and oils.

118. Opium

See Morphine.

119. Oxalates

Gastric lavage with calcium lactate solution, 10 grams (2 tsp) per 100 ml. Ten per cent calcium gluconate intravenously. Give milk and demulcents.

120. Paraldehyde

Gastric lavage or emesis. Artificial respiration and oxygen. Maintain body temperature, fluids, and electrolytes.

121. Paraquat*

Induce vomiting with syrup of ipecac or perform gastric lavage if vomiting has not occurred. If lavage is performed, care must be taken, as paraquat may be corrosive to the esophagus.

Immediately following vomiting or lavage, give approximately 200 to 500 ml of a 30 per cent aqueous suspension of an adsorbent clay (such as Robinson's bentonite U.S.P., or Robinson's fuller's earth U.S.P.) plus an effective dose of cathartic, e.g., magnesium sulfate, to remove paraquat from the entire gastrointestinal tract. Repeat as often as practical (every 2 to 4 hours for several days until paraquat can no longer be detected in blood, urine, or dialysate). If bentonite or fuller's earth is not immediately available, an adsorbent such as powdered activated charcoal should be used until better clays are obtained. Oxygen should be used sparingly and cautiously for dyspnea or cyanosis, because it may aggravate the lung lesions. Forced diuresis should be started as soon as possible to remove paraquat from the blood. If renal function is impaired, hemodialysis or peritoneal dialysis may be of value. Use of forced diuresis and hemodialysis together may aid in hastening removal of paraquat. Monitor the patient's blood urea nitrogen (BUN) and serum creatinine levels, as these are early indicators of systemic poisoning and are useful in determining the patient's progress. Also, obtain daily chest x-rays, arterial oxygen partial pressure, pulmonary function studies, and chest auscultation. Obtain urine, blood, and dialysate samples initially and at least daily to monitor the elimination of paraquat.

For skin contamination, clothing should be removed and the skin thoroughly washed with soap and water for several minutes. If the eyes are involved, they should be irrigated immediately for 10 to 15 minutes and then examined by an ophthalmologist.

122. Parathion (Phosphate Ester Insecticides) (Malathion, Systox, EPN, Diazinon, Guthion, Trithion, TEPP, OMPA, Co-Ral, Phosdrin)

Prompt induction of emesis or gastric lavage with 5 per cent $NaHCO_3$ for ingestion only. Decontaminate by removal of all soiled clothes and thorough washing of skin. Maintain clear airway and respirations with laryngeal intubation and artificial respiration and oxygen. Give atropine, 1 to 2 mg intramuscularly or intravenously, and repeat at 20 to 30 minute intervals, as soon as

---

*Diquat, although it is less toxic, should be treated in a similar fashion.

cyanosis has cleared (chance of ventricular fibrillation). Continue atropine until definite improvement occurs and is maintained (sometimes 2 days or more). The total dosage required may be phenomenal (over 1000 mg). Pralidoxime chloride (Protopam chloride), a cholinesterase reactivator, as 5 per cent solution intravenously. Avoid narcotics, barbiturates, epinephrine, aminophylline, ether, and phenothiazine derivatives, because they further reduce cholinesterase activity and some are respiratory depressants.

123. Pentachlorophenol

Gastric lavage or emesis. Removal of contaminated clothing and thorough washing of skin. Short-acting barbiturates.

124. Pentylenetetrazole (Metrazol)

Delay absorption of intramuscular drug with tourniquet and cryotherapy. Gastric lavage or emesis for ingestion. Short-acting barbiturate for convulsions. Cold packs and alcohol sponging for hyperthermia.

125. Permanganate, Potassium

Thorough lavage of stomach with 3 per cent hydrogen peroxide (10 ml in 100 ml of water). Milk or demulcents. Combat collapse and shock.

126. Phenacetin (Acetophenetidin)

See Acetanilid.

127. Phenol (Derivatives) (Creosote, Guaiacol, Resorcinol, Thymol)

Careful gastric lavage, followed by 60 ml of castor oil, which dissolves phenol and hastens its removal. Activated charcoal. Maintain body temperature, fluids, electrolytes. For skin and mucous membranes, wash thoroughly and follow by application of castor oil or 10 per cent ethyl alcohol. Short-acting barbiturates for convulsions and antibiotics as prophylaxis in pulmonary edema.

128. Phenolphthalein

Gastric lavage or emesis. Activated charcoal. Castor oil given early to hasten the drug through the intestinal tract, but no other solvents because they increase laxative action.

129. Phenothiazine Derivatives

Discontinue drug or reduce dosage. In blood dyscrasias or jaundice do not change to another derivative. Gastric lavage for ingestion of large doses. Antiparkinsonian drugs are rarely necessary. Injectable diphenhydramine hydrochloride (Benadryl) is effective in treatment of extrapyramidal symptoms. Biperiden (Akineton) parenterally or orally. Methylphenidate (Ritalin).

130. Phenytoin (Dilantin Sodium)

Gastric lavage or emesis for ingestion. Discontine use or reduce dosage.

131. Phosphoric Acid

See Table 1.

132. Phosphorus (Red [Nonabsorbed, Nontoxic], Yellow [Volatile and Highly Toxic], Phosphine)

Thorough gastric lavage with potassium permanganate (1:5000) or 3 per cent hydrogen peroxide. Copper sulfate, 0.25 gram in glass of water, forms insoluble copper phosphide. Give 100 ml of mineral oil as a solvent (to prevent absorption and hasten elimination) and repeat in 2 hours. Maintain body temperature, fluids, and electrolytes. Give glucose, vitamin K, and 10 per cent calcium gluconate, if indicated. Exposure to phosphine must be terminated at once, and use of contaminated water for drinking or bathing should be forbidden.

133. Physostigmine (Eserine) (Pilocarpine, Neostigmine, Methacholine [Mecholyl], Muscarine)

Gastric lavage or emesis. Maintain artificial respiration until antidote (propantheline [Pro-Banthine], which is preferable to atropine) can be given; 30 mg intramuscularly every 6 hours may be necessary throughout entire crisis. Maintain airway and remove pulmonary secretion (postural drainage).

134. Picrotoxin

Gastric lavage or emesis. Slow absorption of injected drug by application of cold or tourniquet. Short-acting barbiturate. Cold packs or alcohol sponging for hyperthermia.

135. Procaine

See Cocaine (however, procaine is much less toxic).

136. Pyrethrum (Insecticide Plant)

Gastric lavage or emesis unless kerosene is more suspected than pyrethrum. Demulcents. Short-acting barbiturates for convulsions.

137. Pyribenzamine (Tripelennamine)

See Antihistaminics.

138. Quaternary Ammonium Compounds
(Cationic Detergents)

Gastric lavage with soapy water, milk, or gelatin solution, or emesis. Demulcents or soapy solution. Maintain clear airway; artificial respiration and oxygen. Short-acting barbiturates for convulsions. Atropine recommended without good basis for its use. Avoid alcohol. Thoroughly wash with soap and water for excessive skin contacts.

139. Quinine and Cinchona-like Compounds
(Quinidine, Synthetic Hydrocupreine Compounds [Optochin, Numoquin], Plasmochin, Chloroquine [Aralen], Quinacrine [Atabrine])

Gastric lavage or emesis. Discontinue use of drug. Activated charcoal. Levarterenol for hypotension. Artificial respiration and oxygen.

140. Radiation Syndrome

Remove external clothing and wash clothing and entire body with soap and water. Fresh blood or platelet-enriched plasma. Bone marrow replacement. Antibiotics as prophylaxis for infections.

141. Rotenone

Gastric lavage or emesis if vomiting has not already occurred. Wash thoroughly for skin contact. Short-acting barbiturates. Avoid fats and oils.

142. Ryania

See Rotenone.

143. Sabadilla (Cevadilla)

Demulcents. Activated charcoal. Gastric lavage is usually unnecessary because vomiting occurs early.

144. Salicylate
1. Immediate (emesis or gastric lavage)
   A. Evaluation of severity of intoxication (extrapolation method of Done)
   B. Appraisal of status of dehydration
   C. Determination of acid-base imbalance. Test urine with Phenistix paper and Nitrazene paper
   . D. Determination of electrolyte imbalance.
   E. Draw blood for the following laboratory tests:
      1. Salicylate level
      2. CO_2-combining content
      3. Plasma CO_2 content
      4. pH
      5. Serum electrolyte levels

II. Pending laboratory report
   A. Start intravenous fluids (5 per cent glucose in ⅓ isotonic saline solution)
   B. If dehydration is severe, hydrating solution should be given at the rate of 8 ml per square meter body surface per minute for 30 to 45 minutes
   C. After that time, slow hydrating solution to 2 ml per square meter per minute
   D. Correct bicarbonate and potassium deficits as indicated (average requirement: 5 mEq $NaHCO_3$ per kg and 2 mEq K per kg for 12 hours)
   E. In presence of clinical acidosis and acid urine, $NaHCO_3$ should be given in initial hydrating solution
   F. Body sponging with cool water for hyperpyrexia
III. In life-threatening intoxication, consider exchange transfusion in young children, peritoneal dialysis with 5 per cent albumin solution (Albumisol), or dialysis with artificial kidney
IV. Administer vitamin K and vitamin B complex, the route of administration depending on the condition of the patient
V. Maintenance management
   A. Test each urine voided with Nitrazene paper
   B. Periodic (frequent) determination of:
      1. Blood CO_2-combining power
      2. Blood CO_2 content
      3. Blood pH

145. Santonin

Gastric lavage or emesis. Saline cathartic. Short-acting barbiturates. Avoid opiates.

146. Sea Nettle (Portuguese Man-of-War)

See separate article, page 991.

147. Selenium

Move from occupational environment. Eliminate from diet. Bromobenzene solution, 0.25 to 1 gram in lavage.

148. Silver Nitrate

Dilute with isotonic saline solution (0.9 per cent = 1 tsp salt per 1 pint water) and thorough lavage of stomach; a relatively insoluble and noncorrosive silver chloride is formed in this reaction. Sodium sulfate cathartic (1 oz per cup of water). Milk or demulcents. Shock therapy. Meperidine (Demerol) or codeine for pain.

149. Solanine

Gastric lavage or emesis. Activated charcoal. Pilocarpine. Artificial respiration and circulatory stimulants as necessary.

150. Squill (Red, White)

See Digitalis. Gastric lavage or emesis. Demulcents. Quinidine sulfate. Avoid epinephrine or other stimulants.

151. Strychnine

If symptoms have begun, avoid gastric lavage or emesis. Activated charcoal, followed by gastric lavage if asymptomatic. Short-acting barbiturates. Avoid stimuli and opiates. Artificial respiration and oxygen. Muscle relaxants: diazepam (Valium) is particularly effective.

152. Sulfides (Carbon Disulfide, Soluble Sulfides, Hydrogen Sulfide)

Move from exposure. Artificial respiration and oxygen. Remove swallowed poison by gastric lavage or emesis. Wash skin thoroughly for skin contact and use burn therapy. Antibiotics prevent secondary infection.

153. Sulfonamides

Gastric lavage or emesis for overdosage. Discontinue drug. Alkali and large intake of fluid if renal function is normal. Hemodialysis in severe poisoning.

154. Sulfur Dioxide

Move to fresh air. Artificial respiration and oxygen. Antibiotics and corticosteroids for pneumonitis.

155. Sulfuric Acid

See Hydrochloric Acid.

156. Tear Gases

The most commonly used preparations are chloracetophenone, ethylbromoacetate, bromoacetone, bromobenzyl cyanide, and bromomethyl-ethylketone. *Alpha-chloroacetophenone,* even though called a "gas," is actually a fine powder. In commercial blast-dispersion cartridges, it is mixed half and half with silica anhydride, and a standard shotgun primer is used as a propellant. The mixture is an effective lacrimator in concentrations as low as 2 parts per million (ppm) of air. It can cause extreme irritation and edema of the mucous membranes of the nose and eyes if discharged into the face, and temporary blindness may result. *Mace* contains recrystallized 2-chloroacetophenone (0.9 per cent 1,1,1-trichloroethane), solvents and propellants—Freon, kerosene, methylchloroform, 4.0 per cent.

The eyes should be irrigated for 15 minutes with isotonic solution or water, followed by an anti-inflammatory eye ointment. For clothing and skin contamination the clothes should be removed and a thorough shower taken.

157. Tetrachloroethane

See Carbon Tetrachloride.

158. Thallium

Gastric lavage or emesis. For skin contamination, wash thoroughly. Activated charcoal twice a day, 1 to 2 tbs, and potassium chloride, 3 to 5 grams daily for 5 to 7 days. Dimercaprol (BAL). Dithizon (no preparations marketed for therapeutic use), 10 mg per kg twice a day for 5 days. Maintain body temperature, blood pressure, fluids, and electrolytes. Antibiotics for pneumonitis. Trihexyphenidyl hydrochloride (Artane) for tremors and ataxia.

159. Thiocyanates

Inorganic: Gastric lavage or emesis. Saline cathartic. Give 2 to 4 liters of fluid daily if renal function is normal. Hemodialysis or peritoneal dialysis, if necessary.
Organic (lauryl, ethyl, and methyl thiocyanate. Lethane 60): See Cyanides for treatment.

160. Thiourea

Discontinue use of drug. Antibiotics and corticosteroids for bone marrow depression.

161. Thiram (Tetramethylthiuram Disulfide)

Gastric lavage or emesis. Wash thoroughly for skin contact and remove contaminated clothing. Avoid fats, oils, lipid solvents, and especially alcohol. Artificial respiration and oxygen.

162. Toxaphene

See DDT.

163. Trichloroethylene

See Carbon Tetrachloride.

164. Tricyclic Compounds

When a patient has convulsions, coma, signs of atropinism, and cardiac arrhythmias, one should strongly suspect tricyclic antidepressant poisoning specifically, and intoxication by other anticholinergic drugs and chemicals in general.

Treatment of intoxication from tricyclic antidepressant tranquilizers is supportive and symptomatic, with particular attention paid to the correction of cardiac arrhythmias and maintenance of blood pressure and respiration. Vital signs should be monitored continuously. ECG monitoring is advisable, and severely intoxicated patients should be treated in an intensive care unit.

Cardiac arrhythmias may progress to cardiac arrest owing to ventricular fibrillation or asystole. Death may occur rapidly after a sudden drop of blood pressure and pulse rate. The use of defibrillators and internal or external pacemakers has been advocated. However, in one nonfatal case, an external DC defibrillator produced no alleviation of arrhythmias, and in a fatal case an external pacemaker was tried unsuccessfully. Although documentation is limited, some arrhythmias were controlled in individual patients by use of the parasympathomimetic drugs: physostigmine (drug of choice; readily crosses the blood-brain barrier, 1 mg intravenously), pyridostigmine (Mestinon), neostigmine (Prostigmin), and the beta-adrenergic blocking agent propranolol (Inderal) were also effective. Since it is not possible to predict which patient will respond, it may be necessary to try more than one antiarrhythmic drug. Intravenous phenytoin has had dramatic antiarrhythmic properties and may also be of value in preventing convulsions, which occur frequently. Congestive heart failure is treated by digitalization. However, rapid digitalization should be avoided in a situation in which multiple ventricular ectopic beats are likely to occur. The administration of sodium bicarbonate* and potassium may aid in treating the cardiovascular effects. Convulsions may cause a dangerous increase in the cardiac workload. Agitation, tremors, and convulsions have been successfully treated with parenteral barbiturates. However, use of barbiturates is questionable if drugs that inhibit monoamine oxidase have also been taken by the patient in overdosage or in recent therapy. Also, barbiturates may increase respiratory depression, particularly in children. It is advisable to have equipment available for artificial ventilation and resuscitation. Diazepam (Valium) has been used as an alternative to barbiturates for controlling convulsions, and is considered the drug of choice by some. Hypotension and shock may be treated by intravenous fluids of glucose, saline solution, or plasma, and cautious administration of vasopressor agents such as levarterenol (1-norepinephrine; Levophed), phenylephrine, or metaraminol, which will increase blood pressure without increasing heart rate. Any of these sympathomimetic drugs may induce cardiac arrhythmia and must therefore be used with caution. Other sympathomimetic drugs such as epinephrine and isoproterenol, which stimulate the beta-receptor sites of the heart, should be avoided, because they cause additional increases in the heart rate and may lead to fatal ventricular fibrillation. Respiration must be maintained. Intratracheal artificial respiration is effective and the need for it should be anticipated. Patients should be observed for possible recurrence of respiratory distress after resumption of spontaneous breathing. Various methods have been attempted to hasten excretion of these drugs. They are absorbed quickly from the gastrointestinal tract and are largely bound to plasma proteins. In addition, they are rapidly accumulated in the body tissues, so that high serum concentrations do not occur. They are excreted in the urine largely as glucuronides of the demethylated and hydroxylated metabolites. They are also reportedly secreted into the stomach after absorption. Beneficial effects have been reported from use of exchange transfusion, repeated gastric lavage, and osmotic diuresis. Although evidence is equivocal as to the effectiveness of osmotic diuresis in removing significant amounts of these drugs, it is the general belief that diuresis is beneficial. Osmotic diuresis with mannitol has been employed in the treatment of a number of cases of intoxication with tricyclic antidepressant drugs. In one adult, only 5 per cent of the ingested dose of amitriptyline was recovered in the urine (as amitryptyline and its principal metabolites) after a 10 hour period of forced diuresis with mannitol. Since these drugs also promote urinary retention, catheterization should be considered if diuresis is attempted. Care must also be used to prevent overhydration, which leads to increased cardiac workload. Continuous or repeated gastric lavage has also been recommended to speed excretion. Although continuous gastric lavage was effectively employed in a child intoxicated with imipramine who exhibited coma, convulsions, and cardiac disturbances, it may be unwise to attempt it during convulsive stages. Hemodialysis and peritoneal dialysis are not effective in removing significant amounts of these drugs.

In children the tricyclic drugs are especially treacherous. When a verified ingestion occurs, it probably would be wise to hospitalize the child for monitoring for at least 48 hours, even though the patient may be asymptomatic at the time of admission.

165. Tridione (Trimethadione)

Gastric lavage or emesis for unusual ingestion. Discontinue drug or reduce dosage. Antibiotics and corticosteroids for bone marrow depression.

166. Trinitrotoluene (TNT)

Gastric lavage or emesis. Saline cathartic. Methylene blue for methemoglobinemia. Remove contaminated clothing and wash skin thoroughly. Short-acting barbiturates.

167. Tri-ortho-cresyl Phosphate ("Machine Oil")

Gastric lavage or emesis. Treat as for paralytic poliomyelitis with hydrotherapy, massage,

---

*In one series sodium bicarbonate was the most clinically effective method of treatment of arrhythmias in children; experimental studies support this view.

and orthopedic care. Respirators or rocking bed until sufficient recovery occurs.

168. *Tripelennamine* (Pyribenzamine)

See Anthistaminics.

169. *Turpentine*

Gastric lavage or emesis. Demulcents. Saline cathartic. Stimulants for depression. Artificial respiration and oxygen if necessary.

170. *Veratrum* (Hellebore)

Gastric lavage or emesis. Activated charcoal. Saline cathartic. Atropine every hour to block reflex fall of blood pressure. Phentolamine hydrochloride or other sympathetic blocking agents should be given if hypertension is present.

171. *Vitamins* (Vitamin A, Vitamin D, Vitamin K)

Discontinue use or reduce dosage. Symptomatic and supportive therapy as indicated for hypervitaminosis.

172. *Warfarin* (Coumadin, Panwarfin)

Gastric lavage or emesis. Vitamin K in adequate dosage. Transfusion of fresh blood if hemorrhage is severe.

173. *Xanthines* (Aminophylline, Theophylline, Theobromine, and Caffeine)

Gastric lavage or emesis. Antacids or demulcents. If suppository, remove by enema. Short-acting barbiturates. Oxygen.

174. *Xylene* (Benzene, Toluene, Cumene, and Mesitylene)

Cautious gastric lavage. Fifty milliliters of mineral oil left in stomach. Saline cathartic. Artificial respiration and oxygen. Avoid digestible fats, oils, and epinephrine. Wash thoroughly for skin contact.

175. *Zinc* (Sulfate, Oxide, Phosphide [releases phosphine on contact with water; see Phosphine under Phosphorus])

Gastric lavage or emesis for ingestion. Move patient from source of inhalation. Artificial respiration and oxygen. Antibiotics and corticosteroids for "metal fume fever" and pneumonitis.

SECTION
17

Appendices
and Index

TABLE OF METRIC AND APOTHECARIES' SYSTEMS

(Approved *approximate* dose equivalents are enclosed in parentheses. Use *exact* equivalents in calculations.)

Conversion Factors

METRIC	APOTHECARIES'		METRIC	APOTHECARIES'
1 milligram (mg.)	1/64 grain		3.88 cubic centimeters or grams	1 dram (4 cc. or grams)
64.79 milligrams	1 grain (65 mg.)		31.103 cubic centimeters or grams	1 ounce (30 cc. or grams)
1 gram	15.43 grains (15 grains)		473.167 cubic centimeters	1 pint (500 cc.)
1 cubic centimeter (cc.)	16 minims			

WEIGHTS

METRIC	APOTHECARIES'	METRIC	APOTHECARIES'
0.0001 gram—0.1 mg.—1/640 grain (1/600 grain)		0.057 gram —57 mg.—7/8 grain	
0.0002 gram—0.2 mg.—1/320 grain (1/300 grain)		0.06 gram —60 mg.—9/10 grain (1 grain)	
0.0003 gram—0.3 mg.—1/210 grain (1/200 grain)		0.065 gram —65 mg.—1 grain (60 mg.)	
0.0004 gram—0.4 mg.—1/150 grain		0.07 gram —70 mg.—1-1/20 grains	
0.0005 gram—0.5 mg.—1/120 grain		0.08 gram —80 mg.—1-1/5 grains	
0.0006 gram—0.6 mg.—1/100 grain		0.09 gram —90 mg.—1-1/3 grains	
0.0007 gram—0.7 mg.—1/90 grain		0.097 gram —97 mg.—1-1/2 grains (0.1 gram)	
0.0008 gram—0.8 mg.—1/80 grain		0.12 gram —120 mg.—2 grains	
0.0009 gram—0.9 mg.—1/75 grain		0.2 gram —200 mg.—3 grains	
0.001 gram—1 mg.—1/64 grain (1/60 grain)		0.24 gram —240 mg.—4 grains (0.25 gram)	
0.0011 gram—1.1 mg.—1/60 grain		0.3 gram —300 mg.—4-1/2 grains	
0.0013 gram—1.3 mg.—1/50 grain (1.2 mg.)		0.33 gram —330 mg.—5 grains (0.3 gram)	
0.0014 gram—1.4 mg.—1/48 grain		0.4 gram —400 mg.—6 grains	
0.0016 gram—1.6 mg.—1/40 grain (1.5 mg.)		0.45 gram —450 mg.—7 grains	
0.0018 gram—1.8 mg.—1/36 grain		0.5 gram —500 mg.—7-1/2 grains	
0.0020 gram—2 mg.—1/32 grain (1/30 grain)		0.53 gram —530 mg.—8 grains	
0.0022 gram—2.2 mg.—1/30 grain		0.6 gram —600 mg.—9 grains	
0.0026 gram—2.6 mg.—1/25 grain		0.65 gram —650 mg.—10 grains (0.6 gram)	
0.003 gram—3 mg.—1/20 grain		0.73 gram —730 mg.—11 grains	
0.004 gram—4 mg.—1/16 grain (1/15 grain)		0.80 gram —800 mg.—12 grains (0.75 gram)	
0.005 gram—5 mg.—1/12 grain		0.86 gram —860 mg.—13 grains	
0.006 gram—6 mg.—1/10 grain		0.93 gram —930 mg.—14 grains	
0.007 gram—7 mg.—1/9 grain		1. gram —1000 mg.—15 grains	
0.008 gram—8 mg.—1/8 grain		1.06 grams—1060 mg.—16 grains	
0.009 gram—9 mg.—1/7 grain		1.13 grams—1130 mg.—17 grains	
0.01 gram—10 mg.—1/6 grain		1.18 grams—1180 mg.—18 grains	
0.013 gram—13 mg.—1/5 grain (12 mg.)		1.26 grams—1260 mg.—19 grains	
0.016 gram—16 mg.—1/4 grain (15 mg.)		1.30 grams—1300 mg.—20 grains	
0.02 gram—20 mg.—1/3 grain		1.50 grams—1500 mg.—22 grains	
0.025 gram—25 mg.—3/8 grain		2 grams—2000 mg.—30 grains (1/2 dram)	
0.03 gram—30 mg.—2/5 grain (1/2 grain)		4 grams —1 dram (60 grains)	
0.032 gram—32 mg.—1/2 grain (30 mg.)		5 grams —75 grains	
0.04 gram—40 mg.—3/5 grain (2/3 grain)		8 grams —2 drams (7.5 grams)	
0.043 gram—43 mg.—2/3 grain (40 mg.)		10 grams —2-1/2 drams	
0.05 gram—50 mg.—3/4 grain		15 grams —4 drams	
		30 grams —1 ounce	

LIQUID MEASURES*

METRIC	APOTHECARIES'	METRIC	APOTHECARIES'
0.03 cubic centimeter — 1/2 minim		8 cubic centimeters—2 fluid drams	
0.05 cubic centimeter — 3/4 minim		10 cubic centimeters—2-1/2 fluid drams	
0.06 cubic centimeter —1 minim		15 cubic centimeters—4 fluid drams	
0.1 cubic centimeter —1-1/2 minims		20 cubic centimeters—5-1/2 fluid drams	
0.2 cubic centimeter —3 minims		25 cubic centimeters— 5/6 fluid ounce	
0.25 cubic centimeter —4 minims		30 cubic centimeters—1 fluid ounce	
0.3 cubic centimeter —5 minims		50 cubic centimeters—1-3/4 fluid ounces	
0.5 cubic centimeter —8 minims		60 cubic centimeters—2 fluid ounces	
0.6 cubic centimeter —10 minims		100 cubic centimeters—3-1/2 fluid ounces	
0.75 cubic centimeter —12 minims		120 cubic centimeters—4 fluid ounces	
1 cubic centimeter —15 minims		200 cubic centimeters—7 fluid ounces	
2 cubic centimeters—30 minims		250 cubic centimeters—8 fluid ounces	
3 cubic centimeters—45 minims		360 cubic centimeters—12 fluid ounces	
4 cubic centimeters—1 fluid dram		500 cubic centimeters—1 pint	
5 cubic centimeters—1-1/4 fluid drams		1000 cubic centimeters—1 quart	

* Note: A cubic centimeter (cc.) is the approximate equivalent of a milliliter (ml.). The terms are used interchangeably in general medicine.

TABLES OF HEIGHT AND WEIGHT FOR MEN AND WOMEN*

DESIRABLE WEIGHTS FOR MEN OF AGES 25 AND OVER

Weight in Pounds According to Frame (In Indoor Clothing)

HEIGHT (WITH SHOES ON) 1-INCH HEELS Feet	Inches	SMALL FRAME	MEDIUM FRAME	LARGE FRAME
5	2	112–120	118–129	126–141
5	3	115–123	121–133	129–144
5	4	118–126	124–136	132–148
5	5	121–129	127–139	135–152
5	6	124–133	130–143	138–156
5	7	128–137	134–147	142–161
5	8	132–141	138–152	147–166
5	9	136–145	142–156	151–170
5	10	140–150	146–160	155–174
5	11	144–154	150–165	159–179
6	0	148–158	154–170	164–184
6	1	152–162	158–175	168–189
6	2	156–167	162–180	173–194
6	3	160–171	167–185	178–199
6	4	164–175	172–190	182–204

DESIRABLE WEIGHTS FOR WOMEN OF AGES 25 AND OVER

Weight in Pounds According to Frame (In Indoor Clothing)

HEIGHT (WITH SHOES ON) 2-INCH HEELS Feet	Inches	SMALL FRAME	MEDIUM FRAME	LARGE FRAME
4	10	92– 98	96–107	104–119
4	11	94–101	98–110	106–122
5	0	96–104	101–113	109–125
5	1	99–107	104–116	112–128
5	2	102–110	107–119	115–131
5	3	105–113	110–122	118–134
5	4	108–116	113–126	121–138
5	5	111–119	116–130	125–142
5	6	114–123	120–135	129–146
5	7	118–127	124–139	133–150
5	8	122–131	128–143	137–154
5	9	126–135	132–147	141–158
5	10	130–140	136–151	145–163
5	11	134–144	140–155	149–168
6	0	138–148	144–159	153–173

For girls between 18 and 25, subtract 1 pound for each year under 25.

*Courtesy of the Metropolitan Life Insurance Company.

GLOSSARY OF AMERICAN DRUG NAMES AND INTERNATIONAL SYNONYMS *

United States Adopted Name	British Approved or International Nonproprietary Name	United States Adopted Name	British Approved or International Nonproprietary Name
Acenocoumarol	Nicoumalone	Ethylaminobenzoate	Benzocaine
Acetaminophen	Paracetamol	Ethylestrenol	Ethyloestrenol
Acetarsone	Acetarsol	Evans blue	Azovan blue
Actinomycin	Actinomycin C	Fantridone	Fanthridone
Albuterol	Salbutamol	Fibrinolysin, human	Plasmin
Ambuphylline	Bufylline	Floxacillin	Flucloxacillin
Aminitrozole	Acinitrazole	Flucloronide	Fluclorolone acetonide
Amithizone	Thiacetazone	Flurandrenolide	Flurandrenolone
Amobarbital	Amylobarbitone	Flurogestone	Flugestone
Amoxycillin	Amoxycilline	Fonazine	Dimethothiazine
Amphecloral	Amfecloral	Fructose	Levulose
Anazoline	Anoxynaphthonate	Furosemide	Frusemide
Anisotropine	Octatropine	Gestronorone	Gestronol
Anthralin	Dithranol	Glyburide	Glibenclamide
Antimony sodium gluconate	Sodium stibogluconate	Glycobiarsol	Bismuth glycolylarsanilate
Antipyrine	Phenazone	Glycopyrrolate	Glycopyrronium
Arylam	Sevin	Heptabarbital	Heptabarbitone
Asparaginase	Colaspase	Hexacarbacholine	Carbolonium
Barbital	Barbitone	Hexachlorophene	Hexachlorophane
Bendazac	Bindazac	Hexamarium	Distigmine
Bendroflumethiazide	Bendrofluazide	Hexestrol	Hexoestrol
Benoxinate	Oxybuprocaine	Hexobarbital	Hexobarbitone
Betazole	Ametazole	Hydralazine	Hydrallazine
Biphenamine	Xenysalate	Hydrocortisone	Cortisol
Bismuth subcarbonate	Bismuth oxycarbonate	Hydroxypropyl methylcellulose	Hypromellose
Bromisovalum	Bromeval	Indigotindisulfonate sodium	Indigo carmine
Bunamiodyl	Buniodyl	Inositol niacinate	Inositol nicotinate
Busulfan	Busulphan	Iodochlorhydroxyquin	Clioquinol
Butabarbital	Secbutabarbitone	Iodopyracet	Diodrast
Butethal	Butobarbitone	Iothiouracil	Iodothiouracil
Butyl aminobenzoate	Butesine	Isoflurophate	Dyflos
Calciferol	Ergosterol	Isoproterenol	Isoprenaline
Calcium benzoylpas	Calcium benzamidosalicylate	Isosorbide dinitrate	Sorbide nitrate
Carbachol	Carbamoylcholine	Leucovorin calcium	Calcium folinate
Carbenoxalone	Carbenoxolone	Lidocaine	Lignocaine
Chaulmoogra oil	Hydnocarpus oil	Mechlorethamine	Mustine
Chloroazodin	Chlorazodin	Meclizine	Meclozine
Chlorobutanol	Chlorbutol	Melanotropin	Intermedin
Chloroguanide	Proguanil	Melphalan	Melfalan
Chlorophenothane	Dicophane	Menadione	Menaphthone
Chlorothen	Chloropyrilene	Menotropins	Follicle-stimulating hormone
Colistimethate	Colistin methanesulphomethate	Meparfynol	Methylpentynol
Corticotropin	Corticotrophin	Mepazine	Pecazine
Cosyntropin	Tetracosactrin	Meperidine	Pethidine
Cromolyn	Cromoglycate	Mephenytoin	Methoin
Cyclobarbital	Cyclobarbitone	Mephobarbital	Methylphenobarbitone
Cyclocumarol	Cyclocoumarol	Metaproterenol	Orciprenaline
Daunomycin	Rubidomycin	Methabarbital	Methabarbitone
Deferoxamine	Desferrioxamine	Methacholine	Acetylmethylcholine
Demeclocycline	Demethylchlortetracycline	Methandrostenolone	Methandienone
Desoxycorticosterone	Deoxycortone	Methantheline	Methanthelinium
Dextroamphetamine	Dexamphetamine	Methenamine hippurate	Hexamine hippurate
Dibucaine	Cinchocaine	Methohexital	Methohexitone
Dichloroisoproterenol	Dichloroisoprenaline	Methopholine	Metofoline
Dicumarol	Dicoumarol	Methscopolamine bromide	Hyoscine methobromide
Diethyl dithiolisophthalate	Ditophal	Methylatropine nitrate	Atropine methyl nitrate
Diethylstilbestrol	Stilboestrol	Methylergonovine	Methylergometrine
Diiodohydroxyquin	Diiodohydroxyquinoline	Methyprylon	Methylprylone
Dinoprost tromethamine	Dinoprostone	Mineral oil	Paraffin, liquid
Disodium-p-melaminylphenyl arsonate	Melarsen	Nequinate	Methyl benzoquate
		Niacin	Nicotinic acid
Dromostanolone	Drostanolone	Niacinamide	Nicotinamide
Dyphylline	Diprophylline	Nikethamide	Nicethamide
Echothiophate	Ecothiopate	Nitroglycerin	Glyceryl trinitrate
Epinephrine	Adrenaline	Norepinephrine	Noradrenaline
Ergocalciferol	Calciferol	Norethindrone	Norethisterone
Ergonovine	Ergometrine	Norethynodrel	Noretynodrel
Estradiol	Oestradiol	Normeperidine	Norpethidine
Estrogen	Oestrogen	Nylidrin	Buphenine
Ethenzamide	Etenzamide	Ouabain	Strophanthin
Ethinyl estradiol	Ethinyloestradiol	Oxtriphylline	Choline theophyllinate

GLOSSARY OF AMERICAN DRUG NAMES AND
INTERNATIONAL SYNONYMS* *(Continued)*

United States Adopted Name	British Approved or International Nonproprietary Name	United States Adopted Name	British Approved or International Nonproprietary Name
Peanut oil	Arachis oil	Sulfamethoxypyridazine	Sulphamethoxypyridazine
Penicillin G	Benzylpenicillin	Sulfamoxole	Sulphamoxole
Pentobarbital	Pentobarbitone	Sulfaphenazole	Sulphaphenazole
Pentylenetetrazole	Leptazol	Sulfaproxyline	Sulphaproxyline
Phenobarbital	Phenobarbitone	Sulfasalazine	Sulphasalazine
Physostigmine	Eserine	Sulfasomizole	Sulphasomizole
Phytonadione	Phytomenadione	Sulfathiazole	Sulphathiazole
Polyethylene glycol	Macrogol	Sulfinpyrazone	Sulphinpyrazone
Progestin	Allylestrenol	Sulfisomidine	Sulphasomidine
Proparacaine	Proxymetacaine	Sulfisoxazole	Sulphafurazole
Propoxyphene	Dextropropoxyphene	Sulfomyxin	Sulphomyxin
Pyrilamine	Mepyramine	Tetracaine	Amethocaine
Pyrvinium pamoate	Vipyrnium embonate	Tetramisole	Levamisole
Quinacrine	Mepacrine	Thiabendazole	Mintezol
Riboflavin	Riboflavine	Thialbarbital	Thialbarbitone
Rifampin	Rifampicin	Thiamine	Aneurine
Rolicyprine	Rolicypram	Thimerosal	Thiomersal
Scopolamine	Hyoscine	Thiopental	Thiopentone
Secobarbital	Quinalbarbitone	Thyrotropin	Thyrotrophin
Seperidol	Clofluperol	Thyroxin	Thyroxine
Sodium acetylhydroxyarsanilate	Orsanine	Tilidine	Tilidate
Solasulfone	Solapsone	Triethylenemelamine	Tretamine
Succinylcholine	Suxamethonium	Triflupromazine	Flupromazine
Succinylsulfathiazole	Succinylsulphathiazole	Trihexyphenidyl	Benzhexol
Sulfacetamide	Sulphacetamide	Trimethadione	Troxidone
Sulfadiazine	Sulphadiazine	Trimethaphan	Trimetaphan
Sulfadimethoxine	Sulphadimethoxine	Trimethoprim-sulfamethoxazole	Co-trimoxazole
Sulfaethidole	Sulphaethidole	Troleandomycin	Triacetyloleandomycin
Sulfalene	Sulfametopyrazine	Tromethamine	Trometamol
Sulfameter	Sulphamethoxydiazine	Uracil mustard	Uramustine
Sulfamethazine	Sulfadimidine	Urethan	Urethane
Sulfamethizole	Sulphamethizole	Vinbarbital	Vinbarbitone
Sulfamethoxazole	Sulphamethoxazole	Vitamin A	Retinol

*Modified from Modell, W., Schild, H. O., and Wilson, A.: Applied Pharmacology (American edition). Philadelphia, W. B. Saunders Company, 1976.

LABORATORY REFERENCE VALUES OF CLINICAL IMPORTANCE

prepared by
REX B. CONN, M.D.
Atlanta, Georgia

THE INTERNATIONAL SYSTEM OF UNITS FOR LABORATORY MEASUREMENTS (LE SYSTÈME INTERNATIONAL D'UNITÉS)

Physicians are accustomed to receiving laboratory reports with measurements expressed in metric units such as the gram, liter, or milliliter; however, an extensive modification of the metric system has been adopted by clinical laboratories in many countries, and plans are being formulated to make a similar change in the United States. This adaptation is the International System of Units (Le Système International d'Unités), usually abbreviated S.I. Units. Whereas the metric system utilizes the centimeter, the gram, and the second as basic units, the International System uses the meter, the kilogram, and the second as well as four other basic units.

The overriding consideration for adopting the International System is that it will provide a common language among the various scientific disciplines throughout the world for unambiguous communication regarding all types of measurements. In the medical field, the advantages of conversion are that chemical relationships between various substances will become more readily apparent and there will be an international uniformity in laboratory reporting. The most serious disadvantage in making this conversion is that physicians will have to become accustomed to a new set of figures for almost all laboratory measurements. Because of this inconvenience, as well as a potential for serious misinterpretation of laboratory data, the conversion must be undertaken cautiously and only after a logical plan has been formulated and discussed. There appears to be little question, however, that the International System will be adopted in this country. Clinical laboratories in most western European countries, Canada, and Australia are already using S.I. Units, and American medical journals are adopting the practice of expressing measurements in both conventional and S.I. Units.

The International System

The International System is a coherent approach to all types of measurement which utilizes seven dimensionally independent basic quantities: mass, length, time, thermodynamic temperature, electric current, luminous intensity, and amount of substance. Each of these quantities is expressed in a clearly defined *basic unit* (Table 1).

Two or more basic units may be combined to provide *derived units* (Table 2) for expressing other measurements such as mass concentration (kilograms per cubic meter) and velocity (meters per second). Standardized prefixes (Table 3) for basic and derived units are used to express fractions or multiples of the basic units so that any measurement can be expressed in a value between 0.001 and 1000.

Medical Applications

The most profound change in laboratory reports will result from expressing concentration as amount per volume (moles per liter) rather than mass per volume (milligrams per 100 milliliters). The advantages in the former expression can be seen in the following:

Conventional Units

1.0 gram of hemoglobin
    Combines with 1.37 ml. of oxygen
    Contains 3.4 mg. of iron
    Forms 34.9 mg. of bilirubin

S.I. Units

1.0 mmol of hemoglobin
    Combines with 4.0 mmol of oxygen
    Contains 4.0 mmol of iron
    Forms 4.0 mmol of bilirubin

Chemical relationships between lactic acid and pyruvic acid and the glucose from which both are derived, as well as the relationship between bilirubin and the binding capacity of albumin, are other examples of chemical relationships that will be clarified by using the new system.

There are a number of laboratory and other medical measurements for which the S.I. Units appear to offer little advantage, and some which are disadvantageous because the change would require replacement or revision of instruments such as the sphygmomanometer. The cubic meter is the derived unit for volume; however, it is inappropriately large for medical measurements and the liter has been retained. Thermodynamic

TABLE 1. **Basic Units**

PROPERTY	BASIC UNIT	SYMBOL
Length	metre	m
Mass	kilogram	kg
Amount of substance	mole	mol
Time	second	s
Thermodynamic temperature	kelvin	K
Electric current	ampere	A
Luminous intensity	candela	cd

TABLE 2. Derived Units

DERIVED PROPERTY	DERIVED UNIT	SYMBOL
Area	square metre	m^2
Volume	cubic metre	m^3
	litre	l
Mass concentration	kilogram/cubic metre	kg/m^3
	gram/litre	g/l
Substance concentration	mole/cubic metre	mol/m^3
	mole/litre	mol/l
Temperature	degree Celsius	$C = K - 273.15$

temperature expressed in kelvins is not more informative for medical measurements. Since the Celsius degree is the same as the Kelvin degree, the Celsius scale will be used. Celsius rather than centigrade is the preferred term.

Selection of units for expressing enzyme activity presents certain difficulties. Literally dozens of different units have been used in expressing enzyme activity, and interlaboratory comparison of enzyme results is impossible unless the assay system is precisely defined. In 1964 the International Union of Biochemistry attempted to remedy the situation by proposing the International Unit for enzymes. This unit was defined as the amount of enzyme that will catalyze the conversion of 1 micromole of substrate per minute under standard conditions. Difficulties remain, however, as enzyme activity is affected by the temperature, pH, the type and amount of substrate, the presence of inhibitors, and other factors. Enzyme activity can be expressed in S.I. Units, and the katal has been proposed to express activities of all catalysts, including enzymes. The katal is that amount of enzyme which catalyzes a reaction rate of 1 mole per second. Thus adoption of the katal as the unit of enzyme activity would provide no more information than is obtained when results are expressed in International Units.

Hydrogen ion concentration in blood is customarily expressed as pH, but in S.I. Units it would be expressed in nanomoles per liter. It appears unlikely that the very useful pH scale will be discarded.

Pressure measures, such as blood pressure and partial pressures of blood gases, would be expressed in S.I. Units, using the Pascal, a unit that can be derived from the basic units for mass, length, and time. This change probably will not be adopted in the early phases of the conversion to S.I. Units. Similarly, a proposed change in expressing osmolality in terms of the depression of freezing point is inappropriate, because osmolality may be calculated from vapor pressure as well as freezing point measurement.

Conventions

A number of conventions have been adopted to standardize usage of S.I. Units:

1. No periods are used after the symbol for a unit (kg not kg.), and it remains unchanged when used in the plural (70 kg not 70 kgs).

2. A half space rather than a comma is used to divide large numbers into groups of three (5 400 000 not 5,400,000).

3. Compound prefixes should be avoided (nanometer not millimicrometer).

4. Multiples and submultiples are used in steps of 10^3 or 10^{-3}.

5. The degree sign for the temperature scales is omitted (38 C not 38°C).

6. The preferred spelling is metre not meter, litre not liter.

7. Report of a measurement should include information on the system, the component, the kind of quantity, the numerical value, and the unit. For example: *System,* serum. *Component,* glucose. *Kind of quantity,* substance concentration. *Value,* 5.10. *Unit,* mmol/l.

8. The name of the component should be unambiguous; for example, "serum bilirubin" might refer to unconjugated bilirubin or to total bilirubin. For acids and bases, the maximally ionized form is used in naming the component; for example, lactate or urate rather than lactic acid or uric acid.

Tables of Reference Values

Tables accompanying this article indicate "normal values" for most of the commonly performed laboratory tests. The title of the tables has been changed from the "normal values" of previous years to "reference values" to conform to current usage. The reference value is given in conventional units, the conversion factor is indicated when appropriate, and the value in S.I. Units is calculated from these figures. Notes (pp. 1035 and 1036) are used to provide additional information.

TABLE 3. Standard Prefixes

PREFIX	MULTIPLICATION FACTOR	SYMBOL
atto	10^{-18}	a
femto	10^{-15}	f
pico	10^{-12}	p
nano	10^{-9}	n
micro	10^{-6}	μ
milli	10^{-3}	m
centi	10^{-2}	c
deci	10^{-1}	d
deca	10^1	da
hecto	10^2	h
kilo	10^3	k
mega	10^6	M
giga	10^9	G
tera	10^{12}	T

REFERENCE VALUES IN HEMATOLOGY

	CONVENTIONAL UNITS	FACTOR	S.I. UNITS	NOTES
Acid hemolysis test (Ham)	No hemolysis	—	No hemolysis	
Alkaline phosphatase, leukocyte	Total score 14–100	—	Total score 14–100	
Carboxyhemoglobin	Up to 5% of total	0.01	0.05 of total	a
Cell counts				
Erythrocytes		10^6		
Males	4.6–6.2 million/cu. mm.		4.6–$6.2 \times 10^{12}/l$	
Females	4.2–5.4 million/cu. mm.		4.2–$5.4 \times 10^{12}/l$	
Children (varies with age)	4.5–5.1 million/cu. mm.		4.5–$5.1 \times 10^{12}/l$	
Leukocytes		10^6		
Total	4500–11,000/cu. mm.		4.5–$11.0 \times 10^9/l$	
Differential	*Percentage*	*Absolute*		
Myelocytes	0	0/cu. mm.	10^6	0/1	b
Band neutrophils	3–5	150–400/cu. mm.		150–$400 \times 10^6/l$	
Segmented neutrophils	54–62	3000–580(/cu. mm.		3000–$5800 \times 10^6/l$	
Lymphocytes	25–33	1500–3000/cu. mm.		1500–$3000 \times 10^6/l$	
Monocytes	3–7	300–500/cu. mm.		300–$500 \times 10^6/l$	
Eosinophils	1–3	50–250/cu. mm.		50–$250 \times 10^6/l$	
Basophils	0–0.75	15–50/cu. mm.		15–$50 \times 10^6/l$	
Platelets	150,000–350,000/cu. mm.	10^6	150–$350 \times 10^9/l$	b
Reticulocytes	25,000–75,000/cu. mm.	10^6	25–$75 \times 10^9/l$	
	0.5–1.5% of erythrocytes			
Coagulation tests				
Bleeding time (Duke)	1–5 min.	—	1–5 min	
Bleeding time (Ivy)	Less than 5 min.	—	Less than 5 min	
Clot retraction, qualitative	Begins in 30–60 min.	—	Begins in 30–60 min	
	Complete in 24 hrs.	—	Complete in 24 h	
Coagulation time (Lee-White)	5–15 min. (glass tubes)	—	5–15 min (glass tubes)	
	19–60 min. (siliconized tubes)	—	19–60 min (siliconized tubes)	
Euglobulin lysis time	2–6 hr. at 37°	—	2–6 h at 37 C	a
Factor VIII and other coagulation factors	50–150% of normal	—	0.50–1.5 of normal	
Fibrin split products (Thrombo-Wellco test)	Negative at 1:4 dilution	—	Negative at 1:4 dilution	
Fibrinogen	200–400 mg/100 ml.	0.0293	5.9–11.7 μmol/l	c
Fibrinolysins	0	—	0	
Partial thromboplastin time, activated (APTT)	35–45 sec.	—	35–45 s	
Prothrombin consumption	Over 80% consumed in 1 hr.	0.01	Over 0.80 consumed in 1 h	a
Prothrombin content	100% (calculated from prothrombin time)	0.01	1.0 (calculated from prothrombin time)	a
Prothrombin time (one stage)	12.0–14.0 sec.	—	12.0–14.0 s	
Thromboplastin generation test	Compared to normal control	—	Compared to normal control	
Tourniquet test	Ten or fewer petechiae in a 2.5 cm. circle after 5 min.	—	Ten or fewer petechiae in a 2.5 cm circle after 5 min	
Cold hemolysin test (Donath-Land-steiner)	No hemolysis	—	No hemolysis	
Coombs test				
Direct	Negative	—	Negative	
Indirect	Negative	—	Negative	

Corpuscular values of erythrocytes (values are for adults; in children, values vary with age)

M.C.H. (mean corpuscular hemoglobin)	27–31 picogm.	0.0155	0.42–0.48 fmol	d
M.C.V. (mean corpuscular volume)	80–105 cu. micra	1.0	80–105 fl	a
M.C.H.C. (mean corpuscular hemoglobin concentration)	32–36%	0.01	0.32–0.36	d
Haptoglobin (as hemoglobin binding capacity)	100–200 mg./100 ml.	0.155	16–31 μmol/l	d
Hematocrit				
Males	40–54 ml./100 ml.	0.01	0.40–0.54	a
Females	37–47 ml./100 ml.		0.37–0.47	
Newborn	49–54 ml./100 ml.		0.49–0.54	
Children (varies with age)	35–49 ml./100 ml.		0.35–0.49	
Hemoglobin				
Males	14.0–18.0 grams/100 ml.	0.155	2.17–2.79 mmol/l	d
Females	12.0–16.0 grams/100 ml.		1.86–2.48 mmol/l	
Newborn	16.5–19.5 grams/100 ml.		2.56–3.02 mmol/l	
Children (varies with age)	11.2–16.5 grams/100 ml.		1.74–2.56 mmol/l	
Hemoglobin, fetal	Less than 1% of total	0.01	Less than 0.01 of total	a
Hemoglobin A$_{1c}$	3–5% of total	0.01	0.03–0.05 of total	a
Hemoglobin A$_2$	1.5–3.0% of total	0.01	0.015–0.03 of total	a
Hemoglobin, plasma	0–5.0 mg./100 ml.	0.155	0–0.8 μmol/l	d
Methemoglobin	0–130 mg./100 ml.	0.155	4.7–20 μmol/l	e
Osmotic fragility of erythrocytes	Begins in 0.45–0.39% NaCl	171	Begins in 77–67 mmol/l NaCl	
	Complete in 0.33–0.30% NaCl		Complete in 56–51 mmol/l NaCl	
Sedimentation rate				
Wintrobe: Males	0–5 mm. in 1 hr.	—	0–5 mm/h	
Females	0–15 mm. in 1 hr.	—	0–15 mm/h	
Westergren: Males	0–15 mm. in 1 hr.	—	0–15 mm/h	
Females	0–20 mm. in 1 hr.	—	0–20 mm/h	
(May be slightly higher in children and during pregnancy)				

Bone marrow, differential cell count

	Range	Average		Range	Average	
Myeloblasts	0.3–5.0%	2.0%	0.01	0.003–0.05	0.02	a
Promyelocytes	1.0–8.0%	5.0%		0.01–0.08	0.05	
Myelocytes: Neutrophilic	5.0–19.0%	12.0%		0.05–0.19	0.12	
Eosinophilic	0.5–3.0%	1.5%		0.005–0.03	0.015	
Basophilic	0.0–0.5%	0.3%		0.00–0.005	0.003	
Metamyelocytes	13.0–32.0%	22.0%		0.13–0.32	0.22	
Polymorphonuclear neutrophils	7.0–30.0%	20.0%		0.07–0.30	0.20	
Polymorphonuclear eosinophils	0.5–4.0%	2.0%		0.005–0.04	0.02	
Polymorphonuclear basophils	0.0–0.7%	0.2%		0.00–0.007	0.002	
Lymphocytes	3.0–17.0%	10.0%		0.03–0.17	0.10	
Plasma cells	0.0–2.0%	0.4%		0.00–0.02	0.004	
Monocytes	0.5–5.0%	2.0%		0.005–0.05	0.02	
Reticulum cells	0.1–2.0%	0.2%		0.001–0.02	0.002	
Megakaryocytes	0.3–3.0%	0.4%		0.003–0.03	0.004	
Pronormoblasts	1.0–8.0%	4.0%		0.01–0.08	0.04	
Normoblasts	7.0–32.0%	18.0%		0.07–0.32	0.18	

REFERENCE VALUES FOR BLOOD, PLASMA AND SERUM

(For some procedures the reference values may vary depending upon the method used)

	CONVENTIONAL UNITS	FACTOR	S.I. UNITS	NOTES
Acetoacetate plus acetone, serum				
Qualitative	Negative	—	Negative	
Quantitative	0.3–2.0 mg./100 ml.	10	3–20 mg/l	
Adrenocorticotropin (ACTH), plasma	10–80 picogm./ml.	1.0	10–80 ng/l	
Aldolase, serum	0–11 milliunits/ml. (I.U.) (30°)	1.0	0–11 units/l (30 C)	f
Alpha amino nitrogen, serum	3.0–5.5 mg./100 ml.	0.714	2.1–3.9 mmol/l	
Ammonia, plasma	20–120 mcg./100 ml.	0.554	11–67 μmol/l	
Amylase, serum	Less than 160 Caraway units/100 ml.	—	Less than 160 Caraway units/dl	f
Anion gap	8–16 mEq./l.	1.0	8–16 mmol/l	
Ascorbic acid, blood	0.4–1.5 mg./100 ml.	56.8	23–85 μmol/l	
Base excess, blood	0 ± 2 mEq./liter	1.0	0 ± 2 mmol/l	
Bicarbonate, serum	23–29 mEq./liter	1.0	23–29 mmol/l	
Bile acids, serum	0.3–3.0 mg./dl.	10	3.0–30.0 mg/l	
Bilirubin, serum				
Direct	0.1–0.4 mg./100 ml.	17.1	1.7–6.8 μmol/l	
Indirect	0.2–0.7 mg./100 ml. (Total minus direct)	17.1	3.4–12 μmol/l (Total minus direct)	
Total	0.3–1.1 mg./100 ml.	17.1	5.1–19 μmol/l	
Bromsulphalein (BSP)	Less than 5%	0.01	Less than 0.05	a
(Inject 5 mg./kg. body weight, draw sample at 45 min.)				
Calcium, serum	4.5–5.5 mEq./liter	0.50	2.25–2.75 mmol/l	
	9.0–11.0 mg./100 ml.	0.25	2.25–2.75 mmol/l	
	(Slightly higher in children)		(Slightly higher in children)	
	(Varies with protein concentration)		(Varies with protein concentration)	
Calcium, ionized, serum	2.1–2.6 mEq./liter	0.50	1.05–1.30 mmol/l	
	4.25–5.25 mg./100 ml.	0.25	1.05–1.30 mmol/l	
Carbon dioxide content, serum				
Adults	24–30 mEq./liter	1.0	24–30 mmol/l	
Infants	20–28 mEq./liter	1.0	20–28 mmol/l	
Carbon dioxide tension (Pco$_2$), blood	35–45 mm. Hg	—	35–45 mm Hg	
Carotene, serum	50–300 mcg./100 ml.	0.0186	0.93–5.58 μmol/l	g
Ceruloplasmin, serum	23–44 mg./100 ml.	0.0662	1.5–2.9 μmol/l	h
Chloride, serum	96–106 mEq./liter	1.0	96–106 mmol/l	
Cholesterol, serum				
Total	150–250 mg./100 ml.	0.0259	3.9–6.5 mmol/l	a
Esters	68–76% of total cholesterol	0.01	0.68–0.76 of total cholesterol	
Cholinesterase				
Serum	0.5–1.3 pH units	—	0.5–1.3 pH units	f
Erythrocytes	0.5–1.0 pH unit	—	0.5–1.0 pH unit	f
Copper, serum				
Males	70–140 mcg./100 ml.	0.157	11–22 μmol/l	
Females	85–155 mcg./100 ml.	0.157	13–24 μmol/l	
Cortisol, plasma (8 A.M.)	6–23 mcg./100 ml.	27.6	170–635 nmol/l	

	Conventional value	Conversion factor	SI value	
Creatine, serum	0.2–0.8 mg./100 ml.	76.3	15–61 μmol/l	
Creatine phosphokinase, serum				
Males	0–50 milliunits/ml. (I.U.) (30°) (Oliver-Rosalki)	1.0	0–50 units/l (30 C) (Oliver-Rosalki)	f
Females	0–30 milliunits/ml. (I.U.) (30°)	1.0	0–30 units/l (30 C) (Oliver-Rosalki)	f
Creatine phosphokinase isoenzymes, serum				
CPK-MM	Present	—	Present	
CPK-MB	Absent	—	Absent	
CPK-BB	Absent	—	Absent	
Creatinine, serum	0.7–1.5 mg./100 ml.	88.4	62–133 μmol/l	i
Cryoglobulins, serum	0		0	
Fatty acids, total, serum	190–420 mg/100 ml.	0.0352	7–15 mmol/l	
Ferritin, serum	20–200 nanogm./ml.	1.0	20–200 μg/l	
Fibrinogen, plasma	200–400 mg./100 ml.	0.0293	5.9–11.7 μmol/l	c
Folate, serum	5–21 nanogm./ml.	2.27	11–48 nmol/l	
Follicle stimulating hormone (FSH), plasma				
Males	4–25 milliunits/ml. (I.U.)	1.0	4–25 IU/l	
Females	4–30 milliunits/ml. (I.U.)		4–30 IU/l	
Postmenopausal	40–250 milliunits/ml. (I.U.)		40–250 IU/l	
Gamma glutamyltransferase				
Males	6–32 milliunits/ml. (I.U.) (30°)	1.0	6–32 units/l (30 C)	f
Females	4–18 milliunits/ml. (I.U.) (30°)	1.0	4–18 units/l (30 C)	f
Gastrin, serum	0–200 picogm./ml.	1.0	0–200 ng/l	
Glucose (fasting)				
Blood	60–100 mg./100 ml.	0.0555	3.33–5.55 mmol/l	
Plasma or serum	70–115 mg./100 ml.	0.0555	3.89–6.38 mmol/l	
Growth hormone, serum	0–10 nanogm./ml.	1.0	0–10 μg/l	
Haptoglobin, serum	100–200 mg./100 ml.	0.155	16–31 μmol/l	d
	(As hemoglobin binding capacity)		(As hemoglobin binding capacity)	
Hydroxybutyric dehydrogenase, serum	0–180 milliunits/ml. (I.U.) (30°) (Rosalki-Wilkinson)	1.0	0–180 units/l (30 C) (Rosalki-Wilkinson)	f
	114–290 units/ml. (Wroblewski)	—	114–290 units/ml (Wroblewski)	f
17-Hydroxycorticosteroids, plasma	8–18 mcg./100 ml.	0.0276	0.22–0.50 μmol/l	j
Immunoglobulins, serum				
IgG	550–1900 mg./100 ml.	0.01	5.5–19.0 g/l	
IgA	60–333 mg./100 ml.	0.01	0.60–3.3 g/l	
IgM	45–145 mg./100 ml.	0.01	0.45–1.5 g/l	
Insulin, plasma (fasting)	(Varies with age in children) 5–25 microunits/ml.	1.0	(Varies with age in children) 5–25 milliunits/l	k
Iodine, protein bound, serum	3.5–8.0 mcg./100 ml.	0.0788	0.28–0.63 μmol/l	
Iron, serum	75–175 mcg./100 ml.	0.179	13–31 μmol/l	
Iron binding capacity, serum				
Total	250–410 mcg./100 ml.	0.179	45–73 μmol/l	a
Saturation	20–55%	0.01	0.20–0.55	
17-Ketosteroids, plasma	25–125 mcg./100 ml.	0.0347	0.87–4.34 μmol/l	l
Lactate, blood, venous	0.6–1.8 mEq./liter	1.0	0.6–1.8 mmol/l	
Lactate dehydrogenase, serum	0–300 milliunits/ml. (I.U.) (30°) (Wroblewski modified)	1.0	0–300 units/l (30 C) (Wroblewski modified)	f
	150–450 units/ml. (Wroblewski)	—	150–450 units/ml (Wroblewski)	
	80–120 units/ml. (Wacker)	—	80–120 units/ml (Wacker)	

Table continued on the following page

	CONVENTIONAL UNITS	FACTOR	S.I. UNITS	NOTES
Lactate dehydrogenase isoenzymes, serum				
LDH_1	22–37% of total	0.01	0.22–0.37 of total	a
LDH_2	30–46% of total		0.30–0.46 of total	
LDH_3	14–29% of total		0.14–0.29 of total	
LDH_4	5–11% of total		0.05–0.11 of total	
LDH_5	2–11% of total		0.02–0.11 of total	
Leucine aminopeptidase, serum	14–40 milliunits/ml. (I.U.) (30°)	1.0	14–40 units/l (30 C)	f
Lipase, serum	0–1.5 units (Cherry-Crandall)	—	0–1.5 units (Cherry-Crandall)	f
Lipids, total, serum	450–850 mg/100 ml.	0.01	4.5–8.5 g/l	m
Luteinizing hormone (LH), serum				
Males	6–18 milliunits/ml. (I.U.)	1.0	6–18 IU/l	
Females, premenopausal	5–22 milliunits/ml. (I.U.)	1.0	5–22 IU/l	
midcycle	3 times baseline	—	3 times baseline	
postmenopausal	Greater than 30 milliunits/ml. (I.U.)	1.0	Greater than 30 IU/l	
Magnesium, serum	1.5–2.5 mEq./liter	0.50	0.75–1.25 mmol/l	
	1.8–3.0 mg./100 ml.	0.411		
5'-Nucleotidase, serum	Less than 1.6 milliunits/ml. (I.U.) (30°)	1.0	Less than 1.6 units/l (30 C)	f
Nitrogen, nonprotein, serum	15–35 mg./100 ml.	0.714	10.7–25.0 mmol/l	
Osmolality, serum	285–295 mOsm./kg. serum water	—	285–295 mmol/kg serum water	n
Oxygen, blood				
Capacity	16–24 vol.% (varies with hemoglobin)	0.446	7.14–10.7 mmol/l (varies with hemoglobin)	o
Content Arterial	15–23 vol.%	0.446	6.69–10.3 mmol/l	o
Venous	10–16 vol.%	0.446	4.46–7.14 mmol/l	o
Saturation Arterial	94–100% of capacity	0.01	0.94–1.00 of capacity	a
Venous	60–85% of capacity	0.01	0.60–0.85 of capacity	a
Tension, pO_2 Arterial	75–100 mm. Hg	—	75–100 mm Hg	g
P_{50}, blood	26–27 mm. Hg	—	26–27 mm Hg	g
pH, arterial, blood	7.35–7.45	—	7.35–7.45	
Phenylalanine, serum	Less than 3 mg/100 ml.	0.0605	Less than 0.18 mmol/l	p
Phosphatase, acid, serum	0–7.0 milliunits/ml. (I.U.) (30°)	1.0	0–7.0 units/l (30 C)	f
Phosphatase, alkaline, serum	1.0–5.0 units (King-Armstrong)	—	1.0–5.0 units (King-Armstrong)	f
	10–32 milliunits/ml. (I.U.) (30°)	1.0	10–32 units/l (30 C)	
	5.0–13.0 units (King-Armstrong) (Values are higher in children)	—	5.0–13.0 units (King-Armstrong) (Values are higher in children)	
Phosphate, inorganic, serum				
Adults	3.0–4.5 mg./100 ml.	0.323	1.0–1.5 mmol/l	
Children	4.0–7.0 mg./100 ml.		1.3–2.3 mmol/l	
Phospholipids, serum	6–12 mg./100 ml. (As lipid phosphorus)	0.323	1.9–3.9 mmol/l (As lipid phosphorus)	
Potassium, serum	3.5–5.0 mEq./liter	1.0	3.5–5.0 mmol/l	
Protein, serum				
Total	6.0–8.0 grams/100 ml.	10	60–80 g/l	m
Albumin	3.5–5.5 grams/100 ml.	10	35–55 g/l	
		0.154	0.54–0.85 mmol/l	q

	Conventional	Factor	SI Units	
Globulin	2.5–3.5 grams/100 ml.	10	25–35 g/l	q
Electrophoresis				
Albumin	3.5–5.5 grams/100 ml.	10	35–55 g/l	a
	52–68% of total	0.01	0.52–0.68 of total	
Globulin				
Alpha$_1$	0.2–0.4 gram/100 ml.	10	2–4 g/l	m
	2–5% of total	0.01	0.02–0.05 of total	a
Alpha$_2$	0.5–0.9 gram/100 ml.	10	5–9 g/l	m
	7–14% of total	0.01	0.07–0.14 of total	a
Beta	0.6–1.1 grams/100 ml.	10	6–11 g/l	m
	9–15% of total	0.01	0.09–0.15 of total	a
Gamma	0.7–1.7 grams/100 ml.	10	7–17 g/l	m
	11–21% of total	0.01	0.11–0.21 of total	a
Protoporphyrin, erythrocyte	27–61 mcg./100 ml. packed RBC	0.0178	0.48–1.09 μmol/l packed RBC	
Pyruvate, blood	0.01–0.11 mEq./liter	1.0	0.01–0.11 mmol/l	
Sodium, serum	136–145 mEq./liter	1.0	136–145 mmol/l	
Sulfates, inorganic, serum	0.8–1.2 mg./100 ml.	104	83–125 μmol/l	
Testosterone, plasma				
Males	275–875 nanogm./100 ml.	0.0347	9.5–30 nmol/l	
Females	23–75 nanogm./100 ml.	0.0347	0.8–2.6 nmol/l	
Pregnant	38–190 nanogm./100 ml.	0.0347	1.3–6.6 nmol/l	
Thyroid stimulating hormone (TSH), serum	0–7 microunits/ml.	1.0	0–7 milliunits/l	
Thyroxine, free, serum	1.0–2.1 nanogm./100 ml.	12.9	13–27 pmol/l	
Thyroxine (T$_4$), serum	4.4–9.9 mcg./100 ml.	12.9	57–128 nmol/l	
Thyroxine binding globulin (TBG), serum (as thyroxine)	10–26 mcg./100 ml.	12.9	129–335 nmol/l	
Thyroxine iodine, serum	2.9–6.4 mcg./100 ml.	78.8	229–504 nmol/l	k
Tri-iodothyronine (T$_3$), serum	150–250 nanogm./100 ml.	0.0154	2.3–3.9 nmol/l	
Tri-iodothyronine (T$_3$) uptake, resin (T$_3$RU)	25–38%	0.01	0.25–0.38 uptake	a
Transaminase, serum				
SGOT (aspartate aminotransferase)	0–19 milliunits/ml. (I.U.) (30°) (Karmen modified)	1.0	0–19 units/l (30 C) (Karmen modified)	f
	15–40 units/ml. (Karmen)		15–40 units/ml (Karmen)	
	18–40 units/ml. (Reitman-Frankel)		18–40 units/ml (Reitman-Frankel)	
SGPT (alanine aminotransferase)	0–17 milliunits/ml. (I.U.) (30°) (Karmen modified)	1.0	0–17 units/l (30 C) (Karmen modified)	f
	6–35 units/ml. (Karmen)		6–35 units/ml (Karmen)	
	5–35 units/ml. (Reitman-Frankel)		5–35 units/ml (Reitman-Frankel)	
Triglycerides, serum	40–150 mg./100 ml.	0.01	0.4–1.5 g/l	
		0.0114	0.45–1.71 mmol/l	r
Urate (serum)				
Males	2.5–8.0 mg./100 ml.	0.0595	0.15–0.48 mmol/l	
Females	1.5–7.0 mg./100 ml.	0.0595	0.09–0.42 mmol/l	
Urea				
Blood	21–43 mg./100 ml.	0.167	3.5–7.2 mmol/l	
Plasma or serum	24–49 mg./100 ml.	0.167	4.0–8.2 mmol/l	
Urea nitrogen				
Blood	10–20 mg./100 ml.	0.714	7.1–14.3 mmol/l	
Plasma or serum	11–23 mg./100 ml.	0.714	7.9–16.4 mmol/l	
Vitamin A, serum	20–80 mcg./100 ml.	0.0349	0.70–2.8 μmol/l	
Vitamin B$_{12}$, serum	180–900 picogm./ml.	0.738	133–664 pmol/l	k

REFERENCE VALUES FOR URINE

(For some procedures the reference values may vary depending upon the method used)

	CONVENTIONAL UNITS	FACTOR	S.I. UNITS	NOTES
Acetone and acetoacetate, qualitative	Negative	—	Negative	
Addis count				
Erythrocytes	0–130,000/24 hrs.	—	0–130 000/24 h	
Leukocytes	0–650,000/24 hrs.	—	0–650 000/24 h	
Casts (hyaline)	0–2000/24 hrs.	—	0–2000/24 h	
Albumin				
Qualitative	Negative	—	Negative	
Quantitative	10–100 mg./24 hrs.	—	10–100 mg/24 h	q
Aldosterone	3–20 mcg./24 hrs.	2.77	8.3–55 nmol/24 h	
Alpha amino nitrogen	50–200 mg./24 hrs.	0.0714	3.6–14.3 mmol/24 h	
Ammonia nitrogen	20–70 mEq./24 hrs.	1.0	20–70 mmol/24 h	
Amylase	35–260 Caraway units/hr.	—	35–260 Caraway units/h	f
Bilirubin, qualitative	Negative	—	Negative	
Calcium				
Low Ca diet	Less than 150 mg./24 hrs.	0.025	Less than 3.8 mmol/24 h	
Usual diet	Less than 250 mg./24 hrs.	0.025	Less than 6.3 mmol/24 h	
Catecholamines				
Epinephrine	Less than 10 mcg./24 hrs.	5.46	Less than 55 nmol/24 h	
Norepinephrine	Less than 100 mcg./24 hrs.	5.91	Less than 590 nmol/24 h	
Total free catecholamines	4–126 mcg./24 hrs.	5.91	24–745 nmol/24 h	s
Total metanephrines	0.1–1.6 mg./24 hrs.	5.07	0.5–8.1 µmol/24 h	t
Chloride	110–250 mEq./24 hrs.	1.0	110–250 mmol/24 h	
	(Varies with intake)		(Varies with intake)	
Chorionic gonadotropin	0	—	0	
Copper	0–50 mcg./24 hrs.	0.0157	0–0.80 µmol/24 h	
Creatine				
Males	0–40 mg./24 hrs.	0.00762	0–0.30 mmol/24 h	
Females	0–100 mg./24 hrs.	0.00762	0–0.76 mmol/24 h	
	(Higher in children and during pregnancy)		(Higher in children and during pregnancy)	
Creatinine	15–25 mg./kg. body weight/24 hrs.	0.00884	0.13–0.22 mmol·kg⁻¹ body weight/24 h	
Creatinine clearance				
Males	110–150 ml/min.	—	110–150 ml/min	
Females	105–132 ml/min. (1.73 sq. meter surface area)	—	105–132 ml/min (1.73 m² surface area)	
Cystine or cysteine, qualitative	Negative	—	Negative	
Dehydroepiandrosterone	Less than 15% of total 17-keto-steroids	0.01	Less than 0.15 of total 17-keto-steroids	a
Delta aminolevulinic acid	1.3–7.0 mg./24 hrs.	7.63	10–53 µmol/24 h	

	Conventional	Factor	SI Units	
Estrogens				
Males				
Estrone	3–8 μg./24 hrs.	3.70	11–30 nmol/24 h	
Estradiol	0–6 μg./24 hrs.	3.67	0–22 nmol/24 h	
Estriol	1–11 μg./24 hrs.	3.47	3–38 nmol/24 h	
Total	4–25 μg./24 hrs.	3.60	14–90 nmol/24 h	u
Females				
Estrone	4–31 μg./24 hrs.	3.70	15–115 nmol/24 h	
Estradiol	0–14 μg./24 hrs.	3.67	0–51 nmol/24 h	
Estriol	0–72 μg./24 hrs.	3.47	0–250 nmol/24 h	
Total	5–100 μg./24 hrs.	3.60	18–360 nmol/24 h	u
	(Markedly increased during pregnancy)		(Markedly increased during pregnancy)	
Glucose (as reducing substance)	Less than 250 mg./24 hrs.	—	Less than 250 mg/24 h	
Gonadotropins, pituitary	10–50 mouse units/24 hrs.	—	10–50 mouse units/24 h	
Hemoglobin and myoglobin, qualitative	Negative	—	Negative	
Hemogentisic acid, qualitative	Negative	—	Negative	
17-Hydroxycorticosteroids				
Males	3–9 mg./24 hrs.	2.76	8.3–25 μmol/24 h	j
Females	2–8 mg./24 hrs.		5.5–22 μmol/24 h	
5-Hydroxyindoleacetic acid				
Qualitative	Negative	—	Negative	
Quantitative	Less than 9 mg./24 hrs.	5.23	Less than 47 μmol/24 h	
17-Ketosteroids				l
Males	6–18 mg./24 hrs.	3.47	21–62 μmol/24 h	
Females	4–13 mg./24 hrs.		14–45 μmol/24 h	
	(Varies with age)		(Varies with age)	
Magnesium	6.0–8.5 mEq./24 hrs.	0.5	3.0–4.3 mmol/24 h	
Metanephrines (see Catecholamines)				
Osmolality	38–1400 mOsm./kg. water	—	38–1400 mmol/kg water	n
pH	4.6–8.0, average 6.0	—	4.6–8.0, average 6.0	p
	(Depends on diet)		(Depends on diet)	
Phenolsulfonphthalein excretion (PSP)	25% or more in 15 min.	0.01	0.25 or more in 15 min	a
	40% or more in 30 min.		0.40 or more in 30 min	
	55% or more in 2 hrs.		0.55 or more in 2 h	
	(After injection of 1 ml PSP intravenously)		(After injection of 1 ml PSP intravenously)	
Phenylpyruvic acid, qualitative	Negative	—	Negative	
Phosphorus	0.9–1.3 gm./24 hrs.	32.3	29–42 mmol/24 h	
Porphobilinogen				
Qualitative	Negative	—	Negative	
Quantitative	0–0.2 mg./100 ml.	4.42	0–0.9 μmol/l	
	Less than 2.0 mg./24 hrs.		Less than 9 μmol/24 h	
Porphyrins				
Coproporphyrin	50–250 mcg./24 hrs.	1.53	77–380 nmol/24 h	
Uroporphyrin	10–30 mcg./24 hrs.	1.20	12–36 nmol/24 h	
Potassium	25–100 mEq./24 hrs.	1.0	25–100 mmol/24 h	
	(Varies with intake)		(Varies with intake)	

Table continued on the following page

REFERENCE VALUES FOR URINE (*Continued*)

(For some procedures the reference values may vary depending upon the method used)

	CONVENTIONAL UNITS	FACTOR	S.I. UNITS	NOTES
Pregnanediol				
Males	0.4–1.4 mg./24 hrs.	3.12	1.2–4.4 μmol/24 h	
Females				m
Proliferative phase	0.5–1.5 mg./24 hrs.		1.6–4.7 μmol/24 h	
Luteal phase	2.0–7.0 mg./24 hrs.		6.2–22 μmol/24 h	
Postmenopausal phase	0.2–1.0 mg./24 hrs.		0.6–3.1 μmol/24 h	
Pregnanetriol	Less than 2.5 mg./24 hrs. in adults	2.97	Less than 7.4 μmol/24 h in adults	
Protein				
Qualitative	Negative	—	Negative	
Quantitative	10–150 mg./24 hrs.		10–150 mg/24 h	
Sodium	130–260 mEq./24 hrs.	1.0	130–260 mmol/24 h	
	(Varies with intake)		(Varies with intake)	
Specific gravity	1.003–1.030		1.003–1.030	
Titratable acidity	20–40 mEq./24 hrs.	1.0	20–40 mmol/24 h	
Urate	200–500 mg./24 hrs.	0.00595	1.2–3.0 mmol/24 h	
	(With normal diet)		(With normal diet)	
Urobilinogen	Up to 1.0 Ehrlich unit/2 hrs.	—	Up to 1.0 Ehrlich unit/2 h	
	(1–3 P.M.)		(1–3 P.M.)	
	0–4.0 mg./24 hrs.	—	0–4.0 mg/24 h	
Vanillylmandelic acid (VMA)	1–8 mg./24 hrs.	5.05	5–40 μmol/24 h	
(4-hydroxy-3-methoxymandelic acid)				

REFERENCE VALUES FOR THERAPEUTIC DRUG MONITORING

DRUG	THERAPEUTIC RANGE	TOXIC LEVELS	PROPRIETARY NAMES
Antibiotics			
Amikacin, serum	15–25 mcg./ml.	Peak: >35 mcg./ml.	Amikin
		Trough: >5 mcg./ml.	
Chloramphenicol, serum	10–20 mcg./ml.	>25 mcg./ml.	Chloromycetin
Gentamicin, serum	5–10 mcg./ml.	Peak: >12 mcg./ml.	Garamycin
		Trough: >2 mcg./ml.	
Tobramycin, serum	5–10 mcg./ml.	Peak: >12 mcg./ml.	Nebcin
		Trough: >2 mcg./ml.	
Anticonvulsants			
Carbamazepine, serum	5–12 mcg./ml.	>15 mcg./ml.	Tegretol
Ethosuximide, serum	40–80 mcg./ml.	>150 mcg./ml.	Zarontin
Phenobarbital, serum	10–25 mcg./ml.	Vary widely because of developed tolerance	

Drug	Therapeutic Range	Toxic Level	Trade Names
Phenytoin (diphenylhydantoin), serum	10–20 mcg./ml.	>20 mcg./ml.	Dilantin
Primidone, serum	4–12 mcg./ml.	>15 mcg./ml.	Mysoline
Valproic acid, serum	50–100 mcg./ml.	>200 mcg./ml.	Depakene
Anti-inflammatory agents			
Acetaminophen, serum	10–20 mcg./ml.	>250 mcg./ml.	Tylenol / Datril
Salicylate, serum	100–250 mcg./ml.	>300 mcg./ml.	
Bronchodilator			
Theophylline (aminophylline)	10–20 mcg./ml.	>20 mcg./ml.	
Cardiovascular drugs			
Digitoxin, serum	15–25 nanogm./ml. (Specimen obtained 12–24 hrs. after last dose)	>25 nanogm./ml.	Crystodigin
Digoxin, serum	0.8–2 nanogm./ml. (Specimen obtained 12–24 hrs. after last dose)	>2.4 nanogm./ml.	Lanoxin
Disopyramide, serum	2–4 mcg./ml.	>7 mcg./ml.	Norpace
Lidocaine, serum	1.5–5 mcg./ml.	>7 nanogm./ml.	Anestacon / Xylocaine
Procainamide, serum	4–10 mcg./ml. *8–16 mcg./ml. (*Procainamide + N-Acetyl Procainamide)	>16 mcg./ml. *>20 mcg./ml.	Pronestyl
Propranolol, serum	50–100 nanogm./ml.	Variable	Inderal
Quinidine, serum	2–5 mcg./ml.	>10 mcg./ml.	Cardioquin / Quinaglute / Quinidex / Quinora
Psychopharmacologic drugs			
Amitriptyline, serum	*120–150 nanogm./ml. (*Amitriptyline + Nortriptyline)	*>500 nanogm./ml.	Amitril / Elavil / Endep / Etrafon / Limbitrol / Triavil
Chlordiazepoxide, serum	1–3 mcg./ml.	>5 mcg./ml.	Librium
Desipramine, serum	*150–250 nanogm./ml. (*Desipramine + Imipramine)	*>500 nanogm./ml.	Norpramin / Pertofrane
Diazepam, serum	0.5–2.5 mcg./ml.	>5 mcg./ml.	Valium
Imipramine, serum	*150–250 nanogm./ml. (*Imipramine + Desipramine)	*>500 nanogm./ml.	Antipress / Imavate / Janimine / Presamine / Tofranil
Lithium, serum	0.8–1.5 mEq./liter (Specimen obtained 12 hrs. after last dose)	>2.0 mEq./liter	
Nortriptyline, serum	50–150 nanogm./ml.	>500 nanogm./ml.	Aventyl / Pamelor

REFERENCE VALUES IN TOXICOLOGY

	CONVENTIONAL UNITS	FACTOR	S.I. UNITS	NOTES
Arsenic, blood	3.5–7.2 mcg./100 ml.	0.133	0.47–0.96 μmol/l	
Arsenic, urine	Less than 100 mcg./24 hrs.	0.0133	Less than 1.3 μmol/24 h	
Bromides, serum	0	1.0	0	
Carbon monoxide, blood	Toxic levels:		Toxic levels:	a
	Above 17 mEq./liter		Above 17 mmol/l	
	Up to 5% saturation	—	Up to 0.05 saturation	
	Symptoms occur with 20% satura-		Symptoms occur with 0.20 satura-	
	tion		tion	
Ethanol, blood	Less than 0.005%	217	Less than 1 mmol/l	
Marked intoxication	0.3–0.4%		65–87 mmol/l	
Alcoholic stupor	0.4–0.5%		87–109 mmol/l	
Coma	Above 0.5%		Above 109 mmol/l	
Lead, blood	0–40 mcg./100 ml.	0.0483	0–2 μmol/l	
Lead, urine	Less than 100 mcg./24 hrs.	0.00483	Less than 0.48 μmol/24 h	
Mercury, urine	Less than 10 mcg./24 hrs.	4.98	Less than 50 nmol/24 h	

REFERENCE VALUES FOR CEREBROSPINAL FLUID

	CONVENTIONAL UNITS	FACTOR	S.I. UNITS	NOTES
Cells	Fewer than 5/cu. mm.; all mono-nuclear	—	Fewer than 5/μl; all mononuclear	
Chloride	120–130 mEq./liter	1.0	120–130 mmol/l	
	(20 mEq./liter higher than serum)		(20 mmol/l higher than serum)	
Electrophoresis	Predominantly albumin	—	Predominantly albumin	
Glucose	50–75 mg./100 ml.	0.0555	2.8–4.2 mmol/l	
	(20 mg./100 ml. less than serum)		(1.1 mmol/l less than serum)	
IgG				
Children under 14	Less than 8% of total protein	—	Less than 0.08 of total protein	a,m
Adults	Less than 14% of total protein		Less than 0.14 of total protein	
Pressure	70–180 mm. water		70–180 mm water	g
Protein, total	15–45 mg./100 ml.	0.01	0.150–0.450 g/l	m
	(Higher, up to 70 mg./100 ml., in elderly adults and children)		(Higher, up to 0.70 g/l, in elderly adults and children)	

REFERENCE VALUES FOR GASTRIC ANALYSIS

	CONVENTIONAL UNITS	FACTOR	S.I. UNITS	NOTES
Basal gastric secretion (1 hour)				
Concentration	(Mean ± 1 S.D.)		(Mean ± 1 S.D.)	
Males	25.8 ± 1.8 mEq./liter	1.0	25.8 ± 1.8 mmol/l	
Females	20.3 ± 3.0 mEq./liter		20.3 ± 3.0 mmol/l	
Output	(Mean ± 1 S.D.)		(Mean ± 1 S.D.)	
Males	2.57 ± 0.16 mEq./hr.	1.0	2.57 ± 0.16 mmol/h	
Females	1.61 ± 0.18 mEq./hr.		1.61 ± 0.18 mmol/h	
After histamine stimulation				
Normal	Mean output 11.8 mEq./hr.	1.0	Mean output 11.8 mmol/h	
Duodenal ulcer	Mean output 15.2 mEq./hr.		Mean output 15.2 mmol/h	
After maximal histamine stimulation				
Normal	Mean output 22.6 mEq./hr.	1.0	Mean output 22.6 mmol/h	
Duodenal ulcer	Mean output 44.6 mEq./hr.		Mean output 44.6 mmol/h	
Diagnex blue (Squibb): Anacidity	0–0.3 mg. in 2 hrs.	1.0	0–0.3 mg in 2 h	
Doubtful	0.3–0.6 mg. in 2 hrs.		0.3–0.6 mg in 2 h	
Normal	Greater than 0.6 mg. in 2 hrs.		Greater than 0.6 mg in 2 h	
Volume, fasting stomach content	50–100 ml.	—	0.05–0.1 l	
Emptying time	3–6 hrs.	—	3–6 h	
Color	Opalescent or colorless	—	Opalescent or colorless	
Specific gravity	1.006–1.009	—	1.006–1.009	
pH (adults)	0.9–1.5	—	0.9–1.5	P

GASTROINTESTINAL ABSORPTION TESTS

	CONVENTIONAL UNITS	FACTOR	S.I. UNITS	NOTES
d-Xylose absorption test	After an 8 hour fast, 10 ml./kg. body weight of a 0.05 solution of d-xylose is given by mouth. Nothing further by mouth is given until the test has been completed. All urine voided during the following 5 hours is pooled, and blood samples are taken at 0, 60, and 120 minutes. Normally 0.26 (range 0.16–0.33) of ingested xylose is excreted within 5 hours, and the serum xylose reaches a level between 25 and 40 mg./100 ml. after 1 hour and is maintained at this level for another 60 minutes.		No change	
Vitamin A absorption	A fasting blood specimen is obtained and 200,000 units of vitamin A in oil is given by mouth. Serum vitamin A level should rise to twice fasting level in 3 to 5 hours.		No change	

REFERENCE VALUES FOR FECES

	CONVENTIONAL UNITS	FACTOR	S.I. UNITS	NOTES
Bulk	100–200 grams/24 hrs.	—	100–200 g/24 h	
Dry matter	23–32 grams/24 hrs.	—	23–32 g/24 h	
Fat, total	Less than 6.0 grams/24 hrs.	—	Less than 6.0 g/24 h	
Nitrogen, total	Less than 2.0 grams/24 hrs.	—	Less than 2.0 g/24 h	
Urobilinogen	40–280 mg./24 hrs.	—	40–280 mg/24 h	
Water	Approximately 65%	0.01	Approximately 0.65	a

REFERENCE VALUES FOR SEMEN ANALYSIS

	CONVENTIONAL UNITS	FACTOR	S.I. UNITS	NOTES
Volume	2–5 ml.; usually 3–4 ml.	—	2–5 ml; usually 3–4 ml	
Liquefaction	Complete in 15 min.	—	Complete in 15 min	
pH	7.2–8.0; average 7.8	—	7.2–8.0; average 7.8	p
Leukocytes	Occasional or absent	—	Occasional or absent	
Count	60–150 million/ml.	—	60–150 million/ml	
	Below 60 million/ml. is abnormal	—	Below 60 million/ml is abnormal	
Motility	80% or more motile	—	0.80 or more motile	a
Morphology	80–90% normal forms	—	0.80–0.90 normal forms	a

PANCREATIC (ISLET) FUNCTION TESTS

Glucose tolerance tests		
Oral	Patient should be on a diet containing 300 grams of carbohydrate per day for 3 days prior to test. After ingestion of 100 grams of glucose or 1.75 grams glucose/kg. body weight, blood glucose is not more than 160 mg./100 ml. after 60 minutes, 140 mg./100 ml. after 90 minutes, and 120 mg./100 ml. after 120 minutes. Values are for blood; serum measurements are approximately 15% higher.	
Intravenous	Blood glucose does not exceed 200 mg./100 ml. after infusion of 0.5 gram of glucose/kg. body weight over 30 minutes. Glucose concentration falls below initial level at 2 hours and returns to preinfusion levels in 3 or 4 hours. Values are for blood; serum measurements are approximately 15% higher.	
Cortisone-glucose tolerance test	The patient should be on a diet containing 300 grams of carbohydrate per day for 3 days prior to test. At 8½ and again 2 hours prior to glucose load patient is given cortisone acetate by mouth (50 mg. if patient's ideal weight is less than 160 lb., 62.5 mg. if ideal weight is greater than 160 lb.). An oral dose of glucose, 1.75 grams/kg. body weight, is given and blood samples are taken at 0, 30, 60, 90, and 120 minutes. Test is considered positive if true blood glucose exceeds 160 mg./100 ml. at 60 minutes, 140 mg./100 ml. at 90 minutes, and 120 mg./100 ml. at 120 minutes. Values are for blood; serum measurements are approximately 15% higher.	

REFERENCE VALUES FOR IMMUNOLOGIC PROCEDURES

	CONVENTIONAL UNITS		FACTOR	S.I. UNITS	NOTES
Syphilis serology (RPR and VDRL)	Negative			No change	
Mono screen	Negative			No change	
R.A. test (latex)	1:40	Negative		No change	
	1:80–1:160	Doubtful			
	1:320	Positive			
Rose test	1:10	Negative		No change	
	1:20–1:40	Doubtful			
	1:80	Positive			
Anti-streptolysin O titer	Normal up to 1:128. Single test usually has little significance. Rise in titer or persistently elevated titer is significant.			No change	
Anti-hyaluronidase titer	Less than 1:200. Significant if rising titer can be demonstrated at weekly intervals.			No change	
C-reactive protein	Negative			No change	
Anti-nuclear antibody	One specimen is sufficient, unless the result is inconsistent with the clinical impression. Most patients with active lupus have high ANA titers (160 or greater); some have lower titers (20–40). Patients with inactive lupus may have a negative test. Antinuclear antibodies are occasionally present in patients with no evidence of systemic lupus, usually in lower titers (20–40).			No change	
Febrile agglutinins	Titers of 1:80 or greater may be significant, particularly if subsequent samples show rise in titer.			No change	
Tularemia agglutinins	1:80	Negative		No change	
	1:160	Doubtful			
	1:320	Positive			
Proteus OX-19 agglutinins	Titers of 1:80 or greater may be significant, particularly if subsequent samples show rise in titer.			No change	
Complement fixation tests	Titers of 1:8 or less are usually not significant. Paired sera showing rise in titer of more than two tubes are usually considered significant.			No change	
C3 Test	80–140 mg./100 ml.		0.01	0.80–1.40 g/l	
C4 Test	11–75 mg./100 ml.		0.01	0.11–0.75 g/l	q

1034

NOTES

a. Percentage is expressed as a decimal fraction.

b. Percentage may be expressed as a decimal fraction; however, when the result expressed is itself a variable fraction of another variable, the absolute value is more meaningful. There is no reason, other than custom, for expressing reticulocyte counts and differential leukocyte counts in percentages or decimal fractions rather than in absolute numbers.

c. Molecular weight of fibrinogen = 341,000 daltons.

d. Molecular weight of hemoglobin = 64,500 daltons. Because of disagreement as to whether the monomer or tetramer of hemoglobin should be used in the conversion, it has been recommended that the conventional grams per deciliter be retained. The tetramer is used in the table; values given should be multiplied by 4 to obtain concentration of the monomer.

e. Molecular weight of methemoglobin = 64,500 daltons. See note d above.

f. Enzyme units have not been changed in these tables because the proposed enzyme unit, the katal, has not been universally adopted (1 International Unit = 16.7 nkat).

g. It has been proposed that pressure be expressed in the Pascal (1 mm Hg = 0.133 kPa); however, this convention has not been universally accepted.

h. Molecular weight of ceruloplasmin = 151,000.

i. "Fatty acids" includes a mixture of different aliphatic acids of varying molecular weight. A mean molecular weight of 284 has been assumed in calculating the conversion factor.

j. Based upon molecular weight of cortisol 362.47.

k. The practice of expressing concentration of an organic molecule in terms of one of its constituent elements originated when measurements included a heterogeneous class of compounds (nonprotein nitrogenous compounds, iodine-containing compounds bound to serum proteins). It was carried over to expressing measurements of specific substances (urea, thyroxine), but the practice should be discarded. For iodine and nitrogen 1 mole is taken as the monoatomic form, although they occur as diatomic molecules.

l. Based upon molecular weight of dehydroepiandrosterone 288.41.

m. Weight per volume is retained as the unit because of the heterogeneous nature of the material measured.

n. The proposal that osmolality be reported as freezing point depression using the millikelvin as the unit has not been received with universal enthusiasm. The milliosmole is not an S.I. unit, and the unit used here is the millimole.

o. Volumes per cent might be converted to a decimal fraction; however, this would not permit direct correlation with hemoglobin content, which is possible when oxygen content and capacity are expressed in molar quantities. One millimole of hemoglobin combines with 4 millimoles of oxygen.

p. Hydrogen ion concentration in S.I. units would be expressed in nanomoles per liter; however, this change has not received general approval. Conversion can be calculated as antilog (−pH).

q. Albumin is expressed in grams per liter to be consistent with units used for other proteins.

Concentration of albumin may be expressed in mmol/l also, an expression that permits assessment of binding capacity of albumin for substances such as bilirubin. Molecular weight of albumin is 65,000.

r. Most techniques for quantitating triglycerides measure the glycerol moiety, and the total mass is calculated using an average molecular weight. The factor given assumes a mean molecular weight of 875 for triglycerides.

s. Calculated as norepinephrine, molecular weight 169.18.

t. Calculated as metanephrine, molecular weight 197.23.

u. Conversion factor calculated from molecular weights of estrone, estradiol, and estriol in proportions of 2:1:2.

REFERENCES

1. AMA Drug Evaluations. 4th ed. Chicago, American Medical Association, 1980.
2. Baron, D. N., Broughton, P. M. G., Cohen, M., Lansley, T. S., Lewis, S. M., and Shinton, N. K.: J. Clin. Path. 27:590, 1974.
3. Dybkaer, R.: Am. J. Clin. Path. 52:637, 1969.
4. Goodman, L. S. and Gilman, A.: Pharmacologic Basis of Therapeutics. 5th ed. New York, Macmillan, 1975.
5. Henry, J. B.: Clinical Diagnosis and Management by Laboratory Methods, 16th ed. Philadelphia, W. B. Saunders Company, 1979.
6. Henry, R. J., Cannon, D. C., and Winkleman, J. W.: Clinical Chemistry—Principles and Techniques, 2nd ed. New York, Harper & Row, 1974.
7. International Committee for Standardization in Hematology, International Federation of Clinical Chemistry and World Association of Pathology Societies: Clin. Chem. 19:135, 1973.
8. Lehmann, H. P.: Amer. J. Clin. Path. 65:2, 1976.
9. Miale, J. B.: Laboratory Medicine—Hematology, 5th ed. St. Louis, C. V. Mosby, 1977.
10. Page, C. H., and Vigoureux, P.: The International System of Units (S.I.). U.S. Department of Commerce, National Bureau of Standards, Special Publication 330, 1974.
11. Physicians' Desk Reference. 34th ed. Oradell, N.J., Medical Economics Company, 1980.
12. Scully, R. E., McNeely, B. U., and Galdabini, J. J.: N. Engl. J. Med. 302:37, 1980.
13. Tietz, N. W.: Fundamentals of Clinical Chemistry, 2nd ed. Philadelphia, W. B. Saunders Company, 1976.
14. Wintrobe, M. D., Lee, G. R., Boggs, D. R., Bithell, T. C., Athens, J. W., and Foerster, J.: Clinical Hematology. 7th ed. Philadelphia, Lea & Febiger, 1974.
15. Young, D. S.: N. Engl. J. Med., 292:795, 1975.

Index

Page numbers in *italics* refer to illustrations.

Abdominal aneurysm, 158–159
Abdominal distention and pain, 394–395
Abdominal pregnancy, 871
Abortion, 861–865
  in cholera, 18
Abruptio placentae, 872
Abscess(es), 746
  anal, 389–390
  diverticular, 381
  gingival, 706
  in Crohn's disease, 385
  of brain, 759–762
  of lung, primary, 121–123
Accelerated idioventricular rhythm, in acute myocardial infarction, 228
Accidents. See *Injuries, Trauma.*
Acetaldehyde. See *Methaldehyde.*
Acetaminophen, poisoning from, 994
Acetanilid, poisoning from, 995
Acetic acid, poisoning from, 995
Acetone, poisoning from, 995
Acetylsalicylic acid. See *Salicylates.*
Acid-base imbalance, 498
  hypochloremic, in rickets and osteomalacia, 480
  in severe hypothermia, 983
Acids, corrosive, antidote for, 998
  therapeutic agents to neutralize, 994
Acinetobacter species pneumonia, 130
Acne, occupational, 722
Acne rosacea, 747–748
Acne vulgaris, 655–658
Acoustic neuromas, 835
Acquired diseases of aorta, 157–160
Acromegaly, 509–514
ACTH, abnormal secretion of, lung carcinoma and, 518
  loss of secretory capacity for, 530
Actinic cheilitis, 697
Actinic keratoses, 663, 731
Actinomycetes, thermophilic, and hypersensitivity pneumonitis, 141
Acute adrenal insufficiency, in hypopituitarism, 530
Acute arterial occlusion, 242

Acute chest syndrome, in sickle cell disease, 271
Acute diverticulitis, 381
Acute gastritis, 391
Acute glomerulonephritis, 567
Acute hepatic porphyrias, 342
Acute hepatitis, 397
Acute infectious diarrhea, 421–423
Acute ischemic cerebrovascular disease, 763–766
Acute leukemia, 342
Acute mania, 962
Acute miscellaneous poisoning, 993–1012
Acute myocardial infarction, 223–233
Acute nonspecific pericarditis, 239
Acute-on-chronic renal failure, 588
Acute otitis media, 123–128
Acute pancreatitis, 406–409
Acute peripheral facial paralysis, 812–814
Acute renal failure, 582–588
Acute respiratory failure, 93–99
  and pre-existing obstructive lung disease or asthma, 97
Acute ruptured ectopic pregnancy, 868
Acute (suppurative) thyroiditis, 550
ADA exchange lists, 442–444
Addison's disease, 515
  hyperpigmentation in, 724
Adenocarcinoma, of colon, 419
  of endometrium, 925–927
  of esophagus, 377
  of prostate, 605–607
  of renal pelvis, 600
Adenoma(s), 835
  adrenal, 518
  and acromegaly, 509
  cancer in, 419
  of stomach, 415
Adolescents, atopic dermatitis in, 669
  diabetes mellitus in, 452–459
  epilepsy in, 772–781
  seizure types in, 782
Adrenal adenoma, 518

Adrenocortical carcinoma, 519
Adrenocortical insufficiency, 514–515
Adriamycin, side effects of, 316
Adults, acute head injuries in, 822–829
  atopic dermatitis in, 669
  diabetes mellitus in, 437–452
  epilepsy in, 772–781
  parenteral fluid and electrolyte therapy in, 488–501
  table of heights and weights for, 1015
Adult respiratory distress syndrome, 101
Affective disorders, 956–965
Afibrinogenemia, bleeding in patients with, 286
Agammaglobulinemia, 351
Air embolism, transfusion related, 356
Air pollution, and chronic obstructive pulmonary disease, 103
Airway, establishment of, in cardiac arrest, 164
  management of, in severe hypothermia, 983
Akathisia, antipsychotic drugs and, 968
Albumin, in volume replacement therapy, 351
Alcohol, ethyl, poisoning from, 1004
  methyl, antidote for, 998
  poisoning from, 1006
Alcoholic cirrhosis, 367
Alcohol-disulfiram reaction, 947
Alcoholic hepatitis, 367
Alcoholic neuropathies, 821
Alcoholic pancreatitis, 406
Alcoholics, bacterial pneumonia in, 129
Alcoholism, 943–949
Aldosteronoma, 598
Alimentary hypoglycemia, 471, 472
Alimentary tract, diverticula of, 378–382
Alkalis, caustic, antidote for, 998
  poisoning from, 995
  therapeutic agents to neutralize, 994
Alkyl mercury food poisoning, 31

Allergic cheilitis, 697
Allergic dermatitis, 666–667
Allergic eczematous contact dermatitis, 743
Allergic rhinitis, 643
Allergic transfusion reactions, 354
Allergies, and asthma in adults, 629
  drug, manifestations of, 647
  nasal, due to inhalant factors, 643–646
  to aspirin, 650
  to penicillin, skin testing for, 649
  to insect venom, 651–653
  to insulin, 650
  to radiographic contrast material, 650
Alopecia, 659–662
Alopecia areata, 662
  nail changes in, 717
Alpha-1-antitrypsin deficiency, 369
Alphanaphthylthiourea, poisoning from, 995
Alpha-thalassemia, 266
Alveolar ridges, cancer of, 710
Alveolitis, extrinsic allergic, 141–142
A.M.A. emergency medical identification card, *81*
Amantadine, risks of in pregnant or nursing women, 32
Amebiasis, 1–3
Amebic dysentery, 2
Ameboma, 3
Amebophobia, 1
Amenorrhea, 906–912
  diagnostic scheme for, 906
  hyperprolactinemia in, 531
  oral contraception and, 940
Amenorrhea-galactorrhea syndrome, 531
Aminophylline, dosage guidelines for, 105
  poisoning from, 1012
Amniocentesis, 857
Amodiaquine, toxicity of, 42
Ammonia, poisoning from, 995
Amphetamine, poisoning from, 995
  antidote for, 999
Amphotericin B, toxicity of, 118, 119
Ampullary pregnancy, 870
Amyl acetate. See *Acetone*.
Amyloidosis, in multiple myeloma, 335
Anaerobic soft tissue infections, 22–23
Anal abscess and fistula, 389–390
Anal fissure, 389
Analgesia, effect of on labor, 885
  obstetric, 877–886
Anaphylactic transfusion reactions, 354
Anaphylaxis, 625–628
  emergency treatment of, 649
Anaplastic carcinoma, of thyroid gland, 545
Ancylostoma braziliense, infestation by, 665
Androgen therapy, toxicity of, 254
Androgenetic alopecia, 660
Anemia, antimalarial drugs and, 42
  aplastic, 251–256
  Cooley's, 266
  due to iron deficiency, 256–259
  hemolytic, in lupus erythematosus, 694
  immune hemolytic, 259–261

Anemia (*Continued*)
  in acute childhood leukemia, 311
  in chronic renal failure, 591
  in congenital heart disease, 204
  Mediterranean, 266
  megaloblastic, 263–265
  nonimmune hemolytic, 261–263
  pernicious, 263–265
  sickle cell, 269. See also *Sickle cell disease*.
  spur cell, 263
Anesthesia, and malignant hyperthermia, 989
  effect of on labor, 885
  for cesarean section, 883–884
  for children with congenital heart disease, 205
  in paraplegic patient, 770
  obstetric, 877–886
Anesthetics, local, anaphylactic reactions to, 627
  toxic reactions to, 879
Aneurysms, dissecting, 160
  pericarditis in, 240
  of aorta, 158–160
  of transverse arch, 159
  peripheral arterial, 245
  thoracoabdominal, 160
Angina, Ludwig's, 707
  Prinzmetal's, ventricular premature beats in, 172
  variant, 164
  vasospastic, ventricular premature beats in, 172
Angina pectoris, 160–164
Angiography, in congenital heart disease, 200
Angiomyolipoma, 599
Angular cheilitis, 698
Aniline derivatives, poisoning from, 995
Animal dusts, and hypersensitivity pneumonitis, 141
Animals, small, bites of, rabies from, 58–62
Anionic surfactants, poisoning from, 1003
Anisakiasis, 25
Ankylosing spondylitis, 846–848
Anodontia, 703
Anorectal fistulas, 390
Anovulation, and amenorrhea, 909
Antabuse, 947
Antepartum care, 853–861
Anthrax, malignant lip pustules from, 706
Antianginal agents, 232
Antiarrhythmic agents, for myocardial infarction, 224
Antiepileptic drug interactions, 775
Antifibrinolytic therapy, 279
Antihemophilic factor, cryoprecipitated, therapy with, 350
Antihemophilic factor concentrates, therapy with, 350
Antihistaminics, poisoning from, 995
Antihyperuricemic therapy, 461–462
Antimalarial drugs, toxicity of, 41–42
Antimony, poisoning from, 995
  antidote for, 999

Antiplatelet drugs, for angina pectoris, 163
Antipsychotic drugs, allergic reactions to, 969
  side effects of, 967
Antipyrine. See *Acetanilid*.
Anti-riot gas. See *Tear gases*.
Antithymocytic globulin therapy, anaphylaxis in, 255
Antitoxin, diphtheria, reactions to, 19–20
Antituberculous drugs, side effects of, 148
Antral gastritis, chronic, 392
Anuria, in acute childhood leukemia, 314
Anxiety, 952
Aorta, acquired diseases of, 157–160
  aneurysms of, 158–159
  arteriosclerosis of, 157–158
  atherosclerotic occlusion of, 157
Aphasia, in paraplegia, 770
Aphthous stomatitis, 386, 701
Aplastic anemia, 251–256
Apnea, in low birth weight infant, 891
Apocrine miliaria, 737
Apothecaries' system, table of, 1014
Apresoline, poisoning from, 1005
Arrhythmias, cardiac. See also *Tachycardias*.
  in acute myocardial infarction, 225
  in congenital heart disease, 196–200
  in pericarditis, 237
  in pheochromocytoma, 546
  of congenital heart disease, 192
  ventricular, in acute myocardial infarction, 227
Arsenic, antidote for, 999
Arsenic trioxide, poisoning from, 995
Arsenical keratoses, 732
Arsine gas, poisoning from, 995
Arterial aneurysms, peripheral, 245
Arterial disease, degenerative, 241–246
Arterial embolism, in myocardial infarction, 232
Arterial hypertension, in acute myocardial infarction, 231
Arterial occlusion, acute, 242
Arterial stenosis or occlusion, ischemic stroke secondary to, 765–766
Arteriosclerosis, 241
  of aorta, 157–158
Arteritis, cranial, 793
Arthritis, and neutropenia, 272
  gonococcal, 620
  gouty, 460–461
  in bacterial meningitis, 52
  in Crohn's disease, 386
  rheumatoid, 839–843
Artificial respiration, in cardiac arrest, 164
Ascending aorta, aneurysm of, 158
Ascites, in cirrhosis, 370
Asherman's syndrome, amenorrhea in, 912
L-Asparaginase, side effects of, 316
Aspidium oleoresin, poisoning from, 995
Aspiration, of liver abscess, 3
  of vomitus, during anesthesia, 878
Aspirin. See also *Salicylates*.
  allergy to, 650

Aspirin (*Continued*)
  anaphylactic reactions to, 627
  intolerance to, in allergic rhinitis
    patients, 646
Asplenia, in congenital heart disease,
  205–206
Asterol, poisoning from, 1003
Asthma, acute respiratory failure in,
  97
  in adults, 629–633
  in children, 634–643
  in malignant carcinoid syndrome,
    552
Asthmatics, categories of, 638–642
Astrocytoma, of brain, 835
Asymptomatic bacteriuria, during
  pregnancy, 918
Ataxia, in paraplegia, 770
Atelectasis, 99–101
Atherosclerosis, cholera and, 18
Atopic dermatitis, 668–670
Atrial arrhythmias, in acute myocardial
  infarction, 225
Atrial fibrillation, 167–171
  in congenital heart disease, 199
  in myocardial infarction, 226
  paroxysmal, 182
Atrial flutter, 181
  in congenital heart disease, 199
Atrial tachycardia, éctopic, 181
Atrioventricular block, 173–178
  in acute myocardial infarction, 228
  in congenital heart disease, 199
Atrophic vaginitis, 917
Atropine, and related alkalosis,
    antidote for, 1000
  poisoning from, 995
Atypical psychosis, 957
Auditory hallucinations, 959
Autoimmune thrombocytopenia, 290
Autoimmune thyroiditis, 551
Autoinflation maneuvers, in otitis
    media, 127
Autologous blood donation, 349
Autonomous thrombocytosis, 292–293
Axilla, seborrheic dermatitis of, 674
5-Azacytidine, side effects of, 316
Azotemia, 588
  from irreversible kidney disease, 589
  in typhus fever, 88
  prerenal, 584
  with amphotericin B administration,
    118
Azotemic patient, managing, *592, 593*

Bacille Calmette-Guerin vaccination,
  153
Bacillus cereus food poisoning, 25
Bacteremia, 3–10
  antimicrobial agents for, 7
  in salmonellosis, 73, 74
  treatment of specific types of, 6–10
Bacterial contamination, in blood
  transfusion, 355
Bacterial diseases of the skin, 745–747
Bacterial endocarditis, prophylaxis
  against, 206
Bacterial food poisoning, 25
Bacterial infection(s), and neutropenia,
  272

Bacterial infection(s) (*Continued*)
  of female urinary tract, adult,
    557–559
  in children, 560–561
  of male urinary tract, 555–556
Bacterial meningitis, 44–52
  intravenous dosage regimens used
    in, 46
Bacterial pericarditis, 239
Bacterial pneumonia, 128–132
  in epidemic influenza, 33
  in viral respiratory infections, 156
Bacteriuria, postpartum, and urinary
  retention, during pregnancy,
  920–921
Bacteroides species pneumonia, 130
Bagassosis, 142
Balanitis, 563–564
Balanoposthitis, 563–564
Banana oil. See *Acetone.*
Barbiturates, poisoning from, 995, 996
Barium, poisoning from, 997
Basal cell carcinoma, 663
Basal ganglia, abscess of, 761
Basedow's disease, 533
Bed sores, 666. See also *Decubitus ulcer.*
Bed-wetting. See *Nocturnal enuresis.*
Belching, 394
Bell's palsy, 812–814
Benadryl. See *Antihistaminics.*
Benadryl hydrochloride. See
  Antihistaminics.
Benign prostatic hyperplasia, 576–581
Benign renal tumors, 599
Benzene, poisoning from, 1001, 1012
Benzene hexachloride, poisoning
  from, 1001
Benzine, poisoning from, 1005
Benzol, poisoning from, 1001
Berger's disease, 567
Beriberi, 435–436
Beryllium, poisoning from, 1001
Beta-adrenergic blocking agents, side
    effects of, 162
  toxicity of, 177
Beta-thalassemia, 267
Bifid tongue, 699
Bile salt disorders, 401–402
Biliary cirrhosis, 367
Biliary colic, 364
Biliary obstruction, 401
Biochemical hyperparathyroidism, 526
Birth asphyxia, 865–868
Bismuth, antidote for, 999
  poisoning from, 1001
Bites, small animal, rabies from, 58–62
  spider, 990–991
"Black patch," and delirium, 955
Black widow spider, bites of, 990
Black widow spider venom, antidote
  for, 998–999
Bladder, cancer of, 602–604
  in multiple sclerosis, 802
  pheochromocytoma of, 550
  trauma to, 573
Bladder control training, 562
Blast crisis, in chronic leukemia, 319
Blastomycosis, 119–120
Bleeding. See also *Hemorrhage.*
  breakthrough, oral contraception
    and, 940

Bleeding (*Continued*)
  from esophageal varices, 361
  in diverticulitis, 382
  in hemophiliacs, recommended
    dosages of factor VIII for, 282
  in late pregnancy, 871
  in ulcerative colitis, 432
  oral, in hemophiliacs, 283
  uterine, dysfunctional, 904–906
Bleeding gums, 483
Blepharitis, seborrheic, 674
Blindness, in sickle cell disease, 271
Blisters, of skin, 722
Block, heart. See *Heart block.*
Blood, bacterial disorders of, 3–10
  reference values for, 1022–1025
Blood coagulation disorders, 278
Blood components, therapeutic use of,
    347–351
  in hemophilia, 278–287
Blood cultures, in infective
  endocarditis, 214
Blood donation, autologous, 349
Blood transfusion, adverse reactions
  to, 352–359
  massive, problems with, 355–356
Blood vessels, in acute renal failure,
  585
Blue nevus, 719
Body lice, 723
Bone disease, in primary
  hyperparathyroidism, 525
Bone marrow decompensation, in
  hemolytic anemia, 261
Bone marrow graft, in aplastic anemia,
  255
  in leukemia, 289
Bones, in chronic renal failure, 590
Boric acid, poisoning from, 1001
Botulisms, 1005
Bowel, in multiple sclerosis, 802
Bowen's disease, 665, 732
  of nails, 718
  of vulva, 931
Bradycardia, sinus, in acute myocardial
  infarction, 225
Brain, abscess of, 759–762
    in congenital heart disease, 205
  ischemic vascular disease of,
    763–766
  parenchymatous hemorrhage of,
    762–763
  tumors of, 834–837
Breast feeding, 858
  method of, 893
Breasts, abnormalities of development
  of, 897
  cancer of, 899–902
  carcinoma of, estrogens and, 914
  diseases of, 896–902
  postpartum function of, 887
Breech presentation, anesthesia for
  delivery in, 884
Bridging necrosis, 397
Brill-Zinsser disease, 88
Broad QRS tachycardia, 182
Bromides, antidote for, 1000
  poisoning from, 1001
Bromocriptine, toxicity of, 532
Bronchial hyperreactivity, and asthma
  in adults, 629

Bronchial infections, acute in chronic obstructive pulmonary disease, 102–109
Bronchiectasis, 102–109
Bronchiolitis, 155
Bronchitis, chronic, 102–109
Bronchospasm, 98, 629
Brown recluse spider, bites of, 990
Brucellosis, 10–11
Bubonic plague, 55
Buccal mucosa, carcinoma of, 710
Bullous impetigo, 745
Bundle branch block, in acute myocardial infarction, 228
Burkitt's lymphoma, 321
Burns, 973–980
  chemical, 994
  in children, fluid therapy in, 507
Bursitis, 848–849
Butler's multiple electrolyte solution, 494
Butterfly rash, 673

Cadmium, antidote for, 998
  poisoning from, 1001
Cadmium food poisoning, 25
Caffeine, poisoning from, 1012
Calcific tendinitis, 848–849
Calcium-blocking agents, for angina pectoris, 163
Calcium deficiency, in acute dehydration, 503
Calculi, renal, 612–615
Calluses, 722
Calories, daily requirements of, 493
Camphor, poisoning from, 1001, 1006
Campylobacter fetus food poisoning, 27
Cancer. See also Neoplasms, Tumors, and specific types.
  of bladder, 602–604
  of brain, 836
  of breasts, 897, 899–902
  of colon, in proctocolitis, 433
  of gingiva, 710
  of lung, primary, 109–114
  of mouth, 709
  of renal pelvis, 599–600
  of skin, 663–665
  of thyroid, 543–546
  of uterus, 925–930
  pericarditis secondary to, 241
Candidiasis, cutaneous, 681–682
Cantharidin, poisoning from, 1001
Carbon dioxide, poisoning from, 1001
Carbon dioxide retention, in acute respiratory failure, 93
Carbon disulfide, poisoning from, 1002, 1010
Carbon monoxide poisoning, 483, 977, 1002
Carbon tetrachloride, poisoning from, 1002
Carbuncles, 746
Carcinoid syndrome, malignant, 551–553
Carcinoma, adrenocortical, 519
  cutaneous, 663
  oat cell, 114
  of bladder, 602

Carcinoma (Continued)
  of breast, estrogens and, 914
    recurrent, 901
  of buccal mucosa, 710
  of cervix, 927–930
  of endometrium, 925–927
  of hard palate, 711
  of lips, 710
  of lung, stages of, 111
    T, N, and M categories of, 110
  of penis, 605
  of stomach, 416
    in pernicious anemia, 265
  of testes, 607–610
  of thyroid gland, 543–546
  of urethra, 604
  of vulva, 930–934
  renal tubular, 600
  squamous cell, 600, 732
  ureteral, 600
Cardiac arrest, 164–167
Cardiac arrhythmias, in pheochromocytoma, 546
  in severe hypothermia, 983
Cardiac catheterization, in angina, 163
  in congenital heart disease, 200
Cardiac cirrhosis, 367
Cardiac compression, external, 164–165
  internal, 167
Cardiac conditioning training, 235–236
Cardiac embolus, ischemic stroke secondary to, 764
Cardiac enlargement, in rheumatic fever, 67, 68
Cardiac pseudodisease, prevention of, 208
Cardiac tamponade, in lupus erythematosus, 694
  in pericarditis, 238
Cardiogenic shock, in acute myocardial infarction, 229
Cardiomyopathy, in infants of diabetic mothers, 189
Cardiopulmonary resuscitation, 164
  in acute myocardial infarction, 223
  in cardiac arrest, 164–167
Cardiovascular collapse, in chronic adrenocortical insufficiency, 515
Cardiovascular syphilis, 623
Cardioversion, principles of, 179
Carditis, in bacterial meningitis, 52
  in psittacosis, 57
  in rheumatic fever, 67, 68
Caries, dental, 703
Carotid artery, stenosis or occlusion of, 765–766
Carotid sinus massage, for tachycardia, 179
Carrier state, in amebiasis, 2
  in diphtheria, 21
  in hepatitis, 398
  in salmonellosis, 74
  in streptococcal pharyngitis, 144
  in typhoid, 87
Cataracts, steroid, 36
Catheter, temporary pacing, 174
Cationic detergents, poisoning from, 1009
Cauda equina syndrome, in ankylosing spondylitis, 848

Celiac sprue, 403
Cellulitis, 745
  clostridial, 22
  in acute childhood leukemia, 312
  in chickenpox, 14
  necrotizing, 22
Central diabetes insipidus, 520–522
Central nervous system, in lupus erythematosus, 694
  in non-Hodgkin's lymphomas, 328
  of hemiplegic patient, 767
Cerebral edema, in bacterial meningitis, 50
  in hemiplegic patients, 767
  in relapsing fever, 66
  in viral meningoencephalitis, 798
Cerebral hemorrhage, ischemic stroke secondary to, 764
Cerebrospinal fluid, reference values for, 1030
Cerebrovascular accident, in congenital heart disease, 205
  in sickle cell disease, 271
Cerebrovascular disease, acute ischemic, 763–766
Cerebrovascular occlusion, in meningitis, 52
Cervical adenitis, due to atypical mycobacterium, 153
  tuberculous, 152
Cervical pregnancy, 871
Cervical stenosis, and amenorrhea, 911
Cervicitis, 917
  gonococcal, 619
Cervix, uterine, carcinoma of, 927–930
  uncomplicated gonococcal infections of, 921
Cesarean section, anesthesia for, 883–884
Cevadilla, poisoning from, 1009
Chancre, syphilis, of oral cavity, 707
Chancroid, 617–618
Cheilitis, actinic, 697
  sucking-licking, 697
Cheilitis glandularis apostematosa, 698
Cheilitis granulomatosa, 707
Chemical burns, 994
Chemical food poisoning, 28
Chemosurgery, in cancer of skin, 665
  Mons technique, 663
Chest pain, in pericarditis, 237
Chickenpox, 11–14
Chiclero ulcer, 40
Childbirth, preparation for, 858
Children, asthma in, 634–643
  burns in, fluid therapy in, 507
  cardiac catheterization and angiography in, 200
  dehydration in, 504–506
  delirium in, 955
  diabetes mellitus in, 452–459
  enuresis in, 561–653
  epilepsy in, 781–787
  female, bacterial infections of urinary tract of, 560–561
    urethral meatal stenosis in, 610
  fluid therapy in, 501–508
  head injuries in, 829–834
  hyperthyroidism in, 538
  hypopituitarism of, 529
  hypothyroidism in, 543

Children (*Continued*)
  leukemia in, 309–318
  lymphomas in, 328
  narcotic overdose in, 951
  paroxysmal supraventricular
    tachycardia in, 198
  phosphorus deficiency in, 504
  polycythemia vera in, 341
  seizure types in, 782
  status asthmaticus in, 643
  status epilepticus in, 783
  tuberculosis in, 152
Chloracne, 722
Chloral hydrate. See *Barbiturates.*
Chloramphenicol, adverse effects of,
  70
Chlorates, poisoning from, 1002
Chlordane, poisoning from, 1002
Chlorinated alkalis, poisoning from,
  1002
Chlorinated hydrocarbons, poisoning
  from, antidote for, 999
Chlorine, poisoning from, 1002
Chlorobenzene insecticide, poisoning
  from, 1003
Chloroform, poisoning from, 1002
Chloroquine, toxicity of, 2, 42
Chlorothiazide, poisoning from, 931,
  1002
Cholecystitis, 364–366
Choledocholithiasis, 365
Cholelithiasis, 364–366
  in hemolytic anemia, 261
Cholera, 14–19, 422
  useless and dangerous remedies for,
    18
Cholera bed, *16*
Cholesterol pericarditis, 241
Cholinergic crisis, 806
Cholinesterase inhibiting agents,
    antidote for, 1000
  food poisoning from, 28
Chorea, in rheumatic fever, 68
Chorioamnionitis, 923
Choriocarcinoma, hyperthyroidism in,
  539
Christmas disease, 278
Chromaffin cell tumors, 546
Chromic oxide, poisoning from, 1002
Chromium, poisoning from, 1002
Chronic atopic dermatitis, 669–670
Chronic bronchitis, 102–109
Chronic gastritis, 392
Chronic granulocytic leukemia, 317
Chronic heart block, 178
Chronic hepatitis, 397–398
Chronic hypoparathyroidism, 527–528
Chronic ischemia, 243
Chronic lymphocytic leukemia, 320
Chronic obstructive pulmonary disease
  (COPD), 102–109
Chronic pancreatitis, 409–411
Chronic relapsing polyneuropathy, 822
Chronic renal failure, 588–594
Chronic tophaceous gout, 462
Cicatricial alopecia, 662
Cigarette smoking, in pregnancy, 853
Cinchonism, 41
Circulatory overload transfusion
  reaction, 355
Cirrhosis, 366–372

Citrate toxicity, in blood transfusion,
  355
Cleft lip, 696
Cleft palate, 696
Clonidine, for hypertension, 222
Closed head injury, 823
Clostridial bacteremia, 9
Clostridial cellulitis, 22
Clostridial myonecrosis, 22
Clostridium botulinum food poisoning,
  28
Clostridium perfringens food poisoning,
  25
Clotting factor deficiencies, inherited,
  287
Cluster migraine headache, 792
CNS prophylaxis, in acute childhood
  leukemia, 314
Coagulation abnormalities. See also
  Hemophilia.
  in congenital heart disease, 204
Coal workers' pneumoconiosis,
  138–139
Coated tongue, 699
Cobalt, antidote for, 998
Cocaine, poisoning from, 1002
Coccidioidomycosis, 115–117
Codeine, antidote for, 1000
  poisoning from, 1002, 1006
Colchicine, poisoning from, 1002
Cold, common, 154
  disturbances due to, 981–988
Cold agglutinin disease, 259
Colic, biliary, 364
Colitis, Crohn's, 382–386
  ulcerative, 428–433
    and rectal cancer, 417
Collagen vascular disorders,
  pericarditis in, 240
Colon, diverticular disease of, 380
  obstruction of, 382
  tumors of, 416–421
Colonic amebiasis, 2
Colonoscopic polypectomy, 418
Coma, diabetic, 451–452
  evaluation of, 824–825
  in bacterial meningitis, 50
  in hypothyroidism, 540, 543
Combined headaches, 793
Common cold, 154
Compound nevus, 719
Compressive atelectasis, 100
Congenital alopecia, 659
Congenital erythropoietic porphyria,
  346
Congenital heart disease, 185–209
Congenital nevus, 719
Congenital rubella, 72
Congenital syphilis, 623
Congenital toxoplasmosis, 82, 83
Congestive atelectasis, 101
Congestive heart failure, 209–213
  and ventricular premature beats,
    171
  clinical-hemodynamic subsets, *211*
  in congenital heart disease, 190
  in neonates, 185
  in neonate with congenital heart
    disease, 188
  in rheumatic fever, 67
Conjunctivitis, gonococcal, 619

Connective tissue disorders,
  pericarditis in, 240
Constipation, 372–374
  in multiple sclerosis, 802
Constrictive pericarditis, 237
Contact dermatitis, 666–667, 721
  of vulva, 916
Contraception, 853, 940–942
Contraception methods, for congenital
  heart disease patients, 209
Convulsions. See also *Epilepsy* and
  Seizures.
  due to poisoning, 997
  in pertussis, 91
Cooley's anemia, 266
Copper, antidote for, 998
  poisoning from, 25, 1002
Copperas, poisoning from, 1004
Coproporphyria, 342
Cor pulmonale, in pulmonary
  embolism, 136
  in silicosis, 140
Co-Ral, poisoning from, 1007
Coral snake venom, antidote for, 998
Coronary arteriosclerosis, with
  hypothyroidism, 540
Coronary artery spasm, 164
  in myocardial infarction, 232
Coronary Care Unit, 234
  in acute myocardial infarction, 224
Coronary heart disease, stable,
  ventricular premature beats in,
  172–173
Corpus uteri, carcinoma of, 926
Corrosive gastritis, 391
Corrosive injury to esophagus, 376
Corticosteroid therapy, major side
  effects of, 844
Cosmetics, poisoning from, 1002
Coumadin, poisoning from, 1012
Coumarin derivatives, antidote for,
  1001
Countershock, for atrial fibrillation,
  168–170
CPAP test, for neonate with congenital
  heart disease, 187
Crab lice, 723
Cramps, heat, 989
Cranial arteritis, 793
Craniocerebral trauma, classification
  of, 823
Creeping eruption, 665–666
Creosote, poisoning from, 1008
Crescentic glomerulonephritis, 567
Crohn's disease, 382–386, 390
Croup, 155
Culture-negative endocarditis, 217–218
Cumene, poisoning from, 1012
Curare, poisoning from, 1002
Cushing's syndrome, 515–519
  amenorrhea in, 909
Cutaneous candidiasis, 681–682
Cutaneous horns, 663
Cutaneous larva migrans, 665
Cutaneous leishmaniasis, 40
Cyanide, antidote for, 999
  poisoning from, 1003
Cyanosis, in neonate with congenital
  heart disease, 187
Cyanotic heart disease, polycythemia
  in, 204

Cyclophosphamide, side effects of, 316
Cycloserine, side effects of, 148
Cyclothymic disorders, 959
Cyst passers, 2
Cystinuria, 614
Cystitis, 555, 556
    acute, during pregnancy, 919
Cystosarcoma phylloides, 898
Cysts, 746
    eruption, of teeth, 701
    hydatid, 21–22
    of breasts, 897, 898
Cytosine arabinoside, side effects of,
    316

Dandruff, 673
Darvon, poisoning from, 1006
Daunomycin, side effects of, 316
DC cardioversion, for atrial fibrillation,
    168–170
DDT, poisoning from, 1003
Decortication, in empyema, 121
Decubitus ulcer, 666
Defibrillation, in cardiac arrest, 165
Degenerative arterial disease, 241–246
Dehydration, acute, mineral deficiency
    in, 503
    in children, 504–506
    in cholera, 15, 17
    parenteral therapy in, 496
Dehydroemetine, toxicity of, 1
Delirium, 955–956
Demerol, antidote for, 1000
    poisoning from, 1006
Demulcents, therapeutic agents to
    neutralize, 994
Dental agenesis, 702
Dental caries, 703
Dental extractions, complications of,
    703
Denture stomatitis, 699
Deodorants, poisoning from, 1002
Depigmentation of skin, 722
Depilatories, poisoning from, 1002
Depression, 957
    in paraplegia, 771
    postpartum, 887
de Quervain's disease, 539
Dermal nevus, 719
Dermatitis, atopic, 668–670
    contact, 666–667, 721, 916
    diaper, 669
    gonococcal, 620
    poison ivy, 672–673
    seborrheic, 673–674
    stasis, 674–675
Dermatitis herpetiformis, 667–668
Dermatologic alopecia, 662
Dermatomyositis, 676–677
Dermatophytoses, 679–681
Dermatoses, occupational, 721–722
Dermographism, in urticaria, 753
Descending aorta, aneurysms of, 160
Detergents, poisoning from, 1003,
    1009
DFDT, poisoning from, 1003
Diabetes insipidus, 519–522
Diabetes mellitus, complicating stroke
    in hemiplegic patient, 767

Diabetes mellitus (*Continued*)
    glomerular involvement in, 567
    in adults, 437–452
    in childhood and adolescence,
        452–459
    in chronic pancreatitis, 410
    maternal, infant cardiomyopathy
        form, 189
Diabetic acidosis, in children,
    dehydration in, 506
Diabetic ketoacidosis and coma, in
    adults, 451–452
Diabetic meal plan, 445
Diabetic neuropathies, 821
Diabetics, bacterial pneumonia in, 129
Dialysis, 592–594
Diamthazole, poisoning from, 1003
Diaper dermatitis, 669
Diarrhea, acute infectious, 421–423
Diarrheal disease in children,
    dehydration in, 505
Diazinon, poisoning from, 1007
Dibenzazepines, poisoning from, 1010
DIC. See *Disseminated intravascular
    coagulation.*
Dichlorhydrin. See *Carbon tetrachloride.*
Dichlorophenoxyacetic acid, poisoning
    from, 1003
Dieldrin. See *Chlordane.*
Diet, for Crohn's disease, 382
    for hypertension, 220
    for infants with congestive heart
        failure, 193
    in Coronary Care Unit, 224
Diethylene glycol, poisoning from,
    1004
Diethyltoluamide, poisoning from,
    1003
Diffuse esophageal spasm, 377
Digestion, disorders of, 400–403
Digitalis, antidote for, 998
    poisoning from, 1003
    toxicity of, 106, 177
Digitoxin, poisoning from, 1003
Digoxin, antiarrhythmic effects of, 172
    toxicity of, 191–192
Dihydromorphinone, poisoning from,
    1006
Dilan, poisoning from, 1003
Dilantin. See *Phenytoin.*
Dilaudid, poisoning from, 1006
Dilutional coagulopathy, transfusion
    related, 356
Dimethylaniline, poisoning from, 995
Dimethylphthalate, poisoning from,
    1003
Dimethyl sulfate, poisoning from, 1003
Dimite, poisoning from, 1003
Dinitro-ortho-cresol, poisoning from,
    1003
Dinitrophenol derivatives, poisoning
    from, 1003
Dionin, antidote for, 1000
Dioxane. See *Acetone.*
Diphenhydramine hydrochloride. See
    Antihistaminics.
Diphenylhydantoin sodium. See
    Phenytoin.
Diphtheria, 19–21
    of upper lip, 706
Diplopia, in paraplegia, 771

Disaccharidase deficiencies, 403
Discoid lupus erythematosus, 689,
    691–692
Disorders of the mouth, benign,
    695–709
Disopyramide phosphate, toxicity of,
    177
Dissecting aneurysms, 160
Dissecting aortic aneurysm, pericarditis
    in, 240
Disseminated intravascular
        coagulation, 293–294
    abortion related, 865
    in adult leukemia, 307
    in plague, 55
    in relapsing fever, 65
    in typhus fever, 88
Disulfiram (Antabuse), 947
Dithiocarbamate, poisoning from, 1003
Diuretics, and thrombocytopenia, 291
Diuril, poisoning from, 931, 1002
Diverticular abscess, 381
Diverticular disease, of colon, 380
    symptomatic, 380–381
Diverticulitis, acute, 381
Diverticulum(a), duodenal, 379
    Meckel's, 380
    of alimentary tract, 378–382
    of esophagus, 379
    of stomach, 379
    perforation of, 381
    small intestinal, 379–380
    Zenker's, 378
Diving reflex, 198
Dizziness. See *Vertigo, episodic.*
DMC, poisoning from, 1003
Dolichocolon, 373
Dolophine. See *Morphine.*
Doriden. See *Barbiturates.*
Drug names, American, glossary of,
    with international synonyms,
    1016–1017
Drug related immune hemolysis, 260
Drug related thrombocytopenia, 291
Drug toxicity, heart block from, 177
Drugs, adverse reactions to,
        hypersensitivity, 647–650
    antianginal, 232
    during pregnancy, 854, 857
    inducing ventricular premature
        beats, 172
    nephrotoxicity of, 567
    nonsteroidal antiinflammatory,
        anaphylactic reactions to, 627
    oxidant, and acute hemolysis, 262
Duhring's disease, 667–668
Dumping syndrome, 400
Duodenal diverticula, 379
Duodenum, Crohn's disease of, 384
Dysentery, amebic, 2
Dysfunctional uterine bleeding,
    904–906
Dysgammaglobulinemia, 404
Dyshidrosis, 743, 744
Dyskinesia, antipsychotic drugs and,
    968
Dysmenorrhea, 912–913
Dysphagia, 374–378
Dysthymic disorders, 959
Dystonias, antipsychotic drugs and,
    967

Ear, middle, chronic effusion in, 127
Ear ache, in mumps, 54
Eardrum, ruptured, in otitis media, 125
Early non-insulin-dependent diabetes mellitus, hypoglycemia in, 471, 472
Echinococcosis, 21–22
Eclampsia, 873–877
Ecthyma, 745
Ectopic ACTH production, and adrenocortical hyperplasia and hypercortisolism, 518
Ectopic atrial tachycardia, 181
Ectopic pregnancy, 865–871
Eczema, housewife's, 743
infantile, 668–669
Eczema herpeticum, 682
Edema, pulmonary, in congenital heart disease, 194–195
Edentulism, lip destruction in, 697
Electrolyte imbalance, in acute childhood leukemia, 313
Electrolyte repair solutions, compositions of, 491
Electrolytes, daily requirements of, 493
in cholera, 15
Elliptocytosis, hereditary, and hemolytic anemia, 262
Embolism(s), acute, 242
air, transfusion related, 356
cardiopulmonary resuscitation and, 167
in myocardial infarction, 232
pulmonary, 134–137
in venous thrombosis, 248
Embolus, ischemic stroke secondary to, 764
Emetics, therapeutic agents to neutralize, 994
Emetine, poisoning from, 103
Emetine hydrochloride, toxicity of, 1
Emotions, and asthma, 629
Emphysema, 102–109
Empyema thoracis, 120–121
Encephalitis, in epidemic influenza, 33
in psittacosis, 57
Encephalomyelitis, in chickenpox, 13
Encephalopathy, in pertussis, 91
Endocarditis, bacterial, prophylaxis against, 206
gonococcal, 620
in Q fever, 57
in rat bite fever, 63
infective, 213–219
Endocrine disorders, alopecia in, 659
Endometriosis, 902–904
Endometrium, carcinoma of, 925–927
Endomyometritis, 923
Entamoeba histolytica food poisoning, 26
Enteric fever, in salmonellosis, 73, 74
Enterobacter species pneumonia, 130
Enterococcal bacteremia, 8
Enterococcal infective endocarditis, 215
Enterococcal meningitis, 48
Enterotoxigenic food poisoning, 26
Entrapment neuropathies, 820
Enuresis, childhood, 561–563
Eosinophilic fasciitis, 752
Eosinophilic gastritis, 25
Ependymoma, 835

Ephedrine, poisoning from, 1004
side effects of, 104
Epidemic influenza, 32–34
Epidermoid cancers, 419
Epididymitis, 556, 563
gonococcal, 619
Epidural block obstetric anesthesia, 881
Epidural hematoma, acute, 827
computed tomographic scan of, 825
Epilepsy, in adolescents and adults, 772–781
in brain abscess, 760, 761
in childhood, 781–787
Epileptic seizures, international classification of, 772
Epiphenomena, abscess, of brain, 760–761
Episodic vertigo, 793–796
Epistaxis, in pertussis, 91
in von Willebrand's disease, 286
Epithelial nevi, 719
EPN, poisoning from, 1007
Equanil, poisoning from, 1006
Equine antirabies serum, reactions with, 61
Ergot derivatives, poisoning from, 1004
Erosive gastritis, 391
Erosive lichen planus, 701
Erysipelas, 706, 745
Erythema annulare centrifugum, 668
Erythema marginatum, in rheumatic fever, 68
Erythema multiforme, 677, 701
Erythema nodosum, 386, 677
Erythema nodosum leprosum reaction, 36
Erythemas, 677–678
Erythrasma, 747
Erythroblastopenia, immuno-suppression in, 254
Erythroblastosis fetalis, 275
Erythrocytosis, 336–342
Erythroplasia of Queyrat, 732
Erythropoietic porphyria, 342, 343
Erythropoietic protoporphyria, 689, 691
Escherichia coli bacteremia, 9
Escherichia coli food poisoning, 26, 27
Escherichia coli pneumonia, 130
Eserine, poisoning from, 1008
Esophageal foreign bodies, 377
Esophageal rings and webs, 376
Esophageal varices, bleeding, 361–364
Esophagopharyngitis, radiation induced, 305
Esophagus, diverticula of, 379
obstruction of, 374–378
Espundia, 39
Essential (volatile) oils, poisoning from, 1004
Estrogen, carcinogenic properties of, 913
Ethambutol, side effects of, 148, 149
Ether, poisoning from, 1004
Ethionamide, side effects of, 148
Ethmoiditis, acute, 144
Ethyl alcohol, poisoning from, 1004
Ethylene chlorohydrin, poisoning from, 1004

Ethylene dichloride, poisoning from, 1004
Ethylene glycol, antidote for, 998
poisoning from, 1004
Euphoria, in multiple sclerosis, 802
Eustachian tube dysfunction, 127
Exchange lists, ADA, 442–444
Exchange transfusion, in erythroblastosis fetalis, 275
Exercise, bronchospastic effects of, 629
during pregnancy, 856
for congenital heart disease patients, 207
Exercise conditioning, for angina pectoris patients, 163
Exercise training, following myocardial infarction, 235–236
Exhaustion, heat, 989
Exogenous gastritis, 391
External cardiac compression, 164–165
External hemorrhoids, 387
External otitis, 747
Extramedullary leukemia, 315
Extrapulmonary tuberculosis, 152
Extrinsic allergic alveolitis, 141–142
Eyelid, cancerous lesions of, 664
seborrheic dermatitis of, 674
Eyes, in Graves' disease, 539
in juvenile rheumatoid arthritis, 845

Face, lesions of, in leprosy, 707
seborrheic dermatitis of, 674
Facial paralysis, acute peripheral, 812–814
Factor VIII deficiency, 278
Familial benign pemphigus, 737
Farmer's lung, 142
Fasciitis, necrotizing, 22
Fasting, in obesity, 473
Fatty acid amides, poisoning from, 1003
Febrile seizures, in children, 783
Febrile transfusion reactions, 354
Feces, reference values for, 1032
Feet, inflammatory eruptions of, 743–744
nevoid moles of, 663
Felty's syndrome, and neutropenia, 273
Ferbam, poisoning from, 1003
Ferrous sulfate, poisoning from, 1004
Fetal alcohol syndrome, 853
Fetal depression, obstetric anesthesia and, 879
Fetal distress, delivery in, anesthesia for, 884
Fever, enteric, in salmonellosis, 73
in adult leukemia patient, 306
in bacterial meningitis, 51
in psittacosis, 56
rat bite, 62–63
relapsing, 63–66
rheumatic, 66–69, 144
Rocky Mountain spotted, 69–70
typhoid, 86–87
typhus, 88–89
Fibrillation, atrial, 167–171
in cardiac arrest, 165

Fibrillation (*Continued*)
  ventricular, in acute myocardial
      infarction, 228
    in congenital heart disease, 199
Fibrinolytic system, activators and
    inhibitors of, 294
Fibroadenoma, 898
Fibrocystic disease of breasts, 897
Fibromas, of nails, 718
Fibrosis, progressive massive, 138–139
Fibrous thyroiditis, 551
Figurate erythemas, 678
Fish toxins, food poisoning from, 28
Fissured tongue, 699
Fissures, of lips, 697
Fistula, anal, 389–390
  anorectal, 390
  colonic, 381
  in Crohn's disease, 385
Fistulotomy, 390
Flatus, excessive passage of, 395–396
Fluid replacement therapy, in
    children, 501–508
Fluke infestation, 428
Fluorides, poisoning from, 1004
Fluorine, poisoning from, 1004
    antidote for, 999
Fluoroacetate sodium, poisoning from,
    1005
Fluorosilicates, poisoning from, 1004
Flushing attacks, in malignant
    carcinoid syndrome, 552
Focal glomerulosclerosis, 566
Focal proliferative glomerulonephritis,
    566
Folate deficiency, 264, 265
Folic acid deficiency, and ineffective
    platelet production, 290
Follicular carcinoma, of thyroid, 545
Folliculitis, 746
Food exchange lists, ADA, 442–444
Food impaction, in esophagus, 376
Food poisoning, 23–32, 422, 1005
Food poisoning syndromes,
    gastrointestinal plus neurologic
        symptoms, 28–29
    gastrointestinal plus other systemic
        diseases, 30
    neurologic symptoms alone, 31
    primarily gastrointestinal symptoms,
        25–26
Foot. See *Feet.*
Fordyce's disease, 695–696
Foreign body granulomas, 722
Formaldehyde, antidote for, 998
    poisoning from, 1005
Formalin, antidote for, 998
    poisoning from, 1005
Formula feeding, of normal infants,
    893
Fox-Fordyce disease, 737
Fracture(s), cardiopulmonary
    resuscitation and, 166
  in multiple myeloma patients, 334
  of fused spine, 848
  of skull, in adults, 827
    in children, 832
Fragmentation hemolysis, 262
Freckles, 719, 726
Frontal sinusitis, acute, 143
Frostbite, 985–988

Fulminant hepatitis, 397
Fundal gastritis, chronic, 392
Fungal endocarditis, 217
Fungal pericarditis, 240
Fungus infections, of nail plates,
    714–715
  of skin, superficial, 678–682
Furuncles, 706, 746

Gallstone pancreatitis, 406
Gallstones, 364–366
  in sickle cell disease, 271
Gangrene, gas, 22–23
  nonclostridial anaerobic, 22
  synergistic, 22
Gardnerella vaginalis, infection from,
    916
Gas gangrene, 22–23
Gaseousness, 392–396
Gasoline, poisoning from, 1005
Gastric analysis, reference values for,
    1031
Gastric hypersecretion, 401
Gastric tumors, malignant, 416
Gastric ulcers, 414
Gastritis, 390–392
  eosinophilic, 25
Gastroenteritis, in salmonellosis, 73
Gastrointestinal absorption tests, 1032
Gastrointestinal tract, in scleroderma,
    751
  of hemiplegic patient, 767
Gastrointestinal tract fluid losses,
    parenteral therapy in, 496
Genetic counseling, for parents of
    congenital heart disease patients,
    208
Genital herpes virus infection, 682,
    915
Genitourinary tract, trauma to,
    570–576
Genitourinary tuberculosis, 152,
    594–597
Genitourinary tumors, 597–610
Geographic tongue, 699
Geriatric patients, delirium in, 955
German measles, 71–72
Ghon lesion, of oral cavity, 707
Giardia lamblia, 426
Giardia lamblia food poisoning, 26
Gigantism, 509
Gingivae, benign disorders of, 701–702
  cancer of, 710
Gingival abscess, 706
Gingival stomatitis, herpetic, recurrent,
    701
Gingivitis, 702
Gingivostomatitis, 682
Glasgow coma scale, 824
Glioblastoma multiforme, 835
Glomerulonephritis, 564
Glomerulus, disorders of, 564–568
Glossitis, Moeller's, 699
Glossodynia, 698
Glossopyrosis, 698
Glucose intolerance, in cholera, 17
Glucose-6-phosphate dehydrogenase
    deficiency, and hemolytic anemia,
    263

Glutethimide. See *Barbiturates.*
Goiter, simple, 522–525
  toxic nodular, and hypothyroidism,
    533
Gold, antidote for, 999
  poisoning from, 1005
"Gold paint" pericarditis, 241
Gold therapy, toxicity of, 842, 844
Gonadotropin deficiency, 529
Gonococcal bacteremia, 8
Gonococcal conjunctivitis, 619
Gonococcal infection, 618–620
Gonococcal urethritis, 555
Gonorrhea, 921. See also *Gonococcal
    infection.*
  of mouth, 707
Goodpasture's syndrome, 584
Gout, 459–463
  in pernicious anemia, 265
Grady coma scale, 824
Graft vs. host disease, 256
Graft vs. host reaction, 357
Gram-negative anaerobic bacteremia, 9
Gram-negative bacillary endocarditis,
    217
Gram-positive anaerobic infections, 8
Granulocytic leukemia, chronic, 317
Granulocytopenia, in acute childhood
    leukemia, 312
  in aplastic anemia, 252
Granuloma(s), and hypopituitarism,
    529
  foreign body, 722
  histoplasma, 117
Granuloma inguinale, 620–621, 707
Granuloma venereum, 620–621
Graves' disease, 533
Great saphenous vein stripping
    technique, 249
Green vitriol, poisoning from, 1004
Group A streptococcal bacteremia, 6
Group A streptococcal pneumonia,
    130
Group B streptococcal bacteremia, 8
Group B streptococcal meningitis, 48
Growth hormone deficiency, 528
Growth retardation, in proctocolitis,
    432
Guaiacol, poisoning from, 1008
Guanethidine, for hypertension, 221
Guillain-Barré syndrome, 821
  swine flu vaccine and, 33
Gums, bleeding of, 483
Gunther's disease, 346
Guthion, poisoning from, 1007

Habitual abortion, 863
Hailey-Hailey disease, 737
Hair, ingrowth of, 658
  shedding of, 659
Hair dyes, poisoning from, 1002
Hairy tongue, 699
Halitosis, 704
Hallucinations, auditory, 959
Halo nevi, 719
Hamartoma, 599
Hands, dermatitis of, nail dystrophy
    in, 717
  inflammatory eruptions of, 743–744
  nevoid moles of, 663

Hansen's disease, 34–38
Hard palate, cancer of, 711
Hashimoto's thyroiditis, 539
Hay fever, 643
Head injuries, in adults, acute,
    822–829
  in children, 829–834
Head lice, 723
Headache, 788–793
  post-spinal anesthesia, 885–886
Heart. See also entries under *Cardiac,*
    and specific disorders.
  in acute renal failure, 585
  in ankylosing spondylitis, 848
  in scleroderma, 751
Heart block, 173–178
  in congenital heart disease, 199
  in pericarditis, 237
  in rheumatic fever, 68
Heart disease, congenital, 185–209
    prevention of complications of,
      206
  organic, and supraventricular
      premature beats, 171
Heart failure, congestive, in congenital
    heart disease, 190
  in congenital heart disease, 198
Heart murmurs, in low birth weight
    infants, 892
Heat, disturbances due to, 988–990
Heat cramps, 989
Heat exhaustion, 989
Heat stroke, 989
Heavy metal poisoning, 25
Height, table of, for men and women,
    1015
Hellebore, poisoning from, 1012
Helminth infections, 423–428
Hemarthroses, in hemophiliacs, 281
Hematology, reference values in, 1020
Hematoma(s), epidural, computed
    tomographic scan of, *825*
  epidural and subdural, acute, 827
  of brain, 762–763
  of scrotum, 575
  subungual, 713
Hematuria, in hemophiliacs, 283
  in sickle cell disease, 271
  in urinary tract injury, 572
Hemianopia, in paraplegia, 771
Hemiplegia, rehabilitation of patient
    with, 766–771
Hemochromatosis, 295–296
Hemodialysis, 592
Hemoglobin, abnormal, and hemolytic
    anemia, 263
Hemolytic anemia, immune, 259–261
  in lupus erythematosus, 694
  nonimmune, 261–263
Hemolytic disease of the newborn,
    274–278
Hemophilia, 278–287
Hemophilia A, 278
Hemophilia B, 278
Hemophilus influenzae bacteremia, 10
Hemophilus meningitis, 46
Hemorrhages, at joints, in hemophilia,
    281
  cerebral, 764
  in abortion, 865
  in acute childhood leukemia, 312

Hemorrhages (*Continued*)
  in acute renal failure, 586
  in late pregnancy, 871–873
  in pertussis, 91
  in polycythemia vera, 341
  in relapsing fever, 64
  intestinal, in typhoid fever, 87
  massive, in Crohn's disease, 385
  parenchymatous, of brain, 762–763
  postpartum, 886
  uterine, 905
Hemorrhoids, 387–389
Hemosiderosis, 295–296
  transfusional, 359
Hemostasis, blood component therapy
    for, 349
  drugs which effect, 765
Heparin, antidote for, 1000
  contraindications to, 247
Hepatic amebiasis, 3
Hepatic failure, in relapsing fever, 64
Hepatic porphyria, acute, 342
Hepatitis, acute and chronic, 396–398
  alcoholic, 367
  coagulation disturbances in, 485
  post-transfusion, 357
Hepatitis A food poisoning, 30
Hepatobiliary disease, in Crohn's
    disease, 386
Hepatorenal syndrome, in cirrhosis,
    372
Hereditary elliptocytosis, and
    hemolytic anemia, 262
Hereditary spherocytosis, and
    hemolytic anemia, 262
Heredopathia atactica
    polyneuritiformis, 821
Heroin, antidote for, 1000
  poisoning by, 949
Herpes, genital, 682
  neonatal, 682
Herpes gestationis, 757–758
Herpes keratitis, 683
Herpes labialis, 682
Herpes simplex, 682–684, 690
Herpes zoster, 757
Herpetic gingival stomatitis, recurrent,
    701
Herpetic ulcer, persistent, 683
Herpetic whitlow, 682
Heterologous serum, anaphylactic
    reactions to, 626
Hidradenitis suppurativa, 684–685
High blood pressure. See *Hypertension.*
Hip, aseptic necrosis of, in sickle cell
    disease, 271
His bundle electrocardiography, in
    infants and young children, 201
Histoplasmosis, 117–118
  pericarditis in, 240
Hodgkin's disease, staging classification
    of, 296–298, 302–303
  treatment of, chemotherapy,
    296–302
  radiation, 302–306
Hookworms, 427
Horse serum, hypersensitivity to,
    19–20
Housewife's eczema, 743
Humidifiers, and hypersensitivity
    pneumonitis, 141

Hydatid disease, 21–22
Hydatidiform mole, and
    hyperthyroidism, 539
Hydralazine, poisoning from, 1005
Hydrocephalus, post-traumatic, 834
Hydrochloric acid, poisoning from,
    1005
Hydrogen cyanide, poisoning from,
    1003
Hydrogen fluoride, poisoning from,
    1004
Hydrogen sulfide, poisoning from,
    1010
Hydronephrosis, obstructive, in
    Crohn's disease, 386
Hydrops fetalis, 275
Hydroquinone, poisoning from, 1005
Hydroxychloroquine, toxicity of, 844
1α-Hydroxylase enzyme deficiency,
    479
Hymenoptera stings, anaphylactic
    reactions to, 626
Hymenoptera venom immunotherapy,
    652
Hyperbilirubinemia, exchange
    transfusion in, 275, 276
Hypercalcemia, 526
  in acute childhood leukemia, 313
  in multiple myeloma, 334
  in primary hyperparathyroidism,
    525
Hypercalciuria, 612–615
Hyperchloremic acidosis, 480
Hypercyanotic spells, in congenital
    heart disease, 195–196
Hyperglycemia, in acute pancreatitis,
    407
Hyperkalemia, heart block in, 177
  in acute renal failure, 585
  transfusion related, 356
Hyperkeratosis, retention, 655
Hyperlipidemia, 463
  in acute pancreatitis, 407
Hyperlipoproteinemia, 463–470
Hypermenorrhea, 905
Hypernatremia, in infancy, 506
  parenteral fluid therapy in, 498
Hyperoxic test, for neonate with
    congenital heart disease, 187
Hyperparathyroidism, 525–527
Hyperpigmentation of skin, 722, 724
Hyperprolactinemia, 531–533
  in acromegaly, 509
Hyperpyrexia, in psittacosis, 57
  in relapsing fever, 65
Hypersensitivity pneumonitis,
    141–142
Hypersomatotropism, in acromegaly,
    509
Hypersplenism, and hemolytic anemia,
    262
  platelet pooling in, 290
Hypertension, 219–223
  arterial, in myocardial infarction,
    231
  in chronic renal failure, 591
  in glomerular disorders, 565
  in hemiplegic patient, 767
  pheochromocytoma and, 546
  pregnancy-induced, 873–877
Hypertensive emergencies, 222

Hyperthermia, malignant, anesthesia and, 989
Hyperthyroidism, 533–543
  amenorrhea in, 910
Hyperuricemia, 459–463
  in acute childhood leukemia, 313
  in congenital heart disease, 205
  in hypertension, 221
  in multiple myeloma, 334
Hyperviscosity syndrome, in multiple myeloma, 335
Hypervitaminosis A, 437
Hypervitaminosis D, antidote for, 999
Hypnotherapy, for neurodermatitis, 672
Hypocalcemia, following parathyroidectomy, 526
  in acute childhood leukemia, 312
Hypochlorites, poisoning from, 1002
Hypochromia, in iron deficiency anemia, 256
Hypofibrinogenemia, bleeding in patients with, 286
Hypogammaglobulinemia, 351
Hypoglycemia, in childhood diabetes mellitus, 458
  in cholera, 18
  reactive, 470–472
Hypokalemia, in cholera, 18
  in pernicious anemia, 265
  transfusion related, 356
Hypomagnesemia, in hypoparathyroidism, 527
Hyponatremia, in acute childhood leukemia, 313
  in bacterial meningitis, 51
  in children, 507
  in chronic overhydration, 497
Hypoparathyroidism, 527–528
Hypopigmentation, 725
Hypopituitarism, 528–530
Hypostatic pneumonia, complicating stroke in hemiplegic patient, 766
Hypotension, following obstetric anesthesia, 878
  in pulmonary embolism, 136
  in typhus fever, 88
Hypothalamic pituitary dysfunction, amenorrhea in, 909, 910
Hypothermia, 981–985. See also *Frostbite*.
  transfusion related, 356
Hypothyroidism, 530–531, 540–543
  amenorrhea in, 909
  pericarditis in, 241
  radiation induced, 306
Hypovitaminosis A, 436
Hypovolemia, 347
  in cholera, 17
Hypoxemia, 97
  in acute respiratory failure, 94
Hypoxia, during obstetric anesthesia, 878
  in silicosis, 140

Iatrogenic Cushing's syndrome, 515–516
Idiopathic cryptogenic palsy, 812
Ileitis, regional, 382–386
Immune globulins, therapy with, 351

Immune hemolytic anemia, 259–261
Immune hemolytic reaction, 352
Immunization, against diphtheria, 21
  for congenital heart disease patients, 207
Immunoglobulin deficiencies, 404
Immunologic procedures, reference values for, 1034
Immunosuppression, in erythroblastopenia, 254
Imperforate hymen, and amenorrhea, 911
Impetigo, 706
  in chickenpox, 14
  nonbullous, 745
Incomplete abortion, 862
Incontinence, in multiple sclerosis, 802
  in paraplegia, 771
Indalone, poisoning from, 1003
Induced abortion, 863
  methods of, by gestation age, *864*
Infants, cardiac catheterization and angiography in, 200
  coagulation disturbances in, 484
  hypernatremia in, 506
  low birth weight, care of, 887–893
  myasthenia in, 807
  normal, feeding of, 893–896
  of diabetic mothers, cardiomyopathy in, 189
  paroxysmal supraventricular tachycardia in, 198
  premature, patent ductus arteriosus in, 189
Infantile eczema, 668–669
Infantile spasms, 783
Infarction, lacunar, 765
  myocardial, 223–233
    acute, and supraventricular beats, 171
      heart block complicating, 176–177
    oral contraception and, 941
    pericarditis following, 240
    rehabilitation of patient following, 233–236
    ventricular premature beats in, 173
Infection(s), abortion related, 865
  anaerobic soft tissue, 22–23
  and alopecia, 661
  and hypopituitarism, 529
  bacterial, of urinary tract, in adult females, 557–559
    in female children, 560–561
    in males, 555–556
  enterococcal, 8
  following gynecological surgery, 923
  in acute childhood leukemia, 312
  in adult leukemia patient, 306
  in multiple myeloma patients, 334
  of pelvis, 921–923
  postpartum, 923
  respiratory, viral, 153–156
  staphylococcal, 8
  streptococcal, 6, 8
  systemic, glomerulonephritis in, 568
Infectious mononucleosis, 52–54
Infective endocarditis, 213–219
Inflammatory eruptions of hands and feet, 743–744

Inflammatory polyneuropathy, 821
Influenza, 130
  and chronic obstructive pulmonary disease, 103
  epidemic, 32–34
Influenza A infections, 154
Influenza vaccines, 133
  contraindications to, 33
Ingrown toenail, 712
Inhalation analgesia and anesthesia for obstetric patient, 882–883
Injury. See also *Trauma*.
  head, acute, in adults, 822–829
Inotropic agents, in congestive heart failure, 212
Insect repellents, poisoning from, 1006
Insect stings, allergic reactions to, 651–653
  anaphylactic reactions to, 626, 636–653
Insect venom, antidote for, 999
Insecticides, food poisoning from, 28
  phosphate ester, poisoning from, 1007
  poisoning from, 1003
Insulin(s), 448–450
  allergy to, 650
Interferon, 336
Intermittent acute porphyria, 342
Intermittent claudication, 243
Internal hemorrhoids, 387–389
International classification of epileptic seizures, 772
International system of units for laboratory measurements, 1018
Intertrigo, 737
Intestinal hemorrhage, in typhoid fever, 87
Intestinal obstruction, 405–406
  in Crohn's disease, 386
Intestinal parasites, 423–428
Intestinal perforation, in typhoid fever, 87
Intracerebral hematomas, in children, 834
Intracranial hemorrhage, 282
Intracranial pressure, monitoring of, 827
Intrauterine devices, 942
Intrauterine fetal assessment, 858
Intrauterine growth retardation, 860
Intraventricular block, 173–178
Iodides, poisoning from, 1005
Iodine, poisoning from, 1005
  antidote for, 999
Iodoform, poisoning from, 1005
Ipecac, poisoning from, 1003
Iritis, in ankylosing spondylitis, 848
Iritis-episcleritis, in ulcerative colitis, 432
Iron, poisoning from, antidote for, 998
Iron deficiency anemia, 256–259
  in von Willebrand's disease, 286
Iron overload, in hemolytic anemia, 261
Irregular narrow QRS tachycardia, 181
Ischemia, chronic, 243
Ischemic cerebrovascular disease, acute, 763–766

Ischemic myocardium, protection of, 232
Ischemic optic neuropathy, 810
Isoniazid, poisoning from, 1005
    side effects of, 148
Isopropyl alcohol. See *Ethyl alcohol.*
Isoproterenol, for heart block, 174
Isthmic pregnancy, 870

Jarisch-Herzheimer reaction, 65, 624
Jaundice, in low birth weight infant, 891
    in mononucleosis, 53
Jodbasedow syndrome, 539
Joints, hemorrhages at, in hemophilia, 281
    in scleroderma, 751
Junction nevi, 719
Juvenile nevus, 719
Juvenile plane warts, 755
Juvenile rheumatoid arthritis, 843–845

Kala-azar, 39
Kaposi's varicelliform eruption, 682
Keloids, 685–687
Keratitis, herpes, 683
Keratoacanthoma, 665
Keratoses, actinic, 663, 731
    arsenical, 732
    senile, 663
Keratotic scabies, 749
Kerosene, poisoning from, 1005
Ketoacidosis, in childhood diabetes mellitus, 452–456, 457
    in diabetic adult, 451–452
Kidney(s). See also entries under *Renal.*
    benign tumors of, 599
    damage to, in lupus erythematosus, 694
    in scleroderma, 751
    injury to, 571
    transplantation of, in chronic renal failure, 594
Kidney stones. See *Renal calculi.*
Kidney transplant, acute renal failure following, 588
Klebsiella pneumonia, 130

Labor, anesthesia for, 880
    effect of anesthesia and analgesia on, 885
Laboratory reference values of clinical importance, 1018–1036
Lactase deficiency, 402–403
Lactation, inappropriate, 897
Lactic acidosis, in relapsing fever, 65
Lacunar infarction, ischemic stroke secondary to, 765
Laennec's cirrhosis, 367
Laparotomy, staging, in Hodgkin's disease, 297
Large intestine, Crohn's disease of, 385
Larva migrans, cutaneous, 665

Laryngotracheal obstruction, in diphtheria, 20
Laryngotracheobronchitis, 155
Late benign syphilis, 623
Latent syphilis of indeterminate duration, 623
Lead, poisoning from, 1005
    antidote for, 998
Leaking ectopic pregnancy, 870
Left ventricular failure, in acute myocardial infarction, 229
Legionnaires' disease, antimicrobial therapy for, 130
Legs, ulceration of, in sickle cell disease, 271
Leiomyoma, of stomach, 415
Leishmaniasis, 39–40
Lennox-Gastaut syndrome, 783
Lentigo, 719
Lentigo maligna, 733
Lepromatous lepra reaction, 36
Leprosy, 34–38
    facial lesions of, 707
    sulfone-resistant, 35
    treatment of reactions in, 36
Leptomeningeal infiltration, in non-Hodgkin's lymphomas, 328
Leriche's syndrome, 243
Leukemia, acute, childhood, 309–318
    in adults, 306–309
    in polycythemia vera, 342
    lymphoblastic, 289, 310
    nonlymphocytic, in Hodgkin's disease, 302
    chronic, 317–319
        granulocytic, 317
        lymphocytic, 320
    extramedullary, 315
    meningeal, 309
Leukocyte concentrate, human, therapy with, 350
Leukocytosis, lithium salts induced, 254
Leukokeratosis, 700
Leukoplakia, 700, 733
Lice, 723–724
Lichen planus, 687
    erosive, 701
    in genital area, 737
    nail changes in, 717
Lichen sclerosus, 916
Life support decision tree, for unwitnessed cardiac arrest, *166*
Life support systems in cardiac arrest, 165
Ligamentum arteriosum, aneurysm at, 160
Lingual tonsillitis, 707
Lip pits, 696
Lipid nephrosis, 566
Lips, benign disorders of, 695–698
    carcinoma of, 710
    cleft, 696
    fissures of, 697
    mucoceles of, 696
    trauma of, 696
    vascular tumors of, 696
Liquid measures, metric and apothecaries', table of, 1014
Listeria meningitis, 48
Listeria monocytogenes bacteremia, 9

Liver, cirrhosis of, 366–372
    in chickenpox, 14
Liver abscess, aspiration of, 3
Liver disease, coagulation disturbances in, 485
Liver spots, 663
Local anesthetics, anaphylactic reactions to, 627
    toxic reactions to, 879
Localized atopic dermatitis, 743, 744
Louse borne relapsing fever, 64
Low birth weight infant, care of, 887–893
Lower extremities. See also *Legs* and *Feet.*
    massive deep vein thrombosis of, 246–249
Lown-Ganong-Levine syndrome, and supraventricular premature beats, 171
Ludwig's angina, 707
Lumbar epidural obstetric anesthesia, 881, 882
Lung(s), carcinoma of, T, N, and M categories of, 110
    in ankylosing spondylitis, 848
    in scleroderma, 751
    primary abscess of, 121–23
    primary cancer of, 109–114
Lung cancers, hormone producing, 114
    primary, 109–114
Lung disease, chronic, and supraventricular premature beats, 171
Lupus erythematosus, 690–695
    discoid, 689, 691–692
    pericarditis associated with, 240
Lymphangiectasia, intestinal, 404
Lymphocytic leukemia, chronic, 320
Lymphocytic (autoimmune) thyroiditis, 551
Lymphogranuloma venereum, 621
Lymphoma, Burkitt's, 321
    childhood, 328
    leptomeningeal, 328
    malignant, in controlled Hodgkin's disease, 306
    non-Hodgkin's, 320–329
    T cell, 329–333
Lymphosarcoma, of stomach, primary, 416
    of thyroid gland, 546

Mace. See *Tear gases.*
Machine oil, poisoning from, 1011
Macrocheilia, 698
Macroglossia, 705–706
Magnesium deficiency, in children, 503
Malabsorption, diseases causing, 398
    in chronic pancreatitis, 409
    of vitamin D, 480
Malabsorption syndromes, 398–405
    vitamin K deficiencies in, 485
Malaria, 40–42
    posttransfusion, 358
Malathion, poisoning from, 1007
Maldigestion, diseases causing, 398
Male fern, poisoning from, 995

Malignant carcinoid syndrome, 551–553
Malignant hyperthermia, anesthesia and, 989
Malignant melanoma, 719
Manganese, poisoning from, 1006
Mania, 957
  acute, 962
Marginal gingivitis, chronic, 702
Marihuana, poisoning from, 1006
Mastectomy, 900
Mastitis, 898
Mastodynia, 897
Maxillary sinusitis, acute, 143
Measles, 42–44
  German, 71–72
Measles vaccine, 43
Measures, liquid, metric and apothecaries', table of, 1014
Mecholyl, poisoning from, 1008
Meckel's diverticulum, 380
Median rhomboid glossitis, 699
Mediastinal mass, large, in Hodgkin's disease, 304
Mediterranean anemia, 266
Medullary thyroid carcinoma, 545
Medulloblastoma, 835
Megacolon, acquired, 373
  toxic, 432
    in Crohn's disease, 385
Megaloblastic anemias, 263–265
Melanoma, 663
  malignant, 719
  nail changes in, 718
Melasma, 725
Melkersson-Rosenthal syndrome, 707
Membranes, abnormalities of, and hemolytic anemia, 262
Membranoproliferative glomerulonephritis, 566
Membranous glomerulonephritis, 566
Men, table of desirable heights and weights for, 1015
Meniere's disease, 796–797
Meningeal leukemia, 309
Meningioma, 835
Meningitis, bacterial, 44–52
  gonococcal, 620
  in acute childhood leukemia, 312
  in plague, 55
  in sickle cell disease, 270
  meningococcal, 46
  viral, 797
Meningitis pathogens, 45
Meningococcal bacteremia, 9
Meningoencephalitis, in mumps, 54
  viral, 797–799
Menopause, 913–914
Menthol. See *Phenol*.
Meperidine, poisoning from, 1006
Meperidene hydrochloride. See *Morphine*.
Meprobamate, poisoning from, 1006
6-Mercaptopurine, side effects of, 316
Mercury, antidote for, 999
Mercury compounds, poisoning from, 1006
Mercury salts, antidote for, 1000
Mesangiocapillary glomerulonephritis, 566
Mesangioproliferative glomerulonephritis, 567

Mesitylene, poisoning from, 1012
Metabolic alopecia, 662
Metabolism, disorders of, pericarditis in, 241
Metal poisoning, antidote for, 998
Metaldehyde, poisoning from, 1006
Methacholine, poisoning from, 1008
Methadone, antidote for, 1000
  poisoning by, 1006
Methemoglobinemia, 1000
  in neonate with congenital heart disease, 188
Methotrexate, side effects of, 316
Methoxychlor, poisoning from, 1003
Methyl alcohol, antidote for, 998
  poisoning from, 1006
Methyl bromide, poisoning from, 1006
Methyl salicylate, poisoning from, 1006
Metrazol. See *Pentylenetetrazol*.
Metric system, table of, 1014
Microadenoma, of sella turcica, 516
Microaggregates, in transfusion of whole blood, 358
Microangiopathic hemolytic anemia, 262
Microatelectasis, 99
Microcytosis, in iron deficiency anemia, 256
Microthrombosis, 294
Middle ear, chronic effusion in, 127
Migraine, 788–793
Miliaria, 733–734
Miltown, poisoning from, 1006
Mineral seal oil, poisoning from, 1005
Missed abortion, 862
Mitral regurgitation, acute severe, 229, 230
Mitral valve prolapse, 172
Moeller's glossitis, 699
Molds, and hypersensitivity pneumonitis, 141
Moles, 719–721
Mondor's disease, 898
Mononeuritis and mononeuritis complex, 821
Monosodium glutamate, food poisoning from, 28
MOPP chemotherapy, for Hodgkin's disease, 299–301
Morphea, 752
Morphine, antidote for, 1000
  poisoning from, 1006
Moschcowitz's syndrome, 294
Mothballs, poisoning from, 1006
Mouth. See also *Oral cavity*.
  bleeding of, in hemophiliacs, 283
  disorders of, benign, 695–709
    malignant, 709–711
  gonorrhea of, 707
  infectious diseases of, 706–709
  trench, 707
Mucoceles, of lips, 696
Mucocutaneous leishmaniasis, 39
Mucous membrane, benign pemphigoid of, 701
  precancerous lesions of, 731–733
Multifocal atrial tachycardia, 182
Multiple myeloma, 333–336
Multiple pregnancy, delivery in, anesthesia for, 884
Multiple sclerosis, 799–803
Mumps, 54–55

Muriatic acid, poisoning from, 1005
Murine typhus, 88
Muscarine, poisoning from, 1006, 1008
Muscles, hemorrhages at, in hemophiliacs, 283
  in scleroderma, 751
Muscle tension headaches, 793
Musculoskeletal disease, in Crohn's disease, 386
Mushroom poisoning, 29, 31, 1006
Myasthenia, neonatal, 807
Myasthenia gravis, 803–808
Myasthenic crisis, 806
Mycobacterioses, atypical, 153
  pulmonary (atypical), 153
Mycobacterium tuberculosis, 141
Mycoplasma pneumonia, 133–134
Mycoses, superficial, 678
Mycosis fungoides, 321, 329–333
Mycotic diseases, oral lesions of, 709
Myelitis, in epidemic influenza, 33
  radiation induced, 305
Myelofibrosis, 336
Myeloma, multiple, 333–336
Myocardial failure, in relapsing fever, 64
Myocardial infarction, 223–233
  acute, and supraventricular premature beats, 171
    heart block complicating, 176–177
  oral contraception and, 941
  pericarditis following, 240
  rehabilitation of patient after, 233–236
  ventricular premature beats in, 173
Myocardial rupture, 229
Myocarditis, in diphtheria, 20
Myocardium, ischemic, protection of, 232
Myoma, of uterus, 923–925
Myonecrosis, clostridial, 22
Myringotomy, 124
Myxedema stupor, in hypothyroidism, 540, 543
Myxomatous cysts, of nails, 718

Nails, diseases of, 712–718
  in lichen planus, 717
  overcurvature of, 716
  psoriatic changes in, 717
  tumors of, 718
Nail dystrophy, in Norwegian scabies, 717
Nail plate, fungal infections of, 714–715
Naphtha. See *Kerosene*.
Naphthalene, poisoning from, 1006
Naphthol. See *Phenol*.
Narcotic poisoning, 949–951
  in children, 951
Nasal allergy, due to inhalant factors, 643–646
Nasal polyps, in allergic rhinitis patients, 646
Neck, radical dissection of, acute tetany following, 527
Neck fusion, 848
Necrosis, of hip, aseptic, in sickle cell disease, 271

Necrotizing cellulitis, 22
Necrotizing enterocolitis, in low birth
    weight infant, 891
Necrotizing fasciitis, 22
Neonatal depression, obstetric
    anesthesia and, 879
Neonatal herpes, 682
Neonatal isoimmune
    thrombocytopenia, 291
Neonatal myasthenia, 807
Neonatal seizures, 782
Neonates. See also *Infants; Newborn.*
    cardiac catheterization and
        angiography in, 200
    congenital heart disease in, 188
    congestive heart failure in, 188
    suspected serious heart disease in,
        185
    vitamin K in, 484
Neoplasms. See also *Cancer and
    Tumors.*
    and hypopituitarism, 529
    and neutropenia, 273
    esophageal, 377
    occupationally induced, 722
    of breasts, benign, 898
    pericarditis secondary to, 241
    thyroid, 543–546
Neoplastic alopecia, 660
Neostigmine, poisoning from, 1008
Neotrane, poisoning from, 1003
Nephroblastoma, 601
Nephrogenic diabetes insipidus, 522
Nephrotic syndrome, 564
Nerve block obstetric anesthesia, 881
Neuralgia, postzoster, 757
    trigeminal, 808–809
Neuritis, optic, 809–812
Neuroblastoma, 598
Neurodermatitis, 670–672
Neurofibroma, of stomach, 415
Neurologic deficits, in multiple
    myeloma, 334
Neuromas, acoustic, 835
Neurosyphilis, 623
Neutropenia, 272–274
    radiation induced, 305
Nevi, 719–721
Newborn, congenital heart disease in,
    185–190
    hemolytic disease of, 274–278
    resuscitation of, 865–868
Niacin deficiency, 475
Nickel, antidote for, 999
    poisoning from, 1007
Nickel carbonyl, poisoning from, 1007
Nicotine, antidote for, 1000
    poisoning from, 1007
Nil disease, 566
Nipple discharge, 897
Nipples, supernumerary, 896
Nitrates, poisoning from, 1007
Nitric acid, poisoning from, 1007
Nitrites, poisoning from, 1007
Nitroaniline, poisoning from, 995
Nitrobenzene, poisoning from 1007
Nocturnal enuresis, in children, 561
Nodular adrenocortical hyperplasia,
    519
Nodular scabies, 749
Nonbullous impetigo, 745

"Non-cholera vibrio" food poisoning,
    27
Nonclostridial anaerobic gangrene, 22
Non-Hodgkin's lymphomas, 320–329
Nonimmune hemolytic anemia,
    261–263
Nonionic surfactants, poisoning from,
    1003
Nonoliguric acute renal failure, 588
Nonseminomatous germinal cell
    tumors, 609
Nonspecific urethritis, 555
Nonstenosing plaque disease, 766
Normal infant feeding, 893–896
North American blastomycosis, 119
North and South American snake bite
    venoms, antidotes for, 998
Norwegian scabies, nail dystrophy in,
    717
Nose, cancerous lesions of, 664
Nutritional alopecia, 662
Nutritional deficiency polyneuropathy,
    821

Oak poisoning, 672
Oat cell carcinoma, 114
Obesity, 472–475
Obstetrics and gynecology,
    thrombophlebitis in, 937–940
Obstetric patient, anesthetic care of,
    877–886
Obstructive atelectasis, 100
Obstructive lung disease, acute
    respiratory failure in, 97
Occlusion, arterial, acute, 242
    of aorta, atherosclerotic, 157
Occupational acne, 722
Occupational dermatoses, 721–722
Ocular disease, in toxoplasmosis, 83
Odynophagia, 378
Oil of wintergreen, poisoning from,
    1006
Old World leishmaniasis, 40
Oligomenorrhea, 905
Oliguria, in acute childhood
    leukemia, 314
OMPA, poisoning from, 1007
Onychogryphosis, 715–716
Onycholysis, 715
Onychoschizia, 716
Oophoritis, in mumps, 54
Ophthalmoplegia, 539
Opium. See *Morphine.*
Opium alkaloids, poisoning from,
    1006
Optic neuritis or neuropathy,
    809–812
Oral antidiabetic agents, 446–448
Oral cavity. See also *Mouth.*
    chancre of, 707
    mycotic lesions of, 709
    pigmented lesions of, 700
    syphilis chancre of, 707
    viral lesions of, 709
Oral contraceptives, 940–941
Oral mucosa, benign disorders of,
    699–700
Orchitis, in mumps, 54
Organic phosphate esters, antidote for,
    998

Organic phosphates, food poisoning
    from, 28
Oriental sore, 40
Ornithosis, 56–57
Osmotic diuresis, in diabetes insipidus,
    519
Osteitis fibrosis cystica, in
    hyperparathyroidism, 525
Osteoarthritis, 849–851
Osteodystrophy, renal, 481, 590
Osteomalacia, 476–482
Osteomyelitis, in sickle cell disease, 271
Osteopenia, 485
Osteoporosis, 485–488
Otalgia, in otitis media, 125
Otitis, external, 747
    in bacterial meningitis, 52
Otitis media, acute, 123–128
    in pertussis, 91
    in viral respiratory infection, 156
Ovarian failure, and amenorrhea, 911
Ovarian pregnancy, 870
Ovarian tumors, amenorrhea in, 909
Ovotran, poisoning from, 1003
Ovulation induction, in women with
    hypopituitarism, 530
Oxalates, poisoning from, 1007
    antidote for, 999
Oxygen, for neonate with congestive
    heart failure, 193

Pacemakers, complications of, 175
    for heart block, 174–175
Paget's disease, of vulva, 931
Pain, chest, in pericarditis, 237
    in breasts, 897
    in chronic pancreatitis, 410
    in peripheral neuropathy, 819
    ongoing after acute myocardial
        infarction, 230
Palatal paralysis, in diphtheria, 20
Palate, cleft, 696
    hard, cancer of, 710
Palms, recalcitrant recurrent pustular
    eruption of, 743, 744
Palsy, Bell's, 812–814
Palsy a frigore, 812
Pancreatic exocrine insufficiency, 400
Pancreatic (islet) function tests, 1033
Pancreatitis, acute, 406–409
    chronic, 409–411
Panhypopituitarism, 528
Panmyelosis, 337
Pantopon, antidote for, 1000
    poisoning from, 1006
Panwarfin, poisoning from, 1012
Papillary carcinoma, of thyroid gland,
    544
Papillary hyperplasia, of oral mucosa,
    699
Papilloma, benign, 599
    solitary intraductal, 898
Para-aminosalicylic acid, side effects of,
    149
Paracervical block obstetric anesthesia,
    881
Paradichlorobenzene, poisoning from,
    1006
Paraldehyde, poisoning from, 1007

handwritten margin note: UNASYN 3g/100mℓ Dₓ q 6 hrs
handwritten: P

Paralysis, in bacterial meningitis, 51
  peripheral facial, acute, 812–814
Paraquat, poisoning from, 1007
Parathion, poisoning from, 1007
Parathyroidectomy, acute tetany
    following, 527
  complications of, 526
Parenchymatous hemorrhage of brain,
    762–763
Parkinsonism. See *Parkinson's disease.*
Parkinson's disease, 814–818
  antipsychotic drugs and, 967
Paronychia, 712
Parotitis, paramyxovirus, 54–55
Paroxysmal atrial fibrillation, 182
Paroxysmal cold hemoglobinuria, 260
Paroxysmal hypoxemic spells, in
    congenital heart disease, 195–196
Paroxysmal nocturnal hemoglobinuria,
    263
Paroxysmal supraventricular
    tachycardia, 180
  in acute myocardial infarction, 227
  in congenital heart disease, 198
Parry's disease, 533
Partial epilepsy, 777
Parulis, 706
Patent ductus arteriosus, in premature
    infant, 189
Pear oil. See *Acetone.*
Pediatric tachycardias, 184
Pediculosis, 723–724
  and pruritus ani and vulvae, 738
Pediculosis capitis, 723
Pediculosis corporis, 723
Pediculosis pubis, 723
Pellagra, 475–476
Pelvic sarcoma, 605
Pelvis, fractures of, bladder injury in,
    573
  infections of, 921–923
  inflammatory disease of, 619
    acute, 921–923
Pemphigoid, 726–728
Pemphigus, 726–728
Pemphigus vulgaris, 700
D-Penicillamine, toxicity of, 842–844
Penicillin, allergy to, skin testing for,
    649
  anaphylactic reaction to, 626
Penis, carcinoma of, 605
  trauma to, 575–576
Pentachlorophenol, poisoning from,
    1008
Pentylenetetrazole, poisoning from,
    1008
Peptic stricture, benign, 376
Peptic ulcer, 411–415
  in vitamin C deficiency, 482
Perianal disease, in Crohn's disease,
    385
Pericardial effusion, in pericarditis,
    238
Pericarditis, 237–241
  in acute myocardial infarction, 231
  radiation, 305
Pericholangitis, in proctocolitis, 432
Pericoronitis, 702
Periodontal membrane, benign
    disorders of, 701–702
Peripheral arterial aneurysms, 245

Peripheral neuropathy, 818–822
Peritoneal dialysis, 593
Peritonitis, 381
  spontaneous bacterial, in cirrhosis,
    371
Periungual verrucae, 713–714
Perleche, 698
Permanganate, potassium, poisoning
    from, 1008
Pernicious anemia, 263–265
Persistent fetal circulation, in neonate
    with congenital heart disease, 188
Persistent herpetic ulcer, 683
Pertussis, 89–91
Petroleum distillates, poisoning from,
    1005
Petroleum ether. See *Kerosene.*
Pharyngitis, gonococcal, 619
  streptococcal, 144–145
Phenacetin. See *Acetanilid.*
Phenazone. See *Acetanilid.*
Phenol derivatives, poisoning from,
    1008
Phenolphthalein, poisoning from, 1008
Phenothiazine derivatives, poisoning
    from, 1008
Phenothiazine tranquilizers, poisoning
    from, antidote for, 999
Phenytoin, poisoning from, 1008
Pheochromocytoma, 546–550, 598
Phimosis, and balanoposthitis, 564
Phlebitis, septic, following gynecologic
    surgery, 937
Phlebotomy, in hemochromatosis, 296
  in treatment of polycythemia vera,
    339
Phlegmasia alba dolens, 246
Phlegmasia cerulea dolens, 246
Phosdrin, poisoning from, 1007
Phosphate ester insecticides, poisoning
    from, 1007
Phosphate salts, poisoning from, 1003
Phosphine, poisoning from, 1008
Phosphoric acid, poisoning from, 1008
Phosphorus, poisoning from, 1008
  antidote for, 999
Phosphorus deficiency, in children,
    504
Photoallergic dermatitis, 666–667
Photosensitivity, 686–690
Phototherapy, for mycosis fungoides,
    331
Phototoxic dermatitis, 666–667
Phthalazine derivatives, poisoning
    from, 1005
Physostigmine, antidote for, 1000
  poisoning from, 1008
Picrotoxin, poisoning from, 1008
Pigmentary disturbances, 724–726
Pill. See *Oral contraception.*
Pilocarpine, poisoning from, 1008
Pinworms, 427, 738
Pituitary gland, tumors of, 835
  in acromegaly, 509
Pituitary-dependent Cushing's
    syndrome, 516–518
Pityriasis rosea, 728–729
Pityriasis versicolor, 678
Placenta, rupture of marginal sinus of,
    873
Placenta previa, 872

Plague, 55–56
Plasma, reference values for,
    1022–1025
  single donor, fresh frozen, therapy
    with, 350
Platelet concentrate, human, therapy
    with, 349
Platelet dysfunction, 280
Platelet transfusion, in aplastic anemia,
    253
Platelets, abnormalities of, bleeding
    disorders secondary to, 287–293
  classification of, 288
Pleural diseases, pericarditis in,
    241
Pleural effusions, 120–121
  in lung cancer, 113
  in non-Hodgkin's lymphoma, 329
Pneumococcal bacteremia, 8
Pneumococcal meningitis, 46
Pneumococcal septicemia, in sickle cell
    disease, 270
Pneumoconiosis, coal workers',
    138–139
Pneumonia, bacterial, 128–132
  empyema in, 120
  in acute childhood leukemia, 312
  in chickenpox, 13
  in pertussis, 90
  in plague, 55
  in psittacosis, 57
  in sickle cell disease, 271
  mycoplasma, 133–134
  respiratory tract pathogens as causes
    of, 133
  viral, 132–133
    in epidemic influenza, 33
Pneumonia vaccine, 134
Pneumonitis, hypersensitivity, 141–142
  viral, 155
Poison ivy dermatitis, 672–673
Poisons, chart of antidotes for,
    998–1001
  inhaled, 993
  injected, 993
  oral, 992
Poisoning, acute miscellaneous,
    993–1012
  convulsions due to, 997
  food, 23–32
Poison oak dermatitis, 672
Poison sumac dermatitis, 672
Politzerization, in otitis media, 126
Polyarteritis nodosa, 729–731
Polyarthritis, in rheumatic fever, 67,
    68
Polycystic ovary syndrome, and
    amenorrhea, 909
Polycythemia, in congenital heart
    disease, 204
  in neonate, 188
  relative, 336–342
Polycythemia vera, 336–342
Polydipsia, in diabetes insipidus, 519
  psychogenic, 522
Polymyositis, 676–677
Polyps, nasal, in allergic rhinitis
    patients, 646
  of stomach, 415
Polypectomy, colonoscopic, 418
Polyposis, and rectal cancer, 417

Polyserositis, severe, in lupus erythematosus, 694
Polyuria, in diabetes insipidus, 519
Porphyrias, 342–347
  hepatic, acute, 342
Porphyria cutanea tarda, 346, 689, 691
  phlebotomy in, 296
Porphyria polyneuropathy, 822
Portasystemic encephalopathy, in cirrhosis, 369
Portuguese man-of-war stings, 991–992
Postconcussive syndrome, 829
Postgastrectomy state, malabsorption in, 400–401
Posthitis, 563
Postmenopausal osteoporosis, 486
Postmenopausal vulvar atrophy, 737
Postmyocardial infarction syndrome, 240
Postnecrotic cirrhosis, 368
Postoperative tetany, acute, following surgery, 527
Postpartum bacteriuria and urinary retention during pregnancy, 920–921
Postpartum blues, 887
Postpartum care, 886–887
Postpartum hemorrhage, 886
Postpartum infection, 923
Postperfusion syndrome, 358
Postphlebitic syndrome, 248
Postscabietic pruritus, 749
Post-spinal anesthesia headache, 885–886
Post-sterilization syndrome, 941
Post-transfusion hepatitis, 357
Post-transfusion malaria, 358
Post-transfusion purpura, 291, 357
Post-transfusion syphilis, 358
Post-transplant renal failure, 588
Post-traumatic hydrocephalus, 834
Potassium cyanide, poisoning from, 1003
Potassium deficiency, in acute dehydration, 503
Potassium permanganate, poisoning from, 1008
  antidote for, 999
Potassium salt, poisoning from, 1002
Potato poisoning, 28
Precancerous lesions of the skin and mucous membranes, 731–733
Prednisone, side effects of, 316
Preeclampsia, delivery in, anesthesia for, 884
Preeclampsia hypertension, 873
Pre-excitation, Wolff-Parkinson-White type of, 167
Pre-excitation syndromes, and supraventricular premature beats, 171
Pregnancy, carcinoma of uterus and, 929
  complications of, prevention and treatment of, 860
  confirmation of, 854
  ectopic, 868–871
  hyperthyroidism in, 538
  in lepromatous women, 37
  late, hemorrhage in, 871–873

Pregnancy (Continued)
  multiple, 860
  multiple sclerosis during, 803
  pheochromocytoma in, 550
  plague during, 56
  planned, 853–855
  proctocolitis in, 433
  pruritic urticarial papules and plaques of, 758
  rubella exposure during, 71
  sickle cell disease and, 272
  syphilis in, 623
  toxoplasmosis in, 82, 83
  urinary tract infections during, 918–921
Pregnancy-induced hypertension, 873–877
Premature beats, 171–173
  in congenital heart disease, 196
Premature ventricular beats, 172
Prematurity, delivery in, anesthesia for, 884
Prenatal examination, 854
Prerenal azotemia, 584
Pressure sores, 666
Priapism, in sickle cell disease, 271
Prickly heat, 733–734
Primary biliary cirrhosis, 368
Primary hyperparathyroidism, 525–526
Primary hypophosphatemia, 479
Primary lung abscess, 121–123
Primary lung cancer, 109–114
Prinzmetal's angina, ventricular premature beats in, 172
Probucol, toxicity of, 469
Procainamide, toxicity of, 177
Procaine. See Cocaine.
Proctitis, 431
  gonococcal, 619
Proctocolitis, 428–433
Proctosigmoiditis, 431
Progressive massive fibrosis, 138–139
Prolactin-secreting tumors, 531–533
Prolactin secretion, abnormal, causes of, 531
Propoxyphene, poisoning from, 1006
Propylene glycol, poisoning from, 1004
Prostate, benign hyperplasia of, 576–581
  malignant tumors of, 605–607
  obstruction of, 577
Prostatectomy, 577–578
Prostatic hyperplasia, benign, 576–581
Prostatitis, 555, 581–582
Prosthetic devices, in children with congenital heart disease, 205
Prosthetic valve endocarditis, 218
Proteus bacteremia, indole-positive, 10
Proteus mirabilis bacteremia, 9
Proteus species pneumonia, 130
Protoporphyria, 345
Protozoan food poisoning, 25, 26
Protozoan infections, 425
Pruritic urticarial papules and plaques of pregnancy, 758
Pruritus, 734–736
  postscabietic, 749
Pruritus ani, 736–739
Pruritus vulvae, 736–739

Pseudofolliculitis barbae, 658–659
Pseudomonas aeruginosa bacteremia, 10
Pseudomonas aeruginosa pneumonia, 130
Psittacosis, 56–57
Psoriasis, 738–742
  nail changes in, 717
Psychogenic polydipsia, 522
Psychoneurosis, 951–954
Psychosis, atypical, 957
Psychotherapy, in neurodermatitis, 671
Ptyalism, 704–705
Pudendal nerve block obstetric anesthesia, 881
Puerperal sepsis, 886
Pulmonary disease, labor and, anesthesia in, 885
  pericarditis in, 241
Pulmonary edema, in congenital heart disease, 194–195
Pulmonary embolism, 134–137
  in myocardial infarction, 232
  in venous thrombosis, 248
Pulmonary fibrosis, radiation induced, 305
Pulmonary hypersensitivity transfusion reaction, 355
Pulmonary tuberculosis, 152
Purple foxglove, poisoning from, 1003
Purpura, post-transfusion, 291, 357
  thrombotic thrombocytopenic, 292, 294–295
Purpura fulminans, in chickenpox, 14
Pyelonephritis, 556, 568–570
  acute, during pregnancy, 919
  in sickle cell disease, 271
Pyoderma, with scabies, 749
Pyoderma gangrenosum, 386
Pyrazinamide, side effects of, 148, 149
Pyrethrum, poisoning from, 1008
Pyribenzamine. See Antihistaminics.
Pyrimethamine, toxicity of, 42

Q fever, 57–58
Quaternary ammonium compounds, poisoning from, 1009
Quinidine, toxicity of, 177
Quinidine syncope, 170
Quinine, antidote for, 1000
  toxicity of, 41–42
Quinine and cinchona-like compounds, poisoning from, 1009

Rabies, 58–62
Rabies immune globulin, reactions with, 61
Rabies vaccine, accidental inoculation with, 61
Radiation, consequences of to normal tissue, 305–306
Radiation gastritis, 391
Radiation pericarditis, 240, 305
Radiation syndrome, 1009
Radiodermatitis, chronic, 733
Radiographic contrast material, allergy to, 650
  anaphylactic reactions to, 626
Radioiodine therapy, in hyperthyroidism, 535–537

Radiotherapeutic emergencies, in Hodgkin's disease, 304
Rat bite fever, 62–63
Raynaud's phenomenon, 245, 750
Reactive hypoglycemias, 470–472
Rectosigmoid ameboma, 3
Rectum, tumors of, 416–421
Red blood cells, donor, hemolysis of, 356
transfusion of, 348
Red cell enzymes, abnormalities of, and hemolytic anemia, 263
Red cell mass deficit, use of blood components for, 348
Red cell transfusion, in thalassemia, 266
Refsum's disease, 821
Regional ileitis, 382–386
Rehabilitation of hemiplegic patient, 766–771
Relapsing fever, 63–66
epidemic, 66
Remission maintenance therapy, in adult acute leukemia, 307–308
Renal. See also *Kidney(s)*.
Renal calculi, 612–615
in primary hyperparathyroidism, 526
Renal disease, in sickle cell disease, 271
Renal failure, acute, 582–588
in bacterial meningitis, 51
in children, dehydration in, 505
in cholera, 18
in multiple myeloma, 334
in non-Hodgkin's lymphoma, 329
in psittacosis, 57
Renal injury, 571
Renal osteodystrophy, 481, 590
Renal papillary necrosis, in sickle cell disease, 271
Renal pelvic injuries, 572
Renal pelvic tumors, 599–600
Renal tract obstruction, 584
Renal transplantation, in chronic renal failure, 594
Renal tubular carcinoma, 600
Renal tumors, benign, 599
Resorcinol, poisoning from, 1008
Respiratory distress, in low birth weight infant, 890
Respiratory distress syndrome, adult, 101
Respiratory failure, acute, 93–99
asthma and, 633
in acute pancreatitis, 408
in peripheral neuropathy, 819
Respiratory infections, in congenital heart disease, 205
viral, 153–156
Resuscitation, of newborn, 865–868
Retention hyperkeratosis, 655
Reticulocytopenia, in aplastic anemia, 251
Retinal detachment, in sickle cell disease, 271
Reye's syndrome, in chickenpox, 14
in epidemic influenza, 33
Rh disease, 274
Rh sensitized mother, obstetric management of, 275
Rheumatic fever, 66–69
and streptococcal pharyngitis, 144

Rheumatoid arthritis, 839–843
juvenile, 843–845
Rhinitis, allergic, 643
Rhinoscleroma, 707
Ribs, resection of, in empyema, 121
Rickets, 476–482
Riedel's thyroiditis, 551
Rifampin, side effects of, 148, 149
Right upper quadrant syndrome, in sickle cell disease, 271
Right ventricular failure, in acute myocardial infarction, 229, 230
Rocky Mountain spotted fever, 69–70
Rotenone, poisoning from, 1009
Roundworms, 424, 425, 427
Rubbing alcohol. See *Ethyl alcohol*.
Rubella, 71–72
Rubeola, 42–44
Ruptured eardrum, in otitis media, 125
Russian fly, poisoning from, 1001
Ryania. See *Rotenone*.
Rye staging system, for Hodgkin's disease, 297

Schörls nodes herniation

Sabadilla, poisoning from, 1009
Sacroiliitis, in ankylosing spondylitis, 846
Saddle block obstetric anesthesia, 881
Salicylates, poisoning from, 1009
Salivary glands, benign disorders of, 704
Salmonella bacteremia, 10
Salmonella food poisoning, 26, 27
Salmonella infection, with relapsing fever, 65
Salmonellosis (other than typhoid fever), 73–75
Salmonellosis carrier state, 74
Santonin, poisoning from, 1009
Saphenous veins, stripping of, 249–250
Sarcoidosis, 137–138, 707
Sarcoma, pelvic, 605
Scabies, 748–749
and pruritus ani and vulvae, 738
nodular, 749
Norwegian, nail dystrophy in, 717
Scalds, 973
Scalp, injury to, in adults, 823, 827
in children, 832
seborrheic dermatitis of, 673
Scars, hypertrophic, 685
Schizophrenia, 957, 965–971
Scleroderma, 749–752
in overlap, 752
Sclerosing adenosis, 879
Sclerosing cholangitis/choledochitis, in proctocolitis, 432
Sclerosis, systemic, 749–752
Scorpion stings, 990–991
Scrotum, trauma to, 575
Scrub typhus, 88
Scurvy, 482–483
Sea nettle. See *Portuguese man-of-war stings*.
Seborrheic blepharitis, 674
Seborrheic dermatitis, 673–674
Secondary hyperparathyroidism, 526
Secondary immune hemolytic anemia, 260

Sedation, for neonate with congestive heart failure, 193
Sedatives, therapeutic agents to neutralize, 994
Seizure(s), epileptic. See *Epilepsy*.
in bacterial meningitis, 50
in low birth weight infant, 891
in viral meningoencephalitis, 798
neonatal, 782
Seizure types, in older children and adolescents, 782
Selenium, poisoning from, 1009
Sella turcica, microadenoma of, 516
Semen analysis, reference values for, 1033
Seminoma, 608
Senile keratoses, 663
Sepsis, in acute renal failure, 586
puerperal, 886
Septic arthritis, in bacterial meningitis, 52
Septic cortical thrombophlebitis, 761
Septic phlebitis, following gynecologic surgery, 937
Septic shock, in bacterial pneumonia, 132
Septicemia, pneumococcal, in sickle cell disease, 270
Septicemic plague, 55
Serratia bactercmia, 10
Serratia marcescens pneumonia, 130
Serum, reference values for, 1022–1025
Serum bactericidal titer, in infective endocarditis, 214
Serum sickness, 628
Sex, during pregnancy, 857
Sexuality, contraception, and pregnancy in congenital heart disease patients, 209
Sézary's syndrome, 321, 329–333
Shigella bacteremia, 10
Shigella food poisoning, 27
Shock, cardiogenic, in acute myocardial infarction, 229
following poisoning, 994
in cholera, 17
in meningitis, 49
in pulmonary embolism, 136
in relapsing fever, 65
septic, in bacterial pneumonia, 132
Shunting, in acute respiratory failure, 94
Sialolithiasis, 704
Sick sinus syndrome, 169, 177
in congenital heart disease, 199
Sickle cell disease, 269–272
Sickle cell trait, 269
Silicosis, 140–141
Silver nitrate, antidote for, 1000
poisoning from, 1009
Simple goiter, 522–525
Sino-atrial block, 173–178
Sinus arrhythmia, in congenital heart disease, 196
Sinus bradycardia, in congenital heart disease, 196
in myocardial infarction, 225
Sinus node dysfunction, sinoatrial block and, 177
Sinus tachycardia, 180
in congenital heart disease, 196

Sinusitis, 142–144
  bronchospasm in, 629
  chronic, 144
  in allergic rhinitis patients, 646
  purulent, acute, in viral respiratory
    infections, 156
Skeletal tuberculosis, 152
Skin, atypical mycobacterial infections
    of, 747
  bacterial diseases of, 745–747
  cancer of, 663–665
  mechanically induced alterations of,
    722
  occupationally induced depig-
    mentation of, 722
  pigmented lesions of, 726
  precancerous lesions of, 731–733
  radiation effects on, 305
  superficial fungus infections of,
    678–682
Skull, penetrating wounds of, in
    children, 834
Skull fractures, 827
  in children, 832
Small animals, bites of, rabies from,
    58–62
Small intestine, Crohn's disease of, 384
  diverticula of, 379–380
Smoking, and chronic obstructive
    pulmonary disease, 102
Smooth tongue, 699
Snake bite venoms, North and South
    American, antidotes for, 998
Snuff dipper's keratosis, 700
Sodium carbonate, poisoning from,
    1003
Sodium fluoracetate, antidote for,
    1000
Sodium sulfate, poisoning from, 1003
Solanine, poisoning from, 1009
Solanine food poisoning, 28
Solar keratoses, 663, 731
Solar urticaria, 689, 691
Soles, recalcitrant recurrent pustular
    eruption of, 743, 744
Somogyi phenomenon, 458
Spanish fly, poisoning from, 1001
Spasms, infantile, 783
Spasticity, in paraplegia, 770
Spherocytosis, and hemolytic anemia,
    262
Spider bites, 990–991
Spinal cord compression, in Hodgkin's
    disease, 305
Spine, fused, fracture of, 848
Spleen, enlarged, platelet pooling in,
    290
  in sickle cell disease, 270
  in thalassemia, 267
  in warm antibody autoimmune
    hemolytic anemia, 259
Splenic rupture, in mononucleosis, 53
Splenomegaly, in chronic neutropenia,
    272
Spontaneous abortion, 861–863
Spontaneous bacterial peritonitis, in
    cirrhosis, 371
Sprue, 403
Spur cell anemia, 263
Squamous cell carcinoma, 732
  of renal pelvis, 600

Squill. See *Digitalis.*
Staging classification, in mycosis
    fungoides and Sézary's syndrome,
    329
  in non-Hodgkin's lymphoma, 322,
    323
  of Hodgkin's disease, 296–298,
    302–303
Staphylococcal food poisoning, 25
Staphylococcal infections, 8
Staphylococcal infective endocarditis,
    215–217
Staphylococcal meningitis, 47
Staphylococcal pneumonia, 130
Staphylococcal scalded skin syndrome,
    747
Staphylococcus aureus bacteremia, 8
Staphylococcus epidermidis bacteremia, 8
Staphylococcus epidermidis meningitis, 48
Stasis dermatitis, 674–675
Stasis ulcers, 250, 674–675
Status asthmaticus, 632
  in children, 643
Status epilepticus, in adolescents and
    adults, 773
  in children, 783
Stenosis, arterial, ischemic stroke
    secondary to, 765–766
Sterilization, reversibility of, 941
Steroid cataracts, 36
Stimulants, therapeutic agents to
    neutralize, 994
Stings, insect, allergic reactions to,
    651–653
  anaphylactic reactions to, 626
  Portuguese man-of-war, 991–992
  scorpion, 990–991
Stomach, carcinoma of, in pernicious
    anemia, 265
  Crohn's disease of, 384
  diverticula of, 379
  polyp of, 415
  tumors of, 415–416
Stomatitis, aphthous, 386, 701
  denture, 699
Stomatocytosis, 263
Streptococcal infections, group A, 6
  group B, 8
Streptococcal infective endocarditis,
    215
Streptococcal pharyngitis, 144–145
Streptococcal pneumonia, 130
Streptomycin, side effects of, 148, 149
Stricture, urethral, 610–612
Stroke, acute, in hemiplegic patients,
    766
  heat, 989
  ischemic. See *Acute ischemic
    cerebrovascular disease.*
  oral contraception and, 941
Strongyloides stercoralis, 427
Strongyloidiasis, 427
Strychnine, antidote for, 1000
  poisoning from, 1010
Stupor, myxedema, in hypothyroidism,
    540, 543
Subacute thyroiditis, 550
Subdural hematoma, acute, 827
  in children, 833
Subgaleal hematomas, in children, 833
Subungual hematomas, 713

Subungual verrucae, 713–174
Sucking-licking cheilitis, 697
Sudden death survivors, recurrent
    ventricular fibrillation in, 173
Suicide, in depressed persons, 958
Sulfides, soluble, poisoning from, 1010
Sulfonamides, poisoning from, 1010
Sulfur dioxide, poisoning from, 1010
Sulfuric acid, poisoning from, 1010
Sumac poisoning, 672
Sunburn, 687–690
Superficial mycoses, 678
Superior vena cava blockage, in lung
    cancer, 113
Superior vena cava syndrome, in
    Hodgkin's disease, 304
  in non-Hodgkin's lymphoma, 328
Supernumerary nipples, 896
Supernumerary teeth, 703
Supraventricular premature beats, 171
Supraventricular tachycardia, 180–181
Surgery, acute tetany following, 527
  and hypopituitarism, 529
  fluid requirements during, 495
  gynecologic, elective, preoperative
    and postoperative care for,
    934–937
  infections following, 923
  in benign prostatic hyperplasia,
    577–581
  complications of, 580–581
  in children, fluid therapy in, 507
  in hemophiliacs, 283, 284
Swine flu vaccine, and Guillain-Barré
    syndrome, 33
Synergistic gangrene, 22
Syphilis, 621–624, 921
  post-transfusion, 358
Systemic lupus erythematosus, 690,
    692–695
  renal involvement in, 567
Systemic sclerosis, 749–752
Systox, poisoning from, 1007

Table of heights and weights for men
  and women, 1015
Table of metric and apothecaries'
  systems, 1014
Tachycardia, 178–184
  in cardiac arrest, 165
  paroxysmal supraventricular, in
    acute myocardial infarction, 227
  pediatric, 184
  supraventricular, 180–181
  ventricular, in acute myocardial
    infarction, 228
Tachycardia-bradycardia syndrome,
  177, 184
Tamponade, cardiac, in pericarditis,
  238
Tapeworms, 425, 427
Tardive dyskinesia, antipsychotic drugs
  and, 968
Taste, abnormalities of, 705
T cell lymphoma, 329–333
TDE, poisoning from, 1003
Tear gases, poisoning from, 1010
Teeth, benign disorders of, 702–704
  pigmentation of, 703

Teeth (*Continued*)
supernumerary, 703
trauma to, 703
Temporal arteritis, in hemiplegic
patients, 767
Tendinitis, calcific, 848–849
Tension-vascular headaches, 793
TEPP, poisoning from, 1007
Tertiary hyperparathyroidism, 526
Testis, carcinoma of, 607–610
trauma to, 575
Tetanic uterine contractions, 885
Tetanus, 75–82
prophylaxis against, 75–76
Tetanus antitoxin, 77
Tetrachloroethane, poisoning from,
1010
Tetracyclines, toxicity of, 69
Tetralogy of Fallot, anesthesia for
children with, 205
Tetramethylthiuram disulfide,
poisoning from, 1010
Thalassemia, 265–269
Thalassemia intermedia, 268
Thalidomide, teratogenic effects of, 36
Thallium, antidote for, 999
poisoning from, 1010
Theobromine, poisoning from, 1012
Theophylline, poisoning from, 1012
Theophylline products, dosage
guidelines for, 105
Therapeutic drug monitoring,
reference values for, 1028
Thiacetazone, side effects of, 148
Thiamine deficiency, 435–436
Thiocyanates, poisoning from, 1010
6-Thioguanine, side effects of, 316
Thiourea, poisoning from, 1010
Thiram, poisoning from, 1010
Thoracentesis, in empyema, 120–121
Thoracoabdominal aneurysms, 160
Threatened abortion, 862
Three-day measles, 71–72
Thrombocytopenia, in aplastic anemia,
253
in diphtheria, 20
production abnormalities in, 287
production related, bleeding time
and platelet count in, *291*
Thrombocytopenic purpura, in lupus
erythematosus, 694
Thrombocytosis, 292–293
Thromboembolism, in glomerular
disorders, 565
in proctocolitis, 432
systemic, atrial fibrillation and, 169
Thrombolytic therapy, of pulmonary
embolism, 135
Thrombophlebitis, in brain abscess,
760
in obstetric and gynecologic patients,
937–940
oral contraception and, 941
Thrombosis, acute, 243
deep vein, massive, of lower
extremities, 246–249
in polycythemia vera, 341
Thrombotic thrombocytopenic
purpura, 292, 294–295
Thymol, poisoning from, 1008
Thyroid deficiency, 530–531
Thyroid gland, carcinoma of, 543–546

Thyroid malignancy, 543–546
Thyroid replacement therapy,
complications of, 540
Thyroid storm, 538
Thyroidectomy, acute tetany following,
527
complications of, 535
Thyroiditis, 539, 550–551
Thyrotoxicosis, 539
D-Thyroxine, cardiotoxicity of, 469
Tibial-soleal venous thrombosis, 246
Tick-borne relapsing fever, 64
Tick typhus, 88
Tin food poisoning, 25
Tinea barbae, 679
Tinea capitis, 679
Tinea corporis, 679
Tinea cruris, 680
and vulvar pruritus, 915
Tinea manuum, 681
Tinea nigra, 678
Tinea palmaris, 743, 744
Tinea pedis, 680, 743, 744
Tinea unguium, 715–716
Tinea versicolor, 678
TNT, poisoning from, 1011
Toe webs, bacterial infections of, 746
Toenail, ingrown, 712
Toluene, poisoning from, 1012
Toluidine, poisoning from, 995
Tongue, benign disorders of, 698–699
cancer of, 711
hypomobility of, 706
Tonsillitis, lingual, 707
Tonsillopharyngitis, in mononucleosis,
53
Tooth. See *Teeth.*
Tooth eruption cysts, 701
Tooth substance, loss of, 703
Tophaceous gout, chronic, 462
Torsade des pointes tachycardia, 183
Total spinal obstetric anesthesia, 882
Toxaphene. See *DDT.*
Toxemia, in typhoid fever, 87
Toxemia patient, delivery in,
anesthesia for, 884
Toxic alopecia, 661
Toxic megacolon, 432
in Crohn's disease, 385
Toxicology, reference values in, 1030
Toxoplasmosis, 82–83
Tracheobronchial compression, in
Hodgkin's disease, 304
Tracheostomy, in tetanus, 79
Traction headaches, 793
Transfusion, blood, adverse reactions
to, 352–359
Transfusional hemosiderosis, 359
Transport of neonate with congenital
heart disease, 186
Transverse arch of aorta, aneurysms
of, 159
Trauma, and optic neuropathies, 812
to genitourinary tract, 570–576
to head, in adults, 822–829
to kidneys, 571
to lips, 696
to teeth, 703
Traumatic alopecia, acquired, 660
Traumatic pericarditis, 240
Trematode infestation, 428
Trench mouth, 707

Trichinellosis, 84
Trichinosis, 30
Trichloroethylene. See *Carbon
tetrachloride.*
Trichomonas vaginalis, infection from,
917
Trichostrongylus infection, 427
Trichotillomania, 661
Tricyclic compounds, poisoning from,
1010
Tridione, poisoning from, 1011
Trigeminal neuralgia, 808–809
Trimethadione, poisoning from, 1011
Trinitrotoluene, poisoning from, 1011
Tri-ortho-cresyl phosphate, poisoning
from, 1011
Tripelennamine. See *Antihistaminics.*
Trithion, poisoning from, 1007
Tropical sprue, 403
Tubal pregnancy, 868–871
Tuberculosis, 145–153
amenorrhea derived from, 912
childhood, 152
genitourinary, 594–597
in silicosis, 141
oral involvement in, 707
Tuberculous cervical adenitis, 152
Tuberculous meningitis, 152
Tuberculous pericarditis, 239
Tubular necrosis, acute, 582
Tularemia, 85
oral involvement in, 707
Tumor(s). See also *Cancer, Neoplasms,*
and specific types.
ACTH secreting, 518
adrenocortical, removal of,
cardiovascular collapse following,
515
brain, 834–837
chromaffin cell, 546
genitourinary, 597–610
nonseminomatous germinal cell, 609
of colon and rectum, 416–421
of nails, 718
of stomach, 415, 416
of uterus, benign, 923
malignant, 925–930
of vulva, malignant, 930–934
pituitary, 516
and amenorrhea-galactorrhea
syndrome, 531
in acromegaly, 509
prolactin-secreting, 531–533
renal, benign, 599
testicular, 607–610
thyroid, 543–546
vascular, of lips, 696
Wilms', 601
Turpentine, poisoning from, 1012
Typhoid fever, 10, 86–88
carrier state of, 87
Typhus fever, 88–89
with relapsing fever, 65

Ulcer, Chiclero, 40
decubitus, 666
gastric, 414
peptic, 411–415
in vitamin C deficiency, 482
stasis, 250, 674–675

Ulceration, of leg, in sickle cell disease, 271
Ulcerative colitis, 428–433
  and rectal cancer, 417
Universal antidote, 1001
Universal colitis, 431
Uremia, 592–594
  chronic, 588
Uremic bone disease, 590
Ureteral carcinoma, 600
Ureters, trauma to, 572
Urethra, carcinoma of, 604
  trauma to, 573–575
Urethral meatal stenosis, 610
Urethral stricture, 610–612
Urethritis, 555
  gonococcal, 619
  in prostatitis, 582
  nonspecific, 555
Urinary tract, adult female, bacterial infections of, 557–559
  infections of during pregnancy, 918–921
  male, bacterial infections of, 555–556
  of female children, bacterial infections of, 560–561
  trauma to, 570–576
Urine, reference values for, 1026–1028
Urine retention, in hemiplegic patient, 767
  in multiple sclerosis, 802
Urticaria, 752–755
Uta, 39
Uterine bleeding, dysfunctional, 904–906
Uterus, cancer of, 925–930
  carcinoma of, 926
  myoma of, 923–925
  trauma to, during abortion, 865
Uveitis, asymptomatic, in juvenile rheumatoid arthritis, 845

Vaginal delivery, anesthesia for, 880
Vaginal discharge, without infection, 917
Vaginitis, gonococcal, 619
Varicella, 11–14
Varices, esophageal, bleeding, 361–364
Varicose veins, 249–250
  during pregnancy, 861
Variegate porphyria, 342
Vasa previa, 873
Vascular disease, and hypopituitarism, 529
Vascular headaches, 788–793
Vasculitides, renal involvement in, 568
Vasculitis, acute, in lupus erythematosus, 694

Vasospastic angina, ventricular premature beats in, 172
Vasospastic arterial disease, 245
Veins, saphenous, stripping of, 249–250
  varicose, 249–250
Vena cava, inferior, interruption of, 136–137
Vena caval interruption, for venous thrombosis, 249
Venous thrombosis, following gynecological surgery, 939
  tibial-soleal, 246
Ventilation-perfusion abnormalities, in acute respiratory failure, 94
Ventricular arrhythmias, in acute myocardial infarction, 227
Ventricular fibrillation, in acute myocardial infarction, 228
  in congenital heart disease, 199
Ventricular premature beats, in acute myocardial infarction, 227
Ventricular tachycardia, 183
  in acute myocardial infarction, 228
  in congenital heart disease, 198–199
Verapamil, toxicity of, 177
Veratrum, poisoning from, 1012
Verruca acuminata, 756
Verrucae, periungual and subungual, 713–714
Vertebral arteries, stenosis of, 766
Vertigo, episodic, 793–796
Vibrio cholerae food poisoning, 26
Vibrio parahemolyticus food poisoning, 27
Vincent's disease, 707
Vincristine sulfate, side effects of, 316
Viral diseases, oral lesions of, 709
Viral hepatitis, 396–397
Viral influenza, 155
Viral meningoencephalitis, 797–799
Viral pneumonia, 132–133
  in epidemic influenza, 33
Viral pneumonitis, 155
Viral respiratory infections, 153–156
Visceral leishmaniasis, 39
Vitamin B_1, deficiency of, 435–436
Vitamin B_{12}, deficiency of, 264, 265
  and ineffective platelet production, 290
  sensitivity to, 265
Vitamin C, deficiency of, 482–483
Vitamin D, deficiency of, 478–479
  malabsorption of, 480
  metabolism of, 477
Vitamin D dependent rickets, 479
Vitamin D metabolites, nomenclature of, 477
Vitamin D refractory rickets, 479–480
Vitamin K, deficiency of, 483–485

Vitamins, daily requirements of, 494
  poisoning from, 1012
Vitiligo, 725
Vocational training of congenital heart disease patients, 208
Von Willebrand's disease, 278, 285
Vulva, atrophy of, postmenopausal, 737
  carcinoma of, 930–934
  contact dermatitis of, 916
  dystrophies of, 916, 930
  pruritus of, 738
Vulvitis, Candida, 915
Vulvovaginitis, 914–918

Wandering atrial pacemaker, 196
Warfarin, poisoning from, 1012
Warm antibody autoimmune hemolytic anemia, 259
Warts, 755–757
Water, daily requirement of, 493
Water diuresis, in diabetes insipidus, 519
Weight, table of, for men and women, 1015
Weights, metric and apothecaries', table of, 1014
Whipple's disease, 403
Whipworm, 427
White arsenic, poisoning from, 995
Whooping cough, 89–91
Wilms' tumor, 601
Wilson's disease, 368
Withdrawal dyskinesia, antipsychotic drugs and, 968
Wolff-Parkinson-White syndrome, and supraventricular premature beats, 171
  tachycardias in, 184
Wolff-Parkinson-White type pre-excitation, 167
Women, table of desirable heights and weights for, 1015

Xanthine, poisoning from, 1012
  toxicity of, 104
Xerostomia, 704–705
Xylene, poisoning from, 1012

Yersinia enterocolitica food poisoning, 27

Zenker's diverticulum, 378
Zinc, poisoning from, 25, 1012
Zollinger-Ellison syndrome, 401